DISORDERS OF HEMOGLOBIN

Genetics, Pathophysiology, and Clinical Management

The first comprehensive reference on the genetic and acquired disorders of hemoglobin in more than a decade, *Disorders of Hemoglobin* stands out as the definitive work on the genetics, pathophysiology, and clinical management of this wide range of disorders. The editors have gathered world authorities on the science and clinical management of thalassemias, sickle cell disease, and other inherited and acquired hemoglobinopathies to create the authoritative textbook for researchers and clinicians.

Divided into eight sections, coverage spans the molecular and genetic basis of hemoglobinopathies and thalassemias, their epidemiology and genetic selection, and the diagnosis and special treatments of β and α thalassemias, sickle cell disease, HbE, unstable hemoglobins, M hemoglobin disorders, and acquired and secondary disorders of hemoglobin. Clinical features of all disorders are anchored to the scientific and pathophysiologic events that precede them providing clinicians with a clear scientific background of the disorders they treat and scientists with an essential link between their research and its clinical manifestation.

Disorders of Hemoglobin is the only single-source reference of its kind for hematologists, internists, pediatricians, clinical investigators, and geneticists worldwide.

Martin H. Steinberg was Associate Chief of Staff for Research at the G.V. "Sonny" Montgomery VA Medical Center in Jackson, Mississippi, and is now Professor of Medicine and Pediatrics at Boston University and Director of the Center of Excellence in Sickle Cell Disease at Boston Medical Center. He is a member of the American Society for Clinical Investigation and the Association of American Physicians, and he was president of the Southern Society for Clinical Investigation.

Bernard G. Forget is Professor of Internal Medicine and Genetics and Chief, Section of Hematology, at the Yale University School of Medicine, New Haven, Connecticut. He is a member of several professional organizations, including the American Society of Hematology, the American Society for Clinical Investigation, and the Association of American Physicians.

Douglas R. Higgs is Professor of Molecular Haematology and Director of the MRC Molecular Haematology Unit in the Institute of Molecular Medicine, University of Oxford, United Kingdom. The Unit's work focuses on various aspects of molecular hemopoieses. His own research is concerned with the mechanisms by which globin gene expression is normally regulated and how this is perturbed in inherited and acquired human genetic diseases.

Ronald L. Nagel is Irving D. Karpas Professor of Medicine, Professor of Physiology and Biophysics, and Head, Division of Hematology at Albert Einstein College of Medicine in Bronx, New York. Dr. Nagel is a member of the American Society for Clinical Investigation and the Association of American Physicians.

Disorders of Hemoglobin

Genetics, Pathophysiology, and Clinical Management

Edited by

MARTIN H. STEINBERG

Boston University School of Medicine, Boston, Massachusetts
University of Mississippi School of Medicine, Jackson, Mississippi

BERNARD G. FORGET

Yale University School of Medicine, New Haven, Connecticut

DOUGLAS R. HIGGS

MRC Institute of Molecular Medicine, Oxford, United Kingdom

RONALD L. NAGEL

Albert Einstein College of Medicine, New York, New York

Foreword

H. FRANKLIN BUNN

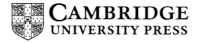

PUBLISHED BY THE PRESS SYNDICATE OF THE UNIVERSITY OF CAMBRIDGE
The Pitt Building, Trumpington Street, Cambridge, United Kingdom

CAMBRIDGE UNIVERSITY PRESS
The Edinburgh Building, Cambridge CB2 2RU, UK
40 West 20th Street, New York, NY 10011-4211, USA
10 Stamford Road, Oakleigh, VIC 3166, Australia
Ruiz de Alarcón 13, 28014 Madrid, Spain
Dock House, The Waterfront, Cape Town 8001, South Africa

http://www.cambridge.org

First published 2001

Printed in the United States of America

Typefaces Sabon 10/12 pt. and Franklin Gothic   *System* QuarkXPress™   [HT]

A catalog record for this book is available from the British Library.

Library of Congress Cataloging in Publication Data

Disorders of hemoglobin : genetics, pathophysiology, and clinical management / edited
by Martin H. Steinberg ... [et al.]
      p.   cm.
    Includes bibliographical references and index.
    ISBN 0-521-63266-8 (HB)
     1. Hemoglobinopathy. I. Steinberg, Martin H.
    [DNLM: 1. Hemoglobinopathies. 2. Anemia, Sickle Cell. 3. Thalassemia. WH 190
D612 2001]
    RC641.7.H35 D575 2001
    616.1′51—dc21   00-046749

ISBN 0 521 63266 8 hardback

Contents

Contributors

Emanuele Angelucci
Department of Hematology, Hospital of Pesaro,
Pesaro, Italy

Lennette J. Benjamin
Division of Hematology, Montefiore Hospital,
Bronx, New York

Edward J. Benz, Jr.
Department of Medicine, Johns Hopkins Hospital,
Baltimore, Maryland

Luigi F. Bernini
Department of Genetics, Sylvius Laboratory,
University of Leiden, Leiden, The Netherlands

Yves Beuzard
Hôpital Saint Louis, Paris, France

Gerd A. Blobel
Abramson Research Center, Children's Hospital
of Philadelphia, Philadelphia, Pennsylvania

Donald K. Bowden
Department of Paediatrics, Monash Medical Centre,
Monash University, Clayton, Australia

Carlo Brugnara
Department of Laboratory Medicine and Pathology,
The Children's Hospital, Harvard Medical School,
Boston, Massachusetts

H. Franklin Bunn
Hematology Division, Brigham and Women's Hospital,
Harvard Medical School, Boston, Massachusetts

Antonio Cao
Instituto de Clinica e Biologia dell'Eta Evolutiva,
Universita degle Studi di Cagliari, Cagliari, Italy

Alan R. Cohen
Division of Hematology, Children's Hospital
of Philadelphia, Philadelphia, Pennsylvania

Lucia De Franceschi
Hôpital Saint Louis, Paris, France

Elaine Dzierzak
Department of Cell Biology, Erasmus University
Medical Faculty, Rotterdam, The Netherlands

James R. Eckman
Division of Hematology/Oncology, Emory University
School of Medicine, Grady Memorial Hospital,
Atlanta, Georgia

Mary E. Fabry
Hematology Division, Albert Einstein College
of Medicine, New York, New York

Frank Ferrone
Department of Physics and Atmospheric Sciences,
Drexel University, Philadelphia, Pennsylvania

Bernard G. Forget
Departments of Internal Medicine and Genetics,
Hematology Section, Yale University School
of Medicine, New Haven, Connecticut

Suthat Fucharoen
Thalassemia Research Center, Institute of Science
and Technology for Research and Development,
Siriraj Hospital, Mahidol University, Nakornpathom,
Thailand

Richard J. Gibbons
Nuffield Department of Clinical Biochemistry,
John Radcliffe Hospital, University of Oxford,
Oxford, United Kingdom

Ross Hardison
Department of Biochemistry and Molecular Biology,
Center for Gene Regulation, Pennsylvania State
University, University Park, Pennsylvania

Robert P. Hebbel
Department of Medicine, University of Minnesota
Medical School, Minneapolis, Minnesota

Douglas R. Higgs
MRC Institute of Molecular Medicine,
John Radcliffe Hospital, University of Oxford,
Oxford, United Kingdom

Shu-Ching Huang
Department of Medicine, Johns Hopkins Hospital,
Baltimore, Maryland

Ernst R. Jaffé
Division of Hematology, Albert Einstein College
of Medicine, Bronx, New York

Panagoula Kollia
First Department of Medicine, University of Athens
School of Medicine, Laikon General Hospital,
Athens, Greece

Stephen A. Liebhaber
HHMI, University of Pennsylvania School
of Medicine, Philadelphia, Pennsylvania

Dimitris Loukopoulos
First Department of Medicine, University of Athens
School of Medicine, Laikon General Hospital,
Athens, Greece

Guido Lucarelli
Department of Hematology, Hospital of Pesaro,
Pesaro, Italy

Anna Rita Migliaccio
Department of Hematology, University of
Washington, Seattle, Washington

Narla Mohandas
Life Sciences Division, Lawrence Berkeley Laboratory,
University of California, Berkeley, Berkeley, California

Ronald L. Nagel
Division of Hematology, Albert Einstein College
of Medicine, New York, New York

Arthur W. Nienhuis
St. Jude Children's Research Hospital, Memphis,
Tennessee

Kwaku Ohene-Frempong
Division of Hematology, The Children's Hospital
of Philadelphia, Philadelphia, Pennsylvania

J. M. Old
Institute of Molecular Medicine, Radcliffe Hospital,
Oxford University, Oxford, United Kingdom

Nancy Olivieri
Hematology/Oncology Department, Toronto General
Hospital and The Hospital for Sick Children,
Toronto, Canada

Thalia Papayannopoulou
Department of Hematology, University
of Washington, Seattle, Washington

Max. F. Perutz
Medical Research Council, Cambridge,
United Kingdom

Orah S. Platt
Children's Hospital, Boston, Massachusetts

John B. Porter
Department of Haematology, University College,
London, United Kingdom

Eliezer A. Rachmilewitz
Hadassah Medical Organization, Jerusalem, Israel

Helen M. Ranney
Alliance Pharmaceutical Corporation, La Jolla,
California

Griffin P. Rodgers
National Institutes of Health, Bethesda, Maryland

Maria Cristina Rosatelli
Instituto di Clincal e Biologia dell'Eta Evolutiva,
Universita degli Studi di Cagliari, Cagliari, Italy

Stanley L. Schrier
Division of Hematology, Stanford University Medical
School, Stanford, California

Graham Serjeant
MRC Laboratories, University of the West Indies,
Kingston, Jamaica

Brian P. Sorrentino
St. Jude Children's Research Hospital,
Memphis, Tennessee

George Stamatoyannopoulos
Medical Genetics, University of Washington, Seattle,
Washington

Martin H. Steinberg
Departments of Medicine and Pediatrics, Boston
University, Boston, Massachusetts

Swee Lay Thein
Guy's, King's and St. Thomas' School of Medicine,
London, United Kingdom

Christiane Vermylen
Centre d'Hematologie Pediatrique, Cliniques
Universitaires Saint-Luc, Bruxelles, Belgium

David J. Weatherall
Institute of Molecular Medicine, John Radcliffe
Hospital, Oxford University, Oxford, United
Kingdom

Mitchell J. Weiss
Abramson Research Center, Children's Hospital
of Philadelphia, Philadelphia, Pennsylvania

W. G. Wood
Institute of Molecular Medicine, John Radcliffe
Hospital, University of Oxford, Oxford, United
Kingdom

Foreword

H. FRANKLIN BUNN

Each year the journal *Science* selects a "Molecule of the Year" in recognition of a substance that has been of particular importance in contemporary chemistry and biology. As we pass into a new millennium, it seems appropriate to reflect on what might be the most apt choice for the grand prize "Molecule of the 20th Century." There are compelling grounds for giving the honor to hemoglobin.

By the end of the 19th century, it was well established that hemoglobin was a composite of protein and heme that could reversibly bind oxygen and that this substance was found in almost all living creatures. The turn of the century marked the dawn of quantitative physiology, biochemistry, and the application of the scientific method to medicine. All three of these developing disciplines owe their early impetus to hemoglobin and the lessons learned from this remarkable molecule. Physiologists from Scandinavia (Bohr and Krogh) and England (Barcroft, the Haldanes, and Roughton) made accurate equilibrium and kinetic measurements of oxygen–hemoglobin binding as a function of pH and thereby provided a mechanistic understanding of the reciprocal transport of oxygen from lung to tissues and of acid waste from tissues to lung. These early contributions set the stage for an appreciation of how the homeostasis of the organism depends upon the orderly integration of its organ systems.

The fledgling science of biochemistry was given a jump start by the studies of Adair and Svedberg, which established that hemoglobin is a uniform protein with a large but narrowly defined molecular weight and was therefore, like sodium chloride and glucose, a *bona fide* molecule. Hemoglobin and its cousin myoglobin were the first proteins whose structures were solved at high resolution by X-ray crystallography by Perutz and Kendrew, respectively, thereby providing an opportunity for detailed exploration of structure–function relationships. Hemoglobin was the first multisubunit protein to be understood at the molecular level and therefore was the model system used by Monod, Changeux, and Wyman for establishing the principles of allostery, which dictate the regulation of a broad range of enzymes, receptors, transcription factors, and so on.

The linkage of specific diseases to abnormalities of specific molecules began with Pauling's demonstration in 1949 that patients with sickle cells have hemoglobin with an altered surface charge. Within 8 years, Ingram demonstrated that sickle hemoglobin differs from normal hemoglobin only by a substitution of valine for glutamic acid in the sixth residue of the β-globin subunit. This was the first example of how an abnormal gene can change the structure of a protein and, therefore, verified in a most satisfying way, the Beadle-Tatem one gene–one enzyme hypothesis.

During the last quarter of the twentieth century, with the development of recombinant DNA technology and genomics, hemoglobin has again been at the vanguard. Indeed the human globin genes were among the first to be molecularly cloned and sequenced. This soon led to the identification of a wide range of globin gene mutants responsible for the α and β thalassemias. Understanding the mechanisms by which these genotypes impair globin biosynthesis provided insight into the diverse clinical manifestations encountered in patients with different types of thalassemia. In addition, the evolving knowledge of human globin genes enabled Kan to develop molecular techniques for antenatal diagnosis and polymorphism-based population studies, both of which were then applied to many other disorders.

To date more than 700 hemoglobin variants have been discovered and characterized. Study of these variants, so amply documented in this book, established the principle of how a mutant genotype alters the function of the protein it encodes, which, in turn, can lead to a distinct clinical phenotype. This linkage is at the heart of how molecular genetics impacts our understanding of pathophysiologic mechanisms.

Thus, hemoglobin has held center stage in the biomedical discoveries of the twentieth century, and there is no indication that the pace has slackened.

This book begins with authoritative and up-to-date coverage of all aspects of hemoglobin, beginning with overviews of erythropoiesis, globin gene regulation, and structure-function relationships. Subsequent sections of the book are devoted to in-depth coverage of the thalassemias, sickle cell disease, and other hemoglobinopathies. A recurrent theme is how understanding pathophysiology at the molecular level has informed the design and development of novel rationally based therapy. The creative energy that is currently bearing down on all aspects of hemoglobin research is well represented by the impressive list of basic and clinical investigators who have contributed to this book. As in any field at the "cutting edge" of science, controversies enrich the scientific dialogue among hemoglobinologists. In carefully reading chapters on closely related topics, the thoughtful reader will adopt a policy of *caveat emptor*, appreciating that strongly held opinions need to be vetted by both experimentation and alternative hypotheses. This proviso notwithstanding, *Disorders of Hemoglobin* offers authoritative and comprehensive coverage of one of the most exciting and fruitful areas at the interface of bioscience and clinical medicine.

Introduction

For the soul of the flesh is the blood—Leviticus, third book of Torah

"The true colour of life is the colour of the body, the colour of the covered red, the implicit and not explicit red of the living heart and the pulses. It is the modest colour of the unpublished blood" (Meynell, 1914)—and hemoglobin colors the blood, often insufficiently or with properties that are catastrophic. Thalassemias and the hemoglobinopathies are man's most common genetic diseases. Whether it is in nonindustrialized developing countries, where the prevalence of these disorders is highest and where they damage the public health, or in industrialized countries, where they are studied at the molecular level and are treated with the latest wonders of modern medicine, the human and economic tolls of these inherited disorders are high. From the days of Malpighi, Leeuwenhoek, Boyle, and Lavoisier through Bohr, Pauling, Perutz, Ingram, Watson, and Crick, studies of the erythrocyte and its contents have propelled the revelation of nature's biological mysteries (see Chapter 1).

No longer is blood "unpublished." With the literature of hemoglobin, including its biophysics, chemistry, molecular biology, and disorders, already measured in gigabytes of disc storage and beyond the capacity of anybody to encompass, we must—in the ritual apologia of editors and authors—defend yet another contribution to the burden of scientist and physician. These past two decades have been a golden age of biology. Our understanding of hemoglobin dis-

orders at the molecular, clinical, and therapeutic levels has been the result of the largess of this era. It has been 15 years since Bunn and Forget published their dual-authored text on hemoglobin and suggested that the current understanding of hemoglobin might be peaking (Bunn and Forget, 1986). Their book, less than 700 pages long, summarized the basic and clinical science of that day. Since then, our knowledge of the molecular basis of erythropoiesis, hemoglobin gene regulation, and thalassemia has burgeoned. Transgenic animal models have been developed that allow new insights into sickle cell disease and thalassemia, providing useful test-beds for innovative treatments. Bone marrow transplantation has become a prime treatment for severe β thalassemia, and hydroxyurea has altered the management and lives of patients with sickle cell anemia. Still, much remains to be done at both the basic and clinical levels. We still do not know how globin gene switching is regulated and how these switches can be manipulated for clinical gain. Iron chelation is unwieldy and often ineffective. Gene therapy remains a glimmer on the horizon. For the sake of our patients and the scientific enterprise we hope that future books about hemoglobin will regard our present contribution as a standard for its time but antediluvian.

Hemoglobin is a subject of interest for basic scientists, translational scientists, and clinicians. We have tried to cover the molecular, cellular, genetic, and clinical aspects of this subject with topical reviews of the science and practical recommendations for diagnosis and treatment. In each chapter we have attempted to summarize what has been learned in the past, place this in the context of the most recent information, and focus on the newest available material. In the first section, we deal with the fundamental aspects of hemoglobin, beginning with the developmental erythropoiesis in lower animals and man, stem cell biology and erythroid progenitor cells, transcriptional control of globin gene expression, and the evolution of globin genes. Focusing on hemoglobin, the specific features of globin gene structure, translational control of hemoglobin synthesis, and the structure and function of normal hemoglobin are recounted. We also include a chapter on the cellular and molecular basis of hemoglobin gene switching, a topic of potential vital therapeutic importance. Concluding this section is a discussion of hemoglobins of the embryo and fetus, minor hemoglobins of adults, and recombinant hemoglobins. The next three sections deal with the diagnosis, pathophysiology, and treatment of β thalassemias and related disorders, α thalassemias, and sickle cell disease. In these sections pathophysiology, clinical features, and molecular mechanisms are discussed.

Hemoglobin disorders are spread throughout the world, and we have attempted to provide a non-parochial view of their clinical spectrum and problems. Section Four begins with a discussion of malaria and how it is responsible for the polymorphic frequency of the thalassemias and major hemoglobinopathies. The distribution and geographic heterogeneity of sickle hemoglobinopathies and the thalassemias illustrate how genetic and environmental factors influence the phenotype of these disorders.

Laboratory diagnostic approaches, transgenic animal models, antenatal diagnosis, and population screening start Section Five. Newer views of the use and misuse of blood transfusion and iron chelation, the employment of "hemoglobin switching" agents to increase fetal hemoglobin production, and bone marrow transplantation for both β thalassemia and sickle cell anemia follow. This section concludes with a look toward the future of gene therapy and discusses innovative strategies for treating sickle cell anemia and thalassemia. Since the beginning of scientific medicine, hemoglobin and its disorders have been in the vanguard of biology, genetics, and medicine. The future of treatment is bright.

Thalassemia and sickle cell anemia are not the sole clinically important hemoglobin disorders. HbE disorders are widespread in Southeast Asia and are a major public health issue. Although rare, unstable hemoglobins, methemoglobins, and hemoglobin variants with altered oxygen affinity often present challenging diagnostic and therapeutic problems and have contributed to our understanding of normal hemoglobin. Many mutant hemoglobins have no clinical phenotype but illustrate interesting biological, genetic, or laboratory features. These conditions are discussed in Section Six.

Finally, not all hemoglobin disorders are genetic disorders intrinsic to the hemoglobin molecule. Acquired disorders of hemoglobin, or dyshemoglobinemias—genetically mediated or due to exogenous agents—are discussed in the final section.

We dedicate this volume to the early pioneers in the field, those who have devoted their life's work to this subject, and to patients who have struggled with hemoglobinopathies and thalassemias. Our families have also born the burden of this work and their support should not be underestimated. Susan and Liza Steinberg have survived with equanimity the mood swings between elation and foreboding that accompanied the beginning optimism, the drudgery of writing and editing, and finally the publication. Claudia and Marta Nagel have seen many a disrupted weekend. Bernadette Forget provided much appreciated support and encouragement.

We thank Richard Barling and Jo-Ann Strangis at Cambridge University Press for stimulating us to begin this project and whipping us continually, but gently, until it was completed. Our many contributors responded to our urgings with understanding and good humor. Our debt to them cannot be overstated. Bristol-Myers Squibb Oncology/Immunology provided very generous support for the editing done by Miriam Blood, Ph.D. We are indebted to Frank Bambarola who made this possible.

References

Bunn, H.F., and Forget, B.G. (1986). *Hemoglobin: Molecular, Genetic and Clinical Aspects*. Philadelphia: W.B. Saunders.

Meynell, A. (1914). *Essays, The True Colour of Life*.

1

Hemoglobin: A Historical Perspective

HELEN M. RANNEY

Isaac Newton's observation, "If I have seen farther than others, it is because I have stood on the shoulders of giants" is as applicable in the history of hemoglobin as it is in numeracy where it has recently been invoked (Steen, 1990). Scientists recognize the creativity of the preceding generation, but memories of the giants more remote in time or place slowly fade. Only rarely is a giant like Gregor Mendel discovered after a lapse of generations.

Builders of the new biology acknowledge that the modern structure has been erected on foundations laid by the giants of earlier eras. Some date the beginning of modern biology and biomedical science to 1953, the year when the three-dimensional structure of DNA was described (Fig. 1.1) (Watson & Crick, 1953). Earlier studies that showed DNA to be the genetic material and disclosed its chemical composition paved the way to that discovery, the most important one in biology in the last century. The Watson-Crick model had a beautiful system of transmission of hereditary material and of controlling the structure and metabolism of cells by dictating protein structure; this was the beginning of a biology not dreamed of two decades earlier.

The content of an historical perspective generally reflects the interests of the writer and this one is no exception. The still unfinished story of the origin, structure and function of hemoglobin continues to engage great scientists and each year brings new insights. This chapter details accounts of research in hemoglobin before 1970.

William Harvey's *De Motu Cordis* of 1628, inaugurating research in cardiac physiology, utilized the anatomic descriptions of arteries and veins published in 1543 by Vesalius, a giant of the previous century. Harvey noted that these vessels contained only blood; the capillaries connecting the arterial and venous systems were described by Malpighi in 1661. More relevant to hemoglobin was Malpighi's incidental observation of the blood globules/corpuscles, erythrocytes, in 1665.

The development of the microscope revolutionized research in blood and blood diseases. The simplest (i.e., single lens) microscopes had small fields, but magnifications of 300 to 400 times could be achieved. The quality of the image depended on the skillful grinding of the lens and the illumination. Malpighi obviously had access to simple microscopes, but the best microscopes of the seventeenth century were those of van Leeuwenhoek, a Dutch tradesman who was a skilled lens grinder and an energetic self-taught microscopist (Ford, 1998; Wintrobe, 1980). In 1678, the Royal Society published van Leeuwenhoek's letter, transmitted by 2 physician friends, describing the red cells of the blood. In many subsequent communications to the Royal Society, van Leeuwenhoek described red cells in considerable detail, including measurements of their diameters.

The mid-seventeenth century also witnessed the initial observations from which the function of the pulmonary circulation would be deduced. In 1660, Robert Boyle (of Boyle's Law) noted that air was necessary to support the combustion of a burning candle or the life of an animal; when he pumped air out of a chamber in which he had placed a burning candle or a mouse, the candle was extinguished or the mouse died. Richard Lower, like Boyle a founding member of the Royal Society, used Robert Hooke's experimental (open chest) animal preparation to demonstrate the change in color of blood as it passed through the lungs (Lower, 1669). In 1674, John Mayow, also an experimentalist, concluded that some part of air was used in combustion or respiration, although most of air was inert (West, 1998). Mayow's observations were largely forgotten. Nearly a century passed before Lavoisier, following the isolation of oxygen by Scheele and Priestley, formulated a unifying theory for Boyle's observations on the requirement of air to support the flame of the candle or the life of the mouse; in each of these experiments oxygen was consumed and carbon

No. 4356 April 25, 1953 N A T U R E

MOLECULAR STRUCTURE OF NUCLEIC ACIDS

A Structure for Deoxyribose Nucleic Acid

WE wish to suggest a structure for the salt of deoxyribose nucleic acid (D.N.A.). This structure has novel features which are of considerable biological interest.

A structure for nucleic acid has already been proposed by Pauling and Corey[1]. They kindly made their manuscript available to us in advance of publication. Their model consists of three intertwined chains, with the phosphates near the fibre axis, and the bases on the outside. In our opinion, this structure is unsatisfactory for two reasons: (1) We believe that the material which gives the X-ray diagrams is the salt, not the free acid. Without the acidic hydrogen atoms it is not clear what forces would hold the structure together, especially as the negatively charged phosphates near the axis will repel each other. (2) Some of the van der Waals distances appear to be too small.

Another three-chain structure has also been suggested by Fraser (in the press). In his model the phosphates are on the outside and the bases on the inside, linked together by hydrogen bonds. This structure as described is rather ill-defined, and for this reason we shall not comment on it.

We wish to put forward a radically different structure for the salt of deoxyribose nucleic acid. This structure has two helical chains each coiled round the same axis (see diagram). We have made the usual chemical assumptions, namely, that each chain consists of phosphate diester groups joining β-D-deoxyribofuranose residues with 3′,5′ linkages. The two chains (but not their bases) are related by a dyad perpendicular to the fibre axis. Both chains follow right-handed helices, but owing to the dyad the sequences of the atoms in the two chains run in opposite directions. Each chain loosely resembles Furberg's[2] model No. 1; that is, the bases are on the inside of the helix and the phosphates on the outside. The configuration of the sugar and the atoms near it is close to Furberg's 'standard configuration', the sugar being roughly perpendicular to the attached base. There

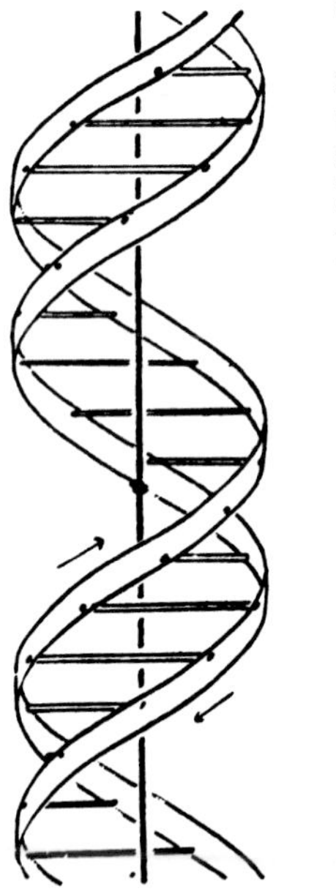

This figure is purely diagrammatic. The two ribbons symbolize the two phosphate—sugar chains, and the horizontal rods the pairs of bases holding the chains together. The vertical line marks the fibre axis

Figure 1.1A. Three articles that dramatically altered research in hemoglobin. Watson and Crick's brief paper (1953) on the molecular structure of nucleic acids changed the direction of biological, biochemical, and biomedical research. It is the cornerstone of our knowledge of the molecular pathology of the diseases of the globin genes, particularly thalassemia.

416   N A T U R E   February 13, 1960   VOL. 185

STRUCTURE OF HÆMOGLOBIN

A THREE-DIMENSIONAL FOURIER SYNTHESIS AT 5·5-Å. RESOLUTION, OBTAINED BY X-RAY ANALYSIS

By Dr. M. F. PERUTZ, F.R.S., Dr. M. G. ROSSMANN, ANN F. CULLIS, HILARY MUIRHEAD
and Dr. GEORG WILL

Medical Research Council Unit for Molecular Biology, Cavendish Laboratory, University of Cambridge

AND

Dr. A. C. T. NORTH

Medical Research Council External Staff, Davy Faraday Research Laboratory,
Royal Institution, London, W.I

VERTEBRATE hæmoglobin is a protein of molecular weight 67,000. Four of its 10,000 atoms are iron atoms which are combined with protoporphyrin to form four hæm groups. The remaining atoms are in four polypeptide chains of roughly equal size, which are identical in pairs[1-3]. Their amino-acid sequence is still largely unknown.

We have used horse oxy- or met-hæmoglobin because it crystallizes in a form especially suited for X-ray analysis, and employed the method of isomorphous replacement with heavy atoms to determine the phase angles of the diffracted rays[4-7]. The Fourier synthesis which we have calculated shows that hæmoglobin consists of four sub-units in a tetrahedral array and that each sub-unit closely resembles Kendrew's model of sperm whale myoglobin[8]. The four hæm groups lie in separate pockets on the surface of the molecule.

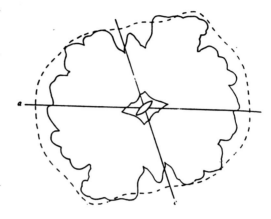

Figure 1.1B. Perutz article (1960) on the three-dimensional structure of hemoglobin. At last the molecule whose awesome function had been so long appreciated could be seen!

dioxide and water were produced (Lavoisier, 1778). Nitrogen, the inert fraction of air, was not changed in the lungs; but the "respirable fraction," oxygen, combined with hemoglobin to yield the characteristic color of oxyhemoglobin. At the end of the eighteenth century, Spallanzini, a brilliant physiologist, identified the peripheral tissues as sites where oxygen is delivered and carbon dioxide taken into the blood (Castiglioni, 1947).

The central role of the cell in the life of plants and animals was not recognized until the nineteenth century. Two names associated with cell theory are Matthias Schleiden, who in 1838 visualized plants as communities of cells with each cell having a separate existence, and Theodor Schwann, who soon thereafter extended the theory to animals (Schwann, 1847). Although the cell theory found rapid acceptance and energized all biological research, disagreement arose about the origin of cells. Both Schleiden and Schwann believed that growth reflected increasing numbers of cells, but both also thought that new cells arose from amorphous material, not from living parent cells. Virchow, the great nineteenth century pathologist, was convinced that cells arise by division of existing cells.

The bone marrow as the site of hematopoiesis was recognized by two investigators, probably simultaneously and certainly independently: Professor Ernst Neumann (Neumann 1868, 1869) and Giulio Bizzozzero (Bizzozzero 1868, 1869) (Fig. 1.2). Both Neumann and Bizzozzero identified nucleated red cells in the marrow as precursors of circulating erythrocytes, and both recognized that red cell production in the marrow was a continuous process in postnatal life. Neumann is generally credited with the discovery, but Bizzozzero, a 22-year-old recent graduate of Pavia, made many important original observations about the marrow. Tavassoli observed that the views of Neumann and Bizzozzero differed in some details and that in each of those instances, Bizzozzero was correct. Tavassoli wrote: "a careful reading of these interesting communications leaves one with the impression that perhaps Bizzozzero might have come to this conclusion even before Neumann but he was unsure of the reception he might receive if his findings were announced" (Tavassoli, 1980). Bizzozzero's model included the marrow as the site of origin of white blood cells as well as red cells. He observed the apparent extrusion of nuclei from normoblasts in the marrow and interpreted large cells containing pigmented granules as sites of red cell destruction.

Sickle Cell Anemia, a Molecular Disease[1]

Linus Pauling, Harvey A. Itano,[2] S. J. Singer,[2] and Ibert C. Wells[3]

*Gates and Crellin Laboratories of Chemistry,
California Institute of Technology, Pasadena, California[4]*

THE ERYTHROCYTES of certain individuals possess the capacity to undergo reversible changes in shape in response to changes in the partial pressure of oxygen. When the oxygen pressure is lowered, these cells change their forms from the normal biconcave disk to crescent, holly wreath, and other forms. This process is known as sickling. About 8 percent of American Negroes possess this characteristic: usually they exhibit no pathological consequences ascribable to it. These people are said to have sicklemia, or sickle cell trait. However, about 1 in 40 (*1*) of these individuals whose cells are capable of sickling suffer from a severe chronic anemia resulting from excessive destruction of their erythrocytes; the term sickle cell anemia is applied to their condition.

that form from normal erythrocytes. In this condition they are termed promeniscocytes. The hemoglobin appears to be uniformly distributed and randomly oriented within normal cells and promeniscocytes, and no birefringence is observed. Both types of cells are very flexible. If the oxygen or carbon monoxide is removed, however, transforming the hemoglobin to the uncombined state, the promeniscocytes undergo sickling. The hemoglobin within the sickled cells appears to aggregate into one or more foci, and the cell membranes collapse. The cells become birefringent (*11*) and quite rigid. The addition of oxygen or carbon monoxide to these cells reverses these phenomena. Thus the physical effects just described depend on the state of combination of the hemoglobin, and only secondarily, if at all, on the cell membrane.

Figure 1.1C. Pauling, Itano, Singer, and Wells' (1949) description of sickle cell anemia as a molecular disease provided a new concept of hereditary diseases.

Despite the clear descriptions of Neumann and Bizzozzero, the normoblasts of the marrow were not generally acknowledged as the parent cells of the circulating red cells for two decades thereafter. Neumann continued to study the marrow; he described bone marrow diseases and supported the erroneous notion that red cells are formed within the marrow microvasculature (as indeed red cells are formed in birds). Hematopoiesis in mammals, however, is extravascular and cells gain access to the circulation through a sinusoidal barrier that is not completely understood. Bizzozzero, who believed that human hematopoiesis was extravascular, subsequently became interested in coagulation and is usually credited with the discovery of platelets and descriptions of their function (Bizzozzero 1882; Spaet, 1980), although others including Osler may have noticed platelets earlier. Bizzozzero became the premier Italian pathologist of the late nineteenth century (Castiglioni, 1947).

Improved compound microscopes had become available in the 1830s. With Ehrlich's introduction of stains for tissues and for blood films, the ready identification of cellular structures placed hematology fore-

most among medical disciplines driven by Schleiden and Schwann's theory of the cell (Ehrlich, 1877). Ehrlich defined the types of leukocytes, indicated that lymphocytes were produced in lymphatic tissues, and suggested that other leukocytes in the blood originated in the bone marrow. He also described the megaloblast of pernicious anemia and distinguished aplastic anemia from other anemias. Ehrlich was a legend in his time not only for his contributions to the morphologic underpinnings of hematology, but also because of his pioneering work in immunology, microbiology, and the chemotherapy of syphilis.

MORPHOLOGY AND HEMATOPOIESIS

The era of morphology, the 50 years that followed the introduction of stained blood smears, did not add much to the understanding of blood or blood diseases. In the United States, few physicians had much skill or interest in clinical microscopy or in clinical chemistry before the Flexner Report of 1911, which described in excruciating detail the inadequacies of most American medical training. The central question of morphologists for the first three decades of the twentieth century was the identification of the parent hematopoietic cell, the stem cell. Much of the following account is taken from Lajtha's excellent summary of that long controversy (Lajtha, 1980). In Ehrlich's dualist theory, lymphocytes origi-

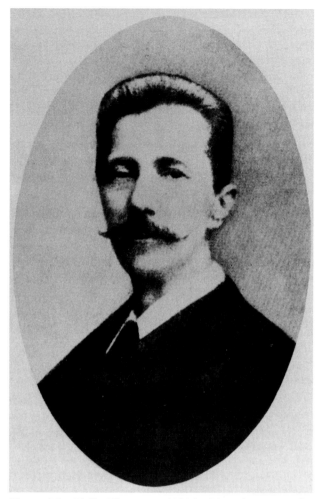

Figure 1.2. Giulio Bizzozzero (1846–1901). At age 22 he described the marrow as the site of erythropoiesis, including hematopoiesis. He recognized normoblasts as red cell precursors, noted extrusion of nuclei from normoblasts, and identified pigmented granules in macrophages as debris from red cell breakdown. In 1868, he published a classic monograph on platelets, describing their structure and function and distinguishing between blood coagulation and hemostasis.

nated in lymphatic tissue and the granulocytes in the bone marrow. His student Pappenheim, however, concluded that a primitive mononuclear cell lacking distinctive features could be totipotential. This monophyletic theory attracted the support of embryologists who think of a single cell as the sole parent of a whole organism. Pappenheim, Maximov, Bloom, Ferrata, and Dantschakoff predicted a single stem cell; Ehrlich, Naegeli, Schilling, and Sabin supported a dualist view. Originally neither camp paid much attention to the parent cell of the erythroid lineage, but in 1909 Pappenheim indicated that the primitive stem cell could also be the ancestral erythroid cell (i.e., a common stem cell could give rise to all blood cells) (Pappenheim, 1909). One distinguished dualist, Naegeli, was an authoritarian Swiss

who held his own opinions in high regard: "In 1900 I described the myeloblast as the precursor of all the white cells in the bone marrow and thereby I established the then shaken dualistic view of Ehrlich on firm grounds" (Lajtha, 1980). The controversy faded after 1930, as investigators appreciated that the answer was beyond the reach of the microscope.

The single common stem cell was established in the 1960s by two separate lines of investigation. Till and McCulloch observed the growth in the spleen of colonies of different types of cells after injection of marrow cells into irradiated mice (Till and McCulloch, 1961). Metcalf in Australia (Bradley and Metcalf, 1966) and Sachs in Israel (Pluznick and Sachs, 1966) devised methods for clonogenic cultures of different cell types (e.g., granulocytes, macrophages, or erythroid cells under different conditions of culture). From these studies, the existence of a common totipotential stem cell was established. Lajtha used highly radioactive tritium-labeled thymidine, which is lethal to dividing cells that incorporate the thymidine into their nuclei, to distinguish types of early progenitor cells; the rate of proliferation of the stem cells was very low (Lajtha et al., 1969).

From many studies emerged the model of the totipotential stem cell. In addition to capacity for self-replication, this cell is capable of generating different hematopoietic cells by transit through stages of "committed" but morphologically indistinguishable cells to "recognizable" cells of known, e.g., myeloid or erythroid lineage. Manifold amplification occurs in both committed and recognizable stages; more than a thousand circulating cells may be derived from a single totipotential cell. The number of totipotential stem cells would be quite small but capable of self-renewal. Changes in the numbers of cells of a given lineage would result mostly from replication of committed progenitor or precursor cells. The effects of growth factors such as erythropoietin are exerted mostly through the committed maturing cell populations.

A modern view of developmental hematopoiesis is presented in Chapter 2. Early observations on erythropoiesis during embryogenesis were made by Kölliker, who found nucleated erythroid cells in the liver (Kölliker, 1846), and Van der Stricht, who later noted the intravascular origin of red cells in embryonic sites (Van der Stricht, 1892). Interest in human embryonic hematopoiesis was stimulated by the finding of two hemoglobins distinct from adult HbA or fetal hemoglobin HbF in small human embryos (Huehns et al., 1961). The correlations of types of hemoglobin with ontogeny of erythropoiesis in mice and humans, constitute an early chapter in developmental molecular genetics. The initial site of erythropoiesis in mammals was thought to be the yolk sac, where at 7 to 8 days of gestation in mice (16 days in humans) primitive cells, hemangioblasts, are formed in the extraembryonic mesenchymal layer, probably with cooperation from the endoderm. Hemangioblasts are almost entirely erythroid and self-assemble to form blood islands; they resemble stem cells and at 10 to 11 days of gestation (mouse), cells from the blood islands of the yolk sac seed the liver to begin a period of mainly hepatic hematopoiesis with detectable hematopoiesis in lymph nodes, spleen, and bone marrow (Moore and Metcalf, 1970).

At the fifth month of gestation in humans, the major site of hematopoiesis shifts from the liver to the marrow. Accompanying the changing sites of erythropoiesis are changes in the globin subunits in both mice and humans. In the mouse genes for embryonic globins are expressed during yolk sac erythropoiesis, and adult α- and β-globin genes are expressed thereafter (Barker, 1968). In humans, as hematopoiesis moves to the liver, embryonic ϵ-globin (β-like) and ζ-globin (α-like) disappear, the synthesis of α-globin rises sharply to a high level where it remains, and the γ-globin chains of HbF replace the embryonic ϵ-globin chains. Synthesis of adult β-globin chains, begun during yolk sac hematopoiesis, persists at low levels during the hepatic phase and rises quickly about the time of birth, as γ-globin chain synthesis declines. The mouse has embryonic and adult hemoglobins but has no hemoglobin corresponding to the HbF of humans. The two hemoglobins observed by Huehns were tetramers, $\alpha_2\epsilon_2$ and $\zeta_2\epsilon_2$, of yolk sac erythropoiesis. The third embryonic hemoglobin tetramer $\zeta_2\gamma_2$ was described later. Recently synthesis of human embryonic hemoglobins in yeast has permitted studies of their crystal structure and oxygen equilibria (Chapter 9).

CHEMISTRY OF HEMOGLOBIN

As hematopoiesis interested experimental pathologists in the mid-nineteenth century, the blood pigment attracted the attention of chemists. Hematin was crystallized from red cells in 1857 by Teichman who noted the presence of iron. Felix Hoppe-Seyler used the term *hemoglobin* to describe the blood pigment. He noted that hemoglobin could be split into hematin and a protein and described the spectrum of oxyhemoglobin (Hoppe, 1862). Stokes at Cambridge then observed the spectral differences between oxygenated and deoxygenated hemoglobin, evidence of the reversible binding of oxygen (Stokes, 1864). The iron content of hemoglobin, found to be 0.33% in several laboratories, indicated a minimum molecular weight of 16,000 daltons. Peters found that 0.975 mole of oxygen bound each mole of iron (Peters, 1912); that is, the iron of each heme bound a single oxygen molecule. By

1929, Hans Fischer had synthesized heme and established its structure as a tetrapyrrole containing iron at its center (Fischer and Orth, 1937). Meanwhile from meticulous measurements of osmotic pressure, Adair concluded that the molecular weight of hemoglobin was 67,000 daltons (Adair, 1924). With the use of the ultracentrifuge, Svedberg found the molecular weight to be 68,000 (Svedberg and Fahraeus, 1926). Thus the work of Adair, Svedberg, and Peters revealed that hemoglobin contained four subunits each of which was capable of reversible binding with oxygen. Pauling deduced the "bent" arrangement of the oxygen atoms in binding to heme iron (Pauling and Coryell, 1936).

FUNCTION OF HEMOGLOBIN: HEMOGLOBIN AS AN OXYGEN TRANSPORT PROTEIN

Although the function of hemoglobin in oxygen transport was recognized by Lavoisier in the late 1700s, the relationships of oxygen supply and altitude sickness were not obvious. In 1569, Joseph de Acosta, a Jesuit priest, described altitude sickness as a syndrome of breathlessness, dizziness, vomiting, and fainting and related it to high altitudes where "the elements of the air are in this place so thin and delicate that it is not suitable for human breathing" (Erslev 1980; West 1998). Acosta's observations and publication in 1590 preceded by nearly 200 years the discoveries of Priestley and Lavoisier. Needless to say, Acosta's idea did not have wide circulation or acceptance.

Experiences of balloonists in the nineteenth century suggested the possible role of oxygen lack in altitude sickness. Bert, who designed and built altitude chambers in which the effects of high and low air pressure were observed, showed in 1878 that altitude sickness was related to oxygen lack (Bert, 1943). Bert has been called the "father of aviation medicine"; his work led to arrangements for oxygen supplies for mountain climbers and for balloonists (Olmstead, 1952). Bert and others believed that the polycythemia of dwellers at high altitudes was an adaptation that had evolved over many generations. That notion was conclusively refuted by Viault, who traveled from Lima at sea level to Morococha at 15,000 ft. Within a few weeks, his red cell count had risen from 5 to 8 million cells/mm^3. Similar changes were noted in others after brief sojourns at high altitudes (Viault, 1890).

The signal that stimulates erythropoiesis at high altitudes was puzzling. The theory of Miescher (1893) that hypoxia stimulates the marrow, was accepted, although Carnot and Deflandre suggested an alternative hypothesis. They found a remarkable rise in the red cell counts of rabbits receiving serum from anemic rabbits. They proposed that a factor, *hematopoietine*, in the blood of the anemic animals stimulated the marrow of the recipients (Carnot and Deflandre, 1906). Other laboratories repeated the studies and in the words of Allen Erslev, "the results from most studies were either too fantastic to believe or too insignificant to trust" (Erslev, 1980), and the existence of hematopoietine was not seriously considered until the measurements of marrow PO_2 in polycythemia made Miescher's hypothesis untenable (Berk et al., 1948).

In 1950, Kurt Reissman inaugurated the series of studies then pursued in many laboratories that led to the identification of the humoral factor of Carnot and Deflandre. Reissmann established a cutaneous connection carrying microvasculature between two rats, one of which breathed a low PO_2 gas mixture and the other, room air. In 39 such parabiotic rat pairs, the rat breathing room air exhibited an erythropoietic response closely resembling that of the connected hypoxemic animal (Fig. 1.3) (Reissmann, 1950). Reissmann's experiment supported the exis-

tence of the humoral factor now designated erythropoietin. Erslev repeated the experiment of Carnot and Deflandre using larger amounts of serum from anemic animals. They noted striking increases in reticulocytes after administration of "anemic" plasma (Erslev, 1953). Erythropoietin was purified to homogeneity from the urine of patients with aplastic anemia by Goldwasser (Mikake et al., 1977). Goldwasser isolated small quantities of purified erythropoietin and established its structure; this provided the basis for cloning and commercial production of erythropoietin years later.

NORMAL HEMOGLOBIN: FUNCTION AND STRUCTURE

In 1904, Christian Bohr described the sigmoid shape of the O_2 dissociation curve of hemoglobin (Bohr, 1904), and in a second paper with Hasselbalch and Krogh noted that carbon dioxide reduced the oxygen affinity (Bohr et al., 1904), an effect later shown to reflect proton binding. Bohr's sigmoid curve supplanted that of Hüfner who believed that oxygen–hemoglobin binding was a simple bimolecular combination described by a hyperbolic curve (Hüfner, 1884). Data supporting the sigmoid oxygen dissociation curve were obtained with manometric techniques (Barcroft, 1928). In 1910, well before the molecular weight of hemoglobin was established, A.V. Hill, a mathematician analyzing the physical basis of the hemoglobin-oxygen equilibria, concluded that the sigmoid curve was the result of the formation of aggregates of oxygen binding units and of cooperative interactions among those aggregates (Hill, 1910). Roughton and Hartridge, like Hill, members of the Barcroft laboratory, concluded from the kinetics of oxygen binding to and dissociation from hemoglobin that the reactions of oxygen with hemoglobin occurred much faster than the time needed for the red cell to traverse the microcirculation (Hartridge and Roughton, 1923, 1925).

Concepts of the structure of hemoglobin lagged behind knowledge of its function for many years. The great chemist Emil Fischer isolated three amino acids—valine, hydroxyproline, and proline—from protein hydrolysates. He developed a method to synthesize peptides as large as 18 amino acids and coined the term *polypeptide* between 1899 and 1907. Although Fischer did not appreciate the

Figure 1.3. Reissman's observations (1950) on a pair of parabiotic rats, one of which was hypoxic (broken line) while the attached partner breathed room air (solid line). The increase in hemoglobin and reticulocytes (shown in top two frames) of the rat breathing room air paralleled increases observed in the hypoxic partner. This experiment reopened the possibility of humoral control of erythropoiesis, suggested in 1906 by Carnot and Deflandre.

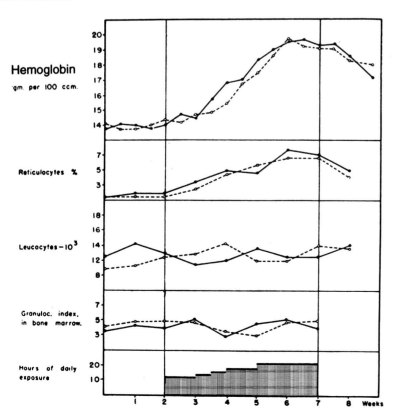

potentially large size of some proteins, he recognized that the identity and sequence of the amino acids determined the characteristics of proteins. In 1920, Staudinger, a pioneer in macromolecular chemistry, argued that these large molecules contained valency bonds and were homogeneous. Svedberg provided solid evidence of a defined structure of proteins: hemoglobin was a single homogeneous molecule with a molecular weight of 68,000; Bernal and Crowfoot developed a model of pepsin derived from x-ray crystallographic data (Bernal and Crowfoot, 1934). Pauling's descriptions of the helical structure of many proteins and of the nature of the peptide bond strengthened the evidence that proteins were compounds of defined chemical structure.

The concept of linked functions of hemoglobin originally formulated by Henderson (Henderson, 1928) was expanded by Wyman (Wyman, 1964): when hemoglobin binds oxygen, CO_2 and protons are released. The tension of CO_2 will affect the extent of oxygen binding, and extent of oxygen binding will affect CO_2 tension. In another ligand-linked function of hemoglobin, Roughton demonstrated binding of CO_2 to hemoglobin in a carbamino linkage (Ferguson and Roughton, 1934). Much larger amounts of CO_2 are transported in carbamino linkage in hemoglobin free ox studied by Roughton than in hemoglobins that bind 2,3-biphosphoglycerte (2,3-BPG) (Bunn, 1971), which binds to hemoglobin at the same site as the carbamino linkage. Oxygenation-linked binding of chloride and phosphate, like that of protons, was recognized in 1961 (Rossi-Fanelli et al., 1961). The structural implications of the sigmoid curve that describes the hemoglobin-oxygen equilibria were recognized by Pauling, who suggested that each step in the binding of oxygen to hemoglobin changed the structure of hemoglobin to increase the oxygen affinity of the unliganded hemes (Pauling, 1935)(Fig. 1.4). Pauling concluded that the four hemes, Adair's binding sites, were at the corners of a square on the surface of the hemoglobin molecule and ascribed the changing oxygen affinity with oxygenation to "heme-heme interaction." In Pauling's model, oxygenation of one heme would directly affect a neighboring heme; the need for the reaction pathway among the hemes was not evident until the three-dimensional model of the hemoglobin molecule was obtained by Perutz (Perutz et al., 1960). That model revolutionized thinking about the structure and function of hemoglobin (Fig. 1.1B) (Chapter 8).

As models based on the x-ray crystallographic analyses of liganded and unliganded hemoglobin (Muirhead et al., 1967) emerged from Perutz' laboratory, discerning the structural basis of hemoglobin function became an adventure in protein

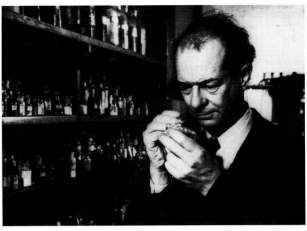

Figure 1.4. Linus Pauling (1901–1994). A renowned scientist of the twentieth century whose work on the nature of the chemical bond was key to understanding the structure of proteins. His interest in hemoglobin, evident from early considerations of the nature of the iron–oxygen bond and of heme–heme interactions found expression in the identification of a molecular lesion as the cause of sickle cell anemia. (Courtesy of the Archives, California Institute of Technology.)

chemistry. The hydrophobic siting of the hemes separated from each other by some distance, the helical arrangement of 75 percent of the amino acids, and the relationships of the subunits were visualized with increasing clarity as x-ray crystallographic data at higher resolution were obtained. The subunits interact with each other by relatively weak forces; deoxyhemoglobin is further stabilized by intersubunit salt bonds formed by the four C-terminal residues, as well as by hydrogen bonds. Liganding the heme leads to changes in the protein: rotation of one $\alpha\beta$-dimer relative to its partner, movement at the $\alpha_1\beta_2$ contacts, and breaking of the C-terminal salt bridges (Perutz, 1970).

Two alternative structural mechanisms were proposed for the cooperative (allosteric) nature of the oxygen equilibria. The first mechanism is the two-state model of Monod, Wyman, and Changeux (the MWC model), in which hemoglobin is in either the liganded, R (relaxed), conformation, or unliganded T (tense) conformation (Monod et al., 1965a). The second is the sequential model of Koshland in which binding to each subunit changes its tertiary structure and that conformation change affects the oxygen affinity of unliganded subunits (Koshland et al., 1966). Koshland's sequential model was a more direct heir to Pauling's formulation of heme-heme interaction. Whereas the MWC model has two states, R and T, the Koshland model has several intermediate states that reflect stages of liganding. Many different experimental methods have been applied to studies of the partially oxygenated intermediates:

kinetic experiments by Quentin Gibson (Parkhurst, 1979), nuclear magnetic resonance by Chien Ho (Ho, 1992), and oxygenation of valency hybrid hemoglobins (e.g., $\alpha^{+CN}\beta_2$ studied by many investigators including Cassoly [Cassoly and Gibson, 1972] and Ackers [Ackers, 1998]). A modified two-state MWC model has received the most support even as allostery continues to attract the interest of physical chemists and biochemists.

With the advent of the three-dimensional model of Perutz, the structural basis of the ligand-linked functions could be investigated in molecular detail. Reinhold and Ruth Benesch (Benesch and Benesch, 1967) and Chanutin and Curnish (Chanutin and Curnish 1967) independently described another ligand-linked function: the binding of 2,3-BPG to deoxyhemoglobin was associated with decreased oxygen affinity. Diphosphoglycerate binds to the central cavity of the deoxyhemoglobin tetramer (Arnone, 1972), increasing the bonds of the T state. Increased 2,3-BPG in red cells was associated with hypoxia (e.g., anemias, ascent to high altitudes), conditions that would benefit from increased oxygen delivery. The right shift of the oxygen dissociation curve mediated by increased 2,3-BPG did not increase oxygen delivery in the presence of significantly decreased arterial oxygen saturation. Decreased binding of 2,3-BPG by Hb^{3}F (as compared with HbA) provided the explanation for the increased oxygen affinity of fetal red cells despite the near equivalence in oxygen affinity of purified fetal and adult hemoglobins (Bauer et al., 1968).

RECOGNITION OF THE HEMOLYTIC ANEMIAS AND THE MEASUREMENT OF THE RED CELL LIFE SPAN

During the nineteenth and early twentieth centuries, physicians noted cases of anemia resulting from hemolysis and distinguished between intrinsic and extrinsic causes of accelerated red cell destruction. Dacie pointed out that the clear descriptions of the hemolytic anemias published in that period are concerned with disorders that are quite uncommon; initial recognition of hemolysis depended on the presence of hemoglobinuria (Dacie, 1980). Although the first such description, that of paroxysmal cold hemoglobinuria, is generally credited to Dressler in 1854, Dacie noted that paroxysmal cold hemoglobinuria "seems likely to have been the diagnosis in the patient described by Elliotson in the *Lancet* in 1832 who passed bloody urine 'whenever the east wind blew'" (Dacie, 1980). Paroxysmal cold hemoglobinuria was associated with now rare congenital syphilis. The Donath Landsteiner serum antibody in paroxysmal cold hemoglobinuria binds to red cells in the cold and with a labile factor (complement) results in hemolysis on warming (Donath and Landsteiner, 1904).

THE LIFE SPAN OF THE CIRCULATING RED CELL

Winifred Ashby, a graduate student at the Mayo Clinic, found between 1919 to 1921 that normal human red cells survive in the circulation for about 100 days. Ashby transfused blood group O red cells to recipients of blood group A and followed the fate of the donor group O cells in blood samples from the recipient at intervals after the transfusion (Ashby, 1919, 1921). Ashby was a pioneer, whose contributions were original, important, and unrecognized for decades. Peyton Rous in a 1923 review noted that about 1/15 (6% to 7%) of the red cells were thought to be destroyed each day (Rous, 1923). In regard to Ashby's findings of a red cell life span of 100 days, Rous concluded that "more facts were needed," despite the fact that three of Ashby's articles on red cell life span had been published in a highly respected journal and she had collected a great deal of data on 100 patients. Ashby's studies received little attention until World War II, when the technique was used extensively to evaluate methods for blood preservation for civilian and military casualties. Using Ashby's method, Sheila Callender calculated an average erythrocyte life span of 120 days for normal group O red cells given to three previously phlebotomized medical students (Callender et al., 1945).

During the 1940s, as World War II ended, methods that were to revolutionize medical research were introduced. At Columbia, Rittenberg, Shemin, and London used the heavy isotope ^{15}N to measure red cell life span in healthy human subjects (Shemin and Rittenberg, 1946), and patients with polycythemia, sickle cell anemia, and pernicious anemia (London et al., 1949). Isotopic glycine was administered orally and the specific activity of heme measured in serial red cell samples during the ensuing weeks. With isotopes the survival of both abnormal and normal cells could be safely studied without danger of transmitting infection. In normal persons, the erythrocyte life span was about 120 days, and the red cells appeared to die as a function of cell age. In polycythemia vera, a normal red cell life span, with increased red cell production, and in pernicious anemia a moderately shortened red cell life span were found. In sickle cell anemia, the accelerated destruction of red cells appeared to be random and unrelated to red cell age. The method of measuring an incorporated isotopic amino acid, while providing the most accurate measurements of survival of both normal and defective red cells, was labor intensive. The introduction of ^{51}Cr for measuring red cell survival (Gray and Sterling, 1950) replaced both the Ashby and the ^{15}N methods in clinical use.

THE SYNTHESIS OF HEME

For studies of the synthesis of heme, David Shemin utilized the observations that young red cells, both mammalian and avian, synthesize heme and globin in vitro (London et al., 1948, 1950; Shemin et al., 1948) and used the newly available ^{14}C for isotopic labeling. The in vitro systems measuring synthesis by incubating young red cells or their subcellular fractions with isotopes would be widely used for studies of synthesis not only of heme but also of globin and of other cellular components. Modifications of those methods were later used for studies of the molecular mechanisms of synthesis. Shemin's group found that the initial step in the biosynthesis of heme in mammals is the condensation of glycine with succinyl CoA to form δ-aminolevulinate. Two molecules of δ-aminolevulinate condense to form the monopyrrole, porphobilinogen (Shemin, 1954). Several investigators contributed to the delineation of the further steps in the synthesis of heme from the linear array of the tetrapyrrole that includes four molecules of porphobilinogen. The discovery of the enzymes of heme synthesis was rapidly followed by the identification of abnormalities of specific enzymes in each of the long known and little understood porphyrias.

Observing the regulatory effects of heme on both heme and protein synthesis, London confirmed repression of heme synthesis and stimulation of globin synthesis by the addition of hemin (London et al., 1964). These and subsequent observations emphasized the tight regulation of normal hemoglobin synthesis: globin chains and heme are produced in each cell only in the requisite amounts to form hemoglobin tetramers.

DISORDERS RESULTING FROM DEFECTS IN THE STRUCTURE OR SYNTHESIS OF HEMOGLOBIN

Diseases caused by defects in the globin gene are the most common lethal genetic defects in the world. Sickle cell disease and thalassemia were described as clinical entities characterized by abnormal red cells many years before their hereditary transmission was recognized. Discoveries in the molecular pathogenesis of sickling and thalassemia often preceded or paralleled discoveries about normal hemoglobin function and globin genes (Fig. 1.1C). Both sickle cell disease and thalassemia were first described in the medical literature in the United States; the sickle hemoglobin gene was obviously brought by the Atlantic slave trade (Curtin, 1969) and thalassemia by immigrants from

Mediterranean countries and later by refugees from Southeast Asia (Chapter 26).

Sickle Cell Disease

While clinical illnesses resembling sickle cell disease were known in West Africa for centuries, the nature of those diseases is uncertain. Most infants with sickle cell anemia would not have survived in Africa beyond the first few years of life, and heterozygotes would not have been symptomatic. If erythrocyte sickling was the cause of the diseases described, then it was probably one of the genetic variants of sickle cell disease or a mild form of sickle cell anemia.

The first medical description of sickle cell disease was published in 1910 by James Herrick who described thin, sickle-shaped red cells in a student from the Caribbean who complained of breathlessness and palpitations and was hospitalized for back and muscle pain (Herrick, 1910). Herrick suggested that the illness might be related to the abnormal-appearing red cells. Within the next few years, similar illnesses in African Americans were reported by others. Conley has written an excellent review of the early history of sickling (Conley, 1980). In 1917 Emmel sealed under a coverslip a drop of blood of a patient with sickle cell anemia; after several days all the red cells were sickled. Emmel also noted sickled cells in the patient's father (Emmel, 1917). Neither Emmel nor succeeding investigators distinguished between the asymptomatic and the anemic individuals with sickle cells, although several, among them Sydenstricker in Georgia (Sydenstricker, 1923), found sickling in asymptomatic parents of patients with sickle cell anemia. Many thought that this asymptomatic sickle state could progress to sickle cell anemia.

Some of the delay in recognizing the relationships of sickling in healthy individuals was related to the unskilled use of Emmel's sickle cell preparations. Sydenstricker found "latent sickling" in only 13 of 300 African Americans tested. In 1947, Neel was unable to discern a pattern of inheritance from the published data (Neel, 1947), but in 1949 he performed tests on the parents of patients with sickle cell anemia and showed that asymptomatic sickle cell trait is the heterozygous state for a gene that in the homozygous state is manifest as sickle cell anemia (Neel, 1949).

Two physicians are preeminent in the early descriptions of the clinical manifestations of sickle cell disease. Sydenstricker had long been interested in sickle cell disease; he described the disease in children, introduced the term *crisis* for the acute illness, noted the variability of the manifestations over time in a given patient, observed that he had seen no patients older than 30 years old, and reported the first autopsy, all in the 1920s. The other physician identified with the early clinical and pathologic descriptions of sickle cell disease is Lemuel Diggs (Diggs, 1933), who for more than 50 years beginning in 1930 made many important observations about sickling. On testing more than 2,500 African Americans in Memphis, Diggs arrived at a carrier frequency of 8.3%, the same range reported in later studies. He noted that newborns had lower frequency and slower rates of sickling and distinguished between sickle cell anemia and sickle cell trait, observing that children with the trait had neither symptoms nor anemia. A pathologist, Diggs reported blood vessel occlusion and other autopsy findings in sicklers. Later he described the morphology of the sickling process, including irreversibly sickled cells, and suggested that sickled cells could not navigate the microcirculation.

Hahn and Gillespie reported reversibility of sickling on ligand binding (Hahn and Gillespie, 1927). Hahn noted many sickle cells in the bottom of a test tube of blood from a child with sickle cell anemia. Thinking this might be related to low oxygen tension, he and Gillespie examined, with a microscope in a device of their design, a drop of the child's blood under differing oxygen pressures. The red cells sickled when the PO_2 dropped to about 45 mm Hg and resumed their normal shape on exposure to higher oxygen pressures or to carbon monoxide. The authors suggested that with anoxemia, cells would sickle in vivo.

In 1940, while fixing shed blood in formalin/saline, Sherman, a medical student, found greater numbers of sickle cells in the venous than in the arterial blood of patients with sickle cell anemia and noted the absence of sickle cells in venous blood from patients with sickle cell trait (Sherman, 1940). In vitro much lower oxygen pressures were needed to induce sickling in red cells of sickle cell trait than in cells from patients with sickle cell anemia. Sherman suggested that damage to red cells during sickle-unsickle cycles in the circulation leads to the hemolytic anemia. Sherman also noted deoxygenation-dependent birefringence of sickled cells, an observation that was later to interest Pauling in his analysis of the hemoglobin in sickle cell anemia.

William Castle had noted increased viscosity of sickle cells on deoxygenation (Ham and Castle, 1940) and discussed the oxygenation dependence of sickling in a conversation with Linus Pauling in 1945. The dependence of sickling on deoxygenation suggested to Pauling that the defect lay in the hemoglobin (Pauling, 1954). Four years later, Pauling and Itano found that hemoglobin from a patient with sickle cell anemia (sickle hemoglobin or HbS) differed in electrophoretic mobility from normal hemoglobin and that hemoglobin from a subject with sickle trait was a mixture of HbS and HbA. Their landmark article (Pauling et al., 1949) introduced

a new concept not only of sickle cell disease but also of other hereditary diseases. (Fig. 1.1C).

In retrospect, changes in globin unrelated to sickle hemoglobin were already known if little appreciated. The increased alkali resistance of HbF had been discovered in 1866 in Germany by Körber, a graduate student (Körber, 1926). Felix Haurowitz observed that crystals of horse deoxyhemoglobin disintegrated on exposure to oxygen, suggesting that oxyhemoglobins and deoxyhemoglobins have different molecular structures (Haurowitz, 1938). Methemoglobinemia resulting from a dominantly inherited abnormality in globin had been described in 1948 as a disease of hemoglobin (Hörlein and Weber, 1948).

As the story of the identification of sickle cell disease as a disease of hemoglobin unfolded, the probable role of hemoglobin seems obvious. Yet of the many hematologists in medical schools at that time, only one is known to have been pursuing hemoglobin as a cause of sickling. Janet Watson in Brooklyn confirmed Diggs' observations on the paucity of sickle cells in newborns and postulated that sickling occurred when the HbF had been replaced by HbS that possessed the sickling property (Watson et al., 1948).

Pauling's observations were rapidly translated into clinical hematology. By 1953, a simple method of paper electrophoresis for clinical laboratories was in widespread use and many "new" hemoglobins were identified. HbC was found with HbS in clinically mild sickle cell disease, and the genes for HbS and HbC were found to be alleles (Ranney, 1954). HbC trait was found in 2 to 3 percent of African Americans, and homozygous HbC disease described by several groups (Ranney et al., 1953; Spaet et al., 1953) was a compensated hemolytic state often with splenomegaly and with abundant target cells on blood smears. HbE was common in Southeast Asia (Chernoff et al., 1956). The minor basic component of normal hemoglobin, HbA_2, and its increase in patients with thalassemia were identified by Henry Kunkel in the mid-1950s (Kunkel et al., 1957). Hermann Lehmann carried out numerous surveys of the occurrence of sickling and of hemoglobins C, D, and E in several areas of the world and was the first to describe many different human hemoglobin variants (Lehmann and Huntsman, 1974).

The genetic implications of the association of the geographic distribution of sickling with that of falciparum malaria in Africa (Beet, 1949) were discussed by J.B.S. Haldane (Haldane, 1949). The best analysis of the possible protective effect of malaria in sickling was that of Allison, who observed striking differences in the occurrence of malaria and in the parasite counts of individuals with sickle cell trait versus individuals without HbS at defined times after exposure to falciparum malaria (Allison, 1954). Allison concluded that in areas where falciparum infection is hyperendemic, children with sickle trait had a lower mortality from malaria than did children with normal hemoglobin (Chapter 30).

While it was clear from the studies of iron-oxygen binding and molecular weight, that hemoglobin has four subunits, the source of the increased net charge of HbS observed by Pauling was obscure. Vernon Ingram at Cambridge separated the tryptic digests of sickle and normal hemoglobin, first by electrophoresis and then by chromatography, to obtain a peptide map or "fingerprint" of each hemoglobin. Two findings were evident from the fingerprints: (1) sickle and normal hemoglobin differed in only one peptide, and (2) although 60 arginine and lysine residues (sites of tryptic cleavage) were present in each hemoglobin molecule, only 30 peptides were found, indicating that hemoglobin is composed of two identical half-molecules. The differences in the peptides of HbS and HbA resulted from the replacement of a normal glutamic acid by valine in the N-terminal tryptic peptide (Ingram 1956, 1957). Reexamination of N-terminal sequences of hemoglobin by two groups (Rhinesmith et al., 1957, 1958; Braunitzer, 1958) disclosed two different sequences, designated α and β. The N-terminal α sequence was Val-Leu-Ser and β, Val-His-Leu. The structures of the other two normal non-α-globin chains, δ and γ, were established by Ingram (Ingram and Stretton, 1961) and Schroeder (Schroeder et al., 1963), respectively. These chemical studies fit well with the x-ray crystallographic analyses of Perutz (Perutz et al., 1960), who showed that hemoglobin contains two pairs of unlike polypeptide chains.

The presence of four hemoglobins in the blood of rare individuals provided evidence for the presence of two separate globin genes. Family studies indicated that these genes were certainly not closely linked and were probably on separate chromosomes (Smith and Torbert 1958; Atwater et al., 1960). Some years later, Deisseroth localized the α genes to chromosome 16 (Deisseroth et al., 1977) and the β gene to chromosome 11 (Deisseroth et al., 1978).

SOME OTHER STRUCTURAL VARIANTS OF HEMOGLOBIN

As numerous new hemoglobin variants were described, the following became evident:

1. Many had no clinical manifestations.
2. Some, notably HbC, had few clinical findings except when associated with HbS.
3. A few had altered oxygen affinity; increased oxygen affinity was associated with polycythemia, decreased affinity with anemia.
4. Some were unstable and associated with Heinz body hemolytic anemia, often with sensitivity to certain drugs or infections, reminiscent of glucose-6-phosphate dehydrogenase deficiency.
5. Some were associated with microcytosis, thalassemia-like red cells (e.g., HbE and Hb Lepore).
6. A few had the cyanosis of methemoglobinemia, designated as hemoglobins M; in these hemoglobins one of the two heme-linked histidines was replaced by tyrosine in either α- or β-polypeptide chain.

The M hemoglobins resulting from mutations in the globin genes were dominantly inherited in contrast with the recessive methemoglobinemia studied by Quentin Gibson in Belfast in 1948. Gibson concluded that the defect in two affected Scottish brothers was in the enzyme that catalyzes the reaction between coenzyme I NAD and methemoglobin. He also concluded that methylene blue improved the methemoglobinemia via the hexose monophosphate shunt rather than the Embden-Meyerhof pathway (Gibson, 1948). Although none of the other more than 200 hemoglobin variants approaches the clinical importance of sickle cell hemoglobin and thalassemia, some, like the M hemoglobins, have provided unique insights into the structural basis of the reactions of hemoglobin with ligands (Perutz et al., 1972; Pulsinelli et al., 1973) (Chapters 44 and 46). Others such as HbC$_{Harlem}$ with amino acid substitutions, β^{6Val} and β^{73Asn} (Bookchin et al., 1967), indicated probable contacts of HbS in the fiber of deoxyHbS, and still others directed attention to the role of specific amino acid residues in the stability of the hemoglobin molecule.

Pauling and Itano speculated on, but did not experimentally address, the ligand-dependent conformational change that would result in the alignment of deoxygenated hemoglobin S molecules; nor did knowledge of the amino acid substitution of HbS disclose the molecular interactions that lead to sickling. In dilute solutions, the properties of sickle cell hemoglobin and normal hemoglobin do not differ much. The central importance of the solubility or polymerization of deoxygenated sickle hemoglobin was recognized immediately after the publication of Pauling (Pauling et al., 1949). In a classic experiment, John Harris observed, in solutions of deoxygenated sickle hemoglobin at concentrations of 10 g/DL or greater, the appearance of bi-refringent polymers, or tactoids, associated with an increase in viscosity (Harris, 1950). Harris concluded that the sickling of the red cells and the accompanying loss of deformability were the results of formation of polymers of deoxyHbS. The illustrations from Harris' article are reproduced in Pauling's Harvey Lecture (Pauling, 1954).

Karl and Lily Singer measured the concentration at which gelation (polymerization) occurred (minimum gelling concentration) in deoxygenated mixtures of HbS with other hemoglobins (Singer and Singer, 1953). Hemoglobin from a patient with HbSC disease gelled at lower total hemoglobin concentration than did hemoglobin from a subject with sickle cell trait. In contrast, mixtures of HbS with HbF gelled only at higher concentrations. The findings of the Singers were in accord with the clinical findings that patients with HbSC disease had mild sickle cell disease, whereas individuals with sickle cell trait were asymptomatic. (It is now known that the solubilities of deoxygenated mixtures of HbC or HbA with HbS are about the same: red cells in HbS/C disease have larger proportions of HbS than in sickle cell trait, and the total intracellular hemoglobin concentration is higher (Chapter 27). The minimum gelling concentration has been replaced by measurement of the "concentration at saturation," the hemoglobin concentration of the supernatant after sedimentation of the gel.

Early electron micrographs of deoxygenated sickle cells revealed long solid rodlike structures parallel to the long axis of deoxygenated sickle cells (White, 1968; Bertles and Dobler, 1969). In later studies (Josephs et al., 1976; Garrell et al., 1979), the usual fiber has fourteen twisted strands, four inner and ten outer, arranged in seven pairs, although other arrangements may be found. In timed measurements during deoxygenation of sickle cells, these polymers appear before the cell membrane becomes rigid and with reoxygenation, polymers melt as membrane flexibility is restored (Hahn et al., 1976). The oxygen equilibria of high concentrations of sickle hemoglobin reflect the presence of polymerized hemoglobin in the deoxy state. The dissociation curve is right-shifted for the portion of the curve at which the oxygen saturation is below 50 percent.

The sites of molecular interactions in the deoxyHbS fiber were first deduced by Wishner and Love from analysis of x-ray crystallography of the deoxyHbS fiber at 5Å (Wishner et al., 1975) and from the known effects of different amino acid residues at $\beta76$, $\beta73$, and $\beta121$ on gelling of HbS (Bookchin et al., 1967) or from the study of patients with compound heterozygous forms of sickle cell disease (McCurdy, 1960). On deoxygenation, binding of β^{6val} of HbS to a complementary site, a hydrophobic pocket lined by Ala 70, Phe 85 and Leu 88 of a neighboring β chain is the key event in polymer formation. Other complementary intermolecular binding sites were identified in later studies (see Chapter 26).

The intracellular crystals found in red cells containing HbC were beautifully described by Diggs (Diggs et al., 1954), who found them on blood smears from an Italian American youth whose spleen was removed.

These crystals are found in oxygenated red cells containing HbC (Chapter 27).

The rate of appearance of sickle polymers on deoxygenation has important implications for pathogenesis and therapy of sickle cell disease. The existence of a delay time in polymer formation was appreciated by the investigators who studied the gelation of HbS, but its importance was not appreciated until the quantification by Eaton and Hofrichter and Ferrone (Ferrone et al., 1985; Eaton and Hofrichter, 1990), which indicated that (1) delay time in the appearance of polymers is inversely proportional to approximate the 30th to 50th power of the initial HbS concentration and (2) a double nucleation mechanism accounts for both the enormous concentration dependence of polymerization and the explosive appearance of polymers. Delay of polymerization until the red cell has traversed the microcirculation would minimize vascular occlusion. Because the traditional estimate for capillary transit time is 1 second (although there are few direct measurements in different organs to substantiate this time), a few seconds of delay would allow red cells to reach the large-caliber veins and return to the lungs. Decreasing the intracellular concentration of HbS, for example, by increasing the amount of HbF would delay polymerization (Chapter 20).

HETEROGENEITY IN SICKLING

Deoxygenation-dependent sickle fiber formation results from the single base mutation, $A \rightarrow T$, in the sixth codon of the β-globin gene. That mutation appears to be the sole constant of sickling. Even the DNA neighboring that codon differs in different individuals (Chapter 26). Different haplotypes of the β^s gene, indicating that separate mutations gave rise to HbS, were first described by Kan (Kan and Dozy, 1978); extensive studies by Nagel and Labie during the 1980s indicated that the β^s mutation arose at least four times in Africa and once in the Near East (Pagnier et al., 1984). A clinically mild form of sickle cell anemia with increased amount of HbF known for many years in Saudi Arabia (Perrine et al., 1978) turned out to be associated with the fifth, "Arab-India" haplotype. The circulating red cells in a patient with sickle cell anemia are remarkably heterogeneous. Differing amounts of HbF are present when cells leave the marrow and the heterogeneity of the distribution of HbF in the red cells increases as cells with higher HbF undergo fewer sickle-unsickle cycles and survive longer than their less fortunately endowed fellow travelers (Reed et al., 1965). Some circulating red cells are young, the exposure of red cells to sickle-unsickle cycles varies, and the corpuscular hemoglobin concentrations of older cells with little HbF vary a great deal (Fabry and Nagel, 1982), suggesting variable loss of cell water. While its shape is dictated by the polymer formation within it, the membrane also has a role in the sickling process that is not entirely clear. In 1952, Tosteson and colleagues found that on deoxygenation, sickle red cells not only become viscous, but also lose potassium and gain sodium (Tosteson et al., 1952) (Chapter 22). These deoxygenated leaky sickle cells may ultimately lose some intracellular sodium and water. If on oxygenation, cells fail to rehydrate fully, the mean corpuscular concentration of HbS increases and with it acceleration of sickling on deoxygenation.

Many factors affect cell density: the age of the cells, the amount of HbF, the amount of 2,3 BPG, and the changing concentration of sickle hemoglobin. The demonstration of adherence of sickle cells to human umbilical cord endothelial cells (Hebbel and Yamada, 1980) and to the endothelium in a flowing system (Kaul et al., 1989) suggests that cellular adhesivity may be yet another source of heterogeneity in sickle cells.

THE THALASSEMIAS

Thalassemias are hereditary disorders of hemoglobin synthesis. Thomas Cooley, a pediatrician in Detroit, first described the clinical syndrome of thalassemia (Cooley and Lee 1925; Cooley et al., 1927). The "new" clinical syndrome was distinct from a heterogeneous group of childhood anemias with splenomegaly designated since the 1890s as von Jacsch's anemia. Cooley's patients had anemia, splenomegaly, icterus, circulating normoblasts, and bone changes; he described the appearance resulting from enlargement of the facial bones as "mongoloid" facies. Of seven patients, three, including two siblings, were of Italian descent, one was "probably Syrian," one was English, one was Greek, and one was described only as "mulatto." The patients ranged in age from 11 months to 5 years; pallor and abdominal enlargement were common presenting symptoms. Hemoglobin values clustered about 35 percent (i.e., 4 to 5 g/DL); nucleated red cells and fragmented erythrocytes were prominent on stained blood smears. Red cells were resistant to hypotonic lysis, distinguishing this entity from hereditary spherocytosis. Because splenectomy had been known to "cure" hereditary spherocytosis for 12 or more years, it is not surprising that attention was devoted to the possible role of the spleen. A $2^1/_2$-year-old patient received a single dose of "deep roentgen-ray therapy" to the spleen on April 4, 1924, and after stormy course died on May 15, 1924. A few months later a 5-year-old Italian-American patient with typical findings of thalassemia survived splenectomy, however without notable improvement.

Cooley's initial article generated considerable attention. In the second article, he abandoned his earlier idea that the anemia was myelophthisic and concluded that the evidence favored hemolysis. The bone lesions he had thought to be pathognomonic for the syndrome in 1925 were mimicked in hereditary spherocytosis and in sickle cell anemia, "which, if it really is a disease entity, is also a form of hemolytic icterus." Cooley thought that the disease was congenital but not hereditary, a belief more credible in the era of congenital syphilis and rickets than today.

Most of the case reports that appeared during the next few years described this disease in Italian Americans. Whipple and Bradford reviewed the clinical and autopsy findings on several cases including identical twins concordant for the syndrome. They concluded that this was an hereditary disease in people of Mediterranean descent; hence they chose the name thalassemia (Whipple and Bradford, 1932, 1936). In addition Whipple emphasized the deposition of tissue iron resembling hemochromatosis in adults. The mongoloid facies was attributed to bone overgrowth coupled with the pigmentation of hemochromatosis. Cooley's original patients had received little transfused blood, but treatment with transfusions was increasingly common after 1927. Whipple observed abundant iron in children who had received few or no transfusions as well as in those who received multiple transfusions (Whipple and Bradford, 1936).

In the mid-1920s Rietti described a syndrome in Italy of mild hemolytic jaundice with microcytic red cells that were resistant to osmotic lysis (Rietti, 1925). Other Italian physicians, particularly Greppi and Micheli, described the same syndrome, but no one related this mild anemia to the anemia described by Cooley (described by Chini and Valeri, 1949). That Cooley's anemia or thalassemia major was first described in the United States rather than Italy reflects the regional immigration patterns to the United States and the distribution of medical care and the distribution of genes for thalassemia in Italy. More than 3 million Italians, more than three fourths of whom were from southern Italy, emigrated to the United States between 1901 and 1920. Many of the southern Italians came from impoverished rural areas, and it was estimated that nearly half the Italian immigrants of that era were illiterate (Nelli, 1980). In the United States, the Italian immigrants joined other Italians in cities such as Detroit. Immigrants from southern Italy where thalassemia was most common had little contact with the medical knowledge and skills of northern Italy.

The recognition of Cooley's anemia as a genetic disease is generally attributed to the Greek physician, Caminopetros (Caminopetros, 1938), although Caminopetros' articles appeared at about the same time as those of Whipple and Bradford (Whipple and Bradford 1932, 1936). In the 1940s, many American (Valentine and Neel, 1944) and Italian hematologists (Chini and Valeri, 1949) studied families with thalassemia. By 1949, it was generally accepted that thalassemia major or Cooley's anemia was the homozygous state for a gene that in the heterozygous state, thalassemia minor, accounted for the syndrome described earlier by the Italian hematologists. Screening for thalassemia (by resistance of red cells to osmotic lysis) in Mediterranean countries; Southeast Asia, particularly Thailand; and India and Turkey indicated that thalassemia was both widespread and variable in its manifestations. Increased HbF in thalassemia was noted by Vecchio (Vecchio, 1946). Alexander Rich suggested among other possibilities that thalassemia might result from impaired synthesis of HbA with compensatory continuing synthesis of HbF (Rich, 1952).

Studies of families of patients who were heterozygous for both sickling and thalassemia provided insights about the genetics and nature of thalassemia (Chapter 28). In most such families, genes for sickling and thalassemia appeared to be allelic or closely linked, and analysis of the hemoglobin of patients with sickle-thalassemia usually showed about 70 percent HbS with the remainder HbF and HbA (Sturgeon et al., 1952). Because in sickle cell trait, a single sickle cell gene accounts for less than 50 percent of the hemoglobin, the obvious explanation was that thalassemia impaired the synthesis of HbA. However, in some patients, sickling and thalassemia did not seem to interact in this fashion; instead the hereditary microcytosis of thalassemia might accompany the usual hemoglobin pattern of sickle cell trait, 20 to 40 percent HbS and 60 to 80 percent HbA. In his description of HbA_2 in normal red cells and increased HbA_2 in patients with thalassemia, Henry Kunkel observed that parents of a few patients with thalassemia had normal levels of HbA_2 (Kunkel et al., 1957).

The first "abnormal" hemoglobin in thalassemia was described by Rigas, who found HbH in blood from two Chinese patients with thalassemia (Rigas et al., 1955). Many patients with HbH were soon thereafter found in Thailand and in Greece. Their anemia was more severe than that of most patients with thalassemia minor, and the abnormal HbH was found neither in the parents nor in the children of the patients. HbH was later found to be a tetramer of normal β-globin chains; it has a high oxygen affinity and lacks the allosteric properties of hemoglobins, with two pairs of unlike chains (Benesch et al., 1961). A tetramer of γ-globin chains, designated Hb Bart's, with similar oxygen equilibria, was found in cord blood samples in Greece (Fessas and Papaspyrou, 1957) and in London (Ager and Lehmann, 1958). In Indonesia, Lie-Injo found that nearly all the hemoglobin of a stillborn infant with hydrops was Hb Bart's (Lie-Injo and Hie, 1959). Hemoglobin Bart's was quickly recognized as a common cause of hydrops fetalis in Southeast Asia; its high oxygen affinity would not support life in the perinatal period. Small amounts (< 10 percent) of Hb Bart's were found in the cord blood of infants with thalassemia minor.

Whereas HbH and Hb Bart's were tetramers of structurally normal β and γ chains, two structurally abnormal hemoglobins were found in association with thalassemia, Hb Lepore and HbE (Chapters 14 and 43). Hb Lepore results from misalignment of the δ- and β-globin genes during meiotic crossing over. In Lepore hemoglobin, the initial portion of the Lepore chain has a δ- and the remainder a β-globin chain sequence (Baglioni, 1962). Different examples of Hb Lepore with different sites of crossing over have been found. The structure of the Lepore hemoglobins, together with that of another fusion polypeptide chain in Hb Kenya, provided evidence for the order of genes, γ δ β, in the β-globin genelike cluster (Huisman et al., 1972). Delineation of the structure of Hb Kenya was but one of many important contributions made by Titus Huisman to our knowledge of normal and abnormal globin genes and their products.

The second structurally abnormal hemoglobin associated with a thalassemic phenotype is HbE, in which lysine replaces glutamic acid at β26. HbE, common in Southeast Asia, particularly in Burma, Cambodia, and Laos, is second in worldwide frequency only to HbS. Although few manifestations except for microcytosis were associated with HbE, either in the heterozygous or in the homozygous state, the compound resulting from the presence of a single gene for HbE together with a single gene for β thalassemia results in an illness clinically indistinguishable from Cooley's anemia (Chernoff et al., 1956).

The recognition that hemoglobin contained two types of polypeptide chains was translated into the idea of distinct α and β thalassemia by Ingram and Stretton (Ingram and Stretton, 1959), who defended the hypothesis that undetected amino acid substitutions were the basis of thalassemia. The idea that the rate of synthesis of globin was determined by the primary structure of the hemoglobin had been proposed by Itano (Itano, 1957) and Pauling (Pauling, 1954). Both Itano and Pauling and Ingram and Stratton thought that thalassemia was probably the result of an undetected amino acid substitution that interfered with the synthesis of normal globin. Itano and Pauling called attention to their original formulation of this hypothesis in a brief and caustic note in *Nature* (Itano and Pauling, 1961) in response to the detailed analysis of Ingram and Stretton (Ingram and Stretton, 1959). Ingram and Stretton had also considered the "tap" hypothesis — that mutations in DNA adjacent to the globin gene locus might "turn down or off" globin synthesis but favored the undetected amino acid substitution, which involved (they thought) fewer assumptions. Many futile attempts were made to find abnormal hemoglobins as a cause of thalassemia (Chapters 13 and 17); neither Ingram nor Itano and Pauling mentioned HbE, although its thalassemic phenotype had already been described (Chernoff et al., 1956).

Measurement of Synthesis of Globin Chains

Both London (London et al., 1950) and Borsook (Kruh and Borsook, 1956) had observed synthesis of globin in vitro after incubating reticulocytes with radioactive amino acids. With modifications of those methods and thalassemic reticulocytes, Paul Marks found normal ribosomal function with impaired synthesis of normal hemoglobin (Marks and Burka, 1964), and Heywood found unequal labeling of α- and β-globin chains (Heywood et al., 1964).

A major contribution to clinical research in thalassemia was the development of a fairly simple chromatographic method for separating globin chains (Clegg et al., 1966). Thalassemic blood was incubated with isotopic leucine; labeled globin was then separated on an ion-exchange urea column. Good recovery of the separated polypeptides α, β, γ, and δ was observed, and by measuring the specific radioactivity of each chain, the amounts of each synthesized during the incubation period could be determined. The thalassemias were shown to have imbalanced globin-chain synthesis: α thalassemia had decreased production of α-globin chains and β thalassemia of β-globin chains. Two questions were evident: (1) How did this unbalanced synthesis produce the syndrome that Cooley described? (2) What was the molecular basis of the unbalanced chain synthesis?

Sturgeon and Finch followed the fate of radioactive iron given to patients with thalassemia major. They showed markedly ineffective erythropoiesis (i.e., the production of defective red cell precursors that never circulate because they die in the bone marrow (Sturgeon and Finch, 1957) (Chapter 10). Thalassemic red cells that circulated had shortened survival. Ineffective erythropoieisis accounted for the enlargement of bone marrow and resulting bony abnormalities, and handling the breakdown products of defective circulating red cells led to splenomegaly. By 1957, patients with thalassemia major were being transfused regularly, and their iron overload reflected in large part the iron received in transfusions.

Phaedon Fessas of Athens suggested in 1963 the source of injury to thalassemic red cells and their precursors. In β thalassemia, the normal α-globin chains, finding no β-globin chains with which to mate, precipitate on the membrane of the developing or mature erythroid cell (Fessas, 1963). The precipitated chains wreak oxidative damage to the membrane, leading to cell death. If γ-globin chains are present, the α chains combine with them to form HbF. A similar mechanism was postulated for α thalassemia, except that the β-globin chains are more soluble and more thermostable than α globin and circulate in red cells in significant quantities as HbH (Chapter 16). Precipitated HbH is easily recognized as inclusion bodies in red cells after incubation with a supravital stain. This "garbage in the red cell" description of pathogenesis was developed further by Nathan and Gunn, who suggested that α or β chains might have different effects on the membrane (Nathan and Gunn, 1966). Interactions of α- or β-globin chains with different membrane proteins were described in the 1990s (Advani et al., 1992).

Determining the cause of the unbalanced synthesis almost immediately involved the approaches of molecular biology. Cell-free systems had been developed in which RNA and the processes of chain initiation, elongation, and termination could be studied. In 1961, Howard Dintzis showed that the synthesis of hemoglobin begins at the N-terminal residue (Dintzis, 1961). Two groups reported the synthesis of normal hemoglobin in heterologous cell-free systems to which thalassemic mRNA had been added (Nienhuis and Anderson 1971; Benz and Forget, 1971). The same chain imbalance that had characterized globin synthesis in the reticulocytes from which the messenger mRNA was isolated was found in the heterologous systems. The thalassemic messenger mRNA, therefore, was responsible for decreased polypeptide chain synthesis. The variable nature of the defective thalassemic mRNA was studied when reverse transcriptase (Temin and Mizutani 1970; Baltimore 1970) made cDNA-mRNA hybridization possible (Kacian et al., 1973; Houseman et al., 1973; Forget et al., 1974). A decreased amount of hybridizable β-globin chain mRNA was found in β-thalassemia and of α-mRNA in α-thalassemia. Some β-globin gene mutations completely suppressed the synthesis of β chains, whereas in others, small amounts of β-globin chains were synthesized. The two types of mutations were called β^0 and β^+ types of thalassemia, respectively.

The types of gene mutations resulting in thalassemia would be understood only from knowledge of the fine structure of the globin genes, knowledge that grew rapidly as techniques for sequencing DNA were developed. The important discovery of the intervening sequences (IVS) in the globin genes was made by two groups, one by gene cloning and electron microscopy of mouse β-globin cDNA and genomic DNA (Tilghman et al., 1978) and the other group by mapping the rabbit β-globin gene (Jeffreys and Flavell, 1977). Splicing, the post-transcriptional excision of the IVS from RNA and annealing to form mRNA, has proved to be the site of many thalassemic mutations, particularly those of β-thalassemia.

Alpha Thalassemia

After discovery by Schroeder and Huisman that the gene for the γ chain of HbF is duplicated (Schroeder et al., 1968), a second α-globin gene was sought. A duplicated α-globin locus would explain the smaller proportions (± 20 percent) of the abnormal hemoglobin in individuals with α-chain variants. The inheritance of HbH, which is not found in the parents of the patient, would be readily explained by the presence of the three and of Hb Bart's hydrops by four defective α-globin genes (Lehmann and Carrell, 1968). Although codon 136 of the two γ-globin genes differed, one coding for glycine and the other for alanine, the coding sequences of the two α-globin genes were identical. A few years later, the duplicated α-gene loci were demonstrated directly by sequencing DNA adjacent to the coding sequences.

HbH, together with a small component (± 3 percent) of an abnormal basic hemoglobin designated Hb Constant Spring, was found by Milner in Jamaica in two siblings with thalassemia (Clegg et al., 1971). The minor component represented an elongated α-globin, the product of a defective α-globin gene carrying a mutation of the normal termination codon. In Hb Constant Spring, thirty-one amino acids not normally expressed are added at the C-terminus of the α-globin chain. About half the Southeast Asian patients with HbH disease have Hb Constant Spring. Four other Constant Spring-like variants with α-globin chain elongation and different mutations of the termination codon have been described. The most common genetic defects of the α-globin genes are deletions of variable length in different populations. The most frequent nondeletional defect is chain elongation, notably Hb Constant Spring, but many other molecular defects are represented in the ± 15 percent of α-thalassemias that are nondeletional.

Beta Thalassemia

The syndrome described by Cooley represented defective synthesis of β-polypeptide chains. In contrast with the deletions that account for most of the α thalassemias, point mutations affecting any one of the steps of globin gene expression, transcription, processing of mRNA precursor, translation, or stability of the polypeptide chain account for most of the β-thalassemias (Chapter 11). Molecular diagnosis is facilitated by the small number of mutations that is common in each racial/ethnic group exhibiting a high frequency of β thalassemia. Within these groups, however, thalassemia major often results from compounds (i.e., different thalassemia mutations in each of the two β-globin genes) (Chapter 36).

Of particular note is the thalassemic phenotype associated with HbE. The mutation of HbE at codon 26 activates a cryptic splice site. Alternative splicing at that site yields an mRNA that is not translated. The mRNA from the normal splice site is translated to globin with lysine (instead of glutamic) at β26, the amino acid substitution of HbE.

Deletions in the β-globin gene cluster, much less common than in the α-globin genes, are generally identified by the presence of increased proportions of HbF (Chapter 14). An example is hereditary persistence of fetal hemoglobin (HPFH), first found in Africa (Edington and Lehmann, 1955) and studied in Baltimore (Conley et al., 1963). The hemoglobin of patients homozygous for HPFH (who are clinically quite well) is entirely HbF; heterozygotes (or compounds) for both HbS and HPFH have about 70 percent HbS with the remainder HbF. In red cells of these compound heterozygotes, HbF is uniformly distributed. Each erythrocyte has about the same complement of HbF. Patients heterozygous for HbS and HPFH do not have symptoms of sickle cell disease despite the presence of 70 percent HbS-evidence of the protective effect of HbF uniformly distributed (Bradley et al., 1961) (Chapter 28).

Both α- and β-thalassemias are seen in the populations of Southeast Asia. The profile of thalassemia in the western United States changed profoundly with the influx of refugees from Southeast Asia after the fall of Saigon in 1975. During the next dozen years, α-thalassemia was found in arriving refugees from Vietnam, Cambodia, and Laos. Hemoglobin E, and consequently HbE-β thalassemia, were infrequent among the Vietnamese but common among Cambodians and Laotians. As in Southeast Asia, Hemoglobin Constant Spring was found in nearly half the patients with HbH, and the majority of patients with transfusion-dependent thalassemia in California had HbE-β-thalassemia.

TREATMENT OF HEMOGLOBINOPATHIES

Improved supportive treatment has accounted for significant prolongation of life in both sickle cell disease and thalassemia. In sickle cell anemia, high fluid intake to combat cellular dehydration, judicious use of antibiotics for infections, transfusions when anemia becomes severe, and for some patients regular transfusions are essential components of management. The high death rate from infections, particularly pneumococcal infections in children with sickle cell anemia (Powars, 1975), was the basis of the studies that led to the recommendation that children with sickle cell anemia receive prophylactic penicillin (Gaston et al., 1986). Although the advances in the treatment of thalassemia have not yet reflected the vast gains in knowledge of its cellular and molecular pathogenesis, patients with those diseases are obviously much better off now than they were in 1960. Maintaining the hemoglobin at 9 to 10 g/dL by transfusions and removal of iron by chelation has dramatically improved both quality of life and the life expectancy for patients with thalassemia major, and stem cell transplantation can be curative.

FETAL HEMOGLOBIN IN THERAPY

The switch from fetal to adult hemoglobin, from the synthesis of γ-globin chains to the synthesis of β-globin chains that occurs at about the time of birth, has long engaged the attention of physician-scientists interested in diseases of the globin gene (Chapter 38). If the switch could be prevented and the synthesis of γ chains maintained throughout life, the manifestations of sickling and of many of the thalassemias would be prevented. Preventing the switch remains the aim of research programs both in gene therapy (Chapter 41) and pharmacologic modification of hemoglobin synthesis.

A RETROSPECTIVE NOTE

Many major contributions to our present knowledge of hemoglobin were made by investigators who were young in years and/or junior in the academic hierarchy. Among them, in addition to Giulio Bizzozzero, were James Watson, Winifred Ashby, E. Vernon Hahn, Elizabeth Gillespie, E. Körber, Irving Sherman, and John Harris. Most articles by these young scientists were brief, the investigator was usually the sole author, and any co-authors were likely to be contemporaries rather than mentors. Acknowledgments of financial support if included were brief. Perhaps the systems of biomedical research of the last half of the twentieth century have resulted in less independence, recognition, or motivation for young investigators than did the systems or lack of systems of earlier eras.

THE FUTURE OF DISORDERS OF THE GLOBIN GENES

The World Health Organization anticipated in 1995 the annual birth of 294,475 infants with serious "homozygous" hemoglobinopathies. Of these, 2 percent would be born in America, 73 percent in Africa, and 24 percent in Asia (Table 1.1). The prevalence of the hemoglobinopathies is highest in regions of the world where the fewest resources are available for treatment. Clinical research in the hemoglobinopathies is now approached with short-term and long-term goals, but the short-term goals developed for the United States and Europe will not find worldwide application for a long time. The present treatment of the hemoglobinopathies in the United States and Europe is reminiscent of what Lewis Thomas called the "half-technologies,"—cumbersome, expensive, and only partially effective. His examples included the iron lung as contrasted with vaccination for poliomyelitis. For most patients with hemoglobinopathies, transfusion and chelation of iron, bone marrow transplantation, and treatment with expensive drugs such as hydroxyurea constitute treatment as remotely possible as the iron lung.

Table 1.1. Global Distribution of Hereditary Globin Defects

Region	Population (millions)	Annual births (thousands)	Defective gene	Annual births pathologic*	Percent of world total pathologic*
Africa	664.00	29,802	β	216,439	73.50
America	731.20	17,174	β	5,181	1.76
Asia	3,149.94	83,847	β	57,875	24.13
Asia			α	13,186	
Europe	780.50	11,053	β	1,620	0.55
Oceania	26.82	524	β	174	0.08
TOTAL	5,346.00	142,040		294,475	100.00

* Pathologic indicates symptomatic hemoglobinopathy.
Modified from Angastiniotis et al., 1995.

Long-term goals in therapy of the hemoglobinopathies include the control of the switch from α- to β-globin synthesis or transfer to patients of normal globin genes with significant rates of expression. Although both of these goals are attainable, neither is immediately at hand. When better technologies emerge, we hope that they may somehow benefit the millions of people with hemoglobinopathies who do not have access to the present half technologies.

ACKNOWLEDGMENTS

In preparing this chapter the author has relied heavily on *Blood, Pure and Eloquent*, M. Wintrobe, ed.; *Hemoglobin, Molecular Genetic and Clinical Aspects* by Bunn and Forget; and *A History of Medicine* by Castiglioni. A few of the older references, not readily available, were copied from these excellent books.

References

Ackers, GK. (1998). Deciphering the molecular code of hemoglobin allostery. *Adv. Protein Chem.* 51: 183–253.

Adair, GS. (1924). A comparison of the molecular weights of the proteins. *Proc. Camb. Philos. Soc. Biol. Sci.* 1: 75–78.

Advani, R, Sorenson, S, Shinar, E, et al. (1992). Characterization and comparison of the red blood cell membrane damage in severe human α- and β-thalassemia. *Blood* 79: 1058–1063.

Ager, JAM and Lehmann, H. (1958). Observations on some "fast" haemoglobins: K, J, N, and Bart's. *Br. Med. J.* 1: 929–931.

Allison, AC. (1954). Protection afforded by sickle-cell trait against subtertian malarial infection. *Br. Med. J.* 1: 290–294.

Angastiniotis, M, Modell, B, Englezos, P, et al., (1995). Prevention and control of haemoglobinopathies. Bull. World Health Organ 73(3): 375–386.

Arnone, A. (1972). X-ray diffraction study of binding of 2, 3 diphosphoglycerate to human deoxyhemoglobin. *Nature* 237: 146–149.

Ashby, W. (1919). The determination of the length of life of transfused blood corpuscles in man. *J. Exp. Med.* 29: 267–281.

Ashby, W. (1921). Study of transfused blood. II. Blood destruction in pernicious anemia. *J. Exp. Med.* 34: 147–166.

Atwater, J, Schwartz, IR, and Tocantins, LM. (1960). A variety of human hemoglobin with four distinct electrophoretic components. *Blood* 15: 901–908.

Baglioni, C. (1962). The fusion of two peptide chains in hemoglobin Lepore and its interpretation as a genetic deletion. *Proc. Natl. Acad. Sci. USA* 48: 1880–1886.

Baltimore, D. (1970). RNA-dependent DNA polymerase in virions of RNA tumour viruses. *Nature* 221: 1209–1211.

Barcroft, J. (1928). *The respiratory function of the blood. Part I.* Cambridge: Cambridge University Press.

Barker, JE. (1968). Development of the mouse hematopoietic system. 1. Types of hemoglobin produced in embryonic yolk sac and liver. *Dev. Biol.* 18: 14–29.

Bauer, C, Ludwig, I, and Ludwig, M. (1968). Different effects of 2,3-diphosphoglycerate and adenosine triphosphate on the oxygen affinity of adult and foetal human hemoglobin. *Life Sci.* 7: 1339–1343.

Beet, EA. (1946). Sickle cell disease in the Balovale District of Northern Rhodesia. *East Afr. Med. J.* 23: 75–86.

Benesch, RE, Ranney, HM, Benesch, R, and Smith, GM. (1961). The chemistry of the Bohr effect. II. Some properties of hemoglobin H. *J. Biol. Chem.* 236: 2926–2929.

Benesch, RF and Benesch, R. (1967). The effect of organic phosphates from the human erythrocyte in the allosteric properties of hemoglobin. *Biochem. Biophys. Res. Commun.* 26: 162–167.

Benz, EJ and Forget, BG. (1971). Defect in messenger RNA for human hemoglobin synthesis in beta thalassemia. *J. Clin. Invest.* 50: 2755–2760.

Berk, L, Burchenal, JH, Wood, T, and Castle, WB. (1948). Oxygen saturation of sternal marrow blood with special reference to pathogenesis of polycythemia vera. *Proc. Soc. Exp. Biol. Med.* 69: 316–320.

Bernal, JD and Crowfoot, D. (1934). X-ray photographs of crystalline pepsin. *Nature* 133: 794–795.

Bert, P. (1943). *La pression barométrique.* Paris: Masson 1878. English translation by MA Hitchcock and FA Hitchcock, Columbus, OH. College Book Co., 1943. Reprinted by the Underseas Medical Society, Bethesda, MD, 1978.

Bertles, JF and Dobler, J. (1969). Reversible and irreversible sickling: A distinction by electron microscopy. *Blood* 33: 884–898.

Bizzozzero, G. (1868). Sulla funzione ematopoetica del midollo delle ossa. *Zentralbl. Med. Wissensch.* 6: 885.

Bizzozzero, G. (1869). Sulla funzione ematopoetica del midollo delle ossa. Seconda communicazione preventia. *Zentralbl. Med. Wissensch.* 10: 149–150.

Bizzozzero, G. (1882). Ueber einen neuen formbestandtheil des Blutes und dessen Rolle ber der Thrombose und der Blutgerinnung. *Virchows Arch. Pathol. Anat. Physiol.* 90: 261–332.

Bohr, C. (1904). Theoretische Behandlung der quantitativen Vehältnisse der Kohlensäurebindung des Hämoglobins. *Zentralbl. Physiol.* 17: 713–715.

Bohr, C, Hasselbalch, L, and Krogh, A. (1904). Ueber einen in biologischer Bezichung wichtigen Einfluss, den die Kohlensäurespannung des Blutes auf dessen Sauerstoffbendung ubt. *Skand. Arch. Physiol.* 16: 402–412.

Bookchin, RM, and Nagel, RL. (1970). The effect of β^{73Asn} on the interactions of sickling hemoglobins. *Biochem. Biophys. Acta.* 221: 373–375.

Bookchin, RM, Nagel, RL, and Ranney, HM. (1967). Structure and properties of hemoglobin C_{Harlem}: A human hemoglobin variant with amino acid substitutions in two residues of the b-polypeptide chain. *J. Biol. Chem.* 242: 248–255.

Bradley, TB, Brawner, JN, and Conley, CL. (1961). Further observations on an inherited anomaly characterized by persistence of fetal hemoglobin. *Bull. Johns Hopkins Hosp.* 108: 242–257.

Bradley, TR and Metcalf, D. (1966). The growth of mouse bone marrow cells in vitro. *Austr. J. Exp. Biol. Med. Sci.* 44: 287–299.

Braunitzer, G. (1958). Vergleichende untersuchungen zur Primärstruktur der Protein-komponente Einiger Hämoglobine. *Z. Physiol. Chem.* 312: 72–84.

Bunn, HF. (1971). Differences in the interaction of 2,3-diphosphoglycerate with certain mammalian hemoglobins. *Science* 172: 1049–1050.

Callender, S, Powell, EO, and Witts, L. (1945). The life span of the red cell in man. *J. Pathol. Bacteriol.* 57: 129–139.

Caminopetros, J. (1938). Recherches sur l'anemie erythroblastique infantile des peuples de la Méditerranée Orientale. Etude anthropologique, étiologique et pathogénique. La transmission héréditaire del la maladie. *Ann. de Médecine* 43: 104–125.

Carnot, P and Deflandre, C. (1906). Sur l'activité hémopoiétique de sérum au cours de la régénération du sang. *C.R. Acad. Sci. (Paris)* 143: 384–386.

Cassoly, R and Gibson, QH. (1972). The kinetics of ligand binding to hemoglobin valency hybrids and the effect of anions. *J. Biol. Chem.* 247: 7332–7341.

Castiglioni, A. (1947). *A history of medicine.* New York: Alfred A. Knopf.

Chanutin, A, and Curnish, RR. (1967). Effect of organic and inorganic phosphates on the oxygen equilibrium of human erythrocytes. *Arch. Biochem. Biophys.* 121: 96–102.

Chernoff, Al, Minnich, V, NaNakorn, S et al. (1956). Studies on hemoglobin E. The clinical, hematologic and genetic characteristics of the hemoglobin E syndromes. *J. Lab. Clin. Med.* 47: 455–489.

Chini, V and Valeri, CM. (1949). Mediterranean hemopathic syndromes. *Blood* 4: 989–1013.

Clegg, JB, Naughton, MA, and Weatherall, DJ. (1966). Abnormal human hemoglobins. Separation and characterization of α- and β-chains by chromatography, and the determination of two new variants. *J Mol Biol* 19: 91–108.

Clegg, JB, Weatherall, DJ, and Milner, PF. (1971). Haemoglobin Constant Spring—a chain termination mutant? *Nature* 234: 337–340.

Conley, CL. (1980). Sickle-cell anemia—the first molecular disease. In Wintrobe MM, editor. *Blood: Pure and eloquent.* New York: McGraw-Hill.

Conley, CL, Weatherall, DJ, Richardson, SN, Shepard, MK, et al. (1963). Hereditary persistence of fetal hemoglobin: A study of 79 affected persons in 15 negro families in Baltimore. *Blood* 21: 261–281.

Cooley, TB and Lee, P. (1925). A series of cases of splenomegaly in children with anemia and peculiar bone changes. *Trans Am Pediatr Soc* 37: 29.

Cooley, TB, Witwer, ER, and Lee, P. (1927). Anemia in children with splenomegaly and peculiar changes in bones: report of cases. *Am J Dis Child* 34: 347–363.

Curtin, PD. (1969). *The Atlantic slave trade.* Madison: University of Wisconsin Press.

Dacie, JV. (1980). The life span of the red blood cell and circumstances of its premature death in blood. In Wintrobe

MM, editor. *Blood: Pure and eloquent.* New York: McGraw-Hill.

Deisseroth, A, Nienhuis, A, Lawrence, et al. (1978). Chromosomal localization of human β-globin gene on human chromosome 11 in somatic cell hybrids. *Proc Natl Acad Sci USA* 75: 1456–1460.

Deisseroth, A, Nienhuis, A, Turner, P et al. (1977). Localization of the human α globin structural gene to chromosome 16 in somatic cell hybrids by molecular hybridization assay. *Cell* 12: 205–218.

Diggs, LW. (1933). The incidence and significance of the sickle cell trait. *Ann Intern Med* 7: 769–778.

Diggs, LW, Kraus, AP, Morrison, DB, and Rudnicki, RPT. (1954). Intraerythrocytic crystals in a white patient with hemoglobin C in the absence of other types of hemoglobin. *Blood* 9: 1172–1184.

Dintzis, HM. (1961). Assembly of the peptide chains of hemoglobin synthesis. *Science* 141: 123–130.

Donath, J, and Landsteiner, K. (1904). Ueber paroxysmale Hämoglobinurie. *Munch Med Wochenschr* 51: 1590–1593.

Eaton, WA, and Hofrichter, J. (1990). Sickle cell hemoglobin polymerization. *Adv Protein Chem* 40: 63–279.

Edington, GM, and Lehmann, H. (1955). Expression of the sickle cell gene in Africa. *Br Med J* 1:1308–1311 and 2:1238.

Ehrlich, P. (1877). Beitrag zur Kenntnis der Anilinfarbungen und ihrer Verwendung in der mikroskopischen Technik. *Arch Mikr Anat* 13: 263–277.

Emmel, VE. (1917). A study of the erythrocytes in a case of severe anemia with elongated and sickle-shaped red blood corpuscles. *Arch Intern Med* 20: 586–598.

Erslev, AJ. (1953). Humoral regulation of red cell production. *Blood* 8, 349–387.

Erslev, AJ. (1980). Blood and mountains. In Wintrobe, MM, editor. *Blood: pure and eloquent.* New York: McGraw-Hill.

Fabry, ME and Nagel, RL. (1982). Heterogeneity of red cells in the sickler: A characteristic with practical clinical and pathophysiological implications. *Blood Cells* 8: 9–15.

Ferguson, JKW and Roughton, FJW. (1934). The chemical relationships with physiological importance of carbamino compounds of CO_2 with haemoglobin. *J Physiol (London)* 83: 87–102.

Ferrone, FA, Hofrichter, J, and Eaton, WA. (1985). Kinetics of sickle hemoglobin polymerization. I. Studies using temperature-jump and laser photolysis technique. *J Mol Biol* 183: 592–610.

Fessas, P. (1963). Inclusion of hemoglobin in erythroblasts and erythrocytes of thalassemia. *Blood* 21: 21–32.

Fessas, P and Papaspyrou, A. (1957). A new fast hemoglobin associated with thalassemia. *Science* 126: 1119.

Fischer, H and Orth, H. (1937). *Die Chemie des Pyrrols.* Leipzig: Akademische Verlagsgeselshaft, vol I, 1934, vol II, 1937.

Ford, BJ. (1998). The earliest views. *Sci Am* 278(4): 50–53.

Forget, BG, Baltimore, D, Benz, EJ et al. (1974). Globin messenger RNA in the thalassemia syndrome. *Ann NY Acad Sci* 232: 76–87.

Garrell, RL, Crepeau, RH, and Edelstein, SJ. (1979). Cross-sectional views of hemoglobin S fibers by electron microscopy and computer modeling. *Proc Natl Acad Sci USA* 76: 1140–1144.

Gaston, MH, Verter, JI, and Woods, G. (1986). Prophylaxis with oral penicillin in children with sickle cell anemia. *N Engl J Med* 314: 1593–1599.

Gibson, QH. (1948). The reduction of methemoglobin in red blood cells and studies on the cause of idiopathic methemoglobinemia. *Biochem J* 42: 13–23.

Gray, SJ and Sterling, K. (1950). Tagging of red cells and plasma proteins with radioactive chromium. *J Clin Invest* 29: 1604–1613.

Hahn, EV and Gillespie, EB. (1927). Sickle cell anemia. Report of a case greatly improved by splenectomy. Experimental study of sickle cell formation. *Arch Intern Med* 39: 233–254.

Hahn, JA, Messer, MJ, and Bradley, TB. (1976). Ultrastructure of sickling and unsickling in time-lapse studies. *Br J Haematol* 34: 559–565.

Haldane, JBS. (1949). The rate of mutation of human genes. In *Proceedings of the VIII International Congress on Genetics and Heredity.* Suppl. 35, p. 367.

Ham, TH and Castle, WB. (1940). Relation of increased hypotonic fragility and of erythrostasis to mechanism of hemolysis in certain anemias. *Trans Assoc Am Physicians* 55: 127–132.

Harris, JW. (1950). Studies on the destruction of red blood cells. VIII. Molecular orientation in sickle cell hemoglobin solutions. *Proc. Soc. Exp. Biol. Med.* 75: 197–201.

Hartridge, H and Roughton, FJW. (1923). The kinetics of haemoglobin. II. The velocity with which oxygen dissociates from its combination with haemoglobin. *Proc. R. Soc. A.* 104: 395–429.

Hartridge, H and Roughton, FJW. (1925). The kinetics of haemoglobin. III. The velocity with which oxygen combines with reduced haemoglobin. *Proc. R. Soc. A.* 107: 654–683.

Haurowitz, F. (1938). Das Gleichgewicht zwischen Hämoglobin und Sauerstoff. *Hoppe-Seyler's Z. Physiol. Chem.* 254: 127–132.

Hebbel, RP and Yamada, O. (1980). Abnormal adherence of sickle erythrocytes to cultured vascular endothelium: Possible mechanism for microvascular occlusion in sickle cell disease. *J. Clin. Invest.* 65: 154–160.

Henderson, LJ. (1928). *Blood: a study in general physiology.* New Haven: Yale University Press.

Herrick, JB. (1910). Peculiar elongated and sickle-shaped red blood corpuscles in a case of severe anemia. *Arch. Intern. Med.* 6: 517–521.

Heywood, JD, Karon, M, and Weissman, S. (1964). Amino acids: Incorporation into alpha- and beta-chain of hemoglobin by normal and thalassemic reticulocytes. *Science* 146: 530–531.

Hill, AV. (1910). The possible effects of aggregation of the molecules of hemoglobin on its dissociation curve. *J. Physiol.* 40: 4.

Ho, C. (1992). Proton nuclear magnetic resonance studies on hemoglobin: Cooperative interactions and partially ligated intermediates. *Adv. Protein. Chem.* 43: 153–312.

Hoppe, F. (1862). Über das Verhalten des Blutfarbstoffes im Spectrum des Sonnenlichtes. *Virchows Arch. Pathol. Anat. Physiol.* 23: 446–449.

Hörlein, H and Weber, G. (1948). Über chronische familiäre Methämoglobinämie und eine neue Modifikation des Methämoglobins. *Dtsch. Med. Wochenschr.* 73: 476–478.

Houseman, D, Forget, BG, Skoultchi, A, and Benz, EJ. (1973). Quantitative deficiency of chain specific messenger ribonucleic acids in the thalassemia syndromes. *Proc. Natl. Acad. Sci. USA* 70: 1809–1813.

Huehns, ER, Flynn, FV, Butler, EA, and Beaven, GH. (1961). Two new haemoglobin variants in the very young human embryo. *Nature* 189: 496–497.

Hüfner, G. (1884). Ueber das oxyhämoglobin des Pferdes. *Z. Physiol. Chem.* 8: 358–365.

Huisman, THJ, Wrightstone, RN, Wilson, JB, et al. (1972). Hemoglobin Kenya, the product of a fusion of γ and β polypeptide chains. *Arch. Biochem. Biophys.* 153: 850–853.

Ingram, VM. (1956). A specific chemical difference between the globins of normal human and sickle-cell anaemia haemoglobin. *Nature* 178: 792–794.

Ingram, VM. (1957). Gene mutations in human haemoglobin: the chemical difference between normal and sickle haemoglobin. *Nature* 180: 326–328.

Ingram, VM, and Stretton, AOW. (1959). Genetic basis of the thalassemia diseases. *Nature* 184: 1903–1909.

Ingram, VM, and Stretton, AOW. (1961). Human haemoglobin A_2: Chemistry, genetics and evolution. *Nature* 190: 1079–1084.

Itano, HA. (1957). The human hemoglobins: Their properties and genetic control. *Adv Protein Chem.* 12: 216–268.

Itano, HA and Pauling, L. (1961). Thalassemia and the abnormal human haemoglobins. *Nature* 191: 398–399.

Jeffreys, AJ and Flavell, RA. (1977). The rabbit β-globin gene contains a large insert in the coding sequence. *Cell* 12: 1097–1198.

Josephs, R, Jarosch, HS, and Edelstein, SJ. (1976). Polymorphism of sickle haemoglobin fibers. *J. Mol. Biol.* 102: 409–426.

Kacian, DL, Gambino, R, Dow, LW et al. (1973). Decreased globin messenger RNA in thalassemia detected by molecular hybridization. *Proc. Natl. Acad. Sci. USA* 70: 1886–1890.

Kan, YW and Dozy, AM. (1978). Polymorphism of DNA sequence adjacent to human β-globin structural gene: Relationship to sickle mutation. *Proc. Natl. Acad. Sci. USA* 75: 5631–5635.

Kaul, DK, Fabry, ME, and Nagel, RL. (1989). Microvascular sites and characteristics of sickle cell adhesion to vascular endothelium in shear flow conditions: Pathophysiological implications. *Proc. Natl. Acad. Sci. USA* 86: 3356–3360.

Kölliker, A. (1846). Ueber die Blutkörperchen eines menschlichen Embryo und die Entwicklung der Blütkorperchen bei Sängethieren. *Z. Rat. Med. (Zurich)* 4: 112–159.

Körber, E. (1926). Inaugural dissertation: "Über differenzen Blutfarbstoffes." Dorpat, 1866. Cited by Bischoff, H. *Z. Exp. Med.* 48: 472.

Kruh, J and Borsook, H. (1956). Hemoglobin synthesis in rabbit reticulocytes in vitro. *J. Biol. Chem.* 220: 905–915.

Kunkel, HG, Ceppellini, R, Muller-Eberhard, U, and Wolf, J. (1957). Observations on the minor basic hemoglobin components in the blood of normal individuals and patients with thalassemia. *J. Clin. Invest.* 36: 1615–1616.

Lajtha, LG. (1980). The common ancestral cell in blood. In Wintrobe, MM, editor. *Blood: Pure and eloquent.* New York: McGraw-Hill.

Lajtha, LG, Pozzi, LV, Schofield, R, and Fox, M. (1969). Kinetic properties of hematopoietic stem cells. *Cell Tissue Kinet.* 2: 34–49.

Lavoisier, AL. (1778). Sur la nature du principe qui se combine avec less métaux pendant leur calcination, et qui en augmente le poids (a). *Histoire de l'academie royale des Sciences, 1775,* 520–526.

Lehmann, H and Carrell, RW. (1968). Difference between α- and β-chain mutants of human haemoglobin and between α- and β-thalassaemia. Possible duplication of the α-chain gene. *Br. Med. J.* 4: 748–750.

Lehmann, H and Huntsman, RG. (1974). *Man's haemoglobins.* Amsterdam: North Holland Pub. Co. 479 p.

Lie-Injo, LE and Hie, JB. (1960). Hydrops foetalis with a fast moving hemoglobin. *Br. Med. J.* ii: 1649–1650.

London, IM, Bruns, GP, and Karibian, D. (1964). The regulation of hemoglobin synthesis and pathogenesis of some hypochromic anemias. *Medicine (Baltimore)* 43: 789–802.

London, IM, Shemin, D, and Rittenberg, D. (1948). The in vitro synthesis of heme in the human red blood cell of sickle cell anemia. *J. Biol. Chem.* 173: 797–798.

London, IM, Shemin, D, and Rittenberg, D. (1950). The synthesis of heme in vitro by the immature non-nucleated mammalian erythrocyte. *J. Biol. Chem.* 183: 749–755.

London, IM, Shemin, D, West, R, and Rittenberg, D. (1949). Heme synthesis and red blood cell dynamics in normal humans and in subjects with polycythemia vera, sickle cell anemia, and pernicious anemia. *J. Biol. Chem.* 179: 463–484.

Lower, R. (1669). *Tractatus de corde.* (Latin). Translated by KJ Franklin. In Gunther, RT, *Early science at Oxford.* Vol IX. Oxford: Clarendon Press, 1932.

Marks, PA and Burka, ER. (1964). Hemoglobin synthesis in human reticulocytes: A defect in globin formation in thalassemia major. *Ann. N.Y. Acad. Sci.* 119: 513–522.

McCurdy, PR. (1960). Clinical and physiological studies in a Negro with sickle cell-hemoglobin D disease. *N. Engl. J. Med.* 262: 961–964.

Mikake, T, Hung, CK-H, and Goldwasser, E. (1977). Purification of human erythropoeitin. *J. Biol. Chem.* 252: 5558–5564.

Monod, J, Wyman, J, and Changeux, JP. (1965). On the nature of allosteric transitions: A plausible model. *J. Mol. Biol.* 12: 88–118.

Moore, MAS and Metcalf, D. (1970). Ontogeny of the hematopoietic system: Yolk sac origin of in vivo and in vitro colony forming cells in the developing mouse embryo. *Br J. Haematol.* 18: 279–296.

Muirhead, H, Cox, JM, Mazzarella, L, and Perutz, MF. (1967). Structure and function of haemoglobin III. A three-dimensional Fourier synthesis of human deoxy-

haemoglobin at 5.5 Å resolution. *J. Mol. Biol.* 28: 117–156.

Nathan, DG and Gunn, RB. (1966). Thalassemia: The consequences of unbalanced hemoglobin synthesis. *Am. J. Med.* 41: 815–830.

Neel, JV. (1947). The clinical detection of the genetic carriers of inherited disease. *Medicine (Baltimore)* 26: 115–153.

Neel, JV. (1949). The inheritance of sickle cell anemia. *Science* 110: 64–66.

Nelli, HS. (1980). Italians. In Thernstrom, S, editor. *Harvard encyclopedia of American ethnic groups.* Cambridge: Belknap Press of Harvard University.

Neumann, E. (1868). Ueber die Bedeutung des Knochenmarkes für die Blutbildung. *Zentralbl. Med. Wissensch.* 6: 689.

Neumann, E. (1869). Du role de la moelle des os dans la formation du sang. *C. R. Acad. Sci. (Paris)* 68: 1112–1113.

Nienhuis, AW and Anderson, WF. (1971). Isolation and translation of hemoglobin messenger RNA from thalassemia, sickle cell anemia and normal human reticulocytes. *J. Clin. Invest.* 50: 2755–2760.

Olmstead, JMD. (1952). Father of aviation medicine. *Sci. Am.* 186: 66–72.

Pagnier, J, Mears, JG, Dunda-Belkhodja, O et al. (1984). Evidence for the multicentric origin of the sickle cell hemoglobin gene in Africa. *Proc. Natl. Acad. Sci. U.S.A.* 81: 1771–1773.

Pappenheim, A. (1909). Meeting of the German Hematologic Society. *Folia Hematol. (Leipz)* 8: 399–409.

Parkhurst, LJ. (1979). Hemoglobin and myoglobin ligand kinetics. *Annu. Rev. Phys. Chem.* 30: 503–546.

Pauling, L. (1935). The oxygen equilibrium of hemoglobin and its structural interpretation. *Proc. Natl. Acad. Sci. U.S.A.* 21: 186–191.

Pauling, L. (1954). Abnormality of hemoglobin molecules in hereditary hemolytic anemias. In *The Harvey lectures 1954–1955,* Series 49. New York: Academic Press.

Pauling, L and Coryell, CD. (1936). The magnetic properties and structure of hemoglobin, oxyhemoglobin and carbonmonoxyhemoglobin. *Proc. Natl. Acad. Sci. U.S.A.* 22: 210–216.

Pauling, L, Itano, HA, Singer, SJ, and Wells, IC. (1949). Sickle cell anemia: A molecular disease. *Science* 110: 543–548.

Perrine, RP, Pembrey, ME, John, P et al. (1978). Natural history of sickle cell anemia in Saudi Arabs. A study of 270 subjects. *Ann. Intern. Med.* 88: 1–6.

Perutz, MF. (1970). Stereochemistry of cooperative effects in haemoglobin. *Nature* 228: 726–739.

Perutz, MF, Pulsinelli, PD, and Ranney, HM. (1972). Structure and subunit interaction of haemoglobin M Milwaukee. *Nature* 237: 259–263.

Perutz, MF, Rossmann, MG, Cullis, AF et al. (1960). Structure of haemoglobin: A three-dimensional Fourier synthesis at 5.5Å resolution obtained by x-ray analysis. *Nature* 185: 416–422.

Peters, RA. (1912). Chemical nature of specific oxygen capacity of hemoglobin. *J. Physiol.* 44: 131–149.

Pluznick, DH and Sachs, L. (1966). The induction of clones of normal mast cells by a substance from conditioned medium. *Exp. Cell Res.* 43: 553–563.

Powars, DR. (1975). The natural history of sickle cell disease—The first 10 years. *Semin. Hematol.* 12: 267–285.

Pulsinelli, PD, Perutz, MF, and Nagel, RI. (1973). Structure of hemoglobin M Boston: a variant with a five coordinated ferric heme. *Proc. Natl. Acad. Sci. U.S.A.* 70: 3870–3874.

Ranney, HM. (1954). Observations on the inheritance of sickle cell hemoglobin and hemoglobin C. *J. Clin. Invest.* 33: 1634–1641.

Ranney, HM, Larson, DL, and McCormack, GHJ. (1953). Some clinical biochemical and genetic observations on hemoglobin C. *J. Clin. Invest.* 32: 1277–1284.

Reed, LJ, Bradley, TB, and Ranney, HM. (1965). The effect of amelioration of anemia on the synthesis of fetal hemoglobin in sickle cell anemia. *Blood* 25: 37–48.

Reissmann, KR. (1950). Studies on the mechanism of erythropoietic stimulation in parabiotic rats during hypoxia. *Blood* 5: 372–380.

Rhinesmith, HS, Schroeder, WA, and Martin, N. (1958). The N-terminal sequence of the β chains of normal adult human hemoglobin. *J. Am. Chem. Soc.* 80: 3358–3361.

Rhinesmith, HS, Schroeder, WA, and Pauling, L. (1957). A quantitative study of the hydrolysis of human dinitrophenyl (DNP) globin: The number and kind of polypeptide chains in normal adult human hemoglobin. *J. Am. Chem. Soc.* 79: 4682–4686.

Rich, A. (1952). Studies on the hemoglobin of Cooley's anemia and Cooley's trait. *Proc. Natl. Acad. Sci. U.S.A.* 38: 187–196.

Rietti, F. (1925). Ittero emolitico primitivo. *Atti. Accad. Sci. Med. Nat. Ferrara* 2: 14–17.

Rigas, DA, Koler, RD, and Osgood, EE. (1955). New hemoglobin possessing a higher electrophoretic mobility than normal adult hemoglobin. *Science* 121: 372.

Rossi-Fanelli, A, Antonini, E, and Caputo, A. (1961). Studies on the relations between the molecular and functional properties of hemoglobin. II. The effect of salts on the oxygen equilibrium of human hemoglobin. *J. Biol. Chem.* 236: 397–400.

Rous, P. (1923). Destruction of the red blood corpuscles in health and disease. *Physiol. Rev.* 3: 75–105.

Schroeder, WA, Huisman, THJ, Shelton, R et al. (1968). Evidence for multiple structural genes for the α-chain of human fetal hemoglobin. *Proc. Natl. Acad. Sci. U.S.A.* 60: 537–544.

Schroeder, WA, Shelton, JH, Shelton, JB et al. (1963). The amino acid sequence of the g chain of human fetal hemoglobin. *Biochemistry* 2: 992–1008.

Schwann, T. (1847) *Microscopical researches into the accordance in the structure and growth of animals and plants.* London: Sydenham Society.

Shemin, D. (1954–1955). The biosynthesis of porphyrins. In *The Harvey Lectures*, Vol. 49. New York: Academic Press.

Shemin, D, London, IM, and Rittenberg, D. (1948). The in vitro synthesis of heme from glycine by the nucleated red blood cell. *J. Biol. Chem.* 173: 798–800.

Shemin, D and Rittenberg, D. (1946). The life span of the human red blood cell. *J. Biol. Chem.* 166: 627–636.

Sherman, IJ. (1940). The sickling phenomenon, with special reference to the differentiation of sickle cell anemia from the sickle cell trait. *Bull. Johns Hopkins Hosp.* 67: 309–324.

Singer, K and Singer, L. (1953). Studies on abnormal hemoglobins. VIII. The gelling phenomenon of sickle cell hemoglobin: Its biologic and diagnostic significance. *Blood* 8: 1008–1023.

Smith, EW and Torbert, JV. (1958). Study of two abnormal hemoglobins with evidence of a new genetic locus for hemoglobin formation. *Bull. Johns Hopkins Hosp.* 102: 38–45.

Spaet, TH. (1980). Platelets: the blood dust. In Wintrobe MM, editor. *Blood: pure and eloquent.* New York: McGraw-Hill.

Spaet, TH, Alway, RH, and Ward, G. (1953). Homozygous hemoglobin C. *Pediatrics* 12: 483–490.

Steen, LAS. (1990). On the shoulders of giants. In *New approaches to numeracy.* Washington, DC: National Academy Press.

Stokes, GG. (1864). On the reduction and oxidation of the coloring matter of the blood. *Proc. R. Soc.* 13: 355–1864.

Sturgeon, P and Finch, CA. (1957). Erythrokinetics in Cooley's anemia. *Blood* 12: 64–73.

Sturgeon, P, Itano, HA, and Valentine, WN. (1952). Chronic hemolytic anemia associated with thalassemia and sickling trait. *Blood* 7: 350–357.

Svedberg, T and Fahraeus, R. (1926). A new method for the determination of the molecular weight of the proteins. *J. Am. Chem. Soc.* 48: 430–438.

Sydenstricker, VP. (1923). Sickle cell anemia. Report of 2 cases in children, with necropsy in one case. *Am. J. Dis. Child.* 26: 132–154.

Tavassoli, M. (1980). Bone marrow: The seedbed of blood. In Wintrobe, M, editor. *Blood: Pure and eloquent.* New York: McGraw-Hill.

Temin, HM and Mizutani, S. (1970). RNA-dependent DNA polymerase in virions of Rous sarcoma virus. *Nature* 226: 1211–1213.

Tilghman, SM, Tiemeier, DC, Seidman, JG, et al. (1978). Intervening sequence of DNA identified in the structural portion of the mouse β globin gene. *Proc. Natl. Acad. Sci. U.S.A.* 75: 725.

Till, JE and McCulloch, EA. (1961). Direct measurement of the radiation sensitivity of normal mouse bone marrow cells. *Radiat. Res.* 14: 213–222.

Tosteson, DC, Shea, E, and Darling, RC. (1952). Potassium and sodium of red blood cells in sickle cell anemia. *J. Clin. Invest.* 31: 406–411.

Valentine, WN and Neel, JV. (1944). Hematologic and genetic study of transmission of thalassemia. *Arch Intern. Med.* 74: 185–196.

Van der Stricht, O. (1892). Nouvelles recherches sur la genese des globules rouges et des globules blanc du sang. *Arch. Biol. (Liege)* 12: 199–344.

Vecchio, F. (1946). Sulla resistenza della emoglobina alla denaturazione alcalina in alcune sindromi emopatiche. *Pediatria (Napoli)* 54: 545–549.

Viault, F. (1890). Sur l'augmentation considerable du nombre des globules rouge dans le sang chez les habitants des hautes plateaux de l'amerique du sud. *C.R. Acad. Sci. (Paris)* 119: 917–918.

Watson, J, Stahman, AW, and Bilello, FP. (1948). The significance of the paucity of sickle cells in newborn Negro infants. *Am. J. Med. Sci.* 215: 419–423.

Watson, JD and Crick, FHC. (1953). Molecular structure of nucleic acids. A structure for deoxyribose nucleic acid. *Nature* 171: 737–738.

West, JB. (1998). *High life* New York: Oxford University Press.

Whipple, GH and Bradford, WL. (1932). Racial or familial anemia of children associated with fundamental disturbances of bone and pigment metabolism (Cooley – von Jaksch). *Am. J. Dis. Child.* 44: 336–365.

Whipple, GH and Bradford, WL. (1936). Mediterranean disease-thalassemia (erythroblastic anemia of Cooley): Associated pigment abnormalities simulating hemochromatosis. *J. Pediatr.* 9: 279–311.

White, JG. (1968). The fine structure of sickle cell hemoglobin in situ. *Blood* 31: 561–579.

Wintrobe, MM. (1980). Milestones on the path of progress. In Wintrobe, MM, editor. *Blood: Pure and eloquent.* New York: McGraw-Hill.

Wishner, BC, Ward, KB, Lattmann, EE, and Love, WE. (1975). Crystal structure of sickle deoxyhemoglobin at 5Å resolution. *J. Mol. Biol.* 98: 179–194.

Wyman, J. (1964). Linked functions and reciprocal effects in hemoglobin: A second look. *Adv. Protein Chem.* 19: 223–286.

SECTION I

THE MOLECULAR, CELLULAR, AND GENETIC BASIS OF HEMOGLOBIN DISORDERS

BERNARD F. FORGET
DOUGLAS R. HIGGS

Over the last 30 years, we have become familiar with the way in which different types of hemoglobin are expressed at different stages of development. In the human embryo the main hemoglobins include Hb Portland ($\zeta_2\gamma_2$), Hb Gower I ($\zeta_2\varepsilon_2$), and Gower II ($\alpha_2\varepsilon_2$). In the fetus, HbF ($\alpha_2\gamma_2$) predominates, and in the adult HbA ($\alpha_2\beta_2$) makes up the majority of hemoglobin in red cells. However, these simple facts belie the complexity of the cellular and molecular processes that bring about these beautifully coordinated changes in the patterns of globin gene expression throughout development.

To try to understand these phenomena, we must consider the individual components including (1) the origins of erythroid cells in development, (2) the processes by which erythroid cells differentiate to mature red cells at each developmental stage, and (3) the molecular events that produce the patterns of gene expression we observe.

The hemopoietic system probably originates from multipotent cells identified in a part of the embryo that lies close to the dorsal aorta in the region near the site of where the kidneys first develop, the so-called aorta-gonads-mesonephros (AGM) region. Although there is still some uncertainty about the details, it appears that the blood islands in the yolk sac, where embryonic erythropoiesis occurs, are derived from cells originating in the AGM region (primitive hemopoiesis). Similarly, it is thought that the cells destined to pro-vide fetal- (liver) and adult- (bone marrow) derived red cells also originate from AGM cells (definitive hemopoiesis). Red cells made in the yolk sac are quite different from those made in the liver and bone marrow and predominantly contain embryonic hemoglobins, although they also contain smaller amounts of HbF. In the first trimester of pregnancy, fetal cells, derived predominantly from hemopoiesis in the liver, contain mainly HbF with small amounts of embryonic hemoglobin. There are no circumstances in which expression of embryonic globins persist at high levels or become substantially reactivated in fetal or adult life, although low levels of ζ-globin chains are present in the most severe from of α thalassaemia. Until approximately the time of birth, fetal cells continue to make predominantly HbF, but between 30 and 40 weeks postconception switch to make HbA. In contrast to the situation in embryonic cells, there are many conditions in which HbF synthesis persists or becomes reactivated in adult red cells. The simplest explanation for all of these observations is that the switch from embryonic to fetal/adult patterns of hemoglobin synthesis involves the replacement of embryonic cells (with one program of expression) by definitive cells (with a different program of expression). In contrast, the switch from fetal to adult hemoglobin expression takes place in definitive cells, representing a true change in the molecular program within a single lineage.

At present we do not know when the embryonic and fetal programs are established in the developing hemopoietic cells. Furthermore, we do not fully understand the mechanisms that initiate and maintain the programs of globin gene expression. Perhaps the greatest progress toward such an understanding has been to identify key regulatory molecules, including transcription factors, cofactors, and chromatin-associated proteins that play important roles in specifying the formation of erythroid cells from multipotent hemopoietic stem cells. Of greatest importance in this area has been the characterization of the tissue-restricted zinc finger proteins (GATA-1 and GATA-2), their cofactors (FOG1 and FOG2), the b-Zip family of proteins (NF-E2, Nrf1, Nrf2, Nrf3, Bach1, and Bach2), and the erythroid Krüppel-like factors (EKLF and FKLF). Experiments in which GATA-1, GATA-2, and FOG1 have been deleted from the mouse genome show that these proteins play a major role in establishing the erythroid lineage and allowing differentiation to mature red cells.

A major focus of our interest over the last 20 years has been to understand how these developmental programs are played out on the α- and β-globin gene clusters. We now know that in mammals, the globin

Martin H. Steinberg, Bernard G. Forget, Douglas R. Higgs, and Ronald L. Nagel, editors. *Disorders of Hemoglobin: Genetics, Pathophysiology, and Clinical Management.* © 2001 Cambridge University Press. All rights reserved.

genes in each cluster are arranged along the chromosome in the order in which they are expressed in development: the α-globin genelike cluster on chromosome 16 (ζ-α$_2$-α$_1$-) and the β-globin genelike cluster on chromosome 11 (ε-γ^G-γ^A-δ-β-), suggesting that gene order may be important in unfolding this program. Expression of each gene cluster is dependent on remote regulatory elements. In the α-globin gene-like cluster there is a single regulatory element (RE or HS −40), which lies 40 kb upstream of the α-globin gene complex. In the β-globin gene cluster there are four elements, collectively referred to as the β-globin locus control region (β-LCR) lying 5 to 20 kb upstream of the locus. Again, many details remain unknown, but it appears that the ζ and ε genes are switched on in embryonic cells and are largely off in definitive cells in which they cannot be substantially reactivated. By contrast, there appears to be competition between the α genes and β genes for activation in definitive cells with the balance tipped toward γ expression in fetal life and β expression in adult life. However, the situation is complex and both competition and autonomous silencing of the genes appear to play a role in the switching process. The balance between α- and β-globin gene expression may be altered in vivo (in hereditary persistence of fetal hemoglobin) and in experimental systems. Changes in the repertoire or amounts of transcription factors may influence the switch from γ to β gene expression. For example, without EKLF the β genes cannot be fully activated during development. Alternatively, alterations in the arrangement of the β-LCR and the genes with respect to each other may alter switching. The precise molecular mechanisms underlying these changes are still poorly understood but it seems unlikely that changes in the patterns of globin gene expression are only brought about through changes in the repertoire of *trans* acting factors present in embryonic, fetal, and adult red cells, as originally proposed, but may be influenced by other epigenetic changes in the chromosome (e.g. chromatin structure and modification, replication timing, and methylation).

Despite our continuing interest and frustrated attempts to understand how the entire globin clusters are regulated, we do know a lot about the structure and function of individual genes. The globin genes have provided the paradigm for understanding the general arrangement of mammalian genes including their promoters, exons, introns, and processing signals. Furthermore, the mechanisms by which these genes are transcribed into pre-RNA, processed into mature RNA, and translated into protein are now understood in detail. This brings us full circle to the beginnings of modern molecular biology by establishing the structure and function of the proteins expressed by globin genes. Hemoglobin was one of the first proteins whose amino acid sequence and crystal structure were solved, which in turn led to a complete understanding of how it captures, transports, and releases oxygen. Given the large number of natural mutants of hemoglobin that have now been identified, it also provides an unsurpassed example of how mutations can give rise to "molecular diseases," the best example still being sickle cell disease.

Even with this apparent depth of knowledge, however, there are still surprises. We know from theory and experiment that embryonic hemoglobins and fetal hemoglobins have a higher affinity for oxygen than adult hemoglobin. Traditionally we have assumed that this quality enables the developing fetus to acquire oxygen more efficiently from the maternal circulation, a seemingly important consideration. However, we have known for many years that the infants of mothers whose blood contains mainly fetal (high affinity) hemoglobin are entirely normal. Similarly, thanks to experimental work in model systems, we know that mice, who by design only make embryonic hemoglobin throughout fetal and adult development survive normally and thrive as adults. Presumably the complex system of hemoglobin switching that keeps investigators so busy has been molded in subtle ways by natural selection. Why do we pursue this subject with such enthusiasm? There are two main reasons. First, the globin system still provides the most thoroughly studied and comprehensively understood example of mammalian gene expression. If there are undiscovered general principles that govern the regulation of mammalian genes, then analysis of globin gene expression is likely to elucidate them. Second, understanding how these genes are controlled offers the best hope of developing strategies to ameliorate or cure the many thousands of severely affected patients who inherit defects in the structure or production of the α- and β-like globins that make up embryonic, fetal, and adult hemoglobins.

The following nine chapters trace the genesis of hemoglobin, from the earliest appearance of erythroid cells during development, through the nuclear factors that govern its synthesis, to the evolution of globin genes, their organization, and switching, to the production of hemoglobin and its functions in the erythrocyte.

2

A Developmental Approach to Hematopoiesis

ELAINE DZIERZAK

During mammalian embryonic development, the first morphologically recognizable and earliest blood cells to appear are those of the erythroid lineage. The early unbalanced production of erythroid lineage cells in the extraembryonic yolk sac appears to be requisite for the development of the early and midgestation vertebrate embryo. In contrast, studies of the adult hematopoietic hierarchy show the abundant production of immature progenitors, numerous lineage committed progenitors, and at least eight distinct functional lineages of terminally differentiated cells. This complex adult system arises from pluripotential hematopoietic stem cells harbored in the bone marrow. Thus, four important features of developmental hematopoiesis to consider are (1) the embryonic origin of the cells that make up the embryonic hematopoietic compartment, (2) the embryonic origin of the cells that make up the adult hematopoietic compartment, (3) the lineage relationships between the hematopoietic cells of the embryonic and adult compartments, and (4) the migration of hematopoietic cells generated in the embryo and colonization of the hematopoietic organs of the adult. Although the erythroid lineage provided the first clear indications that differences exist between embryonic and adult hematopoiesis, this chapter focuses on the embryonic beginnings and lineage relationships of not only erythroid cells, but of the stem cells, prog-

enitors, and all the lineages of the hematopoietic hierarchy. We will explore the ontogeny of hematopoietic cell formation, the colonization of hematopoietic tissues, and the molecular programming of the hematopoietic system during development in nonmammalian and mammalian vertebrates.

ONTOGENY OF THE HEMATOPOIETIC SYSTEM

In general, developmental studies have led to a better understanding of the basic biology and differentiation of the cells in many of the adult organs. Several vertebrate and invertebrate animal models have shown that the cellular interactions and molecular programs governing development are conserved throughout evolution. The conservation of developmental principles also applies to the generation of the hematopoietic system. Thus, our current knowledge of the embryonic origins of the adult hematopoietic system in mammals has relied heavily on nonmammalian vertebrate models (Dieterlen-Lievre and Le Douarin, 1993; Zon, 1995). Wide support has been generated for at least two independent origins of hematopoiesis in the conceptus and the colonization theory of hematopoiesis. How this applies to human embryonic hematopoiesis is bridged through the recent extensive analysis of mouse models for mammalian embryonic hematopoiesis (Dzierzak and Medvinsky, 1995; Dzierzak et al., 1998). The variety of in vivo and in vitro hematopoietic assays and the ability to create mouse mutants for many hematopoietic-related genes have significantly expanded our knowledge of mammalian blood development. These studies, particularly on the molecular level, bring hope for novel clinical therapies of blood cell deficiencies and malignancies. From this evolutionary perspective, what have been mainly descriptive analyses of embryonic hematopoiesis in humans may now be envisioned as an active and dynamic process.

Initiation and Appearance of Hematopoietic Cells

Mesoderm. Blood is one of the earliest tissues to develop during embryogenesis. The hematopoietic system is derived from the mesodermal germ layer of undifferentiated cells. Thus, the early stage of human hematopoiesis has been referred to as the "mesoblastic" period (Miale, 1982). The mesoderm forms through an inductive interaction between the ectodermal and endodermal germ layers during the mid-blastula stage (Fig. 2.1A). Much of our knowledge of

Martin H. Steinberg, Bernard G. Forget, Douglas R. Higgs, and Ronald L. Nagel, editors. *Disorders of Hemoglobin: Genetics, Pathophysiology, and Clinical Management.* © 2001 Cambridge University Press. All rights reserved.

mesoderm induction comes from studies of amphibian embryos in which the manipulation, grafting,
and culture of embryos is facilitated by their large
size and development outside the mother.
Nieuwkoop (Nieuwkoop, 1969) was the first to
show that culture of the amphibian mid-blastula
stage animal pole (ectoderm) alone leads to the
production of epidermis, whereas co-culture of the
animal pole with the vegetal pole (endoderm) leads
to the generation of mesodermal structures such as
muscle, notochord, heart, pronephros, and blood
(Fig. 2.1B). Cell lineage mapping studies show that
mesodermal cells are formed from the ectodermal
component that receives signals from the underlying
endodermal component of the embryo (Dale et al.,
1985; Nieuwkoop and Ubbels, 1972).

   Most recently, several mesoderm-inducing factors
have been identified through the use of the animal
cap assay, in which animal poles of frog embryos
cultured in the presence of members of the transforming growth factor-β (TGF-β) family such as
BMP-4, activin or Vg1, or members of the fibroblast
growth factor (FGF) family (Green et al., 1992;
Green and Smith, 1990; Smith, 1993) form mesodermal cells. The different and overlapping dorsal-ventral distribution of these factors by endodermal cells
suggests that they act as morphogenic gradients.
This, in combination with the extensive rearrangement of cells during gastrulation, forms the different
classes of mesoderm: dorsal, paraxial, lateral, and
ventral. For example, ventral endodermal cells/fac-
tors induce the formation of mesoderm, which can
differentiate into erythrocytes (Dale et al., 1985;
Sargent et al., 1986). Indeed, genes for numerous
other secreted factors (as well as transcription factors and adhesion molecules) are expressed in the
mesoderm during gastrulation, and these proteins
may play a role in the maintenance and/or the patterning of mesoderm (reviewed in Stennard, 1997).
Mesoderm induction is the first step leading to the
specification of cells for the development of the
hematopoietic system, and two spatially separated
mesodermal compartments (intraembryonic and
extraembryonic) have been shown to independently
initiate hematopoiesis.

   The similarities found in the germ layer fate maps
of fish (Kimmel et al., 1990), amphibian (Smith,
1993), avian (Vakaet, 1985), and mammalian
(Lawson et al., 1991) embryos suggest that the
mechanisms of mesoderm induction and patterning
are well conserved during gastrulation within vertebrate species. Indeed, the extraembryonic mesoderm
of the yolk sac from which the first embryonic erythrocytes are formed in the higher vertebrates, chick,
and the mouse, coincides with the location of the

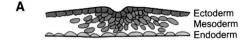

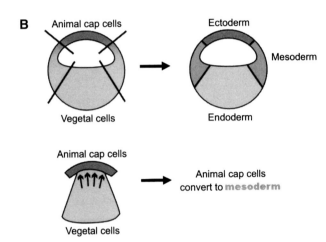

Figure 2.1. Germ layer development in vertebrate embryos. (**A**)
Mesoderm arises from an inductive interaction between ectoderm and endoderm. (**B**) Experimental scheme in *Xenopus*
embryos (Nieuwkoop), which shows that mesodermal cells
arise from the ectoderm (animal fragment) under the inductive
influence of the endodermal vegetal fragment.

blood-forming cells in fish and frog embryos
(Conlon and Beddington, 1995; Smith, 1993).
However, the timing of mesoderm induction and the
cells yielding the mesoderm-inducing signals are not
yet well established in fish and avian embryos, and
these issues have been even more difficult to address
in mouse embryos.

Extraembryonic Yolk Sac Hematopoiesis. The earliest formation of mature blood cells is from ventral
mesodermal cells within the extraembryonic yolk sac
(Fig. 2.2A). The migration of mesodermal precursors
to this extraembryonic site is highly conserved
between amphibian, avian, and mammalian species.
Mesodermal cells form aggregates while in contact
with the extraembryonic endoderm, leading to their
differentiation into blood islands (Risau, 1991).
Differentiation to primitive erythrocytes occurs
within the core of the blood island, while a surrounding layer of differentiating endothelial cells is
established (Fig. 2.2B). In the human conceptus, the
yolk sac blood islands are detectable by histologic
sectioning at about 16 to 20 days of gestation
(Kelemen et al., 1979; Rifkind et al., 1980), and in

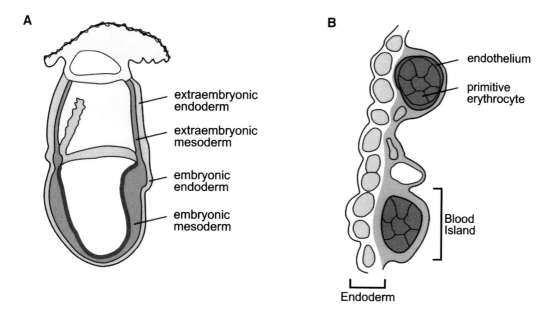

Figure 2.2. Early mammalian embryogenesis. (A) A schematic of an E7.5 mouse embryo showing extraembryonic endoderm and mesoderm, which form the yolk sac, and the endoderm and mesoderm of the embryo body. (B) Yolk sac blood islands in the early stage mammalian embryo.

the mouse conceptus at embryonic day 7.5 (E7.5) (Russell and Bernstein, 1966). The close temporal and spatial association of the cells of the vasculature and the hematopoietic system within the yolk sac has led to a long history of speculation concerning a common precursor, the hemangioblast (His, 1990; Murray, 1932; Sabin, 1920; Wagner, 1980). Indeed many cell surface markers such as flk-1 (Shalaby et al., 1995), CD31 (Baldwin et al., 1994), and CD34 (Tavian et al., 1996; Wood et al., 1997; Young et al., 1995) have been found to be commonly expressed on hematopoietic cells and endothelial cells (Choi et al., 1998; Nishikawa et al., 1998a). Recently, gene targeting experiments for the flk-1 receptor tyrosine kinase protein (the receptor for vascular endothelial growth factor [VEGF]) have resulted in mice deficient for both endothelial and hematopoietic lineages (Shalaby et al., 1997, 1995). These experiments suggest a common hemangioblast precursor, or dual roles, for flk-1 (see gene requirement section) in both endothelial and hematopoietic lineages. Most recently, it has been suggested that in addition to a common hemangioblast precursor, lymphohematopoietic endothelial cells exist in the E9.5 yolk sac (Nishikawa et al., 1998b).

Intraembryonic Hematopoiesis. In mammalian species, it has long been thought that the fetal liver is the first intraembryonic site harboring hematopoi-

etic cells (Moore and Metcalf, 1970). The colonization theory of mammalian hematopoiesis directed most thinking toward the exclusive generation of hematopoietic cells within the extraembryonic yolk sac and their subsequent migration to and colonization of the fetal liver (which does not generate its own hematopoietic cells). However, it has been recently accepted that, within the body of the early stage mammalian embryo, there is a distinct mesodermally derived region capable of autonomously producing hematopoietic cells (Cumano et al., 1996; Dzierzak and Medvinsky, 1995; Dzierzak et al., 1998; Godin et al., 1993; Medvinsky and Dzierzak, 1996; Medvinsky et al., 1996; Medvinsky et al., 1993; Moore and Metcalf, 1970). At early developmental stages, this region is identified as the paraaortic splanchnopleura (PAS) and consists of the mesodermal region adjacent to the endoderm, the paired dorsal aortae, and the surrounding mesenchyme (Fig. 2.3A). With subsequent stages of organogenesis, this intraembryonic region differentiates into urogenital tissue and consists of the aorta-gonads-mesonephros (AGM) and the surrounding mesenchyme (Fig. 2.3B).

Experiments performed in nonmammalian vertebrates have made unique contributions to our understanding of extraembryonic and intraembryonic hematopoiesis and set an important precedent for a nonyolk sac intraembryonic site of hematopoietic development. In the mid-1970s, amphibian and avian embryo culture and grafting approaches were used to extensively study cell fate, morphogenesis, and organogenesis. In the avian species, interspecific grafts between quail and chick embryos or intraspecific grafts between different strains of chicks were

A

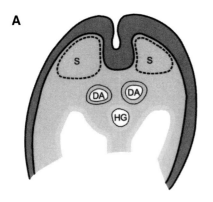

PAS (E8.5-9)

B

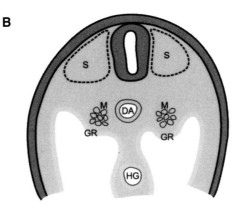

AGM (E10-11)

Figure 2.3. Schematic cross-sections of mouse embryos. (**A**) This section shows the paraaortic splanchnopleura (PAS) at E8.5–9, which contains multipotential progenitors and neonatal repopulating progenitors but no adult repopulating hematopoietic stem cells. (**B**) This section through an E10–11 mouse embryo shows the aorta-gonad-mesonephros (AGM) region. The first adult hematopoietic stem cells are autonomously generated here, although it is uncertain where these cells are localized within this tissue. Hematopoietic cell clusters are found on the ventral wall of the dorsal aorta. DA, dorsal aorta; GR, genital ridge; HC, hematopoietic cluster; HG, hindgut; M, mesonephros; S, somites.

used to create chimeras in which the embryonic origins of adult blood cells were determined (Dieterlen-Lievre, 1975; Dieterlen-Lievre and Le Douarin, 1993). Nucleolar or immunohistochemical markers determined from which grafted tissue the differentiated adult blood cells were derived. For example, yolk sac chimeras were constructed by grafting a quail embryo body onto the extraembryonic area of a chick blastodisc (Fig. 2.4A). The combined results of many such chimeric experiments (Beaupain et al., 1979; Dieterlen-Lievre, 1975; Dieterlen-Lievre and Martin, 1981; Martin et al., 1978) led to the following conclusions: (1) the first emergence of hematopoietic cells is extraembryonic, in the yolk sac; (2) slightly later, hematopoietic cells emerge both extraembryonically and intraembryonically; and (3) intraembryonically derived hematopoietic cells are the permanent contributors to the adult hematopoietic system, whereas extraembryonically derived hematopoietic cells become extinct. Furthermore, multipotential hematopoietic progenitors as assayed in in vitro clonal cultures are associated with the dorsal aortae of avian embryos, but not other embryonic tissues (Cormier and Dieterlen-Lievre, 1988). Interestingly, hematopoietic cell clusters are observed on the ventral wall of the dorsal aorta (Dieterlen-Lievre, 1975).

The close association of hematopoietic cells to endothelial cells has led investigators to examine whether hematopoietic cells differentiate from endothelial cells. Most convincing results have come from chick embryos in which labeling of aortic endothelial cells was performed by specific uptake of lipophilic fluorescent dye (DiI) conjugated to low density lipoprotein (LDL) during pre-hematopoietic stages (Jaffredo et al., 1998). The labeled endothelial cells lining the ventral wall of the dorsal aorta gave rise to intraaortic hematopoietic clusters 1 day later, demonstrating a precursor/progeny relationship between endothelial cells and hematopoietic clusters.

Similarly, chimeric embryo studies in amphibians have shown independent, intraembryonic, and extraembryonic mesodermally derived sites of hematopoiesis (Kau and Turpen, 1983; Maeno et al., 1985; Turpen et al., 1981). Using DNA content as a marker, chimeric frog embryos were generated by reciprocal grafting of the ventral blood island region (region analogous to avian and mammalian yolk sac) and the dorsal lateral plate (region analogous to the avian intraembryonic region surrounding the dorsal aortae) from diploid and triploid embryos (Fig. 2.4B). Again, the ventral mesodermal yolk sac analog produces the first hematopoietic cells, and slightly later, the dorsal mesodermal intrabody compartment generates adult hematopoietic cells. However, unlike with birds, some ventrally derived hematopoietic cells persist to adult stages and can contribute to red and white blood cell populations (Kau and Turpen, 1983; Maeno et al., 1985). Recent *Xenopus* embryo grafting experiments have revealed that during early stages, both ventral blood islands and dorsal lateral plate are bipotential with respect to primitive and definitive hematopoiesis. Commitment to primitive and definitive lineages is suggested to occur by environmentally regulated specification in these respective regions during the relatively early neurula stage (Turpen et al., 1997).

A

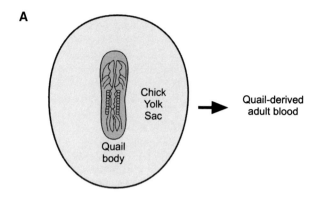

B

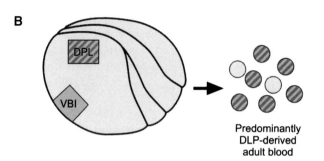

Figure 2.4. Nonmammalian vertebrate embryo grafting experiments used for determining the origin of the adult hematopoietic system. (**A**) A schematic diagram of the avian embryo grafting strategy in which quail embryo bodies were grafted onto chick yolk sacs at the precirculation stage of development. (**B**) A schematic diagram of the amphibian embryo grafting strategy in which genetically marked dorsal lateral plate (DLP) or ventral blood island (VBI) regions were transplanted onto unmarked frog embryos.

However, the results of another study on the AML1 transcription factor in *Xenopus* suggest a previously unsuspected dorsal contribution to the ventral blood island (Tracey et al., 1998). Thus, the early origins remain controversial. The specific localization of intrabody hematopoiesis has been associated with the dorsal aortae and pronephros, with the most abundant hematopoiesis in the pronephros (Turpen and Knudson, 1982).

How precisely do these features apply to mammalian hematopoietic ontogeny? The origins of the adult hematopoietic system in the mammalian embryo are complicated to study because in utero development prohibits direct grafting experiments during appropriate gestational stages. Furthermore, the early joining (E8.5) of the yolk sac and intrabody blood vessels (Cumano et al., 1996) prevents the discrimination of extraembryonically versus intraembryonically derived hematopoietic cells. Only

recently has the careful dissection of the lateral mesodermally derived PAS/AGM region revealed the presence of colony forming units-spleen (CFU-S) erythroid-myeloid progenitors (Medvinsky et al., 1993), B lymphoid progenitors (Godin et al., 1993), and multipotent hematopoietic progenitors for erythroid, myeloid, and lymphoid lineages (Godin et al., 1995) in the preliver E9 mouse embryo body. At slightly later stages of mouse embryogenesis (E10), potent adult-type hematopoietic stem cells are found in the AGM region, which has now begun differentiation into the organs of the urogenital system (Medvinsky and Dzierzak, 1996; Muller et al., 1994). Similar to birds, there appears to be a close spatial and temporal association of the endothelial and hematopoietic lineages in this intrabody site. In a wide range of species that includes mice and humans (Dieterlen-Lievre, 1975; Emmel, 1916; Garcia-Porrero et al., 1995; Jordan, 1918; Medvinsky et al., 1996; Minot, 1910; Tavian et al., 1996), hematopoietic foci appear as clusters adhering tightly along the ventral wall of the dorsal aorta. The expression of cell surface markers, CD34 and CD31 (Tavian et al., 1996; Wood et al., 1997) and the hematopoietic transcription factor AML-1 (North et al., 1999) is shared between the hematopoietic cluster and endothelial cells. Although E9.5 embryo body cells with a putative endothelial cell phenotype can produce lympho-hematopoietic cells in culture (Nishikawa et al., 1998b), it has not yet been shown that endothelial cells of the dorsal aorta possess lymphohematopoietic potential. In conclusion, the early PAS and the slightly later derivative, the AGM region play an important role as an early and potent intraembryonic site of hematopoiesis.

The Embryonic Hematopoietic Hierarchy

The complex lineage relationships of the cells within the adult mammalian hematopoietic hierarchy are well known and have been elaborated for many years by in vivo and in vitro differentiation assays (Metcalf, 1984). These assays, as shown mainly with mouse and in some cases with human cells, measure the functional progression of cells at or near the base and/or branch points of the hematopoietic system to the terminally differentiated cells of at least eight distinct functional blood lineages. The stem cells and progenitors measured by in vitro hematopoietic assays such as CFU-C, FTOC, stromal co-cultures CAFC and LT-CIC, and in vivo transplantation approaches for CFU-S and LTR-HSC (Table 2.1) have led to a placement of these cells within a conceptual hierarchy for adult hematopoiesis (Fig. 2.5). Markers for cell surface molecules expressed on dis-

Table 2.1. Assays for Hematopoietic Cells in the Mouse Embryo

Cell type	Hematopoietic assay	Method	Blood lineage	Reference
Erythroid-myeloid restricted progenitors	CFU-C	In vitro culture for 5 to 14 days in semi-solid medium + hematopoietic growth factors	Erythroid, myeloid	Metcalf, 1984
Erythroid-myeloid restricted progenitors	CFU-S	In vivo transplantation into lethally irradiated adult recipients leading to macroscopic spleen colonies at 8 to 16 days	Erythroid, myeloid	Moore and Metcalf, 1970; Medvinsky et al., 1993
T lymphoid progenitor	Fetal thymic organ culture (FTOC)	In vitro culture with T-depleted thymus for 9 to 21 days	T lymphoid	Liu and Auerbach, 1991a; Godin et al., 1995
B lymphoid progenitor	Stromal co-culture	In vitro 14-day culture with stromal cells +/– IL-7	B lymphoid	Ogawa et al., 1988; Godin et al., 1995
Erythroid-myeloid-lymphoid multi-potential progenitor	Single cell multi-potential assay (SMA)	A two-step in vitro culture with S17 stromal cells and hematopoietic growth factors	B and T lymphoid, myeloid and erythroid	Godin et al., 1995
Neonatal repopulating progenitor	Neonatal trans-plantation	In vivo transplantation into neonatal conditioned or hematopoietic-deficient recipients yielding long-term multilineage repopulation	All hematopoietic lineages	Muller and Dzierzak, 1993; Yoder et al., 1997a
Adult repopulating HSCs	Adult transplantation	In vivo transplantation into lethally irradiated adult recipients producing long-term, high level hemato-poietic repopulation	All hematopoietic lineages	Moore and Metcalf, 1970; Muller et al., 1994

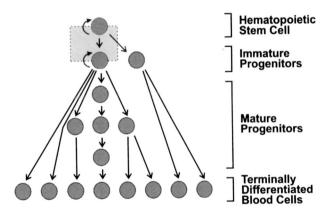

Figure 2.5. Adult hematopoietic hierarchy as envisioned in mammalian species. All adult hematopoietic cells are thought to arise from hematopoietic stem cells at the foundation of this hierarchy. Precursor-progeny relationships in this hierarchy have been established through numerous in vitro and in vivo hematopoietic assays (Table 2.1).

Hematopoietic Stem Cell

Immature Progenitors

Mature Progenitors

Terminally Differentiated Blood Cells

tinct hematopoietic lineages, as well as more undifferentiated hematopoietic cells, have also been instrumental in assigning the direct precursor-progeny relationships and the placement of cells within the conceptual adult hierarchy. Thus, the adult hierarchy is represented as possessing only a unidirectional progression, with restrictive events occurring throughout hematopoietic differentiation. Exceptions are noted in the stem cell and some progenitor cells in which self-renewal events occur. One daughter cell is maintained as a stem cell or progenitor while the other daughter cell proceeds through the hierarchical differentiation scheme.

Until recently, much less was known about the embryonic hematopoietic hierarchy (Dzierzak, 1995; Dzierzak et al., 1998). Whereas the adult mammal has only the bone marrow as the primary tissue harboring hematopoietic activity, the embryo is vastly different; it must de novo generate the entire hematopoietic system, it generates these cells within a

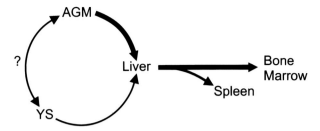

Figure 2.6. Sites of hematopoiesis during mammalian embryonic to adult development and possible migration and colonization events.

short span of time in at least two mesodermally derived microenvironments (yolk sac and PAS/AGM), and promote the sequential migration, colonization, and maintenance of hematopoietic cells in yet other microenvironments (spleen, liver) before they are finally localized in the bone marrow of the adult (Fig. 2.6). Additionally, the function of the hematopoietic cells produced during embryogenesis may differ from their function in the adult. Thus, different subsets of hematopoietic cells may be found in the embryo and adult. Before we can begin to understand the lineage relationships between the hematopoietic cells produced in the mammalian embryo and the pluripotential stem cells at the base of the adult hematopoietic hierarchy, it is important to establish what hematopoietic cells are present during ontogeny. A description of the types of hematopoiesis, terminally differentiated cells, committed progenitors, immature progenitors, and hematopoietic stem cells existing within the mouse, and in some cases the human conceptus, is provided here.

Erythropoiesis. Histologic sectioning reveals that cells of the erythroid lineage are the earliest to be found in human and mouse embryos. Primitive erythroblasts are the first observed in the blood islands of the human at E16–20 (Kelemen et al., 1979) and mouse yolk sac at E7.5 (Russell and Bernstein, 1966) and are the main differentiated cells in the early development of the mammalian species. In human embryos, up to 100 percent of all nucleated blood cells at 4 to 8 weeks of gestation are erythropoietic. These cells are found in the chorial and umbilical vessels, liver sinusoids, and other intraembryonic blood vessels. A switch to enucleated definitive erythropoietic cells is observed between 7 and 10 weeks of gestation in the blood, and slightly earlier in the fetal liver (Kelemen et al., 1979) (Fig. 2.7). Similarly, in the mouse, nucleated primitive erythropoietic cells predominate in the yolk sac and fetal liver until a switch from primitive to definitive cell types occurs between E10 and E12 (Kovach et al., 1967; Rifkind et al., 1969).

In both species, the switch from primitive to definitive erythropoiesis is characterized by changes in the expression of the developmentally regulated fetal and adult globin genes (reviewed in Maniatis et al., 1981; Russell, 1979 and chapter 7) (Figure 2.7). It is now clear that individual erythroid progenitors from embryonic stem (ES) cell differentiation cultures can give rise to both fetal and adult erythroid cells (Kennedy et al., 1997) and that single fetal liver cells can switch from a fetal to adult globin gene expression program (Wijgerde et al., 1995). However, the general populations of mature erythroid cells may be derived from developmentally separate stem cell populations in the embryo (Ingram, 1972; Nakano et al., 1996; Wong et al., 1986). Recently, it has been shown that mouse fetal liver/adult bone marrow cells positive for the receptor tyrosine kinase c-kit differ in erythroid potential from yolk sac/fetal liver c-kit negative cells. In accordance with this finding, administration of anti-c-kit antibodies inhibit fetal liver hematopoieisis but not yolk sac erythropoiesis (Ogawa et al., 1991). Such results on the differential regulation of primitive and definitive erythropoiesis suggest the presence of at least two distinct progenitor/stem cell populations. Additional molecular differences in primitive and definitive erythropoietic programs, particularly in the requirements for erythropoietic growth factors and transcription factors, are well documented and are covered in the following section.

Figure 2.7. Organization and developmental patterns of expression of the human globin genes. A schematic of the chromosomal organization of the genes of the human β-globin locus. Arrows indicate the DNase 1 hypersensitive sites of the LCR (locus control region) an important region for globin gene regulation. The time course of developmental globin gene regulation and the sites of erythropoiesis are shown.

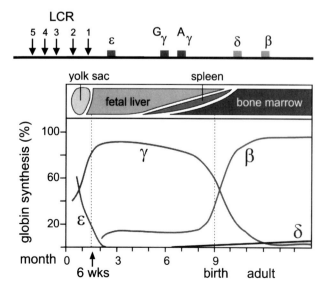

Myelopoiesis. The first cells of the monocyte-macrophage lineage appear in human conceptuses at 4 to 5 weeks of gestation (Kelemen et al., 1979). Monocytes are routinely represented in human embryos at about a 1 to 4 percent frequency in nucleated blood populations after 11 weeks of gestation. Interestingly, macrophages can be found in early human blood smears only until about 14 weeks of gestation. This finding is consistent with findings in the mouse that two separate lineages of macrophages are thought to develop in ontogeny: primitive macrophages and the monocytic lineage of macrophages (Naito, 1993; Naito et al., 1996). In the mouse, primitive macrophages (which begin to appear at E9 in the yolk sac) are thought to arise from a local hematopoietic progenitor and not a monocytic progenitor. These primitive macrophages colonize other embryonic tissues through the circulation. In contrast, adult macrophages do not circulate through the blood, and these cells of the monocytic lineage begin to appear in the fetal liver and yolk sac at E10. Thus, it has been suggested that adult macrophages are the progeny of AGM-derived monocytic precursors, whereas primitive macrophages are yolk sac-derived (Bonifer et al., 1998; Bruijn, 1997).

Lymphopoiesis. The production of lymphoid cells begins in the human at 7 to 10 weeks of gestation (Kelemen et al., 1979). Small lymphocytes are found in the blood: 0.2 percent of nucleated cells at weeks 9 to 10 and 14 percent after 14 weeks. Large lymphocytes represent 3 to 5 percent of nucleated blood cells after 11 weeks of gestation. No lymphoid cells are found in the yolk sac, although the presence of lymphoid progenitors has not been investigated. Lymphopoiesis begins in the human fetal liver, thymus, gut-associated lymphoid tissue, and lymph plexuses around 7 weeks of gestation; the bone marrow lymphocytes are found only at week 12.

Extensive analyses on the development of lymphoid progenitors have been performed in the mouse. Although no functional lymphocytes are found in the mouse conceptus at early gestational stages, lymphoid progenitors have been found to be present. E8.5 yolk sac has been shown to contain T-lymphoid progenitors when cultured in T-cell-depleted fetal thymic explants (Eren et al., 1987; Liu and Auerbach, 1991a, 1991b). B-lymphoid activity was first reported in the embryo body (E9.5) and subsequently the yolk sac (E10) of the mouse conceptus by co-culturing such cells in the presence of stromal cells (Ogawa et al., 1988). More recently, dissection of the PAS/AGM region has revealed the presence of an AA4.1-positive progenitor for the B1a lineage of B cells as early as E8.5 (Godin et al., 1995; Godin et al., 1993). A two-step culture system with E7.5 mouse embryo tissues has shown a multipotential lymphoid

progenitor in the intraembryonic PAS, but not in the yolk sac. Only beginning at E8.5 does the yolk sac acquire such multipotential lymphoid activity (Cumano et al., 1996), suggesting that PAS-generated multipotential lymphoid progenitors may migrate to the yolk sac at E8.5 when the intraembryonic and extraembryonic circulation are fused. Alternatively, the yolk sac may be capable of autonomously producing such progenitors, but 1 day later than the PAS. At slightly later stages, multipotent B progenitors are found in the circulation at E10, reach a maximum at E12, and are undetectable in the blood at E14 (Delassus and Cumano, 1996). B-cell precursors are detected in the fetal liver at E14, and in the embryonic marrow at E15.

Differing lymphoid lineage potentials have been observed in adult mouse bone marrow and fetal liver hematopoietic stem cell-enriched populations. In the T-lymphoid lineage, fetal liver, but not bone marrow hematopoietic stem cells, produces $V\gamma3$ and $V\gamma4$ T cell receptor positive subsets (Ikuta et al., 1990). Such T cells can also be cultured from yolk sac after E8.5 (Liu and Auerbach, 1991a, 1991b). Similarly in the B-lymphoid lineage, the B1a subset of cells is produced by fetal liver (Hayakawa et al., 1985; Herzenberg et al., 1986), yolk sac (Cumano et al., 1993), and PAS (Godin et al., 1993), but not by adult bone marrow. It is interesting to propose that the distinct B1a B-cell subset, as well as $V\gamma3$–4 T cell subsets, may be the product of a special subset of developmentally regulated progenitors or hematopoietic stem cells in the PAS of the early embryo. It is not yet known whether such lymphoid subsets and progenitors exist in human embryos.

Erythroid-Myeloid Progenitors: CFU-C. The early presence of hematopoietic progenitors within the developing mouse yolk sac was established using in vitro culture approaches developed initially for measuring the hematopoietic potential of adult mammalian bone marrow. The culture of yolk sac cells in semisolid medium in the presence of colony-stimulating factors revealed the presence of erythroid and granulocyte-macrophage progenitors beginning at E7 (Johnson and Barker, 1985; Moore and Metcalf, 1970). BFU-E and CFU-Mix are also found in the yolk sac at E8 (Johnson and Barker, 1985) and mast cell precursors at E9.5 (Sonoda et al., 1983). The recent use of an organtypic culture step before hematopoietic differentiation confirms the presence of erythroid-myeloid progenitors within the yolk sac beginning at E7.5 (Cumano et al., 1996).

In the human, yolk sac hematopoiesis covers the period from mid-week 3 in gestation to week 8. BFU-Es have been found at early stages in the yolk sac but begin to decrease in frequency at week 5, when the fetal liver BFU-E frequency increases (Migliaccio et al., 1986), thus suggesting a colonization of the fetal liver by yolk sac progenitors. Along with erythroid progenitors, the yolk sac and embryo body contain clonogenic myeloid progenitors and erythroid-myeloid multipotent progenitors at 25 to 50 days of human gestation (Huyhn et al., 1995). At 4 to 5 weeks of gestation, a discrete population of several hundred cells bearing the cell surface phenotype of immature hematopoietic cells (CD45+, CD34+, CD31+, CD38−) is found adhering to the ventral endothelium of the dorsal aorta (Peault, 1996; Tavian et al., 1996). These clusters are similar to those described in the chick and mouse. When these cell clusters are co-cultured with bone marrow stromal cells and assayed in methylcellulose for CFU-Cs, they yield many progenitors and large multilineage hematopoietic colonies (Tavian et al., 1996).

Erythroid-Myeloid Progenitors: CFU-S.

To determine whether the progenitors within the more immature hematopoietic compartment of the adult hierarchy are present early during embryonic development, complex in vivo transplantation analyses for CFU-S have been performed in mouse irradiation chimeras. CFU-S are immature erythroid-myeloid progenitors that yield macroscopic colonies on the spleens of lethally irradiated mice 9 to 14 days after transplantation (Till and McCulloch, 1961). Beginning at E9, statistically significant numbers of CFU-S are found both in the yolk sac and PAS/AGM (Medvinsky, 1993; Moore and Metcalf, 1970). It is difficult to determine from which tissue these in vivo progenitors originate because the vascular connection between the yolk sac and embryo body is made at E8.5. The absolute numbers of CFU-S from the developing mouse embryo up to late E10 reveal that the AGM region contains more CFU-S than the yolk sac (Medvinsky et al., 1996; Medvinsky et al., 1993). When an organ culture step is used before in vivo transplantation of yolk sac or AGM, the numbers of AGM CFU-S increase substantially, but only a slight increase in yolk sac CFU-S number is observed (Medvinsky and Dzierzak, 1996). These results suggest that both the yolk sac and AGM can autonomously generate CFU-S, but the AGM region is a more potent generator.

Erythroid-Myeloid-Lymphoid Multipotential Progenitors.

Within the mouse embryo, these in vitro progenitors are found at E7.5 within the intrabody PAS/AGM region by a two-step culture system, 1 full day earlier than in the yolk sac (Cumano et al., 1996). Results of temporal studies suggest that preliver intrabody hematopoiesis is more complex and potent than extraembryonic yolk sac blood formation, and such PAS-generated multipotent

progenitors may seed the yolk sac after the circulation is established at E8.5. The multipotential progenitors in the E8-9 PAS have also been tested in vivo for CFU-S and adult repopulating hematopoietic stem cell activity. In vivo, these cells do not repopulate lethally irradiated adult recipient mice either short or long term after transplantation, suggesting that they are not fully competent CFU-S or hematopoietic stem cells. However, they are good candidates for a prestem cell population.

Neonatal Repopulating Cells.

Recently, an in vivo repopulating multilineage hematopoietic progenitor has been described with the use of a transplantation model that is less stringent than that of the lethally irradiated adult recipient mouse. Neonatal mice from pregnant dams treated with busulfan (for myeloablation so as to enhance engraftment) were injected with yolk sac or PAS/AGM cells directly into the fetal liver at birth. E9 yolk sac cells could give rise to multilineage engraftment for long periods post-transplantation (Yoder et al., 1997a). Furthermore, when E9 CD34+c-kit+ cells from E9 yolk sac and E9 PAS/AGM were transplanted in this manner, both were capable of multilineage engraftment and secondary engraftment into adult lethally irradiated recipient mice (Yoder et al., 1997a). However, neither of these sorted populations could repopulate primary adult lethally irradiated recipients or engraft the hematopoietic system of the primary neonatal recipient to 100 percent. The authors concluded that the yolk sac contains 37-fold more neonatal repopulating cells than the PAS/AGM, suggesting that the yolk sac may be the source of definitive hematopoietic stem cells that colonize the fetal liver. Previous studies have suggested that the early stage yolk sac cells can indeed lead to long-term hematopoiesis when transferred into embryonic recipients, either transplacentally (Toles et al., 1989) or into the yolk sac cavity (Weissman I, 1978). These studies showed donor yolk sac-derived cells in the erythroid and lymphoid lineages, respectively, of fully developed adults. Taken together, these studies show that neonatal/fetal repopulating cells are long-lived multilineage progenitors but are not fully competent adult-type hematopoietic stem cells, suggesting that they lack a homing receptor necessary to migrate to adult bone marrow and the necessary high proliferative potential to fully repopulate.

Hematopoietic Stem Cells.

At the base of the adult hematopoietic hierarchy are hematopoietic stem cells of the adult bone marrow and fetal liver, as defined by the high level, multilineage, long-term repopulation of irradiated adult mouse recipients. The presence of differentiated hematopoietic cells and many restricted, multipotent, and in vivo immature hematopoietic progenitors in the PAS/AGM region and yolk sac of the early stage mouse embryo leads to the prediction (within the context of the adult hematopoietic hierarchy) that hematopoietic stem cells should be present from the onset of embryonic hematopoiesis at E7.5. In mouse embryos, however, the first adult repopulating hematopoietic stem cells are found only beginning at E10 in the AGM region sac (Medvinsky and Dzierzak, 1996; Muller et al., 1994) and at E11 in the yolk sac (Huang and Auerbach, 1993; Medvinsky and Dzierzak, 1996; Moore and Metcalf, 1970; Muller et al., 1994). Organ explant culture before in vivo transplantation has revealed that the AGM region is the first tissue to autonomously and exclusively generate hematopoietic stem cells (Medvinsky and Dzierzak, 1996). The yolk sac may subsequently be seeded by AGM-generated hematopoietic stem cells, or alternatively the yolk sac may be capable of autonomously generating its own hematopoietic stem cells. The localization of the first adult-type hematopoietic stem cells has been shown in the anterior AGM region at E10 by organ culture sub-dissection analysis (Medvinsky and Dzierzak, 1996). Although stem cell activity has not yet been tested, evidence for hematopoietic cell localization to other portions of the AGM exists. The ventral wall of the dorsal aorta contains hematopoietic clusters (Garcia-Porrero et al., 1995; Medvinsky et al., 1996; North et al., submitted; Wood et al., 1997); primordial germ cells from the gonad in a special coculture system are capable of hematopoietic differentiation (Rich, 1995); and hematopoietic stem cell marker Sca-1 is expressed on pro/mesonephros cells (Miles et al., 1997). Currently, attempts to further localize the first functional hematopoietic stem cells to the aorta, the aortic clusters, gonads, or pro/mesonephros are in progress. Nonetheless, the initiation of hematopoietic stem cells in the AGM at E10 in the mouse, together with data on the origins of the adult hematopoietic system in non-mammalian vertebrates, strongly suggests that the hematopoietic stem cells founding the mammalian adult hematopoietic hierarchy are AGM-derived.

Comparisons of Adult and Embryonic Hierarchies.
These data from the E7 to E10 mouse embryo showing (1) the earliest appearance of differentiated erythroid lineage cells and erythroid-myeloid progenitors in the yolk sac and multipotent erythroid-myeloid-lymphoid progenitors in the PAS, (2) the slightly later appearance of CFU-S in the yolk sac and AGM, and (3) the relatively late appearance of hematopoietic stem cells in the AGM strongly suggest that the embryonic hematopoietic hierarchy is constructed differently from that in the adult (Dzierzak and Medvinsky, 1995). The appearance of highly differentiated and mature blood cells before adult repopulating cells suggests a stepwise progression or acquisition of imma-

ture, undifferentiated phenotypes culminating in the generation of a pool of stem cells for the hematopoietic system. This stepwise progression occurs in a complete reversal to our notion of the adult hematopoietic hierarchy. Such a reversed embryonic hierarchy (Fig. 2.8) may be essential to the developing embryo to rapidly produce differentiating erythropoietic cells. Only afterwards does this lead to the generation of progenitors and hematopoietic stem cells that harbor or acquire properties consistent with multilineage potential, high proliferative potential and adhesion molecules necessary for providing hematopoietic activity throughout fetal and adult life.

In general, the sequential appearance of the differentiated lineages of hematopoietic cells and progenitors in the human embryo (Fig. 2.9) is consistent with what has been observed in the mouse embryo.

Figure 2.8. The embryonic/developmental hematopoietic hierarchy. The temporal appearance of hematopoietic cells in the mouse embryo is indicated and the reverse orientation of the cells compared with the appearance of differentiated, mature, and immature cells/progenitors in the adult suggest that the hematopoietic hierarchy in the embryo is unique. Although it has been thought that these embryonic activities derive from a hematopoietic stem cell, as in the adult, their appearance does not correspond sequentially to classical hierarchy. Thus, it is possible and likely that embryonic hematopoietic cells derive independently early in gestation (beginning at E7.5) and the adult hierarchy also develops independently but at later embryonic stages beginning at E10.5.

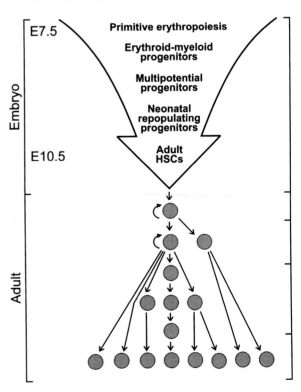

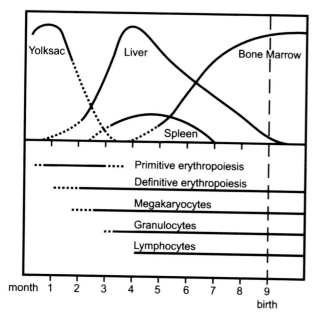

Figure 2.9. The temporal activity of hematopoietic sites and the appearance of the distinct hematopoietic lineages in the human embryo. These closely correspond to the sites and appearance of hematopoietic cells in the mouse embryo.

Hematopoietic progenitors, as assayed by in vitro cultures, have been seen in the yolk sac, as well as in the eviscerated embryo body (Huyhn et al., 1995; Peault, 1996). Studies of less differentiated human progenitors and hematopoietic stem cells await adaptation of suitable assays.

HEMATOPOIETIC MIGRATION AND COLONIZATION DURING DEVELOPMENT

For many years, it was widely accepted that the human adult hematopoietic system was derived from the first hematopoietic cells in the yolk sac that migrated and colonized the liver rudiment at fetal stages, and the bone marrow cavities at later stages (Moore and Owen, 1967). This notion led to controversy and speculation that mammalian hematopoietic development was fundamentally different from that of nonmammalian vertebrates. However, the recent observation, that the intrabody PAS/AGM region of the mouse embryo contains potent hematopoietic stem cells and progenitors, has shifted the paradigm of the origins of the mammalian hematopoietic system (Fig. 2.6). Our current understanding of mammalian developmental hematopoiesis now strongly suggests that the fundamental features of hematopoietic origin and colonization are conserved in all vertebrate classes. However, hematopoietic migration and colonization have been definitively shown only in nonmammalian vertebrates

by grafting experiments that allowed dynamics of marked cells from the yolk sac and intrabody region to be followed within the developing embryo. In mammals, in the absence of embryo grafting or single cell marking experiments, it is difficult to determine whether the intrabody PAS/AGM region is responsible for all adult hematopoietic cells (as in the avian species) or whether both this intraembryonic site and the extraembryonic yolk sac contribute to adult hematopoiesis (as in the amphibian species). An historical basis for these observations and experimental results of many developmental biologists and basic research scientists is provided here and compared with the available information from human embryos.

Vertebrate Models in the Study of Hematopoietic Colonization

Avian. Until 1965, the hematopoietic populations found in adult vertebrates were thought to originate intrinsically in tissues such as the liver, spleen, bone marrow, thymus, and bursa of Fabricius (found only in avian species). The results of experiments of Moore and Owen (Moore and Owen, 1967), in which parabiosed chick embryos were examined, suggested that these tissues were colonized by blood-borne cells. Definitive proof that the hematopoietic cells in adult tissues are extrinsically derived comes from the quail-chick and chick-chick chimera models. In these embryo grafting experiments, the precise colonization pattern of adult hematopoietic tissues at different stages of development and the sites of cell origin could be determined. Initial experiments focused on the colonization of the grafted thymus and spleen rudiments with embryonic hematopoietic precursors (Dieterlen-Lievre, 1975; Martin et al., 1978). Each tissue rudiment provided the stroma or microenvironment for the seeding and differentiation of extrinsic precursors. It was found that several short periodic waves of lymphoid precursors enter the thymus, whereas a single long wave of precursors enters and colonizes the bursa (Le Douarin et al., 1984). Although these studies did not show the site where the progenitors emerged, they suggested the emergence of progenitors at several discrete developmental times and limited times of receptivity of the tissue rudiments.

Similarly, the ontogeny of the multilineage hematopoietic system was examined in embryo grafting experiments in which yolk sac chimeras were made (reviewed in Dieterlen-Lievre and Le Douarin, 1993) and references therein) (Fig. 2.4A). The sites of de novo hematopoietic cell emergence were determined to be both the yolk sac and the intraembryonic region containing the dorsal aorta. However, only very briefly in early stages of embryogenesis do yolk sac-borne erythrocytes predominate in the blood. Subsequently, intrabody-borne erythrocytes rapidly predominate, and red cells from the yolk sac disappear completely by the hatching stage. At least two generations of hemoglobin-producing cells were observed; the first from yolk sac-derived cells and the second from yolk sac- as well as intrabody-derived cells. The role of the intrabody as the originating source of adult blood was confirmed in adult birds that were raised as yolk sac chimeras. During embryonic stages a small number of intrabody-derived cells can be found in the yolk sac, and likewise a small number of yolk sac-derived macrophage-like (microglial) cells can be found intraembryonically in the eye and in the brain (Pardanaud et al., 1987). These cellular exchanges are thought to occur through the circulation of small populations or subsets of hematopoietic cells that may serve a specialized, short-lived function.

Recently, another avian embryonic site, the allantois, was examined for hematopoietic potential (Caprioli et al., 1998). The prevascularized quail allantoic bud was grafted in the coelom of a chick host. Cells of both the hematopoietic and endothelial lineages were found in the bone marrow of the host, suggesting that the bone marrow is seeded by hemangioblasts and/or hematopoietic and endothelial precursors that arise in situ in the allantois. Hence, the allantois- as well as the paraaortic-derived cells of the avian embryo seed the adult blood system.

Amphibians. Waves of colonization are also observed in the amphibian model system. Embryo grafting experiments show that the larval liver is colonized by intrabody-derived hematopoietic cells (Chen and Turpen, 1995). The liver is thought to be seeded by intrabody cells that migrate through the interstitium because intrabody cells are not found in the circulation. Interstitial migration of cells is thought to be an efficient means of cell distribution within the amphibian embryo body and occurs even before the completion of the vascular network (Turpen et al., 1981). Near the time of metamorphosis, intrabody-derived hematopoietic clones fluctuate in their contribution to the liver and some ventral blood island-derived clones are detected (Bechtold et al., 1992; Chen and Turpen, 1995) but do not become the predominant cell type.

Mammalian. The first experiments probing hematopoietic migration and colonization in mammals were performed by Moore and Metcalf (Moore and Metcalf, 1970) in the E7 mouse conceptus. In these studies, whole mouse embryo bodies were cultured for 2 days in the presence and absence of a yolk sac. Then fetal livers were dissected and analyzed for granulocyte-macrophage colony formation. Only embryo bodies that retained their yolk sac were able to give rise to hematopoietic cells in the liver, suggesting that the yolk sac is the only embryonic site producing hematopoietic cells that colonize the liver rudiment. This experiment, as well as those examining the kinetics of CFC production in the yolk sac and fetal liver, suggests a dependence of early fetal hepatic hematopoiesis on an influx of exogenous yolk sac-derived cells (Johnson and Barker, 1985; Moore and Metcalf, 1970; Wong et al., 1986). Indeed Cudennec et al. (Cudennec et al., 1981) have shown that the fetal liver is populated by yolk sac-derived erythroid cells when these tissues are cultured adjacent to each other. However, these experiments were performed only on early tissues and did not take into account the multiple waves of hematopoietic cell generation and migration seen in the nonvertebrate species, particularly those that give rise to the adult hematopoietic system. Additionally, the analysis of the mouse embryo body for hematopoietic activity did not focus on the intraembryonic region surrounding the dorsal aortae, gonads, and pro/mesonephros.

At this time, it is still difficult to culture mouse embryos for the periods necessary to create chimeras and examine the origins of the adult hematopoietic system. As described in the previous section, current analyses probe the spatial and temporal genesis of the adult hematopoietic system in the mouse embryo using in vitro and in vivo hematopoietic assays. It appears that extensive cellular exchange, migration, and colonization is occurring. Owing to the high absolute numbers of CFU-S observed in the E10 (Medvinsky et al., 1996; Medvinsky et al., 1993), it appears that CFU-S generated in the AGM migrate to and colonize the fetal liver. This is supported by organ explant studies, in which the number of CFU-S in cultured AGM explants is greatly increased compared with CFU-S numbers in cultured yolk sacs (Medvinsky and Dzierzak, 1996). Thus, the AGM region appears to be the major generator of CFU-S that colonize the fetal liver.

Similarly, the major purveyor of the hematopoietic stem cells colonizing the fetal liver is thought to be the AGM region. The AGM region is the first tissue to initiate adult repopulation stem cell activity at E10, as shown by direct transplantation studies (Muller et al., 1994) and by transplantation after organ explant cultures (Medvinsky and Dzierzak, 1996). Hematopoietic stem cell activity follows shortly afterwards in the yolk sac at E11 and subsequently in the fetal liver. Taken together, waves of migrating hematopoietic cells colonize the fetal liver—first more differentiated progenitors beginning at E9 (28 somite pair stage) followed by immature progenitors such as

CFU-S and adult type hematopoietic stem cells at late E10. It is unclear by what means hematopoietic cells in the mouse embryo migrate between tissues. However, data on B lymphopoiesis suggest migration occurs through the circulation (Delassus and Cumano, 1996). Only after direct experimentation with the marking of single cells within a whole embryo can definitive conclusions be drawn on the migration of yolk sac or AGM-derived hematopoietic cells and the colonization of the fetal liver.

MOLECULAR ASPECTS OF PRIMITIVE AND DEFINITIVE HEMATOPOIESIS

The molecular basis for the generation of the hematopoietic system in the embryo and the adult is of great interest and importance. Two bodies of data on the cellular level predict some differences in the molecular programming of the primitive (embryonic) and definitive (adult) hematopoietic systems of mammals: (1) the description of distinct functional subsets of hematopoietic cells within each of the blood lineages of embryos as compared to adults (for example, the Vγ3-Vγ4 T-cell subset, primitive macrophages, and B1, a B-cell subset); and (2) the presence of at least two (yolk sac and PAS/AGM) spatially independent origins of hematopoiesis in the mammalian embryo. Not only do these findings suggest differential programs of maturation to functional blood cells, but also dissimilarity in the programs at the progenitor/stem cell level. Interestingly, these differences can also be implied for mesodermal precursors existing in the spatially separate microenvironments of the yolk sac (ventral mesoderm) compared with the intraembryonic PAS/AGM (lateral mesoderm).

On the macromolecular level, research with human and mouse cells has shown that chromosomal telomere length decreases as cells divide. It has been found that enriched adult human hematopoietic stem cells have shorter telomeres than fetal hematopoietic stem cells, suggesting that stem cells are not as dormant as once thought (Lansdorp, 1998). These molecular changes have not yet been found to directly affect hematopoietic function, but replication history may indeed have some influence on differentiation. On the micromolecular level of the individual gene, study on the human β-globin locus has revealed a strict developmental regulation of ε, γ, and β genes in embryonic and adult erythropoiesis (Grosveld et al., 1998). After more than 20 years of research, the regulation of this complex of genes is still a focus of intense investigation. Thus, an understanding of developmental genetic influences should help determine how the primitive and definitive hematopoietic repertoires of cells are generated.

The relatively recent application of gene targeting in ES cells for the generation of mutant mice has uncovered critical roles for numerous genes in the early stages of hematopoietic development. Thus, the availability of mouse genetic mutants, in which hematopoiesis is perturbed, is of enormous value in the study of the origins and genetic programming of the embryonic and adult hematopoietic systems. Gene targeting technology has revealed two types of hematopoietic defects: genes that profoundly affect primitive and definitive hematopoiesis, and genes that act differentially, having a profound effect on definitive but not primitive hematopoiesis. Several of the null or nonfunctional mutations that result in yolk sac anemia and early embryonic lethality at E9–10 suggest a critical requirement for yolk sac hematopoiesis (mainly primitive erythropoiesis) in the midgestational mouse embryo. The ability to generate chimeric mice with homozygous mutant ES cells has revealed additional roles for most of these genes at the later definitive developmental stages. In contrast, a number of hematopoietic mutant strains have been found to be defective only in definitive hematopoiesis, with embryonic lethality occurring at E11–16. Thus, the genetic programs of primitive and definitive hematopoiesis are overlapping but also divergent.

In general, both classes of hematopoietic mutants can be further grouped according to their suggested roles in (1) specification for the hematopoietic lineage, (2) progenitor/stem cell function, (3) migration, or (4) terminal differentiation. Included within these groups are genes that encode transcription factors, growth and differentiation factors, signaling molecules, and adhesion/homing molecules. A brief summary and grouping of several genes that play profound roles in primitive and/or definitive hematopoiesis follows (also see Table 2.2).

Genes Affecting Specification for the Hematopoietic Lineage

Hematopoietic specification occurs shortly after the onset of mesoderm formation. Molecular studies in nonmammalian vertebrates have greatly enriched our understanding of the numerous steps required in the specification of hematopoietic cells from mesoderm. The effects of various factors of the TGF-β superfamily and FGF family of genes in mesoderm and blood formation (Dale et al., 1992; Smith, 1993) have been revealed in the *Xenopus* embryo model. The TGF-β superfamily member, BMP-4, acts as a ventralizing molecule within the mesoderm (the region known to form hematopoietic cells). BMP-4 also induces the expression of Mix. 1, a gene that has been shown to

Table 2.2. Gene Specific Requirements in Hematopoiesis as Revealed by Targeted Mutagenesis in Mice

Affects	Gene	Phenotype	Reference
Hematopoietic specification	BMP-4	Lethal at gastrula stage, no mesodermal differentiation. Later embryonic lethal, decreased YS mesoderm formation and decreased YS erythropoiesis.	Winnier et al., 1995
	TGF-β1	Lethal at E9.5–11.5, defects in hematopoiesis and in vascular network formation.	Dickson et al., 1995
	flk-1	Lethal at E8.5–9.5, defective in YS blood island and vessel formation, severe decrease in YS hematopoietic progenitor cell number, and deficient in definitive hematopoiesis.	Shalaby et al., 1995; Shalaby et al., 1997
	SCL	Lethal at E9.5, deficient in primitive and definitive hematopoiesis and defective in angiogenesis.	Robb et al., 1995; Shivdasani et al., 1995; Porcher et al., 1996; Robb et al., 1996
Hematopoietic progenitor/stem cell formation/ function	GATA-2	Lethal at E10.5, severe FL anemia. Relatively normal YS hematopoiesis but decrease in CFU-C.	Tsai et al., 1994
	GATA-3	Lethal at E11.5, decrease in FL hematopoiesis and in CFU-S number but no T lymphoid cell formation	Pandolfi et al., 1995; Ting et al., 1996
	CBFα2 (AML 1) and CBFβ	Lethal at E11.5–12.5, complete absence of FL hematopoiesis and aortic hematopoietic clusters.	Okuda et al., 1996; Sasaki et al., 1996; Wang et al., 1996a; Wang et al., 1996b
	c-myb	Lethal at E5, FL anemia, granulocyte-macrophage progenitors and adult erythroid cell numbers decreased.	Mucenski et al., 1991; Lin et al., 1996b
	c-kit/SCF	Severe mutants lethal at E16, deficiencies in hematopoietic cells, CFU-S, primordial germ cells and melanocytes.	Reviewed in Bernstein, 1993; Witte, 1990
	LIF	Adults viable, decreased numbers of clonogenic progenitors and CFU-S.	Escary et al., 1993
	IL-6	Adults viable, decrease in CFU-S numbers and potency of hematopoietic stem cells.	Bernad et al. 1994
	flk2/flt3	Adults viable, defects in proliferative potential of immature hematopoietic progenitors.	Mackarehtschian et al., 1995
Migration	β1-integrin	Preimplantation lethal. Chimeras show normal YS and circulating blood but no hematopoietic cells in FL, thymus, or bone marrow.	Fassler and Meyer, 1995; Stephens et al., 1995; Hirsch et al., 1996
	α4-integrin	Early embryonic lethal. Chimeras show defects in B and T cell homing to adult but not fetal hematopoietic sites.	Arroyo et al., 1996
Terminal differentiation (erythroid)	GATA-1	Lethal at E10, severe YS anemia, defect localized to proerythroblast.	Pevny et al., 1991; Fujiwara et al., 1996
	Jak2	Lethal at E12.5, normal primitive erythropoiesis but absence of FL definitive erythropoiesis, BFU-E and CFU-E.	Neubauer et al., 1998; Parganas et al., 1998
	EKLF	Lethal at E14-15, severe FL anemia. FL BFU-E and CFU-E numbers are normal, but these cells do not mature.	Nuez et al., 1995; Perkins et al., 1995
	EPO/EPOR	Lethal at E14–16, severe FL anemia. FL contains BFU-E and CFU-E, but progenitor number is decreased.	Lin et al., 1996a; Wu et al., 1995

induce hematopoiesis in the *Xenopus* animal cap assay (Mead et al., 1996; Turpen et al., 1997). In chicken embryos, overexpression of BMP-4 has been found to influence mesodermal subtype formation (Tonegawa et al., 1997). Thus, graded expression patterns of mesoderm specific genes probably define unique subsets of mesoderm (Stennard and Gurdon, 1997). Ectopic injection of RNA encoding the SCL hemato-poietic transcription factor gene, which is known to play a role in mouse embryonic hematopoiesis (as noted later), specifies normally nonhematopoietic pronephric mesoderm to become hematopoietic. Thus, graded expression of hematopoietic specification factors may also define the normal spatial borders of hematopoiesis in the different mesodermally derived regions of the embryo.

Because of the results observed in nonmammalian vertebrates, BMP-4 is expected to play a role in early stages of mouse hematopoiesis. This factor was shown to induce the in vitro hematopoietic differentiation of ES cells (Johansson and Wiles, 1995). Indeed, gene targeting supports a role for BMP-4 in hematopoietic specification in mouse embryos. Mouse embryos deficient for BMP-4 usually die at the time of gastrulation, with little or no mesodermal differentiation (Winnier et al., 1995). The few BMP-4-deficient embryos that do survive to slightly later ontogenic stages show profound decreases in mesoderm formation and erythropoiesis in the yolk sac, indicating a strict requirement for BMP-4 in the formation of the ventral-most mesoderm. To determine whether hematopoietic potential exists throughout the mouse mesoderm, in vitro CFU-C assays with BMP-4 have been performed on various portions of the epiblast (Kanatsu and Nishikawa, 1996). BMP-4 influenced hematopoietic cell formation from the presumptive anterior head fold, normally a nonhematopoietic portion of the mouse embryo. Thus, the expression pattern of BMP-4 is important in hematopoietic specification.

Subsequent to, and perhaps overlapping with, early mesodermal induction events, other growth factors, receptors, and transcription factors are critical to hematopoietic specification. TGF-β1 is one of the crucial factors and flk-1 one of the crucial receptors. Within the yolk sac blood islands, there is a juxtaposition of cells of the vascular system and those of the hematopoietic system (His, 1990). This close association of cells, together with shared cell surface markers (Garcia-Porrero et al., 1998; Newman et al., 1990; North et al., submitted; Young et al., 1995), has led many investigators to the hypothesis of a common progenitor, the hemangioblast. Gene targeting experiments have shown a clear requirement for these genes in the formation of both of these tissues in the yolk sac. In the TGF-β1 homozygous null con-

dition, perinatal lethality occurs in 50 percent of the embryos between E9.5 and E11.5 (Dickson et al., 1995). The initial differentiation of endothelial cells from mesoderm occurs, but there is no organization of these cells into a vascular network. Defects in yolk sac vasculogenesis and hematopoiesis appear to be responsible for embryonic death, although the severity of the endothelial and hematopoietic cell defects do not always correlate. Thus, the effects of TGF-β1 may be indirect, and the examination of TGF-β1 chimeric mice will determine whether the effect is cell autonomous and whether this factor similarly influences definitive hematopoiesis and the adult vascular network.

Mouse embryos deficient in the flk-1 receptor tyrosine kinase exhibit more severe and consistent defects than TGF-β1-deficient embryos. All flk-1-deficient embryos die between E8.5 and E9.5 (Shalaby et al., 1995). They are defective in the production of yolk sac blood islands and vessel formation, and the numbers of hematopoietic progenitors are dramatically reduced. A LacZ marker gene inserted in the flk-1 gene allowed tracking of endothelial and hematopoietic cell formation in embryos. Embryos lacking functional flk-1 expressed the LacZ marker appropriately in the developing mesoderm. However, these expressing cells accumulated in the amnion instead of in the areas of blood island formation, suggesting the requirement for flk-1 as early as the formation and/or migration of the yolk sac mesodermal cells. Studies on flk-1 null ES chimeric adults have shown a similar requirement for flk-1 in the formation of the adult hematopoietic system (Shalaby et al., 1997). The gene for vascular endothelial growth factor (VEGF) has also been mutated. The generation of chimeric embryos with VEGF +/− ES cells results in embryonic lethality at E11, defective vasculogenesis, and a substantially reduced number of yolk sac red blood cells (Carmeliet et al., 1996; Ferrara et al., 1996). Recently VEGF, the ligand for flk-1, has been reported to direct the in vitro differentiation of ES cells to both endothelial and hematopoietic lineages (Choi et al., 1998). Although a putative hemangioblast has been isolated from ES cells, it is not yet determined whether flk-1 acts at the level of the hemangioblast or the two separate differentiated lineages derived from this putative precursor.

The SCL gene is known to play a pivotal role in the production of all hematopoietic cells in the embryo as shown by gene targeting to the germline (Robb et al., 1995; Shivdasani et al., 1995). In addition, it is required for adult hematopoiesis as shown by the generation of SCL −/− ES cell chimeric mice (Porcher et al., 1996; Robb et al., 1996). The SCL gene was initially isolated from a chromosomal translocation in a human T-leukemic cell line, thus predicting some role for it in hematopoiesis. Unlike TGF-β1 and flk-1, SCL is not required for all endothelial cell and vascular formation; yolk sac capillaries are initiated but vitelline vessel formation is blocked and subsequent angiogenesis in the yolk sac is defective. A transgenic rescue of the hematopoietic defects in SCL –/– embryos confirms that SCL is necessary for embryonic angiogenesis (Visvader et al., 1998). Mutation of the LMO2 gene also results in an identical phenotype to SCL –/– embryos (Warren et al., 1994 and Yamada et al., 1998). It has been found that the LMO2 protein heterodimerizes, with the SCL protein forming a transcriptional regulatory complex.

Genes Affecting Definitive Hematopoietic Progenitor/Stem Cell Formation/Function

The multifocal distribution of blood islands within the yolk sac suggests that primitive hematopoiesis is initiated from numerous precursors. The individual foci appear to have a low proliferative potential, contributing to the relatively small pool of circulating erythrocytes in the embryo. In contrast, in the adult, large numbers of hematopoietic cells are produced from a relatively small number of definitive hematopoietic progenitors (Berger and Sturm, 1996) that possess high proliferative potential compared with yolk sac (Moore and Metcalf, 1970). Thus, genes involved in the proliferative/clonogenic potential of hematopoietic progenitors should be readily apparent in gene-targeted mutant embryos and result in defective fetal liver but relatively normal yolk sac hematopoiesis. In addition, it can be predicted that genes involved in the generation, maintenance, or self-renewal of definitive hematopoietic progenitors/stem cells may also yield this phenotype. Examples of genes in this category, as determined by gene targeting studies, are the transcription factors GATA-2, GATA-3, core binding factor (CBF) and myb, and the receptor tyrosine kinase c-kit and its ligand steel factor (SCF).

GATA-2 is a member of GATA transcription factor family of genes. The GATA factors are highly conserved among all vertebrate species. Along with GATA-1 and GATA-3, studies in mammalian cell lines have shown that GATA-2 plays a role in transcriptional regulation within the hematopoietic system (Jippo et al., 1996; Labbaye et al., 1995). More specifically, GATA-2 is thought to act in hematopoietic stem cells and progenitors, owing to its specific expression pattern. Gene targeting of the GATA-2 locus in ES cells results in a complete deficiency of this

transcription factor in vivo, which leads to death in homozygous mutant embryos beginning at E10.5 (Tsai et al., 1994). The overwhelming phenotypic characteristic of such embryos is severe fetal liver anemia. Yolk sac erythropoiesis appears relatively normal, with embryonic erythrocytes slightly reduced in number. However, in vitro clonogenic progenitors (CFU-Cs) within the yolk sac are decreased 100-fold. When chimeric mice are generated with GATA-2 –/– ES cells, no hematopoietic contribution of these cells is observed in fetal liver or in the adult hematopoietic system. Thus, GATA-2 is strictly required for definitive hematopoiesis but not embryonic erythropoiesis, suggesting the defect occurs at the level of the clonogenic potential hematopoietic progenitors.

Similarly, homozygous deficiency for GATA-3 results in embryonic lethality in midgestation beginning at E11 (Pandolfi et al., 1995) and severe aberration in fetal liver hematopoiesis. However, CFU-C numbers are decreased only by a factor of 10 in fetal liver, whereas yolk sac CFU-C numbers are normal. Studies in which GATA-3 –/– ES cells were used to generate chimeric mice show that no T-lineage cells, but some differentiated myeloid lineage cells, are derived from the GATA-3 null cells (Ting et al., 1996). Thus, GATA-3 is required for the production of T-lymphoid lineage cells. The low level contribution of the GATA-3 null cells to the myeloid lineage suggests a role for GATA-3 in the proliferative potential of progenitors.

The CBF transcription factor genes are the most frequent targets of chromosomal rearrangements in human leukemias and were thus suggested to function in the hematopoietic system. CBFα2 and CBFβ form a heterodimeric factor that interacts through the CBFα2 DNA binding domain to bind the core enhancer motif present in a number of hematopoietic specific genes. To test for the function of the CBF transcription factors in normal hematopoiesis, CBFα2 (AML 1) and CBFβ targeted mutations were generated in ES cells. Homozygous mutant embryos for either CBFα2 or CBFβ genes (Okuda et al., 1996; Sasaki et al., 1996; Wang et al., 1996a; Wang et al., 1996b) were subject to embryonic lethality after E11.5, and a complete absence of fetal liver-derived hematopoiesis was found. Yolk sac vessels appear normal in these embryos, with only nucleated large primitive erythrocytes found. Hematopoietic progenitors in the E11.5 fetal liver and E10.5 yolk sac were absent. Mouse chimeras produced with CBFα2 –/– ES cells showed no contribution of the deficient cells to adult hematopoiesis. Hence, this factor appears to act at the level of proliferation, generation, or maintenance of definitive hematopoietic progenitor and/or stem cells. Recently, a LacZ gene has been inserted into the CBFα2 locus (North et al., in press). LacZ-positive hematopoietic clusters and endothelial cells are found in the dorsal aorta and vitelline artery. LacZ-positive intraaortic clusters are absent in CBFα2-deficient embryos, indicating a requirement for this transcription factor in the formation of these hematopoietic cells.

C-myb gene is a proto-oncogene transcription factor that is known to regulate transcription of a number of hematopoietic-specific genes. It defines immature hematopoietic cells and is downregulated as hematopoietic cells differentiate. Targeted disruption of the c-myb gene resulted in the first description of a gene affecting definitive fetal liver hematopoiesis, but not embryonic yolk sac hematopoiesis. Homozygous mutant embryos die at E15, most likely from fetal liver anemia that becomes apparent at E13 (Mucenski et al., 1991). Multipotential granulocyte-macrophage progenitors and adult erythrocytes are decreased (Lin et al., 1996b), but other hematopoietic lineages and adult chimeric mice must be examined to determine whether a progenitor or stem cell is affected.

Many natural mutations for the receptor tyrosine kinase c-kit, and its ligand steel factor (SCF) have been found in mice. W and Sl strains of mice (Bernstein, 1993; Witte, 1990) exhibit deficiencies in hematopoiesis, primordial germ cells, and melanocytes; and the most severe mutations result in embryonic lethality beginning at E16. Yolk sac erythropoiesis is not affected, but CFU-S progenitors and mast cells are absent. SCF has been shown to act as a proliferative (Ogawa et al., 1988; Okada et al., 1991) or antiapoptotic (Hassan and Zander, 1996) agent in hematopoietic progenitors and CFU-S. Thus, c-kit/SCF signaling is required for normal definitive hematopoiesis and may play a role in clonogenicity of early hematopoietic progenitors or, as in primordial germ cells and melanocytes, in progenitor migration.

The mouse adult hematopoietic system can arise from a single hematopoietic stem cell (Lemischka et al., 1986). Thus the adult hematopoietic system does not require the complete function of all hematopoietic stem/progenitors simultaneously, and a balance between self-renewal and proliferation of these cells must be maintained. Mice lacking growth factors IL-6 or LIF or the receptor tyrosine kinase flk2/flt3 fall into this group in which definitive hematopoietic stem/progenitor cell function is compromised. Unlike GATA-2, GATA-3, CBF, c-myb, and c-kit, these mutations in the homozygous condition do not result in embryonic lethality or the absence of definitive hematopoietic cells. Instead, in adult mutant mice, a subtle phenotype is observed. LIF-deficient adults have decreased numbers of clonogenic prog-enitors, including CFU-S progenitors (Escary et al., 1993). It is not yet known whether hematopoietic stem cell numbers are affected. In IL-6-deficient animals, a decrease in both CFU-S progenitor number and the potency of hematopoietic stem cells is observed (Bernad et al., 1994). These results suggest that LIF is required in the microenvironment as a maintenance factor, and IL-6 plays a role in the maintenance of self-renewal. In contrast, a deficiency of flk2/flt3 (which is expressed on a subset of hematopoietic stem cells) does not affect CFU-S or pre-CFU-S numbers (Mackarehtschian et al., 1995). Instead, defects in myeloid and lymphoid reconstitution are revealed in transplantation experiments, suggesting effects on the proliferative potential of immature hematopoietic progenitors.

Genes Affecting Hematopoietic Cell Migration

In the adult mouse, integrins have been found to play a role in the differentiation and migration of hematopoietic cells. β1 integrin-specific polyclonal antibodies have been found to block the formation of CFU-S, presumably by blocking the adhesion of these progenitors to the spleen stroma (Williams et al., 1991). Likewise, α4 integrin acts at the level of adhesion of hematopoietic progenitors to the bone marrow (Arroyo et al., 1996). Subsequent to the generation of hematopoietic cells in the extraembryonic and intraembryonic sites during early to midgestation, these cells colonize the secondary hematopoietic territories: fetal liver, spleen, thymus, and bone marrow. There is convincing evidence that integrins play an important role in the embryo in the colonization of secondary hematopoietic territories.

Mouse embryos lacking β1 integrin die during preimplantation stages of gestation (Fassler and Meyer, 1995; Stephens et al., 1995); thus chimeric embryos with β1 integrin −/− ES cells were generated to examine its role during later stages of hematopoietic ontogeny (Hirsch et al., 1996). Although the yolk sac was found to contain normal numbers of hematopoietic cells derived from the β1 integrin −/− ES cells, the fetal liver did not contain any β1 integrin-deficient hematopoietic cells. The clonogenic potential of the yolk sac hematopoietic cells was normal, and such cells were found in the circulation of embryos until E15. These results strongly suggest that β1 integrin is required for the successful migration of hematopoietic cells to the fetal liver. Additionally, and in accordance with a role for β1 integrin in adult hematopoietic cell migration, no β1 integrin-deficient hematopoietic cells were found in the thymus, bone marrow, or blood of chimeric mice.

Gene targeting has also been performed with the α4 integrin gene. Again, an early embryonic lethal phenotype was found (Arroyo et al., 1996). The chimeric studies with these deficient ES cells show a defect in the homing of B and T lymphocytes to adult hematopoietic territories, but not to the fetal liver. Monocytes and natural killer cells develop normally; therefore, not all hematopoietic cells are affected. Studies of the role of $\alpha 4$ integrin in early stage yolk sac and fetal liver hematopoiesis are needed.

Genes Affecting Lineage Specificity and Terminal Differentiation

Several genes examined in gene targeting experiments appear to be involved at the point of lineage commitment in the differentiating hematopoietic system or in the lineage-specific differentiation program. Briefly, for lymphoid cells, the Ikaros gene is required for specification to this lineage (other genes affecting lymphoid and myeloid differentiation are reviewed in Singh, 1996). In Ikaros-deficient mice, both fetal T and B cells are absent (Wang et al., 1996). However, whereas B cells remain absent in the adult, after birth T-cell precursors appear and undergo aberrant differentiation into CD4+ T cells. Also, natural killer cells, some $\gamma\delta$ T cells, and thymic dendritic cells are also affected, suggesting different requirements for Ikaros in fetal and adult lymphoid progenitors.

Many examples of essential genes in the erythroid lineage differentiation program have been identified by gene targeting experiments. One of the most essential erythroid-specific transcription factors is GATA-1 (Fujiwara et al., 1996; Pevny et al., 1991). Embryos mutant for GATA-1 exhibit an embryonic lethal phenotype at about E10 from severe yolk sac anemia. No mature erythrocytes are found in the vessels of the embryo or yolk sac. Through in vitro culture experiments, the defect has been localized to the proerythroblast, which is incapable of differentiating to mature erythroid cells. As demonstrated by ES cell chimera experiments, this transcription factor is also required for the differentiation of proerythroblasts to definitive erythrocytes in the fetal liver and the adult.

Jak2 is a member of the Janus kinase family of genes that play an important role in signal transduction through hematopoietic cell cytokine receptors (Ihle and Kerr, 1995). Targeted disruption of the Jak2 gene results in embryonic lethality at E12.5 and a surprising absence of definitive erythropoiesis (Neubauer et al., 1998; Parganas et al., 1998). Primitive erythropoiesis is normal, but fetal liver lacks any detectable BFU-E or CFU-E, suggesting a requirement for Jak2 in the generation or function of progenitors. Multipotential hematopoietic cells and adult transplantable hematopoietic stem cells are present in the fetal liver, indicating that Jak2 defines an essential and early developmental checkpoint in definitive erythropoiesis and is required for signaling through a variety of cytokine receptors.

Similar to the general phenotype of Jak2 mutant embryos, mutations of the EKLF transcription factor gene (Nuez et al., 1995; Perkins et al., 1995), erythropoietin gene, or erythropoietin receptor gene (Lin et al., 1996a; Wu et al., 1995) result in embryonic lethality owing to a lack of definitive erythropoiesis. Fatal anemia occurs during the switch to adult erythropoiesis in the fetal liver at around E14–16; this is slightly later than the lethal phenotype observed in the Jak2 mutants. Yolk sac hematopoiesis appears to be normal, and does not strictly require EKLF, EPO, or the EPOR. In contrast to the requirement for Jak2 in the generation of BFU-E and CFU-E, these progenitors are normal in EKLF-deficient fetal livers. EPO- and EPOR-deficient fetal livers contain BFU-E and CFU-E, but their numbers are decreased. These results show that EKLF is essential for the final steps of definitive erthropoiesis in the fetal liver and that EPO and EPOR are critical in the survival of the late CFU-E progenitors, their irreversible differentiation, or both in the fetal liver.

A Molecular Hierarchy in Developmental Hematopoiesis?

Gene targeting studies in the mouse have indicated that molecular regulation of hematopoiesis during ontogeny is complex. A growing number of genes are emerging as essential for development of the hematopoietic lineage: genes involved in hematopoietic specification, in the generation of primitive and definitive hematopoietic progenitors, in the migration of hematopoietic cells to hematopoietic territories, and in specific lineage commitment and differentiation. Although these genes can be generally classed according to important developmental checkpoints, a number of biological functions can be directed by single lineage specific factors in different cells and during different stages of ontogeny. Additionally, it is important to be aware that although a specific gene product may be interpreted to act in a common progenitor, it may also function independently downstream in each lineage.

The hierarchical organization of the hematopoietic system on the cellular level suggests hierarchical relationships on the molecular level. Clearly, the molecular programs of primitive and definitive hematopoietic cells are overlapping in their requirements for some mesodermal inducing genes, hematopoietic specification genes, and even genes for terminal differentiation. Although yolk sac hematopoiesis does not require the establishment of self-renewing, long-term repopulating hematopoietic stem cells, the adult hematopoietic system does. Thus, gene-targeting experiments reveal that the definitive hematopoietic program is more complex, requiring many more genes to promote the establishment of the complete adult hierarchy of hematopoietic cells, which possess features such as high proliferative potential and self-renewing activity. It is tempting to speculate that these differences in the primitive and definitive molecular programs directing hematopoiesis may have a basis in the two anatomically separate and independent sites of hematopoietic generation in the embryo: the yolk sac and the PAS/AGM. These tissues should be examined in the mutants created by gene targeting, and attempts should be made to identify novel molecules involved in the definitive hematopoietic program by differential cloning methods.

Implications of Embryonic Hematopoiesis for Potential Clinical Application in Human Blood-Related Therapies

During the last few years, significant progress has been made in the field of developmental hematopoiesis. The previous dogma concerning the origins of the adult hematopoietic system in the yolk sac and subsequent colonization of the fetal liver and adult bone marrow by yolk sac-generated cells has given way to a new understanding of multiple and independent sites of hematopoietic generation in the early and midgestation mammalian embryo. The initiation of the first multipotential hematopoietic progenitors and adult-type hematopoietic stem cells is now known to occur in the intraembryonic PAS/AGM. Taken together with the high number of these cells and the kinetics of initiation before their appearance in the yolk sac and fetal liver, these data suggest that the PAS/AGM region is the major source of the definitive hematopoietic system of the adult.

Novel Hematopoietic Signaling Molecules. Studies in neonatal and adult mouse transplantation models have suggested that some hematopoietic progenitors and stem cells found in the mouse conceptus can bypass certain ontogenic stages and secondary hematopoietic territories (Dzierzak et al., 1998). For example, E9 yolk sac and PAS hematopoietic progenitors appear to require a sojourn through the fetal liver, because these cells can multilineage repopulate the adult hematopoietic system when transplanted into a neonatal recipient, but not an adult recipient (Yoder et al., 1997a). In contrast, E10 AGM cells do not require exposure to the fetal liver, because they can fully repopulate an adult recipient (Medvinsky and Dzierzak, 1996; Muller et al., 1994). Thus, understanding of the incremental

maturation of hematopoietic-specified cells to definitive adult hematopoietic cells in both the primary and secondary hematopoietic territories of developing mouse embryos will give insight into the best types of hematopoietic cells for human transplantations in the clinical setting. The ability to create mouse mutants by gene targeting technology has expanded our knowledge of some of the genes required at developmental checkpoints in hematopoiesis. Further studies into the embryonic localization and specific microenvironments required for hematopoietic progenitor/stem cells should allow the isolation of novel molecules that may be useful in the manipulation of human hematopoietic cells in a clinical setting. A report has already described the cloning of a phosphotase, KG1 from human AGM CD34+ hematopoietic cells (Labastie et al., 1998). Such subtractive cloning strategies hold promise for the isolation of novel inducing, expansion, and maintenance factors for hematopoietic progenitor/stem cells.

Reprogramming. In the mouse it is known that fetal liver cells repopulate lethally irradiated adult recipients more effectively than adult bone marrow (Harrison et al., 1997; Pawliuk et al., 1996). Controversy already exists concerning the use of human cord blood, fetal liver cells or adult bone marrow cells in various transplantation scenarios (Broxmeyer et al., 1992; Gluckman, 1995). Both the quality and quantity of hematopoietic progenitors and stem cells must be understood to maximize clinical strategies. In this context, it is worth considering whether transplantation of embryonic or fetal hematopoietic progenitors/stem cells will allow the more complete and robust generation of the hematopoietic system in humans. An in vitro culture system suggests that although mouse fetal hematopoietic stem cells can produce a specific T-cell subset important in the skin, adult stem cells cannot (Ikuta et al., 1990). Thus, restrictions in hematopoietic stem cell programming appear to occur with developmental age.

The subject of reprogramming somatic cells has been an important focus of research for many years. For example, although it has been possible to produce mice from cultured pluripotential ES cells (cells from E3.5 mouse blastocysts), it has been generally thought that somatic cells become restricted in potency and thus cannot contribute to the germline. However, it has now been shown that somatic cells of sheep and mice can be reprogrammed and contribute to the germline (Wakayama et al., 1998; Wilmut et al., 1997). A recent report has more specifically investigated the mechanism of developmental genetic switches in successive generations of hematopoietic stem cells. Enriched murine adult bone marrow hematopoietic stem cells containing a human β-globin locus transgene were injected into mouse blastocysts (Geiger et al., 1998). Chimeric embryos were examined and expression of the human ε- and γ-globin transgenes was found in the E10.5 yolk sac and AGM, and in the E11.5 and E12.5 yolk sac and fetal liver, suggesting that the embryonic and fetal microenvironments can reprogram adult hematopoietic stem cells to express embryonic and fetal genes. Thus, it may be possible to reprogram hematopoietic stem cells to an advantageous earlier ontogenic stage. Because a decrease in telomere length appears to correlate with proliferative history of hematopoietic stem cells in the human, however, (Lansdorp, 1998), it will be important to examine whether such cells retain a high proliferative capacity in a transplantation scenario.

In Vitro Production of Transplantable Hematopoietic Stem Cells.
In mammalian developmental biology, mouse ES cells have long provided a useful in vitro culture system for studying the differentiation of hematopoietic, endothelial, muscle, and neuronal cell lineages. This model system provides access to developmentally early populations of cells with relatively normal functional characteristics. In vitro hematopoietic differentiation of ES cells increased our understanding of early genetic events in the onset of primitive and definitive blood development and has provided an easily accessible source of hematopoietic progenitors for analysis of growth factor requirements and gene expression patterns (Keller, 1995; Muller and Dzierzak, 1993). In many aspects of cellular and molecular hematopoietic development, ES cell hematopoietic differentiation cultures mimic in vivo development of the hematopoietic system, particularly at the early yolk sac stage. All lineages of hematopoietic cells can be produced: erythroid, myeloid, and lymphoid. Also, a common precursor for primitive and definitive hematopoiesis and a common precursor for endothelial and hematopoietic lineages have been described in such cultures. However, some limitations of the ES cell culture system are revealed when such cells are tested in in vivo transplantation experiments for the production of CFU-S and long-term multilineage repopulation. Although low level, long-term multilineage progenitors have been found after in vivo neonatal transplantation of differentiated ES cells (Hole et al., 1996; Muller and Dzierzak, 1993), neither CFU-S nor adult-type hematopoietic stem cells have been found when injected into lethally irradiated adult recipients (Muller and Dzierzak, 1993). These results, together with the strong evidence for the PAS/AGM region as the source of the adult hematopoietic system, suggest that ES cultures lack some of the elements necessary for definitive hematopoietic progenitor and stem cell production. It is possible that the PAS/AGM region provides a spatial microenvironment for the generation of these adult cell types. Thus, future goals are directed toward the introduction of ES cells into PAS/AGM microenvironments. This work, in combination with the recent isolation of human ES cells (Shamblott et al., 1998), holds promise for the in vitro isolation, growth, and expansion of human transplantable hematopoietic stem cells for clinical use.

Gene Therapy for Human Blood-Related Syndromes.
The long-term goals of most hematopoietic research are directed toward therapies of human blood-related genetic diseases, leukemias, and viral infections. Advances in this field have been slow and have relied on small improvements in cell isolation techniques, growth factor cocktail combinations, retroviral vectors, and stromal cell lines (Bodine, 1998; van Hennik et al., 1998). The emerging thought is that a better understanding of stem cell biology and development may lead to better approaches for stem cell manipulation. As hematopoietic stem cells are first generated in limited numbers in the intrabody AGM region of the mouse, examination of the specific microenvironment and precursors to these stem cells, as described throughout this chapter, may yield insight into how hematopoietic stem cells may be expanded without undergoing differentiation. Cells of the AGM microenvironment may be useful in co-culture with adult hematopoietic stem cells for expansion, and in co-culture with ES cells to induce the production of adult transplantable hematopoietic stem cells. Thus, a merging of developmental aspects of hematopoiesis with genetic manipulation may indeed lead to a new paradigm in gene therapy for efficient clinical applications.

References

Arroyo, AG, Yang, JT, Rayburn, H, and Hynes, RO. (1996). Differential requirements for alpha4 integrins during fetal and adult hematopoiesis. *Cell* 85: 997–1008.

Baldwin, HS, Shen, HM, Yan, HC et al. (1994). Platelet endothelial cell adhesion molecule-1 (PECAM-1/CD31): Alternatively spliced, functionally distinct isoforms expressed during mammalian cardiovascular development. *Development* 120: 2539–2553.

Beaupain, D, Martin, C, and Dieterlen-Lievre, F. (1979). Are developmental hemoglobin changes related to the origin of stem cells and site of erythropoiesis? *Blood* 53: 212–225.

Bechtold, TE, Smith, PB, and Turpen, JB. (1992). Differential stem cell contributions to thymocyte succession during development of *Xenopus laevis*. *J. Immunol.* 148: 2975–2982.

Berger, CN and Sturm, KS. (1996). Estimation of the number of hematopoietic precursor cells during fetal mouse development by covariance analysis. *Blood* 88: 2502–2509.

Bernad, A, Kopf, M, Kulbacki, R et al. (1994). Interleukin-6 is required in vivo for the regulation of stem cells and committed progenitors of the hematopoietic system. *Immunity* 1: 725–731.

Bernstein, A. (1993). Receptor tyrosine kinases and the control of hematopoiesis. *Semin. Dev. Biol.* 4: 351–358.

Bodine, DM. (1998). Stem-cell gene therapy: problems and solutions. The 2nd Conference on Stem Cell Gene Therapy: Biology and Technology, Rosario Resort, Orcas Island, WA, USA, 31 March-2 June 1998. *Trends Genet.* 14: 346–347.

Bonifer, C, Faust, N, Geiger, H, and Muller, A. (1998). Developmental changes in the differentiation capacity of haematopoietic stem cell. *Immunol. Today* 19: 236–241.

Broxmeyer, HE, Hangoc, G, Cooper, S et al. (1992). Growth characteristics and expansion of human umbilical cord blood and estimation of its potential for transplantation in adults. *Proc. Natl. Acad. Sci. U. S. A.* 89: 4109–4113.

Bruijn, MD. (1997). Macrophage progenitor cells in mouse bone marrow. In W. van Ewijk, ed. *Immunology.* Rotterdam: Erasmus University.

Caprioli, A, Jaffredo, T, Gautier, R et al. (1998). Blood-borne seeding by hematopoietic and endothelial precursors from the allantois. *Proc. Natl. Acad. Sci. U. S. A.* 95: 1641–1646.

Carmeliet, P, Ferreira, V, Breier, G et al. (1996). Abnormal blood vessel development and lethality in embryos lacking a single VEGF allele. *Nature* 380: 435–439.

Chen, XD and Turpen, JB. (1995). Intraembryonic origin of hepatic hematopoiesis in *Xenopus laevis*. *J. Immunol.* 154: 2557–2567.

Choi, K, Kennedy, M, Kazarov, A et al. (1998). A common precursor for hematopoietic and endothelial cells. *Development* 125: 725–732.

Conlon, F and Beddington, R. (1995). Mouse gastrulation from a frog's perspective. *Semin. in Develop. Biol.* 6: 249–256.

Cormier, F. and Dieterlen-Lievre, F. (1988). The wall of the chick embryo aorta harbours M-CFC, G-CFC, GM-CFC and BFU-E. *Development* 102: 279–285.

Cudennec, CA, Thiery, JP, and Le Douarin, NM. (1981). In vitro induction of adult erythropoiesis in early mouse yolk sac. *Proc. Natl. Acad. Sci. U. S. A.* 78: 2412–2416.

Cumano, A, Dieterlen-Lievre, F, and Godin, I. (1996). Lymphoid potential, probed before circulation in mouse, is restricted to caudal intraembryonic splanchnopleura. *Cell* 86: 907–916.

Cumano, A, Furlonger, O, and Paige, CJ. (1993). Differentiation and characterization of B-cell precursors detected in the yolk sac and embryo body of embryos beginning at the 10- to 12-somite stage. *Proc. Natl. Acad. Sci. U. S. A.* 90: 6429–6433.

Dale, L, Howes, G, Price, BM, and Smith, JC. (1992). Bone morphogenetic protein 4: A ventralizing factor in early Xenopus development. *Development* 115: 573–585.

Dale, L, Smith, JC, and Slack, JM. (1985). Mesoderm induction in *Xenopus laevis*: A quantitative study using a cell lineage label and tissue-specific antibodies. *J. Embryol. Exp. Morphol.* 89: 289–312.

Delassus, S and Cumano, A. (1996). Circulation of hematopoietic progenitors in the mouse embryo. *Immunity* 4: 97–106.

Dickson, MC, Martin, JS, Cousins, FM et al. (1995). Defective haematopoiesis and vasculogenesis in transforming growth factor-beta 1 knock out mice. *Development* 121: 1845–1854.

Dieterlen-Lievre, F. (1975). On the origin of haemopoietic stem cells in the avian embryo: An experimental approach. *J. Embryol. Exp. Morphol.* 33: 607–619.

Dieterlen-Lievre, F and Le Douarin, NM. (1993). Developmental rules in the hematopoietic and immune systems of birds: How general are they? *Semin. Dev. Biol.* 4: 325–332.

Dieterlen-Lievre, F and Martin, C. (1981). Diffuse intraembryonic hemopoiesis in normal and chimeric avian development. *Dev. Biol.* 88: 180–191.

Dzierzak, E, Muller, A, Sinclair, A et al. (1995). Hematopoietic stem cell development in the mouse embryo. In Stamatoyannopoulos, G, editor. *Molecular biology of hemoglobin switching.* Andover: Intercept.

Dzierzak, E, and Medvinsky, A. (1995). Mouse embryonic hematopoiesis. *Trends Genet.* 11: 359–366.

Dzierzak, E, Medvinsky, A, and de Bruijn, M. (1998). Qualitative and quantitative aspects of haemopoietic cell development in the mammalian embryo. *Immunol. Today* 19: 228–236.

Emmel, V. (1916). The cell clusters in the dorsal aorta of mammalian embryos. *Am. J. Anat.* 19: 401–412.

Eren, R, Zharhary, D, Abel, L, and Globerson, A. (1987). Ontogeny of T cells: development of pre-T cells from fetal liver and yolk sac in the thymus microenvironment. *Cell Immunol.* 108: 76–84.

Escary, JL, Perreau, J, Dumenil, D et al. (1993). Leukaemia inhibitory factor is necessary for maintenance of haematopoietic stem cells and thymocyte stimulation. *Nature* 363: 361–364.

Fassler, R and Meyer, M. (1995). Consequences of lack of beta 1 integrin gene expression in mice. *Genes Dev.* 9: 1896–1908.

Ferrara, N, Carver-Moore, K, Chen, H et al. (1996). Heterozygous embryonic lethality induced by targeted inactivation of the VEGF gene. *Nature* 380: 439–442.

Fujiwara, Y, Browne, CP, Cunniff, K et al. (1996). Arrested development of embryonic red cell precursors in mouse embryos lacking transcription factor GATA-1. *Proc. Natl. Acad. Sci. U. S. A.* 93: 12355–12358.

Garcia-Porrero, JA, Godin, IE, and Dieterlen-Lievre, F. (1995). Potential intraembryonic hemogenic sites at pre-liver stages in the mouse. *Anat Embryol (Berl)* 192: 425–435.

Garcia-Porrero, JA, Manaia, A, Jimeno, J et al. (1998). Antigenic profiles of endothelial and hemopoietic lineages in murine intraembryonic hemogenic sites. *Dev Comp Immunol* 22: 303–319.

Geiger, H, Sick, S, Bonifer, C, and Muller, AM. (1998). Globin gene expression is reprogrammed in chimeras generated by injecting adult hematopoietic stem cells into mouse blastocysts. *Cell* 93: 1055–1065.

Gluckman, E. (1995). Advantages of using foetal and neonatal cells for treatment of hematological diseases in human. In Gluckman, E and Coulombel, L, editors. *Ontogeny of hematopoiesis. Aplastic anemia.* Paris: Colloque INSERM/John Libbey Eurotext Ltd.

Godin, I, Dieterlen-Lievre, F, and Cumano, A. (1995). Emergence of multipotent hemopoietic cells in the yolk sac and paraaortic splanchnopleura in mouse embryos, beginning at 8.5 days postcoitus. *Proc. Natl. Acad. Sci. U. S. A.* 92: 773–777.

Godin, IE, Garcia-Porrero, JA, Coutinho, A. et al. (1993). Para-aortic splanchnopleura from early mouse embryos contains B1a cell progenitors. *Nature* 364: 67–70.

Gordon, JB, Harper, R, Mitchell, P, and Lemaike, P. (1999). Activin Signallins and response to a morphogen gradient. *Nature* 371: 487–497.

Green, JB, New, HV, and Smith, JC. (1992). Responses of embryonic *Xenopus* cells to activin and FGF are separated by multiple dose thresholds and correspond to distinct axes of the mesoderm. *Cell* 71: 731–739.

Green, JB and Smith, JC. (1990). Graded changes in dose of a *Xenopus* activin A homologue elicit stepwise transitions in embryonic cell fate [see comments]. *Nature* 347: 391–394.

Grosveld, F, De Boer, E, Dillon, N et al. (1998). The dynamics of globin gene expression and gene therapy vectors. *Ann. N. Y. Acad. Sci.* 850: 18–27.

Harrison, DE, Zhong, RK, Jordan, CT et al. (1997). Relative to adult marrow, fetal liver repopulates nearly five times more effectively long-term than short-term. *Exp. Hematol.* 25: 293–297.

Hassan, HT and Zander, A. (1996). Stem cell factor as a survival and growth factor in human normal and malignant hematopoiesis. *Acta Haematol.* 95: 257–262.

Hayakawa, K, Hardy, RR, Herzenberg, LA, and Herzenberg, LA. (1985). Progenitors for Ly-1 B cells are distinct from progenitors for other B cells. *J. Exp. Med.* 161: 1554–1568.

Herzenberg, LA, Stall, AM, Lalor, PA et al. (1986). The Ly-1 B cell lineage. *Immunol Rev.* 93: 81–102.

Hirsch, E, Iglesias, A, Potocnik, AJ et al. (1996). Impaired migration but not differentiation of haematopoietic stem cells in the absence of fetal integrins. *Nature* 380: 171–175.

His, W. (1990). Lecithoblast und Angioblast der Wirbeltiere. Abhandl. Math-Phys. *Ges. Wiss.* 26: 171–328.

Hole, N, Graham, GJ, Menzel, U, and Ansell, JD. (1996). A limited temporal window for the derivation of multilineage repopulating hematopoietic progenitors during embryonal stem cell differentiation in vitro. *Blood* 88: 1266–1276.

Huang, H and Auerback, R. (1993). Identification and characterization of hematopoietic stem cells from the yolk sac of the early mouse embryo. *Proc. Natl. Acad. Sci. U. S. A.* 90: 10110–10114.

Huyhn, A, Dommergues, M, Izac, B et al. (1995). Characterization of hematopoietic progenitors from human yolk sacs and embryos. *Blood* 86: 4474–4485.

Ihle, JN, and Kerr, IM. (1995). Jaks and Stats in signaling by the cytokine receptor superfamily. *Trends Genet.* 11: 69–74.

Ikuta, K, Kina, T, MacNeil, I et al. (1990). A developmental switch in thymic lymphocyte maturation potential occurs at the level of hematopoietic stem cells. *Cell* 62: 863–874.

Ingram, VM. (1972). Embryonic red blood cell formation. *Nature* 235: 338–339.

Jaffredo, T, Gautier, R, Eichmann, A, and Dieterlen-Lievre, F. (1998). Intraaortic hemopoietic cells are derived from endothelial cells during ontogeny. *Development* 125: 4575–4583.

Jippo, T, Mizuno, H, Xu, Z et al. (1996). Abundant expression of transcription factor GATA-2 in proliferating but not in differentiated mast cells in tissues of mice: demonstration by in situ hybridization. *Blood* 87: 993–998.

Johansson, BAWM. (1995). Evidence for involvement of activin A and bone morphogenetic protein 4 in mammalian mesoderm and hematopoietic development. *Mol. Cell. Biol.* 15: 141–151.

Johnson, GR and Barker, DC. (1985). Erythroid progenitor cells and stimulating factors during murine embryonic and fetal development. *Exp. Hematol.* 13: 200–208.

Jordan, H. (1918). A study of a 7mm human embryo: With special reference to its particular spirally twisted form, and its large aortic cell-clusters. *Anat. Rec.* 14: 479–492.

Kanatsu, M, and Nishikawa, SI. (1996). In vitro analysis of epiblast tissue potency for hematopoietic cell differentiation. *Development* 122: 823–830.

Kau, CL and Turpen, JB. (1983). Dual contribution of embryonic ventral blood island and dorsal lateral plate mesoderm during ontogeny of hemopoietic cells in *Xenopus laevis. J. Immunol.* 131: 2262–2266.

Kelemen, E, Calvo, W, and Fliedner, T. (1979). *Atlas of human hemopoietic development*. Berlin: Springer-Verlag.

Keller, GM. (1995). In vitro differentiation of embryonic stem cells. *Curr. Opin. Cell Biol.* 7: 862–869.

Kennedy, M, Firpo, M, Choi, K et al. (1997). A common precursor for primitive erythropoiesis and definitive haematopoiesis. *Nature* 386: 488–493.

Kimmel, CB, Warga, RM, and Schilling, TF. (1990). Origin and organization of the zebrafish fate map. *Development* 108: 581–594.

Kovach, J, Marks, P, Russell, E, and Epler, H. (1967). Erythroid cell development in fetal mice: ultrastructural characteristics and hemoglobin synthesis. *J. Mol. Biol.* 25: 131–142.

Labastie, MC, Cortes, F, Romeo, PH et al. (1998). Molecular identity of hematopoietic precursor cells emerging in the human embryo. *Blood* 92: 3624–3635.

Labbaye, C, Valtieri, M, Barberi, T et al. (1995). Differential expression and functional role of GATA-2, NF-E2, and GATA-1 in normal adult hematopoiesis. *J. Clin. Invest.* 95: 2346–2358.

Lansdorp, P. (1998). Self-renewal of stem cells. In Monroe, J. and Rothenberg, E., editors. *Molecular Biology of B-cell and T-cell Development*. Totowa, N.J.: Humana Press.

Lawson, KA, Meneses, JJ, and Pedersen, RA. (1991). Clonal analysis of epiblast fate during germ layer formation in the mouse embryo. *Development* 113: 891–911.

Le Douarin, NM, Dieterlen-Lievre, F, and Oliver, PD. (1984). Ontogeny of primary lymphoid organs and lymphoid stem cells. *Am. J. Anat.* 170: 261–299.

Lemischka, IR, Raulet, DH, and Mulligan, RC. (1986). Developmental potential and dynamic behavior of hematopoietic stem cells. *Cell* 45: 917–927.

Lin, CS, Lim, SK, D'Agati, V., and Costantini, F. (1996a). Differential effects of an erythropoietin receptor gene disruption on primitive and definitive erythropoiesis. *Genes Dev.* 10: 154–164.

Lin, HH, Sternfeld, DC, Shinpock, SG, et al. (1996b). Functional analysis of the c-myb proto-oncogene. *Curr. Top. Microbiol. Immunol.* 211: 79–87.

Liu, CP and Auerbach, R. (1991a). In vitro development of murine T cells from prethymic and preliver embryonic yolk sac hematopoietic stem cells. *Development* 113: 1315–1323.

Liu, CP and Auerbach, R. (1991b). Ontogeny of murine T cells: Thymus-regulated development of T cell receptor-bearing cells derived from embryonic yolk sac. *Eur. J. Immunol.* 21: 1849–1855.

Mackarehtschian, K, Hardin, JD, Moore, KA et al. (1995). Targeted disruption of the flk2/flt3 gene leads to deficiencies in primitive hematopoietic progenitors. *Immunity* 3: 147–161.

Maeno, M, Tochinai, S, and Katagiri, C. (1985). Differential participation of ventral and dorsolateral mesoderms in the hemopoiesis of *Xenopus*, as revealed in diploid-triploid or interspecific chimeras. *Dev. Biol.* 110: 503–508.

Maniatis, T, Fritsch, E, Lauer, J, and Lawn, R. (1981). Molecular genetics of human hemoglobins. *Annu. Rev. Genet.* 14: 145–178.

Martin, C, Beaupain, D, and Dieterlen-Lievre, F. (1978). Developmental relationships between vitelline and intra-embryonic haemopoiesis studied in avian 'yolk sac chimaeras.' *Cell Differ.* 7: 115–130.

Mead, PE, Brivanlou, IH, Kelley, CM, and Zon, LI. (1996). BMP-4-responsive regulation of dorsal-ventral patterning by the homeobox protein Mix. 1. *Nature* 382: 357–360.

Medvinsky, A, and Dzierzak, E. (1996). Definitive hematopoiesis is autonomously initiated by the AGM region. *Cell* 86: 897–906.

Medvinsky, AL. (1993). Ontogeny of the mouse hematopoietic system. *Semin. Dev. Biol.* 4: 333–340.

Medvinsky, AL, Gan, OI, Semenova, ML, and Samoylina, NL. (1996). Development of day-8 colony-forming unit-spleen hematopoietic progenitors during early murine embryogenesis: Spatial and temporal mapping. *Blood* 87: 557–566.

Medvinsky, AL, Samoylina, NL, Muller, AM, and Dzierzak, EA. (1993). An early pre-liver intraembryonic source of CFU-S in the developing mouse. *Nature* 364: 64–67.

Metcalf, D. (1984). *The hemopoietic colony stimulating factors.* Amsterdam: Elsevier Science Publishers B. V.

Miale, J. (1982). *Laboratory medicine hematology* (6th ed.). St. Louis: Mosby.

Migliaccio, G, Migliaccio, AR, Petti, S et al. (1986). Human embryonic hemopoiesis. Kinetics of progenitors and precursors underlying the yolk sac-liver transition. *J. Clin. Invest.* 78: 51–60.

Miles, C, Sanchez, M-J, Sinclair, A, and Dzierzak, E. (1997). Expression of the Ly-6E.1 (Sca-1) transgene in adult hematopoietic stem cells and the developing mouse embryo. *Development* 124: 537–547.

Minot, C. (1910). Development of the blood, the vascular system and the spleen. In Keibel, J and Mall, F, editors. *Human embryology.* Philadelphia: JB Lippincott.

Moore, MA and Metcalf, D. (1970). Ontogeny of the haemopoietic system: Yolk sac origin of in vivo and in vitro colony forming cells in the developing mouse embryo. *Br. J. Haematol.* 18: 279–296.

Moore, MA and Owen, JJ. (1967). Experimental studies on the development of the thymus. *J Exp Med* 126: 715–726.

Mucenski, ML, McLain, K, Kier, AB et al. (1991). A functional c-myb gene is required for normal murine fetal hepatic hematopoiesis. *Cell* 65: 677–689.

Muller, A and Dzierzak, E. (1993). ES cells as a model of embryonic hematopoiesis? *Semin. Dev. Biol.* 4: 341–350.

Muller, AM and Dzierzak, EA. (1993). ES cells have only a limited lymphopoietic potential after adoptive transfer into mouse recipients. *Development* 118: 1343–1351.

Muller, AM, Medvinsky, A, Strouboulis, J et al. (1994). Development of hematopoietic stem cell activity in the mouse embryo. *Immunity* 1: 291–301.

Murray, P. (1932). The development in vitro of the blood of the early chick embryo. *Proc. Roy. Soc. London* 11: 497–521.

Naito, M. (1993). Macrophage heterogeneity in development and differentiation. *Arch. Histol. Cytol.* 56: 331–351.

Naito, M, Umeda, S, Yamamoto, T et al. (1996). Development, differentiation, and phenotypic heterogeneity of murine tissue macrophages. *J. Leukoc. Biol.* 59: 133–138.

Nakano, T, Kodama, H, and Honjo, T. (1996). In vitro development of primitive and definitive erythrocytes from different precursors. *Science* 272: 722–724.

Neubauer, H, Cumano, A, Muller, M et al. (1998). Jak2 deficiency defines an essential developmental checkpoint in definitive hematopoiesis. *Cell* 93: 397–409.

Newman, PJ, Berndt, MC, Gorski, J, White, GCD et al. (1990). PECAM-1 (CD31) cloning and relation to adhesion molecules of the immunoglobulin gene superfamily. *Science* 247: 1219–1222.

Nieuwkoop, P. (1969). The formation of mesoderm in Urodelean amphibians. I. Induction by the endoderm. *Roux Arch. Entw. Mech. Org.* 162: 341–373.

Nieuwkoop, P and Ubbels, G. (1972). The formation of mesoderm in Urodelean amphibians. IV. Quantitative evidence for the purely 'ectodermal' origin of the entire mesoderm and of the pharyngeal endoderm. *Roux Arch. Entw. Mech. Org.* 169: 185–199.

Nishikawa, SI Nishikawa, S, Kawamoto, H, Yoshida, H et al. (1998a). In vitro generation of lymphohematopoietic cells from endothelial cells purified from murine embryos. *Immunity* 8: 761–769.

Nishikawa, S-I, Nishikawa, S, Hirashima, M et al. (1998b). Progressive lineage analysis by cell sorting and culture identifies FLK+VE-cadherin+ cells at a diverging point of endothelial and hematopoietic lineages. *Development* 125: 1747–1757.

North, T, Gu, T-L, Stacy, T et al. (1999). Cbfα is required for the formation of intraaortic hematopoietic clusters. *Development* 126: 2563–2575.

Nuez, B, Michalovich, D, Bygrave, A et al. (1995). Defective haematopoiesis in fetal liver resulting from inactivation of the EKLF gene. *Nature* 375: 316–318.

Ogawa, M, Matsuzaki, Y, Nishikawa, S et al. (1991). Expression and function of c-kit in hemopoietic progenitor cells. *J. Exp. Med.* 174: 63–71.

Ogawa, M, Nishikawa, S, Ikuta, K et al. (1988). B cell ontogeny in murine embryo studied by a culture system with the monolayer of a stromal cell clone, ST2: B cell progenitor develops first in the embryonal body rather than in the yolk sac. *EMBO J.* 7: 1337–1343.

Okada, S, Nakauchi, H, Nagayoshi, K et al. (1991). Enrichment and characterization of murine hematopoietic stem cells that express c-kit molecule. *Blood* 78: 1706–1712.

Okuda, T, van Deursen, J, Hiebert, SW et al. (1996). AML1, the target of multiple chromosomal translocations in human leukemia, is essential for normal fetal liver hematopoiesis. *Cell* 84: 321–330.

Pandolfi, PP, Roth, ME, Karis, A et al. (1995). Targeted disruption of the GATA3 gene causes severe abnormalities in the nervous system and in fetal liver haematopoiesis [see comments]. *Nat. Genet.* 11: 40–44.

Pardanaud, L, Altmann, C, Kitos, P et al. (1987). Vasculogenesis in the early quail blastodisc as studied with a monoclonal antibody recognizing endothelial cells. *Development* 100: 339–349.

Parganas, E, Wang, D, Stravopodis, D et al. (1998). Jak2 is essential for signaling through a variety of cytokine receptors. *Cell* 93: 385–395.

Pawliuk, R, Eaves, C, and Humphries, RK. (1996). Evidence of both ontogeny and transplant dose-regulated expansion of hematopoietic stem cells in vivo. *Blood* 88: 2852–2858.

Peault, B. (1996). Hematopoietic stem cell emergence in embryonic life: Developmental hematology revisited. *J. Hematother.* 5: 369–378.

Perkins, AC, Sharpe, AH, and Orkin, SH. (1995). Lethal beta-thalassaemia in mice lacking the erythroid CACCC-transcription factor EKLF. *Nature* 375: 318–322.

Pevny, L, Simon, MC, Robertson, E et al. (1991). Erythroid differentiation in chimaeric mice blocked by a targeted mutation in the gene for transcription factor GATA-1. *Nature* 349: 257–260.

Porcher, C, Swat, W, Rockwell, K et al. (1996). The T cell leukemia oncoprotein SCL/tal-1 is essential for development of all hematopoietic lineages. *Cell* 86: 47–57.

Rich, IN. (1995). Primordial germ cells are capable of producing cells of the hematopoietic system in vitro. *Blood* 86: 463–472.

Rifkind, R, Bank, A, Markes, P et al. (1980). *Fundamentals of hematology* (2nd ed.). Chicago: Year Book Medical Publishers.

Rifkind, R, Chui, D, and Epler, H. (1969). An ultrastructural study of early morphogenetic events during the establishment of fetal hepatic erythropoiesis. *J. Cell Biol.* 40: 343–365.

Risau, W. (1991). Embryonic angiogenesis factors. *Pharmacol. Ther.* 51: 371–376.

Robb, L, Elwood, NJ, Elefanty, AG et al. (1996). The scl gene product is required for the generation of all hematopoietic lineages in the adult mouse. *EMBO J.* 15: 4123–4129.

Robb, L, Lyons, I, Li, R et al. (1995). Absence of yolk sac hematopoiesis from mice with a targeted disruption of the scl gene. *Proc. Natl. Acad. U. S. A.* 92: 7075–7079.

Russell, ES. (1979). Hereditary anemias of the mouse: A review for geneticists. *Adv. Genet.* 20: 357–459.

Russell, ES and Bernstein, SE. (1966). Blood and blood formation. In Green, EL, editor. *Biology of the laboratory mouse,* New York: McGraw-Hill.

Sabin, F. (1920). Studies on the origin of blood vessels and of red blood corpuscles as seen in the living blastoderm of chicks during the second day of incubation. Carnegie Inst. Wash. Pub. #272, *Contrib. Embryol.* 9: 214.

Sargent, TD, Jamrich, M, and Dawid, IB. (1986). Cell interactions and the control of gene activity during early development of *Xenopus laevis. Dev. Biol.* 114: 238–246.

Sasaki, K, Yagi, H, Bronson, RT et al. (1996). Absence of fetal liver hematopoiesis in mice deficient in transcriptional coactivator core binding factor beta. *Proc. Natl. Acad. Sci. U. S. A.* 93: 12359–12363.

Shalaby, F, Ho, J, Stanford, WL et al. (1997). A requirement for Flk1 in primitive and definitive hematopoiesis and vasculogenesis. *Cell* 89: 981–990.

Shalaby, F, Rossant, J, Yamaguchi, TP, Gertsenstein, M et al. (1995). Failure of blood-island formation and vasculogenesis in Flk-1-deficient mice. *Nature* 376: 62–66.

Shamblott, MJ, Axelman, J, Wang, S, Bugg, EM et al. (1998). Derivation of pluripotent stem cells from cultured human primordial germ cells. *Proc. Natl. Acad. Sci. U. S. A.* 95: 13726–13731.

Shivdasani, RA, Mayer, EL, and Orkin, SH. (1995). Absence of blood formation in mice lacking the T-cell leukaemia oncoprotein tal-1/SCL. *Nature* 373: 432–434.

Singh, H. (1996). Gene targeting reveals a hierarchy of transcription factors regulating specification of lymphoid cell fates. *Curr. Opin. Immunol.* 8: 160–165.

Smith, J.C. and Albano, R.M. (1993). Mesoderm induction and erythroid differentiation in early vertebrate development. *Semin. Dev. Biol.* 4: 315–324.

Sonoda, T, Hayashi, C, and Kitamura, Y. (1983). Presence of mast cell precursors in the yolk sac of mice. *Dev. Biol.* 97: 89–94.

Stennard F, Ryan, K, and Gurdon, JB. (1997). Markers of vertebrate mesoderm induction. *Curr. Opini. Genet. Dev.* 7: 620–627.

Stephens, LE, Sutherland, AE, Klimanskaya, IV et al. (1995). Deletion of beta 1 integrins in mice results in inner cell mass failure and peri-implantation lethality. *Genes Dev.* 9: 1883–1895.

Tavian, M, Coulombel, L, Luton, D et al. (1996). Aorta-associated CD34+ hematopoietic cells in the early human embryo. *Blood* 87: 67–72.

Till, J and McCulloch, E. (1961). A direct measurement of the radiation sensitivity of normal mouse bone marrow cells. *Radiat. Res.* 14: 213–222.

Ting, CN, Olson, MC, Barton, KP, and Leiden, JM. (1996). Transcription factor GATA-3 is required for development of the T-cell lineage. *Nature* 384: 474–478.

Toles, JF, Chui, DH, Belbeck, LW et al. (1989). Hemopoietic stem cells in murine embryonic yolk sac and peripheral blood. *Proc. Natl. Acad. Sci. U. S. A.* 86: 7456–7459.

Tonegawa, A, Funayama, N, Ueno, N, and Takahashi, Y. (1997). Mesodermal subdivision along the mediolateral axis in chicken controlled by different concentrations of BMP-4. *Development* 124: 1975–1984.

Tracey, WD, Jr, Pepling, ME, Horb, ME et al. (1998). A *Xenopus* homologue of aml-1 reveals unexpected patterning mechanisms leading to the formation of embryonic blood. *Development* 125: 1371–1380.

Tsai, FY, Keller, G, Kuo, FC et al. (1994). An early haematopoietic defect in mice lacking the transcription factor GATA-2. *Nature* 371: 221–226.

Turpen, JB, Kelley, CM, Mead, PE, and Zon, LI. (1997). Bipotential primitive-definitive hematopoietic progenitors in the vertebrate embryo. *Immunity* 7: 325–334.

Turpen, JB and Knudson, CM. (1982). Ontogeny of hematopoietic cells in Rana pipiens: Precursor cell migration during embryogenesis. *Dev. Biol.* 89: 138–151.

Turpen, JB, Knudson, CM, and Hoefen, PS. (1981). The early ontogeny of hematopoietic cells studied by grafting cytogenetically labeled tissue anlagen: Localization of a prospective stem cell compartment. *Dev. Biol.* 85: 99–112.

Vakaet, L. (1985). Morphogenetic movements and fate maps in the avian blastoderm. In Edelman, GM, editor. *Molecular determinants of animal form.* New York: Alan R. Liss.

van Hennik, PB, Verstegen, MM, Bierhuizen, MF et al. (1998). Highly efficient transduction of the green fluorescent protein gene in human umbilical cord blood stem cells capable of cobblestone formation in long-term cultures and multilineage engraftment of immunodeficient mice. *Blood* 92: 4013–4022.

Visvader, JE, Fujiwara, Y, and Orkin, SH. (1998). Unsuspected role for the T-cell leukemia protein SCL/tal-1 in vascular development. *Genes Dev.* 12: 473–479.

Wagner, R. (1980). Endothelial cell embryology and growth. *Adv. Microcirc.* 9: 45–97.

Wakayama, T, Perry, AC, Zuccotti, M et al. (1998). Full-term development of mice from enucleated oocytes injected with cumulus cell nuclei [see comments]. *Nature* 394: 369–374.

Wang, JH, Nichogiannopoulou, A, Wu, L et al. (1996a). Selective defects in the development of the fetal and adult lymphoid system in mice with an Ikaros null mutation. *Immunity* 5: 537–549.

Wang, Q, Stacy, T, Binder, M et al. (1996b). Disruption of the Cbfa2 gene causes necrosis and hemorrhaging in the central nervous system and blocks definitive hematopoiesis. *Proc. Natl. Acad. Sci. U. S. A.* 93: 3444–3449.

Wang, Q, Stacy, T, Miller, JD et al. (1996c). The CBFbeta subunit is essential for CBFalpha2 (AML1) function in vivo. *Cell* 87: 697–708.

Warren, AJ, Colledge, WH, Carlton, MB et al. (1994). The oncogenic cysteine-rich LIM domain protein rbtn2 is essential for erythroid development. *Cell* 78: 45–57.

Weissman I, Papaioannou, V. and Gardner, R. (1978). *Fetal hematopoietic origins of the adult hematolymphoid system.* Cold Spring Harbor: Cold Spring Harbor Laboratory.

Wijgerde, M, Grosveld, F, and Fraser, P. (1995). Transcription complex stability and chromatin dynamics in vivo. *Nature* 377: 209–213.

Williams, DA, Rios, M, Stephens, C, and Patel, VP. (1991). Fibronectin and VLA-4 in haematopoietic stem cell-microenvironment interactions. *Nature* 352: 438–441.

Wilmut, I, Schnieke, AE, McWhir, J et al. (1997). Viable offspring derived from fetal and adult mammalian cells [see comments] [published erratum appears in *Nature* 1997 Mar 13;386(6621):200]. *Nature* 385: 810–813.

Winnier, G, Blessing, M, Labosky, PA, and Hogan, BL. (1995). Bone morphogenetic protein-4 is required for mesoderm formation and patterning in the mouse. *Genes Dev.* 9: 2105–2116.

Witte, ON. (1990). Steel locus defines new multipotent growth factor [published erratum appears in Cell 1990 *Cell* 63: 5–6].

Wong, PM, Chung, SW, Reicheld, SM, and Chui, DH. (1986). Hemoglobin switching during murine embryonic development: evidence for two populations of embryonic erythropoietic progenitor cells. *Blood* 67: 716–721.

Wood, HB, May, G, Healy, L et al. (1997). CD34 expression patterns during early mouse development are related to modes of blood vessel formation and reveal additional sites of hematopoiesis. *Blood* 90: 2300–2311.

Wu, H, Liu, X, Jaenisch, R, and Lodish, HF. (1995). Generation of committed erythroid BFU-E and CFU-E progenitors does not require erythropoietin or the erythropoietin receptor. *Cell* 83: 59–67.

Yoder, MC, Hiatt, K, Dutt, P et al. (1997a). Characterization of definitive lymphohematopoietic stem cells in the day 9 murine yolk sac. *Immunity* 7: 335–344.

Yamada, Y, Warren, AJ, Dobson, C et al. (1998). The T cell leukemia LIM protein Lmoz is necessary for adult mouse hematopoiesis. *Proc. Natl. Acad. Sci. U. S. A.* 95: 3890–3895.

Yoder, MC, Hiatt, K, and Mukherjee, P. (1997b). In vivo repopulating hematopoietic stem cells are present in the murine yolk sac at day 9.0 postcoitus. *Proc. Natl. Acad. Sci. U. S. A.* 94: 6776–6780.

Young, PE, Baumhueter, S, and Lasky, LA. (1995). The sialomucin CD34 is expressed on hematopoietic cells and blood vessels during murine development. *Blood* 85: 96–105.

Zon, LI. (1995). Developmental biology of hematopoiesis. *Blood* 86: 2876–2891.

3

Erythropoiesis

ANNA RITA MIGLIACCIO
THALIA PAPAYANNOPOULOU

INTRODUCTION

Erythropoiesis is a highly regulated, multistep process, the end product of which is the erythrocyte or red blood cell. One vital function of erythrocytes is to deliver oxygen to the different tissues of the body and remove carbon dioxide. In adults, the number of circulating red cells is constant and represents the balance between two ongoing processes, destruction of old red cells—mainly in the spleen—and the generation of new red cells within the bone marrow.

Erythropoiesis begins when a multipotent hematopoietic stem cell undergoes erythroid unilineage commitment and continues throughout the proliferation and terminal maturation of the erythroid committed progenitor cells (Ogawa, 1993). During this process, distinct cellular compartments are formed characterized by a progressive decline in proliferation and a parallel increase in differentiation potential. The erythroid committed progenitor compartment is composed of cells that are not morphologically recognizable but can be defined functionally in vitro through their progeny (Ogawa, 1993). By contrast, the erythroid precursor cell compartment is composed of morphologically recognizable, maturing erythroid cells at different stages of maturation. Thus, the erythroid compartment, like those in other lineages, has an aging structure and contains early and late progenitor and precursor cells (Fig. 3.1).

Because of its functional importance, erythropoiesis is the main differentiated lineage that appears during ontogeny in the blood islands of the yolk sac (Edmonds, 1966; Moore and Metcalf, 1970). Later, different anatomic sites such as the fetal liver and finally the bone marrow, are recruited for erythropoiesis. (Moore and Metcalf, 1970; Steiner, 1973; Migliaccio, G. et al., 1993). During most of intrauterine life hematopoiesis and erythropoiesis take place in the fetal liver, which remains a predominantly erythroid organ. Changes in sites of hematopoiesis are also associated with profound differences in the stem cell differentiation program and in the phenotypic and functional properties of cells developing in these different sites (Peschle et al., 1981; Muench et al., 1994; Huyhn et al., 1995). Hematopoietic cytokines expressed or sequestered by microenvironmental cells at each site ensure proliferation and differentiation of erythroid cells by establishing, in concert with intrinsic transcriptional factors (see Chapter 4), distinct patterns of gene expression (Stamatoyannopoulos and Nienhuis, 1987). Furthermore, adhesion receptors on hematopoietic cells and their counterreceptors in the microenvironment ensure patterns of migration, firm adherence, and colonization of respective hematopoietic sites (Papayannopoulou et al., 1991). In this chapter we highlight regulatory aspects of erythropoiesis in adults and during embryonic and fetal life. Our focus remains the physiologic control of human erythropoiesis at the cellular level.

CELLULAR COMPARTMENTS OF ERYTHROPOIESIS

Erythropoiesis and hematopoiesis rely on the functional properties and the resilience of a few cells, stem cells, which in the adult are found in high concentration only in the bone marrow. Stem cells, despite efforts to purify them with arguable successes, are still largely defined as functional entities. Their distinctive properties are the ability to self-renew and simultaneously to produce multipotential hematopoietic functional cells for the life of the organism (Morrison et al., 1995). These stem cell properties are revealed in transplantation experiments in animal models. Recently, xenogeneic transplants have been introduced for the study of human stem cells McCune et al., 1988; Dick, 1996; Zanjani et al., 1994), but the relationship of populations studied in these animals to the true stem cell existing in humans has yet to be validated. Several other surrogate assays have been used in vitro to study stem cells. They include long-term culture-initiating cells (LTC-IC), (Sutherland et al., 1989; Petzer et al., 1996), cobblestone area forming cells

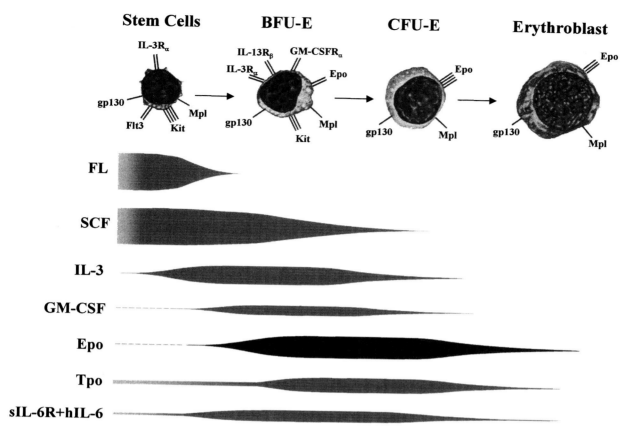

Figure 3.1. Diagrammatic scheme of adult erythroid differentiation: Cellular compartments (top panel) and the in vitro influence of growth factors (bottom panel). The level of expression of the corresponding receptors during the cytogeny of erythroid cells is indicated by bars on the cell surface. The growth factors listed influencing proliferation and/or differentiation along the erythroid pathway are: Flt3 ligand and SCF; IL-3 and GM-CSF, EPO and thrombopoietin (TPO). Human stem cells require either SCF or Flt3 ligand to survive and proliferate in culture. Optimal growth of adult erythroid bursts requires the presence of at least three different growth factors: SCF, IL-3 (or, in humans, GM-CSF) and EPO. Formation of erythroid bursts and of CFU-e-derived colonies is influenced by TPO and EPO. TPO also influences the survival of more primitive cells, and in the presence of other factors, induces proliferation of single murine stem cells and of human CD34+ cells in liquid culture. Recently, the combination of IL-6 with its soluble binding receptor (sIL-6R-IL-6) or a fusion molecule called hyper IL-6 has been shown to induce proliferation of stem cells and sustain terminal erythroid differentiation of progenitor cells in the apparent absence of EPO. It should be noted that, although hematopoietic cells do not express the IL-6 receptor, they constitutively express gp130, its signal partner. For a complete list of the factors acting on erythroid differentiation in vitro, see Table 3.2. For full color reproduction, see color plate 3.1.

(CAFC) (Ploemacher et al., 1991), blast cell colony-forming cells (bcc) (Leary and Ogawa, 1987), high proliferative potential cells (HPPC) (McNiece et al., 1989), and colony-forming cells, granulocytic, erythroid, eosinophilic, megakaryocyte, and macrophage (CFU-GEEMM) (Fauser and Messner, 1979). However, these assays have limitations and may reflect properties of an immediate progeny of the stem cell rather than the true stem cells.

In contrast to stem cells, which are very rare (1 in 10^4 to 10^5 bone marrow cells), the committed progenitor compartment is found in larger numbers (Table 3.1) and can be studied in vitro in clonogenic assays. Thus, different subclasses of progenitor cells can be revealed in vitro and their characterization and response to growth factors can be studied in detail (Fig. 3.1 and Tables 3.1 and 3.2). The earliest progenitor cell with erythroid potential in semisolid culture is a CFU-mix (CFU-GEMM), which can form several lineages, including the erythroid, in several combinations (Fauser and Messner, 1979). More abundant are the unipotent or unilineage progenitor cells, that is, the ones committed to a single lineage (Table 3.1). In erythropoiesis, the earliest erythroid committed progenitor is the erythroid burst forming unit (BFU-e), which generates colonies containing several thousand erythroid cells (Gregory and Eaves, 1977; Mladenovic and Adamson, 1982). Subclasses of BFU-e,

Table 3.1. Human Adult Erythroid Progenitors: General Properties

Properties	Day 14 GM	GEEMM	BFU-e	CFU-e
Incidence				
CFU/10^5 bone marrow cells	40–120	2–5 (137–200)*	40–120	200–600
CFU/10^5 light-density blood cells	10–40	2–5 (10–18)*	10–40	0.1–0.5
Density (g/ml)	<1.077	<1.077	<1.077	>1.077
Cycling status				
Bone marrow	30–40	15–20	30–40	60–80
Peripheral blood	0–5	0–5	0–5	n.d.[†]
Colony size (cells/colony)	1,000–10,000	>10,000	1,000–5000	50–200
Replating potential (progenitor cells per colony)	>100 CFU	>200 CFU	>100 CFU	0
Surface antigens[‡]				
CD34+	++	+++	++	+/–
AC133	++	++	++	+/–
CD38–	++	+	++	+/–
CD33	+++	++	+	+/–
CD45-RA	+++	++	+	+/–
HLA-DR (-DP, -DQ)	+++	+++	+++	+
FAS	+++	+	++	+++
CD71	+/–	+	++	+++
Ep-1	+/–	+	+	++
ABH, iI (blood group antigen)	+/–	+/–	++	+++
CD36	+/–	+/–	+	++
Glycophorin A	+/–	+/–	+/–	++
23.6 (SFL 23.6)	+/–	+/–	+/–	++

Colony growth stimulated with IL-3, GM-CSF and G-CSF (CFU-GM) or EPO (BFU-e, CFU-GEEMM).
* Values in parentheses were obtained when SCF was added.
[†] n.d., not detectable.
[‡] +++,++,+,+/– indicate levels of expression very high, high, low, and low/absent, respectively.

with less proliferative potential and shorter maturation time in culture, lie between the primitive BFU-e and the most mature progenitor, the erythroid colony-forming unit (CFU-e), which generates colonies that contain up to 50 erythroblasts within the first week in culture (Eaves and Eaves, 1978). Studies in mice have shown that the number of progenitor cells within the bone marrow and that circulate, is genetically determined (Phillips et al., 1992; Jordan and Van Zant, 1998) and is constant in a specific strain (Bol, 1980). It is further believed that the relationship between the early and late progenitors remains constant so that one can indirectly estimate the most primitive cells present in a normal human tissue by evaluating the number of later types of progenitors present in that tissue. Whether this is valid in humans is debatable (Spitzer et al., 1980; Migliaccio, A.R., et al., 1996).

When clonogenic assays became available, studies were initiated to purify progenitor cells by physical or immunologic means using positive or negative selection. With the advent of monoclonal antibodies several reagents became available that have aided this effort. Among them, antibodies to CD34+ antigen (Civin et al., 1984; Tindle et al., 1985; Andrews et al., 1986) appear to hold a dominant place for both stem and progenitor cell identification and purification. CD34+ is a highly O-glycosylated cell surface glycoprotein the function of which is not understood (Krause et al., 1996). Deletion of the CD34+ gene in the mouse does not induce an abnormal phenotype except for a slightly lower progenitor cell content in the embryonic and adult tissues (Cheng et al., 1996). The human CD34+ is recognized by several different monoclonal antibodies (i.e., MY10, 12.8, and HPCA 1) with varying epitope distribution (Steen and Egeland, 1998) and is expressed in all hematopoietic progenitors and vascular endothelial cells. Thus, estimates based on the number of hematopoietic cells positive for CD34+ and their progenitor content has been made in a given tissue or in the blood (Table 3.3). Furthermore, subsets of CD34+ cells have been recognized as representing different subclasses of progenitor cells (Table 3.1). For example, the CD38– antigen expression among CD34+ cells has been used to discriminate late from more primitive progenitors, which lack CD38– antigen expression (Terstappen et al., 1991). Support of using CD34+-based strategy

Table 3.2. Factors Enhancing (↑) or Inhibiting (↓) Erythroid Development In Vitro

	Target cells and specific response
Positive effects	
Flk3-ligand	CFU-GEEMM: ↑ survival, proliferation
G-CSF, IL-1	CFU-GEEMM: ↑ differentiation (synergistic)
SCF	CFU-GEEMM, BFUe: ↑ survival, ↑ proliferation, ↑ limited self-replication, ↑ differentiation
IL-3	Stem cells: ↓ lymphoid potential; BFU-e: ↑ survival, ↑ proliferation
GM-CSF	BFU-e: ↑ survival, ↑ proliferation
IL-9, IL-11	BFU-e: ↑ proliferation (synergistic)
EPO	BFU-e: ↑ proliferation (synergistic); CFU-E: ↑, survival, ↑ proliferation, ↑ differentiation
TPO	CFU-GEEMM, BFU-e, and CFU-e: ↑ survival, ↑ proliferation, ↑ differentiation
sIL-6-R/IL-6	CFU-GEEMM, BFU-e, and CFU-e: ↑ proliferation, ↑ differentiation
Insulin, IGF-I, II	CFU-GEEMM, BFU-e, and CFU-e: ↑ proliferation
Transferrin	CFU-GEEMM, BFU-e, and CFU-e: ↑ proliferation
Metallo-proteinase inhibitor (EPA)	BFU-e: ↑ proliferation, ↑ differentiation
Activin A	CFU-e: ↑ differentiation
Steroid hormones	BFU-e: ↑ proliferation, ↓ differentiation
Butyric acid	CFU-e: ↑ differentiation, ↑ HbF expression
Retinoic acid	↑ Differentiation
Hemin	BFU-e, CFU-e: ↑ differentiation
Negative effects	
TNF-α	CFU-GEEMM and BFU-e: ↑ apoptosis
IFN-γ	CFU-GEEMM and BFU-e: ↑ apoptosis
Sialomucins (CD43, 147, 162)	↑ apoptosis, ↑ growth arrest
TGF-β	CFU-GEEMM and BFU-e: ↓ proliferation, ↑ differentiation
PGE-1	CFU-GEEMM and BFU-e: ↓ proliferation, ↓ differentiation

Table 3.3. Frequency* of CD34+/CD38− Cells in the Blood at Different Ontogenetic Stages (Fetus, Neonate, and Adult) and in the Adult Bone Marrow

	Fetal blood	Cord blood	Neonatal blood[†]	Adult blood	Adult marrow
CD34+*	30.7	31.0	6.0	0.01	18.9
CD34+, CD38−	1.04	1.81	0.3	<0.01	0.60

* The results are given as percent of the cells in the lymphocyte gate.
[†] 48 hours after delivery.
Source: Modified from Li et al., 1999.

the autologous and allogeneic setting (Berenson et al., 1991; Schiller et al., 1995). Recent transplantation studies in the mouse (Osawa et al., 1996) and in xeno-transplantation of human cells into fetal sheep (Zanjani et al., 1998) have also shown the presence of long-term repopulating cells among the murine and human CD34+ low or null cells of adult marrow. However, in xenotransplants of human cells in NOD/SCID mice the CD34+ low/null fraction does not repopulate mice unless cultured for several days in the presence of specific growth factors (Bhatia et al., 1998). Since high numbers of CD34+ cells are generated in these cultures, CD34+ low/null cells may represent CD34+ low stem cell precursors.

Expression of surface antigens by erythroid committed progenitor cells is largely similar to other progenitors, but some distinct differences have been noted. For example, BFU-e are negative for the CD45− RA antigen, whereas most myeloid progenitor cells are positive (Lansdorp et al., 1990; Fritsch et al., 1993). Similarly, BFU-e are low or negative for the CD33 and the AC133 antigens that are uniformly positive in myeloid progenitors (Andrews et al., 1986; Yin et al., 1997). Furthermore, a tendency among erythroid progenitors to express high levels of transferrin receptors (Iacopetta et al., 1982; Sawyer and Krantz, 1986) or possibly specific receptor isoforms for erythroid cells is present (Cotner et al., 1989).

Although BFU-e have few distinguishing features from their counterparts in myeloid lineage, later progenitors acquire more distinctive erythroid features (Table 3.1). Thus, the CFU-e appears to be glycophorin A positive (Robinson et al., 1981) throughout their maturation and they acquire carbohydrate antigens characteristic for mature erythrocytes, such as I antigen (Fukuda et al., 1980; Hann et al., 1983) and other less characterized antigens (Yokochi et al., 1984; Gupta et al., 1985). Recently, the activation of the expression of blood group antigens has been analyzed during the transition from

for stem cell purification has been provided recently in transplantation experiments, in which the engraftment kinetics have been correlated with the total number of CD34+ cells infused or a specific CD34+ subset both in

BFU-e to erythroblasts (Southcott et al., 1999): The first antigen to be expressed at the BFU-e level is the glycoprotein (gp) Kell followed by Rh gp, Landersteiner Wiener (LW) gp, glycoprotein A, Band 3, Lutheran (Lu) gp, and, at last at the erythroblast level, Duffy gp. A list of properties between early and late erythroid committed cells is presented in Table 3.1.

Besides phenotypic properties, the response of erythroid progenitor cells to hematopoietic growth factors distinguishes them from other progenitor types (Fig. 3.1). Several growth factors influence the survival, growth, and differentiation of erythroid progenitor cells in vitro and in vivo (Metcalf, 1993). Their effects depend on whether the progenitor is early or late, whether used alone or in combination, on their relative concentration, on the cellular environment (composition of accessory cells, presence of stromal support, etc.), and the sources of culture media. Factors that exert mostly proliferative effects on erythroid cells are stem cell factor (SCF or Steel factor or kit ligand), interleukin 3 (IL-3), granulocyte-macrophage colony-stimulating factor (GM-CSF), and, in certain progenitor types, erythropoietin (EPO) (Fig. 3.1 and Table 3.2). Recent evidence also suggests that thrombopoietin may exert a redundant control on erythroid differentiation being capable of partial replacement of EPO (Kieran et al., 1996; Papayannopoulou et al., 1996).

Among the growth factors mentioned, a large body of experimental data suggests that SCF is very important for erythropoiesis, as it can influence multiple facets of erythropoiesis, from survival and proliferation to partial differentiation (Broudy, 1997). Mice with mutations of SCF or its receptor, kit, have anemia, the severity of which correlates with kit kinase activity (Russell, 1979; Besmer, 1991). Viable mutants, such as the Steel Dickey mouse (Sl/Sl^d) or the white spotted mouse, W/W^v, have normal levels of hematopoietic stem cells but reduced levels of BFU-e and CFU-e (Barker and Starr, 1991). Spleen colonies, CFU-S, generated by normal cells within the spleen of Steel mutants (Wolf, 1974) or by W/W^v cells within the spleen of normal animals (Barker and Starr, 1991) contain predominantly blast cells and granulocytes, while normally erythroid cells predominate in normal spleens. This shows that while commitment to expansion and differentiation toward nonerythroid lineages occurs normally, this process is curtailed in mice with aberrant SCF/kit kinase activity. In humans, kit mutations have been described in heterozygotes with piebaldism (Fleischman et al., 1996; Schinzel et al., 1997; Spritz and Beighton, 1998). Despite the melanocyte defects, no hematopoietic abnormalities have been found in these individuals but homozygotes have not been described. Other evidence suggesting the importance of kit in erythropoiesis are studies where anti-kit receptor antibodies in vivo pro-

duced anemia in mice (Rico-Vargas et al., 1994; Broudy et al., 1996). Furthermore, studies using antisense oligonucleotides in vitro to inhibit the expression of kit from human CD34$^+$ cells have shown that the generation of erythroid progenitor cells from CD34$^+$ cells purified from adult marrow or cord blood requires a functional kit (Migliaccio, AR et al., 1993). Influx of new BFU-e from an earlier compartment was greatly reduced, suggesting that while maintenance of already generated in vivo and their subsequent differentiation might be at least partially SCF dependent, the generation of BFU-e from an earlier compartment is largely SCF dependent (Migliaccio AR et al., 1993).

Besides SCF, optimal growth of early erythroid progenitors in culture requires the presence of additional hematopoietic growth factors, such as IL-3, GM-CSF, EPO (Migliaccio, G et al., 1988; Sonoda et al., 1988), and factors necessary for any cell growth in vitro such as the insulin family of growth factors and transferrin (Dainiak and Kreczko, 1985; Akahane et al., 1987; Migliaccio, G et al., 1990b). In cultures of T cells and fibroblasts, IGF-1 is required to bypass the restriction point in mid G1 while transferrin is required to enter the S phase, probably because the enzymatic activity of the DNA polymerase is limited by the iron concentration within the cell (Hirschman and Garfinkel, 1977). None of these factors on its own induces proliferation of progenitor cells and the combination of them is required for optimal growth of erythroid bursts. For example, simultaneous presence of EPO with GM-CSF is necessary to protect the survival of human BFU-e, the proliferation of which later can be detected in the presence of EPO (Migliaccio, G et al., 1990b). If addition of EPO is delayed, the formation of erythroid bursts in these cultures is restored, but the appearance of the colonies is also delayed for a time equal to the time that EPO was delayed (Migliaccio, G et al., 1990b). More mature progenitor cells such as CFU-e, in contrast to BFU-e, require only EPO and insulin-like growth factors for complete differentiation in culture (Iscove et al., 1980).

EPO is the main physiologic regulator of the number of red cells in vivo, since genetic abrogation of EPO expression in mice leads to profound anemia and fetal death at 13.5 days of gestation (Wu et al., 1995a; Lin et al., 1996). The numbers of BFU-e and generation of CFU-e in the liver of these fetuses are normal, suggesting that both defects impair only the final stages of erythroid differentiation. Since erythroblasts with signs of apoptosis are present in fetal liver (Wu et al., 1995a; Lin et al., 1996), the defect is due to the inability of erythroblasts to survive (Koury and Bondurant, 1990) and not necessarily to differentiate (Fairbairn et al., 1993). It is still debated whether the effect of EPO on erythroid cells is only to prevent apoptosis or to induce in addition proliferation and differentiation of these cells

(Enver et al., 1998; Metcalf, 1998; Papayannopoulou et al., 1999). In the absence of EPO, erythroid cells undergo apoptosis either in G1 or in the S phase of the cycle without growth arrest in a specific phase of the cycle (Kelley et al., 1994). As survival is a cellular function dominant over proliferation, the effects of EPO on proliferation (and differentiation) may have been underestimated in vitro. In fact, fetal murine CFU-e that constitutively express either Bcl-2 or Bcl-XLC genes that specifically suppress apoptosis survive but do not form colonies without EPO (Chida et al., 1999). Other indirect evidence of a link between EPO and cell cycle progression has been provided by the 60 percent to 80 percent suicide index of CFU-e (Table 3.1). The suicide index measures the percentage of the cells in the S phase of the cycle sensitive to ^{3}H-thymidine. Maximal proliferation rates occur when all the cells in a population are undergoing synchronized proliferation and correspond to the relative time, that is about 30 percent, cells spend in S phase. To measure a suicide index higher than 30 percent implies that a cell population is spending relatively more time in the S phase of the cycle. Growth factor-dependent erythroid cell lines undergo a cycle characterized by a long S phase and a very short G1 phase when growing in the presence of EPO (Shimada et al., 1993; Dolznig et al., 1995). However, the relationship between EPO and cell cycle progression during erythroid differentiation might be more complicated because only cell lines with a prolongation of the G1 phase of the cycle in response to EPO (Carroll et al., 1995), become committed to erythroid differentiation (Liboi et al., 1993). On the other hand, erythroblasts exposed to a high EPO are arrested in G2 (Fibach and Rachmilewitz, 1993).

Although all committed erythroid progenitors are at least partially dependent on EPO for proliferation and differentiation in vitro (Migliaccio G et al., 1988; Migliaccio, G et al., 1990b), most primitive BFU-e and most intermediate stage BFU-e in vivo are insensitive to endogenous levels of EPO (Adamson, 1968). Thus, with sustained anemia in experimental animals the frequency and cell cycle characteristics (15 percent to 20 percent in S phase) of the more primitive BFU-e are unaltered. Simultaneously the number and cycling characteristics of more mature BFU-e and the numbers of CFU-e are increased three to six times the control value (Adamson, 1968). Similarly, reduction of endogenous EPO levels by physiologic manipulations, such as hypertransfusion, results in a substantial decline in the numbers of mature BFU-e and especially CFU-e, with no effect on the number of primitive BFU-e.

EPO triggers its biological effect by binding to a specific receptor present on the cell membrane (D'Andrea et al., 1989; Jones et al., 1990). EPO-R numbers on cells of the erythroid lineage correlate with the corresponding in vitro responsiveness to EPO. BFU-e express approximately 25 to 55 high-affinity EPO binding sites per cell, while CFU-e and proerythroblasts have 300 to 400 high-affinity sites (Sawada et al., 1988; Landschulz et al., 1989; Broudy et al., 1991). Following several divisions of the CFU-e, EPO-R numbers decline and they are virtually absent on late normoblasts and reticulocytes. The increased expression of EPO-R on erythroid cells with the progression of differentiation contrasts with the declining number of receptors of early-acting growth factors such as SCF (Papayannopoulou et al., 1991; Katayama et al., 1993; Orlic et al., 1995; de Jong et al., 1997; Kimura et al., 1997) or IL-3 (Park et al., 1989; Ashihara et al., 1997; McKinstry et al., 1997) on these cells. Beyond the erythroid cells, EPO receptor expression has been found in cells of the megakaryocytic lineage (Fraser et al., 1989) and in endothelial cells (Anagnostou et al., 1994). Erythroid- and myeloid-specific EPO-R mRNA encoding soluble forms of EPO-R have been recently isolated by reverse transcriptase (RT)-PCR (Barron et al., 1994). These mRNAs are expressed at high levels in normal bone marrow stromal cells and may be involved in establishing erythroid or myeloid permissive environments by modulating the local EPO concentrations within the bone marrow (Broxmeyer et al., 1983). Also, two forms of Epo-R, a full-length (EpoR-F) and a truncated form (EpoR-T) are expressed in erythroid cells (Shimizu et al., 1999). Whereas the EpoR-F is predominant in more mature cells, the truncated form (EpoR-T) has been shown in mice to act as a dominant negative regulator of EpoR-F mediated signals (Nakamura et al., 1998), possibly modulating anti-apoptotic or proliferation events depending on EPO levels. Furthermore, a special relationship between the EpoR and SCF has been documented in cell lines genetically engineered to express c-kit. These cells do not proliferate in the presence of SCF unless they are co-transfected with erythropoietin receptors (Wu et al., 1995b). In the doubly transected cell lines c-kit and EPO receptors are closely associated on the cell membrane, and EPO-R becomes phosphorylated upon stimulation with SCF, the kit ligand. It would appear, therefore, that SCF may trigger amplification of the erythroid progenitor cell compartment by establishing a specific interaction with EPO receptor.

ONTOGENY OF ERYTHROPOIESIS

The ontogenetic development of the human erythroid system encompasses a series of well-coordinated events in embryonic and early fetal life (Kelemen et al., 1979; Moore, 1982). Although the timing of these changes is distinct for each species, parallel changes apply to all mammals. Developmental aspects of erythropoiesis are discussed in Chapter 2.

The first detectable hematopoietic cells in the human embryo are found in the yolk sac at 3 to 4 weeks of gestation (Kelemen and Janossa, 1980). Macrophages are first seen and soon afterwards, many primitive erythroblasts are present. Both are derived from extra embryonic mesoderm (Kelemen and Janossa, 1980). They are released into newly formed vascular channels from 4 weeks onward. Blood circulation is incomplete until 6 weeks of gestation when the heart is formed (Kelemen et al., 1979; Moore, 1982). After 6 weeks, yolk sac erythropoiesis declines and the liver becomes the main hematopoietic organ (Migliaccio, G et al., 1986). At 5 weeks, the only hematopoietic cells detectable in the liver rudiment are the yolk sac megaloblasts present in the sinusoids (Petti et al., 1985). However, some blastlike cells and mesenchymal cells are present in the liver parenchyma. By 6 weeks, many macrophages found most frequently within the sinusoidal walls are observed. At 7 to 8 weeks erythroid cells are first detected in the liver parenchyma within the sinusoidal walls. These cells are initially organized in discrete nests of definitive erythroblasts, but are rapidly expanded to colonize the rest of the parenchyma. Definitive erythroblasts are not released into the circulation until after the 8th week (Peschle et al., 1985). Until then all the circulating red cells are the yolk sac-derived megaloblasts. Besides erythroid cells, which predominate in the liver parenchyma, macrophages, granulocytes, and megakaryocytes begin to appear (Migliaccio, G et al., 1986).

Cultures from different hematopoietic sites during ontogeny have provided additional insights into the ontogeny of erythropoiesis and hematopoiesis. Cultures of yolk sac cells generate colonies of differ-

ent hematopoietic lineages (Muench et al., 1994; Migliaccio, G et al., 1986). Thus, small CFU-e-like colonies, consisting of embryonic erythroblasts with brilliant red color (Stamatoyannopoulos et al., 1987), or larger colonies of mixed type containing both erythroid and nonerythroid components (Muench et al., 1994) are present. Myeloid or megakaryocytic colonies are also seen. The small CFU-e-like colonies appearing early in culture are composed of primitive erythroblasts (Stamatoyannopoulos et al., 1987), whereas the rest of the colonies are the progeny of definitive progenitors present in yolk sac (Peschle et al., 1984; Stamatoyannopoulos et al., 1987; see also Fig. 3.2). Adult hemoglobin is synthesized by erythroid cells in these colonies in the mouse (Keller et al., 1993). The picture of yolk sac cells in culture generating both primitive and definitive erythropoiesis contrasts with the primitive erythropoiesis

Figure 3.2. Erythropoiesis during human ontogeny. Diagram of the anatomic sites (indicated in red) of erythropoiesis and the corresponding globin patterns (bottom) of erythroid cells during development. Globin patterns expressed by erythroid cells in vivo, or by the erythroid progeny of BFU-e in vitro. Note that in yolk sac the in vivo pattern reflects that of primitive erythroblasts, whereas in vitro it is that of the erythroid progeny of definitive lineage BFU-e. In fetal liver stages, the in vivo and in vitro patterns are stable and show minor differences. In the adult stage, the reactivation of fetal globin synthesis under in vitro conditions is shown. The globin pattern expressed by progenitor cells from cord blood is intermediate between those of fetal and adult cells. A tendency for increase in HbA synthesis in vitro has been found, as the in vitro pattern reflects the globin program of progenitors further along in their switch than the red cells present in vivo. For full color reproduction, see color plate 3.2.

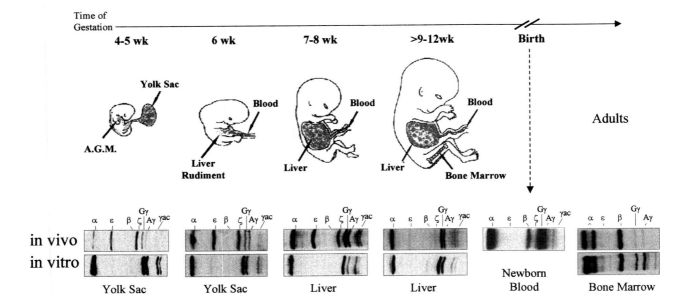

that is solely expressed in vivo (Fig. 3.2). Whether both primitive and definitive cells are derived from a single progenitor is currently debated. A common progenitor for both primitive and definitive erythroid cells has been detected by in vitro cultures of embryonic stem (ES) cells (Kennedy et al., 1997). However, no single cells producing both primitive and definitive progeny in vitro have been isolated and opposing views have been published (Nakano et al., 1996). Furthermore, whether definitive progenitors are generated in situ, in the yolk sac, or migrate from intraembryonic sites, is also debatable (Keller et al., 1999). Early work has shown the autonomous presence of definitive progenitors in the yolk sac (Weissman et al., 1977, 1978; Huang and Auerbach, 1993). However, recent studies have shown that definitive hematopoietic stem cells capable of reconstituting multiple lineages in sublethally irradiated adult recipients are first detected within the intraembryonic aorta-gonad-mesonephros region (AGM) (see Chapter 2) and not in the yolk sac (Medvinsky et al., 1993; Rich, 1995). In vitro generation of definitive progenitors by undifferentiated primordial cells contained in these sites provided convincing evidence

for the presence of intraembryonically generated stem cells (Medvinsky and Dzierzak, 1996; Mukouyama et al., 1998). Whether these migrate subsequently to the yolk sac or the yolk sac cells are generated in situ, remains currently an open question (Fig. 3.3). This debate was recently revived when definitive stem cells were found in high concentrations in yolk sac as early as 9 to 10 days post coitus (dpc) and could reconstitute multiple lineages in conditioned newborn recipient mice (Yoder et al., 1997; Yoder and Hiatt, 1997). Thus, the observation that the yolk sac stem cells were unable to colonize adult recipients (Medvinsky et al., 1993) suggests that it was not the absence of these cells but the requirements of a specific environment for their homing and development that was vital.

When human fetal liver cells are used for cultures, all types of progenitor cells (Rowley et al., 1978; Hassan et al., 1979; Peschle et al., 1981; Hann et al., 1983) can be detected. From 6 weeks p.c. and from 12 weeks p.c. are also found in the developing bone marrow (Hann et al., 1983). In the liver, the number of progenitor cells doubles almost every other day to meet the hematopoietic needs of an exponentially growing fetus (see Fig. 3.4). Although progenitor cells with the potential to differentiate along all types of hematopoietic lineages are clearly present in the fetal liver (Rowley et al., 1978; Hassan et al., 1979; Peschle et al., 1981; Hann et al., 1983), differentiation in this organ in vivo is primarily erythroid (Migliaccio, G et al., 1986). Definitive hematopoietic stem cells (HSC) persist in the liver, however, during adult life. In fact, limited numbers of definitive HSC can be purified from adult liver of the mouse (Taniguchi et al., 1996) and hematopoietic chimerism is occasionally associated with liver transplantation in humans (Nagler et al., 1994).

Figure 3.3. Current models of ontogeny of hematopoiesis. Early mesodermally derived cells with both endothelial and hematopoietic potential have been described using cells from yolk sac or intraembryonic sites. Although yolk sac harbors cells giving rise to primitive erythroblasts in vivo, as well as definitive progenitors giving rise to differentiated definitive cells in vitro, AGM contains only definitive lineage multipotent progenitors. Evidence from embryonic stem (ES) cell differentiation in vitro suggests that a single colony can give rise to both definitive and primitive erythroid cells. However, other data and the molecular requirements of primitive cells suggest otherwise. The surface phenotype of definitive progenitors in AGM, FL, and adult bone marrow is shown.

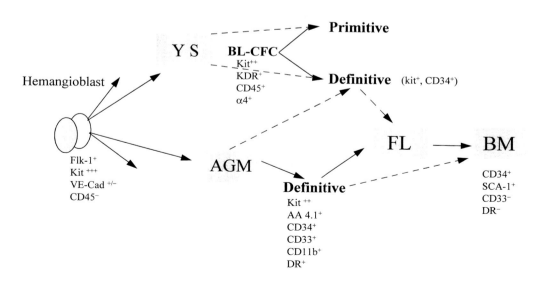

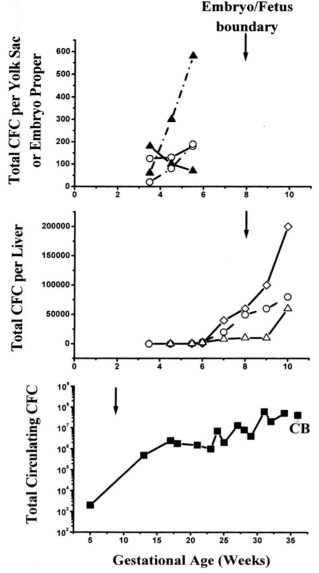

Figure 3.4. Total number of definitive progenitor cells present in the embryo proper (---) and in the yolk sac (—) [top panel], in the liver (middle panel) or circulating in the blood (bottom panel) during human ontogeny. The values of definitive CFU-GEEMM (○), of HPP-CFC (△, ▲) and of CFU-e (◇) are presented separately for FL and YS, but the values of CFU-GEEMM and HPPC (■) were pooled for fetal blood. (Modified from Migliaccio, G et al., 1986 and Eddleman et al., 1996, with permission. The fetal data are from A.R. Migliaccio, unpublished observation, calculated according to the average fetal blood volume reported in Zhang and Bowes, 1995.)

Presence of definitive multilineage progenitors in the AGM long before development of the liver is established (Huyhn et al., 1995) is also associated with the appearance of CD34+ cells in this area (Tavian et al., 1996). Whether definitive progenitors present in AGM and later in fetal liver have different characteristics

(i.e., expression of CD34+ or Sca-1 or AA4.1 in the murine model, see Fig. 3.3) than the definitive cells present in yolk sac cannot be determined as conflicting data are available (Marcos et al., 1997; Wood et al., 1997; Petrenko et al., 1999).

Little is known about the early development of the fetal bone marrow. Progenitor cells (Hann et al., 1983) and hematopoietic CD34+ cells (Charbord et al., 1996) have been detected in the marrow as early as 12 weeks p.c. Similar numbers of CD34+ cells and progenitor cells are present within the bone marrow and the fetal liver at the same gestational age (Wilpshaar et al., 1998). In contrast to fetal bone marrow, however, much more is known about the composition of progenitor cells circulating in fetal blood (Tchernia et al., 1981; Linch et al., 1982; Eddleman et al., 1996; Shields and Andrews, 1998). This is due to easier blood access for diagnostic purposes (Hohlfield et al., 1994).

CD34+ cells represent about 30 percent of the cells in the lymphocyte gate of fetal and perinatal blood when fluorescence-activated cell sorting (FACS) is used (Table 3.3). Further, the 1 percent to 2 percent frequency of CD34+/CD38− cells in fetal-neonatal blood is comparable to the frequency of these cells in adult bone marrow and is 100-fold higher than their frequency in adult blood (Eddleman et al., 1996; Shields and Andrews, 1998). Thus, in contrast to adult blood, it is not surprising that progenitor cells can be detected by culturing directly very small quantities of fetal perinatal blood (Eddleman et al., 1996). Most progenitor cells detected in fetal-neonatal blood are very immature, because they lead to mixed erythroid/myelomonocytic/megakaryocytic colonies, usually composed of more than 5,000 cells and visible to the naked eye (Table 3.4). When cells from these colonies are replated, they can generate secondary mixed colonies in secondary culture plates (Eaves, 1993; Migliaccio, AR et al., 1994). By contrast, only a few progenitor cells producing pure erythroid colonies (day 10 BFU-e) or small erythroid colonies (CFU-e) and myelomonocytic colonies (day 8 CFU-GM) are detected (Table 3.4). As the number of progenitors present in adult blood is too low to be detected by directly plating a small amount of blood, comparison of progenitor frequency between adult and fetal-neonatal blood has to rely on findings that use mononuclear cells containing most of the progenitor cells. The mononuclear fraction of neonatal and fetal cord blood contains at least ten times more progenitor cells of all types than the corresponding fraction of the adult blood (370 ± 123 vs. 17 to 40 CFU-C/10^5 mononuclear cells, respectively) (Lu et al., 1993; Migliaccio, AR et al., 1994). While most progenitor cells in the fetal-neonatal fraction generate large mixed colonies, in adult blood, either pure erythroid colonies

Table 3.4. Progenitor Cell Content in Unfractionated Blood at Different Ontogenetic Stages

	Number of colonies* ± SEM per ml of blood			
	BFU-e	HPP/GM	GEEMM	Total
Fetal blood* (13–30 wk)	500 ± 100 (4%)	14,700 ± 200 (74%)	3,500 ± 800 (22%)	18,000 ± 1,600 (100)
Cord blood (at birth)	2,700 ± 100 (7%)	26,100 ± 500 (61%)	12,200 ± 200 (32%)	40,900 ± 600 (100)
Infant blood (3 mo old)	[130] (16%)	[650] (78%)	[50] (6%)	[830] (100)
Adult blood	[1,120 ± 200] (62%)	[587±166] (32%)	[106 ± 80] (6)	[1,813 ± 446] (100)

* Colony growth was measured in FBS-supplemented (40%) cultures stimulated with SCF, IL-3, G-CSF, G-CSF, and EPO. The values in parentheses represent the relative distribution (in percent) of each progenitor among the total number of progenitor cells. The values for fetal and cord blood were obtained by culturing directly aliquots of whole blood. The values for neonatal and adult blood, in brackets, are calculated from cultures of mononuclear cells on the basis of the mononuclear cell recovery per given volume of blood. Note that the majority of the myelomonocytic colonies detected from fetal/cord blood and from infant and adult blood were HPP or GM colonies, respectively.

Modified from Migliaccio, G. et al, 1996.

(BFU-e) or myeloid (CFU-GM) colonies are found with far fewer CFU-Mix cells (Table 3.4).

Throughout ontogeny the number of progenitor cells circulating in the fetal blood remains very high (Fig. 3.4). It has been calculated that at any given time, approximately the same number of progenitor cells is present in the liver, in the bone marrow, and in the blood (Eaves, 1993; Wilpshaar et al., 1998). For example, at 17 weeks of gestation, about 5×10^6 progenitor cells are present in any one of these tissues. The number of progenitor cells circulating in the blood (Fig. 3.4) sharply decreases 24 hours after birth (Li et al., 1999) and continues to decline with age in adults (Egusa et al., 1998). At birth, one-third the progenitor cells of a fetus are present in the blood and, since half the fetal blood is in the cord and in the placenta, one-sixth of all the progenitor cells of a fetus are also discarded at birth. These considerations have prompted the collection of blood from the cord and the placenta after the delivery (Rubinstein et al., 1995) and its use as an alternative source of stem cells for related and unrelated transplantation (Rubinstein et al., 1993; Cairo and Wagner, 1997). The success of the transplants with cord blood (Rubinstein et al., 1998), the high progenitor cell content in fetal blood at all ages (Fig. 3.4), and the simplicity of its collection make the use of fetal blood a valuable resource for stem cells for transplantation and for purposes of gene therapy.

DISTINCT FEATURES OF FETAL AND ADULT ERYTHROPOIESIS

Besides their development within a distinct anatomic site, progenitors developing in the fetal liver display a composite phenotypic and functional profile, which is unlike their adult counterparts (Table 3.5). Unique cell cycling rates (Peschle et al., 1981), kinetics of

proliferation and differentiation in culture (Lansdorp et al., 1993), sensitivity to different growth factors (Migliaccio and Migliaccio, 1988; Emerson et al., 1989; Zandstra et al., 1998), and activation of a set of different globin genes (Stamatoyannopoulos and Nienhuis, 1987) distinguish fetal from adult erythroid cells. Differences in the transplantation potential of fetal and adult stem cells (Zanjani et al., 1992; Harrison et al., 1997; Hogan et al., 1997) and of their respective hematopoietic microenvironments have also been documented. In vivo and in vitro differences between fetal and adult erythropoiesis include the following.

Globin Synthesis Patterns

Globin gene expression in erythroid cells during the different stages of ontogeny represents one of the best studied differences between erythroid cells from the various ontogenetic stages (Stamatoyannopoulos and Nienhuis, 1987). Detailed time-related switches in globin synthetic profiles have been described (see Fig. 3.2). Erythroid cells in the yolk sac synthesize mainly embryonic hemoglobins, such as Gower I, Gower II, and hemoglobin Portland (see Chapter 9) (Peschle et al., 1984; Stamatoyannopoulos et al., 1987). These hemoglobins are likely synthesized sequentially, suggesting an early switch between the two α-like chains from ζ- to α-globin chain, followed by a switch between the two β-like chains, from ε- to β-globin chain. Although both switches begin during the embryonic stage of erythropoiesis, they are completed during the early stages of fetal liver hematopoiesis (Peschle et al., 1985; Stamatoyannopoulos et al., 1987). Thus, early embryonic erythroblasts of the yolk sac contain only embryonic globins and do not coexpress any adult globin chains (Stamatoyannopoulos et al., 1987a). As

Table 3.5. Differences Among Fetal, Neonatal, and Adult Hematopoietic Stem and Progenitor Cells*

Cell characteristics	Fetal cells	Neonatal cells	Adult cells
LTR:STR in vivo*	1:2.5–8.9	n.d.	1:0.8–1.14
hSRU in NOD/SCID mice	High	High	Low
	hGF-independent	hGF-independent	hGF-dependent
hSRU in fetal sheep	High	High	Low
Average telomere length (CD34+ cells)	12.8 ± 0.35 kb	12.3 ± 0.4 kb	8.4 ± 0.3 kb
Expansion potential	High	High	Low
	1–2 GF-dependent	2–3 GF-dependent	3–4 GF-dependent
Frequency (LTC-IC/bcc/ CFU-Mix)	High	High	Low
CFC in circulation	High	High	Low
CFC			
% in cycle	High	High	Low
Doubling time	20 ± 2 h	26 ± 2 h	32 ± 2 h
Time to terminal diff.	10 d	14 d	16 d
BFU-e			
Response to EPO	100%	30–60%	1–3%
Response to KL	100%	10–30%	1–3%
Inhibition by IFN-γ	0	n.d.	80–100%
Surface phenotype (CD34+ cells)			
CD117 (c-kit)	+++	++	+
HLA-DR	++	+	+/–
CD33	++	+/–	–
CD38⁻	(++)	–	–
$\alpha_2\beta_1$	++	n.d.	+/–

Abbreviations: hSRU, human SCID repopulating units; CFC, progenitor cell of all types.
* Ratio between long-term repopulating (LTR) and short-term repopulating (STR) in vivo.

erythropoiesis moves to fetal liver, a subset of erythroblasts expresses both embryonic and fetal globins (Peschle et al., 1984; Stamatoyannopoulos et al., 1987a). Embryonic erythroblasts have a unique morphology and size and at their final stages do not extrude their nucleus, remaining nucleated like amphibians or avian erythroid cells.

Fetal hemoglobin is the major hemoglobin synthesized during fetal life and a small amount of HbA is also present (Fig. 3.2). This pattern remains stable until about the 30th week of fetal life when there is a progressive increase in adult hemoglobin and a parallel slow decline in fetal hemoglobin until birth. At birth, approximately equal amounts of adult and fetal hemoglobin are synthesized (Fig. 3.2). The final adult erythroid hemoglobin pattern of HbA and less than 1 percent HbF is not reached until several months after birth. The switch from fetal to adult hemoglobin is accomplished through changing programs within the same population of cells and does not involve gradual changes in cell populations (Stamatoyannopoulos et al., 1987b). Unrelated to birth, it is strictly related to gestational age. Switches in globin gene activity have been attributed to formation and activation of specific transcriptional complexes within cells at specific stages of ontogeny (Fraser and Grosveld, 1998). These selective transcriptional forces could dictate differences in globin gene activity; however, the detailed molecular mechanisms involved remain elusive. Globin gene switching is discussed in Chapter 7.

In vivo patterns of globin chain synthesis of erythroid cells at different ontogenetic stages are largely reproduced in vitro, in semisolid or suspension cultures in the presence of appropriate growth factors (Fig. 3.2). Deviations from in vivo patterns include enhancement of HbF when adult cells are cultured under specific culture conditions or of adult hemoglobin with cord blood cell cultures, in which the globin program of progenitor cells further advanced in their switching is expressed (Constantoulakis et al., 1990; Migliaccio, AR et al., 1990a).

Fetal liver progenitors are more stable in their globin patterns and generate in vitro progeny that synthesizes mostly HbF like the differentiated erythroid cells in vivo, and this pattern is not influenced by culture conditions (Papayannopoulou et al., 1982). Only minor variations, such as some increase in HbA, are seen with time in culture. The stable pattern of fetal globin synthesis characterizing the fetal erythroid cells can be reproduced by fusion of fetal erythroblasts to adult origin murine erythroid cells (Papayannopoulou et al., 1986a). Such heterospecific hybrid cells upon induction continue to execute their predominantly fetal program within the adult erythroid environment. Although late progenitors and erythroblasts display stable programs, stem cells, when educated under different environments, such as an adult environment, may behave differently. Thus, adult stem cells injected into mouse blastocysts and implanted in pregnant mice could direct the synthesis of embryonic hemoglobins during the yolk sac stage of hematopoiesis in the developing mouse (Geiger et al., 1998), suggesting some facultative plasticity in globin programs of stem cells. Rigorous proof, however, of donor-type embryonic globin within morphologically identified embryonic erythroblasts is lacking. Furthermore, in the frog it has been shown that within a narrow window of time, cells from the dorsal lateral plate (DLP), the equivalent of intraembryonic site AGM of definitive stem cell generation, can differentiate into either embryonic or definitive progenitors, depending on the environment in which they are implanted (Turpen et al., 1997). Unfortunately, no human data exist about long-term erythroid repopulation by fetal stem cells. Although observations during the first 2 months following transplantation suggest that fetal progenitors synthesize typically fetal globin patterns (Papayannopoulou et al., 1986b), evidence from permanent erythroid reconstitution by fetal stem cells has not been documented (O'Reilly et al., 1984).

Proliferation/Cell Cycle Kinetics

Fetal progenitors in vitro have distinct kinetics of proliferation and differentiation (Table 3.5). Their average doubling time is about 20 hours compared with 32 hours for the adult cells (Peschle et al., 1981). Because of this, they reach terminal maturation and optimal size much earlier in culture than adult cells under the same conditions (Peschle et al., 1981). Their replicative potential, defined as the ability of progenitors to form a certain colony size in vitro, is also higher and is reached earlier in culture (Peschle et al., 1981). Fetal progenitors also seem to undergo a limited number of self-replicative divisions and cells from primary colonies can be replated in secondary cultures that in turn can generate tertiary colonies with the same wide spectrum of phenotypes (Lu et al., 1993; Migliaccio, G et al., 1996). Serum deprived fetal CD34+ cells stimulated with SCF and IL-3 can be replated 3 to 4 times in culture. Similar colonies raised from adult cells under identical conditions can be replated only once (Migliaccio, G et al., 1996). Each high proliferative potential (HPP) colony from fetal progenitors can generate another 150 CFU-Mix in secondary cultures. Self-replicating divisions occur during the first 10 days early in culture but similar divisions in adult cells happen during the third week in culture.

Although details about hematopoietic regulation within the fetal liver microenvironment are lacking, abundant evidence suggests that this environment exerts distinct regulation compared with the adult environment. Most of this evidence derives from mice with targeted ablation of certain transcriptional factors or other molecules that have shown that fetal liver hematopoiesis is unaffected at a time when bone marrow hematopoiesis, either prenatally or after birth, is largely abrogated. For example, mice with ablation of transcriptional factor TEL show normal embryonic erythropoiesis and normal in vitro colony formation from definitive progenitors, both in the yolk sac and intraembryonic sites, but die at 11.5 dpc because of failure to maintain a developing vascular network (Wang et al., 1997). In chimeric mice, however, although TEL is dispensable for fetal liver hematopoiesis, it is specifically required for bone marrow hematopoiesis as early as the immediate postnatal period (Wang et al., 1998). Apparently TEL −/− progenitors exit the fetal liver, migrate, and home, but fail to colonize the bone marrow microenvironment. Therefore, TEL −/− cells are cell autonomous in their inability to interact with bone marrow microenvironment. Analogous results have been obtained with PU-1 −/− animals, in which erythroid and megakaryocytic lineage within the fetal liver was not affected, but myeloid lineage and subsequent development and establishment of adult bone marrow hematopoiesis is largely abolished (Scott et al., 1997; Fisher et al., 1999). Not only differences in specific sites but within specific lineages developed in these sites have been documented. Furthermore, mice that are lacking stromal cell derived factor 1 (SDF-1), or its receptor, CXCR-4, in hematopoietic cells show impairment of bone marrow hematopoiesis (Zucali et al., 1975; Nagasawa et al., 1996). Detailed evaluation of chimeric mice with CXCR4 −/− cells suggest that this factor is not as important for the homing of early progenitors as for the expansion and retainment of intermediate precursors within the marrow (Kawabata et al., 1999; Ma et al., 1999). Other examples with specific impact on the adult bone marrow environment are the Nrf-1 (Chan et al., 1998), and the jumonji (Kitajima et al., 1999) or the tenascin-C (Ohta et al., 1998) knockouts, which show more quantitative reduction rather than ablation of bone marrow hematopoiesis.

One of the most intriguing questions is how erythropoiesis is favored in fetal liver and why it is suppressed at the later stages. Apart from intrinsic differences in fetal cells or their adhesive interactions with their environment alluded to above, hormonal differences between fetal liver and bone marrow could play a role. Whereas the adult kidney is the main EPO-synthesizing organ, the liver is the predominant source of EPO in the fetus (Koury et al., 1991), although the kidney also contributes (Moritz et al., 1997). It is unclear whether EPO levels produced in the fetus are higher than in adults and some studies suggest that EPO levels are lower in the fetus (Forestier et al., 1991). Either EPO is more efficient at stimulating erythropoiesis during fetal development, or synergy with other factors is important. In this context, it is notable that SCF/kit is expressed by hepatic cells surrounding hematopoietic cells providing a more favorable environment for erythropoiesis compared to bone marrow (Fujio et al., 1994, 1996).

Hepatocyte growth factor (HGF) stimulates erythroid colonies in vitro in synergy with kit ligand (Galimi et al., 1994). HGF receptor mRNA is highly expressed in embryonic erythroid cells and in the embryonic liver of the mouse (Galimi et al., 1994). Thrombopoietin or activin, the latter formed by the placenta, could also potentiate the effect of EPO on BFU-e and CFU-e formation (Yu et al., 1981; Era et al., 1997). The IGF family of factors could also contribute to this effect. But why is erythropoiesis suppressed in the liver during the later stages? The switch from the erythroid to the hepatic phase of the fetal liver may be mediated by oncostatin-M (Kinoshita et al., 1999), which is produced by CD45$^-$ hematopoietic cells in the developing liver, while its receptor is predominantly expressed by hepatocytes (Kamiya et al., 1999). In contrast to the stimulatory function of oncostatin-M on hematopoietic cells of the AGM region (Mukouyama et al., 1998), oncostatin-M inhibits the growth of hematopoietic progenitors from fetal liver (Kinoshita et al., 1999). Nevertheless, mice that do not express gp-130, one of the common subunits for oncostatin-M, IL-6, and LIF receptor (Yoshida et al., 1996), display defects in maturation of the hepatocytes and decreased erythropoiesis, perhaps as an indirect result of improper liver development. Increasing glucocorticoid concentrations in fetal liver near term may also exert an effect on the suppression of erythropoiesis (Moritz et al., 1997). Removal of the pituitary by the decapitation of rat fetuses resulted in increased liver erythropoiesis at day 21 compared with controls (Moritz et al., 1997). Similar results were found in fetuses of bilaterally adrenalectomized mice treated with cortisol. These findings suggest that in sheep fetuses, increasing levels of glucocorticoids in the liver may decrease hepatic erythropoiesis.

Hematopoietic cells have their permanent home in the bone marrow. Bone marrow stroma is the best understood of all sites that support hematopoiesis. Five stages are recognized during the development of the complex marrow structure necessary for colonization and support of hematopoiesis (Charbord et al., 1996). In the first stage (stage one: 6.6 to 8.5 gestational weeks) the cartilagenous rudiments are formed and CD34$^+$ endothelial cells are observed in the perichondral mesenchyme. Stages two and three (8.5 to 10.5 weeks) are characterized by active chondrolysis and formation of a vascular bed without detectable hematopoiesis. At mid-diaphysis, however, specific structures are beginning to be formed and

consist of small chambers of connective tissue, framed by a loose network of CD45$^-$ cells organized around an arteriole and separated from the surrounding sinus by a lining of CD34$^+$ endothelial cells. Finally, at stage four (10.5 to 15 weeks) the first hematopoietic cells consisting of CD15$^+$ myelocytes and very rare glycophorin positive immature erythroblasts are recognized. These specific structures are transient and are not recognized from 16 weeks onward (stage five) when the organization of the long bones is complete with fully calcified areas interspersed with areas of dense hematopoiesis (Charbord et al., 1996). Granulopoiesis predominates during all the stages of bone marrow development.

The bone marrow microenvironment and its extracellular matrix have been the subject of recent reviews (Torok-Storb, 1988; Long, 1992; Klein, 1995; Yoder and Williams, 1995; Papayannopoulou and Craddock, 1997; Furusawa, et al., 1998). Only differences concerning hematopoietic cell regulation within bone marrow compared with the fetal liver environment will be emphasized here. Bone formation and the establishment of bone architecture precede the appearance of hematopoietic cells within the bone marrow and seem important for their development. This has been documented in experiments using ectopic transplantation of marrow, where remodeling of bone has been observed, followed by the ability to support hematopoietic cells (Eaves and Eaves, 1978). A major difference between bone marrow and fetal liver erythropoiesis is the preferential differentiation and presence of progenitors of the granulomonocytic lineage in the bone marrow in contrast to fetal liver (Hann et al., 1983). As other areas of hematopoiesis, such as yolk sac, AGM, and fetal liver, do not produce G-CSF and GM-CSF (Azoulay et al., 1987; Metcalf et al., 1995), cytokines important for myeloid differentiation, it is believed that their presence within the bone marrow is instrumental for the further development of granulomonocytic cells. Partial reconstruction of several stromal elements and extracellular matrix in vitro is believed to be present in murine long-term culture systems that support hematopoiesis for several months (Dexter, 1979) and in the human long-term culture systems that support hematopoiesis for several weeks (Hocking and Golde, 1980). Transplantation experiments in mice have also shown that the expression of hematopoietic cell cytoadhesion molecules and their counter-receptors on the marrow microenvironment are important for engraftment (Hardy, 1995; Yoder and Williams, 1995; Papayannopoulou and Craddock, 1997). According to this line of evidence, the integrin and its endothelial ligand VCAM-1, in cooperation with selectins, play a major role in bone marrow homing of hematopoietic cells

(Papayannopoulou et al. 1995; Mazo, et al., 1998; Frenette, et al., 1998). Emerging information from xenotransplantation models—SCID/NOD mouse or the fetal sheep for human cells—also points to the importance of these molecules for homing of human cells (Zanjani et al., 1999). In addition, in the SCID/NOD model the importance of the receptor, CXCR4, for engraftment has been emphasized (Peled et al., 1999). As human CD34+ cells respond chemotactically to SDF-1, it may not be surprising that SDF-1/CXCR4 −/− mice show no maintenance of hematopoiesis in the marrow (Zucali et al., 1975; Nagasawa et al., 1996), pointing to the SDF-1 as the major factor for anchoring hematopoietic cells and keeping them within the marrow microenvironment (Kawabata et al., 1999; Ma et al., 1999).

Many questions regarding the migration and colonization of transfused cells to the bone marrow remain to be clarified. Discrepancies between in vitro and in vivo data exist and limitations of gene knock-out studies in mice also exist. Bone marrow microenvironment is a complex structure and the cooperation among many signaling molecules and their receptors modulate its function.

References

Adamson, JW. (1968). The erythropoietin-hematocrit relationship in normal and polycythemic man: Implications of marrow regulation. *Blood* 32: 597–609.

Akahane, K, Tojo, A, Urabe, A, and Takaku, F. (1987). Pure erythropoietic colony and burst formations in serum-free culture and their enhancement by insulin-like growth factor I. *Exp. Hematol.* 15: 797–802.

Anagnostou, A, Liu, Z, Steiner, M et al. (1994). Erythropoietin receptor mRNA expression in human endothelial cells. *Proc. Natl. Acad. Sci. U.S.A.* 91: 3974.

Andrews, RG, Singer, JW, and Bernstein, ID. (1986). Monoclonal antibody 12-8 recognizes a 115-kd molecule present on both unipotent and multipotent hematopoietic colony-forming cells and their precursors. *Blood* 67: 842–845.

Andrews, RG, Singer, JW, and Bernstein, ID. (1989). Precursors of colony-forming cells in humans can be distinguished from colony-forming cells by expression of the CD33 and CD34 antigens and light scatter properties. *J. Exp. Med.* 169: 1721–1731.

Ashihara, E, Vannucchi, AM, Migliaccio, G, and Migliaccio, AR. (1997). Growth factor receptor expression during in vitro differentiation of partially purified populations containing murine stem cells. *J. Cell. Physiol.* 171: 343–356.

Azoulay, M, Webb, CG, and Sachs, L. (1987). Control of hematopoietic cell growth regulators during mouse fetal development. *Mol. Cell. Biol.* 7: 3361–3364.

Barker, JE and Starr, E. (1991). Characterization of spleen colonies derived from mice with mutations at the W locus. *J. Cell. Physiol.* 149: 451–458.

Barron, C, Migliaccio, AR, Migliaccio, G, Jiang, Y et al. (1994). Alternatively spliced mRNAs encoding soluble isoforms of the erythropoietin receptor in murine cell lines and bone marrow. *Gene* 147: 263–268.

Berenson, RJ, Bensinger, WI, Hill, RS et al. (1991). Engraftment after infusion of CD34+ marrow cells in patients with breast cancer or neuroblastoma. *Blood* 77: 1717–1722.

Besmer, P. (1991). The kit ligand encoded at the murine Steel locus: A pleiotropic growth and differentiation factor. *Curr. Opin. Cell Biol.* 3: 939–946.

Bhatia, M, Bonnet, D, Murdoch, B et al. (1998). A newly discovered class of human hematopoietic cells with SCID-repopulating activity [see comments]. *Nat. Med.* 4: 1038–1045.

Bol, SJL. (1980). The recognition of early developmental stages in haematopoiesis. University of Delft, The Netherlands.

Broudy, VC. (1997). Stem cell factor and hematopoiesis. *Blood* 90: 1345–1364.

Broudy, VC, Lin, N, Brice, M et al. (1991). Erythropoietin receptor characteristics on primary human erythroid cells. *Blood* 77: 2583–2590.

Broudy, VC, Lin, NL, Priestley, GV et al. (1996). Interaction of stem cell factor and its receptor c-kit mediates lodgment and acute expansion of hematopoietic cells in the murine spleen. *Blood* 88: 75–81.

Broxmeyer, HE, Lu, L, Platzer, E et al. (1983). Comparative analysis of the influences of human gamma, alpha and beta interferons on human multipotential (CFU-GEMM), erythroid (BFU-E) and granulocyte-macrophage (CFU-GM) progenitor cells. *J. Immunol.* 131: 1300–1305.

Cairo, MS and Wagner, JE. (1997). Placental and/or umbilical cord blood: An alternative source of hematopoietic stem cells for transplantation. *Blood* 90: 4665–4678.

Carroll, M, Zhu, Y, and D'Andrea, AD. (1995). Erythropoietin-induced cellular differentiation requires prolongation of the G1 phase of the cell cycle. *Proc. Natl. Acad. Sci. U.S.A.* 92: 2869–2873.

Chan, JY, Kwong, M, Lu, R et al. (1998). Targeted disruption of the ubiquitous CNC-bZIP transcription factor, Nrf-1, results in anemia and embryonic lethality in mice. *EMBO J.* 17: 1779–1787.

Charbord, P, Tavian, M, Humeau, L, and Peault, B. (1996). Early ontogeny of the human marrow from long bones: An immunohistochemical study of hematopoiesis and its microenvironment [see comments]. *Blood* 87: 4109–4119.

Cheng, J, Baumhueter, S, Cacalano, G et al. (1996). Hematopoietic defects in mice lacking the sialomucin CD34. *Blood* 87: 479–490.

Chida, D, Miura, O, Yoshimura, A, and Miyajima, A. (1999). Role of cytokine signaling molecules in erythroid differentiation of mouse fetal liver hematopoietic cells: Functional analysis of signaling molecules by retrovirus-mediated expression. *Blood* 93: 1567–1578.

Civin, CI, Strauss, LC, Brovall, C et al. (1984). Antigenic analysis of hematopoiesis. III. A hematopoietic progenitor cell surface antigen defined by a monoclonal antibody raised against KG-1a cells. *J. Immunol.* 133: 157–165.

Constantoulakis, P, Nakamoto, B, Papayannopoulou, T, and Stamatoyannopoulos, G. (1990). Fetal calf serum contains activities that induce fetal hemoglobin in adult erythroid cell cultures. *Blood* 75: 1862–1869.

Cotner, T, Gupta, AD, Papayannopoulou, T, and Stamatoyannopoulos, G. (1989). Characterization of a novel form of transferrin receptor preferentially expressed on normal erythroid progenitors and precursors. *Blood* 73: 214–221.

D'Andrea, AD, Lodish, HF, and Wong, GG. (1989). Expression cloning of the murine erythropoietin receptor. *Cell* 57: 277–285.

Dainiak, N and Kreczko, S. (1985). Interactions of insulin, insulinlike growth factor II, and platelet-derived growth factor in erythropoietic culture. *J. Clin. Invest.* 76: 1237–1242.

de Jong, MO, Westerman, Y, Wagemaker, G, and Wognum, AW. (1997). Coexpression of Kit and the receptors for erythropoietin, interleukin 6 and GM-CSF on hemopoietic cells. *Stem Cells* 15: 275–285.

Dexter, TM. (1979). Haemopoiesis in long-term bone marrow cultures. A review. *Acta Haematol.* 62: 299–305.

Dick, JE. (1996). Human stem cell assays in immune-deficient mice. *Curr. Opin. Hematol.* 3: 405–409.

Dolznig, H, Bartunek, P, Nasmyth, K, et al. (1995). Terminal differentiation of normal chicken erythroid progenitors: Shortening of G1 correlates with loss of D-cyclin/cdk4 expression and altered cell size control. *Cell Growth Differ.* 6: 1341–1352.

Eaves, CJ. (1993). Peripheral blood stem cells reach new heights [editorial; comment]. *Blood* 82: 1957–1959.

Eaves, CJ, and Eaves, AC. (1978). Erythropoietin (Ep) dose-response curves for three classes of erythroid progenitors in normal human marrow and in patients with polycythemia vera. *Blood* 52: 1196–1210.

Eddleman, KA, Chervenak, FA, George-Siegel, P, et al. (1996). Circulating hematopoietic stem cell populations in human fetuses: Implications for fetal gene therapy and alterations with in utero red cell transfusion. *Fetal Diagn. Ther.* 11: 231–240.

Edmonds, RH. (1966). Electron microscopy of erythropoiesis in the avian yolk sac. *Anat. Rec.* 154: 785–805.

Egusa, Y, Fujiwara, Y, Syahruddin, E et al. (1998). Effect of age on human peripheral blood stem cells. *Oncol. Rep.* 5: 397–400.

Emerson, SG, Thomas, S, Ferrara, JL, and Greenstein, JL. (1989). Developmental regulation of erythropoiesis by hematopoietic growth factors: Analysis on populations of BFU-E from bone marrow, peripheral blood, and fetal liver. *Blood* 74: 49–55.

Enver, T, Heyworth, CM, and Dexter, TM. (1998). Do stem cells play dice? *Blood* 92: 348–351.

Era, T, Takahashi, T, Sakai, K et al. (1997). Thrombopoietin enhances proliferation and differentiation of murine yolk sac erythroid progenitors. *Blood* 89: 1207–1213.

Fairbairn, LJ, Cowling, GJ, Reipert, BM, and Dexter, TM. (1993). Suppression of apoptosis allows differentiation and development of a multipotent hemopoietic cell line in the absence of added growth factors. *Cell* 74: 823–832.

Fauser, AA and Messner, HA. (1979). Identification of megakaryocytes, macrophages, and eosinophils in colonies of human bone marrow containing neutrophilic granulocytes and erythroblasts. *Blood* 53: 1023–1027.

Fibach, E and Rachmilewitz, EA. (1993). Stimulation of erythroid progenitors by high concentrations of erythropoietin results in normoblasts arrested in G2 phase of the cell cycle. *Exp. Hematol.* 21: 184–188.

Fisher, RC, Lovelock, JD and Scott, EW. (1999). A critical role for PU. 1 in homing and long-term engraftment by hematopoietic stem cells in the bone marrow. *Blood* 94: 1283–1290.

Fleischman, RA, Gallardo, T and Mi, X. (1996). Mutations in the ligand-binding domain of the kit receptor: An uncommon site in human piebaldism. *J Invest. Dermatol.* 107: 703–706.

Forestier, F, Daffos, F, Catherine, N et al. (1991). Developmental hematopoiesis in normal human fetal blood. *Blood* 77: 2360–2363.

Fraser, JK, Tan, AS, Lin, FK, and Berridge, MV. (1989). Expression of specific high-affinity binding sites for erythropoietin on rat and mouse megakaryocytes. *Exp. Hematol.* 17: 10–16.

Fraser, P and Grosveld, F. (1998). Locus control regions, chromatin activation and transcription. *Curr. Opin. Cell Biol.* 10: 361–365.

Frenette, PS, Subbarao, S, Mazo, IB et al. (1998). Endothelial selectins and vascular cell adhesion molecule-1 promote hematopoietic progenitor homing to bone marrow. *Proc. Natl. Acad. Sci. U.S.A.* 95: 14423–14428.

Fritsch, G, Buchinger, P, Printz, D et al. (1993). Rapid discrimination of early CD34+ myeloid progenitors using CD45-RA analysis. *Blood* 81: 2301–2309.

Fujio, K, Evarts, RP, Hu, Z et al. (1994). Expression of stem cell factor and its receptor, c-kit, during liver regeneration from putative stem cells in adult rat. *Lab. Invest.* 70: 511–516.

Fujio, K, Hu, Z, Evarts, RP et al. (1996). Coexpression of stem cell factor and c-kit in embryonic and adult liver. *Exp. Cell Res.* 224: 243–250.

Fukuda, M, Fukuda, MN, Papayannopoulou, T, and Hakomori, S. (1980). Membrane differentiation in human erythroid cells: Unique profiles of cell surface glycoproteins expressed in erythroblasts in vitro from three ontogenic stages. *Proc. Natl. Acad. Sci. U.S.A.* 77: 3474–3478.

Furusawa, T, Yanai, N, Hara, T et al. (1998). Integrin-associated protein (IAP, also termed CD47) is involved in stroma-supported erythropoiesis. *J. Biochem. (Tokyo)* 123: 101–106.

Galimi, F, Bagnara, GP, Bonsi, L et al. (1994). Hepatocyte growth factor induces proliferation and differentiation of multipotent and erythroid hemopoietic progenitors. *J. Cell Biol.* 127: 1743–1754.

Geiger, H, Sick, S, Bonifer, C et al. (1998). Globin gene expression is reprogrammed in chimeras generated by injecting adult hematopoietic stem cells into mouse blastocysts. *Cell* 93: 1055–1065.

Gregory, CJ, and Eaves, AC. (1977). Human marrow cells capable of erythropoietic differentiation in vitro: Definition of three erythroid colony responses. *Blood* 49: 855–864.

Gupta, AD, Samoszuk, MK, Papayannopoulou, T, and Stamatoyannopoulos, G. (1985). SFL 23.6: A monoclonal antibody reactive with CFU-E, erythroblasts, and erythrocytes. *Blood* 66: 522–526.

Hann, IM, Bodger, MP, and Hoffbrand, AV. (1983). Development of pluripotent hematopoietic progenitor cells in the human fetus. *Blood* 62: 118–123.

Hardy, CL. (1995). The homing of hematopoietic stem cells to the bone marrow. *J. Am. Med. Sci.* 309: 260–266.

Harrison, DE, Zhong, RK, Jordan, CT et al. (1997). Relative to adult marrow, fetal liver repopulates nearly five times more effectively long-term than short-term. *Exp. Hematol.* 25: 293–297.

Hassan, MW, Lutton, JD, Levere, RD et al. (1979). In vitro culture of erythroid colonies from human fetal liver and umbilical cord blood. *Br. J. Haematol.* 41: 477–484.

Hirschman, SZ and Garfinkel, E. (1977). Ionic requirements of the DNA polymerase associated with serum hepatitis B antigen. *J. Infect. Dis.* 135: 897–910.

Hocking, WG and Golde, DW. (1980). Long-term human bone marrow cultures. *Blood* 56: 118–124.

Hogan, CJ, Shpall, EJ, McNulty, O et al. (1997). Engraftment and development of human CD34(+)-enriched cells from umbilical cord blood in NOD/LtSz-scid/scid mice. *Blood* 90: 85–96.

Hohlfeld, P, Forestier, F, Kaplan, C et al. (1999). Fetal thrombocytopenia: A retrospective survey of 5,194 fetal blood samplings. *Blood* 84: 1851–1856.

Huang, H and Auerbach, R. (1993). Identification and characterization of hematopoietic stem cells from the yolk sac of the early mouse embryo. *Proc. Natl. Acad. Sci. U.S.A.* 90: 10110–10114.

Huyhn, A, Dommergues, M, Izac, B et al. (1995). Characterization of hematopoietic progenitors from human yolk sacs and embryos. *Blood* 86: 4474–4485.

Iacopetta, BJ, Morgan, EH, and Yeoh, GC. (1982). Transferrin receptors and iron uptake during erythroid cell development. *Biochem. Biophys. Acta* 687: 204–210.

Iscove, NN, Guilbert, LJ, and Weyman, C. (1980). Complete replacement of serum in primary cultures of erythropoietin-dependent red cell precursors (CFU-E) by albumin, transferrin, iron, unsaturated fatty acid, lecithin and cholesterol. *Exp. Cell Res.* 126: 121–126.

Jones, SS, D'Andrea, AD, Haines, LL, and Wong, GG. (1990). Human erythropoietin receptor: Cloning, expression, and biologic characterization. *Blood* 76: 31–35.

Jordan CT and Van Zant, G. (1998). Recent progress in identifying genes regulating hematopoietic stem cell function and fate. *Curr. Opin. Cell Biol.* 10: 716–720.

Kamiya, A, Kinoshita, T, Ito, Y et al. (1999). Fetal liver development requires a paracrine action of oncostatin M through the gp130 signal transducer. *EMBO J.* 18: 2127–2136.

Katayama, N, Shih, JP, Nishikawa, S et al. (1993). Stage-specific expression of c-kit protein by murine hematopoietic progenitors. *Blood* 82: 2353–2360.

Kawabata, K, Ujikawa, M, Egawa, T et al. (1999). A cell-autonomous requirement for CXCR4 in long-term lymphoid and myeloid reconstitution. *Proc. Natl. Acad. Sci. U.S.A.* 96: 5663–5667.

Kelemen, E, Calvo, W, and Fliedner, TM. (1979). *Atlas of human hemopoietic development.* New York: Springer.

Kelemen, E and Janossa, M. (1980). Macrophages are the first differentiated blood cells formed in human embryonic liver. *Exp. Hematol.* 8: 996–1000.

Keller, G, Kennedy, M, Papayannopoulou, T, and Wiles, MV. (1993). Hematopoietic commitment during embryonic stem cell differentiation in culture. *Mol. Cell Biol.* 13: 473–486.

Keller, G, Lacaud, G, and Robertson, S. (1999). Development of the hematopoietic system in the mouse. *Exp. Hematol.* 27: 777–787.

Kelley, LL, Green, WF, Hicks, GG et al. (1994). Apoptosis in erythroid progenitors deprived of erythropoietin occurs during the G1 and S phases of the cell cycle without growth arrest or stabilization of wild-type p53. *Mol. Cell. Biol.* 14: 4183–4192.

Kennedy, M, Firpo, M, Choi, K et al. (1997). A common precursor for primitive erythropoiesis and definitive haematopoiesis. *Nature* 386: 488–493.

Kieran, MW, Perkins, AC, Orkin, SH, and Zon, LI. (1996). Thrombopoietin rescues in vitro erythroid colony formation from mouse embryos lacking the erythropoietin receptor. *Proc. Natl. Acad. Sci. U.S.A.* 93: 9126–9131.

Kimura, T, Sakabe, H, Tanimukai, S et al. (1997). Simultaneous activation of signals through gp130, c-kit, and interleukin-3 receptor promotes a trilineage blood cell production in the absence of terminally acting lineage-specific factors. *Blood* 90: 4767–4778.

Kinoshita, T, Sekiguchi, T, Xu, MJ et al. (1999). Hepatic differentiation induced by oncostatin M attenuates fetal liver hematopoiesis. *Proc. Natl. Acad. Sci. U.S.A.* 96: 7265–7270.

Kitajima, K, Kojima, M, Nakajima, K et al. (1999). Definitive but not primitive hematopoiesis is impaired in jumonji mutant mice. *Blood* 93: 87–95.

Klein, G. (1995). The extracellular matrix of the hematopoietic microenvironment. *Experientia* 51: 914–926.

Koury, MJ, and Bondurant, MC. (1990). Erythropoietin retards DNA breakdown and prevents programmed death in erythroid progenitor cells. *Science* 248: 378–381.

Koury, ST, Bondurant, MC, Koury, MJ, and Semenza, GL. (1991). Localization of cells producing erythropoietin in murine liver by in situ hybridization [see comments]. *Blood* 77: 2497–2503.

Krause, DS, Fackler, MJ, Civin, CI, and May, WS. (1996). CD34: Structure, biology, and clinical utility [see comments]. *Blood* 87: 1–13.

Landschulz, KT, Noyes, AN, Rogers, O, and Boyer, SH. (1989). Erythropoietin receptors on murine erythroid colony-forming units: Natural history. *Blood* 73: 1476–1486.

Lansdorp, PM, Sutherland, HJ, and Eaves, CJ. (1990). Selective expression of CD45 isoforms on functional subpopulations of CD34+ hemopoietic cells from human bone marrow. *J. Exp. Med.* 172: 363–366.

Lansdorp, PM, Dragowska, W, and Mayani, H. (1993). Ontogeny-related changes in proliferative potential of human hematopoietic cells. *J. Exp. Med.* 178: 787–791.

Leary, AG, and Ogawa, M. (1987). Blast cell colony assay for umbilical cord blood and adult bone marrow progenitors. *Blood* 69: 953–956.

Li, K, Liu, J, Fok, TF, et al. (1999). Human neonatal blood: Stem cell content, kinetics of CD34+ cell decline and ex vivo expansion capacity. *Br. J. Haematol.* 104: 178–185.

Liboi, E, Carroll, M, D'Andrea, AD, and Mathey-Prevot, B. (1993). Erythropoietin receptor signals both proliferation and erythroid-specific differentiation. *Proc. Natl. Acad. Sci. U.S.A.* 90: 11351–11355.

Lin, CS, Lim, SK, D'Agati, V, and Costantini, F. (1996). Differential effects of an erythropoietin receptor gene disruption on primitive and definitive erythropoiesis. *Genes Dev.* 10: 154–164.

Linch, DC, Knott, LJ, Rodeck, CH, and Huehns, E.R. (1982). Studies of circulating hemopoietic progenitor cells in human fetal blood. *Blood* 59: 976–979.

Long, MW. (1992). Blood cell cytoadhesion molecules. *Exp. Hematol.* 20: 288–301.

Lu, L, Xiao, M, Shen, RN et al. (1993). Enrichment, characterization, and responsiveness of single primitive CD34 human umbilical cord blood hematopoietic progenitors with high proliferative and replating potential. *Blood* 81: 41–48.

Ma, Q, Jones, D, and Springer, TA. (1999). The chemokine receptor CXCR4 is required for the retention of B lineage and granulocytic precursors within the bone marrow microenvironment. *Immunity* 10: 463–471.

Marcos, MA, Morales-Alcelay, S, Godin, IE et al. (1997). Antigenic phenotype and gene expression pattern of lymphohemopoietic progenitors during early mouse ontogeny. *J. Immunol.* 158: 2627–2637.

Mazo IB, Gutierrez-Ramos, JC, Frenette, PS et al. (1998). Hematopoietic progenitor cell rolling in bone marrow microvessels: Parallel contributions by endothelial selections and vascular cell adhesion molecule 1 [published erratum appears in *J Exp Med* 1998 Sep 7; 188(5):1001]. *J. Exp. Med.* 188:465–474.

McCune, JM, Namikawa, R, Kaneshima, H et al. (1988). The SCID-hu mouse: Murine model for the analysis of human hematolymphoid differentiation and function. *Science* 241: 1632–1639.

McKinstry, WJ, Li, CL, Rasko, JE et al. (1997). Cytokine receptor expression on hematopoietic stem and progenitor cells. *Blood* 89: 65–71.

McNiece, IK, Stewart, FM, Deacon, DM et al. (1989). Detection of a human CFC with a high proliferative potential. *Blood* 74: 609–612.

Medvinsky, A and Dzierzak, E. (1996). Definitive hematopoiesis is autonomously initiated by the AGM region. *Cell* 86: 897–906.

Medvinsky, AL, Samoylina, NL, Muller, AM, and Dzierzak, EA. (1993). An early pre-liver intraembryonic source of CFU-S in the developing mouse. *Nature* 364: 64–67.

Metcalf, D. (1993). Hematopoietic regulators: Redundancy or subtlety? *Blood* 82: 3515–3523.

Metcalf, D, Willson, TA, Hilton, DJ et al. (1995). Production of hematopoietic regulatory factors in cultures of adult and fetal mouse organs: Measurement by specific bioassays. *Leukemia* 9: 1556–1564.

Metcalf, D. (1998). Lineage commitment and maturation in hematopoietic cells: The case for extrinsic regulation. *Blood* 92: 345–347.

Migliaccio, AR and Migliaccio, G. (1988). Human embryonic hemopoiesis: Control mechanisms underlying progenitor differentiation in vitro. *Dev. Biol.* 125: 127–134.

Migliaccio, AR, Migliaccio, G, Brice, M et al. (1990a). Influence of recombinant hematopoietins and of fetal bovine serum on the globin synthetic pattern of human BFUe. *Blood* 76: 1150–1157.

Migliaccio, AR, Migliaccio, G, Mancini, G et al. (1993). Induction of the murine "W phenotype" in long-term cultures of human cord blood cells by c-kit antisense oligomers. *J. Cell. Physiol.* 157: 158–163.

Migliaccio, AR, Baiocchi, M, Durand, B et al. (1994). Stem cell factor and the amplification of progenitor cells from CD34+ cord blood cells. *Blood Cells* 20: 129–138.

Migliaccio, AR, Adamson, JW, Rubinstein, P, and Stevens, CE. (1996). Placental/cord blood stem cell transplantation: Correlation between the progenitor cell dose and time to myeloid engraftment in 55 unrelated transplants. *Blood* 88 (10): 286a. (Abstract).

Migliaccio, G, Migliaccio, AR, Petti, S et al. (1986). Human embryonic hemopoiesis. Kinetics of progenitors and precursors underlying the yolk sac–liver transition. *J. Clin. Invest.* 78: 51–60.

Migliaccio, G, Migliaccio, AR, and Adamson, JW. (1988). In vitro differentiation of human granulocyte/macrophage and erythroid progenitors: Comparative analysis of the influence of recombinant human erythropoietin, G-CSF, GM-CSF, and IL-3 in serum-supplemented and serum-deprived cultures. *Blood* 72: 248–256.

Migliaccio, G, Migliaccio, AR, and Adamson, JW. (1990b). The biology of hematopoietic growth factors: Studies in vitro under serum-deprived conditions. *Exp. Hematol.* 18: 1049–1055.

Migliaccio, G, and Migliaccio, AR. (1993). Kinetics of hematopoiesis in the human yolk sac. In Nogales, FF, editor. *The human yolk sac and yolk sac tumor.* Heidelberg: Springer-Verlag, p. 70.

Migliaccio, G, Baiocchi, M, Hamel, N et al. (1996). Circulating progenitor cells in human ontogenesis: Response to growth factors and replating potential. *J. Hematother.* 5: 161–170.

Mladenovic, J and Adamson, JW. (1982). Characteristics of circulating erythroid colony-forming cells in normal and polycythaemic man. *Br. J. Haematol.* 51: 377–384.

Moore, KL. (1982). *The developing humans.* Philadelphia: WB Saunders.

Moore, MA and Metcalf, D. (1970). Ontogeny of the haemopoietic system: Yolk sac origin of in vivo and in vitro colony forming cells in the developing mouse embryo. *Br. J. Haematol.* 18: 279–296.

Moritz, KM, Lim, GB, and Wintour, EM. (1997). Developmental regulation of erythropoietin and erythropoiesis. *Am. J. Physiol.* 273: R1829–R1844.

Morrison, SJ, Uchida, N, and Weissman, IL. (1995). The biology of hematopoietic stem cells. *Annu. Rev. Cell Dev. Biol.* 11: 35–71.

Muench, MO, Cupp, J, Polakoff, J, and Roncarolo, MG. (1994). Expression of CD33, CD38, and HLA-DR on CD34+ human fetal liver progenitors with a high proliferative potential. *Blood* 83: 3170–3181.

Mukouyama, Y, Hara, T, Xu, M et al. (1998). In vitro expansion of murine multipotential hematopoietic progenitors from the embryonic aorta-gonad-mesonephros region. *Immunity* 8: 105–114.

Nagasawa, T, Hirota, S, Tachibana, K et al. (1996). Defects of B-cell lymphopoiesis and bone-marrow myelopoiesis in mice lacking the CXC chemokine PBSF/SDF-1. *Nature* 382: 635–638.

Nagler, A, IIan, Y, Amiel, A et al. (1994). Systemic chimerism in sex-mismatched liver transplant recipients detected by fluorescence in situ hybridization. *Transplantation* 57: 1458–1461.

Nakamura, Y, Takano, H, Osawa, M et al. (1998). Impaired erythropoiesis in transgenic mice overexpressing a truncated erythropoietin receptor. *Exp. Hematol.* 26: 1105–1110.

Nakano, T, Kodama, H, and Honjo, T. (1996). In vitro development of primitive and definitive erythrocytes from different precursors. *Science* 272: 722–724.

O'Reilly, RJ, Brochstein, J, Dinsmore, R, and Kirkpatrick, D. (1984). Marrow transplantation for congenital disorders. *Semin. Hematol.* 21: 188–221.

Ogawa, M. (1993). Differentiation and proliferation of hematopoietic stem cells. *Blood* 81: 2844–2853.

Ohta, M, Sakai, T, Saga, Y et al. (1998). Suppression of hematopoietic activity in tenascin-C-deficient mice. *Blood* 91: 4074–4083.

Orlic, D, Anderson, S, Biesecker, LG et al. (1995). Pluripotent hematopoietic stem cells contain high levels of mRNA for c-kit, GATA-2, p45 NF-E2, and c-myb and low levels or no mRNA for c-fms and the receptors for granulocyte colony-stimulating factor and interleukins 5 and 7. *Proc. Natl. Acad. Sci. U.S.A.* 92: 4601–4605.

Osawa, M, Hanada, K, Hamada, H, and Nakauchi, H. (1996). Long-term lymphohematopoietic reconstitution by a single CD34- low/negative hematopoietic stem cell. *Science* 273: 242–245.

Papayannopoulou, T and Craddock, C. (1997). Homing and trafficking of hemopoietic progenitor cells. *Acta Haematol.* 97: 97–104.

Papayannopoulou, T, Craddock, C, Nakamoto, B et al. (1995). The VLA4/VCAM-1 adhesion pathway defines contrasting mechanisms of lodgement of transplanted murine hemopoietic

Papayannopoulou, T, Kurachi, S, Nakamoto, B et al. (1982). Hemoglobin switching in culture: Evidence for a humoral factor that induces switching in adult and neonatal but not fetal erythroid cells. *Proc. Natl. Acad. Sci. U.S.A.* 79: 6579–6583.

Papayannopoulou, T, Brice, M, and Stamatoyannopoulos, G. (1986a). Analysis of human hemoglobin switching in MELxHuman fetal erythroid cell hybrids. *Cell* 46: 469–476.

Papayannopoulou, T, Nakamoto, B, Agostinelli, F et al. (1986b). Fetal to adult hemopoietic cell transplantation in humans: Insights into hemoglobin switching. *Blood* 67: 99–104.

Papayannopoulou, T, Brice, M et al. (1991). Isolation of c-kit receptor-expressing cells from bone marrow, peripheral blood, and fetal liver: Functional properties and composite antigenic profile. *Blood* 78: 1403–1412.

Papayannopoulou, T, Brice, M, Farrer, D, and Kaushansky, K. (1996). Insights into the cellular mechanisms of erythropoietin-thrombopoietin synergy. *Exp. Hematol.* 24: 660–669.

Papayannopoulou, T, Abkowitz, J, and D'Andrea, AD. (1999). Biology of erythropoiesis, erythroid differentiation and maturation. In Hematology, 3rd edition. Hoffman, R, editor. pp. 202–219. Philadelphia: Churchill Livingstone.

Park, LS, Waldron, PE, Friend, D, Sassenfeld, HM et al. (1989). Interleukin-3, GM-CSF, and G-CSF receptor expression on cell lines and primary leukemia cells: Receptor heterogeneity and relationship to growth factor responsiveness. *Blood* 74: 56–65.

Peled, A, Petit, I, Kollet, O et al. (1999). Dependence of human stem cell engraftment and repopulation of NOD/SCID mice or CXCR4. *Science* 283: 845–848.

Peschle, C, Migliaccio, AR, Migliaccio, G et al. (1981). Identification and characterization of three classes of erythroid progenitors in human fetal liver. *Blood* 58: 565–572.

Peschle, C, Migliaccio, AR, Migliaccio, G et al. (1984). Embryonic–fetal Hb switch in humans: Studies on erythroid bursts generated by embryonic progenitors from yolk sac and liver. *Proc. Natl. Acad. Sci. U.S.A.* 81: 2416–2420.

Peschle, C, Mavilio, F, Care, A et al. (1985). Haemoglobin switching in human embryos: Asynchrony of $\zeta \to \alpha$ and $\varepsilon \to \gamma$-globin switches in primitive and definite erythropoietic lineage. *Nature* 313: 235–238.

Petrenko, O, Beavis, A, Klaine, M et al. (1999). The molecular characterization of the fetal stem cell marker AA4. *Immunity* 10: 691–700.

Petti, S, Testa, U, Migliaccio, AR et al. (1985). Embryonic hemopoiesis in human liver: Morphological aspects at sequential stages of ontogenic development. In Gale, RP, Tourain, JL, Lucarelli, G, editors. *Fetal liver transplantation.* New York: Alan R. Liss, p. 57.

Petzer, AL, Hogge, DE, Landsdorp, PM et al (1996). Self-renewal of primitive human hematopoietic cells (long-term-culture-initiating cells) in vitro and their expansion in defined medium. *Proc. Natl. Acad. Sci. U.S.A.* 93: 1470–1474.

Phillips, RL, Reinhart, AJ, and Van Zant, G. (1992). Genetic control of murine hematopoietic stem cell pool sizes and cycling kinetics. *Proc. Natl. Acad. Sci. U.S.A.* 89: 11607–11611.

Ploemacher, RE, van der Sluijs, JP, van Beurden, CA et al. (1991). Use of limiting-dilution type long-term marrow cultures in frequency analysis of marrow-repopulating and spleen colony-forming hematopoietic stem cells in the mouse. *Blood* 78: 2527–2533.

Rich, IN. (1995). Primordial germ cells are capable of producing cells of the hematopoietic system in vitro. *Blood* 86: 463–472.

Rico-Vargas, SA, Weiskopf, B, Nishikawa, S, and Osmond, DG. (1994). c-kit expression by B cell precursors in mouse bone marrow. Stimulation of B cell genesis by in vivo treatment with anti-c-kit antibody. *J. Immunol.* 152: 2845–2852.

Robinson, J, Sieff, C, Delia, D et al. (1981). Expression of cell-surface HLA-DR, HLA-ABC and glycophorin during erythroid differentiation. *Nature* 289: 68–71.

Rowley, PT, Ohlsson-Wilhelm, BM, and Farley, BA. (1978). Erythroid colony formation from human fetal liver. *Proc. Natl. Acad. Sci. U.S.A.* 75: 984–988.

Rubinstein, P, Rosenfield, RE, Adamson, JW, and Stevens, CE. (1993). Stored placental blood for unrelated bone marrow reconstitution. *Blood* 81: 1679–1690.

Rubinstein, P, Dobrila, L, Rosenfield, RE, et al. (1995). Processing and cryopreservation of placental/umbilical cord blood for unrelated bone marrow reconstitution. *Proc. Natl. Acad. Sci. U.S.A.* 92: 10119–10122.

Rubinstein, P, Carrier, C, Scaradavou, A et al. (1998). Outcomes among 562 recipients of placental-blood transplants from unrelated donors [see comments]. *N. Engl. J. Med.* 339: 1565–1577.

Russell, ES. (1979). Hereditary anemias of the mouse: A review for geneticists. *Adv. Genet.* 20: 357–459.

Sawada, K, Krantz, SB, Sawyer, ST, and Civin, CI. (1988). Quantitation of specific binding of erythropoietin to human erythroid colony-forming cells. *J. Cell. Physiol.* 137: 337–345.

Sawyer, ST and Krantz, SB. (1986). Transferrin receptor number, synthesis, and endocytosis during erythropoietin-induced maturation of Friend virus-infected erythroid cells. *J. Biol. Chem.* 261: 9187–9195.

Schiller, G, Vescio, R, Freytes, C et al. (1995). Transplantation of CD34+ peripheral blood progenitor cells after high-dose chemotherapy for patients with advanced multiple myeloma. *Blood* 86: 390–397.

Schinzel, A, Braegger, CP, Brecevic, L et al. (1997). Interstitial deletion, del(4)(q12q21.1), owing to de novo unbalanced translocation in a 2 year old girl: Further evidence that the piebald trait maps to proximal 4q12. *J. Med. Genet.* 34: 692–695.

Scott, EW, Fisher, RC, Olson, MC et al. (1997). PU.1 functions in a cell-autonomous manner to control the differentiation of multipotential lymphoid-myeloid progenitors. *Immunity* 6: 437–447.

Shields, LE, and Andrews, RG. (1998). Gestational age changes in circulating CD34+ hematopoietic stem/progenitor cells in fetal cord blood. *Am. J. Obstet. Gynecol.* 178: 931–937.

Shimada, Y, Migliaccio, G, Ralph, H et al. (1993). Erythropoietin-specific cell cycle progression in erythroid subclones of the interleukin-3-dependent cell line 32D [published erratum appears in *Blood* 1993, June 1;81(11):3168]. *Blood* 81: 935–941.

Shimizu, R, Komatsu, N, and Miura, Y. (1999). Dominant negative effect of a truncated erythropoietin receptor (EPOR-T) on erythropoietin-induced erythroid differentiation: Possible involvement of EPOR-T in ineffective erythropoiesis of myelodysplastic syndrome. *Exp. Hematol.* 27: 229–233.

Sonoda, Y, Yang, YC, Wong, GG et al. (1983). Analysis in serum-free culture of the targets of recombinant human

hemopoietic growth factors: Interleukin 3 and granulocyte/macrophage-colony-stimulating factor are specific for early developmental stages. *Proc. Natl. Acad. Sci. U.S.A.* 85: 4360–4364.

Southcott, MJ, Tanner, MJ, and Anstee, DJ. (1999). The expression of human blood group antigens during erythropoiesis in a cell culture system. *Blood* 93: 4425–4435.

Spitzer, G, Verma, DS, Fisher, R et al., (1980). The myeloid progenitor cell—its value in predicting hematopoietic recovery after autologous bone marrow transplantation. *Blood* 55: 317–323.

Spritz, RA and Beighton, P. (1998). Piebaldism with deafness: Molecular evidence for an expanded syndrome. *Am. J. Med. Genet.* 75: 101–103.

Stamatoyannopoulos, G, Constantoulakis, P, Brice, M et al. (1987a). Coexpression of embryonic, fetal, and adult globins in erythroid cells of human embryos: Relevance to the cell-lineage models of globin switching. *Dev. Biol.* 123: 191–197.

Stamatoyannopoulos, G and Nienhuis, AW. (1987b). Hemoglobin switching. In Stamatoyannopoulos, G, Nienhuis, AW, Leder, P, and Majerus, P, editors. *Molecular basis of blood diseases.* Philadelphia: WB Saunders, pp. 66–105.

Steen, R and Egeland, T. (1998). CD34 molecule epitope distribution on cells of haematopoietic origin. *Leuk. Lymphoma* 30: 23–30.

Steiner, R. (1973). On the kinetics of erythroid cell differentiation in fetal mice. II. DNA and hemoglobin measurements of individual erythroblasts during gestation. *J. Cell. Physiol.* 82: 219–230.

Sutherland, HJ, Eaves, CJ, Eaves, AC et al. (1989). Characterization and partial purification of human marrow cells capable of initiating long-term hematopoiesis in vitro. *Blood* 74: 1563–1570.

Taniguchi, H, Toyoshima, T, Fukao, K, and Nakauchi, H. (1996). Presence of hematopoietic stem cells in the adult liver [see comments]. *Nat. Med.* 2: 198–203.

Tavian, M, Coulombel, L, Luton, D et al. (1996). Aorta-associated CD34+ hematopoietic cells in the early human embryo. *Blood* 87: 67–72.

Tchernia, G, Mielot, F, Coulombel, L, and Mohandas, N. (1981). Characterization of circulating erythroid progenitor cells in human newborn blood. *J. Lab. Clin. Med.* 97: 322–331.

Terstappen, LW, Huang, S, Safford, M et al. (1991). Sequential generations of hematopoietic colonies derived from single nonlineage-committed CD34+CD38– progenitor cells. *Blood* 77: 1218–1227.

Tindle, RW, Nichols, RA, Chan, L et al. (1985). A novel monoclonal antibody BI-3C5 recognises myeloblasts and non-B non-T lymphoblasts in acute leukaemias and CGL blast crises, and reacts with immature cells in normal bone marrow. *Leuk. Res.* 9:1–9.

Torok-Storb, B. (1988). Cellular interactions. *Blood* 72: 373–385.

Turpen, JB, Kelley, CM, Mead, PE, and Zon, LI. (1997). Bipotential primitive-definitive hematopoietic progenitors in the vertebrate embryo. *Immunity* 7: 325–334.

Wang, LC, Kuo, F, Fujiwara, Y et al. (1997). Yolk sac angiogenic defect and intra-embryonic apoptosis in mice lacking the Ets-related factor TEL. *EMBO J.* 16: 4374–4383.

Wang, LC, Swat, W, Fujiwara, Y et al. (1998). The TEL/ETV6 gene is required specifically for hematopoiesis in the bone marrow. *Genes Dev.* 12: 2392–2402.

Weissman, IL, Baird, S, Gardner, RL et al. (1977). Normal and neoplastic maturation of T-lineage lymphocytes. *Cold Spring Harbor Symp. Quant. Biol.* 41 Pt 1, 9–21.

Weissman, IL, Papaioannou, VE, and Gardner, RL. (1978). Fetal hematopoietic origins of the adult hematolymphoid system. In Anonymous. *Differentiation of normal and neoplastic hematopoietic cells.* New York: Cold Spring Harbor Laboratory Press, pp. 33–43.

Wilpshaar, J, Joekes, EC, Lim, FTH et al. (1998). Magnetic resonance imaging to characterize the human hematopoietic stem cell compartment during fetal development. *Blood* 92 (Abstract).

Wolf, NS. (1974). Dissecting the hematopoietic microenvironment. I. Stem cell lodgment and commitment, and the proliferation and differentiation of erythropoietic descendants in the S1-S1d mouse. *Cell Tissue Kinet.* 7: 89–98.

Wood, HB, May, G, Healy, L et al. (1997). CD34 expression patterns during early mouse development are related to modes of blood vessel formation and reveal additional sites of hematopoiesis. *Blood* 90: 2300–2311.

Wu, H, Liu, X, Jaenisch, R, and Lodish, HF. (1995a). Generation of committed erythroid BFU-E and CFU-E progenitors does not require erythropoietin or the erythropoietin receptor. *Cell* 83: 59–67.

Wu, H, Klingmuller, U, Besmer, P, and Lodish, HF (1995b). Interaction of the erythropoietin and stem-cell-factor receptors. *Nature* 377: 242–246.

Yergeau, DA, Hetherington, CJ, Wang, Q et al. (1997). Embryonic lethality and impairment of haematopoiesis in mice heterozygous for an AML1-ETO fusion gene. *Nat. Genet.* 15: 303–306.

Yin, AH, Miraglia, S, Zanjani, ED et al. (1997). AC 133, a novel marker for human hematopoietic stem and progenitor cells. *Blood* 90: 5002–5012.

Yoder, MC and Hiatt, K (1997). Engraftment of embryonic hematopoietic cells in conditioned newborn recipients. *Blood* 89: 2176–2183.

Yoder, MC and Williams, DA. (1995). Matrix molecule interactions with hematopoietic stem cells. *Exp. Hematol.* 23: 961–967.

Yoder, MC, Hiatt, K, Dutt, P et al. (1997). Characterization of definitive lymphohematopoietic stem cells in the day 9 murine yolk sac. *Immunity* 7: 335–344.

Yokochi, T, Brice, M, Rabinovitch, PS et al. (1984). Monoclonal antibodies detecting antigenic determinants with restricted expression on erythroid cells: From the erythroid committed progenitor level to the mature erythroblast. *Blood* 63: 1376–1384.

Yoshida, K, Taga, T, Saito, M et al. (1996). Targeted disruption of gp130, a common signal transducer for the interleukin 6 family of cytokines, leads to myocardial and hematological disorders. *Proc. Natl. Acad. Sci. U.S.A.* 93: 407–411.

Yu, J, Shao, LE, Lemas, V et al. (1981). Importance of FSH-releasing protein and inhibin in erythroid differentiation. *Nature* 330: 765–767.

Zandstra, PW, Conneally, E, Piret, JM, and Eaves, CJ. (1998). Ontogeny-associated changes in the cytokine responses of primitive human haemopoietic cells. *Br. J. Haematol.* 101: 770–778.

Zanjani, ED, Pallavicini, MG, Ascensao, JL et al. (1992). Engraftment and long-term expression of human fetal hemopoietic stem cells in sheep following transplantation in utero. *J. Clin. Invest.* 89: 1178–1188.

Zanjani, ED, Silva, MR, and Flake, AW. (1994). Retention and multilineage expression of human hematopoietic stem cells in human-sheep chimeras. *Blood Cells* 20: 331–338.

Zanjani, ED, Almeida-Porada, G, Livingston, AG et al. (1998). Human bone marrow CD34– cells engraft in vivo and undergo multilineage expression that includes giving rise to CD34+ cells [see comments]. *Exp. Hematol.* 26: 353–360.

Zanjani, ED, Flake, AW, Almeida-Porada, G et al. (1999). Homing of human cells in the fetal sheep model: Modulation by antibodies activating or inhibiting VLA-4 dependent function. *Blood* 94: 2515–2522.

Zhang, J, Bowes and WAJ. (1995). Birth weight for gestational age patterns by race, sex, and parity in the United States population. *Obstet. Gynecol.* 86: 200–208.

Zucali, JR, Stevens, V, and Mirand, EA. (1975). In vitro production of erythropoietin by mouse fetal liver. *Blood* 46: 85–90.

4

Nuclear Factors that Regulate Erythropoiesis

GERD A. BLOBEL
MITCHELL J. WEISS

Studies of erythroid transcription factors originate from efforts to identify and characterize the numerous tissue-specific and ubiquitous proteins that bind *cis* regulatory motifs within the globin gene loci (Chapters 5, 6, and 15). In addition to elucidating mechanisms of globin gene regulation and erythroid development, this highly focused approach has led to the discovery of nuclear factors that function in a wide range of developmental processes. Experimental approaches and insights gained through studies of the globin loci have broad implications for understanding how transcription factors regulate the expression of individual genes and work together to coordinate cellular differentiation.

Erythrocyte formation in the vertebrate embryo occurs in several distinct waves (Brotherton et al., 1979; Wood, 1982) (see also Chapter 2). The first erythrocytes, termed *primitive* (EryP), arise in the extraembryonic yolk sac at mouse embryonic day 7.5 (E7.5) and week 3 to 4 in the human embryo. Later, erythropoiesis shifts to the fetal liver where adult-type (EryD, definitive) erythrocytes are produced. Finally, at birth, blood formation shifts to the bone marrow, and also the spleen in mice. Primitive and definitive erythrocytes are distinguished by their unique cellular morphology, cytokine responsiveness, transcription factor requirements, and patterns of gene expression (Mucenski et al., 1991; Ogawa et al., 1993; Wu et al.,

1995; Chyuan-Sheng et al., 1996; Wang et al., 1996; Okuda et al., 1996). Most notably, the expression of individual globin genes is developmentally regulated (Chapter 2 and 7). Understanding the temporal control of β-like globin genes during mammalian development is of general interest to the study of gene regulation in higher eukaryotes and could eventually lead to new approaches to reactivate the human fetal γ globin genes in individuals affected with β-chain hemoglobinopathies, such as sickle cell anemia and β thalassemia.

The primary *cis*-acting determinants of individual globin gene expression reside in the promoter regions immediately upstream of each gene and act in concert with the β-globin locus control region (β-LCR) (Chapters 5, 6, and 15). The β-LCR encompasses about twenty kilobases of DNA situated upstream of the β-globin cluster. Originally identified as a cluster of erythroid-specific DNAse hypersensitive sites, the β-LCR is now known to be essential for high-level erythroid expression of β–globin genes (Grosveld et al., 1987; Tuan et al., 1985, 1989; Forrester et al., 1987). Detailed analysis of globin gene promoters and the β-LCR has revealed a number of conserved DNA motifs important for globin expression. Among these motifs, the best studied are the "GATA," "CACCC," and "TGA(C/G)TCA"(NF-E2/AP-1-like) elements (Fig. 4.1). Perhaps not surprisingly, identical motifs also function in the promoters and enhancers of many other erythroid genes such as heme biosynthetic enzymes, red cell membrane proteins and α globin. One or several cognate transcription factors have been discovered to bind each of these *cis* elements in erythroid cells.

GENERAL PRINCIPLES

General studies of transcription factors have conveyed several important concepts and experimental approaches applicable to studies of erythroid nuclear proteins.

Transcription factors are modular proteins with distinct domains mediating DNA binding, transcriptional activation, repression, and protein interactions (Mitchell and Tjian, 1989). However, these distinctions are not absolute as a single domain may have more than one function. For example, GATA and Krüppel zinc fingers mediate both DNA binding and protein interactions. Typically, domains are analyzed by determining the effects of various mutations and "domain swaps" on the ability to activate synthetic promoter-reporter constructs in transient transfection

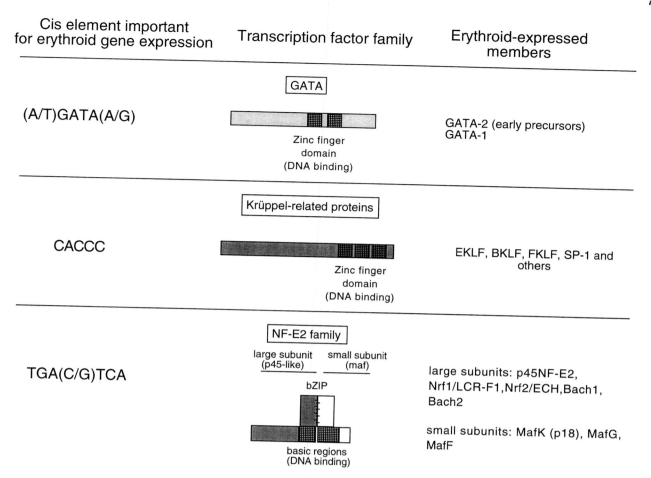

Cis element important for erythroid gene expression	Transcription factor family	Erythroid-expressed members
(A/T)GATA(A/G)	GATA — Zinc finger domain (DNA binding)	GATA-2 (early precursors) GATA-1
CACCC	Krüppel-related proteins — Zinc finger domain (DNA binding)	EKLF, BKLF, FKLF, SP-1 and others
TGA(C/G)TCA	NF-E2 family — large subunit (p45-like) small subunit (maf) — bZIP — basic regions (DNA binding)	large subunits: p45NF-E2, Nrf1/LCR-F1,Nrf2/ECH,Bach1, Bach2 — small subunits: MafK (p18), MafG, MafF

Figure 4.1. *Cis*-acting elements and corresponding transcription factor families important for erythroid gene expression.

assays using heterologous cells, such as 3T3 or COS. Such studies are useful, but fail to provide the native chromosomal and cellular context in which a lineage-specific factor normally operates. In this regard, the availability of more biologically relevant cellular models has complemented the use of conventional promoter-reporter studies.

Transcription factors function within multiprotein complexes (Ptashne and Gann, 1997; Kadonaga, 1998). Defining these complexes in erythroid cells is critical to understanding the mechanisms that underlie globin gene expression and erythroid differentiation. Several approaches, including the yeast two-hybrid screen to identify interacting proteins and biochemical purification of high molecular weight complexes, are beginning to delineate transcription factor networks in erythroid cells.

Posttranslational alterations, such as phosphorylation (Hunter and Karin, 1992) and acetylation (Gu and Roeder, 1997; Hung et al., 1999; Zhang and Bieker 1998, Boyes et al., 1998d) can modulate tran-

scription factor function. These chemical modifications establish another level of control through which gene expression may be fine-tuned in response to changes in the nuclear environment and/or extracellular signals. Examples relevant to erythroid biology are discussed later.

An important function of transcriptional activators and repressors is to modify chromatin (Kadonaga, 1998; Wolffe and Pruss, 1996; Felsenfeld, 1996). Accordingly, it is believed that in erythroid cells, the β-LCR interacts with nuclear proteins to maintain an "open" chromatin state, which renders the locus more accessible to basal transcription factors (Higgs, 1998). How erythroid transcription factors regulate chromatin and DNA accessibility is an active area of research. In vitro studies of chromatin-assembled DNA templates demonstrate that erythroid transcription factors, either independently or in the context of multiprotein complexes, can alter nucleosome structure. In addition, recent evidence suggests that erythroid nuclear proteins can modify histones indirectly by recruiting ubiquitously expressed histone acetyltransferases, leading to a more transcriptionally active chromatin state (as noted below).

ELUCIDATING GENE FUNCTION BY TARGETED MUTAGENESIS

The advent of targeted gene disruption using homologous recombination in embryonic stem (ES) cells and mice has been instrumental in assessing transcription factor function by providing a means to inactivate or "knock out" genes of interest and examine the biological consequences. Murine ES cells derived from the inner cell mass of blastocyst stage mouse embryos provide the basis for gene targeting strategies (Robertson,

Figure 4.2. (A) Experimental strategies for studying gene knockouts. (B) In vitro differentiation of embryonic stem cells to obtain pure hematopoietic colonies. (Reprinted from Weiss and Orkin, 1995a with permission from Elsevier Science, Copyright 1995.)

1986; Evans and Kaufman, 1981; Martin, 1981). ES cells can be maintained in a totipotent state in culture and contribute to somatic and germ line tissues when introduced into blastocysts by microinjection. The first step toward studying a gene of interest is to disrupt a single allele by homologous recombination in ES cells to create a heterozygous, or "single knockout" state (Capecchi, 1989; Smithies et al., 1985). Several complementary experimental approaches are then available for further study (Fig. 4.2).

First, genetically altered ES cells may be injected into host blastocysts to produce chimeric mice, which may transmit the mutant allele to progeny. Through interbreeding of heterozygous offspring, homozygous null animals can be created for analysis. One limitation of this approach is that mutations causing early embryonic

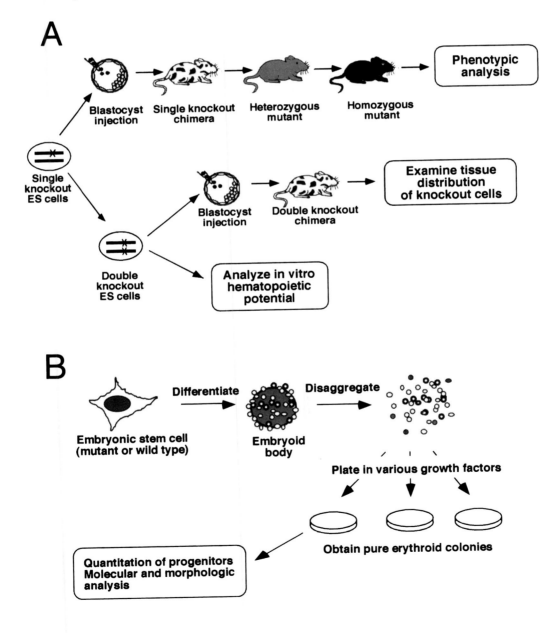

death can obscure the analysis of later developmental events. For example, direct examination of definitive hematopoiesis is difficult to assess in embryos that die before development of the fetal liver. Another potential problem in interpreting the phenotypes of knockout animals is failure to determine whether observed defects are cell autonomous or an indirect consequence of lesions in other cell types (non-cell autonomous). Both of these problems may be circumvented through chimera analysis or in vitro ES cell differentiation assays (see later). In addition, recent technology now permits developmental stage and tissue-specific gene targeting (Rossant and McMahon, 1999; Gu et al., 1994).

Second, heterozygous mutant ES cells can be converted to a homozygous-null state (Riele et al., 1990; Mortensen et al., 1992). These mutant ES cells may be injected into wild-type host blastocysts to create chimeric animals in which the ability of the mutant donor ES cells to contribute to various tissues is assessed using polymorphic markers. For loci that are encoded on the X chromosome, such as GATA-1 (see later), a single targeting event renders male ES cells null for the gene of interest. Failure of homozygous (or hemizygous for X-linked genes) null ES cells to contribute to a specific cell type or tissue indicates a cell-autonomous requirement for the disrupted gene in the formation of that tissue.

Finally, the hematopoietic potential of double knockout ES cells may be examined by in vitro techniques (Fig. 4.2B). Under appropriate conditions, ES cells form embryoid bodies, spherical aggregates containing numerous differentiated cell types, including mature hematopoietic cells that can be studied directly (Doetschman et al., 1985). In addition, embryoid bodies may be disaggregated into a single cell suspension and analyzed for hematopoietic progenitors using standard methylcellulose-based colony assays (Keller et al., 1993) Wild-type and genetically manipulated ES cells can also be induced to form hematopoietic lineages by cocultivation on the stromal line OP9 (Nakano et al., 1994; Suwabe et al., 1998).

GATA-1 AND GATA-2

The abundant erythroid nuclear protein GATA-1 was identified through its ability to bind the (T/A)GATA(A/G) consensus motif found in regulatory regions of virtually all erythroid-specific genes including globins, heme biosynthetic enzymes, red cell membrane proteins, and transcription factors (Tsai et al., 1989; Evans and Felsenfeld, 1989) (also see Chapters 5 and 6). An interesting example of a medically relevant GATA-target gene is the Duffy blood group antigen, which encodes the receptor for *Plasomdium vivax* malaria and various chemokines. In a subset of Duffy-

negative individuals, loss of erythroid Duffy gene expression is caused by a mutation that impairs promoter activity by disrupting a GATA consensus motif (Tournamille et al., 1995).

Although generally viewed as a positive regulator of erythroid gene expression, GATA-1 also appears to function as a repressor (as discussed later). For example, there is evidence that GATA-1 negatively regulates human ε-globin gene expression by interacting with one or more silencer elements within the 5′ flanking region of the ε gene (Li et al., 1998; Raich et al., 1995). The GATA-1 cofactor FOG, which synergizes with GATA-1 during erythroid and megakaryocytic differentiation (as noted later), can also inhibit certain GATA-1-dependent promoters (Fox et al., 1999). In addition, GATA-1 negatively regulates myeloid gene expression by binding and inhibiting the transcription factor PU.1 (Zhang et al., 1999), and represses expression of the nuclear proteins GATA-2 and c-*myb* in erythroid cells through unknown mechanisms (Weiss et al., 1994a).

GATA-1 recognizes DNA through two related, tandemly arranged zinc fingers of the configuration Cys-X2-Cys-X17-Cys-X2-Cys. The carboxyl (C) finger is necessary and sufficient for DNA binding, whereas the amino (N) finger stabilizes protein-DNA interactions at a subset of sites, in particular those that contain two GATA motifs arranged as direct or inverted repeats (Martin and Orkin, 1990a; Whyatt et al., 1993; Trainor et al., 1996; Yang and Evans, 1992). Nuclear magnetic resonance analysis of the carboxyl terminal finger of chicken GATA-1 bound to DNA revealed a core structure containing zinc coordinated by four cysteines that interacts with the major groove, and a carboxyl-terminal tail that stabilizes binding by wrapping around into the minor groove (Omichinski et al., 1993).

The GATA Multigene Family

The discovery of GATA-1 led to the identification of several related proteins with highly conserved zinc finger domains, but little homology outside of this region (Kelley et al., 1993; Arceci et al., 1993; Jiang and Evans, 1996; Laverriere et al., 1994; Yamamoto et al., 1990; Zon et al., 1991; Detrich et al., 1995) (reviewed in Orkin, 1992, and Weiss and Orkin, 1995a). GATA proteins are present throughout eukaryotic evolution. Six vertebrate GATA proteins, named in the order of their discovery, have been described.

GATA-1 and GATA-2 are particularly relevant for erythroid development. Both are expressed in multipotential progenitors, although GATA-2 to a greater extent (Sposi et al., 1992; Leonard et al., 1993). Concurrent with erythroid differentiation, GATA-2 expression declines as that of GATA-1 increases. In addition, GATA-1 and GATA-2 are coexpressed in megakaryocytes, mast cells, and eosinophils (Martin et al., 1990b; Romeo et al., 1990; Zon et al., 1993). Outside of the hematopoietic system, GATA-1 is expressed in the Sertoli cells of testes in young mice (Ito et al., 1993; Yomogida et al., 1994). GATA-2 is found in a variety of embryonic and adult tissues including placenta, blood vessel endothelial cells, and specific areas of the nervous system (Ng et al., 1994; Kornhauser et al., 1994; Ma et al., 1997; Dorfman et al., 1992; Nardelli et al., 1999).

GATA-3, the only other hematopoietic-expressed family member, is found in the lymphoid system, where it is essential for T-cell formation (Ting et al., 1996; Hendriks et al., 1999), and has additional roles in specification of the Th2 subtype (Zheng and Flavell, 1997). GATA-3 is also found in chicken erythrocytes and in the nervous system, where it exhibits an essential developmental role (Pandolfi et al., 1995). GATA-4 through GATA-6 are expressed in distinct but overlapping embryonic and adult tissues including heart, gonads, and various endoderm-derived lineages (Morrisey et al., 1996, 1997, 1998; Koutsourakis et al., 1999).

GATA-1 is Required for Terminal Erythroid Maturation and Platelet Formation

An important role for GATA-1 was predicted by its high level expression in erythroid precursors and the presence of functional GATA motifs in numerous erythroid expressed genes. This expectation was borne out by gene targeting studies showing that GATA-1 is essential for the production of mature erythrocytes. In chimeric mice, GATA-1⁻ donor ES cells contribute to all tissues examined except red blood cells; reintroduction of GATA-1 cDNA into the mutant ES cells restores their ability to contribute circulating red blood cells (Pevny et al., 1991; Simon et al., 1992). These experiments demonstrate an essential, cell autonomous role for GATA-1 in the production of mature definitive erythrocytes.

To study the effects of GATA-1 loss in vivo, the gene-disrupted allele was transmitted through the mouse germ line (Fujiwara et al., 1996). GATA-1⁻ embryos exhibit extreme pallor at E9.5 and die between E10.5 and E11.5 with no other obvious morphologic abnormalities (Fig. 4.3A, left and middle panels). Examination of the peripheral blood smear reveals immature and dying primitive erythroblasts (Fig. 4.3A, right panels). Although early death of GATA-1⁻ embryos precludes direct examination of definitive hematopoiesis, developmentally arrested, dying definitive erythroid precursors are observed in hematopoietic colonies derived from yolk sac of the mutant embryos.

In vitro differentiation of GATA-1⁻ ES cells was used to pinpoint the block in definitive erythropoiesis (Weiss and Orkin, 1995b; Weiss et al., 1994b). GATA-1⁻ ES cells generate normal numbers of EryD colonies, but cells within the mutant colonies exhibit maturation arrest at the proerythroblast stage and die by apoptosis (Fig. 4.3B). GATA-1 may protect maturing erythroblasts from cell death by inducing (directly or indirectly) production of the antiapoptosis protein bcl-x$_L$ (Gregory et al., 1999). Myeloid colonies from GATA-1⁻ mice and ES cells are normal in number and appearance.

Together, the studies described here indicate that GATA-1 is dispensable for establishment of the erythroid lineage, but required for survival and terminal maturation of committed primitive and definitive erythrocytes. The failure of GATA-1⁻ erythroid precursors to progress beyond the proerythoblast stage is not simply a consequence of premature death, as evidenced by the differentiation block of G1E cells (for GATA-1⁻ Erythroid), an immortal erythroid line derived from in vitro differentiation of GATA-1⁻ ES cells (Weiss et al., 1997). G1E cells proliferate as immature erythroblasts, yet complete differentiation upon restoration of GATA-1 function. These findings emphasize the critical role for GATA-1 in proerythroblast maturation (beyond simply preventing cell death) and provide an experimental tool to analyze GATA-1 function in an erythroid context (as noted later) (Gregory et al., 1999; Weiss et al., 1997; Tsai and Orkin, 1997; Crispino et al., 1999).

In addition to its role in erythroid development, GATA-1 is also essential for normal megakaryocytopoiesis and platelet formation (Pevny et al., 1994; Shivdasani et al., 1997; Vyas et al., 1999). Mice with megakaryocyte-selective GATA-1 deficiency exhibit prolonged bleeding times with quantitative and qualitative platelet defects and accumulation of abnormal, developmentally arrested megakaryocytes in the bone marrow and spleen (Vyas et al., 1999a).

An Early Hematopoietic Requirement for GATA-2

Ablation of the GATA-2 gene reveals an important role in the expansion and maintenance of multipotential hematopoietic progenitors and possibly stem cells. GATA-2⁻/⁻ embryos exhibit severe anemia and die at E10.5–11.5 (Tsai et al., 1994). Mature circulating primitive erythrocytes are present, but severely reduced in number. In adult chimeric mice, GATA-2⁻/⁻ ES cells fail to contribute efficiently to all lymphoid and myeloid hematopoietic tissues, suggesting a cell autonomous defect in the ability of mutant stem cells to colonize or expand within the hematopoietic system of the mature host. In vitro analysis of GATA-2⁻/⁻ ES cells and yolk sac from GATA-2⁻/⁻ mice reveals a

A

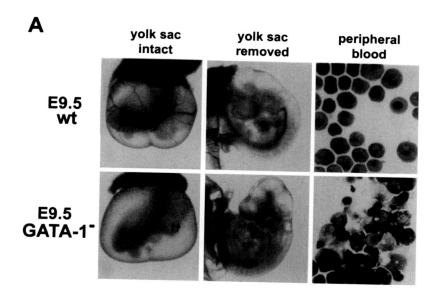

B

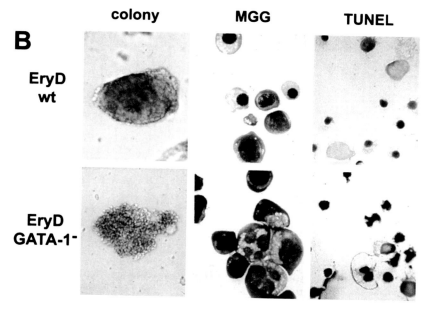

Figure 4.3. Loss of GATA-1 blocks erythroid maturation. (**A**) Impaired primitive erythropoiesis in GATA-1⁻ embryos. (**B**) Developmental arrest and apoptosis of cells within definitive erythroid (EryD) colonies generated by in vitro differentiation of GATA-1⁻ ES cells. (Modified from Fujiwara et al., 1996, and Weiss and Orkin 1995b. Copyright 1995 and 1996, National Academy of Sciences, U.S.A. Photographs in panel A provided by Yuko Fujiwara and Stuart Orkin.) For full color reproduction, see color plate 4.3.

mitting survival into late gestation, at which point the embryos died of probable obstructive hydronephrosis (Zhou et al., 1998). These experiments reveal an additional critical role for GATA-2 in morphogenesis of the urinary tract and provide an example of how problems of early embryonic lethality can be circumvented by tissue-specific rescue to reveal otherwise concealed phenotypes of animals with targeted mutations.

marked reduction of all definitive hematopoietic precursors and a selective defect in mast cell production (Tsai and Orkin, 1997; Tsai et al., 1994).

Recently, a transgenic approach was used to selectively rescue erythropoiesis in GATA-2⁻/⁻ embryos, per-

Gain of Function Experiments Using GATA Proteins

Gain of function studies show that GATA proteins are capable of influencing hematopoietic cell fate determination in a number of experimental systems. In this

regard, GATA-1 and GATA-2 exhibit distinct but over-laping biological activities. Some degree of functional redundancy among these related proteins is not surprising as they recognize similar DNA consensus motifs. Thus, forced expression of either GATA-1, GATA-2, or GATA-3 induces megakaryocytic differentiation in the early myeloid cell line 416B (Visvander and Adams, 1993). GATA-1 can also convert transformed avian myelomonocytic cell lines into either eosinophils, erythroblasts, or thromboblasts (megakaryocyte-like cells), depending on the level of GATA-1 expressed (Kutessa et al., 1995). GATA-2, but not GATA-1 (or GATA-3), inhibits differentiation of chicken erythroid progenitors (Briegel et al., 1993). In mice, retroviral transfer of GATA-1 into hematopoietic stem cells followed by bone marrow transplantation causes modest expansion of the erythroid progenitor pool and a concurrent mild decrease in myeloid precursors (Farina et al., 1995). In similar experiments, forced expression of GATA-2 blocks expansion and differentiation of hematopoietic stem cells in vivo (Persons et al., 1999). Thus, although GATA-1 and GATA-2 share some common effects, enforced expression of GATA-2 tends to impede hematopoietic maturation, while GATA-1 appears to promote differentiation along specific lineage pathways, including erythroid.

Shared and Unique Functions for GATA Proteins During Erythroid Development

Unexpectedly, numerous presumptive GATA target genes, including globins, the erythropoietin receptor, and erythroid transcription factors such as erythroid krüppel-like factor (EKLF) and SCL (stem cell leukemia, tal-1, tcl-5) (see later), are expressed in definitive GATA-1⁻ proerythroblasts (Weiss et al., 1994b). These observations may be explained by the finding that GATA-2 is upregulated approximately fifty-fold in the mutant cells. It is possible, therefore, that GATA-2 substitutes for the loss of GATA-1 to regulate the expression of some erythroid GATA targets. During normal development, GATA-2 may help to initiate the erythroid program in early progenitors and subsequently be replaced by GATA-1 during terminal maturation. Derepression of GATA-2 in GATA-1⁻ erythroblasts suggests that GATA-1 negatively regulates GATA-2 (either directly or indirectly) during normal erythroid maturation. Thus, GATA-1 and GATA-2 appear to act sequentially and coordinately during erythroid maturation.

Why GATA-1⁻ proerythroblasts die despite what appears to be partial compensation by GATA-2 remains an open question. One possibility is that unidentified GATA-1-specific target genes are critical for terminal maturation, consistent with qualitative

biological differences observed between these two related transcription factors (see the previous discussion). Alternatively, the quantity of GATA-2 may be insufficient to completely rescue GATA-1⁻ erythroblasts. Consistent with this possibility, high GATA-1 protein dosage is critical for normal erythropoiesis (Takahashi et al., 1997; McDevitt et al., 1997).

Structure-Function Analysis of GATA-1

GATA-1 acts as a potent transcriptional activator when cotransfected into heterologous cells (such as COS or 3T3) with a reporter gene containing a promoter with one or more GATA motifs (Martin and Orkin, 1990a; Evans and Felsenfeld, 1991). In this assay, several domains of murine GATA-1 are required for activity (Martin and Orkin, 1990a). In particular, the amino terminus contains an acidic domain that is required for transactivation of reporter constructs and functions as an independent activator when fused to a heterologous GAL4 DNA binding domain. The C-finger, which is required for DNA binding, is also essential for transactivation of GATA reporter constructs. The N-finger, not required for DNA binding (see previous discussion), is dispensable for activation of reporter genes that contain simple GATA motifs.

A strikingly different view emerges from structure-function analyses that exploit the ability of GATA-1 to influence hematopoietic lineage selection or maturation. Remarkably, the GATA-1 zinc finger region alone is sufficient to induce megakaryocytic differentiation of 416B cells (Visvader et al., 1995) and restore erythropoiesis in GATA-1⁻ embryoid bodies (Blobel et al., 1995). Therefore, the amino terminal activation domain of GATA-1, critical for transcriptional activity in promoter-reporter assays, is dispensable for at least some activities in hematopoietic cells. These findings demonstrate that structure-function relationships within the GATA-1 protein are context-dependent and reveal potent biological activity within the zinc finger region. Further dissection of the GATA-1 DNA binding domain demonstrates that the N-finger is essential for activity in erythroid cells (Weiss et al., 1997). One critical role of the N-finger is to mediate the interaction between GATA-1 and an essential cofactor, FOG (friend of GATA-1, see later). The N-finger may also be necessary to stabilize in vivo DNA interactions at a subset of bipartite GATA-1 motifs (see the previous discussion), including one present in the GATA-1 promoter.

Posttranslational Modifications of GATA-1

Murine GATA-1 is phosphorylated constitutively on six serine residues within the amino terminus. An additional serine, at position 310, which lies in a conserved region near the carboxyl boundary of the DNA binding domain, is phosphorylated on chemically induced differentiation of murine erythroleukemia (MEL) cells. Extensive mutagenesis experiments have shown that phosphorylation at these sites does not significantly influence DNA binding, DNA bending, or transcriptional activation by GATA-1 (Crossley and Orkin, 1994). Phosphorylation of GATA-1 has been reported to influence DNA binding in human K562 cells, although the functional significance of this observation is unclear (Partington and Patient, 1999).

GATA-1 is acetylated in vivo at two highly conserved lysine-rich motifs present at the C-terminal tails of both fingers, adjacent to regions that contact DNA. Acetylation within these regions is mediated by interaction with the ubiquitous transcriptional cofactors CREB-binding protein (CBP) and its relative, p^{300} (Hung et al., 1999; Boyes et al., 1998). Acetylation of GATA-1 appears to be functionally important as mutation of the acetylated lysine motifs reduces the ability of GATA-1 to rescue erythroid maturation in G1E cells (Hung et al., 1999). It has been proposed that acetylation augments the affinity of GATA-1 for DNA (Boyes et al., 1998), although a different study suggests that this may not be the major mechanism by which this modification regulates GATA-1 activity in vivo (Hung et al., 1999).

GATA-1-Interacting Proteins

GATA-1 participates in erythroid gene activation (and probably repression) through interactions with numerous erythroid-specific and ubiquitous nuclear factors. For instance, GATA-1 physically interacts with zinc finger proteins such as GATA-1 itself, other GATA factors, EKLF, and SP1 (Crossley et al., 1995; Merika and Orkin, 1995; Gregory et al., 1996; Fischer et al., 1993). In each case, protein interactions occur through the zinc finger regions of the respective proteins and potentiate GATA-1 transcriptional activity at defined promoters. These interactions provide a possible mechanism for communication between erythroid gene promoters and more distant regulatory regions (Chapter 7). For example, promoters of genes within the β-globin locus and the core elements of the LCR each contain CACCC and GATA motifs. Interactions between proteins bound to these elements could facilitate direct communication via looping between the LCR and specific globin genes (see later discussion and Chapter 7).

The GATA-1 protein interactions discussed previously underscore the complexity and multifaceted nature of its zinc finger motifs. This notion was further validated by Tsang and co-workers who used the yeast two hybrid screen to search for proteins that specifically interact with the N-finger of GATA-1 (Tsang et

al., 1997). They identified a novel nuclear protein named FOG that contains nine zinc fingers, several of which interact with the GATA-1 N-finger surface that faces away from DNA (Fox et al., 1998, 1999; Crispino et al., 1999; Kowalski et al., 1999). Physical interaction with FOG potentiates the action of GATA-1 in erythroid and megakaryocytic cells where FOG is normally coexpressed (Crispino et al., 1999; Tsang et al., 1997). Disruption of the FOG gene produces an erythroid defect similar to that of GATA-1 loss, albeit not as severe, suggesting the possibility of both FOG-dependent and independent functions of GATA-1 in red blood cells. In contrast, FOG$^{-/-}$ mice and ES cells exhibit a complete block to megakaryocytopoiesis, indicating that GATA-1-independent functions for FOG exist in megakaryocytes (Tsang et al., 1998). The mechanism of FOG actions is likely to be complex; for example, FOG can either activate or repress transcription, depending on promoter and cell context (Fox et al., 1999; Tsang et al., 1997). Recently, a related GATA-interacting protein, FOG-2, has been identified (Lu et al., 1999; Svensson et al., 1999; Tevosian et al., 1999; Holmes et al., 1999). FOG-2 is expressed in nonhematopoietic tissues, such as heart and brain, where it is presumed to modulate the actions of other GATA family members.

Tissue-restricted nuclear factors must communicate with generalized transcriptional machinery. For GATA-1, this "bridge" may be provided in part by its interaction with the general coactivator CBP and the highly related protein p^{300}. The zinc finger region of GATA-1 physically interacts with CBP in vitro and in vivo, and CBP, as well as p^{300}, potentiate the action of GATA-1 (Boyes et al., 1998a; Blobei et al., 1998). CBP/p^{300} could augment GATA-1 in several important ways (Shikama et al., 1997). First, CBP/p^{300} interact with numerous ubiquitous transcription factors via dedicated domains and, therefore, may provide a link between GATA-1 and the basal transcriptional machinery. Second, CBP/p^{300} possess intrinsic and associated histone acetyltransferase activity. Histone acetylation is associated with an "open" chromatin configuration characteristic of the β-globin locus in erythroid cells. Hence, GATA-1 could alter chromatin configuration by recruiting CBP/p^{300} to induce regional histone acetylation. It is worth noting, however, that GATA-1 itself is capable of disrupting histone-DNA contacts independent of CBP (Boyes et al., 1998). Finally, CBP-mediated acetylation of GATA-1 may be of functional importance in erythroid cells (Hung et al., 1999; Boyes et al., 1998a) (see previous discussion). CBP also interacts with a number of other erythroid transcription factors (as noted later) and, therefore, may participate in the formation of large multiprotein complexes.

In the instances discussed previously, interaction partners of GATA-1 largely potentiate its activity. In contrast, physical association with the Ets family transcription factor, PU.1, has a negative effect on GATA-1 action. PU.1 is normally expressed in multipotential progenitors, myeloid cells, and B lymphocytes, and is required for normal myelopoiesis and lymphopoiesis (reviewed in Fisher and Scott, 1998). Inappropriate expression of PU.1 by retroviral insertion (Moreau-Gachelin et al., 1989) and transgenesis (Moreau-Gachelin et al., 1996) causes erythroleukemia, and forced expression of PU.1 blocks differentiation in erythroid cell lines and primary progenitors (Rao et al., 1997; Quang et al., 1995; Yamada et al., 1997; Delgado et al., 1998). Hence, it has been postulated that downregulation of PU.1 is essential for normal erythropoiesis. An underlying mechanism for this hypothesis stems from recent observations that PU.1 binds GATA-1 and inhibits its transcriptional activity (Rekhtman et al., 1999; Yamada et al., 1998). Moreover, overexpression of GATA-1 relieves the PU.1-induced block to chemical-induced maturation of erythroleukemia cells. Conversely, GATA-1 (and GATA-2) inhibit PU.1 transactivation activity, possibly by displacing the PU.1 coactivator, c-Jun (Zhang et al., 1999). Together, these data suggest that GATA-1 and PU.1 oppose each other's actions and that their relative stochiometry may influence differentiation decisions in uncommitted myeloerythroid progenitors.

STEM CELL LEUKEMIA (SCL, TAL-1, TCL-5)

The SCL gene was originally identified via chromosomal rearrangements involving 11p13 in acute T-cell leukemias (reviewed in Begley and Green, 1999). SCL is a member of the basic helix-loop-helix (bHLH) class of transcription factors that recognizes a cognate DNA element termed E boxes (consensus CANNTG) in association with ubiquitously expressed heterodimeric partners, such as E2A. Gene-targeting studies show that SCL is critical for the development of all primitive and definitive blood lineages and for organization of the yolk sac vasculature (Robb et al., 1995, 1996; Shivdasani et al., 1995; Porcher et al., 1996; Visvader et al., 1998). These and other data indicate that SCL functions in the earliest hematopoietic stem cell, and possibly the hemangioblast, a bipotential hematopoietic-endothelial cell precursor (Chapter 2).

Several lines of evidence also suggest a dedicated role for SCL in erythroid development. First, SCL is expressed at a relatively high level in erythroid precursors and erythroid cell lines (Visvader et al., 1991; Mouthon et al., 1993; Green et al., 1991). Second, forced expression of SCL stimulates erythroid differentiation of murine erythroleukemia cells and the multipotential myeloid cell line, TF-1 (Hoang et al., 1996; Aplan et al., 1992). Third, conserved, functionally important E box motifs found within the HS2 core of the β-globin LCR are occupied by SCL in erythroid cells (Elnitski et al., 1997).

In erythroid cells, SCL/E2A is associated with a larger protein complex consisting of GATA-1 and two non-DNA binding nuclear proteins, Lmo-2 and Ldb-1 (Wadman et al., 1997). This complex can bind DNA via a bipartite motif consisting of GATA and E box sites, separated by about one full helical turn of DNA. While the in vivo significance of this oligomeric protein complex is unclear, it is intriguing that composite GATA-E-box motifs are present in gene regulatory regions of two erythroid transcription factors: GATA-1 itself and ELKF (Anderson et al., 1998; Vyas et al., 1999).

EKLF AND OTHER CACCC BOX-BINDING PROTEINS

Functionally important GC-rich elements, also referred to as CACCC boxes, are found in many erythroid gene regulatory elements including several of the globin gene promoters and the LCR (Chapters 5 and 6). The importance of an intact CACCC box in the β-globin gene promoter is underscored by the observation that certain thalassemias are associated with mutations in these elements (Orkin et al., 1982, 1984; Kulozik et al., 1991). CACCC boxes, which vary somewhat in their sequence, are recognized by a diverse set of at least 16 transcription factors that share a related DNA binding domain composed of three zinc fingers with homology to the *Drosophila melanogaster* Krüppel protein (for review see Philipsen and Suske, 1999; Turner and Crossley, 1999; Cook et al., 1999). These factors include the Sp-1 family, and proteins related to EKLF.

EKLF is of particular interest to studies of globin gene regulation because its expression is restricted mainly to erythroid cells, with low level expression in mast cells (Miller and Bieker, 1993; Southwood et al., 1996). No expression has been detected in myeloid or lymphoid cells, or outside the hematopoietic system. EKLF binds to the β globin CACCC box with high affinity and mutations found in CACCC boxes of β thalassemia patients abrogate EKLF binding (Feng et al., 1994).

EKLF is Required for β Globin Gene Expression

The presence of numerous erythroid factors that bind CACCC elements (Fig. 4.4) suggested the possibility of considerable functional redundancy at a given promoter or enhancer in vivo. Therefore, it was surprising to discover that targeted disruption of the EKLF gene leads to selective loss of β globin

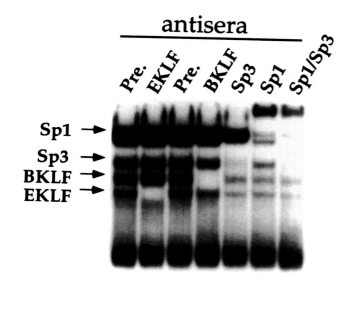

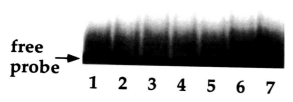

Figure 4.4. Gel mobility shift experiment showing multiple CACCC box binding proteins in erythroid cells. In this assay, CACCC binding proteins present in nuclear extracts of murine erythroleukemia cells bind a radiolabeled oligonucleotide containing a single CACCC box, retarding its electrophoretic mobility. Migration of individual protein-DNA complexes is altered by incubation with specific antisera, as shown (Pre, preimmune serum). Note the presence of four major complexes, the most prominent one being Sp-1. Despite the low abundance of erythroid Krüppel-like factor (EKLF) in this assay, loss of EKLF function leads to a pronounced defect in β-globin gene transcription, which cannot be compensated for by other CACCC box-binding factors (see text). Although gel mobility shift experiments such as this identify factors that can bind to a CACCC box in vitro, they do not permit conclusions as to which factor(s) binds to a given CACCC box-containing promoter in vivo. (Photograph provided by Merlin Crossley.)

expression with resultant anemia and embryonic lethality of homozygous null animals at E14-E16 (Perkins et al., 1995; Nuez et al., 1995) (Fig. 4.5). EKLF$^{-/-}$ definitive erythrocytes exhibit molecular and morphologic features typical of severe β thalassemia including hypochromia, poikilocytosis, and markedly elevated α/β globin synthesis ratio with Heinz body formation and ineffective erythropoiesis.

Primitive erythropoiesis appears to be normal in the mutant mice, although there is a selective loss of the low, but normally detectable, levels of adult type β globin in E11 yolk sac (Perkins et al., 1995). Expression of embryonic β-like globin genes (βH1 and ε), the α-like globin genes (α and ζ), and other erythroid genes with functional CACCC boxes in their regulatory regions are essentially unaffected, suggesting that other factors, such as Sp-1 or FKLF (as noted later), might act at those promoters. Together, these results indicate that EKLF is a highly promoter-specific activator in erythroid cells.

A Role for EKLF in β Globin Switching

Selective loss of adult β-globin gene expression in mutant embryos suggested that EKLF might participate in the switch from γ to β globin in humans. Indeed, when transgenic mice bearing a human globin gene locus were crossed with EKLF-deficient mice, the resulting EKLF-deficient fetal liver cells displayed dramatically reduced human β globin levels with a concomitant increase in the levels of γ globin (Wijgerde et al., 1996; Perkins et al., 1996). In addition, mice heterozygous for EKLF-deficiency showed delayed completion of the human γ- to β-globin switch (Wijgerde et al., 1996) whereas overexpression of EKLF in transgenic mice accelerated it (Tewari et al., 1998). These studies are consistent with a model in which the γ- and β-globin gene promoters compete for the action of the LCR. In this model EKLF might contribute to a more stable interaction between the LCR and the β-globin promoter and therefore accelerate shutoff of γ. It is important to note, however, that γ-globin gene silencing can also occur independent of a competing β promoter (Dillon and Grosveld, 1991).

Loss of EKLF also leads to reduced DNase 1 hypersensitivity at HS3 and the β-globin promoter of both the human and endogenous globin genes (Wijgerde et al., 1996). This suggests that EKLF might contribute to changes in the chromatin configuration at selected sites at the globin gene locus. The changes in chromatin structure might facilitate binding of transcription factors to DNA, or increase the interaction between the β-globin promoter and the LCR. Alternatively, they might merely be a consequence of promoter/LCR interactions and transcriptional activity. The observation that EKLF associates with factors that have chromatin remodeling activity (as noted later) supports the former model.

Specificity of EKLF Action

An important issue is how EKLF activates gene expression with such promoter selectivity, given that

E15 EKLF -/-   E15 wild type

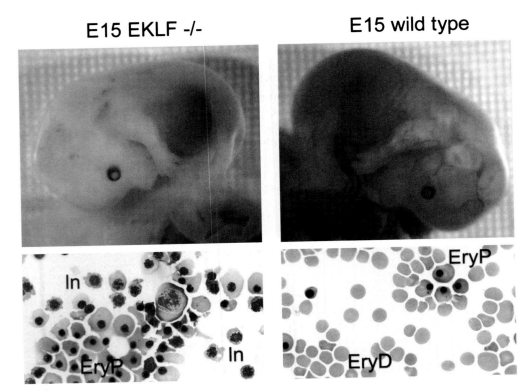

Figure 4.5. Impaired definitive erythropoiesis in erythroid Krüppel-like factor (ELKF)⁻/⁻ embryos. Affected embryos are extremely pale, but otherwise structurally normal (top panels). Peripheral blood smears are shown in the bottom panels. In E15 wild-type mice, there are mainly fetal liver-derived enucleated definitive erythrocytes (EryD) and a few yolk sac-derived primitive erythrocytes (EryP). The blood of EKLF⁻/⁻ littermates contains an increased proportion of normal appearing primitive erythrocytes but few mature definitive erythrocytes. Definitive erythroid cells consist mainly of immature nucleated late normoblasts (In) with irregular, poorly hemoglobinized cytoplasm. Rare circulating enucleated definitive erythrocytes exhibit pallor, microcytosis and poikilocytosis (not shown). (Photographs provided by Andrew Perkins.) For full color reproduction, see color plate 4.5.

conserved, functionally important CACCC boxes are present in all β-like globin genes (except for δ) and numerous nonglobin genes. Early biochemical studies suggest that selectivity might be explained by the higher affinity of EKLF for the β-globin CACCC box compared with the γ-globin CACCC box (Donze et al., 1995). However, in GAL4 fusion constructs, the activation domain of EKLF, but not Sp-1, can activate a β-globin-containing reporter construct in erythroid cells, suggesting that DNA binding affinity is not the sole determinant of EKLF specificity (Bieker and Southwood, 1995). In agreement with this interpretation, when the β- and γ-globin CACCC boxes are switched, EKLF still activates only the β- and not the γ-globin gene promoter (Asano and Stamatoyannopoulos, 1998). Thus promoter con-

text, as well as differences in DNA binding affinities, could determine the specificity of EKLF action.

Another study examined the enhancer activity of a mutant HS3 construct where a critical CACCC box had been altered such that both Sp-1 and EKLF binding were abolished (Gillemans et al., 1998). Subsequently, mutant Sp-1 and EKLF constructs capable of recognizing the altered CACCC box were coexpressed with HS3-dependent reporter constructs in transgenic mice. The results showed that mutant EKLF, but not mutant Sp-1, could activate the HS3-reporter gene, demonstrating that EKLF is likely the critical regulator of HS3-dependent β-globin expression in vivo (Gillemans et al., 1998). In addition, expression of mutant EKLF increased DNase1 hypersensitivity at HS3 in these mice, which, together with the knockout studies, showed a causal role for EKLF in the establishment of HS3 in vivo.

Specific activation of the β-globin gene promoter by EKLF is likely determined by promoter architecture and by other nuclear proteins bound next to EKLF. For example, the erythroid transcription factor GATA-1 physically interacts with Sp-1 and EKLF and synergizes with them during gene activation (Merika and Orkin, 1995; Gregory et al., 1996; Fischer et al., 1993) (see also previous discussion). It is also noteworthy that the activation domains of EKLF and Sp-1 share no obvious homology, the former being proline-rich and the latter being glutamine-rich, suggesting that they interact with different coactivator/adaptor molecules.

Posttranslational Modifications of EKLF

Terminal differentiation of MEL cells is accompanied by a dramatic increase in α- and β-globin gene expression, whereas EKLF protein levels remain largely unchanged (Bieker and Southwood, 1995). This raises the possibility that EKLF activity might be subject to regulation by posttranslational modifications. Indeed, EKLF is phosphorylated at its N-terminal activation domain, and mutation of the phosphorylation site leads to reduced activity (Ouyang et al., 1998). Furthermore, EKLF is also acetylated by CBP and p[300], two highly related transcriptional cofactors with acetyltransferase activity (Zhang and Bieker, 1998). CBP and p[300] bind to EKLF and stimulate its activity in transient transfection assays. Whether these modifications play a role in regulating EKLF activity during differentiation of erythroid cells remains to be determined.

EKLF and Chromatin Structure

Direct evidence for a role in modifying chromatin came from studies showing that ELKF interacts with a complex, the EKLF coactivator-remodeling complex 1 (E-RC1), which contains components of the mammalian SWI/SNF complex, an ATP-dependent chromatin remodeling machine (Armstrong et al., 1998). E-RC1 is required for EKLF-dependent formation of a DNase1 hypersensitive, transcriptionally active, chromatinized β-globin promoter template in vitro.

Another mechanism by which EKLF functions might involve the recruitment of CBP and p[300] is similar to what has been described for GATA-1 (see previous discussion) and NF-E2 (as noted later). In addition to acetylating EKLF, CBP/p[300] acetylates, histones, providing a potential mechanism by which EKLF regulates chromatin structure. Furthermore, CBP and p[300] might link EKLF to components of the basal transcription machinery (Shikama et al., 1997).

EKLF-related Transcription Factors

If EKLF acts at the β-globin gene promoter to participate in its stage-specific activation, what factors control expression of the embryonic and fetal globin genes at their respective CACCC boxes? One candidate is fetal Krüppel-like factor (FKLF). FKLF was isolated from a human fetal liver library based on its homology to EKLF, and is expressed in erythroid cells (Asano et al., 1999). FKLF activates the ε- γ- and β-globin gene promoters in transient transfection assays, with the ε-globin and γ-globin gene promoters showing the strongest response. This suggests that FKLF might be important for embryonic/fetal globin gene expression in vivo. In contrast to the globin genes, reg-ulatory regions of several other erythroid expressed genes that contain functional CACCC boxes are not activated by FKLF (Asano et al., 1999).

TIEG2, a protein identical to FKLF, was independently isolated as a TGF-β-inducible gene and shown to repress transcription and inhibit cell proliferation (Cook et al., 1998). In addition, these authors showed that TIEG2/FKLF is expressed ubiquitously in adult tissues, suggesting that it might serve functions other than globin gene expression. Therefore, the exact roles of TIEG2/FKLF depend on cell type and promoter context, similar to what has been described for EKLF.

Another major CACCC box-binding activity found in embryonic yolk sac and fetal liver erythroid cells has been identified as the basic Krüppel-like factor (BKLF) (Crossley et al., 1996). BKLF is a widely expressed protein that activates or represses transcription depending on cell and promoter context. Repression by BKLF is at least in part mediated through the association with a corepressor termed CtBP (Turner and Crossley, 1998). Of note, EKLF-deficient erythroid cells display dramatically reduced BKLF levels (Perkins et al., 1995; Crossley et al., 1996), suggesting that EKLF might regulate BKLF expression. In light of the complexity of proteins bound to the β-globin CACCC box, this finding underscores the difficulty in directly linking a transcription factor to a specific target gene in vivo, and in interpreting the phenotype of a gene knockout experiment on a molecular level. Targeted mutation of BKLF does not dramatically alter globin gene expression, suggesting that the ELKF null phenotype is not solely attributable to secondary loss of BLKF (Perkins et al., 1997). However, the role of BKLF, if any, in regulating β-globin gene expression remains to be determined.

Sp1, which was the first CACCC binding factor to be cloned, is expressed in a wide variety of cell types. Mice lacking Sp1 die at approximately day 10 of embryogenesis, displaying a multitude of defects (Marin et al., 1997). Given the relative abundance of Sp-1 in erythroid cells, it was somewhat of a surprise that embryonic α- and β-like globin genes are expressed normally. This suggests the possibility of compensatory expression of related factors, or that Sp1 plays no role in globin gene regulation in vivo.

It is clear from the above studies that a formidable effort is required to establish which transcription factor operates at any given CACCC box. Combined gene knockouts might be one approach to address this issue. Of equal importance will be to determine the mechanisms by which CACCC factors regulate transcription. The identification of novel interacting proteins and their analysis in vivo and in vitro will contribute to the understanding of the function of CACCC box binding proteins.

NF-E2 AND RELATED PROTEINS

The study of *cis*-acting regulatory elements in the β-LCR identified extended AP-1-like elements [(T/C)GCTGA(G/C)TCA(T/C)], now called Maf recognition elements (MAREs), as functionally important components of DNase 1 hypersensitive sites (HS) 2 and 3 (Chapters 5 and 6). Whereas GATA elements are mostly associated with the position independence conferred by the LCR, the presence of MARE binding sites correlates with the enhancer activity of the LCR (Talbot and Grosveld, 1991). Factors binding to MAREs directly contribute to the formation of DNase 1 hypersensitivity, suggesting a role of MARE-binding proteins in chromatin modification (Gong et al., 1996; Stamatoyannopoulos et al., 1995; Boyes and Felsenfeld, 1996; Pomerantz et al., 1998). MAREs are also found in a few nonglobin genes such as the porphobilinogen deaminase and ferrochelatase genes (Mignotte et al., 1989a; Taketani et al., 1992). Careful analysis of these elements showed that they are bound by an erythroid-specific transcription factor, NF-E2 (Mignotte et al., 1989a, 1989b). Affinity purification of NF-E2 from erythroleukemia cells revealed that it consists of two subunits, p45 and p18 (now referred to as MafK) (Andrews et al., 1993a, 1993b; Ney et al., 1993). Both subunits contain a basic-zipper (b-Zip) domain, which mediates dimerization and DNA binding. p45 is expressed predominantly in erythroid cells and megakaryocytes, whereas p18 is found in a variety of cell types.

It is now appreciated that both p45 and p18 belong to multiprotein families that are expressed in distinct but overlapping patterns, generating a large number of possible combinations of NF-E2-related complexes on DNA in different cell types.

The p45 Family of Proteins

p45 is the founding member of the growing family of proteins that contain a region termed the CNC domain with high similarity to the *Drosophila* Cap'*n*'Collar protein. This family includes Nrf-1 (LCRF1, TCF11), Nrf-2 (ECH), Nrf-3, Bach1, and Bach2. These proteins bind DNA as obligate heterodimers with Maf proteins (see later) and are unable to homodimerize (for reviews see Blank and Andrews, 1997; Motohashi et al., 1997).

Expression of p45 is restricted to the hematopoietic system (Andrews et al., 1993a; Ney et al., 1993). Erythroid cells and megakaryocytes express high levels of p45 mRNA, whereas little or no p45 mRNA is found in macrophages, B and T cells. This expression pattern suggests that p45 is a critical regulator of globin gene expression. Consistent with this idea, the erythroid cell line CB3, which lacks both functional alleles of p45, expresses very low levels of α and β globin. The introduction of an intact p45 gene restores globin gene expression (Lu et al., 1994; Kotkow and Orkin, 1995). Surprisingly, however, targeted inactivation of the p45 gene in mice has little effect on erythropoiesis or globin gene expression, whereas megakaryocytes display a pronounced defect in maturation resulting in severe thrombocytopenia and usually fatal hemorrhage (Shivdasani and Orkin, 1995; Shivdassani et al., 1995b).

Given the large body of evidence implicating MARE elements in globin gene transcription, the minimal effect of p45 gene disruption on erythropoiesis suggested the potential for compensation by other CNC family members. However, homozygous disruption of the Nrf-2 gene does not lead to reduced globin gene expression in mice (Chan et al., 1996), and the combined loss of Nrf-2 and p45 is no more severe than the p45 knockout alone (Kuroha et al., 1998; Martin et al., 1998). Disruption of the Nrf-1 gene causes anemia and embryonic lethality, but the defect in erythropoiesis is not cell-autonomous (Farmer et al., 1997; Chan et al., 1998). Thus, the exact contribution of each CNC-b-Zip protein to globin gene expression in vivo remains to be determined.

Bach1 and Bach2 are additional p45-related molecules that bind to MAREs as heterodimers with Maf family members (Oyake et al., 1996). Bach1 is expressed in hematopoietic cells starting at the earliest progenitor stages, suggesting it might fulfill a role distinct from that of p45, which is expressed only at later stages of differentiation (Oyake et al., 1996; Igarashi et al., 1998). The roles of Bach1 or Bach2 in globin gene expression in intact erythroid cells are unknown.

The Maf Family

Purification and cloning of the small subunit of NF-E2 revealed that it belongs to the Maf family of proteins. The Maf proteins, which share homology with the c-Maf proto-oncoprotein, are divided into two groups, the large and the small Maf molecules. The small Maf proteins (MafF, MafG, and MafK) heterodimerize with CNC-b-Zip family and exhibit distinct temporal and spatial expression patterns. MafG and MafK are highly expressed in megakaryocytes and erythroid cells, with a predominance of MafG in megakaryocytes and MafK in erythroid cells (Blank and Andrews, 1997; Motohashi et al., 1997). Small Maf proteins lack an activation domain and are thought to activate transcription as heterodimers with CNC-b-Zip (p45-like) molecules. Small Maf proteins can also form homodimers on DNA and repress transcription, presumably by competing with activating heterodimers or AP-1-like molecules for DNA binding (Igarashi et al., 1994).

To investigate the role of MafK in hematopoiesis (p18), the gene was inactivated by homologous recombination. Surprisingly, MafK$^{-/-}$ mice develop normally and display no obvious defect in erythroid maturation, globin gene expression, or platelet formation (Kotkow and Orkin, 1996). NF-E2-like DNA binding activity is still detected in fetal liver erythroid cells from MafK$^{-/-}$ mice, consistent with the presence of other Maf family members. MafK-deficient mice were bred with p45-deficient mice to generate compound homozygous mice deficient for both MafK and p45, with no effect on erythropoiesis (Kotkow and Orkin, 1996). Thus, other members of the p45 and MafK gene families can provide sufficient NF-E2-like activity in vivo. Targeting of the MafG gene produces no obvious defects in erythropoiesis, but does cause a defect in megakaryocytic differentiation, similar to, but not as pronounced as, that observed in the p45 knockout mice (Shavit et al., 1998).

Mechanisms of NF-E2 Action

Structure/function analysis of p45 in transient transfection experiments and in gene complementation assays using CB3 cells revealed that full NF-E2 activity requires an intact N-terminal activation domain and the CNC domain (Kotkow and Orkin, 1995; Bean and Ney, 1997). The N-terminus of p45 interacts with a number of proteins, some of which likely mediate the activation function of NF-E2. These include the transcriptional integrators CBP and p^{300} (Cheng et al., 1997), ubiquitin ligase (Gava et al., 1997; Mosser et al., 1998), and the TBP-associated factor TAF$_{II}$130 (Amrolia et al., 1997).

As is the case for GATA-1 and EKLF (see previous discussion), the implications for NF-E2/CBP/p^{300} interactions are twofold. First, CBP and p^{300} might participate in linking NF-E2 with basal transcription factors (for a review see Shikama et al., 1997). Direct communication between p45 and the basal transcription machinery is also suggested by the ability of p45 to interact with TAF$_{II}$130 (Amrolia et al., 1997). Such bridging mechanisms could promote looping between the LCR and the globin gene promoters. Second, recruitment of CBP/p^{300} and associated histone acetyltransferase activity to the LCR and other erythroid gene regulatory elements could lead to "open" chromatin structure through histone acetylation. That NF-E2 can disrupt chromatin structure on in vitro assembled chromatinized templates containing the β-globin LCR HS2 site suggests an additional role for NF-E2 in chromatin modification (Armstrong and Emerson, 1996). This ATP-dependent chromatin opening activity facilitates binding of GATA-1 to its nearby sites. Whether this activity also contains histone acetyltransferases is not known.

The N-terminus of p45 harbors two PPXY motifs that mediate interaction with several ubiquitin ligases (Gavva et al., 1997; Mosser et al., 1998). Mutations in these motifs reduce transcriptional activity of NF-E2 (Mosser et al., 1998). It has been hypothesized that ubiquitin ligases might contribute to ubiquitination of nearby histones, thus regulating chromatin structure.

The onset of high level globin gene expression is coordinated with differentiation and cell cycle arrest. Thus, it is likely that transcription factors involved in globin gene expression are subject to regulation by cellular signaling pathways controlling proliferation and terminal differentiation. Consistent with this idea, NF-E2 is a downstream target of regulation by the MAP kinase pathway. Activation of the MAP kinase pathway in MEL cells leads to an increase both in DNA binding and transcriptional activity of NF-E2 (Nagai et al., 1998). In addition, NF-E2 binding sites are required for MAP kinase inducibility of the HS2 region within the LCR (Versaw et al., 1998). NF-E2 p45 has been shown to be phosphorylated by protein kinase A; the physiologic significance of this finding is unclear (Casteel et al., 1998).

In summary, similar to the CACCC binding proteins discussed previously, MARE-binding factors are a heterogeneous group of proteins with distinct but overlapping functions and expression patterns. As an additional complexity, MARE factors activate transcription as heterodimers, leading to increased diversity through combinatorial associations. The major future challenge is to determine which combinations of MARE-binding proteins act at a given gene regulatory element in vivo. In particular for erythroid biology, it will be important to learn the full complement of NF-E2-like proteins that normally act at the β-globin locus and in the background of various targeted mutations of MARE-binding protein subunits.

STAGE SELECTOR ELEMENT/STAGE SELECTOR PROTEIN

One model to account for developmental regulation of gene expression within the β-globin locus is based on the principle that individual globin genes compete for β-LCR enhancer activity, which is available only to a single gene at any given time (Trimborn et al., 1999; Wijgerde et al., 1995; Choi and Engel, 1988). These competitive interactions are believed to be influenced by variations in the relative concentrations and/or posttranslational modifications of transcription factors that are expressed at all developmental stages

(Minie et al., 1992; Kenezetic and Felsenfeld, 1993) such as those discussed in the previous sections.

In addition, it is likely that erythroid stage-specific nuclear factors also influence the timing of individual globin gene expression. One potential example is human stage selector protein (SSP), which recognizes a DNA motif, termed stage selector element (SSE), found in the proximal γ-globin gene promoter. SSE was identified through its ability to allow the γ promoter to function in preference to a linked β-globin gene in plasmid constructs containing the HS-2 portion of the β-LCR (Jane et al., 1992). SSP DNA binding activity appears to be relatively restricted to fetal erythroid cells. Thus, it is believed that γ-globin synthesis is stimulated in part by expression of SSP, which binds SSE to impart a competitive advantage for recruitment of the LCR to the γ promoter. However, the SSE is neither necessary nor sufficient for competitive inhibition of β-globin gene expression in immortalized erythroid cell lines (Jane et al., 1992; Sargent et al., 1999a, 1999b). Therefore it is particularly important to determine the extent to which this element influences γ-gene expression in vivo.

SSP is a heterodimeric protein consisting of the widely expressed transcription factor CP2 and an unknown partner of approximately 40–45 KDa (Jane et al., 1995). As CP2 alone does not bind well to the SSE, the heterodimeric partner is presumed to confer both tissue specificity and DNA binding activity. Identification of this partner should allow further elucidation of the biological significance of the SSE/SSP complex. For example, it will be interesting to determine whether enforced expression of the SSP complex in β-globin-expressing definitive erythroid cells is capable of reactivating γ-globin synthesis.

SUMMARY AND PERSPECTIVE

Studies of globin gene regulation provide a paradigm for the investigation of tissue-specific and developmental control of eukaryotic gene expression. Therefore, it is no surprise that pursuit of the nuclear factors that coordinate globin gene transcription has produced a complexity of information with important implications for erythropoiesis in general and a variety of other developmental processes. For example, GATA-1 regulates the entire program of terminal erythropoiesis as well as megakaryocyte maturation, presumably by controlling many known and unknown target genes. Moreover, discovery of GATA-1 led to the identification of several related proteins important for the formation of hematopoietic stem cells, T lymphocytes, heart, nervous system, and a number of endodermally derived tissues. NF-E2, originally believed to be red blood cell specific, was shown by

knockout studies to be largely dispensable for globin synthesis and erythroid development, yet critical for platelet formation. Moreover, studies of NF-E2 have focused attention on the large family of MARE binding proteins, which participate in numerous processes including cognitive development and formation of early embryonic mesoderm. Likewise, the discovery and characterization of several Krüppel-related proteins with diverse functions have been motivated largely by studies of globin regulation.

Discovery of numerous tissue-restricted and widely expressed transcription factors that function in red blood cells provides a solid foundation for understanding globin gene expression and erythroid differentiation. The current challenge is to better understand the mechanistic basis for transcription factor function in the intact organism. Presumably, insights will be gained through continued investigation of the dynamic developmental stage and tissue-specific regulatory networks that exist between erythroid nuclear factors, basal transcription machinery, and chromatin. A speculative model depicting one subset of potential interactions is shown in Figure 4.6A. In this example, erythroid DNA binding proteins interact with each other, as well as with the general coactivator, CBP (or p^{300}). CBP/p^{300}, in turn, could modify histones and individual transcription factors through acetylation and might also link promoter/enhancer bound proteins with components of the basal transcriptional machinery. Similar models based on demonstrated interactions between erythroid nuclear factors and chromatin remodeling machinery (Armstrong et al., 1998; Gong et al., 1996; Armstrong and Emerson, 1996) can also be envisioned.

Although the concept of transcription factor networks is generally applicable, many questions specifically pertain to erythroid biology. For example, do nuclear multiprotein complexes contribute to the hypothesized formation of a loop between the LCR and globin gene promoters (Fig. 4.6B)? How do the relative concentrations of related factors such as GATA-1/GATA-2, ELKF/FKLF/BKLF, and MARE-binding factors at a given developmental stage influence globin expression and erythroid differentiation?

In addition, it is important to examine the hierarchical order by which transcription factors regulate each other's expression. For example, GATA-1-mediated repression of GATA-2, may be prerequisite for terminal erythroid maturation (Weiss and Orkin, 1995a). GATA-1 appears to positively regulate expression of the EKLF gene (Crossley et al., 1994), and EKLF is required for full expression of BKLF (Perkins et al., 1995; Crossley et al., 1996). Such cross-regulation imposes a tissue-restricted and developmental order on the erythroid gene expression program. Analysis of cis-acting regulatory regions of erythroid

A

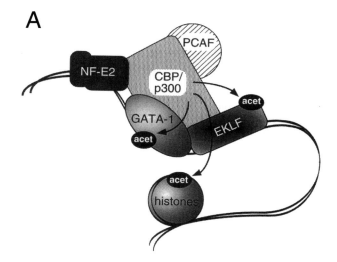

B

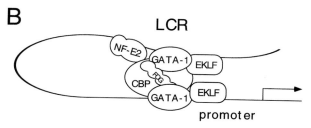

Figure 4.6. Erythroid transcription factor networks. (**A**) A hypothetical model in which GATA-1, erythroid Krüppel-like factor (EKLF) and NF-E2 cooperate in recruiting an acetyl-transferase-containing complex, containing CBP/p^{300} and p^{300}/CBP-associated factor (PCAF), to the locus control regions (LCR), leading to histone and transcription factor acetylation. Histone acetylation might lead to changes in chromatin structure, and acetylation of transcription factors might regulate DNA binding or transcriptional activity (see text for details). (**B**) A proposed model in which transcription factors and their coactivators participate in the generation of a loop between the LCR and a globin gene promoter. Within this context, developmental stage-specific differences in the abundance of various nuclear factors and/or posttranslational protein modifications could regulate hemoglobin switching by favoring particular promoter-LCR interactions.

transcription factor genes is beginning to unravel how their expression is regulated.

Ultimately, one goal of this basic knowledge is to manipulate gene expression to treat human disease. The realization that transcriptional cofactors such as CBP/p^{300} have enzymatic activity raises the possibility of developing compounds that alter specific activity or substrate specificity. For example, the drug butyrate, which is used to activate fetal globin gene expression in patients with sickle cell anemia or β thalassemia (Chapter 38) inhibits histone deacetylases (Candido et al., 1978), thereby presumably derepressing γ globin via increased acetylation of histones, and possibly

transcription factors. More potent agents with similar activity are now being studied (McCaffrey et al., 1997). Histone deacetylase inhibitors have also been shown to reactivate silenced globin transgenes delivered by retroviral vectors designed for gene therapy (Chen et al., 1997). Together, these results define an interface through which basic studies of gene regulation might ultimately impinge on clinical management of hematologic disorders.

ACKNOWLEDGMENTS

We thank Stuart Orkin, Merlin Crossley, and Steven Liebhaber for reviewing this chapter.

References

Amrolia, PJ, Ramamurthy, L, Saluja, D et al. (1997). The activation domain of the enhancer binding protein p45NF-E2 interacts with TAFII130 and mediates long-range activation of the alpha- and beta-globin gene loci in an erythroid cell line. *Proc. Natl. Acad. Sci. U.S.A.* 94: 10051–10056.

Andrews, NC, Erdjument-Bromage, H, Davidson, M et al. (1993a). Erythroid transcription factor NF-E2 is a haematopoietic-specific basic-leucine zipper protein. *Nature* 362: 722–728.

Andrews, NC, Kotkow, KJ, Ney, PA et al. (1993b). The ubiquitous subunit of erythroid transcription factor NF-E2 is a small basic-leucine zipper protein related to the v-maf oncogene. *Proc. Natl. Acad. Sci. U.S.A.* 90: 11488–11492.

Anderson, KP, Crable, SC, and Lingrel, JB. (1998). Multiple proteins binding to a GATA-E box-GATA motif regulate the erythroid Kruppel-like factor (EKLF) gene. *J. Biol. Chem.* 273: 14347–14354.

Aplan, PD, Nakahara, K, Orkin, SHO, and Kirsch, IR. (1992). The SCL gene product: A positive regulator of erythroid differentiation. *EMBO J.* 11: 4073–4081.

Arceci, RJ, King, AAJ, Simon, MC et al. (1993). Mouse GATA-4: A retinoic acid-inducible GATA-binding transcription factor expressed in endodermally derived tissues and heart. *Mol. Cell. Biol.* 13: 2235–2246.

Armstrong, JA and Emerson, BM. (1996). NF-E2 disrupts chromatin structure at human beta-globin locus control region hypersensitive site 2 in vitro. *Mol. Cell. Biol.* 16: 5634–5644.

Armstrong, JA, Bieker, JJ, and Emerson, BM. (1998). A SWI/SNF-related chromatin remodeling complex, E-RC1, is required for tissue-specific transcriptional regulation by EKLF in vitro. *Cell* 95: 93–104.

Asano, H, Li, XS, and Stamatoyannopoulos, G. (1999). FKLF, a novel Kruppel-like factor that activates human embryonic and fetal beta-like globin genes. *Mol. Cell. Biol.* 19: 3571–3579.

Asano, H and Stamatoyannopoulos, G. (1998). Activation of beta-globin promoter by erythroid Kruppel-like factor. *Mol. Cell. Biol.* 18: 102–109.

Bean, TL and Ney, PA. (1997). Multiple regions of p45 NF-E2 are required for β-globin gene expression in erythroid cells. *Nucleic Acids Res.* 25: 2509–2515.

Begley CG and Green, AR. (1999). The SCL gene: From case report to critical hematopoietic regulator. *Blood* 93: 2760–2770.

Bieker, JJ and Southwood, CM. (1995). The erythroid Kruppel-like factor transactivation domain is a critical component for cell-specific inducibility of a beta-globin promoter. *Mol. Cell. Biol.* 15: 852–860.

Blank, V and Andrews, NC. (1997). The Maf transcription factors: Regulators of differentiation. *Trends Biochem. Sci.* 22: 437–441.

Blobel, GA, Simon, MC, and Orkin, SH. (1995). Rescue of GATA-1-deficient embryonic stem cells by heterologous GATA-binding proteins. *Mol. Cell. Biol.* 15: 626–633.

Blobel, GA, Nakajima, T, Eckner, R et al. (1998). CREB-binding protein cooperates with transcription factor GATA-1 and is required for erythroid differentiation. *Proc. Natl. Acad. Sci. U.S.A.* 95: 2061–2066.

Boyes, J and Felsenfeld, G. (1996). Tissue-specific factors additively increase the probability of the all-or-none formation of a hypersensitive site. *EMBO J.* 15: 2496–2507.

Boyes, J, Byfield, P, Nakatani, Y, and Ogryzko, V. (1998a). Regulation of activity of the transcription factor GATA-1 by acetylation. *Nature* 396: 594–598.

Boyes, J, Omichinski, J, Clark, D et al. (1998b). Perturbation of nucleosome structure by the erythroid transcription factor GATA-1. *J. Mol. Biol.* 279: 529–544.

Briegel, K, Lim, K-C, Plank, C et al. (1993). Ectopic expression of a conditional GATA-2/estrogen receptor chimera arrests erythroid differentiation in a hormone-dependent manner. *Genes Dev.* 7: 1097–1109.

Brotherton, TW, Chui, DHK, Gauldie, J, and Patterson, M. (1979). Hemoglobin ontogeny during normal mouse fetal development. *Proc. Natl. Acad. Sci.* 76: 2853–2857.

Candido, EP, Reeves, R, and Davie, JR. (1978). Sodium butyrate inhibits histone deacetylation in cultured cells. *Cell* 14: 105–113.

Capecchi, MR. (1989). Altering the genome by homologous recombination. *Science* 244: 1288–1292.

Casteel, D, Suhasini, M, Gudi, T et al. (1998). Regulation of the erythroid transcription factor NF-E2 by cyclic adenosine monophosphate-dependent protein kinase. *Blood* 91: 3193–3201.

Chan, JY, Kwong, M, Lu, R et al. (1998). Targeted disruption of the ubiquitous CNC-bZIP transcription factor, Nrf-1, results in anemia and embryonic lethality in mice. *EMBO J.* 17: 1779–1787.

Chan, K, Lu, R, Chang, JC, and Kan, YW. (1996). NRF2, a member of the NFE2 family of transcription factors, is not essential for murine erythropoiesis, growth, and development. *Proc. Natl. Acad. Sci. U.S.A.* 93: 13943–13948.

Chen, WY, Bailey, EC, McCune, SL et al. (1997). Reactivation of silenced, virally transduced genes by inhibitors of histone deacetylase. *Proc. Natl. Acad. Sci. U.S.A.* 94: 5798–5803.

Cheng, X, Reginato, MJ, Andrews, NC, and Lazar, MA. (1997). The Transcriptional Integrator CREB-binding protein mediates positive cross talk between nuclear hormone receptors and the hematopoietic bZip protein p45/NF-E2. *Mol. Cell. Biol.* 1: 1407–1416.

Choi, O-RB and Engel, JD. (1988). Developmental regulation of β-globin gene switching. *Cell* 56: 17–26.

Chyuan-Sheng, L, Lim, S-K, D'Agati, V, and Costantini F. (1996). Differential effects of an erythropoietin receptor gene disruption on primitive and definitive erythropoiesis. *Genes Dev* 10: 154–164.

Cook, T, Gebelein, B, Mesa, K et al. (1998). Molecular cloning and characterization of TIEG2 reveals a new subfamily of transforming growth factor-beta-inducible Sp1-like zinc finger-encoding genes involved in the regulation of cell growth. *J. Biol. Chem.* 273: 25929–25936.

Cook, T, Gebelein, B, and Urrutia, R. (1999). Sp1 and its likes: Biochemical and functional predictions for a growing family of zinc finger transcription factors. *Ann. N.Y. Acad. Sci.* 880: 94–102.

Crispino, JD, Lodish, MB, MacKay, JP, and Orkin, SH. (1999). Use of altered specificity mutants to probe a specific protein-protein interaction in differentiation: The GATA-1:FOG complex. *Mol. Cell* 3: 219–228.

Crossley, M, Tsang, AP, Bieker, JJ, and Orkin, SH. (1994). Regulation of the erythroid Kruppel-like factor (EKLF) gene promoter by the erythroid transcription factor GATA-1. *J. Biol. Chem.* 269: 15440–15444.

Crossley, M and Orkin, SH. (1994). Phosphorylation of the erythroid transcription factor GATA-1. *J. Biol. Chem.* 269: 16589–16596.

Crossley, M, Merika, M, and Orkin, SH. (1995). Self-association of the erythroid transcription factor GATA-1 mediated by its zinc finger domains. *Mol. Cell. Biol.* 15: 2448–2456.

Crossley, M, Whitelaw, E, Perkins, A et al. (1996). Isolation and characterization of the cDNA encoding BKLF/TEF-2, a major CACCC-box-binding protein in erythroid cells and selected other cells. *Mol. Cell. Biol.* 16: 1695–1705.

Delgado, MD, Gutierrez, P, Richard, C et al. (1998). Spi-1/PU.1 proto-oncogene induces opposite effects on monocytic and erythroid differentiation of K562 cells. *Biochem. Biophys. Res. Commun.* 252: 383–391.

Detrich, HWr, Kieran, MW, Chan, FY et al. (1995). Intraembryonic hematopoietic cell migration during vertebrate development. *Proc. Natl. Acad. Sci. U.S.A.* 92: 10713–10717.

Dillon, N and Grosveld, F. (1991). Human gamma-globin genes silenced independently of other genes in the beta-globin locus. *Nature* 350: 252–254.

Doetschman, TC, Eistetter, H, Katz, M et al. (1985). The in vitro development of blastocyst-derived embryonic stem cell lines: Formation of visceral yolk sac, blood islands, and myocardium. *J. Embryol. Exp. Morphol.* 87: 27–45.

Donze, D, Townes, TM, and Bieker, JJ. (1995). Role of erythroid Kruppel-like factor in human gamma- to beta-globin gene switching. *J. Biol. Chem.* 270: 1955–1959.

Dorfman, DM, Wilson, DB, Bruns, GA, and Orkin, SH. (1992). Human transcription factor GATA-2. Evidence for regulation of preproendothelin-1 gene expression in endothelial cells. *J. Biol. Chem.* 267: 1279–1285.

Elnitski, L, Miller, W, and Hardison, R. (1997). Conserved E boxes function as part of the enhancer in hypersensitive site 2 of the beta-globin locus control region. Role of basic helix-loop-helix proteins. *J. Biol. Chem.* 272: 369–378.

Evans, T and Felsenfeld, G. (1989). The erythroid-specific transcription factor Eryf1: A new finger protein. *Cell* 58: 877–885.

Evans T and Felsenfeld, G. (1991). *trans*-Activation of a globin promoter in nonerythroid cells. *Mol. Cell. Biol.* 11: 843–853.

Evans, MJ and Kaufman, MH. (1981). Establishment in culture of pluripotent cells from mouse embryos. *Nature* 292: 154–156.

Farina, SF, Girard, LJ, Vanin, EF et al. (1995). Dysregulated expression of GATA-1 following retrovirus-mediated gene transfer into murine hematopoietic stem cells increases erythropoiesis. *Blood* 86: 4124–4133.

Farmer, SC, Sun, CW, Winnier, GE et al. (1997). The bZIP transcription factor LCR-F1 is essential for mesoderm formation in mouse development. *Genes Dev.* 11: 786–798.

Felsenfeld, G. (1996). Chromatin unfolds. *Cell* 86: 13–19.

Feng, WC, Southwood, CM, and Bieker, JJ. (1994). Analyses of beta-thalassemia mutant DNA interactions with erythroid Kruppel-like factor (EKLF), an erythroid cell-specific transcription factor. *J. Biol. Chem.* 269: 1493–1500.

Fischer, K-D, Haese, A, and Nowock, J. (1993). Cooperation of GATA-1 and Sp1 can result in synergistic transcriptional activation or interference. *J. Biol. Chem.* 268: 23915–23923.

Fisher, RC and Scott, EW. (1998). Role of PU.1 in hematopoiesis. *Stem Cells* 16: 25–37.

Forrester, WC, Takegawa, S, Papayannopoulou, T et al. (1987). Evidence for a locus activation region: The formation of developmentally stable hypersensitive sites in globin-expressing hybrids. *Nucleic Acids Res.* 15: 10159–10177.

Fox, AH, Kowalski, K, King, GF et al. (1998). Key residues characteristic of GATA N-fingers are recognized by FOG. *J. Biol. Chem.* 273: 33595–33603.

Fox, AH, Liew, C, Holmes, M et al. (1999). Transcriptional cofactors of the FOG family interact with GATA proteins by means of multiple zinc fingers. *EMBO J.* 18: 2812–2822.

Fujiwara, Y, Browne, CP, Cunniff, K et al. (1996). Arrested development of embryonic red cell precursors in mouse embryos lacking transcription factor GATA-1. *Proc. Natl. Acad. Sci. U.S.A.* 93: 12355–12358.

Gavva, NR, Gavva, R, Ermekova, K et al. (1997). Interaction of WW domains with hematopoietic transcription factor p45/NF-E2 and RNA polymerase II. *J. Biol. Chem.* 272: 24105–24108.

Gillemans, N, Tewari, R, Lindeboom, F et al. (1998). Altered DNA-binding specificity mutants of EKLF and Sp1 show that EKLF is an activator of the beta-globin locus control region in vivo. *Genes Dev.* 12: 2863–2873.

Gong, QH, McDowell, JC, and Dean, A (1996). Essential role of NF-E2 in remodeling of chromatin structure and transcriptional activation of the epsilon-globin gene in vivo by 5′ hypersensitive site 2 of the beta-globin locus control region. *Mol. Cell. Biol.* 16: 6055–6064.

Green, AR, Salvaris, E, and Begley, CG. (1991). Erythroid expression of the helix-loop-helix gene, SCL. *Oncogene* 6: 475–479.

Gregory, RC, Taxman, DJ, Seshasayee, D et al. (1996). Functional interaction of GATA1 with erythroid Kruppel-like factor and Sp1 at defined erythroid promoters. *Blood* 87: 1793–1801.

Gregory, T, Yu, C, Ma, A et al. (1999). GATA-1 and erythropoietin cooperate to promote erythroid cell survival by regulating bcl-xL expression. *Blood* 94: 87–96.

Grosveld, F, van Assendelft, GB, Greaves, DR, and Kollias, G. (1987). Position-independent, high-level expression of the human beta-globin gene in transgenic mice. *Cell* 51: 975–85.

Gu, W and Roeder, RG. (1997). Activation of p53 sequence-specific DNA binding by acetylation of the p53 C-terminal domain. *Cell* 90: 595–606.

Gu, H, Marth, JD, Orban, PC et al. (1994). Deletion of a DNA polymerase β gene segment in T cells using cell type-specific gene targeting. *Science* 265: 103–106.

Hendriks, RW, Nawijn, MC, Engel, JD et al. (1999). Expression of the transcription factor GATA-3 is required for the development of the earliest T cell progenitors and correlates with stages of cellular proliferation in the thymus. *Eur. J. Immunol.* 29: 1912–1918.

Higgs, DR. (1998). Do LCRs open chromatin domains? *Cell* 95: 299–302.

Hoang, T, Paradis, E, Brady, G et al. (1996). Opposing effects of the basic helix-loop-helix transcription factor SCL on erythroid and monocytic differentiation. *Blood* 87: 102–111.

Holmes, M, Turner, J, Fox, A et al. (1999). hFOG-2, a novel zinc finger protein, binds the co-repressor mCtBP2 and modulates GATA-mediated activation. *J. Biol. Chem.* 274: 23491–23498.

Hung, HL, Lau, J, Kim, AY et al. (1999). CREB-binding protein acetylates hematopoietic transcription factor GATA-1 at functionally important sites. *Mol. Cell. Biol.* 19: 3496–3505.

Hunter, T and Karin, M. (1992). The regulation of transcription by phosphorylation. *Cell* 70: 375–387.

Igarashi, K, Kataoka, K, Itoh, K et al. (1994). Regulation of transcription by dimerization of erythroid factor NF-E2 p45 with small Maf proteins. *Nature (London)* 367: 568–572.

Igarashi, K, Hoshino, H, Muto, A et al. (1998). Multivalent DNA binding complex generated by small Maf and Bach1 as a possible biochemical basis for beta-globin locus control region complex. *J. Biol. Chem.* 273: 11783–11790.

Ito, E, Toki, T, Ishihara, H et al. (1993). Erythroid transcription factor GATA-1 is abundantly transcribed in mouse testis. *Nature* 362: 466–468.

Jane, SM, Ney, PA, Vanin, EF et al. (1992). Identification of a stage selector element in the human gamma-globin gene promoter that fosters preferential interaction with the 5′ HS2 enhancer when in competition with the beta-promoter. *EMBO* 11: 2961–2969.

Jane, SM, Nienhuis, AW, and Cunningham, JM. (1995). Hemoglobin switching in man and chicken is mediated by a heteromeric complex between the ubiquitous transcription factor CP2 and a developmentally specific protein [published erratum appears in *EMBO J.* 1995 Feb 15;14(4):854]. *EMBO J.* 14: 97–105.

Jiang, Y and Evans, T. (1996). The *Xenopus* GATA-4/5/6 genes are associated with cardiac specification and can regulate cardiac-specific transcription during embryogenesis. *Dev. Biol.* 174: 258–270.

Kadonaga, JT. (1998). Eukaryotic transcription: An interlaced network of transcription factors and chromatin-modifying machines. *Cell* 92: 307–313.

Keller, G, Kennedy, M, Papayannopoulou, T, and Wiles, MV. (1993). Hematopoietic differentiation during embryonic stem cell differentiation in culture. *Mol. Cell. Biol.* 13: 472–486.

Kelley, C, Blumberg, H, Zon, LI and Evans, T. (1993). GATA-4 is a novel transcription factor expressed in endocardium of the developing heart. *Development* 118: 817–827.

Knezetic, JA and Felsenfeld, G. (1993). Mechanism of developmental regulation of alpha pi, the chicken embryonic alpha-globin gene. *Mol. Cell. Biol.* 13: 4632–4639.

Kornhauser, JM, Leonard, MW, Yamamoto, M et al. (1994). Temporal and spatial changes in GATA transcription factor expression are coincident with development of the chicken optic tectum. *Mol. Brain Res.* 23: 100–110.

Kotkow, K and Orkin, SH. (1995). Dependence of globin gene expression in mouse erythroleukemia cells on the NF-E2 heterodimer. *Mol. Cell. Biol.* 15: 4640–4647.

Kotkow, KJ and Orkin, SH. (1996). Complexity of the erythroid transcription factor NF-E2 as revealed by gene targeting of the mouse p18 NF-E2 locus. *Proc. Natl. Acad. Sci. U.S.A.* 93: 3514–3518.

Koutsourakis, M, Langeveld, A, Patient, R et al. (1999). The transcription factor GATA6 is essential for early extraembryonic development [corrected and republished in Development 1999 May; 126(9):723–32]. *Development* 126: 723–732.

Kowalski, K, Czolij, R, King, GF et al. (1999). The solution structure of the N-terminal zinc finger of GATA-1 reveals a specific binding face for the transcriptional co-factor FOG. *J. Biomol. NMR* 13: 249–262.

Kulessa, H, Frampton, J, and Graf, T. (1995). GATA-1 reprograms avian myelomonocytic cell lines into eosinophils, thromboblasts, and erythroblasts. *Genes Dev.* 9: 1250–1262.

Kulozik, AE, Bellan-Koch, A, Bail, S et al. (1991). Thalassemia intermedia: Moderate reduction of beta globin gene transcriptional activity by a novel mutation of the proximal CACCC promoter element. *Blood* 77: 2054–2058.

Kuroha, T, Takahashi, S, Komeno, T et al. (1998). Ablation of Nrf2 function does not increase the erythroid or megakaryocytic cell lineage dysfunction caused by p45 NF-E2 gene disruption. *J. Biochem.* 123: 376–379.

Laverriere, AC, MacNeill, C, Mueller, C et al. (1994). GATA-4/5/6, a subfamily of three transcription factors transcribed in developing heart and gut. *J. Biol. Chem.* 269: 23177–23184.

Leonard, M, Brice, M, Engel, JD, and Papayannopoulou, T. (1993). Dynamics of GATA transcription factor expression during erythroid differentiation. *Blood* 82: 1071–1079.

Li, J, Noguchi, CT, Miller, W et al. (1998). Multiple regulatory elements in the 5′-flanking sequence of the human epsilon-globin gene. *J. Biol. Chem.* 273: 10202–10209.

Lu, JR, McKinsey, TA, Xu, H et al. (1999). FOG-2, a heart- and brain-enriched cofactor for GATA transcription factors. *Mol. Cell. Biol.* 19: 4495–4502.

Lu, S-J, Rowan, S, Bani, MR, and Ben-David Y. (1994). Retroviral integration within the Fli-2 locus results in inactivation of the erythroid transcription factor NF-E2 in Friend erythroleukemias: Evidence that NF-E2 is essential for globin gene expression. *Proc. Natl. Acad. Sci. U.S.A.* 91: 8398–8402.

Ma, GT, Roth, ME, Groskopf, JC et al. (1997). GATA-2 and GATA-3 regulate trophoblast-specific gene expression in vivo. *Development* 124: 907–914.

Marin, M, Karis, A, Visser, P et al. (1997). Transcription factor Sp1 is essential for early embryonic development but dispensable for cell growth and differentiation. *Cell* 89: 619–628.

Martin, GR. (1981). Isolation of a pluripotent cell line from early mouse embryos cultured in medium conditioned by teratocarcinoma cells. *Proc. Natl. Acad. Sci. U.S.A.* 78: 7634–7638.

Martin, DIK, and Orkin, SH. (1990a). Transcriptional activation and DNA binding by the erythroid factor GF-1/NF-E1/Eryf 1. *Genes Dev.* 4: 1886–1898.

Martin, DI, Zon, LI, Mutter, G, and Orkin, SH. (1990b). Expression of an erythroid transcription factor in megakaryocytic and mast cell lineages. *Nature* 344: 444–447.

Martin, F, van Deursen, JM, Shivdasani, RA et al. (1998). Erythroid maturation and globin gene expression in mice with combined deficiency of NF-E2 and nrf-2. *Blood* 91: 3459–3466.

McCaffrey, PG, Newsome, DA, Fibach, E et al. (1997). Induction of gamma-globin by histone deacetylase inhibitors. *Blood* 90: 2075–2083.

McDevitt, MA, Shivdasani, RA, Fujiwara, Y et al. (1997). A "knockdown" mutation created by cis-element gene targeting reveals the dependence of erythroid cell maturation on the level of transcription factor GATA-1. *Proc. Natl. Acad. Sci. U.S.A.* 94: 6781–6785.

Merika, M and Orkin, SH. (1995). Functional synergy and physical interactions of the erythroid transcription factor GATA-1 with the *Krüppel* family proteins Sp1 and EKLF. *Mol. Cell. Biol.* 15: 2437–2447.

Mignotte, V, Eleouet, JF, Raich, N, and Romeo, P-H. (1989a). *Cis-* and *trans-*acting elements involved in the regulation of the erythroid promoter of the human porphobilinogen deaminase gene. *Proc. Natl. Acad. Sci. U.S.A.* 86: 6548–6552.

Mignotte, V, Wall, L, deBoer, E et al. (1989b). Two tissue-specific factors bind the erythroid promoter of the human porphobilinogen deaminase gene. *Nucl. Acids Res.* 17: 37–54.

Miller, IJ and Bieker, JJ. (1993). A novel, erythroid cell-specific murine transcription factor that binds to the CACCC element and is related to the Kruppel family of nuclear proteins. *Mol. Cell. Biol.* 13: 2776–2786.

Minie, ME, Kimura, T, and Felsenfeld G. (1992). The developmental switch in embryonic rho-globin expression is correlated with erythroid lineage-specific differences in transcription factor levels. *Development* 115: 1149–1164.

Mitchell, PJ and Tjian, R. (1989). Transcriptional regulation in mammalian cells by sequence-specific DNA binding proteins. *Science* 245: 371–378.

Moreau-Gachelin, F, Wendling F, Molina, T et al. (1996). Spi-1/PU.1 transgenic mice develop multistep erythroleukemias. *Mol. Cell. Biol.* 16: 2453–2463.

Moreau-Gachelin, F, Ray, D, Mattei, MG et al. (1989). The putative oncogene Spi-1: Murine chromosomal localization and transcriptional activation in murine acute erythroleukemias [published erratum appears in *Oncogene* 1990 Jun;5(6):941]. *Oncogene* 4: 1449–1456.

Morrisey, EE, Ip, HS, Lu, MM, and Parmacek, MS. (1996). GATA-6: A zinc finger transcription factor that is expressed in multiple cell lineages derived from lateral mesoderm. *Dev. Biol.* 177: 309–322.

Morrisey, EE, Ip, HS, Tang, Z et al. (1997). GATA-5: A transcriptional activator expressed in a novel temporally and spatially-restricted pattern during embryonic development. *Dev. Biol.* 183: 21–36.

Morrisey, EE, Tang, Z, Sigrist, K et al. (1998). GATA6 regulates HNF4 and is required for differentiation of visceral endoderm in the mouse embryo. *Genes Dev.* 12: 3579–3590.

Mortensen, RM, Conner, DA, Chao, S et al. (1992). Production of homozygous mutant ES cells with a single targeting construct. *Mol. Cell. Biol.* 12: 2391–2395.

Mosser, EA, Kasanov, JD, Forsberg, EC et al. (1998). Physical and functional interactions between the trans-activation domain of the hematopoietic transcription factor NF-E2 and WW domains. *Biochemistry* 37: 13686–13695.

Motohashi, H, Shavit, JA, Igarashi, K et al. (1997). The world according to Maf. *Nucleic Acids Res.* 25: 2953–2959.

Mouthon, M-A, Bernard, O, Mitjavila, M-T et al. (1993). Expression of tal-1 and GATA-binding proteins during human hematopoiesis. *Blood* 81: 647–655.

Mucenski, ML, McLain, K, Kier, AB et al. (1991). A functional c-myb gene is required for normal fetal hematopoiesis. *Cell* 65: 677–689.

Nagai, T, Igarashi, K, Akasaka, J et al. (1998). Regulation of NF-E2 activity in erythroleukemia cell differentiation. *J. Biol. Chem.* 273: 5358–5365.

Nakano, T, Kodama, H, and Honjo T. (1994). Generation of lymphohematopoietic cells from embryonic stem cells in culture. *Science* 265: 1098–1101.

Nardelli, J, Thiesson, D, Fujiwara, Y et al. (1999). Expression and genetic interaction of transcription factors GATA-2 and GATA-3 during development of the mouse central nervous system. *Dev. Biol.* 210: 305–321.

Ney, PA, Andrews, NC, Jane, SM et al. (1993). Purification of the human NF-E2 complex: cDNA cloning of the hematopoietic cell-specific subunit and evidence for an associated partner. *Mol. Cell. Biol.* 13: 5604–5612.

Ng, YK, George, KM, Engel, JD, and Linzer, DI. (1994). GATA factor activity is required for the trophoblast-specific transcriptional regulation of the mouse placental lactogen I gene. *Development* 120: 3257–3266.

Nuez, B, Michalovich, D, Bygrave, A et al. (1995). Defective haematopoiesis in fetal liver resulting from inactivation of the EKLF gene. *Nature (London)* 375: 316–318.

Ogawa, M, Nishikawa, S, Yoshinaga, K et al. (1993). Expression and function of c-Kit in fetal hemopoietic progenitor cells: Transition from the early c-Kit-independent to the late c-Kit-dependent wave of hemopoiesis in the murine embryo. *Development* 117: 1089–1098.

Okuda, T, van Deursen, J, Hiebert, SW et al. (1996). AML 1, the target of multiple chromosomal translocations in human leukemia, is essential for normal fetal liver hematopoiesis. *Cell* 84: 321–330.

Omichinski, JG, Clore, GM, Schaad, O et al. (1993). NMR structure of a specific DNA complex of Zn-containing DNA binding domain of GATA-1. *Science* 261: 438–446.

Orkin, SH. (1992). GATA-binding transcription factors in hematopoietic cells. *Blood* 80: 575–581.

Orkin, SH, Kazazian, HHJ, Antonarakis, SE et al. (1982). Linkage of beta-thalassaemia mutations and beta-globin gene polymorphisms with DNA polymorphisms in human beta-globin gene cluster. *Nature (London)* 296: 627–631.

Orkin, SH, Antonarakis, SE, and Kazazian, HHJ. (1984). Base substitution at position-88 in a beta-thalassemic globin gene. Further evidence for the role of distal promoter element ACACCC. *J. Biol. Chem.* 259: 8679–8681.

Ouyang, L, Chen, X, and Bieker, JJ. (1998). Regulation of erythroid Kruppel-like factor (EKLF) transcriptional activity by phosphorylation of a protein kinase casein kinase II site within its interaction domain. *J. Biol. Chem.* 273: 23019–23025.

Oyake, T, Itoh, K, Motohashi, H et al. (1996). Bach proteins belong to a novel family of BTB-basic leucine zipper transcription factors that interact with MafK and regulate transcription through the NF-E2 site. *Mol. Cell. Biol.* 16: 6083–6095.

Pandolfi, PP, Roth, ME, Karis, A et al. (1995). Targeted disruption of the GATA3 gene causes severe abnormalities in the nervous system and in fetal liver haematopoiesis [see comments]. *Nat. Genet.* 11: 40–44.

Partington, GA and Patient, RK. (1999). Phosphorylation of GATA-1 increases its DNA-binding affinity and is correlated with induction of human K562 erythroleukaemia cells. *Nucleic Acids Res.* 27: 1168–1175.

Perkins, AC, Sharpe, AH, and Orkin, SH. (1995). Lethal β-thalassaemia in mice lacking the erythroid CACCC-transcription factor EKLF. *Nature* 375: 318–322.

Perkins, AC, Gaensler, KM, and Orkin, SH. (1996). Silencing of human fetal globin expression is impaired in the absence of the adult beta-globin gene activator protein EKLF. *Proc. Natl. Acad. Sci. U.S.A.* 93: 12267–12271.

Perkins, AC, Yang, H, Crossley, PM et al. (1997). Deficiency of the CACC-element binding protein BKLF leads to a progressive myeloproliferative disease and impaired expression of SHP-1. *Blood* 90 (suppl. 1):575a.

Persons, DA, Allay, JA, Allay, ER et al. (1999). Enforced expression of the GATA-2 transcription factor blocks normal hematopoiesis. *Blood* 93: 488–499.

Pevny L, Simon MC, Robertson E et al. (1991). Erythroid differentiation in chimaeric mice blocked by a targeted mutation in the gene for transcription factor GATA-1. *Nature* 349: 257–260.

Pevny, L, Chyuan-Sheng, L, D'Agati, V et al. (1994). Development of hematopoietic cells lacking transcription factor GATA-1. *Development* 121: 163–172.

Philipsen, S and Suske, G. (1999). A tale of three fingers: The family of mammalian Sp/XKLF transcription factors. *Nucleic Acids Res.* 27: 2991–3000.

Pomerantz, O, Goodwin, AJ, Joyce, T, and Lowrey CH. (1998). Conserved elements containing NF-E2 and tandem GATA binding sites are required for erythroid-specific chromatin structure reorganization within the human β-globin locus control region. *Nucleic Acids Res.* 26: 5684–5691.

Porcher, C, Swat, W, Rockwell, K et al. (1996). The T cell leukemia oncoprotein SCL/tal-1 is essential for development of all hematopoietic lineages. *Cell* 86: 47–57.

Ptashne, M and Gann, A. (1997). Transcriptional activation by recruitment. *Nature* 386: 569–577.

Quang, CT, Pironin, M, von Lindern, M et al. (1995). Spi-1 and mutant p53 regulate different aspects of the proliferation and differentiation control of primary erythroid progenitors. *Oncogene* 11: 1229–1239.

Raich, N, Clegg, CH, Grofti, J et al. (1995). GATA1 and YY1 are developmental repressors of the human epsilon-globin gene. *EMBO J.* 14: 801–809.

Rao, G, Rekhtman, N, Cheng, G et al. (1997). Deregulated expression of the PU.1 transcription factor blocks murine erythroleukemia cell terminal differentiation. *Oncogene* 14: 123–131.

Rekhtman, N, Radparvar, F, Evans, T, and Skoultchi, AI. (1999). Direct interaction of hematopoietic transcription factors PU.1 and GATA-1: Functional antagonism in erythroid cells. *Genes Dev.* 13: 1398–1411.

te Riele, H, Maandag, ER, Clarke, A et al. (1990). Consecutive inactivation of both alleles of the pim-1 proto-oncogene by homologous recombination in embryonic stem cells. *Nature* 348: 649–651.

Robb, L, Lyons, I, Li, R et al. (1995). Absence of yolk sac hematopoiesis from mice with a targeted disruption of the scl gene. *Proc. Natl. Acad. Sci. U.S.A.* 92: 7075–7079.

Robb, L, Elwood, NJ, Elefanty, AG et al. (1996). The scl gene is required for the generation of all hematopoietic lineages in the adult mouse. *EMBO J.* 15: 4123–4129.

Robertson, E. (1986). Pluripotential stem cell lines as a route into the mouse germ line. *Trends Genet.* 2: 9–13.

Romeo, P-H, Prandini, M-H, Joulin, V et al. (1990). Megakaryocytic and erythrocytic lineages share specific transcription factors. *Nature* 344: 447–449.

Rossant, J and McMahon, A. (1999). "Cre"-ating mouse mutants—a meeting review on conditional mouse genetics. *Genes Dev.* 13: 142–145.

Sargent, TG, DuBois, CC, Buller, AM, and Lloyd JA. (1999a). The roles of 5′-HS2, 5′-HS3, and the gamma-globin TATA, CACCC, and stage selector elements in suppression of beta-globin expression in early development. *J. Biol. Chem.* 274: 11229–11236.

Sargent, TG, Buller, AM, Teachey, DT et al. (1999b). The gamma-globin promoter has a major role in competitive inhibition of beta-globin gene expression in early erythroid development. *DNA Cell Biol.* 18: 293–303.

Shavit, JA, Motohashi, H, Onodera, K et al. (1998). Impaired megakaryopoiesis and behavioral defects in mafG-null mutant mice. *Genes Dev.* 12: 2164–2174.

Shikama, N, Lyon, J, and LaThangue, NB. (1997). The p300/CBP family: Integrating signals with transcription factors and chromatin. *Trends Cell. Biol.* 7: 230–236.

Shivdasani, RA and Orkin SH. (1995). Erythropoiesis and globin gene expression in mice lacking the transcription factor NF-E2. *Proc. Natl. Acad. Sci. U.S.A.* 1995; 92. 8690–8694.

Shivdasani, RA, Mayer, EL, and Orkin, SH. (1995a). Absence of blood formation in mice lacking the T-cell leukemia oncoprotein tal-1/SCL. *Nature* 373: 432–434.

Shivdasani, RA, Rosenblatt, MF, Zucker-Franklin, DC et al. (1995b). Transcription factor NF-E2 is required for platelet formation independent of the actions of thrombopoietin/MGDF in megakaryocyte development. *Cell* 81: 695–701.

Shivdasani, RA, Fujiwara, Y, McDevitt, MA, and Orkin, SH. (1997). A lineage-selective knockout establishes the critical role of transcription factor GATA-1 in megakaryocyte growth and platelet development. *EMBO J.* 16: 3965–3973.

Simon, MC, Pevny, L, Wiles, M et al. (1992). Rescue of erythroid development in gene targeted GATA-1⁻ mouse embryonic stem cells. *Nat. Genet.* 1: 92–98.

Smithies, O, Gregg, RG, Boggs, SS et al. (1985). Insertion of DNA sequences into the human chromosomal beta-globin locus by homologous recombination. *Nature* 317: 230–234.

Southwood, CM, Downs, KM, and Bieker, JJ. (1996). Erythroid Kruppel-like factor exhibits an early and sequentially localized pattern of expression during mammalian erythroid ontogeny. *Dev. Dyn.* 206: 248–259.

Sposi, NM, Zon, LI, Care, A et al. (1992). Cycle-dependent initiation and lineage-dependent abrogation of GATA-1 expression in pure differentiating hematopoietic progenitors. *Proc. Natl. Acad. Sci. U.S.A.* 89: 6353–6357.

Stamatoyannopoulos, JA, Goodwin, A, Joyce, T, and Lowrey, CH. (1995). NF-E2 and GATA binding motifs are required for the formation of DNase I hypersensitive site 4 of the human β-globin locus control region. *EMBO J.* 14: 106–116.

Suwabe, N, Takahashi, S, Nakano, T, and Yamamoto, M. (1998). GATA-1 regulates growth and differentiation of definitive erythroid lineage cells during in vitro ES cell differentiation. *Blood* 92: 4108–4118.

Svensson, EC, Tufts, RL, Polk, CE, and Leiden, JM. (1999). Molecular cloning of FOG-2: A modulator of transcription factor GATA-4 in cardiomyocytes. *Proc. Natl. Acad. Sci. U.S.A.* 96: 956–961.

Takahashi, S, Onodera, K, Motohashi, H et al. (1997). Arrest in primitive erythroid cell development caused by promoter-specific disruption of the GATA-1 gene. *J. Biol. Chem.* 272: 12611–12615.

Taketani, S, Inazawa, J, Nakahashi, Y et al. (1992). Structure of the human ferrochelatase gene. Exon/intron gene organization and location of the gene to chromosome 18. *Eur. J. Biochem.* 205: 217–222.

Talbot, D and Grosveld, F. (1991). The 5′HS2 of the globin locus control region enhances transcription through the interaction of a multimeric complex binding at two functionally distinct NF-E2 binding sites. *EMBO J.* 10: 1391–1398.

Tevosian, SG, Deconinck, AE, Cantor, AB et al. (1999). FOG-2: A novel GATA-family cofactor related to multitype zinc-finger proteins Friend of GATA-1 and U-shaped. *Proc. Natl. Acad. Sci. U.S.A.* 96: 950–955.

Tewari, R, Gillemans, N, Wijgerde, M et al. (1998). Erythroid Kruppel-like factor (EKLF) is active in primitive and definitive erythroid cells and is required for the function of 5′HS3 of the beta-globin locus control region. *EMBO J.* 8: 2334–2341.

Ting, CN, Olson, MC, Barton, KP, and Leiden, JM. (1996). Transcription factor GATA-3 is required for development of the T-cell lineage. *Nature* 384: 474–478.

Tournamille, CYC, Cartron, J, and Le Van Kim, C. (1995). Disruption of a GATA-motif in the Duffy gene promoter abolishes erythroid gene expression in Duffy-negative individuals. *Nat. Genet.* 10: 224–228.

Trainor, CD, Omichinski, JG, Vandergon, TL et al. (1996). A palindromic regulatory site within vertebrate GATA-1 promoters requires both zinc fingers of the GATA-1 DNA-binding domain for high-affinity interaction. *Mol. Cell. Biol.* 16: 2238–2247.

Trimborn, T, Gribnau, J, Grosveld, F, and Fraser, P. (1999). Mechanisms of developmental control of transcription in the murine alpha- and beta-globin loci. *Genes Dev.* 13: 112–124.

Tsai, FY and Orkin, SH. (1997). Transcription factor GATA-2 is required for proliferation/survival of early hematopoietic cells and mast cell formation, but not for erythroid and myeloid terminal differentiation. *Blood* 89: 3636–3643.

Tsai, SF, Martin, DIK, Zon, LI et al. (1989). Cloning of cDNA for the major DNA-binding protein of the erythroid lineage through expression in mammalian cells. *Nature* 339: 446–451.

Tsai, F-Y, Keller, G, Kuo, FC et al. (1994). An early hematopoietic defect in mice lacking the transcription factor GATA-2. *Nature* 371: 221–226.

Tsang, AP, Visvader, JE, Turner, CA et al. (1997). FOG, a multitype zinc finger protein, acts as a cofactor for transcription factor GATA-1 in erythroid and megakaryocytic differentiation. *Cell* 90: 109–119.

Tsang, AP, Fujiwara, Y, Hom, DB, and Orkin, SH. (1998). Failure of megakaryopoiesis and arrested erythropoiesis in mice lacking the GATA-1 transcriptional cofactor FOG. *Genes Dev.* 12: 1176–1188.

Tuan, D, Solomon, W, Li, Q, and London, IM. (1985). The "beta-like-globin" gene domain in human erythroid cells. *Proc. Natl. Acad. Sci. U.S.A.* 82: 6384–6388.

Tuan, DY, Solomon, WB, London, IM, and Lee, DP. (1989). An erythroid-specific, developmental-stage-independent enhancer far upstream of the human "beta-like globin" genes. *Proc. Natl. Acad. Sci. U.S.A.* 86: 2554–2558.

Turner, J and Crossley, M. (1999). Mammalian Kruppel-like transcription factors: More than just a pretty finger. *Trends Biochem. Sci.* 24: 236–240.

Turner, J and Crossley, M. (1998). Cloning and characterization of mCtBP2, a co-repressor that associates with basic Kruppel-like factor and other mammalian transcriptional regulators. *EMBO J.* 17: 5129–5140.

Versaw, WK, Blank, V, Andrews, NM, and Bresnick, EH. (1998). Mitogen-activated protein kinases enhance long-range activation by the beta-globin locus control region. *Proc. Natl. Acad. Sci. U.S.A.* 95: 8756–8760.

Visvader, J and Adams, JM. (1993). Megakaryocytic differentiation induced in 416B myeloid cells by GATA-2 and GATA-3 transgenes or 5-azacytidine is tightly coupled to GATA-1 expression. *Blood* 82: 1493–1501.

Visvader, J, Begley, CG, and Adams, JM. (1991). Differential expression of the Lyl, SCL, and E2a helix-loop-helix genes within the hemopoietic system. *Oncogene* 6: 187–194.

Visvader, JE, Crossley, M, Hill, J et al. (1995). The C-terminal zinc finger of GATA-1 or GATA-2 is sufficient to induce megakaryocytic differentiation of an early myeloid cell line. *Mol. Cell. Biol.* 15: 634–641.

Visvader, JE, Fujiwara, Y, and Orkin, SH. (1998). Unsuspected role for the T-cell leukemia protein SCL/tal-1 in vascular development. *Genes Dev.* 12: 473–479.

Vyas, P, Ault, K, Jackson, CW et al. (1999a). Consequences of GATA-1 deficiency in megakaryocytes and platelets. *Blood* 93: 2867–2875.

Vyas, P, McDevitt, MA, Cantor, AB et al. (1999b). Different sequence requirements for expression in erythroid and megakaryocytic cells within a regulatory element upstream of the GATA-1 gene. *Development* 126: 2799–2811.

Wadman, IA, Osada, H, Grutz, GG et al. (1997). The LIM-only protein Lmo2 is a bridging molecule assembling an erythroid, DNA-binding complex which includes the TAL1, E47, GATA-1 and Ldb1/NLI proteins. *EMBO J.* 16: 3145–3157.

Wang, Q, Stacy, T, Binder, M et al. (1996). Disruption of the Cbfa2 gene causes necrosis and hemorrhaging in the central nervous system and blocks definitive hematopoiesis. *Proc. Natl. Acad. Sci. U.S.A.* 93: 3444–3449.

Weiss, MJ and Orkin, SH. (1995a). GATA transcription factors: Key regulators of hematopoiesis. *Exp. Hematol.* 23: 99–107.

Weiss, MJ and Orkin, SH. (1995b). Transcription factor GATA-1 permits survival and maturation of erythroid precursors by preventing apoptosis. *Proc. Natl. Acad. Sci. U.S.A.* 92: 9623–9627.

Weiss, MJ, Keller, G, and Orkin, SH. (1994a). Novel insights into erythroid development revealed through in vitro differentiation of GATA-1− embryonic stem cells. *Genes Dev.* 8: 1184–1197.

Weiss, MJ, Yu, C, and Orkin, SH. (1997). Erythroid-cell-specific properties of transcription factor GATA-1 revealed by phenotypic rescue of a gene-targeted cell line. *Mol. Cell. Biol.* 17: 1642–1651.

Whyatt, DJ, deBoer, E, and Grosveld, F. (1993). The two zinc finger-like domains of GATA-1 have different DNA binding specificities. *EMBO J.* 12: 4993–5005.

Wijgerde, M, Grosveld, F, and Fraser, P. (1995). Transcription complex stability and chromatin dynamics in vivo. *Nature* 377: 209–213.

Wijgerde, M, Gribnau, J, Trimborn, T et al. (1996). The role of EKLF in human β-globin gene competition. *Genes Dev.* 10: 2894–2902.

Wolffe, AP and Pruss, D. (1996). Targeting chromatin disruption: Transcription regulators that acetylate histones. *Cell* 84: 817–819.

Wood, WG. (1982). Erythropoiesis and haemoglobin production during development. In Jones CT, editor. *Biochemical development of the fetus and neonate.* New York: Elsevier Biomedical Press.

Wu, H, Liu, X, Jaenisch, R, and Lodish HF. (1995). Generation of committed erythroid BFU-E and CFU-E progenitors does not require erythropoietin or the erythropoietin receptor. *Cell* 83: 59–67.

Yamada, T, Kondoh, N, Matsumoto, M et al. (1997). Overexpression of PU.1 induces growth and differentiation inhibition and apoptotic cell death in murine erythroleukemia cells. *Blood* 89: 1383–1393.

Yamada, T, Kihara-Negishi, F, Yamamoto, H et al. (1998). Reduction of DNA binding activity of the GATA-1 transcription factor in the apoptotic process induced by overexpression of PU.1 in murine erythroleukemia cells. *Exp. Cell Res.* 245: 186–194.

Yamamoto, M, Ko, LJ, Leonard, MW et al. (1990). Activity and tissue-specific expression of the transcription factor NF-E1 multigene family. *Genes Dev.* 4: 1650–1662.

Yang, H-Y and Evans, T. (1992). Distinct roles for the two cGATA-1 Finger Domains. *Mol. Cell. Biol.* 12: 4562–4570.

Yomogida, K, Ohtani, H, Harigae, H et al. (1994). Developmental stage- and spermatogenic cycle-specific expression of the transcription factor GATA-1 in mouse sertoli cells. *Development* 120: 1759–1766.

Zhang, W and Bieker, JJ. (1998). Acetylation and modulation of erythroid Kruppel-like factor (EKLF) activity by interaction with histone acetyltransferases. *Proc. Natl. Acad. Sci. U.S.A.* 95: 9855–9860.

Zhang, P, Behre, G, Pan, J et al. (1999). Negative cross-talk between hematopoietic regulators: GATA proteins repress PU.1. *Proc. Natl. Acad. Sci. U.S.A.* 96: 8705–8710.

Zheng, W and Flavell, RA. (1997). The transcription factor GATA-3 is necessary and sufficient for Th2 cytokine gene expression in CD4 T cells. *Cell* 89: 587–596.

Zhou, Y, Lim, KC, Onodera, K et al. (1998). Rescue of the embryonic lethal hematopoietic defect reveals a critical role for GATA-2 in urogenital development. *EMBO J.* 17: 6689–6700.

Zon, LI, Mather, C, Burgess, S et al. (1991). Expression of GATA-binding proteins during embryonic development in *Xenopus laevis. Proc. Natl. Acad. Sci. U.S.A.* 88: 10642–10646.

Zon, LI, Yamaguchi, Y, Yee, K et al. (1993). Expression of mRNA for the GATA-binding proteins in human eosinophils and basophils: Potential role in gene transcription. *Blood* 81: 3234–3241.

5

Organization, Evolution, and Regulation of the Globin Genes

ROSS HARDISON

Hemoglobin genes are ancient, dating back perhaps as far as the origins of cellular life. The familiar class of hemoglobins used for oxygen transport illustrates only one function of hemoglobins. This chapter reviews some of the principal events in the evolution of vertebrate globin gene clusters within the context of their long history. This evolutionary framework provides some insights into important issues such as the origin and function of the locus control regions (LCR), the contrasting chromatin structure of α- and β-like globin gene clusters, and the prospects for targeting δ- or γ-globin gene expression in therapies for β-globin gene defects.

BROAD DISTRIBUTION OF HEMOGLOBINS IN THE BIOSPHERE

Hemoglobins similar to human HbA are found in erythrocytes of all vertebrates (Dickerson and Geis, 1983). Each is a heterotetramer with two subunits related to the α-globin gene subfamily (referred to here as α-like globins) and two subunits related to the β-globin gene subfamily (β-like globins). Globin polypeptides bind heme, which in turn allows the hemoglobin in erythrocytes to bind oxygen reversibly and transport it from the lungs to respiring tissues. In all species studied, different α-like and β-like globin chains are synthesized at progressive stages of development to produce hemoglobins characteristic of primitive (embryonic) and defini-

tive (fetal and adult) erythroid cells (Bunn and Forget, 1986). However, the vertebrate hemoglobins comprise only a small part of the hemoglobin family (Fig. 5.1). A close relative, the monomeric myoglobin, stores oxygen in tissues such as muscle (Wittenberg and Wittenberg, 1987). As illustrated by the summary phylogenetic tree in Figure 5.1, the amino acid sequences of the α- and β-globin chains and myoglobin are related to each other, indicating a common ancestor in early vertebrates approximately 500 million years ago (Goodman et al., 1987). The three-dimensional structure of myoglobin was one of the first protein structures ever solved, revealing a series of α-helices that form the heme-binding pocket. This structure, the globin fold, is seen in myoglobin, α-globin, and β-globin; it is characteristic of all members of the hemoglobin family of proteins (Dickerson and Geis, 1983).

Hemoglobins are also used for oxygen transport in invertebrates (Riggs, 1991; Dixon et al., 1992; Sherman et al., 1992). Many nonvertebrates have gigantic extracellular hemoglobins, in some species formed by as many as 200 monodomain subunits in a multimeric protein, and in others by covalent linkage into long polypeptide chains (reviewed in Terwilliger, 1998). The invertebrate hemoglobins are homologous to the vertebrate hemoglobins, and they form a distinct branch in a phylogenetic tree of hemoglobins (Fig. 5.1.). Hemoglobins are present in plants, both the leghemoglobins with specialized functions in root nodules (Brisson and Verma, 1982; Appleby, 1984) and the broadly distributed, nonsymbiotic hemoglobins (Andersson et al., 1996). The genes for plant and invertebrate hemoglobins have a similar structure. Both groups of genes have three introns separating four exons, with at least two introns in identical positions (Fig. 5.2). The similarities in gene structure and the amino acid sequences of the encoded proteins strongly support the hypothesis of a common ancestor to both groups of hemoglobins, showing that the evolutionary history of hemoglobin genes predates the divergence of plants and animals, roughly 1.3 billion years ago (Feng et al., 1997). It is likely the middle intron was lost before the divergence of the vertebrate globin genes, all of which have only two introns.

Given that the hemoglobins in the major groups of multicellular organisms—plants, invertebrates and vertebrate animals—are used for storage and transport of oxygen, one might have expected hemoglobins to be absent from unicellular organisms. It was thought that simple diffusion was sufficient to provide adequate oxygen inside the cells of unicellular, free-living organisms. However, hemoglobins have now been characterized in several species of eubacteria, the fungus *Saccharomyces*

Martin H. Steinberg, Bernard G. Forget, Douglas R. Higgs, and Ronald L. Nagel, editors. *Disorders of Hemoglobin: Genetics, Pathophysiology, and Clinical Management.* © 2001 Cambridge University Press. All rights reserved.

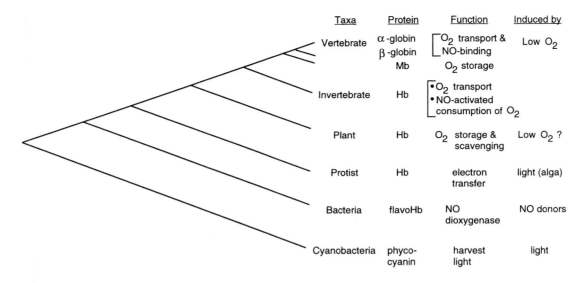

Taxa	Protein	Function	Induced by
Vertebrate	α-globin β-globin Mb	⌈O₂ transport & ⌊NO-binding O₂ storage	Low O₂
Invertebrate	Hb	•O₂ transport •NO-activated consumption of O₂	
Plant	Hb	O₂ storage & scavenging	Low O₂ ?
Protist	Hb	electron transfer	light (alga)
Bacteria	flavoHb	NO dioxygenase	NO donors
Cyanobacteria	phyco- cyanin	harvest light	light

Figure 5.1. Broad distribution and diverse functions of hemoglobins. The phylogenetic tree on the left is a summary of trees generated by aligning amino acid sequences of hemoglobins from species representative of each taxa (using CLUSTAL W) and computing trees based on parsimony (PAUP) and analysis of distance measures by Neighbor joining and UPGMA. The latter two used the MEGA suite of programs (Kumar et al., 1993). Trees of the same topology were generated by all three methods. The summary tree shows that topology but is not drawn to scale. This and subsequent trees indicate the relative time of the divergences; nodes more to the left indicate a relatively earlier time. Functions and induction agents are also listed. More details and references have been reviewed (Hardison, 1998).

cerevisiae, and protists such as the alga *Chlamydomonas* and the protozoan *Paramecium* (reviewed in Hardison, 1996; Hardison, 1998) These hemoglobins from unicellular organisms play roles distinctly different from those of vertebrate hemoglobins. The familiar functions in oxygen transport and storage require *reversible* binding of oxygen, which occurs only when the iron in the heme stays in the reduced (+2) oxidation state (i.e., when it is a ferrous ion). Biochemical analysis has shown that hemoglobins from *Chlamydomonas* (Couture and Guertin, 1996), *Saccharomyces* (Zhu and Riggs, 1992), and the bacterium *Alcaligenes* (Cramm et al., 1994) can participate in electron transfer reactions in vitro, with the heme-bound iron changing cyclically between the +2 and +3 oxidation states. The latter two hemoglobins are actually two-domain proteins, one domain binding heme and the other binding a flavin cofactor, which usually plays a role in redox reactions. Recent studies clearly show that the hemoglobins in unicellular organisms have enzymatic functions and are not oxygen-transporting proteins. The flavohemoglobins from the enteric bacteria *Escherichia coli* and *Salmonella typhimurium* (Crawford and Goldberg, 1998: Gardner et al, 1998; Hausladen et al., 1998) and from yeast (Liu et al., 2000) are enzymes protecting these microorgan-

isms from the highly reactive free radical compound nitric oxide. Each of these flavohemoglobins is a nitric oxide dioxygenase, catalyzing the conversion of nitric oxide to nitrate. Other functions have also been proposed for bacterial hemoglobins. For instance, the hemoglobin from *Vitreoscilla* can serve as a terminal electron acceptor during respiration in vivo (Dikshit et al., 1992).

Hemoglobins involved in catalytic conversions of nitric oxide and oxygen are not limited to microorganisms. A hemoglobin found in the perienteric fluid of the parasitic worm *Ascaris lumbricoides* also catalyzes reactions between oxygen and nitric oxide, producing nitrate (Minning et al., 1999). However, the chemical mechanism is different from that of the microbial flavohemoglobins, and Minning et al. (1999) propose that this hemoglobin functions to remove oxygen from the perienteric fluid via a series of reactions driven by nitric oxide.

In mammals, hemoglobins not only transport oxygen, but they also help regulate nitric oxide levels. Gow et al. (1998) show that at physiological concentrations, nitric oxide will bind to a cysteine in hemoglobin to form a S-nitrosohemoglobin. This binding is favored in oxyhemoglobin, and retains the bioactivity of nitric oxide. Nitric oxide can subsequently be released from deoxyhemoglobin (Jia et al., 1996; Stamler et al., 1997). Since nitric oxide is a major regulator of blood pressure, these new findings indicate that hemoglobin is involved in the control of blood pressure in ways that may facilitate efficient delivery of oxygen to tissues. Furthermore, the interplay between binding of oxygen and nitric oxide to hemoglobin and effects on vasodilation and constriction may have therapeutic applications (e.g. Bonaventura et al., 1999; Galdwin et al., 1999; Nagel, 1999).

The variety of functions now found for hemoglobins raises the issue of whether the microbial proteins are

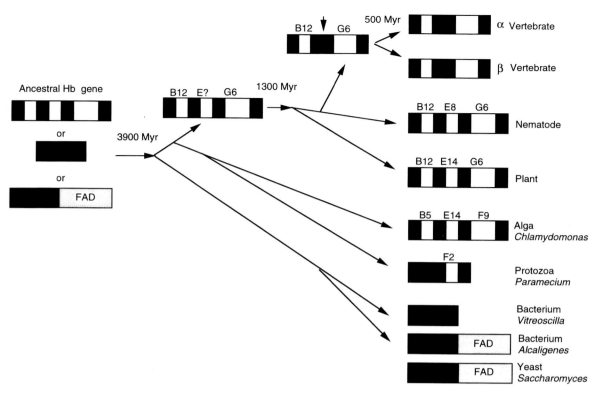

Figure 5.2. Intron/exon structure during evolution of hemoglobin genes. The structures of illustrative contemporary hemoglobin genes are shown on the right, with exons denoted by dark boxes and introns by white boxes. The position in the hemoglobin α-helical structure of the amino acid encoded at the site of interruption is indicated over the intron, and the loss of the central intron in the ancestor to vertebrates is marked by a vertical arrow. The evolutionary pathway is indicated by the other arrows. This "tree" is a gene tree, and grouping of of a yeast hemoglobin gene with bacterial hemoglobin genes may reflect a horizontal gene transfer. Estimated times of divergence in millions of years (Myr) are given at selected nodes.

truly homologous to the hemoglobins from plants and animals. The amino acid sequence comparisons certainly support a common ancestor to all these sequences, as illustrated in the summary phylogenetic tree (Fig. 5.1). Despite the low percentage identity (e.g., 25 percent) between the more dissimilar members of the family, different types of phylogenetic analysis generate trees of the same topology. The three-dimensional structures strongly support the conclusion that all these hemoglobins share a common ancestor. The structures of the bacterial hemoglobins from *Vitreoscilla* (Tarricone et al., 1997) and *Alcaligenes* (Ermler et al., 1995) both have the globin fold first characterized in vertebrate myoglobin. Indeed, hemoglobins may be part of a larger family of hemoproteins. For instance, the light-harvesting biliprotein, C-phycocyanin, from the cyanobacterium *Mastigocladus laminosus* has a three-dimensional structure similar to that of a globin (Schirmer et al., 1985).

Although this is not a heme-binding protein per se, it does bind a linear tetrapyrrole pigment derived from heme. The structural comparisons indicate that genes for at least some other hemoproteins share a common ancestor with hemoglobin genes (Fig. 5.1).

These observations all indicate that the gene encoding hemoglobin is truly ancient; that is, it appears to have been present in the ancestor to eubacteria and eukaryotes, which is the earliest proposed divergence since the origin of cellular organisms. This divergence has been dated at approximately 3.9 billion years ago (Feng et al., 1997). At this early time, very little oxygen was present in the earth's atmosphere. Hence the primordial function of hemoglobin may have had little to do with molecular oxygen (Hardison, 1998). The enzymatic functions of hemoglobins found in contemporary microorganisms and nematodes, involving nitric oxide metabolism, provide some insight into the early functions of hemoglobins (Durner et al., 1999). Mining et al. (1999) describe a scenario in which hemoglobins present in contemporary bacteria, which catalyze the enzymatic detoxification of nitric oxide, representing an ancestral function. These ancestral hemoglobins may have evolved into enzymes that catalyze the nitric oxide-mediated consumption of oxygen, as now observed as a "deoxygenase" in *Ascaris*. The deoxygenase may have evolved into contemporary mammalian hemoglobins with their limited enzymatic function but the ability to bind and transport both oxygen and nitric oxide.

Because the separation between archaebacteria and eukaryotes appears to have occurred after the divergence of eubacteria and eukaryotes, one may anticipate finding homologs to hemoglobins in archae as well. An automated analysis of genome sequences has included an archaebacterial gene (from *Methanococcus jannaschii*) in an orthologous group (Tatusov et al., 1997) containing proteins related to hemoglobins (see http://www.ncbi.nlm.nih.gov/COG/). Further investigation of this and other archaebacterial genes related to hemoglobins, revealed from the whole genome sequencing, should provide even more insights into the origin and range of functions of hemoglobins.

An issue that has received much attention is the age of the introns and whether they separate genes into exons that encode distinct protein domains (Gilbert, 1978). The three introns of globin genes in plants and invertebrates, dating back approximately 1.3 billion years, are between the segments of the gene encoding measurable domains of protein structure (Go, 1981). This has lent support to the model that introns are old and are the remnants of a process that combined exons to generate genes with new structures and functions (Gilbert, 1978). However, the hemoglobin genes from protists have introns in positions unique to many of the species, and those of eubacteria have no introns (Fig. 5.2). Attempts to explain this degree of heterogeneity as the result of differential loss of introns require a large number of introns to be proposed in the ancestral gene. An alternative explanation is that at least some of the introns in the protist hemoglobin genes arose by insertion of new introns in each lineage, consistent with the "introns late" model (Stoltzfus et al., 1994). Thus it seems unlikely that all the introns in contemporary hemoglobin genes were present in the ancestral gene (i.e., preceding the divergence of eubacteria, archaebacteria, and eukaryotes), and hence the "introns early" hypothesis is not adequate to explain all of the introns. However, this does not rule out the possibility that some introns, perhaps those still in hemoglobin genes in multicellular organisms, were in the ancestral gene.

EVOLUTION OF α- AND β-GLOBIN GENE CLUSTERS IN VERTEBRATES

Human hemoglobins are encoded at two separate loci, the β-like globin gene cluster on chromosome 11p15.5 (Deisseroth et al., 1978) and the α-like globin gene cluster close to the terminus of chromosome 16p (Deisseroth et al., 1977). As shown in Figure 5.3, the genes in each cluster are in the same transcriptional orientation and are arranged in the order of their expression during development, with the active β-like globin genes arranged 5'-ϵ (embryonic)-[G]-γ (fetal)-[A]γ (fetal)-δ (minor adult)-β (major adult)-3' (Fritsch et al., 1980) and the active α-like globin genes arranged 5'-ζ (embryonic)-α_2 (fetal and adult)-α_1 (fetal and adult)-3' (Lauer et al., 1980). (Lower levels of the γ and α

globins are also produced in embryonic red cells.) This section reviews some of the key events in the evolution of this arrangement of globin genes.

The effective transport of oxygen between tissues by hemoglobin is accomplished by highly cooperative binding of oxygen when its concentration is high (e.g., in the lungs), followed by cooperative dissociation when its concentration is low (e.g., in respiring tissues in the periphery). In vertebrates, this cooperativity is accomplished by the interactions between the α- and β-globin subunits of hemoglobin (Chapter 9). Vertebrate hemoglobins are kept at high concentrations inside erythrocytes, specialized cells devoted to the task of oxygen transport. Thus the divergence of the ancestral globin gene into the α-globin and β-globin genes (Fig. 5.3), and expression of these genes at a high level only in erythroid cells, were key steps in the evolution of cooperativity in hemoglobin and efficient oxygen transport in vertebrates. These goals have been accomplished by different mechanisms in other evolutionary lineages. For instance, the basis for cooperativity in nonvertebrate hemoglobins is quite different, in many cases involving reversible dissociation of hemoglobin subunits upon oxygenation (Riggs, 1998).

Vertebrate α- and β-globin genes likely arose by the duplication and subsequent divergence of an ancestral globin gene in early vertebrates. This would have generated a linked set of α- and β-globin genes (Fig. 5.3), which is the arrangement seen in contemporary globin gene clusters of the teleost zebrafish *Danio rerio* (Chan et al., 1997) and in the amphibian *Xenopus* (Hosbach et al., 1983). The α-globin gene cluster is thought to have separated from the β-globin gene cluster before the divergence of birds and mammals, because these gene clusters are on separate chromosomes in both groups of animals (Deisseroth et al., 1976; Hughes et al., 1979). Gene duplication and divergence continued independently in each of these lineages to generate the contemporary gene clusters. This is illustrated by the avian and mammalian β-globin gene clusters, which contain multiple genes expressed differentially in development (Fig. 5.3). In both species the ϵ-globin gene is expressed in embryos and the β-globin gene is expressed in adults. However, the sequence of each chicken β-like globin gene is equally similar to each human gene (Goodman et al., 1987; Reitman et al., 1993), so that, for example, chicken ϵ-globin is no more similar to human ϵ-globin than to human β-globin. This indicates that the gene duplications generating these β-globin gene clusters occurred after the species diverged.

Much is now known about the organization of α- and β-globin gene clusters in contemporary mammals, which can be understood in terms of descent from common gene clusters in an ancestral eutherian mammal. Figure 5.4 shows β-globin gene clusters in species from five orders of eutherian mammals and a marsu-

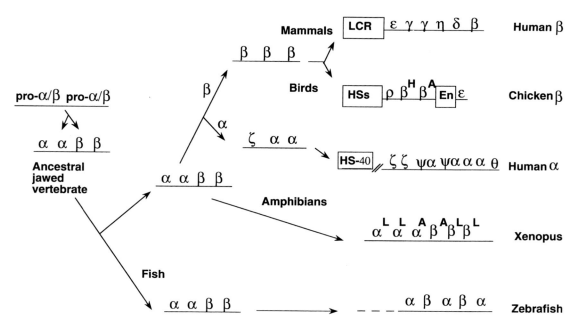

Figure 5.3. Evolutionary pathways for α- and β-globin gene clusters in vertebrates. Each gene is indicated simply by a Greek letter. Contemporary gene clusters are on the right (Hardison, 1991 and references therein), and the deduced course of evolution to them is shown by a series of arrows. The ancestor to α- and β-globin genes is indicated as pro-α/β. LCR, locus control region; HS-40, the distal major control region of mammalian α-globin genes; HSs, DNase hypersensitive sites; En, enhancer.

pial. Analysis of DNA sequences showed that a given globin gene in one species is usually more related to a gene in another mammal than to other globin genes in the same species (Hardison, 1983; Goodman et al., 1984; Hardies et al., 1984; Hardison, 1984; Townes et al., 1984). This indicated that these genes are *orthologous* (i.e., they are similar because of descent from the same gene in the last common ancestor to the two species). The exceptions to this observation could be explained by gene duplications within a single mammalian lineage for example, the duplication of γ-globin genes in the ancestor to simian primates to produce *paralogous* genes (similar because of duplication of the ancestor), such as the ^{G}γ- and ^{A}γ-globin genes in humans (Shen et al., 1981; Fitch et al., 1991). Finding orthologs to ε-, γ-, η-, δ-, and β-globin genes, in that order, in virtually all eutherian mammals suggested that the ancestral eutherian had at least this set of genes (Fig. 5.4). This hypothesis was strongly supported by the observation of substantial regions of sequence similarity outside the coding regions of the genes, in the introns and flanking regions (Hardies et al., 1984; Hardison, 1984; Margot et al., 1989; Shehee et al., 1989; Hardison and Miller, 1993). As will be discussed more extensively later, some but not all of these matching sequences are strong candidates for

regulatory function. The long regions of matching sequences outside functional regions, which were thus not subject to any obvious selection, were key observations in establishing this model for evolution of the mammalian globin gene clusters. Deletions, conversions, and duplications of both single genes and blocks of genes have occurred in each mammalian order to generate the current gene clusters (reviewed in Collins and Weissman, 1984; Hardison, 1991).

The proposed ε- γ- η- δ- β-globin gene cluster in the ancestral eutherian mammal was generated by earlier gene duplications. Estimates based on rates of divergence indicated that the ε-, γ-, and η-globin genes arose from duplications of one ancestral gene, whereas the δ- and β-globin genes arose by duplication of a different gene, perhaps before the divergence of eutherian and metatherian (marsupials and monotreme) mammals (Goodman et al., 1984; Hardison, 1984). This prediction was verified by genomic analysis of marsupials (Koop and Goodman, 1988; Cooper et al., 1996), which have two genes in their β-globin gene clusters, one most related to eutherian ε-globin genes and the other most related to β-globin genes. Thus the model shown in Figure 5.4 is robust, in that it has been supported not only by deductions from analysis of contemporary species, but also by tests of predictions made by the model.

One important ramification of this model is that orthologous genes have not retained the same time of expression during development in all mammalian orders. The γ-globin gene in most mammals is expressed in embryonic erythroid cells, but in simian primates, including humans, it is expressed predominantly in fetal erythroid cells. Concomitantly with the fetal recruitment of the γ-globin gene, expression of the β-globin gene has

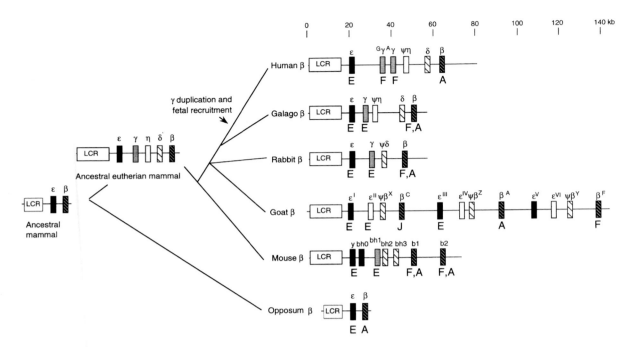

Figure 5.4. Pathways to contemporary mammalian β-globin gene clusters. Genes are indicated by boxes, and orthologous genes have the same type of fill. The presumptive presence of an LCR in marsupials is indicated by the gray outline (R. Hope, personal communication). The stage of expression is indicated as E, embryonic; F, fetal; and A, adult. References are in the text and in reviews (Collins and Weissman, 1984; Hardison, 1991).

been delayed in higher primates so that in humans, it is expressed primarily in postnatal life. In other mammals, the β-globin gene is expressed in both fetal and adult erythroid cells. In goats, the γ-globin gene has been deleted, and subsequent expansion of the gene cluster by triplication of a four-gene set (Townes et al., 1984) allowed expression of the resulting paralogous β-globin genes in fetal life (β^F), adult life (β^A), or under conditions of erythropoietic stress (β^C). The δ-globin gene is expressed at low levels in adult humans, is silent in some mammals, and is expressed at high levels in others. In contrast, the ε-globin gene in each mammalian species is expressed only in embryonic erythroid cells derived from the yolk sac. Within the β-globin gene clusters of mammals, conservation of stage-specific expression is seen only for this gene, which is located closest to the distal LCR (see later and Chapter 6). Perhaps the embryonic restriction of ε-globin gene expression is related to this spatial relationship, with active expression in the embryonic lineage owing to its proximity to the LCR, followed by silencing in the fetal and adult (definitive) lineage of erythroid cells (Chapter 7). Both the proximity to the LCR and the embryonic restriction to expression are conserved in all mammalian ε-globin genes examined.

The β-globin gene clusters of humans and mice are embedded within a large cluster of olfactory receptor genes, or ORGs (Bulger et al., 1999). This arrangement suggests that the β-globin genes transposed into a pre-existing array of ORGs. A related ORG is found on the 3′ side of the chicken β-globin gene cluster (Bulger et al., 1999), but an erythroid-specific folate receptor gene is located on the 5′ side, separated from the β-globin gene cluster by an insulator (Prioleau et al., 1999). The 3′ breakpoints of at least two deletions causing hereditary persistence of fetal hemoglobin (HPFH) in humans are close to ORGs located 3′ to the β-globin genes (Kosteas et al., 1997; Feingold et al., 1999). The ORG close to the HPFH-1 breakpoint is an open chromatin domain in human erythroid cells (Elder et al., 1990). Enhancer sequences from this ORG are brought into proximity of the β-globin genes by HPFH-1 deletion, and this may play a role in the increased expression of β-globin genes in adults carrying this deletion (Feingold and Forget, 1989).

The evolution of α-globin gene clusters in contemporary mammals is not as well understood as that of β-globin gene clusters, in part because less information is available on gene organization and sequence in nonhuman mammals, and in part because the rate of sequence change in this gene cluster appears to be higher than in the β-globin gene cluster (Hardison et al., 1991). Figure 5.5 summarizes the arrangement of α-like globin gene clusters in representatives of five orders of eutherian mammals. Orthologous relationships have been assigned primarily on the basis of DNA sequence matches outside the genes (Hardison and Gelinas, 1986; Sawada and Schmid, 1986; Wernke and Lingrel, 1986; Flint et al., 1988), even though such matches are considerably more limited than in the mammalian β-globin gene clusters. Since a variant of the arrangement 5′-ζ-ζ-

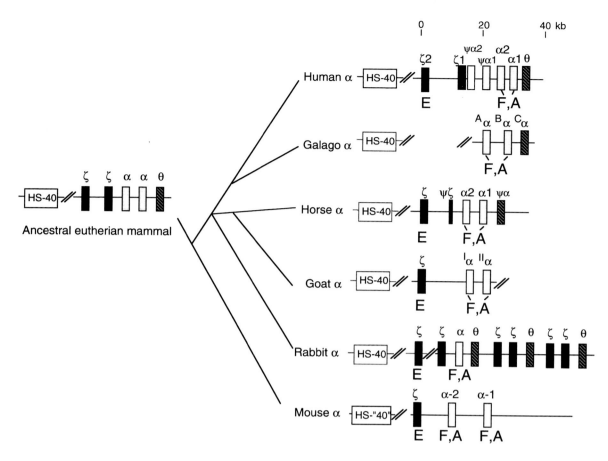

Figure 5.5. Pathways to contemporary mammalian α-globin gene clusters. Genes are indicated by boxes, and orthologous genes have the same type of fill. The presumptive presence of a homolog to HS-40 (the distal major control region) in mammals besides human and mouse is indicated by the gray outline. References are in the text and in reviews (Collins and Weissman, 1984; Hardison, 1991; Hardison and Miller, 1993).

α-α-θ-3′ is found in all contemporary mammals examined, it is likely that these genes were present in this order in the gene cluster of the ancestral eutherian mammal. The timing of expression is well conserved among these mammals. The ζ-globin genes are expressed only in embryonic erythroid cells, whereas the α-globin genes are expressed in all erythroid cells, albeit at lower levels at the embryonic stage (Rohrbaugh and Hardison, 1983; Leder et al., 1985; Peschle et al., 1985). The θ-globin genes are still not well understood. The human θ-globin gene is transcribed at low levels but does not encode any known polypeptide found in human hemoglobins (Hsu et al., 1988; Kim et al., 1989; Leung et al., 1989). A θ-globin gene is found in every mammalian α-like globin gene cluster examined (Fig. 5.5), and given that gene deletions can occur in this locus (see later), one would anticipate the loss of nonfunctional genes in at least some mammalian lineages. The retention of the θ-globin genes is suggestive of some functional importance, but perhaps not for encoding a globin polypeptide.

Although no examples of recruitment for expression at different developmental stages are seen in the α-like globin gene clusters, some genes have lost their function during evolution. In particular, based on upstream sequence matches, the human ψα1-globin pseudogene appears to be orthologous to an active α-

globin gene in goats and horse (Fig. 5.5). The inactivation of ψα1-gene is accompanied by the loss of a CpG island that encompasses its homologs (Bird et al., 1987). The orthologous relationships in Figure 5.5 indicate that the α2- and α1-globin genes in humans result from a duplication only in primates (i.e., distinct from the duplication proposed to generate the pair of α-globin genes in the ancestral eutherian mammal). The more recent duplication in primates has left a long region of sequence similarity surrounding the α-globin genes (Hess et al., 1984), and unequal crossovers within that region of homology cause some forms of α thalassemia (Chapter 17). Not all mammals have retained a pair of active α-globin genes. Rabbits are the exception, with only one α-globin gene (Cheng et al., 1986). Curiously, this gene cluster has expanded by block duplications of a ζ-ζ-θ gene triad (Cheng et al., 1987), similar to the expansion of the β-like globin gene cluster in goats (Townes et al., 1984) (Fig. 5.4).

All the vertebrate globin gene clusters examined to date encode subunits of hemoglobins differentially expressed in embryonic and adult erythroid cells (Fig. 5.3). Likewise, hemoglobin synthesis is developmentally regulated in some invertebrates (Terwilliger, 1998) and different plant leghemoglobins are made at progressive stages of nodulation (Hyldig-Nielsen et al., 1982; Lee et al., 1983). Even species as distant from human as *Chlamydomonas* (Couture et al., 1994) and *Paramecium* (Yamauchi et al., 1995) have multiple hemoglobin genes. Thus the ability to express different hemoglobins at particular developmental stages (i.e., hemoglobin switching) is very old, predating the plant-animal divergence, and possibly being much older. In Figure 5.3, multiple globin genes are shown in the ancestral gene clusters. It is likely that they were differentially expressed during development in these ancestral species.

DIFFERENCES IN GENOMIC CONTEXT AND REGULATION OF THE MAMMALIAN α-GLOBIN AND β-GLOBIN GENE CLUSTERS

The separation of α- and β-globin gene clusters to different chromosomes has allowed them to diverge into strikingly different genomic contexts, with paradoxical consequences for our understanding of their regulation. Given that all contemporary vertebrates have developmentally regulated hemoglobin genes encoding proteins used for oxygen transport in erythrocytes, it would have been reasonable to expect that the molecular mechanisms of globin gene regulation would be conserved in vertebrates. Certainly, the coordinated and balanced expression of α- and β-globin genes to produce the heterotypic tetramer $\alpha_2\beta_2$ in erythrocytes should be a particularly easy aspect of regulation to explain. Because the two genes would have been identical after the initial duplication in the ancestral vertebrate, with identical regulatory elements, it is parsimonious to expect selection to keep the regulatory elements very similar.

However, much has changed between the α- and β-like globin gene clusters since their duplication. Not only are they now on separate chromosomes in birds and mammals, but in mammals they are in radically different genomic contexts (Fig. 5.6). The β-globin gene clusters are A+T rich, with no CpG islands (reviewed in Collins and Weissman, 1984), whereas the α-like globin gene clusters are highly G+C rich, with multiple CpG islands (Fischel-Ghodsian et al., 1987). [A+T rich means the DNA has a high mole fraction of the nucleotides adenylic acid (A) and thymidylic acid (T), whereas G+C rich means the DNA has a high mole fraction of the nucleotides guanidylic acid (G) and cytidylic acid (C). CpG islands are segments of DNA in which the frequency of the dinucleotide CpG approaches that expected from the individual frequencies of the nucleotides C and G. In vertebrate genomes, the effects of DNA methylation have reduced the frequency of CpG to low levels except in these CpG islands.] Tissue-specific gene expression is frequently correlated with an increased accessibility of the chromatin only in expressing cells, and hence "opening" of a chromatin domain is a key step in activation of many tissue-specific genes. This is the case for β-like globin genes of mammals (Groudine et al., 1983; Forrester et al., 1990), but not the α-like globin genes, which are in constitutively open chromatin (Craddock et al., 1995). In keeping with the presence of CpG islands, the α-globin gene cluster is not methylated in any cell types (Bird et al., 1987), whereas the β-globin gene cluster is subject to tissue-specific DNA methylation (van der Ploeg and Flavell, 1980). Thus the mammalian α-globin genes have several characteristics associated with constituively expressed "housekeeping" genes.

The differences between α-globin gene clusters and β-globin gene clusters extend to their replication as well. Many tissue-specific genes, including the human and mouse β-globin genes, are replicated early in S phase only in cells expressing them, whereas the human α-globin genes are replicated early in all cells (Epner et al., 1981; Furst et al., 1981; Calza et al., 1984; Goldman et al. 1984, Dhar et al., 1988). The human β-globin gene cluster is replicated from a single origin close to the promoter of the β-globin gene (Kitsberg et al., 1993, Aladjem et al., 1998). The activity of this origin early in S phase in erythroid cells requires an open chromatin structure (Forester et al., 1990; Aladjem et al., 1995). In contrast, a large 325 kb G+C-rich isochore containing the human α-globin genes and several constitutively expressed genes is replicated early in S phase in both erythroid and nonerythroid cells (Smith and Higgs, 1999). This study also showed that multiple origins of replication must be present in this G+C-rich isochore, in contrast to the single origin found in the β-globin gene cluster. Although the two gene clusters differ in the types of cells in which they are replicated early and in the number of replication origins, early replication is associated with open chromatin at both loci.

Thus the strikingly different genomic contexts of the two gene clusters affect several aspects of DNA and chromatin metabolism, including timing of replication, extent of methylation, and the type of chromatin into which the loci are packaged. Rather than selecting for similarities to insure coordinate and balanced expression, the processes of evolution at these two loci have made them quite different.

The α- and β-globin gene clusters also have important differences in their *cis*-regulatory elements. Both have distal control elements—the LCR for β-globin genes (reviewed in Grosveld et al., 1993; Hardison et al., 1997b) and HS-40 for the α-globin genes (Higgs et al., 1990)—which are required for high-level expression of the respective globin genes in transgenic mice, indepen-

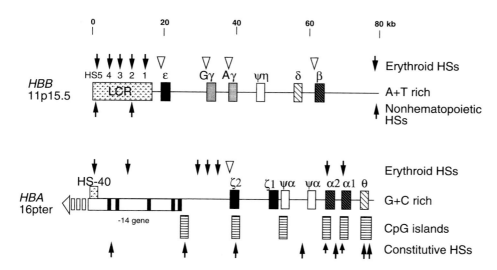

Figure 5.6. Differences in chromatin structure of α- and β-globin gene clusters of humans. Globin genes and distal control regions are shown as filled boxes. HS-40 is located within an intron (white box) of the −14 gene (exons of this gene are shown as black boxes), located upstream of the ζ-globin gene and transcribed in the opposite orientation. Developmentally stable DNase hypersensitive sites (HSs) are shown as filled arrows, and those that occur at specific developmental stages (when the associated gene is expressed) are shown as white triangles. CpG islands are shown as boxes with horizontal lines. None are in the β-globin gene. HBB, β-globin gene; HBA, α-globin gene. References are in the text.

dent of the position of chromosomal integration. However, they differ in the range of functions associated with them. The β-globin LCR or sequences 5′ to it have been implicated in tissue-specific chromosomal domain opening (Forrester et al., 1987; Forrester et al., 1990), whereas no such function has been implicated for HS-40, as expected for a regulator in constitutively open chromatin. The distal regulatory elements also differ dramatically in size, with the β-globin LCR containing 17 kb with 5 DNase hypersensitive sites in chromatin (Tuan et al., 1985; Forrester et al., 1987; Grosveld et al., 1987; Dhar et al., 1990), compared to about 0.4 kb and a single DNase hypersensitive site in chromatin for the α-globin HS-40 (Jarman et al., 1991).

Indeed, the α-globin HS-40 is most similar to a single hypersensitive site, HS2, from the β-globin LCR. Both will confer inducible, high level expression on reporter genes in transfected cells (e.g., Tuan et al., 1985; Ney et al., 1990; Pondel et al., 1992; Ren et al., 1993), in addition to their effects in transgenic mice (Fraser et al., 1990; Higgs et al., 1990; Morley et al., 1992). As illustrated in Figure 5.7, these two enhancers share binding sites for some, but not all, transcription factors (e.g., Talbot et al., 1990; Jarman et al., 1991; Strauss et al., 1992; Reddy et al., 1994). Both contain *Maf*-response elements, or MAREs (Motohashi et al., 1997), to which transcriptional activator proteins of the basic leucine

zipper class can bind. A particular subfamily of proteins related to AP1, such as NFE2, LCRF1/Nrf1, and Bach1, bind to this site (reviewed in Orkin, 1995; Baron, 1997) (Chapter 4). All are heterodimers containing a Maf protein as one subunit, which is the basis for the name. Other binding sites in common are GATA, to which GATA1 and its relatives bind (Evans et al., 1990), and the CACC motif, to which a family of Zn-finger proteins including erythroid Krüppel-like factor (EKLF) can bind (Miller and Bieker, 1993). These binding sites are occupied in vivo (Strauss et al., 1992; Reddy et al., 1994) and all contribute to the function of the enhancers (Strauss et al., 1992; Caterina et al., 1994; Reddy et al., 1994; Rombel et al., 1995). Other functional sites, such as the E boxes in HS2 (Lam and Bresnick, 1996; Elnitski et al., 1997), are not found in common. Each of these binding sites is conserved in homologous regulatory elements in mammals (reviewed in Gourdon et al., 1995; Hardison et al., 1997b). In general, binding sites for many of the proteins implicated in activation of globin gene expression are present in both HS-40 and HS2 of the β-globin LCR, but their number and arrangement differ in the two enhancers (Fig. 5.7). It is currently not possible to assess whether this limited similarity occurs via divergence from a common ancestral regulatory element or by convergence from different ancestral elements.

The proximal regulatory elements in α- and β-globin genes also differ in important ways (Fig. 5.8). The promoters do contain two binding sites in common—the TATA motif, to which the general transcription factor TFIID binds, and the CCAAT motif, to which several families of *trans*-activators, such as CP1, can bind (Efstratiadis et al., 1980). However, the other protein binding sites in the human α- and β-globin genes are completely different (deBoer et al., 1988; Rombel et al., 1995). In addition, the CpG island encompassing the 5′ flanking region and much of the gene is a key component of the *cis*-regulatory elements for the α-globin gene

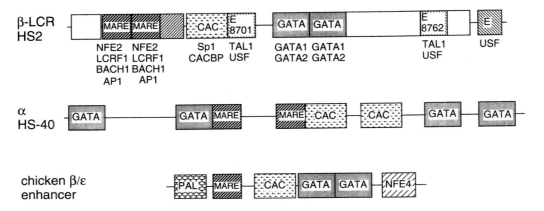

Figure 5.7. Conserved motifs in distal regulatory elements. Similar protein binding sites have the same fill, and proteins implicated in acting at a given site are listed below that motif in the β-LCR HS2 line; the same proteins have been implicated at similar motifs in the other regulatory elements. Boxes without labels are conserved sequences of untested function.

of rabbits and humans, possibly through its effects on chromatin structure (Pondel et al., 1995; Shewchuk and Hardison, 1997); again, no CpG island is found at any of the β-like globin genes.

The differences in genomic context between α- and β-globin genes have been seen for nonhuman mammals as well (Bernardi et al., 1985), indicating an origin before the divergence of eutherian mammals. The high G+C content and presence of CpG islands are characteristic of α-globin gene clusters from goats (Wernke and Lingrel, 1986), horses (Flint et al., 1988), and rabbits (Hardison et al., 1991), whereas the β-globin gene clusters from nonhuman mammals are rich in A+T (e.g., Margot et al., 1989; Shehee et al., 1989). The only apparent exception is the mouse α-globin gene cluster, which to date has not been completely characterized. However, the sequenced mouse α-globin gene is not in a

CpG island (Nishioka and Leder, 1979). Indeed, the mouse genome shows a general depletion in CpG islands (Antequera, 1993; Matsuo et al., 1993). The loss of the CpG island is correlated with a chromosomal rearrangement that moved the α-globin locus from the terminus of a chromosome, where it is in human (Flint et al., 1997) and rabbit (Xu and Hardison, 1991), to an internal location in mouse (Tan and Whitney, 1993). It

Figure 5.8. Conserved features of globin gene promoters. Binding sites for the human globin genes are shown; similar protein binding sites have the same fill. Those sites conserved in other mammals have a dark outline; those not conserved have a gray outline. The figure is not drawn to scale, but relative positions are indicated; the genes themselves are truncated. The chicken β-globin gene promoter is shown for comparison; no information about evolutionary conservation is presented for this gene. This figure summarizes work from a large number of authors (e.g., Efstratiadis et al., 1980; Lacy and Maniatis, 1980; Hardison, 1983; Antoniou et al., 1988; Barnhart et al., 1988; deBoer et al., 1988; Wall et al., 1988; Martin et al., 1989; Puruker et al., 1990; Stuve and Myers, 1990; Macleod and Plumb, 1991; McDonagh et al., 1991; Yu et al., 1991; Gong and Dean, 1993; Motamed et al., 1993; Peters et al., 1993; Yost et al., 1993; Lloyd et al., 1994; Rombel et al., 1995).

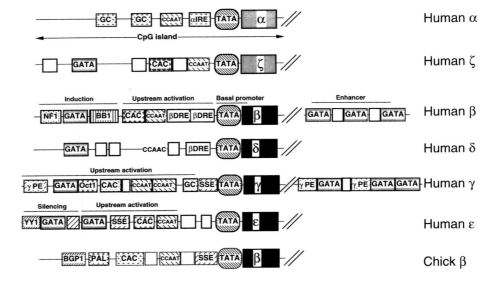

is possible that position of the α-globin locus close to the end of the chromosome, in a large region high in G+C content (Flint et al., 1997), is critical to maintenance of the CpG islands.

Despite these many differences between α- and β-globin gene clusters in mammals, the appropriate genes are still expressed coordinately between the two loci, resulting in balanced production of α- and β-like globins needed for the synthesis of normal hemoglobins. The full mechanism that accomplishes this task still eludes our understanding.

ORIGIN AND LOCATION OF THE LCR IN BIRDS AND MAMMALS

In contrast to the differences between the α- and β-globin gene clusters of mammals, tissue-specific opening of a chromatin domain occurs in β-globin gene clusters of both mammals and birds. In fact, the association between accessible chromatin and gene activation was first observed with the chicken globin genes (Weintraub and Groudine, 1976). Further studies of the avian gene clusters carefully mapped the limits of the open domain in chromatin to a region of 33 kb, extending about 10 kb on each side of the set of four globin genes (Clark et al., 1993; Hebbes et al., 1994). The limits of the open domain for the human β-globin gene cluster have not been determined. The open domain at the 5' end encompasses at least the LCR, which extends 20 kb 5' to the ε-globin gene, and an erythroid HS has been mapped as far as 70 kb 3' to the β-globin gene (Elder et al., 1990), indicating an open domain of at least 150 kb.

LCRs have been mapped in β-globin gene clusters in both chickens and all mammals examined to date. The LCRs in mammals are homologous (Moon and Ley, 1990; Li et al., 1991; Hug et al., 1992; Jimenez et al., 1992; Hardison et al., 1993; Hardison et al., 1997b; Slightom et al., 1997), with long segments of high sequence similarity found both inside and outside the cores of the LCR HSs (Fig. 5.9). All are located 5' to the ε-globin gene (Fig. 5.4). Sequences similar to HS2 and HS3 of the β-globin LCR are also found in marsupials and monotremes (R. Hope, personal communication), indicating that the LCR predates the divergence of placental and nonplacental mammals, about 173 Myr ago (Kumar and Hedges, 1998). In contrast, the major LCR activity in chickens maps to an enhancer located between the β^A- and ε-globin genes (Reitman et al., 1990). Four additional HSs are 5' to the ρ-globin gene, and together they produce a modest enhancement in expression (Reitman et al., 1995). Despite their analogous location at the 5' ends of the gene cluster, they do not have the pronounced effects associated with the HSs in the mammalian LCR. In fact, comparison of the DNA sequences of the β-globin gene clusters of chicken and human fails to reveal any statistically significant align-

ments outside the coding regions of some of the exons (Reitman et al., 1993; Hardison, 1998). No clear homologies are present in either the distal regulatory elements (LCRs and enhancers) or in the promoters. However, enhancer sequences are conserved between mammals and chickens at other loci, such as *SCL/TAL1* (Gottgens et al., 2000). Enhancers of *Hox* gene clusters are conserved between human and puffer fish (Aparicio et al., 1995). A full explanation of the lack of homology in the regulatory regions of the chicken and human β-globin gene clusters awaits better understanding of their evolutionary history, which is still under study.

Even though the pairwise alignments of chicken and human β-globin gene regulatory regions did not reveal sufficiently long matching segments to be significant, a comparison of the protein-binding sites in these regulatory regions shows that some of the same proteins are used in both species. For instance, the chicken β/ε enhancer has a MARE, a CACC motif, and a GATA site (Evans et al., 1990), motifs also found in HS2 of the β-globin LCR and the α-globin HS-40 (Fig. 5.7). All three have a group of binding sites in the order MARE, CACC, GATA; but the number and spacing of the sites differ in the three enhancers. The inability to detect these similar regulatory regions using nucleotide identities as the basis for a similarity score illustrates the need to develop software that finds similar patterns of protein binding sites in comparisons of DNA sequences.

CONSERVED SEQUENCES IN THE PROXIMAL REGULATORY REGIONS OF MAMMALIAN α- AND β-LIKE GLOBIN GENES

Unlike the absence of extragenic sequence matches in comparisons of β-globin gene clusters of chickens and humans, or α- and β-globin gene clusters of humans, comparisons of homologous gene clusters of eutherian mammals reveal many informative sequence matches. As illustrated in Figure 5.9 when DNA sequences of the human (Collins and Weissman, 1984; Li et al., 1985) and mouse (Shehee et al., 1989) β-globin gene clusters are compared, extensive matches are seen outside the coding regions, including the 5' flanking regions and in the distal LCR. Pairwise comparisons of the human gene cluster with that from galago (Table et al., 1992) or rabbit (Margot et al., 1989) show even more sequence matches (Hardison and Miller, 1993). When sequences from several species are aligned simultaneously, one can detect *conserved* blocks of sequences (Miller et al., 1994), or phylogenetic footprints (Tagle et al., 1988; Gumucio et al., 1996), that are clearly changing more slowly than the surrounding sequences. The well-conserved sequences are reliable guides to functional regions (e.g., Gumucio et al., 1992; Gumucio et al., 1993; Elnitski et al., 1997).

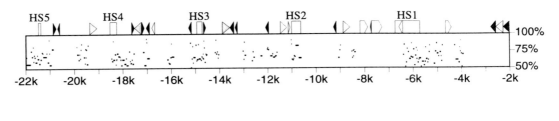

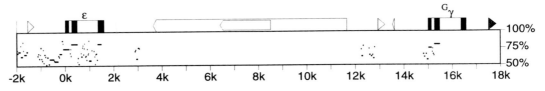

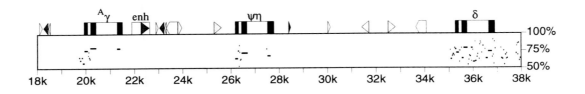

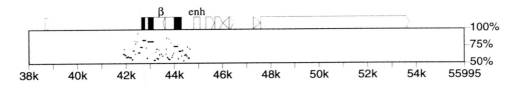

The multiple sequence alignments can be used to find conserved protein binding sites throughout the mammalian β- and α-globin gene clusters. A detailed map of the human β-globin gene clusters is shown in Figure 5.10, along with the positions of all matches to consensus binding sites for selected proteins. Binding sites that are conserved in all available sequences are denoted by longer vertical lines. This analysis illustrates dramatically the restriction of conserved MARE to the HSs 2 and 3 in the LCR. Conserved CACC motifs are also found in HS2 and HS3, and conserved GATA sites are in four HSs of the LCR, with HS3 containing three such sites. In keeping with its high content of A+T, the β-globin gene cluster has an abundance of GATA sites but almost no GC boxes, which are binding sites for Sp1. Only a small subset of the matches to binding sites are conserved in other mammals, and these conserved sites tend to be in the 5' flanking regions (but as much as a 1000 bp away from the genes) and in the LCR.

The results of this type of analysis in the proximal regulatory regions of mammalian α- and β-like globin genes are summarized in Figure 5.8. The conserved sites are outlined with thicker lines. Only two binding sites, the TATA box and CCAAT box (Efstratiadis et al., 1980), are found in all these globin genes. A set of binding sites is distinctive to each type of gene. For

Figure 5.9. Positions and degree of similarity of alignments between human and mouse β-globin gene clusters. This percent identity plot, or pip (Hardison et al., 1997a), shows a detailed map of the human β-globin gene cluster along the top horizontal axis, with the positions of segments that align with the mouse sequence shown as horizontal lines in the plot. The vertical position in the plot is the percent identity of each aligning segment. The HSs in the LCR are appropriately labeled white boxes, globin genes are shown with black exons and white introns, and the 3' enhancers are labeled enh. Interspersed repeats were identified using Repeat Masker (U. of Washington) and are indicated as follows: white arrowed boxes, L1 repeats; black arrowed boxes, L2 repeats; light gray triangles, Alu repeats; black triangles, MIR repeats; darker gray triangles or arrowed boxes, other repeats, like LTR repeats, and DNA transposons. One factor in the limited amount of matching sequences in the region between the δ- and β-globin genes is the insertion of an HMG14 pseudogene for the gene between βh3 and the β-major globin gene in mouse (S. Philipsen, personal communication).

instance, βDRF (Stuve and Myers, 1990), EKLF (Miller and Bieker, 1993; Donze et al., 1995; Nuez et al., 1995; Perkins et al., 1995), and BB1-binding protein (Antoniou et al., 1988; Macleod and Plumb, 1991) have been implicated only in the regulation of the β-globin gene. All are conserved in mammals. EKLF binds to a CACC motif, and similar but distinctive CACC motifs are also found in a comparable posi-

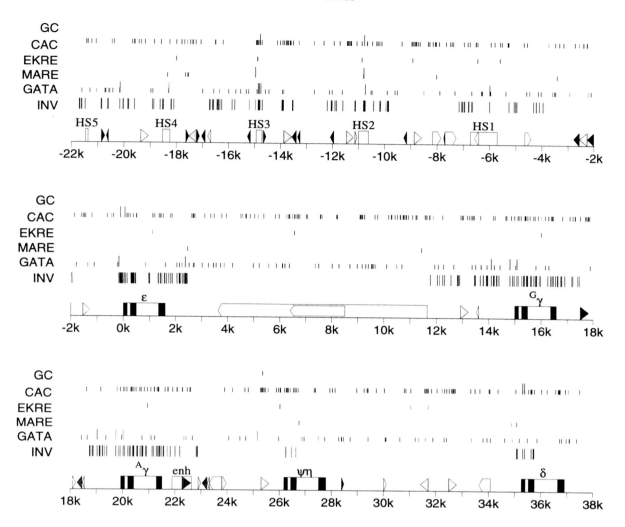

Figure 5.10. Distribution and conservation of sequence motifs throughout mammalian β-globin gene clusters. A detailed map of the gene cluster is shown on the numbered line, using the same conventions as in Figure 5.9. Results of analysis of a multiple alignment of β-globin gene cluster sequences (available at the Globin Gene Server, http://globin.cse.psu.edu) are shown above this map. The positions of invariant blocks at least six columns long are on the line labeled INV (this is one criterion for conserved sequences). Matches to the following sequence motifs or their reverse complement are indicated as labeled: GATA = WGATAR; MARE (maf-response element) = TGASTCA; EKRE (EKLF-response element) = CCNCACCC; CACC (core of site for binding Kruppel class Zn finger proteins) = CACC; GC (binding site for Sp1) = CCGCCC. Motifs that are conserved in other species in the alignment (at least three of them) are denoted by *long* vertical lines; those that are not conserved are denoted by *short* vertical lines.

tion in the 5′ flanks of the γ- and ε-globin genes, again conserved in orthologous mammalian genes. The specificity of EKLF in regulating the β-globin gene raises the intriguing possibility that other, related proteins binding to CACC motifs, perhaps active only at one developmental stage, are regulating γ- and ε-globin genes and recently, fetal Krüppel-like factors

(FKLF), have been described (Chapters 4, 7, and 15). A GATA site is conserved at about the same position in both γ- and ε-globin gene 5′ flanking regions; these have been implicated in positive regulation of the respective genes (Martin et al., 1989; Gong and Dean, 1993). The comparable region for β-globin does not have a conserved GATA site (Hardison et al., 1994). Even conserved DNA sequence motifs in paralogous genes may serve as binding sites for different proteins. A CCAAT motif located at about −80 in all the vertebrate globin gene promoters can be bound by a heteromeric complex called CP1, NF-Y, or CBF (Hooft van Huijsduijnen et al., 1990 and references therein). However, preparations of CP1 bind much more strongly to the CCAAT box in the α-globin gene promoter than in the β-globin gene promoter (Cohen et al., 1986). Also, multiple additional proteins bind to the CCAAT box, some of which have been implicated in the activation of β-globin gene expression (deBoer et al., 1988; Delvoye et al., 1993).

Thus, sequence alignments of these groups of orthologous genes in different eutherian mammals reveal protein-binding sites important for regulated expression.

The differences in the arrays of proteins functioning at ε-, γ-, β- and α-globin genes indicate that a distinct battery of proteins functions in the promoter for each type of gene. Indeed, this is consistent with the observation that *cis*-acting sequences needed for stage-specific regulation of expression map close to the genes (Trudel and Costantini, 1987 and references therein). In contrast to the conservation of sites in the 5' proximal regions, the enhancers located 3' to the $^A\gamma$- and β-globin genes (Bodine and Ley, 1987; Wall et al., 1988; Puruker et al., 1990) are not well conserved among mammals (Fig. 5.8), indicative of a function peculiar to higher primates. One such function discussed in more detail later is the expression of the γ-globin genes in fetal life.

RISE AND FALL OF THE δ-GLOBIN GENE: NEW PROSPECTS FOR THERAPY

HbA$_2$ ($\alpha_2\delta_2$) can inhibit the polymerization of deoxy-HbS in patients with sickle cell disease (Nagel et al., 1979; Poillon et al., 1993) (Chapter 10). Because low levels of the minor HbA$_2$ are present in all adult erythrocytes (Heller and Yakulis, 1969), strategies to increase synthesis of δ-globin should have a pancellular effect on the decrease in sickling, a possible advantage over the strategies to increase synthesis of γ-globin, which is expressed only in a subpopulation of erythrocytes. Examination of δ-globin gene sequences in other mammals provides some important insights into sequence changes that can activate or silence its expression.

The evolutionary history of the δ-globin gene is complex, with recombinations and mutations resulting in the loss, silencing, or expression at a range of levels in different mammals. Even identifying β-like globin genes that are orthologous to the human δ-globin gene is complicated, because the human gene itself is a hybrid of a 5' region closely related to the β-globin gene fused to a 3' region that is distinctive for the δ-globin gene (Spritz et al., 1980; Martin et al., 1983). This is the result of a gene conversion event (Fig. 5.11), with the β-globin gene serving as the donor of the DNA sequences to the 5' region during the recombination (Martin et al., 1983). Thus for comparisons with other mammalian globin gene clusters, matching sequences in the 3' portion are most useful for assignments of orthologous relationships with the human δ-globin gene (Fig. 5.4). Further analysis reveals a striking tendency for the δ-globin genes to undergo gene conversions with β-globin genes (Fig. 5.11); this has occurred independently in several primates, rabbits (Lacy and Maniatis, 1980; Hardison and Margot, 1984), and mice (Hardies et al., 1984).

Expression of the δ-globin genes varies over a wide range in primates. In contrast to the low level expression in humans, the δ-globin gene is silent in Old World monkeys (Martin et al., 1983). It is expressed at a low level in a New World monkey, the spider monkey (Spritz and Giebel, 1988), and at a high level (up to 40% of total fetal and postnatal hemoglobin) in the prosimian primates galago and tarsier (Tagle et al., 1991). In the galago, the δ-globin gene has undergone an extensive gene conversion that effectively replaces it with β-globin gene sequences (i.e., extending from 800 bp 5' to the CCAAT box to near the end of exon 3). This shows that the δ-globin gene locus can be activated to high level expression, if the promoter is appropriately modified (in this case replacing the δ-globin gene promoter with the β-globin gene promoter).

Comparison of the promoter sequences in the silenced or low-level expression δ-globin genes and the highly expressed β-globin genes has revealed several mutations associated with low level expression (Lacy and Maniatis, 1980; Martin et al., 1983; Tang et al., 1997). Two prominent changes in the δ-globin gene promoters are the mutation of the CCAAT box to a CCAAC and the loss of the proximal CACC box, which is the binding site for EKLF in β-globin gene promoters (Fig. 5.8). Site-directed mutagenesis experiments have shown that these alterations in the δ-globin gene promoter do cause lower level expression. Directed mutations that restore the CCAAT box or insert a CACC motif will activate δ-globin reporter gene expression in transfected erythroid cells (Donze et al., 1996; Tang et al., 1997). Thus strategies can be pursued to construct novel transcriptional activators that will recognize the altered binding sites in the wild-type δ-globin gene (expressed at a low level) to attempt to increase the level of expression in erythroid cells. Success in this endeavor may lead to new strategies for therapy for patients with sickle cell disease; however, studies in transgenic animals have shown that expression of high levels of HbA$_2$ may have deleterious effects on the erythrocyte (Nagel et al., 1995).

RECRUITMENT TO FETAL EXPRESSION OF THE γ-GLOBIN GENE IN HIGHER PRIMATES

Increased concentrations of HbF ($\alpha2\gamma2$) in erythrocytes will ameliorate the symptoms of both sickle cell disease and thalassemia (Chapters 7, 15, 24, 38). Thus considerable effort has gone into understanding the fetal-specific expression of the human γ-globin genes and mutations that cause its continued expression in adult life, leading to the syndrome of hereditary persistence of fetal hemoglobin (Chapters 7 and 15). This section provides an evolutionary context for these studies, emphasizing the efficacy of phylogenetic comparisons for generating hypotheses about *cis*-regulatory elements.

As discussed previously, most eutherian mammals (including prosimians) express the γ-globin gene only in embryonic red cells, but anthropoid primates (monkeys, apes and humans) express it abundantly in fetal red cells. The appearance of this new pattern of fetal expression

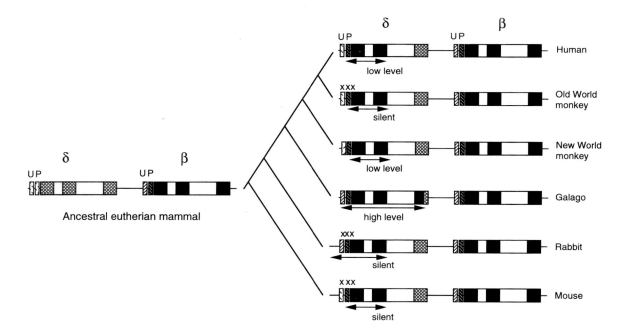

Figure 5.11. Gene conversion, silencing, and activation of δ-globin genes during mammalian evolution. The ancestral pair of δ- and β-globin genes are shown with fills distinctive for the exons and introns of each gene. The basal promoter is indicated by the box labeled P, the upstream activating sequence indicated by the box labeled U (shown in more detail in Fig. 5.8). The extent of each gene conversion is shown by the double-headed arrow. The x's indicate mutations that silence the gene.

coincides with the duplication of the γ-globin genes in an ancestral simian, which leads to the hypothesis that the duplication allowed the changes that caused the fetal recruitment (Fitch et al., 1991; Hayasaka et al., 1993). Concomitantly, expression of the β-globin gene is delayed until just before birth in the anthropoid primates. In other mammals, β-globin gene expression initiates and predominates in the fetal liver, arguing that fetal expression of the β-globin gene is the ancestral state. Note that these changes in pattern of expression in anthropoid primates are in the definitive erythroid cell lineage (derived from fetal liver and adult bone marrow), but they do not necessarily require changes in expression in the primitive erythroid cell lineage derived from embryonic yolk sac cells (Chapter 2).

Further analysis reveals some heterogeneity in the timing of expression of γ-globin genes in anthropoid primates (Fig. 5.12). As in humans, two γ-globin genes are found in apes and Old World monkeys (Slightom et al., 1987; Slightom et al., 1988), and presumably these are actively expressed in fetal erythroid cells. Duplicated γ-globin genes are also found in New World monkeys, but there is a tendency to inactivate one of the copies, either by partial deletion or by mutations that decrease expression (reviewed in Chiu et al., 1997). Fetal erythrocytes

from three species of New World monkeys contain both γ and β globins (Johnson et al., 1996); thus fetal recruitment of γ-globin gene expression predates the divergence between New World and Old World monkeys (about 48 million years ago) but follows the simian-prosimian split (about 60 million years ago). The switch in synthesis from γ globin to β globin appears to occur earlier in New World monkeys than in Old World monkeys and apes. Thus the γ-globin genes in New World monkeys may represent an intermediate state in which the change in timing of expression has not completely shifted to that seen in humans.

The cis-elements close to the γ-globin gene are key determinants of fetal versus embryonic expression because in otherwise identical constructs, a prosimian γ-globin gene is expressed embryonically in transgenic mice, whereas a human γ-globin gene is expressed fetally (TomHon et al., 1997). One would like to identify alterations in the regulatory regions of anthropoid γ-globin genes that are associated with this change in stage-specificity (i.e., sequences that are conserved in anthropoid primates but are different in prosimians and nonprimate mammals. Blocks of aligned sequences with such properties are called differential phylogenetic footprints (Gumucio et al., 1994). This approach led to the identification of a stage selector element (SSE) in the human γ-globin gene promoter (Fig. 5.8). The SSE is a binding site for a factor called the stage-selector protein, or SSP, which has been implicated in the differential expression of γ- and β-globin genes (Jane et al., 1992). SSP is a heterodimer (Jane et al., 1995) between CP2 (Lim et al., 1992) and another protein. Interestingly, the NFE4 protein implicated in the stage-specific expression of the chicken β-

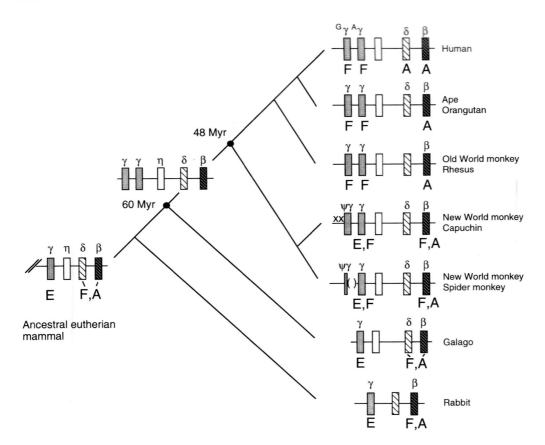

Figure 5.12. Recruitment of the γ-globin gene to fetal expression in simian primates. The portion of the β-globin gene clusters from γ-globin through β-globin genes is shown, along with the deduced gene duplication in the ancestor to anthropoid primates. Conventions and abbreviations are as in other figures.

globin gene (Foley and Engel, 1992) also contains CP2 as part of a heterodimer (Jane et al., 1995). Further analysis has revealed an additional DNA sequence that binds several proteins implicated in fetal silencing of the γ-globin gene (Gumucio et al., 1994).

The enhancers located 3′ to the Aγ- and β-globin genes may also be involved in the changes in timing of expression in anthropoid primates. The 3′ ᴬγ-globin gene enhancer is not conserved in prosimians or nonprimate mammals (Figs. 5.9 and 5.10); in fact two of the GATA1-binding sites (Puruker et al., 1990) were brought in via a transposable element (Fig. 5.10). Thus the presence of this enhancer correlates with the fetal recruitment of γ-globin gene expression. The 3′ β-globin gene enhancer is characterized by several GATA sites (Wall et al., 1988), but these are not conserved in nonanthropoid mammals (Fig. 5.10). Experiments in transgenic mice revealed effects of this enhancer primarily on developmental timing (Trudel and Costantini, 1987; Antoniou et al., 1988; Perez-Stable and Costantini, 1990). It is possible that the 3′ enhancers, as well as promoter regions, contain cis-regulatory elements impor-

tant in the fetal recruitment of γ-globin genes and the delay in expression of the β-globin gene. Increased understanding of the role and mechanism of action of proteins implicated in activation of γ-globin gene expression (Fig. 5.8), such as SSP, γPE (Lloyd et al., 1994), GATA1 (Martin et al., 1989; Puruker et al., 1990; McDonagh et al., 1991), and proteins binding to the CACC and CCAAT motifs, could lead to novel strategies to increase γ-globin production in sickle cell disease and thalassemia.

ACKNOWLEDGMENTS

I thank Webb Miller for producing Figures 9 and 10. Work in this laboratory is supported by the National Institutes of Health, grant RO1DK27635, and the National Library of Medicine, grants RO1LM05110 and RO1LM05773.

References

Aladjem, MI, Groudine, M, Brody, LL et al. (1995). Participation of the human β-globulin locus control region in initiation of DNA replication. *Science* 270: 815-819.
Aladjem, MI, Rodewald, LW, Kolman, JL, and Wahl, GM. (1998). Genetic dissection of a mammalian replicator in the human beta-globin locus. *Science* 281: 1005-1009.

Andersson, CR, Jensen, EO, Llewellyn, DJ et al. (1996). A new hemoglobin gene from soybean: A role for hemoglobin in all plants. *Proc. Natl. Acad. Sci. U.S.A.* 93: 5682–5687

Antequera, FBA. (1993). Number of CpG islands and genes in human and mouse. *Proc. Natl. Acad. Sci. U.S.A.* 90: 11995–11999.

Antoniou, M, deBoer, E, Habets, G, and Grosveld, F. (1988). The human β-globin gene contains multiple regulatory regions: Identification of one promoter and two downstream enhancers. *EMBO J.* 7: 377–384.

Aparicio, S, Morrison, A, Gould, A et al. (1995). Detecting conserved regulatory elements with the model genome of the Japanese puffer fish, *Fugu rubripes. Proc. Natl. Acad. Sci. U.S.A.* 92: 1684–1688.

Appleby, CPA. (1984). Leghemoglobin and Rhizobium respiration. *Annu. Rev. Plant Physiol.* 35: 443–478.

Barnhart, K, Kim, C, Banerji, S, and Sheffery, M. (1988). Identification and characterization of multiple erythroid cell proteins that interact with the promoter of the murine α-globin gene. *Mol. Cell. Biol.* 9: 3215–3226.

Baron, MH. (1997). Transcriptional control of globin gene switching during vertebrate development. *Biochim. Biophys. Acta* 1351: 51–72.

Bernardi, G, Olofsson, B, Filipski, J et al. (1985). The mosaic genome of warm-blooded vertebrates. *Science* 228: 953–958.

Bird, A, Taggart, M, Nicholls, R, and Higgs, D. (1987). Non-methylated CpG-rich islands at the human α-globin locus: Implications for evolution of the α-globin pseudogene. *EMBO J.* 6: 999–1004.

Bodine, D and Ley, T. (1987). An enhancer element lies 3′ to the human A gamma globin gene. *EMBO J.* 6: 2997–3004.

Bonaventura, C, Feruzzi, G, Tesh, S, and Stevens, RD. (1999). Effects of S-nitrosation on oxygen binding by normal and sickle cell hemoglobin. *J. Bio. Chem.* 274: 24742–24748.

Brisson, N and Verma DP. (1982). Soybean leghemoglobin gene family: Normal, pseudo, and truncated genes. *Proc. Natl. Acad. Sci. U.S.A.* 79: 4055–4059.

Bulger, M, von Doorninck, JH, Saitoh, N et al. (1999). Conservation of sequence and structure flanking the mouse and human beta-globin genes are embedded within an array of odorant receptor genes. *Proc. Natl. Acad. Sci. U.S.A.* 96: 5129–5134.

Bunn, HF, and Forget, BG. (1986). Animal hemoglobins. *Hemoglobin: Molecular, genetic and clinical aspects.* Philadelphia: W. B. Saunders Co.

Calza, RE, Eckhardt, LA, Giudice, T, and Schildkraut CL. (1984). Changes in gene position are accompanied by a change in time of replication. *Cell* 36: 689–696.

Caterina, JJ, Ciavatta, DJ, Donze, D et al. (1994). Multiple elements in human β-globin locus control region 5′ HS2 are involved in enhancer activity and position-independent transgene expression. *Nucl. Acids Res.* 22: 1006–1011.

Chan, F, Robinson, J, Brownlie, A et al. (1997). Characterization of adult alpha- and beta-globin genes in the zebrafish. *Blood* 89: 688–700.

Cheng, J, Raid, L, and Hardison, RC. (1986). Isolation and nucleotide sequence of the rabbit globin gene cluster pseudoZ-alpha1-pseudoA. *J. Biol. Chem.* 261: 839–848.

Cheng, J, Raid, L, and Hardison, RC. (1987). Block duplications of α_ζ-ζ-α-τ gene set in the rabbit α-like globin gene cluster. *J. Biol. Chem.* 262: 5414–5421.

Chiu, CH, Schneider, H, Slightom, JL et al. (1997). Dynamics of regulatory evolution in primate β-globin gene clusters: cis-mediated acquisition of simian γ fetal expression patterns. *Gene* 205: 47–57.

Clark, D, Reitman, M, Studitsky, V et al. (1993). Chromatin structure of transcriptionally active genes. *Cold Spring Harb. Symp. Quant. Biol.* 58: 1–6.

Cohen, RB, Sheffery, M, and Kim, CG. (1986). Partial purification of a nuclear protein that binds to the CCAAT box of the mouse α1-globin gene. *Mol. Cell. Biol.* 6: 821–832.

Collins, FS and Weissman, SM. (1984). The molecular genetics of human hemoglobin. *Prog. Nucl. Acids Res. Mol. Biol.* 31: 315–462.

Cooper, S, Murphy, R, Dolman, G et al. (1996). A molecular and evolutionary study of the beta-globin gene family of the Australian marsupial *Sminthopsis crassicaudata. Mol. Biol. Evol.* 13: 1012–1022.

Couture, M, Chamberland, H, St.-Pierre, B et al. (1994). Nuclear genes encoding chloroplast hemoglobins in the unicellular green alga *Chlamydomonas eugametos. Mol. Gen. Genet.* 243: 185–197.

Couture, M and Guertin, M. (1996). Purification and spectroscopic characterization of a recombinant chloroplastic hemoglobin from the green unicellular alga *Chlamydomonas eugametos. Eur. J. Biochem.* 242: 779–787.

Craddock, CF, Vyas, P, Sharpe, JA et al. (1995). Contrasting effects of alpha and beta globin regulatory elements on chromatin structure may be related to their different chromosomal environments. *EMBO J.* 14: 1718–1726.

Cramm, R, Siddiqui, RA, and Friedrich, B. (1994). Primary structure and evidence for a physiological function of the flavohemoprotein of *Alcaligenes eutrophus. J. Biol. Chem.* 269: 7349–7354.

Crawford, MJ and Goldberg, DE. (1998). Role for the *Salmonella* flavohemoglobin in protection from nitric oxide. *J. Biol. Chem.* 273: 12543–12547.

deBoer, E, Antoniou, M, Mignotte, V et al. (1988). The human β-globin promoter: Nuclear protein factors and erythroid specific induction of transcription. *EMBO J.* 7: 4203–4212.

Deisseroth, A, Nienhuis, A, Turner, P et al. (1977). Localization of the human alpha globin structural gene to chromosome 16 in somatic cell hybrids by molecular hybridization assay. *Cell* 12: 205–218.

Deisseroth, A, Nienhuis, AW, Lawrence, J et al. (1978). Chromosomal localization of the human beta globin gene to human chromosome 11 in somatic cell hybrids. *Proc. Natl. Acad. Sci., U.S.A.* 75: 1456–1460.

Deisseroth, A, Velez, R, and Nienhuis, AW. (1976). Hemoglobin synthesis in somatic cell hybrids: independent segregation of the human alpha- and beta-globin genes. *Science* 191: 1262–1263.

Delvoye, NL, Destroismaisons, NM, and Wall, LA. (1993). Activation of the β-globin gene promoter by the locus control region correlates with binding of a novel factor to the CCAAT bos in murine erythroleukemia cells but not in K562 cells. *Mol. Cell. Biol.* 13: 6969–6983.

Dhar, V, Mager, D, Iqbal, A, and Schildkraut, CL. (1988). The co-ordinate replication of the human β-globin gene domain reflects its transcriptional activity and nuclease hypersensitivity. *Mol. Cell. Biol.* 8: 4958–4965.

Dhar, V, Nandi, A, Schildkraut, CL, and Skoultchi, AI. (1990). Erythroid-specific nuclease-hypersensitive sites flanking the human β-globin gene cluster. *Mol. Cell. Biol.* 10: 4324–4333.

Dickerson, RE, and Geis, I. (1983). *Hemoglobin: Structure, function, evolution and pathology.* Menlo Park, CA: Benjamin/Cummings Publishing Co.

Dikshit, RP, Dikshit, KL, Liu, Y, and Webster, DA. (1992). The bacterial hemoglobin from *Vitreoscilla* can support aerobic growth of *Escherichia coli* lacking terminal oxidases. *Arch. Biochem. Biophys.* 293: 241–245.

Dixon, B, Walker, B, Kimmins, W, and Pohajdak, B. (1992). A nematode hemoglobin gene contains an intron previously thought to be unique to plants. *J. Mol. Evol.* 35: 131–136.

Donze, D, Jeancake, P, and Townes, T. (1996). Activation of delta-globin gene expression by erythroid Krupple-like factor: A potential approach for gene therapy of sickle cell disease. *Blood* 88: 4051–4057.

Donze, D, Townes, TM, and Bieker, JJ. (1995). Role of erythroid kruppel-like factor in human γ- to β-globin gene switching. *J. Biol. Chem.* 270: 1955–1959.

Durner, J, Gow, AJ, Stamler, JS, and Glazebrook, J. (1999). Ancient origins of nitric oxide in signaling in biological systems. *Proc. Natl. Acad. Sci. U.S.A.* 96: 14206-14207.

Efstratiadis, A, Posakony, JW, Maniatis, T et al. (1980). The structure and evolution of the human β-globin gene family. *Cell* 21: 653–668.

Elder, JT, Forrester, WC, Thompson, C et al. (1990). Translocation of an erythroid-specific hypersensitive site in deletion-type hereditary persistence of fetal hemoglobin. *Mol. Cell Biol.* 10: 1382–1389.

Elnitski, L, Miller, W, and Hardison, R. (1997). Conserved E boxes function as part of the enhancer in hypersensitive site 2 of the β-globin locus control region: Role of basic helix-loop-helix proteins. *J. Biol. Chem.* 272: 369–378.

Epner, E, Rifkin, RA, and Marks, PA. (1981). Replication of alpha and beta globin DNA sequences occurs during early S phase in murine erythroleukemia cells. *Proc. Natl. Acad. Sci. U.S.A.* 78: 3058-3062.

Ermler, U, Siddiqui, RA, Cramm, R, and Friedrich, B. (1995). Crystal structure of the flavohemoglobin from *Alcaligenes eutrophus* at 1.75 Angstrom resolution. *EMBO J.* 14: 6067–6077.

Evans, T, Felsenfeld, G, and Reitman, M. (1990). Control of globin gene transcription. *Annu. Rev. Cell Biol.* 6: 95–124.

Feingold, EA and Forget, BG. (1989). The breakpoint of a large deletion causing hereditary persistence of fetal hemoglobin occurs within an erythroid DNA domain remote from the beta-globin gene cluster. *Blood* 74: 2178–2186.

Feingold, EA, Penny, LA, Nienhuis, AW, and Forget, BG. (1999). An olfactory receptor gene is located in the extended human β-globin gene cluster and is expressed in erythroid cells. *Genomics* 61: 15–23.

Feng, DF, Cho, G, and Doolittle, RF. (1997). Determining divergence times with a protein clock: Update and reevaluation. *Proc. Natl. Acad. Sci. U.S.A.* 94: 13028–13033.

Fischel-Ghodsian, N, Nicholls, RD, and Higgs, DR. (1987). Unusual features of CpG-rich (HTF) islands in the human α-globin complex: Association with nonfunctional pseudogenes and presence within the 3′ portion of the ζ genes. *Nucl. Acids Res.* 15: 9215–9225.

Fitch, DH, Bailey, WJ, Tagle, DA et al. (1991). Duplication of the gamma-globin gene mediated by L1 long interspersed repetitive elements in an early ancestor of simian primates. *Proc. Natl. Acad. Sci. U.S.A.* 88: 7396–7400.

Flint, J, Taylor, AM, and Clegg, JB. (1988). Structure and evolution of the horse zeta globin locus. *J. Mol. Biol.* 199: 427–437.

Flint, J, Thomas, K, Micklem, G et al. (1997). The relationship between chromosome structure and function at a human telomeric region. *Nat. Genet.* 15: 252–257.

Foley, KP and Engel, JD. (1992). Individual stage selector element mutations lead to reciprocal changes in β- vs. ε-globin gene transcription: Genetic confirmation of promoter competition during globin gene switching. *Genes Dev.* 6: 730–744.

Forrester, W, Takegawa, S, Papayannopoulou, T et al. (1987). Evidence for a locus activating region: The formation of developmentally stable hypersensitive sites in globin-expressing hybrids. *Nucl. Acids Res.* 15: 10159–10177.

Forrester, WC, Epner, E, Driscoll, MC et al. (1990). A deletion of the human β-globin locus activation region causes a major alteration in chromatin structure and replication across the entire β-globin locus. *Genes Dev.* 4: 1637–1649.

Fraser, P, Hurst, J, Collis, P, and Grosveld, F. (1990). DNase I hypersensitive sites 1, 2 and 3 of the human β-globin dominant control region direct position-independent expression. *Nucl. Acids. Res.* 18: 3503–3508.

Fritsch, E, Lawn, R, and Maniatis, T. (1980). Molecular cloning and characterization of the human beta-like globin gene cluster. *Cell* 19: 959–972.

Furst, A., Brown, EH, Braunstein, JD, and Schildkraut, CL. (1981). Alpha-globin sequences are located in a region of early-replicating DNA in murine erythroleukemia cells. *Proc. Natl. Acad. Sci. U.S.A.* 78: 1023-1027.

Gardner, PR, Gardner, AM, Martin, LA, and Salzman, AL. (1998). Nitric oxide dioxygenase: an enzymatic function for flavohemoglobin. *Proc. Natl. Acad. Sci. U.S.A.* 95: 10378–10383.

Gilbert, W. (1978). Why genes in pieces? *Nature* 271: 501.

Gladwin, MT, Schechter, AN, Shelhamer, JH et al. (1999). Inhaled nitric oxide augments nitric oxide transport on sickle cell hemoglobin without affecting oxygen affinity. *J. Clin. Invest.* 104: 937–945.

Go, M. (1981). Correlation of DNA exonic regions with protein structural units in haemoglobin. *Nature* 291: 90–92.

Goldman, MA, Holmquist, GP, Gray, MC et al. (1984). Replication timing of genes and middle repetitive sequences. *Science* 224: 686-692.

Gong, QH and Dean, A. (1993). Enhancer-dependent transcription of the ε-globin promoter requires promoter-bound GATA-1 and enhancer-bound AP-1/NF-E2. *Mol. Cell Biol.* 13: 911–917.

Goodman, M, Czelusniak, J, Koop, B et al. (1987). Globins: A case study in molecular phylogeny. *Cold Spring Harb. Symp. Quant. Biol.* 52: 875–890.

Goodman, M, Koop, BF, Czelusniak, J et al. (1984). The η-globin gene: Its long evolutionary history in the β-globin gene families of mammals. *J. Mol. Biol.* 180: 803–824.

Gottgens, B, Barton, LM, Gilbert, JG et al. (2000). Analysis of vertebrate *SCL* loci identifies conserved enhancers. *Nat. Biotechnol.* 18: 181–186.

Gourdon, G, Sharpe, JA, Higgs, DR, and Wood, WG. (1995). The mouse α-globin locus regulatory element. *Blood* 86: 766–775.

Gow, AJ and Stamler, JS. (1998). Reactions between nitric oxide and haemoglobin under physiological conditions. *Nature* 391: 169–173.

Grosveld, F, Antoniou, M, Berry, M et al. (1993). The regulation of human globin gene switching. *Philos. Trans. R. Soc. Lond.* 339: 183–191.

Grosveld, F, van Assendelft, GB, Greaves D, and Kollias, G. (1987). Position-independent, high-level expression of the human β-globin gene in transgenic mice. *Cell* 51: 975–985.

Groudine, J, Kohwi-Shigematsu, T, Gelinas, R et al. (1983). Human fetal to adult hemoglobin switching: Changes in chromatin structure of the β-globin gene locus. *Proc. Natl. Acad. Sci. U.S.A.* 80: 7551–7555.

Gumucio, D, Shelton, D, Zhu, W et al. (1996). Evolutionary strategies for the elucidation of *cis* and *trans* factors that regulate the developmental switching programs of the β-like globin genes. *Mol. Phylogenet. Evol.* 5: 18–32.

Gumucio, DL, Heilstedt-Williamson, H, Gray, TA et al. (1992). Phylogenetic footprinting reveals a nuclear protein which binds to silencer sequences in the human γ and ε globin genes. *Mol. Cell. Biol.* 12: 4919–4929.

Gumucio, DL, Shelton, DA, Bailey, WJ et al. (1993). Phylogenetic footprinting reveals unexpected complexity in trans factor binding upstream from the ε-globin gene. *Proc. Natl. Acad. Sci. U.S.A.* 90: 6018–6022.

Gumucio, DL, Shelton, DA, Blanchard-McQuate, K et al. (1994). Differential phylogenetic footprinting as a means to identify base changes responsible for recruitment of the anthropoid γ gene to a fetal expression pattern. *J. Biol. Chem.* 269: 15371–15380.

Hardies, SC, Edgell, MH, and Hutchison III, CA. (1984). Evolution of the mammalian β-globin gene cluster. *J. Biol. Chem.* 259: 3748–3756.

Hardison, R. (1998). Hemoglobins from bacteria to man: Evolution of different patterns of gene expression. *J. Exp. Biol.* 201: 1099–1117.

Hardison, R, Chao, KM, Schwartz, S et al. (1994). Globin gene server: A prototype E-mail database server featuring extensive multiple alignments and data compilation. *Genomics* 21: 344–353.

Hardison, R, Krane, D, Vandenbergh, D et al. (1991). Sequence and comparative analysis of the rabbit α-like globin gene cluster reveals a rapid mode of evolution in a G+C rich region of mammalian genomes. *J. Mol. Biol.* 222: 233–249.

Hardison, R and Miller, W. (1993). Use of long sequence alignments to study the evolution and regulation of mammalian globin gene clusters. *Mol. Biol. Evol.* 10: 73–102.

Hardison, R, Oeltjen, J, and Miller, W. (1997a). Long human-mouse sequence alignments reveal novel regulatory elements: A reason to sequence the mouse genome. *Genome Res.* 7: 959–966.

Hardison, R, Slightom, JL, Gumucio, DL et al. (1997b). Locus control regions of mammalian β-globin gene clus-

ters: Combining phylogenetic analyses and experimental results to gain functional insights. *Gene* 205: 73–94.

Hardison, R, Xu, J, Jackson, J et al. (1993). Comparative analysis of the locus control region of the rabbit β-like globin gene cluster: HS3 increases transient expression of an embryonic ε-globin gene. *Nucl. Acids Res.* 21: 1265–1272.

Hardison, RC. (1983). The nucleotide sequence of the rabbit embryonic globin gene β4. *J. Biol. Chem.* 258: 8739–8744.

Hardison, RC. (1984). Comparison of the β-like globin gene families of rabbits and humans indicates that the gene cluster 5′ ε-γ-δ-β_3′ predates the mammalian radiation. *Mol. Biol. Evol.* 1: 390–410.

Hardison, RC. (1991). Evolution of globin gene families. In Selander, RK, Whittam, TS, and Clark AG, editors. *Evolution at the molecular level* Sunderland, MA: Sinauer Associates, Inc.

Hardison, RC. (1996). A brief history of hemoglobins: Plant, animal, protist and bacteria. *Proc. Natl. Acad. Sci. U.S.A.* 93: 5675–5679.

Hardison, RC and Gelinas, R. (1986). Assignment of orthologous relationships among mammalian α-globin genes by examining flanking regions reveals a rapid rate of evolution. *Mol. Biol. Evol.* 3: 243–261.

Hardison, RC and Margot, JB. (1984). Rabbit globin pseudogene pseudobeta2 is a hybrid of delta- and beta-globin gene sequences. *Mol. Biol. Evol.* 1: 302–316.

Hausladen, A, Gow, AJ, and Stamler, JS. (1998). Nitrosative stress: metabolic pathway involving the flavohemoglobin. *Proc. Natl. Acad. Sci. U.S.A.* 95: 14100–14105.

Hayasaka, K, Skinner, C, Goodman, M, and Slightom, J. (1993). The γ-globin genes and their flanking sequences in primates: findings with nucleotide sequences of capuchin monkey and tarsier. *Genomics* 18: 20–28.

Hebbes, TR, Clayton, AL, Thorne AW, and Crane-Robinson, C. (1994). Core histone hyperacetylation co-maps with generalized DNase I sensitivity in the chicken β-globin chromosomal domain. *EMBO J.* 13: 1823–1830.

Heller, P and Yakulis, V. (1969). The distribution of hemoglobin A_2. *Ann. N.Y. Acad. Sci.* 165: 54–59.

Hess, J, Schmid, C, and Shen, C. (1984). A gradient of sequence divergence in the human adult alpha-globin duplication units. *Science* 226: 67–70.

Higgs, D, Wood, W, Jarman, A et al. (1990). A major positive regulatory region located far upstream of the human α-globin gene locus. *Genes Dev.* 4: 1588–1601.

Hooft van Huijsduijnen, R, Li, XY, Black, D et al. (1990). Co-evolution from yeast to mouse: cDNA cloning of the two NF-Y (CP-1/CBF) subunits. *EMBO J.* 9: 3119–3127.

Hosbach, HA, Wyler, T, and Weber, R. (1983). The *Xenopus laevis* globin gene family: Chromosomal arrangement and gene structure. *Cell* 32: 45–53.

Hsu, S, Marks, J, Shaw, J et al. (1988). Structure and expression of the human theta 1 globin gene. *Nature* 331: 94–96.

Hug, BA, Moon, AM, and Ley, TJ. (1992). Structure and function of the murine β-globin locus control region 5′ HS-3. *Nuclic. Acids Res.* 21: 5771–5778.

Hughes, S, Stubblefield, E, Payvar, F et al. (1979). Gene localization by chromosome fractionation: Globin genes are on at least two chromosomes and three estrogen-inducible genes are on three chromosomes. *Proc. Natl. Acad. Sci. U.S.A.* 76: 1348–1352.

Hyldig-Nielsen, JJ, Jensen, EO, Paludan, K et al. (1982). The primary structures of two leghemoglobin genes from soybean. *Nucleic Acids Res.* 10: 689–701.

Jane, S, Nienhuis, A, and Cunningham, J. (1995). Hemoglobin switching in man and chicken is mediated by a heteromeric complex between the ubiquitous transcription factor CP2 and a developmentally specific protein. *EMBO J.* 14: 97–105.

Jane, SM, Ney, PA, Vanin, EF et al. (1992). Identification of a stage selector element in the human γ-globin gene promoter that fosters preferential interaction with the 5′ HS2 enhancer when in competition with the β-promoter. *EMBO J.* 11: 2961–2969.

Jarman, A, Wood, W, Sharpe, J et al. (1991). Characterization of the major regulatory element upstream of the human α-globin gene cluster. *Mol. Cell. Biol.* 11: 4679–4689.

Jia, L, Bonaventura, C, Bonaventura, J, and Stamler, JS. (1996): S-nitrosohaemoglobin: a dynamic activity of blood involved in vascular control. *Nature* 380: 221–226.

Jimenez, G, Gale, KB, and Enver, T. (1992). The mouse β-globin locus control region: Hypersensitive sites 3 and 4. *Nucl. Acids Res.* 20: 5797–5803.

Johnson, RM, Buck, S, Chiu, C-H et al. (1996). Fetal globin expression in New World monkeys. *J. Biol. Chem.* 271: 14684–14691.

Kim, J, Yu, C, Bailey, A et al. (1989). Unique sequence organization and erythroid cell-specific nuclear factor-binding of mammalian theta 1 globin promoters. *Nucleic Acids Res.* 17: 5687–5700.

Kitsberg, D, Selig, S, Keshet, I, and Cedar, H. (1993). Replication structure of the human beta-globulin gene domain. *Nature* 366: 588-590.

Koop, B, and Goodman, M. (1988). Evolutionary and developmental aspects of two hemoglobin beta-chain genes (epsilon M and beta M) of opossum. *Proc. Natl. Acad. Sci. U.S.A.* 85: 3893–3897.

Kosteas, T, Palena, A, and Anagnou, NP. (1997). Molecular cloning of the breakpoints of the hereditary persistence of fetal hemoglobin type-6 (HPFH-6) deletion and sequence analysis of the novel juxtaposed region from the 3′ end of the β-globin gene cluster. *Hum. Genet.* 100: 441–445.

Kumar, S, and Hedges, SB. (1998). A molecular timescale for vertebrate evolution. *Nature* 392: 917–920.

Kumar, S, Tamura, K, and Nei, M. (1993). *MEGA: Molecular evolutionary genetic analysis, version 1.01.* University Park, PA: The Pennsylvania State University.

Lacy, E, and Maniatis, T. (1980). Nucleotide sequence of the rabbit pseudogene ιβ1. *Cell* 21: 545–553.

Lam, L, and Bresnick, EH. (1996). A novel DNA binding protein, HS2NF5, interacts with a functionally important sequence of the human β-globin locus control region. *J. Biol. Chem.* 271: 32421–32429.

Lauer, J, Shen, C, and Maniatis, T. (1980). The chromosomal arrangement of human alpha-like globin genes: Sequence homology and alpha-globin gene deletions. *Cell* 20: 119–130.

Leder, A, Weir, L, and Leder, P. (1985). Characterization, expression and evolution of the mouse embryonic zeta-globin gene. *Mol. Cell. Biol.* 5: 1025–1033.

Lee, JS, Brown, GG, and Verma, DPS. (1983). Chromosomal arrangement of leghemoglobin genes in soybeans. *Nucleic Acids Res.* 11: 5541–5552.

Leung, S, Whitelaw, E, and Proudfoot, N. (1989). Transcriptional and translational analysis of the human theta globin gene. *Nucleic Acids Res.* 17: 8283–8300.

Li, Q, Powers, PA, and Smithies, O. (1985). Nucleotide sequence of 16-kilobase pairs of DNA 5′ to the human ε-globin gene. *J. Biol. Chem.* 260: 14901–14910.

Li, Q, Zhou, B, Powers, P et al. (1991). Primary structure of the goat β-globin locus control region. *Genomics* 9: 488–499.

Lim, LC, Swendeman, SL, and Sheffery, M. (1992). Molecular cloning of the alpha-globin transcription factor CP2. *Mol. Cell. Biol.* 12: 828–835.

Liu, L, Zelig, M, Hausladen, A et al. (2000). Protection from nitrosative stress by yeast flavohemoglobin. *Proc. Natl. Acad. Sci. U.S.A.*, in press.

Lloyd, JA, Case, SS, Ponce, E, and Lingrel, JB. (1994). Positive transcriptional regulation of the human γ-globin gene: γPE is a novel nuclear factor with multiple binding sites near the gene. *J. Biol. Chem.* 269: 26–34.

Macleod, K and Plumb, M. (1991). Derepression of mouse β-major-globin gene transcription during erythroid differentiation. *Mol. Cell. Biol.* 11: 4324–4332.

Margot, JB, Demers, GW, and Hardison, RC. (1989). Complete nucleotide sequence of the rabbit β-like globin gene cluster: Analysis of intergenic sequences and comparison with the human β-like globin gene cluster. *J. Mol. Biol.* 205: 15–40.

Martin, DIK, Tsai, S-F, and Orkin, SH. (1989). Increased gamma-globin expression in a nondeletion HPFH mediated by an erythroid-specific DNA-binding factor. *Nature* 338: 435–438.

Martin, SL, Vincent, KA, and Wilson, AC. (1983). Rise and fall of the delta globin gene. *J. Mol. Biol.* 164: 513–528.

Matsuo, K, Clay, O, Takahashi, T et al. (1993). Evidence for erosion of mouse CpG islands during mammalian evolution. *Somat. Cell Mol. Genet.* 19: 543–555.

McDonagh, KT, Lin, HJ, Lowrey, CH et al. (1991). The upstream region of the human γ-globin gene promoter: Identification and functional analysis of nuclear protein binding sites. *J. Biol. Chem.* 266: 11965–11974.

Miller, IJ, and Bieker, JJ. (1993). A novel, erythroid cell-specific murine transcription factor that binds to the CACCC element and is related to the *Kruppel* family of nuclear factors. *Mol. Cell. Biol.* 13: 2776–2786.

Miller, W, Boguski, M, Raghavachari, B et al. (1994). Constructing aligned sequence blocks. *J. Computat. Biol.* 1: 51–64.

Minning, DM, Gow, AJ, Bonaventura, J et al. (1999). Ascaris haemoglobin is a nitric oxide-activated 'deoxygenase'. *Nature* 401: 497–502.

Moon, AM, and Ley, TJ. (1990). Conservation of the primary structure, organization, and function of the human and mouse β-globin locus-activating regions. *Proc. Natl. Acad. Sci. U.S.A.* 87: 7693–7697.

Morley, BJ, Abbott, CA, Sharpe, JA et al. (1992). A single β-globin locus control region element (5′ hypersensitive site 2) is sufficient for developmental regulation of human globin genes in transgenic mice. *Mol. Cell. Biol.* 12: 2057–2066.

Motamed, K, Bastiani, C, Zhang, Q et al. (1993). CACC box and enhancer response of human embryonic ε globin promoter. *Gene* 123: 235–240.

Motohashi, H, Shavit, JA, Igarashi, K et al. (1997). The world according to Maf. *Nucleic Acids Res.* 25: 2953–2959.

Nagel, R, Bookchin, R, Johnson, J et al. (1979). Structural bases of the inhibitory effects of hemoglobin F and hemoglobin A2 on the polymerization of hemoglobin S. *Proc. Natl. Acad. Sci. U.S.A.* 76: 670–672.

Nagel, RL. (1999). Can we just say NO to sickle cell anemia? *J. Clin. Invest.* 104: 847–848.

Nagel RL, Sharma A, Kumar R, and Fabry ME. (1995). Severe red cell abnormalities in transgenic mice expressing high levels of normal human delta chains. *Blood* 86, 251a.

Ney, P, Sorrentino, B, McDonagh, K, and Nienhuis, A. (1990). Tandem AP-1-binding sites within the human β-globin dominant control region function as an inducible enhancer in erythroid cells. *Genes Dev.* 4: 993–1006.

Nishioka, Y, and Leder, P. (1979). The complete sequence of a chromosomal mouse alpha-globin gene reveals elements conserved throughout vertebrate evolution. *Cell* 18: 875–882.

Nuez, B, Michalovich, D, Bygrave, A et al. (1995). Defective haematopoiesis in fetal liver resulting from inactivation of the EKLF gene. *Nature* 375: 316–318.

Orkin, SH. (1995). Transcription factors and hematopoietic development. *J. Biol. Chem.* 270: 4955–4958.

Perez-Stable, C, and Costantini, F. (1990). Role of fetal Gγ-globin promoter elements and the adult β-globin 3′ enhancer in the stage-specific expression of globin genes. *Mol. Cell. Biol.* 10: 1116–1125.

Perkins, AC, Sharpe, AH, and Orkin, SH. (1995). Lethal β-thalassaemia in mice lacking the erythroid CACCC-transcription factor EKLF. *Nature* 375: 318–322.

Peschle, C, Mavilio, F, Care, A et al. (1985). Hemoglobin switching in human embryos: Asynchrony of zeta-alpha and epsilon-gamma-globin switches in primitive and definite erythropoietic lineage. *Nature* 313: 235–238.

Peters, B, Merezhinskaya, N, Diffley, JFX, and Noguchi, CT. (1993). Protein-DNA interactions in the ε-globin gene silencer. *J. Biol. Chem.* 268: 3430–3437.

Poillon, W, Kim, B, Rodgers, G et al. (1993). Sparing effect of hemoglobin F and hemoglobin A2 on the polymerization of hemoglobin S at physiologic ligand saturations. *Proc. Natl. Acad. Sci. U.S.A.* 90: 5039–5043.

Pondel, M, Murphy, S, Pearson, L et al. (1995). Sp1 functions in a chromatin-dependent manner to augment human alpha-globin promoter activity. *Proc. Natl. Acad. Sci. U.S.A.* 92: 7237–7241.

Pondel, MD, George, M, and Proudfoot, NJ. (1992). The LCR-like α-globin positive regulatory element functions as an enhancer in transiently transfected cells during erythroid differentiation. *Nucl. Acids Res.* 20: 237–243.

Prioleau, MN, Nony, P, Simpson, M, and Felsenfeld, G. (1999). An insulator element and condensed chromatin region separate the chicken beta-globulin locus from an independently regulated erythroid-specific folate receptor gene. *Embo. J.* 18: 4035–4048.

Puruker, M, Bodine, D, Lin, H et al. (1990). Structure and function of the enhancer 3′ to the human Aγ-globin gene. *Nucleic Acids Res.* 18: 407–7415.

Reddy, PMS, Stamatoyannopoulos, G, Papayannopoulou, T, and Shen, CKJ. (1994). Genomic footprinting and sequencing of human β-globin locus: Tissue specificity and cell line artifact. *J. Biol. Chem.* 269: 8287–8295.

Reitman, M, Grasso, JA, Blumentahl, R, and Lewit, P. (1993). Primary sequence, evolution and repetitive elements of the *G. gallus* (chicken) β-globin cluster. *Genomics* 18: 616–626.

Reitman, M, Lee, E, and Westphal, H. (1995). Function of upstream hypersensitive sites of the chicken β-globin gene cluster in mice. *Nucl. Acids Res.* 23: 1790–1794.

Reitman, M, Lee, E, Westphal, H, and Felsenfeld, G. (1990). Site-independent expression of the chicken βA-globin gene in transgenic mice. *Nature* 348: 749–752.

Ren, S, Luo, X-N, and Atweh, G. (1993). The major regulatory element upstream of the α-globin gene has classical and inducible enhancer activity. *Blood* 81: 1058–1066.

Riggs, AF. (1991). Aspects of the origin and evolution of non-vertebrate hemoglobins. *Am. Zool.* 31: 535–545.

Riggs, AF. (1998). Self-association, cooperativity and super-cooperativity of oxygen binding by hemoglobins. *J. Experimental Biol.* 201: 1073–1084.

Rohrbaugh, ML, and Hardison, RC. (1983). Analysis of rabbit beta-like globin gene transcripts during development. *J. Mol. Biol.* 164: 395–417.

Rombel, I, Hu, K-Y, Zhang, Q et al. (1995). Transcriptional activation of human α-globin gene by hypersensitive site-40 enhancers: Function of nuclear factor-binding motifs occupied in erythroid cells. *Proc. Natl. Acad. Sci. U.S.A.* 92: 6454–6458.

Sawada, I, and Schmid, C. (1986). Primate evolution of the alpha-globin gene cluster and its Alu-like repeats. *J. Mol. Biol.* 192: 693–709.

Schirmer, T, Bode, W, Huber, R et al. (1985). X-ray crystallographic structure of the light harvesting biliprotein C-phycocyanin from the thermophilic cyanobacterium *Mastigocladus laminosus* and its resemblance to globin structures. *J. Mol. Biol.* 184: 257–277.

Shehee, R, Loeb, DD, Adey, NB et al. (1989). Nucleotide sequence of the BALB/c mouse β-globin complex. *J. Mol. Biol.* 205: 41–62.

Shen, S-H, Slightom, JL, and Smithies, O. (1981). A history of the human fetal globin gene duplication. *Cell* 26: 191–203.

Sherman, DR, Kloek, AP, Krishnan, BR et al. (1992). *Ascaris* hemoglobin gene: Plant-like structure reflects the ancestral globin gene. *Proc. Natl. Acad. Sci. U.S.A.* 89: 11696–11700.

Shewchuk, BM and Hardison, RC. (1997). CpG islands from the α-globin gene cluster increase gene expression in an integration-dependent manner. *Mol. Cell. Biol.* 17: 5856–5866.

Slightom, J, Bock J, Tagle, D et al. (1997). The complete sequences of the galago and rabbit β-globin locus control regions: Extended sequence and functional conservation outside the cores of DNase hypersensitive sites. *Genomics* 39: 90–94.

Slightom, J, Koop, B, Xu, P, and Goodman, M. (1988). Rhesus fetal globin genes: Concerted gene evolution in the descent of higher primates. *J. Biol. Chem.* 263: 12427–12438.

Slightom, J, Theisen, TW, Koop, B, and Goodman, M. (1987). Orangutan fetal globin genes: Nucleotide sequences reveal multiple gene conversions during hominid phylogeny. *J. Biol. Chem.* 262: 7472–7483.

Smith, ZE and Higgs, DR. (1999). The pattern of replication at a human telomeric region (16p13.3); its relationship to chromosome structure and gene expression. *Hum. Mol. Gen.* 8: 1373–1386.

Spritz, R, DeRiel, J, Forget, B, and Weissman, S. (1980). Complete nucleotide sequence of the human δ-globin gene. *Cell* 21: 639–646.

Spritz, R and Giebel, L. (1988). The structure and evolution of the spider monkey delta-globin gene. *Mol. Biol. Evol.* 5: 21–29.

Stamler, JS, Jia, L, Eu, JP et al. (1997). Blood flow regulation by S-nitrosohemoglobin in the physiological oxygen gradient. *Science* 276: 2034–2037.

Stoltzfus, A, Spencer, DF, Zuker, M et al. (1994). Testing the exon theory of genes: The evidence from protein structure. *Science* 265: 202–207.

Strauss, EC, Andrews, NC, Higgs, DR, Orkin, SH. (1992). In vivo footprinting of the human α-globin locus upstream regulatory element by guanine and adenine ligation-mediated polymerase chain reaction. *Mol. Cell. Biol.* 12: 2135–2142.

Stuve, LL and Myers, RM. (1990). A directly repeated sequence in the β-globin promoter regulates transcription in murine erythroleukemia cells. *Mol. Cell. Biol.* 10: 972–981.

Tagle, D, Slightom, J, Jones, R, and Goodman, M. (1991). Concerted evolution led to high expression of a prosimian primate delta globin gene locus. *J. Biol. Chem.* 266: 7469–7480.

Tagle, D, Stanhope, MJ, Siemieniak, DR et al. (1992). The β-globin gene cluster of the prosimian primate *Galago crassicaudatus*: Nucleotide sequence determination of the 41-kb cluster and comparative sequence analysis. *Genomics* 13: 741–760.

Tagle, DA, Koop, BF, Goodman, M et al. (1988). Embryonic ε and γ globin genes of a prosimian primate *(Galago crassicaudatus)*: Nucleotide and amino acid sequences, developmental regulation and phylogenetic footprints. *J. Mol. Biol.* 203: 7469–7480.

Talbot, D, Philipsen, S, Fraser, P, and Grosveld, F. (1990). Detailed analysis of the site 3 region of the human β-globin dominant control region. *EMBO J.* 9: 2169–2178.

Tan, H and Whitney, JI. (1993). Genomic rearrangement of the alpha-globin gene complex during mammalian evolution. *Biochem. Genet.* 31: 473–484.

Tang, DC, Ebb, D, Hardison, RC, and Rodgers, GP. (1997). Restoration of the CCAAT box and insertion of the CACCC motif activate δ-globin gene expression. *Blood* 90: 421–427.

Tarricone, C, Galizzi, A, Coda, A et al. (1997). Unusual structure of the oxygen-binding site in the dimeric bacterial hemoglobin from *Vitreoscilla* sp. *Structure* 5: 497–507.

Tatusov, R, Koonin, E, Lipman, D. (1997). A genomic perspective on protein families. *Science* 278: 631–637.

Terwilliger, NB. (1998). Functional adaptations of oxygen-transport proteins. *J. Exp. Biol.* 201: 1085–1098.

TomHon, C, Zhu, W, Millinoff, D et al. (1997). Evolution of a fetal expression pattern via cis-changes near the γ-globin gene. *J. Biol. Chem.* 272: 14062–14066.

Townes, TM, Fitzgerald, MC, and Lingrel, JB. (1984). Triplication of a four-gene set during evolution of the goat β-globin locus produced three gene now expressed differentially during development. *Proc. Natl. Acad. Sci. U.S.A.* 81: 6589–6593.

Trudel, M and F. Costantini. (1987). A 3′ enhancer contributes to the stage-specific expression of the human β-globin gene. *Genes & Devel.* 1: 954–961.

Tuan, D, Solomon, W, Li, Q, and London, IM. (1985). The β-like globin gene domain in human erythroid cells. *Proc. Natl. Acad. Sci. U.S.A.* 82: 6384–6388.

van der Ploeg, LHT and Flavell, RA. (1980). DNA methylation in the human γ-δ-β globin locus in erythroid and non-erythroid tissues. *Cell* 19: 947–958.

Wall, L, deBoer, E, Grosveld, F. (1988). The human β-globin gene 3′ enhancer contains multiple binding sites for an erythroid-specific protein. *Genes Dev.* 2: 1089–1100.

Weintraub, H and Groudine, M. (1976). Chromosomal subunits in active genes have an altered conformation. *Science* 193: 848–856.

Wernke, SM and Lingrel, JB. (1986). Nucleotide sequences of the goat embryonic α globin gene (ζ) and evolutionary analysis of the complete α globin cluster. *J. Mol. Biol.* 192: 457–471.

Wittenberg, BA and Wittenberg, JB. (1987). Myoglobin-mediated oxygen delivery to mitochondria of isolated cardiac myocytes. *Proc. Natl. Acad. Sci. U.S.A.* 84: 7503–7507.

Xu, J and Hardison, RC. (1991). Localization of the α-like globin gene cluster to region q12 of rabbit chromosome 6 by *in situ* hybridization. *Genomics* 9: 362–365.

Yamauchi, K, Tada, H, and Usuki, I. (1995). Structure and evolution of *Paramecium* hemoglobin genes. *Biochim. Biophys. Acta* 1264: 53–62.

Yost, SE, Shewchuk, B, and Hardison, R. (1993). Nuclear protein binding sites in a transcriptional control region of the rabbit α-globin gene. *Mol. Cell. Biol.* 13: 5439–5449.

Yu, CY, Motamed, K, Chen, J et al. (1991). The CACC box upstream of human embryonic ε globin gene binds Sp1 and is a functional promoter element in vitro and in vivo. *J. Biol. Chem.* 266: 8907–8915.

Zhu, H and Riggs, AF. (1992). Yeast flavohemoglobin is an ancient protein related to globins and a reductase family. *Proc. Natl. Acad. Sci. U.S.A.* 89: 5015–5019.

6

Molecular Genetics of the Human Globin Genes

BERNARD G. FORGET

NUMBER AND CHROMOSOMAL LOCALIZATION OF HUMAN GLOBIN GENES

Before precise knowledge of globin gene organization by gene mapping and gene cloning procedures was gained, a general picture of the number and arrangement of the normal human globin genes emerged from the genetic analysis of normal and abnormal hemoglobins and their pattern of inheritance. The number and subunit composition of different normal human hemoglobins (Fig. 6.1) suggested that at least one different globin gene must be present for each of the different globin chains: α, β, γ, δ, ε, and ζ. Evidence then accumulated, from the study of hemoglobin variants and the analysis of the biochemical heterogeneity of the chains in fetal hemoglobin (HbF), that the α- and γ-globin genes were duplicated. Persons were identified whose red cells contained more than two structurally different α-globin chains that could be best explained by duplication of the α-globin gene locus, and the characterization of the structurally different $^G\gamma$ and $^A\gamma$ globin chains of HbF imposed a requirement for duplication of the γ-globin gene locus.

From the study of the pattern of inheritance of hemoglobin variants from persons carrying both an α chain and a β chain variant, the α- and β-globin genes must clearly be on different chromosomes or widely separated if on the same chromosome. α- and β-chain hemoglobin variants were always observed to segregate independently in offspring of doubly affected parents (reviewed in Weatherall and Clegg, 1981). Linkage of the various β-like globin genes to one another was established from the study of interesting hemoglobin variants that contained fused globin chains, presumably resulting from nonhomologous crossover between different β-like globin gene loci. Characterization of Hb Lepore (Baglioni, 1962), with its δβ fusion chain, established that the δ-globin gene was linked to and located on the 5′ (or N-terminal) side of the β-globin gene. Analysis of Hb Kenya (Kendall et al., 1973), with its $^A\gamma\beta$ fusion chain, provided evidence for linkage of the $^A\gamma$ gene, and presumably the $^G\gamma$ gene as well, to the 5′-side of the δ- and β-globin genes.

Thus, the general concept of the arrangement of the globin genes that emerged from these various genetic analyses can be represented as illustrated in Figure 6.1. It was also assumed, but unsupported by genetic evidence, that the embryonic α-like (ζ) and β-like (ε) globin genes were likely to be linked to the loci for their adult counterparts.

By using rodent-human somatic hybrid cells containing only one or a few human chromosomes, Deisseroth and colleagues (1977 and 1978) clearly established that the human α- and β-globin genes resided on different chromosomes and that the α genes were on chromosome 16, whereas the β-like genes were found on chromosome 11. The latter results were obtained by solution hybridization assays of total cellular DNA from the various somatic hybrid cells hybridized to radioactive cDNAs synthesized from α- and β-globin mRNAs by use of the enzyme reverse transcriptase.

These results were later confirmed and extended by various groups using the gene mapping procedure of Southern blot analysis with DNA from various hybrid cell lines containing different translocations or deletions of the involved chromosomes.

These studies led to the regional localization of the globin gene loci on their respective chromosomes: the β-globin gene cluster to the short arm of chromosome 11, and the α-globin gene cluster to the short arm of chromosome 16. These chromosomal assignments were further confirmed and refined by in situ hybridization of radioactive cloned globin gene probes to metaphase chromosomes and by fluorescence-based in situ hybridization (FISH). Thus, the β-globin gene cluster was assigned to 11p 15.5 and the α-globin gene cluster to 16p 13.3.

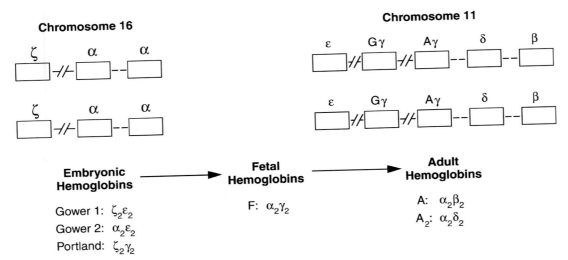

Figure 6.1. Model of the human globin gene system based on genetic information available before the actual cloning of the genes. The various hemoglobins expressed at different stages of development are indicated below the model. (From Forget, BG. [1995]. Hemoglobin synthesis and the thalassemias. In Handin, RI, Lux, SE, and Stossel, TP, editors. *Blood: Principles and practice of hematology.* Philadelphia: JB Lippincott.)

Detailed Chromosomal Organization of the Human Globin Genes

A precise picture of the chromosomal organization of the α- and β-like human globin gene clusters, with respect to the number of structural loci and intergene distances, was obtained by a number of different techniques: (1) restriction endonuclease mapping of genomic DNA using the gel blotting procedure of Southern and, (2) gene isolation by recombinant DNA technology. Sets of overlapping genomic DNA fragments spanning the entire α- and β-globin gene clusters were obtained by gene cloning, initially in bacteriophage λ and larger fragments in cosmid vectors. Detailed analysis of these recombinant DNA clones led to the determination of the gene organization illustrated in Figure 6.2. Some results were expected, such as the finding of single δ- and β-globin gene loci and duplication of the α- and γ-globin gene loci. In addition, single loci for the embryonic ζ and ε

globin chains were found linked to the α- and β-globin gene clusters, respectively.

An unexpected finding was the presence in the globin gene clusters of additional genelike structures with structural homology to the authentic globin genes: one in the β-gene cluster, between the γ- and δ-globin genes, and three in the α-gene cluster, between the ζ- and authentic α-globin genes. These structures have been called pseudogenes. They are characterized by the presence of one or more mutations that render them incapable of encoding a functional globin chain. These pseudogenes appear to have arisen by gene duplication events within the globin gene clusters followed by mutation and inactivation of the duplicated gene and subsequent accumulation of additional mutations through loss of selective pressure.

Figure 6.2. Structure of the human α- and β-globin gene loci based on information obtained by gene cloning and DNA sequence analysis. The vertical arrows indicate the positions of developmentally stable, erythroid-specific DNase I-hypersensitive sites located in the locus control region (LCR) of the β-gene cluster and HS-40 of the α-gene cluster. The fine structure of the genes (exon-intron organization) is shown in Figure 6.3. (From Forget, BG. [1995]. Hemoglobin synthesis and the thalassemias. In Handin, RI, Lux, SE, and Stossel, TP, editors. *Blood: Principles and practice of hematology.* Philadelphia: JB Lippincott.)

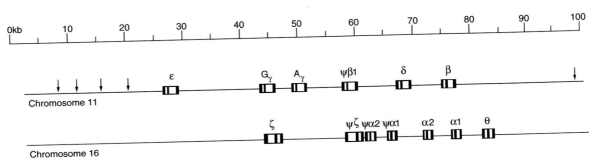

Another α-like globin gene has been identified and characterized in the α-globin gene cluster: the θ gene located to the 3′ or C-terminal side of the duplicated α-globin genes (Hsu et al., 1988). This gene is evolutionally related to and expressed with the α-globin genes (Ley et al., 1989; Albitar et al., 1989). mRNA transcripts are present only at very low levels (less than 1% of α), and no hemoglobin containing the θ-globin chains has been identified. Furthermore, the predicted structure (translated amino acid sequence) of the θ-globin chain suggests that functioning normally as a hemoglobin subunit is unlikely (Clegg, 1987).

GLOBIN GENE STRUCTURE

Intervening Sequences or Introns

The coding region of the globin genes of humans and other animals is interrupted at two positions by considerable stretches of noncoding DNA called intervening sequences or introns. In the β-like globin genes, the intervening sequences interrupt the sequence between codons 30 and 31 and between codons 104 and 105; in the α-globin gene family, the intervening sequences interrupt the coding sequence between codons 31 and 32 and between codons 99 and 100 (Fig. 6.3). Although the precise codon position numbers at which the interruption occurs differ between the α- and β-like globin genes, the introns occur at precisely the same position relative to the regions of the primary structure of the α- and β-globin chains that are homologous and can be aligned if one assumes that the α- and β-globin gene families originally evolved from a single ancestral globin gene (Chapter 5). The first intervening sequence (IVS-1) is shorter than the second interven-

ing sequence (IVS-2) in both α- and β-globin genes, but IVS-2 of the human β-globin gene is much larger than that of the α-globin gene.

The pattern of intron sizes of the ζ-like globin genes differs from that of the other α-like globin genes. Whereas the introns in the α and ψα genes are small (fewer than 150 base pairs [bp]), those of the ζ and ψζ genes are larger. Furthermore, IVS-1 is much larger than IVS-2—eight to ten times larger than the IVS-1 of any other globin gene (Fig. 6.2).

The presence of intervening sequences that interrupt the coding sequences of structural genes imposes a requirement for some cellular process to remove these sequences in the mature mRNA. Intervening sequences are transcribed into globin (and other) precursor mRNA molecules, but they are subsequently excised and the proper ends of the coding sequences relegated to yield the mature mRNA. This posttranscriptional processing of mRNA precursors has been termed *splicing* and is illustrated schematically in Figure 6.4A.

A crucial prerequisite for the proper splicing of globin (and other) precursor mRNA molecules is the presence of specific nucleotide sequences at the junctions between coding sequences (exons) and intervening sequences (introns). Comparison of these sequences in many different genes has permitted the derivation of two different

Figure 6.3. Fine structure of the human α- and β-globin genes. The black blocks represent the coding regions of the gene; the cross-hatched blocks at either end represent the 5′ and 3′ untranslated sequences; the open blocks represent the intervening sequences (introns) IVS-1 and IVS-2, which interrupt the coding sequences of the genes. The numbers above the diagram indicate the amino acid codon positions of the coding sequence. (From Bunn, HF and Forget, BG. [1986]. *Hemoglobin: molecular, genetic and clinical aspects*. Philadelphia: WB Saunders.)

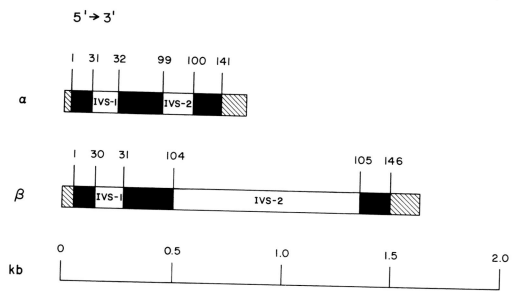

A

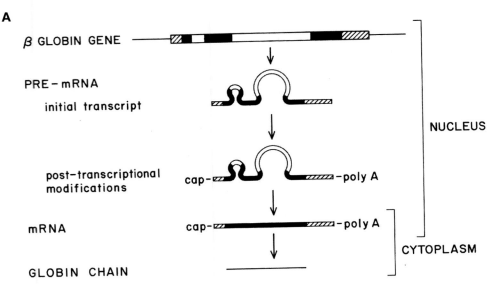

Figure 6.4A. Schematic representation of the process of β-globin gene expression. Overall process, including gene transcription, posttranscriptional processing of the mRNA, transport of mRNA from nucleus to cytoplasm, and mRNA translation. (From Bunn, HF and Forget, BG. [1986]. *Hemoglobin: molecular, genetic and clinical aspects.* Philadelphia: WB Saunders.)

Figure 6.4B. Steps involved in excision of an intron.

B

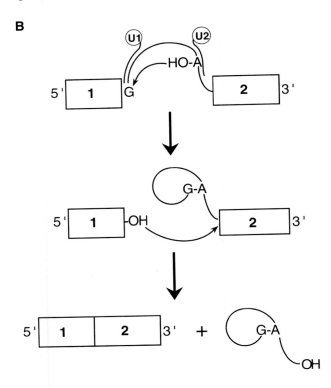

"consensus" sequences, which are universally found at the 5′ (donor) and 3′ (acceptor) ends, respectively, of introns (Mount, 1982; Padgett et al., 1986). The consensus sequences thus derived are the following:

$$(5') \ (C/A) \ AG \, ^- \, GT \ (A/G) \ AGT$$
$$----- \ (T/C)_n \ N \ (C/T) \ AG \, ^- \, G(3'),$$

where "N" represents any nucleotide and "n" a variable number of primidine nucleotides, equal to or greater than 11. The vertical arrows show the splice site junctions within the consensus sequences where cleavage or splicing actually occurs. The 5′-sequence is sometimes called the donor splice site and the 3′-sequence, the acceptor splice site. The underlined dinucleotides GT and AG, at the 5′ and 3′ ends, respectively, of the intron, are essentially invariant and are thought to be absolutely required for proper splicing: the so-called GT-AG rule. Rare examples have been described in which GC instead of GT is found at the donor splice site junction. The importance or significance of these consensus sequences is underscored by the fact that mutations that alter these normal consensus sequences, or mutations that create similar consensus sequences at new sites in a globin gene, lead to abnormal processing of globin mRNA precursors and constitute the molecular basis for many types of thalassemia (Chapters 12 and 17).

The mechanism by which introns are excised from pre-mRNAs involves a cellular organelle called the spliceosome (Madhani and Guthrie, 1994; Nilsen, 1994; Staley and Guthrie, 1998). The spliceosome is a large macromolecular complex consisting of five RNA species (called small nuclear RNAs or snRNAs: U1, U2, U4, U5, and U6) and many different proteins. In the presplicing complex, U1 RNA binds to the 5′ end of the intronic sequence, whereas U2 RNA binds to a sequence called the branch site near the 3' end of the intronic sequence. The excision is a two-step ATP-independent process involving two trans-esterification reactions. Because of the first reaction, the 5' end of the intronic sequence forms a covalent bond with the region of the intron called the branch site, found approximately 18 to 37 nucleotides from the 3' end of the intron, forming a lariat-like or branched RNA structure (Fig. 6.4B). This bond involves the G of the GU dinucleotide of the 5' donor site and the A residue in the branch site recognition sequence ACT(TT/CC) or ATC(TT/CC). Following the second transesterification reaction, the lariat is released and the two adjacent exons joined (Fig. 6.4B).

Conserved Functional Sequences of Mature Globin mRNAs

Transcripts of the human globin genes represented in mature globin mRNA contain sequences at both extremities of the mRNA, beyond the information required to encode the globin polypeptide chains. These additional untranslated nucleotides account for about 30 percent of the total length of globin mRNA. The 3' (C-terminal) untranslated sequences are two to three times the length of the 5' (N-terminal) untranslated sequences. The lengths of these sequences in the major human globin mRNAs are illustrated in Figure 6.5. Besides the nucleotides transcribed from the globin gene, the globin mRNA contains additional nucleotides added to it within the cell nucleus after transcription: a methylated guanylic acid (m^7G) cap structure at the 5'-end of the mRNA, and many adenylic acid residues forming a poly(A) tail at the 3'-end of the mRNA. How these untranslated sequences function in globin and other

mRNAs is not completely known. The 5'-methylated cap structure seems important for the initiation of polypeptide chain synthesis through its interaction with specific initiation factors. The poly(A) tail of mRNAs appears to contribute to the stability of the mRNA.

Two general consensus sequences are at or near the extremities of these untranslated sequences and are important for the efficient processing of mRNA transcripts. The cap site in globin (and most eukaryotic) mRNAs is usually at an A residue preceded in genomic DNA by a C. The DNA sequence to either side of the CA is generally rich in pyrimidines. The cap site consensus sequence seems important not only for accurate initiation of transcription and 5' processing of the mRNA, but also for serving as a promoter element, called the initiator or Inr element (Smale and Baltimore, 1989), which can influence both the efficiency and accuracy of transcription initiation. This is especially true for certain genes that lack a TATA box in their promoters (see the next section). At least one β thalassemia mutation involves a base substitution in the cap site consensus sequence.

The one common feature of the 3'-noncoding sequence of globin and other mRNAs is the presence of the hexanucleotide AAUAAA (AATAA in the DNA) about 20 nucleotides upstream of the poly(A) tail (reviewed in Wickens, 1990; Wahle and Keller, 1996; Proudfoot, 1996). It was initially assumed, and subsequently shown experimentally, that this consensus sequence forms a necessary signal for the proper processing and polyadenylation of the 3'-end of mRNA transcripts. Base substitutions in this consensus sequence have also been responsible for certain types of thalassemia because of faulty processing and polyadenylation of globin mRNA transcripts. It appears that the AAUAAA is a signal, not only for poly(A) addition, but also—perhaps more importantly—for the proper cleavage, before polyadenylation, of the primary RNA transcripts of globin (and other) genes that normally extend well beyond the site

Figure 6.5. Relative sizes of translated and untranslated regions of the major human globin messenger RNAs. (From Forget, BG. [1979]. Molecular genetics of human hemoglobin synthesis. *Ann. Intern. Med.* 91:605–616).

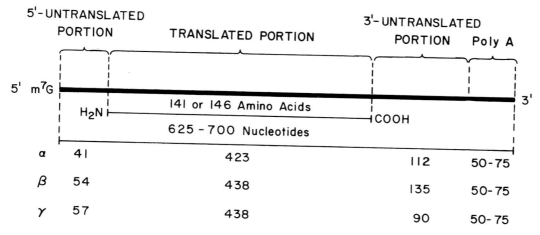

of polyadenylation. The nucleotide immediately preceding the site of poly(A) addition in globin and other mRNAs is usually C and GC is the most common, although not invariant, dinucleotide at this site.

Translation of globin (and other eukaryotic) mRNAs starts at the initiator codon ATG, which is generally the first ATG encountered in any reading frame of the mature mRNA. The initiator ATG, like ATG codons elsewhere in the mRNA, encodes the amino acid methionine, which is present at the N-terminus of all nascent polypeptide chains. During the process of peptide chain elongation, the N-terminal methionine is cleaved from nascent globin chains and is thus absent from the full-length chains. The nature of the first two amino acids encoded immediately after the initiator methionine is important in determining whether the N-terminal methionine is cleaved from a nascent peptide chain. Generally, if the second amino acid is also a methionine or is a charged residue, or if the third amino acid is a proline, the N-terminal methionine is retained (Boissel et al., 1985). Some human β-globin chain variants in which such amino acid replacements have occurred at codon positions 2 or 3 have retained the initiator methionine at the N-terminus of the full-length mutant globin chain (Chapter 45).

Surrounding the initiator ATG are sequences important for the efficiency of peptide chain initiation. Comparison of the nucleotide sequence of many eukaryotic mRNAs has revealed the presence of a conserved consensus sequence flanking the initiator ATG, the so-called Kozak consensus sequence: CC(A/G)CCATGG (Kozak, 1989). Its most important features are the presence of a purine (A or G) at position −3, then the presence of a G at position +4 (where position +1 is the A of the initiator ATG). The consensus sequence presumably facilitates efficient binding of the mRNA to ribosomes. One form of α thalassemia is due to a base substitution changing the purine to a pyrimidine at position −3 of the consensus sequence. Other α and β thalassemia mutations are due to base substitutions in the ATG itself, resulting in a complete block to normal globin chain initiation (Chapters 12 and 17).

Termination of globin chain synthesis occurs when one of the three possible chain termination codons (UAA, UAG, or UGA) is encountered in the mRNA sequence. Point mutations in the termination codon result in the insertion of a novel amino acid residue at that position and translation of the normally untranslated 3′ portion of the mRNA into an abnormally elongated peptide chain until a new in-phase termination codon is encountered. Several different termination codon mutations are the cause of hemoglobin variants associated with α thalassemia (Chapter 17).

The synthesis of normal globin chains requires that the triplet codons of the mRNA encoding each amino

acid of the peptide chain be arrayed in the proper uninterrupted alignment. Nucleotide insertions or deletions other than those in multiples of three will lead to a shift in the reading frame (frameshift) of mRNA translation and the synthesis of a novel peptide sequence until a new in-phase termination codon is encountered, which usually occurs within a short distance. The mutant globin chain thus encoded usually accumulates in markedly reduced amounts, because either the mutant globin chain itself or its mRNA is unstable, resulting in a thalassemia phenotype. Many different forms of α and β thalassemia are the result of frameshift mutations. Point mutations (nonsense mutations) can also change a normal amino acid codon to a chain termination codon, resulting in the synthesis of truncated, unstable globin chain and a thalassemia phenotype. A number of nonsense mutations have also been documented as causes of α and β thalassemia (Chapters 12 and 17).

Conserved Sequences in 5′-Flanking DNA of Globin Genes

The DNA flanking the 5′-extremity of the globin genes contains several sequences that are common to all these genes and are situated at similar distances from the site of initiation of transcription of the genes (cap site) (Fig. 6.6). The first preserved sequence is ATAA, situated approximately 30 nucleotides from the cap site. A second preserved sequence is CCAAT,

Figure 6.6. Model of the structure of a typical globin gene showing specific sequences and *cis*-acting elements that are important for the regulation of gene expression. The same conventions are used as in Figure 6.3. The following elements and consensus sequences are shown: LCR, locus control region; consensus sequences of the promoter, CACCC, CCAAT, ATA; cap site, CA; initiator codon, ATG; consensus dinucleotide at exon-intron junctions, 5′ GT ... AG 3′; termination codons TGA, TAA or TAG; polyadenylation signal, AATAAA; and enhancer element, E. The bottom line shows the consensus binding sequences, for the erythroid-specific factor GATA-1, found within the LCR, promoter, and enhancer. (From Forget, BG. [1995]. Hemoglobin synthesis and the thalassemias. In Handin, RI, Lux, SE, and Stossel, TP, editors. *Blood: Principles and practice of hematology.* Philadelphia: JB Lippincott.)

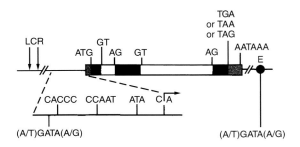

situated approximately 70 to 80 nucleotides from the cap site. In both γ-globin genes, the CCAAT sequence is duplicated. With the human δ-globin gene, three CCAAT-like sequences are found, but neither has the perfect canonical sequence; the closest is CCAAC. A third preserved 5'-flanking sequence is more variable in location and is found 80 to 140 nucleotides from the cap site. It has the general structure CACCC or the inverted form GGGTG and is duplicated in the 5'-flanking DNA of the β gene. For the δ-globin gene, the proximal CACCC sequence is missing. The abnormalities of CCAAT and CACCC sequences of the δ-globin gene are thought to be responsible in great part for its normally low level of transcription: correction by site-directed mutagenesis of the CCAAT sequence and insertion of a β-like CACCC sequence into the promoter confer a high level of expression to the δ gene (Donze et al., 1996; Tang et al., 1997). The detailed topography of the various conserved sequences in the promoters of the different human globin gene promoters is shown in Figure 5.8 (see Chapter 5).

Site-directed mutagenesis or deletion of these preserved sequences, followed by testing the modified genes in various expression systems, including transgenic mice, has shown the importance of these sequences for the efficiency and accuracy of gene transcription. Their importance for normal globin gene expression is also underscored by the fact that decreased expression of the β-globin genes in certain forms of β thalassemia is due to base substitutions in these sequences, specifically in and around the ATA box and the proximal and distal CACCC box of the β-globin gene (Chapter 12). These various promoter sequences are common to many other nonglobin eukaryotic genes and form binding sites for the general transcription apparatus of the cell: RNA polymerase II (Lewin, 1990; Kadonaga, 1998) and other associated transcription factors that are ubiquitously expressed (Mitchell and Tjian, 1989).

The 5' flanking DNA of many, but not all, globin genes also contains one or more copies of a consensus sequence having the motif (A/T)GATA(A/G), which is the binding site of a hematopoietic-specific transcription factor called GATA-1 (Martin et al., 1989; Tsai et al., 1989) (reviewed by Engel et al., 1991; Orkin 1992, 1995a, 1995b; Weiss and Orkin 1995a). GATA-1 sites are also present in globin gene enhancers and locus control regions (LCRs) (see next section). The importance of GATA-1 for gene expression in erythroid cells is underscored by the fact that chimeric mice that developed from male embryonic stem (ES) cells with a disruption of their single X-linked GATA-1 gene failed to produce erythroid cells of the ES cell lineage (Pevny et al., 1991). Normal definitive erythropoiesis was totally absent in hemizygous mice derived from these mutated ES cells, thus resulting in an embryonic lethal pheno-

type (Fujiwara et al., 1996). Using in vitro tissue culture systems for hematopoietic differentiation of ES cells, and/or of yolk sac progenitors of GATA-1⁻ embryos, it has been shown that GATA-1⁻ ES cells or erythroid progenitor cells can differentiate to the proerythroblast stage of erythroid cell maturation (Simon et al., 1992; Pevny et al., 1991; Weiss et al., 1994), but the cells then fail to differentiate terminally and they undergo apoptosis (Weiss and Orkin, 1995b). The ability of the mutant ES cell line to undergo normal erythroid differentiation in vitro was restored after transfer of a functional GATA-1 gene to the cells (Simon et al., 1992; Blobel et al., 1995; Weiss et al. 1997).

Using various mutants of GATA-1 to rescue erythroid differentiation of GATA-1 ES⁻ cells, it was subsequently shown that the N-terminal (non-DNA binding) zinc finger of GATA-1 was essential for the effect, suggesting that it might be the binding site for a second trans-acting factor essential for erythroid differentiation. This factor was subsequently isolated and named Friend of GATA-1, or FOG (Tsang et al., 1997). Homozygous disruption of the FOG gene leads to an embryonic lethal phenotype similar to that of the GATA-1 gene disruption, with severe anemia, partial block of terminal erythroid differentiation, and failure of megakaryocytopoiesis (Tsang et al., 1998; see also Chapter 4). Evidence exists that GATA-1 forms several different multimeric protein complexes with other transcription factors: with CBP/p300 (Blobel et al., 1998); with EKLF and Sp1 (Merika and Orkin, 1995; Gregory et al., 1996); and a pentameric complex with SCL/tal1, Rbtn2/Lmo2, the LIM-binding protein Ldb-1/NL1 and helix-loop-helix (HLH) proteins such as the E2A proteins, E12 and E47 (Wadman et al., 1997) (Chapter 4). The pentameric complex binds to a DNA element consisting of one or two GATA sites flanking an E box motif, the general consensus site for basic HLH proteins (Wadman et al., 1997; Anderson, et al., 1998).

In the γ-globin gene promoters, two GATA-1 binding sites flank the octameric consensus sequence ATTTGCAT for a ubiquitous octamer binding transcription factor (OCT-1), which is related to the lymphoid-specific octamer binding transcription factor (OCT-2) involved in immunoglobulin gene regulation (Mitchell and Tjian, 1989). A base substitution involving one of the GATA-1 consensus sequences of the γ-globin gene promoter is associated with a form of nondeletion hereditary persistence of fetal hemoglobin (HPFH) (Chapter 15).

Orkin and co-workers have also characterized a hematopoietic-specific trans-acting factor, called NF-E2, that binds to the LCR of the β-globin gene cluster and a related sequence in the cluster called HS-40 (see next section) (Andrews et al., 1993a). The NF-E2 binding site of the DNase I hypersensitive site 2 (HS2) of the β-globin gene-like cluster LCR is important for the functional ability of the LCR to enhance globin gene expression (Ney et al., 1990a, 1990b; Talbot and Grosveld, 1991). The promoter of the gene encoding the heme synthetic enzyme porphobilinogen deaminase also contains a consensus binding site for NF-E2 (Mignotte et al., 1989). NF-E2 is a heterodimer consisting of an erythroid/megakaryocytic-specific subunit of 45 kDa (p45) and a ubiquitously expressed subunit of 18 kDa (p18) (Andrews et al., 1993b), both of which are members of the basic region-leucine zipper (bZip) family of transcription factors. The ubiquitously expressed p18 subunit is a member of the Maf family of transcription factors and the binding site for the complex is referred to as a MARE (maf-recognition element), which is used by proteins related to AP1. Disruption of the p45 gene in mice results in a major defect of megakaryocytopoiesis, but only a minor defect in erythropoiesis, resulting in a mild hypochromic anemia (Shivdasani and Orkin, 1995). One possible explanation for the lack of a more dramatic effect of p45 deficiency on globin gene expression is the finding of other genes encoding p45-related proteins such as LCRF1/Nrf1, Nrf2/ECH, Bach 1, and Bach 2. These may compensate for the absence of p45 NF-E2 gene expression (Chan et al., 1993; Caterina et al., 1994; Moi et al., 1994; Chui et al., 1995; Oyake et al., 1996; Itoh et al., 1995).

In the extended proximal CACCC sequence of the β-globin gene promoter is a binding site for yet another erythroid-specific transcription factor called EKLF (erythroid Krüppel-like factor) (Miller and Bieker, 1993). This transcription factor is a member of the large family of zinc finger transcription factors that includes the ubiquitous factor Sp1 (Mitchell and Tjian, 1989) that can bind CACCC motifs besides its more usual G + C rich consensus sequence. EKLF binds preferentially to the β-globin gene promoter compared to its binding activity to other globin gene promoters, and β-thalassemic point mutations of the proximal CACCC/EKLF binding sequence result in markedly decreased binding of EKLF in gel mobility shift assays (Feng et al., 1994). Disruption of the EKLF gene in mice results in a β-thalassemic phenotype (Nuez et al., 1995; Perkins, et al., 1995), but does not cause a generalized defect in erythropoiesis, as does disruption of the GATA-1 gene. Thus, EKLF may be a quasi β-globin gene-specific transcription factor, and it has been called by some a *hemoglobin switching factor* (Donze et al., 1995). However, although EKLF is necessary for full activity of the β-globin gene, it is not sufficient to cause the γ- to β-globin gene switch, because it is present and fully functional in embryonic erythroid tissues before switching occurs (Guy et al., 1998). Therefore, the γ- to β-globin gene switch is regulated by mechanisms other than differential expression or

function of EKLF during development. More recently, Asano et al. (1999) have identified another EKLF-like factor, called FKLF (fetal Krüppel-like factor), which is preferentially expressed in fetal erythroid cells and appears to selectively activate the transcription of embryonic and fetal β-like globin genes.

Additional transcription factors have been identified that appear to have preferential activity on the expression of one or another globin gene. These include the stage-specific selector protein (SSP) complex that binds a G + C rich region in the −50 region of the γ-globin gene promoter (Jane et al., 1995; Zhou et al., 1999) and is analogous to a similar factor, called NF-E4, that is involved in embryonic to definitive globin gene switching in the chicken (Gallarda et al., 1989) (see Chapter 7); and a multimeric protein complex called the PYR complex, which contains proteins of the SWI/SNF family of chromatin-modifying factors. These latter factors bind to a polypyrimidine region 5′ to the δ-globin gene and appear to influence the timing of human γ- to β-globin gene switching in a transgenic mouse model (O'Neill et al., 1999).

Enhancers and Other *cis*-Acting Sequences That Influence Globin Gene Expression

Enhancer elements are *cis*-acting DNA sequences close to a gene that confer to the gene a high level of expression, frequently in a tissue-specific or developmentally specific manner. Originally described in viral genomes, enhancer elements were subsequently discovered in many chromosomal genes, either in 5′ or 3′ flanking DNA or in introns (Khoury and Gruss 1993). Typically, enhancers are functional in a position- and orientation-independent fashion when tested in various gene transfer-expression systems. How enhancers act is not completely understood. Enhancers are known to bind various ubiquitous and tissue-specific *trans*-acting protein factors with resulting alterations in the configuration of the local chromatin such as the creation of sites that are hypersensitive to various nucleases such as DNase I (Svaren and Chalkley, 1990). Such perturbations in the structure or configuration of chromatin are probably associated with activation of transcription of the adjacent gene through various protein-protein interactions (Lewin, 1990; Ptashne and Gann, 1990).

A well-defined, tissue-specific, and developmental stage-specific enhancer element has been identified and characterized in the 3′ flanking DNA of the β-globin gene in humans and in other animal species, particularly the chicken (Kollias et al., 1987; Trudel et al., 1987; Behringer et al., 1987; Trudel and Costantini, 1987; Antoniou et al., 1988). This element confers a high level of gene expression specifically in adult erythroid cells and contains multiple binding sites for the erythroid-specific transcription factor GATA-1 (Wall et al., 1988). A less well-defined enhancer element has also been identified in the 3′ flanking DNA of the human $^A\gamma$-globin gene (Bodine and Ley, 1987). Analogous enhancer elements have not been identified in proximity to the human α-globin genes, although an enhancer has been found in the 3′-flanking DNA of the chicken α-globin gene (Knezetic and Felsenfeld, 1989). In contrast to such positive regulatory sequences, which are found adjacent to adult and fetal globin genes, negative regulatory sequences in 5′- or 3′-flanking DNA have been shown to influence the expression of the human embryonic ε- and ζ-globin genes (Cao et al., 1989; Watt, et al., 1993; Liebhaber et al., 1996; Li, Q et al., 1998; Li, J., et al., 1998; Wang and Liebhaber, 1999). Putative negative regulatory elements have also been identified in the 5′ flanking DNA of the human β- and γ-globin genes. (Berg et al., 1989; Stamatoyannopoulos et al., 1993).

Another important group of cis-acting DNA elements is present at some distance from the globin genes that they influence, within regions of chromatin that are particularly hypersensitive to digestion by DNase I in erythroid cell nuclei. A number of major DNase I hypersensitive sites were originally identified by Tuan et al. (1985) and Forrester et al. (1986) in the human β-globin gene locus, in DNA located between 6 kb and 18 kb 5′ to the ε-globin gene. An additional site was found in the DNA approximately 20 kb 3′ to the β-globin gene. In contrast to DNase I hypersensitive sites in promoter regions of the individual globin genes, which are usually present only at developmental stages when the particular globin gene is expressed, these remote hypersensitive sites were present in erythroid cells at all developmental stages. The human β-globin gene locus contains four 5′ erythroid-specific, developmentally stable DNase I hypersensitive sites (HSs) (5′ HS 1, 2, 3 & 4). A fifth site (5′ HS5) is not erythroid-specific and is thought to act as an "insulator" element (Li and Stamatoyannopoulos, 1994). More recently, two additional HSs sites (5′ HS6 and HS7) have been identified (Bulger et al., 1999). The presence and sequences of these DNase I HSs at the 5′ end of the β gene locus are conserved in all mammalian animal species examined to date, but not in the chicken, where the 3′β enhancer sequence appears to be the evolutionarily and functionally corresponding sequence (Chapter 5).

The functional significance of the 5′ HSs of the human β locus in vivo was initially suggested by the fact that naturally occurring deletions of these sites (see section on γδβ thalassemia in Chapter 15) are associated with total silencing of any remaining downstream structurally intact β-like globin genes, and these globin genes remain in a DNase I-resistant chromatin configuration in erythroid cells (Forrester et al., 1990). The smallest deletion with this phenotype (Hispanic γδβ thalassemia) encompasses 35kb, including 5′ HS2 through HS5. The suspected functional importance of this region of DNA was then demonstrated experimentally by Grosveld et al. (1987) and subsequently by other investigators in experiments involving transfer of human globin genes into transgenic mice. When DNA containing the DNase I HSs normally located 5′ to the ε gene were linked to a human β-globin gene used to produce transgenic mice, the expression of the transferred β-globin gene was virtually equivalent, on a per copy basis, to that of the endogenous murine β-globin gene and did not vary significantly with the site of integration of the transgene (i.e., there was erythroid-tissue specific, position-independent, and copy number-dependent high level of gene expression) (Grosveld et al., 1987). Similar results were also obtained in mouse erythroleukemia (MEL) cells. Previous gene transfer-expression studies in transgenic mice and MEL cells using human β-globin genes without these HSs resulted in low levels of expression of the transferred gene. The expression level without the HSs was, on average, less than 10 percent of that of the endogenous murine β-globin gene and frequently varied depending on the site of integration of the transferred gene. Because of its functional properties, this region of DNA was initially called the locus activating region (Forrester et al., 1987) or the dominant control region (Talbot et al., 1989), but subsequently renamed the locus control region (LCR) (Orkin, 1990).

A similar region (HS-40) has also been identified in the α-globin gene cluster in the DNA located between 28 kb and 65 kb 5′ to the ζ-globin gene. This region was essential for obtaining high levels of human α-globin gene expression in transgenic mice (Higgs et al, 1990) (Chapter 17). Naturally occurring deletions involving this region of DNA were also associated with various forms of α thalassemia in which the α-globin genes themselves were structurally intact (Chapter 17). The critical region was subsequently narrowed down to a 0.35 kb segment of DNA located 40 kb upsteam of the ζ-globin gene (HS-40) (Jarman et al., 1991). The α HS-40 and β 5′ HS2 share many features in common such as conservation of many sequence motifs (see Fig. 5.7), and their ability to serve as strong enhancers of globin gene expression in transient and stable transfection assays and in transgenic mice. However, there are several differences between HS-40 and the β-cluster LCR (reviewed by Higgs et al., 1998): (1) the HS-40 consists of a single element in contrast to the multiple elements in the β-LCR complex; (2) the HS-40 does not confer a copy number-dependent level of expression to transgenes; (3) the level of expression of HS-40/α globin transgenes is not equivalent to that of the endogenous murine genes; (4) deletion of HS-40 does not affect long-range chromatin structure in the α-globin gene cluster; and (5) deletion of HS-40 does not affect the timing of replication of the α-gene cluster during the cell cycle.

The conserved sequence motifs in αHS-40, β5′ HS2 and the other β5′ HSs consist of consensus sequences and functional in vitro binding sites in gel mobility shift assays for ubiquitous and hematopoietic-specific transcription factors, such as GATA-1, EKLF (and other CACCC binding proteins), Sp1, AP-1, and NF-E2 (Moi and Kan, 1990; Philipsen et al., 1990; Ikuta and Kan, 1991; Strauss and Orkin, 1992) (see also Fig. 5.7 and Chapter 5). These factor binding sites have been shown by in vivo footprinting experiments to be protected or "occupied" in the chromatin of erythroid cell nuclei, strongly suggesting that transcription factors are bound to these sites in erythroid cells *in vivo* (Strauss et al., 1992; Reddy et al., 1994; Zhang et al., 1993). The ubiquitous factor AP-1 and the erythroid-specific factor NF-E2 share a very similar DNA binding consensus sequence; evidence shows that competitive binding of these two factors occurs at a duplicated MARE consensus sequence in HS2 of the β cluster LCR, which is critical for the activity of the β LCR (Ney et al., 1990a; Talbot and Grosveld, 1991; Liu et al., 1992). A duplicated MARE in αHS-40 also serves as a binding site for NF-E2 (Jarman et al., 1991; Strauss et al., 1992) and is important for the function of HS-40 (Zhang et al., 1993).

Each of the βLCR HS sequences can individually influence the expression of β-like globin genes in transgenic mice. HS2 and HS3 have a particularly strong positive regulatory effect on globin gene expression. HS2 acts as a strong enhancer in transient transfection assays, and this effect is mediated by a core element that contains a duplicated MARE that serves as a binding site for NF-E2. HS3 is particularly effective in rendering surrounding chromatin DNase I sensitive or "open." Although initial experiments suggested some selectivity of different HS sites for regulatory effects on the γ- versus the β-globin gene during development (reviewed by Engel, 1993), the current consensus is that the entire LCR, with its bound *trans*-acting factors acts as a holocomplex in mediating its effects on globin gene expression (Fraser et al., 1993; Ellis et al., 1996; Wijgerde et al., 1995; Milot et al., 1996).

When transgenic mice carrying the β-LCR linked to a globin gene are generated, the DNA region containing the transgene becomes DNase I sensitive in erythroid cells, and the globin gene is expressed at high levels. Thus, the β LCR has long been considered not only to function simply as a traditional enhancer element, but also to possess chromatin-opening (or activating) properties. However, recent LCR deletion experiments using homologous recombination in an erythroid cell line and also in β LCR knockout mice in vivo have shown that the negative effect of LCR loss on globin gene expression can occur without the loss of DNase I sensitive, open chromatin in the β cluster (Reik et al., 1998; Epner et al., 1992). Thus, other regions of the β cluster, outside the LCR region, may be sufficient for maintaining an open chromatin configuration (reviewed by Higgs, 1998).

The general molecular processes or mechanisms by which the LCRs carry out their effects on globin gene expression from their remote locations are not known. The prevailing model is a "looping" mechanism, by which the LCR holocomplex, including its bound *trans*-acting protein factors, would form a loop and interact in a combinatorial manner, through protein-protein interactions, with the promoter and/or enhancer regions of the target globin genes and their bound transcription factor complexes. In this model, high levels of expression of the globin gene(s) that are in contact with the LCR holocomplex at a particular time in development are facilitated: the ε- and ζ-globin genes in yolk sac-derived erythroid cells, α- and γ-globin genes during fetal development, and the α- and β-globin genes in adult erythroid cells. Many articles have examined the implications of this looping model in the regulation of the fetal to adult hemoglobin switch (Stamatoyannopoulos, 1991; Epner et al., 1992; Dillon and Grosveld, 1993; Grosveld et al., 1993; Orkin 1990, 1995b; Townes and Behringer, 1990; Hardison et al., 1997; Fraser and Grosveld, 1998) (Chapter 7). An alternative hypothesis is the "tracking" model in which RNA transcripts originating from the LCR would extend to and include globin gene transcripts and form very long pre-mRNA molecules (Tuan et al., 1992; Kong et al., 1997).

References

Albitar, M, Peschle, C, and Liebhaber, SA. (1989). θ, ζ, and ε globin messenger RNAs are expressed in adults. *Blood* 74: 629–637.

Anderson, KP, Crable, SC, and Lingrel, JB. (1998). Multiple proteins binding to a GATA-E box-GATA motif regulate the erythroid Kruppel-like factor (EKLF) gene. *J. Biol. Chem.* 273: 14347–14354.

Andrews, NC, Erdjument-Bromage, H, Davidson, MB et al. (1993a). Erythroid transcription factor NF-E2 is a haematopoietic-specific basic-leucine zipper protein. *Nature* 362: 722–728.

Andrews, NC, Kotkow, KJ, Ney, PA et al. (1993b). The ubiquitous subunit of erythroid transcription factor NF-E2 is a small basic-leucine zipper protein related to the v-maf oncogene. *Proc. Natl. Acad. Sci. U.S.A.* 90: 11488–11492.

Antoniou, M, deBoer, E, Habets, G, and Grosveld, F. (1988). The human β-globin gene contains multiple regulatory regions: Identification of one promoter and two downstream enhancers. *EMBO J.* 7: 377–384.

Asano, H, Li, XS, and Stamatoyannopoulos, G. (1999). FKLF, a novel Kruppel-like factor that activates human embryonic and fetal beta-like globin genes. *Mol. Cell. Biol.* 19: 3571–3579.

Baglioni, C. (1962). The fusion of two peptide chains in hemoglobin Lepore and its interpretation as a genetic deletion. *Proc. Natl. Acad. Sci. U.S.A.* 48: 1880–1886.

Behringer, RR, Hammer, RE, Brinster, RL, and Palmiter, RD. (1987). Two 3′ sequences direct adult erythroid-specific expression of human β-globin genes in transgenic mice. *Proc. Natl. Acad. Sci. U.S.A.* 84: 7056–7060.

Berg, PE, Williams, DM, Quian, RL et al. (1989). A common protein binds to two silencers 5′ to the human β-globin gene. *Nucleic Acids Res.* 17: 8833–8852.

Blackwood, EM and Kadonaga, JT. (1998). Going the distance: A current view of enhancer action. *Science* 281: 60–63.

Blobel, GA, Simon, MC, and Orkin SH. (1995). Rescue of GATA-1-deficient embryonic stem cells by heterologous GATA-binding proteins. *Mol. Cell. Biol.* 15: 626–633.

Blobel, GA, Nakajima, T, Eckner, R et al. (1998). CREB-binding protein cooperates with transcription factor GATA-1 and is required for erythroid differentiation. *Proc. Natl. Acad. Sci. U.S.A.* 95: 2061–2066.

Bodine, DM and Ley TJ. (1987). An enhancer element lies 3′ to the human Aγ globin gene. *EMBO J.* 6: 2997–3004.

Bohl, KS, Li, C, and Tuan, D. (1997). Transcription of the HS2 enhancer toward a *cis*-linked gene is independent of the orientation, position, and distance of the enhancer relative to the gene. *Mol. Cell. Biol.* 17: 3955–1965.

Boissel, J-P, Kasper, TJ, Shah, SC et al. (1985). Amino-terminal processing of proteins: Hemoglobin South Florida, a variant with retention of initiator methionine and Nᵃ-acetylation. *Proc. Natl. Acad. Sci. U.S.A.* 82: 8448–8452.

Bulger, M, Hikke von Doorninck, J, Saitoh, N et al. (1999). Conservation of sequence and structure flanking the mouse and human b-globin loci: The β-globin genes are embedded within an array of odorant receptor genes. *Proc. Natl. Acad. Sci. U.S.A.* 96: 5129–5134.

Bungert, J, Tanimoto, K, Patel, S et al. (1999). Hypersensitive site 2 specifies a unique function within the human β-globin locus control region to stimulate globin gene transcription. *Mol. Cell. Biol.* 19: 3062–3072.

Cao, SX, Gutman, PD, Dave, HP et al. (1989). Identification of a transcriptional silencer in the 5′-flanking region of the human ε-globin gene. *Proc. Natl. Acad. Sci. U.S.A.* 86: 5306–5309.

Caterina, JJ, Donze, D, Sun, C-W et al. (1994). Cloning and functional characterization of LCR-F1: A bZIP transcription factor that activates erythroid-specific, human globin gene expression. *Nucleic Acids Res.* 22: 2383–2291.

Chan, JY, Han, X-L, and Kan, YW. (1993). Cloning of Nrf1, and NF-E2-related transcription factor, by genetic selection in yeast. *Proc. Natl. Acad. Sci. U.S.A.* 90: 11371–11375.

Chui, DH, Tang, W, and Orkin, SH. (1995). cDNA cloning of murine Nrf2 gene, coding for a p45 NF-E2 related transcription factor. *Biochem. Biophys. Res. Commun.* 209: 40–46.

Clegg, JB. (1987). Can the product of the θ gene be a real globin? *Nature* 329: 465–466.

Deisseroth, A, Nienhuis, A, Turner, P et al. (1977). Localization of the human α-globin structural gene to chromosome 16 in somatic cell hybrids by molecular hybridization assay. *Cell* 12: 205–218.

Deisseroth, A, Nienhuis, AW, Lawrence, J et al. (1978). Chromosomal localization of human β-globin gene on human chromosome 11 in somatic cell hybrids. *Proc. Natl. Acad. Sci. U.S.A.* 75: 1456–1460.

Dillon, N and Grosveld, F. (1993). Transcriptional regulation of multigene loci: Multilevel control. *Trends Genet.* 9: 134–137.

Donze D, Townes, TM, and Bieker, JJ. (1995). Role of erythroid Kruppel-like factor in human γ- to β- globin gene switching. *J. Biol. Chem.* 270: 1955–1959.

Donze, D, Jeancake, P, and Townes, T. (1996). Activation of delta-globin gene expression by erythroid Kruppel-like factor: A potential approach for gene therapy of sickle cell disease. *Blood* 88: 4051–4057.

Ellis, J, Tan-Un, KC, Harper, A et al. (1996). A dominant chromatin-opening activity in 5′ hypersensitive site 3 of the human beta-globin locus control region. *EMBO J.* 15: 562–568.

Engel JD, George KM, Ko, LJ et al. (1991). Transcription factor regulation of hematopoietic lineage cells. *Semin. Hematol.* 28: 158–169.

Engel, JD. (1993). Developmental regulation of human β-globin gene transcription: A switch of loyalties? *Trends Genet.* 9: 304–309.

Epner, E, Kim, CG, and Groudine, M. (1992). What does the locus control region control? *Curr. Biol.* 2: 262–264.

Feng, WC, Southwood, CM, and Bieker, JJ. (1994). Analyses of b-thalassemia mutant DNA interactions with erythroid Kruppel-like factor (EKLF), an erythroid cell-specific transcription factor. *J. Biol. Chem.* 269: 1493–1500.

Forrester, WC, Thompson, C, Elder, JT, and Groudine, M. (1986). A developmentally stable chromatin structure in the human β-globin gene cluster. *Proc. Natl. Acad. Sci. U.S.A.* 83: 1359–1363.

Forrester, WC, Takegawa, S, Papayanopoulou, T et al. (1987). Evidence for a locus activating region: The formation of developmentally stable hypersensitive sites in globin-expressing hybrids. *Nucleic Acids Res.* 15: 10159–10177.

Forrester, WC, Epner, E, Driscoll, MC et al. (1990). A deletion of the human β-globin gene locus activation region causes a major alteration in chromatin structure and replication across the entire β-globin locus. *Genes Dev.* 4: 1637–1649.

Fraser, P, Pruzina, S, Antoniou, M, and Grosveld, F. (1993). Each hypersensitive site of the human β-globin locus control region confers a different developmental pattern of expression on the globin genes. *Genes Dev.* 7: 106–113.

Fraser, P, and Grosveld, F. (1998). Locus control regions, chromatin activation and transcription. *Curr. Opin. Cell Biol.* 10: 361–365.

Fujiwara, Y, Browne, CP, Cunniff, K et al. (1996). Arrested development of embryonic red cell precursors in mouse embryos lacking transcription factor GATA-1. *Proc. Natl. Acad. Sci. U.S.A.* 93: 12355–12358.

Gallarda, JL, Foley, KP, Yang, ZY, and Engel, JD. (1989). The beta-globin stage selector element factor is erythroid-specific promoter/enhancer binding protein NF-E4. *Genes Dev.* 3: 1845–1859.

Gourdon, G, Sharpe, JA, Higgs, DR, and Wood, WG. (1995). The mouse α-globin locus regulatory element. *Blood* 86: 766–775.

Gregory, RC, Taxman, DJ, Seshasayee, D et al. (1996). Functional interaction of GATA1 with erythroid Kruppel-like factor and Sp1 at defined erythroid promoters. *Blood* 87: 1793–1801.

Grosveld, F, Blom van Assendelft, G, Greaves, DR, and Kollias, G. (1987). Position-independent, high-level expression of the human β-globin gene in transgenic mice. *Cell* 51: 975–985.

Grosveld, F, Antoniou, M, Berry, M et al. (1993). The regulation of human globin gene switching. *Philos. Trans. R. Soc. Lond.* 339: 183–191.

Guy, L-G, Mei, Q, Perkins, AC et al. (1998). Erythroid Kruppel-like factor is essential for β-globin gene expression even in absence of gene competition, but is not sufficient to induce the switch from γ-globin to β-globin gene expression. *Blood* 91: 2259–2263.

Hardison, R, Slightom, JL, Gumucio, DL et al. (1997). Locus control regions of mammalian β-globin gene clusters: Combining phylogenetic analyses and experimental results to gain functional insights. *Gene* 205: 73–94.

Higgs, DR. (1998). Do LCRs open chromatin domains? *Cell* 95: 299–302.

Higgs, DR, Wood, WG, Jarman, AP et al. (1990). A major positive regulatory region located far upstream of the human α-globin gene locus. *Genes Dev.* 4: 1588–1601.

Higgs, DR, Sharpe, JA, and Wood, WG. (1998). Understanding α globin gene expression: A step towards effective gene therapy. *Semin. Hematol.* 35: 93–104.

Hsu, S-L, Marks, J, Shaw, J-P et al. (1988). Structure and expression of the human α_1 globin gene. *Nature* 331: 94–96.

Ikuta, T and Kan, YW. (1991). In vivo protein-DNA interactions at the β-globin gene locus. *Proc. Natl. Acad. Sci. U.S.A.* 88: 10188–10192.

Itoh K, Igarashi K, Hayashi N et al. (1995). Cloning and characterization of a novel erythroid cell-derived CNC family transcription factor heterodimerizing with the small Maf family proteins. *Mol. Cell. Biol.* 15: 4184–4193.

Jane, SM, Nienhuis, AW, and Cunningham, JM. (1995). Hemoglobin switching in man and chicken is mediated by a heteromeric complex between the ubiquitous transcription factor CP2 and a developmentally specific protein. *EMBO J.* 14: 97–105.

Kadonaga, J. (1998). Eukaryotic transcription: An interlaced network of transcription factors and chromatin-modifying machines. *Cell* 92: 307–313.

Kendall, AG, Ojwang, PJ, Schroeder, WA, and Huisman THJ. (1973). Hemoglobin Kenya, the product of a γ-β fusion gene: Studies of the family. *Am. J. Hum. Genet.* 25: 548–563.

Khoury, G and Gruss, P. (1983). Enhancer elements. *Cell* 33: 313–314.

Knezetic, JA and Felsenfeld, G. (1989). Identification and characterization of a chicken α-globin enhancer. *Mol. Cell. Biol.* 9: 893–901.

Kollias, G, Hurst, J, deBoer, E, and Grosveld, F. (1987). The human β-globin gene contains a downstream developmental specific enhancer. *Nucleic Acids Res.* 15: 5739–5747.

Kozak, M. (1989). The scanning model for translation: An update. *J. Cell Biol.* 108: 229–241.

Lewin, B. (1990). Commitment and activation at Pol II promoters: A tale of protein-protein interactions. *Cell* 61: 1161–1164.

Ley, TJ, Maloney, KA, Gordon, JI, and Schwarty, AL. (1989). Globin gene expression expression in erythroid human fetal liver cells. *J. Clin. Invest.* 83: 1032–1038.

Li, J, Noguchi, CT, Miller, W et al. (1998). Multiple regulatory elements in the 5'-flanking sequence of the human ε-globin gene. *J. Biol. Chem.* 273: 10202–10209.

Li, Q and Stamatoyannopoulos, G. (1994). Hypersensitive site 5 of the human β locus control region functions as a chromatin insulator. *Blood* 84: 1399–1401.

Li, Q, Blau, CA, Clegg, CH et al. (1998). Multiple ε-promoter elements participate in the developmental control of ε-globin genes in transgenic mice. *J. Biol. Chem.* 273: 17361–17367.

Liebhaber, SA, Wang, Z, Cash, FE et al. (1996). Developmental silencing of the embryonic ζ-globin gene: concerted action of the promoter and the 3'-flanking region combined with stage-specific silencing by the transcribed segment. *Mol. Cell. Biol.* 16: 2637–2646.

Liu, D, Chang, JC, Moi, P et al. (1992). Dissection of the enhancer activity of β-globin 5' DNase I-hypersensitive site 2 in transgenic mice. *Proc. Natl. Acad. Sci. U.S.A.* 89: 3899–3903.

Madhani, HD and Guthrie, C. (1994). Dynamic RNA-RNA interactions in the spliceosome. *Annu. Rev. Genet.* 28: 1–26.

Martin, D, Tsai, S, and Orkin, S. (1989). Increased γ-globin expression in a non-deletion HPFH is mediated by an erythroid-specific DNA-binding factor. *Nature* 338: 435–438.

Merika, M and Orkin, SH. (1995). Functional synergy and physical interactions of the erythroid transcription factor GATA-1 with the Kruppel family proteins Sp1 and EKLF. *Mol. Cell. Biol.* 15: 2437–2447.

Mignotte, V, Wall, L, deBoer, E et al. (1989). Two tissue-specific factors bind the erythroid promoter of the human porphobilinogen deaminase gene. *Nucleic Acids Res.* 17: 37–54.

Miller U and Bieker JJ. (1993). A novel, erythroid cell-specific murine transcription factor that binds to the CACCC element and is related to the Kruppel family of nuclear proteins. *Mol. Cell. Biol.* 13: 2776–2786.

Mitchell, PJ and Tjian R. (1989). Transcriptional regulation in mammalian cells by sequence-specific DNA binding proteins. *Science* 245: 371–378.

Moi, P and Kan, YW. (1990). Synergistic enhancement of globin gene expression by activator protein-1-like proteins. *Proc. Natl. Acad. Sci. U.S.A.* 87: 9000–9004.

Moi, P, Chan, K, Asunis, I et al. (1994). Isolation of NF-E2 like basic leucine zipper transcriptional activator that binds to the tandem NF-E2/AP1 repeat of the b-globin locus control region. *Proc. Natl. Acad. Sci. U.S.A.* 91: 9926–9930.

Mount, SM. (1982). A catalogue of splice junction sequences. *Nucleic Acids Res.* 10: 459–472.

Ney, PA, Sorrentino, BP, McDonagh, KT, and Nienhuis, AW. (1990a). Tandem AP-1-binding sites within the human β-globin dominant control region function as an inducible enhancer in erythroid cells. *Genes Dev.* 4: 993–1006.

Ney, PA, Sorrentino, BP, Lowrey, CH, and Nienhuis, AW. (1990b). Inducibility of the HS II enhancer depends on binding of an erythroid specific nuclear protein. *Nucl. Acids Res.* 18: 6011–6017.

Nilsen, TW. (1994). RNA-RNA interactions in the spliceosome: Unraveling the ties that bind. *Cell* 78: 1–4.

Nuez, B, Michalovich, D, Bygrave, A et al. (1995). Defective haematopoiesis in fetal liver resulting from inactivation of the EKLF gene. *Nature* 375: 316–318.

O'Neill, D, Yang, J, Erdjument-Bromage, H et al. (1999). Tissue-specific and developmental stage-specific DNA binding by a mammalian SWI/SNF complex associated with human fetal-to-adult globin gene switching. *Proc. Natl. Acad. Sci. U.S.A.* 96: 349–54.

Orkin, SH. (1990). Globin gene regulation and switching: Circa 1990. *Cell* 63: 665–672.

Orkin, SH. (1992). GATA-binding transcription factors in hematopoietic cells. *Blood* 80: 575–581.

Orkin, SH. (1995a). Tanscription factors and hematopoeitic development. *J. Biol. Chem.* 270: 4955–4958.

Orkin, SH. (1995b). Regulation of globin gene expression in erythroid cells. *Eur. J. Biochem.* 231: 271–281.

Oyake, T, Itoh, K, Motohashi, H et al. (1996). Bach proteins belong to a novel family of BTB-basic leucine zipper transcription factors that interact with MafK and regulate transcription through the NF-E2 site. *Mol. Cell. Biol.* 16: 6083–6095.

Padgett, RA, Grabowski, PJ, Konaroka, MM et al. (1986). Splicing of messenger RNA precursors. *Annu. Rev. Biochem.* 55: 1119–1150.

Perkins, AC, Sharpe, AH, and Orkin, SH. (1995). Lethal β-thalassemia in mice lacking the erythroid CACCC-transcription factor EKLF. *Nature* 375: 318–322.

Pevny, L, Simon, MC, Robertson, E et al. (1991). Erythroid differentiation in chimeric mice blocked by a targeted mutation in the gene for transcription factor GATA-1. *Nature* 349: 257–260.

Philipsen, S, Talbot, D, Fraser, P, and Grosveld, F. (1990). The β-globin dominant control region: Hypersensitive site 2. *EMBO J.* 9: 2159–2167.

Proudfoot, N. (1996). Ending the message is not so simple. *Cell* 87: 779–781.

Ptashne, M and Gann, AAF. (1990). Activators and targets. *Nature* 346: 329–331.

Reddy, PMS, Stamatoyannopoulos, G, Papayannopoulou, T, and Shen, C-KJ. (1994). Genomic footprinting and sequencing of human β-globin locus: Tissue specificity and cell line artifact. *J. Biol. Chem.* 269: 8287–8295.

Reik, A, Telling, A, Zitnik, G et al. (1998). The locus control region is necessary for gene expression in the human β-globin locus but not the maintenance of an open chromatin structure in erythroid cells. *Mol. Cell. Biol.* 18: 5992–6000.

Rombel, I, Hu, K-Y, Zhang, Q et al. (1995). Transcriptional activation of human α-globin gene by hypersensitive site-40 enhancers: function of nuclear factor-binding motifs

occupied in erythroid cells. *Proc. Natl. Acad. Sci. U.S.A.* 92: 6454–6458.

Shivdasani, RA and Orkin, SH. (1995). Erythropoiesis and globin gene expression in mice lacking the transcription factor NF-E2. *Proc. Natl. Acad. Sci. U.S.A.* 92: 8690–8694.

Simon, MC, Pevny, L, Wiles, MV et al. (1992). Rescue of erythroid development in gene targeted GATA-1 mouse embryonic stem cells. *Nat. Genet.* 1: 92–98.

Smale, ST and Baltimore, D. (1989). The "initiator" as a transcription control element. *Cell* 57: 103.

Staley, JP and Guthriue C. (1998). Mechanical devices of the spliceosome: Motors, clocks, springs, and things. *Cell* 92: 315–326.

Stamatoyannopoulos, G. (1991). Human hemoglobin switching. *Science* 252: 383.

Stamatoyannopoulos, G, Josephson, B, Zhang, J-W, and Li, Q. (1993). Developmental regulation of human γ-globin genes in transgenic mice. *Mol. Cell. Biol.* 13: 7636–7644.

Strauss, EC and Orkin, SH. (1992). In vivo protein-DNA interactions at hypersensitive site 3 of the human β-globin locus control region. *Proc. Natl. Acad. Sci. U.S.A.* 89: 5809–5813.

Strauss, EC, Andrews, NC, Higgs, DR, and Orkin, SH. (1992). In vivo footprinting of the human α-globin locus upstream regulatory element by guanine and adenine ligation-mediated polymerase chain reaction. *Mol. Cell. Biol.* 12: 2135–2142.

Svaren, J and Chalkley, R. (1990). The structure and assembly of active chromatin. *Trends Genet.* 6: 52.

Talbot, D and Grosveld, F. (1991). The 5′ HS2 of the globin locus control region enhances transcription through the interaction of a multimeric complex binding at two functionally distinct NF-E2 binding sites. *EMBO J.* 10: 1391–1398.

Talbot, D, Collis, P, Antoniou, M et al. (1989). A dominant control region from the human β-globin locus conferring integration site-independent gene expression. *Nature* 338: 352–355.

Talbot, D, Philipsen, S, Fraser, P, and Grosveld, F. (1990). Detailed analysis of the site 3 region of the human β-globin dominant control region. *EMBO J.* 9: 2169–2178.

Tang, DC, Ebb, D, Hardison, RC, and Rodgers, GP. (1997). Restoration of the CCAAT box and insertion of the CACCC motif activate δ-globin gene expression. *Blood* 90: 421–427.

Townes, TM and Behringer, RR. (1990). Human globin locus activation region (LAR): Role in temporal control. *Trends Genet.* 6: 219–223.

Trudel, M and Costantini, F. (1987). A 3′ enhancer contributes to the stage-specific expression of the human β-globin gene. *Genes Dev.* 1: 954–961.

Trudel, M, Magram, J, Bruckner, L, and Constantini F. (1987). Upstream Gγ-globin and downstream β-globin sequences required for stage-specific expression in transgenic mice. *Mol. Cell. Biol.* 7: 4024–4029.

Tsai, S, Martin, D, Zon, L et al. (1989) Cloning of the cDNA for the major DNA-binding protein of the erythroid lineage through expression in mammalian cells. *Nature* 339: 446–451.

Tsang AP, Visvader JE, Turner, CA et al. (1997). FOG, a multitype zinc finger protein, acts as a cofactor for transcription factor GATA-1 in erythroid and megakaryocytic differentiation. *Cell* 90: 109–119.

Tsang, AP, Fujiwara, Y, Hom, DB, and Orkin, SH. (1998). Failure of megakaryopoiesis and arrested erythropoiesis in mice lacking the GATA-1 transcriptional cofactor FOG. *Genes Dev.* 12: 1176–1188.

Tuan, D, Solomon, W, Li, Q, and London, IM. (1985). The "β-like-globin" gene domain in human erythroid cells. *Proc. Natl. Acad. Sci. U.S.A.* 82: 6384–6388.

Tuan, D, Kong, S, and Hu, K. (1992). Transcription of the hypersensitive site HS2 enhancer in erythroid cells. *Proc. Natl. Acad. Sci. U.S.A.* 89: 11219–11223.

Wadman, IA, Osada, H, Grutz, GG et al. (1997). The LIM-only protein Lmo2 is a bridging molecule assembling an erythroid, DNA-binding complex which includes the TAL1, E47, GATA-1 and Ldb1/NLI proteins. *EMBO J.* 16: 3145–3157.

Wahle, E and Keller, W. (1996). The biochemistry of polyadenylation. *Trends Biochem. Sci.* 21: 247–251.

Wall, L, deBoer, E, and Grosveld, F. (1988). The human β-globin gene 3′ enhancer contains multiple binding sites for an erythroid-specific protein. *Genes Dev.* 2: 1089–1100.

Wang, Z and Liebhaber, SA. (1999). A 3′-flanking NK-kB site mediates developmental silencing of the human z-globin gene. *EMBO J.* 18: 2218–2228.

Watt, P, Lamb, P, and Proudfoot, NJ. (1993). Distinct negative regulation of the human embryonic globin genes zeta and epsilon. *Gene Exp.* 3: 61–75.

Weatherall, DJ and Clegg, JB. (1981). *The thalassaemia syndromes* (3rd ed). Oxford: Blackwell Scientific Publications.

Weiss, MJ and Orkin, SH. (1995a). GATA transcription factors: Key regulators of hematopoiesis. *Exp. Hematol.* 23: 99–107.

Weiss, MJ and Orkin, SH. (1995b). Transcription factor GATA-1 permits survival and maturation of erythroid precursors by preventing apoptosis. *Proc. Natl. Acad. Sci. U.S.A.* 92: 9623–9627.

Weiss, MJ, Keller, G, and Orkin, SH. (1994). Novel insights into erythroid development revealed through in vitro differentiation of GATA-1 embryonic stem cells. *Genes Dev.* 8: 1184–1197.

Weiss, MJ, Yu, C, and Orkin, SH. (1997). Erythroid-cell-specific properties of transcription factor GATA-1 revealed by phenotypic rescue of a gene-targeted cell line. *Mol. Cell. Biol.* 17: 1642–1651.

Wickens, M. 1990. How the messenger got its tail: Addition of poly(A) in the nucleus. *Trends Biochem. Sci.* 15: 277–281.

Wijgerde, M, Grosveld, F, and Fraser, P. (1995). Transcription complex stability and chromatin dynamics in vivo. *Nature* 377: 209–213.

Zhou, WL, Clouston, DR, Wang, X et al. (1999). Isolation and characterization of human NF-E4, the tissue restricted component of the stage selector protein complex. *Blood* 94(Suppl.1): 614a.

7

Molecular and Cellular Basis of Hemoglobin Switching

GEORGE STAMATOYANNOPOULOS

INTRODUCTION

Hemoglobin switching is characteristic of all animal species that use hemoglobin for oxygen transport. Most species have only one switch, from embryonic to adult globin formation. Humans and a few other mammals have two globin gene switches, from embryonic to fetal globin coinciding with the transition from embryonic (yolk sac) to definitive (fetal liver) hematopoiesis and from fetal to adult globin formation, occurring around the perinatal period (Fig. 7.1; see Chapters 2 and 3). The switch from ε- to γ-globin production begins very early in gestation, as HbF is readily detected in 5-week human embryos (Huehns et al., 1964; Hecht et al., 1966), and it is completed well before the 10th week of gestation (Huehns et al., 1964; Gale et al., 1979). β-globin expression starts early in human development, and small amounts of HbA can be detected by biosynthetic or immunochemical methods even in the smallest human fetuses studied. In these fetuses γ and β globin are present in the same fetal red cell (Papayannopoulou et al., 1983). β-chain synthesis increases to approximately 10 percent of total hemoglobin by 30 to 35 weeks of gestation. At birth, HbF comprises 60 percent to 80 percent of the total hemoglobin. It takes about 2 years to reach the level of 0.5 percent to 1 percent HbF that is characteristic of adult red cells. HbF in the adult is restricted to a few erythrocytes called "F-cells" (see Chapter 10) (Boyer et al., 1975; Wood et al., 1975). Approximately 3 percent to 7 percent of erythrocytes are F-cells (Wood et al., 1975), and each contains approximately 4 to 8 picograms (pg) of HbF (Boyer et al., 1975).

Hemoglobin switching has been the target of intensive investigation for two reasons. First, it provides an excellent model for studying the control of gene activity during development. Indeed, until the late 1970s, hemoglobin switching was the only developmental system that could be investigated in detail at the protein level. Second, understanding of the control of switching is expected to lead to the development of treatments of hemoglobinopathies. The β-chain hemoglobinopathies, sickle cell disease and thalassemia are unique among genetic disorders in that nature has shown an effective means of treatment: the production of HbF that can compensate for the loss of β-chain activity or can decrease the propensity for sickling. Research on the cell and molecular control of switching is expected to lead to discoveries that will cure these disorders through abundant production of HbF in the patient's red cells.

CELLULAR CONTROL OF SWITCHING

Before the era of molecular biology, insights on the cellular mechanisms of hemoglobin switching were obtained through phenomenological observations in human and animal models and from cell biological studies. The observation that human fetuses have different hemoglobin than adults was made more than 100 years ago when it was discovered that the hemoglobin of neonates is alkali resistant. The observation that amphibia have different hemoglobins in the embryonic and adult stages was made in the 1930s when the oxygen affinity of frog and tadpole blood was examined. The two types of hemoglobin were actually separated by Svedberg while he was developing the ultracentrifuge. Hemoglobin switching was more intensely investigated when the introduction of electrophoretic techniques allowed detailed studies of hemoglobin during the development of many species. Several questions on the cellular control of switching were asked during that time and, amazingly, clonal models of switching (see below) were proposed even before it became possible to analyze hemoglobin switching at the protein level. Systematic investigation of the cellular control of switching, however, started only when modern methods of cell biology became available in the 1970s.

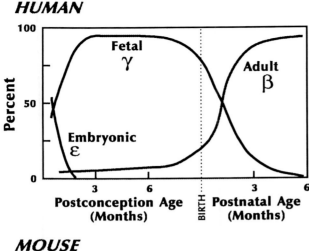

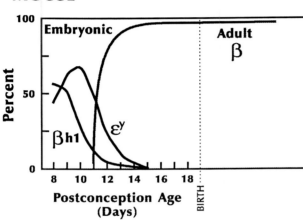

Figure 7.1. Hemoglobin switching in humans and mice. The human ε gene is homologous to murine εy. The γ-globin gene is homologous to βh1 while the β-globin gene is homologous to murine β minor and β major.

Models of Cellular Control

The first models of hemoglobin switching assumed that it represents an epiphenomenon due to replacement of hematopoietic stem cell lineages. The model was eloquently formulated by Vernon Ingram (Ingram, 1972). To explain hemoglobin switching in the mouse or chicken, it was postulated that there is an embryonic stem cell lineage that is committed to embryonic globin gene formation and this is replaced by an adult stem cell lineage committed to expression of the adult globin gene. In the case of the human hemoglobin switch, three lineages were thought to exist: an embryonic, a fetal, and an adult stem cell lineage. The γ- to β-switch was attributed to the replacement of the fetal stem cell lineage by the adult stem cell lineage (Weatherall et al., 1968, 1976; Alter et al., 1976, 1981a, 1981b). The transitions in major erythropoietic sites during ontogeny

(see Chapter 2) seemed to support the clonal hypothesis of switching.

An alternative model was developed in the mid 1970s (Papayannopoulou et al., 1977). It proposed that switching is not due to changes in stem cell populations but to changes in programs of gene expression that occur in the progeny of a single stem cell population. During the differentiation of progenitor cells in the embryo, a program allowing synthesis of embryonic hemoglobin is activated. A fetal program is activated in the progenitor cells of the fetus and an adult program in the progenitor cells of the adult.

Finding out which of the two models (i.e., changes in stem cell populations or changes in programs) is correct was important from the theoretical and the therapeutic point of view. In the 1970s it was thought that it is difficult to manipulate stem cell populations; on the other hand, it was possible that manipulation of gene expression programs can be achieved with pharmacologic means. Therefore, a systematic investigation of the two models was done.

The lineage models assume an absolute restriction of embryonic globins to primitive cells and of adult globins to definitive cells. However, during switching in chickens (Chapman and Tobin, 1979), in the mouse (Brotherton et al., 1979), and in quail-chick chimeras (Le Douarin, 1978; Beaupain et al., 1981), there are cell populations coexpressing both embryonic and adult hemoglobins. One can use the hematopoietic cells of human embryos to produce erythroid colonies, each of which originates from a single progenitor cell; typically, these colonies coexpress ε and γ globins (Peschle et al., 1984; Stamatoyannopoulos et al., 1987). Thus, a single cell can form progeny producing adult as well as embryonic globins against the expectations of the lineage models. Three types of experiments provided the evidence against the lineage model of γ- to β-switch. First, studies of individuals with clonal hemoglobin stem cell disorders (polycythemia vera, chronic myelogenous leukemia, or paroxysmal nocturnal hemoglobinuria) clearly showed that both F-cells and A-cells are produced by a single stem cell clone (summaries in Stamatoyannopoulos and Nienhuis, 1994). Second, studies in culture showed that single-cell origin erythroid colonies from fetuses, neonates, or adults contain both fetal and adult globins (Stamatoyannopoulos and Nienhuis, 1994). Third, direct evidence came from analyses of somatic cell hybrids produced by fusion of mouse erythroleukemia (MEL) cells with human cells. These hybrids initially synthesize only (or predominantly) fetal human globin, and after 20 to 40 weeks in culture they switch to β-globin chain formation. Since each hybrid originates from a single cell, β- to γ-switching can occur in cells of a single lineage (Papayannopoulou et al., 1986).

It is thus clear that hemoglobin switching takes place in the progeny of a single stem cell lineage. It represents changes in transcriptional environments at the level of committed cells rather than changes in stem cell populations "frozen" in a single gene expression program. It is of interest that in spite of the extensive evidence, even today phenotypes of HbF elevations in the adult are attributed by some authors to the continued presence of fetal stem cells in the adult marrow!

Environmental Modulation Versus Developmental Clock

Another question that was asked by investigators 20 years ago was: If switching takes place in the cells of a single lineage, how do these cells know when to switch their globin gene expression program? Many changes occur during development and there is ample evidence that the cell's microenvironment can determine the fate of a cell. Initially, inductive mechanisms were thought to also apply to hemoglobin switching, and several experiments have been done to determine what types of changes within the microenvironment of the developing fetus, especially what hormonal changes, underlie the γ- to β-switch. The summary of this work is that there is no evidence that there exists a specific environmental signal that is responsible for the switch. On the other hand, there is abundant evidence that the environment can modulate the γ- to β-switch. Thus, in sheep, removal of the adrenal inhibits the normal increase in plasma cortisol that precedes birth (Wintour et al., 1985). The γ- to β-switch in such adrenalectomized animals is delayed, although the animals are grossly normal with respect to developmental progression. Administration of cortisol to establish levels approximating those found in fetuses with normal adrenals allows the switch to progress with normal kinetics. Also, external factors can influence the rate of switch in MEL × fetal erythroid hybrids: serum deprivation or addition of dexamethasone in the culture media strikingly accelerates the γ- to β-switch (Zitnik et al., 1993, 1995).

Considerable evidence suggests that the timing of switching is inherently controlled, perhaps through the action of a developmental clock type of mechanism. Three arguments in favor of a clock type of mechanism will be mentioned here. First, in vivo observations in humans indicate that the level of HbF in newborns is related to their age from conception rather than to birth itself (della Torre and Meroni, 1969; Bard et al., 1970). Thus, the switch is independent of the intrauterine or extrauterine status of the individual; rather, the degree of developmental maturity of the fetus determines the rate as well as the timing of γ- to β-switch.

Second, the rate of the switch of the MEL × human fetal erythroid hybrids mentioned earlier, correlates to the age of the fetus from which the human erythroblasts were derived (Papayannopoulou et al., 1986). Thus, hybrids produced using cells of younger fetuses switch more slowly than do hybrids produced using cells of older fetuses, as if the human fetal erythroid cells "know" whether they belong to an early or to a late developmental time, and transmit this information into the hybrid cells. Third, transplantations of hematopoietic cells have been done in sheep to determine whether the environment can influence the rate of switch in the transplanted cells. Adult stem cells were transplanted into fetuses and fetal stem cells into adult animals, and hemoglobin production in the engrafted donor cells was monitored. The adult cells transplanted into fetuses continued to produce adult globin, suggesting that the fetal environment cannot change the program of the adult cells (Zanjani et al., 1982). Transplantation of fetal sheep stem cells into lethally irradiated adult recipients showed that the donor cells switch (Wood et al., 1985). However, the rate of switching of the transplanted fetal cells is dependent on the gestational age of the donor fetus, suggesting that switching reflects the action of a mechanism that in some way can count developmental time.

Presumably a clock determining the rate of switching is set sometime during embryogenesis and proceeds to execute a preset program as development advances. It is difficult at present to test experimentally the molecular basis of this phenomenon. There are several examples of developmental clocks in drosophila, but these clocks represent mostly diurnal variations in a phenotype and have been explained by the periodicity in accumulation of a metabolic product. How a "clock" that can operate for several months (as in the case of human switching) is controlled is difficult to conceive, although hypotheses on how cells can count developmental time have been proposed in the past (Holliday and Pugh, 1975). The available evidence suggests that the clock of switching is located on chromosome 11 (Melis et al., 1987). It acts in *cis* and certain findings (Stanworth et al., 1995), although interpreted by these authors differently, suggest that the clock may be controlled through sequences present in the globin gene clusters.

MOLECULAR CONTROL OF SWITCHING

The last 15 years have witnessed considerable progress in the understanding of molecular control of switching. Several tools have been used. Transgenic mice have provided information on the sequences of the locus that are responsible for developmental control and on the mechanisms that control switching in vivo.

Traditional biochemistry and gene cloning techniques have led to the discovery of *trans* factors that interact with motifs of globin gene promoters and the locus control region (LCR). Essentially, we know today, in general terms, the mechanisms that regulate globin gene activity during development. However, there is a vast amount of specific information that needs to be learned until the phenomenon is completely delineated at the molecular level.

Regulatory Elements of the ε-Globin Gene

In vitro experiments indicate that the CACCC and CCAAT boxes in conjunction with the GATA sites of the ε-globin gene promoter are required for expression (Gong and Dean, 1993; Gong et al., 1991, Walters and Martin, 1992). However, it is not known which factors interact with these sequences in vivo. The CACCC box binds the ubiquitous factor Sp1 (Yu et al., 1991), but inactivation of Sp1 in vivo (Marin et al., 1997) does not result in defective ε gene expression. Two factors belonging to the erythroid Krüppel-like factor (EKLF)/Sp1 family, named as fetal Krüppel-like factor (FKLF) (Asano et al., 1999) and FKLF-2 (Asano et al., 2000), have been shown to interact with the gene CACCC box and activate gene expression in transient assays and in stable transections. The CAAT box of the gene binds CP1; binding of CP1 activates in vitro gene expression. In the region of the CCAAT box of the embryonic and fetal, but not of adult, globin gene promoters there exist direct repeats of a short motif that is analogous to DR-1 binding sites for nonsteroid nuclear hormone receptors (Filipe et al., 1999). In vitro experiments and studies in transgenic mice have demonstrated that COUP-TF, an orphan nuclear receptor, binds to the DR-1 element of the gene promoter and acts as a developmental repressor (Filipe et al., 1999). The promoter also contains a number of GATA sites. Studies in transgenic mice suggest that when GATA-1 binds at −163 or −269 it acts as a gene activator, but when it binds to the −208 site it acts as a repressor (Raich et al., 1995). Several sites that bind to factors that act either as repressors or activators in vitro have been identified in the upstream promoter (Li et al., 1998; Trepicchio et al., 1993).

Regulatory Elements of the γ-Globin Genes

The fact that the promoter contains elements important for developmental control is shown by the point mutations that produce the hereditary persistence of fetal hemoglobin (HPFH) phenotype (see Chapter 15). Most of these HPFH mutations occur in transcription factor binding motifs. Between the CAAT box and the TATA box of the promoter there exists a G-rich sequence designated as stage selector element (SSE). This sequence is conserved in species that express the γ gene in the fetal stage, but diverges in species in which the gene homologue is expressed in embryonic cells (Gumucio et al., 1992). A binding activity, called stage selector protein (SSP) (Jane et al., 1992, 1993), binds to this sequence. SSP is composed of the ubiquitously expressed factor CP2 and a recently cloned protein, NF-E4, which is erythroid specific and activates γ-gene expression in transfection experiments (Jane et al., 1995, Zhou et al., 1999). Several proteins bind to the CAAT box region of the promoter (Gumucio et al., 1988; mantovani et al., 1988, 1989; Fucharoen et al., 1990; McDonagh and Nienhuis, 1991; Berry et al., 1992). CP1, a ubiquitously expressed protein, acts as a positive transcriptional activator in vitro. CAAT displacement protein (CDP) binds to both CAAT boxes, competitively displacing CP1, and, in vitro, acts as a transcriptional repressor (Skalnik et al., 1991). NF-E3 and GATA-1 bind in the CAAT box region (Gumucio et al., 1988; Mantovani et al., 1988; Berry et al., 1992; Ronchi et al., 1995) and are considered to act as gene suppressors, but this hypothesis is not supported by experiments in transgenic mice (Ronchi et al., 1996). Studies in transgenic mice indicate that the CACCC box plays an important role in gene expression at the fetal stage of definitive hematopoiesis when the major synthesis of fetal hemoglobin takes place in humans (Q. Li et al., unpublished). FKLF (Asano et al., 1999) and FKLF-2 (Asano et al., 2000) bind to the CACCC box in vitro but their in vivo role has not yet been determined.

Other developmentally important sites have been revealed in the upstream promoter by HPFH mutants. GATA and octamer 1 sites are located around position −175. The −175 HPFH mutation alters the interaction with GATA-1 and removes the binding site for octamer (McDonagh et al., 1991; Magis and Martin, 1995), but the relevance of these in vitro effects to the HPFH phenotype remains unknown. Several HPFH mutations are located in the −200 region. This region of the promoter is capable of forming a triple stranded structure, which is thought to be the binding site for a repressor complex that is displaced by the transcription factors that bind to the novel sequences created by the HPFH mutations (Ulrich et al., 1992; Bacolla et al., 1995). Other potential binding sites are located further upstream in the promoter (Ponce et al., 1991; Gumucio et al., 1992). Transgenic mice experiments have localized a silencer in the −382 to −730 region (Stamatoyannopoulos et al., 1993). Also, this region contains a butyrate response element (Pace et al., 1996).

An "enhancer" has been located downstream from the $^A\gamma$ gene on the basis of transfection experiments (Bodine and Ley, 1987). This element contains binding sites for transcriptional factors (Purucker et al., 1990; Dickinson et al., 1992) but it has no role in enhancing gene expression (Liu et al., 1998). In transgenic mice, presence of this 3' element protects the γ gene from position effects (Li and Stamatoyannopoulos, 1994; Stamatoyannopoulos et al., 1997), suggesting that its likely role is stabilization of the interaction between the γ-globin gene and the LCR.

Regulatory Elements of the β-Globin Gene

Several factors have been shown to bind in the CAAT box region of the β-globin gene (Antoniou et al., 1988; deBoer et al., 1988; Wall et al., 1996); CP1 behaves as a positive regulator of the CAAT box in vitro. The CACCC box binds several factors in vitro (Hartzog and Myers, 1993) but the protein that is important in vivo is EKLF (Miller and Bieker, 1993; Feng et al., 1994). The β-globin CAC box has a higher binding affinity for EKLF than the ε- or γ-globin CAC boxes (Donze et al., 1995).

An enhancer is located downstream from the poly-A site of the β-globin gene (Behringer et al., 1987; Antoniou et al., 1988; deBoer et al., 1988). Its deletion severely affects gene expression (Liu et al., 1997) indicating that this element plays an important role in β-globin gene expression.

The β-Globin Locus Control Region

This region is described in Chapter 5 of this book. It is located 6 to 25 kb upstream from the ε-globin gene and contains a series of developmentally stable DNAse I hypersensitive sites (HS) (Tuan et al., 1985; Forrester et al., 1986). A larger body of data indicate that the activities of the LCR are mostly localized to the core elements of the HSs, which are approximately 300 bp long. The regions flanking the HS core elements of the LCR are also important for function. The current concept is that the LCR functions as a complex formed by interaction of the transcriptional factors that bind to the individual HS elements.

The unique property of the LCR is its activating function, which "opens" the chromatin domain and provides the possibility for gene transcription. In transgenic mice, the LCR is recognized by its capacity to confer integration position-independent expression on a linked gene (Grosveld et al., 1987; Fraser and Grosveld, 1998). Position effects are always overcome by the LCR in a dominant manner (Milot et al., 1996; Fraser and Grosveld, 1998). Experiments in knockout mice have been recently interpreted to indicate that

the LCR is not required for opening the chromatin domain (Epner et al., 1998; Reik et al., 1998; Bender et al., 2000). Thus, while in β thalassemia mutants due to LCR deletions (Van der Ploeg et al., 1980; Vanin et al., 1983; Curtin et al., 1985; Driscoll et al., 1989; Forrester et al., 1990) there is total inactivation of the β locus chromatin and total absence of transcription of the genes in cis, when the LCR is deleted from the endogenous murine locus by homologous recombination, the globin genes continue to show some low levels of expression, and the chromatin of the β locus remains in the open configuration (Epner et al., 1998; Bender et al., 2000). Why the phenotypes of the LCR deletions in humans and the LCR knock-outs in mice differ is still unknown (Higgs, 1998; Grosveld, 1999). Among the possible reasons are differences in the composition and organization of the murine and the human LCRs. Alternatively, the total silencing of the β locus in the human LCR deletions may not be due to the deletion of the LCR per se, but the juxtaposition to the locus of upstream located heterochromatic regions that silence the genes of the locus.

The DNAse I hypersensitive sites of the LCR have developmental specificity (Fraser et al., 1993). This was recently unequivocally shown in the studies of transgenic mice carrying β locus yeast artificial chromosomes (YAC mice). Deletion of the core element of HS3 in the context of a β locus YAC results in total absence of ε-globin gene expression in day-9 embryonic cells (Navas et al., 1998), suggesting that sequences of the core element of HS3 are necessary for activation of ε-globin gene transcription. γ-gene expression in embryonic cells is normal, suggesting that an HS other than HS3 interacts with the γ promoter in embryonic cells. However, β-globin gene expression is totally absent in fetal liver cells, indicating that the core of HS3 is necessary for γ-gene transcription in the fetal stage of definitive erythropoiesis. These results are also compatible with the possibility that the LCR changes conformation during the course of development (Navas et al., 1998).

Molecular Control of Switching

Major insights on the molecular control of switching have been obtained through studies of transgenic mice. As mentioned earlier, in the mouse there is only one switch during development—the switch from embryonic to definitive globin gene expression, which coincides with the transition from the yolk sac to the definitive, fetal liver, erythropoiesis. The εy and βh1 genes are expressed exclusively in the yolk sac. These genes are silenced in the fetal liver where β major and β minor expression occur. The εy is homologous to human ε while the βh1 is homologous to human γ. Initial studies of transgenic mice carrying human globin transgenes, done before the discovery of the LCR, have shown that the human transgenes are regulated similarly to their murine homologous genes, that is, they display normal developmental regulation (references in Stamatoyannopoulos and Nienhuis, 1994). Thus, the γ genes, like the murine βh1, are expressed only in the yolk sac cells while the β genes are expressed only in the definitive cells, indicating that all the elements required for correct developmental regulation are included in the sequences of the genes or their flanking sequence. With the discovery of the LCR, the question of how the globin genes are developmentally regulated in the presence of this powerful regulatory element arose. Studies in transgenic mice revealed that two mechanisms, gene silencing and gene competition, control hemoglobin switching.

Globin Gene Silencing

The studies of *cis* elements and *trans* factors involved in turning off the gene provide the best example of how globin genes are silenced during development. ε-globin gene expression is totally restricted in the embryonic yolk sac cells and its developmental control is autonomous, that is, all the sequences required for silencing of the ε gene in the cells of definitive erythropoiesis are contained in the sequences flanking the gene (Raich et al., 1990; Shih et al., 1990). Regulatory sequences mediating this autonomous silencing have been mapped to the distal and proximal promoter (Wada-Kiyama et al., 1992; Raich et al., 1995; J. Li et al., 1998; Q. Li et al., 1998).

A negative regulatory element was initially identified in the upstream gene promoter using transfection assays in cultured cells (Cao et al., 1989). This element is located between −182 and −467 bp from the initiation site and contains three binding motifs: a GATA site at −208, a YY1 site at −269, and a CAC motif at −379 (Peters et al., 1993; Raich et al., 1995) (Fig. 7.2). Evidence that this element functions as a silencer was obtained when the deletion of the element resulted in ε gene expression in the red cells of adult transgenic mice (Raich et al., 1992). Subsequently it was found that disruption of either the −208 GATA-1 or the −269 YY1 binding site also results in ε-gene expression in adult transgenic mice (Raich et al., 1995). Presumably, several transcriptional factors interact to form the silencing complex and disruption of any of these factors results in inhibition of silencing. ε-gene silencing, therefore, is combinatorial (Fig. 7.3). The fact that GATA-1 binding at −208 results in gene suppression was subsequently shown using a binary transgenic mouse system. Overexpression of GATA-1 in transgenic mice carrying a human β locus YAC resulted in a specific decrease of human ε-globin expression (Li et al., 1997). The −182 to −467 silencer is not the only element involved in turning off the gene. As mentioned earlier, COUP-TF binding in the DR repeats near the CAAT box has suppressive effects and there is

Figure 7.2. Globin gene silencing. The middle diagram shows the sequence of the upstream gene promoter, which when deleted results in continuation of ε-gene expression in the adult. The lower diagram shows the binding sites for transcriptional factors contained in this silencer.

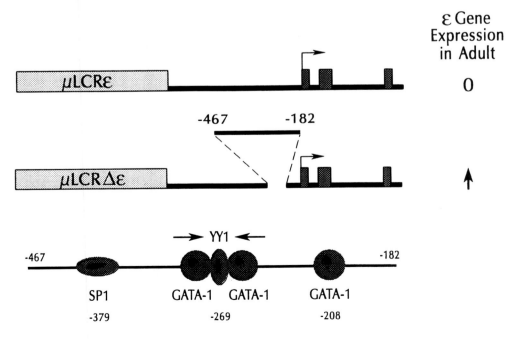

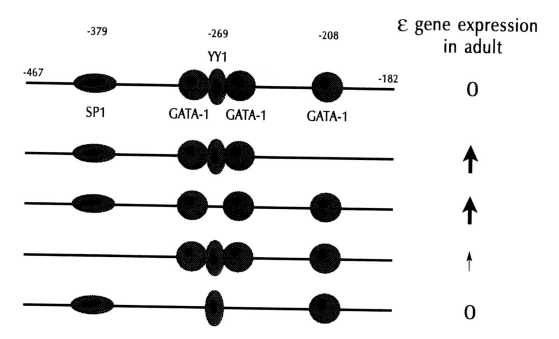

Figure 7.3. Evidence that the silencing of the ε gene is combinatorial. Mutations that affect binding of GATA-1 at –208 or YY1 at –269 or a CACCC binding protein at –379 result in continuation of ε-globin gene expression in the adult. Other transcriptional factors involved in silencing include COUP-TF that binds to the DR-1 element near the gene's CAAT box (see text).

evidence that sequences having silencing properties are located in the further upstream gene promoter.

The mechanism that turns off the γ-globin gene has been more difficult to determine. Initially, the silencing of the γ gene was attributed solely to gene competition (Behringer et al., 1990; Enver et al., 1990). However, other experiments in transgenic mice suggested that the gene turns off solely through an autonomous silencing mechanism (Dillon and Grosveld, 1991). It seems that the latter is correct and that autonomous silencing is the major mechanism whereby the γ genes are turned off during development. The strongest evidence was provided by two types of experiments. The first type were studies in transgenic mice carrying β YAC constructs from which the β gene have been deleted (Peterson et al., 1995). In these mice the γ genes turn off after birth, although the β genes are absent; this argues against the hypothesis that γ-gene silencing is the result of competition by the β gene. The second type of experiment tested the effect of gene order on gene expression. When the globin gene is placed close to the LCR (in front or in the place of the ε gene) it is expressed in the embryonic cells and remains active throughout development (Dillon et al., 1997; Peterson et al., in preparation). When the gene is placed in the same position, it is expressed in the embryonic and the early fetal liver cells but it is turned off postnatally, as expected if γ-gene silencing is autonomous (Peterson et al., in preparation).

Very little is known about the molecular events that lead to the autonomous silencing of the γ gene. Indeed, only one silencing element has been identified so far, and it is located in the upstream γ-gene promoter (Stamatoyannopoulos et al., 1993).

Gene Competition

The initial observation that led to the formulation of the competition model was made in transgenic mice carrying either the β- or the γ-globin gene or both genes linked to the LCR. When the genes were alone, developmental control was lost. When the genes were linked together, developmental control was restored. Such findings led to the proposal that the β-globin gene is regulated through competition with the γ-globin genes and vice versa (Behringer et al., 1990; Enver et al., 1990). The hypothesis is that in the embryonic stage, the LCR interacts with the ε-globin gene; the downstream genes are being turned off competitively. In the fetus, ε is silenced, and the LCR interacts with the Gγ and Aγ genes; the β gene is transcribed less efficiently. In the adult, the γ genes are silenced, and the LCR now interacts with the β-globin gene, the last available gene (Fig. 7.4).

Two conditions influence the probability of interaction of a gene with the LCR: the prevailing transcriptional environment and the distance from the LCR. The trans-acting factors that are likely to facilitate the interaction of the LCR with the ε- or γ-gene promoters

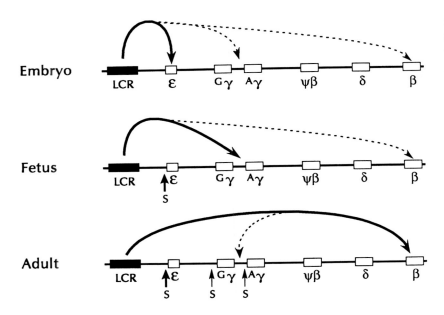

Figure 7.4. Model of the competitive control of hemoglobin switching. "S" indicates the activity of a silencer element.

include the FKLFs and the SSP. EKLF is the factor that participates in the interaction between β-gene promoter and the LCR. In addition to the *trans*-acting factors, gene order and proximity to the LCR are important in determining a gene's competitive advantage for interaction with the LCR (Hanscombe et al., 1991; Peterson and Stamatoyannopoulos, 1993). The closer the gene, the higher this advantage is. Its placement in the 3′ end of the locus explains why the β gene is totally shut off in the embryonic cells when it is placed in its normal chromosomal location, while it is always expressed in the embryo if it is placed close to the LCR.

In situ hybridization methods have allowed the visualization of the interaction of globin genes with the LCR (Wijgerde et al., 1995; Fraser and Grosveld, 1998). This element interacts with only one promoter of the locus at a given time, and switching essentially represents a change in frequency of interaction of the LCR with either the γ- or the β-gene promoter.

Control of HbF in the Adult

One of the most interesting characteristics of human γ- to β-switching is its leakiness and the continuation of synthesis of small amounts of HbF in the adult. This has been known since the time the alkali denaturation method was used for HbF quantitation, but its significance was only realized when immunofluorescent methods were used to stain peripheral blood smears. These methods were first applied in the mid-1960s and they were rediscovered in the 1970s. It was then real-

ized that this residual γ-globin expression is restricted to a minority of cells, the F-cells. The question was then raised of how these F-cells are formed. Initially, clonal hypotheses (reviewed earlier in this chapter) were proposed to explain the F-cells: They were the progeny of fetal stem cell clones. Major insights into the understanding of the control of HbF in the adult were obtained through analyses of HbF expression in erythroid cultures and through observations in patients with activated erythropoiesis.

The first clue on mechanisms came from studies in erythroid cultures, which showed that high levels of HbF are characteristic of colonies produced by adult origin erythroid burst-forming units (BFU-e) (Papayannopoulou et al., 1976, 1977). In these colonies HbF was not uniformly distributed but the clones were usually composed of erythroblasts that contained both HbF and HbA, and those that contain only HbA. These observations indicated that the production of F-cells was related to the phenomenon of erythroid cell differentiation (Papayannopoulou et al., 1977).

The second clue on mechanisms came from the realization that rapid regeneration of the erythroid marrow induces F-cell production (reviewed in Stamatoyannopoulos et al., 1985). For example, increased F-cell production is characteristic of bone marrow regeneration following bone marrow transplantation (Alter et al., 1976) (this phenomenon was initially attributed to the selection of a "fetal" stem cell clone) and of the recovery from the aplastic phase of erythroblastopenia of childhood (Papayannopoulou et al., 1980), following chemotherapeutic ablation of bone marrow (Sheridan et al., 1976) and following acute hemolysis (Papayannopoulou et al., 1980). Experimental acute bleeding in baboons or in humans activated γ-globin production (DeSimone et al., 1978; Nute et al., 1980; Papayannopoulou et al., 1980). Proof that acute erythropoietic stress can induce HbF production was obtained when baboons were treated with high doses of recombinant erythropoietin and responded with striking elevation of F-cell production (Al-Khatti et al., 1987; Umemura et al., 1988).

It should be mentioned that in contrast to the consistent activation of HbF in acute erythropoietic expansion, with the exception of hemoglobinopathies and congenital hypoplastic anemias, there is no elevation of HbF in most patients with chronic anemias (Ellis and White, 1960). Administration of low doses of erythropoietin to baboons increases the hematocrit but fails to induce HbF (Al-Khatti et al., 1987). Following acute bleeding there is a surge of F-reticulocyte production, but when chronic anemia is instituted the number of F-reticulocytes falls (Nute et al., 1980; Stamatoyannopoulos et al., 1985). The difference in the rates of F-cell formation between acute and chronic erythropoietic stress provided strong evidence that the kinetics of erythroid regeneration determine whether a cell will become an F-cell or an A-cell.

The mechanism proposed to explain these phenomena assumes that early progenitors encode a program allowing expression of fetal globin genes, but this program is changed to one allowing only adult globin expression during the downstream differentiation of erythroid progenitor cells (Fig. 7.5) (Papayannopoulou et al., 1977; Stamatoyannopoulos and Papayannopoulou, 1979). Presumably, the earlier progenitor cells contain *trans*-acting factors that favor γ-globin expression, whereas the late progenitors have *trans*-acting factors that favor β-globin expression. F-cells are produced when earlier progenitors become committed prematurely (Stamatoyannopoulos and Papayannopoulou, 1979). In acute erythropoietic stress, the accelerated erythropoiesis will increase the chance of premature commitment of early progenitors, resulting in an increment in production of F-cells. Experimental evidence in support of the hypothesis was obtained by sequential daily measurements of erythroid progenitor pools in baboons treated with high doses of recombinant erythropoietin (Umemura et al., 1988). The major effect of erythropoietin is an acute expansion of the late erythroid progenitors and a mobilization of BFU-e. An increase in F-programmed erythroid colony-forming units (CFU-e; F-CFU-e) accounts for almost all the expansion of CFU-e. The increase in F-CFU-e is followed by a striking increase in F-positive erythroid clusters, which precedes the appearance of F reticulocytes in the circulation (Umemura et al., 1988).

THE CONCEPTUAL BASIS OF PHARMACOLOGIC INDUCTION OF FETAL HEMOGLOBIN SYNTHESIS

The development of methods of pharmacologic induction of HbF synthesis was a direct consequence of the studies on the cellular control of HbF in the adult. Cytotoxic drugs were initially used to test, in experimental animals, hypotheses of cellular control of HbF in the adult. Their application in clinical medicine followed.

The origin of the use of cytotoxic drugs for HbF induction can be traced to the debate about the mechanism whereby 5-azacytidine stimulates HbF production. In order to test the hypothesis that DNA demethylation can activate gene expression, DeSimone et al. (1982) treated anemic juvenile baboons with

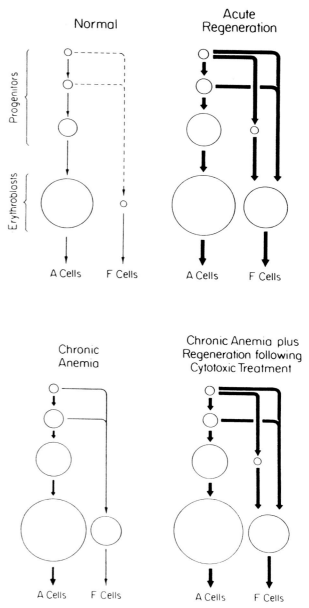

Figure 7.5. Model of regulation of fetal hemoglobin and F-cell production in the adult following acute erythroid regeneration or treatment with cytotoxic drugs such as hydroxyurea.

escalating doses of 5-azacytidine; a striking augmentation of HbF production occurred. Induction of HbF was subsequently demonstrated in patients with homozygous β thalassemia (Ley et al., 1982). At this stage debate started. This cytotoxic compound is expected to kill the most actively cycling erythroid cells. The resulting decrease in late erythroid progenitor cells could trigger rapid erythroid regeneration and induce F-cell formation. Therefore, it was argued, the induction of HbF was not simply due to the demethylating effect of 5-azacytidine but to its cytotoxicity that triggers secondary erythroid regeneration. Measurements of erythroid progenitor cell pools in baboons treated with 5-azacytidine supported this hypothesis (Torrealba de Ron et al., 1984).

To test whether cytoreduction and the ensuing secondary erythroid regeneration were the cause of HbF induction by 5-azacytidine, it was asked whether other cytotoxic compounds producing similar perturbations of erythropoiesis but not DNA demethylation would also induce F-cell formation (Papayannopoulou et al., 1984). Baboons treated with cytotoxic doses of ara-C responded with striking elevations of F-reticulocytes with kinetics indistinguishable from those elicited by 5-azacytidine (Papayannopoulou et al., 1994). Induction of γ globin also occurred in monkeys or baboons treated with hydroxyurea (Letvin et al., 1984; Papayannopoulou et al., 1984). Vinblastine, an M stage-specific agent that arrests cells in mitosis, also produces perturbations of erythropoiesis and stimulates HbF synthesis in baboons (Veith et al., 1985). Following these studies, hydroxyurea was used for induction of HbF in humans (see Chapter 38). Although other hypotheses for the mechanisms of action of hydroxyurea have been proposed, it is fair to say that the regeneration mechanism of action is almost uniformly accepted, although the origins of the conceptual explanation of this phenomenon are usually forgotten (Fibach et al., 1993; Platt and Falcone, 1995; Steinberg et al., 1997).

The pharmacologic induction of HbF through the mechanism of late progenitor cell cytotoxicity is practically at a dead end regarding drug discovery. It is unlikely that a compound better than hydroxyurea can be found. The molecular or cell biological basis of this mechanism remains unexplored. This is regrettable because considerable new knowledge about the relationship of progenitor cell cycling and globin gene expression could have been gained by molecular analyses of this phenomenon.

Short Chain Fatty Acids

The seminal observation that led to the discovery that these compounds are HbF inducers was that the γ- to β-switch is delayed in infants of diabetic mothers (Perrine et al., 1985). Perrine hypothesized that a metabolite in the blood of diabetic mothers was responsible for this finding and, using experiments in clonal erythroid cultures, she showed that γ-aminobutyric acid, which is elevated in the blood of diabetic mothers, is a fetal hemoglobin inducer (Perrine et al., 1987). Subsequent studies showed that butyrate stimulated globin production in adult baboons (Constantoulakis et al., 1988), and it induced γ globin in erythroid progenitors from adult animals or

patients with sickle cell anemia (Constantoulakis et al., 1988; Perrine et al., 1989). Several other short chain fatty acids were found to increase HbF in adult BFU-e cultures and in baboons (Stamatoyannopoulos et al., 1994; Liakopoulou et al., 1995). Derivatives of short chain fatty acid such as phenylbutyrate (Dover et al., 1994) and valproic acid (Collins et al., 1994; Liakopoulou et al., 1995) induce HbF in vivo. Increased levels of HbF were also recorded in patients showing accumulation of short chain fatty acids (Little et al., 1995; Peters et al., 1998). Butyrate and short chain fatty acid derivatives were used in clinical trials (see Chapter 38).

The induction of HbF by short chain fatty acids is very interesting from the practical and biological points of view. The practical significance lies with the fact that there is a very large number of short chain fatty acid derivatives that are potential inducers of HbF. Therefore, there are ample opportunities for discovering HbF inducers that can be administered orally and are more potent than butyrate. Recent studies with short carbon chain acids such as phenylacetic and phenylalkyl acids (Torkelson et al., 1996) support this premise.

The biological interest stems from the mechanisms of activation of γ-gene expression by short chain fatty acids. The prevailing hypothesis is that they exert their effect through inhibition of histone deacetylase. Histone acetyltransferases catalyze histone acetylation through the transfer of acetyl groups to the amino residues of lysine side chains of the core histones (Kuo et al., 1996; Mizzen et al., 1996; Ogryzko et al., 1996). It is believed that histone acetylation leads to gene activation by weakening the binding of histone to nucleosomal DNA, which makes the DNA subsequently accessible to transcription factors (Vettese-Dadey et al., 1996). Conversely, histone deacetylases are believed to largely mediate gene repression, as deacetylation of histones would allow the histone to bind more tightly to the nucleosomal DNA and displace transcription factors. Thus, the HbF induction observed with compounds having histone deacetylase inhibition activity may occur through mechanisms involving increased histone acetylation levels. However, the exact mechanism whereby the short chain fatty acids affect gene transcription remains unknown. Studies in transgenic mice are compatible with the assumption that the stimulation of HbF synthesis reflects inhibition of silencing rather than activation of transcription (Pace et al., 1994) but the evidence is indirect. It is obvious that the delineation of the mechanisms of stimulation of HbF synthesis by short chain fatty acids will provide new insights into the control of silencing or activation of gene expression.

References

Al-Khatti, A, Veith, RW, Papayannopoulou, Th et al. (1987). Stimulation of fetal hemoglobin synthesis by erythropoietin in baboons. *N. Engl. J. Med.* 317: 415–420.

Alter, BP, Rappeport, JM, Huisman, THJ et al. (1976). Fetal erythropoiesis following bone marrow transplantation. *Blood* 48: 843–853.

Alter, BP, Jackson, BT, Lipton, JM, Piasecki, GJ et al. (1981a). Control of simian fetal hemoglobin switch at the progenitor cell level. *J. Clin. Invest.* 67: 458–466.

Alter, BP, Jackson, BT, Lipton, JM, Piasecki, GJ et al. (1981b). Three classes of erythroid progenitors that regulate hemoglobin synthesis during ontogeny in the primate. In Stamatoyannopoulos, G and Nienhuis, AW editors. *Hemoglobins in development and differentiation.* New York: Alan R. Liss, pp. 331–340.

Antoniou, M, deBoer, E, Habets, G, and Grosveld, F. (1988). The human β-globin gene contains multiple regulatory regions: Identification of one promoter and two downstream enhancers. *EMBO J.* 7: 377–384.

Asano, H, Li, XS, and Stamatoyannopoulos, G. (1999). FKLF, a novel Krüppel-like factor that activates human embryonic and fetal β-like globin genes. *Mol. Cell. Biol.* 19: 3571–3579.

Asano, H, Li, XS, and Stamatoyannopoulos, G. (2000). FKLF-2: A novel *Krüppel*-like transcriptional factor that activates globin and other erythroid lineage genes. *Blood* 95: 3578–3584.

Bacolla, A, Ulrich, MJ, Larson, JE et al. (1995). An intramolecular triplex in the human gamma-globin 5'-flanking region is altered by point mutations associated with hereditary persistence of fetal hemoglobin. *J. Biol. Chem.* 270: 24556–24563.

Bard, H, Makowski, EL, Meschia, G, and Battaglia, F. C. (1970). The relative rates of synthesis of hemoglobins A and F in immature red cells of newborn infants. *Pediatrics* 45: 766–772.

Beaupain, D, Martin, C, and Dieterlen-Lievre, F. (1981). Origin and evolution of hemopoietic stem cells in the avian embryo. In Stamatoyannopoulos, G and Nienhuis, AW, editors. *Hemoglobins in development and differentiation.* New York: Alan R. Liss, pp. 161–169.

Behringer, RR, Hammer, RE, Brinster, RL et al. (1987). Two 3' sequences direct adult erythroid-specific expression of human β-globin genes in transgenic mice. *Proc. Natl. Acad. Sci. U.S.A.* 84: 7056–7060.

Behringer, RR, Ryan, TM, Palmiter, RD et al. (1990). Human γ- to β-globin gene switching in transgenic mice. *Genes Dev.* 4: 380–389.

Bender, MA, Bulger, M, Close, J, and Groudine, M. (2000). β-globin gene switching and DNase I sensitivity of the endogenous β-globin locus in mice do not require the locus control region. *Mol. Cell* 5: 387–393.

Berry, M, Grosveld, F, and Dillon, NA. (1992). A single point mutation is the cause of the Greek form of hereditary persistence of foetal haemoglobin. *Nature* 358: 499–502.

Bodine, DM, and Ley, TJ. (1987). An enhancer element lies 3' to the human ^Aγ globin gene. *EMBO J.* 6: 2997–3004.

Boyer, SH, Belding, TK, Margolet, L, and Noyes, AN. (1975). Fetal hemoglobin restriction to a few erythrocytes (F cells) in normal human adults. *Science* 188: 361–363.

Brotherton, TW, Chui, DHK, Gauldie, J, and Patterson, M. (1979). Hemoglobin ontogeny during normal mouse fetal development. *Proc. Natl. Acad. Sci. U.S.A.* 76: 2853–2857.

Cao, SX, Gutman, PD, Davie, HP, and Schechter, AN. (1989). Identification of a transcriptional silencer in the 5'-flanking region of the human ε-globin gene. *Proc. Natl. Acad. Sci. U.S.A.* 86: 5306–5309.

Chapman, BS and Tobin, AJ. (1979). Distribution of developmentally regulated hemoglobins in embryonic erythroid populations. *Dev. Biol.* 69: 375–387.

Collins, AF, Dover, GJ, and Luban, NL. (1994). Increased fetal hemoglobin production in patients receiving valproic acid for epilepsy. *Blood* 84: 1690–1691.

Constantoulakis, P, Papayannopoulou, Th, and Stamatoyannopoulos, G. (1988). γ-Amino-N-butyric acid stimulates fetal hemoglobin in the adult. *Blood* 72: 1961–1967.

Curtin, P, Pirastu, M, Kan, YW et al. (1985). A distant gene deletion affects β-globin gene function in an atypical β-thalassemia. *J. Clin. Invest.* 76: 1554–1558.

deBoer, E, Antoniou, M, Mignotte, V et al. (1988). The human β-globin promoter; nuclear protein factors and erythroid specific induction of transcription. *EMBO J.* 7: 4203–4212.

della Torre, L and Meroni, P. (1969). Studi sul sangue fetole nota I: Livelli di emoglobina fetale e adulta nella gravidanza fisio-logica; relazione con la maturita fetal. *Ann. Ostet. Ginecol.* 91: 148.

DeSimone, J, Biel, SI, and Heller, P. (1978). Stimulation of fetal hemoglobin synthesis in baboons by hemolysis and hypoxia. *Proc. Natl. Acad. Sci. U.S.A.* 75: 2937–2940.

DeSimone, J, Heller, P, Hall, L, and Zwiers, D. (1982). 5-Azacytidine stimulates fetal hemoglobin synthesis in anemic baboons. *Proc. Natl. Acad. Sci. U.S.A.* 79: 4428–4431.

Dickinson, LA, Joh, T, Kohwi, Y, and Kohwi-Shigematsu, T. (1992). A tissue-specific MAR/SAR DNA-binding protein with unusual binding site recognition. *Cell* 70: 631–645.

Dillon, N and Grosveld, F. (1991). Human gamma-globin genes silenced independently of other genes in the beta-globin locus. *Nature* 350: 252–254.

Dillon, N, Trimborn, T, Strouboulis, J et al. (1997). The effect of distance on long-range chromatin interactions. *Mol. Cell* 1: 131–139.

Donze, D, Townes, TM, and Bieker, JJ. (1995). Role of erythroid Kruppel-like factor in human γ- to β-globin gene switching. *J. Biol. Chem.* 270: 1955–1959.

Dover, GJ, Brusilow, S, and Charache, S. (1994). Induction of fetal hemoglobin production in subjects with sickle cell anemia by oral sodium phenylbutyrate. *Blood* 84: 339–343.

Driscoll, MC, Dobkin, CS, and Alter, BP. (1989). β-Thalassemia due to a de novo mutation deleting the 5'β -globin gene activation-region hypersensitive sites. *Proc. Natl. Acad. Sci. U.S.A.* 86: 7470–7474.

Ellis, MJ and White, JC. (1960). Studies on human foetal haemoglobin. II. Foetal haemoglobin levels in healthy children and adults and in certain haematological disorders. *J. Haematol.* 6: 201.

Enver, T, Raich, N, Ebens, AJ et al. (1990). Developmental regulation of human fetal-to-adult globin gene switching in transgenic mice. *Nature* 344: 309–313.

Epner, E, Reik, A, Cimbora, D et al. (1998). The β-globin LCR is not necessary for an open chromatin structure or developmentally regulated transcription of the native mouse beta-globin locus. *Mol. Cell.* 2: 447–455.

Feng, WC, Southwood, CM, and Bieker, JJ. (1994). Analyses of beta-thalassemia mutant DNA interactions with erythroid Kruppel-like factor (EKLF), an erythroid cell-specific transcription factor. *J. Biol. Chem.* 269: 1493–1500.

Fibach, E, Burke, LP, Schechter, AN et al. (1993). Hydroxyurea increases fetal hemoglobin in cultured erythroid cells derived from normal individuals and patients with sickle cell anemia or β-thalassemia. *Blood* 81: 1630–1635.

Filipe, A, Li, Q, Deveaux, S et al. (1999). Regulation of embryonic/fetal globin genes by nuclear hormone receptors: A novel perspective on hemoglobin switching. *EMBO J.* 18: 687–697.

Forrester, WC, Thompson, C, Elder, JT, and Groudine, M. (1986). A developmentally stable chromatin structure in the human beta-globin gene cluster. *Proc. Natl. Acad. Sci. U.S.A.* 83: 1359–1363.

Forrester, WC, Epner, E, Driscoll, MC et al. (1990). A deletion of the human β-globin locus activation region causes a major alteration in chromatin structure and replication across the entire β-globin locus. *Genes Dev.* 4: 1637–1649.

Fraser, P, and Grosveld, F. (1998). Locus control regions, chromatin activation and transcription. *Curr Opin. Cell Biol.* 10: 361–365.

Fraser, P, Pruzina, S, Antoniou, M, and Grosveld, F. (1993). Each hypersensitive site of the human beta-globin locus control region confers a different developmental pattern of expression on the globin genes. *Genes Dev.* 7: 106–113.

Fucharoen, S, Shimizu, K, and Fukumaki, Y. (1990). A novel C-T transition within the distal CCAAT motif of the ᴳγ-globin gene in the Japanese HPFH: Implication of factor binding in elevated fetal globin expression. *Nucleic Acids Res.* 18: 5245–5253.

Gale, RE, Clegg, JB, and Huehns, ER. (1979). Human embryonic haemoglobins Gower 1 and Gower 2. *Nature* 280: 162–164.

Gong, Q, and Dean, A. (1993). Enhancer-dependent transcription of the ε-globin promoter requires promoter-bound GATA-1 and enhancer-bound AP-1/NF-E2. *Mol. Cell. Biol.* 13: 911–917.

Gong, Q-H, Stern, J, and Dean, A. (1991). Transcriptional role of a conserved GATA-1 site in the human ε-globin gene promoter. *Mol. Cell. Biol.* 11: 2558–2566.

Grosveld, F. (1999). Activation by locus control regions? *Curr. Opin. Genet. Dev.* 9: 152–157.

Grosveld, F, van Assendelft, GB, Greaves, DR, and Kollias, G. (1987). Position-independent, high-level expression of the human β-globin gene in transgenic mice. *Cell* 51: 975–985.

Gumucio, DL, Rood, KL, Gray, TA et al. (1988). Nuclear proteins that bind the human γ-globin gene promoter: Alterations in binding produced by point mutations associated with hereditary persistence of fetal hemoglobin. *Mol. Cell. Biol.* 8: 5310–5322.

Gumucio, DL, Heilstedt-Williamson, H, Gray, TA et al. (1992). Phylogenetic footprinting reveals a nuclear protein which binds to silencer sequences in the human ε and γ globin genes. *Mol. Cell. Biol.* 12: 4919–4929.

Hanscombe, O, Whyatt, D, Fraser, P, Yannoutsos, N et al. (1991). Importance of globin gene order for correct developmental expression. *Genes Dev.* 5: 1387–1394.

Hartzog, GA and Myers, RM. (1993). Discrimination among potential activators of the β-globin CACCC element by correlation of binding and transcriptional properties. *Mol. Cell. Biol.* 13: 44–56.

Hecht, F, Motulsky, AG, Lemire, RJ, and Shepard, TE. (1966). Predominance of hemoglobin Gower 1 in early human embryonic development. *Science* 152: 91–92.

Higgs, DR. (1998). Do LCRs open chromatin domains? *Cell* 95: 299–302.

Holliday, R and Pugh, JE. (1975). DNA modification mechanisms and gene activity during development. *Science* 187: 226–232.

Huehns, ER, Dance, N, Beaven, GH et al. (1964). Human embryonic haemoglobins. *Nature* 201: 1095.

Ingram, VM. (1972). Embryonic red cell formation. *Nature* 235: 338–339.

Jane, SM, Ney, PA, Vanin, EF et al. (1992). Identification of a stage selector element in the human γ-globin gene promoter that fosters preferential interaction with the 5′ HS2 enhancer when in competition with the β-promoter. *EMBO J.* 11: 2961–2969.

Jane, SM, Gumucio, DL, Ney, PA et al. (1993). Methylation enhanced binding of Sp1 to the stage selector element of the human γ-globin gene promoter may regulate developmental specificity of expression. *Mol. Cell. Biol.* 13: 3272–3281.

Jane, SM, Nienhuis, AW, and Cunningham, JM. (1995). Hemoglobin switching in man and chicken is mediated by a heteromeric complex between the ubiquitous transcription factor CP2 and a developmentally specific protein. *EMBO J.* 14: 97–105.

Kuo, MH, Brownell, JE, Sobel, RE et al. (1996). Transcription-linked acetylation by Gen5p of histones H3 and H4 at specific lysines. *Nature* 383: 269–272.

Le Douarin, N. (1978). Ontogeny of hematopoietic organs studied in avian embryo interspecific chimeras. In Clarkson, B, Marks, PA, and Till, J, editors. *Differentiation in normal and neoplastic hemopoietic cells.* New York: Cold Spring Harbor, pp. 5–31.

Letvin, NL, Linch, DC, Beardsley, GP et al. (1984). Augmentation of fetal-hemoglobin production in anemic monkeys by hydroxyurea. *N. Engl. J. Med.* 310: 869–873.

Ley, TJ, DeSimone, J, Anagnou, NP et al. (1982). 5-Azacytidine selectively increases γ globin synthesis in a patient with β⁺ thalassemia. *N. Engl. J. Med.* 307: 1469–1475.

Li, J, Noguchi, CT, Miller, W et al. (1998). Multiple regulatory elements in the 5′ flanking sequence of the human epsilon-globin gene. *J. Biol. Chem.* 273: 10202–10209.

Li, Q and Stamatoyannopoulos, JA. (1994). Position independence and proper developmental control of γ-globin gene expression require both a 5′ locus control region and a downstream sequence element. *Mol. Cell. Biol.* 14: 6087–6096.

Li, Q, Clegg, C, Peterson, K et al. (1997). Binary transgenic mouse model for studying the trans control of globin gene switching: Evidence that GATA-1 is an in vivo repressor of human epsilon gene expression. *Proc. Natl. Acad. Sci. U.S.A.* 94: 2444–2448.

Li, Q, Blau, CA, Clegg, CH et al. (1998). Multiple ε-promoter elements participate in the developmental control of ε-globin genes in transgenic mice. *J. Biol. Chem.* 273: 17361–17367.

Liakopoulou, E, Blau, CA, Li, Q et al. (1995). Stimulation of fetal hemoglobin production by short chain fatty acids. *Blood* 86: 3227–3235.

Little, JA, Dempsey, NJ, Tuchman, M, and Ginder, GD. (1995). Metabolic persistence of fetal hemoglobin. *Blood* 85: 1712–1718.

Liu, Q, Bungert, J, and Engel, JD. (1997). Mutation of gene-proximal regulatory elements disrupts human epsilon-, gamma- and beta-globin expression in yeast artificial chromosome transgenic mice. *Proc. Natl. Acad. Sci. U.S.A.* 94: 169–174.

Liu, Q, Tanimoto, K, Bungert, J, and Engel, JD. (1998). The A-gamma globin 3′ element provides no unique function(s) for human β-globin locus gene regulation. *Proc. Natl. Acad. Sci. U.S.A.* 95: 9944–9949.

Magis, W and Martin, DI. (1995). HMG-I binds to GATA motifs: Implications for an HPFH syndrome. *Biochem. Biophys. Res. Commun.* 214: 927–933.

Mantovani, R, Malgaretti, N, Nicolis, S et al. (1988). The effects of HPFH mutations in the human γ-globin promoter on binding of ubiquitous and erythroid specific nuclear factors. *Nucleic Acids Res.* 16: 7783–7797.

Mantovani, R, Superti-Furga, G, Gilman, J, and Ottolenghi, S. (1989). The deletion of the distal CCAAT box region of the Aγ-globin gene in Black HPFH abolishes the binding of the erythroid specific protein NFE3 and of the CCAAT displacement protein. *Nucleic Acids Res.* 17: 6681–6691.

Marin, M, Karis, A, Visser, P et al. (1997). Transcription factor Sp1 is essential for early embryonic development but dispensable for cell growth and differentiation. *Cell* 89: 619–628.

McDonagh, KT, and Nienhuis, AW. (1991). Induction of the human γ-globin gene promoter in K562 cells by sodium butyrate: Reversal of repression by CCAAT displacement protein. *Blood* 78: 255a.

McDonagh, KT, Lin, HJ, Lowrey, CH et al. (1991). The upstream region of the human γ-globin gene promoter. Identification and functional analysis of nuclear protein binding sites. *J. Biol. Chem.* 266: 11965–11974.

Melis, M, Demopulos, G, Najfeld, V et al. (1987). A chromosome 11-linked determinant controls fetal globin expression and the fetal-to-adult globin switch. *Proc. Natl. Acad. Sci. U.S.A.* 84: 8105–8109.

Miller, IJ, and Bieker, JJ. (1993). A novel, erythroid cell-specific murine transcription factor that binds to the CACCC element and is related to the Kruppel family of nuclear proteins. *Mol. Cell. Biol.* 13: 2776–2786.

Milot, E, Strouboulis, J, Trimborn, T et al. (1996). Heterochromatin effects on the frequency and duration of LCR-mediated gene transcription. *Cell* 87: 105–114.

Mizzen, CA, Yang, XJ, Kokubo, T et al. (1996). The TAF(II)250 subunit of TFIID has histone acetyltransferase activity. *Cell* 87: 1261–1270.

Navas, PA, Peterson, KR, Li, Q et al. (1998). Developmental specificity of the interaction between the locus control region and embryonic or fetal globin genes in transgenic mice with an HS3 core deletion. *Mol. Cell. Biol.* 18: 4188–4196.

Nute, PE, Papayannopoulou, Th, Chen, P, and Stamatoyannopoulos, G. (1980). Acceleration of F-cell production in response to experimentally induced anemia in adult baboons *(Papio cynocephalus)*. *Am. J. Hematol.* 8: 157–168

Ogryzko, VV, Schiltz, RL, Russanova, V et al. (1996). The transcriptional coactivators p300 and CBP are histone acetyltransferases. *Cell* 87: 953–995.

Pace, B, Li, Q, Peterson, K, and Stamatoyannopoulos, G. (1994). γ-amino butyric acid cannot reactivate the silenced γ gene of the locus βYAC transgenic mouse. *Blood* 84: 4344–4353.

Pace, BS, Li, Q, and Stamatoyannopoulos, G. (1996). In vivo search for butyrate responsive sequences using transgenic mice carrying Aγ gene promoter mutants. *Blood* 88: 1079–1083.

Papayannopoulou, Th, Brice, M, and Stamatoyannopoulos, G. (1976). Stimulation of fetal hemoglobin synthesis in bone marrow cultures from adult individuals. *Proc. Natl. Acad. Sci. U.S.A.* 73: 2033–2037.

Papayannopoulou, Th, Brice M, and Stamatoyannopoulos, G. (1977). Hemoglobin F synthesis in vitro: Evidence for control at the level of primitive erythroid stem cells. *Proc. Natl. Acad. Sci. U.S.A.* 74: 2923–2927.

Papayannopoulou, Th, Vichinsky, E, and Stamatoyannopoulos, G. (1980). Fetal Hb production during acute erythroid expansion. I. Observations in patients with transient erythroblastopenia and postphlebotomy. *Br. J. Haematol.* 44: 535–546.

Papayannopoulou, Th, Shepard, TH, and Stamatoyannopoulos, G. (1983). Studies of hemoglobin expression in erythroid cells of early human fetuses using anti-β and anti-α-globin chain fluorescent antibodies. In Stamatoyannopoulos, G and Nienhuis, AW, editors. *Globin gene expression and hemopoietic differentiation*. New York: Alan R. Liss, pp. 421–430.

Papayannopoulou, Th, Torrealba de Ron, A, Veith, R et al. Arabinosylcytosine induces fetal hemoglobin in baboons by perturbing erythroid cell differentiation kinetics. *Science* 224: 617–619.

Papayannopoulou, Th, Brice, M, and Stamatoyannopoulos, G. (1986). Analysis of human globin switching in MEL × human fetal erythroid cell hybrids. *Cell* 46: 469–476.

Perrine, SP, Green, MF, and Faller, DV. (1985). Delay in the fetal globin switch in infants of diabetic mothers. *N. Engl. J. Med.* 312: 334–338.

Perrine, SP, Miller, BA, Greene, MF et al. (1987). Butyric acid analogues augment gamma globin gene expression in neonatal erythroid progenitors. *Biochem. Biophys. Res. Commun.* 148: 694–700.

Perrine, SP, Miller, BA, Faller, DV et al. (1989). Sodium butyrate enhances fetal globin gene expression in erythroid progenitors of patients with Hb SS and thalassemia. *Blood* 74: 454–459.

Peschle, C, Migliaccio, AR, Migliaccio, G et al. (1984). Embryonic to fetal Hb switch in humans: Studies on erythroid bursts generated by embryonic progenitors from yolk sac and liver. *Proc. Natl. Acad. Sci. U.S.A.* 81: 2416–2420.

Peters, A, Rohloff, D, Kohlmann, T et al. (1998). Fetal hemoglobin in starvation ketosis of young women. *Blood* 91: 691–694.

Peters, B, Merezhinskaya, N, Diffley, JFX, and Noguchi, CT. (1993). Protein-DNA interactions in the ε-globin gene silencer. *J. Biol. Chem.* 268: 3430–3437.

Peterson, KR and Stamatoyannopoulos, G. (1993). Role of gene order in developmental control of human γ- and β-globin gene expression. *Mol. Cell. Biol.* 13: 4836–4843.

Peterson, KR, Li, QL, Clegg, CH et al. (1995). Use of yeast artificial chromosomes (YACs) in studies of mammalian development: Production of β-globin locus YAC mice carrying human globin developmental mutants. *Proc. Natl. Acad. Sci.* 92: 5655–5659.

Platt, OS. and Falcone, JF. (1995). Membrane protein interactions in sickle red blood cells: Evidence of abnormal protein 3 function. *Blood* 86: 1992–1998.

Ponce, E, Lloyd, JA, Pierani, A et al. (1991). Transcription factor OTF-1 interacts with two distinct DNA elements in the ᴬγ-globin gene promoter. *Biochemistry* 30: 2961–2967.

Purucker, M, Bodine, D, Lin, H et al. (1990). Structure and function of the enhancer 3′ to the human ᴬγ globin gene. *Nucleic Acids Res.* 18: 7407–7415.

Raich, N, Enver, T, Nakamoto, B et al. (1990). Autonomous developmental control of human embryonic globin gene switching in transgenic mice. *Science* 250: 1147–1149.

Raich, N, Papayannopoulou, T, Stamatoyannopoulos, G, and Enver, T. (1992). Demonstration of a human ε-globin gene silencer with studies in transgenic mice. *Blood* 79: 861–864.

Raich, N, Clegg, CH, Grofti, J, Romeo, PH et al. (1995). GATA1 and YY1 are developmental repressors of the human epsilon-globin gene. *EMBO J.* 14: 801–809.

Reik, A, Telling, A, Zitnik, G et al. (1998). The locus control region is necessary for gene expression in the human beta-globin locus but not the maintenance of an open chromatin structure in erythroid cells. *Mol. Cell. Biol.* 18: 5992–6000.

Ronchi, AE, Bottardi, S, Mazzucchelli, C et al. (1995). Differential binding of the NFE3 and CP1/NFY transcription factors to the human gamma- and epsilon-globin CCAAT boxes. *J. Biol. Chem.* 270: 21934–21941.

Ronchi, A, Berry, M, Raguz, S et al. (1996). Role of the duplicated CCAAT box region in γ-globin gene regulation and hereditary persistence of fetal haemoglobin. *EMBO J.* 15: 143–149.

Sheridan, BL, Weatherall, DJ, Clegg, JB et al. (1976). The patterns of fetal haemoglobin production in leukaemia. *Br. J. Haematol.* 32: 487–506.

Shih, DM, Wall, RJ, and Shapiro, SG. (1990). Developmentally regulated and erythroid-specific expression of the human embryonic β-globin gene in transgenic mice. *Nucleic Acids Res.* 18: 5465–5472.

Skalnik, DG, Strauss, EC, and Orkin, SH. (1991). CCAAT displacement protein as a repressor of the myelomonocytic-specific gp91-phox gene promoter. *J. Biol. Chem.* 266: 16736–16744.

Stamatoyannopoulos, G and Nienhuis, AW. (1994). Hemoglobin switching. In Stamatoyannopoulos, G, Nienhuis, AW, Majerus, P, and Varmus, H, editors. *Molecular basis of blood diseases*, 2nd Ed. Philadelphia: WB Saunders Co. pp. 107–154.

Stamatoyannopoulos, G and Papayannopoulou, Th. (1979). Fetal hemoglobin and the erythroid stem cell differentiation process. In Stamatoyannopoulos, G and Nienhuis, AW, editors: *Cellular and molecular regulation of hemoglobin switching*. New York: Grune & Stratton, pp. 323–349.

Stamatoyannopoulos, G, Blau, CA, Nakamoto, B et al. (1974). Fetal hemoglobin induction by acetate, a product of butyrate catabolism. *Blood* 84: 3198–3204.

Stamatoyannopoulos, G, Veith, R, Galanello, R, and Papayannopoulou, Th. (1985). Hb F production in stressed erythropoiesis: Observations and kinetic models. *Ann. N.Y. Acad. Sci.* 445: 188–197.

Stamatoyannopoulos, G, Constantoulakis, P, Brice, M et al. (1987). Coexpression of embryonic, fetal, and adult globins in erythroid cells of human embryos: Relevance to the cell-lineage models of globin switching. *Dev. Biol.* 123: 191–197.

Stamatoyannopoulos, G, Josephson, B, Zhang, JW, and Li, Q. (1993). Developmental regulation of human gamma-globin genes in transgenic mice. *Mol. Cell. Biol.* 13: 7636–7644.

Stamatoyannopoulos, J, Clegg, CH, and Li, Q. (1997). Sheltering of γ-globin expression from position effects requires both an upstream locus control region and a regulatory element 3′ to the ᴬγ-globin gene. *Mol. Cell. Biol.* 17: 240–247.

Stanworth, SJ, Roberts, NA, Sharpe, JA et al. (1995). Established epigenetic modifications determine the expression of developmentally regulated globin genes in somatic cell hybrids. *Mol. Cell. Biol.* 15: 3969–3978.

Steinberg, MH, Lu, Z-H, Barton, FB et al. and the Multicenter Study of Hydroxyurea. (1997). Fetal hemoglobin in sickle cell anemia: Determinants of response to hydroxyurea. *Blood* 89: 1078–1088.

Torkelson, S, White, B, Faller, DV et al., (1996). Erythroid progenitor proliferation is stimulated by phenoxyacetic and phenylalkyl acids. *Blood Cells Mol. Dis.* 22: 150–158.

Torrealba de Ron, A, Papayannopoulou, Th, Knapp, MS et al. (1984). Perturbations in the erythroid marrow progenitor cell pools may play a role in the augmentation of Hb F by 5-azacytidine. *Blood* 63: 201–210.

Trepicchio, WL, Dyer, MA, and Baron, MH. (1993). Developmental regulation of the human embryonic β-like globin gene is mediated by synergistic interactions among multiple tissue- and stage-specific elements. *Mol. Cell. Biol.* 13: 7457–7468.

Tuan, D, Solomon, W, Li, O, and London, IM. (1985). The "β-like-globin" gene domain in human erythroid cells. *Proc. Natl. Acad. Sci. U.S.A.* 82: 6384–6388.

Ulrich, MJ, Gray, WJ, and Ley, TJ. (1992). An intramolecular DNA triplex is disrupted by point mutations associated with hereditary persistence of fetal hemoglobin. *J. Biol. Chem.* 267: 18649–18658.

Umemura, T, Al-Khatti, A, Papayannopoulou, Th, and Stamatoyannopoulos, G. (1988). Fetal hemoglobin synthesis in vivo: Direct evidence for control at the level of erythroid progenitors. *Proc. Natl. Acad. Sci. U.S.A.* 85: 9278–9282.

Van der Ploeg, LH, Konings, A, Oort, M et al. (1980). γ-β-thalassemia studies showing that deletion of the γ- and δ-genes influence β-globin gene expression in man. *Nature* 283: 637–642.

Vanin, EF, Henthorn, PS, Kioussis, D et al. (1983). Unexpected relationships between four large deletions in the human β-globin gene cluster. *Cell* 35: 701–709.

Veith, R, Papayannopoulou, Th, Kurachi, S, and Stamatoyannopoulos, G. (1985). Treatment of baboon with vinblastine: Insights into the mechanisms of pharmacologic stimulation of Hb F in the adult. *Blood* 66: 456–459.

Vettese-Dadey, M, Grant, PA, Hebbes, TR et al. (1996). Acetylation of histone H4 plays a primary role in enhancing transcription factor binding to nucleosomal DNA in vitro. *EMBO J.* 15: 2508–2518.

Wada-Kiyama, Y, Peters, B, and Noguchi, CT. (1992). The ε-globin gene silencer. *J. Biol. Chem.* 267: 11532–11538.

Wall, L, Destroismaisons, N, Delvoye, N, and Guy, LG. (1996). CAAT/enhancer-binding proteins are involved in beta-globin gene expression and are differently expressed in murine erythroleukemia and K562 cells. *J. Biol. Chem.* 271: 16477–16484.

Walters, M, and Martin, DIK. (1992). Functional erythroid promoters created by interaction of the transcription factor GATA-1 with CACCC and AP-1/NFE-2 elements. *Proc. Natl. Acad. Sci. U.S.A.* 89: 10444–10448.

Weatherall, DJ, Edwards, JA, and Donohoe, WTA. (1968). Haemoglobin and red cell enzyme changes in juvenile myeloid leukaemia. *Br. Med. J.* 1: 679–681.

Weatherall, DJ, Clegg, JB, and Wood, WG. (1976). A model for the persistence or reactivation of fetal haemoglobin production. *Lancet* 2: 660–663.

Wijgerde M, Grosveld, F, and Fraser, P. (1995). Transcription complex stability and chromatin dynamics in vivo. *Nature* 377: 209–213.

Wintour, EM, Smith, MB, Bell RJ et al. (1985). The role of fetal adrenal hormones in the switch from fetal to adult globin synthesis in the sheep. *J. Endocrinol.* 104: 165–170.

Wood, WG, Stamatoyannopoulos, G, Lim, G, and Nute, PE. (1975). F-cells in the adult. Normal values and levels in individuals with hereditary and acquired elevations of Hb F. *Blood* 46: 671–682.

Wood, WG, Bunch, C, Kelly, S et al. (1985). Control of haemoglobin switching by a developmental clock? *Nature* 313: 320–323.

Yu, C-Y, Motamed, K, Chen, J et al. (1991). The CACC box upstream of human embryonic ε globin gene binds Sp1 and is a functional promoter element in vitro and in vivo. *J. Biol. Chem.* 266: 8907–8915.

Zanjani, ED, McGlave, PB, Bhakthavathsalan, A, and Stamatoyannopoulos, G. (1979). Sheep fetal haematopoietic cells produce adult haemoglobin when transplanted in the adult animal. *Nature* 280: 495–496.

Zanjani, ED, Lim, G, McGlave, PB et al. (1982). Adult haematopoietic cells transplanted to sheep fetuses continue to produce adult globins. *Nature* 295: 244–246.

Zhou, WL, Clouston, DR, Wang, X et al. (1999). Isolation and characterization of human NF-E4, the tissue restricted component of the stage selector protein complex. *Blood* 94 (Suppl 1): 614a (abstract).

Zitnik, G, Li, Q, Stamatoyannopoulos, G, and Papayannopoulou, Th. (1993). Serum factors can modulate the developmental clock of γ- to β-globin gene switching in somatic cell hybrids. *Mol. Cell. Biol.* 13: 4844–4851.

Zitnik, G, Peterson, K, Stamatoyannopoulos, G, and Papayannopoulou, Th. (1995). Effects of butyrate and glucocorticoids on γ- to β-globin gene switching in somatic cell hybrids. *Mol. Cell. Biol.* 15: 790–795.

8

Posttranscriptional Factors Influencing the Hemoglobin Content of the Red Cell

SHU-CHING HUANG
EDWARD J. BENZ, JR.

BACKGROUND

Transcriptional induction is the major mechanism responsible for the high levels of globin mRNA production during erythropoiesis. Transcriptional activities of the individual globin genes are also the primary determinants of the approximately equal output of α- and β-like globin chains in red cell progenitors. Changes in transcription of these genes account for most of the developmental changes in the predominance of embryonic, fetal, and adult hemoglobins (Chapters 5, 7, and 15). Selective processing, stabilization, and translation ability of individual globin mRNAs play a secondary but nonetheless important role in these processes. Modifications of the final hemoglobin content of both normal red cells and red cells in patients with hemoglobinopathies arise from mechanisms affecting the metabolism of globin mRNA and protein after transcription and biosynthesis. For example, red cells of patients co-inheriting sickle cell trait and α-thalassemia trait typically contain 15 to 30 percent sickle hemoglobin (HbS), instead of the 50 percent HbS predicted from gene dosage and transcription rates (Chapter 29). Similarly, the absence of δ-globin mRNA from normal reticulocytes is due to its posttranscriptional instability (Chapter 6), whereas some mutations causing β thalassemia are dominantly inherited because of the impact of the mutation on the posttranslational stability of the newly synthesized hemoglobin (Chapter 14). Understanding normal human hemoglobin production and the pathophysiology of some hemoglobinopathies thus requires knowledge of normal posttranscriptional events and their disruptions in hemoglobinopathies.

This chapter surveys the major features of posttranscriptional metabolism of globin mRNA and the posttranslational behavior of individual globin chains and hemoglobin tetramers. These factors can be organized into three major categories: (1) events in posttranscriptional mRNA metabolism that modulate the amount of normal mRNA accumulating in the cytoplasm, which include processing of the pre-messenger RNA, transport of mature messenger RNA (mRNA) to the cytoplasm, and stability of normal and abnormal cytoplasmic mRNAs; (2) factors that affect the translational activity of the individual globin mRNAs; translational activity determines the numbers of new globin protein molecules synthesized from each globin mRNA molecule; and (3) the assembly of newly synthesized globin chains into hemoglobin tetramers and the stability of the resulting globins and hemoglobins in erythrocyte cytoplasm. Because each broad area of mRNA and protein metabolism is a complex field of research, a detailed review is beyond the scope of this chapter. Therefore, we provide a brief survey and overview of only the most relevant features of normal pre-mRNA splicing; mRNA transport, translation, stability; globin chain assembly into hemoglobin tetramers; and the stabilities of globin chains and hemoglobin tetramers. We also describe the impact of informative globin gene mutations on the hemoglobin phenotype and clinical features of selected hemoglobinopathies.

POSTTRANSCRIPTIONAL FACTORS AFFECTING THE QUANTITATIVE ACCUMULATION OF MATURE CYTOPLASMIC MESSENGER RNA

Intranuclear Processing, Stability, and Export of mRNAs to the Cytoplasm

The major posttranscriptional events in globin gene expression (Fig. 8.1) can be separated into the following: (1) intranuclear mRNA processing, consisting largely of splicing of the mRNA precursor, polyadenylation of the nascent pre-mRNA, and the addition of the 5′ cap; (2) intranuclear mRNA stability or turnover, about which virtually nothing is known; (3) transport of processed mRNA from nucleus to cytoplasm, about which rudimentary information is avail-

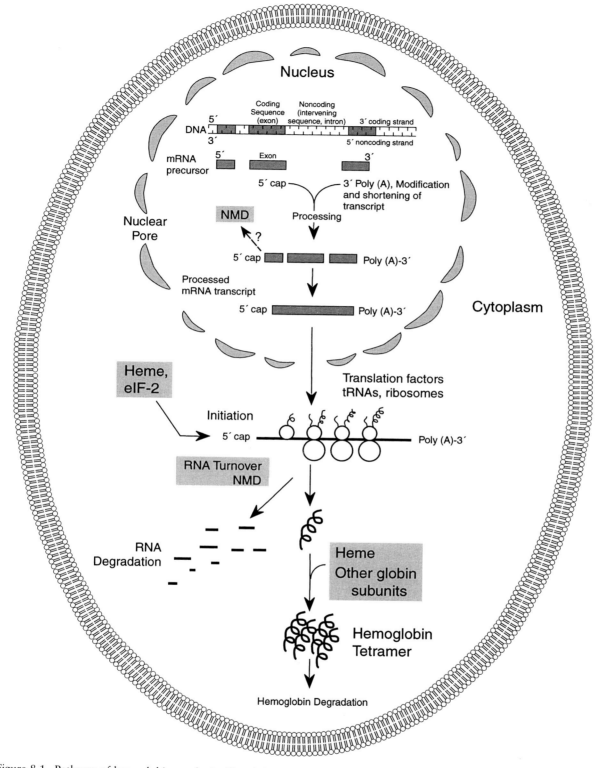

Figure 8.1. Pathway of hemoglobin synthesis. The globin gene is transcribed in the nucleus into an mRNA precursor, which is then spliced into mature mRNA and transported to the cytoplasm where it is translated into globin. The newly synthesized globin chain combines with heme and other globin subunits to form hemoglobin, which is normally degraded very slowly if at all. Key posttranscriptional control points for hemoglobin accumulation are indicated by shading: mRNA turnover, the control of mRNA translation initiation by heme, and the effect of heme and other globin subunits on assembly of the tetramer. NMD, nonsense mediated decay of mutant mRNAs bearing premature terminator codons. See text for details. (Adapted from Berliner and Benz, 1999.)

able; (4) translation of the mRNA into protein in the cytoplasm; (5) cytoplasmic stability or turnover in the cytoplasm; and (6) posttranslational assembly and stability of the translated polypeptides. Of these, mRNA processing, transport, and stability affect the quantitative accumulation of mature cytoplasmic mRNAs. Translational activity and the fate of translated polypeptides are considered in subsequent sections.

Although subdividing posttranscriptional mRNA metabolism into the preceding steps is convenient, the distinctions are arbitrary; in reality, these steps merge and relate to each other in complex ways that make them interdependent. For example, missplicing of transcripts can yield structurally altered mRNAs whose subsequent fate depends on the metabolic machineries controlling mRNA export or stability. An unproven conjecture is that lacking active stabilization mechanisms, mRNA molecules failing to proceed smoothly through all of the posttranscriptional steps of mRNA metabolism will be degraded. Nonetheless, considering splicing, intranuclear turnover and transport, and mRNA stability as discrete entities is useful. Only variable mRNA stability has been shown to have a significant impact, at least for generation of the normal hemoglobin phenotype.

Splicing of pre-mRNA transcripts is nearly universal among eukaryotic genes (see Benz and Huang, 1996, and Berliner and Benz, 1999, for reviews). The splicing mechanism removes transcribed introns and ligates exons together in the precise register needed for translation (Fig. 8.1). Only a few examples of nonspliced mRNAs exist. Splicing, described in Chapter 6, occurs on ribonucleoprotein complexes called spliceosomes. Spliceosomes consist of small nuclear RNAs and their protein-binding partners, often called snRNPs. Many components of spliceosomes have been characterized structurally and their general functions delineated. However, the precise biochemical mechanisms governing the normal patterns of splicing and the regulation of tissue-specific alternative splicing of pre-mRNA transcripts remain incompletely understood.

Selective (or "alternative") splicing appears to play little, if any, role in the normal handling of globin gene transcripts. Each mammalian globin gene contains two introns; every intron is flanked by canonical splice signal sequences, which are strongly recognized by the splicing apparatus (Benz and Huang 1996; Berliner and Benz, 1999). Alternative splicing of normal globin pre-mRNA does not occur, and splicing of all transcripts is 100 percent efficient. Transcription, rather than splicing, is the primary determinant of the amount of mature mRNA generated for export to the cytoplasm. However, globin gene expression is unusual in the sense that splicing out of at least one intron may be absolutely required for the generation of cytoplasmic mRNA

(Hamer and Leder, 1979). Similarly, polyadenylation and addition of the 5' cap seem rapid and quantitative on globin mRNAs. No selective regulatory steps exercised on the individual globin mRNAs at the level of export from nucleus to cytoplasm are present. Thus, intranuclear metabolism of globin pre-mRNAs appears to have little impact on the relative amounts of individual globins accumulating in normal red cells.

Intranuclear globin mRNA metabolism is relevant to understanding how pathologic transcripts are generated in some thalassemic patients. Mutations that alter the signals affecting normal splicing, polyadenylation, or capping are obvious examples (Chapters 12 and 17). Both the amounts and the structures of transcripts resulting from these mutations are often complex and not readily explained by the location or nature of the individual mutations. Further understanding of splicing, polyadenylation, and capping in the nucleus is needed to understand why these aberrant transcripts arise in larger or smaller amounts. Less obvious, but especially interesting, is the potential role of intranuclear mechanisms in modulating the accumulation of thalassemic mRNAs that carry mutations that abolish mRNA translation. As discussed later, the nucleus may play a role in marking, or even degrading, transcripts incapable of normal translation via a mechanism called nonsense-mediated decay. Cytoplasmic mRNA stability has the greatest impact on the development of the normal hemoglobin phenotype at different stages of differentiation and ontogeny.

Cytoplasmic Stability of Mature mRNA

Differential pre-mRNA splicing, other nuclear processing steps, and export of mRNA to the cytoplasm do not appear to affect the erythrocyte hemoglobin profile at various stages of normal differentiation and development. However, selective stabilization or destabilization of globin and nonglobin mRNAs and differential stability of the individual normal globin mRNAs have considerable impact. The transition from embryonic to adult α-like globins, the decline of γ-globin chain synthesis in reticulocytes compared with erythroblasts, and the disappearance of γ-globin biosynthesis in reticulocytes are three prime examples. In addition, the phenomenon of nonsense-mediated decay and the molecular mechanisms leading to thalassemia in patients with Hemoglobin Constant Spring clearly show the important role of mRNA stability in hemoglobinopathies (Chapter 17).

Differential mRNA stability is a critical factor that allows globin mRNA—virtually absent in the early proerythroblast—to account for more than 90 percent of the total mRNA in circulating reticulocytes. The dramatic activation of globin gene transcription at the onset of erythroblast maturation is the critical mechanism responsible for the absolute increase in new globin mRNA molecules produced. However, it has been known for more than 20 years that transcription alone cannot account for the extraordinarily selective accumulation of globin mRNAs during erythroblast development. Aviv et al. (1976) and Bastos et al. (1977) showed that the large pools of preexisting nonglobin mRNAs in early erythroid cells would continue to account for a large percentage of the total mRNA in late erythroid cells if transcription were the only step altered during maturation. Simple addition of new globin mRNA molecules to the mixture—even in the large numbers generated by induced transcription—could not, during the few days of erythroblast maturation, provide for the 90 to 95 percent predominance of globin mRNA at the late stages of differentiation. Rather, one must invoke a mechanism by which nonglobin mRNAs are progressively degraded while globin mRNAs are selectively stabilized in erythroid cell cytoplasm. In other words, the highly specialized devotion of the protein biosynthetic machinery to hemoglobin production during erythropoiesis must perforce involve the selective stabilization of globin mRNAs and/or destabilization of other mRNAs.

Many studies have shown that mRNA stability is an important regulatory mechanism by which the relative concentrations of mRNAs can be modulated in specialized cell types, during differentiation or development, or in response to physiologic or noxious stimuli. Also, the stabilities, or half-lives, of different mRNAs vary widely (Ross, 1995; Liebhaber, 1997). Most eukaryotic mRNAs have half-lives between minutes and a few hours. Some, including, those encoding cell cycle control factors and proto-oncogenes have half-lives of minutes. At the other end of the spectrum are globin mRNAs in erythroblasts, with estimated half-lives of 30 to 50 hours (Aviv et al., 1976; Ross, 1995; Russell et al., 1997; Volloch and Housman, 1981). These mRNAs are thus extraordinarily stable.

The mechanisms governing differential mRNA stability are under active investigation. In cases that have been thoroughly studied, mRNAs of differing stabilities appear to differ primarily in the type of signature sequences present in the 3′ untranslated sequences (3′UTR). For example, many highly labile mRNAs share sequence motifs marked by multiple repetitions of the dinucleotide AU (refer to Liebhaber, 1997, for review). On the other hand, α-globin mRNA, the most thoroughly studied of the highly stable mRNAs, possesses a sequence motif remarkable for being pyrimidine ("CU") rich in its 3′ UTR (Weiss and Liebhaber, 1994, 1995; Wang et al., 1995a). These sequence motifs are recognized by RNA binding proteins, which, in turn,

modulate the interaction of the mRNAs with the degradative machinery present in the cytoplasm (Fig. 8.2). This machinery consists of several interrelated catabolic pathways, primarily characterized in yeast (Culbertson, 1999; Caapoinigro and Parker, 1996; LeGrandeur and Parker, 1998; Tarun and Sachs, 1996).

A particularly common degradative pathway in yeast appears to involve nucleolytic shortening of the poly(A) tail, subsequent removal of the 5′ CAP structure by a decapping enzyme, and finally, dissolution of the "naked" mRNA by a 5′–3′ exonuclease (Culbertson, 1999). This pathway is less well characterized in other species, but deadenylation is clearly a prominent mechanism used in mammalian cells as well (Jacobson and Peltz, 1996). Other pathways that have been detected are probably less prominent. These include direct endonucleolytic cleavage at specific sequence sites in the 3′ UTR (Culbertson, 1999; Jacobson and Peltz, 1996) and direct 5′ decapping, without a requirement for deadenylation. The latter mechanism appears to be especially relevant to erythroid cells because it mediates the phenomenon of nonsense-mediated decay.

Molecular Basis for the Unusually Long Half-Life of Globin mRNAs

Examination of the molecular basis for variable mRNA stability has become a vast field, generating complex hypothetical mechanisms whose relevance to hemoglobin homeostasis is not yet clear. Several excellent reviews have been published (Liebhaber, 1997; Russell et al., 1997; Culbertson, 1999; Jacobson and Peltz, 1996). α-Globin mRNA stability, studied extensively by Leibhaber and co-workers (Liebhaber and Russell, 1998), has contributed the most useful insights about the stable accumulation of globin mRNAs during the later stages of erythropoiesis. The other globin mRNAs, less thoroughly characterized, presumably use a similar mechanism.

The key element contributing to the long half-life of α-globin mRNA is a sequence motif, about 20 bases long, embedded in the 3′ UTR (Fig. 8.2). This sequence is pyrimidine-rich (CU-rich). Leibhaber's group (Makeyev et al., 1999; Chkheidze et al., 1999) has provided convincing evidence that this motif interacts with specific RNA-binding proteins, which they called α CPs. An exciting recent finding has been that α CPs are identical to a family of RNA binding proteins called hnRNP E1 and E2 (hnRNP = heterogenous nuclear ribonucleoproteins) (Ostareck-Lederer et al., 1998). The α-globin mRNA binding proteins are thus members of the KH domain-bearing family of hnRNP (Wang et al., 1995b). The prototype of this protein, hnRNP K, appears to mediate intranuclear processing

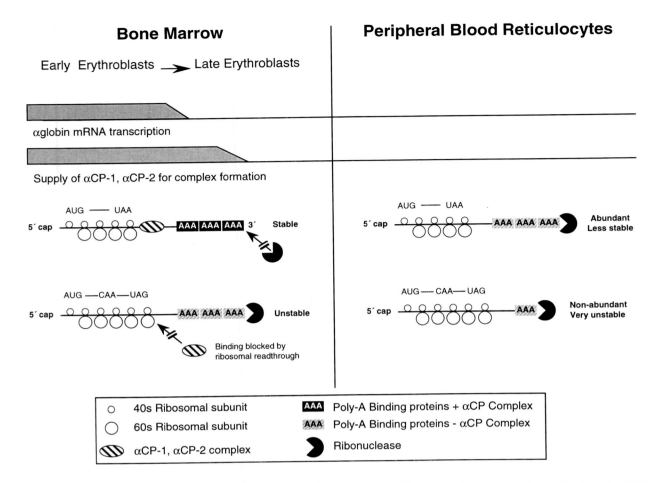

Figure 8.2. Molecular stabilization of α-globin mRNA and its disruption in the hemoglobin Constant Spring (HbCS) form of α thalassemia. Synthesis of α-globin mRNA and the levels of the α CP stabilizing proteins both decline during the mid stages of erythroblast maturation, leaving both more susceptible to degradation in late erythroblasts and circulating reticulocytes, because α CP binding enhances stabilization of the Poly (A) tail by Poly (A) binding proteins. The upper mRNA lines show normal α mRNA; the lower, α^{CS} mRNA, in which α CP binding is blocked by ribosomal read through the α CP binding sites, thus rendering α^{CS} mRNA less stable, even in early erythroblasts. (Adapted from Morales et al., 1997.)

of RNA transcripts, and, possibly, transport from nucleus to cytoplasm or nuclear-cytoplasmic shuttling. hnRNPs E1 and E2 are closely related proteins that were independently identified as RNA binding proteins involved in the translational silencing of reticulocyte 15-lipoxygenase (LOX), and in the replication and cap-independent translation of poliovirus RNA (Ostareck-Lederer et al., 1998). The interaction of hnRNP E1 and E2 and hnRNP K with 15 LOX mRNA blocks the translation of LOX mRNA until the very end-stages of erythropoiesis. This translational silencing is important because LOX catalyzes the degradation of mitochondria, which are required by

erythroblasts until the time of enucleation. hnRNP E1 and E2 thus clearly play a critical function in modulating relative levels of relevant mRNA accumulation and activity during erythropoiesis.

hnRNP E1 and E2 share at least 80 percent homology and are identical, respectively, to α CP1 and α CP2. (Makeyev et al., 1999; Chkheidze et al., 1999; Ostarek-Lederer et al., 1998). The KH domains appear to promote direct binding interactions with the target RNA sequence. Once bound to mRNA, they can promote a variety of effects, depending on the recruitment to the RNP complex of additional proteins that stabilize, destabilize, or modulate the translational potential target mRNA species.

hnRNPs E1 and E2 also appear to serve analogous functions in a variety of nonerythroid tissues. Holcik and Liebhaber (1997) have identified, by DNA database search, at least three other mRNAs containing the pyrimidine-rich 3′ UTR motif. Each of these is a long-lived mRNA; in each case, the high degree of stability appears to depend on the formation of complexes with hnRNP E1 and E2. Studies of α-globin mRNA have thus uncovered a more generalized system for stabilizing mRNAs intended for long-term survival in the cytoplasm.

Less is known about the precise molecular mechanisms governing the long-term stabilities of other human globin mRNAs. Clearly, the key sequence elements also reside in the 3' UTR. Thus, if the 3' UTR of β-globin mRNA is substituted for the 3' UTR of the highly labile G-CSF mRNA, the G-CSF mRNA is stabilized (refer to Ross, 1995; Liebhaber, 1997). Russell and Liebhaber (1996) have shown that the 3' UTR contains stability determinants that maintain β-globin mRNA stability when coupled to the α-globin 3' UTR, but that these elements are different. Two separate mutations necessary for extensive read-through of the 3' UTR were needed to destabilize the β-globin 3' UTR, and destabilization was, curiously, independent of translation, at least at distances less than ten nucleotides into the 3' UTR.

Realizing that some individual globin mRNAs vary considerably in stability is important, although all of them are much longer lived than "typical" mRNA species. For example, δ-globin mRNA is less stable than β-globin mRNA; δ mRNA is virtually absent from circulating reticulocytes, although it accounts for 3 to 5 percent as much mRNA as β-globin mRNA in early erythroblasts. This may be because the half-life of δ mRNA was only 3.5 hours under conditions yielding a half-life of 16.5 hours for β-globin mRNA (Chapter 10) (Ross and Pizarro, 1983). γ- Globin mRNA also appears to be at least slightly less stable than β-globin mRNA (Ross and Sullivan, 1985). Similarly, ζ-globin mRNA is much less stable than α-globin mRNA (Russell et al., 1998a; Liebhaber et al., 1996). Even though the silencing of ζ-globin gene transcription accounts for much of the disappearance of ζ-globin after the first few weeks of gestation, reduced stability of ζ-globin mRNA is necessary for its complete disappearance. Differential mRNA stability thus plays an important role in modifying the final hemoglobin content of normal human red cells.

Hemoglobin Constant Spring, a Form of Thalassemia Caused by Altered mRNA Stability

Study of the molecular basis of α-globin mRNA turnover has provided a molecular explanation for the thalassemic phenotype associated with Hemoglobin Constant Spring (HbCS). As noted in Chapter 17, HbCS contains mutant α-globin chains (α^{CS}) carrying a single base change that converts the normal translation termination codon into a sense codon, thus permitting translational read-through beyond the normal stop signal. The primary translated protein product is an elongated globin chain, 172 amino acids long, rather than the normal 141. The α^{CS} protein is sufficiently stable and functional to allow assembly of an intact, functioning hemoglobin tetramer.

The thalassemic phenotype associated with HbCS is due to a 98 to 99 percent reduction in accumulation of α^{CS} mRNA (Liebhaber and Kan, 1981; Hunt et al., 1982). To a first approximation, transcription of the gene, posttranscriptional handling, and export to the cytoplasm all seem normal; but α^{CS} mRNA has a half-life of only 20 hours, compared with the 60-hour half-life of normal α-globin mRNA (Weiss and Liebhaber, 1994).

Morales et al. (1997) presented convincing evidence that the molecular basis for the extremely low accumulation of α^{CS}-globin mRNA is directly related to the fact that ribosomes read through the translation termination codon, disrupting the normal conformation of the 3' UTR (Fig. 8.2). Ribosomal read-through interferes with the formation of the ribonucleoprotein stabilizing complex mediated by hnRNPs E1 and E2. These studies have also revealed an interesting feature of the subsequent pattern of α^{CS} mRNA degradation. The pathway appears to involve quantal shortening of the poly(A)-tail with a periodicity of 20 to 25 A residues. This shortening appears to occur primarily during the earlier stages of erythroblast maturation. This quantal poly(A) shortening mechanism appears to apply to normal α mRNA as well, but occurs far more slowly, presumably because the stabilizing hnRNP complex interferes with this catabolic process (Fig. 8.2). In reticulocytes, on the other hand, both α^{CS} mRNA and normal α mRNA are degraded more rapidly but at identical rates, indicating, presumably, that the hnRNP E1/E2 complex components are no longer present in sufficient amounts to support formation of the stabilizing complex on normal α mRNA.

Alteration in the stability of mutant globin mRNAs carrying premature terminator codons also plays a role in determining the final molecular and physiologic phenotype of various forms of thalassemia. These modulations are mediated by nonsense-mediated decay, a generalized mechanism present in all eukaryotic cells. Since nonsense-mediated decay represents a special case directly tied to the molecular pathology of mutant genes, it is now considered in more detail.

NONSENSE-MEDIATED DECAY OF NONTRANSLATED mRNAs: A MECHANISM FOR PROTECTING CELLS FROM THE TRANSLATION OF ABNORMAL PROTEIN PRODUCTS

Hemoglobinopathies have often provided the first opportunities to apply evolving techniques of molecular genetics to clinical medicine, one reason that study of hemoglobin carries importance beyond the clinical impact of these disorders worldwide. The discovery of introns and pre-mRNA splicing in eukaryotic single-copy genes is one example. Another is the discovery of nonsense-mediated decay, a basic cellular mechanism uncovered during studies of the unusual behavior of some thalassemic mutant globin mRNAs in human erythroid cells.

Mutations creating premature translation termination codons are a common cause of thalassemia and other genetic disorders (Chapters 12 and 17). One prediction about the cytoplasmic fate of the mRNA of a nonsense mutation is that the mRNA would be present in normal amounts but would support the translation of only the truncated globin fragment that could be assembled before the ribosome encounters the premature termination codon. However, early efforts to identify the predicted protein fragments, even in short-term pulse-labeling studies, were unsuccessful (refer to Benz and Forget, 1974, 1975 for reviews). This led to the hypothesis that RNAs must exist on polyribosomes to be stable in the cytoplasm, and that mRNAs uncovered beyond the point of premature translation termination would be degraded. Evidence in support of this view, however, could never be convincingly assembled.

The first suggestions that nontranslatable mutant mRNAs were handled in a distinct and complex way by cells arose from studies of β^0 thalassemias, where no β globin is produced. In a series of patients with β^0 thalassemia, significantly reduced but readily detectable levels of β mRNA were present in both erythroblasts and reticulocytes (Benz et al., 1978; Temple et al., 1977). In many of these patients, β^0 thalassemia was subsequently shown to be due to mutations that created premature termination, or nonsense, codons (Chang and Kan, 1979).

Background and General Features

One mutation, particularly common in the Mediterranean region, creates a premature termination codon at position 39 of the β-globin chain. Levels of β-globin mRNA in this mutation were reduced to 5 to 10 percent of normal (Takeshita et al., 1984). However, the same low level was detected in both erythroblasts, reticulocytes, and in nuclear and cytoplasmic mRNA, suggesting that the small amounts of mRNA detected were relatively stable. Neither a progressive decline in mRNA in the transition from nucleus to cytoplasm, nor a progressive loss of the mRNA during the enucleated reticulocyte phase was found (Takeshita et al., 1984). Pulse labeling studies showed that the reduced steady state levels of β-globin mRNA were achieved within 20 minutes of transcription but remained stable afterwards. Transfection of cells with a suppressor tRNA capable of recognizing the premature termination codon, thus permitting translation of the β-globin peptide, restored β mRNA to nearly normal levels.

These studies implicated an intranuclear step in mRNA metabolism that recognized premature translation termination and caused reduced accumulation of stable mRNA in the cytoplasm. Paradoxically, however, the impact of suppressor tRNAs implies the requirement for translation, a process clearly confined to the cytoplasm. Studies of many premature termination codons in a variety of mutant globin and nonglobin mRNAs subsequently established that reduced amounts of relatively stable cytoplasmic mRNA were a general feature associated with nonsense mutations (Maquat, 1995; Ruiz-Echevarria et al., 1996). Examples were found throughout nature, ranging from yeast to human disease-causing mutations, and could be shown by deliberate construction of nonsense mutations in heterologous gene expression systems (Daar and Maquat, 1988; Baserga and Benz, 1992; Peltz et al., 1994).

Many confounding and confusing aspects of these phenomena existed. For example, the amounts of mRNA remaining in the cytoplasm varied widely, depending on the particular mRNA, the location of the mutation, and the cell system used for evaluation (Maquat, 1995; Daar and Maquat, 1998; Baserga and Benz, 1988). Some forms of thalassemia resulting from nonsense mutations *result* in accumulation of nearly normal amounts of mRNA (Baserga and Benz, 1992; Hall and Thien, 1994). Many forms result in the accumulation of 2 to 20 percent of the normal levels of mRNA, and a few result in undetectable levels of mRNA. Transfection of these mutant genes into heterologous (nonerythroid) cells results in a reduction in mRNA level that is frequently less severe than that in erythroid cells (Baserga and Benz, 1992).

This wide variation in β-globin mRNA levels reflects the existence of a highly conserved and complex mechanism to prevent the accumulation of prematurely terminated mRNAs incapable of translating their complete encoded proteins. This process is called *nonsense-mediated decay* (Fig. 8.3). It apparently exists to ensure that cells will not manufacture the potentially harmful truncated proteins that would result from accumulation of mRNAs and their foreshortened protein products (Culbertson, 1999; Jacobson and Peltz, 1996; Hall and Thien, 1994; Thien et al., 1990; Cooper, 1993; Kugler et al., 1995).

Truncated proteins may be harmful to the cell. Recombinant DNA technology has allowed the construction of many truncated forms of many metabolically important proteins. This method is commonly used to establish structure/function relationships of different domains within the protein. Many of these foreshortened proteins behave as dominant negative mutations;

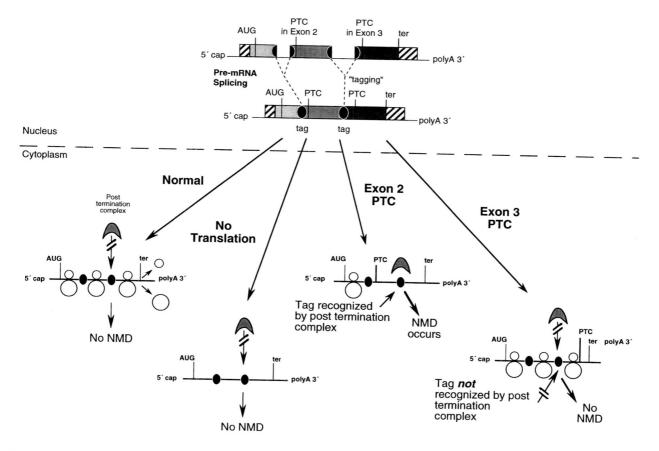

Figure 8.3. A model of nonsense-mediated decay (see text for details). The exon-intron junctions are "tagged" or masked during intranuclear processing. Nonsense-mediated decay occurs only when translation both occurs *and* is prematurely terminated *before* the last tag is encountered. (Based on Thermann et al., 1998.)

they can sustain some binding interactions with their intracellular partners but cannot participate fully in the relevant metabolic processes (refer to Culbertson, 1999; Jacobson and Peltz, 1996). They thus behave as partial agonists, resulting in disruption of the critical pathway and, often, derangement of cell function. Nonsense-mediated decay ensures that these messenger mRNAs are destroyed before they can generate significant amounts of the harmful abnormal proteins.

In mammalian cells, available evidence suggests that the nucleus is involved in reducing the nonsense codon-bearing mRNAs to their final steady state level, but that translation of the mRNA is an obligate step for the degradation (Fig. 8.3) (Takeshita et al., 1984; Baserga and Benz, 1992; Kugler et al., 1995; Urlaub et al., 1989; Kessler and Chasin, 1996; Belgrader et al., 1994; Belgrader and Maquat, 1994; Cheng and Maquat, 1993). Moreover, the location of the mutation seems relevant in complex ways that relate to pre-

mRNA splicing, another intranuclear event. For example, the pre-mRNA must contain introns to experience nonsense-mediated decay in heterologous expression systems. Insertion of nonsense codons in strategic locations in some genes can alter the pattern of splicing (Zhang et al., 1998a, 1998b; Cheng et al., 1994; Dietz et al, 1993). Conversely, and of particular relevance to thalassemias, is the consistent observation that termination codons in the terminal exon do not result in nonsense-mediated decay (Fig. 8.3). (Hall and Thien, 1994; Thien et al., 1990). Nagy and Maquat (1998) and Cheng et al. (1990) have shown that mutations occurring more than 55 to 60 bases 3' of the 3'-most intron (i.e., at least 55 to 60 bases into the terminal exon of the gene) do not undergo nonsense-mediated decay.

Nonsense-mediated decay accounts for the reduced, but detectable, levels of the relevant globin mRNA detected in forms of α and β thalassemia due to premature translation termination codons that occur in exon 1 or exon 2 of the relevant globin gene. However, Hall and Thien (1994) showed that many nonsense mutations occurring in the third exon of the globin genes, particularly the β-globin gene, were associated with accumulation of normal or nearly normal levels of β-globin mRNA, allowing translation of substantial amounts of the truncated peptides (Chapter 14). In addition, some frame shift mutations that resulted in premature translation termination in the third exon were also associated with high levels of β-globin mRNA and production of truncated globin chains. These foreshortened chains lack amino acid sequences essential for stable formation of soluble tetramers and precipitate and form inclusion bodies, even in heterozygotes. They behave as dominant-negative mutant proteins, interacting with other globin chains to form highly unstable molecular species causing a severe thalassemia phenotype in heterozygotes. Truncated peptides exhibiting abnormal behavior in subsequent steps of the metabolism of the affected protein have subsequently been identified in other disease states (Culbertson, 1999). Nonsense-mediated decay or, more properly, the imperfections in nonsense-mediated decay, are thus important to the clinical phenotype of some forms of thalassemia.

In aggregate, these studies support the notion that all eukaryotes possess the ability to detect and degrade transcripts containing a premature termination codon. This mechanism likely governs the expression of some normal, and mutant, transcripts. It is widely appreciated, for example, that genes vary widely in the efficiency with which their pre-mRNAs are spliced. Many "normal" genes contain inefficiently utilized splicing sites. Some of these are used to generate alternatively spliced mRNA and protein products. A few, such as the CYH2 transcript in yeast, may be generally inefficiently spliced (Culbertson, 1999; Jacobson and Peltz, 1996). Some mRNA generated from this gene routinely retains at least one exon containing an inframe termination codon. These aberrant transcripts are degraded by a nonsense-mediated decay pathway.

Increasingly apparent is that some mRNA species, even after completion of intranuclear processing and transport to the cytoplasm, contain more than one translatable open reading frame (ORF). In most of these cases, a short upstream open reading frame (UORF) is followed by the longer ORF that codes for the intended protein product (Culbertson, 1999; Jacobson and Peltz, 1996; Nagy and Maquat, 1998; Hentze and Kulozik, 1999). Nonsense-mediated decay may mandate lower levels of mRNAs with UORFs, thus serving as a normal mechanism for gene regulation. Nonsense-mediated decay has also been postulated to play a role in minimizing expression of transcripts from pseudogenes.

Role of the Nucleus in Nonsense-Mediated Decay

In mammalian cells, the most controversial and puzzling aspect of nonsense-mediated decay remains the paradoxical involvement of both intranuclear and cytoplasmic translational steps. The pathway for nonsense-mediated decay, as discussed later, has been at least partly characterized in yeast, where there is no evidence for nuclear involvement. However, several investigators using several different gene systems have identified the nucleus as the primary site for reduction in the levels of the mRNA. The demonstration by Nagy and Maquat (1998) and Thermann et al. (1998), that nonsense-mediated decay occurs only if the nonsense mutation is located "upstream" (i.e., to the 5′ side) of a position approximately 50 to 60 nucleotides before the junction between the penultimate and ultimate 3′ exon clearly implicates a relationship of nonsense-mediated decay to splicing and intranuclear processing (Fig. 8.3). On the other hand, suppressor tRNAs can clearly reverse nonsense-mediated decay; moreover, cytoplasmic translation is obligatory for nonsense-mediated decay by use of translation inhibitors or mutations that abolish translation initiation (refer to Jacobson and Peltz, 1996; Takeshita et al., 1984; Gozalbo and Hohmann, 1990; Stephenson and Maquat, 1996).

Several models have been developed to reconcile these conflicting features. Some propose that pre-mRNA can be "scanned" for premature termination codons during the actual process of RNA splicing (Takeshita et al., 1984), but no mechanism by which the scanning could be accomplished is apparent. Other models suggest that newly processed mRNA is immediately translated by polyribosomes as it exits the nucleus; translation itself is proposed to be necessary to "spool" the RNA from nucleus to cytoplasm (Urlaub et al., 1989). If premature termination occurs, exit from the nucleus is blocked, and the RNA is presumably degraded at the nuclear-cytoplasmic interface. This clever formulation is attractive, as it would reconcile the nuclear and cytoplasmic components of the process. However, it is unclear how ribosome scanning would "recognize" the position of the last exon after processing is already complete, or how the ribosome would "know" whether the first termination codon encountered was a normal or premature codon.

Thermann et al. (1998) have proposed that the junction of the penultimate and extreme 3′ exon is "marked" or "tagged" during the process of RNA splicing (Fig. 8.3). The fully spliced mRNA is then transported to cytoplasm, where the tag can be recognized during translation on ribosomes. Normal translation termination would occur at the first termination codon encountered after the tag. If the translation termination codon is encountered before the tag, nonsense-mediated decay would be initiated. This model reconciles the requirement for translation with a clearly documented involvement of splicing in the nucleus, but does not explain the observation that nuclear levels of these mRNAs are also reduced. Proponents of the model raise the possibility that "nuclear mRNA levels" may be deceiving because of difficulty eliminating the possibility of cytoplasmic mRNA contamination from these preparations; it is also possible that distinct fractions of cytoplasmic mRNA—possibly those on which the ribosomal scanning for "tags" occurs—may be perinuclear and thus co-isolated with the nucleus. Perhaps the process of nonsense-mediated decay itself could generate a signal that is carried back to the nucleus for intranuclear or perinuclear degradation.

Metabolic Pathways of Nonsense-Mediated Decay in Yeast

Resolution of the issues surrounding metabolism of mutant globin mRNAs will require complete characterization of the metabolic pathways of nonsense-mediated decay. Progress has been made in yeast. Several genes encoding the nonsense-mediated decay pathways have been cloned and their products characterized. Initial results in mammalian cells suggest that the pathways are highly conserved.

At least three *trans*-acting factors participate in yeast nonsense-mediated decay. The genes encoding these factors have been called UPF1, UPF2, and UPF3. Their protein products, Upf1p, Upf2p, and Upf3p, appear to interact with one another on ribosomes to initiate nonsense-mediated decay (refer to Culbertson, 1999; He et al., 1997 for reviews).

Yeast mRNAs are susceptible to nonsense-mediated decay only if the premature termination codon occurs within the first two thirds of the ORF. Nonsense-mediated decay in yeast requires the presence of a consensus "destabilizing" sequence downstream of the premature termination codon (Zhang et al., 1995). This consensus sequence, TGYYGATGYYYYY, must be to the 3' side of a termination codon in order for the termination codon to be recognized as premature (Zhang et al., 1995). This sequence is widely distributed in the yeast genome. At a time when about 2,000 yeast genes had been sequenced, nearly 400 (20 percent) contained an exact match of this sequence near the 3' end of the ORF.

The present model (Czaplinski et al., 1998; Ruiz-Echevarria et al., 1998) for nonsense-mediated decay in yeast states that ribosomes traversing the mRNA and translating nascent polypeptide chains will, when they encounter a termination codon, release a "scanning complex," presumably containing the Upf1-3p proteins. The complex travels downstream toward the 3' end in search of the consensus destabilizing sequence motif. If no such motif is encountered, the termination codon is taken to be normal, and the nor-

mal process of translation termination proceeds (release of the completed polypeptide chain and dissociation and recycling of the ribosomal subunits and translation factors). However, if the termination codon is premature (defined in this model as located before the destabilizing sequence motif), the nonsense-mediated decay proteins will, on encountering the destabilizing signal, provoke the decapping and degradation of the mRNA in a 5'→3' direction.

This model provides one means by which "premature" translation stop signals could be distinguished from normal signals. It does not provide a mechanism for relating translation to intranuclear events, nor does it explain how nonsense-mediated decay differs from normal translation termination, which requires the presence of termination signals near the normal termination codon. This mechanism also provides no evident understanding of the clearly demonstrated phenomenon in mammalian cells by which mRNAs containing premature termination codons appear to be able to accumulate in detectable, albeit reduced, amounts.

Nonsense-Mediated Decay Pathways in Mammalian Cells

A major difference between nonsense-mediated decay in yeast and mammals is that a role for the nucleus has clearly been shown in the mammalian pathways, whereas the role of the nucleus in yeast is completely unclear. One *trans*-acting factor homologous to the yeast UPF protein families has been cloned and characterized from mammalian sources. Called RENT-1, it is homologous to the UPF1 gene and appears to support all of the same activity when complemented into yeast cells (Perlick et al., 1996). Immunolocalization studies suggest both a cytoplasmic and a nuclear localization. More detailed analysis revealed that the "nuclear" localization actually resulted from its presence in unique cytoplasmic invaginations that have recently been shown to penetrate deep into the nucleus. This finding might offer insight into the way in which components localized inside the nucleus might have better access to the cytoplasmic translation machinery.

It is unclear whether the nonsense-mediated decay pathway identified in yeast and the homolog that appears to exist in mammalian cells are the only mechanisms by which nonsense-mediated decay occurs. Also, unknown is the percentage of genes susceptible to nonsense-mediated decay. That only about 20 percent of known genes in yeast contained the downstream element required for recognition of premature stop codons suggests that nonsense-mediated decay might be restricted to a specific subset of mRNAs or that multiple pathways exist, each associated with its own recognition mechanism.

Also requiring clarification is the mechanism that allows intranuclear events to "anticipate" the translation potential of pre-mRNAs (Fig. 8.3). Recently, an increasing number of RNA-binding proteins have been shown to shuttle between nucleus and cytoplasm; transfer RNA-like elements have been located in the nucleus (refer to Culbertson, 1999). Data have been presented to suggest that some mRNAs might emerge from the nucleus 5' end first, where they would be available for a "first round" of translation (refer to Jacobson and Peltz, 1996). Coupling of intranuclear and cytoplasmic events could occur at this transitional stage. Existing methods for recovery of separate cytoplasmic and nuclear RNAs would probably not be able to distinguish consistently between RNA species clearly found inside the nucleus and those at the interface between nucleus and cytoplasm.

In summary, the unexpectedly low but persistent levels of mRNAs carrying premature termination codons in patients with β thalassemia suggested that a mechanism must exist for the regulated catabolism of abnormal transcripts unable to be translated into complete proteins. Further study of this and other abnormal transcripts has led to the discovery of a highly complicated pathway—nonsense-mediated decay—which is likely to be the prototype of several mechanisms ensuring stable accumulation only of those mRNAs that can generate the proteins intended by the normal coding sequence of the gene. Nonsense-mediated decay is clearly an imperfect surveillance mechanism, as exemplified by the fact that some mutations occurring close to the normal termination point in the β-globin genes can escape degradation. Their mutant β globins disrupt normal hemoglobin solubility and assembly, causing unusually severe thalassemia trait. The conservation of nonsense-mediated decay across all eukaryotic species suggests a critical general mechanism for ensuring the fidelity of the mRNA products of genes.

FACTORS AFFECTING THE ACTIVITY OF GLOBIN mRNAs

The essential biological activity of cytoplasmic mRNA is translation of the information encoded in the codons of its ORF into the amino acid sequence of the polypeptide chain encoded by that reading frame. Translation occurs on polyribosomes, which read the nucleotide sequence of the mRNA in "ticker tape" fashion so that each ribosome generates a nascent polypeptide chain as it traverses the mRNA. The overall process is extremely complex (see Benz and Forget, 1974, 1975; Preiss and Hentze, 1999 for background information).

Translation requires the recruitment, utilization, and release of a bewildering array of ribosomal subunits, proteinaceous factors, transfer RNAs, the mRNA itself, and critical cofactors, such as guanosine triphosphate (GTP) and adenosine triphosphate (ATP), magnesium, and possibly other factors. These interactions must be extraordinarily precise with regard to spatial relationships, timing, and sequence. Clearly, many of these steps, perhaps all, are susceptible to regulatory intervention. Translation efficiency can be modulated by embedded sequence motifs in mRNA that alter interaction with the actual translational apparatus, or modifications of the translational factors that interact with these sequences. Regulation of the rate of translation of individual messages is now widely appreciated to be a critical mechanism used by cells for differentiation, entry into, or exit from, the cell cycle, as well as adaptation to physiologic or pathologic perturbations. In many situations, including critical steps in iron and heme metabolism in erythroid cells, translational regulation is the predominant means by which the amount of protein produced from a gene is determined, whatever the level of the particular mRNA.

Initiation: Rate Limiting Step in mRNA Translation

Most students of mRNA translation regard the overall process as consisting of three major steps (Kozak, 1991; Pain, 1996; Sachs et al., 1991). Initiation is the process by which the small ribosomal subunit (40S) becomes attached to the mRNA near its 5' end, usually at a site called the internal ribosomal entry site (IRES), for which canonical consensus sequences have been identified. To bind the IRES, the 40S subunit must first bind to a ternary complex consisting of a proteinaceous translation initiation factor called eIF-2α, GTP, and the specialized initiator methionyl-tRNA (Fig. 8.4). This quartenary complex is called the 43S preinitiation complex. It then binds to message, positioning the initiator tRNA in apposition to the AUG initiator codon, and facilitating binding of the large ribosomal subunit (60S) to constitute the complex of an intact 80S ribosome surrounding the initiation region of a single strand of mRNA (Fig. 8.4). Elongation is the subsequent process by which the 80S ribosome progressively positions each transfer RNA in apposition to the next codon in sequence on the mRNA strand and facilitates the formation of peptide bonds between the amino acid residues bound to the charged tRNAs. The ribosome "ratchets" itself one codon further along the sequence, releasing the spent tRNA and retaining the growing peptide in position for entry of the next tRNA and addition of the next amino acid. During elongation, the mRNA sequence is

Abundant Heme Supply

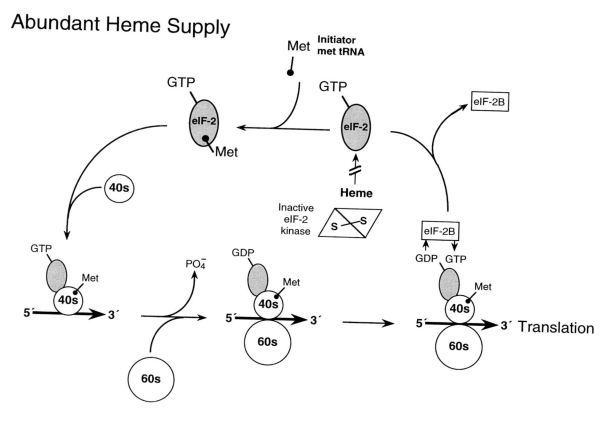

Figure 8.4. Normal cycle of eIF2 translation initiation in heme-replete cells (see text for details). EIF2 forms the critical 43S preinitiation complex by complexing with GTP, met-tRNA, and the 40S ribosomal subunit. Initiation begins by binding of the 60S subunit with hydrolysis of GTP to GDP. Recycling of eIF-2 requires the exchange of GDP for GTP-mediated by eIF2B. eIF2 must then dissociate from eIF2B for reutilization. This cycle functions only when eIF2 is in the *nonphosphorylated* state. Heme is critical because the eIF2 kinase remains inactivated when bound to heme by sulfhydryl oxidation. (Based on Chen and London, 1995.)

read in "ticker tape" fashion. The methionine invariably present as the first incorporated residue is cleaved from most mammalian proteins during elongation. Elongation continues until an inframe translation termination codon is encountered. Termination is the phase by which elongation is ended and the completed polypeptide chain is released from the ribosome, with subsequent dissociation and recycling of the ribosomal subunits for new rounds of initiation and elongation.

All three major steps in translation require the reversible binding of specialized initiation, elongation, or termination and release factors (Pain, 1996; Sachs et al., 1991). In most cells producing large amounts of protein, such as erythroblasts the supplies of these factors and ribosomal subunits are limited. These components must be used repeatedly to support multiple rounds of translation on each mRNA template. Reversible attachment with subsequent recycling is thus critical. Clearly, normal translation also requires adequate supplies of the various transfer RNA moieties and the amino acids with which they are charged. Amino acid starvation, the use of certain amino acid analogs that "freeze" the ribosome on the mRNA, or certain antibiotics such as puromycin or erythromycin, which inhibit ribosomal translocation, damage cells because they deplete the effective supply of components of the protein synthetic machinery by "locking them" on stalled mRNA sequences.

Translation initiation, especially when regarded as including events up to and including formation of the first peptide bond, is generally regarded as the rate-limiting step in mRNA translation under most physiologic conditions (Pain, 1996). It is the initiation step of globin translation that is most relevant to modification of the hemoglobin phenotype in humans. Therefore, only this aspect of translation is considered further.

Different normal mRNAs initiate translation at considerably different rates. It appears that differences in the inherent translational efficiency of mRNAs depend almost entirely on variations in the 5′ untranslated sequences and perhaps the first few codons surrounding the AUG initiation codon (Kozak, 1991). Messenger RNAs lacking a 5′ cap are translated at a much lower efficiency than capped mRNAs; however, capping may not be an important mechanism for differential translational regulation, as almost all mRNAs appear to contain cap structures that are equally effective for enhancing translation initiation. Variable efficiencies in translation initiation appear to depend instead on sequence elements near the 5′ end of the mRNA. These include the "strength" of consensus sequences surrounding the initiator AUG codon ("Kozak" boxes) and the first few codons downstream, and the degree to which 5′ UTR sequences favor the formation of stable secondary structures, such as hairpin loops (Kozak, 1991). The former sequence element appears to affect the likelihood that a particular methionine codon will be recognized as an initiator codon, whereas the formation of hairpin loops appears to impair the efficiency with which the 43S ribosomal initiator subunit complex finds and binds to the IRES. Usually, the first inframe AUG codon encountered as the ribosome scans from the 5′ end of the mRNA is selected for translation initiation; however, many exceptions to this rule have been described.

Two features of the initiation scheme just outlined are relevant to mammalian hemoglobin production during erythroblast maturation. The first involves differences in the 5′ UTR sequences between α- and β-globin mRNAs. The second reflects the coordination of heme and globin synthesis mediated by the impact of heme on the supply of 43S initiator complexes available for globin mRNA translation.

α and β mRNA are Present in Different Amounts in Normal Erythroblasts and are Translated at Different Rates

Equal α- and β-globin chain synthesis during normal adult erythroid maturation is generally regarded as an axiomatic feature for the normal production of large amounts of hemoglobin tetramers without deleterious accumulation of individual unpaired globin subunits. However, no clear-cut mechanism to ensure coordinated transcription of the α- and non-α-globin genes at nearly identical rates is known; α mRNA, whether by virtue of higher rates of transcription or greater stability, accumulates in slight excess compared with β mRNA during normal adult erythropoiesis. α-Globin mRNA tends to be 25 to 50 percent more abundant than β mRNA in normal erythroid cells (refer to Benz and Forget, 1974, 1975). Yet, rates of biosynthesis of α- and β-globin chains in bone marrow erythroblasts and reticulocytes are virtually equal. Only a small pool, accounting for at most 5 percent of the total globin produced, accumulates as excess free α-globin chains.

The near equivalence of globin polypeptide production in the face of a relative excess of α mRNA occurs

because β-globin mRNA is more efficiently translated than α-globin mRNA. The magnitude of the difference *is* sufficient to counterbalance almost exactly the differences in quantitative supply of the individual mRNAs (Lodish and Jacobsen, 1972; Lodish, 1971, 1974). Ample evidence supports the notion that β mRNA is translated more efficiently because its 5′ UTR interacts more effectively with the initiation complex. The 5′ UTR of α-globin mRNA has a higher GacC content; intramolecular base pairing to form hairpin loops tends to result in the formation of more stable loops in areas rich in G and C residues. The highly stable hairpin loops, in turn, are unfavorable for the efficient attachment and movement to the site of initiation in the initiation complex. The normal balance of α- and β-globin polypeptide synthesis is thus highly dependent on the evolution of different 5′ UTRs in the α- and β-globin mRNAs (Nienhuis and Benz, 1977; Liebhaber et al., 1992).

Similar factors may also play a role in determining the relative output of α-globin chains attributable to the α1 and α2 gene loci. As noted in Chapter 17, the transcriptional output from these two loci is unequal, with α2 predominating by a 2.5- to 3.5-fold higher level of mRNA synthesis. Mutations affecting the α2 locus thus have a greater impact on total α globin production. Liebhaber and Kan (1982) have suggested that partial "compensation" of this transcriptional inequality might occur by more efficient translation of mRNA from the α1 locus. However, subsequent work has called into question the quantitative significance of differential mRNA α1 and α2 translation rates (Shakin and Liebhaber, 1986). Similarly, no direct evidence presently suggests that variations in the 5′ UTRs of the other globin mRNAs differentially influence their translation, other than the suggestion that ζ, δ, and γ mRNAs, like β mRNA, have more favorable 5′ UTRs for translation initiation. This makes theoretical sense because balance between total non-α-globin and α-globin peptide chain synthesis is critical throughout development.

The different translational efficiencies of α- and β-globin mRNAs also play a role in mechanisms leading to unequal synthesis of α- and β-globin chains in certain pathologic conditions, such as iron deficiency. Thorough understanding of the relationship of translation initiation to these phenomena, however, requires consideration of the mechanisms by which iron supply, heme production, and globin chain synthesis appear to interact.

Impact of Heme Deficiency on Translation Initiation in Developing Reticulocytes

Heme and globin biosynthesis are coordinated during erythroid maturation. That heme deficiency suppresses synthesis of de novo globin polypeptide chains has been known for decades (Sassa, 1983; Kruh and Borsook, 1956; Bruns and London, 1965; Waxman and Rabinovitz, 1965; Grayzel et al, 1960). Heme and globin production are coordinated so that their accumulation is nearly equal. Accumulation of excess heme or of free globin chains is highly noxious to erythroblasts. Yet, no apparent transcriptional mechanism ensures that the mRNAs responsible for encoding heme biosynthetic enzymes and globin are produced in amounts appropriate to generate equal amounts of heme, α globin, and non-α globin.

Heme is required for the conversion of globin chains into hemoglobin tetramers (Fig. 8.1). However, for nearly 30 years it has been known that heme also exerts other effects on the biogenesis of globin. This was first appreciated during early efforts to develop cell-free systems capable of synthesizing globin from endogenous polyribosomes or by the addition of exogenous mRNA to cell preparations of reticulocyte lysates. (Benz and Forget, 1974; Waxman and Rabinovitz, 1965; Bonanou-Tzedaki et al., 1984) Reticulocyte lysates were chosen because of their ease of preparation and the readily detectable rates of globin biosynthesis in intact reticulocytes (refer to Benz and Forget, 1974 for review). However, these extracts incorporated radiolabeled amino acids into globin for only about 5 minutes. Cessation of globin synthesis was accompanied by disaggregation of polyribosomes into inactive 80S particles. No completely new globin chains were synthesized during the brief period that the lysates were active; amino acids were simply incorporated into preexisting nascent chains, allowing for their completion. Addition of exogenous globin mRNAs or nonglobin mRNAs to these extracts did not result in new protein biosynthesis. Remarkably, supplementation of these lysates with hemin (the oxidized [Fe^{+++}] form of heme) restored the ability of the lysates to support initiation of new rounds of protein synthesis and to use exogenous mRNAs as templates for the de novo synthesis of their encoded polypeptides. Protein synthesis could also be sustained for more than 1 hour at 37° C.

These observations strongly implicated heme as a major modulator of the rate of initiation of globin mRNA translation, at least in reticulocytes. This effect was generalized; nonglobin mRNA templates and globin mRNA could be initiated efficiently only in heme-supplemented lysates (e.g., Chinchar et al., 1989). Heme supplementation also had a substantial, if less dramatic, impact on translation initiation in cell-free systems derived from nonerythroid cells (Soreq, 1985).

Much effort was expended during the 1970s and 1980s to identify the translational factors modulated by the heme supply and to characterize the modulating agents. These studies have culminated in the recognition that heme depletion results in the accumulation of the so-called "heme-regulated inhibitor" (Chen and London, 1995). (An older name for this entity was the heme-controlled repressor.) Heme-regulated inhibitor is a kinase that specifically phosphorylates the translation initiation factor eIF-2α, whose role in the initiation of mRNA translation is critical.

Heme-regulated inhibitor accumulates at high levels and is activated when heme deficiency develops. It phosphorylates eIF-2α, which results in generalized inhibition of translation initiation by a complex mechanism (Fig. 8.4) that has recently been described and reviewed (Chen and London, 1995; deHaro et al., 1996). Understanding this mechanism requires a more detailed consideration of the mechanism of action of eIF-2α (deHaro et al., 1996). In the nonphosphorylated state, eIF-2α forms a ternary complex with GTP and initiator met tRNA, to form the 43S preinitiation complex described earlier. During the binding of the 43S complex to mRNA and subsequent joining of the 60S ribosomal subunit, eIF-2α-GTP is hydrolyzed to eIF-2α-guanosine diphosphate (GDP), an inactive complex. To be recycled for additional rounds of protein synthesis, eIF-2α requires the exchange of bound GDP for GTP; this step requires the participation of another initiation factor, eIF-2B, which has also been called "GDP exchange factor" or "reversing factor" (Chen and London, 1995).

Reversing factor normally exchanges the spent GDP for a fresh GTP molecule and then dissociates, making the regenerated eIF-2α-GTP available for a new round of translation. eIF-2B is present in cells in much smaller amounts than eIF-2α. The phosphorylated eIF-2α-GDP complex binds eIF-2B with a very high affinity, forming a virtually irreversible bond. Therefore, when the level of phosphorylated eIF-2α becomes sufficiently high, it sequesters all of the available eIF-2B. The supply of eIF-2B needed to catalyze recycling of eIF-2α is depleted. No regeneration of eIF-2α-GTP occurs, and new rounds of protein initiation are effectively stopped.

This mechanism explains why heme deficiency results in generalized inhibition of protein initiation in reticulocyte lysates. It also accounts for the fact that complete inhibition of translation initiation occurs when only 20 to 30 percent of the total supply of eIF-2α is phosphorylated by the heme-dependent eIF-2α kinase. This amount is sufficient to serve as an effective "sump" to bind up and sequester the entire lesser supply of eIF-2B (Fig. 8.5). The remaining nonphosphorylated eIF-2α molecules are rendered useless because they are unable to participate in a recycling interaction with eIF-2B.

Heme Depleted State

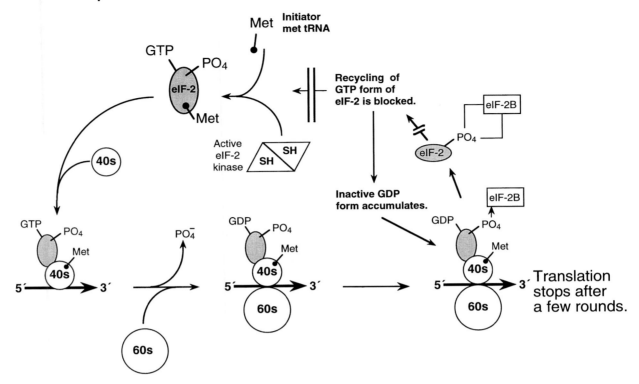

Figure 8.5. Effect of heme depletion on eIF-2-mediated translation initiation (see text and Fig. 8.4 for background). In the absence of heme, eIF-2 kinase is active, and eIF-2 becomes phosphorylated. The phosphorylated form binds irreversibly to eIF-2B so that recycling cannot occur for new rounds of translation. (Based on Chen and London, 1995.)

Hemin prevents the phosphorylation of eIF-2α. It inactivates heme-regulated inhibitor by inhibiting its autophosphorylation and by promoting intersubunit disulfide bond formation. In the absence of heme, heme-regulated inhibitor exists as a functional dimer. Hemin converts the noncovalent dimer to a covalently linked dimer joined by disulfide linkages. The disulfide linkages and the inactive state are reversible upon hemin depletion.

The phenomenon of heme-mediated translational suppression in erythroid cells was originally thought to be a curious aspect of globin gene expression, of restricted general interest or applicability. However, the heme-dependent eIF-2α kinase (heme-regulated inhibitor) is a member of a large kinase family exerting important effects on gene expression in a much more general way (reviewed by Kaufman, 1999; Silverman and Williams, 1999). A second member, called PKR, is activated indirectly by double-stranded RNA, which in turn induces interferon. The suppression of de novo protein synthesis by double-stranded RNA or its

agent, interferon, is a major widespread response by which interferon appears to respond to cellular attack of double-stranded RNA viruses. An eIF-2α kinase called GCN4 is activated by amino acid starvation in yeast. This slows the consumption of limited supplies of amino acids. Heme-regulated eIF-2α kinase interacts with heatshock proteins, particularly HSP90, and this interaction modulates its activity. Controversy currently exists about whether HSP90 exerts its influence primarily through interaction with eIF-2α kinase or by interaction with heme itself. Interactions with HSP70 and p59 have also been shown.

The heme-dependent eIF-2α kinase was once thought to be widely expressed because immunologically cross-reacting proteins and cross-hybridizing mRNA species were detected in a variety of tissues. More precise analysis has recently suggested that heme-regulated inhibitor itself is restricted to hematopoietic cells and, perhaps, liver, spleen, and kidney (Olmstead et al., 1993; Pal et al., 1991). (In this regard, it is interesting that liver is another major site of heme biosynthesis and accumulation, and that liver, spleen, and kidney can serve as sites of erythropoiesis [e.g., the kidney in fish] at certain times of development.) The cross-reacting materials detected in earlier studies now appear to be family members, although they are not PKR or GCN4. The levels of eIF-2α kinase appear to rise during erythroid differentiation.

Although the effect of heme-regulated inhibitor and translation factor phosphorylation on globin biosynthesis has been shown most dramatically for elF-2α kinase and its relationship to heme, heme-regulated inhibitors appear to interdict mRNA translation at one other step in response to noxious stimuli. elF-4 is an initiation factor that binds the cap structure and unwinds the 5' untranslated region of mRNA. This facilitates entry of the preinitiation complex at the IRES. elF-4 also seems susceptible to modulation by phosphorylation (Soneberg and Gingras, 1998). elF-4 can also localize in the nucleus and may have direct or indirect effects on gene transcription (Lejbkowicz et al., 1992).

Because heatshock proteins and initiation factor kinases appear to mediate a variety of inhibitory effects on translation provoked by a wide range of toxic substances, including benzene, thermal stress, amino acid starvation, and double-stranded RNA, the phenomenon of heme-deficient inhibition of globin synthesis seems to reflect a general molecular response to injury. Study of globin mRNA translation has thus helped identify and characterize fundamental mechanisms through which cells respond to stress by reducing protein biosynthesis.

Relationship of the Translatability of α- and β-Globin mRNAs to the Supply of Heme and Iron

Numerous reports over several decades have shown that heme or iron deficiency results in a mild "α-thalassemia-like" state (White et al., 1971; White and Harvey, 1972; White and Ali, 1973; Ben-Basselt et al., 1974; White and Hoffbrand, 1974; El-Hazmi and Lehmann, 1978; Piddington and White, 1974; Kan et al., 1969; Tavill et al., 1968; Franco et al., 1979; Walford and Deacon, 1980; Zago and Boltura, 1982; Peters et al., 1983). Biosynthesis of α-globin chains is selectively depressed in iron deficiency anemia, sideroblastic anemias, lead poisoning, and the anemia of chronic disease. These conditions are associated, for a variety of pathophysiologic reasons, with inadequate supplies of iron and/or heme for erythroblasts during critical phases of maturation.

One can expect a reduced content of heme in the erythroblast to cause an increase in elF-2α kinase activity, causing increased levels of phosphorylated elF-2α and reduced levels of elF-2B. As a result, the availability of recycled elF-2α for translation initiation is reduced, and the supply of elF-2α becomes rate-limiting for initiation of new rounds of protein synthesis. β-Globin mRNA translation is normally initiated more efficiently than α-globin mRNA because it interacts more efficiently with the 43S preinitiation complex. Because the supply of these complexes will be rate limiting, the rate of both α- and β-mRNA translation will decrease. However, α-globin mRNA translation will decline more significantly because α mRNA cannot compete as effectively for the limited supply of preinitiation complexes as can β mRNA. Thus, a mild deficiency of α-globin biosynthesis develops, accounting for the "mild α-thalassemia-like" phenotype.

Normal erythroid cells contain a small pool of excess free α-globin chains. As discussed later, the existence of this pool implies that newly synthesized non-α-globin chains will have access to an abundant binding partner for immediate formation of hemoglobin tetramers. In heme-deficient erythroid cells, the reduced synthesis of α globin results in loss of this pool, so that newly synthesized non-α-globin chains must compete for a limiting supply of α-globin binding partners.

FACTORS THAT INFLUENCE THE GENERATION OF COMPLETE HEMOGLOBIN TETRAMERS FROM NEWLY SYNTHESIZED GLOBIN CHAINS

To form soluble functioning hemoglobin molecules, nascent globin chains must bind heme and associate to form the characteristic α_2:non-α_2 tetramers. This process is called hemoglobin assembly. Tetramers containing heme form from nascent nonheme-containing globin chains by rapid nonenzymatic binding interactions driven largely by the primary amino acid sequences of the globin chains. Nascent chains fold, probably cotransitionally, forming hydrophobic heme-binding pockets and exposing more hydrophilic exterior surfaces. Hemoglobin can form from nascent globin chains without benefit of chaperone proteins because these reactions can be accomplished in solution and in bacteria transfected with globin genes (Wakasugi et al., 1997). However, the possibility that chaperones play a role in normal hemoglobin assembly in vivo has not been eliminated.

Normal Hemoglobin Assembly

Nascent globin chains appear to bind to heme cotranslationally (Komar et al., 1997) and are probably released from the ribosome in the form of nearly completely folded globin. A single α-globin chain forms a dimer with a single non-α-globin chain to form, in the case of HbA, α:β dimers [$\alpha + \beta \rightarrow (\alpha\beta)$]. Two heterodimers then join to form the fully functioning tetramers ($2(\alpha\beta) \rightarrow \alpha_2\beta_2$). In mammals, the tetramer is the highest order structure normally formed during the process of hemoglobin assembly. The limitation of hemoglobin aggregation to the tetramer state is critical for hemoglobin solubility and normal red cell homeostasis. However, higher order aggregation of hemoglobins into very large molecules is physiologically normal in some other species, particularly cold water fish (Manning et al., 1998).

The structural basis for normal assembly into heme-liganded globin, globin heterodimers, and completed tetramers is still under investigation. Recombinant hemoglobin production systems in heterologous cellular or cell-free hosts have made it possible to mutate almost any desired residue and assess the effects of the mutation on hemoglobin assembly. Before this process was possible, progress was limited by access to naturally occurring mutations and by differences among normal human and nonhuman hemoglobins available for comparative analysis. Numerous structural features of each globin chain influence the affinity of chains for heme and for one another and, in all likelihood, the rate and stability of dimer and tetramer formation (Manning et al., 1998, 1999). Many amino acid residues in the globin chains contribute to normal folding, heme liganding, and subunit interaction; these are considered in other chapters.

Hydrophobic interactions at points of α/β chain contact contribute to the affinity and reversibility of dimer and tetramer formation, but the primary driving forces are electrostatic. α-Globin chains are more positively charged than most non-α chains. Among the non-α chains, those that are more negatively charged have a higher affinity for α globin than those that are more positively charged. In competitive mixing experiments (McDonald et al., 1984), the more negatively charged globins preferentially form tetramers at the expense of the more positively charged non-α globin species. Mixed heterodimers and heterotetramers (e.g., $\alpha_2\beta\gamma$, $\alpha_2\gamma\delta$) do not form in a stable fashion, except as a minute percentage of the total hemoglobin. Like dimers have a much higher affinity for each other than unlike dimers.

The important role played by electrostatic charge in dimer and tetramer formation is relevant to understanding the hemoglobin content in red blood cells from many patients heterozygous for hemoglobinopathies. The relative amounts of normal adult hemoglobin, HbA, and various hemoglobin variants, particularly HbS and HbC, are frequently not those expected on the basis of gene dosage, net transcription of α- and non-α-globin mRNAs, and translation of the mRNAs into nascent globin chains. For example, one would expect that the red cells of patients with sickle cell trait would contain 50 percent HbA and 50 percent HbS, on the basis of gene dosage and initial rates of globin biosynthesis. However, the HbS content of patients heterozygous for HbS varies considerably but rarely exceeds 40 to 45 percent of normal hemoglobin (McDonald et al., 1984; Bunn 1997; Embury and Vichinsky, 1999; Forget, 1999). There is now strong evidence to support the view that deviations from the predicted level of a mutant hemoglobin are due to differences in the relative affinities of the normal and variant non-α chains for α chains during hemoglobin assembly.

Impact of Competitive Tetramer Assembly on Hemoglobin Phenotypes

γ-Globin chains are the most negatively charged among the normal and among most of the frequently encountered abnormal non-α-globin chains. In increasing order of positive charge, the normal globin chains can be arrayed as follows: $\gamma > \beta^A > \beta^S > \beta^C = \delta$ (McDonald et al., 1984). Thus, γ chains should have the greatest, and β^C or δ chains the least, affinity for α chains. Consequently, assembly and stability of hemoglobin tetramers should be arrayed in descending order as follows: HbF>HbA>HbS>HbC or HbA$_2$. In a series of competitive mixing experiments, McDonald and co-workers (1984) verified these predictions; moreover, mutant hemoglobins with known alterations in charge were positioned along this array in a manner predicted by the model.

In normal red cells, these effects on the net accumulation of hemoglobins in the steady state are slight, because of the existence, as noted earlier, of a small pool of excess free α chains. Virtually every newly synthesized non-α chain thus has access to adequate numbers of α chains for tetramer formation. However, in circumstances that limit the supply of free α chains, such as co-inheritance of α thalassemia or heme deficiency, these non-α globins must compete for a limited supply of α-globin chains. The inadequate numbers of α-globin chains will reduce the accumulation of every hemoglobin type, producing hypochromia and microcytosis. Hemoglobins containing the more positively charged non-α subunits, such as hemoglobins S, C, and A$_2$, will be reduced more dramatically because their non-α chains will compete less well for the limited supply of α globin. In patients with α thalassemia, who also inherit β^S or β^C globin, the concentration of HbS or HbC will be relatively lower (Chapters 27 and 29) (Embury and Vichinsky, 1999).

These predictions have been borne out by clinical studies (Embury and Vichinsky, 1999). In patients with four intact normally functioning α-globin genes (wild type), the ratio of HbS:HbA was 60:40. In α-thalassemic patients, the HbA:HbS ratio was 65:35 in patients with three loci, 71:29 in patients with two functioning α-globin genes, and 79:21 in patients with only a single functional α-globin gene.

Interestingly, the HbS:HbA ratio is not 50:50, even in patients with a completely normal α-globin gene profile. This consistent finding probably indicates that the pool of free α-globin chains becomes limiting even at normal rates of α-globin production, perhaps during the later stages of erythropoiesis. This same event may explain why HbS levels may be slightly higher than HbC levels in patients with HbSC disease, the HbC level is less than 50 percent in patients with HbC trait, and some negatively charged β-globin gene variants such as HbJ may exceed 50 percent of the hemolysate. Therefore, the electrostatic model for assembly of hemoglobin tetramers from subunits is heuristically useful in a clinical context because it provides a rational way to interpret the quantitative amounts of various hemoglobins in patients with complex hemoglobinopathies. However, it is highly unlikely that electrostatic charge alone provides a complete explanation for the molecular process of hemoglobin assembly. The importance of other factors, such as hydrophobic contact points, is dramatically borne out by the fact that many mutations that profoundly impair formation of stable hemoglobin tetramers do not alter the net charge of the affected globin chain (Chapter 44 and 45).

On the basis of the electrostatic model, elevated levels of HbF would be expected in patients with α-thalassemia trait. Although slight elevations in HbF in patients with α-thalassemia syndromes have been reported, this finding has not been confirmed (Embury et al., 1982; Higgs et al., 1982).

Once formed, hemoglobin tetramers are extraordinarily stable. The vast majority survive throughout the entire circulating life span of the erythrocyte. Proteolytic enzymes capable of degrading hemoglobin and its subunits do, however, exist in normal erythrocytes. These proteolytic systems have not yet been completely characterized. It is clear, however, that at least one set of proteases is ATP and ubiquitin-dependent (Etlinger and Goldberg, 1977); that another is independent of these agents (Fagan et al., 1986); and that the proteolytic machinery is capable of selectively removing free α globin, α-globin proteolytic fragments, and oxidized hemoglobins, leaving normally assembled tetramers relatively unscathed (Fagan et al., 1986). Proteolysis of excess α globin accumulating during erythroblast maturation in patients with β-thalassemia trait probably explains why α-globin inclusions are not seen in these patients, despite a nearly 50 percent deficit in β-globin production. Further characterization of these proteolytic mechanisms would be of considerable interest, because this information could clarify a number of puzzling clinical phenomena, such as the variability in the severity of β thalassemia intermedia in patients who seem to inherit combinations of thalassemic β-globin genes associated with the same net impairment in β-globin chain production. As discussed elsewhere, dominant forms of β

thalassemia resulting from the production of highly unstable β-globin chains, and the curious clinical phenotype associated with HbE-β thalassemia (Chapter 43), could also be modulated by varying proteolytic susceptibility of the structurally abnormal molecules formed as a result of these mutations. Variations in proteolytic sensitivity would affect the rate of inclusion body formation and thereby clinical severity (Chapters 13 and 45).

Numerous posttranslational modifications of mature hemoglobin tetramers are known to occur, including glycosylation, acetylation, sulfation, and lig-and binding to 2,3 BPG. These modifications, discussed in other chapters of this book, are useful as clinical markers in conditions such as diabetes and for understanding the physiology of oxygen binding and release under different normal and pathologic conditions. However, for our purposes, it is sufficient to note that posttranslational modifications of this sort do not have any known impact on the hemoglobin content of normal cells or the clinical behavior of hemoglobinopathies.

ASPECTS OF HEME BIOSYNTHESIS AND IRON METABOLISM PARTICULARLY RELEVANT TO THE HEMOGLOBINOPATHIES

Heme is an indispensable component of hemoglobin, as is iron of heme. Heme consists of a protoporphyrin IX complexed to a divalent (reduced, or ferrous) iron ion; the oxidized form of heme, called hemin, is identical except that the iron residue is in the trivalent state in hemin. Coordination exists between the levels of heme and globin during erythropoiesis. Adequate supplies of heme are necessary for posttranslational assembly of hemoglobin tetramers and for translation of globin mRNA. Heme production is correspondingly modulated by the rates of globin and hemoglobin production in an obscure but readily detectable manner. Levels of heme, for example, are depressed in patients with thalassemia syndromes who do not produce adequate amounts of hemoglobin (Forget, 1999). The supply of iron, in turn, modulates the rate of heme synthesis, as discussed later. The net effect of these complex interactions is to ensure that neither iron, free porphyrins, heme, nor free globin chains accumulate to any appreciable degree during erythroblast maturation. Each of these components is insoluble in the concentrations that would normally accumulate during erythropoiesis unless they were incorporated into hemoglobin. Each is known to exert a variety of toxic effects on cells. The interactions among these pathways thus ensure that only intact, soluble, functioning hemoglobin tetramers accumulate to any significant degree in developing erythrocytes.

This section focuses primarily on relevant aspects of the pathways of intracellular heme biosynthesis. Iron homeostasis has been extensively studied in recent years, and its metabolism involves regulation by several fascinating mechanisms. However, its impact on hemoglobin production may be mediated largely through its eventual effects on the levels of heme accumulation. For a more comprehensive and detailed review of these subjects, the reader is referred to recent excellent reviews on heme (Ponka et al., 1998; Wiley and Moore, 1999) and on iron by Brittenham (1999), which are the source materials for these sections. The summary that follows focuses on aspects most relevant to hemoglobin homeostasis.

Relevant Aspects of Heme Biosynthesis

Heme is an essential component of vital proteins besides hemoglobin, including many of the cytochromes; it is synthesized in all cell types that possess mitochondria. These cells, however, account for only a small percentage of total heme synthesis in the body. Eighty-five percent of total body heme is produced in erythroid marrow for hemoglobin synthesis, and much of the remainder in the liver, where production of cytochromes for enzyme complexes such as the p450 system is especially abundant.

The genes responsible for each of the ten enzymes needed for heme biosynthesis have been cloned and characterized. Most studies of the biosynthesis and regulation of the biosynthetic pathways have compared the two major sites of production: hepatocytes and erythroid cells.

Heme biosynthesis begins with the condensation of glycine and succinyl CoA to form 5-δ aminolevulinate (ALA) (Fig. 8.6). The reaction is catalyzed by the intramitochondrial enzyme, ALA synthase, which requires a cofactor, pyridoxal phosphate (vitamin B_6). ALA synthase is synthesized in the cytoplasm and must be transported into the mitochondrion for this first intramitochondrial step in the pathway to occur. ALA then travels to the cytoplasm, where it is converted into porphobilinogen by the enzyme porphobilinogen deaminase to form the first recognizable monoporphyrin. Subsequent enzymes convert porphobilinogen into tetrapyrroles, which are condensed into the porphyrin ring and further modified. A late intermediate, coproporphyrinogen III is then reimported into the mitochondrion where it is enzymatically and successively oxidized to protoporphyrin IX. The final step of heme formation is mediated by the enzyme ferrochelatase, which inserts iron into protoporphyrin IX to complete the heme molecule.

Heme biosynthesis requires the importation of enzymes, substrates, and iron into the mitochondrion,

and the export of ALA and the completed heme molecule into the cytoplasm (Fig. 8.7). That the initial enzymatic reaction in the pathway and the terminal step are both localized in mitochondria provides an elegant feedback control mechanism because much of the regulation of heme biosynthesis appears to depend on end-product inhibition of ALA synthase, as described later. It is not clear whether the initial product is heme or whether hemin is first produced and then reduced by cytochrome b_3, an enzyme important for detoxifying methemoglobin.

Recent investigations have shown clear differences between the regulation of hepatic and erythroid cell heme biosynthesis. In both cases, end-product inhibition (feedback repression) appears to be the primary mechanism of control. In both liver and bone marrow, the first enzymatic step is the target of regulation, and ALA synthase is the rate-limiting step in the entire enzymatic pathway. In both types of cells, ALA synthase is under negative feedback control by heme, which acts at several levels to reduce ALA synthase activity when the concentration of heme rises above threshold levels.

ALA synthase consists of a family of two isoenzymes (Fig. 8.7). ALA synthase 1 is prominent in liver and many nonerythroid tissues. ALA synthase 2 is largely limited to erythroid cells. Each form is encoded by a different gene. The gene for ALA synthase 1 maps to chromosome 3, and the gene for ALA synthase 2, to the X chromosome. Mutations in ALA synthase 2 account for the syndrome of X-linked sideroblastic anemia. The critical role played by the ALA synthase 2 gene and its mRNA and protein products in the coordination of heme biosynthesis with the supply of iron and of globin is apparent by examination of its structure. Of the eleven exons present in the gene, exons 5 to 11 encode the catalytic domain of the enzyme, including a critical lysine needed for binding to pyridoxal phosphate. Exon 1 codes for a portion of the 5′ UTR that contains a distinctive IRE. The IRE is recognized by iron-binding proteins whose affinity for the IRE is modified by the supply of iron, resulting in altered stability of ALA synthase 2 mRNA, as discussed later. Exons 1 and 2 encode a cleavable amino acid sequence in the enzyme that targets ALA synthase 2 for mitochondrial import. Its recognition and utilization are modulated by the supply of heme.

The mechanisms by which heme regulates its own biosynthesis via ALA synthase in liver and erythroid cell mechanisms are shown in Figure 8.7. This diagram also describes the interrelationships between heme and iron in the developing erythroblasts. Regulation of heme biosynthesis in the liver has evolved to serve the need for heme in proteins with rapid turnover; hepatic

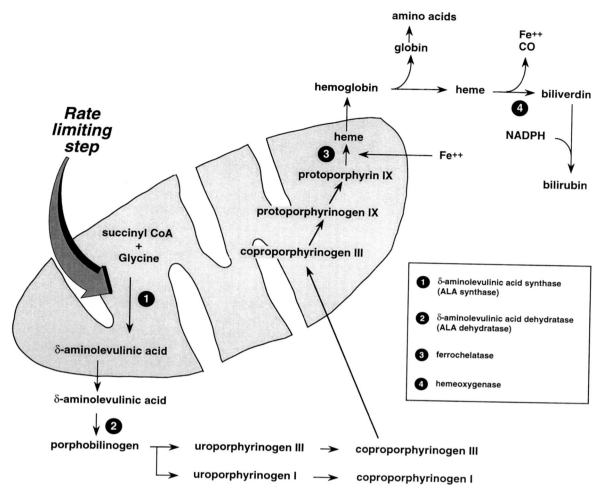

Figure 8.6. Heme synthesis and degradation (see text for details). The key regulated steps involving the four listed enzymes are indicated by numbers 1 through 4. Step 1 is rate limiting, as shown in more detail in Figure 8.7.

heme levels fluctuate from hour to hour, depending on physiologic conditions.

Heme regulates its own biosynthesis in liver by negative feedback inhibition at three levels: inhibition of transcription of the pre-mRNA, destabilization and accelerated degradation of the mRNA, and inhibition of the transport of the newly synthesized proenzyme from cytosol into the mitochondrion. These comprehensive effects provide for rapid and reversible modification of the rate of heme biosynthesis in response to changing conditions. Heme control in erythrocytes appears to be adapted to a slower, more long-term modulation and coordination of the supply of heme, iron, and globin. This rate is appropriate because the vast majority of heme produced on a moment-by-moment basis in normal red cell progenitors will be incorporated into hemoglobin, where it will survive

intact for the 120-day life span of the erythrocyte. Fluctuations in the levels of heme and globin, except under extreme conditions, are much less likely to occur in these cells than in hepatocytes.

Heme synthesis is stimulated by iron and repressed in the face of inadequate iron supply (Fig. 8.7). A major mechanism by which sensitivity to iron supply is achieved involves the translation efficiency of ALA synthase 2 mRNA. The IRE of this mRNA is bound to a repressor protein (IRP, described later) when iron supplies are low. The majority of the iron-binding repressor protein exists in the apoprotein state when iron is scarce. As iron supply rises, the repressor protein progressively binds more iron, altering its conformation and lessening its binding affinity for the IRE. When the repressor is bound to the IRE, ALA synthase 2 mRNA is translationally suppressed. Release of binding by rising iron stores thus permits more efficient translation of ALA synthase 2 mRNA, a situation favoring increased heme biosynthesis. The rate of formation of the porphyrin ring of heme thus rises in iron-replete states and falls in iron-depleted states.

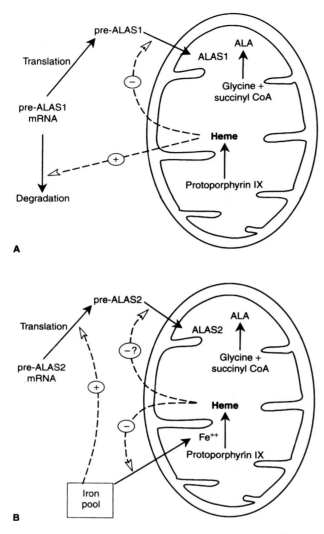

Figure 8.7. Regulation of ALA synthase by heme and iron in hepatic (A) and erythroid (B) cells (see text for details). Panel A shows the effect of iron and heme supplies on ALAS 1, which is ubiquitous but especially abundant in liver. Heme stimulates mRNA degradation and inhibits translocation into the mitochondrion, thus feedback inhibiting heme synthesis. Panel B shows ALAS 2, abundant only in erythroid cells. Iron stimulates translation, thus promoting heme production. Heme inhibits iron transport to mitochondria, thus feedback inhibiting ferro chelatase, and may also inhibit movement to ALAS 2 into the mitochondrion.

As heme accumulates above threshold levels in erythroblasts, it suppresses its own synthesis in at least two ways. First, importation of ALA synthase 2 into the mitochondrion is thought to be inhibited by high levels of heme in a manner analogous to that seen in hepatocytes. Second, by an incompletely understood mechanism, high levels of heme inhibit the uptake of iron into erythroblasts from iron-transferrin complexes in the external milieu. However, in contrast to

its effects in liver, heme does not appear to exert direct transcriptional control on the ALA synthase 2 gene. The promoter for the ALA synthase 2 locus contains erythroid-specific regulatory elements, including GATA-1 (Chapter 4). Transcription of ALA synthase 2 increases dramatically during the early phases of erythroblast maturation, in keeping with the need for increased production of protoporphyrin during erythropoiesis. Heme appears to have no effect on ALA synthase 2 mRNA transcription.

Porphobilinogen deaminase, the second enzyme in the pathway, may also serve as a control point sensitive to abnormal accumulation of intermediate tetrapyrrole products. Porphobilinogen deaminase exhibits relatively low endogenous activity in cells, and also consists of erythroid-specific and more generalized isoforms. Both forms arise from a single gene by differential use of alternative promoters. The upstream promoter is used in all cells, including erythroid cells. The downstream promoter is erythroid specific and generates an mRNA product that is also alternatively spliced, yielding a smaller protein isoform (40 to 42 kD, as opposed to 42 to 44 kD in nonerythroid cells). Activity of the downstream promoter is induced during erythropoiesis; this promoter is highly sensitive to many of the same transcription factors that stimulate globin gene activity.

Heme content in erythroblasts appears to depend primarily on end-product repression of the early steps of its biosynthesis, including suppression of iron import and reduction in the effective activities of ALA synthase 2 and porphobilinogen deaminase. It is also likely that accumulation of excess heme is prevented by accelerated catabolism. Heme oxygenase is the rate-limiting step in the heme degradation pathway. Transcription of the mRNA for heme oxygenase is accelerated by free heme.

The detailed information that has become available about the interrelatedness of the iron and heme supply on globin mRNA translation and heme biosynthesis has illuminated understanding of the ways that heme can modulate the intracellular supply of iron and the rate of globin production. However, how diminished globin biosynthesis—induced experimentally or in patients with thalassemia—suppresses the rate of heme production is less well understood. No evidence suggests that heme biosynthesis or iron incorporation is directly sensitive to the levels of intact hemoglobin tetramers, free globin chains, or unassembled intermediates of hemoglobin. Rather, the best available explanation is that free heme must begin to accumulate in cells with inadequate pools of globin available for its incorporation. This free heme would then be expected to inhibit its own biosynthesis by the mechanism just described. Whether this or

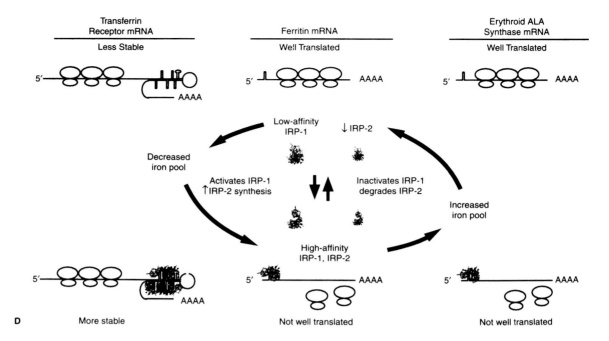

Figure 8.8. The effect of iron on iron uptake, storage, and incorporation into heme. This cycle is described in detail in the text. The globular structures indicate iron response proteins (IRP) 1 and 2.

other mechanisms are ultimately found to be responsible, sensitivity of heme biosynthesis to the supply of globin clearly exists. Iron assimilation into erythroblasts, heme synthesis, globin biosynthesis, and hemoglobin assembly are thus coordinated by a complex set of largely posttranscriptional events.

Modulation of the Supply of Iron in Developing Erythroblasts

Iron is absolutely essential for the formation of heme and hemoglobin. It is, however, an extraordinarily toxic substance when it accumulates as free ions or in low-molecular-weight iron complexes. The challenge for the developing erythroblasts is thus to assimilate the extraordinarily large amounts of iron needed to generate normal mature red cells without accumulating low-molecular-weight iron compounds. This appears to be accomplished by the coordination of the supply of intracellular iron with the metabolism and translational activity of critical mRNAs. These mRNAs encode proteins that modulate the uptake of iron from the environment, the storage of iron into ferritin complexes, and the utilization of iron for heme biosynthesis. This exquisitely regulated system acts largely at the level of posttranscriptional control of the relevant mRNAs.

A simplified diagram of intracellular iron homeostasis is provided in Figure 8.8. Briefly, each of the three key mRNAs (transferrin receptor mRNA, ferritin mRNA, and ALA synthase 2 mRNA) contains one or more IREs. The IRE is recognized by two iron regulatory proteins, IRP-1 and IRP-2. The mRNAs encoding ferritin and ALA synthase 2 have a single element in their 5′ UTR; transferrin receptor mRNA has multiple elements scattered along its 3′ UTR. When either IRP-1 or IRP-2 binds to the IRE, it stabilizes hairpin loops in the 5′ UTR or 3′ UTR of the mRNAs. Binding to the 5′ UTRs of ferritin mRNA and ALA synthase 2 mRNA inhibits their translation. Binding of IRPs to 3′ UTR of transferrin receptor mRNA stabilizes its half-life; transferrin receptor mRNA levels thus rise. The recently described divalent metal transporter gene-1 (DMT-1, nRAMP 2), which appears to play a key role in iron transport across membranes, also contains an IRE (Andrews et al., 1999).

IRPs regulate the levels of intracellular iron by the effect of iron on their affinity for the IRE sequences or on their quantitative levels in the cytoplasm. When iron is abundant in the cytoplasm, IRP-1 becomes replete with iron, forming an Fe-S cluster that stabilizes the protein in a conformation in which it has enzymatic activity as aconitase but little or no affinity for the mRNA. IRP-1 does not bind mRNA in iron replete cells. Iron supply has essentially no impact on the amount of IRP-1 present in cytoplasm. In contrast, IRP-2 appears to respond to the iron supply primarily by changes in its quantitative availability. In iron-replete cells, IRP-2 is degraded, whereas IRP-2 biosynthesis is stimulated in iron-deficient cells. The net physiologic effect is the same as for IRP-1. In states where iron supplies are abundant in the cell, neither IRP-1 nor IRP-2 is likely to bind to the IRE-IRP-1 because of reduced affinity, and to IRP-2 because of diminished concentration.

Consider the cytoplasm of an iron-deficient cell. Under these circumstances, IRP-1 has a high affinity for the IRE, and IRP-2 supplies are abundant. Thus, the three target mRNAs will be fully bound by the IRPs. As a result, transferrin receptor mRNA will be stabilized, allowing it to synthesize greater numbers of transferrin receptors, leading to an increased uptake of external iron into the cell. Translation of ALA synthase 2 and ferritin mRNAs will be suppressed, reducing the amount of enzyme available for making porphyrins for iron incorporation into heme and the amount of ferritin available for sequestration of iron into ferritin complexes. The net result is an increase in the intracellular concentration of iron and less production of free protoporphyrin and apo-ferritin.

As intracellular iron concentrations reach a threshold level, IRP-1 becomes iron replete and loses its affinity for mRNA; synthesis of IRP-2 declines, and its degradation is accelerated, reducing IRP-2 levels. The net effect is to generate increasing numbers of the target mRNA molecules that do not have either IRP bound to them. As a result, transferrin receptor mRNA will be degraded more rapidly, leading to reduced levels of transferrin receptor synthesis and reduced uptake of new iron molecules into the cell. In contrast, translation of both ferritin and ALA synthase 2 mRNAs will increase, increasing the use of iron for heme biosynthesis and the sequestration of iron into ferritin complexes. The net effect is to reduce the amount of cytosolic iron, increase iron incorporation into heme, and increase ferritin sequestration. This elegant mechanism ensures that iron uptake, use for hemoglobin biosynthesis, and storage are coordinated in a physiologically appropriate way.

The function and metabolism of IRP-1 and IRP-2 are also sensitive to factors other than the iron supply. These include oxidative agents, NO (nitric oxide, a chemical mediator of the inflammatory process), and phosphorylation state. Although the precise mechanisms by which these alterations might influence iron metabolism in pathologic states are still unclear, the susceptibility of IRPs to these key molecules could explain alterations in iron use in diseases such as the anemia of chronic disease, or the accumulation of iron deposits or ringed sideroblasts in response to a variety of pharmacologic agents. Ferritin levels also appear to vary during erythroblast maturation, as does the relative accumulation of its "L" and "H" subunits. Erythroblast ferritin levels are severely depressed in iron deficiency, as expected, but also in states of severe chronic inflammation. In contrast, in other conditions in which hemoglobin synthesis is reduced, such as thalassemia or sideroblastic anemias, and in hemochromatosis, ferritin levels rise. Once again, although the exact mechanisms are not clear, these changes are almost certainly germane to the characteristically altered utilization of iron and the morphology of erythroblasts in these pathologic states. It should be noted, however, that no abnormality of heme synthesis appears to occur in patients with iron overload.

Impact of Disordered Iron Supply and Heme Biosynthesis on Hemoglobin Production

Besides the effects of heme on hemoglobin synthesis already discussed, three general abnormalities of iron and heme metabolism merit consideration because of their relationship to normal and pathologic hemoglobin content: iron deficiency, iron overload, and "sideroblastic" states. The porphyrias, which are primary disorders of heme biosynthesis resulting from mutations in the biosynthetic enzyme pathways, have, for the most part, little impact on the process of hemoglobin synthesis, except as noted later.

Iron deficiency clearly limits the capacity of developing erythroblasts to produce hemoglobin. One obvious site at which iron deficiency acts is ferrochelatase, where the supply of iron affects the ability of the enzyme to couple iron and protoporphyrin IX to form heme. The reduced supply of iron, by mechanisms already described, also reduces heme biosynthesis. Furthermore, the reduced heme supply results in inhibition of globin mRNA translation by means of the heme-controlled inhibitor. The net effect is diminished hemoglobin synthesis in iron deficiency. Repression of the synthesis of the porphyrin precursor of heme in iron deficiency is imperfect because free porphyrins do accumulate in iron-deficient patients. This phenomenon is used clinically by testing for elevated free erythrocyte protoporphyrin (FEP test) levels in iron deficiency anemia.

Iron overload, caused by either congenital hemochromatosis, transfusional hemosiderosis, or toxic exposures, should theoretically increase the level of iron within erythroid cells. It was once thought that this effect should increase heme oxygenase and inhibit ALA synthase, thus depressing heme levels. However, the elucidation of the IRE-IRP mechanism for regulating iron homeostasis may explain why systemic iron overload appears to have little impact on net heme synthesis. The primary impact may well be mediated by increased ferritin mRNA translation, leading to sequestration of a vast amount of excess iron with maintenance of high levels of ALA synthase translation for maximum available use of iron in the form of heme synthesis.

Sideroblastic anemias are characterized morphologically by the presence of "ringed" sideroblasts in the bone marrow, with or without anemia. Ringed sideroblasts contain perinuclear iron-laden mitochondria and, when stained with Prussian blue, the iron-loaded mitochondria appear as a ring of speckled blue around the nucleus of the erythroblast. Ringed sideroblasts occur when heme synthesis is impaired and/or mitochondrial damage is inflicted by noxious agents. Clinically significant forms of acquired sideroblastic anemia are the myelodysplastic syndromes in which clonal somatic cell mutations possibly impair either heme metabolism or mitochondrial integrity in poorly understood ways. Some toxic agents can cause secondary acquired sideroblastic anemias. The most commonly encountered toxic agent that can generate ringed sideroblasts is alcohol. Alcohol has a direct toxic effect on mitochondria, causing swelling and distortion of cristae. In addition, alcohol provokes folate deficiency, which, in turn, causes inhibition of the activation of pyridoxine to pyridoxal phosphate. Reduced pyridoxal phosphate levels impair the activity of ALA synthase 2. Treatment with folate can reverse the sideroblastosis even before blood alcohol levels fall significantly, suggesting that impaired heme biosynthesis may indeed be of primary importance in the formation of ringed sideroblasts. Lead is also a potent inhibitor of heme biosynthesis, by virtue of its inactivation of several enzymes in the heme biosynthetic pathway. The antibiotic chloramphenicol is a direct inhibitor of mitochondrial protein synthesis and is known to suppress heme biosynthesis. Finally, a large number of antituberculous drugs, notably isoniazid (INH), cycloserine, and pyrazinamide, are known to be potent inhibitors of heme biosynthesis. Like a number of other drugs, including hydralizine, L-dopa, and penicillamine, they almost certainly act by antagonism of the production and/or cofactor activity of pyridoxal phosphate. Pyridoxal phosphate usually reverses the effects in vitro and in vivo. Of these drugs, the most clinically significant is INH, which can produce symptomatic anemia.

The development of ringed sideroblasts probably reflects increased amounts of intracellular iron because of decreased ability to incorporate the iron into heme, coupled with mitochondrial damage. These agents may inflict damage that exceeds the ability of the IRE-IRP mechanisms to reduce iron influx or sequestration by ferritin. Many of the toxic agents responsible for sideroblastic anemia appear to have direct effects on key enzymatic steps in the heme synthetic pathway or on pyridoxal phosphate metabolism. These facts suggest that inhibition of heme synthesis alone is sufficient to produce ringed sideroblasts. The primary impact of these conditions on

hemoglobin synthesis and accumulation appears to be mediated through the reduced supply of heme. Although published reports are sketchy, there does seem to be the expected selective reduction in α-globin production in these patients, producing a mild, usually subclinical, α-thalassemia-like state.

That coordination exists between heme and globin biosynthesis during erythropoiesis has been widely accepted for nearly 50 years. However, only within the last 5 to 10 years have molecular mechanisms mediating this coordination been discovered. How iron and heme supply influence globin biosynthesis is reasonably well defined. Most of this coordination is accomplished at the translational or posttranslational level. Less well understood is the degree to which impaired globin synthesis is sensed directly or indirectly as a signal to reduce iron assimilation and heme production.

SUMMARY

Each of the multiple steps in the biogenesis of hemoglobin is susceptible to regulatory mechanisms and sensitive to disruptive pathologic phenomena. Many of these alter the hemoglobin composition in individual patients. In some cases, posttranscriptional factors alter the severity or character of the clinical phenotypes. The normal production of intact functioning hemoglobin tetramers depends on an adequate supply of iron, and the production of protoporphyrin IX rings and globin chains, and is coordinated to generate amounts appropriate to the iron supply. Coordination is critical so that only intact functioning hemoglobin tetramers are assembled. A small pool of excess free α-globin chains appears to be compatible with cellular homeostasis and is important for ensuring efficient incorporation of all non-α-globin chains into stable hemoglobin tetramers. Iron uptake and heme production appear to be coordinated by the presence of iron-sensitive elements affecting the translation and/or stability of key mRNAs in heme biosynthesis, iron uptake, and iron sequestration. Heme and globin coordination appears to be mediated predominantly through the supply of free heme molecules. If globin is not present in sufficient amounts to use all of the available heme, free heme accumulates and causes a decrease in its own biosynthesis by feedback inhibition.

Nearly equal initial rates of synthesis of α and non-α globins appear to occur despite the fact that α–globin mRNA is present in a 30 to 50 percent excess over non-α-globin mRNAs. This is almost exactly counterbalanced by more efficient translation of the non-α-globin mRNAs, whose 5′ UTRs are more accommodating to entry and activity of the translation initiation apparatus than the 5′ UTRs of α-globin mRNAs. The efficiency of translation of globin mRNAs in erythroid cells depends heavily on an initiation factor, EIF-2α, whose activity and availability are impaired in heme deficiency, thus coupling globin synthesis to the supply of heme. Because of their inherent differences in translational efficiency, α-globin mRNAs are more severely diminished in translational activity by heme deficiency, leading to a mild α-thalassemia phenotype.

A reduced supply of free α-globin chains alters the distribution of hemoglobins in patients with complex hemoglobinopathies, regardless of whether α-globin deficiency is caused by mutations (α thalassemia) or indirectly by states leading to heme deficiency (e.g., iron deficiency, sideroblastic anemias). These situations render the supply of free α globin limiting for hemoglobin assembly, so that different non-α-globin chains must compete with one another for the limited pool of α chains. Reduction in total hemoglobin, producing hypochromia and microcytosis, results. Many mutant non-α-globin chains, such as the β^S and β^C chains, which are more positively charged, cannot compete as efficiently for binding to the more positively charged α-globin chains. As a result, diminution in the levels of HbS or HbC in cells with reduced α-chain pools is selectively more severe than that of HbF or HbA. In patients heterozygous for HbS or HbC, the levels of these hemoglobins will thus be lower than expected on the basis of β^S or β^C gene dosage. Similarly, normal δ globin is more positively charged and competes poorly under these circumstances, thus explaining the low HbA_2 levels seen in iron deficiency. Posttranscriptional and posttranslational steps in the production of hemoglobin are thus critically important for understanding the clinical and pathophysiologic features of many hemoglobinopathies.

References

Andrews NC, Fleming MD, and Gunshin H. (1999). Iron transport across biologic membranes. *Nutr. Rev.* 57: 114–23.

Aviv, H, Volloch, Z, Bastos, R, and Levy, S. (1976). Biosynthesis and stability of globin mRNA in friend erythroleukemia cells. *Cell* 8: 495–503.

Baserga, S and Benz, EJ Jr. (1988). Nonsense mutations in the human beta-globin gene affect mRNA metabolism. *Proc. Natl. Acad. Sci. U.S.A.* 85: 2057–60.

Baserga, S and Benz, EJ Jr. (1992). Beta globin nonsense mutation: Deficient accumulation of mRNA occurs despite normal cytoplasmic stability. *Proc. Natl. Acad. Sci. U.S.A.* 89: 2935–2939.

Bastos, RN, Volloch, Z, and Aviv, H. (1977). Theoretical analysis of a model for globin mRNA accumulation during erythropoiesis. *J. Mol. Biol.* 110: 191–203.

Belgrader, P and Maquat, L.G. (1994). Nonsense but not missense mutations can decrease the abundance of nuclear RNA for the mouse major urinary protein while both types of mutations can facilitate exon skipping. *Mol. Cell Biol.* 14: 6326–6336.

Belgrader, P, Cheng, J, Zhou, X et al. (1994). Mammalian nonsense codons can be cis effectors of nuclear mRNA half-life. *Mol. Cell Biol.* 14: 8219–8228.

Ben-Basselt, I, Mozel, M, and Ramot, B. (1974). Globin synthesis in iron-deficiency anemia. *Blood* 44: 551–555.

Benz, EJ Jr and Forget, BG. (1974). The biosynthesis of hemoglobin. *Semin. Hematol.* 11: 463–523.

Benz, EJ Jr and Forget, BG. (1975). The molecular pathology of the thalassemia syndromes. *Prog. Hematol.* 9: 107–155.

Benz, EJ Jr, Forget, BG, Hillmann, DG et al. (1978). Variability in the amount of β globin mRNA in β° thalassemia. *Cell* 14: 299–308.

Benz EJ Jr and Huang, SC. (1996). The role of tissue specific alternative splicing of pre-mRNA in the biogenesis of the red cell membrane. *Trans. Am. Clin. Climatol. Assoc.* 108: 78–95.

Berliner, N and Benz, EJ Jr. (1999). Anatomy and physiology of the gene. In Hoffmann, R et al. (1999). *Hematology: Basic principles and practice* (3rd ed). New York: Churchill Livingstone.

Bonanou-Tzedaki, SA, Sohi MK, and Arnstein, HR. (1984). The effect of haemin on RNA synthesis and stability in differentiating rabbit erythroblasts. *Eur. J. Biochem.* 144: 589–596.

Brihenham, GM. (1999). Disorders of iron metabolism: Iron deficiency and overload. In Hoffman, R, Benz, EJ Jr, Shattil, SJ et al. (editors). *Hematology: Basic principles and practice.* Philadelphia: Churchill Livingstone.

Bruns, GP and London, IM. (1965). The effect of hemin on the synthesis of globin. *Biochem. Biophys. Res. Commun.* 18: 236.

Bunn, HR. (1997). Pathogenesis and treatment of sickle cell disease. *N. Engl. J. Med.* 337: 762–769.

Caapoinigro, G and Parker, R. (1996). Mechanisms and control of mRNA turnover in *Sacchromyces cerevisiae*. *Microbiol. Revi.* 60: 233–249.

Chang, JC and Kan, YW. (1979). β° Thalassemia, a nonsense mutation in man. *Proc. Natl. Acad. Sci. U.S.A.* 76: 2886–2889.

Chen, JJ and London, IM. (1995). Regulation of protein synthesis. *Trends Biochem. Sci.* 20: 105–108.

Cheng, J, Fogel-Petroux, M, and Maquat, LE. (1990). Translation to near the distal end of the penultimate exon is required for normal levels of spliced triosephosphate isomerase mRNA. *Mol. Cell. Biol.* 10: 5215–5225.

Cheng, J and Maquat, LE. (1993). Nonsense codons can reduce the abundance of nuclear mRNA without affecting the abundance of pre-mRNA or the half-life of cytoplasmic mRNA. *Mol. Cell. Biol.* 13: 1892–1902.

Cheng, J, Belgrader, P, Zhou, X, and Maquat, LE. (1994). Introns are Cis-effectors of the nonsense-codon-mediated reduction in nuclear mRNA abundance. *Mol. Cell. Biol.* 14: 6317–6325.

Chinchar, VG, Turner, LA, and Kumar, G. (1989). Hemin and cyclic AMP stimulate message dependent translation in lysates from friend erythroleukemia cells. *Exp. Haematol.* 17: 405–410.

Chkheidze, AN, Lyakhov, DL, Makeyev, AV et al. (1999). Assembly of the alpha-globin mRNA stability complex reflects binary interaction between the pyrimidine-rich 3 untranslated region determinants and poly(C) binding protein. *Mol. Cell Biol.* 18: 2173–2183.

Cooper, DN. (1993). Human gene mutations affecting RNA processing and translation. *Ann. Med.* 25: 11–17.

Culbertson, MR. (1999). RNA surveillance. *Trends Geneti.* 15: 74–80.

Czaplinski, K, Ruiz-Echevarria, MF, Paushkin, SV, et al. (1998). The surveillance complex interacts with the translation release factors to enhance termination and degrade aberrant mRNAs. *Genes Dev.* 12: 1665–1677.

Daar, IO and Maquat, LE. (1988). Premature translation termination mediates triosephosphate isomerase mRNA degradation. *Mol. Cell Biol.* 8: 802–813.

deHaro, C, Mendez, R, and Santoyo, J. (1996). The eIF-2 alpha kinases and the control of protein synthesis. *FASEB J.* 10: 1378–1387.

Dietz, HC, Valley, D, Francomano, CA et al. (1993). The skipping of constitutive exons in vivo induced by nonsense mutations. *Science* 259: 680–683.

El-Hazmi, MAF and Lehmann, H. (1978). Interaction between iron deficiency and α-thalassaemia: The "in vitro" effect of haemin on alpha-chain synthesis. *Acta Haematol.* 60: 1–9.

Embury, SE and Vichinsky, EP. (1999). Sickle cell disease. In Hoffman R, Benz, EJ Jr, et al. (editors). *Hematology: Basic principles and practice.* Philadelphia: Churchill Livingstone.

Embury, SH, Dozy, AM, Miller, J et al. (1982). Concurrent sickle cell anemia and α thalassemia: Effect on severity of anemia. *N. Engl. J. Med.* 306: 270–274.

Etlinger, JD and Goldberg AL. (1977). A soluble ATP dependent proteolytic system responsible for the degradation of abnormal proteins in reticulocytes. *Proc. Natl. Acad. Sci. U.S.A.* 74: 54–58.

Fagan, JM, Waxman, L, and Goldberg, AL. (1986). Red blood cells contain a pathway for the degradation of oxidant-damaged hemoglobin that does not require ATP or ubiquitin. *J. Biol. Chem.* 261: 5705–5713.

Forget, BG. (1999). The thalassemia syndromes. In Hoffman R, Benz, EJ Jr, et al. (editors). *Hematology: Basic principles and practice.* Philadelphia: Churchill Livingtone.

Franco, RS, Hogg, JW, and Martelo, OJ. (1979). The effect of INH-inhibited heme synthesis on globin synthesis. *J. Lab. Clin. Med.* 93: 679–686.

Gozalbo, D and Hohmann, S. (1990). Nonsense suppressors partially revert the decrease of the mRNA level of a nonsense mutant allele in yeast. *Curr. Genet.* 17: 77–79.

Grayzel, AJ, Norchner P, and London IM. (1960). The stimulation of globin synthesis by heme. *Proc. Natl. Acad. Sci. U.S.A.* 55: 560–564.

Hall, GW and Thien, S. (1994). Nonsense codon mutations in the terminal exon of the β globin gene are not associated with a reduction in β mRNA accumulation: A mechanism for the phenotype of dominant β thalassemia. *Blood* 83: 2031–2037.

Hamer, DH and Leder, P. (1979). Splicing and the formation of stable mRNA. *Cell* 18: 1299–1302.

He, F, Brown, AH, and Jacobson, A. (1997). UpF1p, Nmd 2p, and UpF3p are interacting components of the yeast nonsense mediated mRNA decay pathway. *Mol. Cell Biol.* 17: 1580–1594.

Hentze, MW and Kulozik, AG. (1999). A perfect message with RNA surveillance and nonsense mediated decay. *Cell* 96, 307–310.

Higgs, DR, Aldridge, BE, Lamb, J et al. (1982). The interaction of alpha thalassemia and homozygous sickle cell disease. *N. Engl. J. Med.* 306: 1441–1446.

Holcik, M and Liebhaber, SA. (1997). Four highly stable eukaryotic mRNAs assemble 3 untranslated region RNA-protein complexes sharing *cis* and *trans* components. *Proc. Natl. Acad. Sci. U.S.A.* 94: 2410–2414.

Hunt, DM, Higgs, DR, Winichagoon, P et al. (1982). Haemoglobin constant spring has an unstable α chain messenger RNA. *Brit. J. Haematol.* 51: 405–413.

Jacobson, A and Peltz, SW. (1996). Interrelationships of the pathways of mRNA decay and translation in eukaryotic cells. *Annu. Rev. Biochem.* 65: 693–739.

Kan, YW, Schwartz, E, and Nathan, DG. (1969). Globin chain synthesis in the alpha thalassemia syndromes. *J. Clin. Invest.* 47: 2512–2522.

Kaufman, RJ. (1999). Stress signaling from the lumen of the endoplasmic reticulum: Coordination of gene transcriptional and translational controls. *Genes Dev.* 13: 1211–1233.

Kessler, O and Chasin, LA. (1996). Effects of nonsense mutations on nuclear and cytoplasmic adenine phosphoribosyl transferase RNA. *Mol. Cell Biol.* 16: 4426–4435.

Komar, AA, Kommer, A, Krasheninnikou, IA, and Spirin, AS. (1997). Cotranslational folding of globin. *J. Biol. Chem.* 272: 10696–10651.

Kozak, M. (1991). An analysis of vertebrate mRNA sequences: Intimations of translational control. *J. Cell Biol.* 115: 887–903.

Kruh, J and Borsook, H. (1956). Hemoglobin synthesis in rabbit reticuloctyes in vitro. *J. Biol. Chem.* 220: 905.

Kugler, W, Enssk, J, Hertze, MW, and Kulozik, AE. (1995). Nuclear degradation of nonsense mediated mutated β globin mRNA: A posttranscriptional mechanism to protect heterozygotes from severe clinical manifestations of β thalassemia? *Nucleic Acids Res.* 23: 413–418.

LeGrandeur, TG and Parker, R. (1998). Isolation and characterization of dcp1p, the yeast mRNA decapping enzyme. *EMBO J.* 17: 1487–1496.

Lejbkowicz, F, Goyer, C, Darveau, A et al. (1992). A fraction of the mRNA 5′ cap binding protein, eukaryotic initiation factor 4E, localizes to the nucleus. *Proc. Natl. Acad. Sci. U.S.A.* 89: 9612–9616.

Liebhaber, SA. (1997). mRNA stability and the control of gene expression. *Nucleic Acids Symp. Series* 36: 27–32.

Liebhaber, SA and Kan, YW. (1981). Differentiation of the transcripts originating from the a1 and a2 globin loci in normal and thalassemics. *J. Clin. Invest.* 68: 439–446.

Liebhaber, SA and Russell, JE. (1998). Expression and developmental control of the alpha globin cluster. *Ann. N.Y. Acad. Sci.* 850: 54–63.

Liebhaber, SA and Kan, YW. (1982). Differentiates of mRNA translation balance the expression of the two alpha-globin loci. *J. Biol. Chem.* 257: 11852–11855.

Liebhaber, SA, Cash, F, and Eshleman, SS. (1992). Translation inhibition by an mRNA coding region secondary structure is determined by its proximity to the AUG initiation codon. *J. Mol. Biol.* 226: 609–621.

Lodish, HF. (1971). Alpha and beta globin messenger ribonucleic acid: Different amounts and rates of initiation of translation. *J. Biol. Chem.* 246: 7131–7138.

Lodish, HF. (1974). Model for the regulation of mRNA translation applied to hemoglobin synthesis. *Nature* 251: 385–388.

Lodish, H and Jacobsen, M. (1972). Regulation of hemoglobin synthesis: Equal rates of translation and termination of α and β globin chains. *J. Biol. Chem.* 247: 3622–3629.

Makeyev, AV, Chkheidze, AN, and Liebhaber, SA. (1999). A set of highly conserved RNA binding proteins, alpha CP-1 and alpha CP-2, implicated in mRNA stabilization, are coexpressed from an intronless gene and intron containing paralog. *J. Biol. Chem.* 274: 24849–24857.

Manning, JM, Dunaolin, A, Li, X, and Manning, LR. (1998). Normal and abnormal subunit interactions in hemoglobins. *J. Biol. Chem.* 273: 19359–19362.

Manning, JM, Dunaolin, A, Manning, LR et al. (1999). Remote contributions to subunit interactions: lessons from adult and fetal hemoglobins. *Trends Biochem. Sci.* 24: 211–212.

Maquat, LE. (1995). When cells stop making sense: Effects of nonsense codons on RNA metabolism in vertebrate cells. *RNA* 1: 453–465.

McDonald, MJ, Turei, SM, and Bunn, HF. (1984). Subunit assembly of normal and mutant hemoglobins. *Prog. Clin. Biol. Res.* 165: 3–15.

Morales, J, Russell, JE, and Liebhaber, SA. (1997). Destabilization of human α globin mRNA by translation antitermination is controlled during erythroid differentiation and is paralleled by phased shortening of the poly(A) tail. *J. Biol. Chem.* 272: 6607–6613.

Nagy, G and Maquat, LG. (1998). Azule purtermination codon position within intron containing genes when nonsense affects RNA abundance. *Trends Biochem. Sci.* 23: 198–199.

Nienhuis, AW and Benz, EJ Jr. (1977). Regulation of hemoglobin synthesis during development of the red cell. *N. Engl. J. Med.* 297: 1318–1328.

Olmstead, GA, O'Brien, L, Henshaw, EG, and Panniers, R. (1993). Purification and characterization of eIF-2 alpha kinases from Ehrlich ascites tumor cells. *J. Biol. Chem.* 268: 12552–12559.

Ostareck-Lederer, AL, Ostareck, DH, and Hentze, MW. (1998). Cytoplasmic regulatory functions of the KH domain proteins hnRNP's K and EI/E2. *Trends Biochem Sci.* 23: 409–411.

Pain, VM. (1996). Initiation of protein synthesis in eukaryotic cells. *Eur. J. Biochem.* 236: 747–771.

Pal, JK, Chen, JD, and London, IM. (1991). Tissue distribution and immunoreactivity of eIF2 alpha kinase determined by monoclonal antibodies. *Biochemistry* 30: 2555–2562.

Peltz, SW, He, F, Welch, E, and Jacobson, A. (1994). Nonsense mediated decay in yeast. *Prog. Nucleic Acid Res. Mol. Biol.* 47: 271–298.

Perlick, HA, Medghalchi, SM, Spencer, FA et al. (1996), Mammalian orthologues of a yeast regulator of nonsense transcript stability. *Proc. Natl. Acad. Sci. U.S.A.* 93: 10928–10932.

Peters, RE, May, A, and Jacobs, A. (1983). Globin chain synthesis ratios in sideroblastic anaemia. *Br. J. Haematol.* 53: 201–209.

Piddington, SK and White, JM. (1974). The effect of lead on total globin and alpha- and beta-chain synthesis: In vitro and in vivo. *Br. J. Haematol.* 27: 415–427.

Ponka, P, Beaumont, C, and Richardson, DR. (1998). Function and regulation of transferrin and ferritin. *Semin. Hematol.* 35: 35–54.

Preiss T and Hentze MW. (1999). From factors to mechanisms: Translation and translational control in eukaryotes. *Curr. Opin. Genet. Dev.* 9: 515–521.

Ross, J. (1995). mRNA stability in mammalian cells. *Microbiol. Rev.* 59: 423–450.

Ross J and Pizarro, A. (1983). Human beta and delta mRNA's turnover at different rates. *J. Mol. Biol* 167: 607–614.

Ross, J and Sullivan, TD. (1985). Half lives of beta and gamma globin messenger RNAs and of protein synthetic capacity in cultured human reticulocytes. *Blood* 66: 1149–1160.

Ruiz-Echevarria, MF, Gonzalez, CI, and Peltz, SW. (1998). Identifying the right stop: Determining how the surveillance complex recognizes and degrades an aberrant mRNA. *EMBO J.* 17: 575–589.

Ruiz-Echevarria, MJ, Czaplinski, K, and Peltz, SW. (1996). Making sense of nonsense in yeast. *Trends Biochem. Sci.* 21: 433–438.

Russell, JE, Liebhaber, SA. (1996). The stability of beta-globin mRNA is dependent on structural determinants positioned within its 3′ untranslated region. *Blood* 87: 5314–5323.

Russell, JE, Morales, J, and Liebhaber, SA. (1997). The role of mRNA stability in the control of globin gene expression. *Prog. Nucleic Acids Res. Mol. Biol.* 57: 249–287.

Russell, JE, Lee, AE, and Liebhaber, SA. (1998a). Full developmental silencing of the embryonic zeta-globin gene reflects in stability of its mRNA. *Ann. N.Y. Acad. Sci.* 850: 386–390.

Russell, JE, Morales, J, Makeyev, AV, and Liebhaber, SA. (1998b). Sequence divergence in the 3′ untranslated regions of human zeta and alpha globin mRNAs mediates an influence in their stabilities and contributes to efficient alpha to zeta gene developmental switching. *Mol. Cell. Biol.* 18: 2173–2183.

Sachs, AB, Sarnow, P, and Hentze, MW. (1991). Starting at the beginning, middle and end: Translation initiation in eukaryocytes. *Cell* 89: 831–838.

Sassa, S. (1983). Heme Biosynthesis in erythroid cells: Distinctive aspects of the regulatory mechanism. In Goldwasser, E (editor). *Regulation of hemoglobin biosynthesis.* New York: Elsevier Science Publishing.

Shakin SH and Liebhaber, SA. (1986). Translational profiles of alpha 1, alpha 2, and beta globin, messenger ribonucleic acids in human reticulocytes. *J. Clin. Invest.* 78: 1125–1129.

Silverman, RH and Williams, BRG. (1999). Translational control perks up. *Nature* 397: 208–209.

Sonnenberg, N and Gingras, AC. (1998). The mRNA 5 cap binding protein eIF 4E and control of cell growth. *Curr. Opin. Cell Biol.* 10: 268–275.

Soreq, H. (1985). The biosynthesis of biologically active proteins in mRNA microinjected xenopus in oocytes. *CRC Criti. Rev. Biochem.* 18: 199–238.

Stephenson, LS and Maquat, LE. (1996). Cytoplasmic mRNA for human triosephosphate isomerase is immune to nonsense-mediated decay despite forming polysomes. *Biochimie* 78: 1043–1047.

Takeshita, K, Forget, BG, Scarpa, A, and Benz, EJ Jr. (1984). Intranuclear detection β globin mRNA accumulation due to a premature termination codon. *Blood* 64: 13–22.

Tarun, SZ and Sachs, A. (1996). Association of the yeast poly(A) binding protein with translation initiation factor eIF-4G. *EMBO J.* 15: 168–7177.

Tavill, AS, Grayzel, AI, London, IM et al. (1968). The role of heme in the synthesis and assembly of hemoglobin. *J. Biol. Chem.* 243: 4987–4999.

Temple, GF, Chang, JC, and Kan, UW. (1977). Authentic β Globin mRNA Sequences in homozygous β° thalassemia. *Proc. Natl. Acad. Sci. U.S.A.* 73: 3047–3051.

Thermann, P, Nev-Yilik, G, Deters, A et al. (1998). Binary specification of nonsense codons by splicing and cytoplasmic translation. *EMBO J.* 17: 3484–3494.

Thien, SL, Hesketh, C, Taylor, B et al. (1990). Molecular basis for dominantly inherited inclusion body β thalassemia. *Proc. Natl. Acad. Sci. U.S.A.* 87: 3924–3928.

Urlaub, G, Mitchell, PJ, Ciudad, CJ, and Chasin, LA. (1989). Nonsense mutations in the dihydrofolate reductase gene affect RNA processing. *Mol. Cell Biol.* 9: 2868–2880.

Volloch, Z and Housman, D. (1981). Stability of globin mRNA in terminally differentiating murine erythroleukemia Cells. *Cell* 23: 509–514.

Wakasugi, K, Ishimori, K, and Morishina, I. (1997). Module substituted hemoglobins: Artificial exon shuffling among myoglobin, hemoglobin alpha- and beta-subunits. *Biophys. Chem.* 68: 265–273.

Walford, DM and Deacon, R. (1980). Globin chain biosynthesis in iron deficiency. *Br. J. Haematol.* 44: 201.

Wang, X, Kiledijan, M, Weiss, IM, and Liebhaber, SA. (1995a). Detection and characterization of a 3′ untrans-

lated region ribonucleoprotein complex associated with human alpha globin mRNA stability. *Mol. Cell Biol.* 15: 1769–1777.

Wang, X, Kiledjan, M, Weiss, IM, and Liebhaber, SA. (1995b). Identification of two KH domain proteins in the alpha-globin mRNP stability complex. *EMBO J.* 14: 4357–4364.

Waxman, HS and Rabinovitz, M. (1965). Iron supplementation in vitro and the state of aggregation and function of reticulocyte vibosomes in hemoglobin synthesis. *Biochem. Biophys. Res. Commun.* 19: 538.

Weiss, IM and Liebhaber, SA. (1994). Erythroid specific determinants of alpha globin mRNA stability. *Mol. Cell Biol.* 14: 8123–8132.

Weiss, IM and Liebhaber, SA. (1995). Erythroid cell-specific mRNA stability elements in the alpha 2-globin 3 nontranslated region. *Mol. Cell Biol.* 15: 2457–2465.

White, JM and Ali, MA. (1973). Globin synthesis in sideroblastic anaemia. *Br. J. Haematol.* 24: 481–489.

White, JM and Harvey, DR. (1972). Defective synthesis of α and β globin chains in lead poisoning. *Nature* 236: 71–73.

White, JM and Hoffbrand, AV. (1974). Haeme deficiency and chain synthesis. *Nature* 248: 88.

White, JM, Brain, MC, and Ali, MA. (1971). Globin synthesis in sideroblastic anaemia. I. Alpha and beta peptide chain synthesis. *Br. J. Haematol.* 20: 263–275.

Wiley, JS and Moore, MR. (1999). Heme biosynthesis and its disorders. In Hoffman R, Benz, EJ Jr, et al (editors). *Hematology: Basic principles and practice.* Philadelphia: Churchill Livingstone.

Zago, MA and Bottura, C. (1982). Bone marrow and peripheral blood globin chain biosynthesis in iron deficiency. *Blut* 44: 159–164.

Zhang, S, Ruiz-Echevarria, MJ, Quan, Y, and Peltz, SW. (1995). Identification and characterization of a sequence motif involved in nonsense mediated mRNA decay. *Mol. Cell Biol.* 15: 2231–2244.

Zhang, J, Sun, X, Qian, Y et al. (1998a). At least one intron is required for the nonsense-mediated decay of triosephosphate isomerase mRNA: A possible link between nuclear splicing and cytoplasmic transplantion. *Mol. Cell Biol.* 18: 5272–5283.

Zhang, J, Sun, X, Qian, Y, and Maquat, LE. (1998b). Intron function in the nonsense mediated decay of β globin mRNA: Indications that pre-mRNA splicing in the nucleus can influence mRNA translation in the cytoplasm. *RNA* 4: 801–815.

9

Molecular Anatomy and Physiology of Hemoglobin

MAX F. PERUTZ

HEMOGLOBIN AND MYOGLOBIN AND THEIR REACTION WITH OXYGEN

Hemoglobin is the protein of the red blood cells that allows vertebrates to transport oxygen from the lungs to the tissues and that helps the return transport of carbon dioxide from the tissues back to the lungs. More may have been written about hemoglobin than about any other molecule. Physicists, crystallographers, chemists of all kinds, zoologists, physiologists and geneticists, pathologists, and hematologists have all contributed to a vast literature. In the erratic ways that scientific research shares with other human endeavors, the multifarious work of that great throng has provided us with an enormous store of knowledge from which one can extract data on subjects as diverse as the quantum chemistry of iron and the buoyancy of fish. This chapter concentrates mainly on the relation between three-dimensional structure and physiologic function in humans. For more extensive treatments the reader is referred to the monographs and reviews listed at the end of the chapter (Barcroft, 1914; Antonini and Brunori, M, 1971; Antonini et al., 1981; Bunn and Forget, 1985; Dickerson and Geis, 1983; Fermi and Perutz, 1981; Garby and Madden, 1977; Ho, 1982; Imai, 1982; Lehmann and Huntsman, 1974; Perutz and Lehmann, 1968; Lehmann and Kynoch, 1976; Perutz, 1998) The reader should start with Sir Joseph

Barcroft's classic, The *Respiratory Function of the Blood* (Barcroft, 1914).

The hemoglobin molecule is made up of four polypeptide chains, two α chains of 141 amino acid residues each and two β chains of 146 residues each (Bunn and Forget, 1985; Dickerson and Geis, 1983; Fermi and Perutz, 1981). The α and β chains have different sequences of amino acids, but fold up to form similar three-dimensional structures. Each chain harbors one heme, which gives blood its red color. The heme consists of a porphyrin ring with an atom of iron, like a jewel, at its center (Fig. 9.1). A single polypeptide chain combined with a single heme is called a subunit of hemoglobin or a monomer of the molecule. In the complete molecule four subunits are closely joined, as in a three-dimensional jigsaw puzzle, to form a tetramer.

In red muscle there is another protein, myoglobin, which is similar in constitution and structure to a β subunit of hemoglobin, but made up of only one polypeptide chain and one heme. Myoglobin combines with the oxygen released by red cells, stores it, and transports it to the mitochondria, where the oxygen generates chemical energy by the combustion of glucose to carbon dioxide and water. Myoglobin was the first protein whose three-dimensional structure was determined; it was solved by my colleague John C. Kendrew and his collaborators.

Myoglobin is the simpler of the two molecules. This protein, with its 2,500 atoms, exists for the sole purpose of allowing its single atom of iron to form a loose chemical bond with a molecule of oxygen (O_2). Why does nature go to so much trouble to accomplish what is apparently such a simple task? Like most compounds of iron, heme by itself combines with oxygen irreversibly to yield ferric heme, but when ferrous heme is embedded in the folds of the globin chain, it is protected so that its reaction with oxygen is reversible. The effect of the globin on the chemistry of the heme has been explained only recently with the discovery that the irreversible oxidation of heme proceeds by way of an intermediate compound in which an oxygen molecule forms a bridge between the iron atoms of two hemes. In myoglobin and hemoglobin, the folds of the polypeptide chain prevent the formation of such a bridge by isolating each heme in a separate pocket. Moreover, in the protein the iron is linked to a nitrogen atom of the amino acid histidine, which donates a negative charge that enables the iron to form a loose bond with oxygen.

An oxygen-free solution of myoglobin or hemoglobin is purple like venous blood. When oxygen is bubbled through it, it turns scarlet like arterial blood. If these proteins are to act as oxygen carriers, then hemoglobin must be capable of taking up oxygen in the lungs, where it is plentiful, and giving it up to myoglobin in the capillaries of muscle, where it is less plentiful. Myoglobin in turn must pass the oxygen on to the mitochondria, where it is scarcer still.

THE OXYGEN EQUILIBRIUM

A simple experiment shows that myoglobin and hemoglobin can accomplish this exchange, because there is an equilibrium between free oxygen and oxygen bound to heme iron. Suppose a solution of myoglobin is placed in a tonometer, where a large volume of gas can be mixed with it and where its color can be measured through a spectroscope. The spectroscope measures the proportion of oxymyoglobin in the solution on injection of oxygen. The results are plotted on a graph, with the partial pressure of oxygen on the horizontal axis and the percentage of oxymyoglobin on the vertical axis. It is a rectangular hyperbola that is steep at the start, when all the myoglobin molecules are free, and then flattens out at the end, when free myoglobin molecules have become so scarce that only a high pressure of oxygen can saturate them (Fig. 9.2).

Figure 9.1. Iron protoporphyrin IX. The arabic numbers are those adopted in Antonini and Brunori (1971) and Baldwin and Chothia (1979). The Roman numbers are from Fermi and Perutz (1981) and Fermi (1975), and the letters are from Sober, 1968. (From Perutz, MF. [1979]. Regulation of oxygen affinity of hemoglobin. Influence of the structure of the globin on the heme iron. *Ann. Rev. Biochem.* 48:327.)

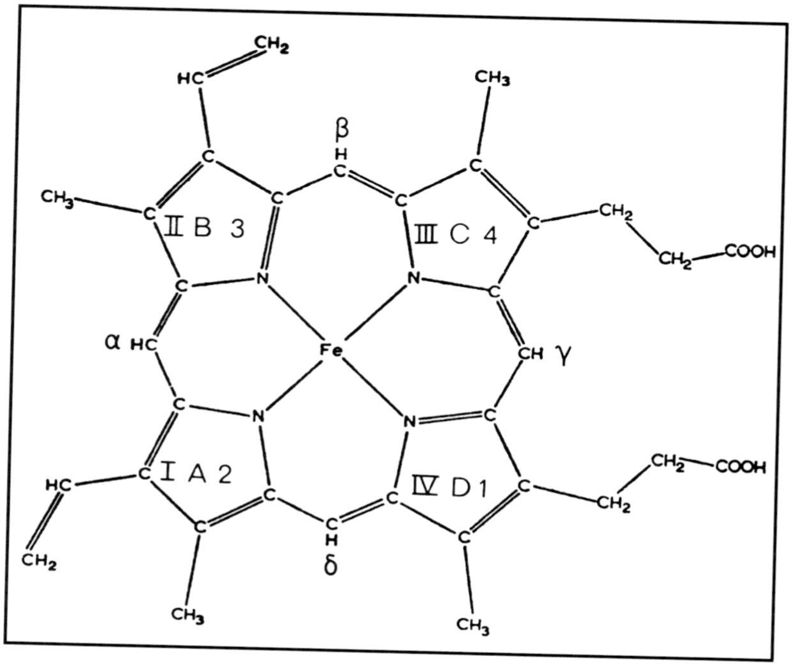

Equilibrium Curves and Hill's Coefficient

The equilibrium between myoglobin and oxygen can be represented by the equation:

$$[Mb] + [O_2] \overset{K}{\leftrightarrow} [MbO_2]$$

The square brackets mean concentrations and K is the equilibrium constant. If we define the fractional saturation with oxygen Y by the equation:

$$Y = \frac{[MbO_2]}{[Mb] + [MbO_2]}$$

then the equilibrium is best represented by a graph in which the logarithm of Y divided by 1-Y is plotted against the logarithm of the partial pressure of oxygen. The hyperbola now becomes a straight line at 45° to the axes (Fig. 9.3). The equilibrium constant between myoglobin, oxymyoglobin, and oxygen is an association constant defined as $K = \dfrac{Y}{(1-Y) \, PO_2}$. Hence, K has the dimension $(mm \ Hg)^{-1}$. In Figure 9.3, the intercept of the line with the vertical axis drawn at $\log PO_2 = 0$ gives the log of the equilibrium constant K. K^{-1} is the partial pressure of oxygen at which exactly half the myoglobin molecules have taken up oxygen (p^{50}). The greater the affinity of the protein for oxygen, the lower the pressure needed to achieve half-saturation and the larger the equilibrium constant. The 45° slope remains unchanged, but lower oxygen affinity shifts the line to the right, while higher affinity shifts it to the left.

If the same experiment is done with blood or with a solution of hemoglobin, an entirely different result is obtained. The curve rises gently at first, then steepens and finally flattens out as it approaches the myoglobin curve (Fig. 8.2). This sigmoid shape signifies that the molecule's appetite for oxygen grows with the eating. Conversely, the loss of oxygen by some of the hemes lowers the oxygen affinity of the remaining hemes. The distribution of oxygen among the hemoglobin molecules in a solution therefore follows the biblical parable of the rich and the poor: "For unto every one that hath shall be given, and he shall have abundance: but from him that hath not shall be taken away even that which he hath." This phenomenon suggests communication between the four hemes in each molecule, and physiologists have therefore called it heme-heme interaction.

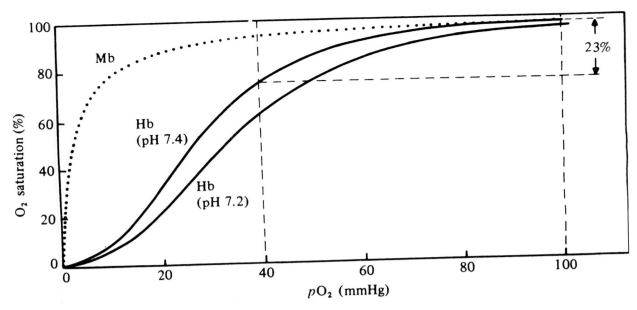

Figure 9.2. Oxygen equilibrium curves of human red cell and sperm whale myoglobin. The curves for the red cells were determined at 37°C with fresh human blood that was 150 times diluted with isotonic phosphate buffers (0.15 mol/L KH_2PO_4 + 0.15 M Na_2HPO_4). The curve for myoglobin was determined at 37°C, with 60 μmol/L myoglobin dissolved in 0.1 mol/L potassium phosphate buffer (pH 7.4). At pH 7.4, the oxygen saturation of the red cells is 98 percent at the arterial blood (PO_2 = 100 mm Hg), and 75 percent at the mixed venous blood (PO_2 = 40 mm Hg), so that oxygen corresponding to a 23 percent difference in saturation is transported by circulating red cells. (From Imai, 1982.)

Figure 9.3. Logarithmic plot of oxygen equilibrium curve of human myoglobin at pH 8.0 and 20°. Y = fractional saturation with oxygen.

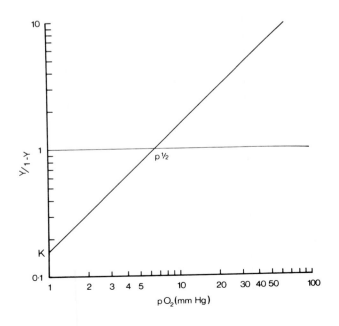

A better picture of the underlying mechanism of heme-heme interaction is obtained in a logarithmic graph (Fig. 9.4). The equilibrium curve then begins with a straight line at 45° to the axes, because at first oxygen molecules are so scarce that only one heme in each hemoglobin molecule has a chance of catching one, and all the hemes therefore react independently, as in myoglobin. As more oxygen flows in, the four hemes in each molecule begin to interact, and the curve steepens. The tangent to its maximum slope is known as Hill's coefficient (n), after the English physiologist A. V. Hill, who first attempted a mathematical analysis of the oxygen equilibrium. The normal value of Hill's coefficient in the blood of healthy human subjects under standard physiologic conditions is 3.0; without heme-heme interaction it becomes (unity). The curve ends with another line at 45° to the axes, because oxygen has now become so abundant that only the last heme in each molecule is likely to be free, and all the hemes in the solution react independently once more. Continuation of the 45° lines to the ordinate gives the logarithms of the equilibrium constants for the combination with oxygen of the first and the fourth hemes, K_1 and K_4. K_2, and K_3 can be found only by curve fitting.

Heterotropic Ligands

Hill's coefficient and the oxygen affinity of hemoglobin depend on the concentrations of several factors in the red blood cell: hydrogen ions, carbon dioxide, chloride ions, and 2,3-biphosphoglycerate (BPG). They are known as the heterotropic ligands, as opposed to oxygen and carbon monoxide, which are called homotropic ligands. Increasing the concentration of any of these

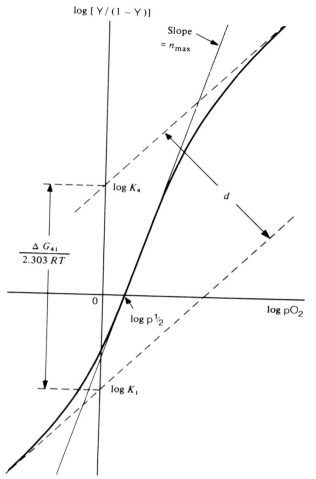

Figure 9.4. Logarithmic (Hill) plot of oxygen equilibrium curve of human hemoglobin. Y = fractional saturation with oxygen, K_1 and K_4 are the equilibrium constants of the first and fourth heme with oxygen. N_{max} is Hill's coefficient. ΔG_{41} is the free energy of cooperativity per heme. (From Imai, 1982.)

heterotropic ligands shifts the oxygen equilibrium curve to the right, toward lower oxygen affinity, and makes it more sigmoid (Fig. 9.5). None of these factors influence either the oxygen equilibrium curve of myoglobin or the individual chains of hemoglobin.

Effect of Temperature

The reaction of heme-iron with oxygen is exothermic; the oxygen affinity of hemoglobin drops with rising temperature. This means that during heavy exercise, a raised temperature in the muscles promotes the release of oxygen. Being intrinsic to the reaction of the heme iron with oxygen, high temperature also lowers the oxygen affinity of free α and β chains and of $\alpha\beta$ dimers. In fact, their oxygen affinity is more temperature sensitive than that of the $\alpha_2\beta_2$ tetramer, because

some of the heat given off by the hemes' reaction with oxygen is absorbed by heme-heme interaction.

Physiologic Significance of Cooperative Effects

What is the purpose of these extraordinary effects? Why is it not good enough for the red cell to contain a simple oxygen carrier such as myoglobin? Such a carrier would not allow enough of the oxygen in the red cell to be unloaded to the tissues, nor would it allow enough carbon dioxide to be carried to the lungs by the blood plasma.

The cooperativity of oxygen binding and release, the effects of the heterotropic ligands, and the effects of the temperature conspire to maximize the difference in fractional oxygen saturation between arterial and venous blood. The partial pressure of oxygen in arterial blood is normally 90 to 100 mm Hg, and in mixed venous blood 35 to 40 mm Hg. Under standard conditions (pH 7.4, PCO_2 = 40 mm Hg, [BPG] = 5 mmol/L packed red cells, Hb CO = 1 percent and temperature = 37° C) in whole blood from apparently healthy subjects, these partial pressures correspond to oxygen saturation of 98 to 100 percent in arterial and 66 to 73 percent in venous blood. Under these circumstances only one fourth to one third of the total oxygen carried is released in the tissues; the fractional saturation with oxygen in muscular veins during heavy exercise is believed to be lower.

The more pronounced the sigmoid shape of the equilibrium curve, the greater the fraction of oxygen that can be released. Several factors conspire to this purpose. Oxidation of nutrients by the tissues liberates lactic acid and carbonic acid; these acids shift the curve to the right and make it more sigmoid. Another important regulator of the oxygen affinity is 2,3 BPG. The number of 2,3 BPG molecules in the red cell is about the same as the number of hemoglobin molecules (280 million) and probably remains fairly constant during circulation. Shortage of oxygen causes more 2,3 BPG to be made, which helps to release more oxygen. The human fetus has a hemoglobin with the same α chains as the adult, but with γ instead of β chains with a lower affinity for 2,3 BPG. This gives fetal hemoglobin a higher oxygen affinity and facilitates the transfer of oxygen from the maternal circulation to the fetal circulation (Chapter 10).

THE BOHR EFFECT AND THE TRANSPORT OF CARBON DIOXIDE

If protons lower the oxygen affinity of hemoglobin, then oxygen must lower the affinity for protons. Liberation of oxygen causes hemoglobin to combine with protons and vice versa; at physiologic pH about two protons are taken up for every four molecules of oxygen released

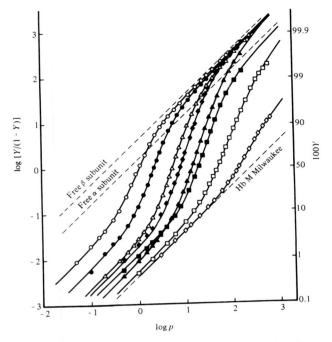

Figure 9.5. Hill plots of oxygenation of human adult hemoglobin (HbA) under representative sets of effector conditions. Temperature = 25°C; hemoglobin concentration = 0.6 mol/L on a heme basis in 0.05 mol/L bis-tris buffer for pH 7.4 and pH 6.5, and in 0.05 MTris buffer for pH 9.1; ● = pH 9.1, 2.6 mM Cl⁻; ○ = pH 9.1, 0.1 mol/L Cl⁻; Δ = pH 7.4, 0.1 mol/L Cl⁻; ▲ = pH 7.4, 0.1 mol/L Cl⁻, 2 mol/L DPG; ◆ = pH 7.4, 0.1 mol/L Cl⁻ 5 percent CO₂; □ = pH 7.4, 0.1 mol/L Cl⁻, 2 mol/L IHP; ■ = pH 6.5, 0.1 mol/L Cl⁻; ◇ = pH 6.5, 0.1 mol/L Cl⁻, 2 mol/L IHP. IHP (inositolhexaphosphate) is a synthetic effector that lowers the oxygen affinity of both R and T structures. HbM Milwaukee is an abnormal hemoglobin with the substitution Val E77 (67)β → Glu. In the presence of IHP it remains in the T structure even when the hemes are fully oxygenated. (From Imai, 1982.)

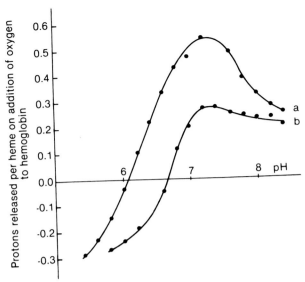

Figure 9.6. Full discharge of protons on uptake of oxygen by (a) normal human hemoglobin A and (b) half discharge of protons by hemoglobin from which the C-terminal histidines of the β chains have been cleaved with carboxypeptidase B (des His 146 β hemoglobin). Note the reversal of the alkaline Bohr effect at pH 6.0 in HbA and at pH 6.7 in des His hemoglobin, and the halving of the alkaline Bohr effect in the latter. (From Kilmartin, JV and Wootton, JF [1970]. Inhibition of Bohr effect after removal of C-terminal histidines from haemoglobin β chains. Nature 228:766.)

and are liberated again when oxygen is taken up (Fig. 9.6). This is known as the Bohr effect (after the Danish physiologist Christian Bohr who discovered it early in the twentieth century), and it is the key to the mechanism of carbon dioxide transport. The carbon dioxide released by respiring tissues is too insoluble to be transported efficiently, but it can be rendered more soluble by combining with water to form a bicarbonate ion and a proton.

$$CO_2 + H_2O \leftrightarrow HCO_3^- + H^+$$

In the absence of hemoglobin, this reaction would be brought to a halt by the excess of protons produced. Deoxyhemoglobin acts as a buffer, mopping up the protons and tipping the balance toward the formation of soluble bicarbonate. In the lungs the process is reversed. There, as oxygen binds to hemoglobin, protons are cast off, driving carbon dioxide out of solution

so that it can be exhaled. The reaction between carbon dioxide and water is catalyzed by carbonic anhydrase, an enzyme in the red cells that speeds up the reaction to a rate of about half a million molecules per second, one of the fastest of all known biological reactions. The uptake of protons on liberation of oxygen and the release of protons on uptake of oxygen are known as the alkaline Bohr effect, because they occur only above pH 6. Below pH 6 protons are released on liberation of oxygen (Fig. 9.6). This is known as the acid Bohr effect. It is enhanced by both 2,3 BPG and chloride.

The Bohr effect is measured either by determining the pH dependence of p^{50} $\frac{d \log p^{50}}{d \, pH}$ or the change of pH on oxygen binding of an unbuffered hemoglobin solution, $\frac{d \, pH}{d \log Y}$. In human hemoglobin in 0.1 MCl⁻ without 2,3 BPG at 20° C, either measurement gives a value of about −0.5. 2,3 BPG enhances the Bohr effect.[1]

In the absence of chloride, the alkaline Bohr effect is halved. The chloride-independent part of the alkaline Bohr effect was found to be due exclusively to a change

[1] p^{50} is the partial pressure of oxygen where half the hemoglobin is saturated with oxygen.

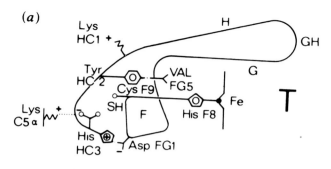

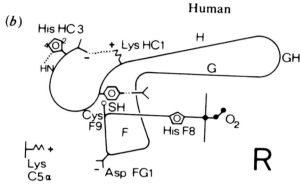

Figure 9.7. Contribution of His HC3(146)β to the alkaline Bohr effect. The C-terminal salt bridge between the imidazole of histidine HC3(146)β and aspartate FG1(94)β in the deoxyhemoglobin (T) structure raises the pKa of the imidazole to 8.0. In oxyhemoglobin (R) the α carboxyl of histidine HC3(146)β forms a salt bridge with lysine HC1(144)β; the imidazole of the histidine accepts a hydrogen bond from its own main chain NH; as a consequence its pKa drops to 7.1 or lower. (From Perutz, MF et al. [1985]. The pKa values of two histidine residues in human haemoglobin, the Bohr effect, and the dipole moments of α-helices. *J. Mol. Biol.* 183:491.)

in pK$_a$ of His HC3 β, which donates a hydrogen bond to Asp FG1 β in deoxyhemoglobin and accepts one from its own main-chain NH in oxyhemoglobin (Fig. 9.7). In 0.2 mol/L NaCl, titration of the proton resonances of that histidine yielded pK$_a$s of 7.1 in HbCO and of 8.0 in deoxyHb (19), but the pK$_a$ of 7.1 in HbCO became controversial when another nuclear magnetic resonance (NMR) study seemed to show that in bis/tris buffers with minimal Cl$^-$ it becomes as high as 7.9 (Russu et al., 1980). However, the resonance assigned to His HC3 in that study was later shown to belong to His FG4; its pK$_a$ is abnormally high because it caps the carboxyl end of a helix (Shih et al., 1993). Discovery of the correct resonance for His HC3 has confirmed its original low pK$_a$. (Busch et al., 1991).

The chloride-dependent part of the alkaline Bohr effect used to be attributed to Val NA1 α and Lys EF6 β, because it was inhibited when the α-amino groups of the valines were carbamylated and the lysines were replaced by neutral residues. Recent work has shown this to be incorrect. Instead, the effect arises through changes in the width of the central cavity (see Fig. 9.11). The cavity is lined with an excess of positively charged side chains that attract chloride ions. Expansion of the cavity in the transition from oxyhemoglobin to deoxyhemoglobin allows entry of more chloride ions. The rise in their pK$_a$s brought about by the chloride ions is responsible for the chloride-dependent part of the Bohr effect (see Fig. 9.18) (Perutz, Shih, and Williamson, 1993).

Recent advances in NMR have opened the possibility of determining the pH in live human muscle from the difference in chemical shift between the ^{31}P signals from phosphocreatine and inorganic phosphate. By this method, muscle at rest was found to have a pH of 7.03 ($\pm$ 0.03). During exercise, liberation of lactic and carbonic acids caused the intracellular pH in the finger flexor muscle of some individuals to drop as low as 6.0. If the pH in the red cell dropped from 7.0 to 6.0, this would double p^{50}; over the middle part of the equilibrium this would increase oxygen delivery from about 30 percent of the oxygen carried to about 70 percent.

$$-\underset{\underset{O}{\|}}{C}-\underset{\underset{|}{}}{CH}-NH_2 + CO_2 \rightleftharpoons -\underset{\underset{O}{\|}}{C}-\underset{\underset{|}{}}{CH}-NHCOO^- + H^+$$

There is a second mechanism for transporting carbon dioxide (CO_2). The gas binds more readily to deoxyhemoglobin than it does to oxyhemoglobin, so that it tends to be taken up when oxygen is liberated and cast off when oxygen is bound. The direct transport of CO_2 by hemoglobin accounts for about 10 percent of the total CO_2 exchanged by the red blood cells during respiration. Under physiologic conditions, human oxyhemoglobin binds about 0.15 mol CO_2 per mole heme, and deoxyhemoglobin binds about 0.40 mol CO_2 per mole heme. CO_2 is bound covalently by the α-amino groups of the globin to form a carbamino compound as shown above. The protons liberated in this reaction oppose the conversion of other molecules of carbon dioxide to bicarbonate by the Bohr effect. Protons entering the red cell draw negatively charged chloride ions in with them, and these ions too are bound more readily by deoxyhemoglobin than by oxyhemoglobin. 2,3 BPG is synthesized in the red cell itself and cannot leak out through the cell membrane. It is strongly bound by deoxyhemoglobin and only very weakly bound by oxyhemoglobin.

ALLOSTERY

Puzzle of Cooperative Effects

Heme-heme interaction and the interplay between oxygen and the heterotropic ligands are known collectively as the cooperative effects of hemoglobin. Their discovery by a succession of able physiologists and biochemists took more than half a century and aroused many controversies. In 1938, Felix Haurowitz of the Charles University in Prague made another vital observation. He discovered that deoxyhemoglobin and oxyhemoglobin form different crystals, as though they were different chemical substances. This difference implied that hemoglobin is not an oxygen tank but a molecular lung, because it changes its structure every time it takes up oxygen or releases it (Haurowitz, 1938).

The discovery of an interaction among the four hemes made it seem obvious that they are touching, but when the structure of hemoglobin was finally solved, the hemes were found to lie in isolated pockets on the surface of the subunits (Perutz et al., 1960). Without contact among them, how could one of them sense whether the others had combined with oxygen? And how could as heterogeneous a collection of chemical agents as protons, chloride ions, carbon dioxide, and biphosphoglycerate influence the oxygen equilibrium curve in a similar way? It did not seem plausible that any of them could bind directly to the hemes, nor that all of them could bind at any other common site. To add to the mystery, none of these agents affected the oxygen equilibrium of myoglobin or of isolated subunits of hemoglobin. We now know that all the cooperative effects disappear if the hemoglobin molecule is merely split in half, but for many years this vital clue was missed.

Analogy Between Hemoglobin and Allosteric Enzymes

Monod, Changeux, and Jacob discovered that the activity of certain enzymes is controlled by switching their synthesis on and off at the gene; they and others then found a second mode of regulation that appeared to operate switches on the enzymes themselves (Monod et al., 1963). In 1965 Monod, Wyman, and Changeux recognized that the enzymes in the latter class have certain features in common with hemoglobin. They are all made of several subunits, so that each molecule includes several sites with the same catalytic activity, just as hemoglobin includes several hemes that bind oxygen, and they all show similar cooperative effects. Monod and his colleagues knew that deoxyhemoglobin and oxyhemoglobin have different structures, which made them suspect that the enzymes too may exist in two (or at least two) structures. They postulated that these structures should be distinguished by the arrangement of the subunits and by the number and strength of the bonds between them (Monod et al., 1965).

Theory of Allostery

The structure with fewer and weaker bonds between the subunits would be free to develop its full catalytic activity (or oxygen affinity); this was therefore labeled R, for "relaxed." The activity would be damped in the structure with more and stronger bonds between the subunits; this form is called T, for "tense." In either of these structures the catalytic activity (or oxygen affinity) of all the subunits in one molecule should always remain equal. This postulate of symmetry allowed the properties of allosteric enzymes to be described by a neat mathematical theory with only three independent variables: K_R and K_T, which in hemoglobin denote the oxygen association constants of the R and T structures, respectively, and L, which stands for the number of molecules in the T structure divided by the number in the R structure, the ratio being measured in the absence of oxygen. The term allostery (from the Greek roots *allos*, "other," and *stereos*, "solid") was coined because the regulator molecule that switches the activity of the enzyme on or off has a structure different from that of the molecule whose chemical transformation the enzyme catalyzes (Fig. 9.8). Baldwin (1975) has written a comprehensive review of the structure and function of hemoglobin in the light of the theory of allostery. In thermodynamic terms, allostery means that oxygen is bound to the R structure more firmly than to the T structure by the equivalent of a free energy:

$$\Delta G = 2.303 \, RT \log K_R/K_T \text{ kcal mol}^{-1},$$

where R is the gas constant and T the absolute temperature (Fig. 9.4). At 20°C, $\Delta G = 1.34 \log K_R/K_T$: at 37°C, $\Delta G = 1.42 \log K_R/K_T$. This means that a change in free energy of 1.34 kcal mol^{-1} at 20° or of 1.42 kcal mol^{-1} at 37°C, corresponding to no more than an average hydrogen bond, produces a tenfold change in K_R/K_T. At 25°C and under conditions otherwise representative of those in the red cell (pH 7.4, 0.1 m Cl$^-$, 2 mmol/L BPG) $\Delta G = 3,600$ calories. This is known as the free energy of cooperativity or heme-heme interaction. Raising of the temperature to 37°C lowers this value by only about 2 percent. A more rigorous definition is given by the equation:

$$\Delta G = 2.303 \, RT \, (\log p^c_m - p^o_m) \text{ kcal mol}^{-1}$$

p_m is defined as that partial pressure of oxygen in which the integral over the upper part of the oxygen equilibrium curve equals that over the lower part of the curve and is called the mean oxygen binding activity.

$$\int_{p=m}^{p=o} y \, d \ln p = \int_{p=m}^{p=o} (1-y) \, d \ln p$$

p^c_m is the mean oxygen binding activity of the cooperative hemoglobin; p^o_m is the mean oxygen binding activity in the absence of cooperativity, for example, the average of free α and β subunits (Minton and Saroff, 1974).

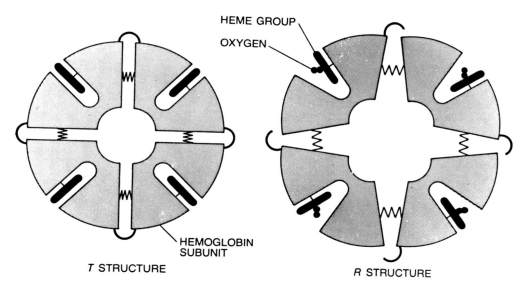

Figure 9.8. Schematic illustrations of allosteric theory. In the molecule on the left, the subunits are constrained by clamps, the springs between them are compressed, and the heme pockets are too narrow to admit oxygen easily. On the right, the clamps have sprung open, the springs are relaxed, and the heme pockets have widened. In each of the two states, the oxygen affinity is independent of the number of oxygen molecules bound. (From Perutz, MF. [1978]. Hemoglobin structure and respiratory transport. *Sci. Am.* 239:92.) 1978.)

Allosteric Interpretation of Cooperative Effects

Monod, Wyman, and Changeux's ingenious theory greatly simplified the interpretation of the cooperative effects. The progressive increase in oxygen affinity illustrated by the parable of the rich and the poor now arises not from any direct interaction between the hemes, but from the increasing ratio of molecules in the R to those in the T structure. Under conditions that mimic physiologic ones as nearly as possible (pH 7.4, 0.1 M Cl⁻, 2 mmol/L BPG), only 1 in 3 million molecules has the R structure in the absence of oxygen, and only 1 in 15,000 has the T structure at full oxygen saturation. The switch from T to R normally takes place when either the second or third molecule of oxygen is bound (MacQuarrie and Gibson, 1971). Heterotropic ligands lower the oxygen affinity by biasing the equilibrium toward the T structure, which would make the transition to the R structure come after three rather than two molecules of oxygen have been bound. Such ligands raise L, the fraction of molecules in the T structure. Usually they also lower the oxygen affinity of the T structure (i.e., they lower K_T while leaving K_R constant).

Table 9.1 illustrates some of the vital features of the cooperative effects. It gives the values of the association constants K and oxygen pressures at half saturation p^{50} for myoglobin, for free α and β chains, and for the hemoglobin tetramer in the T and R states under vari-ous representative conditions. It also gives the free energies of cooperativity ΔG and the values of the allosteric constant L = [T]/[R] in the absence of oxygen and $L = \left(\dfrac{K_T}{K_R}\right)^4 = $ [T]/[R] at oxygen saturation. Note that the oxygen affinities of myoglobin and of the free α and β subunits are similar; they are about 30 times larger than the oxygen affinity of hemoglobin at half saturation and about 160 times larger than the oxygen affinity of the T structure under conditions that mimic physiologic ones (pH 7.4, 0.1 M Cl⁻, 2 mmol/L 2,3 BPG). The affinities of the free α and β subunits are about half that of the R structure under these same conditions, showing that the main effect of cooperativity is to lower the oxygen affinity. 2,3 BPG, chloride, or hydrogen ions all lower K_T and raise both L and ΔG, whereas K_R and $L = \left(\dfrac{K_T}{K_R}\right)^4$ are little affected.

Table 9.1 also shows M, the partition coefficient between carbon monoxide and oxygen, for myoglobin and for free α and β chains.

Note: 1 mm Hg corresponds to a 1.82 μm solution of O_2 in water at 20°C and 760 mm Hg. Hence, $K = \dfrac{1}{1.82 \times p^{50}}$. M is the partition coefficient between O_2 and CO.

A partition coefficient of 250 means that half the hemes are saturated with CO when the molar ratio of CO to O_2 is 1/250. $M = \dfrac{FeCO}{FeO_2} \times \dfrac{PO_2}{PCO}$.

ΔG is the free energy of cooperativity per heme. L gives the concentration ratio of hemoglobin molecules in the T structure to those in the R structure in the absence of oxygen; $L = \left(\dfrac{K_T}{K_R}\right)^4$ gives the same ratio at oxygen saturation.

Table 9.1. Oxygen Equilibria of Myoglobins and Hemoglobins (20°C)

Protein	K (μmol/L^{-1})	p^{50} (mm Hg)	pH	M	Reference
Human myoglobin	0.85	0.65	8.0	39	Antonini et al., 1971
Human α chains	1.2	0.46	7.0	181	Antonini et al., 1971
Human β chains	1.4	0.40	7.0	250	Antonini et al., 1971

	K_T (μmol/L^{-1})	K_R (μmol/L^{-1})	p^{50} (mm Hg)	ΔG (kcal)	L	L(K_T/K_R)^4	Reference
Human hemoglobin A conditions							
pH 7.4, 0.1 mol/L Cl$^-$, 2 mmol/L 2,3 BPG	0.008	3.0	14.0	3.4	3.0×10^6	1.5×10^{-4}	lmai, 1982
pH 7.4, 0.1 mol/L Cl$^-$	0.018	3.9	5.3	3.1	7.3×10^5	3.3×10^{-4}	lmai, 1982
pH 7.4, 0.007 mol/L Cl$^-$	0.093	3.8	2.1	2.2	3.7×10^3	1.3×10^{-3}	lmai, 1982
pH 9.1, 0.1 mol/L Cl$^-$	0.060	3.3	2.2	2.3	2.7×10^3	2.9×10^{-4}	lmai, 1982

Note: 1 mm Hg corresponds to a 1.82 μmol/L solution of O_2 in water at 20°C and 760 mm Hg. Hence, $K = \frac{1}{1.82 \times p^{50}}$. M is the partition coefficient between O_2 and CO. A partition coefficient of 250 means that half the hemes are saturated with CO when the molar ratio of CO to O_2 is $^1/_{250}$. $M = \frac{FeCO}{FeO_2} \times \frac{PO_2}{PCO}$.

ΔG is the free energy of cooperativity per heme. L gives the concentration ratio of hemoglobin molecules in the T structure to those in the R structure in the absence of oxygen; $L \left(\frac{K_T}{K_R} \right)^4$ gives the same ratio at oxygen saturation.

Relative Ligand Affinities of α and β Subunits

For reasons explained later the atomic model of deoxyhemoglobin also suggested that in the T structure, the ligand affinity of the β hemes should be lower than that of the α hemes. For oxygen, this was first verified qualitatively by an NMR study of a series of partially oxygenated hemoglobin solutions. It is now generally accepted that the α hemes have three times greater oxygen affinity than the β hemes.

Comparisons with Other Species

In view of the similarity in tertiary structure between the hemoglobins of different species, one would have expected their oxygen affinities to be similar, but this is not true. There is an 18,000-fold difference between the lowest and highest oxygen equilibrium constants recorded: K = 145 in Ascaris hemoglobin and 0.008 in the T structure of human hemoglobin; the oxygen affinities of certain fish hemoglobins in the T structure are several orders of magnitude lower still. Similarly, there is an 11,000-fold difference between the partition coefficients M of Chironomus and Ascaris hemoglobins. This shows the drastic influence that the detailed structure of the globin exercises on the properties of the heme.

REACTION OF FERROUS IRON WITH OTHER LIGANDS

Carbon monoxide (CO) and nitric oxide (NO) combine with heme iron and have a much higher affinity for it than oxygen, which they are therefore able to displace. If the CO affinity of hemoglobin were as high as that of free ferrous heme, vertebrate life could not exist, because one mole of CO is released for every mole of porphyrin metabolized, and this would suffice to poison the hemoglobin. Steric factors in the heme pocket of hemoglobin lower the CO affinity relative to the oxygen affinity sufficiently to reduce the fraction of hemoglobin poisoned by endogenously produced CO to 1 to 2 percent, but not sufficiently to prevent up to 20 percent of the oxygen combining sites to be blocked by carbon monoxide in heavy smokers, so that less oxygen is carried by the blood. In addition, CO has a more sinister effect. The combination of one of the four hemes in any hemoglobin molecule with CO raises the oxygen affinity of the remaining three hemes by heme-heme interaction. The oxygen equilibrium curve is therefore shifted to the left, which diminishes the fraction of the oxygen carried that can be released to the tissues (Fig. 9.9). Alternatively, to carry the same amount of oxygen to the tissues, the heart has to work harder. The partition coefficient between CO and oxygen of human hemoglobin is 250, which means that at a concentration of one part CO in 250 parts of oxygen, half the heme irons are saturated with CO. The question is sometimes asked why a person who has lost half his or her blood survives, whereas a person who has had half his or her hemoglobin poisoned with CO asphyxiates. The first person's oxygen equilibrium curve is unchanged, whereas the other's is shifted so far to the left that his tissues cannot extract the oxygen that is carried (Chapter 44).

REACTION RATES OF HEMOGLOBIN (PARKHURST, 1979)

Basic Theory

The average length of the capillaries in the human body is about 1 mm, and the linear velocity of flow through them is about 0.5 to 1 mm/sec; thus the time spent by a red cell flowing through a capillary is approximately 1 to 2 seconds. Is this long enough for blood to be saturated with oxygen in the lungs or to deliver it to the tissues? To answer such questions, chemists have developed methods for measuring the rates at which gases combine with and dissociate from myoglobin and hemoglobin. These rates are expressed in terms of the following constants:

O₂	CO
k′-on	1′-on
k-off	1-off

Consider myoglobin that contains only one heme reacting with oxygen according to the equation:

$$Mb + O_2 \overset{k'}{\underset{k}{\leftrightarrow}} MbO_2$$

Figure 9.9. Oxygen equilibrium curves of a nonsmoker at rest and during heavy exercise. Release of carbonic and lactic acids lowers the pH, and the high metabolic rate raises the temperature; both effects shift the curve to the right. In a smoker, binding of carbon monoxide shifts the curve to the left, allowing less oxygen to be released to the tissues. (From Garby and Madden, 1977.)

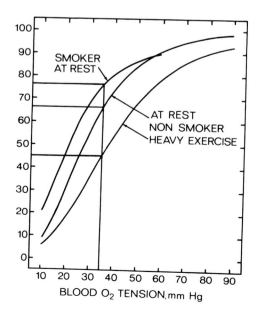

The relative rate constants k′ and k determine the equilibrium constant:

$$K = \frac{[MbO_2]}{[Mb][O_2]} = \frac{k'}{k}$$

k′ has the dimension mol⁻¹ sec⁻¹, and k has the dimension sec⁻¹, so that K has the dimension mol⁻¹.

The rate at which equilibrium is reached is determined by the differential equation:

$$-\frac{d[Mb]}{dt} = \frac{d[MbL]}{dt} = k' = k\,[Mb]\,[L]\,[MbL],$$

where [Mb], [L], and [MbL] are the concentrations of myoglobin, ligand (e.g., oxygen or CO), and liganded myoglobin. Note that the rate of dissociation to deoxymyoglobin is proportional only to the concentration of oxymyoglobin, whereas the rate of formation of oxymyoglobin is proportional to the product of the concentrations of myoglobin and oxygen. In terms of reaction kinetics, the former is called a first-order reaction, and the latter a second-order reaction. However, in a typical experiment, the molar concentration of oxygen or carbon monoxide is many orders of magnitude greater than that of myoglobin, whence to a good approximation their concentrations will remain constant throughout the reaction. We can therefore write k″ = k′ [L] and call this a pseudo-first-order rate constant, as the velocity now depends only on [Mb].

What do these rate constants mean? When oxymyoglobin dissociates into myoglobin and oxygen, the concentration of oxymyoglobin decays exponentially with time. Suppose we wish to find the half-life (t½), the time it takes for the concentration of oxymyoglobin to drop to half its initial value, then:

$$t\frac{1}{2} = \frac{\ln 0.5}{k} = \frac{0.693}{k} \text{ sec}$$

The kinetics of the reactions of hemoglobin with gases are more complex than those of myoglobin because both the on and off rate constants change as successive hemes react, but the values of these constants for the first and the fourth heme can be measured with some confidence and normally represent the reactions of the T and R states, respectively.

What determines the values of these rate constants? Rates of chemical reactions depend on the height of the free-energy barrier that has to be overcome for two molecules to combine into one molecule or one molecule to dissociate into two. This barrier is known as the activation free energy of the reaction ΔG* and is related to its rate constant by the equation:

$$\Delta G^* = -RT\,2.303 \log \frac{kh}{KT},$$

where R is the gas constant, K is the Bolzmann constant, h is Planck's constant, and T is the absolute temperature. By substituting the values of these constants we find that at 20°C, $\Delta G^* = -5.61 \log (1.64 \text{ k} \times 10^{-13})$ kj mol^{-1}. As a rule of thumb, it is useful to remember that each additional kilocalorie of activation energy slows the reaction by a factor of 5.6, or each additional kilojoule by a factor of 1.5.

Physiologic Significance of Reaction Rates

The rate constants tell us that uptake of oxygen is much faster than its release. In the lungs, at a hemoglobin concentration of 20 mmol/L heme and in the presence of an excess of oxygen, half the hemes would become oxygenated in a few microseconds. In the tissues, hemoglobin in the R structure or myoglobin can lose half its oxygen in approximately 50 ms. Both these times are short compared with the 1 to 2 seconds blood takes to traverse the average capillary. However, some capillaries may be shorter than average, or the rate of flow through them may be faster than average, so that the 50 milliseconds required for half dissociation is comparable to the time taken for a red cell to traverse some of the capillaries. Another factor to be considered is the rate of diffusion of oxygen through the membrane of the red cell and the hemoglobin solution inside it. This takes milliseconds, much longer than the uptake of oxygen by hemoglobin, but shorter than its release (Antonini and Brunori, 1971).

Uptake of carbon monoxide by the T structure of hemoglobin is 30 to 120 times slower than that of oxygen, but still fast compared with the time of passage of a red cell through capillaries. On the other hand, the half-time for dissociation of carbon monoxide from the R structure is 77 seconds, or 300 times slower than the time of passage through a capillary, which aggravates CO poisoning, because it prolongs the time needed to replace CO by oxygen and makes the half-life of CO in the blood very long. Its exact value depends on the rate of ventilation. Even when no more CO is being inhaled, the half-life is 3.5 hours in a human at rest; walking reduces it to 2 hours and playing football to 1 hour.

STRUCTURE OF HEMOGLOBIN

The Globin

It has become customary to speak of the primary, secondary, tertiary, and quaternary structure of proteins. Primary refers to the amino acid sequence; secondary to the local conformation of the polypeptide chain, such as a helix or pleated sheet; tertiary to the fold of a single polypeptide chain, such as α or β globin; and quaternary to the assembly of several chains or subunits, such as the hemoglobin tetramer.

Sperm whale myoglobin and horse hemoglobin were the first protein structures to be solved, at a time when their amino acid sequences were still unknown. Not knowing the sequence homologies among the three types of chains we were surprised when our x-ray analyses showed that the fold of the polypeptide chain was the same in myoglobin and in the α and β chains of hemoglobin. Later x-ray analyses revealed the same fold in hemoglobins that occur in the root nodules of a leguminous plant (lupin) (Borisov et al. 1977), in an annelid worm (Glycera) (Padian and Love, 1968), and in the larva of a fly (Chironomus thummii) (Steigemann and Weber, 1979), showing that it is one of the fundamental patterns of nature, evolved to turn heme into an oxygen carrier. The fold is made up of seven or eight α-helical segments and an equal number of nonhelical segments placed at the corners between them and at the ends of the chain (Fig. 9.10). According to a notation introduced by Watson and Kendrew (1961), the helices are named A to H, starting from the amino end; the nonhelical segments that lie between helices are named AB, BC, CD, and so on. The nonhelical segments at the ends of the chain are called NA and HC. Residues within each segment are numbered from the amino end, A1, A2, CD1, CD2, and so on. Evolution has conserved this fold of the chain despite great divergence of the sequence; the only residues common to all hemoglobins are the proximal histidine F8 and phenylalanine CD1, which wedges the heme into its pocket. Most, but not all globins also have a histidine on the distal (oxygen) side of the heme. Ionized residues are excluded from the interior of the globin chains, which is filled largely by hydrocarbon side chains, but some serines and threonines also occur there. The proximal and distal histidines (also called the heme-linked histidines) are potentially polar, but the proximal histidine does not ionize, and the pKa of the distal one is so low (5.5) that the fraction ionized in vivo is negligible (Ikeda-Saito et al., 1978; Asher et al., 1981). Apart from these two histidines and phenylalanine CD1, the only detectable sequence homology between the globins consists of an invariant pattern of internal sites that are occupied by non-polar residues. Helical segments exhibit a periodic pattern of polar and non-polar residues, the former in interior and the latter in exterior positions (Perutz et al., 1965).

Myoglobin has ionized side chains distributed all over its surface, but the surfaces of the α- and β-globin chains have nonpolar patches that allow them to combine to form the $\alpha_2\beta_2$ tetramer. To make a model of the tetramer, each of the subunits must first be joined to its partner around a twofold sym-

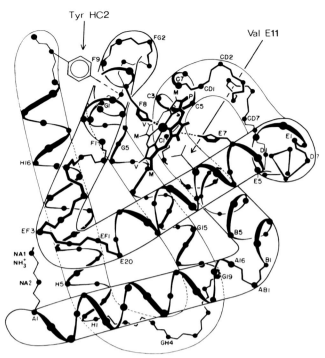

Figure 9.10. Secondary and tertiary structure of the hemoglobins showing α carbons and coordination of the hemes. The diagram shows the proximal histidine F8 linked to the heme iron, the distal residues His E7 and Val Ell, and also Tyr HC2, which are important in the mechanism of the mammalian hemoglobins. The exact numbers of residues in the different segments are the same in all mammals, but vary in other vertebrates and especially in invertebrates. The letters M, V, and P refer to the methyl, vinyl, and propionate side chains of the heme.

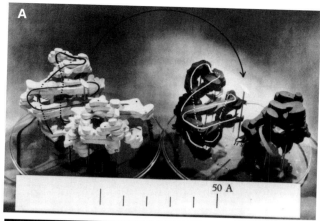

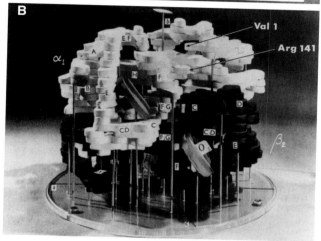

Figure 9.11. Assembly of hemoglobin tetramer. (A) a pair of α subunits (white) and β subunits (black) is placed on either side of the twofold symmetry axis (central rod). (B) The pair of α subunits is then inverted and placed on top of the β subunits to form the complete tetramer. Note the hemes in separate pockets. The white sign at the top marks the twofold symmetry axis running through the central cavity. Rotation by 180° about this axis brings the molecule to congruence with itself.

metry axis that brings one subunit into congruence with the other by a rotation of 180°. One pair of chains is then inverted and placed on top of the other to make a tetramer that would have tetrahedral symmetry if the four chains were identical (Fig. 9.11). A tetrahedron has six edges, and the four subunits are therefore joined by six contacts, which symmetry reduces to four unique ones: $\alpha_1\beta_1 = \alpha_2\beta_2$; $\alpha_1\beta_2 = \alpha_2\beta_1$; $\alpha_1\alpha_2$, and $\beta_1\beta_2$. The $\alpha_1\beta_1$ contact is the most extensive; in oxyhemoglobin it includes 40 amino acid residues and many hydrogen bonds, some of them with caged-in water molecules. The $\alpha_1\beta_1$ contact remains the same in oxyhemoglobin and deoxyhemoglobin, while all the other contacts change.

Central Cavity

The twofold symmetry axis runs through a water-filled cavity at the center of the molecule. This cavity widens on transition from the R to the T structure to form a receptor site between the two β chains for the allosteric effector 2,3 BPG. It is lined by helices H β and by the nonhelical segments NA β and EF β such

that the negative charges of 2,3 BPG are compensated by eight cationic groups of the protein; these make the receptor site both sterically and electrostatically complementary nature to the effector (Arnone, 1972). On transition to the R structure, the EF and H segments close up, and the NA segments move apart, so that the complementary is lost (Fig. 9.12). The channel between the two α chains forms a receptor site for certain drugs (Abraham et al., 1983; Perutz et al., 1986).

THE HEME-LIGAND COMPLEX

Changes in Heme Structure on Ligand Binding

Heme is made up of one atom of ferrous iron at the center of protoporphyrin IX, which is synthesized in the

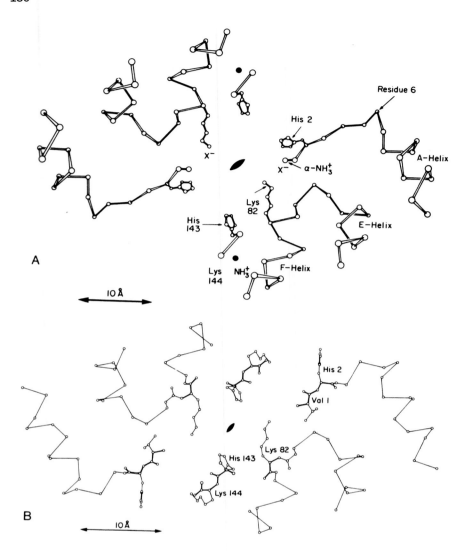

Figure 9.12. (**A**) 2,3 BPG binding site in deoxy HbA. The negative charges of 2,3 BPG are compensated by the positive ones of the eight cationic groups surrounding it. (**B**) The same site in oxyhemoglobin or carbon monoxyhemoglobin. In both (**A**) and (**B**) the N_ε of Lys HC1(144)β is shown in one of its several possible positions. The uncertainty over its position arose because its side chain was not visible on the electron density maps. Note how the gap between the two β chains closes up upon going from the T to the R structure.

bone marrow from glycine and acetate. It is wedged into a pocket of the globin with its hydrocarbon side chains interior and its polar propionate side chains exterior; it is in contact with about 20 side chains of the globin, all hydrophobic apart from the two histidines (Fermi et al., 1984). Around its entrance the heme pocket carries several lysines that are vital for the reduction of methemoglobin by cytochrome b_5, which carries acid groups around the entrance to its heme pocket. Combination between the basic group of hemoglobin

and the acid ones of cytochrome b_5 allows the two proteins to combine with their hemes facing each other edge on, thus bringing them close enough for an electron to jump across. The same mechanism facilitates the reaction of cytochrome c with cytochrome oxidase and reductase (Gacon et al., 1980).

Combination with ligands is accompanied by stereochemical changes at the hemes. These were first discovered by x-ray crystallography of synthetic models. One particularly useful one has been Collman's picket fence complex, which combines reversibly with molecular oxygen and crystallizes in both the deoxy and oxy forms (Figs. 9.13 and 9.14) (Jameson et al., 1980). The accuracy of the bond distances of these structures is greater by an order of magnitude than that attainable in myoglobin and hemoglobin, for which they can serve as standards (Table 9.2) (Fermi et al., 1984; Shaanan, 1980; Phillips, 1980). In hemoglobin and myoglobin the crucial interatomic distances, Fe-N$_{porph}$ and Fe-N$_\varepsilon$, are the same within error as in the picket fence com-

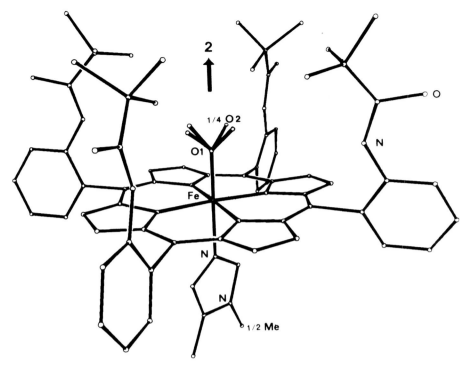

Figure 9.13. The oxygenated picket fence complex: FeII-O_2-tetrapivalamido-phenylporphyrin-N-methylimidazole. The pivalamido side chains have the constitution $(CH_3)_3$-C-CO-NH and form a fence around the iron-bound oxygen. The oxygen is inclined to the heme axis by 129° and is randomly distributed over four equivalent positions, with Fe-O-O projecting on to lines at 45° to the N-Fe-N bonds. The arrow is the twofold symmetry axis. (From Collman JP et al. [1974]. Structure of an iron (II) dioxygen complex: A model for oxygen carrying hemoproteins. *Proc. Natl. Acad. Sci. U.S.A.* 71:1326.)

Figure 9.14. Heme stereochemistry of the deoxygenated picket fence complex. In this structure the proximal base is 2-methylimidazole. The diagram shows only the iron atom, the four nitrogens of the porphyrin, and the proximal base, illustrating the pyramidal coordination of the iron relative to the porphyrin nitrogens. On oxygenation the iron becomes coplanar with the nitrogens. (From Jameson et al., 1980.)

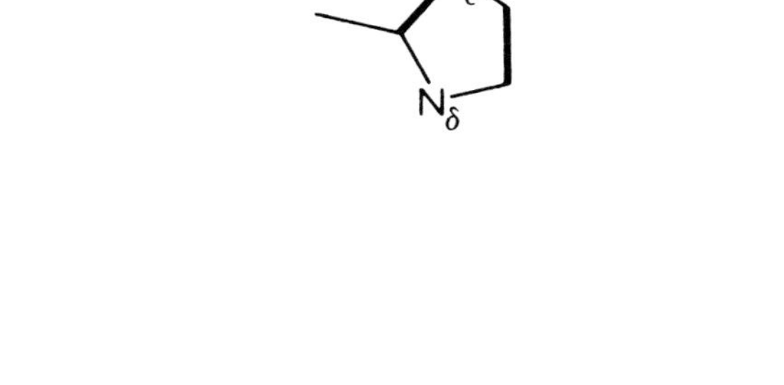

plex, which gives one confidence that they are correct. Fe-N_{porph} shrinks from 2.06Å in the oxygen-free compounds to 1.99Å in the oxy compounds, whereas Fe-N_{ϵ} changes little. P_N-P_C is an index of the doming of the pyrroles, which is seen only in the deoxy compounds. Fe-P_N gives the distance of the iron atoms from the plane of the porphyrin nitrogens; it is +0.4Å within error in all the deoxy compounds, but varies between −0.11Å and +0.18Å in the oxy compounds (+ being toward the proximal histidine). Fe-P_{porph} gives the distance of iron atoms from the mean plane of the porphyrin nitrogens and carbons; it shrinks on oxygenation from 0.58Å to 0.16Å in the α subunits and from 0.50 to 0 in the β subunits. The combination of these changes results in a movement of N_{ϵ} of the proximal histidine toward the mean plane of the porphyrin and carbons by 0.6Å in the α and 0.5Å in the β subunits; this is shown in the first column of Table 9.2 and is one of the vital movements that trigger the T → R transition.

In the α subunits, the distal residues offer no steric hindrance to the binding of oxygen in either the T or the R structure (Fig. 9.15). In the β subunits, on the other hand, the R → T transition is accompanied by a shift and tilting of the heme relative to helix E, which results in obstruction of the ligand site by the γ_2- methyl of valine E11 (Perutz, 1970; Baldwin and Chothia, 1979) and a consequent lowering of the ligand affinity. This feature led me to suggest that in the T structure, the α subunits possess the higher ligand affinity, as indeed they have. The shift of helix E relative to the heme acts as an additional trigger for the R ↔ T transition.

Table 9.2. Heme Stereochemistry of Hemoglobin, Myoglobin, and the Picket Fence Complex

	Distances to/between mean planes				Bond lengths and angles				
	N_ε-P_{porph}	Fe-P_{porph}	Fe-P_N	P_N-P_C	Fe-N_{porph} (mean)	Fe-N_ε	Reference		
Deoxyhemoglobin	(Å)	(Å)	(Å)	(Å)	(Å)	(Å)	Fermi et al., 1984		
α subunit (mean)	2.72(6)	0.58(3)	0.40(5)	0.16(6)	2.08(3)	2.16(6)			
β subunit (mean)	2.58(6)	0.50(3)	0.36(5)	0.10(6)	2.05(3)	2.09(6)			
Deoxymyoglobin	2.67	0.47	0.42		2.03(10)	2.22	Takano, 1977		
Fe(TpivPP) (2-MeIm)	2.665	0.43	0.399	0.14	2.086(4)	2.095(5)	Jameson et al., 1980		

	N_ε-P_{porph}	Fe-P_{porph}	Fe-P_N	P_N-P_C	Fe-N_{porph} (mean)	Fe-N_ε	Fe - O	Fe - O - O	Reference
Oxyhemoglobin						(Å)	(°)		
α subunits	2.1(1)	0.16(8)	0.12(8)	0.04	1.99(5)	1.94(9)	1.66(8)	153.0(7)	Shaanan, 1980
β subunits	2.1(1)	0.00(8)	−0.11(8)	0.06	1.96(6)	2.07(9)	1.87(13)	159.0(12)	Shaanan, 1980
Oxymyoglobin	2.28(6)	0.22(3)	0.18(3)	0.00	1.95(6)	2.07(6)	1.83(6)	115.0(5)	Phillips, 1980
Fe-O_2 (TpivPP) (2-MeIm)	2.107(4)	0.199	0.086	0.03	1.996(4)	2.107(4)	1.898(7)	129.0	Jameson et al., 1977.

P_{porph} is the mean plane of the porphyrin together with the first side chain atoms. P_N is the plane of the porphyrin nitrogens, P_C the mean plane of the porphyrin carbons. (TpivPP) (2-MeIm) stands for tetrapivalamidophenylporphyrin-2-methylimidazole, which is the chemical name of Collman's picket fence complex, shown in Figures 5.13 and 5.14. Figure 5.14 illustrates the meaning of several of the distances listed here.

Stereochemistry of Ligand Binding

In the picket fence complex, the Fe-O-O angle is 129°, in oxymyoglobin 115°, and in oxyhemoglobin 153° and 159°. The differences arise from the stereochemistry of the pocket surrounding the oxygen. In the picket fence complex, there are no distal residues, and there is therefore no steric hindrance to the bound oxygen. In myoglobin the distal histidine, valine, and phenylalanine form a pocket that is exactly tailored to a ligand at an angle of 115°. In hemoglobin the same distal residues are tailored toward larger Fe-O-O angles (Fig. 9.16).

Until quite recently the role of the distal histidine (E7) was unclear. Using neutron diffraction of crys-

Figure 9.15. Stereo view of the active site of the α subunits of human hemoglobin. Full lines, oxy; broken lines, deoxy. Note how the distal histidine moves toward the bound oxygen to form a hydrogen bond with it. Stereoviewers are obtainable from the Lansing Instrument Corporation, Lansing, Michigan. They are also available in the libraries of most university chemistry departments.

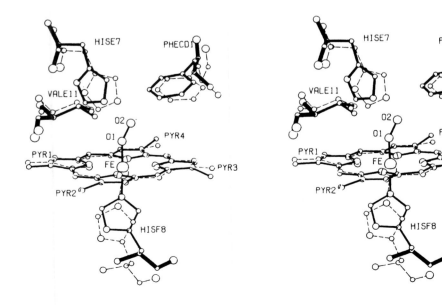

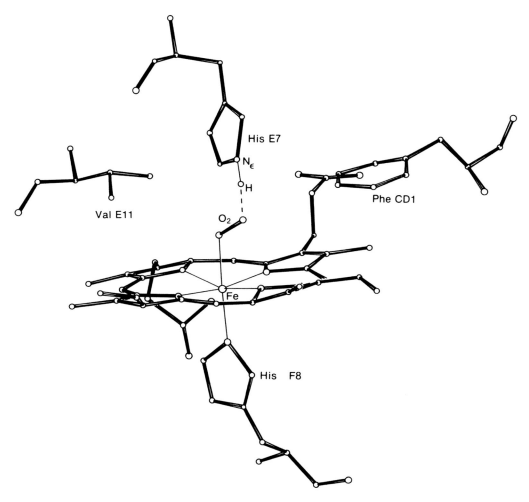

Figure 9.16. Arrangement of proximal and distal histidines in oxymyoglobin, showing the hydrogen bonds between N_ϵ of the distal histidine and the bound oxygen. (From Phillips and Schoenborn, 1981.)

talline oxymyoglobin, Phillips and Schoenborn (1981) showed that its N_ϵ forms a hydrogen bond with the bound oxygen. In oxyhemoglobin, a strong hydrogen bond between the bound oxygen and the distal histidine exists in the α subunits, but only a weak one exists in the β subunits (Shaanan, 1980).

CHANGES IN STRUCTURE OF THE GLOBIN

Quaternary Changes

On transition from the deoxy (T) to the oxy (R) structure, one $\alpha\beta$ dimer rotates relative to the other by 12° to 15°. The rotation is accompanied by a shift of ~1Å along the rotation axis (Fig. 9.17) and makes the two $\alpha\beta$ dimers move relative to each other along the $\alpha_1\beta_2$ and $\alpha_2\beta_1$ contact (Baldwin and Chothia, 1979; Perutz and Ten Eyck, 1971). The contacts form a two-way switch

that ensures that the $\alpha\beta$ dimers click back and forth between no more than two stable positions, so that any intermediates in the reaction of hemoglobin with ligands must have either the quaternary R or T structure. This conclusion is inescapable from the structure (Perutz, 1970; Baldwin and Chothia, 1979), even though it sometimes appears to be at variance with equilibrium and kinetic properties of hemoglobin. It is confirmed by x-ray analysis of hybrids such as (α deoxy)$_2$ – (β oxy)$_2$ (Luisi and Shibayaina, 1989; Breozowski et al., 1984). Caged-in water molecules play an essential part in the network of hydrogen bonds between neighboring subunits (Fermi and Perutz, 1981; Fermi et al., 1984; Shaanan, 1980; Perutz, 1990). Silva et al. (1992) have produced a third quaternary structure by crystallization of human HbCO from 16 percent polyethylene glycol of pH5.8 (Silva et al., 1992). It is related to T and R by a combined rotation and translation of the $\alpha_1\beta_1$ dimer relative to the $\alpha_2\beta_2$ dimer, but the directions and positions of the screw axes are different from those of axes relating to T and R. In the transition from T to R one $\alpha\beta$ dimer turns relative to the other by 13.2°; Janin and Wodak (1993) have shown that in the other T to R tran-

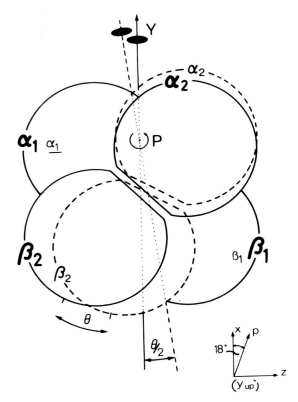

Figure 9.17. Schematic diagram illustrating the change in quaternary structure that accompanies ligation of hemoglobin. Bold symbols and plain lines in the diagram refer to deoxyhemoglobin, and light symbols and broken lines to liganded hemoglobin. Ligation causes little movement of the α_1 and the β_1 subunits relative to each other, or of the α_2 and β_2 subunits relative to each other. In the diagram the liganded and unliganded $\alpha_1\beta_1$ dimers have been superimposed. The position of the liganded $\alpha_2\beta_2$ dimer corresponds to that obtained by moving the unliganded $\alpha_2\beta_2$ dimer as follows: rotating it about an axis P (which is perpendicular to the dyad symmetry axes, marked Y, of both the liganded and unliganded molecules and to the picture plane) by an angle $\varphi = 12°$ to 15° and shifting it along the axis P by 1Å into the page, from the same angle as in A. (From Baldwin and Chothia, 1979.)

sition it turns by nearly 10° beyond R. The translation along the $\alpha_1\beta_2$ and $\alpha_2\beta_1$ contacts also goes beyond R. A similar quaternary structure was found in the abnormal human Hb Ypsilanti (AspG1 $\beta \rightarrow$ Tyr) Janin and Wodak (1993). Both Silva et al. (1992) and Smith et al. suggest that its structure might be an intermediate in the T $\rightarrow$ R transition, but Janin and Wodak (1993) have shown that its quaternary structure is far beyond R, rather than between T and R, which makes this unlikely.

Salt Bridges

The additional bonds between the subunits in the T structure postulated by allosteric theory take mainly the form of salt bridges (Perutz, 1970) (i.e., hydrogen bonds

between oppositely charged ions). One pair of salt bridges is formed by the C-terminal arginines of the α chains, another by the C-terminal histidines of the β chains, and four pairs are formed by 2,3 BPG with cationic groups of the β chains (Figs. 9.18 and 9.19).

$$-NH_3^+ \dots \overset{\displaystyle -O}{\underset{\displaystyle -O}{C}} - \text{ or } >NH_3^+ \dots \overset{\displaystyle -O}{\underset{\displaystyle -O}{C}} - \text{ or } -NH_3^+ \dots Cl^-$$

ALLOSTERIC MECHANISM

How are the stereochemical changes at the heme transmitted to the globin so as to trigger the change from

Figure 9.18. Schematic diagram of $\alpha_1\beta_2$ contact switch showing the dovetailing between the subunits and the two alternative hydrogen bonds between tyrosine C7(42) α_1 and aspartate G1(99) β_2 in deoxyhemoglobin and asparagine G4(102) β_2 and aspartate G1(94) α_1 in oxyhemoglobin. (From Perutz, MF, [1978]. Hemoglobin structure and respiratory transport. *Sci. Am.* 239:92.)

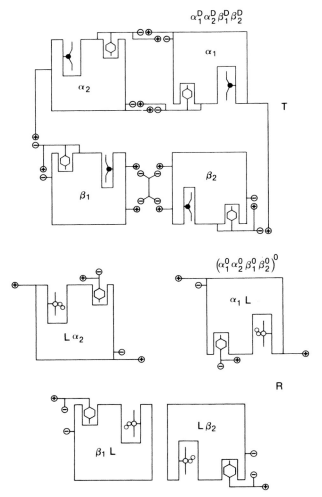

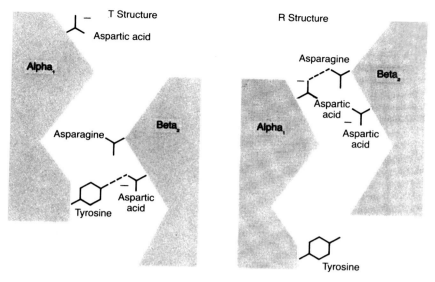

Figure 9.19. Digrammatic sketch of closing of salt bridges by C-terminal residues in deoxy (T) and opening in oxyhemoglobin (R). The molecule with the four negative charges between the β chains of the T structure is diphosphoglycerate.

the R to the T structure? How can we explain the more than a hundredfold drop in oxygen affinity that takes place on transition from the R to the T structure? How close is Monod and co-workers' theory of allostery to the real behavior of hemoglobin? I shall try to answer these questions, in turn, in the next sections.

Control of Oxygen Affinity

The oxygen affinity of the R structure is close to the mean of that of free α and β subunits, so that it does not require explanation. I have proposed that the additional bonds between the subunits in the T structure restrain the movement of the iron atoms toward the plane of the porphyrin that is needed for ligand binding (Perutz, 1970). Paoli et al. (1996, 1997) have confirmed these constraints by x-ray analyses at high resolution of crystals of human Hb suspended in concentrated solutions of polyethylene glycol, which maintained the T structure intact on addition of a variety of heme ligands (Paoli et al., 1996, 1997). They then compared the stereochemistry of the oxygenated heme complex in the T and R structures with that of deoxyhemoglobin in the T structure (Fig. 9.20). In fully oxygenated Hb in the T structure, the Fe-N_ϵ bonds were stretched by 0.36Å in the α and 0.13Å in the β subunits, compared with HbO_2 in the R structure. In the α subunits, combination with oxygen had moved the irons into the porphyrin plane, pulling the F helix with it part of the way; in the β subunits the porphyrins had moved toward the iron and the F helix, thus mak-

ing room for the oxygen as well as allowing the iron to come into the porphyrin plane. The apparent stretching of the Fe-N_ϵ bonds may have concealed an unresolved superposition of six- and five-coordinated oxyhemes.

Five-coordinated hemes have actually been found in Hb^+CN^- and Hb^+F^- in the T structure, where the Fe-N_ϵ-bonds are broken in the α subunits and the irons have moved to the distal side. Rupture of the Fe-N_ϵ-bonds in Hb^+CN^- allowed the α subunits to relax into an exaggerated T-like tertiary structure in the vicinity of the heme. At the β hemes the Fe-N_ϵ bonds have remained intact, but the distal residues have moved relative to the hemes to make room for the cyanide ion. The changes toward an R-like tertiary structure of the β subunits are smaller than those accompanying oxygenation of all four hemes in the T structure. It seems that an R-like tertiary structure of the α subunits restrains the transition toward a T-like tertiary structure of the β subunits, whereas an R-like tertiary structure of the α-subunits promotes it. This is clear evidence of stereochemical interaction between α and β subunits in the quaternary T structure (Paoli et al., 1997).

Behavior Observed Versus Behavior Predicted by Allosteric Theory

Allosteric theory requires hemoglobin to exist in only two thermodynamic states, the T state with the oxygen equilibrium constant K_T, and the R state with the oxygen equilibrium constant K_R, regardless of the number of oxygen molecules or heterotropic ligands bound. Ideally, changes in hydrogen ion, chloride, and 2,3 BPG concentration should affect only the allosteric constant L and leave K_T, and K_R unaltered. In reality, the oxygen affinity of the T structure rises with the number of oxy-

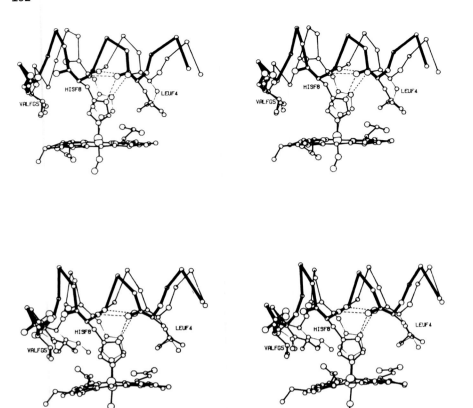

Figure 9.20. Stereo view of the heme groups (edge-on) and sides of oxyhemoglobin (thick lines) and deoxyhemoglobin (thin lines) in the α subunits and the β subunit. Most of the residues in the F helix and the FG corner are shown by α carbons and only a few residues in full. The heme groups of deoxyhemoglobin and oxyhemoglobin were made to overlap, and the other residues were transformed accordingly (only the oxyhemoglobin heme is plotted for clarity). The bifurcated hydrogen bonds N(F8)-O(F4)-NH)(F8) in both deoxyhemoglobin and oxyhemoglobin are shown by broken lines. (From Shaanan, 1980.)

gen molecules bound. Moreover, the concentration of heterotropic ligands alters both K_T and L. K_R, on the other hand, is largely independent of either the number of oxygen molecules bound to the R structure or of the concentration of heterotropic ligands. These properties are understood when we examine the structural changes accompanying the binding of ligands. Binding of oxygen to the α subunits in the T structure induces a change in their tertiary structure similar in kind, but much smaller than those accompanying the T → R transition (Paoli et al., 1996). Conversely, loss of ligands from the R structure induces changes in tertiary structure similar in kind and smaller than those accompanying the R → T transition (Paoli et al., 1997). In the T structure a change in tertiary structure of any one subunit may affect the oxygen affinities of all the other subunits by loosening the constraints placed on them, but owing to the weaker constraints in the R structure, the change in tertiary structure of any one subunit hardly affects the ligand affinities of its neighbors. Study of abnormal or chemically modified hemoglobins shows that weakening of any chemical bond between or even within the subunits relaxes the constraints of the T structure and consequently raises its oxygen affinity (Fermi and Perutz, 1981). Conversely, any tightening of the constraints of the T structure, for example, by an increase in hydrogen ion 2,3 or BPG concentration, lowers its oxygen affinity (Imai, 1982). The tightening of the T structure induced by 2,3 BPG can actually be seen by x-ray analysis: 2,3 BPG and the related allosteric effector inositol hexaphosphate make the A helices of the β chains move toward the center of the molecule, thus clamping them together more firmly (Arnone, 1972; Arnone and Perutz, 1974). Changes such as these are the structural corollary of the decline in K_T with rising 2,3 BPG concentration. Even though hemoglobin takes up only two alternative quaternary structures, the continuous variation of K_T as a function of ligand concentration implies a continuum of thermodynamic states, distinguished by subtle changes in tertiary structure.

FERRIC HEMOGLOBIN

The heme irons are subject to auto-oxidation to ferric hemoglobin or methemoglobin, which cannot combine with oxygen. Erythrocytes contain a scavenging enzyme system that reduces methemoglobin to deoxyhemoglobin. That system is composed of cytochrome b_5 and an NADH-dependent cytochrome b_5, reductase, also known as methemoglobin reductase. In vitro oxyhemoglobin or deoxyhemoglobin are oxidized rapidly by ferricyanide or by sodium nitrite. Conversely, methemoglobin can be reduced with dithionite, ascorbate, or borohydride. Methemoglobin is an indicator dye with a pKa of 8.1, brown at acid and red at alkaline pH. The color change is due to the ionization of the iron-linked water molecule:

$$Fe^{3+} + H_2O \leftrightarrow Fe^{3+} OH^- + H^+$$

The water molecule can be replaced by F^-, OCN^-, SCN^-, N^-_3, imidazole, or CN^-, where F^- is the weakest and CN^- the strongest ligand. Each of these methemoglobin compounds exhibits its characteristic absorption spectrum. In cyanide poisoning, methemoglobin is used as a scavenger. Intravenous injection of sodium nitrite oxidizes some of the ferrous hemoglobin to methemoglobin, which binds cyanide very firmly, thus protecting the enzyme cytochrome oxidase. All liganded forms of hemoglobin have the quaternary R structure, regardless of the nature of the ligand.

SUBUNIT DISSOCIATION

In dilute solution, oxyhemoglobin is partly dissociated into $\alpha\beta$ dimers. In 0.1 mol/L NaCl at 20°C the dissociation constant for the reaction $\alpha_2\beta_2 \leftrightarrow 2\alpha\beta$ is 3µmol/L. In erythrocytes, in which the concentration of hemoglobin tetramer is about 4 mmol/L, dissociation of oxyhemoglobin is negligible; but when measuring oxygen equilibrium curves in solutions of less than 60 µmol/L heme, it must be considered (Ackers et al., 1975). Dissociation into dimers can be detected by measuring the sedimentation velocity of hemoglobin in the ultracentrifuge. It can also be detected by light scattering and by a change in the ultraviolet absorption spectrum. The tetramer-dimer dissociation constant of deoxyhemoglobin is 10^5 to 10^6 times smaller than that of oxyhemoglobin. Owing to the extensive contacts and the many hydrogen bonds between the two subunits in the $\alpha\beta$ dimers, their dissociation constant into free α and β subunits is too small to be measured, but the first order rate constant of dissociation has recently been determined from the rate of exchange of free ^3H-labeled α chains with unlabeled hemoglobin tetramers and has been found to be 4×10^{-3} hours^{-1}, which corresponds to a half life of 173 hours (0.01 mol/L phosphate, pH 7.0, 25°C) (Antonini et al., 1965).

Molecular Dynamics of the Transition of Quaternary Structure

There has been much discussion about molecular dynamics of the transition of quaternary structure, especially over the question of whether the salt bridges open and release protons as successive molecules of oxygen or other ligands combine with the T structure (Perutz, 1970), as I suggested, or whether this happens only during the transition from T to R. My suggestion was inspired by kinetic studies that proved the release of protons to be synchronous and linear with uptake of carbon monoxide (Antonini et al., 1965; Gray 1970). Recent measurements showed the oxygen affinity at less than 1 percent oxygen saturation to be strongly pH dependent, which implies that protons are released on combination of the first oxygen when the molecules still remain in the T structure (Poyart et al., 1978). This has been confirmed by measurements of the oxygen and pH dependence of the tetramer-dimer equilibrium (Chu et al., 1984). In 0.1 mol/L tris or glycine buffers + 0.1 mol/L NaCl at pH 7.4 and 21.5°C in the absence of 2,3 BPG, the numbers of protons released per oxygenation step are 0.64 for the first, 1.62 for the second and third oxygen combined, and only 0.05 for the fourth. Under these conditions, the T to R transition takes place mainly on combination of the third oxygen (MacQuarrie and Gibson, 1971). Because half the protons come from salt bridges, it follows that salt bridges must open and release protons on uptake of oxygen by the T structure, as well as on transition from T to R. 2,3 BPG reduces the number of protons released in the first step (Poyart et al., 1978) but probably increases the number in the fourth, since a greater fraction of the molecules would not change from T to R until the fourth step.

HUMAN FETAL HEMOGLOBIN

The transport of oxygen differs in the embryonic, fetal, and adult stages of development. Early on embryos obtain oxygen from the maternal interstitial fluid and use embryonic hemoglobin (Chapter 10). The developing fetus obtains its oxygen via the placenta, using a hemoglobin known as HbFII ($\alpha_2\gamma_2$). This has the same α chain as the adult form, but its β chain, known as γ, differs from the adult form in 39 positions. There is also a minor component, known as hemoglobin F1, in which the valines 1γ are acetylated. In vivo the oxygen affinities of hemoglobins HbF and HbFI are higher than those of the two adult forms HbA ($\alpha_2\beta_2$) and Hb A_2 ($\alpha_2\delta_2$) which facilitates transfer of oxygen across the placenta from the adult to the fetal circulation (Chu et al., 1984). However, when isolated and stripped of phosphates, the oxygen affinities of the fetal forms become lower than those of the adult forms, especially at acid pH (Antonini et al., 1964; Tyuma and Shimizu, 1970). Their higher oxygen affinity in vivo is due entirely to their lower affinity for the allosteric effector 2,3 BPG. The alkaline Bohr effect of the fetal forms is almost the same as that of HbA and is not influenced by the acetylation of Val 1β, but their acid Bohr effect is halved (Frier and Perutz, 1977), so that below pH 6 their oxygen affinity rises less than that of HbA. Deoxyhemoglobin F is more soluble than deoxyhemoglobin A, which has important implications for the pathology of sickle cell anemia. HbF is recognized most easily by its higher absorption of light at 290 nm; this is due to the presence of two additional tryptophans per tetramer (tyrosine H8(130)β → tryptophan γ). It can also be recognized by its greater resistance to denaturation by alkali.

The structure of deoxyhemoglobin F is similar to that of deoxyhemoglobin A, because most of the 39 amino acid replacements are external and therefore incapable of exercising any influence on the folding of the polypeptide chain. The few internal replacements are accommodated with barely detectable structural changes. The exceptions are the replacements leucine NA3(3)β → phenylalanine γ and glutamate A4(7)β → aspartate γ. The former pushes the amino terminal segment away from the EF corner and from the dyad symmetry axis, whereas the latter draws helix A closer to helix E and the symmetry axis, because residue A4 makes a salt bridge with Lys H10 (132)β (Frier and Perutz, 1977).

The low affinity of Hb F for 2,3 BPG is caused mainly by the substitution histidine H21 (143)β → serine γ, which reduces the cationic 2,3 BPG binding groups from eight to six per tetramer (Fig. 9.11), but the changed conformation of the N-terminal segment and the resultant increase in the distance of valine NA1(1)γ from the dyad symmetry axis may also contribute. In Hb FI, acetylation of valine NA1 (1) γ reduces the number 2,3 BPG binding groups to four, with the result that 2,3 BPG has no measurable effect on its oxygen affinity.

In earlier times fetal hemoglobin was recognized by its resistance to denaturation by alkali. This is due to the replacements Cys G13(112)β → Ser and Tyr H8(130)β → Trp (Perutz, 1974). They have a pKa between 9.5 and 10.5 and therefore become ionized in alkaline solutions above pH ~10, but their charges, buried in the largely nonpolar interior of the globin, are unstable unless they can surround themselves with shells of water molecules. Such shells disrupt the tertiary structure of the globin and initiate denaturation. An expanded discussion of HbF is found in Chapter 10.

MOLECULAR BASIS OF HEMOGLOBIN DISEASES (PERUTZ AND LEHMANN, 1968)

Hemoglobin genes are subject to mutations that alter the structure and synthesis of globin. Several hundred variant human hemoglobins have been isolated and chemically characterized. In most of them the abnormality consists of the replacement of one symmetry-related pair of amino acid residues by another. All these replacements are consistent with single-base substitutions in the DNA coding for the globin chains. Some variant hemoglobins have residues deleted or inserted; in others the chains are cut short or elongated; still others contain hybrids of β and δ or β and γ chains. Although many of the abnormal hemoglobins do not affect the carrier's health, others give rise to symptoms. In more than 30 abnormal hemoglobins, the stereochemical causes of these symptoms have been found by x-ray analysis of the hemoglobins' crystal structure, sometimes combined with spectroscopic analysis of their structure in solution. For lists of abnormal hemoglobins see Bunn and Forget (1985), Fermi and Perutz (1981), Perutz and Lehmann (1968), Lehmann and Kynoch (1976), and also, interesting hemoglobin variants are discussed in detail in many of the following chapters.

References

Abraham, DJ, Perutz, MF, and Phillips, SE. (1983). Physiological and X-ray studies of potential antisickling agents. *Biochemistry* 80: 324.

Ackers, GK, Johnson, ML, Mills, FC et al. (1975). The linkage between oxygenation and subunit dissociation in human hemoglobin. Consequences for the analysis of oxygenation curves. *Biochemistry* 14: 5128.

Antonini, E, and Brunori, M. (1971). *Hemoglobin and myoglobin and their reactions with ligands.* Amsterdam: North Holland Publishing Co.

Antonini, E, Rossi-Bernardi, L, and Chiahcone, E, editors (1981). *Hemoglobins. Methods in enzymology* 76, New York: Academic Press.

Antonini, E, Schuster, TM, Brunori, M, and Wyman, J. (1965). The kinetics of the Bohr effect in the reaction of human hemoglobin with carbon monoxide. *J. Biol. Chem.* 240: PC2262.

Antonini, E, Wyman, J, Brunori, M et al. (1964). The oxygen Bohr effect of human fetal hemoglobin. *Arch. Biochem. Biophys.* 108: 569.

Arnone, A. (1972). X-ray diffraction study of binding of 2,3 diphosphoglycerate to human deoxyhaemoglobin. *Nature* 237: 146.

Arnone, A and Perutz, MF. (1974). Structure of inositol hexaphosphate-human deoxyhaemoglobin complex. *Nature* 249: 34.

Asher, SA, Adams, ML, and Schuster, TM. (1981). Resonance Raman and absorption spectroscopic detection of distal histidine-fluoride interactions in human methemoglobin fluoride and sperm whale metmyoglobin fluoride: Measurements of distal histidine ionization constants. *Biochemistry* 20: 339.

Baldwin, JM. (1975). Structure and function of haemoglobin. *Prog. Biophys. Mol. Biol.* 29: 225.

Baldwin, J and Chothia, C. (1979). Haemoglobin: The structural changes related to ligand binding and its allosteric mechanism. *J. Mol. Biol.* 129: 175.

Barcroft, J. (1914) The *respiratory function of the blood* (1st ed). Cambridge: Cambridge University Press. The second edition appeared in Vol. 1, Lessons from High Altitudes, 1925; Vol. II Haemoglobin. 1928.

Blough, NV and Hoffman, BM. (1984). Carbon monoxide binding to the ferrous chains of [Mn, Fe(II)] hybrid hemoglobins: pH dependence of the chain affinity constants associated with specific hemoglobin ligation pathways. *Biochemistry* 23: 2875.

Blough, NV, Zemel, H, and Hoffman, BM. (1984). Flash photolytic studies of carbon monoxide binding to the ferrous chains of [Mn(II), Fe(II)] hybrid hemoglobins: Kinetic mechanism for the early stages of hemoglobin ligation. *Biochemistry* 23: 2883.

Borisov VV, Sogfenov NI, Pavlovski, AG et al. (1977). Spacial structure of lupin leghemoglobin at 2.8Å resolution. *Dokl. Akad. USSR* 223: 238.

Brzozowski, A, Derewenda, Z, Dodson, E et al. (1984). Bonding of molecular oxygen to the T state human haemoglobin. *Nature* 307: 74, 1984.

Bunn, HF and Forget, BG. (1985). *Hemoglobin: Molecular, genetic and clinical aspects.* Philadelphia: W. B. Saunders.

Burton, AC. (1972). *Physiology and biophysics of the circulation* (2nd ed) Chicago, Year Book Medical Publishers Inc.

Busch, MR, Mace, JE, Ho, NT, and Ho, C. (1991). Roles of the beta 146 histidine residue in the molecular basis of the Bohr effect of haemoglobin: A proton nuclear magnetic resonance study. *Biochemistry* 30: 865.

Chu, AH, Turner, BW, and Ackers, GK. (1984). Effects on the oxygen-linked subassembly in human hemoglobin. *Biochemistry* 23: 604.

Dickerson, RE and Geis, I. (1983). *Hemoglobin: Structure, function, evolution, pathology.* Kenlo Park: Benjamin/Cummings Publishing Co.

Fermi, G. (1975). Three-dimensional Fourier synthesis of human deoxyhaemoglobin at 2.5Å resolution: Refinement of the atomic model. *J. Mol. Biol.* 97: 237.

Fermi, G and Perutz, MF. (1981). *Atlas of molecular structures in biology: Haemoglobin and myoglobin.* Oxford: Clarendon Press.

Fermi, G, Perutz, MF, Shaanan, B, and Fourme, R. (1984). The crystal structure of human deoxyhaemoglobin at 1.74Å resolution. *J. Mol. Biol.* 175: 159.

Frier, JA and Perutz, MF. (1977). Structure of human foetal deoxyhaemoglobin. *J. Mol. Biol.* 114: 385.

Gacon, G, Lostanten, G, Labie, D, and Kaplan, J-C. (1980). Interaction between cytochrome $b5$, and hemoglobin: Involvement of $\beta66$(E10) and $\beta95$(FG2) lysyl residues of hemoglobin. *Proc. Natl. Acad. Sci. U.S.A.* 77: 1917.

Garby, L and Madden, J. (1977). *The respiratory functions of blood.* New York: Plenum Medical Book Co.

Gray, RD. (1970). The kinetics of the alkaline Bohr effect in human hemoglobin. *J. Biol. Chem.* 245: 2914.

Haurowitz, F. (1938). Des Gleichgewicht zwischen Hämoglobin und Sauerstoff. *Hoppe-Seyler's Ztschr. f. physiolog.* Chem. 254: 266.

Ho, C, editor. (1982). *Hemoglobin and oxygen binding.* New York: Elsevier Biomedical.

Ikeda-Saito, MI, Brunori, M, and Yonetani, T. (1978). Oxygenation and EPR spectral properties of Aplysia myoglobins containing cobaltous porphyrins. *Biochim Biophys Acta* 533: 173.

Imai, K. (1982). *Allosteric effects in haemoglobin.* Cambridge: Cambridge University Press.

Jameson, GB, Molinaro, FS, Ibers, JA et al. (1980). Models for the active site of oxygen-binding hemoproteins. Dioxygen binding properties and the structures of (2-methylimidazole)-mesotetra ($\alpha,\alpha,\alpha,\alpha$-o-pivalamidophenyl)-porphyrinatoiron(II)-ethanol and its dioxygen adduct. *J. Am. Chem. Soc.* 102: 3224.

Janin, J and Wodak, SJ. (1993). The quaternary structure of hemoglobin Ypsilanti. *Proteins* 15: 1.

Johnson, ME and Ho, C. (1974). Effects of ligands and organic phosphates on functional properties of human adult hemoglobin. *Biochemistry* 13: 365.

Lehmann, H and Huntsman, RG. (1974). *Man's hemoglobins.* Amsterdam: North Holland Publishing Co.

Lehmann, H and Kynoch, PAM. (1976). *Human hemoglobin variants and their characteristics.* Amsterdam: North Holland Publishing Company.

Luisi, B and Shibayaiua, N. (1989). Structure of haemoglobin in the deoxy quaternary state with ligand bound to the α-hemes. *J. Mol. Biol.* 206: 723.

MacQuarrie, R and Gibson, QH. (1971). Use of fluorescent analogue of 2,3-diphosphoglycerate as a probe of human hemoglobin conformation during carbon monoxide binding. *J. Biol. Chem.* 246: 5833.

Minton, AP and Saroff, HA. (1974). A general formulation of the free energy of interaction in cooperative ligand binding: Application to hemoglobin. *Biophys. Chem.* 2: 296.

Monod, J, Changeux, J-P, and Jacob, F. (1963). Allosteric proteins and cellular control systems. *J. Mol. Biol.* 6: 306, 1963.

Monod, J, Wyman, J, and Changeux, J-P. (1965). On the nature of allosteric transitions: A plausible model. *J. Mol. Biol.* 12: 88.

Padlan, EA and Love, WE. (1968). Structure of the hemoglobin of the marine annelid worm, Glycera dibranchiata at 5.5Å resolution. *Nature* 220: 376.

Paoli, M, Liddington, R, Tame, T et al. (1996). Crystal structure of T-state haemoglobin with oxygen bound at all four haems. *J. Mol. Biol.* 256: 775.

Paoli, M, Liddington, R, Williamson, A, and Dodson, G. (1997). Tension in haemoglobin revealed by Fe-His (F8) bond rupture in the fully ligated T-state. *J. Mol. Biol.* 271: 161.

Parkhurst, LJ. (1979). Hemoglobin and myoglobin ligand kinetics. *Annu. Rev. Phys. Chem.* 30: 503.

Perutz, MF. (1970). Stereochemistry of cooperative effects in haemoglobin. *Nature* 228: 726.

Perutz, MF. (1972). Nature of haem-haem interaction. *Nat. New Biol.* 237: 495.

Perutz, MF. (1974). Mechanism of denaturation of haemoglobin by alkali. *Nature* 247: 341.

Perutz, MF. (1998). The stereochemical mechanism of the cooperative effects in haemoglobin revisited. *Ann. Rev. Biophys. Biomol. Structure* 27: 1.

Perutz, MF and Lehmann, H. (1968). Molecular pathology of haemoglobin. *Nature* 222: 902.

Perutz, MF and Ten Eyck, LF. (1971). Stereochemistry of cooperative effects in hemoglobin. *Cold Spring Harb. Symp. Quant. Biol.* 36: 295.

Perutz, MF, Fermi, G, Abraham, DJ et al. (1986). Hemoglobin as a receptor of drugs and peptides: X-ray studies of the stereochemistry of binding. *J. Am. Chem. Soc.* 108: 1064.

Perutz, MF, Kendrew, JC, and Watson, HC. (1965). Structure and function of haemoglobin. Some relations between polypeptide chain configuration and amino acid sequence. *J. Mol. Biol.* 13: 669.

Perutz, MF, Muirhead, H, Mazzarella, L et al. (1969). Identification of the residues responsible for the alkaline Bohr effect in Haemoglobin. *Nature* 222: 1240.

Perutz, MF, Rossman, MG, Cullis, AF et al. (1970). Structure of haemoglobin. A three-dimensional Fourier synthesis at 5.5Å resolution, obtained by X-ray analysis. *Nature* 185: 416.

Perutz, MF, Shi, PT, and Williamson, D. (1994). The chloride effect in human haemoglobin, a new kind of allosteric mechanism. *J. Mol. Biol.* 239: 555.

Perutz, MF, Shih, DT-b, & Williamson, D. (1993). The chloride effect in human haemoglobin. A new kind of allosteric mechanism. *J. Mol. Biol.* 239, 555–560.

Phillips, SEV. (1980). Structure and refinement of oxymyoglobin at 1.6A resolution. *J. Mol. Biol.* 142: 531.

Phillips, SEV and Schoenborn, B. (1981). Neutron diffraction reveals oxygen-histidine hydrogen bond in oxymyoglobin. *Nature* 292: 81.

Poyart, CF, Bursaux, E, and Bohn, B. (1978). An estimation of the first binding constant of O_2 to human hemoglobin A. *Eur. J. Biochem.* 87: 75.

Roughton, FJW. (1959). Diffusion and simultaneous chemical reaction velocity in haemoglobin solutions and red cell suspensions. *Prog. Biophys. Chem.* 9: 55.

Russu, IM, Ho, NT, and Ho, C. (1980). Role of the β146 histidyl residue in the alkaline Bohr effect of hemoglobin. *Biochemistry* 19: 1043.

Shaanan, B. (1980). The crystal structure of oxyhaemoglobin at 2.1A resolution. *J. Mol. Biol.* 142: 531.

Shi, DT, Luisi, BP, Miyazaki, G et al. (1993). A mutagenic study of the allosteric linkage of histidine of His (HC3) 146 beta in haemoglobin. *J. Mol. Biol.* 230: 1291.

Silva, MM, Rogers, PH, and Arnone, A. (1992). A Third Quaternary structure of human haemoglobin A at 1.7Å resolution. *J. Biol. Chem.* 267: 17248.

Sober, HA, editor. (1968). *Handbook of biochemistry.* Cleveland: Chemical Rubber Company.

Steigemann, W and Weber, E. (1979). Structure of erythrocruorin in different ligand states refined at 1.4Å resolution. *J. Mol. Biol.* 127: 309.

Tanford, C. (1961). *The physical chemistry of macromolecules.* New York: John Wiley & Sons.

Taylor, DJ, Bore, PJ, Styles, P et al. (1983). Bioenergetics of intact human muscle: a ^{31}P nuclear magnetic resonance study. *Mol. Biol. Med.* 1: 177.

Tyuma, I and Shimizu, K. (1970). Effect of organic phosphates on the difference in oxygen affinity between fetal and adult human hemoglobin. *Fed. Proc.* 29: 1112.

Up-to-date lists of abnormal hemoglobins are obtainable from the International Hemoglobin Information Center, Augusta, Georgia, 30921, U.S.A.

Watson, HJ and Kendrew, JC. (1961). Comparisons between the amino-acid sequences of sperm whale myoglobin and of human haemoglobin. *Nature* 190: 670.

10

Hemoglobins of the Embryo and Fetus and Minor Hemoglobins of Adults

RONALD L. NAGEL
MARTIN H. STEINBERG

In intrauterine life and postnatally, erythroblasts express—in a developmentally regulated manner—eight different globin genes, and the blood contains six types of hemoglobin (Fig. 10.1). The organization and evolution of genes encoding human hemoglobin were discussed in Chapter 5, and general features of the structure and function of hemoglobin was covered in Chapter 9. Hemoglobin switching is addressed in Chapter 7. Several hemoglobin species, Gower I, Gower II, and Portland, are found only during the earliest stages of embryogenesis. Although clinically unimportant, the presence of minute quantities of the ζ-globin chain of Hb Portland can be a useful marker of the common Southeast Asian form of α thalassemia-1 (Chapters 17 and 18). Fetal hemoglobin (HbF), the predominant hemoglobin in the fetus, is present in trace quantities in normal adults. Many clinically important conditions affect the concentration of HbF, and HbF plays an important role in the pathophysiology and treatment of sickle cell anemia and the β thalassemias (Chapters 12–14, 24, 26, and 28). HbA_2 is present in adults at levels between 2 and 3 percent of the total hemoglobin. Although HbA_2 is of little apparent physiologic importance, its measurement is a useful diagnostic aid for detecting β thalassemia. This chapter presents the clinical and physiologic features of hemoglobins besides HbA that are found in the embryo, fetus, and adult.

HEMOGLOBIN F

In 1866, Korber found that the hemoglobin in newborns' erythrocytes was resistant to alkaline denaturation (see later), providing the first suggestion that a hemoglobin existed that differed from normal adult hemoglobin (HbA), a supposition proven conclusively by Chernoff and colleagues (1951). HbF ($\alpha_2\gamma_2$) can be differentiated spectrophotometrically from HbA ($\alpha_2\beta_2$) by the presence of a "tryptophan notch" at 252 nm, the consequence of an extra tryptophan in position γ130 (Jope, 1949).

Structure of the γ-Globin Genes and γ-Globin Chains

γ-Globin chains differ from β-globin chains (Fig. 10.2) in either 39 or 40 amino acid residues (depending on whether a glycine or alanine residue is present at γ136) (Schroeder et al., 1963). Two γ-globin genes are closely linked in tandem between the ε and ψβ gene within the β-globin gene like cluster on chromosome 11 (Chapter 5). These genes differ only at position γ136 where a glycine residue is present in the 5′ or $^G\gamma$ gene, and an alanine is present in the 3′, or $^A\gamma$ gene. In addition, a common polymorphism of the $^A\gamma$ gene, where threonine ($^A\gamma^T$) replaces isoleucine ($^A\gamma^I$) at codon γ75 (HbF-Sardinia), is present (Schroeder et al., 1979). This striking similarity in protein sequence and structure of the γ-globin gene reflects their concerted evolution from gene duplication and gene conversion (the nonreciprocal exchange of genetic material between the two linked homologous genes) (Slightom et al., 1980). Gene conversion of the γ-globin genes may be an ongoing process during evolution as suggested by the analysis of chromosomes in which the Bantu haplotype is linked to the β^S gene; a subgroup of these chromosomes has undergone a recent gene conversion, eliminating several sequence differences between the two γ-globin genes (Bouhassira et al., 1989) (Chapter 26). Selection may maintain the sequence of γ-globin chains and the structure of HbF. Because HbF is present through most of the fetal life and functionally critical sequence abnormalities could affect fetal development, maintaining the normal gene sequence could be vitally important.

Protein Conformation

Of the 39 amino acid residue differences between γ- and β-globin chains, 22 are on the molecule's surface. Four critical differences are present in the $\alpha_1\beta_1$ area of

Martin H. Steinberg, Bernard G. Forget, Douglas R. Higgs, and Ronald L. Nagel, editors. *Disorders of Hemoglobin: Genetics, Pathophysiology, and Clinical Management.* © 2001 Cambridge University Press. All rights reserved.

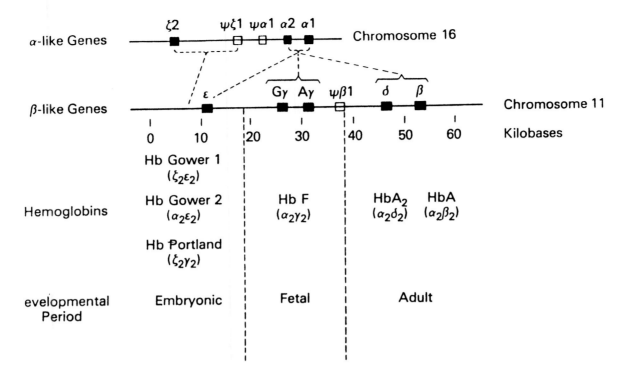

Figure 10.1. Hemoglobins generated by the α- and β-globin gene cluster in a developmentally determined sequential fashion.

contact (the packing contact) that dissociates only under extreme conditions (e.g., very high butyl urea concentration, iodine salts, extreme pH). Two differences, γ112 Thr (β112 Cys) and γ130 Trp (β130 Tyr), in the $\alpha_1\gamma_1$ interface, could be involved in giving the HbF molecule its resistance to alkaline and acid (see later). Sequence differences are not present in the $\alpha_1\beta_2$ area of contact (the sliding contact) that is the center of ligand-dependent conformational changes. Other critical sequence differences are discussed when the anomalous functional properties of HbF are considered.

Crystallographic studies of HbF at 2.5 Å resolution (Frier and Perutz, 1977) showed almost complete isomorphism between HbA and HbF, with the sole difference in the N-terminal portion of the γ-globin chain. This change increases the distance from 2,3 BPG inserted in the central cavity of the hemoglobin molecule to the γ2 His, possibly a secondary contributor to the reduction in 2,3 BPG effect exhibited by HbF, although the results of the crystallographic studies may not be entirely correct (see later). Another aspect of HbF not readily understood is its strong globin-heme interaction and lower rate of dimerization than that of HbA (Bunn and Jandl, 1966).

Based on these findings, HbF appears a more stable and tighter tetramer than HbA and can resist extremes of pH, properties that may endow the HbF molecule

with yet another attribute—providing some protection to neonates and young children from dying from *Plasmodium falciparum* malaria (Chapter 30).

Functional Properties of HbF

Alkaline Resistance. HbF can resist denaturation at alkaline and acid pH, and this forms the basis for one of the most frequently used tests to measure its concentration in blood (Chapter 34). This resistance probably resides in two critical differences from other hemoglobins in primary structure that affect residues buried in the interface between α and γ chains in the $\alpha_1\gamma_1$ dimer. At positions 112 and 130, β^A chains have cysteine and tyrosine residues, respectively, ionizable at alkaline pH, that destabilize the $\alpha_1\beta_1$ dimer, generating easily denaturable monomers. In contrast, in γ-globin chains, threonine and tryptophane at these corresponding positions do not ionize at alkaline pH, making HbF more resistant to high pH.

Ligand Binding. Erythrocytes of newborns with high HbF concentrations have higher oxygen affinity than adult red cells, but in hemolysates of newborn and adult cells, oxygen affinities are identical (Allen, et al., 1953). This finding suggests that HbF and HbA have identical intrinsic oxygen binding properties but interact differentially with intraerythrocytic effectors. 2,3 BPG has decreased binding to HbF (Tyuma and Shamizu, 1969). The primary structural basis of this

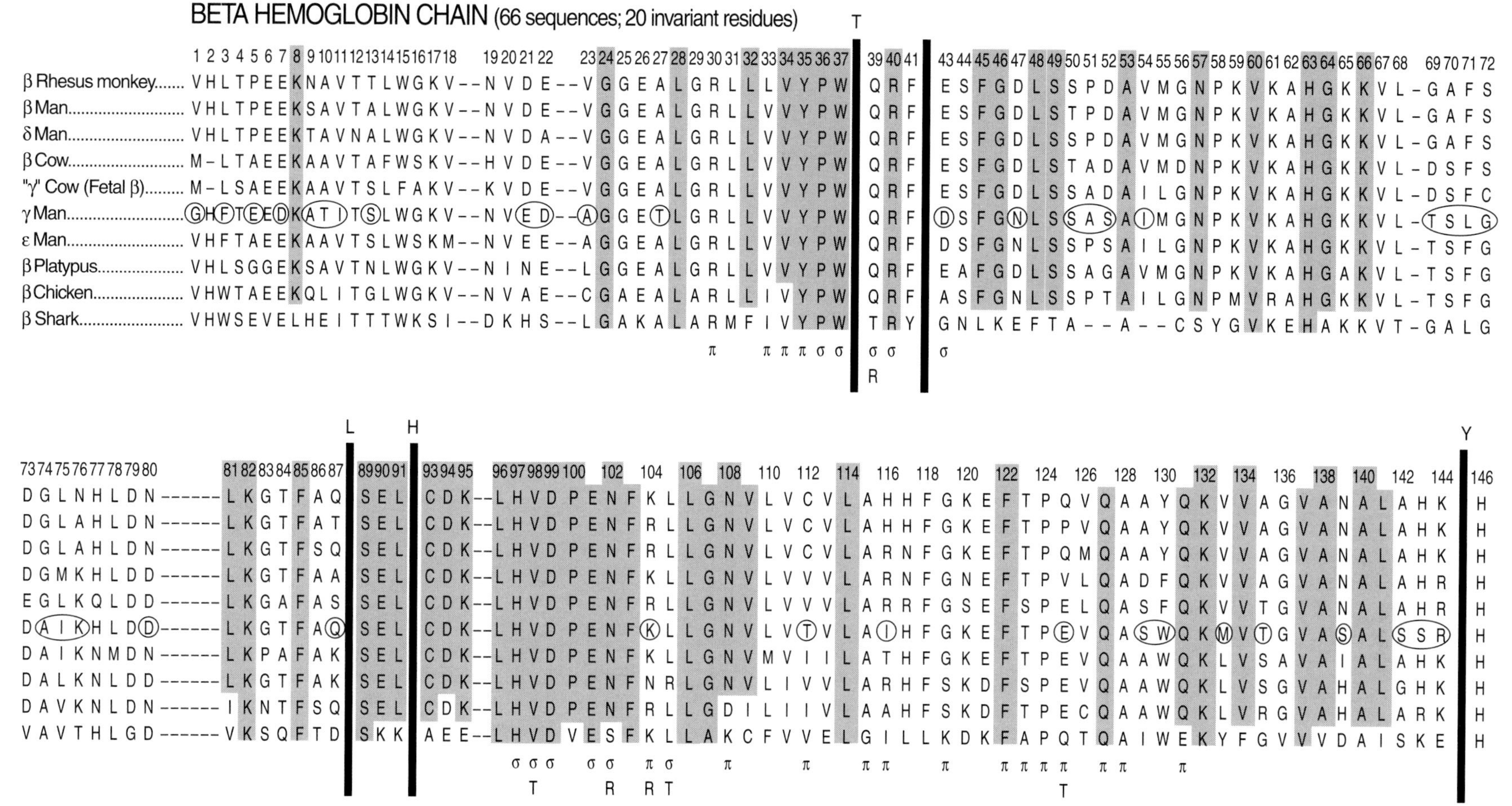

BETA HEMOGLOBIN CHAIN (66 sequences; 20 invariant residues)

Figure 10.2. Protein sequences of the β-globin-like genes in several species. Black bars represent absolutely conserved residues (that is, present in all globins so far tested) thought to be responsible for the myoglobin-type fold. Boxed residues are conserved in most β-like genes depicted.

effect is the replacement of β143 His, a phosphate binding site in the central cavity, with a serine residue in γ143, abolishing an important binding site. Secondary effects, mentioned previously, come from the displacement of the N-terminal portion of the γ-globin chain that alters phosphate binding with γ2 His. Finally, HbF molecules, acetylated at the N-terminus of the γ-globin chain, are incapable of binding 2,3 BPG (Schroeder et al., 1962).

Also impaired in HbF-containing erythrocytes is the Cl^- effect (Poyart et al., 1978). This anion binds in the 2,3 BPG binding site in the central cavity. At low NaCl concentrations—up to 0.05M—HbF has a lower affinity for oxygen than HbA. At higher Cl^- concentrations, this difference disappears. Although not well understood, this effect might be due to the diminution of positive charges in the central cavity, with a reduction in the binding affinity for anions and destabilization of the T state. Increased stability of the T state induced by the absence of anion neutralizing positive charges would favor low ligand affinity.

CO_2 binding by HbF is drastically decreased (Gros and Bauer, 1978). Fewer carbamates are formed at the N-terminus at a wide range of PCO$_2$. The γ chain N-terminus has a pKa of 8.1, higher than that of the β chain pKa of 6.6, making 90 percent of the site protonated at physiologic conditions and unable to bind CO_2.

The alkaline Bohr effect (relation between high pH and ligand affinity) is increased by 20 percent in HbF-containing red cells (Burseaux et al., 1979). This might be a Cl^- effect, because in isolated HbF at low anion concentration, HbF and HbA have an identical Bohr effect, whereas the Bohr effect of HbF increases pari-passu with the Cl^- concentration. A plausible explanation is that the binding of Cl^- at low pH at the β143 His stabilizes the R state. The absence of this Cl^- site would reduce the low pH Bohr effect, because this condition favors the T state. Consequently, the alkaline Bohr effect is favored in HbF.

The question of the interrelationships between the dimer interface, the 2,3 BPG binding site within the central cavity between the γ chains, and the acetylated N-terminal in HbF on dimerization rate has been addressed (Dumoulin et al., 1997). Dimerization rate of HbF was considerably lower than previously estimated—70 times less than HbA; nevertheless, acetylated HbF (HbF$_1$) dimerized at the same rate as HbA. HbA was mutated to make the α1β2 interface HbF-like by substituting the four differences between HbA and HbF in the α1β1 interface of HbA, leaving the rest of the molecule, including the central cavity, unchanged. Surprisingly, this hybrid molecule had decreased binding with 2,3 BPG, much like HbF, although the central cavity was entirely HbA. Dissociation into dimers was intermediate between

HbA and HbF, and not like HbF, although the residues in the α1β2 interface were HbF-like. Inescapably, it appears that both 2,3 BPG binding and dimerization are not simply dependent on critical residues, but that the rest of the molecule contributes strongly to these properties. N-terminal acetylation of γ-globin chains affects dimerization, making HbF$_1$ more like HbA. Understanding these long-range interactions must wait further experimentation.

Physiology of HbF-Containing Cells

How do the modified properties of HbF benefit the fetus and newborn? Perhaps the main feature of fetal circulation—in terms of its differences from postnatal life—is that oxygen loading occurs under more difficult circumstances than postnatal gas exchange. Postnatally, oxygen loading occurs over a gas/liquid interface, whereas in the fetus there is a liquid/liquid interface. Tissues of the fetus function at a high metabolic rate so oxygen loading, rather than oxygen delivery, may be limiting because it is likely that a blood/tissue PO$_2$ gradient exists.

Based on this analysis, the high oxygen affinity of HbF-containing erythrocytes promotes uptake of oxygen in the placenta. It also suggests reasons why enhancement of tissue oxygen delivery by an increased P$_{50}$ is less important and why HbF lacks a 2,3 BPG response. Because of an increased Bohr effect, HbF increases pH when it passes through the intravillous spaces of the placenta because of its release of CO_2. In effect, the Bohr effect accounts for 40 percent of the mother/fetus gas exchange (Burseaux et al., 1979). An increased Bohr effect permits HbF to modulate delivery of O_2 to tissues when needed, even without a 2,3 BPG effect. Fifty percent of oxygen delivery to tissues is accounted for by the increased Bohr effect. An increased Bohr effect could also explain the paradox of mothers with high oxygen affinity hemoglobin variants having neither pregnancy-related complications nor fetal morbidity (Charache et al., 1985). Therefore, the advantage of HbF is not limited to its reduced P$_{50}$; even if this is erased—as with the existence of a high oxygen affinity hemoglobin variant in mothers' blood—the enhanced Bohr effect can compensate. Giardina et al. (1995) have proposed that heat release, which is higher in HbF than in HbA, may also be an important function of HbF in the fetus.

Heterogeneity of HbF

Two nearly identical γ-globin chains are synthesized by the ^{G}γ- and ^{A}γ-globin genes but, in some populations, the ^{A}γ^T polymorphism is also found. Additional heterogeneity is caused by posttranslational acetylation of the γ N-terminal glycine residue in about 10 to 15 percent of newborn HbF (Schroeder, 1980). This is discussed more fully below when we consider minor hemoglobin fractions.

Gender-related and *Trans*-acting Modulation of HbF Levels

Miyoshi et al. (1988) reported that in 300 normal, healthy Japanese adults, the range of HbF (0.17 to 2.28 percent) and HbF-containing erythrocytes, F cells (0.3 to 16.0 percent), was affected by gender (Fig. 10.3). Family studies of 21 probands with high HbF levels and F cells suggested a dominant X-linked pattern of inheritance. In another study of 122 patients with sickle cell anemia, an excess of higher HbF levels was present among females (Nagel, 1991). Mean HbF in males was 6.1 ± 4.3 percent compared with 8.6 ± 7.5 percent in females. Similarly, other investigators also found that HbF was higher among females with sickle cell anemia than males (Morris et al., 1991; Steinberg et al., 1995).

These results suggest, but do not prove, that a factor linked to the X chromosome might influence HbF concentrations in both normal individuals and patients with sickle cell anemia. It has been proposed that females, with two X chromosomes, can be homozygotes for this factor, which presumably escapes X-inactivation, and therefore express higher levels of HbF. Given the estimated gene frequency of this locus, female homozygotes will be infrequent so that large samples will be required to investigate further this phenomenon.

Dover et al. (1992) and Chang et al. (1995) have presented evidence that F cells are increased in females with sickle cell anemia and sickle cell trait and postulated that two genes and three alleles are linked to the X chromosomes (LL, HL, and HH). They have called these alleles the F-cell production or FCP locus (Dover et al., 1992). In one study, this locus accounted for about 40 percent of HbF variability in sickle cell anemia (Chang et al., 1995). HbF production may also be influenced by a gene localized to chromosome 6q (Thein et al., 1994). A possible role of these putative *trans*-acting factors on HbF gene expression has been shown only by linkage analysis, and neither the genes nor their protein products have yet been isolated, although the recent availability of a high resolution map of the X chromosome may hasten the identification of the FCP locus. An RFLP detected by anonymous probes seems to place this locus to the end of the short arm of the X chromosome.

Variation of HbF levels and F cells has also been linked to chromosome 6q22.3–23.2 in an Asian-Indian family (Thein et al., 1994). A total of 210 members of this complex family, in which two different β-thalassemia alleles are present, were studied. Although β thalassemia and the presence of an Xmn I restriction site 5′ to the ^Gγ-globin gene influenced the levels of HbF, linkage analysis using 247 microsatellite markers showed that this "quantitative trait locus"

Figure 10.3. Distribution of F cells in 150 normal men and 150 normal women. The vertical broken lines are at 4.4 percent F cells (Miyoshi et al., 1988).

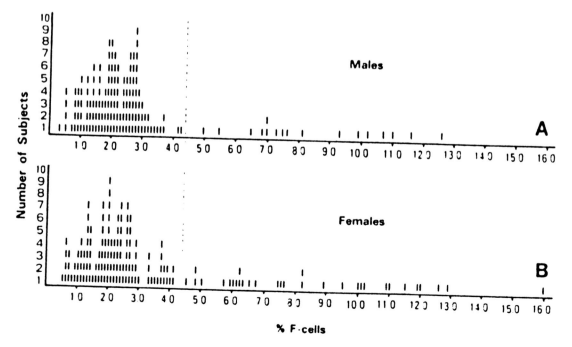

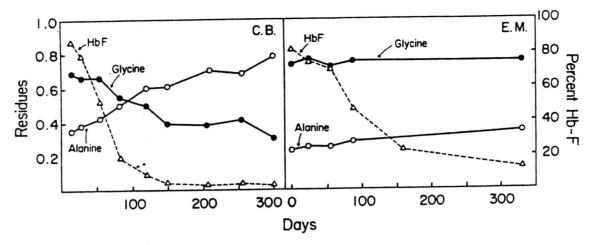

Figure 10.4. $^G\gamma$-globin chains (glycine) are about 70 percent at birth and fall to about 40 percent at age 150 days when $^A\gamma$-globin chains become predominant (left panel). However, a decline in $^G\gamma$-globin gene expression may not always happen (right panel). This is associated with the presence of a -158 C$\rightarrow$T mutation 5′ to the $^G\gamma$-globin gene, and is linked to the Senegal/IX haplotype and the Arab-India haplotype (Chapter 26).

was within 1.5 Mb between markers D6S270 and D6S1626. Several candidate genes within these markers are being studied further (Thein and Craig, 1998). Evidence for another *trans*-acting quantitative trait locus unlinked to chromosome 6 or the X chromosome has been found in an English family (Craig et al., 1997). In studies of monozygotic and dizygotic twins, 15 percent of the variability of F-cell levels could be ascribed to the Xmn 1 restriction site polymorphism 5′ to the $^G\gamma$-globin gene, leaving more than 70 percent to be explained by other genetic modulators (Thein and Craig, 1998; Garner *et al.*, 1998).

The description of a major human erythroid DNA binding protein (GF-1) that can bind a locus in the X chromosome (Xp21–11) (Zon *et al.*, 1990) opens the possibility that this is the determinant related to the excess of high HbF expression in females.

Gene Products of the γ-Globin Genes

The first evidence for the presence of two γ-globin genes in the human genome came from protein analysis that detected both alanine and glycine at γ136 (Schroeder et al., 1968; Huisman et al., 1981; Huisman, 1981). A variant of HbF, originally called HbF Sardinia (Grifoni et al., 1975; Ricco et al., 1976; Saglio et al., 1979), is a common polymorphism of the $^A\gamma$-globin locus where at position 75, an isoleucine residue is replaced by threonine. The $^A\gamma^T$ gene, which is less common than the $^A\gamma^I$ gene, is linked to the Mediterranean haplotype II (Labie et al., 1985) and to the Cameroon haplotype in Africa. These haplotypes are identical but associated with thalassemia in the Mediterranean (Labie et al., 1985) and with the β^S-globin gene in Africa (Lapoumeroulie, et al., 1989). In early life a switch occurs in the expression of the $^G\gamma$- and $^A\gamma$-globin genes (Fig. 10.4). Most individuals have a decrease in $^G\gamma$-globin chains in the first 3 months of life, with a reciprocal rise in $^A\gamma$-globin chains, but a

minority of infants maintain the neonatal pattern of γ-globin chain expression.

Physiology of Hemoglobin Switching

In normal newborns, it takes about 1 year for HbF to decrease from 55 to 85 percent at birth to less than 1 percent, the HbF concentration in most adults (Fig. 10.5) This switch from γ-globin gene expression to β-globin gene expression is discussed in Chapter 15. Fetal cells decrease in number rapidly after birth as shown by the decrease in mean cell volume (MCV), an event followed by the progressive decrease in the number of F cells (Mason et al., 1982). Sickle cell anemia patients have a much delayed switch from γ-globin gene expression to β^S-globin gene expression and from HbF to HbS (Huisman, 1980–1981). A stable HbF level in these patients may not be reached for 10 to 20 years. This delay in the decline of γ-globin gene expression may not be due to anemia per se because thalassemia trait individuals with very slight anemia also exhibit a delay in HbF switching, albeit much more moderate, than sickle cell anemia patients (Schroter and Nafz, 1981) (Fig. 10.6).

Cellular Heterogeneity of HbF

Fetal Cells. HbF makes up close to 100 percent of the hemoglobin in fetal cells (Stockman and Oski, 1978). Normal neonatal blood has an HbF concentration between 55 and 85 percent of the hemolysate.

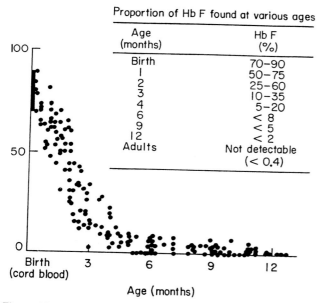

Proportion of Hb F found at various ages

Age (months)	Hb F (%)
Birth	70–90
1	50–75
2	25–60
3	10–35
4	5–20
6	< 8
9	< 5
12	< 2
Adults	Not detectable (< 0.4)

Figure 10.5. Fall in HbF concentration in normal infants from birth to age 1 year.

During the first 10 days of life, hemoglobin synthesis decreases 10-fold from antenatal levels, the bulk of this fall occurring in the first 2 to 3 days after birth (Garby and Sjoli, 1963).

Figure 10.6. Decline in HbF concentration in normal individuals and patients with homozygous (○) and heterozygous (●) β thalassemia. Shaded area is the range for normal controls.

Many characteristics of fetal erythrocytes are similar to those of cells containing HbS, HbC, and HbE. (Table 10.1)

F Cells

HbF is distributed unevenly among nonfetal or "adult" erythrocytes (Kleihauer et al., 1957). HbF, unstable at low pH and eluted from the cell, leaves the remaining HbA that can be stained with acid hematoxylin, forming the basis for the acid-elution or "Betke" test for HbF. Boyer and co-workers delineated the origins, genetics, and physiology of F cells. (Boyer et al., 1975, Dover and Boyer, 1980, 1981; Dover et al., 1977, 1978a, 1978b, 1981).

By definition, F cells contain measurable HbF, implying that the sensitivity of the method used for detecting HbF will accurately determine the number of F cells. Relatively insensitive, the acid-elution method can detect a minimum of 5 to 6 pg of HbF per cell (greater than the average amount of HbF per F cell) (Dover and Boyer, 1980, 1981). Radial immunoprecipitation, where red cells are embedded in an anti-HbF antibody containing agarose gel, can detect 3 pg of HbF per cell (Katsura, 1964). With this technique, the radius of immunoprecipitation surrounding each erythrocyte estimates the HbF concentration of the cell. Fluorescent labeled anti-HbF antibodies can detect F cells on a fixed smear (Hosoi, 1965), but cannot measure directly HbF per F cell. HbF per F cell is then calculated by dividing HbF by the number of F cells and provides an estimate of the average HbF per

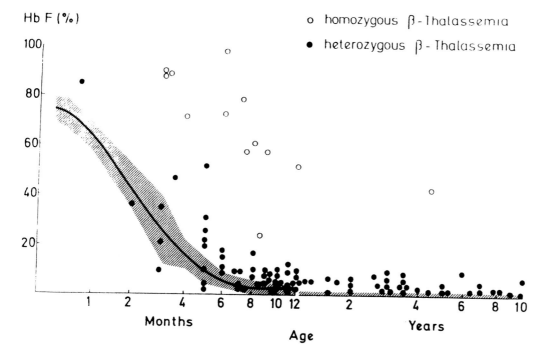

Table 10.1 Characteristics of Neonatal Erythrocytes

1. Increased MCV—about 120 to 130 fl at birth.
2. Decreased erythrocyte life span—60 to 70 days (Premature infants have fetal red cell life spans of 35 to 55 days; adult erythrocyte life span is 120 days) (Nathan and Orkin, 1998).
3. Decreased osmotic fragility—a fraction of these cells are rapidly destroyed in their first few days of life (Sjolin, 1952).
4. Increased numbers of abnormally shaped cells—bowl shapes, keratocytes, knizocytes (Zipursky et al., 1983).
5. Increased numbers of "pocked" cells and cells with vacuoles detected by electron microscopy, reflecting splenic immaturity (Pearson et al., 1978).
6. Increased membrane total lipid, phospholipid, and cholesterol per cell (perhaps a result of macrocytosis).
7. Excess membrane sphingomyelin and decreased lecithin.
8. Enhanced tendency toward lipid peroxidation. (Neerhout, 1968; Younkin et al., 1971; Mollison, 1967)
9. Antigenic differences from adult cells in the Lewis and ABO systems—A and B antigens are weakly expressed—reduced or absent I antigen and presence of i antigen (Mollison, 1967).
10. Increased glucose consumption and activity of many glycolytic enzymes, particularly phosphoglucose isomerase, glyceraldehyde-3-phosphate dehydrogenase, phosphoglycerate kinase, enolase. Decreased activity of phosphofructokinase (Konrad et al., 1972).
11. Tendency toward methemoglobin formation, probably reflecting decreased activity of methemoglobin reductase and increased glutathione stability (Glader and Conrad, 1972).
12. Decreased deformability (Gross and Hathaway, 1972).

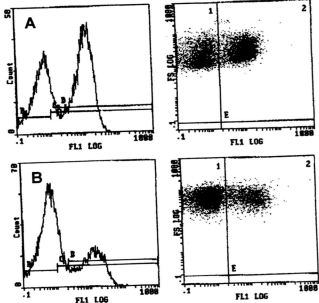

Figure 10.7. Comparison of distribution of γ-globin chains in red cells of by FACS analysis using FITC-labeled antibody specific for human γ-globin supplied by Thomas Campbell and performed by Marsha Mason of EG&G Wallac, a Perkin-Elmer Life Science Company. In this case the examples are of two different sickle cell anemia patients, one with a higher level of HbF (10.4 percent HbF). Panel A or a lower level of HbF (5.4 percent HbF) Panel B. Left panels: number of cells versus fluorescence intensity; right panels: cell size versus fluorescence intensity. Note the presence of two populations of red cells that represent non-F cells and F cells (high fluorescence intensity).

cell. Flow cytometry, using anti-HbF antibodies, is the simplest method of enumerating F cells and can detect cells with an HbF content of 6 pg.

Using radial immunodiffusion, the blood of white adults contained 0.1 to 7.5 percent (1.7 ± 2.2 percent) F cells while using fluorescent antibodies, F cells numbered 2.6 ± 1.6 percent (Katsura, 1964; Hosoi, 1965). Normal African Americans had 2.8 ± 1.6 F cells (Dover and Boyer, 1981). Figure 10.7 shows the separation of F and non-F cells by fluorescence-activated cell sorter (FACS) analysis. Establishing precisely the average concentration of HbF per F cell has been difficult because cells with HbF levels below the limits of detection are not counted. In ten normal individuals,

mature F cells contained an average of 4.4 ± 0.3 pg HbF, with a range between 3.9 and 5.0 pg (Dover and Boyer, 1981). Using another, more sensitive method, HbF was 4.7 pg per F cell. (Hosoi, 1965). In 46 African Americans with sickle cell anemia, the range of F cells was between 2 and 80 percent of erythrocytes and the average HbF per F cell was 6.4 ± 1.6 pg (Dover and Boyer, 1981).

A small group of apparently normal individuals had more than 8 percent F cells in their blood, and in most of these cases, one parent of the proband had similar numbers of F cells. Many of these high F-cell individuals have a form of non-gene deletion hereditary persistence of HbF (Chapter 15). F-cell numbers are affected by age, although this has not been completely studied, and acutely increased erythropoiesis can cause transient increases in HbF and F cells (Chapter 15).

For any level of HbF in the hemolysate, the distribution and concentration of HbF in F-cells can differ among individuals. Patients with sickle cell anemia have individually characteristic distributions of HbF per F cell (Horiuchi et al., 1995). In sickle cell anemia, low levels of HbF in many erythrocytes do not have the same inhibitory effects on HbS polymerization as do higher concentrations of HbF in fewer sickle cells. The more sickle cells carrying polymerization-inhibitory concentrations of HbF, the greater the antipolymerization effect for each percent of HbF increase. Very high concentrations of HbF in few cells is equivalent to an "endogenous" blood transfusion. Lower but still inhibitory concentrations of HbF more widely distributed among sickle (or β thalassemia) cells would have a greater effect on disease severity (Chapter 26).

Most evidence suggests that F cells are not clonal but acquire their particular characteristics stochastically during development. In clonal disorders, including polycythemia vera, paroxysmal nocturnal hemoglobinuria, and Philadelphia chromosome positive chronic granulocytic leukemia, F cells are present in the same proportion as in normal individuals. In adult red cells no relationship exists between F cells and i-antigen, a maker for fetal-like cells (Papayannopoulou et al., 1982).

F Reticulocytes. Using a double-labeling technique that detects both HbF and reticulocytes (F reticulocytes), F reticulocytes in sickle cell anemia numbered 10.6 ± 7.0 percent (2 to 55 percent) (Dover and Boyer, 1981). These observations raised the question of preferential survival of F cells in sickle cell anemia. Preferential survival was suggested by finding more F cells than F reticulocytes in most, but not all, patients. Increased F-cell survival may be the result of inhibition of HbS polymerization by HbF, differential susceptibility of F cells and non-F cells to phagocytosis and endothelial cell adherence, or unknown factors.

Laboratory Detection of HbF

Different methods of measuring HbF can give different results on the same blood sample, and the most precise method for determining HbF varies according to blood HbF concentration (Chapter 34). In 200 normal adults, HbF concentrations were measured by cation-exchange HPLC (Leonova et al., 1996). Normal levels were established between 0.1 and 0.4 percent. Individuals with elevated values of 0.4 to 4.3 percent had $^G\gamma$-globin chain levels measured and extensive DNA sequencing of the β-globin gene cluster locus control region (LCR) and γ-globin gene promoters. Twenty teenagers, randomly selected from the 25 percent of a 200 individual sample with high HbF levels, were mostly females who were homozygous for the C→T variation at position −158 5′ to the $^G\gamma$-globin gene (Gilman, 1988; Labie et al., 1985). One individual was heterozygous for the A→G change at position −161 of the $^G\gamma$-globin gene. Among whites with elevated HbF, a high frequency of the $^G\gamma$−158 C→T polymorphism was present in addition to triplications of the $^G\gamma$ gene. Perhaps mutations in the promoters of the γ-globin gene (Chapter 12) and gene duplications account for the minor elevations of HbF concentration in the normal population.

Medical Conditions Besides Hemoglobinopathies and Thalassemia Associated with High HbF

Pregnancy is associated with a modest increase in HbF in the second trimester. Hydatidiform moles are associated with HbF levels up to 6 percent (Lee et al., 1982). Although hormones secreted during pregnancy have been implicated in these effects, the mechanism of HbF elevation is not clear (Pembrey et al., 1973).

Premature infants and infants of diabetic mothers have a delayed γ→β switch and higher HbF levels than other neonates (Huehns et al., 1964a). This switch is accelerated in Down syndrome and other chromosomal translocations. Controversy exists regarding the relationship of HbF to sudden infant death syndrome (SIDS) (Zielke, et al., 1989; Giulian, et al., 1987; Perry et al., 1997). In most studies carefully controlled for the postconceptual or gestational age—the prime determinant of neonatal HbF level—infants dying with SIDS between 8 and 16 weeks old had significantly higher levels of HbF than control infants (Perry et al., 1997). These levels, measured by different techniques, were between 28 and 65 percent in SIDS infants, whereas controls had HbF concentrations between 12 and 41 percent. Methodologic differences or dissimilarities in patient populations with SIDS are unlikely to account for the discordant results among these studies. If HbF is increased in SIDS infants, perhaps the high O_2 affinity of HbF contributes to chronic hypoxia, a common finding in these patients (Giulian et al., 1987).

Juvenile chronic myeloid leukemia and Fanconi anemia are often accompanied by elevated levels of HbF—up to 30 percent in some cases at age 3 years (Zago, 1987). Highest numbers are associated with C→T mutation at −158 (Xmn I positive) 5′ to the $^G\gamma$-globin gene (Rosatelli et al., 1992). Solid tumors and hematologic malignancies or premalignant states and Kala-Azar and paroxysmal nocturnal hemoglobinuria (particularly when hemolysis is present or red cell survival reduced) can have HbF levels of 5 to 10 percent. The highest levels are found in Di Guglielmo's disease and juvenile myeloid leukemia, where levels higher than 50 percent have been reported (Wood et al., 1989; Weatherall et al., 1975; Boyer et al., 1975; Newman et al., 1973). Other increases in HbF associated with disease are discussed in Chapters 12 and 15.

Mutations of the γ-Globin Genes

Mutations may be found in either the $^{G}\gamma$-globin gene, the $^{A}\gamma$-globin gene, or the $^{A}\gamma^{T}$-globin gene. γ-Globin chain variants will alter a single major hemoglobin band during fetal and neonatal life but, after the first year of life, will alter only the faint HbF band and are rarely detected. Mutations can be present in γ-globin loci of the usual $^{G}\gamma$-$^{A}\gamma$ arrangement, on chromosomes with $^{G}\gamma$-$^{G}\gamma$ loci, and in *cis* or *trans* to the $^{A}\gamma^{T}$-globin gene. Depending on the chromosomal arrangement of the γ-globin genes and many other factors, the levels of $^{G}\gamma$-globin gene variants may range from 5 to 30 percent of total hemoglobin present in neonates, with most accounting for about 25 percent of all hemoglobin. Levels of most $^{A}\gamma$-globin gene variants are about half this amount. This difference is due to the greater expression of the $^{G}\gamma$-globin gene in fetal erythroid cells (Chapter 15). Very few γ-globin gene variants have been subjected to functional studies so that the numbers of mutants reported to have altered properties may be underestimated. A listing of variant γ-globin genes can be found at the Globin Gene Server (http://globin.cse.psu.edu) or Huisman et al. (1998).

Variants of the $^{G}\gamma$ Gene.

Of 39 point mutations of the $^{G}\gamma$-globin gene, two are unstable (**HbF-Poole** γ130 (H8) Trp→Gly; **HbF-La Grange** γ101 (G3)Glu→Lys); two have high oxygen affinity (**HbF Onoda** γ146 (HC3) His→Tyr; **HbF-La Grange**); HbF–M-Osaka has low oxygen affinity; and two are associated with methemoglobinemia (**Hb F-M Fort Ripley** γ92 (F8) His→Tyr; **HbF-M Osaka** γ63 (E7) His→Tyr). The latter two variants were associated with neonatal "cyanosis" that disappeared with maturation. **Hb F-Port Royal** (γ125(H3)Glu→Ala) was found in the African-American population of southeastern United States and was expressed at 14 to 15 percent of total HbF level (Brimhall et al., 1974). Several infants with HbF-Port Royal had a normal $^{G}\gamma$ gene but an $^{A}\gamma$ gene with two nucleotide changes: GAG→GCG at codon 125 (producing a Glu→Ala), GCA→GGA at position (136 producing Ala→Gly). In effect, the "$^{A}\gamma$" gene, was really a $^{G}\gamma$ gene carrying an F-Port Royal mutation, an example of the $^{G}\gamma$-$^{G}\gamma$- gene rearrangement. HbF-Port Royal has been described with other γ-globin gene haplotypes, including the $^{A}\gamma^{T}$ gene and the-$^{G}\gamma$-$^{G}\gamma$-haplotype in *trans* (Huisman, 1997).

$^{G}\gamma$-Globin gene mutations expressed at low levels in newborns are **HbF-Marietta** ($^{G}\gamma$80 (EF4) Asp→Asn) (Nakatsuji et al., 1982) and **HbF-Charlotte** ($^{G}\gamma$75(E19) Ile→Thr) (Plaseska et al., 1990). HbF-Marietta is expressed at 16 percent of total ^{A}HbF, but the arrangement of γ-globin genes is not known. HbF-Charlotte is expressed at 10 percent of total HbF. The same variant has been found in an Italian infant (initially called Hb F-Sassari) and an African-American infant (initially called Hb Waynesboro). These last two cases, found in heterozygotes for the $^{A}\gamma^{T}$ gene, were expressed at 30 percent of HbF. In Hb-F-Charlotte, the mutation was in the 3′ member of a -$^{G}\gamma$-$^{G}\gamma$-haplotype, whereas the other two cases with the same $^{G}\gamma$ mutation occurred in the 5′ member of the locus, accounting for the differences in expression. (Huisman, 1997).

Another HbF mutation that is unstable is **HbF Xinjiang** ($^{A}\gamma^{T}$ 25 (B7)Gly→Arg) (Hu and Ma, 1987), but the degree of its instability is less than Hb Poole (Huisman et al., 1998; Harano et al., 1990; Glader et al., 1989; Hayashi et al., 1969; Lee-Potter et al., 1975). Neonatal cyanosis may accompany methemoglobin-forming variants, and unstable Hb Poole was associated with neonatal hemolytic anemia (Priest et al., 1989).

HbF-Malta-1 (γ117 (G19) His→Arg) migrates between HbS and HbC at alkaline pH. It is present in about 0.3 to 1 percent of Maltese and is linked to the β-globin gene variant, **Hb Valetta** (β87 (F3) Thr→Pro) (Kutlar et al., 1991).

In macerated fetal tissues, an HbF was found that was missing the terminal (γ 141 (HC3) Arg) whose levels increased over time (Kohne et al., 1977). This hemoglobin was called **HbF-Koelliker** because of the strong resemblance to a degraded HbA that lacks the same residue and was called Hb Koelliker. These are not genetic abnormalities but artifacts caused by hemoglobin digestion by the carboxypeptidase B present in macerated tissue.

Mutations of the $^{A}\gamma$ Gene and the $^{A}\gamma^{T}$ Gene (HbF Sardinia).

Twenty-one $^{A}\gamma$-globin gene variants have been described, none with functional abnormalities, although **HbF-Texas-1** (γ5 (A2) Glu→Lys) is acetylated.

HbF-Sardinia ($^{A}\gamma$75 (E19) Ile→Thr, the $^{A}\gamma^{T}$ gene (Grifoni et al., 1975), was a frequent polymorphism without functional or clinical abnormalities. While present at high frequency in many populations, it has a low frequency among Africans and individuals of African descent unless the Cameroon haplotype, found among the Eton people of Central Cameroon, is present (Chapter 26). A reason for the high frequency of this variant has not been established, but its low frequency in most of Africa and high frequency elsewhere suggest that it occurred after man left Africa or that its advantage, if any, is related to a selective pressure not existent in Africa.

Six mutants of this common variant $^{A}\gamma^{T}$ have been described (Huisman, 1992; none are associated with any clinical abnormalities. The best studied of these variants is **Hb F-Yamaguchi** ($^{A}\gamma^{T}$ 80 (EF4) Asp→Asn), which was discovered in a newborn (Fuyuno et al., 1981). Detailed gene mapping revealed the coincidental presence of a −5.1 kb deletion encompassing the 3′ part of the $^{G}\gamma$ gene, the intergenic sequence, and the 5′ part of the $^A\gamma$ gene. This hybrid gene (indicated in some publications as $^G\gamma{\bullet}^A\gamma$) produces an $^A\gamma$-globin gene that expresses at the level of a $^G\gamma$-globin gene in newborns, most likely because of the presence of the $^G\gamma$-globin gene promoter. Interestingly, this hybrid gene, without the Hb Yamaguchi mutation, has been described as γ thalassemia in homozygotes (Sukumaran et al., 1983). Six variants of the $^A\gamma^T$ gene have been described and one, HbF-Xinjiang, is unstable.

HbF-Mauritius (γ23 (B5) Val deleted) is the sole γ-globin chain variant with a deleted residue. The identical deletion in the β-globin chain, **Hb Freiburg**, is associated with hemolytic anemia and cyanosis.

Hb F-Texas, **Hb F-Alexandria**, and **HbF-Ube** have not been localized to a specific γ-globin gene.

γ Thalassemia

γ Thalassemia caused by the types of point mutations that typify β thalassemia have not been described, although it is likely that they exist. Most instances of γ thalassemia are due to gene deletion, and most of these are better classified as γδβ thalassemias or εγδβ thalassemia and have a pathophysiology and phenotype described in Chapters 11 and 12. A γ$^+$ thalassemia phenotype was proposed to result from an IVS II-115 A→G substitution in both the $^A\gamma$-and $^G\gamma$-globin genes and the deletion of an A at position −6 relative to the $^G\gamma$-globin gene polyadenylation site (Bayoumi et al., 1999). However, the IVS II substitutions appear to have gene frequencies of 0.73 for the $^A\gamma$-globin gene and 0.86 for the $^G\gamma$-globin gene, suggesting that they are common polymorphisms.

One "pure" γ thalassemia resulted from an unequal crossover between the $^G\gamma$ and $^A\gamma$-globin genes deleting one γ-globin gene from the affected chromosome and leaving a hybrid γ-globin gene, akin to the Hb Lepore type genes (Chapters 11 and 12; Sukumaran et al., 1983; Zeng et al., 1985). Found in heterozygotes and in two homozygotes, newborns homozygous for this deletion had only 50 percent HbF, all of the $^A\gamma$ type.

HbA$_2$

HbA$_2$ ($\alpha_2\delta_2$), is a minor hemoglobin without an obvious physiologic function (Kunkle and Wallenius, 1995). In normal hemolysates, HbA$_2$ represents between 2 and 3 percent of all hemoglobin.

Evolution of the δ-Globin Gene

Origins of the δ-globin gene are discussed in Chapter 5. HbA$_2$ is present in humans, apes, and New World monkeys, but not Old World monkeys, a finding at variance with the evolutionary data that had humans and Old World monkeys diverging after the divergence of New World monkeys (Boyer, 1972). This inconsistency was resolved with the observation that δ-globin genes are present in Old World monkeys, but have been inactivated by mutation (Martin et al., 1980; Martin et al., 1983).

Comparisons of δ-globin genes among mammals have shown that this locus has not evolved independently, but has done so in concert with the β-globin gene. As shown in Figure 5.11, the δ-globin gene is the product of gene conversion, with the 5′ region related to the β-globin gene and a 3′ portion that is distinct (Hardies, 1984; Koop et al., 1989; Martin et al., 1983). Two variants of the δ-globin gene could have arisen by gene conversion. **HbA$_2$ Flatbush** (δ 22 Ala→Glu) and **HbA$_2$ Coburg** (δ116 Arg→His) both contain a β-globin chain amino acid residue in one of the 10 amino acid residues where these two globins differ and could represent gene conversion events, a hypothesis supported by the frequency that these variants are greater than expected for multiple mutations (Petes, 1982). This hypothesis could be tested in the variant HbA$_2$ Coburg where a gene conversion event would result in a codon 116 change of CGC to CAT, whereas a point mutation would result in a CGC to CAC change. **Hb Parchman** could also be due to gene conversion (δ22 Ala→Glu, 50 Ser→Thr) rather than to a double crossover (δ1-12; β22-50; δ586-146) as proposed initially (Adams et al., 1982).

The δ-Globin Gene and Structure of the δ-Globin Chain

Linked closely to the β-globin gene (Chapter 5) on the short arm of chromosome 11, the general structure of the δ-globin gene is identical to all other expressed globin genes (Chapter 6). δ-Globin chains of HbA$_2$ differ from β-globin chains of HbA by only 10 amino acid residues (Fig. 10.8). Only 31 nucleotide differences are found between the coding regions of the β- and δ-globin genes, and a similar high level of homology is present until 70 base pairs 5′ to the mRNA capping site (Table 10.2). Greater sequence differences in the 5′ noncoding portion are found beyond this point, accounting, in part for the diminished transcription of the δ- compared with the β-globin gene (Fig. 10.9).

δ-Globin Chain Synthesis

Quantitatively, the expression of the δ- and β-globin genes is strikingly different. HbA makes up more than 95 percent of the adult hemolysate, whereas HbA$_2$ accounts for only 2 to 3 percent. HbA$_2$ is syn-

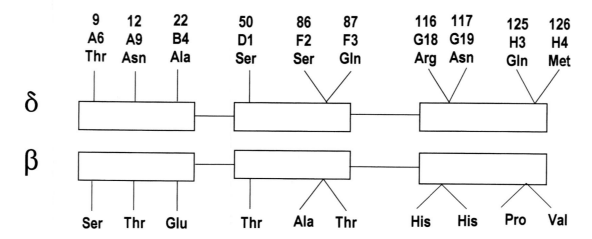

Figure 10.8. Amino acid differences between the human δ- and β-globin chains.

thesized in all erythroid progenitors; therefore its distribution in the blood is pancellular as opposed to the heterocellular distribution of HbF. This is an advantage when consideration is given to raising HbA₂ concentrations as a means to retard HbS polymerization (see later). In bone marrow, δ-globin chains are synthesized at a reduced rate compared with β chains; δ globin is not synthesized in reticulocytes, and reticulocytes contain almost no δ-globin mRNA (Rieder et al., 1965; Roberts et al., 1972). Maturity-fractionated bone marrow erythroblasts showed a progressive decline of δ- in relation to β-globin chain synthesis, as the maturity of the erythroid cell increased. Relative instability of δ-globin mRNA was postulated to be responsible for the premature decline in δ-globin synthesis, and the half-life of δ-globin mRNA was less than one-third that of β-globin mRNA (Wood et al., 1978; Steinberg and Adams, 1991). The instability of δ mRNA may depend on the sequence of its 3′ untranslated region. mRNA instability alone does not account for the vast reduction of

HbA₂ compared with HbA concentration (Ross and Pizarro, 1983; Wood et al., 1978). Translation rates of δ- and β-globin mRNA were similar (Wood et al., 1978). HbA and HbA₂ had almost identical molecular stability, making it unlikely that differential posttranslational survival of the two molecules accounted for the low proportion of HbA₂ (Steinberg and Adams, 1991). These observations suggested that the reduced accumulation of HbA₂ was a result of decreased transcription of the δ-globin gene.

In vitro, transcription of the δ-globin gene was 50 times less efficient than that of the β-globin gene (Humphries, 1982; Proudfoot et al., 1980). Transcription of a hybrid βδ-globin gene was equivalent to that of a normal β-globin gene, but a δβ gene was expressed like a normal δ-globin gene, suggesting that the δ-globin gene promoter was faulty. Two differences between the promoters of the δ-globin gene and β-globin gene seem especially critical. In the δ-globin gene promoter, the conserved CCAAT box is replaced by CCAAC. A CCAAC mutant binds the ubiquitous CCAAT binding protein, CP1, less avidly than the wild type and forms unstable complexes with other possible CCAAT binding proteins,

Table 10.2. Nucleotide Differences in the Coding Portions of the δ-and β-Globin Genes

	2 His	10 Ala	11 Val	30 Arg	31 Leu	66 Lys	68 Leu
β	CAC	GCC	GTT	AGG	CTG	AAA	CTC
δ	CAT	GCT	GTC	AGA	TTA	AAG	CTA
	84 Thr	86 Ala/Ser	87 Thr/Gln	106 Leu	108 Asn	111 Val	116 His/Arg
β	ACC	GCC	ACA	CTG	AAC	GTC	CAT
δ	ACT	TCT	CAG	TTG	AAT	GTG	CGC
	120 Lys	132 Lys	142 Ala	145 Tyr	146 His		
β	AAA	AAA	GCC	TAT	CAC		
δ	AAG	AAG	GCT	TAC	CAT		

Two of the codons that specify amino acid differences between the β- and the δ-globin chain contain two base pair differences and one codon contains three differences. Codon 31 Leu has two base changes.

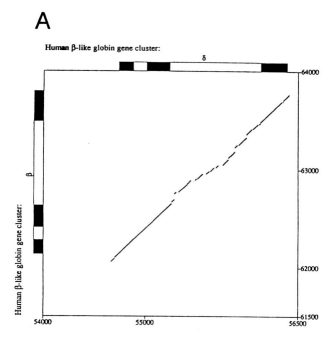

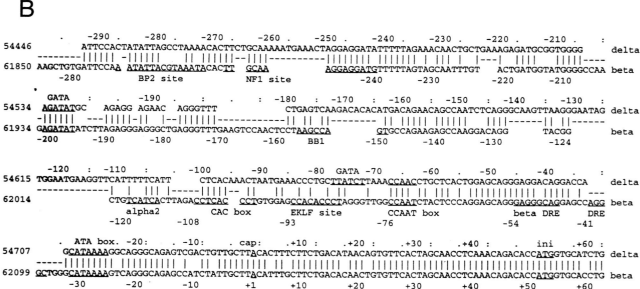

Figure 10.9. Comparisons of the promoters of the β- and δ-globin genes. Panel A shows the alignment of sequences, whereas Panel B shows the pairwise alignment of sequences beginning with –294 and ending at +62 of the δ-globin gene. Vertical lines (I) indicate matches, hyphens (-) indicate gaps to optimize alignment, and spaces indicate mismatches. Transcription factor binding sites are underlined and annotated. (Tang et al., 1997).

reducing β-globin gene promoter activation by the LCR (Delvoye, 1993). The CCAAT box is required for normal transcription of the rabbit β-globin gene. A second major difference between the β- and δ-globin gene promoters is the absence of the proximal

CACC in the δ-globin gene. This sequence forms the binding site for the β-globin gene-specific transcription factor, erythroid Krüppel-like factor (EKLF), the most globin gene-specific of the known erythroid transcription factors (Chapters 4 and 5). Interacting with the β-globin gene promoter, EKLF may influence the γ→β switch (Miller and Bieker, 1993; Perkins et al., 1995).

In vitro studies have shown partial normalization of the transcriptional defect of the δ-globin gene when both the CCAAC and CACC sequences have been "corrected." A mutation in the δ-globin gene promoter, that restored the CCAAC motif to the CCAAT sequence of the β-globin gene promoter, was associated with a 2.4- to 5.6-fold increase in the expression of a reporter gene, depending on the cell line transfected. Introducing EKLF binding sites into the δ-globin gene promoter increased expression 6.5- to 26.8-fold or 35 percent of the total δ and β chains produced according to the conditions of study (Donze, 1996; Tang, 1997).

Mutations in the gene promoter do not totally explain the reduced accumulation of δ-globin mRNA, and additional sites in the δ-globin gene may account for its reduced expression. IVS-II of the δ-globin gene also has been shown to reduce the δ-globin gene transcription by mechanisms that are unclear, but in these studies with stable transformants, an LCR element was not used and the specific roles of the promoter or 3′ untranslated region were untested (LaFlamme et al., 1987). Lepore hemoglobins (Chapters 12 and 14) are products of δβ fusion genes, and the δ-globin gene sequences in their 5′ portion are thought to result in their characteristically reduced rate of synthesis. Yet the Lepore δβ-globin chain is synthesized at a higher rate than the δ-globin chain. The δβ gene contains the β IVS-II, which may explain this observation. Hb Parchman (see previous discussion) is synthesized at the same rate as the normal δ-globin chain (Adams et al., 1982). If, as first postulated, this variant is the result of a double crossover, it should contain a δ-globin gene promoter, a β IVS-I, and a δ IVS-II, supporting the proposition that both the promoter and δ IVS-II contribute to decreased δ-globin gene expression (Kosche et al., 1984, 1985). In contrast, a βδ chain variant, β-like through IVS-1 and then δ-like, was expressed at levels that were greater than the δ-globin gene, but less than the β-globin gene, suggesting that δ IVS-II and 3′ sequences also influence gene expression (Badr et al., 1973). The δ-globin gene IVS-II contains only a single GATA-I binding site, whereas β IVS-II has two GATA-I sites and an Oct-I site, perhaps accounting for the effects of δ IVS-II. Positive and negative regulatory elements may exist in 500 base pairs 5′ to the δ-globin gene (Tang et al., 1997). When β-and δ-gene constructs containing sequences 5′ to the gene were examined in the primitive erythroid environment of K562 cells, a positive regulatory element 5′ to the δ gene was suggested (Ebb et al., 1993).

Functional Aspects of HbA₂

HbA₂ has functional properties nearly identical to HbA; ligand binding curves are similar, although HbA₂ has higher oxygen affinity (de Bruin and Janssen, 1973; Eddison et al., 1964); but Bohr effect, cooperativity, and response to 2,3 BPG are identical to HbA (Bunn and Briehl, 1970). Greater thermal stability of HbA₂ (Kinderlerer et al., 1973) may be due to the δ116 Arg that can form a salt bridge with α114 Pro, increasing even further the stability of the α1β1 packing contact. HbA₂ has slightly increased autoxidation to methemoglobin, and its hemichrome had increased stability (Ranney et al., 1993). These differences could explain its increased membrane binding. HbA₂ inhibits the polymerization of HbS, (Nagel et al., 1979) and δ22 Ala and δ87 Gln may be the important inhibitory sites. When HbA₂ levels are exceptionally high and in the presence of elevated HbF levels, the combination of these two hemoglobins may modulate the phenotype of HbS-β⁰ thalassemia (Chapter 28). When a δ6 Val mutation is introduced into the δ-globin chain in the presence or absence of either or both δ22 Glu and δ87 Thr, the deoxy molecule polymerizes without a delay time in the simple δ6 Val variant and with delay times when other mutations are present (Adachi et al., 1996).

The positive charge of HbA₂ may endow it with properties similar to other positively charged hemoglobins, such as HbC, in its interaction with the erythrocyte membrane (Klipstein and Ranney, 1960; Fischer et al., 1975). HbA₂ has a higher affinity for erythrocyte membrane Band 3 than does HbA (Fischer et al., 1975). Although the interaction of HbC with the membrane is believed to determine the red cell phenotype of HbC trait and HbC disease (Chapter 27), the very low concentration of HbA₂ makes it doubtful that it meaningfully affects cation transport and mean corpuscular hemoglobin concentration (Chapter 22).

It has been suggested that the δ-globin gene is a pseudogene in evolution, destined for the biological scrapheap of history. This analysis presupposes that the sole functional role of all hemoglobins is oxygen transport. If so, HbA₂ is clearly useless, and its mutations have no clinical significance. Alternatively, increased binding of HbA₂ to the membrane might mask another functional role for this hemoglobin. It is not clear whether HbA₂ binds other membrane proteins besides Band 3 and if this has any functional role. The presence of a variant HbA₂ at polymorphic frequencies in the Dogon region of Mali at least hints at some possible selective advantage for this variant.

Mutational Events Involving the δ Gene

A priori, mutation in the δ-globin gene should be as frequent as the β-globin gene. However, far fewer δ-thalassemia-causing mutations and δ-globin chain variants have been described. This anomaly probably has a twofold explanation. First, detecting δ-globin chain hemoglobinopathies is difficult because of the low concentration of δ-globin gene variants, and few clinical or hematologic abnormalities are expected with δ thalassemia. Second, the inconsequential hematologic changes of δ thalassemia provide an insufficient basis for natural selection to protect the carrier from *P. falciparum* malaria.

In individuals heterozygous for stable δ-globin chain variants, the concentration of the HbA$_2$ variant is equivalent to about half the usual HbA$_2$ concentration, and the sum of normal and variant HbA$_2$ is equal to the normal HbA$_2$ level (The Globin Gene Server; http://globin.cse.psu.edu). Homozygotes for these HbA$_2$ variants have normal HbA$_2$ levels. Thirty-four single amino acid substitutions, products of single base changes, have been described for HbA$_2$. More than 40 percent of the reported δ-globin gene variants have been characterized at the DNA level. Like α- and β-globin gene mutants (Chapters 44 and 45), δ-globin gene variants can be unstable and have increased oxygen affinity. Two mutations, **HbA$_2$** Wrens (98 (FG5) Val→Met) (Codrington et al., 1989) and **HbA$_2$** Manzanares (δ121 (GH4) Glu→Val) (Garcia et al., 1983) are unstable. **HbA$_2$** Canada (δ99 (F1)Asp→Asn) (Salkie et al., 1982) has very high affinity for oxygen. Even these functionally abnormal variants are not accompanied by any adverse clinical consequences.

HbA$_2$′ (δ16 Gly→Arg)—sometimes called HbB$_2$—is the most common variant of the δ-globin gene (Ceppellini, 1959; Stamatoyannopoulos et al., 1977; Weatherall et al., 1976). HbA$_2$′ is present in about 1 percent of African Americans, and both homozygotes and heterozygotes are found. In Africa, it has been described in samples from different geographic locations including Ghana. More recently, it has been found at polymorphic frequencies in one cast in the Dogon region of the Republic of Mali (Nagel, personal communication) Although haplotype analysis of the β-like globin gene cluster in individuals from Mali with HbA$_2$′ showed that all unrelated individuals carried this mutation on the same haplotype, samples from unrelated African Americans with this mutation displayed haplotype heterogeneity. It is possible therefore that this mutation arose in Africa unicentrically and distributed itself to other regions of Africa by gene flow.

HbA$_2$′ migrates cathodic to normal HbA$_2$ on alkaline electrophoresis and can also be separated by anion and cation exchange chromatography and high-performance liquid chromatography (HPLC). Its presence can be suspected by finding a split HbA$_2$ band on hemoglobin electrophoresis or HPLC where each fraction is half the total HbA$_2$. It is found both in *cis* and in *trans* to HbS and HbC.

MEASUREMENT OF HbA$_2$

Separation of HbA$_2$ from HbA by electrophoretic and chromatographic methods is simplified by the presence of two additional positive charges in the δ-globin chain but not the β-globin chain. Different methods of measurement, including new and traditional methods of electrophoresis and spectrophometric measurement of eluted fractions, HPLC, column chromatography, and immunologic detection are detailed in Chapter 34. Scanning densitometry of electrophoresis strips is an inaccurate means of measuring Hb A$_2$, and Hb A$_2$ levels are elevated in the presence of HbS when some HPLC hemoglobin separation kits are used.

CLINICAL ASPECTS OF HbA$_2$

Developmental Changes in HbA$_2$ Level

Little δ-globin chain synthesis occurs in utero so that HbA$_2$ does not become easily measurable until late in gestation. In normal newborns, HbA$_2$ concentration is 0.27 ±0.02 percent (Felicetti, 1984). HbA$_2$ levels vary with gestational age and are lowest in the least mature infants (Neumeyer and Betke, 1987). HbA$_2$ levels do not rise synchronously with HbA, but lag behind; the HbA/HbA$_2$ ratio is about 100 by 32 weeks' gestation and 75 by 45 weeks' gestation (Felicetti et al., 1984). "Adult" HbA/HbA$_2$ ratios of about 40:1 are not reached until at least age 6 months. This sluggish response of HbA$_2$ during maturation may reduce its value for the diagnosis of β-thalassemia in young infants (Serjeant, 1978). In the presence of an α-globin variant, such as HbG^{Philadelphia}, the variant α chain combines with the δ chain to form a hemoglobin tetramer with the structure, $\alpha^{Variant}_2\delta_2$ (Huehns, and Shooter, 1961). This tetramer—often called HbG$_2$—usually accounts for less than half the total amount of HbA$_2$. HbG$_2$ is more positively charged than HbA$_2$ because of the positive charge of the α^G chain and is easily separated from HbA$_2$. Extra HbA$_2$ bands are a valuable clue to the presence of variant α-globin chains, although, depending on the charge of the α-globin variant, they may, or may not, separate from the major hemoglobin bands.

Low HbA$_2$ Levels

Low HbA$_2$ values are usually the result of either posttranslational modifications in the assembly of the HbA$_2$ tetramer or reduced synthesis of the δ-globin chain secondary to δ thalassemia. (Table 10.3). Posttranslational causes of reduced HbA$_2$ can result from either acquired or genetic disorders. In either case, the underlying cause of the low HbA$_2$ level is insufficient synthesis of α-globin chains.

Posttranslational Causes of Reduced HbA$_2$. Assembly of hemoglobin tetramers depends on charge differences of the globin chains that form α:non-α

Table 10.3. Low HbA$_2$ Levels

Iron deficiency	Lowest with increasing severity
G-6-PD deficiency	Reports are conflicting; levels probably not reduced (Al-Jawadi, and Al-Hilali 1998)
α thalassemia	Lowest with increasing severity
Myelody splastic syndromes	Only in a minority of cases
Hb Lepore	Half normal in heterozygotes
Gene deletion hereditary persistence of HbF	Half normal in heterozygotes
δβ thalassemia	Half normal in heterozygotes
δ thalassemia	Usually about half of normal
HbA$_2$ variants	Variant may be poorly expressed
Sideroblastic anemia	Due to impaired α-globin synthesis
Juvenile CGL with increased HbF	Only in a minority of cases
Acute myelocytic leukemia	Minor reduction
α-globin gene variants	Hybrid HbA$_2$ may not separate

dimers (for a detailed discussion of hemoglobin assembly, see Chapter 8). Normal α- and β-globin monomers have nearly equivalent positive and negative charges, respectively, and are united by electrostatic attraction. δ-Globin chains are more positively charged than the β-globin chains (or γ-globin chains). Under normal conditions of α-chain sufficiency or slight excess, HbA is formed in preference to HbA$_2$, because αβ dimers assemble more readily than αδ dimers. When the supply of α-globin chain is limited, this effect of monomer charge on dimer formation is exaggerated, as β chains (and γ chains) compete more effectively than δ chains for scarce α globin (Bunn, and McDonald 1983; Bunn, and Forget, 1986; Bunn, 1987; McDonald, et al., 1984).

Acquired conditions that reduce α-globin chain synthesis appear to work through the common mechanism of absolute or functional iron deficiency. Lacking sufficient iron, a repressor of initiation of protein synthesis is formed (Ochoa, 1983). This preferentially affects α-, rather than non-α-globin chain initiation, resulting in a relative deficiency of α chains. Patients with iron deficiency anemia have reduced levels of HbA$_2$. This reduction is greatest in individuals with the most severe iron deficiency (Rai et al., 1987; Wasi et al., 1968; Harthoorn-Lasthuizen et al., 1999). Individuals with anemia, microcytosis, and low levels of HbA$_2$ from iron deficiency might be mistaken for

carriers of some forms of α thalassemia. When iron deficiency and β thalassemia coexist, the HbA$_2$ level has been reported to fall occasionally, although it may remain within the range expected for thalassemia heterozygotes (Galanello et al., 1981). The iron utilization defect associated with sideroblastic anemias may also reduce HbA$_2$ levels (White, 1971).

In the α-thalassemia/myelodysplasia syndrome (Chapter 18), inhibition of α-globin chain synthesis is associated with low HbA$_2$ levels. With acute myeloid leukemia, HbA$_2$ is lower than in acute lymphocytic leukemias (Feuilhade et al., 1981), suggesting that the leukemic clone involves the erythroid lineage. Patients with juvenile chronic granulocytic leukemia may have a hemoglobin pattern similar to fetal erythropoiesis. Fetal hemoglobin levels may soar (see previous discussion), accompanied by low HbA$_2$ values, recapitulating normal neonatal findings and the reciprocity of γ- and δ-globin gene expression (Dover et al., 1977; Sheridan, et al., 1976; Weatherall et al., 1968). Erythroleukemia has also been associated with very low levels of HbA$_2$ without HbH (Markham et al., 1983). These acquired "α thalassemias" bridge the gap between reduced HbA$_2$ secondary to acquired diseases and low HbA$_2$ associated with genetic abnormalities of α-globin synthesis.

α Thalassemia is the common cause of a genetically determined reduction in HbA$_2$ level owing to posttranslational mechanisms. HbA$_2$ concentration varies commensurately with the deficit in α-globin chain synthesis (Weatherall and Clegg, 1981). With the mildest types of α thalassemia, HbA$_2$ values may be indistinguishable from normal. When α-globin production is impaired significantly, the reduction in HbA$_2$ is dramatic. In 21 patients with HbH disease, the HbA$_2$ ranged from 0.5 to 1.8 percent and averaged 0.8 percent (Kutlar et al., 1989). Homotetramers of δ chains have been reported in α thalassemia hydrops fetalis.

Reduced Biosynthesis of δ-Globin Chains—the δ Thalassemias. Thalassemia-inducing mutations may affect the δ-globin gene and can cause reduction of HbA$_2$ levels or even absence of HbA$_2$ (Table 10.4). Early descriptions of δ thalassemia were based on hematologic and family studies and are often unreliable. δ Thalassemias have been reported most often in Japanese, Italian, and Greek populations. Whether this represents their true distribution is not known, as extensive surveys for these barely detectable conditions have not been done. In Italians, and potentially in other ethnic groups where β thalassemia is common, the coexistence of δ thalassemia and β thalassemia may cause the HbA$_2$ to be normal and complicate β thalassemia screening programs (Chapter 36) (Loudianos

Table 10.4. Causes of Increased HbA₂ Levels

Proven cases	Doubtful cases
β Thalassemia	Malaria
Sickle cell anemia-α thalassemia	Sickle cell trait
	Sickle cell anemia
Megaloblastic anemia	Hereditary spherocytosis
Unstable hemoglobinopathies	4–6%, rarely up to 12%, microcytosis
Zidovudine-treated HIV patients	4–5%, microcytosis, ~ HbS-β thalassemia
CDA, type I	Modest increases
Hyperthyroidism	Not uniformly found
Normal individuals	HbA₂ lower than in β thalassemia, macrocytosis
	HbA₂ lower than in β thalassemia, macrocytosis
	HbA₂ lower than in β thalassemia
	Rare, normal RBC indices, no thalassemia

CDA, congenital dyerythropoietic anemia; RBC, red blood cells.

et al., 1990; Weatherall and Clegg, 1981). In Greece, about 5 percent of individuals with β thalassemia may have borderline or normal HbA₂ concentrations. Most of these cases also have δ thalassemia owing to point mutations or the 7.2 kb Corfu deletion (Loudianos et al., 1990). Interactions between α thalassemia and β thalassemia may also result in normal HbA₂ values. β Thalassemia may escape detection if the sole basis of diagnosis is the level of HbA₂.

Uncomplicated δ thalassemia has no clinical repercussions. In δ⁺ thalassemia, both heterozygotes and homozygotes have reduced HbA₂ levels. When the δ-gene is totally inactivated (δ⁰ thalassemia), the heterozygote has half normal HbA₂ levels, and HbA₂ is absent in the homozygote (Fessas and Stametoyannopoulos, 1962). Seventeen δ thalassemia mutations have been reported (the Globin Gene Server; http://globin.cse.psu.edu). They include mutations that reduce or abolish gene transcription, RNA processing mutants, nonsense mutations, frameshifts, and unstable hemoglobin variants. Some cases have been the subject of expression studies to define precisely the mechanisms of thalassemia (Trifillis et al., 1996). A mutation at codon δ27 (GCC→TCC; **HbA₂-Yialousa**) that causes an mRNA splicing defect was also found in *cis* to the β39 nonsense mutation (Oggiano et al., 1994). This mutation has a frequency of 1.2 percent in Sardinians, and when it coexists with β thalassemia, a normal level of HbA₂ is found (Guiso et al., 1996).

A single δ-globin gene deletion has been reported. This 7.2 kb deletion (Corfu) removed most of the δ-globin gene and stopped just 3′ to the ψβ-gene. Although the initial molecular characterization of this deletion suggested that it inactivated the β-globin gene, subsequent studies revealed a β⁺ thalassemia mutation that was responsible for the reduced expression of the β-globin gene in *cis* to this deletion (Galanello et al., 1990; Kulozik et al., 1988). Some instances of low HbA₂ concentrations associated with unstable δ-globin gene variants and classified as δ thalassemias are more logically examples of δ-globin hemoglobinopathies.

When δ-globin gene expression is abolished because of large DNA deletions that remove the β-, and at times the γ-globin genes besides the δ-globin gene, HbA₂ levels are reduced. However, the phenotype is a consequence of impaired β- or γ-globin gene expression (Chapter 12). Heterozygotes for δβ thalassemia, Hb Lepore, and gene deletion hereditary persistence of fetal hemoglobin (HPFH) have half-normal HbA₂ levels; homozygotes have no HbA₂. Although the percentage of HbA₂ may be low when δ-globin gene expression is abolished, the absolute level, expressed as pg HbA₂ per cell, is elevated, reflecting increased synthesis of HbA₂ from the chromosome in *trans* to the gene deletion.

High HbA₂

Heterozygous β thalassemia is the cause of at least 95 percent of the cases of high HbA₂ levels (Table 10.5). Only a few of the point mutations causing β thalassemia are not associated with a raised HbA₂ level. "Normal" or borderline HbA₂ thalassemias have multiple causes including triplicated α-globin loci, β thalassemia with α-globin gene deletion, and δ plus β thalassemia, usually in *trans* but rarely in *cis* (Oggiano et al., 1994). Mean HbA₂ levels in 879 carriers of β thalassemia of diverse ethnic backgrounds were 5.08 ± 0.39 percent (Steinberg et al., 1982). The highest observed value was 6.8 percent. In 184 black patients with β thalassemia trait, the mean HbA₂ level was 4.97 ± 1.07 percent (Steinberg et al., 1982). With the few exceptions mentioned previously, an elevated level of HbA₂, in the presence of microcytic erythrocytes, identifies patients with heterozygous β thalassemia. HbA₂ levels may be higher in heterozygous β⁰ thalassemia and severe β⁺ thalassemia than in mild β⁺ thalassemia because of the greater impairment of β-globin chain synthesis in β⁰ thalassemia (Huisman, 1997; Weatherall and Clegg, 1981; Codrington et al., 1990; Gonzalez-Redondo et al., 1989b; Jankovic et al., 1990; Kutlar and Kutlar, 1990). Average levels of HbA₂ in heterozygotes for 32 different β alleles are

Table 10.5. Mutations Causing δ Thalassemia

Type	Mutation	Substitution	Ethnic group
Transcriptional mutants			
δ°	−77	−	Japanese
δ°	−65	−	Greeks, Cypriots
δ+	−55	−	Greeks, Cypriots
δ+	−36	−	Greeks
RNA processing mutations, splice junction			
δ°	Codon 30 G→C	Arg→Thr	Italians
δ°	IVS I nt 2 T→C	−	Italians
δ°	IVS II nt 897 A→G	−	Greeks, Cypriots
δ+	Codon 11 T→G	Val→Gly	Greeks
δ+	Codon 85 T→C	Phe→Ser	Greeks
δ+	Codon 98 G→A	Val→Met	Blacks
δ+	Codon 116 C→T	Arg→Cys	Greeks, Cypriots
δ+	Codon 141 T→C	Leu→Pro	Greeks, Cypriots
RNA translation mutants			
δ°	Codon 37 G→A	Stop	Sardinians
δ°	Codon 59 −A	Frameshift	Egyptians
δ°	Codon 91 +T	Frameshift	Belgians
Activation of cryptic splicing site			
δ+	Codon 27 G→T	Ala→Ser	Sardinians, Greeks
RNA cleavage and polyadenylation			
?	PolyA +69nts G→A	−	Sardinians
Deletion			
δ°	Corfù, −7.2 Kb	−	Italians; Greeks

From Huisman T, and Carver, 1998.

shown in Figure 10.10 (Huisman, 1997). In mild β-thalassemia mutations, a nominal suppression of β-chain synthesis and minor excess of α-globin chains may lead to less αδ-dimer formation. However, it has been proposed that point mutations in the β-globin gene promoter may alter binding of transcription factors and augment δ-globin gene transcription in *cis* to the mutation (Weatherall and Clegg, 1981). In one patient with the −88 C→T β+thalassemia and HbA2′ in *trans*, the total HbA2 level was about 7 percent; ten heterozygotes with this mutation had HbA2 levels of 5.4 ± 0.4 percent (4.5 to 6.6 percent). In another study, the average HbA2 was 4.9 percent (4.1 to 5.2 percent) in six heterozygotes with this mutation (Steinberg, 1993).

Because of the striking increases of HbF that typify the severe β thalassemias, HbA2 levels in homozygous β thalassemia are variable and of little diagnostic value. However, the level of HbA2 in homozygotes for the promoter mutations −88C→T and −29 A →G averaged 6.6 percent (4.0–9.7 percent) (Huisman, 1997). Transcription of the δ-globin gene appears to vary reciprocally with that of the γ-globin gene. This reciprocity is evident as HbF levels fall rapidly during the last trimester of gestation and

is also observed in the β-thalassemia syndromes (Weatherall and Clegg, 1981). In homozygous β thalassemia, cells with the highest HbF levels have the lowest HbA2 concentrations (Loukopoulos and Fessas, 1965). One dramatic example of the relationship between HbA2 and HbF was seen when chemotherapy for Hodgkin's disease appeared to reactivate HbF synthesis in a patient with β-thalassemia trait and the Swiss type HPFH. HbF level rose from 4.5 to 26 percent, accompanied by a fall in HbA2 from 4.5 to 2.4 percent (Cech et al., 1982). The mechanism of this effect has not been studied but may be a result of gene order on the chromosome and competition for the LCR and transcription factors (Chapter 15).

Increased HbA2 in heterozygous β thalassemia appears to result from both transcriptional and posttranslational effects (Codrington et al., 1990). There is an increase in both the percentage and absolute amount of HbA2 present, with the former about twice as great as the latter. Reduced production of β-globin chains, with a relative excess of α-globin chains, favors the formation of αδ dimers and the assembly of HbA2 tetramers. If part of the cause of elevated HbA2 was due to posttranslational perturbation, the product of each δ-globin gene should contribute equally to this rise; that is, the effect should be present both *cis* and *trans* to the β-thalassemia gene. This has been shown directly in the study of families where a structural variant of the δ-globin chain segregates independently from the β-thalassemia-causing mutation (Codrington et al., 1990; Horton et al., 1961; Lee and Huisman, 1963). Increased δ-globin gene transcription, because of a β-thalassemia-causing mutation, might be expected to occur only in *cis*. The mechanism for the "compensatory" increase in δ-globin chain synthesis is not totally clear but may result from a competition among the β globin-like gene promoters for transcription factors (Codrington et al., 1990).

Recently, 40 individuals with normal MCV and mean cell hemoglobin (MCH) and borderline HbA2 levels between 3 and 3.5 percent were examined to see if δ-globin gene nucleotide sequence changes were present that might account for these hemato-

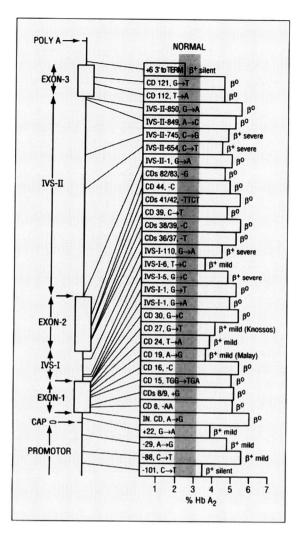

Figure 10.10. HbA$_2$ concentrations according to the β-thalassemia mutation in more than 600 patients (Huisman, 1997).

logic findings (Papapanagiotuo et al., 1998). Four individuals had an A→G substitution at position −65 5′ to the cap site of the δ-globin gene within the normal CCAAC sequence that was now altered to CCAGC. A similar substitution was not found in 200 normal or 100 δ-thalassemia chromosomes. Transient expression studies of the mutated and a wild type δ-globin gene promoter showed that the variant promoter had a twofold increase in expression in K562 and MEL cells, results similar to those observed upon restoration of the CCAAT sequence in the δ-globin gene promoter (see the previous discussion). This work further supports the importance of an enfeebled δ-globin/gene promoter as an explanation of the naturally low levels of HbA$_2$ and provides one explanation for elevated levels of HbA$_2$ without β thalassemia.

Exceptionally High HbA$_2$

Some individuals with β-thalassemia trait have HbA$_2$ concentrations much higher than usual. These exceptionally high HbA$_2$ levels are usually the result of a unique and informative class of small deletions of DNA that usually begin within the β-globin gene and extend 5′, removing the gene promoter (Steinberg and Adams 1991) (Chapter 11). Removing the β-globin gene promoter sequences by the 5′ deletion may increase the likelihood that transcription factors bind the remaining δ- and γ-globin gene promoters, enhancing the transcription of these genes. Alternatively, deletion-induced disruption of higher-order DNA or chromatin structure may make γ- and δ-globin promoters more accessible to the LCR. The absence of a functional β promoter might permit the LCR to interact with the δ-globin gene in *cis*, enhancing its expression. One 3.4 kb deletion had its 5′ terminus between nucleotides −810 and −128 while the 3′ breakpoint was between the Ava II and Xmn I sites 3′ to the β-globin gene so that the β-gene promoter and the 3′ enhancer were lost. In the single heterozygote for this deletion who was examined, the HbA$_2$ level was 6.7 percent. Perhaps the loss of the 3′ enhancer element modulated the rise of HbA$_2$ expected from the removal of the promoter (Sanguansermsri et al., 1990). One deletion of 44 base pairs began in codon 24 or between codons 24 and 25 and extended 26 or 27 bases into IVS-1 (Gonzalez-Redondo et al., 1989a). As the β-gene promoter is left intact, the level of HbA$_2$ should be similar to that seen in the bulk of β thalassemias. Unfortunately, no information is available regarding HbA$_2$ levels in heterozygotes for this deletion. In a Thai family with β⁰ thalassemia caused by a 105 base pair deletion of the 5′ β-globin gene, the deletion began at positions −24 or −25 from the β-globin gene mRNA capping site and extended to position +80 or +81. HbA$_2$ levels were 5.6 and 6.3 percent, levels higher than the average 5.1 percent these investigators found in individuals with point mutations causing β thalassemia. The CACCC, CCAAT, and TATA elements of the β-globin gene promoter remain intact in this deletion, suggesting that the region 3′ to the canonical promoter may influence the interactions of the transcriptional apparatus with the β-globin gene (Nopparatana et al., 1999).

HbA$_2$ levels in heterozygotes for these 5′ β-gene deletion thalassemias have been reported to range from about 7 to 12 percent. Bona fide HbA$_2$ levels that exceed the top of this range have not been reported. Laboratory reports of HbA$_2$ values more than 15 or 20 percent are usually spurious or represent instances of HbC or HbE heterozygosity complicated by α thalassemia or iron deficiency. Another theoretical possibility for exceptionally high levels of HbA$_2$ is the presence of a Miyada-type hemoglobin, where the point of crossing over leads to a globin chain structurally identical to δ globin, although such a gene has not yet been described (Schroeder et al., 1973a).

Miscellaneous Causes of High HbA$_2$

Patients with either sickle cell anemia α thalassemia or HbS-β^0 thalassemia have high HbA$_2$ concentrations (Chapter 28). In the former group of patients, the δ-globin chain competes more effectively than the β^S-globin chain for the limited quantities of α-globin chain.

HbA$_2$ levels may be consistently elevated in hyperthyroidism, although not as markedly as in β thalassemia. (Kendall and Bastomsky, 1981; Krishnamoorthy et al., 1982; Kuhn et al., 1983). Both the percentage and absolute amount of HbA$_2$ are increased, suggesting increased synthesis of the δ-globin chain and an effect of thyroid hormone on δ-globin gene transcription. (Krishnamoorthy et al., 1982). Euthyroidism after treatment is accompanied by a fall in HbA$_2$ and rise in MCV. (Kendall, and Bastomsky, 1981; Kuhn et al., 1983) In untreated, nonanemic, hypothyroidism, HbA$_2$ levels cluster toward the low end of normal (Kendall and Bastomsky, 1981). In hyperthyroidism, the combination of high HbA$_2$ and low MCV can be confused with β thalassemia.

Megaloblastic anemias have been associated with HbA$_2$ concentrations that exceed normal (Alperin et al., 1977; Henshaw et al., 1978). The most severely anemic patients have the highest HbA$_2$ values. (Alperin et al., 1977). However, the incidence of this finding seems low, the amount of the increase above normal is slight, and, in one study, the mean HbA$_2$ levels in the normal and megaloblastic anemia groups were similar (Henshaw et al., 1978). Perhaps the high HbA$_2$ of megaloblastic anemia is a result of more hemoglobin synthesis occurring in less mature erythroid precursors.

Seventy-eight patients infected with the human immunodeficiency (HIV) virus who were taking zidovudine had HbA$_2$ levels of 3.2 ± 0.5 percent compared with 2.7 ± 0.4 percent in HIV-positive control subjects not exposed to this drug (Routy et al., 1993). The MCV was higher in zidovudine-treated patients, but evidence of folic acid or vitamin B$_{12}$ deficiency was lacking. It was speculated that increased HbA$_2$ levels of the treated patients was secondary to drug-induced megaloblastic erythropoiesis.

In fourteen Israeli Bedouins with congenital dyserythropoietic anemia, type I, the mean HbA$_2$ was 3.5 ± 0.5 percent and was between 3.8 and 5.1 percent in four patients (Tamary et al., 1996). MCV was 98 ± 5 fl, but biosynthesis studies showed a deficit of β-globin chain synthesis with a mean α/β synthesis ratio of 1.27, suggesting β thalassemia trait. However, the sequence of the β-globin gene in four individuals was normal.

HbA$_2$ levels may be raised in some examples of unstable hemoglobin (Bradley and Ranney, 1973). An unstable β-globin chain may have difficulty forming αβ dimers increasing αδ dimer assembly.

Four individuals from two Sardinian families had HbA$_2$ levels from 3.9 to 4.2 percent. They had no hematologic abnormalities, balanced globin biosynthesis, and normal α-, β-, and δ-globin gene structures. (Tang, et al., 1992). The authors posited a *trans*-acting effector as a possible explanation for this dominantly transmitted finding.

Malaria infection and elevated HbA$_2$ levels have been linked in some reports (Lie-Injo et al., 1971; Wasi et al., 1971) but not others (Van Ros et al., 1978). The best controlled study casts doubt on such an association (Van Ros et al., 1978). An association of hereditary spherocytosis and very high HbA$_2$ levels has also not been proven (Harmeling and Moguin, 1967).

POSTTRANSLATIONAL MODIFICATION OF NORMAL ADULT, FETAL, AND EMBRYONIC HEMOGLOBINS: THE "MINOR" HEMOGLOBINS

So-called "minor" components of normal hemoglobins are the result of posttranslational hemoglobin modification—usually nonenzymatic glycation (glycosylation), acetylation, or acetaldehyde adduct formation. When associated with HbA they are termed HbA1a1, A1a2, A1b, A1c, and A1d (and its subtypes, A1d1,2, and 3). HbS, HbF, HbC, and other variant hemoglobins also have minor components. These minor hemoglobins are modified by their reactions with glucose, G-6-P, fructose-1, 6-diphosphate, oxidized glutathione, acetaldehyde, and acetate. Separation of minor hemoglobins in neonates and in patients with sickle cell anemia, HbSC disease, HbC disease, and sickle cell trait by HPLC is shown in Figure 10.11. HbA1c is the best studied minor hemoglobin, and its clinical importance dwarfs that of other minor components whose major clinical significance is the confusion and uncertainty they cause in the interpretation of isoelectric focusing gel patterns, HPLC columns, and hemoglobin electrophoresis. Although the full impact of glycated hemoglobin in diabetology is outside the purview of this chapter, we will describe some functional properties of HbA1c and provide a brief description of other minor normal hemoglobin components. In individuals heterozygous for HbS or HbC who have increased concentrations of HbA1c (6 to 9 percent), some methods of quantitation overestimate HbA1c levels (Roberts et al., 1999).

Minor hemoglobins can vary in quantity according to whether diseases such as diabetes or uremia are present and if an individual is exposed to external agents

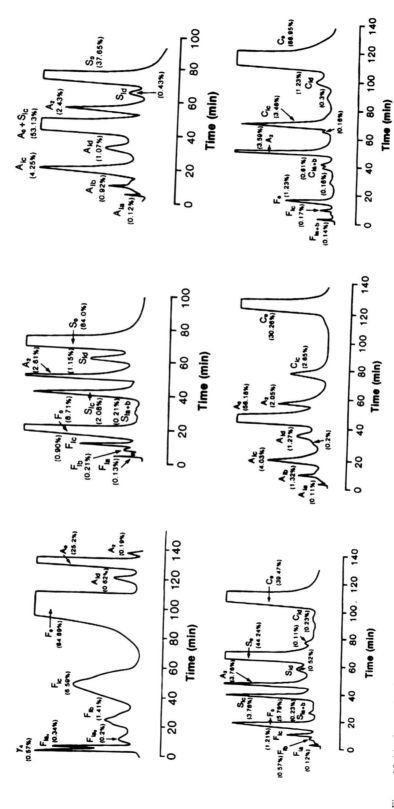

Figure 10.11. Separation by HPLC of the minor hemoglobins from neonates (top left), adults with sickle cell anemia (top center), adults with sickle cell trait (top right), HbSC disease (bottom left), HbC trait (bottom center), and HbC disease (bottom right). (Modified from Abraham et al., 1984) These examples illustrate the complexity of patterns caused by the presence of minor hemoglobins on HPLC separation (and by isoelectric focusing) and the difficulty of knowing, without DNA analysis or protein sequencing, whether one of these minor peaks represents or contains a genetically encoded hemoglobin variant that may be present in trace amounts (Chapters 13 and 17).

217

like penicillin and aspirin. Minor components of normal hemoglobin have been suggested to be "reporters" of physiologic and pathophysiologic events (Bunn, 1984; Bunn and Forget, 1986). One report showed that HbA1c levels in patients with AIDS and with normal glucose concentrations may be increased when compared with normal control subjects (9.1 ± 0.5 vs. 7.4 ± 0.2 percent; $P<.01$); however, a mechanism for this observation is not obvious (Kabadi et al., 1992). An inverse relationship existed between glycohemoglobin concentrations and the CD4 cell count, and AIDS patients with the most advanced disease and lowest CD4 counts had glycohemoglobin levels of about 8 percent (Kabadi and Hood, 1998).

Glycated Hemoglobins

In the mid-1960s, Dr. Samuel Rahbar made a fundamental observation: patients with diabetes often had an extra hemoglobin band visible when their hemoglobin was separated by cellulose acetate electrophoresis. At the time, Bookchin and Gallop (1968), trying to define the structure of HbA1c, had concluded that A1c, one of the many minor components of the hemolysate that Schroeder and Jones (1965) had identified by column chromatography, contained a hexose, establishing that this hemoglobin was a glycated minor component of normal hemoglobin. A connection between HbA1c and the "diabetic band" was made, and the hemolysates of diabetics were found to contain an increase of HbA1c. Cerami's laboratory at Rockefeller University and Bunn's group chemically characterized HbA1c simultaneously and described its implications for the pathophysiology and clinical management of diabetes (see later).

As discussed by Bunn (Bunn, 1981; Bunn and McDonald, 1983; Bunn, 1984; Bunn and Forget, 1986), HbA1c is a result of posttranslational and nonenzymatic glycation of HbA. The most abundant minor hemoglobin component in human red cells,

HbA1c is formed by the rapid nonenzymatic condensation of glucose with the N-terminus of the β-globin chain to form a Schiff base that undergoes a slow Amadori rearrangement to a stable ketoamine linkage (Fig. 10.12). This adduct is increased in patients with diabetes mellitus, and its measurement is a useful index of diabetic glycemic control. Glucose also forms covalent attachments with the ϵ-amino groups of lysine residues of both the α- and the β-globin chain, although these adducts are not readily resolved by electrophoretic and chromatographic techniques. Nonenzymatic glycation also occurs in proteins with long turnover times exposed to high glucose concentrations. Examples are proteins of the red cell membrane, albumin, and lens crystallins. This phenomenon is important in the pathogenesis of diabetes. Nonenzymatic glycation of other tissue proteins (lens crystallin, glomerular proteins, endothelial cell proteins) with the generation of advanced glycation end products (AGEs) may contribute significantly to the long-term complications of diabetes (Bucala and Cerami, 1992). AGEs form spontaneously from glucose-derived Amadori products and accumulate on long-lived tissue proteins—hemoglobin is but one example. They have been implicated in the pathogenesis of aging and diabetes. Using recently developed AGE-specific antibodies, an AGE-modified form of human hemoglobin has been identified (Makita et al., 1992). Hemoglobin-AGE (Hb-AGE) accounts for 0.42 percent of circulating hemoglobin in normal individuals but increases to 0.75 percent in patients with diabetes-induced hyperglycemia. Hemoglobin-AGE measurements may provide an index of long-term tissue modification by AGEs and prove useful in assessing the contribution of advanced glycosylation to a variety of diabetic and age-related complications.

Figure 10.12. Mechanism of HbA1c formation.

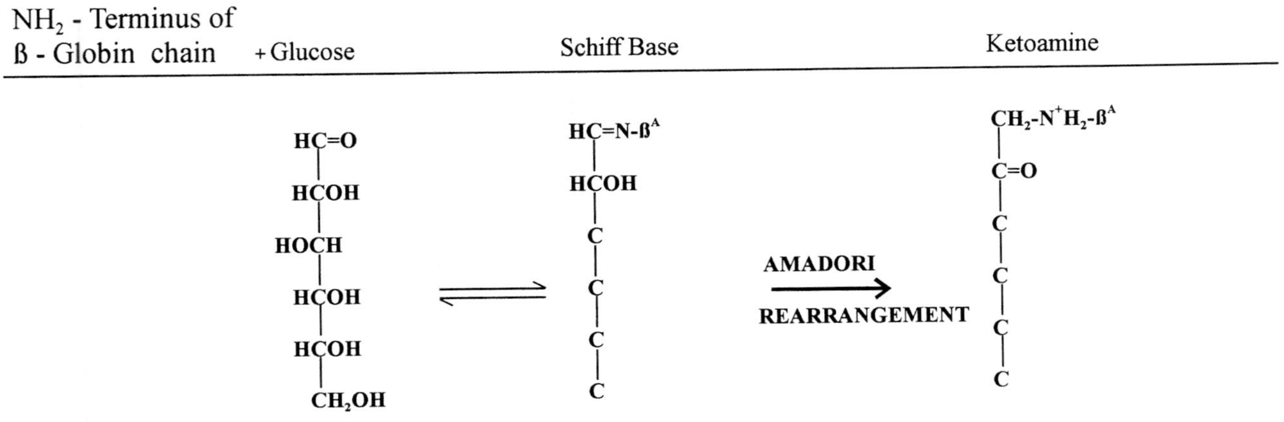

Glycohemoglobin levels can be measured by ion-exchange column chromatography on Bio-Rex 70, affinity chromatography, HPLC, by electrophoresis, and colorimetrically (Goldstein and Little, 1997). Electrospray ionization mass spectrometry to detect the extent of glycation of samples separated by boronate affinity and cation exchange chromatography has provided new insights on modified globin (Peterson et al., 1998). Analyses of clinical samples were consistent with the curvilinear relationship of patient glucose and HbA1c. As glycation increased, the ratio of β- to α-globin chain glycation increased, and the number of glycated sites on the β chain increased, although these were minor components. Several glycated species co-chromatographed with HbA1c on cation exchange chromatography, including species with both glycated α- and β-globin chains, nonglycated α- and glycated β-globin chains, and multiply glycated β-globin chains.

After centrifugation in isopycnic concentrations of dextran to separate the 10 percent youngest and 10 percent oldest erythrocytes of normal and diabetic subjects, the minor hemoglobin components, Hb A1a+b (see later) and HbA1c, were measured (Fitzgibbons et al., 1976). Both normal and diabetic erythrocytes contained increased amounts of Hb A1a+b and Hb A1c in old, compared with young cells, and diabetics had higher levels of all minor components. These results showed that both cell age and diabetes are significant determinants of the amounts of Hbs A1a+b and A1c.

What are the functional properties of HbA1c? Without allosteric effectors, the P-50 of HbA and of HbA1c is similar. HbA1c, because of its blocked N-terminal, has reduced interaction with 2,3 BPG decreasing its P-50. The low-affinity conformation (or T state) of HbA1c is destabilized by the chemical modification per se, and the Bohr effect is reduced compared with nonglycated HbA. The affinity of the T state of HbA1c for 2,3 BPG is about 2.6 times lower than that of the corresponding conformational state of HbA, and the R state is less affected with an affinity of 1.7 times lower (De Rosa et al., 1998). The oxygen affinity of blood of diabetic patients is increased nearly 2 mm Hg but this is not likely to be clinically significant (Bunn and Forget, 1986).

At the structural level, computer modeling studies by De Rosa et al. (1998) show that the two sugar moieties are asymmetrically disposed within the 2,3 BPG binding site. Calculations concerning the interaction with 2,3 BPG show that while in HbA the effector can assume two different stable orientations, in glycated hemoglobin only one orientation is possible. Together, these results show that glycation of the Val 1 residues of both β-globin chains do not impair the binding of 2, 3 BPG but imposes a different mode of binding by changing the internal geometry of the complex and the surface distribution of the positive electrostatic potential within the binding pocket.

Minor hemoglobin components of both HbA and HbF were detected more than 40 years ago (Allen et al., 1958). Garrick et al. (1980) separated the α- and β-globin chains from purified HbA1a1, HbA1a2, and HbA1b by ion-exchange chromatography. The β-globin chains were reducible by sodium borohydride and gave a positive thiobarbituric acid test, suggesting that these components were modified by ketoamine-linked carbohydrate. In addition, phosphate analysis revealed 1.5 phosphate residues associated with each β A1a1 chain and one phosphate residue with each β A1a2 chain. HbA1a1, HbA1a2, and HbA1b were all contaminated by nonglobin proteins. Protein-sequencing showed that the N-termini of β A1a1, β A1a2, and β A1b1 were blocked. In support of this conclusion, analysis of tryptic digests of β A1a2 and A1b2 revealed modified N-terminal peptides, leading the authors to conclude that, like Hb A1c, components HbA1a1, HbA1a2, and HbA1b also contain a sugar moiety linked to the N-terminus of the β-globin chain.

Bio-Rex 70 chromatography in normal and diabetic subjects detects the following minor hemoglobins: A1a1, A1a2, A1b1, A1b2, A1b3, A1c, A1d1, A1d2, and A1d3 (Abraham et al., 1983). Based on colorimetric assay, protein-bound ketoamine was present in all the minor hemoglobins, which was confirmed by chromatographic separation of hemoglobins after reduction with NaB_3H_4. All the minor hemoglobins, except HbA1a1, Hba2, and HbA1b1, were increased twofold in diabetics. HbA1c, whose levels were about 5.0 percent of total hemoglobin in normal subjects and about 9 percent in diabetic patients, and HbA1d3, measuring about 1.9 percent in normal subjects and about 3.2 percent in diabetic patients, were present in the largest amounts. HbA1d3 showed a decrease in oxygen affinity in the presence of 2,3 BPG, whereas HbA1c showed no effect. Separation of globin chains by cellulose acetate electrophoresis at pH 8.6 showed that the cathodal mobility of the α-globin chains of HbA1d3 was slower than those of HbA. Glycation of hemoglobin with [^{14}C]glucose, followed by separation of hemoglobins by two Bio-Rex 70 chromatographic methods, indicated that the minor hemoglobin formed by glycation of the α-globin chain amino-terminus was separable from HbA, whereas the minor hemoglobins formed by the glycation of ε-amino groups chromatographed with HbA.

Early studies with electron paramagnetic resonance (EPR) spectra of the glycated minor hemoglobins A1a1, A1a2, A1b, and A1c and HbA in the nitrosyl form have been obtained in the absence and presence of inositol hexaphosphate. Without inositol hexaphosphate, nitrosyl hemoglobins A1a1, A1a2, and A1b exhibited a triplet hyperfine structure shown to be diagnostic of the low affinity (T) quaternary structure. Addition of inositol hexaphosphate to nitrosyl HbsA, A1c, A1b, and A1a2 developed a triplet hyperfine structure of the EPR spectra; but the magnitude of the hyperfine was decreased in the order of HbA, A1c, A1b, and A1a2. However, inositol hexaphosphate did not affect the EPR spectrum of nitrosyl hemoglobin A1a1. These results accounted qualitatively for the oxygen-binding properties of these glycated minor hemoglobins in the framework of a two-state allosteric model.

Cord blood samples from women with preterm fetuses of gestational ages 30- to 36- weeks and from a control group of term fetuses of 40 weeks' gestational age were analyzed for total glycated hemoglobin and the percentages of the minor hemoglobins F1a+b and F1c (Elseweidy et al., 1984). The absolute levels and the increase due to red cell aging of glycohemoglobins F1a+b and Hb F1c were significantly reduced in the preterm samples compared with the term samples, suggesting decreased hemoglobin glycation in preterm fetus. The acetylated form of HbF1c also showed an increase with red cell aging, indicating posttranslational enzymatic or nonenzymatic acetylation of HbF during the entire life span of red cells. As with glycohemoglobins, the acetylated HbF was also decreased in the preterm newborns. Both erythrocyte age and the time of gestation influence hemoglobin glycation. Hb Bart's, the tetramer of γ-globin chains found in some α thalassemias also has minor components acetylated and glycated (Abraham et al., 1987).

The structure of HbA1b that forms less than 0.5 percent of total hemoglobin has more recently been established. By electrospray ionization of its abnormal β-globin chain, purified Hb A1b had a 70-Da mass increase. Separation of the tryptic digest by reversed-phase liquid chromatography revealed an abnormal β-T1 peptide. Cesium ion bombardment ionization produced a protonated molecular ion, showing an additional $C_3H_2O_2$ residue in normal β-T1. The amino acid sequences of both abnormal and normal β-T1 peptides were identical in terms of their collision activation spectra. Time course hydrolysis of abnormal β-T1 showed a rapid loss of the modifying group, leading to normal β-T1. Mild treatment with acidic methanol showed an additional methylated site compared with normal β-T1. All these results are consistent with a ketamine-linked pyruvic acid at the amino end of the β chain of HbA1b (Prome et al., 1991).

Hemoglobin variants also have glycated minor components, and those of HbS have been best studied. HbS1c and HbSo, a component formed by glycation of the ε-amino groups of lysine, made up 33 percent and 42 percent, respectively, of the total glycohemoglobin in individuals with sickle cell anemia, the remainder being glycated HbF and Hb A_2 (Abraham and Elseweidy, 1986). These modified HbS fractions had higher minimum gelling concentrations, suggesting that HbS polymerization was inhibited, perhaps because of interference with contact points in the polymer by glycated amino acid residues. Diabetics with sickle cell anemia had a twofold increase in glycohemoglobin, but this increase is less than the increase in HbA1c seen in diabetics without sickle cell anemia (Abraham and Rao, 1987). This may be due to very short-lived sickle cells. A direct relationship is found between HbF concentration and the level of glycated hemoglobin in patients with sickle cell anemia (Elseweidy and Abraham, 1984). This is most likely due to the longer life span of cells containing high concentrations of HbF that permits additional time for the slow process of nonenzymatic glycation.

Acetylated Hemoglobin

Hemoglobin acetylation, in contrast to glycation, is usually an enzymatically driven process although, at least in vitro, nonenzymatic acetylation has been reported (Garbutt and Abraham, 1981). A general discussion of hemoglobin and protein acetylation is provided in Chapter 45 where acetylated mutant hemoglobins are discussed. Acetylation is more common in proteins where the N-terminal amino acid is either alanine, serine, and, to a lesser extent, glycine. Hemoglobin requires an unblocked N-terminus to function normally, so that blocked N-terminal residues have been largely excluded by selection. A blocked N-terminal glycine in HbF contributes to its decreased 2,3 BPG binding. Acetylation occurs early in the posttranslational period and involves the acetyltransferase-mediated catalytic transfer of the acetyl moiety from acetyl-CoA to the hemoglobin. Acetylated HbF is called HbF_1. Whether or not there is any functional advantage or disadvantage of HbF_1 is unknown. Feline hemoglobin, where the $\beta1$ residue is serine, is also acetylated and binds 2,3 BPG poorly (Moo-Penn et al., 1977; Taketa et al., 1972).

Acetaldehyde Adducts

Acetaldehyde, a metabolic product of ethanol, forms nonenzymatically mediated adducts with hemoglobin, and about 15 to 25 percent of the adducts are stable to dialysis (Peterson and Nguyen, 1985). No current assay systems are available to detect acetaldehyde adducts in the blood of humans consuming alcohol. Acetaldehyde adducts separate chromatographically with HbA1a and HbA1b. The amount of stable hemoglobin adducts formed is proportional to the amount of acetaldehyde or to the number of intermittent pulses. Acetaldehyde adducts with hemoglobin involve primarily the β-globin chain and at least three different amino acid residues (valine, lysine, and tyrosine) and two modified residues (glucosyl-valine and glucosyl-lysine). The acetaldehyde possibly reacts with the ε-amino group of lysine and α-amino group of valine probably through an initial Schiff base. The secondary amines of glycated valine or glycated lysine residues are also proposed to be at the sites of reaction with acetaldehyde (Schwartz and Gray, 1977). Acetaldehyde adduct formation with tyrosine residues is not as well understood. Only part of the stable hemoglobin-acetaldehyde adducts that were stable after 24 hours of dialysis could be irreversibly fixed by sodium borohydride. This chemistry makes assay for acetaldehyde adducts difficult to develop.

Carbamylated Hemoglobin

Urea is in equilibrium with cyanate and when urea concentrations are high, as in uremia, irreversible covalent adducts of cyanate with the N-terminal amino groups of both α- and β-globin chains form (Bunn and Forget, 1986). Carbamylated hemoglobin levels of up to 4 percent have been found in individuals with untreated uremia but are unlikely to be functionally significant (Fluckiger et al., 1981). Carbamylation of HbS by either urea or cyanate was proposed as a possible treatment for sickle cell anemia about 30 years ago. Unfortunately, a cumbersome ex vivo treatment of blood was needed to modify HbS as in vivo administration of cyanate carbamylated lens proteins forming cataracts.

EMBRYONIC HEMOGLOBINS

In early development, between 4 and 14 weeks of gestation, the human embryo synthesizes three distinct hemoglobins in yolk sac-derived primitive nucleated erythroid cells: $\zeta_2\epsilon_2$ (**Hb Gower I**), $\zeta_2\gamma_2$ (**Hb Portland**), and $\alpha_2\epsilon_2$ (**Hb Gower II**) (Huehns et al., 1964a). ζ- and ε-Globin chains are expressed before the γ- and α-globin chain. By 14 days of development, after the establishment of the placenta, embryonic hemoglobins are replaced by HbF, but ζ- and ε-globin chains can be found in definitive fetal erythrocytes (Luo et al., 1999)(Chapter 2). At 15 to 22 weeks of gestation, 53 percent of fetal cells contained ζ-globin chains and 5 percent had ε-globin chains. At term, cord blood contained 34 percent ζ- and 0.6 percent ε-globin chain positive cells. Erythrocytes from normal adults did not contain embryonic globins.

Embryonic hemoglobins have been studied in erythroid cells of 35- to 56-day-old embryos (Stamato-yannopoulos et al., 1987). Analyses of globins synthesized in vivo and in cultures of erythroid burst-forming units showed that cells of the yolk sac, where primitive erythropoiesis occurs, and cells of the liver, a site of definitive erythropoiesis, produce embryonic, fetal, and adult globins. Similar results have been found with the expression of the adult α-globin gene and the corresponding embryonic α-like chains (ζ-globin gene) coexpressed in the earliest murine erythrocyte progenitors (Leder et al., 1992). From these studies and the recent finding of embryonic hemoglobin in cord blood, it appears that embryonic globin is expressed in both primitive and definitive erythroblasts, although in vastly different quantities. These results are compatible with the postulate that the switch from embryonic to fetal globin synthesis represents a time-dependent change in programs of progenitor cells rather than a change in hemopoietic cell lineages.

Hoffman et al. (1995a) have analyzed embryonic hemoglobins obtained from an in vitro expression system. They found that, lacking any effector of hemoglobin function, including Cl⁻, they all have oxygen affinities and ligand binding rates similar to HbA. In the presence of organic phosphates, the oxygen affinities of $\zeta_2\epsilon_2$ and $\alpha_2\epsilon_2$ are lowered for Gower II to a lesser extent than normal HbA. This showed that the ζ- and ε-globin chains do bind 2,3 BPG. Nevertheless, differences compared with HbA binding of this effector do exist and require explanation (see later). Hb Portland not surprisingly, since its central cavity is formed by γ-globin chains, does not bind organic phosphates well.

The rates of oxygen dissociation from the embryonic hemoglobins have been measured by Hoffmann and Brittain (1996) and seem responsible for the high oxygen-binding affinity associated with the embryonic proteins compared with the adult protein. The pH dependence of the oxygen dissociation rate constants also accounts for the unusual, previously described, Bohr effects characteristic of embryonic hemoglobins.

Bonaventura et al. (1994), were the first to realize that reducing the destabilizing effect of an excess of positive charges in the central cavity by Cl-binding to preserve the physiologic oxygen affinity of hemoglobin is indispensable. Perutz et al. (1993) proposed that Cl⁻binding in embryonic hemoglobins differed from that of HbA. The chloride interactions with embryonic hemoglobins are particularly interesting (Hoffmann et al., 1995b). Hb Portland is completely insensitive to Cl⁻, and Hb Gower I has a small effect and Hb Gower II a chloride effect approaching that of HbA. Chloride binding and the Bohr effect of these hemoglobins follow the allosteric model proposed by Perutz et al. (1993).

For $\alpha_2\epsilon_2$ (Hb Gower II), crystallographic data on the CO form are available (Sutherland-Smith et al., 1998). Compared with HbA and HbF, the tertiary structure of the α-globin chain is unchanged. The ε-globin chain has a structure similar to the β-globin chain with small differences in the N-terminus and A helix. The Cl⁻ binding sites involve the polar residues withing the central cavities (anionic α94, α126 and β101 and the cationic α1, α99, α103, β1, β2, β82, β104 and β143). Of these residues, only β104 Arg is changed to a Lys in the ε-globin chain. This ε-globin Lys residue might be involved in an ionic interaction with ε101 Glu, but whether the pK of Lys is low enough to be un-ionized in physiologic conditions and whether this sequence change can explain the decrease in Cl⁻ binding are uncertain. Other candidate residues that may influence Cl⁻ binding are the sequence changes β77His→ε77Asn, β116 His→ε116Thr, and β125 Pro→ε125 Gly. A better understanding of the consequence of these changes requires knowledge of the T-crystal structure of Hb Gower II. It is possible that the decrease of the Cl⁻ effect is the sum of small aggregated changes and not the result of a single amino acid substitution.

The most distinct change in Hb Gower II compared with HbA is a shift of the N-terminus and the A helix, similar to that seen in HbF. The α helix moves into the central cavity because of a complex disruption of the N-terminal region owing to the sequence changes at β3Leu→ε3Phe, β78Leu→ε78Met, β5Pro→ε5 Ala, β130Tyr→ε130Trp. To definitively establish the mechanism of the decrease in 2,3 BPG binding, it is necessary to know the T-crystal structure of Gower II, which is not yet available, but the A helix shift remains a likely candidate.

The embryonic ε-globin chain has a lysine residue at position 87 compared with a threonine residue in the β-globin chain. Is there a microconformational change at this site? Any change would have to be only solution-active, because crystallography does not support this interpretation.

Hoffmann et al. (1997) have studied the effect of CO_2, adenosine triphosphate (ATP), and lactate ions on the oxygen affinity of the three human embryonic hemoglobins. CO_2 and ATP lower the affinity of both the adult and embryonic hemoglobins for oxygen. Lactate ions do not affect the oxygen equilibrium process over the concentration range studied. The three embryonic hemoglobins have reduced values of CO binding compared with previously reported mammalian fetal or adult hemoglobin (Hoffmann and Brittain, 1998). It is possible that this feature is a protection mechanism by the embryo against CO poisoning.

Using azide that acts as nucleophile oxidant, the three embryonic hemoglobins exhibit lower oxidation rates than the adult protein (Robson and Brittain, 1996). The absolute rates of azide-induced oxidation with the rates of spontaneous autoxidation correlate

with the previously determined oxygen affinities of the embryonic hemoglobins. Heme exchange to human serum albumin was used to measure the relative binding constants for heme for each of the embryonic proteins and to evaluate the tetramer-dimer equilibrium constant for each hemoglobin. High oxygen affinity human embryonic hemoglobins are much less susceptible to anion-induced oxidation, and the heme groups in each of the embryonic globin proteins are more tightly bound than in the corresponding adult protein. This is a similar situation to that of HbF (see the previous discussion).

Using recombinant embryonic hemoglobins generated in a yeast expression system Sutherland-Smith et al. (1998) have crystallized Hb Gower II, in its carbon-monoxy form, and determined its structure by x-ray crystallography at 2.9 A resolution. In the framework of these authors, COHb Gower II hemoglobin tetramer is intermediate between the adult R and R2 states, although closer to R2. The α subunit is identical with α-globin chains of adult and fetal hemoglobins. The embryonic ε subunit is similar to adult β and fetal γ subunits, although with small differences at the N terminus and in the A helix. Amino acid substitutions could be identified that are candidates for the altered response of the Hb Gower II to allosteric effectors, in particular chloride ions. The reduced chloride effect is thought to be the primary cause of the higher affinity of this embryonic hemoglobin compared with the adult molecule. A computer-generated representation of the Gower II hemoglobin tetramer is shown in Figure 10.13.

Two recent advances have occurred in our molecular understanding of embryonic hemoglobins. Zeng, Zhu and Brittain (1999) have established the origin of the suppression of the chloride ion sensitivity in Hb Gower II. Using site-directed mutagenesis the authors have explored three candidate amino acids. The results demonstrate that an Asn at ε77 site (that replaces a His present in the β chains) is unambiguously responsable for the lower chloride sensitivity in Gower II. This is an important functional change since it allows oxygen exchange from the mother to the late embryo under physiological conditions.

Zheng et al (1999) have probed with site-directed mutagenesis the highly conserved α38Thr site, which is replaced by Gln in the ζ chain of Hb Portland. This substitution in adult Hb alters the ligand equilibrium and kinetic properties of the T state of the molecule. Mutation of hemoglobin Portland ζ-chain (the only known non-Thr containing globin) to a Thr residue, shows the reverse change in properties compared to the adult mutation. Nevertheless, in Hb Portland the situation is complicated by significant chain heterogeneity in the T state. Experiments with the HbA mutant Thrα38→Gln, the embryonic Hb Portland mutant

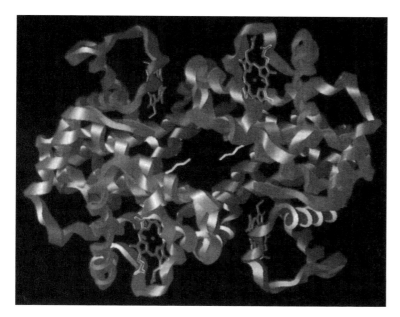

Figure 10.13. A GRASP generated figure of Gower II embryonic hemoglobin tetramer. The ε subunits are in green and the α subunits in blue. The two critical ε104Lys residues (whose side chains are in yellow) point to the center of the central cavity from each ε-globin chain. For full color reproduction, see color plate 10.13.

Glnζ38 Thr, and the wild-type proteins, as well as molecular modeling, the following molecular pathway arises: The naturally occurring Gln at position 38 of the ζ-chain would be expected to have two effects: (1) Alteration of the energetics of the interdigitation change of His97 in the transition from the T to R state; (2) destabilization of the T state by weakening of the Tyr145–Va198 carbonyl interaction, which would be unique to the specific presence of the Gln residue.

Thalassemias and Hemoglobinopathies of the Embryonic Globin Genes

Thalassemic or structural variants of the embryonic ε- and ζ-globin chains resulting from point mutations have not been described at the DNA or protein level, although they are likely to occur. Some large deletions that affect the β- and the α-globin gene clusters remove embryonic genes. The phenotypes of these conditions, when expressed postnatally, derive from loss of the β- or the α-globin genes. Deletion of the ζ- and α-globin genes cause early embryonic loss, presumably because a functional hemoglobin tetramer cannot be synthesized.

References

Abraham, EC and Elseweidy, MM. (1987). Non-enzymatic glycosylation influences Hb S polymerization. *Hemoglobin* 10: 173–183.

Abraham, EC and Rao KR. (1987). Gycosylated hemoglobin in a diabetic patient with sickle cell anemia. *Clin. Physiol. Biochem.* 5: 343–349.

Abraham, EC, Stallings, M, Abraham, A, and Clardy, R. (1983). Demonstration of a minor hemoglobin with modified alpha chains and additional modified hemoglobins in normal and diabetic adults. *Biochim. Biophys. Acta* 744: 335–341.

Abraham, EC, Abraham, A, and Stallins, M. (1984). High-pressure liquid chromatographic separation of glycosylated and acetylated minor hemoglobins in newborn infants and patients with sickle cell disease. *J. Lab. Clin. Med.* 104: 1027–1034.

Abraham, EC, Abraham, A, and Kasten-Jolly, J. (1987). Minor components of Hb Bart's. *Hemoglobin* 11: 329–339.

Adachi, K, Pang, JA, Reddy, LR et al. (1996). Polymerization of three hemoglobin A_2 variants containing Val^{d6} and inhibition of hemoglobin S polymerization by hemoglobin A^2. *J. Biol. Chem.* 271: 24557–24563.

Adams, JG III, Morrison, WT, and Steinberg, MH. (1982). Hb Parchman: A double crossover within a single human gene. *Science* 218: 291–293.

Al-Jawadi, O and Al-Hilali, A. (1998). Haemoglobin A_2 concentration in glucose-6-phosphate-dehydrogenase-deficient patients. *Acta Haematol.* 100: 99–100.

Allen, DW, Wyman J, and Smith, CA. (1953). The oxygen equilibrium of foetal and adult human hemoglobin. *J. Biol. Chem.* 203, 81–85.

Allen, DW, Schroeder, WA, and Balog, J. (1958). Observations on the chromatographic heterogeneity of normal adult and fetal hemoglobin. *J. Am. Chem. Soc.* 80: 1628–1634.

Alperin, JB, Dow, PA, and Petteway, MB. (1977). Hemoglobin A_2 levels in health and various hematologic disorders. *Am. J. Clin. Pathol.* 67: 219–226.

Badr, FM, Lorkin, PA, and Lehmann, H. (1973). Hemoglobin P-Nilotic: Containing a β-δ chain. *Nature New Biology* 242: 107–110.

Bayoumi RA, Dawodu A, Quereshi MM et al. (1999). The association of Hb Khartoum [β124(H2)pro->arg] with γ$^+$–thalassemia is responsible for hemolytic disease in the newborn of a Sudanese family. *Hemoglobin* 23: 33–45.

Bonaventura, C, Arumugam, M, Cashon, R et al. (1994). Chloride masks effects of opposing positive charges in Hb

A and Hb Hinsdale (beta 139 Asn→Lys) that can modulate cooperativity as well as oxygen affinity. *J. Mol. Biol.* 239: 561–568.

Bookchin, RM and Gallop, PM. (1968). Structure of hemoglobin A1c: nature of the N-terminal beta chain blocking group. *Biochem. Biophys. Res. Commun.* 32: 86–93.

Bouhassira, EE, Lachman, H, Labie, D, and Nagel, RL. (1989). A gene conversion located 5′ to the $^A\gamma$ gene is in linkage disequilibrium with the Bantu haplotype in sickle cell anemia. *J. Clin. Invest.* 83: 2070–2073.

Boyer, SH, Noyes, AN, Timmons, CF, and Young, RA. (1972). Primate hemoglobins: Polymorphisms and evolutionary patterns. *J. Hum. Evol.* 1: 515–543.

Boyer, SH, Belding, TK, Margolet, L et al. (1975). Variations in the frequency of fetal hemoglobin-bearing erythrocytes (F-cells) in well adults, pregnant women, and adult leukemics. *Johns Hopkins Med. J.* 137: 105–115.

Bradley, TB and Ranney, HM. (1973). Acquired disorders of haemoglobin. *Prog. Haematol.* 8: 77 85–98.

Bucala, R and Cerami, A. (1992). Advanced glycosylation: Chemistry, biology, and implications for diabetes and aging. *Adv. Pharmacol.* 23: 1–34.

Bunn HF. (1981). Modification of hemoglobin and other proteins by nonenzymatic glycosylation. *Prog. Clin. Biol. Res.* 51: 223–239.

Bunn, HF. (1984). Post-translational modifications of hemoglobin. *Haematologia (Budap)* 17: 179–186.

Bunn, HF. (1987). Subunit assembly of hemoglobin: an important determinant of hematologic phenotype. *Blood* 69: 1–6.

Bunn, HF and Briehl, RW. (1970). The interaction of 2,3-diphosphoglycerate with various human hemoglobins. *J. Clin. Invest.* 49: 1088–1095.

Bunn, HF and Forget, BG. (1986). *Hemoglobin: Molecular, genetic and clinical aspects.* Philadelphia: WB Saunders Company.

Bunn, HF and Jandl, JH. (1966). Exchange of heme among hemoglobin molecules. *Proc. Natl. Acad. Sci. U.S.A.* 56: 974–978.

Bunn, HF and McDonald, MJ. (1983). Electrostatic interactions in the assembly of haemoglobin. *Nature* 306: 498–500.

Burseaux, E, Poyart, C, Guesnon, P, and Teisseire, B. (1979). Comparative effects of CO_2 on the affinity for O_2 of fetal and adult hemoglobins. *Pflugers Arch* 378: 197–102.

Cech, P, Testa, U, Dubart, A et al. (1982). Lasting Hb F reactivation and Hb A_2 reduction induced by the treatment of Hodgkin's disease in a woman heterozygous for beta-thalassemia and the Swiss type of the heterocellular hereditary persistence of Hb F. *Acta Haematol.* 67: 275–284.

Ceppellini, R. (1959). L'emoglobina normale lenta A_2. *Acta Genet. Med. Gemellol.* 8: 47–68.

Chang, YC, Smith, KD, Moore, RD et al. (1995). An analysis of fetal hemoglobin variation in sickle cell disease: The relative contributions of the X-linked factor, β-globin haplotypes, α-globin gene number, gender, and age. *Blood* 85: 1111–1117.

Charache, S, Catalano, P, Burns, S et al. (1985). Pregnancy in carriers of high-affinity hemoglobins. *Blood* 65: 713–718.

Codrington, JF, Kutlar, F, Harris, HF et al. (1989). Hb A_2-Wrens or $\alpha_2\delta^{98}$ (FG5) Val→Met, an unstable δ chain vari-

ant identified by sequence analysis of amplified DNA. *Biochim. Biophys. Acta.* 1009: 87–89.

Codrington, JF, Li, HW, Kutlar, F et al. (1990). Observations on the levels of Hb A_2 in patients with different β-thalassemia mutations and a δ chain variant. *Blood* 76: 1246–1249.

Craig, JE, Rochette, J, Sampietro, M et al. (1997). Genetic heterogeneity in heterocellular hereditary persistence of fetal hemoglobin. *Blood* 90: 428–434.

de Bruin, SH and Janssen, LHM. (1973). Comparison of the oxygen and proton binding behavior of human hemoglobin A and A_2. *Biochim. Biophys. Acta* 295: 490–494.

Delvoye, NL, Destroismaisons, NM, and Wall, LA. (1993). Activation of the β-globin promoter by the locus control region correlates with binding of a novel factor to the CAAT box in murine erythroleukemia cells but not in K562 cells. *Mol. Cell. Biol.* 13: 6969–6983.

De Rosa, MC, Sanna, MT, Messana, I et al. (1998). Glycated human hemoglobin (HbA1c): Functional characteristics and molecular modeling studies. *Biophys. Chem.* 72: 323–335.

Donze, D, Jeancake, PH, and Townes, TM. (1996). Activation of δ-globin gene expression by erythroid Kruppel-like factor: A potential approach for gene therapy of sickle cell disease. *Blood* 88: 4051–4057.

Dover, GJ and Boyer, SH. (1980). Quantification of hemoglobins within individual red cells; Asynchronous biosynthesis of fetal and adult hemoglobins during erythroid maturation in normal subjects. *Blood* 56: 1082–1091.

Dover, GJ and Boyer, SH. (1980–1981). The cellular distribution of fetal hemoglobin: Normal adults and hemoglobinopathies. Human hemoglobins and hemoglobinopathies: A review to 1981. *Texas Reports on Biology and Medicine* 40: 43–52.

Dover, GJ, Boyer, SH, Zinkham, WH et al. (1977). Changing erythrocyte populations in juvenile chronic myelocytic leukemia: Evidence for disordered regulation. *Blood* 49: 355–365.

Dover, GJ, Boyer, SH, Charache, S, and Heintzelman, K. (1978a). Individual variation in the production and survival of F-cells in sickle cell disease. *N. Engl. J. Med.* 299: 1428–1435.

Dover, GJ, Boyer, SH, and Bell, WR, (1978b). Microscopic method for assaying F cell production: Illustrative changes during infancy and in aplastic anemia. *Blood* 52: 664–647.

Dover, GJ, Boyer, SH, and Pembrey, ME (1981). F cell production in sickle cell anemia: Regulation by genes linked to β-hemoglobin locus. *Science* 211: 1441–1444.

Dover, GJ, Smith, KD, Chang, YC et al. (1992). Fetal hemoglobin levels in sickle cell disease and normal individuals are partially controlled by an X-linked gene located at Xp22.2. *Blood* 80: 816–824.

Dumoulin, A, Manning, LR, Jenkins, WT et al. (1997). Exchange of subunit interfaces between recombinant adult and fetal hemoglobins. Evidence for a functional inter-relationship among regions for the tetramer. *J. Biol. Chem.* 272: 31326–31334.

Ebb, D, Chin, K, and Rodgers, GP. (1993). Identification of upstream regulatory elements that repress expression of adult beta-like globin genes in a primitive erythroid environment. *Clin. Res.* 41: 206A.

Eddison, GG, Briehl RW, and Ranney, HM. (1964). Oxygen equilibria of hemoglobin A2 and hemoglobin Lepore. *J. Clin. Invest.* 43: 2323–2326.

Elseweidy, MM, and Abraham, EC. (1984). The relationship between fetal hemoglobin level and glycosylation in sickle cell disease. *Am. J. Hematol.* 16: 375–381.

Elseweidy, MM, Fadel, HE, and Abraham, EC. (1984). Glycosylated and acetylated hemoglobins in relation to gestational age and red cell age. *Hemoglobin* 8: 363–372.

Felicetti, L, Novelletto, A, Benincasa, A, et al. (1984). The HbA/HbA2 ratio in newborns and its correlation with fetal maturity. *Br. J. Haematol.* 56: 465–471.

Fessas, P and Stamatoyannopoulos, G. (1962). Absence of haemoglobin A2 in an adult. *Nature* 196: 1215–1216.

Feuilhade, F, Testa, U, Vainchenker, W et al. (1981). Comparative patterns of i-antigen expression, F-cell frequency and Hb A2 level in acute myeloid leukemia and in acute lymphoid leukemia. *Leuk. Res.* 5: 203–213.

Fischer, S, Nagel, RL, Bookchin, RM et al. (1975). The binding of hemoglobin to membranes of normal and sickle erythrocytes. *Biochim. Biophys. Acta,* 375: 422–433.

Fitzgibbons, JF, Koler, RD, and Jones, RT. (1976) Red cell age-related changes of hemoglobins AIa+b and AIc in normal and diabetic subjects. *J Clin Invest,* 58, 820–4.

Fluckiger R, Harmon, W, Meier, W et al. (1981). Hemoglobin carbamylation in uremia. *N. Engl. J. Med.* 304: 823–827.

Frier, JA and Perutz, M. (1977). Structure of human foetal deoxyhemoglobin. *J Mol Biol* 112: 97–102.

Galanello, R, Ruggeri, R, Addis, M et al. (1981). Hemoglobin A2 in iron deficient beta-thalassemia heterozygotes. *Hemoglobin* 5: 613–618.

Galanello, R, Melis, MA, Podda, A et al. (1990). Deletion delta-thalassemia: the 7.2 kb deletion of Corfu delta beta-thalassemia in a non-beta-thalassemia chromosome [letter]. *Blood* 75: 1747–1749.

Garbutt, GJ and Abraham, EC. (1981) Non-enzymatic acetylation of human hemoglobins. *Biochim. Biophys. Acta* 670: 190–194.

Garby, L and Sjoli, A. (1963). Studies on the erythrokinetics in infancy. *Acta Paediat. (Stockh)* 52: 537–542.

Garcia, CR, Navarro, JL, Lam, H et al. (1983). Hb A2-Manzanares or $\alpha_2\delta_2$ 121 (GH4) Glu→Val, an unstable δ chain variant observed in a Spanish family. *Hemoglobin* 7: 435–442.

Garner, C, Tatu, T, Reittie, J et al. (1998). Twins *en route* to QTL mapping for heterocellular HPFH. *Blood* 92: 694a.

Garrick, LM, McDonald, MJ, Shapiro, R et al. (1980). Structural analysis of the minor human hemoglobin components: Hb AIa1, Hb AIa2 and Hb AIb. *Eur. J. Biochem.* 106: 353–359.

Giardina, B, Messana, I, Scatena, R, and Castagnola, M. (1995). The multiple functions of hemoglobin. *Crit. Rev. Biochem. Mol. Biol.* 30: 165–196.

Gilman, JG. (1988). Expression of G gamma and A gamma globin genes in human adults. *Hemoglobin* 12: 707–716.

Giulian, GG, Gilbert, EF, and Moss, RL. (1987). Elevated fetal hemoglobin levels in sudden infant death syndrome. *N. Engl. J. Med.* 316: 1122–1126.

Glader, BE. (1989). Hemoglobin FM-Fort Ripley: another lesson from the neonate. *Pediatrics* 83: 792–793.

Glader, BE and Conrad, ME. (1972). Decreased glutathione peroxidase in neonatalerythrocytes: Lack of relation to hydrogen peroxide metabolism. *Pediatr. Res.* 6: 900–904.

Goldstein D. and Little RR (1997) Monitoring glycemia in diabetes. Short-term assessment. *Endocrinol Metab Clin North Am* 26: 475–486.

Gonzalez-Redondo, JM, Kattamis, C, and Huisman, THJ. (1989a). Characterization of three types of β^0-thalassemia resulting from a partial deletion of the β-globin gene. *Hemoglobin* 13: 377–392.

Gonzalez-Redondo, JM, Stoming, TA, Kutlar, A et al. (1989b). A C→T substitution at nt -101 in a conserved DNA sequence of the promoter region of the b-globin gene is associated with "silent β-thalassemia". *Blood* 73: 1705–1711.

Grifoni, V, Kumuzora, H, Lehmann, H, and Charlesworth, D. (1975). A new Hb variant: F Sardinia γ75(E19) Isoleucine→Threonine found in a family with Hb G-Philadelphia, β-chain deficiency and a Lepore-like hemoglobin indistinguishable from Hb A2. *Acta Haematol* 53: 347–355.

Gros, G and Bauer, C. (1978). High pK value of the N-terminal amino group of the γ chains causes low CO_2 binding of human fetal hemoglobin. *Biochem Biophys Res Commun* 80: 56–59.

Gross GP and Hathaway WE. (1972). Fetal erythrocyte deformability. *Proc. Soc. Pediatr. Res.* 6: 593–599.

Guang, W, Ma, M, and Qian, D. Hb F-Xin-Jin or $^{G}\gamma^{I}$119(GH2)Gly→Arg A new unstable fetal hemoglobin variant. *Hemoglobin* (in press).

Guiso, L, Frogheri, L, Pistidda, P et al. (1996). Frequency of delta+ 27-thalassaemia in Sardinians. *Clin. Lab. Haematol.* 18: 241–244.

Harano, T, Harano, K, Doi, K et al. (1990). HbF-Onoda or $\alpha_2{}^{G}\gamma_2$146(HC3)His→Tyr, a newly discovered fetal hemoglobin variant in a Japanese newborn. *Hemoglobin* 14: 217–222.

Hardies, SC, Edgell, MH, and Hutchison, CA, III. (1984). Evolution of the mammalian β-globin gene cluster. *J. Biol. Chem.* 259: 3748–3756.

Harmeling, JG and Moquin, RB. (1967). An abnormal elevation of hemoglobin A2 in hereditary spherocytosis. *Am. J. Clin. Pathol.* 47: 454–458.

Harthoorn-Lasthuizen, EJ, Lindemans, J, and Langenhuijsen, MM. (1999). Influence of iron deficiency anaemia on haemoglobin A2 levels: Possible consequences for beta-thalassaemia screening. *Scand. J. Clin. Lab. Invest.* 59: 65–70.

Hayashi, A, Fujita, T, Fujimura, M, and Titani, K. (1979). A new fetal hemoglobin, HbF M Osaka (α_2 γ_2 63 His→Leu). A mutant with high oxygen affinity and erythrocytosis. *A. J. Clin. Pathol.* 172: 1028–1032.

Henshaw, LA, Tizzard, JL, Booth, K, and Beard ME. (1978). Haemoglobin A2 levels in vitamin B12 and folate deficiency. *J. Clin. Pathol.* 31: 960–962.

Hoffmann, OM and Brittain, T. (1996). Ligand binding kinetics and dissociation of the human embryonic haemoglobins. *Biochem. J.* 315: 65–70.

Hoffmann, OM and Brittain, T. (1998). Partitioning of oxygen and carbon monoxide in the three human embryonic hemoglobins. *Hemoglobin* 22: 313–319.

Hoffman, O, Mould, R, and Brittain, T. (1995a). Allosteric modulation of oxygen binding to the three human embryonic haemoglobins. *Biochem. J.* 306: 367–370.

Hoffman, O, Currucan, G, Robson, N, and Brittain, T. (1995b). The chloride effect in the human embryonic haemoglobins. *Biochem. J.* 309: 959–962.

Hoffmann, OM, Brittain, T, and Wells, RM. (1997). The control of oxygen affinity in the three human embryonic haemoglobins by respiration linked metabolites. *Biochem. Mol. Biol. Int.* 42: 553–566.

Horiuchi, K, Osterhout, ML, and Ohene-Frempong, K. (1995). Survival of F-reticulocytes in sickle cell disease. *Biochem. Biophys. Res. Commun.* 217: 924–930.

Horton, B, Payne, RA, Bridges, MT, and Huisman, THJ. (1961). Studies on an abnormal minor hemoglobin component (Hb-B2). *Clin. Chem. Acta* 6: 246–253.

Hosoi, T. (1965). Studies on hemoglobin F within single erythrocytes by fluorescent antibody technique. *Exp. Cell. Res.* 37: 680–683.

Huehns, ER, and Shooter, EM. (1961). The polypeptide chains of haemoglobin-A_2 and haemoglobin-G_2. *J. Mol. Biol.* 3: 257–262.

Huehns, ER, Dance, N, Beaven, GH et al. (1964a). Human embryonic hemoglobins. *Cold Spring Harbor Symp.* 19: 327–331.

Huehns, ER, Hecht, F, Keil, JV, and Motulsky, AG. (1964b). Developmental hemoglobin anomalies in a chromosomal triplication: D_1 trisomy syndrome. *Proc. Natl. Acad. Sci. U.S.A.* 51: 89–97.

Huisman, THJ. (1980–1981). The human fetal hemoglobins. *Texas Rep. Biol. Med.* 40: 29–42.

Huisman, THJ. (1992). Abnormal hemoglobin list. *Hemoglobin* 16: 127–236.

Huisman, THJ. (1997). Levels of Hb A_2 in heterozygotes and homozygotes for beta-thalassemia mutations: Influence of mutations in the CACCC and ATAAA motifs of the beta-globin gene promoter. *Acta Haematol.* 98: 187–194.

Huisman, THJ, Altay, C, Webber, B, et al. (1981). Quantification of three types of γ chain of Hb F by high pressure liquid chromatography; application of this method to the Hb F of patients with sickle cell anemia or the S-HPFH condition. *Blood* 57: 75–82.

Humphries, RK, Ley, T, Turner, P et al. (1982). Differences in human α, β-, δ-globin gene expression in monkey kidney cells. *Cell* 30: 173–183.

Jankovic, L, Efremov, GD, Petkov, G et al. (1990). Two novel polyadenylation mutations leading to beta(+)-thalassemia. *Br. J. Haematol.* 75: 122–126.

Jonxis, JHP, and Huisman, THJ. (1956). The detection and estimation of fetal hemoglobin by means of alkali denaturation test. *Blood* 11: 1009–1015.

Jope, EM.(1949). The ultra-violet spectral absorption of haemoglobin inside and outside the red blood cell. In Roughton, FJW and Kendrew, JC, editors. *Haemoglobin*. London: Butterworth.

Kabadi, UM, and Hood, L. (1998). Increased glycation of hemoglobin in AIDS: Relation to the severity of the disorder. *Diabetes Res.* 33: 37–44.

Kabadi, UM, Gopal, V, Hood, L et al. (1992). Elevated glycosylated hemoglobin concentrations in AIDS. *AIDS* 6: 236–238.

Katsura, S. (1964). A new serological method for the detection of fetal hemoglobin in the single erythrocyte. *Yokohama Med. Bull.* 15: 117–126.

Kendall, AG and Bastomsky, CH. (1981). Hemoglobin A_2 in hyperthyroidism. *Hemoglobin* 5: 571–577.

Kinderlerer, V, Lehmann, H, and Tipton, KF. (1973). Thermal denaturation of human oxyhemoglobins A, A_2, C, and S. *Biochem J* 135: 805–814.

Kleihauer, E, Braun, H, and Betke, K. (1957). Demostration von fetalem hamoglobin in den erythrozyten eines blutausstrichs. *Klin. Wochensshr* 35: 637–642.

Klipstein, FA and Ranney, HM. (1960). Electrophoretic components of the hemoglobin of red cell membranes. *J. Clin. Invest.* 39: 1894–1899.

Kohne, E, Krause, M, Leupold, D, and Kleihauer, E.(1977). Hemoglobin F Koelliker (alpha2 minus 141 (HC 3) Arg gamma2); A modification of fetal hemoglobin. *Hemoglobin* 1: 257–266.

Konrad, PN, Valentine, WN, Paglia DE et al. (1972). Enzymatic activities and glutathione content of erythrocytes in the newborn: Comparison with red cells of older normal subjects and those with comparable reticulocytosis. *Acta Haematol.* 48: 193–201.

Koop, BF, Siemieniak, D, Slightom, JL et al. (1989). Tarsius delta- and beta-globin genes: Conversions, evolution, and systematic implications. *J. Biol. Chem.* 264: 68–79.

Korber, E.(1926). Inaugural dissertation: "Uber differenzen Blutfarbstoffes." *Dorpat*, 1866, cited by Bischoff, H, Z. *Exp. Med.* 48: 472–476.

Kosche, K, Dobkin, C, and Bank, A. (1984). The role of intervening sequences (IVS) in human β globin gene expression. *Blood* 64(Suppl. 1): 58a.

Kosche, KA, Dobkin, C, and Bank, A. (1985). DNA sequences regulating human β globin gene expression. *Nucleic Acids Res.* 13: 7781–7793.

Krishnamoorthy, R, Elion, J, Kuhn, JM et al. (1982). Haemoglobin A_2 is elevated in hyperthyroid patients. *Nouvelle Revue Francaise d´ Hematologie* 24: 39–40.

Kuhn, JM, Rieu, M, Rochette, J et al. (1983). Influence of thyroid status on hemoglobin A_2 expression. *J. Clin. Endocrinol. Metab.* 57: 344–348.

Kulozik, AE, Yarwood, N, and Jones, RW. (1988). The Corfu delta beta zero thalassemia: A small deletion acts at a distance to selectively abolish beta globin gene expression. *Blood* 71: 457–462.

Kunkle, HG and Wallenius, G. (1955). New hemoglobin in normal human blood. *Science* 122: 288.

Kurantsin-Mills, J and Lessin, LS. (1984). Freeze-etching and biochemical analysis of human fetal erythrocyte membranes. *Pediatr. Res.* 18: 1035–1041.

Kutlar, F, Gonzalez-Redondo, JM, Kutlar, A et al. (1989). The levels of ζ, γ, and δ chains in patients with Hb H disease. *Hum. Genet.* 82: 179–186.

Kutlar, A, Kutlar, F, Gu, LG et al. (1990). Fetal hemoglobin in normal adults and beta-thalassemia heterozygotes. *Hum. Genet.* 85: 106–110.

Kutlar, F, Felice, AE, Grech, JL et al. (1991). The linkage of Hb Valletta $\alpha2\beta2^{87(F3)Thr\rightarrow Pro]}$ and Hb F-Malta-I

$[\alpha2\gamma2^{117(G19)His\rightarrow Arg}]$ in the Maltese population. *Hum. Genet.* 86: 591–594.

Labie, D, Pagnier, J, Lapoumeroulie, C et al. (1985). Common haplotype dependency of high $^G\gamma$-globin gene expression and high HbF levels in β-thalassemia and sickle cell anemia patients. *Proc. Natl. Acad. Sci. U.S.A.* 82: 2111–2114.

LaFlamme, S, Acuto, S, Markowitz, D et al. (1987). Expression of chimeric human beta- and delta-globin genes during erythroid differentiation. *J. Biol. Chem.* 262: 4819–4826.

Lapoumeroulie, C, Dunda, O, Trabuchet, G, et al. (1989). A novel sickle gene of yet another origin in Africa: The Cameroon type. *Blood* 74 (Suppl 1): 63a.

Leder, A, Kuo, A, Shen, MM, and Leder, P.(1992). In situ hybridization reveals co-expression of embryonic and adult alpha globin genes in the earliest murine erythrocyte progenitors. *Development* 116: 1041–1049.

Lee, RC and Huisman, THJ. (1963). Study of a family possessing hemoglobin C. Classical thalassemia and the abnormal minor hemoglobin component A₂′. *Am. J. Hum. Genet.* 15: 69–73.

Lee, JC, Hayashi, RH, and Shepard, MK. (1982). Fetal hemoglobin in women with normal and with hydatidiform molar pregnancy. *Am. J. Hematol,* 13: 131–139.

Lee-Potter, JP, Deacon-Smith, RA, Simpkiss, MJ et al. (1975). A new cause of haemolytic anemia in the newborn. A description of an unstable fetal haemoglobin: F Poole, $\alpha2^G\gamma2$ 130 Tryptophan→Glycine. *J. Clin. Pathol.* 28: 317–320.

Leonova, JYE, Kazanetz, EG, Smetanina, NS et al. (1996). Variability in the fetal hemoglobin level of the normal adult. *Am. J. Hematol.* 53: 59–65.

Lie-Injo, LE, Lopez, CG, and Lopez, M. (1971). Hemoglobin A2 in malaria patients. *Trans. R. Soc. Trop. Med. Hyg.* 65: 480–483.

Loudianos, G, Cao, A, Ristaldi, MS et al. (1990). Molecular basis of delta beta-thalassemia with normal fetal hemoglobin level [letter]. *Blood* 75: 526–528.

Loukopoulos, D and Fessas, P. (1965). The distribution of hemoglobin types in thalassemic erythrocytes. *J Clin Invest,* 44, 231–240.

Luo, HY, Liang, XL, Frye, C et al. (1999) Embryonic hemoglobins are expressed in definitive cells. *Blood* 94: 359–361.

Makita, Z, Vlassara, H, Rayfield, E et al. (1992). Hemoglobin-AGE: a circulating marker of advanced glycosylation. *Science* 258: 651–653.

Markham, RE, Butler, F, Goh, K, and Rowley PT. (1983). Erythroleukemia manifesting delta beta-thalassemia. *Hemoglobin* 7: 71–78.

Martin, SL, Vicent, KA, and Wilson, AC. (1983). Rise and fall of the delta globin gene. *J Mol. Biol.* 64: 513–528.

Martin, SL, Zimmer, EA, Kan, YW, and Wilson, AC. (1980). Silent delta-globin gene in Old World monkeys. *Proc. Natl. Acad. Sci. U.S.A.* 77: 3563–3566.

Mason, KP, Grandison, Y, Hayes, RJ et al. (1982). Post-natal level of fetal haemoglobin in homozygous sickle cell disease: Relationship to parental Hb F levels. *Br. J. Haematol.* 52: 455–463.

McDonald, MJ, Turci, SM, and Bunn, HF. (1984). Subunit assembly of normal and variant human hemoglobins. *Prog. Clin. Biol. Res.* 165: 3–15.

Miyoshi, K, Kaneto, Y, Kawai, H et al. (1988). X-linked dominant control of F-cells in normal adult life: Characterization of the Swiss type as hereditary persistence of fetal hemoglobin regulated dominantly by gene(s) on X chromosome. *Blood* 72: 1854–1860.

Mollison, PL. (1967). *Blood transfusion in clinical medicine* (4th ed.) Oxford: Blackwell Scientific Publishers.

Moo-Penn, WF, Bechtel, KC, Schmidt, RM et al. (1977), Hemoglobin Raleigh (β1 Valine→Acetylalanine): Structural and functional characterization. *Biochemistry* 16: 4872–4879.

Morris, J, Dunn, D, Beckford, M et al. (1991). The haematology of homozygous sickle cell disease after the age of 40 years. *Br. J. Haematol.* 77: 382–385.

Nagai K, Enoki Y, Kaneko A, and Hori H. (1980). Functional properties of the glycosylated minor hemoglobins A1a-1, A1a-2 and A1b. EPR evidence for increased stability of the low affinity quaternary structure and decreased susceptibility to organic phosphate. *Biochim. Biophys. Acta.* 623: 376–380.

Nagel, RL. (1991). Severity, pathobiology, epistatic effects, and genetic markers in sickle cell anemia. *Semin. Hematol.* 28: 180–201.

Nagel, RL, Bookchin, RM, Labie, D et al. (1979). Structural basis for the inhibitory effects of hemoglobin F and hemoglobin A₂ on the polymerization of hemoglobin S. *Proc. Natl. Acad. Sci. U.S.A.* 76: 670–672.

Nathan, DG and Orkin, SH. (1998). *Nathan and Oski's hematology of infancy and childhood.* Philadelphia: WB Saunders Co.

Neerhout, RC. (1968). Erythrocyte lipids in the neonate. *Pediatr. Res.* 2: 172–178.

Neumeyer, P and Betke, K. (1987). Haemoglobin A₂ in newborn infants of different maturity. *Euro. J. Pediatr.* 146: 598–600.

Newman, DR, Pierre, RV, and Linman, JW. (1973). Studies on the diagnostic significance of hemoglobin F levels. *Mayo Clin. Proc.* 48: 199–202.

Nopparatana, C, Saechan, V, Nopparatana, C et al. (1999). A novel 105 base pair deletion causing β⁰-thalassemia in members of a Thai family. *Am. J. Hematol.* 61, 1–4.

Ochoa, S. (1983). Regulation of protein synthesis initiation in eucaryotes. *Arch. Biochem. Biophys.* 223: 325–349.

Oggiano, L, Guiso, L, Frogheri, L et al. (1994). A novel Mediterranean "δβ-thalassemia" determinant containing the δ+27 and β°39 point mutations in cis. *Am. J. Hematol.* 45: 81–84.

Papapanagiotuo, E, Kollia, P, Loutradi, A et al. (1998). Functional analysis of the –65 (A→G) nucleotide substitution in the promoter region of the δ-globin gene. *Blood* 92: 531a.

Papayannopoulou, TH, Lawn, RM, Stamatoyannopoulos, G, and Maniatis, T. (1982). Greek ($^A\gamma$) variant of hereditary persistence of fetal haemolobin: Globin gene organization and studies of expression of fetal haemoglobins in clonal erythroid cultures. *Br. J. Haematol.* 50: 387–399.

Pembrey, ME, Weatherall, DJ, and Clegg, JB. (1973). Maternal synthesis of haemoglobin F in pregnancy. *Lancet* 16: 1350–1354.

Perry, GW, Vargas-Cuba, R, and Vertes, RP. (1997). Fetal hemoglobin levels in sudden infant death syndrome. *Arch. Pathol. Lab. Med.* 121: 1048–1054.

Perutz, M, Fermi, G, Poyart, C et al. (1993). A novel allosteric mechanism in haemoglobin. Structure of bovine deoxy-haemoglobin, absence of specific chloride-binding sites and origin of the chloride-linked Bohr effect in bovine and human haemoglobin. *J. Mol. Biol.* 233: 536–545.

Peterson, CM and Nguyen, LB. (1985). Clinical implications of acetaldehyde adducts with hemoglobin. *Prog. Clin. Biol. Res.* 183: 19–30.

Peterson, KP, Pavlovich, JG, Goldstein, D et al. (1998). What is hemoglobin A1c? An analysis of glycated hemoglobins by electrospray ionization mass spectrometry. *Clin. Chem.* 44: 1951–1958.

Petes, TD. (1982). Evidence that structural variants within the human d-globin protein may reflect genetic interactions between the δ- and β- globin genes. *Am. J. Hum. Genet.* 34: 820–823.

Poyart, C, Burseaux, E, Guesnon, P, and Teissiere, B. (1978). Chloride binding and Bohr effect of human fetal erythrocytes and HbF_{II} solutions. *Pflugers Arch.* 37: 169–173.

Priest, JR, Watterson, J, Jones, RT et al. (1989). Mutant fetal hemoglobin causing cyanosis in a newborn. *Pediatrics* 83: 734–736.

Prome, D, Blouquit, Y, Ponthus, C et al. (1991). Structure of the human adult hemoglobin minor fraction A1b by electrospray and secondary ion mass spectrometry. Pyruvic acid as amino-terminal blocking group. *J. Biol. Chem.* 266: 13050–13054.

Proudfoot, NJ, Shander, MHM, Manley, JL et al. (1980). Structure and in vitro transcription of human globin genes. *Science* 209: 1329–1336.

Rai, R, Pati, H, Sehgal, AK et al. (1987). Hemoglobin A_2 in iron deficiency and megaloblastic anemia: relation with severity and etiology of anemia. *Indian Pediatri.* 24: 301–305.

Ranney, HM, Lam, R, and Rosenberg, G. (1993). Some properties of hemoglobin A_2. *Am. J. Hematol.* 42: 107–111.

Ricco, G, Mazza, V, Turi, RM et al. (1976). Significance of a new type of human fetal hemoglobin carrying a replacement isoleucine-threonine at position 75 (E19) of the γ chain. *Hum. Genet.* 32: 305–313.

Rieder, RF and Weatherall, DJ. (1965). Studies on hemoglobin biosynthesis: Asynchronous synthesis of hemoglobin A and hemoglobin A_2, by erythrocyte precursors. *J. Clin. Invest.* 44: 42–50.

Roberts, AV, Weatherall, DJ, and Clegg, JB. (1972). The synthesis of human haemoglobin A_2 during erythroid maturation. *Biochem. Biophys. Res. Commun.* 47: 81–87.

Roberts, WL, Chiasera, JM, and Ward-Cook, KM. (1999). Glycohemoglobin results in samples with hemoglobin C or S trait: A comparison of four test systems. *Clin. Chem.* 45: 906–909.

Robson, N and Brittain, T. (1996). Heme stability in the human embryonic hemoglobins. *J. Inorg. Biochem.* 64: 137–147.

Ross, J and Pizarro, A. (1983). Human beta and delta globin messenger RNA's turn over at different rates. *J. Mol. Biol.* 167: 607–617.

Rosatelli, MC, Altay, C, Oner, R et al. (1992). A beta-globin haplotype and XmnI polymorphism at position G

(gamma)-158 and HbF production in Fanconi's anemia. *Haematologica* 77: 106–109.

Routy, JP, Monte, M, Beaulieu, R et al. (1993). Increase of hemoglobin A_2 in human immunodeficiency virus-1 infected patients treated with zidovudine. *Am. J. Hematol.* 43: 86–90.

Saglio, G, Ricco, G, Mazza, U et al. (1979). Human ^{T}γ globin chain is a variant of ^{A}γ chain (^{A}γ Sardinia). *Proc. Natl. Acad. Sci. U.S.A.* 76: 3420–3424.

Salkie, ML, Gordon, PA, Rigal, WM et al. (1982). HbA2-Canada or $\alpha_2\delta_2$ 99 (G1) Asp→Asn, a newly discovered delta chain variant with increased oxygen affinity occurring in cis to β-thalassemia. *Hemoglobin* 6: 223–231.

Sanguansermsri, T, Pape, M, Laig, M et al. (1990). β°-Thalassemia in a Thai family is caused by a 3.4 kb deletion including the entire β-globin gene. *Hemoglobin* 14: 157–168.

Schroeder, WA. (1980) The synthesis and chemical heterogeneity of human fetal hemoglobin, *Hemoglobin* 4: 431–446.

Schroeder, WA and Jones, RT. (1965). Some aspects of the chemistry and function of human and animal hemoglobins. *Fortschr. Chem. Org. Naturst.* 23: 113–194.

Schroeder, WA, Cua, JT, Matsuda, G, and Fenninger, WD. (1962). Hemoglobin F_1, an acetyl-containing hemoglobin. *Biochem Biophys Acta* 63: 532–536.

Schroeder, WA, Shelton, JR, Shelton, JB, et al. (1963). The amino acid sequence of the γ-chain of human fetal hemoglobin. *Biochemistry* 2: 992–1001.

Schroeder, WA, Huisman, THJ, Shelton, JR et al. (1968). Evidence of multiple structural genes for the γ chain of human hemoglobin. *Proc. Natl. Acad. Sci. U.S.A.* 60: 537–544.

Schroeder, WA, Huisman, THJ, Hyman, C et al. (1973a). An individual with "Miyada"-like hemoglobin indistinguishable from hemoglobin A_2. *Biochem. Genet.* 10: 135–147.

Schroeder WA, Bannister WH, Grech JL et al. (1973b). Non-synchronized suppression of postnatal activity in non-allelic genes which synthesize the gamma chain in human foetal haemoglobin. *Nature New Biology* 244: 89–90.

Schroeder, WA, Huisman, THJ, Efremov, GD et al. (1979). Further studies on the frequency and significance of the ^{T}γ chain of human fetal hemoglobin. *J. Clin. Invest.* 63: 268–275.

Schroter, W and Nafz, C. (1981). Diagnostic significance of hemoglobin F and A_2 levels in homo- and heterozygous beta-thalassemia during infancy. *Helv. Paediatr. Acta* 36: 19–25.

Schwartz, BA and Gray, GR. (1977). Proteins containing reductively aminated disaccharides. Synthesis and chemical characterization. *Arch. Biochem. Biophys.* 181: 542–549.

Serjeant, BE, Mason, KP, and Serjeant, GR. (1978). The development of haemoglobin A_2 in normal negro infants and in sickle cell disease. *Br. J. Haematol.* 39: 259–265.

Sheridan, BL, Weatherall, DJ, Clegg, JB et al. (1976). The pattern of foetal haemoglobin production in leukaemia. *Br. J. Haematol.* 32: 487–506.

Singer, K, Chernoff, AI, and Singer, L. (1951). Studies on abnormal hemoglobins. I. Their demonstration in sickle cell anemia and other hematologic disorders by means of alkali denaturation. *Blood* 6: 428–433.

Sjolin, S. (1952). The resistance of the foetal red blood corpuscles. *Acta Paediatr.* 41: 610–611.

Slightom, JL, Blechl, AE, and Smithies, O. (1980). Human fetal $^G\gamma$- and $^A\gamma$-globin genes: Complete nucleotide sequences suggest that DNA can be exchanged between these duplicated genes. *Cell* 21: 627–638.

Stamatoyannopoulos, G, Weitkamp, LR, Kotsakis, P, and Akrivakis, A. (1977). The linkage relationships of the b and δ hemoglobins genes. *Hemoglobin,* 1: 561–570.

Stamatoyannopoulos, G, Constantoulakis, P, Brice, M et al. (1987). Coexpression of embryonic, fetal, and adult globins in erythroid cells of human embryos: Relevance to the cell-lineage models of globin switching. *Dev. Biol.* 123: 191–197.

Steinberg, MH. (1993). Effects of iron deficiency and the −88 C→T mutation on HbA$_2$ levels in β-thalassemia. *Am. J. Med. Sci.* 305: 312–313.

Steinberg, MH and Adams, JG, III. (1991). Hemoglobin A$_2$: Origin, evolution, and aftermath. *Blood* 78: 2165–2177.

Steinberg, MH, Coleman, MB, and Adams, JG. (1982). Beta-thalassemia with exceptionally high hemoglobin A$_2$. Differential expression of the delta-globin gene in the presence of beta-thalassemia. *J. Lab. Clin. Med.* 100: 548–557.

Steinberg, MH, Hsu, H, and Nagel, RL, et al. (1995). Gender and haplotype effects upon hematological manifestations of adult sickle cell anemia, *Am. J. Hematol.* 48: 175–181.

Stockman, JA 3d and Oski FA. (1978). Erythrocytes of the human neonate. *Curr. Top. Hematol.* 1: 193–232.

Sukumaran, PK, Nakatsuji, T, Gardiner, MB et al. (1983). Gamma thalassemia resulting from the deletion of a gamma-globin gene. *Nucleic Acids Res.* 83: 4635–4643.

Sutherland-Smith, AJ, Baker, HM, Hoffmann, OM et al. (1998). Crystal structure of human embryonic haemoglobin: the carbonmonoxide for Gower II (alpha2epsilon2) haemoglobin at 2.9 Å resolution. J. Mol. Biol, 280, 475–484.

Taketa, F, Attermeir, MH, and Mauk, AG. (1972). Acetylated hemoglobins in feline blood. *J. Biol. Chem.* 247: 33–35.

Tamary, H, Shalev, H, Luria, D et al. (1996). Clinical features and studies of erythropoiesis in Israeli Bedouins with congenital dyserythropoietic anemia type 1. *Blood* 87: 1763–1770.

Tang, TK, Huang, C-S, Huang, M-J et al. (1992). Diverse point mutations result in glucose-6-phosphate dehydrogenase (G6PD) polymorphism in Taiwan. *Blood* 79: 2135–2140.

Tang, C, Ebb D, Hardison, RC, and Rodgers, GP. (1997). Restoration of the CCAAT box or insertion of the CACCC motif activate δ-globin gene expression. *Blood* 90: 421–427.

Thein, SL and Craig, JE. (1998). Genetics of Hb F/F cell variance in adults and heterocellular hereditary persistence of fetal hemoglobin. *Hemoglobin* 22: 401–414.

Thein, SL, Sampietro, M, Rohde, K et al. (1994). Detection of a major gene for heterocellular hereditary persistence of fetal hemoglobin after accounting for genetic modifiers. *Am. J. Hum. Genet.* 54: 214–228.

Trifillis, P, Adachi, K, Yamaguchi, T et al. (1996). Expression studies of δ-globin gene alleles associated with reduced hemoglobin A$_2$ levels in Greek Cypriots. *J. Biol. Chem.* 271: 26931–26938.

Tyuma, I and Shamizu, K. (1969). Different response to organic phosphates of human fetal and adult hemoglobins. *Arch. Biochem. Biophys.* 129: 404–407.

Van Ros, G, Moors, A, De Vlieger, M, and De Groof E. (1978). Hemoglobin A$_2$ levels in malaria patients. *Am. J. Trop. Med. Hyg.* 27: 659–663.

Wasi, P, Disthasongchan, P, and Na-Nakorn, S. (1968). The effect of iron deficiency on the levels of hemoglobin A$_2$ and E. *J. Lab. Clin. Med.* 71: 85–91.

Wasi, P, Kruatrachue, M, Piankijagum, A, and Pravatmeung, P. (1971). Hemoglobin A$_2$ and E levels in malaria. *J. Med. Assoc. Thailand* 54: 559–562.

Weatherall, DJ and Clegg, JB. (1981). *The thalassaemia syndromes.* Oxford: Blackwell.

Weatherall, DJ, Edwards, JA, and Donohoe, WT. (1968). Haemoglobin and red cell enzyme changes in juvenile myeloid leukaemia. *Br. Med. J.* 1: 679–681.

Weatherall, DJ, Clegg, JB, Wood, WG et al. (1975). Foetal erythropoiesis in human leukaemia. *Nature* 257: 710–712.

Weatherall, DJ, Clegg, JB, Milner, PF et al. (1976). Linkage relationships between β- and δ-structural loci and African forms of β thalassaemia. *J. Med. Genet.* 13: 20–26.

White, JM, Brain, MC, and Ali, MAM. (1971). Globin synthesis in sideroblastic anaemia. I. a and b peptide chain synthesis. *Br. J. Haematol.* 20: 263–275.

Wood, WG, Stamatoyannopoulos, G, Lim, G, and Nute, PE. (1975). F-cells in the adult: Normal values and levels in individuals with hereditary and acquired elevations of HbF. *Blood* 46: 671–682.

Wood, WG. (1989). HbF production in adult life. In *Hemoglobin switching.* Part B: *Cellular and molecular mechanisms,* 251–267.

Wood, WG, Old, JM, Roberts, AVS et al. (1978). Human globin gene expression control of β, δ, and βδ chain production. *Cell* 15: 437–446.

Younkin, S, Oski, FA, Barness, LA, et al. (1971). Observations on the mechanism of the hydrogen peroxide hemolysis test and its reversal with phenols. *Am. J. Clin. Nutr.* 24: 7–13.

Zago, MA. (1987). G gamma-levels of the HbF of patients with bone marrow failure syndromes. *Braz. J. Med. Biol. Res.* 20: 363–368.

Zeng, Y-T, Huang, SZ, Nakatsuji, T, and Huisman, TH. (1985). G gamma A gamma-thalassemia and gamma-chain variants in Chinese newborn babies. *Am. J. Hematol.* 18: 235–242.

Zheng T, Brittain T, Watmough NJ, and Weber RE (1999). The role of amino acid α38 in the control of oxygen binding to human adult and embryonic haemoglobin Portland. *Biochem J.* 343: 681–5.

Zheng, T, Zhu, Q, and Brittain, T. (1999). Origin of the suppression of chloride ion sensitivity in human embryonic hemoglobin Gower II. *IUBMB Life* 48: 435–7.

Zielke, HR, Meny, RG, O'Brien, MJ et al. (1989). Normal fetal hemoglobin levels in the sudden infant death syndrome. *N. Engl. J. Med.* 321: 1359–1364.

Zipursky, A, Brown, E, Palko, J, and Brown, EJ. (1983). The erythrocyte differential count in newborn infants. *Am. J. Pediatr. Hematol. Oncol.* 5: 405–510.

Zon LI, Tsai SF, Burgess S et al. (1990). The major human erythroid DNA-binding protein (GF-1): Primary sequence and localization of the gene to the X chromosome *Proc. Natl. Acad. Sci. U.S.A.* 87: 668–672.

SECTION II

THE β THALASSEMIAS

BERNARD G. FORGET

Over the years, study of the thalassemia syndromes has served as a paradigm for gaining insights into the factors that can regulate or disrupt normal gene expression. The thalassemias constitute a heterogeneous group of naturally occurring, inherited mutations characterized by abnormal globin gene expression resulting in total absence or quantitative reduction of α- or β-globin chain synthesis in human erythroid cells. α Thalassemia is associated with absent or decreased production of α chains, while in the β thalassemias, there is absent or decreased production of β chains. In those cases in which some of the affected globin chain is synthesized, early studies demonstrated no evidence of an amino acid substitution. However, in all cases in which genetic evidence was available, the thalassemia gene appeared to be allelic with the structural gene encoding α or β globin. The elucidation of the nature of the various molecular lesions in thalassemia has been a fascinating process, full of surprises. Increase in our knowledge of the molecular basis of β thalassemia has closely followed, and depended on, progress and technical breakthroughs in the fields of biochemistry and molecular biology. In particular, recombinant DNA technology has contributed to a virtual explosion of new information on the precise molecular basis of most forms of thalassemia. The accrual of this knowledge has, to a great degree, paralleled the acquisition of new, detailed information on the structure, organization, and function of the normal human globin genes, as described in the preceding chapters. Historically, as new techniques have been developed for the study of protein synthesis and gene expression, they have been rapidly applied to the study of normal human hemoglobin synthesis and the abnormalities associated with abnormal globin gene expression in thalassemia. As a result, there has gradually emerged a progressively clearer and increasingly complex picture of the molecular pathology of this group of genetic disorders. One major conclusion that was drawn as this mystery unfolded was that a relatively limited number of phenotypes can result from a surprisingly large number of varied genotypes.

The chapters that follow describe in detail the knowledge and progress that have accrued over the last two to three decades on the understanding of the pathophysiology, the molecular genetics, and the clinical manifestations and management of the various β thalassemia syndromes.

There are many primary and secondary causes for the anemia observed in β thalassemia. It is easy to understand how reduced synthesis of α- and β-globin chains of HbA ($\alpha_2\beta_2$) will result in an overall deficit of hemoglobin accumulation in red cells and cause a hypochromic, microcytic anemia with a low mean corpuscular hemoglobin concentration in affected erythrocytes. This is true in both the heterozygous and homozygous states. In the homozygous state, however, another pathophysiologic process worsens the anemia and is responsible for the major clinical manifestations in the syndrome referred to as β thalassemia major or Cooley's anemia. The continued synthesis in normal amounts of normal α-globin chains results in the accumulation, within the erythroid cells, of excessive amounts of these chains. Not finding complementary globin chains with which to bind, these chains form insoluble aggregates and precipitate with the cell causing membrane damage and premature destruction of the red cells. The α-chain aggregates are called inclusion bodies or, perhaps improperly, Heinz bodies. In contrast to true Heinz bodies, which are made up of total precipitated hemoglobin tetramers, these inclusion bodies have been shown convincingly to consist of only α-globin chains, which do have some attached heme in the form of hemichromes. The process of inclusion body formation occurs not only in mature erythrocytes, but in particular in the erythroid precursor cells of the bone marrow. As a result, there is extensive intramedullary destruction of erythroid precursor cells, a process that is called ineffective erythropoiesis.

Martin H. Steinberg, Bernard G. Forget, Douglas R. Higgs, and Ronald L. Nagel, editors. *Disorders of Hemoglobin: Genetics, Pathophysiology, and Clinical Management.* © 2001 Cambridge University Press. All rights reserved.

The severity of the clinical manifestations in β thalassemia generally correlates well with the size of the free α-chain pool and the degree of α- to non-α globin chain imbalance. Therefore, the fortuitous co-inheritance of α thalassemia together with homozygous β thalassemia reduces the degree of α- to non-α globin chain imbalance and leads to a milder clinical course. Similarly, co-inheritance with β thalassemia of conditions that are associated with increased levels of synthesis of chains of HbF ($\alpha_2\gamma_2$) leads to less imbalance between α- and non-α globin chain synthesis, resulting in decreased formation of α-chain inclusion bodies, increased effective production of red cells, and their prolonged survival in the circulation.

The clinical course in most cases of homozygous β thalassemia is severe. Although anemia is not evident at birth, severe hypochromic, microcytic, hemolytic anemia develops during the first year of life and a regular transfusion program must be undertaken to maintain an adequate hemoglobin level. The clinical manifestations of homozygous β thalassemia in childhood have changed considerably over the last two to three decades owing to changes in the philosophy and practice of transfusion therapy. With modern transfusion therapy, most children will develop normally, with little or no skeletal abnormalities, and will have a reasonably good quality of life. In order to avoid iron overload from transfusional hemosiderosis, transfusion therapy is usually coupled with a vigorous program of iron chelation using parenterally administered deferoxamine. Although it is possible to maintain iron balance with such a management program, compliance is often difficult to achieve. Iron overload eventually develops in most patients and is the major cause of morbidity and mortality in young adults. The one therapy that is curative is bone marrow or stem cell transplantation, which is being increasingly practiced when feasible. The hope for the future is the development of effective oral iron chelating agents and improved approaches to gene therapy.

Studies of the molecular basis of β thalassemia have demonstrated that the gene defects responsible for the disorder are quite heterogeneous. In contrast to α thalassemia, where deletions in the α-globin gene cluster account for most of the mutations, the molecular defects associated with β thalassemia are usually point mutations involving only one (or a limited number of) nucleotide(s), but resulting in a major defect of β-globin gene expression either at the transcriptional or post-transcriptional level, including translation. Practically every conceivable type of defect in gene expression has been identified in one form or another of β thalassemia. Over 175 point mutations have been identified. Some deletion types of β thalassemia have also been described. In cases of β thalassemia where β-globin gene expression is not totally absent (so-called β⁺ thalassemia), the β chain that is synthesized is usually structurally normal. However, there is a syndrome called dominant β thalassemia in which a highly unstable, structurally abnormal β-globin chain is synthesized resulting in inclusion body formation in the heterozygous state. Finally, there are a number of β thalassemia-like disorders, called δβ thalassemia and hereditary persistence of fetal hemoglobin (HPFH), that are distinguished from the more typical forms of β thalassemia by the presence of a substantial elevation of HbF in heterozygotes, as well as in homozygotes and compound heterozygotes. These disorders are usually due to deletions of different sizes involving the β-globin gene cluster, although nondeletion types of these disorders have also been identified.

The great heterogeneity of molecular lesions causing β thalassemia may appear at first glance to create insurmountable problems in putting this knowledge to practical use in the form of prenatal diagnosis and genetic counseling. However, the availability of rapid and accurate polymerase chain reaction (PCR)-based assays for the detection of specific mutations in small samples of DNA has resulted in a number of surveys for the detection of the prevalence of different β thalassemic mutations in various population groups. The results of these surveys indicate that a given mutation is usually found only within one racial group and not another. Furthermore, a small number of different mutations, usually five or six, usually accounts for 90 percent or more of the cases of β thalassemia in a given population group. Thus, it is possible to devise efficient and precise prenatal diagnosis programs using DNA-based approaches. Such programs have led to a striking decrease in the number of new births of infants with homozygous β thalassemia in many countries where the disease is prevalent.

11

Pathophysiology of β Thalassemia

ELIEZER RACHMILEWITZ
STANLEY L. SCHRIER

In the thalassemia syndromes, the basic pathophysiology of premature hemolysis of red blood cells in the peripheral circulation and more particularly of extensive destruction of erythroid precursors in the bone marrow and in extramedullary sites (ineffective erythropoiesis) results from the excess of α- or β-globin chains due to the basic genetic defect.

HEMOLYSIS

By the classical hematologist's yardstick, the hemolysis is intracorpuscular—due to abnormalities primarily within the red cell—and extravascular—occurring primarily in the monocyte-macrophage organs with little hemoglobinemia or hemoglobinuria. In addition to abnormal red blood cell sizes and shapes and hypochromia and microcytosis, there are, depending on the phenotype, grossly abnormal shapes with fragmented forms, echinocytes, and inclusions (Fig. 11.1).

Inclusion Bodies

In 1963, Fessas noted "large, single, inclusions" in β thalassemia major normoblasts and red blood cells (Fessas, 1963). Fewer mature red blood cells had inclusions. More inclusions were seen in the red blood cells of splenectomized patients. Fessas thought that these inclusions, which stained like

Heinz bodies, were precipitated hemoglobin and deduced that they represented excess α chains (Fessas, 1963). The hemolysate of red blood cells from these patients contains free α-globin chains (Fessas and Loukopoulos, 1964) lending support to this idea. The importance of this imbalance in globin chain synthesis was emphasized by a study showing that the shortening of ^{51}Cr-labeled red blood cell survival (i.e., the extent of hemolysis) was directly correlated with the excess of α-globin chains in the red blood cells (Vigi et al., 1969). Further proof of the role of excess α-globin chains in producing hemolysis came from more recent studies showing that β thalassemia trait patients who have triplicated α-globin genes develop the classical picture of β thalassemia intermedia (Traeger-Synodinos et al., 1996). Therefore, the driving hypothesis is that the excess α-globin chains are unstable and cannot maintain a stable tetrameric structure. Consequently, an excess of α-globin chains in β thalassemia will aggregate and precipitate early in red blood cell formation, in bone marrow normoblasts, and in mature peripheral blood erythrocytes (Polliack and Rachmilewitz, 1973).

Instability of Hemoglobin Subunits In Vitro and In Vivo

Studies of structure-function relationships in normal adult hemoglobin tetramers, which are composed of two α and β chains, show that the affinity for oxygen is quite different when compared to that of the isolated chains in their native form. Therefore, besides their different functional properties, the behavior of isolated chains following oxidation is quite different from that of the normal hemoglobin tetramer. While oxidation of HbA, which occurs constantly during the life span of red blood cells, results in the formation of methemoglobin, the oxidation of either α- or β-globin subunits results in the ultimate formation of hemichrome, which has a characteristic spectrum in the visible wavelength between 500 and 700 mμ (Fig. 11.2) (Rachmilewitz, 1974). The change to hemichrome was preceded by the appearance of methemoglobin (Fig. 11.2). Hemichromes, which are found following oxidation of either α-, β-, or γ-globin subunits, are unstable and precipitate with time.

The basic structure of hemichromes results from the covalent binding of the distal histidine E7 to the sixth coordination position of the heme iron in a similar axial arrangement as that of the proximal histidine F8 (Fig. 11.3). A better understanding of the structure of hemichromes was obtained using electron paramag-

Martin H. Steinberg, Bernard G. Forget, Douglas R. Higgs, and Ronald L. Nagel, editors. *Disorders of Hemoglobin: Genetics, Pathophysiology, and Clinical Management.* © 2001 Cambridge University Press. All rights reserved.

A

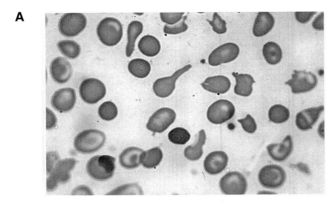

B

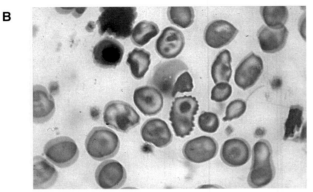

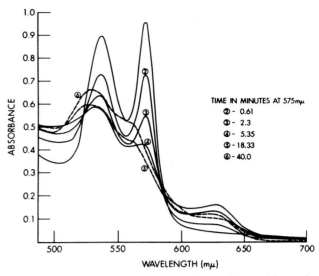

Figure 11.1. Peripheral blood smears of patients with β thalassemia intermedia. (A) Nonsplenectomized patient and (B) splenectomized patient. For full color reproduction, see color plate 11.1.

Figure 11.2. Denaturation of the normal and abnormal hemoglobin molecule. Spectrophotometric changes during the oxidation of oxy α-globin subunits separated by paramercuribenzoate (PMB): The unnumbered curve represents the oxy subunit before the addition of fourfold excess of ferricyanide. Note the transient appearance of methemoglobin with absorption peak at 630 mμ followed by hemichrome (broken lines 5 and 6), with major absorption at 535 mμ and a shoulder at 565 mμ. (From Rachmilewitz, 1974, with permission.)

netic resonance spectroscopy (EPR), which can distinguish between high and low spin forms of ferric heme proteins (Peisach et al., 1971). Consequently, four types of hemichromes have been identified, two reversible and two irreversible, in red blood cells from patients with various forms of thalassemia. Only irreversible hemichromes were found in membrane ghosts of cells containing numerous precipitated globin subunits (Heinz bodies, HbH bodies) (Rachmilewitz et al., 1969) while reversible hemichromes were found in soluble hemoglobin. The formation of irreversible from reversible hemichromes is a time-dependent reaction as observed following spontaneous denaturation of isolated oxidized α- and β-globin chains (Rachmilewitz et al., 1971), which in fact is the situation within thalassemic erythrocytes. One can therefore conclude that there is a similarity between the properties of globin subunits prepared and oxidized in vitro and the behavior of the same subunits in vivo.

Therefore, it seems that the interaction between different and similar globin subunits plays a substantial role in maintaining the stability of the hemoglobin molecule. Because α-globin chains dissociate into monomers more readily than β- or γ-globin chains, they form more hemichromes as compared to the other two

Figure 11.3. Denaturation of the normal and abnormal hemoglobin molecule. The model illustrates the changes in the structure around the heme group of oxidized hemoglobin subunits following removal of the water molecule. The double bond between the iron and the proximal (F8) and distal (E7) histidines is thought to be the structure present in heme proteins which have the characteristic absorption spectrum of hemichromes. (From Rachmilewitz, 1974, with permission.)

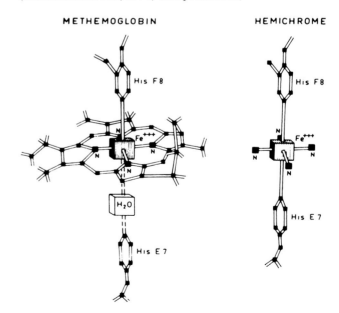

subunits. The reasons for the difference in stability between tetramers of β and γ chains are not known.

Different in vitro kinetics of hemichrome formation and precipitation of the three major hemoglobin chains, α, β, and γ, correspond closely to the instability of the different excess individual subunits in the various types of thalassemic red blood cells. In β thalassemia, α chains precipitate early in the course of hemoglobin synthesis and form inclusion bodies early during differentiation of young nucleated erythroid cells in the bone marrow (Polliack et al., 1974), whereas only very small amounts of soluble α subunits can be detected. Greater stability is exhibited by excess hemoglobin H ($β_4$), which undergoes progressive precipitation with the formation of Heinz bodies, particularly in mature red blood cells (Rachmilewitz et al., 1969) (see Chapter 16). γ-Globin chains, when present in excess, do not form Heinz bodies, in vivo, because they are more stable in solution than β and α chains. This difference may also explain why one cannot expect the amounts of HbH and Hb Bart, calculated on the basis of electrophoretic separation, to be identical when there are equal amounts of β- and γ-globin chains in the red blood cells.

All of these denatured components can affect the material properties of red blood cells that allow these cells of 7 to 8 μm in diameter to elongate, tank tread, and otherwise deform to pass through capillaries of 3 μm in diameter and 2 μm slits in the reticuloendothelial system sinusoids (see Chapter 21). Alternatively, but not exclusively, the surface of the red blood cells can be altered to provide signal recognition by macrophages, which can lead to the removal of the affected cells from the circulation.

Mechanical Properties

Characterization of the mechanical properties of β-thalassemic red blood cells is important because the shapes of the red blood cells are so grossly abnormal and because of the demonstration (Teitel, 1977) that impaired filterability—reduced deformability—correlates with the in vivo shortening of ^{51}Cr-labeled red blood cell survival.

Red Blood Cell Deformability.

Using osmotic gradient ektacytometry (see Chapter 22) red blood cells from nonsplenectomized and splenectomized patients with β thalassemia intermedia were found to be more rigid than normal red blood cells (Schrier et al., 1989). There are three major determinants of red blood cells deformability (see Chapter 22): the ratio of surface area to volume (SA/V), the MCHC or hemoglobin concentration per cell, and the membrane per se. Osmotic gradient ektacytometry permits the analysis of these factors. The red blood cells from nonsplenectomized patients had reduced deformability but the SA/V was in fact increased. Surprisingly, there seemed to be an interaction of hemoglobin with the membrane that contributed to the cellular rigidity and altered the membrane. Red blood cells from splenectomized patients with β thalassemia intermedia were even more rigid in the physiologic range of osmolality. However, the deformability of these cells became almost normal at very low osmolality (150 mOsm). The SA/V was not reduced. Interestingly, there was even more evidence of hemoglobin interaction with the membrane in cells from nonsplenectomized patients and these alterations took place at a normal MCHC of 32.9 (Schrier et al., 1989). This is in striking contrast to the finding in sickle cell anemia where this sort of interaction occurs at pathologically high MCHCs in the high 30s and low 40s (Fortier et al., 1988) (Fig. 11.4).

Membrane Deformability.

Isolated red blood cell membranes were also studied and membranes from nonsplenectomized patients were 2.5 to 3 times more rigid than controls. Osmotic gradient ektacytometry showed that membranes from splenectomized patients were only 1.3 times more rigid than normal (Fig. 11.5). It had been previously shown (Fortier et al., 1988) that even in β thalassemia trait, membrane rigidity was directly correlated with the amount of hemoglobin-spectrin complex formation, which in turn was dependent on the MCHC. It was proposed that these complexes formed in vivo as a consequence of oxidative attack (Fortier et al., 1988).

Membrane Stability.

Isolated membranes from splenectomized β thalassemia patients were very unstable and fragmented readily, whereas membranes from nonsplenectomized patients were either normal or slightly unstable (Fig. 11.5). Interpretation of these changes is complex. It is likely that the spleen removes the red blood cells with the most unstable membranes—those most likely to undergo fragmentation. Thus, in the postsplenectomy state many fragmented red blood cells with unstable membranes survive (Schrier et al., 1989). These cells also have an uncharacterized abnormality that allows their hemoglobin (normal HbA) to interact with the membrane (Schrier et al., 1989) to produce whole red cell rigidity. The explanation for the increased membrane rigidity of nonsplenectomized red blood cells is not apparent.

Biochemical Abnormalities Accompanying Alterations in Mechanical Properties

Red blood cell rigidity. In severe β thalassemia, the SA/V is greater than normal but surprisingly, given the

A

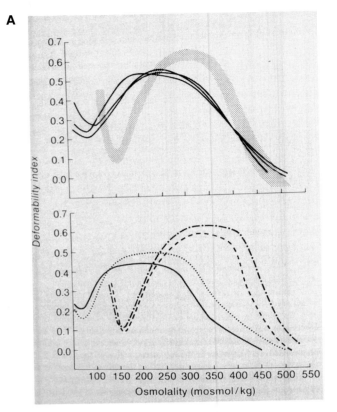

B

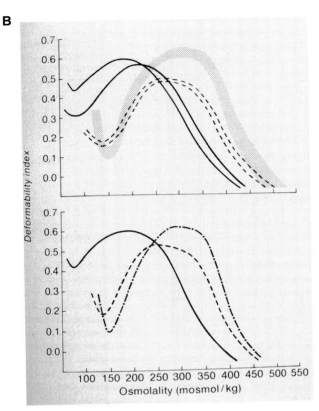

Figure 11.4A. Osmotic deformability profiles of HbH disease erythrocytes. In the top panel are shown the deformability profiles for whole blood from three different individuals. The hatched area represents the variations for normal controls. In the bottom panel are shown the deformability profiles for subpopulations of density-fractionated normal cells: MCHC, 29.6 g/dL (—·—) or 31.5 g/dL (- - -); and HbH disease erythrocytes: MCHC, 29.6 g/dL (····) or 31.5 g/dL (—).

Figure 11.4B. Osmotic deformability profiles of β thalassemia intermedia erythrocytes. In the top panel are shown the deformability profiles for whole blood from two different splenectomized individuals with β thalassemia (—) and two nonsplenectomized individuals with β thalassemia (- - - -). The hatched area represents the variations for normal controls. In the bottom panel are shown the deformability profiles for a subpopulation of cells with a narrowly defined range of cell densities (MCHC, 32.9 g/dL) obtained from whole blood of a normal donor (—·—), a nonsplenectomized β-thalassemic donor (- - - -), and a splenectomized β-thalassemic donor (—). (From Schrier et al., 1989, with permission.)

decrease in hemoglobin per cell, there are populations of dense dehydrated thalassemic red blood cells (Schrier et al., 1989) (see below). Furthermore, at normal MCHC values of 32.9, there is an unexplained strong interaction of normal HbA with the membrane of the thalassemic cells producing erythrocyte rigidity (Schrier et al., 1989). This is more prominent in red blood cells of postsplenectomized subjects with β thalassemia intermedia, suggesting that populations of red blood cells with these characteristics are selectively removed by the spleen. The membrane contributions to red blood cells rigidity are described next.

Membrane rigidity. Isolated β-thalassemic membranes, particularly from nonsplenectomized subjects, are very rigid (Schrier et al., 1989). The membrane skeletons prepared from red blood cells from such patients are grossly abnormal by scanning and transmission electron microscopy (Fig. 11.6).

SDS gel electrophoresis showed these deposits were globin (Rachmilewitz et al., 1985; Shinar et al., 1987). Subsequent studies showed that this membrane skeletal-bound globin was virtually all α globin and that it was partially oxidized (Advani et al., 1992b). The likely explanation for the membrane rigidity rests on the changes produced by binding of partially oxidized α-globin chains to the membrane and its skeleton. These changes could be mass effects or the consequences of oxidant attack (see below). Furthermore, detailed analyses of membrane skeletons showed that they retained about twice as much band 3 (the major red blood cell integral membrane protein (see Chapter 22) as controls. Interaction of band 3 with the skeleton lattice is likely to produce membrane rigidity as is the case when another inte-

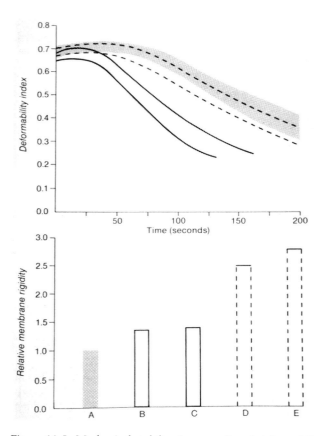

Figure 11.5. Mechanical stability (top panel) and deformability (bottom panel) of membranes from β-thalassemic erythrocytes. Membrane fragmentation curves for resealed ghosts prepared from whole blood samples of two splenectomized (—) and two nonsplenectomized (- - - -) individuals with β- thalassemia are shown in the top panel. The hatched area represents the variations in the fragmentation curves for normal membranes. Relative rigidity of β-thalassemic erythrocyte membranes is illustrated in the bottom panel. The relative rigidity of membranes of erythrocytes from splenectomized individuals is (**B** and **C** are marginally increased) compared to normal (**A**), while those from nonsplenectomized individuals (**D** and **E**) are substantially increased. (From Schrier et al., 1989, with permission.)

gral membrane protein, glycophorin A, is induced to bind to the membrane skeleton (Chasis et al., 1988).

Membrane instability. β thalassemia intermedia membranes are unstable (Schrier et al., 1989), particularly when they are isolated from splenectomized patients. This suggests that the cells with most unstable membranes are removed by the spleen. Since membrane stability depends heavily on the structure-function properties of the membrane skeleton, studies of β thalassemia intermedia skeletal proteins were undertaken.

Protein 4.1, a key component of the skeleton, is defective in β thalassemia intermedia with a 50 percent reduction in the ability of protein 4.1 of β-thalassemic red blood cells to mediate the critical formation of the spectrin-protein 4.1-actin ternary complex (Shinar et al., 1989). A clue to the abnormal function of protein 4.1 in β thalassemia came from studies showing that it had undergone partial oxidation (Advani et al., 1992b). Some authors (Lamchiagdhase et al., 1987) but not others (Shinar et al., 1989) report a defect in formation of spectrin tetramers from spectrin dimers. The skeletal lattice is critically dependent on spectrin tetramer formation. The entire skeletal lattice may be somewhat reduced in density because small amounts of spectrin, actin, and protein 4.1 are found in the first lysate used in the preparation of hypotonic red blood cell membranes. This finding suggested that β-thalassemic membrane skeletal proteins are not assembled normally (Yuan et al., 1995). A decrease in membrane spectrin was directly correlated with the amount of insoluble α chains and was also associated with a decrease in

Figure 11.6. Scanning electron micrograph of red blood cell membrane skeletons from a normal control (**A**) and a splenectomized β thalassemia intermedia patient (**B**). (Original magnification ×6,000) (From Shinar et al., 1987, with permission.)

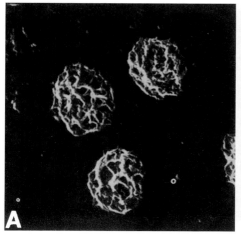

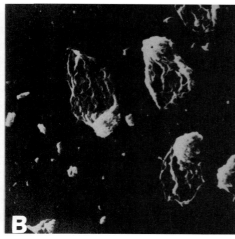

membrane ankyrin, a protein that links the skeleton to the major transmembrane protein band 3 (Rouyer-Fessardt et al., 1989). Furthermore, the very active red cells and red cell membrane associated proteases in β thalassemia could degrade some membrane proteins. This topic is not discussed explicitly in the literature, but anyone who works with β thalassemia red blood cell membranes quickly learns to add "cocktails" of protease inhibitors to virtually all of the preparatory steps to avoid the multiple gel bands indicative of protease action (Yuan et al., 1995).

There is in vitro support for the role of aggregated α chains in producing red cell and membrane rigidity. When purified α-globin chains were resealed within normal red blood cells and then incubated for about 20 hours there was a progressive increase in membrane-associated α chains accompanied by an increase in cell rigidity and the rigidity of isolated membranes (Scott et al., 1990, 1992). Because these changes were associated with loss of membrane thiols and evidence of oxidation of membrane proteins (Scott et al., 1990, 1992, 1993) (see below), it was proposed that the associated iron, heme, and hemichromes of the α-globin chains produced oxidant damage.

OXIDATIVE DENATURATION AND DEGRADATION OF HEMOGLOBIN IN β THALASSEMIA

To perform its major role in oxygen transport, the red cell has to deal with a potentially hazardous burden of hemoglobin, oxygen and iron, and expose itself to oxidative reactions that are associated with cell breakdown (Pryor, 1977). The major danger to the integrity of the red blood cells is the potential ability of its oxidative products to interact and damage their membrane components. Denaturation of oxyhemoglobin results in the formation of methemoglobin, hemichromes, and inclusion bodies (Heinz bodies) (Rachmilewitz, 1974), while degradation of the hemoglobin molecule results in the formation of three different components: denatured globin, heme, and iron. Each one of these metabolites, created in the two different pathways, will alter the normal structure of the red cell membrane, and consequently result in its removal from the circulation (Shinar and Rachmilewitz, 1993).

The most toxic breakdown products of the hemoglobin molecule are hemichromes, which associate tightly with the cytoplasmic domain of protein band 3 (Waugh and Low, 1985) and promote clustering of band 3 in the membrane. It has already been mentioned that in thalassemia, excessive α-, β-, or γ-globin subunits within the red cell are unstable and tend to oxidize readily to hemichromes and precipitate in the membrane. The same mechanism operates not only in the peripheral blood, but also in erythroid precursors

in β thalassemia patients (see below) and may explain, at least in part, the intramedullary hemolysis. The formation of hemichromes as a prime determinant of the severity of the anemia with the consequent clinical manifestations is true not only in thalassemia, but also in unstable hemoglobin variants (Chapter 44) and in sickle cell anemia (Rachmilewitz, 1974).

Following hemoglobin oxidation, the excess globin subunits disintegrate to form excess globin chains that bind to various membrane compounds. In β thalassemia, the precipitation of excess α-globin chains affects the major cytoskeletal protein spectrin, possibly by cross-linking the two proteins (see above). While the impaired structure of spectrin may not result in major alteration in its function, the structure of protein 4.1 has been changed and consequently there is decreased ability of the binding of spectrin (see above) to actin, which is a crucial function to maintain normal cytoskeleton stability (Shinar et al., 1989; Shinar and Rachmilewitz, 1990) (Fig. 11.7). The role of excess α-globin chains in modifying the rheological and mechanical behavior of β-thalassemic red blood cells was provided by Scott (Scott et al., 1990) and by Schrier (Schrier and Mohandas, 1992) in experiments in vitro, which mimic the existing conditions in β thalassemia.

In HbH disease, a severe form of α thalassemia, abnormal interactions were found among ankyrin and spectrin, the cytoplasmic domain of band 3 and the irreversible hemichromes morphologically identified as Heinz bodies (Shinar and Rachmilewitz, 1990) (Fig. 11.7) (see Chapter 16). These changes in ankyrin were not found in β thalassemia, where the excess α chains, being more unstable than the β chains, precipitate early in young nucleated red cells both in the nucleus and cytoplasm before reacting with specific sites on the membrane (Polliack et al., 1974; Shinar et al., 1989). Additional support for the damaging effects of membrane-associated globin on different skeletal proteins was obtained by studying interactions between α- and β-globin chains in normal red cell membranes (Shalev et al., 1988).

Another potential cause for severe toxicity to the red cell membrane is excess iron. Normally, free iron is separated from the cell membrane, thereby preventing iron ions from catalyzing lipid and protein peroxidation via the "Fenton" reaction (Hebbel, 1985) (see Chapter 22). In thalassemia, increased amounts of nonheme iron were identified first morphologically and then chemically (Polliack and Rachmilewitz, 1973; Jacobs et al., 1981), in reticulocytes and normoblasts, which contained large amounts of iron either as free particles or as aggregates of ferritin and/or hemosiderin (Polliack and Rachmilewitz, 1973). High levels of non-transferrin–bound iron, loosely bound to plasma proteins, were found in the

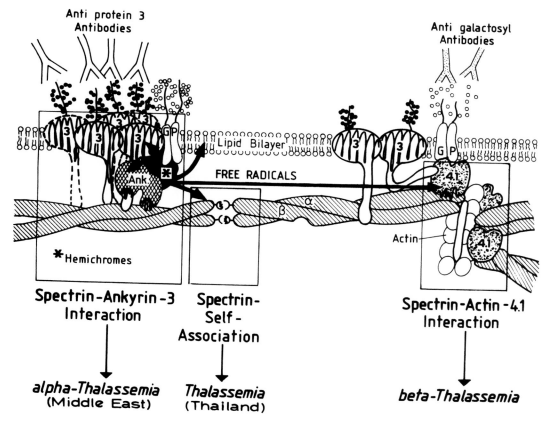

Figure 11.7. Oxidative denaturation of red blood cells in thalassemia. Schematic representation of red blood cell membrane structure. Depicted are the lipid bilayer; the integral membrane proteins, protein 3 (3) and glycophorins (GP); and the membrane skeleton proteins spectrin, actin, ankyrin (Ank), and protein 4.1. Black arrows represent possible routes of oxidative damage generated during hemichrome (HEM) denaturation and directed against different membrane components. The different alterations in cytoskeletal interactions are shown with specific relationships to the different thalassemic syndromes. (From Shinar and Rachmilewitz, 1990, with permission.)

Figure 11.8. Deferiprone (L1) chelates pathologic iron deposits from membranes of intact thalassemic and sickle red blood cells both in vitro and in vivo. Membrane free iron (mean +/− SD) in red blood cells from patients with β thalassemia intermedia before and during treatment with various doses of L1; n, number of patients treated at each L1 dosage. P values refer to differences from red blood cell membrane free iron level before L1 therapy. (From Shalev et al., 1995, with permission.)

plasma of thalassemia patients (Graham et al., 1979). The amounts of intracellular iron were much higher in splenectomized patients and were found to be closely associated with denatured hemoglobin in the membranes, mostly with hemichromes and other aggregates of membrane protein (Repka et al., 1993). Consequently, the orally administered iron chelator deferiprone (L1) (see Chapter 37), which has an enhanced capacity to permeate cell membranes, was able to remove free iron from β-thalassemic red cell membranes in a dose-related fashion (Fig. 11.8). Both in vivo and in vitro, L1 alleviated membrane damage possibly mediated by catalytic iron, such as lipid peroxidation, measured by increased levels of malonyldialdehyde, and hemichrome formation and also reduced the KCl cotransporter activity (Shalev et al., 1995; De Franceschi et al., 1999).

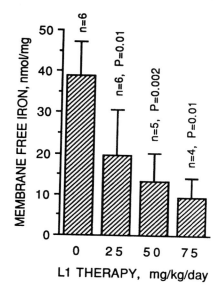

Heme and/or hemin will only be exposed to oxidant stress when the structure of the heme-protecting carrier protein, globin, is altered as occurs in the different hemoglobinopathies, particularly in β thalassemia. Membrane lipids and proteins are the main target of oxidation induced by heme due to its capacity to catalyze the formation of oxygen radicals such as superoxide (Aft and Mueller, 1984; Vincent, 1989). Abnormal heme loss involves the integrity of both α- and β-globin chains in both forms of thalassemia. Although β-globin chains lose heme much faster than α chains, the latter are more likely to autooxidize (Bunn and Jandl, 1968).

Hemin, the oxidized form of heme, is also found during oxidative denaturation of hemoglobin, and like heme, interacts with membrane skeletal proteins leading to the initiation of in situ oxidative damage to the neighboring lipids and proteins of the kind that has been described in β thalassemia (Chiu and Lubin, 1989). However, there is still a need for direct measurements of hemin levels in β-thalassemic red cells and membranes in order to add further support to its role in the severe hemolysis in the thalassemia syndromes.

CELL HYDRATION

Red blood cell hydration plays an important role in determining their deformability (Chapter 22). Hemoglobin concentration is a major determinant of intracellular viscosity. β-thalassemic red blood cells uniformly have a low hemoglobin content even in heterozygotes (Rund et al., 1992). Therefore, it was unexpected to find in β thalassemia trait (Fortier et al., 1988) that 10 percent of erythrocytes had an MCHC greater than 37 and 2 percent of cells had an MCHC greater than 45. Surprisingly, when specific cell density gradient profiles were performed on β thalassemia intermedia red blood cells (Schrier et al., 1989) (Fig. 11.9) there were dense cell populations in both nonsplenectomized and splenectomized subjects. Red cell volume is controlled by a complex interplay between pores, channels, and pumps (Canessa, 1991) (see Chapter 22). One important volume controller is the KCl cotransport system, which normally functions in reticulocytes and appears to be involved in the remodeling process by which reticulocytes lose volume from an MCV of about 110 fl to the MCV of 85 to 95 fl of normal mature red cells. This cotransporter responds to volume and pH in such a way that there is K⁺ efflux with volume loss. The KCl cotransporter stays open in red blood cells containing HbS or HbC, leading to K⁺ efflux followed by water loss that leads to the cellular dehydration seen in sickle cell anemia and HbSC disease (Olivieri et al., 1992) (see Chapter 27). KCl cotransport system is also activated beyond the reticulocyte stage in patients with β tha-

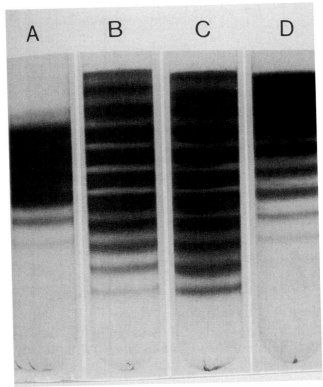

Figure 11.9. Analysis of the density distribution of normal erythrocytes. (A) erythrocytes from a nonsplenectomized individual with β thalassemia intermedia; (B) erythrocytes from a splenectomized individual with β thalassemia intermedia (C); and HbH disease erythrocytes (D) on discontinuous Stractan-density gradients. The gradients covered a density range from 1.065 to 1.130 g/mL in increments of ~0.0045 g/mL. (From Schrier et al., 1989, with permission.)

lassemia intermedia, probably accounting in part for the dehydration that is observed (Schrier et al., 1989; Olivieri et al., 1992; De Franceschi et al., 1999). The onset of red blood cell dehydration could occur as a consequence of the alterations resulting from the extended circulation of red cells, or be induced during intramedullary erythropoiesis. When this question was studied using the Bayer Technicon H-3, it became apparent that in β thalassemia intermedia there were populations of reticulocytes that were already profoundly dehydrated (Fig. 11.10). This finding, in stark contrast to results observed in HbH disease (see Chapter 16), indicates that events within the marrow triggered by α-chain accumulation produced lesions leading to the heterogeneous pattern of cellular dehydration.

CALCIUM TRANSPORT IN THALASSEMIC RED BLOOD CELLS

A high total Ca content was found in thalassemic red blood cells, particularly in splenectomized patients

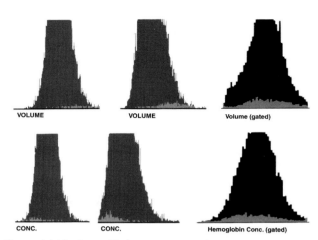

Figure 11.10. Bayer Technicon H-3 analysis of red blood cells from normals (left), β thalassemia intermedia (right), and HbH disease (center). Top row displays MCV (volume) and the bottom row displays MCHC (hemoglobin concentration). The more lightly shaded area at the bottom of each display represents reticulocytes.

(Shalev et al., 1984; Bookchin et al., 1988). However, unlike red blood cells from sickle cell patients, most of the Ca was found in the younger cells, was not mobilized by ionophore, and was apparently tightly bound to organelles in nucleated and other young red cells. The Ca permeability of β-thalassemic cell membranes, however, was found to be normal or minimally increased. and the Ca pump was normal. Most of the cellular Ca was probably compartmentalized in the endocytic inside-out vesicles. Because the levels of [Ca^{++}] were normal in these cells, the high content of total Ca is not associated with the deleterious effects observed with increased levels of [Ca^{++}] in vitro, such as ATP depletion, sodium pump inhibition, or membrane protein cross-linking (Bookchin et al., 1988). Similar results were obtained by another group that studied thalassemic red blood cells from different populations (Rhoda et al., 1987). However, intracellular Ca can activate proteases (Cohen and Gascard, 1992) and in spite of the trapping of the calcium within inside-out vesicles (Bookchin et al., 1988), small but sufficient amounts may be available to produce activation of proteases.

PHAGOCYTOSIS BY MACROPHAGES

Hemoglobin denaturation induces microscopic changes in the external topography of sickle erythrocytes (Waugh et al., 1986). These microscopic clusters, which contain hemichromes and less than 1 percent of the band 3 population of the cell (Kannan et al., 1988), are rapidly opsonized with autologous

IgG and complement. The deposition of IgG and complement at several of the microscopic clusters triggers the recognition and removal of the cell by macrophages. These changes have also been observed in membranes of β-thalassemic red cells (Yuan et al., 1992). Several additional factors may contribute to alterations in thalassemia membrane structure and function. Among them are changes in cell rigidity and deformability, which have been discussed above. Also there is increased exposure of β-galactosyl residues (Galili et al., 1983), which could result from the accelerated removal and distribution of sialic acid residues found in the glycophorin portion of thalassemia cell membranes (Kahane et al., 1978, 1980). Exposed "unmasked" cryptic antigenic sites of galactosyl residues may initiate their binding with naturally occurring antigalactosyl IgG antibodies and consequently their removal by macrophages (Galili et al., 1983).

Multiple factors may contribute to the removal of thalassemic red cells from the circulation. Included among them are changes in cell rigidity, deformability, exposure of galactosyl residues, and the binding of autologous IgG to hemichromes and band 3. All of these factors alter the normal exposure and composition of antigens on the outer surface of the membrane and consequently cause erythrophagocytosis by macrophages.

Using mouse peritoneal macrophages, it was found that red blood cells from splenectomized patients were phagocytized 22-fold higher than cells from normal donors. The phagocytized cells consisted of both mature and nucleated red blood cells (Knyszynski et al., 1979). The cells that seem to be involved in the phagocytosis are monocytes, which attached to threefold as many red blood cells from β^0 thalassemia/HbE disease compound heterozygotes as to normal red cells (Wanachiwanawin et al., 1993). It is possible that the activation of mononuclear phagocytes plays a role in determining the severity of the anemia in β thalassemia because there was also a threefold increase in the percentage of leukocytes expressing the Fc-gamma receptor in β^0 thalassemia/HbE disease.

In serum of patients with HbH disease and β^0 thalassemia/HbE disease there was also an increase in macrophage colony-stimulating factor, which may enhance the effector function of the mononuclear phagocytes on pathologic red cells (Wiener et al., 1996). Membrane phosphatidylserine (PS) is also recognized by macrophages as a signal for attachment and phagocytosis. Normally, PS is confined to the inner surface of the membrane phospholipid bilayer (Chapter 22) and thus does not provide a signal to macrophages. However in some β-thalassemic cells, the membrane phospholipid bilayer is oxidized (Rachmilewitz et al., 1976) and is scrambled such that some PS moves to the outer leaflet (Borenstain et al., 1993). Detailed studies revealed that usually only a small population of β-thalassemic cells, detected by a fluorescently labeled annexin V probe, have exofacial PS, some of which appears to be caused by the oxidation induced by α-globin chain aggregates (Kuypers et al., 1998).

INEFFECTIVE ERYTHROPOIESIS–INTRAMEDULLARY HEMOLYSIS

Events That Take Place in β-Thalassemic Erythroid Precursors

Kinetics. For much of the 1900s—until the use of kinetic studies—β thalassemia was defined as a hereditary hemolytic disease. In Cooley's anemia there had been clinical awareness of the discrepancy between the severity of the anemia and the related extraordinary increase in intra- as well as extramedullary erythropoiesis versus the relatively modest reticulocytosis. These discrepancies were resolved when isotopes came into use in clinical hematology and showed that there was enormous ineffective erythropoiesis in severe β thalassemia (Finch et al., 1970). Using ferrokinetic analysis, it was discovered in normal subjects that 75 percent to 90 percent of ^{59}Fe that entered marrow erythropoiesis appeared in circulating red blood cells in 7 to 10 days. In contrast, in some cases of Cooley's anemia, 15 percent of ^{59}Fe was incorporated in circulating erythrocytes (Finch et al., 1970), indicating that the extent of ineffective erythropoiesis or intramedullary hemolysis could account for as much as 60 percent to 75 percent of total erythropoiesis. In a general hypothesis of β thalassemia pathophysiology, accumulation of excess α-globin chains, either soluble or more likely in aggregated precipitated forms, is the proximate cause for most abnormalities found.

Populations of reticulocytes are found in peripheral blood of patients with β thalassemia intermedia that are already profoundly dehydrated. This would indicate that the defect in volume control occurred during erythropoiesis (see above and Fig. 11.10). Studies described below further focus on observations identifying events occurring during β-thalassemic erythropoiesis that play a major role in the pathophysiology of the disease.

Morphology. Ultrastructural studies revealed several abnormalities in orthochromic normoblasts in patients with Cooley's anemia. These included glycogen accumulation, plasma membrane enfolding, vacuole formation, hyaline figures, and Heinz bodies (Polliack and Rachmilewitz, 1973). Polychromatophilic and orthochromic erythroblasts contained cyto-

plasmic aggregates of electron dense material (Wickramasinghe and Bush, 1975), which on the basis of prior biochemical analysis (Fessas et al., 1966) were thought to be aggregates of α chains. β-thalassemic erythroid precursors containing apparent α-globin chain precipitates had decreased protein synthetic capacities (Wickramasinghe et al., 1973). Iron-loaded mitochondria were also seen, paralleling the ringed sideroblasts seen in the myelodysplastic syndromes where ineffective erythropoiesis also helps account for anemia (Wickramasinghe and Hughes, 1980). Final proof that the aggregates were α-globin chains came from studies using an anti-α-globin monoclonal antibody combined with laser confocal fluorescence microscopy (Yuan et al., 1993) (Fig. 11.11). These studies (Yuan et al., 1993) also confirmed the heterogeneity of the α-globin deposition (Polliack and Rachmilewitz, 1973; Wickramasinghe and Bush, 1975; Wickramasinghe and Hughes, 1980) and showed that large aggregates of α chains occurred as early as the proerythroblast stage. The heterogeneity of the α-chain deposition has been an unresolved problem. One hypothesis was that the erythroid precursors that were capable of turning on fetal globin gene expression and thus synthesizing γ-globin chains would be protected from the deposition of excess unmatched α-globin chains. However this hypothesis was disproved by studies using monoclonal anti-α-globin chain antibody where erythroid precursors with large amounts of α-globin deposits also had large amounts of γ-globin chains (Wickramasinghe and Lee, 1997).

Figure 11.11. Laser confocal immunofluorescence showing the deposition of α-globin chains in β thalassemia major erythroid precursors. The erythroid precursors were fixed on Alcian blue-coated cover slips and permeabilized with 0.5% Triton X-100 in phosphate-buffered saline. The cells were then reacted with monoclonal anti-α-globin chain antibody for 1 hour at room temperature and Texas Red-labeled goat anti-mouse IgG for 30 minutes at room temperature. (From Yuan et al., 1993, with permission.)

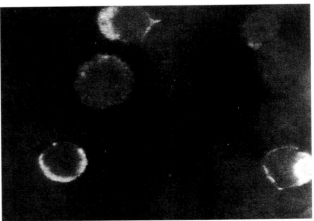

Assembly of Membrane Proteins in β-Thalassemic Erythroid Precursors. The Bone Marrow Transplantation Program at Pesaro, Italy (Chapter 39) provided the opportunity to obtain and study marrow erythroid precursors from patients with Cooley's anemia. Studies were done on isolated erythroid precursors using specific antibodies and the results were analyzed by laser confocal fluorescence microscopy. In normal erythroid precursors, the membrane skeleton proteins, spectrin and band 4.1, as well as the major transmembrane protein band 3 (see Chapter 22) are generally incorporated smoothly and in an orderly rim fashion into membranes (Fig. 11.12). In contrast, in Cooley's anemia erythroid precursors spectrin (Fig. 11.13) and particularly band 4.1 (Fig. 11.14) incorporation was frequently clumped, disorderly, and discontinuous (Aljurf et al., 1996). When double immunofluorescence was performed using antibodies to α-globin chains and also antibodies to spectrin and band 4.1, there was clear evidence of colocalization of α-chain aggregates with abnormal areas of incorporation of spectrin and particularly of band 4.1 into the membrane skeleton (Fig. 11.12). The evidence suggested that α-chain aggregates damage adjacent skeletal proteins either by mass action or by the oxidant injury induced by the α-chain-associated iron, heme, or hemichromes. Additionally, there was evidence of a decrease in band 3 incorporation into β thalassemia erythroid precursor membranes at the proerythroblast and basophilic erythroblast stages. However, band 3 incorporation into polychromatophilic and orthochromic erythroblasts was virtually normal (Aljurf et al., 1996). Band 3 incorporation, when it occurred, was always in a smooth rim pattern and never colocalized with α-globin chain aggregates. Thus, the deficit in band 3 incorporation that occurred early in erythropoiesis is either corrected after further maturation or the erythroid precursors that are deficient in band 3 are destroyed (Aljurf et al., 1996).

Apoptosis (Programmed Cell Death). Intramedullary death of 60 percent to 75 percent of erythroid precursors, as detected by ferrokinetic analysis, led to a conceptual problem. Such a large number of cells dying by necrosis should have left a large morphologically detectable collection of degenerating erythroid precursors. This was not observed and led to the consideration that apoptosis (programmed cell death) could be playing a major role in the ineffective erythropoiesis of β thalassemia. Studies then revealed that accelerated or enhanced apoptosis occurred in Cooley's anemia erythroid precursors as detected by DNA ladder formation (Yuan et al., 1993) (Fig. 11.15), alteration in DNA (Angelucci et al., 1996, 1997), and the movement of PS to the membrane outer leaflet (Angelucci et al., 1996, 1997). Cells undergoing programmed cell death seem to signal this fact to neighboring macrophages and are expeditiously removed by phagocytosis. One of the signals is thought to be the apoptosis-associated movement of PS to the outer membrane leaflet (Fig. 11.16).

Figure 11.12. Normal and thalassemic marrow erythroid precursors in paired experiments were fixed, permeabilized, and reacted with specific antibodies. The cells were first reacted with Texas Red-labeled rabbit polyclonal antibodies to either band 3, band 4.1, or spectrin, and then with monoclonal FITC-labeled anti-α globin. α-Globin reactivity was never detected in normal erythroid precursors because the antibody detects only denatured or aggregated α-globin. Note smooth rim fluorescence in normals. Overlapping green and red fluorescence produced brilliant yellow fluorescence, indicating colocalization. For full color reproduction, see color plate 11.12. (From Aljurf et al., 1996, with permission.)

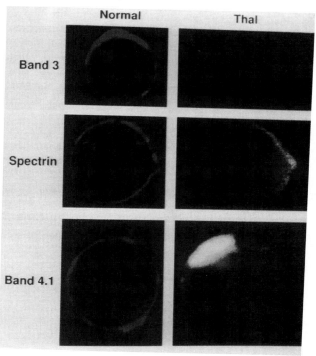

Biochemical and Structural Differences Between β and α Thalassemia and Their Implications on Red Blood Cell Survival

Earlier literature tended to assume that the pathophysiology of α and β thalassemia were quite similar. While there was clearly a difference with regard to which globin chain accumulated in excess, both variants produced a hypochromic microcytic anemia characterized by target cells, increased unconjugated bilirubin, and in the more severe forms, splenomegaly and expansion of erythroid marrow.

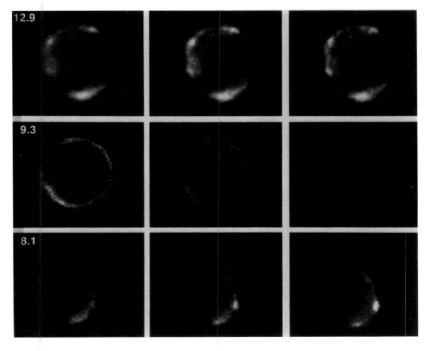

Figure 11.13. Incorporation of spectrin into thalassemic erythroid precursors. The middle three cuts at the cell's maximum diameter (equatorial cuts) are shown. The top row shows three sequential images through a proerythroblast of 12.9 μm diameter, the middle row through a polychromatophilic erythroblast of 9.3 μm diameter and the bottom row is through an orthochromic normoblast of 8.1 μm diameter. For full color reproduction, see color plate 11.13. (From Aljurf et al., 1996, with permission.)

Figure 11.14. Incorporation of band 4.1 into two thalassemic polychromatophilic erythroblasts of 10.4 (top row) and 9.5 (bottom row) μm diameter showing three equatorial cuts spaced at 0.5 μm. Note the very abnormal incorporation as well as band 4.1 overlying the nucleus. For full color reproduction, see color plate 11.14. (From Aljurf et al., 1996, with permission.)

Now it is apparent that the pathophysiologies of α and β thalassemia are very different and it is highly likely that the differences are determined by the biochemical differences of α- and β-globin chains. β-Globin chains have two thiols while α-globin chains have only one. β Globin can form soluble tetramers while α globin does not (see above). Thus, the accumulation of these specific globin chains in erthyroid precursors and on red blood cell membrane skeletons produces very different pathophysiologic manifestations.

Using the power of ferrokinetic studies, it was recognized that in severe β thalassemia there was profound ineffective erythropoiesis with ^{59}Fe red cell utilization values of between 20 percent and 40 percent with occasional values as low as 15 percent (Finch et al., 1970). Comparably, anemic patients with severe α thalassemia have a modest degree of intramedullary erythroid cell death with ^{59}Fe red blood cell utilization values occasionally as low as 50 percent but ranging up to 70 percent.

The mechanical properties of the red blood cell membrane are dramatically different, with β-thalassemic red blood cells showing impressive membrane instability, whereas in severe α thalassemia, the membranes are hyperstable, a situation otherwise encountered only in Southeast Asian ovalocytosis. The differences in membrane stability can be mimicked in vitro by incubating normal erythrocytes with phenylhydrazine and methylhydrazine (Schrier and Mohandas, 1992). When normal RBC are incubated with phenylhydrazine, partially oxidized α-globin chains are deposited on the RBC mem-

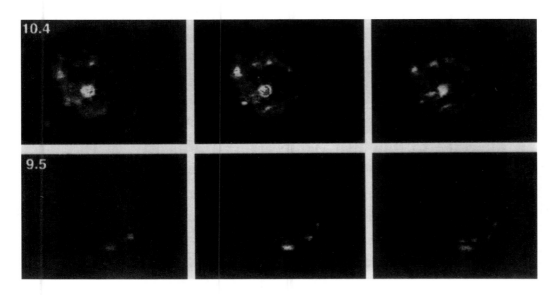

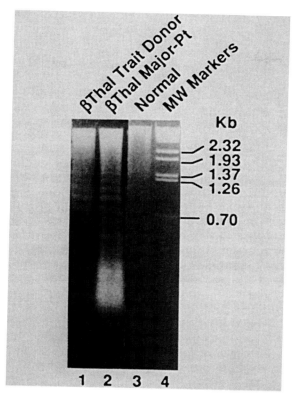

Figure 11.15. Nuclear DNA fragmentation of erythrocyte precursors from a β thalassemia trait donor (lane 1), a β thalassemia major patient (lane 2), and a normal individual (lane 3). Erythrocyte precursors from respective BMs were isolated and 5 million of these cells were lysed in a buffer consisting of 10 mmol/L Tris, pH 7.4; 1 mmol/L EDTA; 0.2% Triton X-100. After centrifugation at 11,000 × g for 30 minutes, the supernatant was collected and the DNA was precipitated with 50 percent isopropanol in 3 mol/L NaCl. After digestion for 1 hour with 1 μg/mL RNase, these samples were loaded onto a 1.5% agarose gel and electrophoresed. The gel was stained with ethidium bromide. (From Yuan et al., 1993, with permission.)

brane skeletons as in severe β thalassemia and also, as in severe β thalassemia, the membranes become unstable. Conversely, incubation of normal RBC with methylhydrazine causes the deposition of partially oxidized β-globin chains on the membrane skeletons as in severe α thalassemia, and the membranes become hyperstable.

Red blood cell hydration is also differently affected by accumulation of excess β globin in α thalassemia or α globin in β thalassemia. α-thalassemic red blood cells are hyperhydrated and their reticulocytes are also hyperhydrated. In marked contrast, β-thalassemic erythrocytes and reticulocytes are occasionally profoundly dehydrated. Whether these divergent patterns of hydration can all be explained by differential effects of the specific globin chains on the KCl cotransporter remains to be determined.

The α- and β-globin chains also seem to have differing capabilities in producing membrane protein oxidation. Excessive globin chains that are bound to the membrane skeleton in α and β thalassemia have undergone partial oxidation as manifested by their loss of free thiols (see above). However, only in β thalassemia is there evidence from at least two sources that protein 4.1 has undergone partial oxidation with concomitant loss of ability to generate the tertiary complex of spectrin, actin, and protein 4.1. This

Figure 11.16. Fluorescence activated cell sorting. Analysis of isolated and purified marrow erythroid precursors from a patient with β thalassemia major (Cooley's anemia). *Left panel:* The erythroid precursors were incubated with the dye Hoechst 33342 (abscissa), which labels cells dying or undergoing apoptosis, and propidium iodide (ordinate), which under these conditions identifies dead cells. *Middle panel:* Erythroid precursors as above, incubated with propidium iodide (ordinate) and FITC labeled annexin V (abscissa), which binds to apoptotic cells expressing phosphatidylserine on their outer surface. *Right panel:* The cells from the two panels above were FACS analyzed simultaneously for FITC annexin V reactivity (abscissa) and Hoechst 33342 reactivity (ordinate). The colored panels indicate apoptotic cells. For full color reproduction, see color plate 11.16.

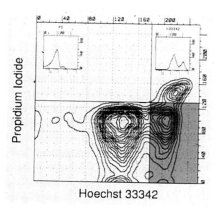

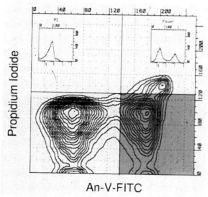

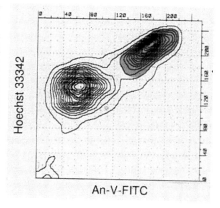

observation suggests that the α-globin chain aggregates that bind to the membrane skeleton in β thalassemia have the ability to produce oxidant damage to adjacent membrane skeletal proteins.

Preliminary data indicate that the effects of specific globin chain accumulation in marrow erythroid precursors also have very different capacities to cause erythroid precursor apoptosis. In severe β thalassemia characterized by accumulation of α-globin chains, the extent of apoptosis is about twice that of α thalassemia variants where there is accumulation of excess β-globin chains. In the murine models of β thalassemia, there is a direct correlation between extent of apoptosis and ineffective erythropoiesis. Thus, it is reasonable to hypothesize that the accumulation of specific globin chains in marrow erythroid precursors have highly specific capabilities of producing apoptosis and thus ineffective erythropoiesis.

Accumulation of a specific partially oxidized globin chain in erythroid precursors and on red cell membrane skeletons produces very specific pathophysiologic alterations, which thereby characterize the differences between α and β thalassemia. A more complete discussion of the pathophysiology of α thalassemia is presented in Chapter 16.

HbE-β THALASSEMIA (SEE CHAPTER 43)

Weatherall and Clegg have indicated that over the next 30 years there will be 100,000 new cases of HbE-β thalassemia (Weatherall and Clegg, 1996). This compound heterozygosity for two relatively mild traits produces remarkable heterogeneity with hemoglobin levels from 2.6 to 13.5 g/dL (Kalpravidh et al., 1995) and an average of 7.7 g/dL. The pathophysiology and heterogeneity of HbE-β thalassemia severity remains a puzzle. Certainly, if the major problem with β thalassemia is accumulation of excess unmatched α chains, then patients with β[0] thalassemia should have clinically more severe disease than patients with β[+] thalassemia. There is a general trend in that direction (Winichagoon et al., 1993; Fucharoen et al., 1996). Similarly, co-inheritance of α thalassemia should result in amelioration and it does to some degree (Winichagoon et al., 1993). Inheritance of a β-thalassemic chromosome with Xmn1 cleavage site at position −158 of the Gγ-globin gene also produces a generally milder disease. Patients who are homozygous for the Xmn1 cleavage site have somewhat higher levels of HbF, which should and does reduce the amount of excess α-globin chains (Fucharoen et al., 1996).

HbE is mildly oxidatively unstable (Rees et al., 1996; Suthipark et al., 1987) and this has led investigators to wonder whether susceptibility to oxidative attack may play a role in the clinical variability and severity of the disease. Red cells from these patients show evidence of oxidative stress in the form of elevated values of superoxide dismutase and glutathione peroxidase with reduced serum levels of vitamins E and C (Teitel, 1977). However, none of these phenomenologically identified events accounts for the heterogeneity of this genotype.

LESSONS FROM MURINE β THALASSEMIA

Some of the critical pathophysiologic events in human β thalassemia have been difficult to pinpoint because of the very complex genetic and environmental background of these patients. Many patients inherit combinations of β[+] and β[0] thalassemia along with HbE and different genotypes of α thalassemia. Also, patients in countries where β thalassemia is prevalent may be exposed to malaria and other infectious agents (Winichagoon et al., 1993).

Thus, there are advantages to the study of inbred strains of murine β thalassemia. One variety has been particularly useful: the Hbb[th-1] mouse has a deletion of the β major globin gene and in the homozygous state, produces only β minor globin and has a phenotype similar to that of human β thalassemia intermedia. It is an excellent analogue of the human disease with increased red blood cell and erythrocyte membrane rigidity, decreased membrane stability, and evidence of red cell dehydration (Sorensen et al., 1990). In these mice, as in humans, α-globin chains were found to be bound to the red cell membrane skeleton and the amount bound correlated strongly with membrane rigidity and with the severity of anemia (Sorensen et al., 1990). The assembly of the membrane proteins 4.1 and spectrin in erythroid precursors is as abnormal as in the human disease (Yuan et al., 1994). The extent of oxidation of globin bound to the membrane skeleton correlates directly with membrane instability (Advani et al., 1992a). Removal of cell membrane iron with deferiprone improves red cell survival and deformability, and, in parallel, reduces the extent of oxidation of membrane thiols (Browne et al., 1997).

Studies of murine β thalassemia provide support for the pathophysiologic importance of oxidized α-globin chain binding to the cell membrane skeleton, and the potentially important role of membrane bound iron as a contributing factor to the oxidation.

THROMBOEMBOLISM – HYPERCOAGULABILITY

Clinical and autopsy studies have shown that patients with severe forms of thalassemia suffer from thromboembolic events (Sonakul et al., 1980; Ruf et al., 1997). Data also suggest the existence of a hypercoagulable state in thalassemia. These include numerous platelet anomalies, shortened platelet survival and low levels of the natural anticoagulants protein C and S, abnormalities that are detectable even in young children (Eldor et al., 1989, 1999). The pathophysiology of the hypercoagulable state in thalassemia is still under investigation. It has been shown that thalassemic red cells, which were used to provide a source of membrane phospholipids, enhanced generation of thrombin in a "prothrombinase" assay (Borenstain et al., 1993). The procoagulant activity of thalassemic cells is due to exposure of anionic phospholipids such as PS, an observation made following the use of the protein annexin V, which has a high affinity for the anionic phospholipids and was able to block the procoagulant effect of thalassemic red blood cells (Helley et al., 1996). In a following study, a highly significant correlation was found between the number of red blood cell-bound annexin V molecules and the fraction of p-selectin (CD62p) positive platelets. Therefore, it seems that the procoagulant surface on thalassemic red blood cells may accelerate the formation of thrombin, which in turn triggers platelet activation (Ruf et al., 1997). It is not known whether the thrombocytosis, which is usually found in splenectomized patients, contributes to the initiation or severity of the hypercoagulability in β thalassemia. Whether these observations justify the use of preventive treatment with antiplatelet aggregants is an issue that has still to be determined by well-controlled clinical trials.

NEW OPTIONS FOR FUTURE THERAPY

HbF Modulators, Erythropoietin

Despite the increasing information of the molecular and cellular pathogenesis of the thalassemia syndromes, allogeneic bone marrow transplantation is the sole curative treatment (Chapter 39). Gene therapy (Chapter 41) still must overcome many obstacles before it can be successfully implemented.

Other therapeutic approaches include the modulation of fetal hemoglobin (HbF) synthesis (Chapter 38). In β thalassemia, a correction of the α/non-α-globin chain synthetic ratio to higher than 0.5, consonant with values seen in β thalassemia trait, could be a practical goal in order to neutralize the effects of the excess of α chains (Rodgers and Rachmilewitz, 1995).

Preliminary clinical trials with rHuEPO were carried out in patients with β thalassemia intermedia; several trials are ongoing using combinations of agents such as hydroxyurea and butyrates capable of inducing HbF synthesis, together with rHuEPO, which has been found to increase the total erythroid cell mass (Rachmilewitz et al., 1995). At this stage, there are not enough data to make any practical recommendations regarding this mode or any other mode of combined therapy with the different agents that have been discussed.

Antioxidants (Chapter 42)

Considerable data have been presented about the mechanism(s) of the premature hemolysis of red blood cells in β thalassemia. One of the major etiologies involves oxidative denaturation of the unstable globin subunits (Shinar and Rachmilewitz, 1993) (Fig. 11.17). In order to substantiate the role of oxidative denaturation in hemolysis, recent experiments were carried out to measure the types and amounts of free oxygen radicals generated in β-thalassemic erythrocytes. In the presence of a prooxidant drug such as primaquine, thalassemic red cells generated twice as much superoxide as normal cells. The excess of superoxide may reduce some oxidized iron in the membrane, initiating a Fenton-type reaction resulting in the formation of hydroxyl free radical (Grinberg et al., 1992). To pursue this hypothesis, hydroxyl free radical fluxes were quantitated by conversion of salicylic acid into its hydroxylated products. While there were no differences in spontaneous hydroxyl radical generation between normal and thalassemic red cells, the addition of ascorbic acid resulted in a marked increase in salicylic acid hydroxylation, which was much more evident in thalassemic compared with normal cells (Grinberg et al., 1995).

These data suggested a potential role for the use of antioxidants to neutralize the deleterious effects of the toxic oxygen species in thalassemic erythrocytes. While serum vitamin E levels were low (less than 0.5 mg/dL) in patients with β thalassemia, a preliminary therapeutic trial with large doses of vitamin E showed a decrease in the levels of malonyldialdehyde, indicating improvement in the degree of lipid membrane peroxidation, but not in the low number of titratable SH groups. In three of seven patients, red blood cell survival was prolonged, but there was no improvement in transfusion requirements (Rachmilewitz et al., 1979).

Plant flavonoids have been studied for their capacity to inhibit oxygen radical formation in chemical and biological systems. One compound, rutin, a quercetin rutinoside, was able to prevent, by 50 percent, primaquine-induced oxyhemoglobin oxidation to methemoglobin in red blood cells, but failed to restore

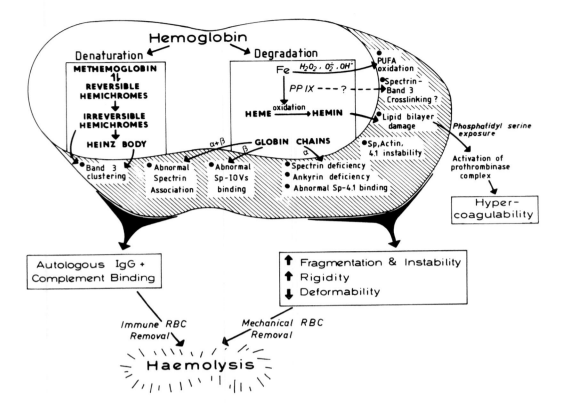

Figure 11.17. Mechanisms leading to red cell membrane dysfunction in hemoglobinopathies. Schematic representation of the chain of events leading to denaturation and degradation of the hemoglobin molecule. Note the alterations in the different red blood cell membrane components, caused by both hemoglobin breakdown products and the irreversibly oxidized species. These changes eventually lead to the immune-mediated and/or mechanical removal of the affected red blood cells from the circulation. Sp, spectrin. (From Shinar and Rachmilewitz, 1993, with permission.)

oxyHb from preformed methemoglobin (Grinberg et al., 1994). Another natural polyphenol is curcumin, which was found to protect hydrogen peroxide-induced lysis and lipid peroxidation of normal red blood cells (Grinberg et al., 1996). Curcumin caused significant inhibition of lipid peroxidation in β-thalassemic red cell ghosts, which was much more pronounced when ascorbic acid was added prior to hydrogen peroxide. It is possible that ferrous iron complexing with curcumin may lead to lower iron reactivity toward hydrogen peroxide and therefore protect thalassemic red cells against iron catalyzed oxidative damage.

Tea polyphenols were evaluated for their antioxidant effect both on normal red blood cells and on β-thalassemic red cell membranes challenged with antioxidants in vitro. Both green and black tea protected cells against primaquine-induced lysis and also against hydrogen peroxide-induced membrane lipid peroxidation and from morphologic alterations observed in scanning electron microscopy. The mechanism of the antioxidant properties of the tea polyphenols is most probably due to the binding of ferric iron to form redox inactive complex of iron polyphenol complex (Grinberg et al., 1997).

SUMMARY

Progress in understanding the pathophysiology of β thalassemia in the last 30 years reflects the major advances in biochemistry, immunology, rheology, and molecular and cellular biology. By the mid-1960s it had become clear that the major cause for erythrocyte destruction in β thalassemia was an excess of α-globin chains, which precipitated and formed intracellular inclusion bodies. More than 30 years later, the accumulated knowledge that has been described in this chapter demonstrates that following this basic pathology, there are many complex pathways, summarized in Figure 11.17, which try to elucidate how and why the precipitated α chains eventually result in destruction of the affected erythroid precursors and red blood cells. The steps involved are precipitation and disintegration of the excess α chains to globin, heme, and iron, and the deleterious effects of each of these breakdown products on the different portions of the red blood cell membrane.

Besides understanding the mechanisms involved, this accumulated information may have practical implications for the treatment of the disease. Although correction of the damage to the red blood cells—primarily mediated by oxygen free radicals—is not a primary event in thalassemia, it is very possible that ameliorating the degree of the oxidant damage to different components of the cell cytosol and membrane will reduce the severity of hemolysis and consequently the severity of the clinical expression of the disease. Such therapeutic approaches are beginning and deserve further attention.

References

Advani, R, Rubin, E, Mohandas, N et al. (1992a). Oxidative red blood cell membrane injury in the pathophysiology of severe mouse β-thalassemia. *Blood* 79: 1064–1067.

Advani, R, Sorenson, S, Shinar, E et al. (1992b). Characterization and comparison of the red blood cell membrane damage in severe human α- and β-thalassemia. *Blood* 79: 1058–1063.

Aft, RL and Mueller, GC. (1984). Hemin-mediated oxidative degradation of proteins. *J. Biol. Chem.* 259: 301–305.

Aljurf, M, Ma, L, and Angelucci, E. (1996). Abnormal assembly of membrane proteins in erythroid progenitors of patients with β-thalassemia major. *Blood* 87: 2049–2056.

Angelucci, E, Lucarelli, G, Yuan, J et al. (1996). Programmed cell death (PCD) and ineffective erythropoiesis in Cooley's anemia. *Blood* 88(10): S2817 (Abstract).

Angelucci, E, Ma, L, Lucarelli, G et al. (1997). The role of iron overload in the extent of programmed cell death (PCD) in patients with Cooley's anemia. *Blood* 90(10): S2839 (Abstract).

Bookchin, RM, Ortiz, OE, Shalev, O et al. (1988). Calcium transport and ultrastructure of red cells in β-thalassemia intermedia. *Blood* 72: 1602–1607.

Borenstain, V, Barenholz, Y, Hy-Am, E et al. (1993). Phosphatidylserine in the outer leaflet of red blood cells from β-thalassemia patients may explain the chronic hypercoagulable state and thrombotic episodes. *Am. J. Hematol.* 44: 33–35.

Browne, PV, Shalev, O, Kuypers, FA et al. (1997). Removal of erythrocyte membrane iron in vivo ameliorates the pathobiology of murine thalassemia. *J. Clin. Invest.* 100: 1459–1464.

Bunn, HF, and Jandl, JH. (1968). Exchange of heme among hemoglobins and between hemoglobin and albumin. *J. Biol. Chem.* 243: 465–475.

Canessa, M. (1991). Red cell volume-related ion transport systems in hemoglobinopathies. *Hematol. Oncol. Clin. North Am.* 5(3): 495–516.

Chasis, JA, Reid, ME, Jensen, RH et al. (1988). Signal transduction by glycophorin A: Role of extracellular and cytoplasmic domains in a modulatable process. *J. Cell Biol.* 107: 1351–1357.

Chiu, DA and Lubin, B. (1989). Oxidative hemoglobin denaturation and red blood cells destruction: The effect of heme on red cell membranes. *Semin. Hematol.* 26: 128–135.

Cohen, CM and Gascard, P. (1992). Regulation and post-translational modification of erythrocyte membrane and membrane-skeletal proteins. *Semin. Hematol.* 29: 244–292.

De Franceschi, L, Shalev, O, Piga, A et al. (1999). Deferiprone therapy in homozygous human β-thalassemia removes erythrocyte membrane free iron and reduces KCl cotransport activity. *J. Lab. Clin. Med.* 133(1): 64–69.

Eldor, A, Krausz, Y Atlan, H et al. (1989). Platelet survival in patients with beta-thalassemia. *Am. J. Hematol.* 32: 94–99.

Eldor, A, Durst, R, Hy-Am, E et al. (1999). A chronic hypercoagulable state in patients with β-thalassaemia major is already present in childhood. *Br. J. Haematol.* 107(4): 739–746.

Fessas, P, Loukopoulos, D, and Kaltsoya, A. (1966). Peptide analysis of the inclusions of erythroid cells in beta-thalassemia. *Biochim. Biophys. Acta* 124(2): 430–432.

Finch, CA, Deubelbeiss, K, Cook, JD et al. (1970). Ferrokinetics in man. *Medicine (Balt.)* 49(1): 17–53.

Fortier, N, Snyder, LM, Garver, F et al. (1988). The relationship between in vivo generated hemoglobin skeletal protein complex and increased red cell membrane rigidity. *Blood* 71: 1427–1431.

Fucharoen, S, Siritanaratkul, N, Winichagoon, P et al. (1996). Hydroxyurea increases hemoglobin E levels and improves the effectiveness of erythropoiesis in β-thalassemia/hemoglobin E disease. *Blood* 87(3): 887–892.

Galilli, U, Korkesh, A, Kahane, I, and Rachmilewitz, EA. (1983). Demonstration of a natural antigalactosyl IgG antibody on thalassemic red blood cells. *Blood* 61: 1258–1264.

Graham, G, Bates, GW, Rachmilewitz, EA, and Hershko, C. (1979). Nonspecific serum iron in thalassemia: Quantitation and chemical reactivity. *Am. J. Hematol.* 6: 207–217.

Grinberg, LN, Shalev, O, Goldfarb, A, and Rachmilewitz, EA. (1992). Primaquine-induced superoxide production by β-thalassemic red blood cells. *Biochem. Biophys. Acta* 1139: 248–250.

Grinberg, LN, Rachmilewitz, EA, and Newmark, H. (1994). Protective effects of rutin against hemoglobin oxidation. *Biochem. Pharmacol.* 48(4): 643–649.

Grinberg, LN, Rachmilewitz, EA, Kitrossky, N, and Chevion, M. (1995). Hydroxyl radical generation in β-thalassemia red blood cells. *Free Radical Biol. Med.* 18: 611–615.

Grinberg, LN, Shalev, O, Tonnesen, H, and Rachmilewitz, EA. (1996). Studies on curcumin and curcuminoids: XXVI. Antioxidant effects of curcumin on the red blood cell membrane. *Int. J. Pharm.* 32: 251–257.

Grinberg, LN, Newmark, H, Kitrossky, N et al. (1997). Protective effects of tea polyphenols against oxidative damage to red blood cells. *Biochem. Pharmacol.* 54: 973–978.

Hebbel, RP. (1985). Auto-oxidation and a membrane associated "Fenton Reagent": A possible explanation for development of membrane lesions in sickle erythrocytes. *Clin. Haematol.* 14: 129–140.

Helley, D, Eldor, A, Girot, R et al. (1996). Comparison of the procoagulant activity of red blood cells from patients with homozygous sickle cell disease and β-thalassemia. *Thromb. Haemost.* 76: 322–327.

Jacobs, A, Peters, SW, Bauminger, ER et al. (1981). Ferritin concentration in normal and abnormal erythrocytes measured by immunoradiometric assay with antibodies to heart and spleen ferritin and Mossbauer spectroscopy. *Br. J. Haematol.* 49: 201–207.

Kahane, I, Polliack, A, Rachmilewitz, EA et al. (1978). Distribution of sialic acids on the red blood cell membrane in β thalassaemia. *Nature* 271: 674–675.

Kahane, I, Ben-Chetrit, E, Shifter, A et al. (1980). The erythrocyte membrane in beta-thalassemia. Lower sialic acid levels in glycophorin. *Biochim. Biophys. Acta* 596: 10–17.

Kalpravidh, RW, Komolvanich, S, Wilairat, P et al. (1995). Globin chain turnover in reticulocytes from patients with β⁰-thalassemia/Hb E disease. *Eur. J. Haematol.* 55: 322–326.

Kannan, R, Labotka, RJ, and Low, PS (1988). Isolation and characterization of the hemichrome-stabilized membrane protein aggregates from sickle erythrocytes. *J. Biol. Chem.* 263: 3766.

Knyszynski, A, Danon, D, Kahane, I, and Rachmilewitz, EA. (1979). Phagocytosis of nucleated and mature β thalassaemic red blood cells by mouse macrophages in vitro. *Br. J. Haematol.* 43: 251–255.

Kuypers, FA, Yuan, J, Lewis, RA et al. (1998). Membrane phospholipid asymmetry in human thalassemia. *Blood* 91: 3044–3051.

Lamchiagdhase, P, Wilairal, P, Sahaphong, S et al. (1987). Defective spectrin dimer self-association in thalassemic red cells. *Eur. J. Haematol.* 38: 246–250.

Lucarelli, G, Galimberti, M, Giardini, C et al. (1998). Bone marrow transplantation in thalassemia—The experience of Pesaro. *Ann. N. Y. Acad. Sci.* 850:270.

Olivieri, O, Vitoux, D, Galacteros, F et al. (1992). Hemoglobin variants and activity of the (K⁺Cl⁻) cotransport system in human erythrocytes. *Blood* 79: 793–797.

Peisach, J, Blumberg, WE, Ogawa, S et al. (1971). The effect of protein conformation on the heme symmetry in high ferric heme proteins as studied by electron paramagnetic resonance. *J. Biol. Chem.* 246: 3342.

Polliack, A and Rachmilewitz, EA. (1973). Ultrastructural studies in beta thalassaemia major. *Br. J. Haematol.* 24: 319–326 (Yearbook of Medicine).

Polliack, A, Yataganas, X, and Rachmilewitz, EA. (1974). Ultra-structure of the inclusion bodies and nuclear abnormalities in β-thalassemic erythroblasts. *Ann. N. Y. Acad. Sci.* 232: 261–282.

Pryor, WA. (1977). Free radicals in biology: The involvement of radical reactions in aging and carcinogens. *Med. Chem.* 5: 331–359.

Rachmilewitz, EA. (1974). Denaturation of the normal and abnormal hemoglobin molecule. *Semin. Hematol.* 11(4): 441–462.

Rachmilewitz, EA, Peisach, J, Bradley, TB Jr, and Blumberg, E. (1969). Role of haemichromes in the formation of inclusion bodies in haemoglobin H disease. *Nature* 222: 248–250.

Rachmilewitz, EA, Peisach, J, and Blumberg, WE. (1971). Studies on the stability of oxyhemoglobin A and its constituent chains and their derivatives. *J. Biol. Chem.* 246: 3356–3366.

Rachmilewitz, EA, Lubin, BH, and Shohet, SB. (1976). Lipid membrane peroxidation in β-thalassemia major. *Blood* 47: 495–505.

Rachmilewitz, EA, Shifter, A, and Kahane, I. (1979). Vitamin E deficiency in β-thalassemia major: Changes in hematological and biochemical parameters after a therapeutic trial with α-tocopherol. *Am. J. Clin. Nutr.* 32: 1850–1858.

Rachmilewitz, EA, Shinar, E, Shalev, O et al. (1985). Erythrocyte membrane alterations in β-thalassemia. *Clin. Haematol.* 14(1): 163–182.

Rachmilewitz, EA, Aker, M, Perry, D, and Dover, G. (1995). Sustained increase in haemoglobin and red blood cells following long-term administration of recombinant human erythropoietin to patients with homozygous beta thalassemia. *Br. J. Haematol.* 90: 341–345.

Rees, DC, Duley, J, Simmonds, HA et al. (1996). Interaction of hemoglobin E and pyrimidine 5′ nucleotidase deficiency. *Blood* 88: 2761–2767.

Repka, T, Shalev, O, Reddy, R et al. (1993). Nonrandom association of free iron with membranes of sickle and β-thalassemic erythrocytes. *Blood* 82: 3204–3210.

Rhoda, MD, Galacteros, F, Beuzard, Y, and Giraud, F. (1987). Ca²⁺ permeability and cytosolic Ca²⁺ concentration are not impaired in β-thalassemic and hemoglobin C erythrocytes. *Blood* 70: 804–808.

Rodgers, G and Rachmilewitz, EA. (1995). Annotations—Novel treatment options in the severe β-globin disorders. *Br. J. Haematol.* 91: 263–268.

Rouyer-Fessardt, P, Garel, M-C, Domenget, C et al. (1989). A study of membrane protein defects and α hemoglobin chains of red blood cells in human β thalassemia. *J. Biol. Chem.* 264: 19092–19098.

Ruf, A, Pick, M, Deutsch, V et al. (1997). In-vivo platelet activation correlates with red cell anionic phospholipid exposure in patients with β-thalassemia major. *Br. J. Haematol.* 98: 51–56.

Rund, D, Filon, D, Strauss, N et al. (1992). Mean corpuscular volume of heterozygotes for β-thalassemia correlates with the severity of mutations. *Blood* 79: 238–243.

Schrier, SL and Mohandas, N. (1992). Globin chain specificity of oxidation-induced changes in red blood cell membrane properties. *Blood* 79: 1586–1592.

Schrier, SL, Rachmilewitz, E, and Mohandas, N. (1989). Cellular and membrane properties of alpha and beta thalassemic erythrocytes are different: Implications for differences in clinical manifestations. *Blood* 74: 2194–2202.

Scott, MD, Rouyer-Fessard, P, Lubin, BH, and Beuzard, Y. (1990). Entrapment of purified α-hemoglobin chains in normal erythrocytes: A model for β-thalassemia. *J. Biol. Chemi.* 265: 17953–17959.

Scott, MD, Rouyer-Fessard, P, Ba, MS et al. (1992). α- and β-haemoglobin chain induced changes in normal erythrocyte deformability: Comparison to β-thalassemia intermedia and Hb H disease. *Br. J. Haematol.* 80: 519–526.

Scott, MD, van den Berg, JJM, Repka, T et al. (1993). Effect of excess α-hemoglobin chains on cellular and membrane oxidation in model β-thalassemic erythrocytes. *J. Clin. Invest.* 91: 1706–1712.

Shalev, O, Mogilner, S, Shinar, E et al. (1984). Impaired erythrocyte calcium homeostasis in β-thalassemia. *Blood* 64: 564–566.

Shalev, O, Shinar, E, and Lux, SE. (1988). Isolated beta globin chains reproduce the defective binding of spectrin to alpha thalassemic inside-out membrane vesicles (IOVS). *Blood* 72 (Suppl. 1): 202a.

Shalev, O, Repka, T, Goldfarb, A et al. (1995). Deferiprone (L1) chelates pathologic iron deposits from membranes of intact thalassemic and sickle red blood cells both in vitro and in vivo. *Blood* 86: 2008–2013.

Shinar, E and Rachmilewitz, EA. (1990). Oxidative denaturation of red blood cells in thalassemia. *Semin. Hematol.* 27: 70–82.

Shinar, E and Rachmilewitz, EA. (1993). Hemoglobinopathies and red cell membrane function. *Bailliere's Clin. Haematol.* 6: 357–369.

Shinar, E, Shalev, O, Rachmilewitz, EA et al. (1987). Erythrocyte membrane skeleton abnormalities in severe β-thalassemia. *Blood* 70: 158–164.

Shinar, E, Rachmilewitz, EA, and Lux, SE. (1989). Differing erythrocyte membrane skeletal protein defects in alpha and beta thalassemia. *J. Clin. Invest.* 83: 404–410.

Sonakul, D, Pacharee, P, Laohapand, T et al. (1980). Pulmonary artery obstruction in thalassaemia. *Southeast Asian J. Trop. Med. Public Health* 11: 516–523.

Suthipark, K, Ong-ajyooth, S, Shumnumsirivath, D et al. (1987). Oxidative stress and antioxidants in β-thalassemia/hemoglobin E. *J. Med. Assoc. Thai.* 70: 270–274.

Teitel, P. (1977). Basic principles of the 'filterability test' (FT) and analysis of erythrocyte flow behavior. *Blood Cells* 3: 55–70.

Traeger-Synodinos, J, Kanavakis, E, Vrettou, E et al. (1996). The triplicated α-globin gene locus in β-thalassaemia heterozygotes: Clinical, haematological, biosynthetic and molecular studies. *Br. J. Haematol.* 95: 467–471.

Vigi, V, Volpato, S, Gaburro, D et al. (1969). The correlation between red-cell survival and excess of α-globin synthesis in β-thalassemia. *Br. J. Haematol.* 16: 25–30.

Vincent, SH. (1989). Oxidative effects of heme and porphyrins on proteins and lipids. *Semin. Hematol.* 26: 105–113.

Wanachiwanawin, W, Siripanyaphinyo, U, Fucharoen, S et al. (1993). Activation of monocytes for the immune clearance of red cells in β⁰-thalassaemia/HbE. *Br. J. Haematol.* 85: 773–777.

Waugh, SM and Low, PS. (1985). Hemichrome binding to band 3: Nucleation of Heinz bodies on the erythrocyte membrane. *Biochemistry* 24: 34–39.

Waugh, SM, Willardson, BM, Kannan, R et al. (1986). Heinz bodies induced clustering of band 3, glycophorin and ankyrin in sickle erythrocytes. *J. Clin. Invest..* 78: 1155–1160.

Weatherall, DJ and Clegg, JB. (1996). Thalassemia—a global public health problem. *Nat. Med.* 2(8): 847–849.

Wickramasinghe, SN and Bush, V. (1975). Observations on the ultrastructure of erythropoietic cells and reticulum cells in the bone marrow of patients with homozygous β-thalassaemia. *Br. J. Haematol.* 30: 395–399.

Wickramasinghe, SN and Hughes, M. (1980). Ultrastructural studies of erythropoiesis in β-thalassaemia trait. *Br. J. Haematol.* 46: 401–407.

Wickramasinghe, SN and Lee, MJ. (1997). Observations on the relationship between gamma-globin chain content and globin chain precipitation in thalassaemic erythroblasts and on the composition of erythroblastic inclusions in HbE/beta-thalassaemia. *Eur. J. Haematol.* 59: 305–309.

Wickramasinghe, SN, Letsky, E, and Moffatt, B. (1973). Effect of α-chain precipitates on bone marrow function in homozygous β-thalassaemia. *Br. J. Haematol.* 25: 123–129.

Wiener, E, Wanachiwanawin, W, Chinprasertsuk, S et al. (1996). Increased serum levels of macrophage colony-stimulating factor (M-CSF) in α- and β-thalassaemia syndromes: Correlation with anaemia and monocyte activation. *Eur. J. Haematol.* 57: 364–369.

Winichagoon, P, Thonglairoam, V, Fucharoen, S et al. (1993). Severity differences in β-thalassemia/haemoglobin E syndromes: Implication of genetic factors. *Br. J. Haematol.* 83: 633–659.

Yuan, J, Angelucci, E, Lucarelli, G et al. (1993). Accelerated programmed cell death (apoptosis) in erythroid precursors of patients with severe β-thalassemia (Cooley's anemia). *Blood* 82: 374–377.

Yuan, J, Bunyaratvej, A, Fucharoen, S et al. (1995). The instability of the membrane skeleton in thalassemic red blood cells. *Blood* 86: 3945–3950.

Yuan, J, Kannan, R, Shinar, E et al. (1992). Isolation, characterization and immunoprecipitation studies of immune complexes from membranes of β-thalassemic erythrocytes. *Blood* 79: 3007–3013.

Yuan, J, Rubin, E, Aljurf, M et al. (1994). Defective assembly of membrane proteins in erythroid precursors of β-thalassemic mice. *Blood* 84: 632–637.

12

Molecular Mechanisms of β Thalassemia

BERNARD G. FORGET

Despite having a relatively limited range of clinical, hematologic, and biochemical phenotypes, the β thalassemias are due to a surprisingly large number of different genetic defects. The review of normal globin gene structure and function presented in Chapter 6 illustrates the many steps of gene expression at which a mutation can result in the absent or markedly decreased production or accumulation of β globin, which characterizes the pathophysiology of β thalassemia (Chapter 11). In contrast to the α thalassemias, which are generally due to deletions in the α-globin gene cluster, the β thalassemias are generally due to point mutations in the β-globin gene. However, deletion forms of β thalassemia have also been identified. This chapter describes the different genetic lesions that result in β thalassemia.

POINT MUTATIONS CAUSING THALASSEMIA

Most mutations that cause β thalassemia are due to point mutations in functionally important regions of the β-globin gene. More than 125 different point mutations have thus far been identified as causes of β thalassemia, although a relatively small number of mutations account for the majority of cases in a given racial group (see the later section on prenatal diagnosis as well as Chapter 35). These point mutations can be classified according to the type or category of defect in gene expression that they cause (Table 12.1). The mutations have been catalogued by Huisman et al. (1997), and the updated listing is accessible electronically through the Globin Gene Server Website (Hardison et al., 1998): http://globin.cse.psu.edu.

Promoter Mutations

As discussed in Chapter 6, a number of conserved sequence motifs in the 5′ flanking DNA of globin (and other) genes constitute important functional elements of the gene promoter and are therefore important for efficient transcription of the gene. Three of these consensus sequences are found in the promoter regions of all globin genes: the CACCC box, the CCAAT box, and the ATAA (or TATA) box. Mutations in two of these three conserved sequence motifs have been identified in different patients with β thalassemia, that is, in the CACCC and ATAA boxes. No mutations of the CCAAT box have been identified as causes of β thalassemia, although mutations in this motif are associated with certain nondeletion forms of HPFH (Chapter 15).

In general, the degree of diminished β-globin synthesis associated with mutations of the β-globin gene promoter is relatively minor. Patients have β⁺ thalassemias, which in the homozygous or compound heterozygous form, are relatively mild and frequently associated with the clinical phenotype of β-thalassemia intermedia. This finding is consistent with studies of transcription of the mutant genes in gene transfer-expression studies in tissue culture cells, which reveal only a mild-to-moderate decrease in transcriptional activity of these genes (Orkin et al., 1983a; Antonarakis et al. 1984; Takihara et al., 1986; Orkin et al., 1984a).

As listed in Table 12.1, there are eight mutations at five different positions of the ATAA box (nucleotides −28 to −32 from the cap site) and nine mutations at five different positions of the proximal CACCC box (nucleotides −86, −87, −88, and −92 from the cap site). One mutation has been identified at position −101 within a second (distal) CACCC element of the β-globin gene promoter. This mutation is extremely mild and is associated in heterozygotes with the silent carrier phenotype characterized by little or no hypochromia and microcytosis of the red blood cells (RBCs). The ATAA box mutations at position −28 (A→G) and −29 (A→G) are relatively common causes of β thalassemia in Chinese and black populations, respectively. Although the −29 mutation results in a relatively mild disorder in blacks (Antonarakis et al., 1984), the same mutation was associated with severe transfusion-dependent tha-

Martin H. Steinberg, Bernard G. Forget, Douglas R. Higgs, and Ronald L. Nagel, editors. *Disorders of Hemoglobin: Genetics, Pathophysiology, and Clinical Management.* © 2001 Cambridge University Press. All rights reserved.

Table 12.1. Mutations Causing β Thalassemia

Mutation	Phenotype β⁰ or β⁺	Racial group	Reference
Promoter Mutations			
ATA Box			
−28 (A → G)	+	Chinese	Orkin et al., 1983a
−28 (A → C)	+	Kurdish	Poncz et al., 1982
−29 (A → G)	+	American black, Chinese	Antonarakis et al., 1984; Huang et al., 1986
−30 (T → C)	+	Chinese	Cai et al., 1989
−30 (T → A)	+	Eastern Mediterranean	Fei et al., 1988
−31 (A → G)	+	Japanese	Takahira et al., 1986
−31 (A → C)	+	Italian	Huisman et al., 1997
−32 (C → A)	+	Taiwanese	Lin et al., 1992
CACCC Box			
−86 (C → G)	+	Lebanese, Thai	Kazazian, 1990; Thein et al., 1990a
−86 (C → A)	+	Italian	Meloni et al., 1992
−87 (C → G)	+	Mediterranean	Orkin et al., 1982a
−87 (C → T)	+	German, Italian	Kulozik et al., 1991
−87 (C → A)	+	Yugoslavian, American black	Efremov et al., 1991; Coleman et al., 1992
−88 (C → A)	+	Kurdish	Rund et al., 1991
−88 (C → T)	+	American black, Asian Indian	Orkin et al., 1984a
−90 (C → T)	+	Portuguese, Ashkenazi Jewish	Faustino et al., 1992; Filon et al., 1994
−92 (C → T)	+	Italian	Kazazian, 1990; Divoky et al., 1993a
−101 (C → T)	+	Italian, Eastern Mediterranean	Gonzalez-Redondo et al., 1989a
Cap Site			
+ 1 (A → C)	+	Asian Indian	Wong et al., 1987
Initiation Codon Mutations			
ATG → AGG	0	Korean, Chinese, No. European	Lam et al., 1990; Koo et al., 1992; Waye et al., 1997a
ATG → ACG	0	Yugoslavian, Swiss	Jankovic et al., 1990a; Beris et al., 1993
ATG → GTG	0	Japanese	Hattori et al., 1991
ATG → ATT	0	Iranian	Nozari et al., 1995
ATG → ATA	0	Italian, Swedish	Saba et al., 1992; Landin et al., 1995
ATG → ATC	0	Japanese	Ohba et al., 1997
Cleavage and Polyadenylation Mutations			
AATAAA → AACAAA	+	American black	Orkin et al., 1985
AATAAA → AATAAG	+	Kurdish	Rund et al., 1991
AATAAA → AATAGA	+	Malaysian	Jankovic et al., 1990b
AATAAA → AATGAA	+	Mediterranean	Jankovic et al., 1990b
AATAAA → A(−AATAA)	+	Arab	Rund et al., 1992
AATAAA → AAAA(−AT)	+	French	Ghanem et al., 1992
Splicing Mutations			
Splice site junction mutations			
IVS-1 position 1 (G → A)	0	Mediterranean	Orkin et al., 1982a
IVS-1 position 1 (G → T)	0	Asian Indian, Chinese	Kazazian et al., 1984a
IVS-1 position 2 (T → G)	0	Tunisian	Chibani et al., 1988

(continued)

Table 12.1 (*continued*)

Mutation	Phenotype β^0 or β^+	Racial group	Reference
Splicing Mutations			
Splice site junction mutations			
IVS-1 position 2 (T → C)	0	American black, Algerian	Gonzalez-Redondo et al., 1989b; Lossi et al., 1989
IVS-1 position 2 (T → A)	0	Algerian	Bouhass et al., 1990
IVS-1 5′-end (−44 bp)	0	Mediterranean	Gonzalez-Redondo et al., 1989c
IVS-1 position 130 (G → A)	0	Egyptian	Deidda et al., 1990
IVS-1 position 130 (G → C)	0	Italian, Turkish, Japanese	Kazazian, 1990; Öner et al., 1990; Yamamoto et al., 1992
IVS-1 3′-end (−17 bp)	0	Kuwaiti	Gonzales-Redondo et al., 1989c
IVS-1 3′-end (−25 bp)	0	Asian Indian	Orkin et al., 1983b
IVS-2 position 1 (G → A)	0	Mediterranean, Tunisian American black, Japanese	Treisman et al., 1982; Chibani et al., 1988 Wong et al., 1986; Hattori et al., 1992
IVS-2 position 1 (G → C)	0	Iranian	Nozari et al., 1993
IVS-2 position 2,3 (−TG and insertion of 11 bp)	0	Iranian	Kaeda et al., 1991
IVS-2 position 849 (A → G)	0	American black	Antonarakis et al., 1984; Atweh et al., 1985
IVS-2 position 849 (A → C)	0	American black	Padanilam and Huisman, 1986
IVS-2 position 850 (G → C)	0	Yugoslavian	Jankovic et al., 1992
IVS-2 position 850 (−G)	0	Italian	Rosatelli et al., 1992a
IVS-2 position 850 (G → A)	0	No. European	Curuk et al., 1995
IVS-2 position 850 (G → T)	0	Japanese	Ohba et al., 1997
Consensus sequence mutations			
IVS-1 position −3 (C → T) (codon 29)	+	Lebanese	Chehab et al., 1987
IVS-1 position −2 (A → G) (codon 30)	0	Sephardic Jewish	Waye et al., 1998
IVS-1 position −1 (G → C) (codon 30) (Hb Kairoran or Monroe)	+	Tunisian, American black	Chibani et al., 1988; Vidaud et al., 1989; Gonzalez-Redondo et al., 1989d
IVS-1 position −1 (G → A) (codon 30)	0	Bulgarian	Kalaydjieva et al., 1989
IVS-1 position 5 (G → C)	+	Asian Indian, Chinese, Melanesian	Kazazian et al., 1984a; Cheng et al., 1984; Hill et al., 1988
IVS-1 position 5 (G → T)	+	Mediterranean, American black	Atweh et al., 1987a; Gonzales-Redondo et al., 1991
IVS-1 position 5 (G → A)	+	Greek,* Algerian	Kulozik et al., 1988; Kattamis et al., 1990; Lapoumeroulie et al., 1986
IVS-1 position 6 (T → C)	+	Mediterranean	Orkin et al., 1982a
IVS-1 position 128 (T → G)	+	Saudi Arabian, Chinese	Wong et al., 1989a; Chiou et al., 1993
IVS-2 position 4,5 (−AG)	0	Portuguese	Faustino et al., 1992
IVS-2 position 5 (G → C)	+ (severe)	Chinese	Jiang et al., 1993
IVS-2 position 837 (T → G)	+ or 0	Asian Indian	Varawalla et al., 1991
IVS-2 position 843 (T → G)	+	Algerian	Beldjord et al., 1988
IVS-2 position 844 (C → G)	+	Italian	Murru et al., 1991
IVS-2 position 848 (C → A)	+	Mediterranean, Iranian, Egyptian, American black	Kattamis et al., 1990; Wong et al., 1989a Gonzalez-Redondo et al., 1988
IVS-2 position 848 (C → G)	+	Japanese	Hattori et al., 1992

(*continued*)

Table 12.1 *(continued)*

Mutation	Phenotype β⁰ or β⁺	Racial group	Reference
Mutations Creating Alternative Splice Sites			
In introns			
IVS-1 position 110 (G → A)	+	Mediterranean	Spritz et al., 1981; Westaway and Williamson, 1981
IVS-1 position 116 (T → G)	0	Mediterranean	Metherall et al., 1986
IVS-2 position 654 (C → T)	+ (severe)	Chinese	Cheng et al., 1984
IVS-2 position 705 (T → G)	0	Mediterranean	Dobkin et al., 1983
IVS-2 position 745 (C → G)	+	Mediterranean	Orkin et al., 1982a
In exons			
Codon 19 (A → G) Hb Malay	+	Malaysian	Yang et al., 1989
Codon 24 (T → A)	+	American black, Japanese	Goldsmith et al., 1983; Hattori et al., 1989
Codon 26 (G → A) Hb E	+	SE Asian	Orkin et al., 1982b
Codon 27 (G → T) Hb Knossos	+	Mediterranean	Orkin et al., 1984b
Mutations Producing Nonfunctional mRNAs			
Nonsense Mutations			
Codon 15 (TGG → TAG)	0	Asian Indian	Kazazian et al., 1984a
Codon 15 (TGG → TGA)	0	Portuguese	Ribeiro et al., 1992
Codon 17 (A → T)	0	Chinese	Chang and Kan, 1979
Codon 22 (G → T)	0	Reunion Islander	Ghanem et al., 1992
Codon 26 (G → T)	0	Thai	Fucharoen et al., 1990a
Codon 35 (C → A)	0	Thai	Fucharoen et al., 1989
Codon 37 (G → A)	0	Saudi Arabian	Boehm et al., 1986
Codon 39 (C → T)	0	Mediterranean, European	Trecartin et al., 1981; Moschonas et al., 1981; Orkin and Goff, 1981; Pergolizzi et al., 1981; Jackson et al., 1981; Gorski et al., 1982; Chehab et al., 1986
Codon 43 (G → T)	0	Chinese	Atweh et al., 1988
Codon 61 (A → T)	0	American black	Gonzalez-Redondo et al., 1988
Codon 90 (G → T)	0	Japanese	Hattori et al., 1992; Fucharoen et al., 1990b
Codon 112 (T → A)	0	Czechoslovakian	Divoky et al., 1993b
Codon 121 (G → T)	Dominant β thal.	Polish, Swiss, British, Japanese	Kazazian et al., 1986; Yamamoto et al., 1992; Fei et al., 1989; Thein et al., 1990b
Codon 127 (C → T)	Dominant β thal.	English	Hall et al., 1991
Frameshift Mutations			
Codon 1 (–G)	0	Mediterranean	Rosatelli et al., 1992b
Codons 2/3/4 (–9 bp, +31 bp)	0	Algerian	Badens et al., 1996
Codon 5 (–CT)	0	Mediterranean	Kollia et al., 1989
Codon 6 (–A)	0	Mediterranean, American black	Gonzales-Redondo et al., 1988; Kazazian et al., 1983; Chang et al., 1983
Codon 8 (–AA)	0	Turkish	Orkin and Goff 1981
Codons 8/9 (+G)	0	Asian Indian, Mediterranean	Kazazian et al., 1984a; Kattamis et al., 1990
Codons 9/10 (+T)	0	Greek	Waye et al., 1994

(continued)

Table 12.1 *(continued)*

Mutation	Phenotype β^0 or β^+	Racial group	Reference
Mutations Producing Nonfunctional mRNAs			
Frameshift Mutations			
Codon 11 (–T)	0	Mexican	Economou et al., 1991
Codons 14/15 (+G)	0	Chinese	Chan et al., 1988
Codons 15 (–T)	0	Malaysian	Fucharoen et al., 1990c
Codon 16 (–C)	0	Asian Indian	Kazazian et al., 1984a
Codons 20/21 (+G)	0	Ashkenazi Jewish	Oppenheim et al., 1993
Codons 22/23/24 (–AAGTTGG)	0	Turkish	Ozcelik et al., 1993
Codon 24 (–G, +CAC)	0	Egyptian	Deidda et al., 1991
Codons 25/26 (+T)	0	Tunisian	Fattoum et al., 1991
Codon 26 (+T)	0	Japanese	Hattori et al., 1998
Codons 27/28 (+C)	0	Chinese	Lin et al., 1991
Codon 28 (–C)	0	Egyptian	El-Hashemite et al., 1997
Codons 28/29 (–G)	0	Japanese, Egyptian	Ohba et al., 1997; El-Hashemite et al., 1997
Codon 31 (–C)	0	Chinese	Ko et al., 1997
Codon 35 (–C)	0	Malaysian	Yang et al., 1989
Codons 36/37 (–T)	0	Kurdish (Iranian)	Rund et al., 1991
Codons 37–39 (–GACCCAG)	0	Turkish	Schnee et al., 1989
Codons 38/39 (–C)	0	Czechoslovakian	Indrak et al., 1991
Codons 38/39 (–CC)	0	Belgian	Heusterspreute et al., 1996
Codon 40 (–G)	0	Japanese	Ohba et al., 1997
Codons 40/41 (+T)	0	Chinese	Ko et al., 1997
Codon 41 (–C)	0	Thai	Fucharoen et al., 1991a
Codons 41/42 (–TTCT)	0	Asian Indian, Chinese	Kazazian et al., 1984a; Kimura et al., 1983
Codons 42/43 (+G)	0	Japanese	Ohba et al., 1997
Codons 42/43 (+T)	0	Japanese	Oshima et al., 1996
Codon 44 (–C)	0	Kurdish	Kinniburgh et al., 1982
Codon 45 (–T)	0	Pakistani	El-Kalla and Mathews, 1997
Codon 47 (+A)	0	Surinamese black	Losekoot et al., 1990
Codons 47/48 (+ATCT)	0	Sikh	Garewal et al., 1994; El-Kalla et al., 1995
Codon 51 (–C)	0	Hungarian	Ringelhann et al., 1993
Codons 53/54 (+G)	0	Japanese	Fucharoen et al., 1990b
Codon 54 (–T)	0	Algerian, Swedish	Landin and Berglund, 1996; Huisman et al., 1997
Codon 54/55 (+A)	0	Asian Indian	Garewal et al., 1994
Codons 56 to 60 (14 bp duplication)	0	No information	Ghaffari et al., 1997
Codons 57/58 (+C)	0	Sikh	El-Kalla and Mathews 1995
Codon 59 (–A)	0	Italian	Meloni et al., 1994
Codon 64 (–G)	0	Swiss	Chehab et al., 1989
Codon 67 (–TG)	0	Filipino	Eng et al., 1993
Codon 71 (+T)	0	Chinese	Chan et al., 1989
Codons 71/72 (+A)	0	Chinese	Cheng et al., 1984
Codons 72/73 (–AGTGA, +T)	0	English	Waye et al., 1997b
Codons 74/75 (–C)	0	Turkish	Basak et al., 1992
Codon 76 (–C)	0	Italian	DiMarzo et al., 1988
Codons 82/83 (–G)	0	Azerbaijani; Czechoslovakian	Schwartz et al., 1989; Indrak et al., 1992
Codons 84/85 (+C)	0	Japanese	Ohba et al., 1997

(continued)

Table 12.1 *(continued)*

Mutation	Phenotype β⁰ or β⁺	Racial group	Reference
Mutations Producing Nonfunctional mRNAs			
Frameshift Mutations			
Codons 84/85/86 (+T)	0	Japanese	Ohba et al., 1997
Codon 88 (+T)	0	Asian Indian	Varawalla et al., 1991
Codon 89/90 (−GT)	0	Korean	Ohba et al., 1997
Codon 94 (+TG) β Agnana	Dominant β thal.	Italian	Ristaldi et al., 1990
Codon 95 (+A)	0	Thai	Winichagoon et al., 1992
Codon 100 (−CTT, +11 bp)	Dominant β thal.	South African	Williamson, et al., 1997
Codons 106/107 (+G)	0	American black	Wong et al., 1987
Codon 109 (−G) β Manhattan	Dominant β thal.	Lithuanian	Kazazian et al., 1992
Codon 114 (−CT, +G) β Geneva	Dominant β thal.	French	Beris et al., 1988
Codons 120/121 (+A)	Dominant β thal.	Filipino	Hopmeier et al., 1996
Codon 123 (−A) β Makabe	Dominant β thal.	Japanese	Fucharoen et al., 1990d
Codons 123–125 (−ACCCCACC) β Khon Kaen	Dominant β thal.	Thai	Fucharoen et al., 1991b
Codon 124 (−A)	Dominant β thal.	Russian	Çürük et al., 1994
Codon 125 (−A)	Dominant β thal.	Japanese	Ohba, et al., 1997
Codon 126 (−T) β Vercelli	Dominant β thal.	Italian	Murru et al., 1991
Codons 126 to 131 (−17 bp) β Westdale	0	Pakistani, Asian Indian	Ahmed et al., 1996, Waye et al., 1995
Codons 128/129 (−4, +5) and codons 132 to 135 (−11 bp)	Dominant β thal.	Irish	Thein et al., 1990b
Codons 131–132 (−GA)	Dominant β thal.	Swiss	Deutsch et al., 1998

Other

5′ Untranslated Sequence

Mutation	Phenotype β⁰ or β⁺	Racial group	Reference
+10 (−T)	+	Greek	Athanassiadou et al., 1994
+22 (G → A)	+	Eastern Mediterranean, Italian	Öner et al., 1991a; Cai et al., 1992
+33 (C → G)	+	Greek Cypriot	Ho et al., 1996
+43 to +40 (−AAAC)	+	Chinese	Huang et al., 1991

3′ Untranslated Sequence

Mutation	Phenotype β⁰ or β⁺	Racial group	Reference
Cap site + 1480 (C → G)	+	Greek	Jankovic et al., 1991
Cap site + 1565 to 1577 (13 bp deletion)	0 or +	Turkish	Basak et al., 1993

IVS-2

Mutation	Phenotype β⁰ or β⁺	Racial group	Reference
Insertion of L1 transposable element	+	Czech	Divoky et al., 1996

(continued)

Table 12.1 *(continued)*

Mutation	Phenotype β^0 or β^+	Racial group	Reference
Structural Variants with β Thalassemia Phenotype			
Missense Mutations			
Codon 28 (Leu → Arg) β Chesterfield	Dominant β thal.	English	Thein et al., 1991
Codon 32 (Leu → Glu) + codon 98 (Met → Val) β Medicine Lake	Dominant β thal.	US Caucasian	Coleman et al., 1995
Codon 60 (Val → Glu) β Cagliari	Dominant β thal.	Italian	Podda et al., 1991
Codon 106 (Leu → Arg) β Terre Haute (formerly β Indianapolis)	Dominant β thal.	N. European, French	Coleman et al., 1991; Girodon et al., 1992; Adams et al., 1979
Codon 110 (Leu → Pro) β Showa-Yakushiji	Dominant β thal.	Japanese	Kobayaski et al., 1987
Codon 114 (Leu → Pro) β Durham NC/β Brescia	Dominant β thal.	Russian, Irish, Italian	Çürük et al., 1995; deCastro et al., 1994; Huisman et al., 1997
Codon 115 (Ala → Asp) β Hradec Kralove	Dominant β thal.	Czech	Divoky et al., 1993
Codon 126 (Val → Gly) β Neapolis/β Dhonburi	+	Italian, Thai, German	Pagano et al., 1997; Divoky et al., 1992
Codon 127 (Gln → Pro) β Houston	Dominant β thal.	British	Kazazian et al., 1992
Codon 127 (Gln → Arg) β Dieppe	Dominant β thal.	French	Girodon et al., 1992
Deletion or Insertion of Triplet Codons			
Codons 24/25 (−GGT)		No information	Huisman et al., 1997
Codons 30/31 (+CGG)	Dominant β thal.	Spanish	Arjona et al., 1996
Codons 33/34 (−GTG) β Korea	Dominant β thal.	Korean	Park et al., 1991
Codons 33–35 (−6 bp) β Dresden	Dominant β thal.	German	Vetter et al., 2000
Codons 108 to 112 (−12 bp)	0	Swedish	Landin and Rudolphi, 1996
Codons 124 to 126 (+CCA)	Dominant β thal.	Armenian	Çürük et al., 1994
Codons 127 to 128 (−AGG) β Gunma	0 or Dominant β thal.	Japanese	Fucharoen et al., 1990e
Codons 134 to 137 (−12bp, +6 bp)	Dominant β thal.	Portuguese	Öner et al., 1991b

*Combined with 7.2 kb deletion of δ-globin gene (Corfu δβ thalassemia).

lassemia in a homozygous Chinese patient (Huang et al., 1986). The cause of this striking difference in phenotype is not known but may be related to different levels of β-globin gene expression associated with the different chromosomal backgrounds on which these apparently identical mutations occurred in the two different racial groups (Huang et al., 1986; Kazazian, 1990; Wong et al., 1987).

As previously discussed in Chapter 6, the cap site or transcription initiation site is part of a conserved sequence motif, which, in the case of genes lacking a TATA box, serves as a promoter element (Inr element) (Smale and Baltimore, 1989). It is not known if the Inr element plays a significant role in transcription of the globin genes that do contain a TATA box. Nevertheless, one mutation of the cap site (+1 A→C) has been found to be associated with a mild form of β thalassemia similar to the silent carrier state (Wong et al., 1987). It is not known whether this mutation causes β thalassemia by decreasing β-globin gene transcription or by decreasing the efficiency of capping (posttranscriptional addition of m^7G) and mRNA translation.

Initiation Codon Mutations

Translation of globin mRNAs begins at the initiation codon AUG (or ATG in DNA), which encodes methionine. The initiator ATG is usually located within a consensus sequence (Kozak consensus) that probably constitutes part of the ribosome binding site of the mRNA (Kozak, 1989). Six different point mutations of the initiator ATG have been identified as causes of $β^0$ thalassemia (Table 12.1). It is theoretically possible for the mutant mRNAs to be initiated at the next downstream ATG. In globin mRNA, the next ATG occurs in a different reading frame at codon positions 21 and 22, and the abnormal translation product would terminate approximately 40 codons further downstream, giving a short missense peptide unrelated to β globin. In addition, this ATG is not located within a good Kozak consensus sequence. The only other inframe ATG in β-globin mRNA is codon 55, and it is part of a better Kozak consensus sequence. Even if Codon 55 were utilized, a nonfunctional and possibly unstable N-terminal truncated β-globin chain would be produced.

Mutations Causing Abnormal Posttranscriptional Modification

As discussed in Chapter 6, the nascent precursor globin mRNA molecule is modified at both of its ends; a methylated (m^7G) cap structure is added at the 5' end, and a poly(A) tail is added at the 3' end of the mRNA. One mutation of the cap site has been described, although it is not known whether the principal effect of the mutation is on transcription or on the capping modification. On the other hand, a number of different β thalassemias have been associated with defective polyadenylation owing to mutations involving the consensus sequence AATAAA required for the cleavage-polyadenylation reaction: four base substitutions at different positions of the consensus sequence and two short deletions (of 2 and 5 bp; see Table 12.1). These mutations markedly decrease the efficiency of the cleavage-polyadenylation process, but do not abolish it completely. Therefore, the associated phenotype is that of $β^+$ thalassemia of typical severity because only about 10 percent of the mRNA is properly modified. The remainder of the transcripts extend far beyond the normal polyadenylation site and are probably cleaved and polyadenylated after the next AATAAA consensus sequences, which occur about 0.9 to 3 kb downstream (Orkin et al., 1985). These elongated transcripts are presumably unstable because they constitute only a minor portion of the mRNA in affected erythroid cells.

Mutations Causing Abnormal Precursor mRNA Splicing

The precursor globin mRNA must be processed posttranscriptionally to remove sequences corresponding to the introns of the gene. The complex, multistep process is referred to as splicing, and the consensus sequences required for efficient and accurate splicing were discussed in Chapter 6. Defects in splicing can be either complete or partial resulting in $β^0$ or $β^+$ thalassemia, respectively; they are described individually in the sections that follow.

Mutations of the Splice Site Junction That Totally Abolish Normal Splicing. The dinucleotides GT and AG are nearly always present at the 5' (donor) and 3' (acceptor) splice junctions, respectively, forming the boundaries of the intervening or intronic sequence (IVS) (Chapter 6). Base substitutions that change one or the other of these invariant dinucleotides, or short deletions that remove them, are associated with total absence of normal pre-mRNA splicing. Therefore, the phenotype is that of $β^0$ thalassemia. Nineteen base substitutions or short deletions involving the invariant dinucleotides of the β-globin gene introns have been identified (Table 12.1): six involving the 5' GT of IVS-1, two involving the 5' GT of IVS-2, four involving the 3' AG of IVS-1, and six involving the 3' AG of IVS-2. In some cases, the mutated intron is totally retained within the mutant mRNA. In other cases, the mutation appears to activate (or facilitate the use of) cryptic splice sites present elsewhere in the intron or, in the case of mutations of the IVS-1 5' splice junctions, in the adjacent exon, thus resulting in partial splicing of the mutant intron or removal of the intron together with a portion of the 5' flanking exon (Antonarakis et al., 1984; Treisman et al., 1982, 1983; Atweh et al., 1985; Cheng et al., 1984). The partially or abnormally spliced mRNA species can sometimes be detected in small amounts in affected erythroid cells. They are presumably unstable or poorly transported from nucleus to cytoplasm to account for their low abundance, and they are nonfunctional because translation of the abnormally spliced or frameshifted mRNAs would usually stop prematurely because of the presence of chain termination (nonsense) codons (see the section on mutations that produce nonfunctional β-globin mRNAs).

Mutations of a Splice Site Consensus Sequence That Partially Block Normal Splicing. The invariant dinucleotides GT and AG, which are present at the 5′ and 3′ splice junctions, respectively, are necessary but not sufficient to ensure efficient and accurate splicing. They are normally part of a larger consensus sequence that contains a number of other conserved sequence features (Chapter 6). Mutations of certain residues in this consensus sequence result in a partial block of normal mRNA splicing, the severity of which varies with the site of the mutation within the consensus sequence. As a group, these mutations are generally associated with a phenotype of β⁺ thalassemia. The mutation at position +6 of the IVS-1 5′ (donor) consensus sequence is particularly mild and is usually associated with β thalassemia intermedia owing to a relatively high level of normal mRNA splicing. In contrast, three different mutations at position +5 of the same consensus sequence result in a severe form of β thalassemia, with a markedly reduced amount of normally spliced β-globin mRNA. Other positions of the donor consensus sequences affected by mutations include positions −1 and −3 from the GT. A total of 16 mutations of the β-globin gene have been described in this category, eight of which involve the 5′ consensus sequence of IVS-1; one involves the 3′ consensus sequence of IVS-1 and two involve the 3′ consensus sequence of IVS-2 (Table 12.1). The 3′ consensus mutations affect nucleotides (of the polypyrimidine tract) at positions −1 and −8 from the acceptor AG.

The pattern of splicing that occurs with mutations of the 5′ consensus sequence of IVS-1 is quite complex. Mutations at this site result in the activation or use of three neighboring alternative or cryptic splice sites, two of which are present in adjacent exon 1 and one of which is located downstream in IVS-1 (Fig. 12.1) (Atweh et al., 1987; Treisman et al., 1983). The alternative splice site that is preferentially utilized over all others is located within exon 1 at codon positions 24

Fig. 12.1. Splicing patterns associated with different thalassemic mutations in exon 1 and IVS-1 of the β-globin gene. The normal and abnormal 5′ (donor) splice sites are indicated by arrowheads. The GT dinucleotide sequences required for the splicing events are indicated by the boxes. The nucleotide base substitutions resulting from the mutations are indicated by circled bold letters. The cross-hatched boxes indicate the portions of exon 1 that are removed from the processed mRNA by alternative splicing; the open box represents the portion of IVS-1 retained in the processed mRNA. (Adapted from Forget, BG. [1995]). Hemoglobin synthesis and the thalassemias. In *Blood: Principles and Practice of Hematology.* R.I. Handin, S.E. Lux, and T.P. Stossel (eds.). J.B. Lippincott Co., Philadelphia, PA., pp. 1525–1590).

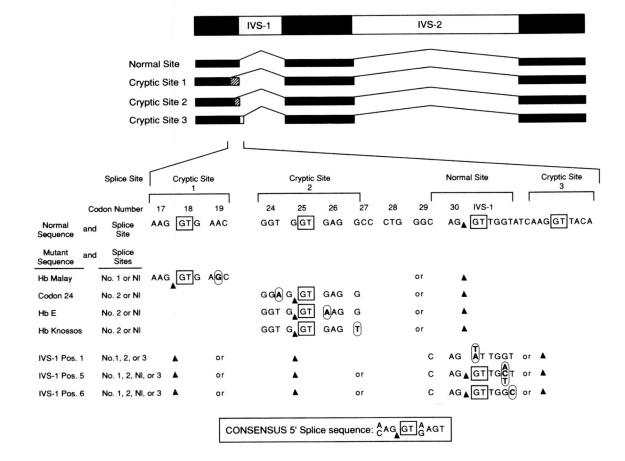

to 27. This cryptic splice site, GTG<u>GT</u>GAGG, consists of a good, though imperfect, match with the generic or canonical consensus sequence (A/C)AG<u>GT</u>(A/G)AGT. Preferential utilization of this same alternative or cryptic splice site also occurs in the case of HbE (Orkin et al., 1982b) as well as two other hemoglobin variants with base substitutions in the same region of the mRNA (Goldsmith et al., 1983; Orkin et al., 1984b) and is presumably responsible for the thalassemia phenotype associated with these disorders (see the later section on mutations that create new alternative splice sites in exons). The resulting abnormally spliced mRNA species have been characterized after gene transfer and expression in tissue culture cells. They are presumably highly unstable in vivo because they are not detectable in erythroid cells of affected patients. Even if these abnormally spliced β-globin mRNAs did accumulate within the cell, the two main species would be nonfunctional because of premature termination owing to frameshift (see the later section on nonfunctional mRNAs).

Mutations That Create New Alternative Splice Sites in Introns.

A third category of splicing mutation is due to base substitutions in introns that generate new splicing signals preferentially used instead of the normal splice sites. Five such mutations have been identified in the β-globin gene: two in IVS-1 and three in IVS-2 (Table 12.1). The associated phenotype may be either β+ or β0 thalassemia, depending on the site and nature of the mutation.

The first base substitution identified in a β-thalassemia gene was at position 110 of IVS-1. This mutation has subsequently been shown to be the most common form of β thalassemia in the Mediterranean population. The mutation is a substitution of G to A that creates an acceptor AG in a favorable consensus sequence environment, 19 bp 5' to the normal acceptor AG of IVS-1 (Fig. 12.2A). Gene transfer and expression studies in tissue culture cells have shown that this newly created alternative splice site is preferentially used in 80 to 90 percent of the transcripts, whereas the normal splice site is used in only 10 to 20 percent of the transcripts (Busslinger et al., 1981; Fukumaki et al., 1982), thus giving the phenotype of β+ thalassemia (Fig. 12.2B). The mutant mRNA is presumably unstable or poorly transported from nucleus to cytoplasm because it is not detected in a significant quantity in affected erythroid cells. Even if it were to accumulate, it would be nonfunctional because the 19 bp segment of retained intronic sequence contains an in-phase termination codon and thus a truncated β-globin peptide would be synthesized.

Another mutation was later identified in a different Mediterranean family, 6 bp farther 3' in IVS-1, at posi-

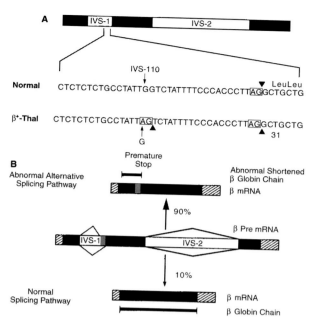

Figure 12.2. Alternative splicing of precursor β-globin mRNA resulting in β+ thalassemia associated with the mutation of IVS-1 position 110. (A) Diagram of the β-globin gene showing the DNA sequence at the 3' end of IVS-1 and the G → A base substitution at position 110, creating an AG dinucleotide within a potential consensus 3' (acceptor) splice site in the β+ thalassemic gene. The arrowheads indicate potential splice sites. (From Forget, BG. [1995]). Hemoglobin synthesis and the thalassemias. In *Blood: Principles and Practice of Hematology*. R.I. Handin, S.E. Lux, and T.P. Stossel (eds.). J.B. Lippincott Co., Philadelphia, PA., pp. 1525–1590).

tion 116 (Metherall et al., 1986). This mutation (T→G) also creates a new acceptor AG in a good consensus sequence, but in this case the phenotype is that of β0 thalassemia. The normal acceptor sequence, although intact, is not used presumably because the new AG occurs at a position that is too proximal to the normal AG and thus totally interferes with its recognition and use as a splice site (Metherall et al., 1986). In a survey of normal acceptor sites, a second AG was virtually never found at positions −5 to −15 from the normal acceptor AG (Mount, 1982); the new AG in the IVS-1 position 116 mutation occurs at positions −13 and −14.

In IVS-2, a mutation at position 654 (C→T) has been identified as a relatively common cause of β0 thalassemia in Chinese (Cheng et al., 1984). The mutation creates a new donor GT splice site within IVS-2. Gene transfer and expression studies revealed that IVS-2 sequences of the mutant precursor β mRNA are partially spliced out in two steps: from the normal 5' donor GT to a cryptic acceptor at position 579 then from the mutant donor site at position 654 to the normal 3' acceptor (Cheng et al., 1984). As a result, a 75 bp segment of IVS-2 sequence is retained in the abnor-

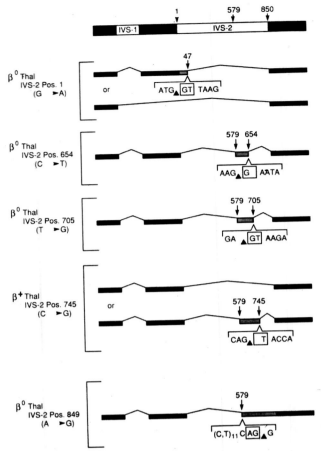

Figure 12.3. Splicing patterns associated with different thalassemic mutations in IVS-2 of the β-globin gene. The nucleotide sequences at the cryptic or alternative splicing sites are indicated with the same conventions as in Figure 12.1. The same cryptic acceptor site at IVS-2 position 579 is used in many of the mutations. The portions of IVS-2 retained in the processed mRNAs are indicated by the gray boxes. (From Forget, BG. [1995]). Hemoglobin synthesis and the thalassemias. In *Blood: Principles and Practice of Hematology*. R.I. Handin, S.E. Lux, and T.P. Stossel (eds.). J.B. Lippincott Co., Philadelphia, PA., pp. 1525–1590).

mally processed mRNA (Fig. 12.3). It is surprising that although the normal splice sites of IVS-2 are intact and located at a considerable distance from the mutation, no normal splicing is observed. A similar phenomenon occurs in the case of the mutation of IVS-2 at position 705 (T→G). There is apparent absence of normal splicing and two-step partial excision of IVS-2: (1) from the normal 5′ GT to the naturally occurring cryptic acceptor at position 579, and (2) from the cryptic donor site created by the mutation at position 705 to the normal 3′ acceptor AG (Dobkin et al., 1983) (Dobkin and Bank, 1985).

In contrast, another mutation of IVS-2 at position 745 also creates a new alternative donor splice site and is associated with a similar two-step excision of IVS-2

with utilization of the cryptic acceptor at position 654 (Treisman et al., 1983). Some normal splicing of IVS-2 occurs; therefore, this mutation results in β⁺ rather than β⁰ thalassemia (Treisman et al., 1983). The β⁰ versus β⁺ phenotype associated with these different mutations must be related to different affinities of the enzymatic splicing complex for a given mutant splice site versus the normal splice sites.

Mutations That Create New Alternative Splice Sites in Exons. Four mutations have been identified in exon 1 that are associated with activation of cryptic or alternative splice sites within exon 1 in a manner analogous to the mutations of the normal IVS-1 5′ consensus sequence (see the previous section on mutations of the splice site consensus sequence that partially block normal splicing). In contrast to the latter group of mutations that activate three cryptic splice sites, the exon mutations activate only the one cryptic splice site that they modify. Three of these mutations are located in codons 24 to 27 (Table 12.1) and activate the previously mentioned cryptic donor site that has a preexisting GT derived from codon 25. The mutations involve the nucleotides at positions −2, +3, and +6 of the consensus sequence (Fig. 12.1). These mutations presumably increase the affinity of the preexisting cryptic splice site for the enzymatic splicing complex so that it is more readily recognized and used. The mutation at codon 24 is silent and does not change the encoded amino acid in the normally spliced β mRNA (Goldsmith et al., 1983).

The mutations at codon positions 26 and 27 do result in the encoding of amino acid replacements by the normally spliced β mRNA and the synthesis of structurally abnormal variant hemoglobins: HbE (Orkin et al., 1982b) and Hb Knossos (Orkin et al., 1984b), respectively. The phenotype associated with these mutations is that of β⁺ thalassemia, because the normal 5′ splice site of IVS-1 is intact and variably used instead of the cryptic site at codon positions 24 to 27. The mutation at codon 24 is associated with a β⁺ thalassemia phenotype of typical severity (Goldsmith et al., 1983). In contrast, HbE and Hb Knossos are associated with relatively mild forms of β⁺ thalassemia (Fessas et al., 1982; Rouabhi et al., 1983). In fact, Hb Knossos is usually associated with the silent carrier state for β thalassemia. HbE, a common hemoglobin variant in Southeast Asia, was long known to be associated with the phenotype of mild β thalassemia with hypochromia, microcytosis, and interaction, with typical β thalassemia resulting in a more severe clinical syndrome (Chapter 43). The basis for the thalassemic phenotype did not become clear until gene cloning and expression studies were done (Orkin et al., 1982b).

A mutation at codon 19 also results in a hemoglobin variant, Hb Malay, which is associated with a mild β+ thalassemia phenotype (Yang et al., 1989). The mutation involves the nucleotide at position +5 of the consensus sequence of a preexisting cryptic donor site at codon positions 17 to 19 of exon 1 (Fig. 12.1). This same cryptic site is also used in the case of mutations of the normal IVS-1 donor consensus sequence (see the previous section on mutations of the splice consensus sequence that partially block normal splicing). Gene expression studies have shown that about 25 percent of the mRNA from the β-Malay gene is abnormally spliced at the alternative splice site (Gonzalez-Redondo et al., 1989e). HbE, Hb Knossos, and Hb Malay are examples of thalassemic hemoglobinopathies discussed in Chapter 14.

Mutations That Produce Nonfunctional β-Globin mRNAs

Nonsense Mutations. Nonsense mutations result from single base substitutions that change a codon for a given amino acid to a chain termination codon and thus cause premature cessation of mRNA translation. There are three possible mRNA chain termination codons: UAA, UAG, and UGA or their DNA codons TAA, TAG, and TGA.

Truncated globin chains should be produced as a result of such mutations, but they are not usually detected, presumably because they are very unstable and rapidly degraded. The phenotype is that of β⁰ thalassemia with total absence of normal β-chain synthesis from the affected gene.

One of the first nonsense mutations to be characterized and extensively studied is the mutation at codon 39 (CAG to TAG). This mutation is the second most common cause of β thalassemia in the Mediterranean population and accounts for most of the cases of β thalassemia in Sardinia. An interesting and poorly understood feature of this and other nonsense mutations is the finding of very low levels of the mutant β-globin mRNA in affected erythroid cells. Initial studies of this phenomenon revealed that the gene was transcribed normally, but there appeared to be defective β-mRNA stability in the nucleus or defective processing and/or transport of the mRNA from nucleus to cytoplasm; mRNA stability in the cytoplasm appeared to be normal (Takeshita et al., 1984; Humphries et al., 1984; Baserga and Benz, 1988, 1992).

Based on a large number of subsequent experimental studies, it now appears that the deficiency of globin mRNA in association with nonsense mutations is due to both posttranscriptional processing and translational mechanisms. The splicing out of intronic sequences from the pre-mRNA apparently marks the mature mRNA in such a manner that if the translational machinery of the cell encounters a nonsense mutation before nucleotides upstream of the last (3'-most) exon-exon splice junction, degradation of the mRNA occurs (Nagy and Maquat, 1998; Thermann et al., 1998; Hentze and Kulozik, 1999). This process, called nonsense-mediated decay, may be a mechanism by which the cell protects itself from the potential noxious effects of dominant negative proteins resulting from the translation of abnormal mRNAs. However, when the nonsense mutations occur in the terminal exon of a gene (such as exon 3 of the globin gene), the protective process does not occur and the abnormal mRNA can accumulate and be translated to produce the abnormal protein, as occurs in cases of dominant β thalassemia (Chapter 14).

In addition to the β39 codon mutation, a number of other nonsense mutations have subsequently been described, ranging in location from codon 15 to codon 127 of the β-globin gene (Table 12.1). In general, the resulting β⁰ thalassemia has a phenotype similar to that associated with the β 39 codon mutation:β⁰ thalassemia with little or no detectable β-globin mRNA. However, the nonsense mutations that occur in exon 3 (gene codons 112, 121, and 127) are associated with an unusually severe phenotype in the heterozygous state, with hemolytic anemia and, in some cases, the formation of inclusion bodies, so-called dominant β thalassemia (Chapter 14). In these cases, there is sufficient accumulation of the abnormal mRNA (owing to absence of nonsense-mediated decay) to result in the synthesis of a highly unstable truncated β-globin chain responsible for the hemolysis. Nevertheless some carriers of the codon 112, 121, and 127 nonsense mutations have the phenotype of typical β-thalassemia trait without hemolysis, perhaps because of enhanced proteolytic capacity of their erythroid cells (Chapter 14).

Frameshift Mutations. Frameshift mutations result from the deletion or insertion of one or more nucleotides (other than multiples of three) in the protein-encoding region of the gene. This causes a change in the normal reading frame of the encoded mRNA at the site of the mutation. Such mutations usually allow the continued translation of the mRNA for some distance, yielding a novel abnormal amino acid sequence, until a chain termination codon is encountered in the new reading frame. Chain termination usually occurs at a position well before the normal termination codon and results in the synthesis of a truncated, unstable mutant globin chain that is presumably rapidly degraded. The frameshift resulting from a 4-bp deletion at codon positions 41 and 42 is a particularly common mutation in persons of Chinese and Asian Indian ancestry (Kazazian et al., 1984a; Kimura et al., 1983). The frameshift resulting from a single base deletion at codon 44 in Kurdish Jewish persons is associated with an unusually short β-globin mRNA half-life of 30 minutes (Maquat et al., 1981). This marked mRNA instability appears to be restricted to erythroid cells, because the abnormal β-globin mRNA is stable after gene transfer and expression in HeLa cells (Maquat and Kinninbugh, 1985). The basis for the mRNA instability is probably the process of non-sense-mediated mRNA decay described previously. A large number of other frameshift mutations have been identified and are listed in Table 12.1.

Although most frameshift mutations are associated with typical β⁰ thalassemia, those that occur relatively far into the coding sequence (in exon 3) are associated with the phenotype of dominant β thalassemia, including moderately severe hemolytic anemia, splenomegaly, and inclusion body formation (Chapter 14). This result occurs presumably because of the absence of nonsense-mediated mRNA decay and the synthesis of mutant β-globin chains, capable of binding heme and producing aggregates that are relatively resistant to proteolytic degradation (Thein et al., 1990; Thein, 1992).

Missense Mutations Resulting in Unstable Globin Chains

Many base substitutions result in amino replacements at residues that are crucial for globin chain stability. The globin chain that is synthesized is so unstable that little or no soluble mutant hemoglobin is detectable. In certain cases, such as Hb Terre Haute (formerly called Hb Indianapolis) (Coleman et al., 1991; Adams et al. 1979), the phenotype may be similar to that of dominant β thalassemia, as seen in cases of nonsense and frameshift mutations involving exon 3 (Chapter 14).

In other cases, simply hypochromia and microcytosis without inclusion body formation or hemolysis are present, presumably because of more rapid and efficient proteolysis of the mutant globin chain. A number of such mutations have been identified in the β-globin gene (Table 12.1). A mild degree of hypochromia can also be associated with a number of additional unstable hemoglobins caused by the progressive loss of intracellular hemoglobin from precipitation and degradation (Adams and Coleman, 1990). In these cases, the β-globin chain that is initially synthesized is stable and assembled into hemoglobin tetramers that become progressively unstable. Variants of this type are not included in Table 12.1.

THE HEMOGLOBIN LEPORE SYNDROMES

Another structurally abnormal hemoglobin associated with a β-thalassemia phenotype (i.e., thalassemic hemoglobinopathy) consists of Hb Lepore. The Hb Lepore syndromes can also be considered as related to the δβ-thalassemia syndromes (Chapter 15) because they are associated with a β-thalassemia phenotype, absence of normal δ- and β-globin gene expression in cis, and usually a modest elevation of HbF. The increase in HbF is not as striking as that seen in typical cases of β thalassemia. Hb Lepore is a structurally abnormal hemoglobin in which the abnormal globin chain is a hybrid or fused globin chain, having the N-terminal amino acid sequence of the normal chain and the C-terminal amino acid sequence of the normal β chain (Baglioni, 1962). The Lepore gene is almost certainly the result of an unequal crossover event or recombination between the highly homologous (but nonidentical) δ- and β-globin genes, with the resulting deletion of the 5′ end of the β gene, the 3′ end of the δ gene and ~ 7 kb of intergene DNA between the δ and β genes (Fig. 12.4). Gene mapping studies have in fact confirmed the expected gene deletion (Flavell et al., 1978; Mears, et al., 1978).

Figure 12.4. Nonhomologous crossing over between δ- and β-globin genes resulting in the formation of the Lepore and anti-Lepore fusion genes. (From Weatherall, DJ and Clegg, JB [1981]). The Thalassaemia Syndromes (3rd ed). Oxford: Blackwell Scientific Publications.)

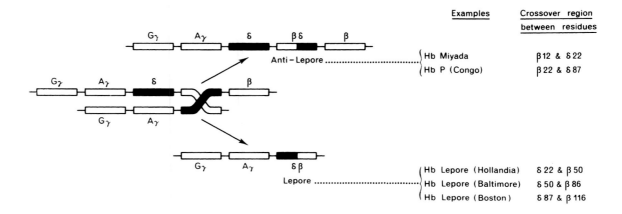

	Examples	Crossover region between residues
Anti-Lepore	Hb Miyada	β 12 & δ 22
	Hb P (Congo)	β 22 & δ 87
Lepore	Hb Lepore (Hollandia)	δ 22 & β 50
	Hb Lepore (Baltimore)	δ 50 & β 86
	Hb Lepore (Boston)	δ 87 & β 116

Three different types of Hb Lepore caused by crossovers at different positions of the genes have been identified. In the most common form, Hb Lepore Boston or Lepore Washington, the recombination event occurred at the 5' end of IVS-2 of the β-globin gene (Baird et al., 1981; Mavilio et al., 1983; Chebloune and Verdier, 1983). The same mutation is found in diverse racial groups and associated with different haplotypes of β-globin gene cluster restriction fragment length polymorphisms (RFLPs) (Lanclos et al., 1987) (see the latter section of this chapter on polymorphisms of the globin gene cluster). Thus, the mutation appears to have arisen independently on more than one occasion. The Hb Lepore gene behaves as a β-thalassemic gene because of the presence of only a low level of synthesis of its gene product (the Lepore β-globin chain) and absence of normal β chain production from the affected chromosome: homozygotes produce no HbA or HbA_2.

The reasons for the low level of synthesis of Hb Lepore are not known. Synthesis may be decreased because of relative instability of the Lepore mRNA. Globin chain synthetic studies reveal that synthesis of the Lepore β chain, like that of the δ chain of the Hb A_2, occurs primarily in bone marrow cells and is virtually absent or much lower in peripheral blood reticulocytes (Wood et al., 1978). In addition, transcription of the Lepore β gene is probably reduced because it shares the same 5'-flanking (promoter) sequences as the δ-globin gene. These sequences, which differ from the corresponding sequences of the β-globin gene (including a mutant CACCC box), are likely to be responsible (at least partly) for the normally low level of δ-globin gene expression (Chapter 10).

Whatever the relative contributions of mRNA instability and decreased gene transcription, Hb Lepore accumulates to a level of about 10 to 15 percent of the total hemoglobin, whereas HbA_2 is rarely increased to levels much greater than 5 percent. The 5'-flanking DNA adjacent to the gene cannot be the only factor that influences the level of expression of the Lepore β gene; otherwise Hb Lepore would be expected to accumulate only to a level similar to that of HbA_2. It is possible that the enhancer elements in IVS 2, exon 3 and the 3' flanking DNA of the β-globin gene, now in proximity to the promoter because of the recombination event, increase the activity of the promoter in the Lepore β fusion gene, especially in the absence of competition from the β-globin promoter for transcription factors (see Chapter 6 and the following section). Other possible mechanisms to explain the differences between steady state amounts of Hb Lepore and HbA_2 include stabilization of the β mRNA by 3' untranslated sequences from the β gene and different affinities of the δ- and δβ-globin chains for association with α–globin chains.

The reciprocal product of Lepore-type recombination events is the anti-Lepore chromosome (Fig. 12.4), which has been identified for all three types of Lepore crossovers. The anti-Lepore syndromes are not associated with a β-thalassemia phenotype because the affected chromosome carries, in addition to the mutant gene, normal β- and δ-globin genes. Similar to the situation observed in the Hb Lepore syndromes, the synthesis of the anti-Lepore globin chain is almost absent in reticulocytes and is essentially limited to bone marrow cells. This phenomenon has been interpreted as evidence of instability of the anti-Lepore globin mRNA and evidence that both the 5'- and 3'-untranslated sequences of β-globin mRNA are important in maintaining its stability. The anti-Lepore gene also lacks the 3' β-globin gene enhancer.

DELETIONS OF THE β-GLOBIN GENE RESULTING IN β⁰ THALASSEMIA

Although most cases of β thalassemia are due to point mutations, a few cases occur in which the cause is a partial or total deletion of the β-globin gene (Fig. 12.5) (reviewed in Huisman et al., 1997). These deletions involve only the β-globin gene and its flanking DNA without affecting any of the other neighboring β-like globin genes. In contrast, β thalassemia and hereditary persistence of fetal hemoglobin (HPFH) are associated with deletions that encompass multiple genes in the cluster (Chapter 15). The thalassemic deletions vary in size between 105 bp and ~67 kb, excluding the smaller intragenic deletions of 17, 25, and 44 bp listed in Table 12.1 under splice site junction mutations. The phenotype associated with these deletions is that of β⁰ thalassemia.

The 0.6-kb deletion involving the 3' end of the β-globin gene is a relatively common cause of β⁰ thalassemia in Asian Indians and accounts for about one third of the cases of β thalassemia in this population (Kazazian et al. 1984a; Spritz and Orkin 1982; Thein et al., 1984). The other β-gene deletions are relatively rare (Anand et al., 1988; Thein et al., 1989; Diaz-Chico et al., 1987; Popovich et al., 1986, Motum, et al., 1992, 1993; Craig, et al., 1992; Lynch et al., 1991; Waye et al., 1991; Dimovski et al., 1993, 1994, 1996; Gilman, 1987; Sanguansermsri et al., 1990; Spiegelberg et al., 1989; Öner et al., 1995; Nopparatana et al., 1995; Gonzalez-Redondo et al., 1989c; Lacerra et al. 1997). Most of these deletions have an interesting phenotype with unusually high levels of HbA_2 in heterozygotes. A common feature of these mutations is the deletion of the promoter region of the β-globin gene. It has been proposed that the unusually high level of HbA_2 may be due to the lack of competition between δ- and β-globin gene promoters for transcription factors, thus allowing more

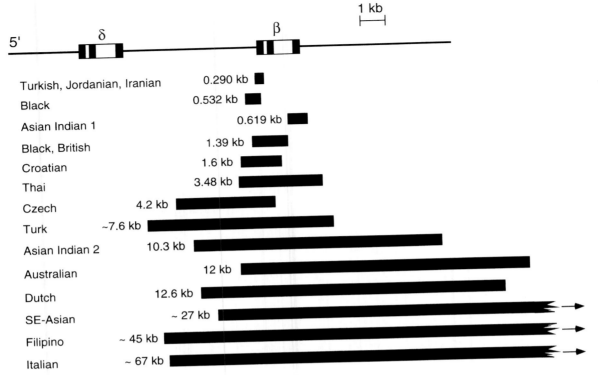

Figure 12.5. Deletions of the β-globin gene and flanking DNA associated with β⁰ thalassemia. The ~7.6 kb Turkish deletion is also associated with a comparable deletion involving the Ψβ gene (Öner et al., 1995). The references reporting the individual deletions are provided in the text and in Huisman et al. (1997).

efficient expression of the δ-globin gene (Popovich et al., 1986). In this regard, the β-gene promoter mutations at position −88, and possibly that at position −29, are also associated with unexpectedly high levels of HbA₂ (Codrington et al., 1990).

UNKNOWN, POSSIBLY DISTANT, MUTATIONS CAUSING β THALASSEMIA

A small number of β-thalassemic patients carry β-globin genes that are entirely normal in structure. The cause of β thalassemia in these cases is presumably a more remote mutation either within the β-globin gene cluster (perhaps in the locus control region [LCR] or the 3′ enhancer of the β-globin gene) or in another gene such as one for a specific transcription factor. The first family of this type to be studied was an Albanian family in which two children had β thalassemia of intermediate severity (β thalassemia intermedia). The mother had typical β-thalassemia trait, whereas the father apparently had the silent carrier trait (Schwartz, 1969). One of the cloned β-globin genes from one of the affected children had a normal DNA sequence except for some sequence variation (−T, +ATA) at position −530 from the cap site (Semenza et al., 1984). This region of DNA is characterized by the presence of variable numbers of repeated AT and T residues in different persons, which is suggestive of a polymorphism (Chebloune et al., 1988; Wong, et al., 1989b; Galanello et al., 1993). Analysis of other β-globin cluster polymorphisms in this family initially indicated that the two affected children had inherited different β-globin gene clusters from their father, suggesting that the β-thalassemia determinant in the father did not reside nearby on chromosome 11 and could even be located on a different chromosome (Semenza et al., 1984). Subsequent analysis of this family revealed that both of the affected children had inherited the same sequence variation at −530, and the difference in the polymorphisms was attributed to a first-generation crossover between the two paternal alleles (Schwartz et al., 1988). It has been proposed that the base changes found in the −530 region of the β-globin gene in this family may be responsible for the β-thalassemia phenotype owing to the increased binding of a putative negative regulatory *trans*-acting factor (Berg et al., 1991). The same changes were also found in three siblings (of a Southern Italian family) who had β-thalassemia intermedia and an otherwise normal β gene (Murru et al., 1990) further suggesting that the sequence variation at position −530 might be functionally significant.

In another Italian family two brothers with β thalassemia intermedia also had the complex rearrangement at −530 (with an otherwise normal β-globin gene) in *trans* to a thalassemic gene with the codon 39 nonsense mutation (Murru et al., 1992). One of the affected brothers had a child with β thalassemia major who inherited the father's codon 39 nonsense mutation (without the −530 rearrangement) and a structurally normal β-globin gene from an apparently normal mother.

In a study of 100 β-thalassemia genes, Kazazian and co-workers (1990) identified nine persons in whom the β-globin gene had a normal DNA sequence from a point 600 nucleotides 5′ to the cap site to a point 200 nucleotides 3′ to the end of the gene, as well as a normal DNA sequence of the 400 bp enhancer region located approximately 0.7 kb 3′ to the gene. These cases appear to represent truly unknown mutations. Other similar cases have also been reported (Huisman et al. 1997; Thein et al., 1993).

POLYMORPHISMS OF THE β-GLOBIN GENE CLUSTER

In contrast to the DNA of exons that shows little or no sequence variability among normal individuals, the DNA between genes and that of introns can vary significantly in its nucleotide sequence from one person to another. An estimated 1 of every 200 to 400 nucleotides of extragenic DNA may be different in any two persons. Such sequence variability has proved to be informative in a number of genetic studies because it provides a type of marker or fingerprint for a person's genome.

Sequence variability is most frequently detected by restriction endonuclease digestion and Southern gel blotting of total cellular DNA followed by hybridization to a labeled DNA probe from the gene region of interest. The generation of DNA fragments of different sizes in different persons provides evidence for sequence variability in the region of DNA tested. This is called *restriction fragment length polymorphism* (RFLP). A large number of such polymorphisms have been identified in the β-globin gene cluster. They are found in intergene and intervening sequence DNA, and one polymorphism is even present in the coding sequence of the β-globin gene but without causing a change in amino acid sequence. Most of these polymorphisms are common and widely distributed among different racial groups. The location and nature of some of these RFLPs are illustrated at the top of Figure 12.6. These different polymorphisms are not associated with each other in a totally random manner, but rather tend to occur in certain groupings or subsets called haplotypes (Antonarakis et al., 1982a, 1985; Orkin and Kazazian, 1984) (see also Chapter 26). The nine major haplotypes of the β-gene cluster are illustrated in Figure 12.6. Orkin and co-workers (1982) first demonstrated that, in Mediterraneans, different specific β-thalassemia mutations were associated with different haplotypes. The determination of haplotypes by gene mapping therefore provided a rela-

tively simple screening test to identify the most probable mutation in an affected person or to help identify the persons with novel mutations. This strategy was successfully applied to a systematic survey of β-thalassemia mutations in different population groups such as Asian Indians, Chinese, and American blacks (Antonarakis et al., 1985; Orkin and Kazazian 1984). Haplotype analysis was also a useful procedure in prenatal diagnosis of β thalassemia by analysis of DNA from amniocentesis samples or chorionic villus biopsies (Chapter 36), prior to the availability of direct DNA-based prenatal diagnosis (Chapter 35).

RFLPs have also been identified in the α-globin gene cluster, and a number of different cluster haplotypes have been defined (Chapter 17).

ASSOCIATION OF RFLP HAPLOTYPES WITH β-THALASSEMIA MUTATIONS AND POPULATION GENETICS OF β THALASSEMIA AND OTHER β-CHAIN HEMOGLOBINOPATHIES.

The prevalence of different haplotypes in Mediterranean β thalassemic patients is shown in Figure 12.6. Follow-up studies of this population using synthetic oligonucleotides, or restriction endonuclease digestion, for direct identification of thalassemic mutations have led to some interesting observations. In general, a given haplotype within this population is usually associated with one specific type of thalassemia. Thus, by haplotype analysis, one can predict, with about 90 percent accuracy, the specific mutation causing β thalassemia in a given person. Exceptions are the following: more than one type of thalassemia mutation can be found within a given haplotype, and a specific type of thalassemia mutation may be associated with two or more different haplotypes in the same population. In Mediterranean β-thalassemic patients with haplotype I, which is the most common haplotype in this population (Fig. 12.6), about 90 percent of cases are associated with the mutation at IVS-1 position 110 (Kazazian et al., 1984b).

Other β-thalassemia mutations are also associated with haplotype I in Mediterraneans: the frameshift mutation at codon 6, Hb Knossos, and even the β codon 39 nonsense mutation. Thus, it cannot be assumed that all Mediterranean β-thalassemic persons with haplotype I have the IVS-1 position 110 mutation. This result is not totally surprising; multiple different independent mutations might be expected to occur on the same chromosomal background if the latter is particularly common in a given normal population, as is haplotype I.

Although there are a number of examples of the association of a given specific β-thalassemia mutation with more than one different haplotype, the most interesting cases consist of the β codon 39 nonsense and β^E globin genes. In the case of the β codon non-

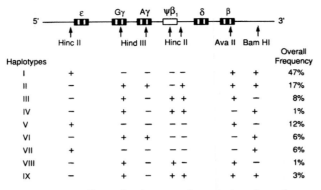

Figure 12.6. Different haplotypes of restriction site polymorphisms in the β-gene cluster and their frequency in Mediterranean individuals with β thalassemia. A plus sign indicates the presence and a minus sign the absence of the particular restriction endonuclease cleavage site. (Adapted from Orkin et al., [1982a] and reproduced from Forget, BG. [1995]. etc. Hemoglobin synthesis and the thalassemias. In *Blood: Principles and Practice of Hematology*. R.I. Handin, S.E. Lux, and T.P. Stossel (eds.). J.B. Lippincott Co., Philadelphia, PA., pp. 1525–1590).

sense mutation, the defect was associated with at least nine different chromosomal backgrounds (Pirastu et al., 1987). For seven of these chromosomes, RFLPs within (or very close to) the β-globin gene itself were identical. Thus, one could explain the observation by a single mutation in an ancestral β-globin gene that then "spread" to other chromosomes by recombination, the crossover site being located between the 5′ side of the β-globin gene and the 3′ side of the polymorphic *Hinc*II sites around the ψβ1 gene (Fig. 12.6). It has been proposed that this region of DNA contains a "hot spot" for recombination (Antonarakis et al., 1982; Chakravarti et al., 1984).

The β codon 39 nonsense mutation has also been identified in β-globin genes with different intragenic polymorphic sites or, in the terminology of Orkin and Kazazian (1984), in different β-globin gene "frameworks." Three (or four) basic β-globin gene frameworks differ by two to five intragenic nucleotide base substitutions (Antonarakis et al., 1985; Orkin and Kazazian, 1984). The occurrence of the same mutation in two different β-gene frameworks, especially in two frameworks differing by five nucleotides (one in exon 1 and four in IVS-2) implies that the identical mutation must have arisen spontaneously at least twice, once in each framework.

Alternatively, if one holds to the theory of a single ancestral mutation, the findings can be explained only by a rare localized interchromosomal recombination event called gene conversion. Such short, discrete recombination or gene conversion events appear to have occurred in the case of the β-globin genes (in IVS-2), as well as in the histocompatibility and

immunoglobulin genes. The HbE mutation in Asian populations has been identified in two different β-globin gene frameworks, differing by four nucleotides (Antonarakis et al., 1982b). This finding must also be explained by the occurrence of independent identical mutations or short gene conversion events. A similar phenomenon has also been observed with the HbS mutation (Chapter 26).

Comparison of haplotypes and β-thalassemic mutations in different populations has provided the interesting finding that the same haplotype is generally associated with different forms of β thalassemia in different populations. In fact, a given β-thalassemia mutation generally appears to be restricted to a particular population, because the same mutation is not usually found in two different racial groups. Of the large number of mutations listed in Table 12.1, only a few have been described in more than one racial group (Kazazian, 1990). In such instances the chromosomal background haplotype or β-globin gene framework (or both) is almost always different in the separate racial groups, indicating that the mutations most likely had independent origins in the different populations (Kazazian, 1990).

SUMMARY AND CONCLUSIONS

Studies of thalassemia have shown that the molecular basis is quite heterogeneous. More than 175 different mutations have been identified. Despite the vast heterogeneity of molecular defects, the biochemical and clinical phenotypes vary within a relatively narrow range. The common denominator is absent or decreased synthesis of β-globin chains, with resulting accumulation of excess α-globin chains that are responsible for the pathophysiology of the disorder. The severity of the phenotype is usually related to the degree of imbalance between α- and non-α-globin chain synthesis (Chapter 11).

A number of additional general conclusions can be drawn from the results of studies on the molecular basis of thalassemia, and these conclusions have implications for the prenatal diagnosis and future prospects for gene therapy of β thalassemia. A given mutation is generally found only within one racial group and not another. β thalassemia is quite common, not only in Mediterranean populations, but also in African, African-American, and Asian populations; however, in these different racial groups, one usually finds a different set of specific mutations. A given mutation also tends to be on the same chromosomal background in different individuals of the same racial group. If one determines polymorphisms in and around a β-thalassemic globin gene, one has a clue to what mutation is likely to be present in that gene. Finally, a small number of mutations usually account for the majority of cases of thalassemia in a given population. For instance, despite the overall high number of different thalassemic mutations, more than 90 percent of all the mutations observed in Mediterraneans can be accounted for by only six different molecular defects, the two most common being the nonsense mutation at codon 39 and the IVS-1 position 110 alternative splicing defect.

Similarly, a limited number of specific mutations are responsible for the majority of cases of thalassemia in other populations (Chapter 31). This finding and the availability of rapid and efficient techniques for DNA-based diagnosis of globin gene mutations (Chapter 35) have greatly facilitated the process of prenatal diagnosis of β thalassemia (Chapter 36).

Studies on the molecular basis of β-thalassemia for gene therapy of the disorder suggest that the heterogeneity of mutations makes it highly impractical to consider mutation-targeted approaches. However, a single effective approach to gene therapy would be the introduction of a functional β-globin gene into hematopoietic stem cells of the homozygous affected individual as a substitute for the defective genes. The transfer of a normal β-globin gene into the hematopoietic stem cells of an affected patient's bone marrow, as well as reinfusion of that transfected or transduced marrow, is one potential approach to gene therapy (Chapter 41).

References

Adams, JG and Coleman, MB. (1990). Structural hemoglobin variants that produce the phenotype of thalassemia. *Semin. Hematol.* 27: 229–238.

Adams, JG III, Boxer, LA, Baehner, RL et al. (1979). Hemoglobin Indianapolis (β112[G14] arginine): An unstable β-chain variant producing the phenotype of severe ββ thalassemia. *J. Clin. Invest.* 63: 931–938.

Ahmed, S, Petrou, M, and Saleem, M. (1996). Molecular genetics of β-thalassaemia in Pakistan: A basis for prenatal diagnosis. *Br. J. Haematol.* 94: 476–482.

Anand, R, Boehm, CD, Kazazian, HH Jr. and Vanin, EF. Molecular characterization of a β⁰ thalassemia resulting from a 1.4 kilobase deletion. *Blood* 72: 636–641.

Antonarakis, SE, Boehm, CD, Giardina, PJ, and Kazazian, HH Jr. (1982a). Nonrandom association of polymorphic restriction sites in the β-globin gene cluster. *Proc. Natl. Acad. Sci. U.S.A.* 79: 137–141.

Antonarakis, SE, Orkin, SH, Kazazian, HH Jr et al. (1982b). Evidence for multiple origins of the βE-globin gene in Southeast Asia. *Proc. Natl. Acad. Sci. U.S.A.* 79: 6608–6611.

Antonarakis, SE, Orkin, SH, Cheng, T-C et al. (1984). β thalassemia in American blacks: Novel mutations in the TATA box and an acceptor splice site. *Proc. Natl. Acad. Sci. U.S.A.* 81: 1154–1158.

Antonarakis, SE, Kazazian, HH Jr, and Orkin, SH. (1985). DNA polymorphism and molecular pathology of the human globin gene clusters. *Hum. Genet.* 69: 1–14.

Arjona, SN, Eloy-Garcia, JM, Gu, L-H et al. (1996). The dominant-thalassaemia in a Spanish family is due to a frameshift that introduces an extra CGG codon (=arginine) at the 5′ end of the second exon. *Br. J. Haematol.* 93: 841–844.

Athanassiadou, A, Papachatzopoulou, A, Zoumbos, N et al. (1994). A novel beta-thalassaemia mutation in the 5′ untranslated region of the beta-globin gene. *Br. J. Haematol.* 88: 207–310.

Atweh, GF, Anagnou, NP, Shearin, J et al. (1985). β thalassemia resulting from a single nucleotide substitution in an acceptor splice site. *Nucl. Acids Res.* 13: 777–790.

Atweh, GF, Wong, C, Reed, R et al. (1987a). A new mutation in IVS-1 of the human β-globin gene causing human β thalassemia due to abnormal splicing. *Blood* 70: 147–151.

Atweh, GF, Zhu, X-X, Brickner, HE et al. (1987b). The β-globin gene on the Chinese β thalassemia chromosome carries a promoter mutation. *Blood* 70: 1470–1474.

Atweh, GF, Brickner, HE, Zhu, XX et al. (1988). A new amber mutation in a β thalassemia gene with non-measurable levels of mutant mRNA *in vivo*. *J. Clin. Invest.* 82: 557–561.

Badens, C, Thuret I, Michel, G et al. (1996). Novel and unusual deletion-insertion thalassemic mutation in exon 1 of the β-globin gene. *Hum. Mutat.* 8: 89–92.

Baglioni, C. (1962). The fusion of two peptide chains in hemoglobin Lepore and its interpretation as a genetic deletion. *Proc. Natl. Acad. Sci. U.S.A.* 48: 1880–1886.

Baird, M, Schreiner, H, Driscoll, C, and Bank, A. (1981). Localization of the site of recombination in formation of the Lepore Boston globin gene. *J. Clin. Invest.* 68: 560–564.

Basak, AN, Özer, A, Özcelik, KB et al. (1992). A novel frameshift mutation: deletion of C in codons 74/75 of the β-globin gene causes β⁰ thalassemia in a Turkish patient. *Hemoglobin* 16: 309–312.

Basak, AN, Özer, A, Kirdar, B, and Akar, N. (1993). A novel 13 bp deletion in the 3′UTR of the beta-globin gene causes beta-thalassemia in a Turkish patient. *Hemoglobin* 17: 551–555.

Baserga, SJ and Benz, EJ Jr. (1988). Nonsense mutations in the human β-globin gene affect mRNA metabolism. *Proc. Natl. Acad. Sci. U.S.A.* 85: 2056–2060.

Baserga SJ and Benz, EJ Jr. (1992). β-Globin nonsense mutation: Deficient accumulation of mRNA occurs despite normal cytoplasmic stability. *Proc. Natl. Acad. Sci. U.S.A.* 89: 2935–2939.

Beldjord, C, Lapoumeroulie, C, Pagnier, J et al. (1988). A novel β-thalassemia gene with a single base mutation in the conserved polypyrimidine sequence at the 3′ end of IVS-2. *Nucl. Acids Res.* 16: 4927–4935.

Berg, PE, Mittelman, M, Elion, J et al. (1991). Increased protein binding to a −530 mutation of the human β-globin gene associated with decreased β-globin synthesis. *Am. J. Hematol.* 36: 42–47.

Beris, P, Miescher, PA, Diaz-Chico, JC et al. (1988). Inclusion-body β-thalassemia trait in a Swiss family is caused by an abnormal hemoglobin (Geneva) with an altered and extended β chain carboxy-terminus due to a modification in codon β114. *Blood* 72: 801–805.

Beris, P, Darbellay, R, Speiser, D et al. (1993). *De novo* initiation codon mutation (ATG→ACG) of the β-globin gene causing β-thalassemia in a Swiss family. *Am. J. Hematol.* 42: 248–253.

Boehm, CD, Dowling, CD, Waber, PG et al. (1986). Use of oligonucleotide hybridization in the characterization of a β⁰-thalassemia gene (β³⁷ ᵀᴳᴳ→ᵀᴳᴬ) in a Saudi Arabian family. *Blood* 67: 1185–1188.

Bouhass, R, Aguercif, M, Trabuchet, G, and Godet, J. (1990). A new mutation at IVS1 nt2(T→A), in β-thalassemia from Algeria. *Blood* 76: 1054–1055.

Busslinger, M, Moschonas, N, and Flavell, RA. (1981). β⁺-thalassemia: aberrant splicing results from a single point mutation in an intron. *Cell* 27: 289–298.

Cai, SP, Zhang, JZ, Doherty, M and Kan,-YW. (1989). A new TATA box mutation detected in prenatal diagnosis. *Am. J. Hum. Genet.* 45: 112–114.

Cai, SP, Eng B, Francombe, WH et al. (1992). Two novel β-thalassemia mutations in the 5′ and 3′ noncoding regions of the β-globin gene. *Blood* 79: 1342–1346.

Chakravarti, A, Buetow, KH, Antonarakis, SE et al. (1984). Nonuniform recombination within the human β-globin gene cluster. *Am. J. Hum. Genet.* 36: 1239–1258.

Chan, V, Chan, TK, Kan, YW, and Todd, D. (1988). A novel β-thalassemia frameshift mutation (codon 14/15) detectable by direct visualization of abnormal restriction fragment in amplified genomic DNA. *Blood* 72: 1420–1423.

Chan, V, Chan, TK, and Todd, D. (1989). A new codon 71 (+T) mutant resulting in β⁰-thalassemia. *Blood* 74: 2304.

Chang, JC, and Kan, YW. (1979). β⁰-thalassemia: A nonsense mutation in man. *Proc. Natl. Acad. Sci. U.S.A.* 76: 2886–2889.

Chang, JC, Alberti, A, and Kan, YW. (1983). A β-thalassemia lesion abolishes the same *Mst* II site as the sickle mutation. *Nucl. Acids Res.* 11: 7789–7794.

Chebloune, Y and Verdier, G. (1983). The delta-beta-crossing-over site in the fusion gene of the Lepore-Boston disease might be localized in a preferential recombination region. *Acta Haematol.* 69: 294–302.

Chebloune, Y, Pagnier, J, Trabuchet, G et al. (1988). Structural analysis of the 5′ flanking region of the β-globin gene in African sickle cell anemia patients: Further evidence for three origins of the sickle cell mutation in Africa. *Proc. Natl. Acad. Sci. U.S.A.* 85: 4431–4435.

Chehab, FF, Honig, GR, and Kan, YW. (1986). Spontaneous mutation in β-thalassemia producing the same nucleotide substitution as that in a common hereditary form. *Lancet* 1: 3–5.

Chehab, FF, Der Kaloustian, V, Khouri, FP et al. (1987). The molecular basis of β-thalassemia in Lebanon: Application to prenatal diagnosis. *Blood* 69: 1141–1145.

Chehab, FF, Winterhalter, KH, and Kan, YW. (1989). Characterization of a spontaneous mutation in β-thalassemia associated with advanced paternal age. *Blood* 74: 852–854.

Cheng, Te, Orkin, SH, Antonarakis, SE et al. (1984). β thalassemia in Chinese: Use of *in vivo* RNA analysis and oligonucleotide hybridization in systematic characterization of molecular defects. *Proc. Natl. Acad. Sci. U.S.A.* 81: 2821–2825.

Chibani, J, Vidaud, M, Duquesnoy, P et al. (1988). The peculiar spectrum of β-thalassemia genes in Tunisia. *Hum. Genet.* 73: 190–192.

Chiou, SS, Chang, TT, Chen, PH et al. (1993). Molecular basis and haematological characterization of β-thalassaemia major in Taiwan, with a mutation of IVS-1 3′ end TAG→GAG in a Chinese patient. *Br. J. Haematol.* 83: 112–117.

Codrington, JF, Li, HW, Kutlar, F et al. (1990). Observations on the level of Hb A₂ in patients with different β-thalassemia mutations and a chain variant. *Blood* 76: 1246–1249.

Coleman, MB, Steinberg, MH, and Adams, JG III. (1991). Hemoglobin Terre Haute [β106 (G8) Arginine]: A posthumous correction to the original structure of Hb Indianapolis. *J. Biol. Chem.* 266: 5798–5800.

Coleman, MB, Steinberg, MH, Harrell, AH (1992). The –87 (C→A) β⁺-thalassemia mutation in a Black family. *Hemoglobin* 16: 399–401.

Coleman, MB, Lu, Z-H, Smith, CM et al. (1995). Two missense mutations in the β-globin gene can cause severe β thalassemia. *J. Clin. Invest.* 95: 503–509.

Craig, JE, Kelly, SJ, Barnetson, R, and Thein, SL. (1992). Molecular characterization of a novel 10.3 kb deletion causing beta-thalassaemia with unusually high Hb A2. *Br. J. Haematol.* 82: 735–744.

Çürük, MA, Molchanova, TP, Postnikov, YV et al. (1994). β thalassemia alleles and unstable hemoglobin types among Russian pediatric patients. *Am. J. Hematol.* 46: 329–332.

Çürük, MA, Howard, SC, Kutlar, A, and Huisman, THJ. (1995). A newly discovered β⁰-thalassemia (IVS-II 850, G→A) mutation in a north European family. *Hemoglobin* 19: 207–211.

DeCastro, CM, Devlin, B, Fleenor, DE et al. (1994). A novel β-globin mutation, Durham-NC[114Leu→Pro], produces a dominant thalassemia-like phenotype. *Blood* 83: 1109–1116.

Deidda, G, Novelletto, A, Hafez, M et al. (1990). A new β-thalassemia mutation produced by a single nucleotide substitution in the conserved dinucleotide sequence of the IVS-1 consensus acceptor site (AG→AA). *Hemoglobin* 14: 431–440.

Deidda, G, Novelletto, A, Hafez, M et al. (1991). A new β-thalassaemia frameshift mutation detected by PCR after selective hybridization to immobilized oligonucleotides. *Br. J. Haematol.* 79: 90–92.

Deutsch, S, Samii, K, Darbellay, R et al. (1998). Nonsense mutations in exon III of β-globin are associated with normal β-thal mRNA production while frameshift mutations lead to a severely decreased amount of β-thal mRNA. *Blood* 92 (Suppl. 1): 334a.

Diaz-Chico, JC, Yang, KG, Kutlar, A et al. (1987). An ~300 bp deletion involving part of the 5′ β-globin gene region is observed in members of a Turkish family with β thalassemia. *Blood* 70: 583–586.

DiMarzo, R, Dowling CE, Wong, C et al. (1988). The spectrum of β-thalassemia mutations in Sicily. *Br. J. Haematol.* 69: 393–397.

Dimovski, AJ, Efremov, DG, Jankovic, L et al. (1993). A β[0]-thalassaemia due to a 1605 bp deletion of the 5′ beta-globin gene region. *Br. J. Haematol.* 85: 143–147.

Dimovski, AJ, Divoky, V, Adekile, AD et al. (1994). A novel deletion of approximately 27 kb including the beta-globin gene and the locus control region 3′HS-1 regulatory sequence: beta zero thalassemia or hereditary persistence of fetal hemoglobin? *Blood* 83: 822–827.

Dimovski, AJ, Baysal, E, Efremov, DG et al. (1996). A large β thalassemia deletion in a family of Indonesian-Malay descent. *Hemoglobin* 20: 277–392.

Divoky, V, Bisse, E, Wilson, JB et al. (1992). Heterozygosity for the IVS-I-5 (G→C) mutation with a G→A change at codon 18 (Val→Met; Hb Baden) in cis and a T→G mutation at codon 136 (Val→Gly: Hb Dhonburi) in trans resulting in a thalassemia intermedia. Biochim. *Biophys. Acta.* 1180: 173–179.

Divoky, V, Baysal, E, Schiliro, G et al. (1993a). A mild type of Hb S-beta(+) thalassemia [–92(C→T)] in a Sicilian family. *Am. J. Hematol.* 42: 225–226.

Divoky, V, Gu, L-H, Indrak, K et al. (1993b). A new β[0]-thalassaemia nonsense mutation (codon 112, T→A) not associated with a dominant type of thalassaemia in the heterozygote. *Br. J. Haematol.* 83: 523–524.

Divoky, V, Svobodova, M, Indrak, K et al. (1993c). Hb Hradec Kralove (Hb HK) or $\alpha_2\beta_2$ 115(G17)Ala→Asp. A severely unstable hemoglobin variant resulting in a dominant β thalassemia trait in a Czech family. *Hemoglobin* 17: 319–328.

Divoky, V, Indrak, K, Ming, M et al. (1996). A novel mechanism of β thalassemia: The insertion of L1 retrotransposable element into β globin IVS II. *Blood* 88(Suppl.1): 148a.

Dobkin, C and Bank A. (1985). Reversibility of IVS 2 missplicing in a mutant human β-globin gene. *J. Biol. Chem.* 260: 16332–16337.

Dobkin, C, Pergolizzi, RG, Bahre, P et al. (1983). Abnormal splice in a mutant β-globin gene not at the site of a mutation. *Proc. Natl. Acad. Sci. U.S.A.* 80: 1184–1188.

Economou, EP, Antonarakis, SE, Dowling, CC et al. (1991). Molecular heterogeneity of β-thalassemia in mestizo Mexicans. *Genomics* 11: 474.

Efremov, DG, Dimovski, AJ, and Efremov, GD. (1991). Detection of β-thalassemia mutations by ASO hybridization of PCR amplified DNA with digoxigenin ddUTP labeled oligonucleotides. *Hemoglobin* 15: 525–533.

El-Hashemite, N, Petrou, M, Khalifa, AS et al. (1997). Identification of novel Asian Indian and Japanese mutations causing beta-thalassaemia in the Egyptian population. *Hum. Genet.* 99: 271–274.

El-Kalla, S and Mathews, AR. (1995). A novel frameshift mutation causing beta thalassemia in a Sikh. *Hemoglobin* 19: 183–189.

El-Kalla, S and Mathews, AR. (1997). A novel beta-thalassemia mutation [codon 45(-T)] in a Pakistani family. *Hemoglobin* 21: 499–503.

Eng, B, Chui, DH, Saunderson, J et al. (1993). Identification of two novel β[0]-thalassemia mutations in a Filipino family: frameshift codon (-TG) and a beta-globin gene deletion. *Hum. Mutat.* 2: 375–379.

Fattoum, S, Guemira, F, Öner, C et al. (1991). β-thalassemia, Hb S-β-thalassemia, and sickle cell anemia among Tunisians. *Hemoglobin* 15: 11–21.

Faustino, P, Osorio-Almeida, L, Barbot, J et al. (1992). Novel promoter and splice junction defects add to the genetic, clinical or geographical heterogeneity of β thalassemia in the Portuguese population. *Hum. Genet.* 89: 573–576.

Fei, YJ, Stoming, TA, Efremov, GD et al. (1988). β-thalassemia due to a T→A mutation within the ATA box. *Biochem. Biophys. Res. Commun.* 153: 741–747.

Fei, YJ, Stoming, TA, Kutlar, A et al. (1989). One form of inclusion body β-thalassemia is due to a GAA→TAA mutation at codon 121 of the β chain. *Blood* 73: 1075–1077.

Fessas, P, Loukopoulos, D, Loutradi-Anagnostou, A, and Komis, G. (1982). "Silent" β-thalassaemia caused by a "silent" β-chain mutant: The pathogenesis of a syndrome of thalassaemia intermedia. *Br. J. Haematol.* 51: 577–583.

Filon, D, Oron, V, Krichevski, S et al. (1994). Diversity of beta-globin mutations in Israeli ethnic groups reflects recent historic events. *Am. J. Hum. Genet.* 54: 836–843.

Flavell, RA, Kooter, JM, deBoer, E et al. (1978). Analysis of the β-δ-globin gene loci in normal and Hb Lepore DNA: direct determination of gene linkage and intergene distance. *Cell* 15: 25–41.

Fucharoen, S, Fucharoen, G, Fucharoen, P and Fukumaki, Y. (1989). A novel ochre mutation in the β-thalassemia gene of a Thai. *J. Biol. Chem.* 264: 7780–7783.

Fucharoen, G, Fucharoen, S, Jetsrisuparb, A, and Fukumaki, Y. (1990a). Molecular basis of HbE-β-thalassemia and the origin of HbE in northeast Thailand: Identification of one novel mutation using amplified DNA from buffy coat specimens. *Biochem. Biophys. Res. Commun.* 170: 698–704.

Fucharoen, S, Katsube, T, Fucharoen, G et al. (1990b). Molecular heterogeneity of β-thalassaemia in the Japanese: Identification of two novel mutations. *Br. J. Haematol.* 74: 101–107.

Fucharoen, S, Fucharoen, G, Ata, K et al. (1990c). Molecular characterization and nonradioactive detection of beta-thalassemia in Malaysia. *Acta. Haematol.* 84: 82–88.

Fucharoen, S, Kobayashi, Y, Fucharoen, G et al. (1990d). A single nucleotide deletion in codon 123 of the β-globin gene causes an inclusion body β-thalassemia trait: a novel elongated globin chain β[Makabe]. *Br. J. Haematol.* 75: 393–399.

Fucharoen, S, Fucharoen, G, Fukumaki, Y et al. (1990e). Three-base deletion in exon 3 of the β-globin gene produced a novel variant (β[Gunma]) with a thalassemia-like phenotype. *Blood* 76: 1894–1896.

Fucharoen, S, Fucharoen, G, Laosombat, V, and Fukumaki, Y. (1991a). Double heterozygosity of the β-Malay and a novel β-thalassmia gene in a Thai patient. *Am. J. Hematol.* 38: 142–144.

Fucharoen, G, Fucharoen, S, Jetsrisuparb, A, and Fukumaki, Y. (1991b). Eight-base deletion in exon 3 of the β-globin gene produced a novel variant (β Khon Kaen) with an inclusion body thalassemia trait. *Blood* 78: 537–539.

Fukumaki, Y, Gosh, PK, Benz, EJ Jr et al. (1982). Abnormally spliced messenger RNA in erythroid cells from patients with β+-thalassemia and monkey cells expressing a cloned β+-thalassemic gene. *Cell* 28: 585–593.

Galanello, R, Meloni, A, Gasperini, D et al. (1993). The repeated sequence $(AT)_X(T)_Y$, upstream to the β-globin gene is a simple polymorphism. *Blood* 81: 1974–1975.

Garewal, G, Fearon, CW, Warren, TC et al. (1994). The molecular basis of beta thalassaemia in Punjabi and Maharashtran Indians includes a multilocus aetiology involving triplicated alpha-globin loci. *Br. J. Haematol.* 86: 372–376.

Ghaffari, G, Lanyon, WG, Haghshenas, M, and Connor, JM. (1997). Molecular characterization of eight β-thalassaemia mutations in the south of Iran. Abstract 49, 6th International Conference on Thalassaemia and the Haemoglobinopathies, Malta.

Ghanem, N, Girodon, E, Vidaud, M et al. (1992). A comprehensive scanning method for rapid detection of beta-globin gene mutations and polymorphisms. *Hum. Mutat.* 1: 229–239.

Gilman, J. (1987). The 12.6 kilobase DNA deletion in Dutch β0 thalassemia. *Br. J. Haematol.* 67: 369–372.

Girodon, E, Ghanem, N, Vidaud, M et al. (1992). Rapid molecular characterization of mutations leading to unstable hemoglobin β-chain variants. *Ann. Hematol.* 65: 188–192.

Goldsmith, ME, Humphries, RK, Ley, T et al. (1983). "Silent" nucleotide substitution in a β+-thalassemia gene activates splice site in coding sequence RNA. *Proc. Natl. Acad. Sci. U.S.A.* 80: 2318–2322.

Gonzalez-Redondo, JH, Stoming, TA, Lanclos, KD et al. (1988). Clinical and genetic heterogeneity in black patients with homozygous β-thalassemia from the southeastern United States. *Blood* 72: 1007.

Gonzalez-Redondo, JM, Stoming, TA, Kutlar, F et al. (1989a). A C→T substitution at nt −101 in a conserved DNA sequence of the promoter region of the β-globin gene is associated with "silent" β-thalassemia. *Blood* 73: 1705–1711.

Gonzalez-Redondo, JM, Stoming, TA, Kutlar, F et al. (1989b). Severe Hb S-β0-thalassaemia with a T→C substitution in the donor splice site of the first intron of the β-globin gene. *Br. J. Haematol.* 71: 113–117.

Gonzalez-Redondo, JM, Kattamis, C, and Huisman, THJ. (1989c). Characterization of three types of β0 thalassemia resulting from a partial deletion of the β-globin gene. *Hemoglobin* 13: 377–392.

Gonzalez-Redondo, JM, Stoming, TA, Kutlar, F et al. (1989d). Hb Monroe or $α_2β_230(B12)$ Arg→Thr, a variant associated with β-thalassemia due to a G→C substitution adjacent to the donor splice site of the first intron. *Hemoglobin* 13: 67–74.

Gonzalez-Redondo, JM, Brickner, HE, and Atweh GF. (1989e). Abnormal processing of β-Malay globin RNA. *Biochem Biophys. Res. Comm.* 163: 8–13.

Gonzalez-Redondo, JM, Kutlar, A, Kutlar, F et al. (1991). Molecular characterization of Hb S(C) β-thalassemia in American blacks. *Am. J. Hematol.* 38: 9–14.

Gorski, J, Fiori, M, and Mach, B. (1982). A new nonsense mutation as the molecular basis for β0-thalassemia. *J. Mol. Biol.* 154: 537–540.

Hall, GW, Franklin, IM, Sura, T, and Thein, SL. (1991). A novel mutation (nonsense β127) in exon 3 of the β globin gene produces a variable thalassaemia phenotype. *Br. J. Haematol.* 79: 342–344.

Hardison, R, Riemer, C, Chui, DHK, et al. (1998). Electronic access to sequence alignments, experimental results and human mutations as an aid to studying globin gene regulation. *Genomics* 47: 429–437.

Hattori, Y, Yamane, A, Yamashiro, Y et al. (1989). Characterization of β-thalassemia mutations among the Japanese. *Hemoglobin* 13: 657–670.

Hattori, Y, Yamashiro, Y, Ohba, Y et al. (1991). A new β-thalassemia mutation (initiation codon ATG→GTG) found in the Japanese population. *Hemoglobin* 15: 317–325.

Hattori, Y, Yamamoto, Ku, Yamashiro, Y et al. (1992). Three β-thalassemia mutations in the Japanese: IVS-II-1 (G→A), IVS-II-848 (C→G), and codon 90 (GAG→TAG). *Hemoglobin* 16: 93–97.

Hattori, Y, Okayama, N, Ohba, Y et al. (1998). A new beta-thalassemia allele, codon 26 (GAG→GTAG), found in a Japanese. *Hemoglobin* 22: 79–82.

Hentze, MW and Kulozik, AE. (1999). A perfect message: RNA surveillance and nonsense-mediated decay. *Cell* 96: 307–310.

Heusterspreute, M, Derclaye, I, Gala, JL et al. (1996). Beta-thalassaemia in indigenous Belgian families: Identification of a novel mutation. *Hum. Genet.* 98: 77–79.

Hill, AV, Bowden, DK, O'Shaughnessy, DF et al. (1988). β-thalassemia in Melanesia: Association with malaria and characterization of a common variant. (IVS-1 nt 5 G→C). *Blood* 72: 9–14.

Ho, PJ, Rochette, J, Fisher, CA et al. (1996). Moderate reduction of β-globin gene transcript by a novel mutation in the 5′ untranslated region: A study of its interaction with other genotypes in two families. *Blood* 87: 1170–1178.

Hopmeier, P, Krugluger, W, Gu, L-H et al. (1996). A newly discovered frameshift at codons 120–121 (+A) of the β gene is not associated with a dominant form of β thalassemia. *Blood* 87: 5393–5394.

Huang, S, Wong, C, Antonarakis, SE et al. (1986). The same TATA box β-thalassemia mutation in Chinese and US blacks: Another example of independent origins of mutation. *Hum. Genet.* 74: 162–164.

Huang, SZ, Xu, YH, Zeng, FY et al. (1991). A novel β-thalassaemia mutation: Deletion of 4 bp (-AAAC) in the 5′ transcriptional sequence. *Br. J. Haematol.* 78: 125–126.

Huisman, THJ, Carver, MFH, and Baysal, E. (1997). A syllabus of thalassemia mutations. The Sickle Cell Anemia Foundation, Augusta, GA, USA (http://globin.cse.psu.edu).

Humphries, RK, Ley, TJ, Anagnou, NP et al. (1984). β0-39 thalassemia gene: A premature termination codon causes β mRNA deficiency without changing cytoplasmic β mRNA stability. *Blood* 64: 23–32.

Indrak, K, Indrakova, J, Kutlar, F et al. (1991). Compound heterozygosity for a β0 thalassemia (frameshift codons

38/39; -C) and a non-deletional Swiss type of HPFH (A→C at nt –110,^{G}γ) in a Czechoslovakian family. *Ann. Hematol.* 63: 111–115.

Indrak, K, Brabec, V, Indrakova, J et al. (1992). Molecular characterization of β-thalassemia in Czechoslovakia. *Hum. Genet.* 88: 399–404.

Jackson, IJ, Freund, RM, Wasylyk, B et al. (1981). The isolation, mapping and transcription *in vitro* of a β⁰-thalassaemia globin gene. *Eur. J. Biochem.* 121: 27–31.

Jankovic, L, Efremov, GD, Josifovska, O et al. (1990a). An initiation codon mutation as a cause of a β-thalassemia. *Hemoglobin* 14: 169–176.

Jankovic, L, Efremov, GD, Petkov, G et al. (1990b). Two novel polyadenylation mutations leading to β⁺-thalassemia. *Br. J. Haematol.* 74: 122–126.

Jankovic, L, Dimovski, AJ, Kollia, P et al. (1991). A C→G mutation at nt position 6 3′ to the terminating codon may be the cause of a silent β-thalassemia. *Int. J. Hematol.* 54: 289–293.

Jankovic, L, Dimovski, AJ, Sukarova, E et al. (1992) A new mutation in the β-globin gene (IVS II-850 G→C) found in a Yugoslavian thalassemia heterozygote. *Haematologica* 77: 119–121.

Jiang, NH, Liang, S, Su, C et al. (1993). A novel beta-thalassemia mutation [IVS-II-5 (G→C)] in a Chinese family from Guangxi Province, P.R. China. *Hemoglobin* 17: 563–567.

Kaeda, JS, Saary, MJ, Saunders, SM et al. (1991). Dominant β thalassemia trait due to a novel insertion. Abstract. Thalassemia Meeting, Nice, France.

Kalaydjieva, L, Eigel, A, and Horst, J. (1989). The molecular basis of beta thalassemia in Bulgaria. *J. Med. Genet.* 26: 614–618.

Kattamis, C, Hu, H, Cheng, G et al. (1990). Molecular characterization of β-thalassaemia in 174 Greek patients with thalassaemia major. *Br. J. Haematol.* 74: 342–346.

Kazazian, HH Jr. (1990). The thalassemia syndromes: molecular basis and prenatal diagnosis in 1990. *Semin. Hematol.* 27: 209–228.

Kazazian, HH Jr, Orkin, SH, Boehm, CD et al. (1983). β-thalassemia due to deletion of the nucleotide which is substituted in sickle cell anemia. *Am. J. Hum. Genet.* 35: 1028–1033.

Kazazian, HH Jr, Orkin, SH, Antonarakis, SE et al. (1984a). Molecular characterization of seven β-thalassemia mutations in Asian Indians. *EMBO J.* 3: 593–596.

Kazazian, HH Jr., Orkin, SH, Markham, AF et al. (1984b). Quantification of the close association between DNA haplotypes and specific β-thalassaemia mutations in Mediterraneans. *Nature* 310: 152–154.

Kazazian, HH Jr, Orkin, SH, Boehm, CD et al. (1986). Characterization of a spontaneous mutation to a β-thalassemia allele. *Am. J. Hum. Genet.* 38: 860–867.

Kazazian, HH Jr, Dowling, CE, Boehm, CD et al. (1990). Gene defects in β-thalassemia and their prenatal diagnosis. *Ann. N.Y. Acad. Sci.* 612: 1–14.

Kazazian, HH Jr, Dowling, CE, Hurwitz, RL et al. (1992). Dominant thalassemia-like phenotypes associated with mutations in exon 3 of the β-globin gene. *Blood* 79: 3014–3018.

Kimura, A, Matsunaga, E, Takihara, Y et al. (1983). Structural analysis of a β-thalassemia gene found in Taiwan. *J. Biol. Chem.* 258: 2748–2749.

Kinniburgh, AJ, Maquat, LE, Schedl T et al. (1982). mRNA-deficient β⁰-thalassemia results from a single nucleotide deletion. *Nucl. Acids Res.* 10: 5421–5427.

Ko, T-M, Tseng, L-H, Hsu, P-M et al. (1997). Molecular characterization of beta-thalassemia in Taiwan and the identification of two new mutations. *Hemoglobin* 21: 131–142.

Kobayashi, Y, Fukumaki, Y, Komatsu, N et al. (1987). A novel globin structural mutant, Showa-Yakushiji (β110 Leu-Pro) causing a β-thalassemia phenotype. *Blood* 70: 1688–1691.

Kollia, P, Gonzalez-Redondo, JM, Stoming, TA et al. (1989). Frameshift codon 5 [FSC-5 (-CT)] thalassemia: A novel mutation detected in a Greek patient. *Hemoglobin* 13: 597–604.

Koo, MS, Kim, SI, Cho, HI et al. (1992). A β-thalassemia mutation found in Korea. *Hemoglobin* 16: 313–320.

Kozak, M. (1989). The scanning model for translation: an update. *J. Cell Biol.* 108: 229–241.

Kulozik, AE, Yarwood, N, and Jones, RW. (1988). The Corfu β⁰ thalassemia: A small deletion acts at a distance to selectively abolish β globin gene expression. *Blood* 71: 457–462.

Kulozik, AE, Bellan-Koch, A, Bail, S et al. (1991). Thalassemia intermedia: Moderate reduction of β-globin gene transcriptional activity by a novel mutation of the proximal CACCC promoter element. *Blood* 77: 2054–2058.

Lacerra, G, DeAngioletti, M, Sabato, V et al. (1997). South-Italy beta⁰-thalassemia: A novel deletion, with 3′ breakpoint in a hsRTVL-H element, associated with beta⁰-thalassemia and HPFH. Abstract 152, 6th International Conference on Thalassaemia and the Haemoglobinopathies, Malta.

Lam, VMS, Xie, SS, Tam, JWO et al. (1990). A new single nucleotide change at the initiation codon (ATG→AGG) identified in amplified genomic DNA of a Chinese β-thalassemic patient. *Blood* 75: 1207–1208.

Lanclos, KD, Patterson, J, Efremov, GD et al. (1987). Characterization of chromosomes with hybrid genes for Hb Lepore-Washington, Hb Lepore-Baltimore, Hb P-Nilotic, and Hb Kenya. *Hum. Genet.* 77: 40–45.

Landin, B, Rudolphi, O, and Ek, B. (1995). Initiation codon mutation (ATG→ATA) of the beta-globin gene causing beta-thalassemia in a Swedish family. *Am. J. Hematol.* 48: 158–162.

Landin, B and Rudolphi, O. (1996). A novel mutation in exon 3 of the β-globin gene associated with β-thalassemia. *Br. J. Haematol.* 93(Suppl 2): 24.

Landin, B and Berglund, S. (1996). A novel mutation in the beta-globin gene causing beta-thalassemia in a Swedish family. *Eur. J. Haematol.* 57: 182–184.

Lapoumeroulie, C, Pagnier, J, Bank, A et al. (1986) β-thalassemia due to a novel mutation in IVS-1 sequence donor site consensus sequence creating a restriction site. *Biochem. Biophys. Res. Comm.* 139: 709–713.

Lin, L-I, Lin, K-S, Lin, K-H, and Cheng, T-Y. (1991). The spectrum of β-thalassemia mutations in Taiwan: Identification of a novel frameshift mutation. *Am. J. Hum. Genet.* 48: 809–812.

Lin, L-I, Lin, K-S, Lin, K-H, and Cheng, T-Y. (1992). A novel −32 (C→A) mutant identified in amplified genomic DNA of a Chinese β-thalassemic patient. *Am. J. Hum. Genet.* 50: 237–238.

Losekoot, M, Fodde, R, van Heeren, H et al. (1990). A novel frameshift mutation [FSC 47 (A+)] causing β-thalassemia in a Surinam patient. *Hemoglobin* 14: 467–470.

Lossi, AM, Milland, M, and Berge-Lefrranc, JL. (1989). A further case of β-thalassemia with an homozygous T→C substitution at the donor splice site of the first intervening sequence of the β-globin gene. *Hemoglobin* 13: 619–621.

Lynch, JR, Brown, JM, Best, S et al. (1991). Characterization of the breakpoint of a 3.5-kb deletion of the beta-globin gene. *Genomics* 10: 509–511.

Maquat, LE, Kinninburgh, AJ, Rachmilewitz EA et al. (1981). Unstable β-globin mRNA in mRNA-deficient $\beta^0\beta$ thalassemia. *Cell* 27: 543–553.

Maquat, LE and Kinninburgh, AJ. (1985). A β^0-thalassemic β-globin RNA that is labile in bone marrow cells is relatively stable in HeLa cells. *Nucleic Acids Res.* 13: 2855–2867.

Mavillo, F, Giampaolo, A, Care A et al. (1983). The crossover region in Lepore Boston hemoglobinopathy is restricted to a 59 base pairs region around the 5′ splice junction of the large globin gene intervening sequence. *Blood* 62: 230–233.

Mears, JG, Ramirez, F, Leibowitz, D et al. (1978). Organization of human δ- and β-globin genes in cellular DNA and the presence of intragenic inserts. *Cell* 15: 15–23.

Meloni, A, Rosatelli, MC, Faa, V et al. (1992). Promoter mutations producing mild β-thalassaemia in the Italian population. *Br. J. Haematol.* 80: 222–226.

Meloni, A, Demurtas, M, Moi, L et al. (1994). A novel beta-thalassemia mutation: Frameshift at codon 59 detected in an Italian carrier. *Hum. Mutat.* 3: 309–311.

Metherall, JE, Collins, FS, Pan, J et al. (1986) β^0-thalassemia caused by a base substitution that creates an alternative splice acceptor site in an intron. *EMBO J.* 5: 2551–2557.

Moschonas, N, deBoer, E, Grosveld, FG et al. (1981). Structure and expression of a cloned β^0-thalassemic globin gene. *Nucl. Acids Res.* 9: 4391–4401.

Motum, PI, Lindeman, R, Hamilton, TJ, and Trent, RJ. (1992). Australian β^0-thalassaemia due to a 12 kb deletion commencing 5′ to the β-globin gene. *Br. J. Haematol.* 82: 107–113.

Motum, PI, Kearney, A, Hamilton, TJ, and Trent, RJ. (1993). Filipino β^0 thalassaemia: a high Hb A_2 β^0 thalassaemia resulting from a large deletion of the 5′ β globin gene region. *J. Med. Genet.* 30: 240–244.

Mount SM. (1982). A catalogue of splice junction sequences. *Nucleic Acids Res.* 10: 459–472.

Murru, S, Loudianos, G, Cao, A et al. (1990). A β-thalassemia carrier with normal sequence within the β-globin gene. *Blood* 76: 2164–2165.

Murru, S, Loudianos, G, Deiana, M et al. (1991). Molecular characterization of β-thalassemia intermedia in patients of Italian descent and identification of three novel β-thalassemia mutations. *Blood* 77: 1342–1347.

Murru, S, Loudianos, G, Porcu, S et al. (1992). A β-thalassaemia phenotype not linked to the β-globin cluster in an Italian family. *Br. J. Haematol.* 81: 283–287.

Nagy, E, and Maquat, LE. (1998). A rule for termination-codon position within intron-containing genes: When nonsense affects RNA abundance. *Trends Biochem. Sci.* 23: 198–199.

Nopparatana, C, Panich, V, Saechan, V et al. (1995). The spectrum of beta-thalassemia mutations in southern Thailand. *Southeast Asian J. Trop. Med. Public Health* 26(Suppl. 1): 229–234.

Nozari, G, Rahbar, S, Rahmanzadeh, S, Golshairgan, A. (1993). Splice junction [IVS-II-1 (G→C)] thalassemia: A new mutation detected in an Iranian patient. *Hemoglobin* 17: 279–283.

Nozari, G, Rahbar, S, Golshaiyzan A, and Rahmanzadeh, S. (1995). Molecular analyses of beta-thalassemia in Iran. *Hemoglobin* 19: 425–431.

Ohba, Y, Hattori, Y, Harano, T et al. (1997). β thalassemia mutations in Japanese and Koreans. *Hemoglobin* 21: 191–200.

Öner, R, Altay, C, Gurgey, A et al. (1990). β-thalassaemia in Turkey. *Hemoglobin* 14: 1–13.

Öner, R, Agarwal, S, Dimovski, AJ et al. (1991a). The G→A mutation at position + 22 3′ to the Cap site of the β-globin gene as a possible cause for a β-thalassemia. *Hemoglobin* 15: 67–76.

Öner, R, Öner, C, Wilson, JB et al. (1991b). Dominant β-thalassaemia trait in a Portuguese family is caused by a deletion of (G)TGGCTGGTGT(G) and an insertion of (G)GCAG(G) in codons 134, 135, 136, and 137 of the β-globin gene. *Br. J. Haematol.* 79: 306–310.

Öner, C, Öner, R, Gurgey, A, and Altay, C. (1995). A new Turkish type of beta-thalassaemia major with homozygosity for two non-consecutive 7.6 kb deletions of the psi beta and beta genes and an intact delta gene. *Br. J. Haematol.* 89: 306–312.

Oppenheim, A, Oron, V, Filon, D et al. (1993). Sporadic alleles, including a novel mutation, characterize beta-thalassemia in Ashkenazi Jews. *Hum. Mutat.* 2: 155–157.

Orkin, SH and Goff, SC. (1981). Nonsense and frameshift mutations in β^0-thalassemia detected in cloned β globin genes. *J. Biol. Chem.* 256: 9782–9784.

Orkin, SH and Kazazian, HH Jr. (1984). The mutation and polymorphism of the human β-globin gene and its surrounding DNA. *Annu. Rev. Genet.* 18: 131A–171.

Orkin, SH, Kazazian, HH Jr, Antonarakis, SE et al. (1982a). Linkage of β-thalassemic mutations and β-globin gene polymorphisms with DNA polymorphisms in the human β-globin gene cluster. *Nature* 296: 627.

Orkin, SH, Kazazian, HH Jr, Antonarakis, SE et al. (1982b). Abnormal RNA processing due to the exon mutation of the β^E-globin gene. *Nature* 300: 768–769.

Orkin SH, Sexton JP, Cheng T-C et al. (1983a). ATA box transcription mutation in β-thalassemia. *Nucleic Acids Res.* 11: 4727–4734.

Orkin, SH, Sexton, JP, Goff, SC et al. (1983b). Inactivation of an acceptor RNA splice site by a short deletion in $\beta\beta$ thalassemia. *J. Biol. Chem.* 258: 7249–7251.

Orkin, SH, Antonarakis, SE, and Kazazian HH, Jr. (1984a). Base substitution at position −88 in a β-thalassemic globin gene: Further evidence for the role of distal promoter element ACACCC. *J. Biol. Chem.* 259: 8679–8681.

Orkin, SH, Antonarakis, SE, Loukopoulos, D. (1984b). Abnormal processing of β^{Knossos} RNA. *Blood* 64: 311–313.

Orkin, SH, Cheng, T-C, Antonarakis, SE et al. (1985). Thalassemia due to a mutation in the cleavage-polyadenylation signal of the human β-globin gene. *EMBO J.* 4: 453–456.

Oshima, K, Harano, T, and Harano, K. (1996). Japanese beta zero-thalassemia: Molecular characterization of a novel insertion causing a stop codon. *Am. J. Hematol.* 52: 39–41.

Ozcelik, H, Basak, AN, Tuzmen, S et al. (1993). A novel deletion in a Turkish beta-thalassemia patient detected by DGGE and direct sequencing: FSC 22–24 (–7 bp). *Hemoglobin* 17: 387–391.

Padanilam, BJ and Huisman, THJ. (1986). The β^0-thalassemia in an American Black family is due to a single nucleotide substitution in the acceptor splice junction of the second intervening sequence. *Am. J. Hematol.* 22: 259–263.

Pagano, L, Carbone, V, Fioretti, G et al. (1997). Compound heterozygosity for Hb Lepore-Boston and Hb Neapolis (Dhonburi) [beta 126(H4)Val→Gly] in a patient from Naples, Italy. *Hemoglobin* 21: 1–15.

Park, SS, Barnetson, R, Kim, SW et al. (1991). A spontaneous deletion of 33/34 Val in exon 2 of the globin gene (Hb Korea) produces the phenotype of dominant thalassaemia. *Br. J. Haematol.* 78: 581–582.

Pergolizzi, R, Spritz, RA, Spence, S et al. (1981). Two cloned β-thalassemia genes are associated with amber mutations at codon 39. *Nucl. Acids Res.* 9: 7065–7072.

Pirastu, M, Galanello, R, Doherty, MA et al. (1987). The same β-globin gene mutation is present on nine different β-thalassemia chromosomes in a Sardinian population. *Proc. Natl. Acad. Sci. U.S.A.* 84: 2882–2885.

Podda, A, Galanello, R, Maccioni, L et al. (1991). Hemoglobin Cagliari (60[E4] VAL→Glu): A novel unstable thalassemic hemoglobinopathy. *Blood* 77: 371–375.

Poncz M, Ballantine M, Solowiejczyk, D et al. (1982). β-thalassemia in a Kurdish Jew. *J. Biol. Chem.* 257: 5994–5996.

Popovich, BW, Rosenblatt, DS, Kendall, AG et al. (1986). Molecular characterization of an atypical β-thalassemia caused by a large deletion in the 5′ β-globin gene region. *Am. J. Hum. Genet.* 39: 797–810.

Ribeiro, ML, Baysal, E, Kutlar, F et al. (1992). A novel β^0-thalassaemia mutation (codon 15, TGG→TGA) is prevalent in a population of central Portugal. *Br. J. Haematol.* 80: 567–568.

Ringelhann, B, Szelenyi, JG, Horanyi, M et al. (1993). Molecular characterization of beta-thalassemia in Hungary. *Hum. Genet.* 92: 385–387.

Ristaldi, MS, Pirastu, M, Murru, S et al. (1990). A spontaneous mutation produced a novel elongated β-globin chain structural variant (Hb Agnana) with a thalassemia-like phenotype. *Blood* 75: 1378–1379.

Rosatelli, MC, Tuveri, T, Scalas, MT et al. (1992a) Molecular screening and fetal diagnosis of β-thalassemia in the Italian population. *Hum. Genet.* 89: 585–589.

Rosatelli, MC, Dozy, A, Faa, V et al. (1992b). Molecular characterization of β-thalassemia in the Sardinian population. *Am. J. Hum. Genet.* 50: 422–426.

Rouabhi, F, Chardin, P, Boissel, JP et al. (1983). Silent β-thalassemia associated with Hb Knossos β27 (B9) Ala→Ser in Algeria. *Hemoglobin* 1983: 7: 555–561.

Rund, D, Cohen, T, Filon, D et al. (1991). Evolution of a genetic disease in an ethnic isolate: β-thalassemia in the Jews of Kurdistan. *Proc. Natl. Acad. Sci. U.S.A.* 88: 310–314.

Rund, D, Dowling, C, Najjar, K et al. (1992). Two mutations in the β-globin polyadenylation signal reveal extended transcripts and new RNA polyadenylation sites. *Proc. Natl. Acad. Sci. U.S.A.* 89: 4324–4328.

Saba, L, Meloni, A, Sardu, R et al. (1992). A novel beta-thalassemia mutation (G→A) at the initiation codon of the beta-globin gene. *Hum. Mutat.* 1: 420–422.

Sanguansermsri, T, Pape, M, Laig, M et al. (1990). β-thalassemia in a Thai family is caused by a 3.4 kb deletion including the entire β-globin gene. *Hemoglobin* 14: 157–168.

Schnee, J, Griese, EV, Eigel, A, and Horst, J. (1989). β-thalassemia gene analysis in a Turkish family reveals a 7 bp deletion in the coding region. *Blood* 73: 2224–2225.

Schwartz, E. (1969). The silent carrier of β-thalassemia. *N. Engl. J. Med.* 281: 1327–1333.

Schwartz, E, Cohen, A, and Surrey, S. (1988). Overview of the β-thalassemias: genetic and clinical aspects. *Hemoglobin* 12: 551–564.

Schwartz, E, Goltsov, AA, Kaboaev, OK et al. (1989). A novel frameshift mutation causing β-thalassemia in Azerbaijan. *Nucleic Acids Res.* 17: 3997.

Semenza, GL, Delgrosso, K, Poncz, M et al. (1984). The silent carrier allele: β-thalassemia without a mutation in the β-globin gene or its immediated flanking regions. *Cell* 39: 123–128.

Smale, ST and Baltimore, D. (1989). The "initiator" as a transcription control element. *Cell* 57: 103–113.

Spiegelberg, R, Aulehla-Scholz, C, Erlich, H et al. (1989). A β-thalassemia gene caused by a 290-base pair deletion: Analysis by direct sequencing of enzymatically amplified DNA. *Blood* 73: 1695–1698.

Spritz, R, and Orkin, SH. (1982). Duplication followed by deletion accounts for the structure of an Indian deletion β^0-thalassemia gene. *Nucleic Acids Res.* 10: 8025–8029.

Spritz, RA, Jagadeeswaran, P, Choudary, PV et al. (1981). Base substitution in an intervening sequence of a β$^+$-thalassemic human globin gene. *Proc. Natl. Acad. Sci. U.S.A.* 78: 2455–2459.

Takeshita, K, Forget, BG, Scarpa, A et al. (1984). Intranuclear defect in β globin mRNA accumulation due to a premature translation termination codon. *Blood* 64: 13–22.

Takihara, Y, Nakamura, T, Yamada, H et al. (1986). A novel mutation in the TATA box in a Japanese patient with β$^+$-thalassemia. *Blood* 67: 547–550.

Thein, SL. (1992). Dominant β thalassaemia: Molecular basis and pathophysiology. *Br. J. Haematol.* 80: 273–277.

Thein, SL, Old, JM, Wainscoat, JS et al. (1984). Population and genetic studies suggest a single origin for the Indian deletion β^0 thalassemia. *Br. J. Haematol.* 57: 271–278.

Thein, SL, Hesketh, C, Brown, JM et al. (1989). Molecular characterization of a high A$_2$ β thalassemia by direct sequencing of single strand enriched amplified genomic DNA. *Blood* 73: 924–930.

Thein, SL, Winichagoon, P, Hesketh, C et al. (1990a). The molecular basis of beta-thalassemia in Thailand: Application to prenatal diagnosis. *Am. J. Hum. Genet.* 47: 369–375.

Thein, SL, Hesketh, C, Taylor, P et al. (1990b). Molecular basis for dominantly inherited inclusion body β-thalassemia. *Proc. Natl. Acad. Sci. U.S.A.* 87: 3924–3928.

Thein, SL, Best, S, Sharpe, J et al. (1991). Hemoglobin Chesterfield (β28 Leu→Arg) produces the phenotype of inclusion body β thalassemia. *Blood* 77: 2791–2793.

Thein, SL, Wood, WG, Wickramasinghe, SN, and Galvin, MC. (1993). β thalassemia unlinked to the β-globin gene in an English family. *Blood* 82: 961–967.

Thermann, R, Neu-Yilik, G, Deters, A et al. (1998). Binary specification of nonsense codons by splicing and cytoplasmic translation. *EMBO J.* 17: 3484–3494.

Trecartin, RF, Liebhaber, SA, Chang, JC et al. (1981). β⁰-thalassemia in Sardinia is caused by a nonsense mutation. *J. Clin. Invest.* 68: 1012–1017.

Treisman, R, Proudfoot, NJ, Shander, M, and Maniatis, T. (1982). A single base change at a splice site in a β⁰-thalassemic gene causes abnormal RNA splicing. *Cell* 29: 903–911.

Treisman, R, Orkin, SH, and Maniatis, T. (1983). Specific transcription and RNA splicing defects in five cloned β-thalassaemia genes. *Nature* 302: 591–596.

Varawalla, NY, Old, JM, and Weatherall, DJ. (1991). Rare β-thalassaemia mutations in Asian Indians. *Br. J. Haematol.* 79: 640–644.

Vetter, B, Neu-Yilik, G, Kohne, E et al. (2000). Dominant β-thalassaemia: a highly unstable haemoglobin is caused by a novel 6 bp deletion of the β-globin gene. *Brit. J. Haemat.* 108: 176–181.

Vidaud, M, Gattoni, R, Stevenin, J et al. (1989). A 5′ splice-region G→C mutation in exon 1 of the human β-globin gene inhibits pre-mRNA splicing: a mechanism for β⁺-thalassemia. *Proc. Natl. Acad. Sci. U.S.A.* 86: 1041–1045.

Waye, JS, Cai, SP, Eng, B et al. (1991). High hemoglobin A₂ β⁰-thalassemia due to a 532-basepair deletion of the 5′ β-globin gene region. *Blood* 77: 1100–1103.

Waye, JS, Eng, B, Olivieri, NF, and Chui, DH. (1994). Identification of a novel β⁰-thalassaemia mutation in a Greek family and subsequent prenatal diagnosis. *Prenat. Diagn.* 14: 929–932.

Waye, JS, Eng, B, Francombe, WH, and Chui, DHK. (1995). Novel seventeen basepair deletion in exon 3 of the β-globin gene. *Hum. Mutat.* 6: 252–253.

Waye, JS, Eng, B, Patterson, M et al. (1997a). De novo mutation of the beta-globin gene initiation codon (ATG→AAG) in a Northern European boy. *Am. J. Hematol.* 56: 179–182.

Waye, JS, Eng, B, Patterson, M et al. (1997b). Novel β⁰-thalassemia mutation in a Canadian woman of British descent (codons 72/73, –AGTGA, +T). *Hemoglobin* 21: 385–387.

Waye, JS, Eng, B, Patterson, M et al. (1998). Novel beta-thalassemia mutation in patients of Jewish descent: [beta 30(B12)Arg→Gly or IVS-I(-2) (A→G)]. *Hemoglobin* 22: 83–85.

Westaway, D and Williamson, R. (1981). An intron nucleotide sequence variant in a cloned β⁺-thalassemia globin gene. *Nucl. Acids Res.* 9: 1777–1788.

Williamson, D, Brown, KP, Langdown, JV, and Baglin, TP. (1997). Mild thalassemia intermedia resulting from a new insertion/frameshift mutation in the β-globin gene. *Hemoglobin* 21: 485–493.

Winichagoon, P, Fucharoen, S, Wilairat, P et al. (1992). Identification of five rare mutations including a novel frameshift mutation causing beta zero-thalassemia in Thai patients with beta zero-thalassemia/hemoglobin E disease. *Biochim. Biophys. Acta* 1139: 280–286.

Wong, C, Antonarakis, SE, Goff, SC et al. (1986). On the origin and spread of β-thalassemia: Recurrent observation of four mutations in different ethnic groups. *Proc. Natl. Acad. Sci. U.S.A.* 83: 6529–6532.

Wong, C, Dowling, CE, Saiki, RK et al. (1987). Characterization of β-thalassemic mutations using direct genomic sequencing of amplified single copy DNA. *Nature* 330: 384–386.

Wong, C, Antonarakis, SE, Goff, SC et al. (1989a). β-thalassemia due to two novel nucleotide substitutions in consensus acceptor site sequences of the β-globin gene. *Blood* 73: 914–918.

Wong, SC, Stoming, TA, Efremov, GD et al. (1989b). High frequencies of a rearrangement (+ATA; –T) at –530 to the β-globin gene in different populations indicate the absence of a correlation with a silent ββ thalassemia determinant. *Hemoglobin* 13: 1–5.

Wood, WG, Old, JM, Roberts, AVS et al. (1978). Human globin gene expression: control of β, δ and δβ chain production. *Cell* 15: 437–446.

Yamamoto, Ku, Yamamoto, Ki, Hattori, Y (1992). Two β-thalassemia mutations: Codon 121 (GAA→TAA) and IVS-I-130 (G→C) in Japan. *Hemoglobin* 16: 295–302.

Yang, KG, Kutlar, F, George, E et al. (1989). Molecular characterization of β-globin gene mutations in Malay patients with Hb E-β-thalassaemia and thalassaemia major. *Br. J. Haematol.* 72: 73–80.

13

Clinical Aspects of β Thalassemia

NANCY F. OLIVIERI
D.J. WEATHERALL

INTRODUCTION

Clinically, either alone or through their interactions with β-globin structural hemoglobin variants, the β thalassemias are by far the most important forms of thalassemia. Their control and management will pose a major drain on health care resources in the new millennium, particularly in emerging countries in which improvements in sanitation and public health measures have dramatically reduced the number of infant deaths from malnutrition and infection, and hence in which babies with these forms of thalassemia increasingly will survive long enough to present for diagnosis and treatment (Weatherall and Clegg, 1996).

In this chapter we describe the clinical and laboratory features of the severe, transfusion-dependent forms of β thalassemia and their carrier states, and discuss what is known of the diverse family of disorders that fall between these extremes, the β thalassemia intermedias. Readers who wish to learn more about the historical development of this field are referred to the monograph of Weatherall and Clegg (2000).

CLASSIFICATION, NOMENCLATURE, AND GENOTYPE/PHENOTYPE RELATIONSHIPS

Despite our increasing knowledge of the molecular pathology of the β thalassemias, it is still useful to retain a broad classification based on their clinical manifestations. The severe, transfusion-dependent forms are designated β thalassemia major, or Cooley's anemia, and the symptomless carrier states, thalassemia minor. The term *thalassemia intermedia* is retained for want of anything better to describe the broad spectrum of different forms of thalassemia in which the clinical manifestations lie between these extremes.

Because of the wide variability of the hemoglobin constitution in all the severe forms of β thalassemia, it has been necessary to resort to describing the different subtypes by the more consistent findings in carriers, particularly the level of HbA_2. Most of the common forms of β thalassemia are associated with increased levels of HbA_2 in heterozygotes. There are, however, varieties in which it is in the normal range. These "normal" HbA_2 varieties of β thalassemia are further subdivided into those in which carriers have typical thalassemic morphology of their red cells, and those in which there are no hematologic changes, the "silent" β thalassemias. Other forms of β thalassemia have been identified in which carriers have unusually high levels of Hbs F or A_2. Finally, there is a group characterized by a dominant rather than the usual recessive from of inheritance. A classification based on this descriptive approach to defining the different forms of β thalassemia is shown in Table 13.1.

β thalassemia major usually results from the compound heterozygous state for two different β-globin gene mutations, or less commonly and usually in populations with a high frequency of consanguineous marriages, from the homozygous state for the same mutation. The majority of the β thalassemias are caused by mutations at the β-globin gene loci, which result in either no output of β-globin chains, β^0 thalassemia, or a reduced output, β^+ thalassemia. Hence compound heterozygotes may be heterozygous for both β^+ and β^0 thalassemia or for two different forms of either β^0 or β^+ thalassemia. The term β^{++} thalassemia is sometimes used to describe β thalassemia with a particularly mild reduction in β-globin chain synthesis.

Because many different mutations underlie the β thalassemias, and those that cause β^+ thalassemia vary in their overall effect on β-chain synthesis, it is not surprising that either alone or through their interactions with structural hemoglobin variants or with α thalassemia, they generate a wide variety of different clinical phenotypes. In the sections that follow the main clinical, laboratory, and diagnostic features of these different forms of β thalassemia are described.

Martin H. Steinberg, Bernard G. Forget, Douglas R. Higgs, and Ronald L. Nagel, editors. *Disorders of Hemoglobin: Genetics, Pathophysiology, and Clinical Management.* © 2001 Cambridge University Press. All rights reserved.

Table 13.1. The Different Phenotypes of
β Thalassemia

β thalassemia major
    β⁰ thalassemia
    β⁺ thalassemia
    (β⁺⁺ thalassemia)
β thalassemia intermedia
β thalassemia minor (trait)
    With raised level of Hb A₂
        Low or slightly elevated level of Hb F
        Unusually high levels of Hb F
        Unusually high levels of Hb A₂
    Normal levels of Hb A₂
        β thalassemia with δ thalassemia
        Mild β thalassemia
        'Silent' β thalassemia
        β thalassemia with α thalassemia
    Symptomatic
        Dominant β thalassemia
        β thalassemia trait with ααα or αααα
β thalassemia with genetic determinant unlinked to
    β globin gene locus

Table 13.2. Age at Presentation of Infants
With Thalassemia Major or Intermedia

Age (years)	Thalassemia major	Thalassemia intermedia
< 1	75 (62%)	4 (11%)
1–2	35 (29%)	11 (30%)
> 2	11 (9%)	22 (59%)
Total	121	37

From Modell, 1984.

THE SEVERE TRANSFUSION-DEPENDENT FORMS OF β THALASSEMIA; β THALASSEMIA MAJOR

The major forms of β thalassemia, still sometimes called Cooley's anemia, are defined as genetic disorders of β-globin chain synthesis in which life can only be sustained by regular blood transfusion.

The early descriptions of severe thalassemia by Cooley and others, reviewed by Weatherall and Clegg (2000), present a picture of the disease as it was, and unfortunately still is, seen in children who have either not been transfused at all or given inadequate transfusion. If children are adequately treated in this way many of the "typical" features of thalassemia do not appear in early childhood and most of the clinical problems, which occur after the first decade, are the result of iron accumulation. For this reason it is necessary to consider this disease in two settings: the inadequately treated child and the child who has been transfused from early in life.

General Clinical Features and Course

Age and Symptoms at Presentation. Since β-chain synthesis replaces γ-chain synthesis during the first months of life it might be expected that β thalassemia would become manifest at about that time. This is usually the case. Severe forms of β thalassemia commonly present during the first year. For example, Kattamis et al. (1975) noted that the mean age at presentation was 13.1 months (±8.1 months), with a range from 2 to 36

months. In reviewing 121 patients, Modell and Berdoukas (1984) found that 60 percent presented within the first year; the mean age at presentation was 6 months (Table 13.2). Similarly, Cao (1988) found that, comparing a group of transfusion-dependent with non-transfusion-dependent β thalassemics, the mean age of presentation of the former was 8.4 ± 9.1 months while in the latter it was 17.4 ± 11.8 months. The mean hemoglobin level at presentation in the transfusion-dependent group was 8.28 g/dL as compared with 9.16 ± 1.2 g/dL in the group with milder disease.

Some infants with severe β thalassemia present later than the first year. Their hemoglobin values are in the 6 to 9 g/dL range and it is not clear whether they are going to fall into the major or intermediate category. However, after observation for several months it is apparent that they are failing to thrive or not growing adequately, and it is clear that they require regular transfusion. The same reasoning applies to even older children who have been categorized as having thalassemia intermedia but in whom poor growth or the development of other complications confirm that they are transfusion-dependent.

A wide variety of symptoms may alert the parents to the fact that the child has a serious illness. Frequently, infants fail to thrive and to gain weight normally and become progressively pale. Feeding problems, diarrhea, irritability, recurrent bouts of infection, progressive enlargement of the abdomen due to splenomegaly, or failure to recover from an infective episode are common presenting symptoms. Less usual presentations include the incidental finding of an enlarged spleen, a fever of unknown origin, or the mother noticing that the infant's urine stains the napkin (diaper) pink or brown (Modell and Berdoukas, 1984). At this stage the infant may look pale but otherwise there may be no abnormal signs. On the other hand, splenomegaly may already be present. Thus an accurate diagnosis depends on the hematologic findings described later in this chapter, together with the demonstration of the β thalassemia trait in both parents.

If a firm diagnosis is made at this stage and the infant is started on a regular blood transfusion regimen, subsequent growth and development may be relatively normal over the next decade. However, if the child is not adequately transfused the typical clinical picture of β thalassemia major develops over the next few years.

Diagnostic Difficulties at Presentation. When babies with β thalassemia major present with failure to thrive and anemia, whether or not splenomegaly is already present, the diagnosis is usually made from the appearances of the peripheral blood film, the finding of an unusually high level of fetal hemoglobin, and the demonstration of the carrier state in both parents. However, infants often present with an acute infective episode and it is not clear the extent to which their anemia reflects infection rather than severe thalassemia. Although the blood picture can be examined first it is often necessary to transfuse them to tide them over this acute episode. All too often the infant is then assumed to be transfusion-dependent, and labeled as having the major form of the illness. However, it is very important to stop transfusions, either immediately or after an interval to allow the child to fully recover, and to observe the steady-state hemoglobin off transfusion. Only in this way is it possible to identify the milder, intermediate forms of the disease that have been exacerbated by intercurrent illness.

Although the diagnosis of β thalassemia major is usually fairly straightforward we have observed a number of cases, particularly in the developing countries, in which difficulties arose. For example, the disease may present with an acute illness, and there are certain infections that can mimic β thalassemia. Malaria causes anemia and splenomegaly, and although the peripheral blood findings are quite different it may be necessary to administer antimalarial agents and carefully reexamine the child to see if the spleen has regressed, and to assess the hematologic findings, before the diagnosis of β thalassemia is confirmed. Occasionally, the anemia and splenomegaly associated with leukemia may superficially resemble β thalassemia; juvenile chronic myeloid leukemia, particularly because of the associated high level of fetal-hemoglobin production, may sometimes cause confusion. Severe iron deficiency can usually be diagnosed from the hematologic picture together with the low serum iron and ferritin values, while the blood pictures associated with other congenital hemolytic anemias are sufficiently different to make them unlikely to be confused with β thalassemia. We have seen several patients with congenital dyserythropoietic anemia who were thought to have β thalassemia; although the blood pictures are quite different the associated splenomegaly and dyserythropoiesis may cause confusion.

Course Through Childhood in Inadequately Transfused Patients. The undertransfused thalassemic child may be growth retarded; some are noticeably smaller than their normal siblings, although, in general, slowing of growth is more marked as puberty approaches. There is pallor of the mucous membranes and skin, a variable degree of icterus, and the dirty gray-brown pigmentation, first noticed by Cooley in his early descriptions of the disease, may develop. These children fail to thrive and show features of a hypermetabolic state, including poor musculature, reduction in body fat, recurrent fever, poor appetite, and lethargy; the neglected child with β thalassemia, with the characteristic protuberant abdomen, poor musculoskeletal development, and spindly legs looks very much like a child with malignant disease (Fig. 13.1). There is a variable degree of hepatosplenomegaly together with skeletal changes that produce a characteristic facial appearance, with bossing of the skull (Fig. 13.2), hypertrophy of the

Figure 13.1. A child with β thalassemia maintained on a low-transfusion regimen. There is massive hepatosplenomegaly and marked wasting of the limbs. The peculiar stance with arching of the back is typical of this condition. (From Weatherall and Clegg, 2000, with permission.)

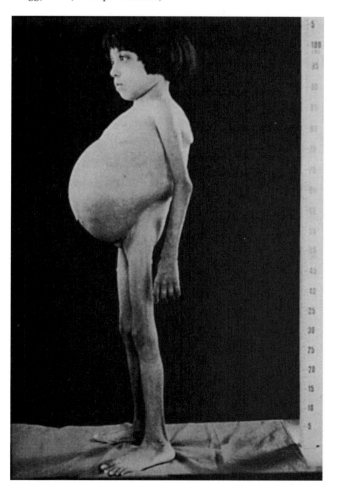

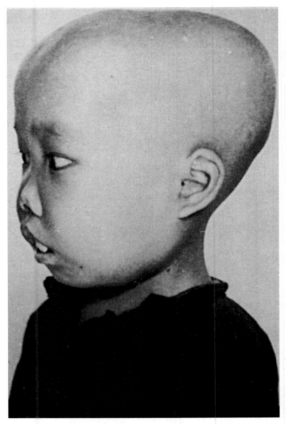

Figure 13.2. Changes in the skull in a child with thalassemia major. (From Weatherall and Clegg, 2000, with permission.)

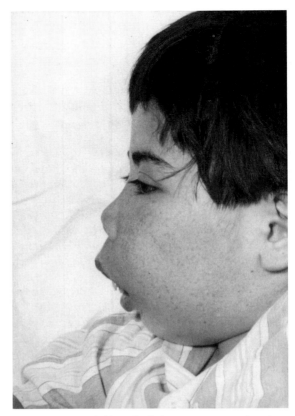

Figure 13.3. A child with thalassemia major showing typical deformities of the jaw and dentition. (From Weatherall and Clegg, 2000, with permission.)

maxilla that tends to expose the upper teeth, prominent malar eminences with depression of the bridge of the nose (Fig. 13.3), puffiness of the eyelids, and a tendency to a mongoloid slant of the eyes. There may also be proximal muscle weakness and a genu valgum. Recurrent ulceration of the legs may occur at any time throughout childhood.

The skeletal changes are mirrored by characteristic radiologic changes of the skull, long bones, and hands. The skull shows dilatation of the diploic space, and the subperiostial bone grows in a series of radiating striations, giving a typical "hair on end" appearance (Fig. 13.4). There is cortical thinning of the long bones with porous rarefaction; similar changes are found in the small bones of the hands and feet (Fig. 13.5). These radiologic changes, noted as early as 1930 by Voght and Diamond, have been the subject of many reviews (Baker, 1964; Middlemis and Raper, 1966; Cammisa and Sabella, 1967). Pathologic fractures are also a major feature of inadequately transfused children (Michelson and Cohen, 1988).

The early childhood of these patients is interspersed with numerous complications. They include recurrent infections associated with worsening of the anemia, and

a variety of complications due to progressive bone deformity, folate deficiency, a bleeding tendency, increasing hypersplenism, gallstones, leg ulcers, and a variety of syndromes due to tumor masses resulting from extramedullary hematopoiesis. If they survive to puberty they often develop similar complications to children who, because they have been adequately transfused, have had a relatively trouble-free childhood.

The Well-Transfused Thalassemic Child. Well-transfused thalassemic children often remain asymptomatic until the age of 10 to 11 years. Their future course then depends on whether they have received adequate iron chelation. If not, they begin to show signs of hepatic, endocrine, and cardiac disturbances resembling those seen in adults with familial hemochromatosis. The first observable changes are often a failure or reduction of the pubertal growth spurt, sometimes associated with delayed sexual maturation. Throughout their teenage life these children suffer from a variety of complications due to different endocrine deficiencies and they nearly all develop cardiac symptoms in the latter half of the second decade.

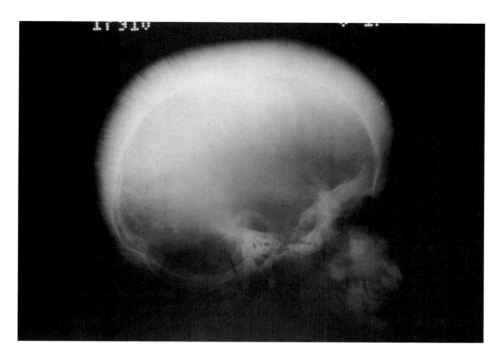

Figure 13.4. The skull in homozygous β thalassemia showing the typical "hair on end" appearance.

Figure 13.5. Radiologic changes in the bones of the hands in thalassemia major.

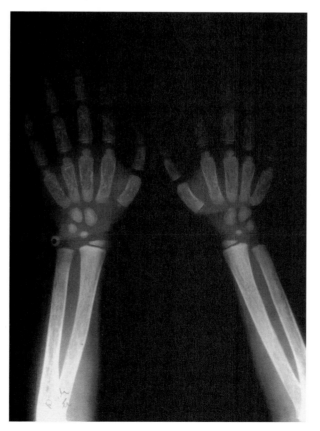

Children who are adequately transfused and are fully compliant with respect to iron chelation may grow and develop normally, enter puberty, and become sexually mature. However, even within this group there is a disappointingly high frequency of growth retardation and retarded sexual maturation.

This subdivision of the course of severe β thalassemia is, of course, rather artificial; many patients are encountered who fall between one or the other group. In the sections that follow we consider the major complications of the severe β thalassemias; in many cases they are also relevant to the intermediate forms, described later in this chapter.

Complications

The frequency and severity of the complications of β thalassemia depend to a large extent on the way that patients are managed, particularly with respect to their steady-state hemoglobin level and effectiveness of chelation therapy. They can all be related to the primary defect in globin-chain synthesis (Fig. 13.6).

Hypersplenism and Plasma-Volume Expansion. All the early literature on thalassemia stresses the occurrence of progressive splenomegaly in the major form of the illness (see Weatherall and Clegg, 2000). Splenectomy for the treatment of thalassemia has also been practiced from the time that the disease was first identified

As soon as there was sufficient experience of children who had been maintained at relatively high hemoglobin levels it became apparent that marked splenomegaly and hypersplenism were being seen much less frequently

(O'Brien et al., 1972; Modell, 1976). In a series of careful measurements of the annual blood requirements of her patients, Modell demonstrated that it was possible to calculate an average annual transfusion requirement to maintain a mean hemoglobin level of approximately 10 g/dL. Patients who exceeded this figure by 50 percent or more almost invariably returned to their "ideal" transfusion requirements after splenectomy (Modell, 1976, 1977; Modell and Berdoukas, 1984). These observations were confirmed by others, who found that children who need more than 200 to 250 mL of packed cells/kg body weight/year to maintain average hemoglobins at about 10 g/dL have significant hypersplenism, and that splenectomy significantly reduces these requirements (Cohen et al., 1989). More recent experience suggests that hypersplenism may usually be avoided by early and regular transfusion, and that many patients reaching adolescence after following a regimen of this type do not require splenectomy (Olivieri and Brittenham, 1997).

Splenic enlargement may cause a variety of complications. Occasionally, there is physical discomfort simply due to the size of the spleen. The formed elements of the blood may be trapped in the splenic pool, producing anemia, thrombocytopenia and some degree of neutropenia. The anemia of hypersplenism has a complex pathophysiology. Several studies have reported red cell mass and survival data in thalassemic children with large spleens (Lichtman et al., 1953; Smith et al., 1955; Reemsta and Elliot, 1956; Blendis et al., 1974). There is invariably some shortening of the autologous red cell survival, trapping of a proportion of the red cells in the splenic red cell pool, and a marked expansion of the total blood volume. In the study of Blendis et al. (1974) the trapped cells in the splenic pool accounted for between 9 percent and 40 percent of the total red cell mass. There is marked expansion of the plasma volume, which has the effect of worsening the anemia and, incidentally, producing a greater load on the myocardium. The reasons for the changes in plasma volume, which occur in patients with splenomegaly associated with other diseases, is not entirely clear. It is not due entirely to splenomegaly or hepatosplenomegaly; the plasma volume may remain significantly expanded after splenectomy for many months (Blendis et al., 1974). One factor that has been incriminated is the expanded bone marrow that may act as a vascular shunt; the latter is thought to result in plasma volume expansion in a number of other settings.

Finally, it should be remembered that a very large spleen constitutes an extensive mass of ineffective hematopoietic tissue as well as a potential pool for the trapping of the formed elements of the blood. Thus, as it enlarges, it increases the metabolic demands of the growing child while, at the same time, causing hemodilution and plasma volume expansion.

Iron Overload. Iron overload has been a recognized feature of severe forms of thalassemia since the first autopsy reports (Whipple and Bradford, 1936). The mechanisms of iron toxicity, its tissue distribution, and the way that it causes organ failure are discussed in Chapter 37, and the methods by which the total body iron burden can be assessed are discussed later in this chapter. Here, we outline the main features of iron accumulation as a background to the description of its effects on individual organs that follow.

It was quite apparent from the results of the first iron absorption studies, and the transfusion histories of thalassemic children in the days before high transfusion regimens were instituted, that iron loading was the result of increased absorption and transfusion, however inadequate. When assessing the results of higher transfusion regimens, Modell (1976) estimated that by the time children maintained asymptomatic at a relatively high hemoglobin level reached the age of 11 years they would have accumulated approximately 28 g of iron. She sug-

Figure 13.6. The pathophysiology of β thalassemia.

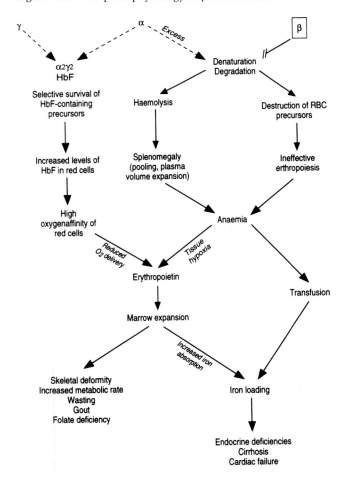

gested that it was only at about this level of iron loading that patients begin to show signs of hepatic, cardiac, and endocrine disturbance, similar to those seen in adults with hereditary hemochromatosis.

Because iron overload was to become the major cause of death in thalassemia it was clearly important to attempt to derive more accurate approaches to assessing the level of iron accumulation that would render patients at risk from life-threatening complications. Letsky et al. (1974) found that there was a good correlation between the serum-ferritin and liver-iron concentrations in β thalassemics maintained on high transfusion regimens. The values in most of their older patients were extremely high and well within the range seen in untreated hereditary hemochromatosis. However, these workers noticed that during the period over which the first 50 to 100 units of blood were transfused there was a steep rise in ferritin levels, after which the rate of increase was less marked. Later studies also indicated that the correlation between transfusion load and serum ferritin may not be so clear-cut (Pippard et al., 1978). Indeed, Worwood et al. (1980) found that a maximum plasma ferritin concentration of about 5,000 µg/L probably reflects the upper physiologic limit of the rate of its synthesis; higher concentrations are now thought to be caused by the release of intracellular ferritin from damaged cells. Several other factors probably determine the level of circulating ferritin, including ascorbate deficiency, infection, hepatic damage, hemolysis, and ineffective erythropoiesis (Roeser et al., 1980; Baynes et al., 1986).

The most clear-cut data that showed that the serum ferritin level cannot be relied on as an accurate assessment of total body iron burden was reported by Olivieri et al. (1995). These workers found that over a wide range of serum ferritin levels and hepatic iron values, there was a wide scatter and, indeed, that the 95 percent prediction intervals in hepatic-iron concentrations for a given plasma ferritin were so broad as to make determination of plasma ferritin a poor predictor of body iron stores.

More recent work, reviewed by Olivieri and Brittenham (1997), has provided more accurate information about the levels of hepatic iron at which patients are at risk of serious complications of iron overload. These studies, which extrapolate from data obtained from patients with genetic hemochromatosis, show that patients with hepatic iron levels of approximately 80 µmol iron/g liver, wet weight, which is about 15 mg iron/g liver, dry weight, are at an increased risk of hepatic disease and endocrine-organ damage. Patients with higher body iron burdens are at particular risk of cardiac disease and early death.

Although in the following sections we shall focus our attention on the consequence of iron loading of the heart, endocrine glands, and liver, it is likely that excess body iron has other, less dramatic pathologic consequences. For example, it is responsible for the curious gray pigmentation that has been a well-recognized feature of the severe forms of thalassemia ever since they were first described. The complex relationship between iron loading and increased susceptibility to infection will be considered further later in this chapter.

Cardiac Complications. The cardiac complications of β thalassemia are the most important factors in determining the survival in both transfused and untransfused patients. While they have been recognized for decades, many aspects of cardiac disease in β thalassemia are still poorly understood. It is clear that they are multifactorial, reflecting chronic anemia, iron overload, the consequences of pulmonary disease, myocarditis, pericarditis, and probably many other mechanisms.

Mechanisms. Many of the cardiological changes observed in undertransfused children with severe thalassemia are part of the adaptive changes to hypoxia that occur in all forms of anemia. They include enhanced left ventricular contractility, an elevated cardiac output, left ventricular hypertrophy, and, ultimately dilatation, and, in cases of profound anemia, all the manifestations of congestive cardiac failure.

The advent of high transfusion regimens rescued many thalassemic children from these distressing complications in early life but, until the development of effective chelation regimens, only bought time until they died of a cardiac death or other complications of iron loading toward the end of the second decade of life (Engle, 1964). There is now good evidence that effective chelation may protect transfusion-dependent patients from developing cardiac disease. However, because many patients do not adhere sufficiently strictly to their chelation programs, and because their expense precludes their use in many developing countries, cardiac disease still remains a major challenge in the management of patients with severe forms of thalassemia.

It should be emphasized that the cardiological complications of thalassemia are not restricted to the effects of anemia and iron loading, although they are by far the most important factors (Table 13.3). More recently it has been recognized that, at least in some countries, patients with thalassemia major may be unusually prone to myocarditis (Kremastinos et al., 1996). In addition, some patients with severe forms of β thalassemia have an additional burden of right-heart strain due to chronic pulmonary hypertension (Grisaru et al., 1990). It has been suggested that this too may be related to iron overload (see later section), but it may also follow recurrent, small pulmonary emboli. Unfortunately, except for data from Thailand

Table 13.3. Cardiac Complications of β Thalassemia

Cardiac failure due to severe anemia
Iron loading of the myocardium
   Cardiac failure with or without arrhythmias
Right-sided failure
   Recurrent pulmonary emboli
   ?Obliterative pulmonary artery disease*
   Lung disease due to iron overload
Pericarditis
Myocarditis

* Thought to be due to platelet aggregation, particularly post-splenectomy in intermediate forms of thalassemia

on the frequent occurrence of this type of complication in splenectomized patients with HbE-β thalassemia (Wasi et al., 1982), there have been few studies that have pursued this possibility. Recently, Hoeper et al. (1999) have suggested that there is an increased risk of pulmonary hypertension in patients who have undergone splenectomy for any cause; autopsy data showed abundant pulmonary thrombotic lesions. The relationship of these changes to persistent thrombocytosis and an increased propensity to thromboembolic disease is discussed later in this chapter.

Children with severe β thalassemia were also prone to recurrent attacks of pericarditis. Smith et al. (1955, 1960) first reported that a benign, transient pericarditis often develops after splenectomy. This complication was later well documented by others (Orsini et al., 1970; Wasi, 1972). Engle (1964) also observed this complication but could find no causal or temporal relationship with splenectomy and suggested that these events may coincide toward the end of the first decade of life. Several workers, notably Orsini et al. (1970), examined the relationship between pericarditis and iron loading but could find no convincing evidence that the two are connected. Over recent years this complication has been seen less frequently.

Pathology. Most of the information on the pathology of the myocardium in β thalassemia comes from autopsy studies, many of which were published in the era before the introduction of iron-chelation therapy. In most cases a diffuse, rust-brown staining of the myocardium was observed, together with right and left ventricular hypertrophy, dilatation, and a greatly increased cardiac weight (see Engle, 1964). In most of the early series, evidence of pericarditis was found (Engle, 1964; Arnett et al., 1975). Interestingly, an autopsy series of 19 patients with cardiac iron loading and anemia due to causes other than thalassemia did not mention pericarditis (Buja and Roberts, 1971).

Estimations of the iron content of the myocardium have shown gross elevations, to as much as 20 times normal. However, they also have underlined the marked variation in cardiac-iron content, in two studies, from 0.9 to 9.2 mg/iron/g of heart, dry weight, for example (Schellhammer et al., 1967; Buja and Roberts, 1971). In an extensive examination of iron-loaded hearts in patients who had received transfusions for conditions other than thalassemia (Buja and Roberts, 1971), iron was present in myocardial fibers as well as in the connective tissue. The endocardium was reported to have an iron concentration equal to less than 50 percent of that in the pericardium; iron was concentrated in the left ventricular septum and free wall, with maximal concentration in the left ventricular epicardium. The preferential deposition of iron in the epicardium, only later involving the remainder of the myocardium, may explain the preservation of systolic ventricular function early in the course of the disease. Attempts to relate the relationship between cardiac function and the degree of iron overload suggest that high concentrations of iron correlate reasonably well with the degree of dysfunction, although, surprisingly, in many patients iron deposition in the conduction system appears to be relatively mild, even in those who die of cardiac arrythmias (Schellhammer et al., 1967; Buja and Roberts, 1971).

Other changes that have been observed at autopsy include extensive myocardial fiber disruption and variable fibrosis (Howell and Wyatt, 1953; Witzleben and Wyatt, 1961; Schellhammer et al., 1967). Witzleben and Wyatt reported findings in two children aged 8 and 10 years, respectively. There was prominent right ventricular hypertrophy and pericarditis, but cardiac fibrosis was absent or minimal, despite the presence of hepatic cirrhosis. Although these studies suggested that iron deposition alone might not be enough to produce a fibrotic reaction, later work showed that iron loading is probably the major factor in generating these changes (Lombardo et al., 1995). Endomyocardial biopsies have demonstrated that interstitial fibrosis correlates reasonably well with persistent electrophysiologic disturbances, at least in primary hemochromatosis (Short et al., 1981).

Pathophysiology. It is clear from the concentrations observed in autopsy studies that the heart can accommodate less iron load than the liver, possibly because cardiac cells have a relatively small amount of storage protein and may be more sensitive to free-iron-induced oxygen radicals. There is some evidence that very low levels of myocardial iron may interfere directly with diastolic function (Spirito et al., 1990), a process that resembles the effect of hypercalcemia, and which is characterized by inadequate relaxation, spontaneous early depolarization, and subsequent failure of contractility (Liu and Olivieri, 1994). The generation of free hydroxyl radicals may result in damage to the lysosomal membrane of cardiac cells and lead to the disruption of the sarcolemmal membrane and inhibition of the mitochondrial respiratory chain (Link et al., 1994, 1996; Hershko et al., 1998a). The effects of iron may be augmented by a number of variables, including the reduction of ferric to ferrous iron and the addition of low concentrations of ascorbic acid; conversely, the effects of iron may be inhibited by high concentrations of ascorbic acid, α-tocopherol, and desferrioxamine (Hershko et al., 1998a,b).

In inadequately transfused patients, the magnitude of the body-iron burden is the chief factor in the development of cardiac disease (Olivieri and Brittenham, 1997). This appears to be true even though lung disease and myocarditis may aggravate iron-induced cardiac disease, as shown in a 5-year study of more than 1,000 thalassemic patients, of whom approximately 5 percent developed serious cardiac disease secondary to myocarditis with no evidence of iron overload (Kremastinos et al., 1996). While the low incidence of iron-induced cardiac disease in this young and well-treated population is not surprising, it should be emphasized that infectious myocarditis may play a role in the development of cardiac disease, and, conversely, that iron-promoted free radical formation may contribute to the pathogenesis of infectious myocarditis.

Clinical Presentations.

Considering this complex pathology it is not surprising that the clinical presentation of cardiac disease in thalassemia is extremely variable. It should be anticipated in any patient over the age of 15 years who has been inadequately transfused and chelated, who has been maintained at a high hemoglobin level with inadequate chelation, and, in particular, who has a hepatic iron concentration in excess of 15 mg/g liver dry weight (Olivieri and Brittenham, 1997). As mentioned in the previous section, the serum ferritin level is an unreliable guide but the liver iron level shows a strong correlation with the likelihood of the onset of cardiac complications.

The clinical descriptions of recent years have never bettered those of Engle (1964). She described a progressive staging for cardiac disease in irregularly transfused patients. In the first stage, observed about the age of 10 years, asymptomatic but progressive cardiac enlargement was noted. This was often followed by attacks of pericarditis at a mean age of approximately 11 years, sometimes associated with large pericardial effusions. This complication was observed in nearly half the patients; no infective cause could be found. The third stage was characterized by the appearance of first-degree heart block, occasional atrial premature beats, and abnormal T waves. Finally, the typical signs of congestive cardiac failure appeared, with features of both right and left ventricular failure in parallel with serious disturbances of rhythm and conduction. The peak incidence of the final stage was between 10 and 15 years. The duration of life after the onset of failure was less than 3 months in over half the patients, and one-third died within a month of the appearance of cardiac failure.

This general pattern of progression of cardiac disease is still observed, although, as mentioned earlier, pericarditis is seen much less frequently. Occasionally the picture may be predominantly of right heart failure (Engle, 1964; Ehlers et al., 1980; Zurlo et al., 1989). As pointed out by Jessup and Manno (1998), in older, adequately chelated patients who are often asymptomatic there may be more subtle abnormalities of both systolic and diastolic function that are multifactorial in origin.

The clinical diagnosis of iron-induced cardiomyopathy is extremely difficult. The symptoms parallel that of left ventricular function, but there may be no abnormalities until the rapid onset of overt cardiac failure. Palpitations may simply be related to anemia or other cardiac abnormalities. Similarly, a poor exercise tolerance may also be related to anemia.

Detection of Cardiac Dysfunction.

The investigation of cardiac function in thalassemia remains problematic. Conduction/rhythm abnormalities correlate poorly with conduction-tissue iron infiltration in autopsy sections of patients who have died of cardiac arrhythmias. Moreover, the subendocardial iron concentration is much less than that found in the epicardial region, so that endomyocardial biopsy may underestimate the degree of iron deposition (Fitchett et al., 1980). As pointed out by Jessup and Manno (1998), there is no particular electrocardiographic finding that is indicative of iron-induced cardiac dysfunction, although they suggest that serial tracings may be useful in that a significant change is often indicative of a process other than increased iron deposition. There is a large literature on the value of echocardiography in the diagnosis of iron loading of the myocardium (Henry et al., 1978; Bahl et al., 1992; Lattanzi et al., 1993; Kremastinos et al., 1996). In general, systolic function, cardiac dimensions, and myocardial wall thickness are normal until there are unequivocal symptoms of cardiac failure. A standardized quantitation of diastolic function is helpful but more difficult to obtain. The measurement of the ventricular end-systolic pressure-dimension ($LVPD_{ES}$) assesses contractility dependent on ventricular loading. This approach showed some abnormalities of function in a proportion of patients with advanced thalassemia (Borow et al., 1982) but does not seem to have been widely studied, or applied.

The most experience has been gained with radionuclide studies of the left- and right-ventricular ejection fraction (EF) by first pass or gated techniques, or with low-dose dobutamine stimulation (Spirito et al., 1990), although they seem to have met with little more success than resting echocardiography. Leon et al. (1979) described the estimation of left-ventricular EF during exercise in 24 patients; the number of transfusions seemed to predict an abnormal exercise LVEF by first pass.

The assessment of the risk of cardiac disease by various methods used for imaging of tissue iron is reviewed by Olivieri and Brittenham (1997). Reasonable correlations between magnetic resonance imaging (MRI) have been observed in a thalassemic-mouse model (Liu et al., 1996), and MRI changes consistent with a reduction of cardiac iron, paralleled by improvement in cardiac function, have been reported in individual patients (Olivieri et al., 1992a). But although it is clear that this technique has the potential to detect iron in the heart, it is uncertain whether it will be possible to apply it to quantitate the concentration of cardiac iron. Other approaches, such as magnetic susceptometry, which provide a direct measurement of hepatic storage iron, have not yet been applied for the evaluation of cardiac iron. Although some abnormalities have been detected by ultrasonic analysis (Lattanzi et al., 1993), this approach has not been widely used or calibrated for the evaluation of cardiac disease in thalassemia.

The measurement of serum atrial natriuretic peptide levels has been reported to be of value in the identification of preclinical cardiac involvement (Derchi et al., 1992), although further experience of this approach is required. Recently, decreased antioxidant activity of apolipoprotein E, related to the frequency of the apolipoprotein E4 allele, has been proposed as a genetic risk for left-ventricular failure in thalassemia (Economou-Petersen et al., 1998).

In a critical review of the current state of assessing cardiac function in iron-loaded patients, Jessup and Manno (1998) emphasize that none of the methods that have been used to assess early myocardial impairment have been rigorously tested in a prospective manner. Indeed, they point out that the combined information obtained from the patient's transfusion record, serial serum ferritin levels, details of their adherence to a chelation regimen, and, most important, hepatic iron concentration, provides as much predictive power as any of the noninvasive tests. Thus, while future research should be directed at a full assessment of these different techniques in patients with well-defined body iron loads, best obtained from hepatic biopsy, for day-to-day practice these simple approaches to the assessment of a patient with cardiac disease are probably as good as any.

Changing Pattern of Cardiac Disease. With the advent of adequate chelation therapy there has been a major change in the frequency of cardiac disease over recent years (Olivieri and Brittenham, 1997). Two long-term trials have shown quite unequivocally that the effective use of desferrioxamine results in long-term survival and the absence of cardiological complications. In one, which used the serum ferritin as a measure of iron loading, those who maintained concentrations of less than 2,500 µg/L had an estimated cardiac-free survival of 91 percent after 15 years; patients in whom most of the serum ferritin concentrations exceeded this figure had an estimated cardiac-disease-free survival after 15 years of less than 20 percent (Olivieri et al., 1994). The other study assessed chelation therapy in terms of hepatic iron storage; values of 80 µmol of iron/g liver weight (15 mg iron/g liver, dry weight) were used as a cut-off point above and below which patients were classified as having received ineffective or effective chelation therapy, respectively. The probability of survival to at least 25 years was only 32 percent among patients above the threshold (Brittenham, 1994).

Lung Disease. Over the last two decades there has been an increasing recognition of the occurrence of chronic lung disease in β thalassemia, which may aggravate cardiac disease. It has been suggested that iron deposition in the lungs may provoke pulmonary hypertension and right-ventricular strain, dilatation, and failure (Koren et al., 1987).

A variety of functional abnormalities have been reported, including small airway obstruction, hyperinflation, and hypoxemia, possibly as the result of several different pathologic processes (Keens et al., 1980; Hoyt et al., 1986; Grisaru et al., 1990; Santamaria et al., 1994). Other studies have described a primarily restrictive pattern of lung disease, with abnormalities consistent with obstructive airways disease (Cooper et al., 1980; Grant et al., 1987; Grisaru et al., 1990; Bacalo et al., 1992; Factor et al., 1994). Studies of total lung capacity have given inconsistent results, as have the effects of transfusion on pulmonary function (Grant et al., 1987; Santamaria et al., 1994).

These abnormalities have been related to autopsy findings, which have shown massive accumulation of hemosiderin in alveolar phagocytes in the perivascular and supporting framework (Witzleben and Wyatt, 1961; Cooper et al., 1980). In some but not all series fibrosis was noted in the majority of cases. In addition, sclerotic vascular lesions and thromboemboli have been observed, and have been attributed to platelet thrombi (Sonakul et al., 1988a,b).

A variety of mechanisms have been proposed to account for this pathology. They include tissue damage due to the generation of free hydroxyl radicals secondary to iron deposition, ferrugination of connective tissue resulting in reduced capillary compliance, and other less well-defined abnormalities of the alveolar capillary membrane (Tai et al., 1996). Abnormal growth and development of the alveolus, secondary either to intrinsic disease or due to frequent transfusions, has also been proposed as a contributing factor (Tai et al., 1996). The additional possibility of pulmonary disease due to recurrent pulmonary thromboembolic episodes resulting from platelet aggregates is discussed in the next section. Because a progressive acute pulmonary syndrome has been described in patients receiving high-dose desferrioxamine (Freedman et al., 1990), it has also been suggested that drug toxicity may also play a role.

In summary, although our knowledge of the evolution and importance of pulmonary disease in β thalassemia is still limited, it seems likely that restrictive lung dysfunction resulting from parenchymal disease may lead to a reduced arterial oxygen saturation. It is possible that his may, in some cases, lead to pulmonary hypertension and right-ventricular strain, and failure. However, until the pathophysiology of this condition is worked out, and the complex interactions between damage to lung tissue and the effects of pulmonary embolic disease are understood, it will be difficult to determine the overall importance of these mechanisms in the generation of cardiopulmonary disease in thalassemia.

Thromboembolic Disease. Because of a variety of abnormalities of platelets and coagulation factors and their antagonists, and the abnormal properties of the red cell membrane, it might be expected that patients with β thalassemia would be at increased risk of thromboembolic disease. In a study that examined the causes of death in thalassemia major, carried out in Italy in 1989, it was found that thromboembolism was the primary cause in four of 159 thalassemic patients (Zurlo et al., 1989). In Israel, Michaeli et al. (1992) reported thromboembolic events, either recurrent arterial occlusion or, more commonly, pulmonary thromboembolism, in 4 percent of patients with thalassemia major. More recently, Pignatti et al., (1988) identified 32 patients with thromboembolic episodes out of a total of 735 patients with β thalassemia, 683 with thalassemia major and 52 with thalassemia intermedia. The most common variety was stroke, which made up half of their cases. Other manifestations included pulmonary embolism, mesenteric or portal thrombosis,

and deep venous thrombosis in either the upper or lower limbs. Two cases of intracardiac thrombosis were observed. In this survey the frequency of thromboembolic events was significantly higher in association with cardiac disease, diabetes, nonspecific liver function abnormalities, and hypothyroidism.

It appears, therefore, that there is a genuine increased risk of thromboembolic disease in patients with β thalassemia. This may be more common in those with β thalassemia intermedia and in those who have undergone splenectomy. The increased propensity to thrombosis in patients with inherited hemolytic anemias has been reviewed recently (Barker and Wandersee, 1999). As well as abnormalities of platelet numbers and function and the potential prethrombotic properties of the abnormal red cell membranes of patients with β thalassemia, it appears that other factors, both genetic and acquired, may contribute toward an increased likelihood of thromboembolic disease (reviewed by Weatherall and Clegg, 2000). For example, as mentioned earlier, thalassemic patients with heart failure have a higher risk of thrombosis if they carry the apolipoprotein E4 allele (Economou-Petersen et al., 1998). Recently, it has been observed that thalassemic patients with hepatitis C may have an increased frequency of anticardiolipin antibodies and lupus anticoagulant, and that this may also be associated with an increased risk of thromboembolic events (Giordano et al., 1998).

Although further work will be required to establish the full spectrum and frequency of thromboembolic disease in β thalassemia, there seems little doubt that this is a genuine problem that may be seen more frequently now that so many patient with this disease are surviving into adult life.

Endocrine Dysfunction

It was recognized many years ago that the iron loading of the tissues that occurs in severe forms of β thalassemia has a particular predilection of the endocrine organs (Ellis et al., 1954; Erlandson et al., 1964a; Fink 1964; Bannerman et al., 1967). Over the years there have been many analyses of endocrine function in thalassemic children over a wide range of ages and body-iron burden (Kuo et al., 1968; Toccafondi et al., 1970a, 1970b; Canale et al., 1974; Lassman et al., 1974a, 1974b; Flynn et al., 1976; McIntosh, 1976; Anoussakis et al., 1977; Costin et al., Landau et al., 1978; Tuchinda et al., 1978 Costin et al., 1979; Kletsky et al., 1979; De Sanctis et al., 1989; Vullo et al., 1990; Perignon et al., 1993; El-Hazmi et al., 1994; Grundy et al., 1994; Italian Working Groups on Endocrine Complications in Nonendocrine Diseases, 1995; Kwan et al., 1995; Jensen et al., 1997; Low, 1997). Although these studies have been carried out in very heterogeneous populations of patients it has become apparent that he most common endocrine abnormalities in the present era are hypogonadotropic hypogonadism, growth hormone deficiency, and diabetes mellitus; the frequencies of hypothyroidism, hypoparathyroidism, and adrenal insufficiency seem to be much lower.

Retarded Growth and Development. Although the all too common problems of growth and development in thalassemic children are multifactorial, and not all related to endocrine deficiency, because recent work has emphasized the importance of hypogonadism in many of these cases, we will consider this topic here.

The early literature on thalassemia major frequently emphasized defective growth and development. This was highlighted in several series that were reported just before or during the period when adequate transfusion regimens were first introduced (Erlandson et al., 1964a,b; Logothetis et al., 1972a,b; Constantoulakis et al., 1975). These workers noted a particular tendency for retarded growth at about the age of 8 to 10 years and pointed out that many children attained a very short final height. They also reported that, although the estimated bone age may be normal in early life, it was frequently delayed after the age of 6 to 7 years (Erlandson et al., 1964a,b). With the introduction of high transfusion regimens many workers reported improvements in the rates of growth (Beard et al., 1969; Modell, 1976) although others were less impressed (Johnsen et al., 1966; Brook et al., 1969; Wolff and Luke, 1969).

In 1984 Modell and Berdoukas reported that early growth failure can often be corrected by raising the hemoglobin level by adequate transfusion or by splenectomy. More recent studies have generally confirmed these observations and suggested that linear growth rates and final heights are related to the hemoglobin levels that have been maintained throughout early life (De Sanctis et al., 1994).

Growth disturbances associated with low transfusion regimens are characterized by lack of weight gain and, in particular, a reduced muscle mass, which often gives the limbs a characteristic sticklike appearance and limits exercise tolerance through weakness. Modell and Berdoukas (1984) observed that undertransfused patients have a much lower level of creatinine excretion in their urine than those maintained on higher transfusion regimens. Since approximately 2 percent of muscle creatin is broken down to creatinine each day, and this provides the only source of urinary creatinine, these studies were compatible with the concept that a low transfusion regimen is associated with a reduced muscle mass and development.

The introduction of high transfusion regimens for thalassemic children did not entirely solve the problem of growth retardation, however. Indeed, as pointed out

by Modell (Modell and Beck, 1974; Modell, 1976) one of the first indications of tissue damage due to iron overload is a failure of the normal pubertal growth spurt. However, this is not the whole story because even children who are well transfused and adequately chelated, and apparently who have normal sexual development, may still show some degree of growth retardation and a reduced final height (Modell and Berdoukas, 1984; Borgna-Pignatti et al., 1985; Kattamis et al., 1990).

The reasons for growth retardation in well-transfused children are extremely complex, multifactorial, and not entirely understood (Table 13.4). Undoubtedly, iron accumulation due to variability in the effectiveness of chelation therapy plays a major role. Here again, several mechanisms may be involved. Delayed pubertal growth has been attributed to iron-induced selective central hypogonadism (Costin et al., 1979; Kletsky et al., 1979; Wang et al., 1989; Landau et al., 1993), or interference by iron with the production of insulin-like growth factor (IGF-1) (Saenger et al., 1980; Herington et al., 1981; Werther et al., 1981). Other mechanisms that have been proposed include impaired growth hormone (GH) response to growth-hormone-releasing hormone (GH-RH) (Pintor et al., 1986), abnormalities in GH secretion (Shehadeh et al., 1990) and, because GH reserves appear to be normal in many patients (Masala et al., 1984; Tolis et al., 1988; Leger et al., 1989), a defect in its receptor, although it has not been possible to demonstrate a lesion of this kind in hepatic tissues.

Several reported studies underline the complexities of these issues. In one, nearly half of a group of patients, most of whom had received regular transfusions and chelation therapy from an early age, had evidence of reduced GH reserve and low IGF-1 levels, with a substantial proportion also demonstrating reduced levels of IGF-BP3, the predominant IGF-1 binding protein, which

---

Table 13.4. Some Suggested Mechanisms of Defective Growth in β Thalassemia

Inadequate transfusion
Iron overload
  Selective central hypogonadism
  Defective production of insulin-like growth factor 1
  Impaired growth hormone response to growth-
    hormone releasing hormone
  Abnormal growth hormone secretion
  Abnormality of growth hormone receptor
  Reduced secretion of adrenal androgen
Zinc deficiency
Free-hemoglobin-induced inhibition of cartilage
  growth
Deferroxamine toxicity

prolongs the serum half-life of IGF peptides, and which is GH dependent. However, the reduction in GH reserve was not shown to be correlated with short height or delay in bone age (Cavallo et al., 1997).

In a similar analysis of 32 patients with thalassemia major, 14 of whom were short in stature, Roth et al. (1997) investigated 13 of the group who exhibited a particularly short stature or reduced growth rate. The stimulated GH secretion in 10 was in the normal range. However, studies of their spontaneous GH secretion during the night revealed that they had markedly reduced amplitudes of their GH peaks (see next section). Low IGF-1 levels were also seen in growth-retarded patients. Stimulation tests showed a marked increase in both IGF-1 and IGF-BP3 levels, indicating intact IGF-1 generation by the liver. After priming with gonadotrophin releasing hormone (GnRH), no change in either estradiol or testosterone levels or in LH or FSH response was observed, suggesting a severe degree of pituitary gonadotrophin insufficiency. These results indicate that low GH secretion and low levels of IGF-1 in thalassemic patients are related to severe neurosecretory dysfunction rather than liver damage. In short, it was apparent that hypogonadotrophic hypogonadism was a major factor, particularly in the growth-retarded patients who had impaired sexual development.

Evidence has also been presented for the existence of a state of partial growth hormone insensitivity due to a postreceptor defect in growth hormone action, which can be overcome with supraphysiologic doses of exogenous growth hormone (Scacchi et al., 1991; Low et al., 1995). Other factors that may play a role include a reduced level of secretion of adrenal androgen (McIntosh, 1976; Sklar et al., 1987), zinc deficiency (Arcasoy et al., 1987), and free-hemoglobin-induced inhibition of cartilage growth (Vassilopoulou-Sellin et al., 1989). Over recent years it has been recognized that short stature, related primarily to disproportionate truncal growth and loss of sitting height, may be caused by desferrioxamine (De Sanctis et al., 1994; Rodda et al., 1995), and may reflect its damaging effect on spinal cartilage (Hatori et al., 1995; Olivieri et al., 1995).

It is clear, therefore, that growth retardation in thalassemia is both multifactorial and extremely common (Table 13.4). In inadequately transfused patients it seems likely that hypoxia plays a role, while in those who are well transfused but inadequately chelated, iron-mediated damage to the hypothalamic/pituitary axis is the main factor. Because of the extreme sensitivity of some of the endocrine organs to iron excess, and the fact that chelating agents such as desferrioxamine in therapeutic doses can inhibit fibroblast proliferation and collagen formation and chelate other metals, even for thalassemic children who have, by all other criteria, received ideal treatment the potential for growth retardation is still considerable.

Delayed Puberty and Defective Function of the Hypothalamic/Pituitary Axis. Arrest or failure of puberty occurs in approximately 50 percent of both male and female patients. In one large series secondary amenorrhea was documented in 23 percent of females and 2 percent of males, and arrested puberty was observed in 16 percent of males and 13 percent of females. Oligomenorrhea or irregular menstrual cycles were reported in approximately 13 percent of females (Italian Working Groups on Endocrine Complications in Non-endocrine Diseases, 1995). While a conflicting literature has accumulated regarding the overall effects of iron chelation on sexual maturation, most recent studies have observed an improvement, with significantly reduced serum ferritin concentrations in those who achieve a normal puberty (Italian Working Groups on Endocrine Complications in Non-endocrine Diseases, 1995; Jensen et al., 1997). However, there have been no studies of this type involving patients whose body-iron loads have been assessed by hepatic biopsy.

While in inadequately treated patients hypogonadism may be a reflection of chronic anemia, deficiency of IGF-1 secondary to liver dysfunction, cirrhosis, diabetes, and low adrenal-androgen production, there is now abundant evidence that, in those who are more adequately managed, the major mechanism involved in failure of sexual maturation is selective central hypogonadism (Kletsky et al., 1979; De Sanctis et al., 1988a; Maurer et al., 1988; Wang et al., 1989; Chatterjee et al., 1993; Landau et al., 1993). Some males tend to have a low baseline testosterone level but their response to human chorionic gonadotrophin is usually normal. Although defective ovarian function has been reported in some cases (De Sanctis et al., 1988a), patients who show retarded sexual development usually demonstrate blunted responses to GnRH rather than to FSH.

The hypothalamic/pituitary axis appears to be particularly vulnerable to the effects of iron loading. This is supported by histologic studies showing selective deposition in pituitary gonadotropes (Bergeron and Kovacs, 1978) and the observation of loss of anterior pituitary volume in iron-loaded patients, demonstrated by MRI scanning (Chatterjee et al., 1998).

Over recent years the importance of linking the function of endocrine organs to circadian cycles has been emphasized. One of the most extensively studied systems is the pulsatile secretion of LSH and FSH, which reflects the intermittent release of GnRH from the hypothalamus. In a long-term prospective study of thalassemic women with secondary amenorrhea, it was found that all of them developed gonadotrophin-pulse abnormalities together with evidence of GnRH-gonadotrophin secretory insufficiency (Chatterjee et al., 1993); over the 10-year period there was a progressive deterioration of hypothalamic pituitary function, and 66 percent of the patients became apulsatile with marked reduction in the levels of GnRH-stimulating gonadotrophin.

These studies emphasize the importance of studying the hypothalamic/pituitary axis in patients with amenorrhea or other evidence of failure of sexual development. Although there were early reports of testicular and ovarian iron loading (Canale et al., 1974), it seems likely that, with improvements in the management of β thalassemia, end-organ unresponsiveness will play a relatively small role in problems of sexual maturation and function in the future.

Thus, although there has been an increase in fertility in men and women with thalassemia over the last decade, it is disappointing that secondary amenorrhea may eventually develop in approximately one-quarter of thalassemic women. This suggests that the anterior pituitary may be particularly susceptible over time to iron-induced damage and that, unlike the heart and liver, the consequences of iron deposition may be irreversible. There are no reports in the literature describing improvement in potency, fertility, or normalization of testosterone levels and sperm counts after reduction of iron load in thalassemia major, although this may occur in primary hemochromatosis. Recent studies have suggested that body iron burdens corresponding to a hepatic iron concentration between 9 and 30 mg/g/liver, dry weight, may be associated with a high risk of development of pituitary failure (Berkovitch et al., 2000). Further studies to quantitate body iron and anterior pituitary function in patients from early in life should provide more secure conclusions with respect to the threshold of risk.

Diabetes Mellitus. Diabetes is relatively common in children who have been inadequately iron chelated and is also observed in those who have been well-transfused and chelated; in an extensive study of transfused and chelated patients it occurred in 4 percent to 6 percent of cases (Italian Working Groups on Endocrine Complications in Non-endocrine Diseases, 1995). It has been attributed to impaired secretion of insulin secondary to chronic pancreatic iron overload (Ellis et al., 1954; Lassman et al., 1974a; Costin et al., 1977; Saudek et al., 1977; Zuppinger et al., 1979; De Sanctis et al., 1988b). There have also been a number of reports of insulin resistance in diabetes (Dandona et al., 1983; Merkel et al., 1988; Dmochowski et al., 1993; Cavello-Perin et al., 1995), although the mechanism is not absolutely clear. It has also been linked

temporally to episodes of acute viral hepatitis (De Sanctis et al., 1986, 1988b).

However, it appears that iron-mediated damage to the pancreas is the major factor in producing diabetes in iron-loaded children; there is a good relationship between the development of diabetes and the severity and duration of iron overload (De Sanctis et al., 1988; Olivieri et al., 1990b). This conclusion is strengthened by consecutive studies over a long period that have shown early and progressive loss of pancreatic β-cell mass, manifested by decreased insulin release in response in secretagogues before the development of significant insulin resistance or diabetes (Karahanyan et al., 1994; Soliman et al., 1996). In addition, there appears to be a reduction in the frequency of diabetes in patients who have been more adequately chelated (Brittenham, 1994).

Hypothyroidism. Mild abnormalities or thyroid function were described in some iron-loaded patients with β thalassemia by Lassman et al. (1974b) and Flynn et al. (1976). These findings have been substantiated in later studies (Sabato et al., 1983; Magro et al., 1990), including patients who had been well managed by transfusion and iron chelation. Grundy et al. (1994) described two adolescents with moderately reduced levels of plasma thyroxine and marked elevations in thyroid-stimulating hormone (TSH); both had clinical features of hypothyroidism. In the study of Jensen et al. (1997) there was a strong correlation between serum ferritin concentrations and the presence of thyroid dysfunction. Although it appears that hypothyroidism is relatively uncommon in transfusion-dependent thalassemia (Vullo et al., 1990), because its clinical onset is so insidious it is very important to bear this complication in mind.

Hypoparathyroidism. Defective parathyroid function has been well documented for many years (Flynn et al., 1976; Costin et al., 1979; Gertner et al., 1979; De Sanctis et al., 1992) and florid, clinical hypoparathyroidism has been described in a few cases (Gabrielle, 1971; Oberklaid and Seshadri, 1975; Flynn et al., 1976; McIntosh, 1976). The symptoms and signs are all attributable to hypocalcemia and hyperphosphatemia. The early signs, which are nonspecific, include neuromuscular irritability, paresthesiae involving the face, fingers, and toes, and abdominal cramps. The full clinical picture of acute irritability, emotional ability, memory impairment, lethargy, and convulsions has been rarely reported in thalassemia. The diagnosis is easily made by the finding of hypocalcemia and hyperphosphatemia, together with a reduction in the level of plasma parathyroid hormone (PTH). In a recent study of 113 transfusion-dependent cases, 12.4

percent showed subnormal PTH levels, suggesting that subclinical hypoparathyroidism may be relatively common (Pratico et al., 1998).

Adrenal Insufficiency. There is much less information about functional adrenal insufficiency in thalassemic patients. What does exist suggests that it is uncommon and that, although there may be measurable abnormalities of adrenal function (Lassman et al., 1974), they are rarely associated with the clinical picture of adrenal failure (Kuo et al., 1968; Canale et al., 1974; McIntosh, 1976; Vullo et al., 1990). Interestingly, there seems to be some dissociation of the different adrenal hormone functions in cases in which defects have been observed. For example, Sklar et al. (1987) observed low levels of adrenal androgen secretion with a normal glucocorticoid reserve. Early suggestions that part of the skin pigmentation in thalassemia might be due to the melanophore-stimulating effect of raised plasma ACTH levels were not confirmed by Costin et al. (1979).

Conclusions. It is clear, therefore, that one of the relative failures of high transfusion and adequate chelation that has otherwise changed the lives of thalassemic patients has been the persistence of endocrine dysfunction, particularly involving the hypothalamic/pituitary axis. Although the reasons are not clear, it is possible that the pituitary is particularly sensitive to even mild degrees of iron overload, and that even chelation regimens that are adequate to retain the function of other organs may simply not always be good enough to protect it.

Bone Disease. The bone changes in inadequately transfused thalassemic children were described earlier in this chapter. As soon as the high transfusion regimens were instituted in the mid-1960s it soon became apparent that the gross skeletal deformities that had been seen earlier could be prevented (Johnston and Roseman, 1967; Piomelli et al., 1969). It seems likely, therefore, that they reflect expansion of the bone marrow mass, a process that can lead to a variety of other distressing symptoms, particularly pathologic fractures (Wolman, 1964; Herrick and Davis, 1975). Similarly, poor dentition (Tas et al., 1976) and attacks of recurrent sinusitis due to inadequate drainage (Hazell and Modell, 1976) are much less common. The pathophysiology of bone disease in thalassemia is not well understood. While it is clear that marrow expansion plays a major role in inadequately treated patients, the osteoporosis that occurs in many patients who have been reasonably well transfused, but in whom there is severe iron loading, may be related to hypogonadism (Fabbri et al., 1991; Anapliotou et al., 1995). Indeed, it is now apparent that even in well-

transfused patients with thalassemia major there may be a relatively high frequency of osteoporosis, at least in part due to this mechanism (Giardina et al., 1995; Vichinsky, 1998; Wonke, 1998).

Jensen et al. (1998) investigated 82 transfusion-dependent patients of both sexes, with a mean age of 27 years. The incidence of osteoporosis was 51 percent. Multivariate analysis showed that hypogonadotropic-hypogonadism, sex, and diabetes were significant risk factors. There was no association between ethnic group, smoking, exercise, calcium supplementation or age at starting chelation therapy or, indeed, the serum ferritin concentration. This study also highlighted some features of osteoporosis in thalassemia that are different from those in the postmenopausal variety. In thalassemia, men are more commonly and more severely affected and their lumbar vertebrae and femoral necks are involved, whereas in women osteoporosis mainly involves the spine. This is surprising because most of the women in this study were receiving hormone replacement therapy. Many of these patients were symptomatic with varying degrees of bone pain.

This study, which confirms the earlier findings of Fabbri et al. (1991), Giuzio et al. (1991), and Anapliotou et al. (1995) in incriminating hypogonadism as an important factor in the development of osteoporosis in thalassemia, further underlines the importance of pituitary failure, even in patients who have been treated adequately.

Recently, there has been considerable interest in the possibility that there may be subsets of individuals who are genetically susceptible to developing osteoporosis (Eisman, 1996). So far very few studies along these lines have been reported in patients with thalassemia. Rees et al. (1998) found that there was a significant correlation between homozygosity of the SS polymorphism of vitamin D receptor and the likelihood of developing osteoporosis of the femoral neck but not the lumbar spine. Jensen et al. (1998) could find no relationship between osteoporosis and polymorphisms of the gene for the estrogen receptor. Hanslip et al. (1998) found a correlation between osteoporosis and a promoter polymorphism of the COLIAI gene in males but not in females. Clearly, this important question needs further study.

Suspicions that β thalassemia minor might be a risk factor for osteoporosis have not been confirmed (Kalef-Exra et al., 1995).

Infection. The notion that thalassemic children are particularly prone to infection has been an accepted part of the thalassemia literature for many years. As symptomatic management improved this concept was questioned (Valassi-Adam et al., 1976) and it was suggested that the incidence of infection in early childhood had been markedly reduced in children maintained at an adequate hemoglobin level (Modell, 1976). In recent years, although there is still an awareness of the dangers of infection, particularly after splenectomy, there has been a major change in emphasis toward concerns about blood-borne infection, notably hepatitis B and C, and human immunodeficiency virus (HIV).

Patterns of Infection with Changing Management. In an extensive retrospective study of the patterns of infection in thalassemic children maintained at different hemoglobin levels, Modell and Berdoukas (1984) concluded that the most serious infections were pneumonia, pericarditis, the sequelae of streptococcal infections, meningitis, peritonitis, and osteomyelitis. Further analysis suggested that pneumonia and septicemia were significantly associated with splenectomy and a low transfusion regimen, and that in patients who had been maintained at a satisfactory hemoglobin level these infections had almost disappeared. They also observed that other serious infections including meningitis, peritonitis, and osteomyelitis are only seen in splenectomized patients and that they have no obvious relationship to anemia. Finally, they noted that pericarditis is also unrelated to anemia and splenectomy but is very clearly related to age, occurring in childhood or later. They suggested that this may reflect a relationship between iron overload and pericarditis. Modell and Berdoukas also provided some comparative information from other countries, indicating that this overall pattern of infection is common in most thalassemic populations. These observations were in keeping with the earlier studies of the dangers of infection in splenectomized thalassemic children (Smith et al., 1962, 1964) and, indeed, in any child who has had the spleen removed early in life (Eraklis et al., 1967; Erikson et al., 1968). In this case the most important organisms are *Streptococcus pneumoniae*, *Hemophilus influenzae*, and *Neisseria meningitidis*.

The widespread use of prophylactic penicillin and appropriate immunization after splenectomy has undoubtedly reduced the frequency of severe infections in splenectomized thalassemic children.

Organisms That Attack Iron-Loaded Patients. Although, as discussed earlier, there has been a great deal of controversy as to whether the frequent attacks of pericarditis in thalassemic children are related to iron loading, no organism has ever been implicated. The only pathogens that have been shown quite unequivocally to occur with an increased frequency in iron-loaded patients are those of the *Yersinia* genus, which normally have a low pathogenicity and an unusually high requirement for iron. They do not secrete siderophores but have receptors for ferrioxamine and become pathogenic in the presence of iron bound to desferrioxamine (Green, 1992). There are numerous reports of severe infections in thalassemic patients due to infections with *Yersinia* spp (Robins-Browne and Prpic, 1985; Gallant et al., 1986; Kelly et al., 1987; Green, 1992). These infections are usually characterized by severe abdominal pain, diarrhea, vomiting, fever, and sore throat. They may also be associated, on occasion, with rupture of the bowel (Mazzoleni, et al., 1991).

Hepatitis B Virus (HBV). It is estimated that about 350 million people worldwide are persistent carriers of hepatitis B. The virus persists in about 10 percent of infected immunocompetent adults. Approximately 25 percent of all patients with chronic hepatitis progress to cirrhosis, about 20 percent of whom develop hepatocellular carcinoma. During the first phase of chronicity, virus replication continues in the liver; markers of this stage include HBV DNA and a soluble antigen, hepatitis Be antigen (HBeAg). In most persons there is immune clearance of infected hepatocytes, associated with seroconversion from HBeAg to anti-HBe.

Because HBV is primarily a blood-borne infection, transfusion-dependent thalassemic children are at particular risk, depending on its prevalence in their community and the effectiveness of donor screening programs. The early experience in Europe was summarized by Schanfield et al. (1975) and by Modell and Berdoukas (1984). At that time, in British, Cypriot, Sardinian, and Greek populations the frequency of antibody positivity ranged from 30 percent to 90 percent with an appropriately low level of those with persistent antigen positivity. Later studies from Greece have shown how the application of adequate screening and vaccination programs results in a major fall in the frequency of HBV infection (Politis, 1989). Although the frequency of HBV infection is now very low in countries in which screening and immunization programs have been established, HBV-related-hepatitis is still seen frequently in parts of the world where these precautions are not taken. The diagnosis of chronic active hepatitis depends on the presence of abnormal liver function tests, particularly elevated transaminases, the appearances on liver biopsy, and, in the early stages, the presence of HBeAg antigens and, later, the presence of anti-HBe. In the early phase there is an HBe-positive viremia that usually becomes negative as the disease progresses.

Hepatitis C Virus (HCV). Following the identification of HCV it soon became clear that this infection is widespread and presents a serious risk to patients with transfusion-dependent thalassemia. The prevalence of anti-HCV in patients with thalassemia major varies in different parts of the world, ranging from 11.7 percent in Turkish Cypriots, through 30 percent in Malaysians and Chinese to nearly 75 percent in Italians (Wonke et al., 1990; Bozkurt et al., 1993; Cancado et al., 1993; Lau et al., 1993; Kaur and Kaur, 1995; Cao et al., 1996; Wonke et al., 1998).

An initial HCV infection is almost invariably anicteric and can only be diagnosed by screening for elevated serum transaminases; jaundice is rare. Unfortunately, only 50 percent of patients recover, and the remainder develop persistent viremia with hepatitis. Of these about one in five develop cirrhosis and run the risk of hepatocellular carcinoma. Antibodies to structural and nonstructural proteins of the virus can be detected at various times after infection. Viremia is detected by polymerase chain reaction (PCR), which can identify HCV-RNA. Patients with chronic active hepatitis are invariably HCV-RNA positive and also have IgG anti-HCV, which is also present after recovery. There is some evidence that the liver damage associated with persistent HCV infection, or response to therapy, may be modified by the presence of excess iron (Clemente et al., 1994; Olynyk and Bacon, 1995; Rubin et al., 1995).

Clearly, therefore, any patient with persistently raised serum transaminases must be screened for HCV using PCR to identify HCV-RNA. If this test is positive it is important to proceed to a liver biopsy to identify those who have histologic changes of chronic active hepatitis. The liver histology shows predominantly chronic persistent hepatitis with a low incidence of periportal, piecemeal necrosis and lobular hepatitis.

Other Forms of Viral Hepatitis. Hepatitis D virus (HDV) only replicates in patients already infected with HBV. Infection is common among HBV carriers in the Mediterranean region and may occur at the same time as HBV. The clinical course is that outlined earlier for HBV infection. Hepatitis E virus (HEV) is enterically transmitted and, like HAV, although it may produce acute hepatitis is not associated with persistent infection. Evidence of infection with HEV was obtained in 2.4 percent of transfusion-dependent thalassemic patients in Athens (Psichogiou et al., 1996) and in 10.7 percent of a similar population in Saudi Arabia (al-Fawaz et al., 1996).

Hepatitis G virus (HGV) was discovered in 1995 (reviewed by Stransky, 1996). It produces a mild form of hepatitis but there is little evidence that patients go on to develop chronic hepatitis. It can be diagnosed by the demonstration of HGV-RNA by PCR in a similar way to HCV. Its prevalence in U.S. blood donors is approximately 1.5 percent. In a study of 40 Italian transfusion-dependent β thalassemics, HGV-RNA was detected in 22 percent of cases. In patients who were also viremic for HCV the clinical manifestations of the co-infection were no different from those of patients with HVC alone. The authors concluded that although HGV is highly prevalent among Italian polytransfused individuals there is no evidence for a clinically significant role in liver disease (Sampietro et al., 1997). Similar conclusions came from a study of Chung et al. (1997) in Taiwan, where the prevalence of HGV-RNA positivity was 14 percent; again the presence of the virus did not seem to be associated with significant hepatitis. In a further follow-up of Italian patients with HGV it was concluded that in over 25 percent of cases the infection resolved within 6 years (Prati et al., 1998). Similar conclusions were reported by Zemel et al. (1998), who found an incidence of HGV infection of 19.4 percent in a population in Tel Aviv; follow-up studies suggested that there is persistent viremia but no significant biochemical evidence of liver damage. The frequency of HGV infections in Southeast Asia seems to be even higher, with reports of frequencies in transfusion-dependent thalassemic children of 32 percent (Poovorawan et al., 1998).

All these studies suggest that HGV infection, while very common, does not seem to be associated with a serious form of hepatitis or long-term liver damage. Although preliminary studies suggested that it might have an ameliorating effect on HCV infections, this question needs much more study. Indeed, more careful, long-term follow-up data on HGV-infected patients are required.

Human Immunodeficiency Viruses. The human immunodeficiency viruses HIV-1 and HIV-2 belong to the lentivirus subfamily of retroviruses. They can both give rise to the acquired immunodeficiency syndrome (AIDS). Globally, HIV-1 is responsible for the worldwide pandemic of AIDS, while HIV-2, though mainly confined to western Africa, is starting to spread rapidly, notably in India. It is currently estimated by the World Health Organization (WHO) that by the year 2000 approximately 40 million people worldwide will be infected. More than 90 percent of them will live in the developing countries in sub-Saharan Africa, south and southwest Asia, Latin America, and the Caribbean. Since these viruses can be transmitted by blood transfusion or perinatally it is clear that thalassemic patients form a high-risk subgroup in any population in which this infection is common.

It should be remembered that most people in the world with HIV infections are asymptomatic. Prospective studies of cohorts of infected people with known dates of seroconversion have suggested that 50 percent to 60 percent of them will develop symptoms and signs of disease within 10 years of infection.

During the asymptomatic phase many individuals show abnormal laboratory tests such as low CD4 lymphocyte counts and hypergammaglobulinemia. It is beyond our scope to deal with the various symptom complexes of AIDS, which have been classified by the Centers for Disease Control and Prevention (CDC) into several subgroups (Table 13.5).

It is not surprising, therefore, that HIV infection has become a major concern for multitransfused patients with thalassemia (Manconi et al., 1998). In the mid-1980s, when it was becoming apparent that HIV infection would pose a serious problem for children who had received regular blood products, a European-Mediterranean WHO Working Group on Hemoglobinopathies together with the Cooleycare Group established a program to coordinate data collection. Work from this group and others has provided valuable information about the change in prevalence of HIV infection after donor screening was established and about the course of the illness in those who were affected (Girot et al., 1991). Early prevalence figures from Italy and Greece ranged from 2.3 percent to 11 percent (De Martino et al., 1985; Politis et al., 1986; Zanella et al., 1986), while the infection rate in transfused thalassemic patients in the United States was reported to be about 12 percent (Robert-Guroff et al., 1987). The European-Mediterranean WHO Working Group carried out a further study of 3,633 patients in 36 centers from 13 countries and found an overall frequency of HIV positivity of 1.56 percent. Further data collected after establishment of screening (reviewed by Girot et al., 1991) revealed a sharp fall in the number of HIV-positive patients, although there is still a very low level of transmission from HIV blood obtained from seronegative donors (Jullien et al., 1988). However, in the period after 1988 an analysis of nearly 3,000 patients in 13 European centers found no HIV-1-positive patients.

The same WHO Working Group started a follow-up study of 75 seropositive thalassemic patients to observe the natural history of HIV infection in thalassemic children (Costagliola et al., 1992). The median follow-up period was 4 years 11 months. At the end of the study, 43 patients were CDC stage II, 23 CDC stage III, and 13 CDC stage IV, including 7 patients with AIDS, of whom 3 had died. The rate of progression to AIDS was not associated with intercurrent infection, splenectomy, age, or sex. For the group, a cumulative AIDS incidence rate of 1.4 percent was observed at 3 years, and of 9 percent at 5 years.

The situation in other parts of the world, where screening started later or has not yet been established, is much less encouraging. In a study of 203 children in New Dehli, Sen et al. (1993) reported a frequency of 8.9 percent for HIV positivity. Kumar et al. (1994) found a frequency of 8.9 percent in a transfusion clinic in Manapur, India. These data provide some indication of the magnitude of the problem that will be posed by HIV infection in thalassemic children in many parts of the world unless urgent steps are taken to institute donor screening. This problem is highlighted by Kumar and Khuranna (1998), who have recently reported on a prospective analysis of the outcome of pregnancies in 123 women with transfusion-dependent β thalassemia, of whom 81 were HIV positive; using the CDC classification, 39 were stage CII and 42 stage AII (see Table 13.5). All 22 preterm babies of mothers with stage CII had positive viral cultures for HIV-1 within 1 week of birth; 10 of these neonates died of AIDS by 8 weeks, and the remaining 12 by 15 months of age. Of 39 CII-stage pregnancies, 5 died undelivered at 32 weeks gestation due to fulminating *Pneumocystis carinii* pneumonia. Although there may be a successful outcome of pregnancies in thalassemic women with asymptomatic HIV disease, AIDS-indicator conditions are associated with an appreciable perinatal and maternal morbidity and mortality.

Malaria. Following early hopes on the part of the WHO that malaria was being contained in many parts of the world, events of the last few years have proved just how unpredictable the control of an important infection can be. The disease has returned to many countries from which it seemed to have disappeared and, even more frighteningly, drug resistance is now widespread. Children with severe forms of thalassemia are subject to attacks of acute malaria like any other child; the protective effect of thalassemia against malaria, reviewed by Weatherall and Clegg (2000), is

---

Table 13.5. Centers for Disease Control (CDC) Classification for HIV Infection

Group I	Acute infection
Group II	Asymptomatic infection
Group III	Persistent, generalised lymphadenopathy
Group IV	Other disease
Subgroup A	Constitutional disease (one or more of: fever for more than one month; weight loss > 10% baseline; diarrhea for more than one month
Subgroup B	Neurological disease
Subgroup C	Secondary infection
	C1 As specified by CDC surveillance definition
	C2 Others
Subgroup D	Secondary cancers
Subgroup E	Other conditions

relative; no form of thalassemia protects any individual completely against the infection. Chronic malaria, as well as exacerbating the anemia of thalassemia, may also increase the degree of splenomegaly.

Thalassemic children are particularly at risk from blood-borne malaria. In a study from India of the blood of children immediately after transfusion, Choudhury et al. (1990) found that in 6.4 percent of cases there was evidence of transfusion-transmitted malaria infection. Thus it is clear that there must be a high frequency of chronic malaria in blood donors in endemic regions.

Another important question regarding malarial infection in thalassemic children relates to the effects of splenectomy on the course of the disease. This complex issue was reviewed by Looareesuwan et al. (1993). Although there have been anecdotal reports suggesting that malaria may be particularly severe in those who have been splenectomized, there is no convincing evidence that this is the case, but this question requires further study.

Severe malaria is not always associated with high parasitemias however. Therefore, in any thalassemic child in a malarious area who presents with fever, drowsiness progressing to coma, renal failure, hemoglobinuria, hypoglycemia, or simply a rapidly worsening anemia, a diagnosis of malaria must be considered, regardless of the number of parasites in the peripheral blood.

Liver Disease. In young adults with thalassemia major liver disease remains a common cause of morbidity and mortality. Although it has been realized for many years that iron overload, acquired through transfusion and increased gastrointestinal absorption, is a major factor in the generation of liver disease, more recently, with the increasing recognition of blood-related viral hepatitis, it has become clear that the pathogenesis of liver damage is extremely complex.

Mechanisms of Liver Damage. Iron produces cellular injury with progression to fibrosis and cirrhosis (Fig. 13.7). This may be mediated in several ways. It promotes free-radical mediated lipid peroxidation and mitochondrial dysfunction (Gutteridge and Halliwell, 1989; Grinberg and Rachmilewitz, 1995; Tsukamoto et al., 1995; Hershko et al., 1998b). The deposition of hemosiderin in lysosomes may lead to fragility and subsequent rupture of their membranes. Iron-promoted catalysis of collagen synthesis or decreased collagen breakdown due to lysosomal blockade following iron overload may promote excess collagen deposition; a similar mechanism has been observed in other storage diseases (Iancu et al., 1977). Furthermore, iron overload may potentiate further iron loading; upregulation of the transport of non–transferrin-bound iron has been observed in cultured hepatocytes (Parkes et al., 1995).

As mentioned earlier, blood-borne viral infection is another major factor in the high frequency of liver disease in thalassemic patients, and iron may potentiate the effects of viral hepatitis. Agents such as alcohol may act synergistically in accelerating the development of liver

Figure 13.7. A liver biopsy obtained at autopsy from a child with thalassemia major showing extensive iron loading. (Perl's stain ×510)

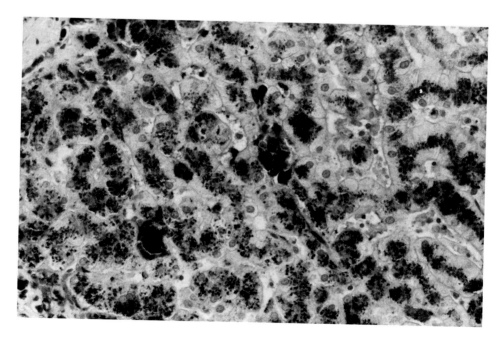

damage. Clearly, therefore, hepatic pathology in patients with thalassemia is extremely complex and many questions about the mechanisms of tissue damage and its pattern of progression remain to be worked out.

Assessment of Iron Loading and Liver Damage.

The methods for assessing body-iron burden in general, and the level of liver iron in particular, are discussed later in this chapter. Hepatic biopsy provides definitive information with respect to quantitative body iron stores (Brittenham, 1994). In addition, it offers the only direct approach for determining both the pattern and extent of liver damage in thalassemic patients.

Early Findings in Inadequately Treated Patients.

Over the last five decades, as survival has extended, severe hepatic fibrosis and siderosis have been regular findings at autopsy (Frumin et al., 1952; Howell and Wyatt, 1953; Ellis et al., 1954; Witzleben and Wyatt, 1961). In the absence of adequate chelation therapy it is an inevitable consequence of iron overload; in most patients fibrosis develops during childhood and progresses to frank cirrhosis during the second decade (Risdon et al., 1975; Iancu et al., 1977; Jean et al., 1984; Aldouri et al., 1987; Maurer et al., 1988).

It appears that pathologic changes in the liver occur very early during the course of the disease. In an early series of studies, the relationship between liver iron content and liver damage was examined in babies of less than 2 years of age (Wollstein and Kreidel, 1930; Koch and Shapiro, 1932; Panizon and Vullo, 1952; Iancu et al., 1977). Hepatic fibrosis of varying degree was reported in 5 of these 16 babies, although the liver iron content was not reported. Importantly, screening tests were of limited clinical value and there was no biochemical evidence of hepatic damage. Consecutive histologic and electron-microscopic changes in liver pathology in early childhood are reported by Iancu et al. (1977).

Early studies in older children (Cooley et al., 1927; Baty et al., 1932; Whipple and Bradford, 1936; Frumin et al., 1952; Panizon and Vullo, 1952; Ellis et al., 1954; Witzleben and Wyatt, 1961) suggested that fibrosis and cirrhosis were common in transfused, nonchelated children after the age of 3 years. The age and iron content at which significant fibrosis and cirrhosis are likely to develop is still unclear. The relationship between liver-iron concentration and transfusional iron overload was best expressed as an exponential, nonlinear function of the transfused iron load (Barry et al., 1974). In these early studies the imperfect correlation between the amount of iron administered by transfusion and the development of fibrosis may be accounted for, in part, by the fact that many children were maintained on low-transfusion regimens that would not have substantially reduced gastrointestinal iron loading.

Later Studies of Factors Influencing the Rate of Development of Liver Disease.

Age, the iron content of the liver, associated hepatitis, and, possibly, splenectomy may all play a role in determining the time at which liver disease is established.

Risdon et al. (1975) suggested that the severity of fibrosis is related to age in a normal linear fashion, but that even when iron accumulation is rapid, severe fibrosis may not be expected before 10 years of age. However, this pattern of fibrosis does not seem to have been consistent between series of transfused, poorly chelated children with thalassemia. One study reported fibrosis as early as 3 years of age, and cirrhosis as early as 8 years; by the age of 16 years, almost all children showed cirrhosis (Jean et al., 1984). Liver biopsies obtained in 51 regularly transfused patients, aged 5 to 36 years (mean, 18 years), showed that only 6 did not have some degree of fibrosis; in 5, cirrhosis was fully developed (Aldouri et al., 1987). Similarly, of 16 patients aged 3 to 17 years, all but 2, both aged 3 years at the time of the biopsy, had moderate to massive fibrosis or cirrhosis; 3 older patients, aged 4 and 5 years, already demonstrated a severe degree of hepatic fibrosis (Maurer et al., 1988). Angelucci et al. (1993) found that fibrosis was established in about 50 percent of transfused, irregularly chelated patients under the age of 6 years, and in 90 percent of similarly treated children over the age of 5 years, an observation that has been confirmed in more recent studies of poorly chelated patients (Thakerngpol et al., 1996).

It has been suggested that, following splenectomy, the iron content of the liver may increase and fibrosis may be accelerated (Witzleben and Wyatt, 1961). However, studies of the iron content of spleens in iron-loaded patients have given inconsistent results. Furthermore, Risdon et al. (1975) could demonstrate no increase in fibrosis in splenectomized patients. Thus, although the question of the relationship between splenectomy and iron loading remains open, the balance of evidence is against this being an important mechanism for potentiating liver damage.

There is extensive evidence that the major factor in the development of fibrosis is the concentration of iron in the liver. Risdon et al. (1975) noted an exponential relationship between iron content and fibrosis in a series of 52 liver biopsies in 19 patients studied over 13 years. The relationship between tissue iron concentration and hepatic cirrhosis was explored in children maintained on a high transfusion regimen who did, or did not, receive intramuscular desferrioxamine, and demonstrated a clear reduction in the degree of fibrosis in the former (Barry et al., 1974). In early attempts to establish a threshold of hepatic iron associated with the development of hepatic damage, it was observed that fibrosis was only present in patients in whom the iron levels exceeded 7.6 mg/g, dry weight (Witzleben and Wyatt, 1961). Later, DeVirgillis et al. (1980) reported chronic persistent hepatitis, or chronic active hepatitis with periportal lesions, but only in patients with liver-iron concentrations exceeding 10 mg/g, dry weight. Aldouri et al. (1987) found a mean hepatic-iron concentration of approximately 12.5 mg/g, dry weight, in patients with moderate or severe fibrosis, although fibrosis was observed in the presence of lower concentration of hepatic iron.

As mentioned earlier, the first clear evidence that fibrosis can be arrested by iron-chelating therapy was obtained by Barry et al. (1974). This effect was observed at a dose that would now be considered inadequate, and at a liver-iron concentration in excess of 20 mg/g, dry weight, a level that was subsequently shown to be associated with a heightened risk of cardiac disease and early death (Brittenham et al., 1994). Arrest of fibrosis was observed in several other small studies (Aldouri et al., 1987; Maurer et al., 1988).

In the absence of prospective clinical trials to evaluate life-long therapy for the prevention of tissue damage in thalassemia, guidance about the risk of hepatic fibrosis has had to be derived from the clinical experience with hereditary hemochromatosis (Olivieri and Brittenham, 1997). Minor iron loading develops in about a quarter of heterozygotes for this condition, although their body iron stores do not seem to increase beyond 2 to 4 times the upper limit of normal, that is, up to approximately 7 mg/g, dry weight. In contrast, homozygotes who have iron burdens exceeding 7 mg/g, dry weight, have a definite increased risk of hepatic fibrosis.

It is clear, however, that the toxic manifestations of iron overload do not depend entirely on the amount of excess iron in the liver. They are also modified by the rate of iron accumulation, the duration of exposure to increased iron, the partition of the iron load between relatively harmless sites in macrophages and more hazardous deposits in parenchymal cells, ascorbate status, which may help to determine this partition effect, the extent of internal redistribution of iron between macrophages and parenchymal sites, and non–iron-related factors, particularly viral hepatitis. In patients with hepatitis C liver damage associated with persistent infection, or response to therapy, may be considerably modified by the presence of excess iron (Clemente et al., 1994; Olynyk and Bacon, 1995; Rubin et al., 1995). It has been reported recently that the use of the oral chelating agent deferiprone may result in progression of hepatic fibrosis (Olivieri et al., 1998).

Assessment of Liver Function. Given the extremely complex and multifactorial nature of liver disease in β thalassemia, assessment of liver function and determining the reasons for abnormalities of liver-function tests may be extremely difficult. As mentioned earlier, there may be significant liver damage due to iron excess without any changes in standard liver function tests. Most patients with β thalassemia, unless their bone marrow is suppressed by transfusion, have elevated serum bilirubin levels, reflecting both ineffective erythropoiesis and a shortened red cell survival. The level of bilirubin is extremely variable and, as mentioned later in this chapter, it is becoming apparent that some patients who remain deeply jaundiced may have an additional genetic defect in bilirubin conjugation. Hepatocellular damage is reflected by a rise in the activity of serum aspartate aminotransferase (AST) and alanine aminotransferase (ALT). Since these enzymes are not specific for the liver, elevated levels must be assessed with caution. Because gallstones occur quite frequently in patients with β thalassemia, particularly of the intermediate variety, a typical picture of obstructive jaundice may occur, with raised levels of serum alkaline phosphatase, 5′ nucleotidase, and γ-glutamyl-transferase.

In assessing patients with suspected liver disease an estimation of the size of the liver may be helpful. A moderate degree of hepatomegaly is quite common in patients who have been maintained at a relatively low hemoglobin level. A large, tender liver should raise the suspicion of an underlying hepatitis or, in grossly iron-loaded patients, cardiac failure. An elevation of the liver enzymes should always be investigated, particularly if the level is rising with time. It is essential to screen for the different forms of hepatitis, as discussed earlier. A liver biopsy should be performed and, where possible, the liver-iron level estimated chemically. The liver should be examined histologically with appropriate stains to demonstrate iron, collagen, and, where applicable, hepatitis antigen.

Exocrine Pancreas. As well as diabetes, described earlier in this chapter, there is increasing evidence that iron may also cause damage to the exocrine pancreas (Gullo et al., 1993). In a combined ultrasonographic and pancreatic-enzyme determination study, the frequency of exocrine pancreatic damage was assessed in 39 consecutive patients with β thalassemia and iron overload. Most of them had markedly increased echogenicity of the pancreas, with decreased size of the gland, as compared with controls. These changes showed a significant correlation with age and the duration of transfusion. Serum concentrations of trypsin and lipase were significantly lower in patients than controls. The lowest values were found in older patients with a longer duration of transfusion therapy, who also had the most marked sonographic changes. Although the functional significance of these findings is not clear, it is possible that, in cases of extreme damage to the exocrine pancreas, malabsorption may occur.

Folic Acid and Vitamin B$_{12}$ Deficiency. The early literature on thalassemia offered clear evidence that in inadequately treated patients folate deficiency is relatively common (Jandl and Greenberg, 1959; Luhby and Cooperman, 1961; Luhby et al., 1961). These findings were confirmed in studies carried out in Thailand (Vatanavicharn et al., 1979). Chanarin (1980) pointed out that the bone marrow may not show features that are absolutely typical of a megaloblastic anemia in patients with thalassemia and coexistent folate deficiency. In several of the early reports it was noted that severe bone pain may follow the administration of folic acid to folate-deficient patients. Folate deficiency is seen less commonly in well-transfused patients although it is still an important problem in those with the intermediate forms of thalassemia.

Vitamin B$_{12}$ levels are usually normal or elevated (Luhby et al., 1969).

Other Vitamin and Trace Metal Deficiencies

Ascorbic Acid. Early studies suggested that leukocyte ascorbic acid concentrations are significantly reduced in patients with severe forms of β thalassemia (Wapnick et al., 1969; Modell and Beck, 1974). Subsequent work confirmed that low ascorbic acid levels are found in iron-loaded thalassemic patients (O'Brien, 1974; Cohen et al., 1981; Chapman et al., 1982). It seems likely that ascorbic acid, because of its role as a biological reducing agent, may well be utilized in combating some of the complex free-radical damage that is mediated by excess iron in the tissues. Its role in this process, and how this may differ at varying tissue concentrations of ascorbate, is reviewed by Gutteridge and Halliwell (1989). Although clinical scurvy must be unusual in iron-loaded patients (Cohen et al., 1981), ascorbate deficiency is of great importance in determining the response to chelating agents such as desferrioxamine. Although the mechanism is uncertain, it seems likely that this effect is mediated by expansion of the chelatable iron pool to which desferrioxamine has access (O'Brien, 1974; Nienhuis, 1981; Bridges and Hoffman, 1986).

Vitamin E Deficiency. It has long been established that severe β thalassemics may be vitamin-E–depleted (Hyman et al., 1974; Modell and Beck, 1974). Hyman and her colleagues found that baseline serum DL-α-tochophoral levels and vitamin E stores were low, and

that serial biopsies of skin, liver, thyroid and testes showed increased deposits of lipofuscin, which are associated with vitamin E deficiency. These findings were corroborated by Rachmilewitz (1976), who suggested that, because of the continual process of peroxidation of thalassemic red cell membranes, low serum vitamin E levels reflect its consumption as an antioxidant rather than a primary defect in vitamin E absorption or metabolism. The antioxidant properties of vitamin E are discussed by Gutteridge and Halliwell (1989). In their studies of the effects of vitamin E supplementation, Rachmilewitz et al. (1979) showed that it was possible to produce a fourfold increase in both serum and red cell vitamin E levels, that the serum vitamin E level dropped rapidly after discontinuation of therapy, that there was a reduction in oxidant stress in red cells due to reduced peroxidative damage, and that in three of seven patients treated there was a significant increase in red cell survival. These findings, while they confirmed the function of vitamin E as an antioxidant in thalassemic red cells, did not define its role, if any, in the treatment of β thalassemia.

Trace Metal Deficiencies. There have been conflicting reports about the levels of certain trace metals in the blood of thalassemic patients, and even less is known about their significance. Erlandson et al. (1965) found increased serum copper and decreased magnesium levels. Prasad et al. (1965) also reported increased serum copper levels and Hyman et al. (1980) confirmed that at least some patients have decreased serum magnesium levels. The significance of these observations is not clear although Hyman et al. suggested that markedly reduced magnesium levels might have a deleterious effect on cardiac function.

Prasad et al. (1965) reported a reduction in serum zinc levels. Again the mechanism is not clear although it appears to be a general feature of hemolytic states, including sickle cell anemia. Low levels of serum zinc were also found in a study in Thailand by Silprasert et al. (1998). Incidentally, this study also confirmed the earlier findings of elevated levels of serum copper, although there was no correlation between copper and zinc levels. These authors point out that, at least in experimental animals with zinc and vitamin A deficiency, there is lack of response to vitamin A that can be corrected by zinc supplementation. Zinc deficiency has also been incriminated in growth retardation, although this has not been documented in thalassemia.

Overall, we know very little about the significance of these changes in the levels of trace elements. Since many chelating agents remove metals other than iron, and even desferrioxamine is not entirely specific for iron, trace metal deficiency may also be exacerbated by treatment.

Gallstones. Gallstone formation is common in undertransfused β thalassemics and in thalassemia intermedia (Dewey et al., 1970).

Secondary Gout. Because of the rapid turnover of red cells in their bone marrow, many patients with β thalassemia who are maintained on a low transfusion regimen are hyperuricemic. Secondary gout has been well documented (Fessas and Loukopoulos, 1974) and gouty arthropathy has been reported (Paik et al., 1970).

Neuromuscular Abnormalities. Neuromuscular complications of thalassemia are not common. Logothetis et al. (1972a) summarized their studies on 138 consecutive patients with thalassemia major who had been maintained on only a moderate transfusion regimen. They noted that walking was delayed beyond 18 months in about one-third of the patients, while speech and intellectual development appeared to proceed normally. Twenty-six of their patients developed a curious myopathic syndrome with proximal weakness, mostly in the lower extremities, and a myopathic electromyographic pattern. This complication was associated with severe skeletal stigmata, suggesting that it occurred in inadequately transfused patients. It does not seem to be a feature of adequately transfused thalassemic children.

In the series of Logothetis et al. 27 patients had histories of episodes suggesting cerebral ischemia, with focal neurologic episodes. Similar episodes were described by Sinniah et al. (1977). Neurosensory deafness has been noted by McIntosh (1976), who described improvement in hearing after commencement of regular blood transfusion and, in the same article, noted that deafness was relatively common in inadequately transfused young thalassemics. This complication was also reported by Hazell and Modell (1976). There is no doubt that severe cranial deformities resulting from massive expansion of the bone marrow can result in symptoms of this kind, or involvement of the optic nerve, but these complications are only seen in patients who have been maintained at extremely low hemoglobin levels.

We discuss the various neurologic syndromes that can follow compression by hematopoietic-cell tumor masses when we describe the complications of thalassemia intermedia. There are several neurologic and sensory complications of desferrioxamine therapy; these are also discussed later.

Intelligence and Behavioral Patterns. Logothetis et al. (1971) evaluated the mental status of 138 consecutive cases of thalassemia major in Greece. Intelligence testing revealed no difference from normal children of the same age and social group. A trend to lower IQ scores was found in those subjected to less vigorous transfusion regimens. Abnormalities of behavior and character were noted in 96 cases and abnormal emotional responses, mainly depression and anxiety, were observed in 67 of the children. In summarizing their experience these workers concluded that their findings were similar to those in any group of children with chronic disease.

More recent studies have utilized the modern techniques of psychology and psychiatry to assess the behavioral and emotional problems of young children with thalassemia. For example, Tsiantis (1990) assessed a group of Greek children using the methods that were pioneered by Michael Rutter and his colleagues (Rutter and Graham, 1968) for studying the reliability and validity of psychiatric assessment of children. Using these strict criteria it was found that approximately 40 percent of the thalassemic children, compared with about 30 percent of a control group of chronically sick children, had an emotional or behavioral disorder that would be classified as requiring some kind of psychiatric help. Problems relating to denial and displacement, which are considered to be maladaptive mechanisms, were particularly common. In a further study of group interactions with the parents of thalassemic children a number of factors were defined that may have contributed to the children's problems: death anxiety; denial; overprotective behavior; and, surprisingly, excessive pressure on the sick child to achieve.

Because of growing concerns about these problems the WHO undertook a large multicenter study in 1985 to evaluate the psychosocial aspects of thalassemia and sickle cell anemia. As an approach to data collection they produced an extremely complex questionnaire. In order to make this more useful for studying thalassemic populations a simpler and more practical program was developed by Ratnip (quoted by Klein et al., 1998). In particular, this attempts to define major psychosocial burdens, but also tries to put them into perspective as seen through the very different eyes of patients and parents. A pilot study carried out on the Toronto thalassemic population using this questionnaire showed just how dangerous it is to generalize about psychosocial problems based on studies in any one group of patients or their relatives. For example, it found that the clinical and psychosocial burdens were not correlated between parents and their children, parents' perception of their child's psychological burden correlated well while the child was young but not when they reached adulthood, the burden experienced by children was affected by that felt by their parents and vice versa, and while the overall psychosocial burden was similarly perceived by children and their parents, the value placed on individual aspects may differ considerably among family members.

These examples of studies of the behavioral problems of thalassemic children and their families, while emphasizing the importance of this aspect of the disease, underline the methodological difficulties that will be encountered when trying to learn more about this important subject.

Pregnancy. Until the era of adequate transfusion and chelation, pregnancy was not observed in patients with severe forms of β thalassemia. However, many patients are now passing through a relatively normal puberty and most centers that look after large numbers of thalassemic patients have had some experience of managing pregnancy in those who are on regular transfusion and chelation therapy.

A number of reports have appeared over recent years of series of successful pregnancies in transfusion-dependent β-thalassemic patients. These have included both spontaneous pregnancies, twin pregnancies, and pregnancies following in vitro fertilization (Seracchioli et al., 1994; Tampakoudis et al., 1997). Presumably because pregnancy would only be likely to occur in women who had been adequately chelated, and therefore in whom it is unlikely that there would be serious hepatic, cardiac, or endocrine complications, most of these pregnancies seem to have gone to term and there have been no major problems. The patients have maintained their usual hemoglobin levels by regular transfusion but have usually avoided chelating drugs during pregnancy.

Autopsy Findings

With one notable exception the recent literature of the thalassemia field has, like that of the rest of medicine, completely neglected the value of the autopsy. The exception is the beautifully illustrated atlas produced by Sonakul (1989).

There are, however, many excellent descriptions of the morbid anatomy of thalassemia in its earlier literature (Whipple and Bradford, 1936; Astaldi et al., 1951; Ellis et al., 1954; Fink, 1964; Modell and Matthews, 1976). Perhaps the most valuable information to come from these reports is the distribution of iron among the different organs. Extensive data, together with the weight of iron per organ, were summarized by Modell and Matthews (1976). Most of the findings at autopsy reflect the various pathologies that have been described in different sections of this chapter. The most striking finding in all these reports is the widespread deposition of iron with varying degrees of organ fibrosis. As might be expected the organs most affected include the liver, spleen, endocrine glands, pancreas, heart, and kidneys. The degree of fibrosis varies widely, and is most marked in the liver and least noticeable in the thyroid gland.

The spleen is enlarged and congested with thickened reticulum. It may contain Gaucher-like cells similar to those seen in the marrow. Detailed studies of the myocardium and conductive tissues are reported by Buja and Roberts (1971) and Modell and Matthews (1976) (see earlier section). As shown most elegantly in the atlas of Sonakul (1989), there may be extensive extramedullary hematopoiesis. This study is also notable for the illustrations of obliterative changes in the small vessels of the lungs seen in some Thai patients with HbE thalassemia and pulmonary hypertension.

Hematologic Findings

Pretransfusion, there is always a severe degree of anemia that is typically hypochromic and microcytic with a low mean cell hemoglobin (MCH) and mean cell volume (MCV). Presumably because of the marked changes in the shape and size of the red cells, red cell indices derived from electronic cell counters do not always reflect the degree of hemoglobinization of the red cells as judged from an inspection of the peripheral blood film. They show marked anisocytosis and poikilocytosis, with many misshapen microcytes, occasional macrocytes, and variable numbers of target cells. Erythroblasts are always present and may reach extremely high levels after splenectomy (Fig. 13.8). The appearances of the red cells are different in splenectomized patients. In particular, large hypochromic cells are found together with small piscine forms that are little more than fragments of stroma. Ragged inclusion bodies can be seen in the cytoplasm of both nucleated and non-nucleated red cells after incubation with methyl violet. Their ultrastructural characteristics have been described in several studies (Rifkind, 1965; Nathan and Gunn, 1966; Polliack and Rachmilewitz, 1973; Zaino and Rossi, 1974). The absolute reticulocyte count is rarely high although it tends to increase after splenectomy. The total white cell count and differential is usually normal but may also increase after splenectomy. A reduction in white cell count, particularly if there is a shift to the right with hyperlobulation of the neutrophils, is indicative of folate deficiency. Severe neutropenia may occur occasionally as part of the picture of hypersplenism. The platelet count is usually normal or slightly elevated, particularly after splenectomy; thrombocytopenia usually reflects hypersplenism or folate deficiency.

The bone marrow shows marked erythroid hyperplasia with a reversal of the myeloid/erythroid ratio. Iron staining reveals an abundance in the reticuloendothelial elements and also in the red cell precursors. On incubation of the marrow with methyl violet it is always possible to demonstrate inclusion bodies in the erythroblasts (Fessas, 1963). Their identification as pre-

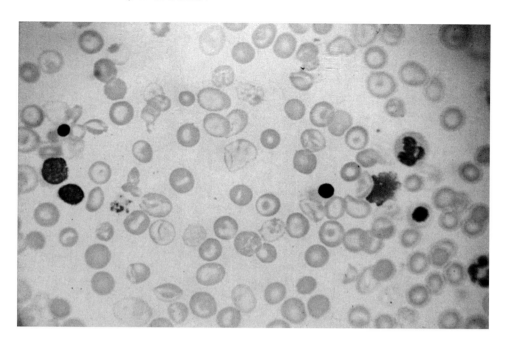

Figure 13.8. The blood smear of a patient with thalassemia major showing the typical morphologic changes. (Wright's stain, ×438) For full color reproduction, see color plate 13.8.

cipitated α chains, kinetics of precipitation, distribution in red cell precursors at different stages of maturation, and ultrastructure, together with the pathophysiologic consequences of α-chain precipitation, are reviewed in detail by Weatherall and Clegg (2000).

The cytoplasm of thalassemic erythroblasts contains an accumulation of glycogen, most marked in the G1 phase of early polychromatic erythroblasts (Yataganas et al., 1973). It has been suggested that this reflects the storage of unutilized energy in cells that are blocked in this phase of the cell cycle. The marrow also shows intense phagocytic activity, with the presence of large foamy cells resembling Gaucher cells (Zaino et al., 1971).

Red Cell Survival and Metabolism. Red cell survival is reduced, with published figures ranging from 7 to 22 days. Several studies have shown that there are two populations of red cells, one that is rapidly destroyed and another with a longer survival (Kaplan and Zuelzer, 1950; Bailey and Prankerd, 1958; Hillcoat and Waters, 1962). The short-lived population appears to be low in HbF and to contain predominantly small amounts of HbA or α-chain precipitates (Gabuzda et al., 1963). Although external scanning suggests that some red cell destruction occurs in the spleen, the main effect of increasing splenomegaly is to trap a large number of red cells with consequent hypervolemia and hemodilution (Prankerd, 1963; Blendis et al., 1974).

There are several distinctive metabolic abnormalities of the red cells; the mechanisms and relationship to red cell membrane damage by excess α chains are discussed elsewhere in this book. The red cell osmotic fragility is markedly decreased. The metabolic changes reflect the marked heterogeneity of the different red cell populations in the peripheral blood. After centrifugation, cells from the "younger," upper layers contain more inclusion bodies, have a lower hemoglobin content, and show a remarkable increase in the rate of flux of potassium, with higher rates of glycolysis and lactate formation and low and unstable levels of ATP (Loukopoulos and Fessas, 1965; Nathan and Gunn, 1966; Nathan et al., 1969). These changes are less marked in the "older," HbF-rich population, underlining the protective effect of increased γ-chain synthesis on both red cell metabolism and survival. Changes in other red cell enzymes and porphyrins are reviewed by Weatherall and Clegg (2000).

Iron Metabolism. As discussed earlier, iron loading is a constant feature of transfusion-dependent β thalassemia. Although the majority of the iron load is derived from blood transfusion, there may, in certain circumstances, be increased gastrointestinal absorption. As will be described later in this chapter, this is certainly the case in the intermediate forms of β thalassemia.

Iron Absorption. The inconsistent results of some iron absorption studies almost certainly relate to the transfusional status of the patients at the time of study. Heinrich et al. (1973) found that inorganic-iron absorption was markedly increased 64 to 300 days after transfusion, whereas it fell into the normal range if carried out 3 to

17 days after transfusion. Presumably, therefore, the level of iron absorption is related to the degree of ineffective erythropoiesis and erythroid hyperplasia; if this is reduced by transfusion iron absorption is also reduced.

Serum Iron. Serum iron is elevated in children with severe β thalassemia, and in older patients the iron-binding capacity is fully saturated. The serum of such patients contains 2 to 7 µmol/L of nonspecifically bound iron that is dializable and can be bound by transferrin from normal sera (Hershko et al., 1978).

Serum Ferritin. The measurement of plasma or serum ferritin is the most commonly used estimate of body iron stores in thalassemia. However, as discussed earlier, it has serious limitations, particularly in severely iron-loaded patients. The wide fluctuations that may occur at high ferritin levels may reflect a variety of mechanisms that alter the concentration independently of body iron load. These include ascorbate deficiency, acute and chronic infection, liver damage, hemolysis, and ineffective erythropoiesis. The 95 prediction intervals for hepatic iron concentration, related to the serum ferritin, are so broad that it is not possible to use the serum ferritin levels as a reliable predicter of body stores (Olivieri and Brittenham, 1997).

Hepatic Iron Concentrations. As discussed earlier, the hepatic iron concentration remains the most effective guide to assessing body iron stores, and the likelihood of tissue damage.

Other Approaches. Although a variety of imaging and related technologies have been applied to the assessment of the degree of iron loading (reviewed by Olivieri and Brittenham, 1997) with the exception of magnetic susceptometry using a superconducting quantum interference device (SQUID), none of them provide measurements of tissue iron that are quantitatively equivalent to those determined directly by hepatic biopsy.

Ferrokinetics and Erythrokinetics. Ferrokinetic and erythrokinetic studies in severe β thalassemia show a marked degree of ineffective erythropoiesis (Malamos et al., 1961; Finch et al., 1970). On the one hand there is evidence of increased red cell production as judged by bone marrow hyperplasia, plasma iron turnover, and fecal urobilinogen production, while effective red cell production as assessed by the hemoglobin level, absolute reticulocyte count, and iron incorporation is not increased, indicating an extreme degree of intramedullary destruction of red cells.

Hemoglobin Constitution. The red cells in all the severe forms of β thalassemia contain increased amounts of HbF. Homozygous $β^0$ thalassemics have only Hbs F and A_2; HbA is absent. The level of HbF in $β^+$ thalassemia homozygotes or compound heterozygotes is variable but is always elevated above normal after the first few months of life. Hemoglobin-A_2 levels are variable and of no diagnostic value. The only other abnormal finding is the presence of free α chains, which can sometimes be demonstrated using appropriate electrophoretic techniques.

Hemoglobin F. The complex and still ill-understood mechanisms for the production of HbF in β thalassemia are reviewed in detail by Weatherall and Clegg (2000). In short, it seems to reflect marked erythroid expansion, which may favor γ-chain synthesis in the postnatal period, together with selective survival of red cell precursors and mature red cells that have relatively higher levels of γ-chain production. This latter mechanism reflects the extreme heterogeneity of the level of γ-chain synthesis between different red cell precursors after birth; those that produce relatively more γ chains, and hence in which the degree of globin-chain balance is less, come under intensive selection in the marrow and blood. By these routes alone, together with the major expansion of the total red cell precursor mass, it is possible to account for between 2 and 2 g/dL HbF without the necessity of invoking other mechanisms. However, as described later in this chapter, there are several genetic factors that undoubtedly modify the HbF response in β thalassemia.

Given the many variables that set the final level of HbF in the peripheral blood it is difficult to make any generalizations about the amount of HbF that is produced in different forms of β thalassemia. This is particularly difficult once patients have started on regular transfusion; in fact recent studies suggest that, in patients with HbE-β thalassemia with HbF levels of over 50 percent, at a posttransfusion hemoglobin level of 9 to 10 g/dL there is very little endogenous production of HbF (Rees et al., 1999). Children homozygous for $β^0$ thalassemia, examined before the first transfusion, have hemoglobin levels of 5 to 8 g/dL, all of which is HbF (Cao, 1988). Similarly, in infants with $β^+$ thalassemia seen before transfusion the HbF levels are almost always in excess of 50 percent of the total hemoglobin (Kattamis et al., 1975). These few observations indicate that some of the very low levels of HbF described in severe forms of β thalassemia must be viewed with extreme caution. In short, through increased production, erythroid expansion, and cell selection it is clear that all forms of severe β thalassemia are associated with high levels of HbF production, probably in most cases well in excess of 50 percent of the total hemoglobin output.

The $^{G}\gamma/^{A}\gamma$ ratios of HbF in severe thalassemia has been reported by Schroeder and Huisman (1970) and Huisman et al. (1974). There was a broad scatter with a mean of about 32, regardless of the findings in the parents.

Hemoglobin A₂. The difficulties in interpreting HbA_2 levels in severe forms of β thalassemia are similar in many ways to those in interpreting the level of HbF. In a series of pretransfusion patients described by Kattamis et al. (1975), the HbA_2 level in 54 homozygotes, of whom 11 were of the β⁺ variety, was 3.0 with a range from 0.8 to 5.5 percent. However, several differential centrifugation studies have shown that the absolute level of HbA_2 in the HbF-rich population is much lower than that in cells that contain predominantly HbA (reviewed by Weatherall and Clegg, 2000). Thus, it is clear that the distribution of HbA_2 is uneven and that the level that is measured in the peripheral blood is an average of cells with widely differing amounts; it is of no diagnostic value.

In Vitro Hemoglobin Synthesis. In vitro globin-chain synthesis studies have provided a clear picture of hemoglobin production in the severe forms of β thalassemia (Weatherall et al., 1965; Bank and Marks, 1966; Bargellesi et al., 1967; Modell et al., 1969; Weatherall et al., 1969). In nonthalassemic reticulocytes α- and β-chain synthesis is almost synchronous and there is only a small pool of free α chains. In reticulocytes or marrow cells from patients with severe β thalassemia there is always marked globin-chain imbalance, with published α/β+γ production ratio ranging from 1.5 to 30. Imbalanced globin-chain synthesis leads to substantial number of free α chains in the cells, which can be demonstrated by both gel filtration and DEAE cellulose chromatography (Modell et al., 1969; Weatherall et al., 1969). The α chains in this pool exist both as monomers and dimers, and either combine with newly made β and γ chains to produce Hbs A and F, respectively, are destroyed by proteolysis, or form hemichromes and become associated with the red cell membrane.

The problems and pitfalls with this approach to measuring globin-chain production in β thalassemia have recently been reviewed in detail (Weatherall and Clegg, 2000). It should be remembered that the excess of α chains that are produced in β thalassemia are unstable and hence in order to obtain an estimate of the absolute amount of globin chain produced in radioactive labeling experiments it is necessary to carry out a time course experiment and extrapolate to zero time. Furthermore, many of the early discrepancies that were reported in α/β+γ-chain production ratios between the peripheral blood and bone marrow were the result of artifacts caused by the contamination of globin chains with nonglobin radioactive proteins produced in the bone marrow.

In short, because of the rapid destruction and turnover of excess α chains, particularly in the bone marrow, and the heterogeneity of cell populations with respect to γ-chain synthesis, the measurement of globin-chain synthesis in the marrow and blood at a single time point does not give information about the *absolute* rates of synthesis of individual chains. Nevertheless, it provides a reasonable indication of the overall severity of the defect in β-globin production. Provided that the various pitfalls associated with the measurements of total counts or specific activities, as outlined in detail by Weatherall and Clegg (2000), are taken into consideration, this approach can be used for diagnostic purposes, or to monitor the effects of different forms of therapy designed to augment γ-chain synthesis, or other modalities, to a reasonable degree of accuracy.

β THALASSEMIA INTERMEDIA

It has been apparent since the earliest descriptions of thalassemia that there are forms characterized by moderate anemia, jaundice, and splenomegaly that, although not as severe as the transfusion-dependent varieties, are clearly worse than the carrier states. In the extensive Italian literature on this subject these conditions have been variously described as La Malattia-di-Rietti-Greppi-Micheli (reviewed by Bannerman, 1961 and Weatherall, 1980), the anemic form of the Mediterranean hematologic disorder (Chini and Valeri, 1949), microcitica costituzionale (Bianco et al., 1952), and thalassemia intermedia (Sturgeon et al., 1955). Over recent years it has been apparent that this clinical picture can result from the interaction of many different thalassemia alleles, either one with another or with those for structural hemoglobin variants. Hence, the term is simply a descriptive title for a particular clinical disorder and has no clear-cut genetic meaning. However, because we are still not at a stage at which we can always describe precisely the genetic interactions that can produce this clinical picture, it seems useful to retain it.

Thalassemia intermedia has been the subject of a number of articles and reviews that focus either on the molecular pathology and pathophysiology in general (Wainscoat et al., 1987; Cao et al., 1990; Weatherall and Clegg, 2000), the molecular basis in certain populations (Antonarakis et al., 1988; Thein et al., 1988; Galanello et al., 1989; Camaschella et al., 1995; Kanavakis et al., 1995; Rund et al., 1997; Ho et al.,

1998), or the clinical features (Pippard et al., 1982; Fiorelli et al., 1988; Camaschella and Cappellini, 1995; Weatherall and Clegg, 2000).

How is β Thalassemia Intermedia Defined?

There is no adequate definition of β thalassemia intermedia. As discussed later in this chapter, the hematologic findings in heterozygous β thalassemia are remarkably uniform, and are characterized by a mild degree of anemia; splenomegaly is extremely unusual. Hence, any thalassemic patient with a hemoglobin level persistently below 9 to 10 g/dL, particularly if there is associated splenomegaly, falls into the intermediate class of β thalassemias. However, it is at the more severe end of the spectrum that the difficulty in definition arises. Some children survive early life with hemoglobin levels in the 5 to 6 g/dL range. Although they are often classified as having thalassemia intermedia, particularly if they present relatively late, many do not thrive or develop normally, and may grow up with gross skeletal deformities. It is now believed that these children should be transfused to avoid these distressing complications. Whether they should be classified as having severe thalassemia intermedia or thalassemia major is, therefore, a question of semantics that is of little importance.

However, some children with β thalassemia have hemoglobin values between 6 and 9 g/dL, grow and develop reasonably well, and reach adult life, and it is also useful to retain the term thalassemia intermedia for this type of patient. However, it should be remembered that they may become transfusion dependent if complications such as hypersplenism develop, or if the disorder is complicated by other factors such as folate deficiency or intercurrent infection. Clearly, the term thalassemia intermedia can cover a broad and shifting clinical spectrum, from almost complete health to a condition characterized by severe growth retardation and skeletal deformity that requires transfusion therapy; it is a diagnosis that can be made only after a considerable period of observation and that often requires revision.

Genetic Interactions That Result in the Phenotype of β Thalassemia Intermedia

The main interactions that are known to modify the phenotype of β thalassemia are summarized in Table 13.6 and Figure 13.9. Other conditions that produce the clinical picture of thalassemia intermedia, the interactions of the β thalassemias with structural hemoglobin variants, the δβ thalassemias and their interactions, and so on, are considered elsewhere in this book. It is still difficult to predict phenotypes from

---

Table 13.6. Thalassemia Intermedia

1. Mild deficit in β globin chain production
   Homozygous mild β^+ thalassemia
   Compound heterozygosity for severe β^0 or β^+ and mild β^+ thalassemia
   Interactions of β^0 with 'silent' β thalassemia
   Homozygosity for 'silent' β thalassemia
2. Reduced globin chain imbalance due to co-inheritance of α and β thalassemia
   Homozygous or compound heterozygous β^0 or β^+ thalassemia with 2 or 3 α gene deletions
   Homozygous or compound heterozygous severe β^0 or β^+ thalassemia with non-deletion α2 gene mutation
   Homozygous or compound heterozygous severe β^+ thalassemia with 1 or 2 α gene deletions
3. Severe β thalassemia with increased capacity for γ chain synthesis
   Homozygous or compound heterozygous β^0 or β^+ thalassemia with heterocellular HPFH
   Homozygous or compound heterozygous β^0 or β^+ thalassemia with particular β globin RFLP haplotype
   Mechanism unknown
4. Deletion forms of δβ thalassemia and HPFH
   Homozygous $(\delta\beta)^0$ or $(^A\gamma\delta\beta)^0$ thalassemia
   Compound heterozygosity for β^0 or β^+ and $(\delta\beta)^0$ or $(^A\gamma\delta\beta)^0$ thalassemia
   Homozygosity for Hb Lepore (some cases)
   Compound heterozygosity for Hb Lepore and β^0 or β^+ thalassemia (some forms)
   Compound heterozygosity for $(\delta\beta)^0$, $^G\gamma^+$ or $^A\gamma\beta^+$ HPFH and β^0 or β^+ thalassemia
   Compound heterozygosity for $(\delta\beta)^0$ thalassemia and $(\delta\beta)^0$ HPFH
5. Compound heterozygosity for β or δβ thalassemia and β chain structural variants
   Hb S, C, E/β or δβ thalassemia
   Many other rare interactions
6. Other β thalassemia alleles or interactions
   Dominant β thalassemia
   β thalassemia trait associated with ααα or αααα globin gene duplications
   Highly unstable β globin chain variants

---

genotypes with certainty; some guidelines are summarized in the following sections.

Interactions of "Silent" or "Mild" β-Thalassemia Alleles.

It is customary to divide the mild β-thalassemia alleles, which can interact with one another or with more severe alleles to produce thalassemia intermedia, into the "silent" and "mild" β^+ thalassemias. Although useful in practice, this is a somewhat artificial classification. Although many of

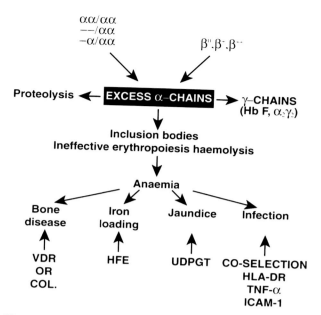

Figure 13.9. Some of the factors that modify the phenotype of β thalassemia. They include variable output from the β-globin genes, different forms of α thalassemia, variation in the level of fetal hemoglobin production, and a variety of secondary genetic modifiers. VDR, vitamin D receptor; OR, estrogen receptor; COL, collagen genes; HFE, primary hemochromatosis gene; UDPGT, UDP-glucuronosyl transferase. Coselection indicates a number of genetic polymorphisms that are, like the thalassemias, modified by malaria resistance. (From Weatherall and Clegg, 2000, with permission.)

the so-called silent alleles show no hematologic changes in individual cases, if large numbers are studied it is apparent that some of them have slightly reduced MCV or MCH values, and slightly elevated HbA$_2$ or α/β globin-chain synthesis ratios. However, there is so much overlap with normal values that, for practical purposes, it is reasonable to classify these extremely mild alleles as "silent," not in the least because they would not be identified by standard screening techniques to detect β-thalassemia carriers. We shall return to this question later in this chapter. It is now apparent that interactions of both silent and mild β-thalassemia alleles may be responsible for some forms of β thalassemia intermedia.

"Silent" β-Thalassemia Interactions. Several of the "silent" β-thalassemia alleles, when co-inherited with more severe β-thalassemia alleles, have been shown to produce the picture of β thalassemia intermedia. For example, the β-101 C→T allele has been observed in the compound heterozygous state with a variety of different β-thalassemia alleles, including codon 39 (C→T), IVS-1-110 (G→A), IVS-1-1 (G→A), IVS-2-745 (C→G), codon 44 (−C−C), and others (Ristaldi et al., 1990; Bianco et al., 1997a,b; Rund et al., 1997).

All these interactions result in mild forms of β thalassemia with steady-state hemoglobin values in the 9 to 12 g/dL range, a marked reduction in the MCV and MCH, elevated HbA$_2$ levels of 4.5 to 6.0, and HbF values ranging from 10 percent to 45 percent. They are a very common cause of β thalassemia intermedia in Mediterranean populations.

Other silent β-thalassemia alleles that interact with more severe alleles to produce β thalassemia intermedia include β CAP+1 (A→C) (Wong et al., 1987), β 5′ UTR+10 (−T) (Athanassiadou et al., 1994), β CAP+33 (C→G) (Ho et al. 1996), and IVS-2-844 (C→G) (Murru et al., 1991).

These silent mutations produce the clinical picture of β-thalassemia trait in their homozygous state. In families in which they interact with severe alleles to produce β thalassemia intermedia it is usual to find one parent with typical β-thalassemia trait, while the other shows no hematologic abnormality.

Interactions of Mild β-Thalassemia Alleles. There are many mild β-thalassemia alleles. However, for most of them there are very few published data about their hematologic characteristics or about the results of their interactions with more severe β-thalassemia alleles (Fig. 13.10).

The β-88 (C→T) allele is relatively common among Africans and African-Americans (Orkin et al., 1984; Gonzalez-Redondo et al., 1988). Its heterozygous phenotype is typical of β-thalassemia trait. The homozygous condition is characterized by a relatively mild form of β thalassemia intermedia, with hemoglobin values in the 9 to 12 g/dL range, HbA$_2$ values in the 4 percent to 8 percent range, and surprisingly high levels of HbF, in the range 40 percent to 72 percent. In the compound heterozygous state with the other common promoter allele in this racial group, β-29 (A→G), the phenotype is also an extremely mild form of β thalassemia intermedia.

The β-87 (C→G) allele has been observed in Mediterranean populations, particularly in Italy and Turkey. The homozygous state is characterized by a mild form of β thalassemia intermedia (Diaz-Chico et al., 1988; Camaschella et al., 1990). This mutation has been observed in the compound heterozygous state with several β-thalassemia alleles including codon 39 (C→T) (Rosatelli et al., 1989), IVS-1-110 (G→A) (Ho et al., 1998). The best characterized of these interactions are with the codon 39 nonsense mutation; these patients have thalassemia intermedia with steady-state hemoglobin levels of about 10 g/dL and fetal hemoglobin values in the 30 percent to 80 percent range.

There have been a few reports of individuals homozygous for the β-31 (A→G) and β-30 (T→A) alleles (Takihara et al., 1986; Fattoum et al., 1991).

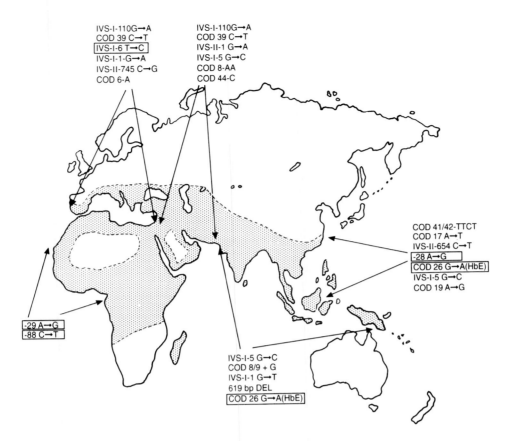

Figure 13.10. The world distribution of the thalassemia alleles. The common mild alleles are shown in boxes. In these populations, many of the intermediate forms of β thalassemia result from the different interactions of these milder alleles. (From Weatherall and Clegg, 2000, with permission.)

These conditions have not been observed in their compound heterozygous state with other β-thalassemia alleles; their homozygous states are characterized by extremely mild forms of β thalassemia intermedia.

The β-29 (A→G) mutation is probably the most common form of β thalassemia in African populations. The homozygous state is characterized by a mild form of β thalassemia intermedia and there have been no reported transfusion-dependent cases (Gonzalez-Redondo et al., 1988; Safaya et al., 1989). Steady-state hemoglobin values range between 10 and 12 g/dL and HbF values between 50 percent and 70 percent. In the compound heterozygous state with the β codon 24 (T→A) allele the clinical picture is, again, a mild form of β thalassemia intermedia, with hemoglobin values in the 9 to 13 g/dL range and HbF levels in the 25 percent to 70 percent range.

In view of the mildness of the promoter mutations it is surprising that the β-29 (A→G) allele, observed in a Chinese family, is described as having a severe, trans-

fusion-dependent phenotype (Huang et al., 1986). Although it has been suggested that the different phenotype to that observed in Black populations with the same mutation may reflect the fact that, in the latter, it is on a chromosome carrying the Xmn-1 $^{G}\gamma$ polymorphism, while this is not the case in the Chinese patient, it is not clear whether this difference alone is suffient to explain the wide difference between the phenotypes in different populations.

Mutations in β codons 19, 26, and 27, in addition to reducing β-globin output, are also associated with the production of the structural hemoglobin variants, Hbs Malay, E, and Knossos, respectively. The homozygous states for Hb Malay and Knossos are characterized by mild forms of thalassemia intermedia, with hemoglobin values in the 9 to 12 g/dL range and moderately elevated levels of HbF. Because of its common occurrence in the Mediterranean region, Hb Knossos has been found in the compound heterozygous state with several severe β thalassemia alleles (Olds et al., 1991; Galacteros et al., 1984; Ho et al., 1998). All these interactions are associated with the clinical picture of a mild to moderate form of β thalassemia intermedia. In the case of compound heterozygosity for Hb Knossos and the IVS-1-110 G→A allele, the disorder has been severe enough to require occasional blood transfusions, and splenectomy.

The β IVS-1-6 (T→C) splice mutation, sometimes called the Portuguese β thalassemia variant, is widespread among the Mediterranean population. Unlike the other mild forms of β thalassemia, the homozygous state for this condition is not always associated with a mild phenotype (Tamagnini et al., 1983; Öner et al., 1990; Scerri et al., 1993; Efremov et al., 1994; Rund et al., 1997; Ho et al., 1998). In the first descriptions of this condition, and in the extensive study of Efremov et al. (1994), it was found that homozygotes had a relatively mild form of thalassemia intermedia; none had required regular transfusion. On the other hand, in a later report from Israel, Rund and her colleagues describe a much more variable clinical phenotype. At one extreme nine patients had baseline hemoglobin levels of 10 to 11 g/dL, none had been splenectomized, and transfusions had either been rare or never required. At the other extreme, however, there were nine patients with baseline hemoglobin levels of 6 to 7 g/dL who were transfused either infrequently or regularly, even though they had undergone splenectomy. This latter group also had growth retardation, pronounced bone changes and thalassemic bone changes, absent puberty, and evidence of iron overload. The reasons for this remarkable clinical heterogeneity are not clear. Because this mutation is so common there have been numerous opportunities for studying its interaction with other β-thalassemia alleles, particularly the more severe forms that are common in the Mediterranean population. The most extensive data relate to interactions with the IVS-1-110 G→A and codon 39 C→T alleles. Overall, it appears that the interactions with β⁰-thalassemia alleles are more severe and result in a picture at the most severe end of the spectrum of β thalassemia intermedia. On the other hand, those with β⁺ mutations are more varied in their phenotype, some of them being described as moderately severe, others mild. Recent studies suggest that many of the latter cases may have, in addition, one or more α-thalassemia alleles (Ho et al., 1998).

Finally, there are several different mutations that involve the poly-A addition site of the β-globin gene. From the limited number of interactions that have been described it seems likely that these are fairly mild alleles. Recently, a homozygote for the AATAAA→AACAAA allele, first described by Orkin et al. (1985), has been encountered (Dr. J. Old, personal communication). This patient has never required transfusion and has a mild form of β thalassemia intermedia with moderate splenomegaly and no skeletal deformities. His steady-state hemoglobin level is approximately 7 to 8 g/dL, with HbF and HbA$_2$ values of 13.3 percent and 9.2 percent, respectively. Other interactions of this family of β-thalassemia alleles are summarized in Weatherall and Clegg (2000).

Interactions between α and β Thalassemia. The extensive literature on the ameliorating effect of the co-inheritance of α thalassemia on the different forms of β thalassemia has been reviewed recently (Weatherall and Clegg, 2000). The concept that defective α-chain synthesis might reduce the severity of β thalassemia by lessening the degree of globin-chain excess was suggested both by biosynthetic studies (Kan and Nathan, 1970), and by direct gene analysis (Weatherall et al., 1980). It was later confirmed by larger population studies (Furbetta et al., 1983; Wainscoat et al., 1983a, 1983b; Winichagoon et al., 1985; Thein et al., 1988; Galanello et al., 1989). From these investigations it was possible to determine, at least in outline, how different α- and β-thalassemia alleles can interact to produce forms of β thalassemia intermedia of varying severity. It appears that, overall, there is a reasonable correlation between the homozygous states for β⁰ or β⁺ thalassemia, together with the homozygous state for α⁺ thalassemia, and a mild phenotype. On the other hand, the loss of a single α-globin gene seems to have minimal phenotypic effect on homozygosity for β⁰ thalassemia, except for a slightly later presentation, and an unpredictable effect on compound heterozygosity for β⁺ or β⁰ thalassemia or homozygosity for β⁺ thalassemia. Reports of the occurrence of homozygous β thalassemia in association with a genotype of HbH disease in the same individual suggests that this rare interaction produces the clinical picture of a severe form of β thalassemia intermedia (Loukopoulos et al., 1978; Furbetta et al., 1979).

Unusual Efficiency of HbF Production in Generating β Thalassemia Intermedia. It has long been realized that variation in the ability to produce HbF in the postnatal period must be a major factor in the generation of the phenotype of β thalassemia intermedia. While many threads of evidence have pointed in this direction, some of the most convincing were early reports of individuals apparently homozygous for β⁰ thalassemia who ran relatively mild clinical courses (Knox-Macaulay et al., 1973; Godet et al., 1977; Bianco et al., 1977a; Cividalli et al., 1978; Weatherall et al., 1980). In the families of some of these patients a determinant for heterocellular hereditary persistence of fetal hemoglobin (HPFH) appeared to be segregating. However, detailed studies of the HbF of parents and relatives sometimes did not always show any evidence for a second determinant of this type (Weatherall et al., 1980). More recent studies, relating HbF production to particular restriction fragment length polymorphism (RFLP) haplotypes in the β-globin gene cluster, together with detailed family studies, suggest that some of the determinants that are associated with an unusually high level of HbF production in β thalassemia lie within the β-globin gene cluster, while others segregate quite independently. Although this work has gone some way to explaining the heterogeneity of HbF production in β thalassemia, in many cases the reasons for unusually high levels of HbF are not clear.

Determinants for Increased HbF Production within the β-Globin Gene Cluster.

A variety of studies have suggested that the β-globin gene RFLP haplotypes associated with the Xmn-1 $^G\gamma$ polymorphism associated with a C→T change at position-158 in the $^G\gamma$-globin gene are associated with an increased propensity for HbF production in β thalassemia (Labie et al., 1985; Thein et al., 1987; Galanello et al., 1989). In both African-Asian and Italian populations this has been the only change found in a number of patients homozygous for β^0 thalassemia whose clinical course has been that of a moderate to severe form of β thalassemia intermedia. This conclusion has been strengthened in more recent comparisons of the β-globin gene RFLP haplotypes of patients with thalassemia major and intermedia (Camaschella et al., 1995; Ho et al., 1998).

A word of caution is necessary, however. In all these studies there has been a wide spectrum of phenotypes associated with homozygosity for the $^G\gamma$ polymorphism. Overall, homozygotes for β^0 of β^+ thalassemia who are also homozygous for this polymorphism have a milder disease, manifested by a late presentation and the picture of a moderately severe form of β thalassemia intermedia. However, this is not always the case and some of them subsequently become transfusion dependent in later life, or even have severe disease from early in childhood. In the study of Ho et al. (1998) there was a wide variation in the phenotypic severity, even among those who fall into the β thalassemia intermedia category. It is also apparent that certain β-thalassemia mutations are, themselves, associated with an increased propensity for fetal hemoglobin production. While this relates particularly to promoter mutations it is also observed in the rare deletional forms of β thalassemia that remove the 5′ end of the β-globin gene (reviewed by Thein, 1993).

Determinants for Increased HbF Production Not Encoding in the β-Globin Gene Complex.

A number of families have been reported in which there is very good evidence that homozygotes or compound heterozygotes for β thalassemia produce unusually high levels of HbF and have the phenotype of β thalassemia intermedia, due to the co-inheritance of a gene for heterocellular HPFH (Cappellini et al., 1981; Thein and Weatherall, 1989). In both the families described in these reports subsequent studies showed that the genetic determinant for heterocellular HPFH did not segregate in the β-globin gene cluster (Gianni et al.,

1983; Thein and Weatherall, 1989). Later studies indicated that the determinant in the large family described by Thein and Weatherall showed strong linkage to chromosome 6, while that in the family originally described by Cappellini et al. does not. Further families have been reported by Ho et al. (1998); again it is clear that heterocellular HPFH is an important factor in the generation of β^0 thalassemia intermedia. It appears, therefore, that there are a number of determinants for a form of heterocellular HPFH that can modify the β-thalassemic phenotype; one is on chromosome 6, but this form of heterocellular HPFH is quite heterogeneous and other varieties exist that are encoded on other chromosomes. The role of the locus on the X chromosome, which seems to be involved in setting the level of F cells in adults (Dover et al., 1992), in determining the level of HbF in β thalassemia is not clear.

Heterozygous β Thalassemia with an Unusually Severe Phenotype.

There are two main mechanisms whereby heterozygous β thalassemia can be associated with the phenotype of β thalassemia intermedia. First, there are cases in which β thalassemia is complicated by the inheritance of chromosomes carying more than the usual number of α-globin genes, ααα or αααα. Second, there are particular β-globin gene mutations that, because of the unusual properties of their products, give rise to severe phenotypes in heterozygotes. The latter are usually referred to as the dominant β thalassemias.

The extensive literature on the ααα and αααα interactions is summarized in detail by Weatherall and Clegg (2000). It is clear that the inheritance of triplicated or quadruplicated α-globin gene arrangements, either in homozygous or heterozygous states, can, together with the heterozygosity for β^0 or β^+ thalassemia, produce a wide spectrum of phenotypes ranging from extremely mild to quite severe forms of β thalassemia intermedia (Galanello et al., 1983; Sampietro et al., 1983; Thein et al., 1984; Camaschella and Cappellini, 1995; Traeger-Synodinos et al., 1996; Bianco et al., 1997b; Ho et al., 1998).

Families with dominantly inherited forms of β thalassemia were first described by Weatherall et al. (1973) and Stamatoyannopoulos et al. (1974). Their relationship to exon 3 mutations are described elsewhere in this book.

Genotype/Phenotype for β Thalassemia Intermedia Relationships: Summary.

Considering the remarkable heterogeneity of the various interactions that can produce the clinical phenotype of β thalassemia intermedia, it is not surprising that this condition has a remarkably variable clinical phenotype. Unfortunately, there are no series of any one interaction of sufficient size to determine how much of the clinical heterogeneity is genetic in origin. Ho et al. (1998) described the findings in eight sibships. Obviously they all shared same β-globin genotypes and gene clusters and only in one case was there a deletion form of α⁺ thalassemia. Yet there were considerable differences among their clinical pictures. The major factor that seemed to account for this discrepancy was the steady-state level of HbF, which was in some, but not all, cases related to the coexistence of a gene for heterocellular HPFH. Clearly there are many factors, particularly those relating to the regulation of HbF production, that modify β thalassemia and that are still not understood. Hence it is extremely difficult to provide anything but an approximate prognostic picture of the likely clinical course for any particular β-thalassemia interaction.

Clinical Features

Presentation and Course During Early Life. One of the hallmarks of β thalassemia intermedia is its late presentation compared with transfusion-dependent forms of the disease (Kattamis et al., 1975; Modell and Berdoukas, 1984; Cao, 1988). Although there is considerable individual variation, overall it is usual for transfusion-dependent patients to come to medical attention in the first year of life, whereas those with thalassemia intermedia tend to present during the second year or later. There are few good published data on the hemoglobin levels over the first few years of life. Although some children maintain a steady-state hemoglobin value that seems to vary little, others do not. While it has been suggested that a fall in hemoglobin over the first few years may reflect increasing hypersplenism (Modell and Berdoukas, 1984) it is not clear whether this is always the case. From our own experience many children with intermediate forms of β thalassemia do not reach a steady-state hemoglobin level for several years and it is very important not to draw conclusions about their likely prognosis without a long period of observation.

The clinical manifestations are extremely variable. In some cases the disorder presents early in life with relatively severe anemia, while in others it may not appear until later due to a complication such as hypersplenism. Many patients have been found to have this condition on routine clinical examination. Growth and development may be normal or there may be a similar pattern of retardation as occurs in undertreated transfusion-dependent β thalassemia. The most common symptoms are those of anemia and mild jaundice. There is always some degree of splenomegaly. Bone changes are variable and range from none at all to the severe skeletal deformities characteristic of transfusion-dependent β thalassemia.

Some infants, who have presented relatively late with hemoglobin values in the 5 to 7 g/dL range, are clearly destined for transfusion from the beginning. When observed over a few months there is failure to thrive, listlessness, proneness to infection, and a poor appetite. Sequential studies over even a short period make it clear that these infants are not developing normally and that they should be considered to have thalassemia major, and treated accordingly. The course for infants who, despite their relatively low hemoglobin levels, are fully active and thriving, is usually one of chronic well-compensated anemia that may be exacerbated during periods of infection or folate deficiency, or with increasing hypersplenism.

Complications

Hypersplenism. Increasing splenomegaly leading to hypersplenism is a relatively common feature of β thalassemia intermedia. In most of the larger series cited earlier, a significant proportion of the patients had undergone splenectomy for worsening of their anemia, thrombocytopenia, or neutropenia.

Iron Loading. There is increasing evidence that although the rate of iron loading is much slower than in transfusion-dependent β thalassemia, patients with β thalassemia intermedia do iron load and this may become of clinical importance in adult life. Bannerman et al. (1967) described a 41-year-old Sicilian patient with β thalassemia intermedia who had gross iron loading with associated cardiac failure, diabetes mellitus, and hypopituitarism. On the other hand, Erlandson et al. (1964a) did not consider that iron loading was a major problem in this disorder. In a later study Pippard et al. (1982) examined the rate of iron loading in 15 patients with this condition. There was a highly significant increase in plasma ferritin levels with age and the majority of patients over 20 years had totally saturated iron-binding capacities. Liver biopsies of three of the older patients showed excessive iron deposition associated with portal cirrhosis in each case. Iron absorption studies, described in a later section, showed that the rate of iron loading from the gastrointestinal tract was approximately three to four times normal.

Later studies confirmed these observations. Cossu et al. (1981) reported an increasing serum ferritin level with age and increased urinary iron excretion in response to deferoxamine. Fiorelli et al. (1990), in attempting to explain some of the variability in the degree of iron loading among 38 adult patients with β thalassemia intermedia, described significant differences between patients who had undergone splenectomy compared with those with intact spleens; the iron burden was considerably greater in the former. This may simply reflect the greater severity and hence more marked marrow expansion and higher rate of iron absorption of these children. While these data are limited, there seems little doubt that iron loading is an important feature of β thalassemia intermedia. It can undoubtedly lead to liver damage and cirrhosis, and to other complications of iron excess. It is not clear how often it causes cardiac damage; as discussed later, there are very few data relating to the cardiac status of older adult patients with this condition.

Endocrine Function. The fact that in many of the larger series of patients with β thalassemia intermedia cited earlier there was a history of a normal puberty and menarche, even though the latter was sometimes delayed, suggests that, overall, endocrine function is often maintained up to and beyond puberty. However, from such limited data as there are it appears that by the time these patients reach the third or fourth decades there is a significant incidence of diabetes mellitus, and other endocrine deficiencies. Of the 15 patients reported by Pippard et al. (1982) 1 was frankly diabetic and 3 showed a reduced first-stage insulin response associated with a high-normal fasting plasma glucose concentration during standard glucose tolerance tests, findings that suggest impairment of pancreatic β-cell function. Similar results were obtained in 3 out of 11 patients studied by De Sanctis et al. (1986). In the series reported by Pippard et al. (1982) all had normal TSH reponses to TRH, and a normal fasting prolactin concentration, but two had a reduced LH response to LHRH. Plasma cortisol response to synacthen was normal in four of five patients tested. McIntosh (1976) described a woman with multiple endocrine deficiencies; replacement therapy was followed by a normal pregnancy.

Cardiac Function. Because of the slower rate of iron loading in β thalassemia intermedia than in transfusion-dependent forms of the disease it would be expected that, if cardiac complications occur at all, they would only be manifest in adult life. Although there have been single case reports of cardiac failure associated with iron loading in this disorder (Bannerman et al., 1967; Mancuso et al., 1985), there is very little information about the dangers of iron loading of the myocardium in this condition.

In the series of patients reported by Pippard et al. (1982), a high proportion complained of exertional dyspnea, palpitations, or both. The electrocardiogram showed only minor abnormalities in a few cases; there were inverted T waves over the right-ventricular leads in one, and evidence of left-ventricular hypertrophy in four of the older paitients. Holter monitoring over a 24-hour period revealed marked abnormalities in eight of the nine patients studied. These included periods of bradycardia and tachycardia, and supraventricular extrasystoles. This was in marked contrast to the absence of rhythm abnormalities in nine cases of well-transfused patients with β thalassemia major, including five over the age of 14 years. Echocardiography showed that four of the older patients with thalassemia intermedia had enlarged diastolic dimensions. However, both the ejection fractions and fractional shortening were normal in all eight cases studied. Fiorelli et al. (1988) described the cardiac status on 18 patients with thalassemia intermedia in Italy. All had cardiomegaly and systolic flow murmurs compatible with the degree of anemia. Their electrocardiograms showed some modifications of the QRS complexes compatible with ventricular hypertrophy. No consistent abnormalities of rhythm or conduction were observed. In five of the patients, echocardiography showed enlarged diastolic dimensions and some rather nonspecific functional alterations. Most of these changes could be ascribed to moderate to severe anemia and none were characteristic of iron loading of the myocardium.

Olivieri et al. (1992b) reported detailed studies on a 29-year-old Italian male who, although he had not received transfusions after the age of 5 years, nevertheless presented with hepatomegaly, abnormal liver function tests, an elevated serum ferritin level, and marked iron loading of the liver as judged by biopsy and quantitative MRI. Before treatment the left-ventricular ejection fraction was 60 percent at rest, with no increase at peak exercise, and there was mild right-ventricular dilatation and abnormalities in diastolic function. These changes did not alter after intensive chelation therapy, except that there was some improvement in the atrial contribution. Although these are relatively mild changes the fact that they altered after treatment suggests that there may have been some functional cardiac anomalies secondary to iron loading.

Clearly, it will be important to try to follow larger series of adult patients with β thalassemia intermedia with consecutive studies of cardiac function; currently there is no way of knowing what proportion of older patients with this condition are at risk from cardiac disease.

Over recent years there has been considerable interest in the syndrome of pulmonary hypertension and right heart failure in patients with HbE β thalassemia, particularly those who have undergone a splenectomy (see Chapter 43). This complication has also been reported in β thalassemia intermedia (Aessopos et al., 1995). In seven patients who presented with congestive cardiac failure and pulmonary hypertension after splenectomy, there was dilatation of the main pulmonary artery with cardiac enlargement, signs of right-ventricular hypertrophy, and a dilated right ventricle, but good left-ventricular function as judged by echocardiography. Right heart catheterization showed markedly raised pulmonary pressure with increased pulmonary vascular resistance. Whether this picture results from platelet aggregation in the pulmonary circulation, as suggested in the case of HbE-β thalassemia, remains to be determined.

Gallstones. Probably as a result of both ineffective erythropoiesis and hemolysis there is a high frequency of pigment stones (Erlandson et al., 1964a; Fiorelli et al., 1988; Goldfarb et al., 1990).

Folic Acid Deficiency. There are many well-documented cases of folate deficiency occurring in patients with β thalassemia intermedia (Erlandson et al., 1964a; Bannerman et al., 1967; Modell and Berdoukas, 1984). The degree of anemia may be profound and patients may present in cardiac failure.

Skeletal Deformities and Bone and Joint Disease. As mentioned earlier, some patients with β thalassemia intermedia develop severe skeletal deformities, similar in every way to those seen in the undertreated transfusion-dependent forms of the disease. Pathologic fractures are also a major feature, particularly in older patients. There is also a particularly distressing complication involving the bones and joints that has been called "thalassemic osteoarthropathy" (Gratwick et al., 1978). This takes the form of a curious periarticular disease characterized by dull aching pains in the ankles, exacerbated by weight-bearing and relieved by rest. Radiologic changes include widening of the medullary spaces, thin cortices with coarse trabeculation, and evidence of microfractures in the region of the joints. Histologic analysis confirmed the presence of the latter and, in addition, showed osteomalacia and increased osteoblastic surface areas with iron deposition in the calcification front and cement lines. We have observed this complication in a number of adult patients with β thalassemia intermedia, at least one of whom required an arthrodesis of the ankle joint for relief of intractable pain. Acetabular protrusion has also been reported in patients with severe bone involvement.

Extramedullary Erythropoiesis. The generation of tumor masses composed of extramedullary erythropoietic tissue is a frequent complication (Erlandson et al., 1964a; Ben-Bassat et al., 1977; Yu et al., 1991). The most common site is in the paraspinal region. Alam et al. (1997) give a valuable summary of the radiologic characteristics of these lesions. Although

they do not usually cause symptoms there have been well-documented case reports of spinal cord compression (David and Balusubramaniam, 1983; Cardia et al., 1994), cauda equina lesions (Mancuso et al., 1993), and hemorrhage causing a massive hemothorax (Smith et al., 1988).

Although these masses are usually identified by conventional radiography (Alam et al., 1997), the diagnosis can be confirmed, particularly if they are in an unusual site, by both computed tomography (CT) and MRI analysis (Papavasiliou et al., 1990). They produce a low-intensity signal similar to that of adjacent marrow of the thoracic spine and are surrounded by a characteristically high-intense rim attributed to a layer of fat surrounding the masses.

More recent CT analyses of adults with β thalassemia intermedia suggest that some degree of extramedullary erythropoiesis is probably quite common; it was detected in 65 percent of these patients. It seems likely that at least some of these lesions may undergo fatty transformation with time, particularly if the hemoglobin level is raised, by splenectomy, for example (Martin et al., 1990).

Infection. Although it is suspected that patients at the severe end of the spectrum of β thalassemia intermedia have increased susceptibility to infection, there are very few supporting data. Such that there are suggest that the pattern of infection is similar to that outlined for transfusion-dependent β thalassemia earlier in this chapter. As is the case in thalassemia major, severe *Yersinia* infection associated with iron chelation, and aplastic or hypoplastic episodes due to parvovirus infection have been recorded (Brownell et al., 1986). There is increasing evidence that those patients who require occasional transfusion are prone to contract hepatitis B and C (Mela et al., 1987). Although there have been attempts at defining specific abnormalities of neutrophil function or of the immune system, as in the case of the more severe forms of β thalassemia there have been no consistent findings. The problem of infection in thalassemia intermedia is discussed in more detail by Weatherall and Clegg (2000).

Hyperuricemia and Gout. Although in several reported series patients with β thalassemia had elevated uric acid levels, secondary gout seems to be uncommon (Gratwick et al., 1978).

Leg Ulcers. This is a relatively common complication of β thalassemia intermedia (Modell and Berdoukas, 1984; Fiorelli et al., 1988; Camaschella and Cappellini, 1995). The cause is unknown; the possible relationship to the rheological properties of the red cells is discussed by Gimmon et al. (1982).

Pregnancy. Because many patients with thalassemia intermedia pass through a normal puberty, pregnancy is not uncommon (Walker et al., 1969; Afifi, 1974). In most of these reports it is stressed that these patients may become quite profoundly anemic during pregnancy, but if they are maintained at a relatively normal hemoglobin level there seems to be no increased rate of fetal loss.

Thromboembolic Disease. The "hypercoagulable state" associated with platelet activation, which correlates with abnormal red cell phospholipid exposure, is reviewed by Ruf et al. (1997). In fact, much of the experimental work that underlies this concept was carried out on the blood of patients with β thalassemia intermedia. In the recent review of thromboembolic complications of β thalassemia from Italy (Pignatti et al., 1998), discussed earlier in this chapter, 5 of the 32 affected patients had thalassemia intermedia. There have been occasional reports of severe thromboembolic disease following splenectomy, but in the series described by Skarsgard et al. (1993) several nonthalassemic patients presented with the same complication. From these limited data it is not possible to assess the overall risk of thrombotic disease, nor is it clear whether it is related to the occurrence of recurrent priapism following splenectomy in patients with this type of thalassemia (Dore et al., 1991).

Hematologic Findings

There is a variable degree of anemia, with hemoglobin values in the 5 to 10 g/dL range. The red cell indices are typically thalassemic and the peripheral blood find-

ings are indistinguishable from those of the more severe forms of β thalassemia. In some of the dominantly inherited forms of β thalassemia, hypochromia is less marked, and poikilocytosis is the main feature (Fig. 13.11). Except when there is hypersplenism the white cell and platelet counts are usually normal. The reticulocyte count is elevated and, following splenectomy, on staining with methyl violet nucleated red cells show ragged inclusions similar to those observed in thalassemia major. The bone marrow shows marked erythroid hyperplasia and, again, many of the red cell precursors contain inclusion bodies.

Red Cell Survival, Ferrokinetics, and Erythrokinetics

Red cell survival studies have shown a moderate reduction in survival times, with $^{51\text{Cr}}$ T1/2 values ranging from 10 to 16 days (Erlandson et al., 1964a; Gallo et al., 1979).

Iron-absorption studies have shown an increase in the rate of iron accumulation (Heinrich et al., 1973; De Alarcon et al., 1979; Pippard et al., 1979, 1982; Pippard and Weatherall, 1984). In the studies of Pippard et al. the patients were in positive balance of between 2.6 and 8.6 mg iron per day. Cavill et al. (1978) found that the marrow turnover was approximately six times normal but that most of this increase

Figure 13.11. A peripheral blood smear from the propositus from the first family to be reported with dominantly inherited β thalassemia (Weatherall et al., 1973). Hypochromia is not a major feature but there is a remarkable degree of poikilocytosis and heavy basophilic stippling. For full color reproduction, see color plate 13.11.

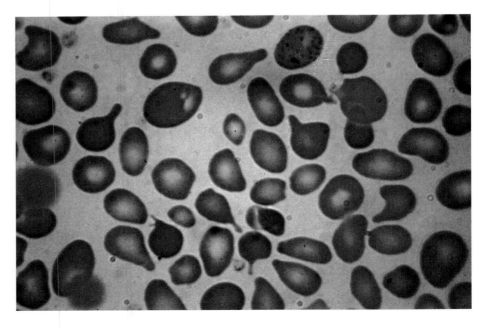

in activity was ineffective. Similar results were reported by Najean et al. (1985).

More recently an estimation of the serum-transferrin-receptor level has been used to assess the degree of erythroid expansion. In a study by Dore et al. (1996) of untransfused patients with a steady-state hemoglobin level of 9.6 g/dL the mean basal transferrin receptor level was 30.3 as compared with 12.8 in a series of age-matched healthy controls.

There have been several studies of serum-erythropoietin levels in β thalassemia intermedia (Dore et al., 1993; Camaschella et al., 1996). As is the case in the transfusion-dependent forms of β thalassemia there have been some inconsistencies. Although, overall, elevated levels have been found, and there was evidence of a reciprocal relationship with the hemoglobin level in one study, there were inappropriately low Epo levels for the degree of anemia. There is also some, although not entirely consistent, evidence of a relationship between the level of Epo and HbF. These results are similar to those described earlier for the more severe forms of β thalassemia. The reasons for the lack of a maximum Epo response in this disease remains to be determined.

Hemoglobin Constitution

Considering the extraordinarily diverse genotypes that underlie the phenotype of β thalassemia intermedia, it is not surprising that it is characterized by a wide range of different hemoglobin constitutions, particularly with respect to the levels of HbF. In the intermediate forms of the β^0 thalassemias the hemoglobin consists entirely of HbF, with HbA_2 values in the low-normal range. However, there is a wide range of HbF levels in the β^+ thalassemia intermedias and it is possible only to make some broad generalizations about how these relate to the underlying genotypes.

In the β^+ thalassemia intermedias that reflect the homozygous state for mild β^+-thalassemia mutations the level of HbF tends to be low compared with those that result from the interaction of two severe alleles. This is exemplified in the homozygous state for the common Mediterranean mutation, IVS-1-6 (T→C), in which the fetal hemoglobin level tends to be in the region of 20 percent of the total, although even here there is considerable scatter (Efremov et al., 1988). The exception to this rule is the homozygous or compound heterozygous states for promoter mutations of the β-globin gene. In this case there tends to be an unexpectedly high level of fetal hemoglobin, usually in excess of 50 percent of the total (Gonzalez-Redondo et al., 1988). In both these conditions homozygotes have, as a rule, increased levels of HbA_2.

In interactions between homozygous or compound heterozygous states for β^+ or β^0 thalassemia and the heterozygous states for α^+ or α^0 thalassemia, the hemoglobin pattern does not seem to alter from that found with the β-thalassemia mutations alone. However, in the interactions between these forms of β thalassemia and the genotype of HbH disease there is quite a different pattern. In this case, while the amounts of Hbs A and F do not differ significantly from those seen with β^+ or β^0 thalassemia alone, there is an unusually high level of HbA_2 and traces of Hb Bart can be demonstrated (Loukopoulos et al., 1978; Furbetta et al., 1979).

Hemoglobin Synthesis

Early studies that provided data on α/non-α globin-chain synthesis ratios in patients with β thalassemia intermedia showed that, overall, the degree of imbalance of globin-chain synthesis was less than that observed in the more severe forms of β thalassemia (Bianco et al., 1977; Gallo et al., 1979). Although there have been sporadic reports since, none has related the degree of globin-chain imbalance to the underlying molecular pathology in sufficient numbers to be able to offer any firm conclusions about the degree of globin-chain imbalance associated with the different combinations of mutations that underlie the intermediate forms of β thalassemia.

THE HETEROZYGOUS FORMS OF β THALASSEMIA

The heterozygous states for the different forms of β thalassemia are summarized in Table 13.1. The most common varieties are associated with an elevated level of HbA_2 and normal or slightly elevated levels of HbF. There is another group that is characterized by normal levels of HbA_2. This is subdivided into Type 1, in which there are no hematologic changes; this corresponds to the "silent" β thalassemias. In Type 2, the hematologic changes are indistinguishable from the β-thalassemia trait with elevated levels of HbA_2. There are other rare groups characterized by unusually high levels of Hbs A_2 or F, or by a much more severe course.

The Common Forms of Heterozygous β Thalassemia

The heterozygous states for most forms of β thalassemia are characterized by mild anemia, characteristic changes in the MCV and MCH, an elevated level of HbA_2, and normal or only slightly elevated levels of HbF.

Clinical Features

Patients heterozygous for β thalassemia are symptom-free; the condition is usually diagnosed as part of a family study, as an incidental finding during an intercurrent illness, or as part of a population survey. Occasionally, and particularly during pregnancy, the mild anemia may bring a carrier to the notice of the physician.

There are no characteristic clinical findings, and palpable splenomegaly is most unusual.

Hematologic Findings

The larger reported series, when adequately analyzed by sex and age, have shown that although there is a considerable scatter in hemoglobin levels, most heterozygous β thalassemics have a significant degree of anemia as compared with controls drawn from the same population (Knox-Macaulay et al., 1973; Castaldi et al., 1974; Mazza et al., 1976). The red cell indices are a valuable diagnostic feature. There is a relatively high red cell count but the cells are small and poorly hemoglobinized and the MCH and MCV are markedly reduced. On the other hand, the MCHC is usually in the normal range or only moderately reduced. There may be a slightly elevated reticulocyte count. The red cells show characteristic morphologic changes; there is microcytosis and hypochromia with variation in the size and shape. The presence of target cells, much stressed by early workers, is very variable and although some are usually found their absence is of little diagnostic value. Basophilic stippling is a frequent finding, particularly in patients with more severe β-thalassemia alleles.

Completely normal hematologic findings in heterozygous β thalassemia are very unusual. They are usually found in individuals with β-thalassemia trait who have co-inherited one or other forms of α thalassemia. These interactions, and their implications for screening programs, are discussed by Weatherall and Clegg (2000).

The bone marrow shows a variable degree of erythroid hyperplasia, in which polychromatic and pyknotic normoblasts predominate. The cytoplasm of the red cell precursors is often ragged and shows basophilic stippling. Iron is usually plentiful and is distributed normally between the reticuloendothelial elements and the red cell precursors. On incubation of the marrow with methyl violet, a few of the red cell precursors show small inclusions, similar to those seen in abundance in homozygous individuals (Yataganas and Fessas, 1969).

Red Cell Survival, Iron Metabolism, and Ferrokinetics

The ^{51}Cr T1/2 of the red cells have given mean values just below the normal range in several reported series (Pearson et al., 1960; Malamos et al., 1961; Gallo et al., 1975; Pippard and Wainscoat, 1987). Serum iron and ferritin estimations have shown that, although there is considerable variability, the mean values are little different from normal (Kattamis et al., 1972; Knox-Macaulay et al., 1973; Pootrakul et al., 1973; Hussain et al., 1976; Pippard and Wainscoat, 1987; Galanello et al., 1990). Iron loading, as evidenced by increased serum iron or ferritin levels, or iron deposition in the tissues, is unusual. In the series described by Knox-Macaulay et al. (1973) five females and four males had iron-binding saturations of 50 percent or more; one 68-year-old woman, who had received oral iron intermittently for 15 years due to a mistaken diagnosis of iron-deficiency anemia, had a totally saturated iron-binding capacity and clinical evidence of iron overload. There have been other reports of iron loading in heterozygous β thalassemics (Bowdler and Huehns, 1963; Tolot et al., 1970). In addition to these isolated case reports, Fargion et al. (1985) described a group of Italian males with very high serum ferritin levels. Whether some of these patients were also carrying the genes for hereditary hemochromatosis is not known.

The rate of iron absorption is either normal or slightly elevated (Crosby and Conrad, 1964; Bannerman et al., 1967). Iron is rapidly removed from the plasma, the rate of plasma iron turnover is increased, but it appears in red cells relatively slowly. In an extensive series of ferrokinetic studies, Pippard and Wainscoat (1987) found that the overall efficiency of erythropoiesis is significantly reduced, with a mean of 76 ± 17 standard deviations of normal. Serum erythropoietin levels are slightly elevated, more so in females than males, but there appears to be no correlation with the hemoglobin level (Vedovato et al., 1993).

These findings suggest that there is a mild degree of ineffective erythropoiesis in β-thalassemia carriers and that the anemia is predominantly due to intramedullary destruction of red cell precursors rather than hemolysis.

Complications

Most patients heterozygous for β thalassemia go through life without any manifestations that can be ascribed to the disease. The only complication of any importance is worsening of the anemia during pregnancy.

Pregnancy. Although it is clear that the hemoglobin level falls to a greater degree during pregnancy than in normal women, the resulting anemia is usually mild; most of the reports of more severe forms of anemia in pregnancy probably reflect the added complications of either iron or folic-acid deficiency (Knox-Macaulay et al., 1973; White et al., 1985; Landman, 1988).

In normal women there is an increase in both plasma volume and red cell mass that commences at the end of the first trimester. Schuman et al. (1973) found that pregnant thalassemic women are unable to increase their red cell mass to the same degree as normal women; there is no difference between them in the degree of expansion of the plasma volume. On average, the decrease in the hemoglobin level between the first and second trimester is comparable with that of normal women, in the range of 7 percent to 10 percent. In the large series of White et al. (1985) and Landman (1988) there were minimal changes in the red cell indices during pregnancy. From these studies it is clear that any pregnant β-thalassemia carrier with a hemoglobin value of less than 8 to 9 g/dL should be investigated for other causes for anemia. Because of the unreliability of serum iron and iron-binding capacity estimations in pregnancy, it is helpful to assess the patient's iron status by the serum ferritin level.

Folic Acid Deficiency. Folic acid deficiency has been reported in heterozygous β thalassemia in nonpregnant persons, but this must be extremely rare (Chanarin et al., 1959; Silva and Varella-Garcia, 1989).

Failure of Diagnosis. In populations in which β thalassemia is not common the trait may be misdiagnosed as iron-deficiency anemia or attract a number of other diagnostic labels. This can lead to a variety of unnecessary investigations, considerable anxiety, and inappropriate treatment with iron.

Life Expectancy

In one extensive study aimed at defining the life span of individuals heterozygous for β thalassemia, no significant differences were found between β-thalassemia heterozygotes and normals (Gallerani et al., 1990). Surprisingly, in a prospective study of 4,401 subjects in Ferrara over a 7-year period of observation by the same group, it was concluded that male β-thalassemia heterozygotes show a significant degree of protection against myocardial infarction (Gallerani et al., 1991). At first sight these observations seem contradictory although it is possible that the relatively small effect on cardiac disease was masked in the life expectancy survey; these observations require further investigation in other populations.

Hemoglobin Constitution

The cardinal finding in the common forms of heterozygous β thalassemia is an elevated level of HbA$_2$.

In most of the larger series the HbA$_2$ levels ranged from 3.5 percent to 7 percent with a mean of approximately 5 percent (reviewed by Weatherall and Clegg, 2000). By relating the percent HbA$_2$ to the MCH it is clear that this reflects an absolute increase in δ-chain production. Studies of patients with β-thalassemia trait who are also heterozygous for δ-chain variants have shown that the increased output is both *cis* and *trans* to the β-thalassemia gene (Ceppellini, 1959; Huisman et al., 1961; Weatherall, 1976; Codrington et al., 1990). The level of HbA$_2$ may be reduced in association with coexistent iron deficiency, but although it has been reported that it may fall into the normal range and is restored to its elevated level after iron therapy (Wasi et al., 1968; Kattamis et al., 1972), this must be unusual. What usually happens is that the level falls but it remains elevated in the β-thalassemia-trait range (Steinberg, 1993).

In most large series the HbF level is elevated in about 50 percent of cases, in the range 1 percent to 2 percent (Beaven et al., 1961). The distribution of HbF within the red cells, as judged either by acid elution or fluorescent antibody techniques, is heterogeneous.

In all the larger reported series of HbF levels a few individuals fall outside the distribution of normal to 2 percent to 3 percent, and have values ranging between 4 percent and 15 percent. Knox-Macaulay et al. (1973) showed that at least some of them have, in addition, determinants for heterocellular HPFH. In one family it was possible to demonstrate independent segregation of β-thalassemia and HPFH genes. Similar families have been reported by Mazza et al. (1976), Wood et al. (1976), and Thein and Weatherall (1989). It seems likely, therefore, that the majority of β-thalassemia heterozygotes with unusually high levels of HbF carry one or more genes for heterocellular HPFH.

There is no evidence that acquired factors alter the level of HbF to any significant degree; the only one that has been adequately documented is pregnancy, during which the normal rise in HbF that occurs at midterm is mirrored in heterozygous β thalassemias by an increase at about the same time. It returns to its basal level some time toward the end of pregnancy (Popat et al., 1977). The level of HbF is not modified by coexistent iron deficiency (Kattamis et al., 1972).

Red Cell Metabolism

One of the characteristic changes of the red cells in β-thalassemia heterozygotes is their decreased osmotic fragility, which in contrast to normal red cells, becomes even more marked after sterile incubation for 24 hours (Selwyn and Dacie, 1954). These altered osmotic properties have formed the basis for several population screening tests.

There have been a variety of studies of membrane function (Gunn et al., 1972; Chapman et al., 1973; Knox-Macaulay and Weatherall, 1974; Vettore et al., 1974). Using radioactive tracers it has been shown that there is an increased flux of K^+, an effect that is accentuated when the cells are incubated for 24 hours at $37°$. This increased permeability to K^+ appears to occur in cells of all ages, although it may be slightly more marked in younger cells. Adenosine triphosphate (ATP) levels are normal or slightly reduced, but on sterile incubation the red cells lose ATP more rapidly than normal; this can be reversed by glucose. It appears that heterozygous β-thalassemic red cells can compensate for their increased cation loss by upregulating the transport-regulated component of glycolysis, and hence can maintain normal ATP levels, but when they are stressed by in vitro incubation this mechanism breaks down.

In some of the studies cited above similar membrane function abnormalities were found in other hypochromic anemias such as iron deficiency. It is likely, therefore, that these abnormalities reflect an under-hemoglobinized red cell as well as globin-chain imbalance. In favor of this concept is the observation that similar changes have been described in cells of α/β thalassemics in which there is minimal globin-chain imbalance (Knox-Macaulay et al., 1972).

These observations suggest a possible mechanism for the further increase in osmotic resistance on sterile incubation of β-thalassemic red cells. With successive loss of K^+ and water, and cellular dehydration, there must be a decrease in red cell volume and hence in osmotic activity. If glucose is added to the incubation this probably provides adequate energy for ATP regeneration and hence for maintaining the Na^+-K^+ pump to counteract excessive loss of K^+ and water from the cells. Further evidence that this is the case is derived from the observation that the increased osmotic resistance can be demonstrated, even in the presence of glucose, by inhibition of the Na^+-K^+ pumps by ouabain or ethacrynic acid (Knox-Macaulay and Weatherall, 1974).

Globin-Chain Synthesis

In vitro hemoglobin synthesis studies indicate that α/β globin-chain production ratios range from about 1.5 to 2.5, both in the bone marrow and in peripheral blood. Reports of more balanced globin-chain synthesis in the bone marrow (Schwartz, 1970; Kan et al., 1972; Gallo et al., 1975) were later found to be based on artifacts produced by the presence of radioactively labeled nonglobin proteins that co-chromatograph with β-globin chains (Chalevelakis et al., 1975, 1976). Hence the measurement of globin-chain synthesis, particularly if peripheral blood reticulocytes are used, provides a valu-

able confirmatory test for heterozygosity for β thalassemia in cases in which the diagnosis is uncertain.

Developmental Changes in Hematologic Findings and Hemoglobin Constitution

The changes in the red cells of infants heterozygous for β thalassemia over the first few months of life are of considerable importance with respect to the diagnosis of the condition over this period. Because of the alterations that occur both in the red cell indices and in the hemoglobin pattern of normal infants over the first year, studies that set out to describe these changes in β-thalassemia heterozygotes must be carefully controlled with a population of normal infants at exactly the same stage of development. Data of this kind have been reported by Galanello et al. (1981) and Wood et al. (1982). Galanello et al. (1991) have produced useful percentile curves for the red cell indices in β-thalassemia heterozygotes in infancy and childhood. Further information on these changes is reported by Metaxatou-Mavromati et al. (1982).

From these studies it is apparent that the hemoglobin values and red cell indices of heterozygous β-thalassemic newborns do not differ significantly from normal. However, by the age of 3 months clear differences emerge, which become highly significant by 6 months and remain so during the rest of development. It appears, therefore, that carrier screening by MCV or MCH determination is feasible from about 3 months onward. Similarly, there is clear distinction in HbA_2 values by 3 months. In all these studies it was observed that the rate of decline of HbF is retarded in β-thalassemia heterozygotes and does not reach its adult level until well into childhood.

Phenotypic Characteristics in Relationship to Different Molecular Forms of β Thalassemia

Limited data have been published that relate the hematologic findings and HbA_2 and F levels to particular mutations in β-thalassemia heterozygotes (Gonzalez-Redondo et al., 1988; Rund et al., 1990; Rosatelli et al., 1992; Stefanis et al., 1994). Although there is some overlap, it is evident that the common, mild β-thalassemia mutations, IVS-1-6 T→C, β-29 A→G, β-87 C→G, and β-88 T→G, for example, have slightly higher hemoglobin levels and, more important, higher MCH and MCV values than the more severe $β^0$- or $β^+$-thalassemia alleles. Other mild alleles for which sufficient data are available, including the forms of β thalassemia associated with Hbs E, Malay, and Knossos, are also associated with MCH and MCV values that are either normal or only slightly reduced. Indeed, the pattern that is emerging is of a continuous spectrum of hematologic findings, ranging from the typical characteristics of β-thalassemia trait associated with severe β^0- or β^+-thalassemia alleles, through milder changes associated with less severe alleles, to complete normality in the "silent" alleles. However, there are insufficient data to make it possible to be dogmatic about what is a "typical" set of red cell indices for a particular allele.

The HbA_2 levels in relationship to underlying mutations have been reviewed by Huisman (1997). Overall, and although there is considerable overlap, several groups can be defined. Carriers of β^0- or severe β^+-thalassemia alleles have HbA_2 levels between 4.5 percent and 5.5 percent, whereas those with mild β^+ alleles have values between 3.6 percent and 4.2 percent. There are exceptions, however. Carriers of β-globin-gene promoter mutations tend to have relatively high levels of HbA_2, even though these are mild β-thalassemia alleles. The highest HbA_2 values in heterozygotes appear to be associated with deletional forms of β thalassemia (see later section and Chapter 12).

The relationship between the underlying mutation and HbF levels in β-thalassemia heterozygotes has been reviewed by Kutlar et al. (1990). These analyses are complicated by the presence or absence of the C→T polymorphism at $-158^{G\gamma}$, which is known to modify both the $^{G\gamma}/^{A\gamma}$ ratio of the HbF and, probably, its level under conditions of erythropoietic stress. However, it appears that β-thalassemia heterozygotes with certain mutations, notably −88 (C→T), −29 (A→G), and IVS-1-1 (C→A), appear to have relatively higher levels of HbF that are independent of the C→T polymorphism at $-158^{G\gamma}$. Carriers of mutations such as IVS-1-6 (T→C), IVS-1-110 (G→A), codon 24 (T→A), codon 39 (C→T), and codons 41–42 (-TCTT) tend to fall into two groups, that is, with high $^{G\gamma}$ and low $^{G\gamma}$ varieties of HbF; neither are associated with high HbF values.

Association with Other Genetic Disorders

Because the heterozygous state for β thalassemia is so common, it is not surprising that it has been found in association with a variety of other genetic disorders.

In many populations glucose-6-phosphate dehydrogenase (G6PD) deficiency and β thalassemia are found at high frequencies and hence they are not infrequently encountered together in the same individual. This interaction was analyzed in Sardinia by Piomelli and Siniscalco (1969). The mean hemoglobin levels in hemizygous G6PD deficient males was 14.1 g/dL, thalassemic males 13.6 g/dL, and males with both conditions 12.5 g/dL. The red cell indices in the thalassemic males were not altered by coexistent G6PD deficiency. In a later study Sanna et al. (1980) found no interaction between the two traits.

Another common occurrence is the co-inheritance of the genetic determinant for Gilbert's syndrome (Galanello et al., 1997; Sampietro et al., 1997). There is a polymorphic variation in the promoter of the bilirubin UDP-glucuronosyl transferase gene (UGT-1); the particular motif is a A(TA)n TAA. Some individuals with Gilbert's syndrome have an additional TA, that is, the arrangement A(TA)7TAA rather than the more usual A(TA)6TAA. It has been found that the expanded variety of promoter polymorphism is found commonly in heterozygous β thalassemics with unusually high bilirubin levels. Interestingly, homozygosity for the (TA)7 motif is not always associated with an elevated bilirubin in otherwise normal persons and hence it is likely that the increased production of bilirubin as a result of the ineffective erythropoiesis in β-thalassemia heterozygotes is sufficient to cause unusually high blood levels.

Several families have been reported in which the genes for hereditary elliptocytosis (HE) and β thalassemia were segregating (Frick, 1970; Ros et al., 1976; Pavri et al., 1977). In these cases there did not seem to be any summation of the effects of the two disorders, although in the family reported by Perillie and Chernoff (1965) there may have been some interaction. Similarly, there have been reports of the interaction of β-thalassemia trait and hereditary spherocytosis (HS) (Cohen et al., 1959; Cunningham and Vella, 1967; Aksoy and Eredem, 1968; Swarup-Mitra et al., 1969). Although it has been reported to cause relatively severe hemolysis it is difficult to determine whether this is a true summation effect; HS is very variable in its expression even within members of the same family. Similarly, in the few reported instances of the co-inheritance of β thalassemia and pyruvate kinase deficiency, the red cell enzyme deficiency has not had any deleterious effect on the phenotype of β-thalassemia trait (Baughan et al., 1968; Zoratto et al., 1969).

Variant Forms of Heterozygous β Thalassemia

The more unusual forms of heterozygous β thalassemia are summarized in Table 13.1. The most common and most important are the normal HbA_2-β thalassemias.

Normal HbA_2-β Thalassemia. Based on the hematologic findings it has been useful to divide the normal HbA_2-β thalassemias into Type 1, in which there are minimal red cell abnormalities and in which the thalassemia allele is clinicaly "silent," and Type 2, in which the hematologic changes are indistinguishable from those of heterozygous β thalassemia with an elevated level of HbA_2 (Kattamis et al., 1979).

"Silent" β Thalassemia. As described by Schwartz (1969), and discussed earlier in this chapter, the importance of the "silent" β thalassemias is that they can interact with more severe β-thalassemia alleles to produce β thalassemia intermedia. Their molecular basis is described in Chapter 12 and the clinical consequences of their interaction with different β-thalassemia alleles are summarized earlier in this chapter. There are no significant hematologic abnormalities but on globin-chain synthesis analysis there is mild imbalance, with α/β-chain production ratios in the 1.2 to 1.3/1 range.

Type 2 Normal HbA2-β Thalassemia. This condition is heterogeneous. One of the most common causes is the compound heterozygous inheritance of both δ and β thalassemia (Silvestroni et al., 1978) (Table 13.7). A variety of different forms of δ^0- or δ^+-thalassemia mutations have been found, either in *cis* or *trans* to β-thalassemia mutations, and in some cases β haplotypes containing β- and δ-thalassemia genes in *cis* have been disseminated throughout populations. For example, in the mild form of β thalassemia, Hb Knossos, carriers have minimal hematologic changes and low levels of HbA2. This phenotype results from a mild β^+-thalassemia mutation (β27 G→T) together with a deletion of an A in codon 59 of the δ gene in *cis*, which completely inactivates it (Olds et al., 1991). The same δ^0 59 (-A) mutation has been found in *cis* to the β^0 39 and β^+ IVS-1-110 mutations in Mediterranean populations (Tzetis et al., 1994), and $\delta^{+}27$ (G→T) has been reported in both *cis* and *trans* to the β^+ IVS-2-745 mutation (Loudianos et al., 1990; Trifillis et al., 1991). While, on average, the HbA2 levels fall into the normal range, there is considerable scatter and in some cases values in the 3 to 3.7 range are observed.

Although the diagnosis of coexistent β and δ thalassemia is best made by analysis of the respective globin genes, some clues can be obtained from family studies. Where the two mutations exist in *cis*, the condition will be transmitted both vertically and laterally. On the other hand, if the two thalassemia mutations are in *trans* they will separate and individuals with both high HbA2- and normal HbA2-β thalassemia may be found in different generations.

When considering the differential diagnosis of normal HbA2-β thalassemia, and if different forms of α thalassemia have been excluded, it is important to remember that there are certain unusual phenocopies of this condition. For example, some forms of εγδβ thalassemia, which involve long deletions of the β-globin gene complex, are characterized by a picture that is indistinguishable from normal HbA2-β thalassemia in heterozygotes. Similarly, the Corfu form of δβ thalassemia, in which a 7.2 kb deletion involves the δ gene but leaves the β gene intact is also associated with this phenotype. This is because the β gene in *cis* to this deletion carries an additional β-thalassemia mutation.

Heterozygous β Thalassemia with Unusually High Levels of HbA2 or HbF. There is a rare group of β thalassemias in which levels of HbA2 in excess of 5 percent to 6 percent are observed. They all seem to result from deletions of the β-globin gene, which remove its 5′ promoter region, including sequences from −125 to +78 relative to the CAP site; in each case the promoter boxes are lost (reviewed by Thein, 1993). The HbA2 levels associated with these β thalassemias may be as high as 8 percent to 9 percent.

These deletion forms of β thalassemia are also associated with unusually high HbF levels in heterozygotes. The first variety to be described, which became known as the Dutch form of β thalassemia (Schokker et al., 1966), was found in a large kindred with 13 heterozygotes; their HbF levels ranged from 5.1 percent to 14.4 percent with a mean value of 8.3 percent. Similar values have been reported in heterozygotes for several other deletional forms of β thalassemia.

Isolated Elevated HbA2 Levels; Heterozygous β Thalassemia with α Thalassemia and Related Conditions. Occasionally, during population screening or family studies, individuals are encountered who have elevated HbA2 levels in the absence of the usual

Table 13.7. Normal Hemoglobin A2 β Thalassemia Type 2 Due to Compound Heterozygosity for β and δ Thalassemia

No.	β thalassemia mutation	δ thalassemia mutation	Hemoglobin A2 level in compound heterozygote
9	IVS-II 745 C→G	δ^{+69} G→A (*cis*)	2.53 – 3.74 (mean – 2.97)
1	IVS-II 745 C→G	$\delta^{+}27$ G→T (probably *cis*)	2.2
1	IVS-II 745 C→G	$\delta^{+}27$ G→T (*trans*)	2.5
1	β39 C→T	$\delta^{+}27$ G→T (*trans*)	3.4
1	IVS-II 745 C→G	$\delta^{+}27$ G→T (*cis*)	3.2
1	β39 C→T	δ^{059} (−A)(*cis*)	3.5
1	IVS-1 110 G→A	δ^{059} (−A)(*cis*)	3.2
1	IVS-16 T→C	$\delta^{+}27$ G→T (*trans*)	2.7

References in Weatherall and Clegg, 2000.

hematologic findings of heterozygous β thalassemia. Since the co-inheritance of α^+ or α^0 thalassemia with β thalassemia may result in normalization of the red cell indices and balanced globin-chain synthesis, leaving a raised HbA_2 as the sole abnormality, it seems likely that many of the reported cases of isolated HbA_2 elevation reflect these interactions (Kanavakis et al., 1982; Melis et al., 1983). However, several families have been described in which there were otherwise normal individuals with raised HbA_2 levels in whom detailed analyses of the α-, β-, and δ-globin genes showed no abnormality (Gasperini et al., 1993).

Heterozygous β Thalassemia with an Unusually Severe Clinical Course.
There are two main mechanisms whereby heterozygous thalassemia may run a more severe course. First, there is the co-inheritance of a chromosome containing additional α-globin genes, either ααα or αααα. The forms of β thalassemia intermedia associated with these genotypes were discussed earlier in this chapter. Second, there are the dominant β thalassemias, which result from mutations that give rise to products that are able to form inclusion bodies in the red cell precursors (Weatherall et al., 1973; Stamatoyannopoulos et al., 1974). These conditions, which give rise to a wide spectrum of forms of β thalassemia intermedia of varying clinical severity, together with the underlying molecular mechanism, are described in Chapter 14.

β Thalassemia Unlinked to the β-Globin Gene Complex.
Several families have been reported in which a form of β-thalassemia trait appears to segregate independently from the β-globin gene complex (Semenza et al., 1984; Schwartz et al., 1988; Murru et al., 1992; Thein et al., 1993). Although subsequent analyses have shown some problems of interpretation in one of these families there seems little doubt from the study of Thein et al. that there is a form of phenotypically characteristic heterozygous β thalassemia that segregates independently of the β-globin genes. It seems likely that this reflects the action of a mutant *trans*-acting factor that is involved with β-globin gene regulation. The red cell indices, HbA_2 levels, and globin-chain synthesis findings are indistinguishable from the forms of β-thalassemia trait associated with mutations in the β-globin genes.

Other β Thalassemias of Unknown Cause.
Most laboratories that have sequenced large numbers of β-globin genes during their studies of families with the phenotype of β thalassemia have amassed varying numbers of cases in which no abnormality has been found. For example, Kazazian (1990) reported that this was the case in 9 of the 100 alleles that his laboratory had sequenced in detail. Since in many cases it has not been possible to carry out the kind of genetic studies required, it is quite possible that at least some of these undefined disorders reflect the type of unlinked forms of β thalassemia described above.

The Problem of Borderline Red Cell Indices or HbA_2 Levels.
In heterozygotes for very mild β-thalassemia alleles, or those for severe alleles who have co-inherited α thalassemia, the red cell indices may be almost normal. The usual levels of the MCH and MCV below which further study is advised, less than 27 pg and 75 fl, respectively, may miss these conditions in screening programs.

In clinical practice it is also not infrequent to encounter individuals with HbA_2 levels that appear to be very marginally raised, that is, in the 3 percent to 3.5 percent range. These cases pose considerable diagnostic and counseling difficulties. What action should be taken? Probably the first thing to do is to repeat the estimation, but if similar values are obtained again, the finding cannot be ignored.

Galanello et al. (1994) have analyzed 125 individuals with HbA_2 values in this range. In 37 cases they were able to detect an underlying molecular defect in the β-, δ-, or α-globin genes. Twenty-three were carriers of mild β-thalassemia alleles, 16 were compound heterozygotes for δ and β thalassemia, two had triplicated α-globin genes, and two had single α-globin gene deletions. The finding of this relatively high percentage of abnormalities, and the fact that many of them can interact with β thalassemia to produce severe phenotypes, suggests that in any screening program, particularly when an individual who has a borderline HbA_2 is planning to have a child with a partner with typical β-thalassemia trait, it is important to investigate the cause for the marginally elevated HbA_2 level.

AVOIDANCE AND POPULATION CONTROL

Because of the changing demography of disease in many countries the thalassemias will be a major health problem in the new millennium (Weatherall and Clegg, 1996). As populations become richer, and standards of nutrition and public health improve, there is a fall in childhood mortality. Hence, an increasing number of babies with genetic diseases such as thalassemia will survive the early months of life and present for treatment. It is essential, therefore, that some form of program for the population control of these diseases is initiated.

It is beyond the scope of this chapter to deal with the complex ethical, economic, and organizational problems of establishing screening programs for the thalassemias. They must be backed up by adequate facilities for counseling and each individual society has to decide whether it wishes to try to reduce the frequency of births of children with serious forms of thalassemia by counseling and marital advice or by establishing a program of prenatal diagnosis. These complex issues are discussed in detail by Weatherall and Clegg (2000) and the extensive experience gained from the successful population programs that have been carried out over the last 20 years in the Mediterranean island populations are reviewed by Cao et al. (1998). The methods that are currently established for prenatal diagnosis of β thalassemia are described in Chapters 35 and 36.

MANAGEMENT

Advances in the management of thalassemia major have greatly improved the prognosis for patients over recent years. While bone marrow transplantation, for those with appropriate donors and in countries in which the facilities exist, now offers the possibility of curing the condition, the mainstays of treatment are still adequate transfusion, backed up with iron-chelation therapy and the judicious use of splenectomy. Some of these topics are dealt with in detail in other chapters. Here we simply outline the principles of management. The broader population, social, and psychological aspects are reviewed elsewhere (Weatherall and Clegg, 2000).

It is very important before embarking on any form of treatment to establish the particular variety of β thalassemia and to obtain a full blood group genotype of the patient. It is also essential to assess the patient carefully over the first few months after the diagnosis is established and not to embark on a transfusion regimen too hastily. Many patients with intermediate forms of β thalassemia, who may not need regular transfusion, embark on a life of unnecessary treatment of this kind, particularly if they present with an unusually low hemoglobin level during a period of intercurrent infection. The important indications for transfusion are not the steady-state hemoglobin level, but the child's well-being, particularly with respect to activity, growth, development, and the early appearance of skeletal changes.

Transfusion and Splenectomy

Transfusion Regimens. Long-term transfusion programs form the cornerstone of treatment for most patients with thalassemia major (Piomelli et al., 1969) (see Chapter 37). Avoidance or reduction of the frequency of transfusions in an effort to ameliorate iron loading does not prevent this complication; when erythropoietic activity is increased more than five-fold, as it may be in severe thalassemia, the amount of iron absorbed surpasses iron loss, resulting in an increase in body iron (Pootrakul et al., 1988). The goals of transfusion, therefore, include not only correction of the anemia but suppression of erythropoiesis and inhibition of increased gastrointestinal absorption of iron. Both "hypertransfusion" and "supertransfusion" regimens, in which pretransfusion hemoglobins are maintained above 10 and 12 g/dL, respectively, prevent most complications of anemia and ineffective erythropoiesis (Fosburg and Nathan, 1990) but are associated with substantial iron loading. Recently, the maintenance of pretransfusion hemoglobin concentrations that did not exceed 9.5 g/dL were found to reduce transfusion requirements and body iron loading, as estimated by serum ferritin concentrations; in parallel, marrow activity did not increase more than threefold over normal, and a lower incidence of endocrine and cardiac complications was observed (Cazzola et al., 1997). These findings will need to be confirmed by extended follow-up.

Type of Red Cell Concentrates. Most centers still use washed or filtered red cells. Early clinical experience of the use of neocytes, young red blood cells separated from older cells by density centrifugation (Piomelli et al., 1978), suggested that a modest extension of the transfusion interval could be achieved (Cohen et al., 1984). Later studies, which used a simpler method of preparation (Simon et al., 1989), confirmed these findings (Kevy et al., 1988). A more recent report observed that the reduction in total annual transfusional iron load during neocyte transfusions varied widely: from less than 10 percent to greater than 25 percent (Spanos et al., 1996). The cost–benefit of neocyte transfusions is unclear; the benefits of reduced iron administration are offset by an up to fivefold increase in preparation expenses over those of standard concentrates (Collins et al., 1994).

Full details of the practical aspects of transfusion therapy are discussed by Weatherall and Clogg (2000).

Splenectomy. In the past, it was quite common to observe an increase in transfusion requirements at about the age of 10 years. In many cases it was apparent that this reflected the effects of hypersplenism (see Modell and Berdoukas, 1984). However, more recent experience suggests that many patients who have received adequate transfusion therapy from an early age do not show this phenomenon and hence splenectomy is now required less often (Olivieri and Brittenham, 1997). Splenectomy has been recommended when transfusion requirements exceed 250 mL (Graziano et al., 1981) or 200 mL packed cells/kg body weight (Cohen et al., 1989). Concerns that it may be associated with acceleration of iron loading in other organs (Okon et al., 1976; Pootrakul et al., 1980) are not supported by one study that reported that the spleen is not a significant repository of transfused iron (Borgna-Pignatti et al., 1984). Because of the risk of infection, splenectomy should be delayed until the age of 5 years. Splenic embolization (Politis et al., 1987) and partial splenectomy (Kheradpir and Albouyeh, 1985; de Montalembert et al., 1989) have been used to preserve splenic function, but an early response has often been followed by recurrence of hypersplenism, and these approaches are not generally recommended.

At least 2 to 3 weeks before splenectomy, patients should be vaccinated with pneumococcal and *Hemophilus influenzae* type B vaccines, and after surgery, daily prophylactic penicillin should be administered, at least during childhood and probably indefinitely. Erythromycin may be substituted for those who are allergic to penicillin.

Iron Chelation

Background. In the absence of iron-chelating therapy, transfusional iron loading is progressive and ultimately fatal (Olivieri and Brittenham, 1997). Cardiac iron loading remains the leading cause of death in thalassemia patients and is still observed in the present era. The beneficial effects of deferoxamine mesylate (DF), the only iron-chelating agent presently licensed for clinical use in most countries, on survival and cardiac disease are reviewed in detail by Olivieri and Brittenham (1997)(see Chapter 37). Two large studies have reported the influence of effective long-term use of DF on the development of clinical cardiac disease (Brittenham et al., 1994; Olivieri et al., 1994). One trial observed that patients who had maintained sustained reduction of body iron, as estimated by a serum ferritin less than 2,500 µg/L over 12 years of follow-up, had an estimated cardiac-disease–free survival of 91 percent, in contrast to patients in whom most determinations of serum ferritin exceeded 2,500 µg/L, whose estimated cardiac-disease–free survival was less than 20 percent (Olivieri et al., 1994). A second study examined the relationship between the development of clinical cardiac disease and the magnitude of the body iron burden determined directly using measurements of hepatic storage iron (Brittenham et al., 1994). Patients who had maintained concentrations of hepatic iron equal to or exceeding 15 mg iron/g liver, dry weight, had a 32 percent probability of survival to the age of 25 years; no cardiac disease developed in those who maintained hepatic iron levels below this threshold. Another study examined the impact of DF on clinical and subclinical cardiac disease, defined as

the presence of an abnormal electrocardiogram or echocardiogram, or both, with or without symptoms of cardiac disease. As in other reports, late commencement of deferoxamine and noncompliance with therapy were associated with an increased risk of heart disease (Richardson et al., 1993).

Assessment and Maintenance of Body Iron Levels
Assessment of Body Iron Levels. Both indirect and direct methods for the assessment of body iron are available (see section on Iron Loading). As discussed earlier, none of the indirect approaches are reliable, and measurement of hepatic iron stores provides the most quantitative, specific, and sensitive method for determining body iron burden in thalassemia major (Pippard, 1989). Hence, it should be considered the reference method for comparison with other techniques. The increasing use of liver biopsy to quantitate body iron has provided new guidelines for the management of iron-chelating therapy that have enhanced our ability to provide a balance between effectiveness and toxicity of DF (Olivieri and Brittenham, 1997). Liver biopsy permits a chemical measurement of the nonheme storage iron concentration, histochemical determination of the pattern of iron accumulation, and evaluation of the extent of inflammation, fibrosis, and cirrhosis. The superconducting quantum interference device (SQUID) magnetometer provides a direct measure of hepatic storage iron that, in the presence of increased body iron stores, provides a measurement of liver iron quantitatively equivalent to that determined at biopsy (Brittenham et al., 1982). It is not generally available, however.

Optimal Body Iron Concentrations in Patients with Thalassemia Major. Data that have accumulated over the past 10 years permit a quantitative approach to the management of iron overload, and provide guidelines for the control of body iron burden in chelated patients. Chelating therapy should not be aimed at maintenance of a normal body iron (about 0.2 to 1.6 mg iron/g liver, dry weight), as this greatly increases the probability of deferoxamine toxicity (Porter and Huehns, 1989). By contrast, maintenance of hepatic iron concentrations exceeding 15 mg iron/g liver, dry weight, is associated with a greatly increased risk of cardiac disease and early death (Brittenham et al., 1994). Slightly lower iron burdens (between about 7 and 15 mg iron/g liver, dry weight) are associated with an increased risk of other complications of iron overload, including hepatic fibrosis, in homozygotes for hereditary hemochromatosis (Loreal et al., 1992; Niederau et al., 1996).

It has been proposed that a conservative goal for chelating therapy is the maintenance of hepatic storage iron concentrations of about 3 to 7 mg iron/g liver, dry weight (Olivieri and Brittenham, 1997), in the range found in asymptomatic heterozygotes for hereditary hemochromatosis (Cartwright et al., 1979). If measurement of hepatic iron is not feasible, the serum ferritin provides an alternative but less reliable means of determining whether the body iron is within an optimal range. As we have seen, a serum ferritin level of 2,500 µg/L, maintained over a period of more than 10 years, may reflect a threshold of increased risk of cardiac disease and early death (Olivieri et al., 1994), but evidence is emerging that the level of body iron that is truly protective with respect to the development of other complications of iron overload may be lower than this (Lai et al., 1995).

The Initiation of Iron-Chelating Therapy. The adverse effects associated with deferoxamine, and the balance between its effectiveness and toxicity, have been recently reviewed (Olivieri and Brittenham, 1997). It has been recommended that initiation of deferoxamine should be guided by the concentration of hepatic iron, obtained by liver biopsy under ultrasound guidance, after approximately 1 year of regular transfusions. If a liver biopsy is not possible at the start of therapy, subcutaneous infusions of deferoxamine, not exceeding 25–35 mg/kg/d, should be initiated after approximately 1 year of regular transfusions. Titration of hepatic iron, as above, should avert the potential toxic effects of deferoxamine (Porter and Huehns, 1989). If the hepatic iron concentration is not regularly assessed, a "toxicity" index, defined as the mean daily dose of deferoxamine (mg/kg) divided by the serum ferritin concentration (g/L) should be calculated for each patient every six months, and should not exceed 0.025 (Porter and Huehns, 1989). Doses of deferoxamine should not usually exceed 50 mg/kg/d, and all patients should undergo regular examination for ophthalmologic or auditory complications.

Alternatives to Subcutaneous Infusions. Regimens of continuous ambulatory intravenous deferoxamine infused through implantable subcutaneous ports, in which the infusion site cannot be manipulated by the patient, overcome the disadvantages of drug preparation and self-administration, eliminate the irritation associated with subcutaneous infusions, and improve compliance (Olivieri et al., 1992). Because this system requires that the site is changed weekly by medical personnel at a clinic visit, it is not popular with many patients. Those unwilling to visit the clinic frequently, and those for whom standard pumps are unwieldly, may benefit from new systems in which the desired concentrations of continuous subcutaneous or intravenous deferoxamine can be infused using a light-

weight, disposable, silent balloon infuser (Baxter) that produces continuous pressure without a battery or other mechanical device (Araujo et al., 1996; Lombardo et al., 1996b).

Deferoxamine "Allergy". Reactions to deferoxamine include acute inflammation, itching, and edema at the site of infusion, increasing in severity, to wheezing, tachypnea, tachycardia, hypotension, and coma. Although these reactions suggest an allergic mechanism, evidence supporting an immunologic basis for this is lacking; direct, IgE-independent activation of dermal mast cells by deferoxamine has been demonstrated (Shalit et al., 1991). These severe reactions may be effectively managed using rapid intravenous desensitization similar to protocols recommended for penicillin-allergic individuals (Miller et al., 1981; Bousquet et al., 1983; Lombardo et al., 1996), followed by long-term, continuous, subcutaneous or intravenous infusion.

Blood-Borne Infections

As discussed earlier, liver disease due to transfusion-transmitted viruses, hepatitis B, C, and HIV, are now a major cause of morbidity and mortality in patients with β thalassemia. Hepatitis B infection is still the most important worldwide, while hepatitis C is a major problem in Europe, North America, and Japan. Since the introduction of HIV donor screening, the risk of acquisition of HIV by transfusion has been greatly reduced in Europe and the United States. In patients becoming HIV seropositive the risk of progression to AIDS appears to be about 9 percent at 5 years. It is beyond our scope to discuss the treatment of HIV infections. Here we will focus on the management of hepatitis C, since this is an important and increasing problem in patients with β thalassemia.

Hepatitis C. Iron overload and infection with hepatitis C virus are cofactors in the evolution of chronic liver disease, a common cause of death after age 15 years in thalassemia major (Zurlo et al., 1989).

Recombinant α-interferon is the only effective therapy for chronic infection with hepatitis C virus (Tin et al., 1991). A recent study of the long-term efficacy of α-interferon in patients with thalassemia major (Di Marco et al., 1997) reported a complete response, defined as both sustained normalization of serum ALT and clearance of HCV-RNA from serum, in 40 percent of patients over a mean follow-up period of 3 years. The rate of relapse was much lower in thalassemic (18 percent) than in nonthalassemic individuals (50 percent). This suggests that in most patients with thalassemia, α-interferon should not be stopped after 3 to 6 months, but should be continued at least until the serum ALT level declines to normal. This, and previous studies (Donohue et al., 1993; Clemente et al., 1994), have highlighted the importance of compliance with deferoxamine during α-interferon therapy. The results of other approaches to improve responses to α-interferon, including its coadministration with ribavirin (Sherlock, 1995; Preston and Wright, 1996), are still awaited.

Other Infections

Although in the past infectious complications were a major problem in thalassemic children, this seems to be less common in those who are maintained on an adequate transfusion and chelation regimen. The one important exception is infections with the *Yersinia* genus of bacteria. The pathophysiology and clinical features were described in a previous section. Treatment with DF should be stopped, stool cultures examined for *Yersinia* spp, and appropriate antibiotic treatment started, either an aminoglycoside or cotrimoxazole.

Bone and Endocrine Disease

The mechanisms of the reduction in bone density in β thalassemia were discussed ealier. It is recommended that bone densitometry, using dual-energy X-ray absorptiometry or in vivo neutron activation, is included in the evaluation of thalassemia patients to guide treatment (Orvieto et al., 1992). Appropriate hormonal replacement therapy in hypogonadal patients, exercise programs, and the administration of elemental calcium and vitamin D may be of benefit. The value of bisphosphonates, calcitonin (Catanan et al., 1995), and fluoride remains to be determined.

Other endocrine disorders are discussed in detail earlier in this chapter. They should be managed by appropriate replacement therapy.

Bone Marrow Transplantation

Bone marrow transplantation from HLA-identical donors has been successfully performed in over 1,000 patients with severe β thalassemia worldwide (Giardini, 1995) (see Chapter 39). Survival and disease-free survival are significantly influenced by three characteristics prior to transplantation: hepatomegaly more than 2 cm below the costal margin, portal fibrosis, and a history of effective chelating therapy. Patients in class I have none of these characteristics; patients in class II have one or two; and patients in class III have all three (Lucarelli et al., 1990). In class III children less than 16 years of age, survival and disease-free survival is 62 percent and 51 percent, respectively, 3 years following transplantation. Increasingly

better outcomes are observed following transplantation of class II patients (86 percent and 82 percent, respectively), while excellent outcomes are observed in class I patients (90 percent and 93 percent, respectively). Transplantation of thalassemic adults over 16 years achieves results approximately equivalent to those observed in class III patients (Lucarelli et al., 1995, 1996). Survival and disease-free survival rates still vary considerably between different centers (Vellodi et al., 1994; Walters and Thomas, 1994; Clift and Johnson, 1997; Roberts et al., 1997). Post-transplant management involves the complications related directly to the transplantation procedure itself, including acute and chronic graft-versus-host disease, and persistence of host hematopoietic cells, that is mixed chimerism. It also includes those unique to the "ex-thalassemic" as a result of the primary disease or the previous treatment, including iron-induced cardiac and endocrine dysfunction and viral hepatitis.

Following transplantation for thalassemia, the probabiiity of the development of moderate chronic graft-versus-host disease is approximately 8 percent, and that of severe, chronic graft-versus-host disease is approximately 2 percent (Gaziev et al., 1997). Mixed chimerism has been described in 28 percent of patients, and is a risk factor for graft failure. Post-transplant, management of hepatic iron loading, using either deferoxamine (Giardini et al., 1995) or phlebotomy (Angelucci et al., 1997), as well as treatment of iron-induced cardiac dysfunction (Mariotti et al., 1997) and viral hepatitis (Giardini et al., 1997), have been shown to arrest or reverse the course of these complications.

Experimental approaches to marrow replacement in patients with thalassemia include cord-blood transplantation (Issagrisil et al., 1995), the use of unrelated phenotypically matched marrow donors (Contu et al., 1994), and in utero transplantation (Westgren et al., 1996).

Thalassemia Intermedia

Patients who are growing and developing adequately without transfusion, and who fall into the β thalassemia intermedia category, should be maintained on folate supplementation and have regular assessment of their iron status, with appropriate chelation therapy if there is evidence of iron loading. In the face of a falling hemoglobin level and progressive splenomegaly, splenectomy may be indicated, although the results are unpredictable. Symptomatic extramedullary hematopoietic masses have been treated with hypertransfusion and X-ray therapy. Recently there has been a report of regression after the administration of hydroxyurea (Saxon et al., 1998).

Experimental Therapies

Bolus Injections of Subcutaneous Deferoxamine. Preliminary studies suggest that deferoxamine administered by twice-daily subcutaneous injections may induce urinary iron excretion equal to the same dose administered by prolonged subcutaneous infusion (Jensen et al., 1995; Borgna-Pignatti and Cohen, 1996). If confirmed, these observations could lead to the implementation of regimens that offer an alternative to prolonged infusions.

Hydroxyethyl Starch Deferoxamine. Attachment of deferoxamine to a hydroxyethyl starch polymer creates a high-molecular-weight chelator with affinity for iron identical to, but with a vascular half-life 10 to 30 times longer than, that of standard deferoxamine (Hallaway et al., 1989). The goal of therapy in chronically transfused patients would be to design similar compounds, a single infusion of which would promote iron excretion over an extended period of time. Pilot studies of this agent have been promising (Olivieri, 1996) and larger trials are planned.

Orally Active Iron Chelators. The expense and inconvenience of deferoxamine has led to a search for an orally active iron chelator. The only agent to reach extended clinical trials is 1,2-dimethyl-3-hydroxypyridin-4-one (deferiprone; L1) (Hider et al., 1982). The effectiveness of deferiprone was initially evaluated using the serum ferritin concentration (Bartlett et al., 1990; Olivieri et al., 1990; Tondury et al., 1990; Agarwal et al., 1992; al-Refaie et al., 1995). Reduction in hepatic iron stores by deferiprone was first demonstrated in a patient with thalassemia intermedia (Olivieri et al., 1992); subsequently, a favorable effect of deferiprone on tissue iron was reported in thalassemia major (Olivieri et al., 1995). Although support for both a long-term open-label study and a randomized trial of deferiprone and deferoxamine was terminated prematurely by the corporate sponsor in 1996, follow-up of hepatic storage iron concentrations in both cohorts have provided information about the long-term effectiveness of deferiprone in thalassemia major. In one-third of patients in a long-term treatment cohort of deferiprone-treated patients (Olivieri et al., 1995), hepatic iron stabilized at, or increased to concentrations, which place patients at risk for cardiac disease and early death (Brittenham et al., 1994). Changes in compliance do not explain the ineffectiveness of long-term deferiprone (Olivieri, 1996).

In a randomized trial of deferiprone and deferoxamine, 38 of 51 patients remained on study at termination; a final hepatic iron concentration was obtained in 37 patients. After 33 months, the hepatic iron level of the deferoxamine-treated patients had not changed significantly from baseline, while in deferiprone-treated patients it increased approximately 100 percent over baseline. Compliance with deferiprone, measured with computerized bottles, was significantly better than with deferoxamine (Olivieri, 1996). These results, supported by the findings of another center, in which the hepatic iron of liver biopsies obtained after an extended period of deferiprone therapy exceeded the threshold for cardiac disease and early death in 50 percent of patients (Hoffbrand et al., 1998), raise concerns that long-term therapy with deferiprone may not provide adequate control of body iron in a substantial proportion of patients with thalassemia major.

During limited toxicity studies of deferiprone in rodents, adrenal hypertrophy, gonadal and thymic atrophy, bone marrow atrophy and pancytopenia, growth retardation, and embryotoxicity have been observed (see Brittenham, 1992; Olivieri et al., 1997); the major previously recognized adverse effects in humans include embryotoxicity, teratogenicity, neutropenia, and agranulocytosis (Hoffbrand, 1996). Recently, chronic coadministration of iron dextran and 1,2-diethyl-3-hydroxypyridin-4-one, a closely related hydroxypyridinone, resulted in increased iron accumulation in the liver and heart, worsening of hepatic fibrosis, and development of cardiac fibrosis in gerbils (Carthew et al., 1994) In guinea pigs, chronic administration of deferiprone was associated with hepatic, myocardial, and musculoskeletal necrosis, even in the absence of iron overload (Wong et al., 1997). In the Toronto long-term treatment cohort a retrospective review indicated that deferiprone treatment was, unexpectedly, associated with progression of hepatic fibrosis. The estimated median time to progression of fibrosis for the entire cohort exceeded 3 years. Hence, before deferiprone can be considered for general clinical use, evaluation of long-term effectiveness and toxicity in prospective, randomized, controlled clinical trials will be necessary (Olivieri and Brittenham, 1997).

Augmentation of Fetal Hemoglobin Production

Since there is abundant evidence that an unusual capacity for producing fetal hemogobin in patients with thalassemia or sickle cell anemia ameliorates the clinical course (reviewed by Wood, 1993), there has been considerable interest over recent years in attempting to find ways of increasing the output of HbF. The approaches that are being tried, and the possible mechanisms for the way in which different agents might stimulate fetal hemoglobin synthesis, are reviewed by Olivieri and Weatherall (1998) and Swank and Stamatoyannopoulos (1998) (see Chapter 38).

Clinical trials aimed at augmentation of fetal hemoglobin synthesis in β thalassemia have included administration of cell-cycle-specific agents, hematopoietic growth factors, and short-chain fatty acids, all of which stimulate γ-globin synthesis by different mechanisms. The compounds of particular interest are hydroxyurea and the butyric acid analogues.

Hydroxyurea. Hydroxyurea has been administered to a total of 46 patients with thalassemia, including 13 with β thalassemia/hemoglobin E. Although in one patient, in whom baseline values were not determined, the requirement for transfusions was eliminated (Arruda et al., 1997), hydroxyurea has generally been ineffective with only modest increases in hemoglobin level or HbF production (Nienhuis et al., 1985; McDonagh et al., 1990; Hajjar and Pearson, 1994; Huang et al., 1994; Cohen et al., 1995; Zeng et al., 1995; Fucharoen et al., 1996). An exception is a patient with Hb Lepore and β^0 thalassemia, in whom increases in fetal and total hemoglobin exceeding 4 g/dL were observed during hydroxyurea therapy (Rigano et al., 1997).

Butyrate Analogues. The butyric acid compounds, derivatives of natural short-chain fatty acids, seemed to offer potential therapy for β thalassemia after it was observed that elevated plasma concentrations of α-amino-N-butyric acid in infants of diabetic mothers delayed the switch from γ- to β-globin production around the time of birth (Bard and Prosmanne, 1985; Perrine et al., 1988). Arginine butyrate was the first butyric acid compound to be administered; in one homozygote for Hb Lepore, a striking increase in the hemoglobin concentration was noted (Perrine et al., 1993). Unfortunately, a larger trial of arginine butyrate in patients with more common forms of β thalassemia did not reproduce these findings (Sher et al., 1995). Evidence supporting the utility of regimens of "pulse" doses of arginine butyrate in β thalassemia (Atweh et al., 1996) is awaited. Further studies were pursued with oral agents including sodium phenylbutyrate and isobutyramide. A pilot trial of sodium phenylbutyrate in 11 adults with β thalassemia (Collins et al., 1995) reported clinical response (defined as a sustained increase in the hemoglobin level exceeding 1 g/dL) in four patients not receiving regular transfusions who had elevated serum erythropoietin levels before treatment. Isobutyramide has been reported to produce a slight increase in γ-globin synthesis in vitro (Perrine et al., 1994) and in vivo (Cappellini et al., 1996).

Combinations of Therapies. Coadministration of erythropoietin with hydroxyurea has induced increases in fetal hemoglobin (Loukopoulos et al., 1995), suggesting that erythropoietin might be usefully combined with agents that exert their effects by cytoreduction and regeneration from the progenitor pool. Combination therapy with butyrate and hydroxyurea in a patient homozygous for Hb Lepore has resulted in long-term, mean steady-state hemoglobin concentrations of 11.5 g/dL, an increase of approximately 6 g/dL in fetal hemoglobin; a similar response has been observed in an affected sibling (Olivieri et al., 1997). The marked elevation of fetal hemoglobin in these siblings, and a response of almost equal magnitude in a compound heterozygote for hemoglobin Lepore and β thalassemia (Rigano et al., 1997), raise the question as to whether the molecular pathology that underlies Hb Lepore may be related in some way to these unusual pharmacologic responses.

Although these attempts to increase the synthesis of fetal hemoglobin in β thalassemia have, with a few exceptions, been disappointing, the handful of spectacular successes offer some encouragement for the future. It is important, therefore, that attempts are made to determine the reasons for the marked variability of response, and, in particular, whether this relates to the underlying mutations, kinetics of erythropoiesis, or the particular dosages and regimens of the drugs that have been used. It is important that work along these lines is pursued. It may not be possible to raise the level of fetal hemoglobin sufficiently to manage patients with severe, transfusion-dependent forms of thalassemia. On the other hand, it is becoming clear that those with the more severe forms of β thalassemia intermedia, many cases of HbE-β thalassemia, for example, might benefit considerably by a modest elevation of their hemoglobin levels, even by a few g/dL. It is still quite possible that this may be achievable by augmentation of fetal hemoglobin production.

References

Aessopos, A, Stamatelos, G, Skoumas, V et al. (1995). Pulmonary hypertension and right heart failure in patients with β-thalassemia intermedia. *Chest* 107: 50–53.

Afifi, AM. (1974). High transfusion regime in the management of reproductive wastage and maternal complications of pregnancy in thalassaemia major. *Acta Haematol.* 52: 331–335.

Agarwal, MB, Gupte, SS, Viswanathan, C et al. (1992). Long-term assessment of efficacy and safety of L1, an oral iron chelator, in transfusion dependent thalassaemia: Indian trial. *Br. J. Haematol.* 82: 460–466.

Aksoy, M and Eredem, S. (1968). Combination of hereditary elliptocytosis and heterozygous beta-thalassaemia: A family study. *J. Med. Genet.* 5: 298–301.

al-Fawaz, I, al-Rasheed, S, al-Mugeiren, M et al. (1996). Hepatitis E virus infection in patients from Saudi Arabia with sickle cell anaemia and β-thalassemia major: Possible transmission by blood transfusion. *J. Virol. Hepatol.* 3: 203–205.

al-Refaie, FN, Hershko, C, Hoffbrand, AV et al. (1995). Results of long-term deferiprone (L1) therapy. A report by the International Study Group on Oral Iron Chelators. *Br. J. Haematol.* 91: 224–229.

Alam, R, Padmanabhan, K, and Rao, H. (1997). Paravertebral mass in a patient with thalassemia intermedia. *Chest* 112: 265–267.

Aldouri, MA, Wonke, B, Hoffbrand, AV et al. (1987). Iron state and hepatic disease in patients with thalassaemia major treated with long term subcutaneous desferrioxamine. *J. Clin. Pathol.* 40: 1352–1359.

Anapliotou, ML, Kastanias, IT, Psara, P et al. (1995). The contribution of hypogonadism to the development of osteoporosis in thalassaemia major: New therapeutic approaches. *Clin. Endocrinol.* 42: 279–287.

Angelucci, E, Baronciani, D, Lucarelli, G et al. (1993). Liver iron overload and liver fibrosis in thalassemia. *Bone Marrow Transplant.* 1: 29–31.

Angelucci, E, Ripalti, M, Baronciani, D et al. (1997). Phlebotomy to reduce iron overload in patients cured of thalassemia by marrow transplantation. *Bone Marrow Transplant.* 19: 123–125.

Anoussakis, C, Alexiou, D, Abatxis, D, and Bechrakis, G. (1977). Endocrinological investigation of pituitary gonadal axis in thalassaemia major. *Acta Paediatr. Scand.* 66: 49–51.

Antonarakis, SE, Kang, J, Lam, VMS et al. (1988). Molecular characterization of β-globin gene mutations in patients with β-thalassemia intermedia in South China. *Br. J. Haematol.* 70: 357–361.

Araujo, A, Kosaryan, M, MacDowell, A et al. (1996). A novel delivery system for continuous desferrioxamine infusion in transfusional iron overload. *Br. J. Haematol.* 93: 835–837.

Arcasoy, A, Cavdar, A, Cin, S et al. (1987). Effects of zinc supplementation on linear growth in beta thalassemia (a new approach). *Am. J. Hematol.* 24: 136.

Arnett, EN, Nienhuis, AW, Henry, WL et al. (1975). Massive myocardial hemosiderosis: A structure-function conference at the National Heart and Lung Institute. *Am. Heart J.* 90: 777–787.

Arruda, VR, Lima, CS, Saad, T, and Costa, FF. (1997). Succesful use of hydroxyurea in β-thalassemia major. *N. Engl. J. Med.* 336: 964.

Astaldi, G, Tolentino, P, and Sacchetti, G. (1951). La talasemia (Morbo di Cooley e forme affini). *Biblioteca 'Haematologica'*. Pavia, Tipografia del libro.

Athanassiadou, A, Papachatzopoulou, A, Zoumbos, N et al. (1994). A novel β-thalassaemia mutation in the 5' untranslated region of the β-globin gene. *Br. J. Haematol.* 88: 307–310.

Atweh, GF, Dover, GJ, Faller, G et al. (1996). Sustained hematologic response to pulse butyrate therapy in beta globin disorders. *Blood* 88 (Suppl.): 652a.

Bacalo, A, Kivity, S, Heno, N et al. (1992). Blood transfusion and lung function in children with thalassemia major. *Chest* 101: 362–370.

Bahl, VK, Malhotra, OP, Kumar, D et al. (1992). Noninvasive assessment of systolic and diastolic left ventricular function in patients with chronic severe anemia: A combined M-mode, two-dimensional, and Doppler echocardiographic study. *Am. Heart J.* 124: 1516–1523.

Bailey, IS and Prankerd, TAJ. (1958). Studies in thalassaemia. *Br. J. Haematol.* 4: 150–155.

Baker, DH. (1964). Roentgen manifestations of Cooley's anemia. *Ann. N. Y. Acad. Sci.* 119: 641–661.

Bank, A and Marks, PA. (1966). Excess α chain synthesis relative to β chain synthesis in thalassaemia major and minor. *Nature* 212: 1198–1200.

Bannerman, RM. (1961). *Thalassemia. A Survey of Some Aspects.* New York Grune & Stratton.

Bannerman, RM, Keusch, G, Kreimer-Birnbaum, M et al. (1967). Thalassemia intermedia, with iron overload, cardiac failure, diabetes mellitus, hypopituitarism and porphyrinuria. *Am. J. Med.* 42: 476–486.

Bard, H and Prosmanne, J. (1985). Relative rates of fetal hemoglobin and adult hemoglobin synthesis in cord blood of infants of insulin-dependent diabetic mothers. *Pediatrics* 75: 1143–1147.

Bargellesi, A, Pontremoli, S, and Conconi, F. (1967). Absence of beta globin synthesis and excess alpha globin synthesis in homozygous β thalassemia. *Eur. J. Biochem.* 1: 73–79.

Barker, JE and Wandersee, NJ. (1999). Thrombosis in heritable hemolytic disorders. *Curr. Opin. Hematol.* 6: 71–75.

Barry, M, Flynn, DN, Letsky, EA, and Risdon, RA. (1974). Long-term chelation therapy in thalassaemia major: Effect on liver iron concentration, liver histology and clinical progress. *Br. Med. J.* 1: 16–20.

Bartlett, AN, Hoffbrand, AV, and Kontoghiorghes, GJ. (1990). Long-term trial with the oral iron chelator 1,2-dimethyl-3-hydroxypyrid-4-one (L1). II. Clinical observations. *Brit. J. Haematol.* 76: 301–304.

Baty, JM, Blackfan, KD, and Diamond, LK. (1932). Blood studies in infants and in children. I. Erythroblastic anemia; a clinical and pathologic study. *Amer. J. Dis. Child.* 43: 667–704.

Baughan, MA, Paglia, DE, Schneider, AS, and Valentine, WN. (1968). An unusual haematological syndrome with pyruvate-kinase deficiency and thalassaemia minor in the kindreds. *Acta Haematol.* 39: 345–358.

Baynes, R, Bezwoda, W, Bothwell, T et al. (1986). The non-immune inflammatory response: Serial changes in plasma iron, iron-binding capacity, lactoferrin, ferritin and C-reactive protein. *Scand. J. Clin. Lab. Invest.* 46: 695–704.

Beard, MJ, Necheles, TF, and Allen, DM. (1969). Clinical experience with intensive transfusion in Cooley's anemia. *Ann. N. Y. Acad. Sci.* 165: 415–422.

Beaven, GH, Ellis, MJ, and White, JC. (1961). Studies in human foetal haemoglobin. III. The hereditary haemoglobinopathies and thalassaemia. *Br. J. Haematol.* 7: 169–186.

Ben-Bassat, I, Hertz, M, Selzer, G, and Ramot, B. (1977). Extramedullary hematopoiesis with multiple tumor-simulating mediastinal masses in a patient with β-thalassemia intermedia. *Isr. J. Med. Sci.* 13: 1206–1210.

Bergeron, C and Kovacs, K. (1978). Pituitary siderosis. A histologic, immunocytologic, and ultrastructural study. *Am. J. Pathol.* 93: 295–309.

Berkovitch, M, Bistritzer, T, Milone, SD et al. (2000). Iron deposition in the anterior pituitary in homozygous beta-thalassemia: MRI evaluation and correlation with gonadal function. *J. Pediatr. Endocrinol. Metab.* 13: 19–184.

Bianco, I, Montalenti, G, Silvestroni, E, and Siniscalco, M. (1952). Further data on genetics of microcythemia or thalassaemia minor and Cooley's disease or thalassaemia major. *Ann. Eugenics* 16: 299–314.

Bianco, I, Cappabianca, MP, Foglietta, E et al. (1997a). Silent thalassemias: Genotypes and phenotypes. *Haematologica* 82: 269–280.

Bianco, I, Lerone, M, Foglietta, E et al. (1997b). Phenotypes of individuals with a β thal classical allele associated either with a β thal silent allele or with α globin gene triplicate. *Haematologica* 82: 513–525.

Blendis, LM, Modell, CB, Bowdler, AJ, and Williams, R. (1974). Some effects of splenectomy in thalassaemia major. *Br. J. Haematol.* 28: 77–87.

Borgna-Pignatti, C and Cohen, AR. (1996). An alternative method of subcutaneous deferoxamine administration. *Blood* 86: 483a.

Borgna-Pignatti, C, de Stefano, P, Bongo, IG et al. (1984). Spleen iron content is low in thalassemia. *Am. J. Pediatr. Hematol. Oncol.* 6: 340–343.

Borgna-Pignatti, C, de Stafano, P, Zonta, L et al. (1985). Growth and sexual maturation in thalassemia major. *J. Pediatr.* 106: 150–155.

Borow, KM, Propper, R, Bierman, FZ et al. (1982). The left ventricular end-systolic pressure-dimension relation in patients with thalassemia major. A new noninvasive method for assessing contractile state. *Circulation* 66: 980–985.

Bousquet, J, Navarro, M, Robert, G et al. (1983). Rapid desensitization for desferrioxamine anaphylactoid reactions. *Lancet* 2: 859–860.

Bowdler, AJ and Huehns, ER. (1963). Thalassaemia major complicated by excessive iron storage. *Br. J. Haematol.* 9: 13–24.

Bozkurt, G, Dikengil, T, Alimoglu, O et al. (1993). Hepatitis C among Turkish Cypriot thalassemic patients. *Fifth International Conference on Thalassemias and Hemaglobinopathies*, Nicosia, Cyprus. (Cited by Wonke et al. 1998.)

Bridges, KR and Hoffman, KE. (1986). The effect of ascorbic acid on the intracellular metabolism of iron and ferritin. *J. Biol. Chem.* 261: 14273–14277.

Brittenham, GM. (1992). Development of iron-chelating agents for clinical use. *Blood* 80: 569–574.

Brittenham, GM. (2000). Disorders of iron metabolism: Iron deficiency and overload. In *Hematology: Basic principles and practice*. Hoffman, R, Benz, Eggr, Shattil, S, Furie, B et al. (eds). New York: Churchill Livingstone. pp. 397–428.

Brittenham, GM, Farrell, DE, Harris, JW et al. (1982). Magnetic-susceptibility measurement of human iron stores. *N. Engl. J. Med.* 307: 1671–1675.

Brittenham, GM, Griffith, PM, Nienhuis, AW et al. (1994). Efficacy of deferoxamine in preventing complications of iron overload in patients with thalassemia major. *N. Engl. J. Med.* 331: 567–573.

Brook, CG, Thompson, EN, Marshall, WC, and Whitehouse, RH. (1969). Growth in children with tha-lassemia major and effect of two different transfusion regimes. *Arch. Dis. Child.* 44: 612–616.

Brownell, AI, McSwiggan, DA, Cubitt, WD, and Anderson, MJ. (1986). Aplastic and hypoplastic episodes in sickle cell disease and thalassaemia. *J. Clin. Pathol.* 39: 121–124.

Buja, LM and Roberts, WC. (1971). Iron in the heart: Etiology and clinical significance. *Am. J. Med.* 51: 209–221.

Camaschella, C and Cappellini, MD. (1995). Thalassemia intermedia. *Haematologica* 80: 58–68.

Camaschella, C, Alfarano, A, Gottardi, E et al. (1990). The homozygous state for the −87 C→G β+ thalassaemia. *Br. J. Haematol.* 75: 132–133.

Camaschella, C, Mazza, U, Roetto, A et al. (1995). Genetic interactions in thalassemia intermedia: Analysis of β-mutations, α-genotype, γ promoters, and β-LCR hypersensitive sites 2 and 4 in Italian patients. *Am. J. Hematol.* 48: 82–87.

Camaschella, C, Gonella, S, Calabrese, R et al. (1996). Serum erythropoietin and circulating transferrin receptor in thalassemia intermedia patients with heterogeneous genotypes. *Haematologica* 81: 397–403.

Cammisa, M and Sabella, G. (1967). Clinico-radiological considerations on the pathogenesis of bone changes in thalassemia major. *Nunt. Radiol.* 33: 77–101.

Canale, VC, Steinherz, P, New, M, and Erlandson, M. (1974). Endocrine function in thalassemia major. *Ann. N. Y. Acad. Sci.* 232: 333–345.

Cancado, RD, Guerra, LGM, Rosenfeld, MOJA et al. (1993). Prevalence of hepatitis C virus antibody in beta thalassemic patients. Fifth International Conference on Thalassemia and Hemoglobinopathies, Nicosia, Cyprus. (Cited by Wonke et al. 1998.)

Cao, A. (1988). Diagnosis of β-thalassemia intermedia at presentation. *Birth Defects: Original Articles Series* 23: 219–226.

Cao, ADG, Podda, A, and Galanello, R. (1990). Molecular pathology of thalassemia intermedia. *Eur. J. Intern. Med.* 1: 227–236.

Cao, A, Galanello R, Rosatelli, MC et al. (1996). Clinical experience of management of thalassemia: The Sardinian experience. *Semin. Hematol.* 33: 66–75.

Cao, A, Galanello, R, and Rosatelli, MC. (1998). Prenatal diagnosis and screening of the haemoglobinopathies. *Clin. Haematol.* 11: 215–238.

Cappellini, MD, Fiorelli, G, and Bernini, LF. (1981). Interaction between homozygous β⁰ thalassaemia and the Swiss type of hereditary persistence of fetal haemoglobin. *Br. J. Haematol.* 48: 561–572.

Cappellini, MD, Graziadei, G, Ciceri, L et al. (1996). Phase II open study of oral isobutyramide in patients with thalassemia intermedia. *Blood* 88: 311a.

Cardia, E, Toscano, S, La Rosa, G et al. (1994). Spinal cord compression in homozygous β-thalassemia intermedia. *Pediatr. Neurosurg.* 20: 186–189.

Carthew, P, Smith, AG, Hider, RC et al. (1994). Potentiation of iron accumulation in cardiac myocytes during the treatment of iron overload with the hydroxypyridinine iron chelator CP94. *Biometals* 7: 267–271.

Cartwright, GE, Edwards, CQ, Kravitz, K et al. (1979). Hereditary hemochromatosis: Phenotypic expression of the disease. *N. Engl. J. Med.* 301: 175–179.

Castaldi, G, Zavagli, G, Ambroso, G et al. (1974). Anaemia in beta-thalassaemia carriers. *Br. Med. J.* 1: 518.

Catanan, D, Akar, N, and Arcasoy, A. (1995). Effects of calcitonin therapy on osteoporosis in patients with thalassemia. *Acta Haematol.* 93: 20–24.

Cavallo, L, Gurrado, R, Gallo, F et al. (1997). Growth deficiency in polytransfused beta-thalassaemia patients is not growth hormone dependent. *Clin. Endocrinol.* 46: 701–706.

Cavello-Perin, P, Pacini, B, Cerutti, F et al. (1995). Insulin resistance and hyperinsulinemia in homozygous β-thalassemia. *Metabolism* 44: 281–286.

Cavill, I, Ricketts, C, Jacobs, A, and Letsky, E. (1978). Erythropoiesis and the effect of transfusion in homozygous beta-thalassaemia. *N. Engl. J. Med.* 298: 776–778.

Cazzola, M, Borgna-Pignatti, C, Locatelli, F et al. (1997). A moderate transfusion regimen may reduce iron loading in β-thalassemia major without producing excessive expansion of erythropoiesis. *Transfusion* 37: 135–140.

Ceppellini, R. (1959). Discussion. Biochemistry of human genetics. *Ciba Foundation Symposium.* Boston: Little, Brown. pp. 133–134.

Chalevelakis, G, Clegg, JB, and Weatherall, DJ. (1975). Imbalanced globin chain synthesis in heterozygous β-thalassemia bone marrow. *Proc. Natl. Acad. Sci. U.S.A.* 72: 3853–3857.

Chalevelakis, G, Clegg, JB, and Weatherall, DJ. (1976). Globin synthesis in normal human bone marrow. *Br. J. Haematol.* 34: 535–557.

Chanarin, I. (1980). *The Megaloblastic Anaemias.* Oxford: Blackwell Scientific Publications.

Chanarin, I, Dacie, JV, and Mollin, DL. (1959). Folic-acid deficiency in haemolytic anaemia. *Br. J. Haematol.* 5: 245–256.

Chapman, RWG, Hussein, MAM, Gorman, A et al. (1982). Effect of ascorbic acid deficiency on serum ferritin concentrations in patients with β-thalassaemia major and iron overload. *J. Clin. Pathol.* 35: 487–491.

Chapman, SJ, Allison, JV, and Grimes, AJ. (1973). Abnormal cation movements in human hypochromic red cells incubates *in vitro*. *Scand. J. Haematol.* 10: 225–231.

Chatterjee, R, Katz, M, Cox, TF, and Porter, JB. (1993). A prospective study of the hypothalmic-pituitary axis in thalassaemic patients who developed secondary amenorrhoea. *Clin. Endocrinol.* 39: 287–296.

Chatterjee, R, Katz, M, Oatridge, A et al. (1998). Selective loss of anterior pituitary volume with severe pituitary-gonadal insufficiency in poorly compliant male thalassemic patients with pubertal arrest. *Ann. N. Y. Acad. Sci.* 850: 479–482.

Chini, V and Valeri, CM. (1949). Mediterranean hemopathic syndromes. *Blood* 4: 989–1013.

Choudhury, NV, Dubey, ML, Jolly, JG et al. (1990). Post-transfusion malaria in thalassaemia patients. *Blut* 61: 314–316.

Chung, JL, Kao, JH, Kong, MS et al. (1997). Hepatitis C and G virus infections in polytransfused children. *Eur. J. Pediatr.* 156: 546–549.

Clemente, MG, Congia, M, Lai, ME et al. (1994). Effect of iron overload on the response to recombinant interferon-alfa treatment in transfusion-dependent patients with tha-lassemia major and chronic hepatitis C. *J. Pediatr.* 125: 123–128.

Clift, RA and Johnson, FL. (1997). Marrow transplants for thalassemia: The USA experience. *Bone Marrow Transplant.* 19: 57–59.

Codrington, JF, Li, HW, Kutlar, F et al. (1990). Observations on the levels of Hb A$_2$ in patients with different β thalassemia mutations and a δ chain variant. *Blood* 76: 1246–1249.

Cohen, A, Cohen, IJ, and Schwartz, E. (1981). Scurvy and altered iron stores in thalassemia major. *N. Engl. J. Med.* 304: 158–160.

Cohen, A, Gayer, E, and Mizanin, J. (1989). Long-term effect of splenectomy on transfusion requirements in thalassemia major. *Am. J. Hematol.* 30: 254–256.

Cohen, AR, Schmidt, JM, Martin, MB et al. (1984). Clinical trial of young red cell transfusions. *J. Pediatr.* 104: 865–868.

Cohen, AR, Martin, MB, and Schwartz, E. (1995). Hydroxyurea therapy in thalassemia intermedia. *Sickle cell disease and thalassemia: New trends in therapy.* Colloque INSERM. pp. 193–194.

Cohen, F, Zuelzer, WW, Neel, JV, and Robinson, AR. (1959). Multiple inherited erythrocyte abnormalities in an American Negro family: Hereditary spherocytosis, sickling and thalassemia. *Blood* 14: 816–827.

Collins, AF, Dias, GC, Haddad, S et al. (1994). Evaluation of a new neocyte transfusion preparation vs. washed cell transfusion in patients with homozygous beta thalassemia. *Transfusion* 34: 517–520.

Collins, AF, Pearson, HA, Giardina, P et al. (1995). Oral sodium phenylbutyrate therapy in homozygous beta thalassemia. *Blood* 85: 43–49.

Constantoulakis, M, Panagopoulos, G, and Augoustaki, O. (1975). Stature and longitudinal growth in thalassemia major. A study of 229 Greek patients. *Clin. Pediatr.* 14: 355–362.

Contu, L, La Nasa, G, Arras, M et al. (1994). Successful unrelated bone marrow transplantation in thalassemia. *Bone Marrow Transplant.* 13: 329–331.

Cooley, TB, Witwer, ER, and Lee, P (1927). Anemia in children with splenomegaly and peculiar changes in bones; report of cases. *Am. J. Dis. Child.* 34: 347–363.

Cooper, DM, Mansell, AL, Weiner, MA et al. (1980). Low lung capacity and hypoxemia in children with thalassemia. *Am. Rev. Respir. Dis.* 121: 639–646.

Cossu, P, Toccafondi, C, Vardeu, F et al. (1981). Iron overload and desferrioxamine chelation therapy in beta-thalassemia intermedia. *Eur. J. Pediatr.* 137: 267–271.

Costagliola, DG, Girot, R, Rebulla, P, and Lefrère, JJ. (1992). Incidence of AIDS in HIV-1 infected thalassaemia patients. *Br. J. Haematol.* 81: 109–112.

Costin, G, Kogut, MD, Hyman, C, and Ortega, JA. (1977). Carbohydrate metabolism and pancreatic islet-cell function in thalassemia major. *Diabetes* 26: 230–240.

Costin, G, Kogut, MD, Hyman, CB, and Ortega, JA. (1979). Endocrine abnormalities in thalassemia major. *Am. J. Dis. Child.* 133: 497–502.

Crosby, WH and Conrad, ME. (1964). Iron imbalance in thalassaemia minor. A preliminary report. *Ann. NY Acad. Sci.* 119: 616–623.

Cunningham, TA and Vella, F. (1967). Combination of spherocytosis and a variant of beta thalassaemia ('isolated raised Hb A₂'). *J. Med. Genet.* 4: 109.

Dandona, P, Hussain, MAM, Varghese, Z et al. (1983). Insulin resistance and iron overload. *Ann. Clin. Biochem.* 20: 77–79.

David, CV and Balusubramaniam, P. (1983). Paraplegia with thalassemia. *Aust. N. Z. J. Med.* 53: 283–284.

De Alarcon, PA, Donovan, ME, Forbes, GB et al. (1979). Iron absorption in the thalassemia syndromes and its inhibition by tea. *N. Engl. J. Med.* 300: 5–8.

De Martino, M, Quarta, G, Melpignano, A et al. (1985). Antibodies to HTLV III and the lymphadenopathy syndrome in multi-transfused beta-thalassemia patients. *Vox Sange* 41: 230–233.

de Montalembert, M, Gitor, R, Revillon, Y et al. (1989). Partial splenectomy in homozygous β thalassemia. *Arch. Dis. Child.* 65: 304–307.

Derchi, G, Bellone, P, Forni, GL et al. (1992). Cardiac involvement in thalassemia major: Altered atrial natriuretic peptide levels in asymptomatic patients. *Eur. Heart J.* 13: 1368–1372.

De Sanctis, V, D'Ascola, G, and Wonke, B. (1986). The development of diabetes mellitus and chronic liver disease in long term chelated β-thalassemic patients. *Postgrad. Med. J.* 62: 831–836.

De Sanctis, V, Vullo, C, Katz, M et al. (1988a). Gonadal function in patients with beta thalassemia major. *J. Clin. Pathol.* 41: 133–137.

De Sanctis, V, Zurlo, MG, Senesi, E et al. (1988b). Insulin dependent diabetes in thalassemia. *Arch. Dis. Child.* 63: 58–62.

De Sanctis, V, Vullo, C, Katz, M et al. (1989). Endocrine complications in thalassemia major. *Prog. Clin. Biol. Res.* 309: 77–83.

De Sanctis, V, Vullo, C, Bagni, B, and Chiccoli, L. (1992). Hypoparathyroidism in β-thalassemia major. Clinical and laboratory observations in 24 patients. *Acta Haematol.* 88: 105–108.

De Sanctis, V, Katz, M, Vullo, C et al. (1994). Effect of different treatment regimes on linear growth and final height in β-thalassemia major. *Clin Endocrinol.* 40: 791–798.

De Virgillis, S, Sanna, G, Carnacchia, G et al. (1980). Serum ferritin, liver iron stores and liver histology in children with thalassemia. *Arch. Dis. Child.* 55: 43–45.

Dewey, KW, Grossman, H, and Canale, VC. (1970). Cholelithiasis in thalassemia major. *Radiology* 96: 385–388.

Di Marco, V, Lo Iacono, O, Almasio, P et al. (1997). Long-term efficacy of α-interferon in β-thalassemics with chronic hepatitis C. *Blood* 90: 2207–2212.

Diaz-Chico, JC, Yang, KG, Stoming, TA et al. (1988). Mild and severe β-thalassemia among homozygotes from Turkey: Identification of the types by hybridization of amplified DNA with synthetic probes. *Blood* 71: 248–251.

Dmochowski, K, Finegood, DT, Francombe, WH et al. (1993). Factors determining glucose tolerance in patients with thalassemia major. *J. Clin. Endocrinol. Metab.* 77: 478–483.

Donohue, SM, Wonke, B, Hoffbrand, AV et al. (1993). Alpha interferon in the treatment of chronic hepatitis C infection in thalassaemia major. *Br. J. Haematol.* 83: 491–497.

Dore, F, Bonfigli, S, Pardini, S et al. (1991). Priapism in thalassemia intermedia. *Haematologica* 76: 523.

Dore, F, Bonfigli, S, Gaviano, E et al. (1996). Serum transferrin receptor levels in patients with thalassemia intermedia during rHuEPO administration. *Haematologica* 81: 37–39.

Dore F, Bonfigli S, Gaviano, E et al. 1993. Serum erythropoietin levels in thalassemia intermedia. *Ann. Hematol.* 67: 183–186.

Dover, GJ, Smith, KD, Chang, YC et al. (1992). Fetal hemoglobin levels in sickle cell disease and normal individuals are partially controlled by an X-linked gene located at Xp22.2. *Blood* 80: 816–824.

Economou-Petersen, E, Aessopos, A, Kladi, A et al. (1998). Apolipoprotein E epsilon4 allele as a genetic risk factor for left ventricular failure in homozygous beta-thalassemia. *Blood* 92: 3455–3459.

Efremov, DG, Efremov, GD, Zisovski, N et al. (1988). Variation in clinical severity among patients with Hb Lepore-Boston——thalassemia is related to the type of β-thalassemia. *Br. J. Haematol.* 68: 351–355.

Efremov, D, Dimovsky, A, Baysal, E et al. (1994). Possible factors influencing the haemoglobin and fetal haemoglobin levels in patients with β-thalassaemia due to a homozygosity for the IVS-1-6 (T-C) mutation. *Br. J. Haematol.* 86: 824–830.

Ehlers, KH, Levin, AR, Markenson, AL et al. (1980). Longitudinal study of cardiac function in thalassemia major. *Ann. N. Y. Acad. Sci.* 344: 397–404.

Eisman, JA. (1996). Vitamin D receptor gene variants: Implications for therapy. *Curr. Opin. Genet. Dev.* 6: 361–365.

El-Hazmi, MA, Warsy, AS, and Al Fawaz, I. (1994). Iron-endocrine pattern in patients with beta-thalassaemia. *J. Trop. Pediatr.* 40: 219–224.

Ellis, JT, Schulman, I, and Smith, CH. (1954). Generalized siderosis with fibrosis of liver and pancreas in Cooley's (Mediterranean) anemia; with observations on the pathogenesis of the siderosis and fibrosis. *Am. J. Pathol.* 30: 287–309.

Engle, MA. (1964). Cardiac involvement in Cooley's anemia. *Ann. N. Y. Acad. Sci.* 119: 694–702.

Eraklis, AJ, Kevy, SV, Diamond, LK, and Gross, RE. (1967). Hazard of overwhelming infection after splenectomy in childhood. *N. Engl. J. Med.* 276: 1225–1229.

Erikson, WD, Burgert, EO, and Lynn, HB. (1968). The hazard of infection following splenectomy in children. *Am. J. Dis. Child.* 116: 1–12.

Erlandson, ME, Brilliant, R, and Smith, CH. (1964a). Comparison of sixty-six patients with thalassemia major and thirteen patients with thalassemia intermedia: Including evaluations of growth, development, maturation and prognosis. *Ann. N. Y. Acad. Sci.* 119: 727–735.

Erlandson, ME, Golubow, J, Wehman, J, and Smith, CH. (1964b). Metabolism of iron, calcium and magnesium in homozygous thalassemia. *Ann. N. Y. Acad. Sci.* 119: 769–775.

Erlandson, ME, Golubow, J, and Smith, CH. (1965). Bivalent cations in homozygous thalassemia. *J. Pediatr.* 66: 637–648.

Fabbri, G, Petraglia, F, Segre, A et al. (1991). Reduced spinal bone density in young women with amenorrhoea. *Eur. J. Obstet. Gynecol. Reprod. Biol.* 41: 117–122.

Factor, JM, Pottipati, SR, Rappaport, I et al. (1994). Pulmonary function abnormalities in thalassemia major and the role of iron overload. *Am. J. Respir. Crit. Care Med.* 149: 1570–1574.

Fargion, S, Piperno, A, Panaiotopoulos, N et al. (1985). Iron overload in subjects with β-thalassaemia trait: Role of idiopathic haemochromatosis gene. *Br. J. Haematol.* 61: 487–490.

Fattoum, S, Guemira, F, Öner, C et al. (1991). β-thalassemia, Hb S-β-thalassemia and sickle cell anemia among Tunisians. *Hemoglobin* 15: 11–21

Fessas, P. (1963). Inclusions of hemoglobin in erythroblasts and erythrocytes of thalassemia. *Blood* 21: 21–32.

Fessas, P and Loukopoulos, D. (1974). The β thalassaemias. *Clin. Haematol.* 3: 411–435.

Finch, CA, Deubelbeiss, K, Cook, JD et al. (1970). Ferrokinetics in man. *Medicine (Balt.).* 49: 17–53.

Fink, HE. (1964). Transfusion hemochromatosis in Cooley's anemia. *Ann. N. Y. Acad. Sci.* 119: 680–685.

Fiorelli, G, Sampietro, M, Romano, M et al. (1988). Clinical features of thalassemia intermedia in Italy. *Birth Defects: Original Articles Series* 23: 287–295.

Fiorelli, G, Fargion, S, Piperno, A et al. (1990). Iron metabolism in thalassemia intermedia. *Haematologica* 75: 89–85.

Fitchett, DH, Coltart, DJ, Littler, WA et al. (1980). Cardiac involvement in secondary haemochromatosis: A catheter biopsy study and analysis of myocardium. *Cardiovasc. Res.* 14: 719–724.

Flynn, DM, Fairney, A, Jackson, D, and Clayton, BE. (1976). Hormonal changes in thalassemia major. *Arch. Dis. Child.* 51: 828–836.

Fosburg, MT and Nathan, DG. (1990). Treatment of Cooley's anemia. *Blood* 76: 435–444.

Freedman, MH, Olivieri, NF, Grisaru, D et al. (1990). Pulmonary syndrome in patients receiving intravenous deferoxamine infusions. *Am. J. Dis. Child.* 144: 565–569.

Frick, P. (1970). Congenital elliptocytosis. Elliptocytosis and thalassemia in the same family. *Schweiz. Med. Wschr.* 100: 1009–1012.

Frumin, AM, Waldman, S, and Morris, P. (1952). Exogenous hemochromatosis in Mediterranean anemia. *Pediatrics* 9: 290–294.

Fucharoen, S, Siritanaratkul, N, Winichagoon, P et al. (1996). Hydroxyurea increases hemoglobin F levels and improves the effectiveness of erythropoiesis in β-thalassemia/hemoglobin E disease. *Blood* 87: 887–892.

Furbetta, M, Galanello, R, Ximenes, A et al. (1979). Interaction of alpha and beta thalassaemia genes in two Sardinian families. *Br. J. Haematol.* 41: 203–210.

Furbetta, M, Tuveri, T, Rosatacelli, C et al. (1983). Molecular mechanism accounting for milder types of thalassemia major. *J. Pediatr.* 103: 35–39.

Gabrielle, O. (1971). Hypoparathyroidism associated with thalassemia. *South. Med. J.* 64: 115–116.

Gabuzda, TG, Nathan, DG, and Gardner, FH. (1963). The turnover of hemoglobins A, F and A_2 in the peripheral blood of three patients with thalassemia. *J. Clin. Invest.* 42: 1678–1688.

Galacteros, F, Delanoe-Garin, J, Monplaisir, N et al. (1984). Two new cases of heterozygosity for hemoglobin Knossos $\alpha_2\beta_2$ Ala→Ser detected in the French West Indies and Algeria. *Hemoglobin* 8: 215–228.

Galanello, R, Melis, MA, Ruggeri, R, and Cao, A. (1981). Prospective study of red blood cell indices, hemoglobin A_2 and hemoglobin F in infants heterozygous for β-thalassemia. *J. Pediatr.* 99: 105–108.

Galanello, R, Ruggeri, R, Paglietti, E et al. (1983). A family with segregating triplicated alpha globin loci and beta thalassemia. *Blood* 62: 1035–1040.

Galanello, R, Dessi, E, Melis, MA et al. (1989). Molecular analysis of β^0-thalassaemia intermedia in Sardinia. *Blood* 74: 823–827.

Galanello, R, Turco, MP, Barella, S et al. (1990). Iron stores and iron deficiency anemia in children heterozygous for β-thalassemia. *Haematologica* 75: 319–322.

Galanello, R, Lilliu, F, Bertolino, F, and Cao, A. (1991). Percentile curves for red cell indices of β^0-thalassaemia heterozygotes in infancy and childhood. *J. Pediatr.* 150: 413–415.

Galanello, R, Barella, S, Ideo, A et al. (1994). Genotype of subjects with borderline hemoglobin A_2 levels: Implication for β-thalassemia carrier screening. *Am. J. Hematol.* 46: 79–81.

Galanello, R, Perseu, L, Melis, MA et al. (1997). Hyperbilirubinaemia in heterozygous β-thalassaemia is related to co-inherited Gilbert's syndrome. *Br. J. Haematol.* 99: 433–436.

Gallant, T, Freedman, MH, Vellend, H, and Francombe, WH. (1986). Yersinia sepsis in patients with iron overload treated with deferoxamine [letter]. *N. Engl. J. Med.* 314: 1643.

Gallerani, M, Cicognani, I, Ballardini, P et al. (1990). Average life expectancy of heterozygous β thalassemia subjects. *Haematologica* 75: 224–227.

Gallerani, M, Scapoli, C, Cicognani, I et al. (1991). Thalassaemia trait and myocardial infarction: Low infarction incidence in male subjects confirmed. *J. Intern. Med.* 230: 109–111.

Gallo, E, Pich, PG, Ricco, G et al. (1975). The relationship between anemia, fecal stercobilinogen, erythrocyte survival and globin synthesis in heterozygotes for β-thalassemia. *Blood* 46: 692–698.

Gallo, E, Massaro, P, Miniero, R et al. (1979). The importance of the genetic picture and globin synthesis in determining the clinical and haematological features of thalassaemia intermedia. *Br. J. Haematol.* 41: 211–221.

Gasperini, D, Cao, A, Paderi, L et al. (1993). Normal individuals with high Hb A_2 levels. *Br. J. Haematol.* 84: 166–168.

Gaziev, D, Polchi, P, Galimberti, M et al. (1997). Graft-versus-host disease following bone marrow transplantation for thalassemia: An analysis of incidence and risk factors. *Transplantation* 63: 854–860.

Gertner, JM, Broadus, AE, Anast, CS et al. (1979). Impaired parathyroid response to induced hypocalcemia in thalassemia major. *J. Pediatr.* 95: 210–213.

Gianni, AM, Bregni, M, Cappellini, MD et al. (1993). A gene controlling fetal hemoglobin expression in adults is not linked to the non-α globin cluster. *EMBO J.* 2: 921–926.

Giardina, PJ, Schneider, R, Lesser, M et al. (1995). Abnormal bone metabolism in thalassemia. In *Endocrine disorders in thalassemia*. Ando, S and Brancati, E (eds.). Berlin: Springer. pp. 38–46.

Giardini, C. (1995). Ethical issue of bone marrow transplantation for thalassemia [editorial]. *Bone Marrow Transplant.* 15: 657–658.

Giardini, C, Galimberti, M, Lucarelli, G et al. (1997). α-Interferon treatment of chronic hepatitis C after bone marrow transplantation for homozygous β-thalassemia. *Bone Marrow Transplant.* 20: 767–771.

Gimmon, Z, Wexler, MR, and Rachmilewitz, EA. (1982). Pathogenesis of juvenile leg ulcers in β-thalassaemia major and intermedia. *Plast. Reconstr. Surg.* 69: 320–323.

Giordano, P, Galli, M, Del Vecchio, GC et al. (1998). Lupus anticoagulant, anticardiolipin antibodies and hepatitis C virus infection in thalassaemia. *Br. J. Haematol.* 102: 903–906.

Girot, R, Lefrère, JJ, Schettini, F et al. (1991). HIV infection and AIDS in thalassemia. *Thalassemia 1991. Proceedings of the 5th Annual Meeting of the COOLEYCARE Group*, Athens, Centro trasfusionale Ospedale Maggiore Policlinico Dio Milano Editore. pp. 69–79.

Giuzio, E, Bria, M, Bisconte, MG et al. (1991). Osteoporosis in patients affected with thalassemia. Our experience. *Chir. Organi. Mov.* 76: 369–374.

Godet, J, Verdier, G, Nigon, V et al. (1977). β⁰-thalassemic from Algeria; genetic and molecular characterization. *Blood,* 50: 463–468.

Goldfarb, A, Grisaru, D, Gimmon, Z et al. (1990). High incidence of cholelithiasis in older patients with homozygous β-thalassemia. *Acta Haematol.* 83: 120–122.

Gonzalez-Redondo, JH, Stoming, TA, Lanclos, KD et al. (1988). Clinical and genetic heterogeneity in Black patients with homozygous β-thalassemia from the Southeastern United States. *Blood* 72: 1007–1014.

Grant, GP, Graziano, JH, Seaman, C, and Mansell, AL. (1987). Cardiorespiratory response to exercise in patients with thalassemia major. *Am. Rev. Respir. Dis.* 136: 92–97.

Gratwick, GM, Bullough, PG, Bohne, WHO et al. (1978). Thalassemia osteoarthropathy. *Ann. Intern. Med.* 88: 494–501.

Graziano, JH, Piomelli, S, Hilgartner, M et al. (1981). Chelation therapy in beta-thalassemia major. III. The role of splenectomy in achieving iron balance. *J. Pediatr.* 99: 695–699.

Green, NS. (1992). Yersinia infections in patients with homozygous beta-thalassemia associated with iron overload and its treatment. *Pediatr. Hematol. Oncol.* 9: 247–254.

Grinberg, LN and Rachmilewitz, EA. (1995). Oxidative stress in β-thalassemic red blood cells and potential use of antioxidants. *Sickle Cell Disease and Thalassaemia: New Trends in Therapy.* Colloque INSERM/John Libby Eurotext Ltd. pp. 519–524.

Grisaru, D, Rachmilewitz, EA, Mosseri, M et al. (1990). Cardiopulmonary assessment in beta-thalassemia major. *Chest* 98: 1138–1142.

Grundy, RG, Woods, RA, Savage, MO, and Evans, JPM. (1994). Relationship of endocrinopathy to iron chelation status in young patients with thalassaemia major. *Arch. Dis. Child.* 71: 128–132.

Gullo, L, Corcioni, E, Brancati, C et al. (1993). Morphologic and functional evaluation of the exocrine pancreas in beta-thalassemia. *Pancreas* 8: 176–180.

Gunn, RB, Silvers, ND, and Rosse, WF. (1972). Potassium permeability in β-thalassemia minor red blood cells. *J. Clin. Invest.* 51: 1043–1050.

Gutteridge, JMC and Halliwell, B. (1989). Iron toxicity and oxygen radicals. *Clin. Haematol.* 2: 195–256.

Hajiar, FM and Pearson, HA. (1994). Pharmacologic treatment of thalassemia intermedia with hydroxyurea. *J. Pediatr.* 125: 490–492.

Hallaway, PE, Eaton, JW, Panter, SS, and Hedlund, BE. (1989). Modulation of deferoxamine toxicity and clearance by covalent attachment to biocompatible polymers. *Proc. Natl. Acad. Sci. U.S.A.* 86: 10108–10112.

Hanslip, JI, Prescott, E, Lelloz, M et al. (1998). The role of the Sp1 polymorphism in the development of osteoporosis in patients with thalassemia major. *Brit. J. Haemat.* 101(Suppl. 1): 26 (Abstract 21).

Hatori, M, Sparkman, J, Teixeira, CC et al. (1995). Effects of deferoxamine on chondrocyte alkaline phosphatase activity: peroxidant role of deferoxamine in thalassemia. *Calcif. Tissue Int.* 57: 229–236.

Hazell, JW and Modell, CB. (1976). E.N.T. complications in thalassaemia major. *J. Laryngol. Otol.* 90: 877–881.

Heinrich, HC, Gabbe, EE, Oppitz, KH et al. (1973). Absorption of inorganic and food iron in children with heterozygous and homozygous beta-thalassemia. *Z. Kinderheilkd.* 115: 1–22.

Henry, WL, Nienhuis, AW, Wiener, M et al. (1978). Echocardiographic abnormalities in patients with transfusion-dependent anemia and secondary myocardial iron deposition. *Am. J. Med.* 64: 547–555.

Herington, AC, Werthe, GA, and Matthews, RNB. (1981). Studies on the possible mechanism for deficiency of non-suppressible insulin-like activity in thalassemia major. *J. Clin. Endocrinol. Metab.* 52: 393–398.

Herrick, RT and Davis, GL. (1975). Thalassemia major and non-union of pathologic fractures. *J. La. State Med. Sci.* 127: 341–347.

Hershko, C, Graham, G, Bates, CW, and Rachmilewitz, ES. (1978). Non-specific serum iron in thalassemia: An abnormal serum iron fraction of potential toxicity. *Br. J. Haematol.* 40: 255–263.

Hershko, C, Konijn, AM, and Link, G. (1998a). Iron chelators for thalassaemia. *Br. J. Haematol.* 101: 399–406.

Hershko, C, Link, G, and Cabantchik, I. (1998b). Pathophysiology of iron overload. *Ann. N. Y. Acad. Sci.* 850: 191–201.

Hider, RC, Kontoghiorghes, GJ, and Silver, J. (1982). U.K. Patent: GB-2118176.

Hillcoat, BL and Waters, AH. (1962). The survival of ^{51}Cr labelled autotransfused red cells in a patient with thalassaemia. *Aust. Med. J.* 11: 55–58.

Ho, PJ, Rochette, J, Fisher, CA et al. (1996). Moderate reduction of β-globin gene transcript by a novel mutation in the 5′ untranslated region: A study of its interaction with other genotypes in two families. *Blood* 87: 1170–1178.

Ho, PJ, Hall, GW, Luo, LY et al. (1998). Beta thalassaemia intermedia: Is it possible to predict phenotype from genotype? *Br. J. Haematol.* 100: 70–78.

Hoeper, MM, Niedermeyer, J, Hoffmeyer, F et al. (1999). Pulmonary hypertension after splenectomy. *Ann. Intern. Med.* 130: 506–509.

Hoffbrand, AV. (1996). Oral iron chelation. *Semin. Hematol.* 33: 1–8.

Hoffbrand, AV, al-Refaie, F, Davis, B et al. (1998). Long-term trial of deferiprone in 51 transfusion-dependent iron overloaded patients. *Blood* 91: 295–300.

Howell, J and Wyatt, JP. (1953). Development of pigmentary cirrhosis in Cooley's anaemia. *Arch. Pathol.* 55: 423–431.

Hoyt, RW, Scarpa, N, Wilmott, RW et al. (1986). Pulmonary function abnormalities in homozygous β-thalassemia. *J. Pediatr.* 109: 452–455.

Huang, S-Z, Wong, C, Antonarakis, SE et al. (1986). The same TATA box β-thalassemia mutation in Chinese and U.S. blacks: Another example of independent origins of mutation. *Hum. Genet.* 74: 162–164.

Huang, S-Z, Ren, ZR, Chen, M-J et al. (1994). Treatment of β-thalassemia with hydroxyurea. Effects of HU on globin gene expression. *Sci. China B.* 37: 1350–1359.

Huisman TH. (1997). Levels of Hb A2 in heterozygotes and homozygotes for beta-thalassemia mutations: Influence of mutations in the CACCC and ATAAA motifs of the beta-globin gene promoter. *Acta. Haematol.* 98: 187–194.

Huisman, THJ, Punt, K, and Schaad, JDG. (1961). Thalassemia minor associated with hemoglobin B₂ heterozygosity. *Blood* 17: 747.

Huisman, THJ, Schroeder, WA, Efremov, GD et al. (1974). The present status of the heterogeneity of fetal hemoglobin in β-thalassemia; an attempt to unify some observations in thalassemia and related conditions. *Ann. N. Y. Acad. Sci.* 232: 107–124.

Huisman, THJ, Carver, MFH, and Baysal, E. (1997). *A Syllabus of Thalassemia Mutations.* Augusta, The Sickle Cell Anemia Foundation.

Hussain, MAM, Green, N, Flint, DM et al. (1976). Subcutaneous infusion and intramuscular injection of desferrioxamine in patients with transfusional iron overload. *Lancet* 2: 1278–1280.

Hyman, CB, Landing, B, Alfin-Slater, R et al. (1974). D1-alpha-tocopherol, iron and lipofuscin in thalassemia. *Ann. N. Y. Acad. Sci.* 232: 211–220.

Hyman, CB, Ortega, JA, Costin, G, and Takahashi, M. (1980). The clinical significance of magnesium depletion in thalassaemia. *Ann. N. Y. Acad. Sci.* 344: 436–443.

Iancu, TC, Neustein, HB, and Landing, BH. (1977). The liver in thalassaemia major: Ultrastructural observations. *Iron Metabolism. Ciba Symposium No. 51.* Amsterdam, Excerpta Medica. pp. 293–316.

Issagrisil, S, Visuthisakchai, S, Suvatte, V et al. (1995). Brief report: Transplantation of cord-blood stem cells into a patient with severe thalassemia. *N. Engl. J. Med.* 332: 367–369.

Italian Working Groups on Endocrine Complications of Non-Endocrine Diseases. (1995). Multi-centre study on prevalence of endocrine complications in thalassemia major. *Clin. Endocrinol.* 42: 581–586.

Jandl, JH and Greenberg, MS. (1959). Bone marrow failure due to relative nutritional deficiency in Cooley's hemolytic anemia. *N. Engl. J. Med.* 260: 461–468.

Jean, G, Terzoli, S, Mauri, R et al. (1984). Cirrhosis associated with multiple transfusions in thalassemia. *Arch. Dis. Child.* 59: 67–70.

Jensen, PD, Jensen, FT, Christensen, T, and Ellegaard, J. (1995). Evaluation of transfusional iron overload before and during iron chelation by magnetic resonance imaging of the liver and determination of serum ferritin in adult non-thalassaemic patients. *Br. J. Haematol.* 89: 880–889.

Jensen, CE, Tuck, SM, Old, J et al. (1997). Incidence of endocrine complications and clinical disease severity related to genotype analysis and iron overload in patients with β-thalassaemia. *Eur. J. Haematol.* 59: 76–81.

Jensen, CE, Tuck, SM, Agnew, JE et al. (1998). High prevalence of low bone mass in thalassaemia major. *Br. J. Haematol.* 103: 911–915.

Jessup, M and Manno, CS. (1998). Diagnosis and management of iron-induced heart disease in Cooley's anemia. *Ann. N. Y. Acad. Sci.* 850: 242–250.

Johnsen, JK, Ibbotson, RN, and Horwood, JM. (1966). Thalassaemia minor in Australians of North European extraction: A report of five families. *Aust. Med. J.* 15: 245–250.

Johnston, FE and Roseman, JM. (1967). The effects of more frequent transfusions upon bone loss in thalassemia major. *Pediatr. Res.* 1: 479–483.

Jullien, AM, Courouce, AM, Richard, D et al. (1988). Transmission of HIV blood from seronegative donors. *Lancet* 2: 1248–1249.

Kalef-Exra, J, Challa, A, Chaliasos, N et al. (1995). Bone minerals in beta-thalassemia minor. *Bone* 16: 651–655.

Kan, YW and Nathan, DG. (1970). Mild thalassemia: The result of interactions of alpha and beta thalassemia genes. *J. Clin. Invest.* 49: 635–642.

Kan, YW, Nathan, DG, and Lodish, HF. (1972). Equal synthesis of α and β globin chains in erythroid precursors in heterozygous β thalassemia. *J. Clin. Invest.* 51: 1906–1909.

Kanavakis, E, Wainscoat, JS, Wood, WG et al. (1982). The interaction of α thalassaemia with heterozygous β thalassaemia. *Br. J. Haematol.* 52: 465–473.

Kanavakis, E, Traeger-Synodinos, J, Tzetis, M et al. (1995). Molecular characterization of homozygous (high Hb A₂) β-thalassemia intermedia in Greece. *Pediatr. Hematol. Oncol.* 12: 37–45.

Kaplan, E and Zuelzer, WW. (1950). Erythrocyte survival studies in childhood. ll. Studies in Mediterranean anemia. *J. Lab. Clin. Med.* 36: 517–523.

Karahanyan, E, Stoyaniva, A, Moumdzhiev, I, and Ivanov, I. (1994). Secondary diabetes in children with thalassaemia major (homozygous thalassaemia). *Folia Med. Plovdiv.* 35: 29–34.

Kattamis, C, Lagos, P, Metaxatou-Mavromati, A, and Matsaniotis, N. (1972). Serum iron and unsaturated iron-binding capacity in the β-thalassaemia trait: Their relation to the levels of haemoglobins A, A$_2$ and F. *J. Med. Genet.* 9: 154–159.

Kattamis, C, Ladis, V, and Metaxatou-Mavromati, A. (1975). Hemoglobins F and A$_2$ in Greek patients with homozygous β and β/δβ thalassaemia. In *Abnormal haemoglobins and thalassaemia: Diagnostic aspects.* Schmidt, RM (ed.). New York: Academic Press. pp 209–228.

Kattamis, C, Metaxatou-Mavromati, A, Wood, WG et al. (1979). The heterogeneity of normal Hb A$_2$-β thalassaemia in Greece. *Br. J. Haematol.* 42: 109–123.

Kattamis, C, Ou, H, Cheng, G et al. (1990). Molecular characterization of β-thalassaemia in 174 Greek patients with thalassaemia major. *Br. J. Haematol.* 74: 342–346.

Kaur, P and Kaur, B. (1995). Thalassemia in Penang. *Proceedings of the First Asian Congress on Thalassemia,* Penang, Malaysia. pp. 70–72 (Cited by Wonke et al. 1998.)

Kazazian, HH. (1990). The thalassemia syndromes: Molecular basis and prenatal diagnosis in 1990. *Semin. Hematol.* 27: 209–228.

Keens, TG, O'Neal, MH, Ortega, JA et al. (1980). Pulmonary function abnormalities in thalassemia patients on a hyper-transfusion program. *Pediatrics* 65: 1013–1017.

Kelly, DA, Price, E, Jani, B et al. (1987). Yersinia entercolitis in iron overload. *J. Pediatr. Gastroenterol. Nutr.* 6: 643–645.

Kevy, SV, Jacobson, MS, Fosburg, M et al. (1988). A new approach to neocyte transfusion: Preliminary report. *J. Clin. Apheresis* 4: 194–197.

Kheradpir, MH and Albouyeh, M. (1985). Partial splenectomy in the treatment of thalassaemia major. *Kinderchirurgie* 40: 195–198.

Klein, N, Sen, A, Rusby, J et al. (1998). The psychosocial burden of Cooley's anemia in affected children and their parents. *Ann. N. Y. Acad. Sci.* 850: 512–513.

Kletsky, OA, Costin, G, Marrs, RP et al. (1979). Gonadotrophin insufficiency in patients with thalassemia major. *J. Clin. Endocrinol. Metab.* 48: 901–905.

Knox-Macaulay, HHM and Weatherall, DJ. (1974). Studies of red-cell membrane function in heterozygous β thalassaemia and other hypochromic anaemias. *Br. J. Haematol.* 28: 277–297.

Knox-Macaulay, HHM, Weatherall, DJ, Clegg, JB et al. (1972). Clinical and biosynthetic characterization of αβ-thalassaemia. *Br. J. Haematol.* 22: 497–512.

Knox-Macaulay, HHM, Weatherall, DJ, Clegg, JB, and Pembrey, ME. (1973). Thalassaemia in the British. *Br. Med. J.* 2: 150–155.

Koch, LA and Shapiro, B. (1932). Erythroblastic anemia; review of cases reported showing roentgenographic changes in bones and 5 additional cases. *Am. J. Dis. Child.* 44: 318–335.

Koren, A, Garty, I, Antonelli, D, and Katzuni, E. (1987). Right ventricular cardiac dysfunction in β-thalassemia major. *Am. J. Dis. Child.* 141: 93–96.

Kremastinos, DT, Tiniakos, G, Theodorakis, GN et al. (1996). Myocarditis in beta-thalassemia major. A cause of heart failure. *Circulation* 91: 66–71.

Kumar, RM and Khuranna, A. (1998). Pregnancy outcome in women with beta-thalassemia major and HIV infection. *Eur. J. Obst. Gynecol. Reprod. Biol.* 77: 163–169.

Kumar, RM, Uduman, S, Hamo, IM et al. (1994). Incidence and clinical manifestations of HIV-1 infection in multi-transfused thalassaemia Indian children. *Trop. Geogr. Med.* 46: 163–166.

Kuo, B, Zaino, E, and Roginsky, MS. (1968). Endocrine function in thalassemia. *J. Clin. Endocrinol. Metab.* 28: 805–808.

Kutlar, A, Kutlar, F, Gu, L-G et al. (1990). Fetal hemoglobin in normal adults and β-thalassemia heterozygotes. *Hum. Genet.* 85: 106–110.

Kwan, EYW, Lee, ACW, Li, AMC et al. (1995). A cross-sectional study of growth, puberty and endocrine function in patients with thalassaemia major in Hong Kong. *J. Paediatr. Child Health* 31: 83–87.

Labie, D, Pagnier, J, Lapoumeroulie, C et al. (1985). Common haplotype dependency of high ^{G}γ-globin gene expression and high Hb F levels in β-thalassemia and sickle cell anemia patients. *Proc. Natl. Acad. Sci. U.S.A.* 82: 2111–2114.

Lai, E, Belluzzo, N, Muraca, MF et al. (1995). The prognosis for adults with thalassemia major: Sardinia. *Blood* 86: 251a.

Lai, ME, DeVirgiliis, S, Argiolu, F et al. (1993). Evaluation of antibodies to hepatitis C virus in a long-term prospective study of post-transfusion hepatitis among thalassemic children: Comparison between first and second-generation assay. *J. Pediatr. Gastroenterol. Nutr.* 16: 458–464.

Landau, H, Spitz, IM, Cividalli, C, and Rachmilewitz, EA. (1978). Gonadotrophin, thyrotrophin and prolactin reserve in β thalassemia. *Clin. Endocrinol.* 9: 163–173.

Landau, H, Matoth, I, Landau-Cordova, Z et al. (1993). Cross-sectional and longitudinal study of the pituitary-thyroid axis in patients with thalassemia major. *Clin. Endocrinol.* 38: 55–61.

Landman, H. (1988). *Haemoglobinopathies and Pregnancy.* Groningen: Van Denderen Printing.

Lassman, MN, Genel, M, Wise, JK, Hendler, R, and Felig, P. (1974a). Carbohydrate homeostasis and pancreatic islet cell function in thalassemia. *Blood* 80: 65–69.

Lassman, MN, O'Brien, RT, Pearson, HA et al. (1974b). Endocrine evaluation in thalassemia major. *Ann. N. Y. Acad. Sci.* 232: 226.

Lattanzi, F, Bellotti, P, Picano, E et al. (1993). Quantitative ultrasonic analysis of myocardium in patients with thalassemia major and iron overload. *Circulation* 87: 748–754.

Lau, YL, Chow, CB, Lee, AC et al. (1993). Hepatitis C virus antibody in multiply transfused Chinese with thalassaemia. *Bone Marrow Transplant.* 12: 26–28.

Leger, J, Girot, R, Crosnier, H et al. (1989). Normal growth hormone (GH) response to GH-releasing hormone in children with thalassemia major before puberty: A possible age-related effect. *J. Clin. Endocrinol. Metab.* 69: 453–456.

Leon, MB, Borer, JS, Bacharach, SL et al. (1979). Detection of early cardiac dysfunction in patients with severe beta-thalassemia and chronic iron overload. *N. Engl. J. Med.* 301: 1143–1148.

Letsky, EA, Miller, F, Worwood, M, and Flynn, DM. (1974). Serum ferritin in children with thalassaemia regularly transfused. *J. Clin. Pathol.* 27: 652–655.

Lichtman, HC, Watson, RJ, Feldman, F et al. (1953). Studies on thalassemia. I. An extracorpuscular defect in thalassemia major. II. The effects of splenctomy in thalassemia major with an associated acquired hemolytic anemia. *J. Clin. Invest.* 32: 1229–1235.

Link, G, Pinson, A, and Hershko, C. (1994). The ability of orally effective iron chelators dimethyl- and diethyl-hydroxypyrid-4-one and of deferoxamine to restore sarcolemmal thiolic enzyme activity in iron-loaded heart cells. *Blood* 83: 2692–2697.

Link, G, Tirosh, R, Pinson, A, and Hershko, C. (1996). Role of iron in the potentiation of anthracycline toxicity: Identification of heart cell mitochondria as the site of iron-anthracycline interaction. *J. Lab. Clin. Med.* 127: 272–278.

Liu, P, Henkelman, M, Joshi, J et al. (1996). Quantitation of cardiac and tissue iron by nuclear magnetic resonance in a novel murine thalassemia-cardiac iron overload model. *Can. J. Cardiol.* 12: 155–164.

Liu, P and Olivieri, N. (1994). Iron overload cardiomyopathies: New insights into an old disease. *Cardiovasc. Drugs Ther.* 8: 101–110.

Logothetis, J, Haritos-Fatouros, M, Constantoulakis, M et al. (1971). Intelligence and behavioral patterns in patients with Cooley's anemia (homozygous beta-thalassemia); a study based on 138 consecutive cases. *Pediatrics* 48: 740–744.

Logothetis, J, Constantoulakis, M, Economidou, J et al. (1972a). Thalassemia major (homozygous beta-thalassemia): A survey of 138 cases with emphasis on neurological and muscular aspects. *Neurology* 22: 294–304.

Logothetis, J, Loewensen, RB, Augoustaki, O et al. (1972b). Body growth in Cooley's anemia (homozygous beta-thalassemia) with a correlative study as to other aspects of the illness in 138 cases. *Pediatrics* 50: 92–99.

Lombardo, T, Tamburino, C, Bartoloni, G et al. (1995). Cardiac iron overload in thalassemic patients: An endomyocardial biopsy study. *Ann. Hematol.* 71: 135–141.

Lombardo, T, Ferro, G, Frontini, V, and Percolla, S. (1996a). High-dose intravenous desferrioxamine (DFO) delivery in four thalassemic patients allergic to subcutaneous DFO administration. *Am. J. Hematol.* 51: 90–92.

Lombardo, T, Frontini, V, Ferro, G et al. (1996b). Laboratory evaluation of a new delivery system to improve patient compliance with chelation therapy. *Clin. Lab. Haematol.* 18: 13–17.

Looareesuwan, S, Suntharasamai, P, Webster, HK, and Ho, M. (1993). Malaria in splenectomized patients: Report of four cases and review. *Clin. Infect. Dis.* 16: 361–366.

Loreal, O, Deugnier, Y, Moirand, R et al. (1992). Liver fibrosis in genetic hemochromatosis. Respective roles of iron and non-iron related factors in 127 homozygous patients. *J. Hepatol.* 16: 122–127.

Loudianos, G, Cao, A, Ristaldi, MS et al. (1990). Molecular basis of δβ-thalassemia with normal fetal hemoglobin. *Blood* 75: 526–528.

Loukopoulos, D and Fessas, P. (1965). The distribution of hemoglobin types in thalassemic erythrocytes. *J. Clin. Invest.* 44: 231–240.

Loukopoulos, D, Loutradi, A, and Fessas, P. (1978). A unique thalassaemia syndrome: Homozygous α-thalassaemia + homozygous β-thalassaemia. *Br. J. Haematol.* 39: 377–389.

Loukopoulos, D, Voskaridou, E, and Stamoulakatou, A. (1995). Clinical trials with hydroxyurea and recombinant human erythropoietin. In *Molecular Biology of Hemoglobin Switching*. Stamatoyannopoulos, G (ed.). Andover: Intercept, pp. 365–372.

Low, LC. (1997). Growth, puberty and endocrine function in β-thalassaemia major. *J. Pediatr. Endocrinol. Metab.* 10: 175–184.

Low, LC, Kwan, EYW, Lim, YJ et al. (1995). Growth hormone treatment of short Chinese children with β-thalassaemia major without growth hormone deficiency. *Clin. Endocrinol.* 42: 359–363.

Lucarelli, G, Galimberti, M, Polchi, P et al. (1990). Bone marrow transplantation in patients with thalassemia. *N. Engl. J. Med.* 322: 417–421.

Lucarelli, G, Giardini, C, and Baronciani, D. (1995). Bone marrow transplantation in β-thalassemia. *Semin. Hematol.* 32: 297–303.

Lucarelli, G, Clift, RA, Galimberti, M et al. (1996). Marrow transplantation for patients with thalassemia: Results in class 3 patients. *Blood* 87: 2082–2088.

Luhby, AL and Cooperman, JM. (1961). Folic acid deficiency in thalassaemia major. *Lancet* 2: 490–491.

Luhby, AL, Cooperman, JM, Feldman, R et al. (1961). Folic acid deficiency as a limiting factor in the anemias of thalassemia major. *Blood* 18: 786.

Luhby, AL, Cooperman, JM, Lopez, R, and Giorgio, AJ. (1969). Vitamin B_{12} metabolism in thalassemia major. *Ann. N. Y. Acad. Sci.* 165: 443–460.

Magro, S, Puzzonia, P, Consarino, C et al. (1990). Hypothyroidism in patients with thalassemia syndromes. *Acta Haematol.* 84: 72–76.

Malamos, B, Belcher, EH, Gyftaki, E, and Binopoulos, D. (1961). Simultaneous studies with Fe^{59} and Cr^{51} in congenital haemolytic anaemias. *Nucl. Med.* (Stuttgart) 2: 1–20.

Manconi, PE, Dessi, C, Sanna, G et al. (1998). Human immunodeficiency virus infection in multi-transfused patients with thalassaemia major. *Eur. J. Pediatr.* 147: 304–307.

Mancuso, L, Iacona, MA, Marchi, S et al. (1985). Severe cardiomyopathy in a woman with intermediate beta-thalassemia. Regression of cardiac failure with desferrioxamine. *G. Ital. Cardiol.* 15: 916–920.

Mancuso, P, Zingale, A, Basile, L et al. (1993). Cauda equina compression syndrome in a patient affected by thalassemia intermedia: Complete regression with blood transfusion therapy. *Childs Nerv. Sys.* 9: 440–441.

Mariotti, E, Agostini, E, Angelucci, E et al. (1997). Reversal of the initial cardiac damage in thalassemic patients treated with bone marrow transplantation and phlebotomy. *Bone Marrow Transplant.* 19: 139–141.

Martin, J, Palacio, A, Petit, J, and Martin, C. (1990). Fatty transformation of thoracic extramedullary hematopoiesis following splenectomy: CT features. *J. Comput. Assist. Tomogr.* 14: 477–478.

Masala, A, Meloni, T, Gallisai, D et al. (1984). Endocrine functioning in multitransfused prepubertal patients with homozygous beta-thalassemia. *J. Clin. Endocrinol. Metab.* 58: 667–670.

Maurer, HS, Lloyd-Still, JD, Ingrisano, C et al. (1988). A prospective evaluation of iron chelation therapy in children with severe β-thalassemia: A six-year study. *Am. J. Dis. Child.* 142: 287–292.

Mazza, U, Saglio, G, Cappio, FC et al. (1976). Clinical and haematological data in 254 cases of beta-thalassaemia trait in Italy. *Br. J. Haematol.* 33: 91–99.

Mazzoleni, G, de Sa, D, Gately, J, and Riddell, RH. (1991). Yersinia entercolotica infection with ileal perforation associated with iron overload and deferoxamine therapy. *Dig. Dis. Sci.* 36: 1154–1160.

McDonagh, KT, Orringer, EP, Dover, GJ, and Nienhuis, AW. (1990). Hydroxyurea improves erythropoiesis in a patient with homozygous beta thalassemia. *Clin. Res.* 38: 346A.

McIntosh, N. (1976). Endocrinopathy in thalassaemia major. *Arch. Dis. Child.* 51: 195–201.

Mela, QS, Cacace, E, Ruggiero, V et al. (1987). Virus infection in β-thalassaemia intermedia. *Birth Defects Orig. Artic. Ser.* 23: 557–564.

Melis, MA, Pirastu, M, Galanello, R et al. (1983). Phenotypic effect of heterozygous α and β0-thalassemia interaction. *Blood* 62: 226–229.

Merkel, PA, Simonson, DC, Amiel, SA et al. (1988). Insulin resistance and hyperinsulinemia in patients with thalassemia major treated by hypertransfusion. *N. Engl. J. Med.* 318: 809–814.

Metaxotou-Mavromati, AD, Antonopoulou, HK, Laskari, SS et al. (1982). Developmental changes in hemoglobin F levels during the first two years of life in normal and heterozygous β-thalassemia infants. Pediatrics 69: 734–738.

Michaeli, J, Mittelman, M, Grisaru, D, and Rachmilewitz, EA. (1992). Thromboembolic complications in beta thalassemia major. *Acta Haematol.* 87: 71–74.

Michelson, J and Cohen, A. (1988). Incidence and treatment of fractures in thalassemia. *J. Orthop. Trauma* 2: 29–32.

Middlemis, JH and Raper, AB. (1966). Skeletal changes in the haemogobinopathies. *J. Bone Joint Surg.* 48: 693.

Miller, KB, Rosenwasser, LJ, Bessette, JA et al. (1981). Rapid desensitisation for desferrioxamine anaphylactic reaction. *Lancet* 1: 1059.

Modell, CB. (1976). Management of thalassaemia major. *Br. Med. Bull.* 32: 270–276.

Modell, CB. (1977). Total management in thalassaemia major. *Arch. Dis. Child.* 52: 489–500.

Modell, CB and Beck, J. (1974). Long-term desferrioxamine therapy in thalassemia. *Ann. N. Y. Acad. Sci.* 232: 201–210.

Modell, CB and Berdoukas, VA. (1984). *The Clinical Approach to Thalassaemia.* New York: Grune & Stratton.

Modell, CB, Latter, A, Steadman, JH, and Huehns, ER. (1969). Haemoglobin synthesis in β-thalassaemia. *Br. J. Haematol.* 17: 485–501.

Modell, CB and Matthews, R. (1976). Thalassemia in Britain and Australia. *Birth Defects: Original Article Series.* New York: Liss. pp. 13–29.

Murru, S, Loudianos, G, Deiana, M et al. (1991). Molecular characterization of β-thalassemia intermedia in patients of Italian descent and identification of three novel β-thalassemia mutations. *Blood* 77: 1342–1347.

Murru, S, Loudianos, G, Porcu, S et al. (1992). A β-thalassaemia phenotype not linked to the β-globin cluster in an Italian family. *Br. J. Haematol.* 81: 283–287.

Najean, Y, Deschryver, F, Henni, T, and Girot, R. (1985). Red cell kinetics in thalassaemia intermedia: Its use for a prospective prognosis. *Br. J. Haematol.* 59: 533–539.

Nathan, DG and Gunn, RB. (1966). Thalassemia: The consequences of unbalanced hemoglobin synthesis. *Am. J. Med.* 41: 815–830.

Nathan, DG, Stossel, TB, Gunn, RB et al. (1969). Influence of hemoglobin precipitation on erythrocyte metabolism in alpha and beta thalassemia. *J. Clin. Invest.* 48: 33–41.

Niederau, C, Fischer, R, Purschel, A et al. (1996). Long-term survival in patients with hereditary hemochromatosis. *Gastroenterology* 110: 1304–1307.

Nienhuis, AW. (1981). Vitamin C and iron. *N. Engl. J. Med.* 304: 170–171.

Nienhuis, AW, Ley, TJ, Humphries, RK, and Young, NS. (1985). Pharmacological manipulation of fetal hemoglobin synthesis in patients with severe beta thalassemia. *Ann. N. Y. Acad. Sci.* 445: 198–211.

O'Brien, RT. (1974). Ascorbic acid enhancement of desferrioxamine induced urinary iron excretion in thalassemia major. *Ann. N. Y. Acad. Sci.* 232: 221–225.

O'Brien, RT, Pearson, HA, and Spencer, RP. (1972). Transfusion induced decrease in spleen size in thalassemia major: Documentation by radioisotope scan. *J. Pediatr.* 81: 105–107.

Oberklaid, F and Seshadri, R. (1975). Hypoparathyroidism and other endocrine dysfunction complicating thalassaemia major. *Med. J. Aust.* 1: 304–306.

Okon, E, Levij, IS, and Rachmilewitz, EA. (1976). Splenectomy, iron overload and liver cirrhosis in beta-thalassemia major. *Acta Haematol.* 56: 142–150.

Olds, RJ, Sura, T, Jackson, B et al. (1991). A novel δ0 mutation in cis with Hb Knossos: A study of different genetic interactions in three Egyptian families. *Br. J. Haematol.* 78: 430–436.

Olivieri, NF. (1996a). Long-term follow-up of body iron in patients with thalassemia major during therapy with the orally active iron chelator deferiprone (L1). *Blood* 88: 310a.

Olivieri, NF. (1996b). Randomized trial of deferiprone (L1) and deferoxamine (DFO) in thalssemia major. *Blood* 88: 651a.

Olivieri, NF and Brittenham, GM. (1997). Iron-chelating therapy and the treatment of thalassemia. *Blood* 89: 739–761.

Olivieri, NF, Koren, G, Hermann, C et al. (1990). Comparison of oral iron chelator L1 and desferrioxamine in iron-loaded patients. *Lancet* 336: 1275–1279.

Olivieri, NF and Weatherall, DJ. (1998). The therapeutic reactivation of fetal haemoglobin. *Hum. Mol. Gene.* 7: 1655–1658.

Olivieri, NF, Ramachandran, S, Tyler, B et al. (1990b). Diabetes mellitus in older patients with thalassemia major: Relationship to severity of iron overload and presence of microvascular complications. *Blood* 76: 72a.

Olivieri, NF, Berriman, AM, Davis, SA et al. (1992a). Continuous intravenous administration of deferoxamine in adults with severe iron overload. *Am. J. Hematol.* 41: 61–63.

Olivieri, NF, Koren, G, Matsui, D et al. (1992b). Reduction of tissue iron stores and normalization of serum ferritin during treatment with the oral iron chelator L1 in thalassemia intermedia. *Blood* 79: 2741–2748.

Olivieri, NF, Nathan, DG, MacMillan, JH et al. (1994). Survival of medically treated patients with homozygous β thalassemia. *N. Engl. J. Med.* 331: 574–578.

Olivieri, NF, Brittenham, GM, Matsui, D et al. (1995). Iron-chelation therapy with oral deferiprone in patients with thalassemia major. *N. Engl. J. Med.* 332: 918–922.

Olivieri, NF, Rees, DC, Ginder, GD et al. (1997). Treatment of thalassaemia major with phenylbutyrate and hydroxyurea. *Lancet* 350: 491–492.

Olivieri, NF, Brittenham, GM, McLaren, CE et al. (1998). Long-term safety and effectiveness of iron chelation therapy with deferiprone for thalassemia major. *N. Engl. J. Med.* 339: 417–423.

Olynyk, JK and Bacon, BR. (1995). Hepatitis C. Recent advances in understanding and management. *Postgrad. Med. J.* 98: 79–81.

Öner, R, Altay, C, Aksoy, M et al. (1990). β-thalassemia in Turkey. *Hemoglobin* 14: 1–13.

Orkin, SH, Antonarakis, SE, and Kazazian, HHJ. (1984). Base substitution at position -88 in a β-thalassemic globin gene. Further evidence for the role of distal promoter element ACACCC. *J. Biol. Chem.* 259: 8679–8681.

Orkin, SH, Cheng, T-C, Antonarakis, SE, and Kazazian, HH. (1985). Thalassaemia due to a mutation in the cleavage-polyadenylation signal of the human β-globin gene. *EMBO J.* 4: 453–456.

Orsini, A, Louchet, E, Raybaud, C et al. (1970). Les pericardites de la maladie de Cooley. *Pediatrie* 15: 831–842.

Orvieto, R, Leichter, I, Rachmilewitz, EA, and Margulies, JY. (1992). Bone density, mineral content, and cortical index in patients with thalassemia major and the correlation to their bone fractures, blood transfusions, and treatment with desferrioxamine. *Calc. Tissue Int.* 50: 397–399.

Paik, CH, Alavi, L, Dunea, G, and Weiner, L. (1970). Thalassemia and gouty arthritis. *J. Am. Med. Assoc.* 213: 296–297.

Panizon, F and Vullo, C. (1952). Sulla envoluzione della siderosi e fibrosi epatica nella malattia di Cooley. Studio bioptico su 20 casi. *Acta Paediatr. Lat.* 10: 71.

Papavasiliou, C, Gouliamos, A, Vlahos, L, Trakadas, S et al. (1990). CT and MRI of symptomatic spinal involvement by extramedullary haemopoiesis. *Clin. Radiol.* 42: 91–92.

Parkes, JG, Randell, EW, Olivieri, NF, and Templeton, DM. (1995). Modulation by iron loading and chelation of the uptake of non-transferrin-bound iron by human liver cells. *Biochim. Biophy. Acta* 1243: 373–380.

Pavri, RS, Baxi, AJ, Grover, S, and Parande, RA. (1977). Study of glycolytic intermediates in hereditary elliptocytosis with thalassemia. *J. Postgrad. Med.* 23: 189–192.

Pearson, HA, McFarland, W, and King, ER. (1960). Erythrokinetic studies in thalassemia trait. *J. Lab. Clin. Med.* 56: 866.

Perignon, F, Brauner, R, Souberbielle, JC et al. (1993). Growth and endocrine function in thalassemia major. *Arch. Fr. Pediatr.* 50: 657–663.

Perillie, PE and Chernoff, AI. (1965). Heterozygous beta-thalassemia in association with hereditary elliptocytosis. *Blood* 25: 494–501.

Perrine, SP, Rudolph, A, Faller, DV et al. (1988). Butyrate infusions in the ovine fetus delay the biologic clock for globin gene switching. *Proc. Natl. Acad. Sci. U.S.A.* 85: 8540–8542.

Perrine, SP, Ginder, GD, Faller, DV et al. (1993). A short-term trial of butyrate to stimulate fetal-globin-gene expression in the β-globin disorders. *N. Engl. J. Med.* 328: 81–86.

Perrine, SP, Dover, GH, Daftari, P et al. (1994). Isaobutyramide, an orally bioavailable butyrate analogue, stimulates fetal globin gene expression *in vitro* and *in vivo*. *Br. J. Haematol.* 88: 555–561.

Pignatti, CB, Carneli, V, Caruso, V et al. (1998). Thromboembolic events in beta thalassemia major: An Italian multicenter study. *Acta Haematol.* 99: 76–79.

Pintor, C, Cella, SG, Manso, P et al. (1986). Impaired growth hormone (GH) response to GH-releasing hormone in thalassemia major. *J. Clin. Endocrinol. Metab.* 62: 263–267.

Piomelli, S, Danoff, SJ, Becker, MH et al. (1969). Prevention of bone malformations and cardiomegaly in Cooley's anemia by early hypertransfusion regimen. *Ann. N. Y. Acad. Sci.* 165: 427.

Piomelli, S, Seaman, C, Reibman, J et al. (1978). Separation of younger red cells with improved survival *in vivo*: An approach to chronic transfusion therapy. *Proc. Natl. Acad. Sci. U.S.A.* 75: 3474–3478.

Piomelli, S and Siniscalco, M. (1969). The haematological effects of glucose-6-phosphate dehydrogenase deficiency and thalassaemia trait: Interaction between the two genes at the phenotype level. *Br. J. Haematol.* 16: 537–549.

Pippard, MJ. (1989). Measurement of iron status. *Progr. Clin. Biol. Res.* 309: 85–92.

Pippard, MJ, Callender, ST, and Weatherall, DJ. (1978). Intensive iron-chelation therapy with desferrioxamine in iron loading patients. *Clin. Sci. Mol. Med.* 54: 99–106.

Pippard, MJ and Wainscoat, JS. (1987). Erythrokinetics and iron status in heterozygous β thalassaemia, and the effect of interaction with α thalassaemia. *Br. J. Haemat.* 66: 123–127.

Pippard, MJ, Warner, GT, Callender, ST, and Weatherall, DJ. (1979). Iron absorption and loading in β-thalassaemia intermedia. *Lancet* 2: 819–821.

Pippard, MJ, Rajagopalan, B, Callender, ST, and Weatherall, DJ. (1982). Iron loading, chronic anaemia, and erythroid hyperplasia as determinants of the clinical features of β-thalassaemia intermedia. In *Advances in red blood cell biology*. Weatherall, DG, Fiorelli, G and Govini, S. (eds) New York: Raven Press. pp. 103–113.

Pippard, MJ and Weatherall, DJ. (1984). Iron absorption in non-transfused iron loading anaemias: Prediction of risk for iron loading, and response to iron chelation treatment, in β thalassaemia and congenital sideroblastic anaemias. *Haematologica* 17: 17–24.

Politis, C. (1989). Complications of blood transfusion in thalassemia. In *Advances and controversies in thalassemia therapy: Bone marrow transplantation and other approaches.* Buckner, CD, Gale, RP and Lucarelli, G (eds). New York: Alan R. Liss. pp. 67–76.

Politis, C, Roumeliotou, A, Germenis, A, and Papaevangelou, G. (1986). Risk of acquired immune deficiency syndrome in multi-transfused patients with thalassemia major. *Plasma Ther. Transfus. Technol.* 7: 41–43.

Politis, C, Spigos, DG, Georgiopoulou, P et al. (1987). Partial splenic embolisation for hypersplenism of thalassaemia major: Five year follow-up. *Br. Med. J.* 294: 665–667.

Polliack, A and Rachmilewitz, EA. (1973). Ultrastructural studies in β-thalassaemia major. *Br. J. Haematol.* 24: 319–326.

Pootrakul, P, Wasi, P, and Na-Nakorn, S. (1973). Haematological data in 312 cases of β thalassaemia trait in Thailand. *Br. J. Haematol.* 24: 703–712.

Pootrakul, P, Rugkiatsakul, R, and Wasi, P. (1980). Increased transferrin iron saturation in splenectomized thalassaemia patients. *Br. J. Haematol.* 46: 143–145.

Pootrakul, P, Kitcharoen, K, Yansukon, P et al. (1988). The effect of erythroid hyperplasia on iron balance. *Blood* 71: 1124–1129.

Poovorawan, Y, Theamboonlers, A, Chongsrisawat, V, and Jantaradsamee, P. (1998). Prevalence of infection with hepatitis G virus among various groups in Thailand. *Ann. Trop. Med. Parasitol.* 92: 89–95.

Popat, N, Wood, WG, Weatherall, DJ, and Turnbull, AC. (1977). The pattern of maternal F-cell production during pregnancy. *Lancet* 2: 377–379.

Porter, J and Huehns, ER. (1989). The toxic effects of desferrioxamine. *Clin. Haematol.* 2: 459–474.

Prankerd, TAJ. (1963). The spleen and anaemia. *Br. Med. J.* 2: 517–524.

Prasad, AS, Diwany, M, Gabr, M et al. (1965). Biochemical studies in thalassemia. *Ann. Intern. Med.* 62: 87–96.

Prati, D, Zanella, A, Bosoni, P, Rebulla, P et al. (1998). The incidence and natural course of transfusion-associated GB virus C/hepatitis G virus infection in a cohort of thalassemic patients. The Cooleycare Cooperative Group. *Blood* 91: 774–777.

Pratico, G, Di Gregorio, F, Caltabiano, L, Palano, GM et al. (1998). Calcium phosphate metabolism in thalassemia. *Pediatr. Med. Chir.* 20: 265–268.

Preston, H and Wright, TL. (1996). Interferon therapy for hepatitis C. *Lancet* 348: 973–974.

Psichogiou, M, Tzala, E, Boletis, J, Zakopoulou, N et al. (1996). Hepatitis E virus infection in individuals at high risk of transmission of non-A, non-B hepatitis and sexually[???]

Rachmilewitz, EA. (1976). The role of intracellular hemoglobin precipitation, low MCHC and iron overload on red blood cell membrane peroxidation in thalassemia. *Birth Defects: Original Articles Series.* New York: Liss. p. 123.

Rachmilewitz, EA, Shifter, A, and Kahane, I. (1979). Vitamin E deficiency in β-thalassaemia major: Changes in hematological and biochemical parameters after a therapeutic trial with α-tocopherol. *Am. J. Clin. Nutr.* 32: 1850–1858.

Reemsta, K and Elliot, RH. (1956). Splenectomy in Mediterranean anemia: An evaluation of long-term results. *Ann. Surg.* 144: 999–1007.

Rees, DC, Basran, RK, Hum, B et al. (1998). Genetic influences on bone disease in thalassemia. *Blood* 92 (Suppl. 1): 532.

Rees, DC, Clegg, JB, and Weatherall, DJ. (1999). Why are haemoglobin F levels raised in Hb E/β thalassaemia? *Blood,* 94: 3199–3204.

Richardson, ME, Matthews, RN, Alison, JF et al. (1993). Prevention of heart disease by subcutaneous desferrioxamine in patients with thalassaemia major. *Aust. N. Z. J. Med.* 23: 656–661.

Rifkind, RA. (1965). Heinz body anemia: An ultrastructural study. II. Red cell sequestration and destruction. *Blood* 26: 433–448.

Rigano, P, Manfré, L, La Galla, R et al. (1997). Clinical and hematologic response to hydroxyurea in patients with Hb Lepore/β-thalassemia. *Hemoglobin* 21: 219–226.

Risdon, AR, Barry, M, and Fynn, DM. (1975). Transfusional iron overload: The relationship between tissue iron concentration and hepatic fibrosis in thalassemia. *J. Pathol.* 116: 83–95.

Ristaldi, MS, Pirastu, M, Murru, S et al. (1990). A spontaneous mutation produced a novel elongated β^0 globin chain structural variant (Hb Agnana) with a thalassemia-like phenotyope. *Blood* 75: 1378–1380.

Robert-Guroff, M, Giardina, PJ et al. (1987). HTLV III neutralizing antibody development in transfusion-dependent seropositive patients with β-thalassemia. *J. Immunol.* 138: 3731–3736.

Roberts, IAG, Darbyshire, PJ, and Will, AM. (1997). B.M.T. for children with β-thalassemia major in the U.K. *Bone Marrow Transplant.* 19 (Suppl. 2): 60–61.

Robins-Browne, RM and Prpic, JK. (1985). Effects of iron and desferrioxamine in infections with *Yersinia enterocolitica. Infect. Immunol.* 47: 774–779.

Rodda, CP, Reid, ED, Johnson, S et al. (1995). Short stature in homozygous β-thalassaemia is due to disproportionate truncal shortening. *Clin. Endocrinol.* 42: 587–592.

Roeser, HP, Halliday, JW, and Sizemore, DEA. (1980). Serum ferritin in ascorbic acid deficiency. *Br. J. Haematol.* 45: 457–466.

Ros, G, Seynhaeve, V, and Fiasse, L. (1976). Beta+-thalassaemia, haemoglobin A and hereditary elliptocytosis in a Zairian family. Ischaemic costal necroses in a child with sickle-cell beta+ thalassaemia. *Acta Haematol.* 56: 241–252.

Rosatelli, C, Oggiano, L, Leoni, GB et al. (1989). Thalassemia intermedia resulting from a mild beta-thalassemia mutation. *Blood* 73: 601–605.

Rosatelli, C, Leoni, GB, Tuveri, T et al. (1992). Heterozygous β-thalassemia: Relationship between the hematological phenotype and the type of β-thalassemia mutation. *Am. J. Hematol.* 39: 1–4.

Roth, C, Pekrun, A, Bartz, M et al. (1997). Short stature and failure of pubertal development in thalassaemia major: Evidence for hypothalamic neurosecretory dysfunction of growth hormone secretion and defective pituitary gonadotropin secretion. *Eur. J. Pediatr.* 156: 777–783.

Rubin, RB, Barton, AL, Banner, BF, and Bonkovsky, HL. (1995). Iron and chronic viral hepatitis: Emerging evidence for an important interaction. *Dig. Dis.* 13: 223–238.

Ruf, A, Pick, M, Deutsch, V et al. (1997). *In vivo* platelet activation correlates with red cell anionic phospholipid exposure in patients with β-thalassaemia major. *Br. J. Haematol.* 98: 51–56.

Rund, D, Filon, D, Dowling, C et al. (1990). Molecular studies of β-thalassemia in Israel. Mutational analysis and expression studies. *Ann. N. Y. Acad. Sci.* 612: 98–105.

Rund, D, Oron-Karni, V, Filon, D et al. (1997). Genetic analysis of β-thalassemia intermedia in Israel: Diversity of mechanisms and unpredictability of phenotype. *Am. J. Hematol.* 54: 16–22.

Rutter, M and Graham, P. (1968). The reliability and validity of psychiatric assessment of the child: Interview with the child. *Br. J. Psychiatry* 114: 581–592.

Sabato, A, De Sanctis, V, Atti, G et al. (1983). Primary hypothyroidism and the low T3 syndrome in thalassemia major. *Arch. Dis. Child.* 58: 120–127.

Saenger, P, Schwartz, E, Markenson, AL et al. (1980). Depressed serum somatomedin activity in beta-thalassemia. *J. Pediatr.* 96: 214–218.

Safaya, S, Rieder, RF, Dowling, CE et al. (1989). Homozygous β-thalassemia without anemia. *Blood* 73: 324–328.

Sampietro, M, Cazzola, M, Cappellini, MD, and Fiorelli, G. (1983). The triplicated alpha-gene locus and heterozygous beta thalassaemia: A case of thalassaemia intermedia. *Br. J. Haematol.* 55: 709–710.

Sampietro, M, Lupica, L, Perrero, L et al. (1997). The expression of uridine diphosphate glucuronosyltransferase gene is a major determinant of bilirubin level in heterozygous β-thalassaemia and in glucose-6-phosphate dehydrogenase deficiency. *Br. J. Haematol.* 99: 437–439.

Sanna, G, Frau, F, Melis, MA et al. (1980). Interaction between glucose-6-phosphate dehydrogenase deficiency and thalassaemia genes at phenotype level. *Br. J. Haematol.* 44: 555–561.

Santamaria, F, Villa, MP, Werner, B et al. (1994). The effect of transfusion on pulmonary function in patients with thalassemia major. *Pediatr. Pulmon.* 18: 139–143.

Saudek, CD, Hemm, RM, and Peterson, CM. (1977). Abnormal glucose tolerance in beta-thalassemia major. *Metabolism* 26: 43–52.

Saxon, BR, Rees, D, and Olivieri, NF. (1998). Regression of extramedullary haemopoiesis and augmentation of fetal haemoglobin concentration during hydroxyurea therapy in β thalassaemia. *Br. J. Haematol.* 101: 416–419.

Scacchi, M, Damesi, L, De Martin, M et al. (1991). Treatment with biosynthetic growth hormone of short thalassaemic patients with impaired growth hormone secretion. *Clin. Endocrinol.* 35: 335–339.

Scerri, CA, Abela, W, Galdies, R et al. (1993). The β+ IVS, I-NT no. 6 (T→C) thalassaemia in heterozygotes with an associated Hb Valletta or Hb S heterozygosity in homozygotes from Malta. *Br. J. Haematol.* 83: 669–671.

Schanfield, MS, Scalise, G, Economidou, I et al. (1975). Immunogenetic factors in thalassemia and hepatitis B infection. A multicentre study. *Dev. Biol. Stand.* 30: 257–269.

Schellhammer, PF, Engle, MA, and Hagstrom, JWC. (1967). Histochemical studies of the myocardium and conduction system in acquired iron-storage disease. *Circulation* 35: 631–637.

Schokker, RC, Went, LN, and Bok, J. (1966). A new genetic variant of beta-thalassaemia. *Nature* 209: 44–46.

Schroeder, WA and Huisman, THJ. (1970). Nonallelic structural genes and hemoglobin synthesis. *XIIth International Congress of Hematology. Plenary Sessions.* Lehmanns, Munich.

Schuman, JE, Tanser, CL, Peloquin, R, and de Leeuw, NKM. (1973). The erythropoietic response to pregnancy in β thalassaemia minor. *Br. J. Haematol.* 25: 249–260.

Schwartz, E. (1969). The silent carrier of beta thalassaemia. *N. Engl. J. Med.* 281: 1327–1333.

Schwartz, E. (1970). Heterozygous beta thalassemia: Balanced globin synthesis in bone marrow cells. *Science* 167: 1513–1514.

Schwartz, E, Cohen, A, and Surrey, S. (1988). Overview of the β thalassemias: Genetic and clinical aspects. *Hemoglobin* 12: 551–564.

Selwyn, JG and Dacie, JV. (1954). Autohemolysis and other changes resulting from the incubation in vitro of red cells from patients with congenital hemolytic anemia. *Blood* 9: 414.

Semenza, GL, Delgrosso, K, Poncz, M et al. (1984). The silent carrier allele: β thalassemia without a mutation in the β-globin gene or its immediate flanking regions. *Cell* 39: 123–128.

Sen, S, Mishra, NM, Giri, T et al. (1993). Acquired immunodeficiency syndrome (AIDS) in multitransfused children with thalassemia. *Ind. Pediatr.* 30: 455–460.

Seracchioli, R, Porcu, E, Colombi, C et al. (1994). Transfusion-dependent homozygous β-thalassaemia major: Successful twin pregnancy following *in vitro* fertilization and tubal embryo transfer. *Hum. Reprod.* 9: 1964–1965.

Shalit, M, Tedeschi, A, Miadonna, A, and Levi-Shaffer, A. (1991). Desferal (desferrioxamine)—a novel activator of connective tissue-type mast cells. *J. Allergy Clin. Immunol.* 6: 854–860.

Shehadeh, N, Hazani, A, Rudolf, MCJ et al. (1990). Neurosecretory dysfunction of growth hormone secretion in thalassaemia major. *Acta Paediatr. Scand.* 79: 790–795.

Sher, GD, Ginder, G, Little, JA et al. (1995). Extended therapy with arginine butyrate in patients with thalassemia and sickle cell disease. *N. Engl. J. Med.* 332: 106–110.

Sherlock, S. (1995). Antiviral therapy for chronic hepatitis C viral infection. *J. Hepatol.* 23: 3–7.

Short, EM, Winkle, RA, and Billingham, ME. (1981). Myocardial involvement in idiopathic hemochromatosis. Morphologic and clinical improvement following venisection. *Am. J. Med.* 70: 1275–1279.

Silprasert, A, Laokuldilok, T, and Kulapongs, P. (1998). Zinc deficiency in β-thalassemic children. *Birth Defects: Original Articles Series* 23: 473–476.

Silva, AE and Varella-Garcia, M. (1989). Plasma folate and vitamin B$_{12}$ levels in β-thalassemia heterozygotes. *Braz. J. Med. Biol. Res.* 22: 1225–1226.

Silvestroni, E, Bianco, I, Graziani, B, and Carboni, C. (1978). Heterozygous β-thalassaemia with normal haemoglobin pattern. *Acta Haematol.* 59: 332–340.

Simon, TL, Sohmer, P, and Nelson, EF. (1989). Extended survival of neocytes produced by a new system. *Transfusion* 29: 221–225.

Sinniah, D, Vegnaendra, V, and Kammaruddin, A. (1977). Neurological complications of beta-thalassaemia major. *Arch. Dis. Child.* 52: 977–979.

Skarsgard, E, Doski, J, Jaksic, T et al. (1993). Thrombosis of the portal venous system after splenectomy for pediatric hematologic disease. *J. Pediatr. Surg.* 28: 1109–1112.

Sklar, CA, Lew, LQ, Yoon, DJ, and David, R. (1987). Adrenal function in thalassemia major following long-term treatment with multiple transfusions and chelation therapy. Evidence for dissociation of cortisol and adrenal androgen secretion. *Am. J. Dis. Child.* 141: 327–330.

Smith, CH, Schulman, I, Ando, RE, and Stern, G. (1955). Studies in Mediterranean (Cooley's) anemia. I. Clinical and hematologic aspects of splenectomy with special reference to fetal hemoglobin synthesis. *Blood* 10: 582–599.

Smith, CH, Erlandson, ME, Stern, G, and Scholman, I. (1960). The role of splenectomy in the management of thalassemia. *Blood* 15: 197–211.

Smith, CH, Erlandson, ME, Stern, G, and Hilgartner, MW. (1962). Postsplenectomy infection in Cooley's anemia. An appraisal of the problem in this and other blood disorders, with consideration of prophylaxis. *N. Engl. J. Med.* 266: 737–743.

Smith, CH, Erlandson, ME, and Hilgartner, H. (1964). Postsplenectomy infection in Cooley's anemia. *Ann. N. Y. Acad. Sci.* 119: 748–757.

Smith, PR, Manjoney, DL, Teitcher, JB et al. (1988). Massive hemothorax due to intrathoracic extramedullary hematopoiesis in a patient with thalassemia intermedia. *Chest* 94: 658–660.

Sonakul, D. (1989). *Pathology of Thalassaemic Diseases.* Thailand: Amarin Printing Group.

Sonakul, D, Pacharee, P, and Thakerngpol, K. (1988a). Pathologic findings in 76 autopsy cases of thalassemia. *Birth Defects: Original Articles Series* 23: 157–176.

Sonakul, D, Suwananagool, P, Sirivaidyapong, P, and Fucharoen, S. (1988b). Distribution of pulmonary thromboembolic lesions in thalassemic patients. *Birth Defects: Original Articles Series* 23: 375–384.

Spanos, T, Ladis, V, Palamidou, F et al. (1996). The impact of neocyte transfusion in the management of thalassaemia. *Vox Sanger* 70: 217–223.

Spirito, P, Lupi, G, Melevendi, C, and Vecchio, C. (1990). Restrictive diastolic abnormalities identified by Doppler echocardiography in patients with thalassemia major. *Circulation* 82: 88–94.

Stamatoyannopoulos, G, Woodson, R, Papayannopoulou, T et al. (1974). Inclusion-body β-thalassemia trait. A form of β thalassemia producing clinical manifestations in simple heterozygotes. *N. Engl. J. Med.* 290: 939–943.

Stefanis, L, Kanavakis, E, Traeger-Synodinos, J et al. (1994). I: Hematologic phenotype of the mutations IVS1-n6 (T→C), IVS1-n110 (G→A), and CD39 (C→T) in carriers of beta-thalassemia in Greece. *Pediatr. Hematol. Oncol.* 11: 509–517.

Steinberg, MH. (1993). Case report: Effects of iron deficiency and the -88 C→T mutation on Hb A$_2$ levels in β-thalassaemia. *Am. J. Med. Sci.* 305: 312–313.

Stransky, J. (1996). The discovery of hepatitis G virus. *Cas. Lek. Cesk.* 135: 99–101.

Sturgeon, P, Itano, HA, and Bergren, WR. (1955). Genetic and biochemical studies of 'intermediate' types of Cooley's anaemia. *Br. J. Haematol.* 1: 264–277.

Swank, RA and Stamatoyannopoulos, G. (1998). Fetal gene reactivation. *Curr. Opin. Genet. Dev.* 8: 366–370.

Swarup-Mitra, S, Ghosh, SK, and Chatterjea, JB. (1969). Haemolytic anaemia due to interaction of genes for spherocytosis and beta-thalassaemia. *Ind. J. Med. Res.* 57: 1842–1845.

Tai, DYH, Wang, YT, Lou, J et al. (1996). Lungs in thalassaemia major parients receiving regular transfusion. *Eur. Respir.* 9: 1389–1394.

Takihara, Y, Nakamura, T, Yamada, H et al. (1986). A novel mutation in the TATA box in a Japanese patient with β⁺-thalassemia. *Blood* 67: 547–550.

Tamagnini, GP, Lopes, MC, Castanheira, ME et al. (1983). β⁺ thalassaemia—Portuguese type: Clinical, haematological and molecular studies of a newly defined form of β thalassaemia. *Br. J. Haematol.* 54: 189–200.

Tampakoudis, P, Tsatalas, C, Mamopoulos, M et al. (1997). Transfusion-dependent homozygous β-thalassaemia major: Successful pregnancy in five cases. *Eur. J. Obstet. Gynecol. Reprod. Biol.* 74: 127–131.

Tas, I, Smith, P, and Cohen, T. (1976). Metric and morphologic characteristics of the dentition in beta thalassaemia major in man. *Arch. Oral Biol.* 21: 583–586.

Thakerngpol, K, Fucharoen, S, Boonyaphipat, P et al. (1996). Liver injury due to iron overload in thalassemia: Histopathologic and ultrastructural studies. *Biometals* 9: 177–183.

Thein, SL. (1993). β-thalassaemia. *Baillière's Clinical Haematology. International Practice and Research: The Haemoglobinopathies.* London: Baillière Tindall. pp. 151–176.

Thein, SL, Al-Hakim, I, and Hoffbrand, AV. (1984). Thalassaemia intermedia: A new molecular basis. *Br. J. Haematol.* 56: 333–337.

Thein, SL, Sampietro, M, Old, JM et al. (1987). Association of thalassaemia intermedia with a beta-globin gene haplotype. *Br. J. Haematol.* 65: 370–373.

Thein, SL, Hesketh, C, Wallace, RB, and Weatherall, DJ. (1988). The molecular basis of thalassaemia major and thalassaemia intermedia in Asian Indians: Application to prenatal diagnosis. *Br. J. Haematol.* 70: 225–231.

Thein, SL and Weatherall, DJ. (1989). A non-deletion hereditary persistence of fetal hemoglobin (HPFH) determinant not linked to the β-globin gene complex. In Stamatoyannopoulos, G and Nienhuis, AW, editors, *Hemoglobin switching, part B: Cellular and molecular mechanisms.* New York: Alan R. Liss. pp. 97–112.

Thein, SL, Wood, WG, Wickramasinghe, SN, and Galvin, MC. (1993). β-thalassemia unlinked to the β-globin gene in an English family. *Blood* 82: 961–967.

Tin, F, Magrin, S, Crax, A, and Pagliaro, L. (1991). Interferon for non-A, non-B chronic hepatitis: A meta-analysis of randomized clinical trials. *J. Hepatol.* 13: 192–199.

Toccafondi, R, Maioli, M, and Meloni, T. (1970a). The plasma HGH and 11-OHCS response to insulin induced hypoglycaemia in children affected by thalassaemia major. *Riv. Clin. Med.* 70: 102–109.

Toccafondi, R, Maioli, M, and Meloni, T. (1970b). Plasma insulin response to oral carbohydrate in Cooley's anemia. *Riv. Clin. Med.* 70: 96–101.

Tolis, G, Politis, C, Kontopoulou, I, Poulatzas, N et al. (1988). Pituitary somatotropic and corticotropic function in patients with β-thalassaemia on iron chelation therapy. *Birth Defects* 23: 449–452.

Tolot, F, Bocquet, B, and Baron, M. (1970). Hemochromatosis and pigmentary cirrhosis in minor thalassemia in adults. *J. Med. Lyon* 51: 655–660.

Tondury, P, Kontoghiorghes, GJ, Ridolfi-Luthy, A et al. (1990). L1 (1,2- dimethyl-3-hydroxyprid-4-one) for oral iron chelation in patients with beta-thalassaemia major *Br. J. Haematol.* 76: 550–553.

Traeger-Synodinos, J, Kanavakis, E, Vrettou, C et al. (1996). The triplicated α-globin gene locus in β-thalassaemia heterozygotes: Clinical, haematological, biosynthetic and molecular studies. *Br. J. Haematol.* 95: 467–471.

Trifillis, P, Ioannou, P, Schwartz, E, and Surrey, S. (1991). Identification of four novel δ-globin gene mutations in Greek Cypriots using polymerase chain reaction and automated fluorescence-based DNA sequence analysis. *Blood* 78: 3298–3305.

Tsiantis, J. (1990). Family reactions and relationships in thalassemia. *Ann. N. Y. Acad. Sci.* 612: 451–461.

Tsukamoto, H, Horne, W, Kamimura, S et al. (1995). Experimental liver cirrhosis induced by alcohol and iron. *J. Clin. Invest.* 96: 620–630.

Tuchinda, C, Punnakanta, L, and Angsusingha, K. (1978). Endocrine disturbances in thalassemia children. *J. Med. Assoc. Thai.* 61: 55–56.

Tzetis, M, Traeger-Synodinos, J, Kanavakis, E et al. (1994). The molecular basis of normal Hb A$_2$ (type 2) β-thalassemia in Greece. *Hematol. Pathol.* 8: 25–34.

Valassi-Adam, H, Nassika, E, Kattamis, C, and Matsaniotis, N. (1976). Immunoglobulin levels in children with homozygous beta-thalassemia. *Acta Paediatr. Scand.* 65: 23–27.

Vassilopoulou-Sellin, R, Oyedeji, CO, Foster, PL et al. (1989). Haemoglobin as a direct inhibitor of cartilage growth *in vitro*. *Horm. Metab. Res.* 21: 11.

Vatanavicharn, S, Anuvatanakulchai, M, Na-Nakorn, S, and Wasi, P. (1979). Serum erythrocyte folate levels in thalassaemia patients in Thailand. *Scand. J. Haematol.* 22: 241–245.

Vedovato, M, Salvatorelli, G, Taddei-Masieri, M, and Vullo, C. (1993). Epo serum levels in heterozygous β-thalassemia. *Haematologia (Budapest)* 25: 19–24.

Vellodi, A, Picton, S, Downie, CJC et al. (1994). Bone marrow transplantation for thalassemia: Experience of two British centres. *Bone Marrow Transplant.* 13: 559–562.

Vettore, L, Falezza, GC, Cetto, GL, and de Matteis, MC. (1974). Cation content and membrane deformability of heterozygous beta-thalassemia red blood cells. *Br. J. Haematol.* 27: 429–437.

Vichinsky, EP. (1998). The morbidity of bone disease in thalassemia. *Ann. N. Y. Acad. Sci.* 850: 344–348.

Voght, EC and Diamond, LK. (1930). Congenital anemias, roentgenologically considered. *Am. J. Roentgenol.* 23: 625.

Vullo, C, De Sanctis, V, Katz, M, Wonke, B et al. (1990). Endocrine abnormalities in thalassemia. *Ann. N. Y. Acad. Sci.* 612: 293–310.

Wainscoat, JS, Kanavakis, E, Wood, WG et al. (1983a). Thalassaemia intermedia—the interaction of α and β thalassaemia. *Br. J. Haematol.* 53: 411–416.

Wainscoat, JS, Kanavakis, E, Wood, WG et al. (1983b). Thalassemia intermedia in Cyprus—the interaction of α- and β-thalassaemia. *Br. J. Haematol.* 53: 411–416.

Wainscoat, JS, Thein, SL, and Weatherall, DJ. (1987). Thalassaemia intermedia. *Blood Rev.* 1: 273–279.

Walker, EH, Whelton, MJ, and Beaven, GH. (1969). Successful pregnancy in a patient with thalassaemia major. *J. Obstet. Gynaecol. Br. Commonw.* 76: 549–553.

Walters, MC and Thomas, ED. (1994). Bone marrow transplantation for thalassemia: The United States experience. *Am. J. Pediatr. Hematol. Oncol.* 16: 1–17.

Wang, C, Tso, SC, and Todd, D. (1989). Hypogonadotropic hypogonadism in severe beta-thalassemia: Effect of chelation and pulsatile gonadotrophin-releasing hormone therapy. *J. Clin. Endocrinol. Metab.* 68: 511–516.

Wapnick, AA, Lynch, SR, Charlton, RW et al. (1969). The effect of ascorbic acid deficiency on desferrioxamine-induced iron excretion. *Br. J. Haematol.* 17: 563–568.

Wasi, P. (1972). Adverse effects of splenomegaly. *J. Med. Assoc. Thailand* 55: 685–688.

Wasi, P, Disthasongchan, P, and Na-Nakorn, S. (1968). The effect of iron deficiency on the levels of hemoglobins A$_2$ and E. *J. Lab. Clin. Med.* 71: 85–91.

Wasi, P, Fucharóen, S, Younghchaiyud, P, and Sonakul, D. (1982). Hypoxemia in thalassemia. *Birth Defects: Original Articles Series* 18: 213–217.

Weatherall, DJ. (1980). Towards an understanding of the molecular biology of some common inherited anemias: the story of thalassemia. In *Blood, Pure and Eloquent*. Wintrobe, MM (ed). New York: McGraw-Hill. pp. 373–414.

Weatherall, DJ and Clegg, JB. (1996). Thalassaemia—a global public health problem. *Nat. Med.* 2: 847–849.

Weatherall, DJ and Clegg, JB. (2000). *The Thalassaemia Syndromes*. Oxford: Blackwell Science. In press.

Weatherall, DJ, Clegg, JB, Milner, PF et al. (1976). Linkage relationships between β- and δ-structural loci and African forms of beta thalassaemia. *J. Med. Genet.* 13: 20–26.

Weatherall, DJ, Clegg, JB, and Naughton, MA. (1965). Globin synthesis in thalassemia: An *in vitro* study. *Nature* 208: 1061–1065.

Weatherall, DJ, Clegg, JB, Na-Nakorn, S, and Wasi, P. (1969). The pattern of disordered haemoglobin synthesis in homozygous and heterozygous β-thalassaemia. *Br. J. Haematol.* 16: 251–267.

Weatherall, DJ, Clegg, JB, Knox-Macaulay, HHM et al. (1973). A genetically determined disorder with features both of thalassaemia and congenital dyserythropoietic anaemia. *Br. J. Haematol.* 24: 681–702.

Weatherall, DJ, Clegg, JB, Wood, WG et al. (1980). The clinical and molecular heterogeneity of the thalassaemia syndromes. *Ann. N. Y. Acad. Sci.* 344: 83–100.

Werther, GA, Matthews, RN, Burger, HG, and Herington, AC. (1981). Lack of response of nonsuppressible insulin-like activity to short term administration of human growth hormone in thalassemia major. *J. Clin. Endocrinol. Metab.* 53: 806–809.

Westgren, M, Ringden, O, Eik-Nes, S et al. (1996). Lack of evidence of permanent engraftment after *in utero* fetal stem cell transplantation in congenital hemoglobinopathies. *Transplantation* 61: 1176–1179.

Whipple, GH and Bradford, WL. (1936). Mediterranean disease-thalassemia (erythroblastic anemia of Cooley); associated pigment abnormalities simulating hemochromatosis. *J. Pediatr.* 9: 279–311.

White, JM, Richards, R, Byrne, M et al. (1985). Thalassaemia trait and pregnancy. *J. Clin. Pathol.* 38: 810–817.

Winichagoon, P, Fucharoen, S, Weatherall, DJ, and Wasi, P. (1985). Concomitant inheritance of α-thalassaemia in β⁰-thalassaemia/Hb E. disease. *Am. J. Hematol.* 20: 217–222.

Witzleben, CL and Wyatt, JP. (1961). The effect of long-survival on the pathology of thalassaemia major. *J. Pathol. Bacteriol.* 82: 1–12.

Wolff, JA and Luke, KH. (1969). Management of thalassemia: A comparative program. *Ann. N. Y. Acad. Sci.* 165: 423–426.

Wollstein, M and Kreidel, KV. (1930). Familial hemolytic anemia of childhood—von Jaksch. *Am. J. Dis. Child.* 39: 115–130.

Wolman, IJ. (1964). Transfusion therapy in Cooley's anemia: Growth and health as related to long-range hemoglobin levels, a progress report. *Ann. N. Y. Acad. Sci.* 119: 736–747.

Wong, A, Alder, V, Robertson, D et al. (1997). Liver iron depletion and toxicity of the iron chelator deferiprone (L1, CP20) in the guinea pig. *Biometals* 10: 247–256.

Wong, C, Dowling, CE, Saiki, RK et al. (1987). Characterization of β-thalassaemia mutations using direct genomic sequencing of amplified single copy DNA. *Nature* 330: 384–386.

Wonke, B. (1998). Annotation: Bone disease in β-thalassaemia major. *Br. J. Haematol.* 103: 897–901.

Wonke, B, Hoffbrand, VA, Brown, D, and Dusheiko, G. (1990). Antibody to hepatitis C virus in multiply transfused patients with thalassaemia major. *J. Clin. Pathol.* 43: 638–640.

Wonke, B, Hoffbrand, AV, Bouloux, P et al. (1998). New approaches to the management of hepatitis and endocrine disorders in Cooley's anemia. *Ann. N. Y. Acad. Sci.* 850: 232–241.

Wood, WG, Weatherall, DJ, and Clegg, JB. (1976). Interaction of heterocellular hereditary persistence of foetal haemoglobin with β thalassaemia and sickle cell anaemia. *Nature* 264: 247–249.

Wood, WG, Weatherall, DJ, Hart, GH et al. (1982). Hematologic changes and hemoglobin analysis in β thalassemia heterozygotes during the first year of life. *Pediatr. Res.* 16: 286–289.

Worwood, M, Cragg, SJ, McLaren, C et al. (1980). Binding of serum ferritin to concanavalia A: Patients with homozygous β thalassaemia and transfusional iron overload. *Br. J. Haematol.* 46: 409–416.

Yataganas, X and Fessas, P. (1969). The pattern of hemoglobin precipitation in thalassemia and its significance. *Ann. N. Y. Acad. Sci.* 165: 270–287.

Yataganas, X, Gahrton, G, Fessas, P et al. (1973). Proliferative activity and glycogen accumulation of erythroblasts in β-thalassaemia. *Br. J. Haematol.* 24: 651–659.

Yu, YC, Kao, EL, Chou, SH et al. (1991). Intrathoracic extramedullary hematopoiesis simulating posterior mediastinal mass—report of a case in a patient with beta-thalassemia intermedia. *Kao Hsiung I Hsueh Ko Hsueh Tsa Chih* 7: 43–48.

Zaino, EC, Rossi, MB, Pham, TD, and Azar, HA. (1971). Gaucher's cells in thalassemia. *Blood* 38: 457–462.

Zaino, EC and Rossi, MB. (1974). Ultrastructure of the erythrocytes in β-thalassemia. *Ann. N. Y. Acad. Sci.* 232: 238–260.

Zanella, A, Mozzi, F, Ferroni, P, and Sirchia, G. (1986). Anti-HTLV III screening in multi transfused thalassaemia patients. *Vox Sang.* 50: 192.

Zemel, R, Dickman, R, Tamary, H et al. (1998). Viremia, genetic heterogeneity, and immunity to hepatitis G/GB-C virus in multiply transfused patients with thalassemia. *Transfusion* 38: 301–306.

Zeng, YT, Huang, SZ, Ren, ZR et al. (1995). Hydroxyurea therapy in β-thalassaemia intermedia: Improvement in haematological parameters due to enhanced β-globin synthesis. *Br. J. Haematol.* 90: 557–563.

Zoratto, E, Norelli, MT, and Lumare, A. (1969). Hemolytic anemia caused by association of a double anomaly beta-thalassaemia and deficiency of G6PD. *Minerva Pediatr.* 21: 605–610.

Zuppinger, K, Molinari, B, Hirt, A et al. (1979). Increased risk of diabetes mellitus in beta-thalassaemia major. *Hel. Paediatr. Acta.* 4: 197–207.

Zurlo, MF, De Stefano, P, Borgna-Pignatti, C et al. (1989). Survival and causes of death in thalassaemia major. *Lancet* 2: 27–30.

14

Structural Variants with a β-Thalassemia Phenotype

SWEE LAY THEIN

INTRODUCTION

Structural variants with a β-thalassemia phenotype are often called "thalassemic hemoglobinopathies." Historically, they comprise a distinctive set of hemoglobin mutants with amino acid substitutions, additions, or deletions in the β-globin chain and a thalassemic phenotype characterized in the heterozygote by hypochromic microcytic red blood cells, basophilic stippling, and elevated HbA_2 levels. Included in this classification, but not discussed in this chapter, are the δβ fusion hemoglobins (Lepore hemoglobins) and the RNA processing mutants HbE (β26 GAG→AAG), Hb Knossos (β27 GCC→TCC), and Hb Malay (β19 AAC→AGC). RNA processing mutants are associated with a thalassemic phenotype because the base substitution causing the amino acid replacement also causes alternative splicing of precursor β-globin mRNA, leading to a reduction of normal splicing; mechanisms underlying the reduced synthesis of Hb Lepore are not definitely known (see Chapter 12). HbE is a major thalassemic hemoglobinopathy particularly prevalent in Southeast Asia, reaching a frequency of 75 percent in Northeast Thailand (see Chapter 43). Its interaction with β thalassemia accounts for a large proportion of thalassemia major in that part of the world. Hb Lepore and HbE disorders, like classical β thalassemias, are inherited as Mendelian recessives; heterozygotes are clinically asymptomatic and the inheritance of two mutant alleles—as homozygotes or compound heterozygotes with another β-thalassemia allele—is required to produce clinical disease.

Thalassemic hemoglobinopathies also include an increasing number of β-globin chain structural variants associated with a β-thalassemia phenotype due to a different molecular mechanism. Some β-globin chain variants are synthesized in normal amounts but are highly unstable and unable to form stable tetramers, resulting in a quantitative deficiency of β-globin chains. Unlike the typical β thalassemias, the hyperunstable β-globin chain variants cause a disease phenotype even in heterozygotes who produce normal chains as well—thus the alternative term, "dominantly inherited β thalassemia."

Probably first recognized in an Irish family in 1973, this unusual type of β thalassemia was accompanied by moderately severe anemia, intermittent jaundice, splenomegaly, and gross abnormalities of the erythrocytes. It was transmitted through three generations as a single β-globin allele in a dominant fashion (Weatherall et al., 1973). Apart from the usual features of heterozygous β thalassemia such as increased levels of HbA_2 and increased α/β-globin chain biosynthesis ratios, there was morphologic evidence of severe dyserythropoiesis. Large inclusion bodies were observed in bone marrow erythroblasts and in nucleated red cells of the peripheral blood of two family members who had been splenectomized. Similar clinical features associated with inclusions in bone marrow erythroblasts and peripheral red blood cells after splenectomy were observed in a Swiss-French family by Stamatoyannopoulos et al. (1974) and the term "inclusion body β thalassemia" was proposed. However, since such intraerythroblastic inclusions are also found in severe forms of typical β thalassemia, this term is not appropriate and the designation "dominantly inherited β thalassemia" is preferred, as this nomenclature also differentiates these disorders from the typical recessive forms of β thalassemia prevalent in the tropical and subtropical regions.

Mutations functionally similar to those causing the dominantly inherited β thalassemias affect the α-globin genes and probably other globin genes (see Chapters 10 and 17). In the case of the α-globin genes, the phenotype is less severe and usually that of α-thalassemia trait because only one of four α-globin genes is involved, and the redundant β-globin chains are able to form $β^4$ tetramers. If the δ-globin gene is affected, no clinical phenotype is present.

Martin H. Steinberg, Bernard G. Forget, Douglas R. Higgs, and Ronald L. Nagel, editors. *Disorders of Hemoglobin: Genetics, Pathophysiology, and Clinical Management.* © 2001 Cambridge University Press. All rights reserved.

MOLECULAR BASIS

In the original Irish family, the molecular lesion was a complex rearrangement involving two deletions of 4 and 11 bp interrupted by an insertion of 5 bp in exon 3 of the β-globin gene. This caused a reading frameshift and predicted synthesis of an elongated β-globin chain variant with an abnormal carboxy terminal (Thein et al., 1990). In the Swiss-French family, a base substitution (GAA→TAA) converted codon β121 to a stop codon, leading to a β chain of 120, rather than 146, amino acids (Fei et al., 1989).

Numerous dominantly inherited β-thalassemia alleles associated with similar clinical features have now been identified in families of disparate ethnic origins. At the molecular level, they fall into four groups (Table 14.1; Fig. 14.1): missense mutations, deletions or insertions of intact codons, single base substitutions leading to premature termination of translation (nonsense mutations), and mutations causing frameshifts or aberrant splicing resulting in elongated or truncated β-globin chain variants with abnormal carboxy terminal ends.

Missense Mutations

An example of a missense mutation causing β thalassemia intermedia is Hb Terre Haute (β106 Leu→Arg) (Coleman et al., 1991), which was initially described as Hb Indianapolis (β112 Cys→Arg) (Adams et al., 1979). In two patients heterozygous for this mutation, globin-chain biosynthesis studies showed an α:non-α ratio of approximately 1.0 in bone marrow erythroblasts compared with a ratio of approximately 2.0 in peripheral blood reticulocytes. Although the variant β-globin chain was synthesized at a level almost equal to that of the normal β-globin chain, most of it was rapidly precipitated on the red cell membrane. The half-life of this globin variant was less than 10 minutes, and the abnormal hemoglobin was not detectable by standard techniques. Other examples of hyperunstable β-globin chain variants include Hb Chesterfield, Hb Cagliari, Hb Showa-Yakushiji, Hb Durham NC/Brescia, and Hb Houston (Thein et al., 1991; Podda et al., 1991; Kobayashi et al., 1987; de Castro et al., 1994; Çürük et al., 1994; Kazazian et al., 1992). Globin chain biosynthesis studies including short-term incubation and pulse chase experiments showed a rapid decline of the variants β^{Houston} and β^{Cagliari}, suggesting that these variants were highly unstable and rapidly catabolized. Yet, in others such as Hb Showa-Yakushiji (β110 Leu→Pro) and Hb Durham NC (β114 Leu→Pro), an abnormal β-globin chain was not seen at 2.5 minutes or at any of the later time points. In the example of Hb Chesterfield, an abnormal peak in the position

expected for the β-globin chain variant but without detectable corresponding protein was demonstrated by globin-chain biosynthesis studies.

Among this group of missense mutations associated with unusually severe thalassemia, hemoglobin electrophoresis failed to detect any of the abnormal hemoglobins except Hb Cagliari, which was identified postsplenectomy on isoelectric focusing (IEF) and formed 9 percent of the total hemoglobin. These observations again suggest the synthesis of β-globin chain variants that are highly unstable and rapidly degraded after synthesis. It should be noted that the "real" Hb Indianapolis (β112 Cys→Arg) was reported in two families (Spanish and Italian) in whom affected members had evidence of mild hemolytic anemia with 2 percent to 4 percent reticulocytosis (Baiget et al., 1986; De Biasi et al., 1988). Hb Indianapolis was mildly unstable; on IEF, the variant β-globin chain formed 38 percent to 45 percent of the total β-globin chains.

A phenotype of mild heterozygous β thalassemia has been reported in association with two β-globin chain variants, Hb North Shore (β134 Val→Glu) and Hb K Woolwich (β132 Lys→Gln) (Lang et al., 1974; Smith et al., 1983). Heterozygotes for Hb North Shore had microcytosis, increased levels of HbA$_2$, and a mild deficit of β-globin synthesis (α/β chain synthesis ratio, 1.35). The imbalanced α/β ratio was evident after a 15-minute pulse chase experiment and remained stable during 120 minutes of chase, suggesting a suboptimal synthesis rather than posttranslational degradation. Hb North Shore was mildly unstable compared with normal hemoglobin. Heterozygotes for Hb K Woolwich also have mild microcytosis and increased levels of HbA$_2$ with defective synthesis of the β-globin chain variant. In both cases, the mechanism for the thalassemia phenotype is not clear. Both β-globin chain variants were identified by peptide mapping before current molecular biology techniques were available.

Deletion or Insertion of Intact Codons

β-globin chain variants due to a gain or loss of intact codons are often highly unstable (see Chapter 44). Although structural β-globin chain variants were predicted by DNA sequence analysis, in all cases no trace of abnormal hemoglobin could be detected by the standard techniques of IEF, HPLC, or heat stability tests. Because entire codons are deleted or inserted, the reading frame remains in phase, and the remaining amino acids are normal. Both Hb Korea and Hb Gunma have 145 amino acid residues each; in Hb Gunma, the β127–128 Gln-Ala dipeptide is replaced by a proline residue due to the deletion of three bases (AGG) (Fucharoen et al., 1990), while in Hb Korea,

Table 14.1. Structural Variants Associated with a β-Thalassemia Phenotype

Mutations	Site	β variant	Phenotype	Ethnic group	References
I Missense mutations					
1) CD 28 (CTG→CGG) Leu→Arg	Exon 1	βChesterfield*	Thal intermedia, inclusion bodies	English	(Thein et al., 1991)
2) CD 32 (CTG→CAG) Leu→Glu in *cis* with CD 98 (GTG→ATG) Val to Met; Hb Köln	Exon 2	βMedicine Lake*	Severe thalassemia	U.S. Caucasian	(Coleman et al., 1995)
3) CD 60 (GTG→GAG) Val to Glu	Exon 2	βCagliari*	Thal intermedia, inclusion bodies	Italian	(Podda et al., 1991)
4) CD 106 (CTG→CGG) Leu→Arg	Exon 3	βTerre Haute	Thal intermedia	N. European, French	(Adams et al., 1979; Coleman et al., 1991; Girodon et al., 1992)
5) CD 110(CTG→CCG) Leu to Pro	Exon 3	βShowa-Yakushii	Thal intermedia	Japanese	(Kobayashi et al., 1987; Ohba et al., 1997)
6) CD 114(CTG→CCG) Leu to Pro	Exon 3	βDurham NC/β Brescia*	Thal trait/thal intermedia	U.S. Irish, Italian	(Çürük et al., 1994; de Castro et al., 1994)
7) CD 115 (GCC→GAC) Ala to Asp	Exon 3	βHradec Kralove	Thal intermedia	Czech	(Divoky et al., 1993)
8) CD 127 (CAG→CCG) Gln to Pro	Exon 3	βHouston	Thal intermedia	U.S. English	(Kazazian et al., 1992)
9) CD 127 (CAG→CGG) Gln→Arg	Exon 3	βDieppe	Thal intermedia	French	(Girodon et al., 1992)
10) CD 132 Lys→Gln	Exon 3	βK Woolwich	Thal trait	West Indian	(Lang et al., 1974)
11) CD 134 Val→Glu	Exon 3	βNorth Shore	Thal trait	Finnish	(Smith et al., 1983)
II Deletion or insertion of intact codons → destabilization					
1) CD 30–31 (+CGG) +Arg	Exon 1/2		Thal intermedia, inclusion bodies	Spanish	(Arjona et al., 1996)
2) CD 32–34 (–GGT) Val-Val to Val	Exon 2	βKorea*	Thal intermedia	Korean	(Park et al., 1991)
3) CD 33–35 (–6) Val-Val-Try→Asp	Exon 2	βDreaden	Thal intermedia	German	(Vetter et al., 2000)
4) CD 108–112 (–12bp) Asn-Val-Leu-Val-Cys to Ser	Exon 3		Thal trait	Swedish	(Landin and Rudolphi, 1996)
5) CD 124–126 (+CCA) +Pro	Exon 3		Thal intermedia	Armenian	(Çürük et al., 1994)
6) CD 127–128 (–AGG) Gln-Ala to Pro	Exon 3	βGunma	Thal trait/thal intermedia	Japanese	(Fucharoen et al., 1990a)
7) CD 134–137 (–12, +6) Val-Ala-Gly-Val to Gly-Arg	Exon 3		Thal intermedia	Portuguese	(Öner et al., 1991)
III Premature termination					
1) CD 121 (GAA→TAA) Glu to Term (120aa)†	Exon 3		Thal trait/thal intermedia, inclusion bodies	N. European, Japanese	(Stamatoyannopoulos et al., 1974; Kazazian et al., 1986; Fei et al., 1989; Thein et al., 1990; Ohba et al., 1997)
2) CD 127 (CAG→TAG) Gln to Term (127aa)	Exon 3		Thal trait/thal intermedia	English	(Hall et al., 1991)

IV Frameshifts or aberrant splicing → elongated or truncated variants with abnormal carboxy terminal

1)	IVSII: 2,3 (+11, −2)	IVSII		Thal trait/thal intermedia	Iranian	(Kaeda et al., 1992)
2)	IVSII: 4, 5 (−AG) → aberrant splicing	IVSII		Thal intermedia, inclusion bodies	Portuguese	(Faustino et al., 1992; Faustino et al., 1998)
3)	CD 94 (+TG) → 156aa	Exon 2	β^{Agnana}*	Thal intermedia, inclusion bodies	S. Italian	(Ristaldi et al., 1990)
4)	CD 100 (−CTT, +TCTGAGAACTT) → 158aa	Exon 2		Thal trait/thal intermedia	S. African	(Williamson et al., 1997)
5)	CD 109 (−G) → 156aa	Exon 3	β^{Manhattan}	Thal intermedia	Lithuanian	(Kazazian et al., 1992)
6)	CD 114 (−CT, +G) → 156aa	Exon 3	β^{Geneva}	Thal intermedia, inclusion bodies	Swiss-French	(Beris et al., 1988)
7)	Cd 120–121 (+A) → 138aa	Exon 3		Thal trait	Filipino	(Hopmeier et al., 1996)
8)	CD 123 (−A) → 156aa	Exon 3	β^{Makabe}	Thal intermedia, inclusion bodies	Japanese	(Fucharoen et al., 1990; Ohba et al., 1997)
9)	CD 123–125 (−ACCCCACC) → 135aa	Exon 3	β$^{Khon\ Kaen}$‡	Severe thal intermedia with HbE	Thai	(Fucharoen et al., 1991)
10)	CD 124 (−A) → 156aa	Exon 3		Thal intermedia	Russian	(Çürük et al., 1994)
11)	CD 125 (−A) → 156aa	Exon 3		Thal intermedia	Japanese	(Ohba et al., 1997)
12)	CD 126 (−T) → 156aa	Exon 3	β^{Vercelli}*	Thal intermedia, inclusion bodies	N. Italian	(Murru et al., 1991)
13)	CD 126–131 (−17 bp) → 132aa	Exon 3	β^{Westdale}‡	Severe thal intermedia with HbE, thal major in homozygote	Asian Indian, Pakistani	(Waye et al., 1995; Ahmed et al., 1996)
14)	CD 128–129 (−4, +5, −11) → 153aa	Exon 3		Thal intermedia, inclusion bodies	Irish	(Weatherall et al., 1973; Thein et al., 1990)
15)	CD 131–132 (−GA) → 138aa	Exon 3		Thai intermedia, inclusion bodies	Swiss	(Deutsch et al., 1998)

* Spontaneous mutations.

† Several families reported including one spontaneous mutation.

‡ Difficult to evaluate phenotypes of heterozygotes as only homozygote and compound heterozygotes reported.

Note: Structural variants such as the δβ fusion hemoglobins and RNA processing mutations (HbE; etc.) are described in Chapters 12 and 43.

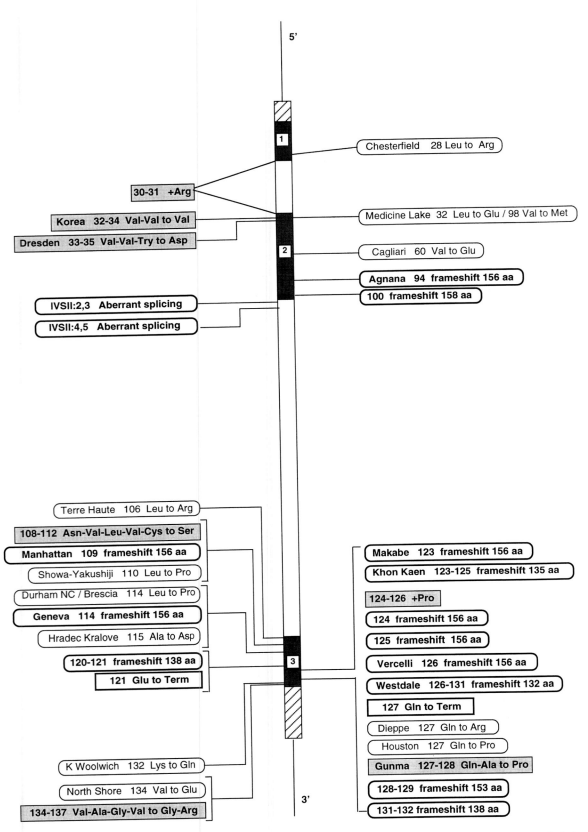

Figure 14.1. The β-globin gene with the location of the various mutations that cause structural variants with a β-thalassemia phenotype. Note the concentration of mutations in exon 3.

the Val-Val dipeptide in the region of codons 32–34 is replaced by a single valine due to the deletion of three bases (GGT) (Park et al., 1991). Two β-globin chain variants have an extra residue, insertion of Arg in codons 30–31 in a Spanish family (Arjona et al., 1996) and insertion of a single proline in codons 124–126 in an Armenian patient (Cürük et al., 1994). A deletion of 12 nucleotides resulting in the replacement of serine for Asn-Val-Leu-Val-Cys in codons 108–112 was described in a Swedish woman (Landin and Rudolphi, 1996). Unlike the other affected individuals who had varying severities of thalassemia intermedia, the clinical phenotype of this woman was consistent with a thalassemia trait.

One mechanism that could explain the lack of detection of these structural β-globin chain variants is that the amino acids affected are involved in α1β1 contacts. In the normal β-globin chain, β30 Arg (B 12), β33 Val (B 15), β34 Val (B 16), β108 Asn (G 10), β112 Cys (G 14), β124 Pro (H2), β125 Pro (H3), β127 Gln (H5), and β128 Ala (H6) are essential for α1β1 dimer formation (Bunn and Forget, 1986). Deletion or substitution of these critical amino acids would be likely to prevent the formation of αβ subunits and, effectively, lead to a functional loss of half of the β-globin chains. Several β-globin chain variants due to the deletions or insertions of one or more intact codons with the remainder of the subunit being normal, have been described (Huisman et al., 1998). None of the variants associated with the clinical phenotype of congenital hemolytic anemia or methemoglobinemia affect the residues involved in α1β1 or α2β2 contacts (see Chapters 44 and 46).

The third example in this category involved a deletion of 12 nucleotides and an insertion of six nucleotides, leading to the substitution of the normal Val-Ala-Gly-Val by Gly-Arg in codons 134–137 and a β-globin subunit that was two amino acids shorter than normal. Affected individuals of this Portuguese family had moderately severe anemia, splenomegaly, and leg ulcers (Öner et al., 1991)

These deletion-insertion mutants probably arose by a mechanism of frameshift mutagenesis during DNA replication (Streisinger et al., 1966). In each case, there is a repeated sequence of two to six nucleotides flanking the deleted nucleotides. The process of frameshift mutagenesis could also explain the internal repetition of six nucleotides in the Portuguese family (Öner et al., 1991).

Premature Termination (Nonsense Mutation)

Probably the most common of the dominantly inherited β-thalassemia alleles is a GAA→TAA change at codon 121, which leads to the synthesis of a truncated β-globin chain (Fig. 14.2). Although substantial amounts of mutant β-globin mRNA could be demonstrated in individuals with such mutations, showing the presence of the truncated β-globin variant has been difficult (Hall and Thein, 1994). In a recent study, the predicted truncated variant was detected indirectly and was highly unstable (Ho et al., 1997); globin biosynthesis studies showed a large difference between the total radioactivity incorporated into newly synthesized chains and the total amount of protein (Fig. 14.3). In a previous study of another case of the β121 GAA→TAA mutation, the truncated β-globin chain was estimated to comprise only 0.05 percent to 0.1 percent of the total non-α globin and even then fractions from 10 HPLC runs had to be pooled to isolate enough protein for peptide analysis (Adams et al., 1990).

Elongated or Truncated Variants with Abnormal Carboxy Terminal Ends

With two exceptions, the elongated or truncated β-globin gene variants in this group have arisen from frameshift mutations that generated distal or premature termination codons (Fig. 14.2). Despite the altered charge created by the abnormal carboxy terminal end, the abnormal β-globin variants were not detected in any of the cases by hemoglobin electrophoresis or globin biosynthesis studies. However, in all cases an imbalanced synthesis of α- and β-globin chains was present.

Elongated β-globin subunits could also arise from aberrant splicing of precursor mRNA, as recently described in a deletion of two nucleotides affecting the IVS-II consensus donor splice site (Faustino et al., 1998). Three species of abnormal β-globin mRNAs were detected, two shorter than normal and a third, 45 nucleotides longer than normal. The latter is predicted to lead to the production of a β-globin chain variant with an insertion of 15 amino acids between exons 2 and 3 (Fig. 14.3). In vitro translation studies showed an abnormal peptide of a higher molecular weight than the normal globin chain, suggesting that it is the translation product of the elongated aberrant β-globin mRNA. A phenotype of unusually severe β thalassemia with inclusion bodies in peripheral normoblasts after splenectomy was observed in five generations of this Portuguese family and the disorder was transmitted in a dominant fashion. Abnormal β-globin mRNA species have also been reported in an Iranian man heterozygous for a mutation that involved an insertion of eleven nucleotides and a deletion of two nucleotides at positions 2 and 3 of the IVS-II consensus donor splice site of the β-globin gene (Kaeda et al., 1992). This patient had hypochromic

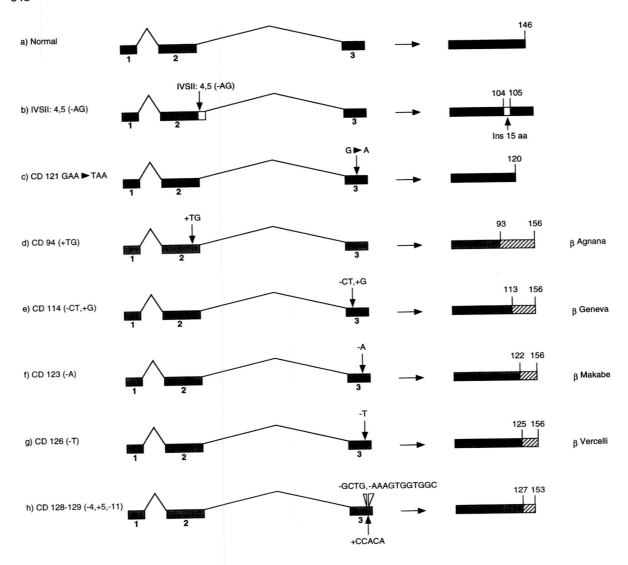

Figure 14.2. Some of the hyperunstable elongated or truncated β-globin variants. (a) Normal β-globin pre-mRNA splicing pattern and β-globin mRNA; (b) deletion of AG in the consensus donor splice site activates a cryptic donor site downstream introducing 15 residues in the aberrant β-globin gene product; (c) a truncated β-globin variant of 120 amino acids is predicted from the β121 nonsense codon; (d) through (h) various frameshift mutations with their predicted elongated β-globin chain variants. While heme binding is intact in these variants—a majority of contact sites are concentrated in exon 2, the α1β1 contacts, which are concentrated in the terminal exon, are abolished.

microcytic anemia, a hemoglobin concentration of 9.5 g/dL—less than normally encountered in typical β-thalassemia trait—with marked anisopoikilocytosis and prominent basophilic stippling. Truncated β-globin chain variants of 101 and 107 residues were predicted, the latter with an abnormal carboxy terminal end of three amino acids.

PATHOPHYSIOLOGY

A common feature underlying thalassemic hemoglobinopathies is their extreme instability due either to impaired heme binding or abnormal subunit interactions. In many cases, the variants can be detected only when newly synthesized, while in others, they are not detectable but predicted from the DNA sequence. The predicted synthesis is supported by the presence of substantial amounts of mutant β-globin gene mRNA in the peripheral blood reticulocytes, comparable in amounts to that of the other, normal, β-globin allele (Hall and Thein, 1994; Ho et al., 1997).

Hb Chesterfield and Hb Cagliari clearly demonstrate that the nature of the amino acid substitution as well as its position in the β-globin chain is a critical determinant of the stability of the variant and the resulting phenotype. Replacing β28 leucine by an arginine residue (Hb Chesterfield) creates an internal ionized group. Such groups surround themselves with

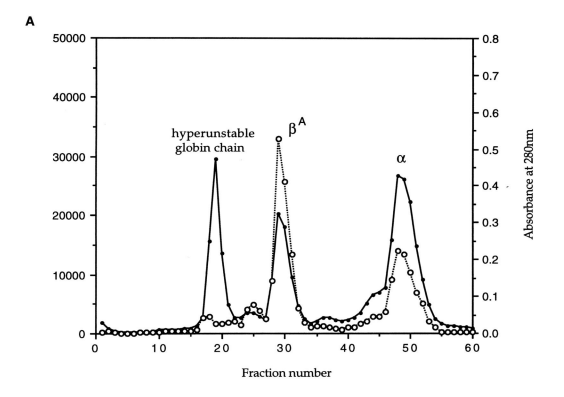

A

B

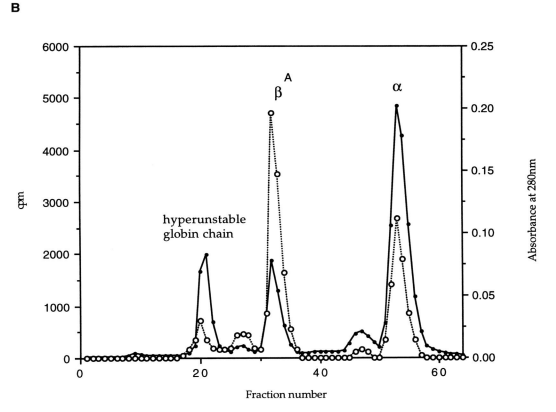

Figure 14.3. Globin-chain biosynthesis studies in a patient heterozygous for the β121 GAA→TAA allele. (**A**) peripheral blood and (**B**) bone marrow, following incubation with ^{3}H-leucine for 60 minutes. Solid line shows the incorporated radioactivity and the dotted line, the protein concentrations (absorbance at 280 nm). (Figures generously provided by from Dr. David Rees.)

water molecules making them so bulky that the tertiary fold of the protein bursts apart, preventing the abnormal β-globin chain from combining with α-globin chains to form a hemoglobin tetramer and leading to ineffective erythropoiesis. In contrast, Hb Genova (β28 Leu→Pro) (Sansone et al., 1967) produces the phenotype of severe congenital hemolytic anemia associated with Heinz bodies in the erythrocytes. It appears that the replacement of β28 leucine, by proline, although causing a profound distortion of the B helix, seems less destructive than the replacement by Arg, because β28 Pro is stable enough to allow the formation of viable tetramers (Hb Genova), which then fall apart in the peripheral circulation, injure the cell, and cause hemolytic anemia. A different replacement, β28 Leu→Gln (Hb St. Louis), is also unstable but produces a distinctly different clinical phenotype of severe hemolytic anemia associated with methemoglobinemia (Thillet et al., 1976). In this case, β28 (B 10) glutamine and the distal histidine (E7) swing toward each other, stabilizing a water molecule in the normally hydrophobic heme pocket resulting in thermal instability and methemoglobin formation. Similarly, while the replacement β60 Val (nonpolar) with Glu (polar) (Hb Cagliari) causes ineffective erythropoiesis and thalassemia intermedia, β60 Val→Ala (Hb Collingwood) (Williamson et al., 1983) and β60 Val→Leu (Hb Yatsushiro) (Kagimoto et al., 1978), which are more conservative substitutions (neutral for hydrophobic amino acids), result in moderately unstable β-globin variants and no clinical phenotype.

One suggestion is that the alterations arising from the missense mutations in β$^{\text{Terre-Haute}}$ (106 Leu→Arg), β$^{\text{Showa-Yakushigi}}$ (110 Leu→Pro), and β$^{\text{Durham NC}}$ (114 Leu→Pro) destabilize the heme pocket and affect the ability to bind heme (de Castro et al., 1994). Such β-globin gene variants would be unstable and degraded before αβ dimer formation. The other missense mutants, β$^{\text{Hradec Kralove}}$, β^{Houston}, and β^{Dieppe}, which are associated with unusually severe thalassemia phenotypes, affect residues involved in α1 β1 contact at codons 115 and 127.

A comparison of the frameshift and premature termination mutants in the β-globin gene showed that those associated with dominantly inherited β thalassemia intermedia occur in the 3′ third of exon 2 and in exon 3, the terminal exon (Fig. 14.1), while the vast majority (71/75) of the in-phase termination mutants that are recessively inherited terminate in exon 1 or 2. A mechanism that explains why mutations that occur in exon 3 give rise to a severe phenotype is related to the positional effect of premature termination on mRNA accumulation (Maquat, 1995; Thermann et al., 1998; Zhang et al., 1998b). Studies have shown that premature termination in exons 1 or 2 is associated with minimal amounts of mutant β-globin mRNA and therefore the quantitative reduction of β-globin is typical of recessive β thalassemia (Baserga and Benz, 1992; Enssle et al., 1993; Hall and Thein, 1994). In contrast, mutants that terminate more toward the carboxyl end of the β-globin chain in exon 3 are associated with substantial amounts of β-globin mRNA and the predicted synthesis of these abnormal β-globin chain variants. Truncated chains of 120 residues arising from the β121 GAA→TAA mutation lack the H helix, and are not capable of forming tetramers with α-globin chains (Fig. 14.2).

Molecular mechanisms distinguishing premature termination codons that do not elicit a reduction in mRNA abundance from premature termination, or nonsense codons that do elicit a reduction in mRNA abundance, were further explained in recent studies by Thermann et al. (1998) and Zhang et al. (1998b). Their results suggest that the position of the termination codon relative to the downstream exon-exon junction (after splicing) is critical. Nonsense codons present 54 bp or more upstream of the 3′-most intron of the β-globin gene, intron 2, reduce the abundance of nucleus-associated mRNA to 10 percent to 15 percent of normal. Cytoplasmic mRNA is also reduced to 10 percent to 15 percent of normal, indicating that decay does not take place once the mRNA is released from the nucleus into the cytoplasm.

These findings are remarkably consistent with studies of transcripts that encode triose phosphate isomerase where nonsense codons located less than 50 to 55 bp upstream of intron 6, the 3′-most intron of the triose phosphate isomerase gene, fail to mediate mRNA decay (Zhang et al., 1998a). On this basis, Nagy and Maquat (1998) have proposed that only those termination codons located more than 50 to 55 nucleotides upstream of the 3′-most exon-exon junction (measured after splicing) mediate a reduction in mRNA abundance. It is suggested that the mechanisms by which this is executed involve the interactions of sequence elements and the cytoplasmic translation-termination complex to trigger nonsense mediated decay (NMD). An example of such sequence elements is provided by the downstream elements (DSE) found in yeast, the functional equivalent in mammals being the 3′-most exon-exon junction which is marked by a 'tag' (measured after splicing). Because DSEs downstream of a premature termination codon (PTC) within the reading frame are required to trigger NMD, premature stop codons near the 3′ end of the gene, in exon 3 in the β-globin gene, are less likely to trigger NMD (Hentze and Kulozik, 1999) (see Chapter 8).

In-phase termination mutants exemplify how shifting the position of a nonsense codon can alter the phenotype of recessive inheritance associated with haplo insufficiency, to a dominant negative effect due to the synthesis of an abnormal deleterious protein (Maquat, 1995, 1996).

Similarly, frameshift mutations that occur later in the sequences tend to lead to accumulation of the mutant message and the synthesis of elongated β-globin variants (Fig. 14.2). These elongated variants have abnormal carboxy-terminal ends made up of hydrophobic sequences causing their instability. Furthermore, these β-globin variants would not be able to form αβ dimers as most of the α1β1 contact residues would have been removed (Bunn and Forget, 1986). Since the heme contact site codons—mostly located in exon 2—are retained, these elongated variants should have some tertiary structure, be less susceptible to proteolytic degradation, and presumably, form the characteristic inclusion bodies. Prominent inclusions were noted in individuals heterozygous for Hb Geneva, Hb Makabe, Hb Agnana, Hb Vercelli, and the frameshift mutation at codon 128—the original Irish family reported by Weatherall et al. (1973). In contrast, other elongated β-globin gene variants such as Hb Cranston and Hb Tak, where the frameshift mutations occur close to the C terminus, have normal amino acids through to codon 146 in Hb Tak (Flatz et al., 1971) and codon 144 in Hb Cranston (Bunn et al., 1975). In these cases, the formation of viable tetramers is still possible and heterozygotes have minimal phenotypic consequences.

CLINICAL FEATURES AND LABORATORY FINDINGS

Thalassemic hemoglobinopathies have a gradation of clinical severity ranging from a just detectable clinical phenotype to transfusion dependency. In a few cases, heterozygotes have a phenotype consistent with thalassemia trait, as reported for Hb North Shore and Hb K Woolwich. The variant hemoglobin in both cases was stable enough to be detectable on alkaline cellulose acetate electrophoresis. Heterozygotes for the mutation that involved codons 108 to 112 (Landin and Rudolphi, 1996) and another due to a frameshift caused by the insertion of an A between codons 120–121 have also been reported to be clinically asymptomatic with a phenotype of thalassemia trait (Hopmeier et al., 1996). A variable thalassemia phenotype has been observed in heterozygotes for the premature termination mutations at codons 121 and 127. The β121 GAA→TAA allele was originally reported as a de novo mutation in a child of Greek-Polish ancestry (Kazazian et al., 1986). Evaluating the clinical phenotype in this case is difficult as the child who had thalassemia major was a compound heterozygote for the β121 allele and another β-thalassemia mutation.

Since then, the mutation has been described in several families. Some heterozygotes have clinical phenotypes consistent with thalassemia trait while others clearly have severe thalassemia intermedia with inclusion bodies. In an unusual case, the severity of disease was aggravated by the co-inheritance of a triplicated α-globin gene locus and the α-globin gene haplotype ααα/αα. The proband, a heterozygote for β121 GAA→TAA and a triplicated α-globin gene, was transfusion dependent despite splenectomy, while her mother, who was heterozygous for β121 GAA→TAA with a normal α-globin genotype, had the phenotype of thalassemia trait (Thein et al., 1990).

Variable phenotypes have been described in affected members of the same family who were heterozygous for a different premature termination codon, CAG→TAG at β127 (Hall et al., 1991); the proband had thalassemia intermedia needing splenectomy while her sister and mother, heterozygotes for the same mutation, were asymptomatic. All three members of the family had normal α-globin genotypes. Phenotypic variability may be a consequence of the differences in the proteolytic capacities of the erythroid cells from the thalassemia intermedia patients and the asymptomatic cases, from known modifiers of the phenotype such as α thalassemia or triplicated α-globin genes, or from unknown epistatic modifiers (see Chapter 26).

Most patients present with moderate anemia and splenomegaly. A proportion of these patients are also jaundiced. Like typical β-thalassemia heterozygotes, affected individuals have poorly hemoglobinized small red cells with elevated levels of HbA_2 and variable increases of HbF. Mean corpuscular volume (MCV) and the mean red cell hemoglobin (MCH) as measured by the Coulter Counter may not be representative since there is often severe anisopoikilocytosis. Red cell morphology is more abnormal than in typical β-thalassemia trait and basophilic stippling is prominent. ^{51}Cr red cell half-life shows a shorter survival than that observed in patients with typical β-thalassemia trait, implying that ineffective erythropoiesis is a major factor in the increased severity of disease in these patients. Reticulocytes are often increased (4 percent 10 percent); postsplenectomy, levels of more than 40 percent have been observed in some cases (Beris et al., 1988; Thein et al., 1990). Unlike typical congenital Heinz body hemolytic anemia, an abnormal unstable hemoglobin cannot be detected on hemoglobin electrophoresis—except in the variants with a mild phenotype such as Hb North Shore and Hb K Woolwich—or by the heat denaturation and isopropanol stability tests. Globin-chain biosynthesis studies of both bone marrow samples and peripheral blood reticulocytes show imbalanced α/β synthesis ratios typical of those found in β-thalassemia trait. In the majority of cases, while the abnormal β-globin variant is not detectable, there is a significant pool of free α-globin chains that, presumably, form the characteristic cytoplasmic inclusions (Weatherall et al., 1973). Marked erythroid hyperplasia with dyserythropoiesis is found in the bone marrow and after methyl violet staining, large inclusion bodies are seen in normoblasts. These inclusions are also observed in peripheral blood nucleated red blood cells after splenectomy (Fig. 14.4). Peptide mapping indicated that these inclusions are composed of precipitated α- and β-globin chains (Weatherall et al., 1973; Stamatoyannopoulos et al., 1974; Beris et al., 1988), a finding recently confirmed in two cases of the β121 GAA→TAA mutation by immunoelectron microscopy using mouse monoclonal antibodies against human α- and β-globin chains (Ho et al., 1997) (Fig. 14.5). These observations support the hypothesis that both hyperunstable β-globin chains and the redundant excess α-globin chains were responsible for the underlying pathology of ineffective erythropoiesis (Adams et al., 1979). By contrast, the intra-erythroblastic inclusions found in homozygous β thalassemia consisted only of precipitated α-globin chains (Fig. 14.5).

Hyperunstable β-globin chain variants belong to a phenotypic class of their own. Unlike the other thalassemic hemoglobinopathies, the variant globin is usually undetectable using the usual means of hemoglobin detection due to extreme instability, but in vitro labeling studies show that there is near normal synthesis. They share the hallmarks of heterozygous β thalassemia with increased levels of HbA₂, varying degrees of hypochromia and microcytosis, and α/β-globin chain synthesis imbalance. Underlying the pathophysiology of these defects in heterozygotes is whether a β-globin chain variant is synthesized, its stability, its ability to bind heme and to form αβ dimers

Figure 14.5. Electron micrographs of erythroblastic inclusions from sections of bone marrow immunogold labeled with mouse monoclonal antibody against α-globin chains and β-globin chains in (A) a patient heterozygous for the β121 GAA→TAA allele. The inclusions show a positive reaction with antibodies against both α- and β-globin chains. In (B) a patient with β thalassemia major. The inclusions show a positive reaction with antibody against α-globin chains but no reaction with antibody against β-globin chains. (Photographs generously provided by Professor S. Wickramasinghe.)

Figure 14.4. Peripheral blood smear of a splenectomized patient with Hb Chesterfield stained by (A) Giemsa and (B) methyl violet, showing inclusions.

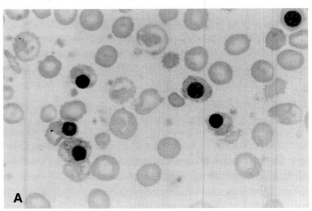

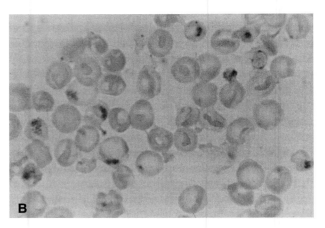

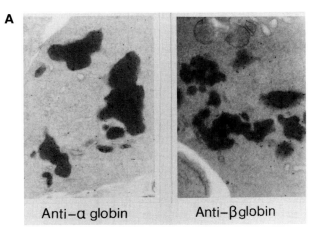

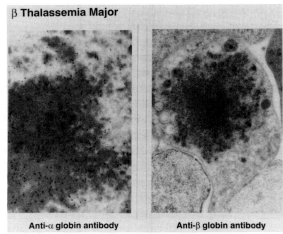

and tetramers, and the stability of the tetramers (Fig. 14.6). At one end of the spectrum are the typical β-thalassemia traits due to a simple reduction in β-globin chains characterized by an asymptomatic clinical state and hypochromic microcytic red cells, while the other end of the spectrum is formed by the congenital Heinz body hemolytic anemias with peripheral hemolysis due to instability of the hemoglobin tetramers. The most severely unstable β-globin gene variants fail to form functional tetramers and precipitate intracellularly with the concomitant excess α-globin chains leading to ineffective erythropoiesis. They resemble β thalassemia intermedia due to their ineffective erythropoiesis while they also bear resemblance to the congenital Heinz body hemolytic anemias with the variable amount of peripheral hemolysis.

Unlike the typical recessive β thalassemia, which is prevalent in malaria-endemic regions, the hyperunstable β-globin chain variants associated with a thalassemia phenotype are rare, occurring in dispersed geographic regions including Northern and Eastern Europe, Japan, and Korea, where the gene frequency of β thalassemia is very low (Thein, 1993). It was postulated that the low frequency of the "dominant" β-thalassemia mutations is due to the lack of positive selection by malaria as is the case for the recessive forms (Kazazian et al., 1992). Family studies have shown that many of these hyperunstable or dominantly inherited β-thalassemia variants are de novo events. Hence, it is important that the disorder be suspected in any patient with a thalassemia intermedia phenotype even if both parents are hematologically normal and the patient is from an ethnic background where β thalassemia is rare.

MANAGEMENT

Because of the extreme variability of these disorders, management has to be clinically guided. Most patients are asymptomatic. Splenectomy has been found to be beneficial in a few patients with chronic anemia and transfusion dependency, and cholecystectomy was necessary in a few cases because of gallstones (Ristaldi et al., 1990; Hall et al., 1991; Podda et al., 1991; Thein et al., (1991). Some of these patients continue to be transfusion dependent postsplenectomy, although at less frequent intervals. As in thalassemia intermedia, iron loading is an important problem despite minimal blood transfusions. It results from excessive iron absorption and iron is distributed mainly in the parenchymal tissues (Thein et al., 1990). Iron overload together with the extensive extramedullary hematopoiesis is typical of a hematologic disorder characterized by ineffective erythropoiesis.

To add to the iron overload, many of these patients have also been treated with oral iron due to an erroneous diagnosis of iron-deficiency anemia. Hence, these patients should be carefully monitored by an annual measurement of serum ferritin. Iron chelation should be considered for patients with progressive iron loading. Genetic counseling and prenatal diagnosis should be offered when feasible because compound heterozygosity with β thalassemia could result in transfusion-dependent thalassemia major.

Figure 14.6. Pathophysiology underlying the β-globin gene defects in the heterozygous state. On the left, the pathophysiology in typical β-thalassemia trait, in the center a hyperunstable β-globin chain variant, and on the right, an unstable hemoglobin causing hemolytic anemia.

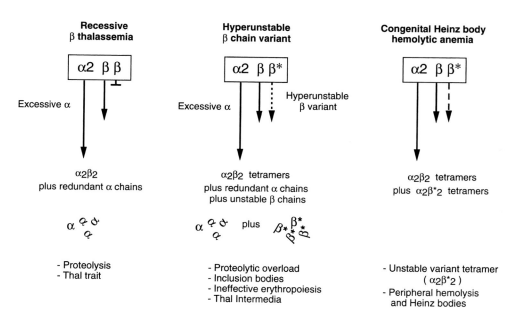

References

Adams, JGI, Boxer, LA, Baehner, RL et al. (1979). Hemoglobin Indianapolis (β112[G14] Arginine). An unstable β chain variant producing the phenotype of severe β-thalassemia. *J. Clin. Invest.* 63: 931–938.

Adams, JGI, Steinberg, MH, and Kazazian, HHJ. (1990). Isolation and characterization of the translation product of a β-globin gene nonsense mutation (β121 GAA→TAA). *Br. J. Haematol.* 75: 561–567.

Ahmed, S, Petrou, M, and Saleem, M. (1996). Molecular genetics of β-thalassaemia in Pakistan: a basis for prenatal diagnosis. *Brit. J. Haemat.* 94: 476–482.

Arjona, SN, Maldonado Eloy-Garcia, J, Gu, LH et al. (1996). The dominant β-thalassaemia in a Spanish family is due to a frameshift that introduces an extra CGG codon (=arginine) at the 5′ end of the second exon. *Br. J. Haematol.* 93: 841–844.

Baiget, M, Gornez Pereira, CI, Jue, DL et al. (1986) A case of hemoglobin Indianapolis [β112(G14) Cys→Arg] in an individual from Cordoba, Spain. *Hemoglobin* 10: 483–494.

Baserga, SJ and Benz, EJ Jr. (1992). β-globin nonsense mutation: Deficient accumulation of mRNA occurs despite normal cytoplasmic stability. *Proc. Nat. Acad. Sci. U.S.A.* 89: 2935–2939.

Beris, P, Miescher, PA, Diaz-Chico, J et al. (1988). Inclusion-body β-thalassemia trait in a Swiss family is caused by an abnormal hemoglobin (Geneva) with an altered and extended β chain carboxy-terminus due to a modification in codon β114. *Blood* 72: 801–805.

Bunn, HF and Forget, BG. (1986). *Hemoglobin: Molecular, Genetic and Clinical Aspects.* Philadelphia: W.B. Saunders.

Bunn, HF, Schmidt, GJ, Haney, DN et al. (1975). Hemoglobin Cranston, an unstable variant having an elongated β chain due to non-homologous crossover between two normal β chain genes. *Proc. Nat. Acad. Sci. U.S.A.* 72: 3609–3613.

Coleman, MB, Steinberg, MH, and Adams JG III. (1991). Hemoglobin Terre Haute Arginine β106. *J. Biol. Chemi.* 266: 5798–5800.

Cürük, MA, Molchanova, TP, Postnikov, YV et al. (1994). β-Thalassemia alleles and unstable hemoglobin types among Russian pediatric patients. *Am. J. Hemat.* 46: 329–332.

De Biasi, R, Spiteri, D, Caldora, M et al. (1988). Identification by fast atom bombardment mass spectrometry on Hb Indianapolis [β112(G14)Cys→Arg] in a family from Naples, Italy. *Hemoglobin* 12: 323–336.

de Castro, CM, Devlin, B, Fleenor, DE et al. (1994). A novel β-globin mutation, β Durham-NC [β114 Leu→Pro], produces a dominant thalassemia-like phenotype. *Blood* 83: 1109–1116.

Deutsch, S, Samii, K, Darbellay, R et al. (1998). Nonsense mutations in exon III of β-globin are associated with normal β-thal mRNA production while frameshift mutations lead to a severely decreased amount of β-thal mRNA. *Blood* 92 (Suppl. 1): 334a.

Divoky, V, Svobodova, M, Indrak, K et al. (1993). Hb Hradec Kralove (Hb HK) or α2β2115(G17)Ala → Asp. A severely unstable hemoglobin variant resulting in a dominant β-thalassemia trait in a Czech family. *Hemoglobin* 17: 319–328.

Enssle, J, Kugler, W, Hentze, MW, and Kulozik, AE. (1993). Determination of mRNA fate by different RNA polymerase II promoters. *Proc. Nat. Acad. Sci. U.S.A.* 90: 10091–10095.

Faustino, P, Osorio-Almeida, L, Barbot, J et al. (1992). Novel promoter and splice junction defects add to the genetic, clinical or geographical heterogeneity of β-thalassaemia in the Portuguese population. *Hum. Genet.* 89: 573–576.

Faustino, P, Osório-Almeida, L, Romão, J et al. (1998). Dominantly transmitted β-thalassaemia arising from the production of several aberrant mRNA species and one abnormal peptide. *Blood* 91: 685–690.

Fei, YJ, Stoming, TA, Kutlar, A et al. (1989). One form of inclusion body β-thalassemia is due to a GAA→TAA mutation at codon 121 of the β chain. *Blood* 73: 1075–1077.

Flatz, G, Kinderlerer, JL, Kilmartin, JV, and Lehmann, H. (1971). Haemoglobin Tak: A variant with additional residues at the end of the β-chains. *Lancet* 1: 732–733.

Fucharoen, S, Fucharoen, G, Fukumaki, Y et al. (1990a). Three-base deletion in exon 3 of the β-globin gene produced a novel variant (β Gunma) with a thalassemia-like phenotype. *Blood* 76: 1894–1896.

Fucharoen, S, Kobayashi, Y, Fucharoen, G et al. (1990b). A single nucleotide deletion in codon 123 of the β-globin gene causes an inclusion body β-thalassaemia trait: a novel elongated globin chain β^Makabe. *Brit. J. Haemat.* 75: 393–399.

Fucharoen, G, Fucharoen, S, Jetsrisuparb, A et al. (1991). Eight-base deletion in exon 3 of the β-globin gene produced a novel variant (β Khon Kaen) with an inclusion body β-thalassaemia trait. *Blood* 78: 537–539.

Girodon, F, Ghanem, N, Vidaud, M et al. (1992). Rapid molecular characterization of mutations leading to unstable hemoglobin β-chain variants. *Ann. Hematol.* 65: 188–192.

Hall, GW, Franklin, IM, Sura, T et al. (1991). A novel mutation (nonsense β127) in exon 3 of the β globin gene produces a variable thalassaemia phenotype. *Br. J. Haematol.* 79: 342–344.

Hall, GW and Thein, SL. (1994). Nonsense codon mutations in the terminal exon of the β-globin gene are not associated with a reduction in β-mRNA accumulation: A mechanism for the phenotype of dominant β-thalassaemia. *Blood* 83: 2031–2037.

Hentze, MW and Kulozik, AE. (1999). A perfect message: RNA surveillance and nonsense-mediated decay. *Cell* 96: 307–310.

Ho, PJ, Wickramasinghe, SN, Rees, DC et al. (1997). Erythroblastic inclusions in dominantly inherited β thalassaemias. *Blood* 89: 322–328.

Hopmeier, P, Krugluger, W, Gu, LH et al. (1996). A newly discovered frameshift at codons 120–121 (+A) of the β gene is not associated with a dominant form of β-thalassemia. *Blood* 87: 5393–5394.

Huisman, THJ, Carver, MFH, and Efremov, GD. (1998). *A Syllabus of Human Hemoglobin Variants* (2nd ed.). Augusta, GA: The Sickle Cell Anemia Foundation.

Kaeda, JS, Saary, MJ, Sauders, TJ et al. (1992). Dominant β thalassaemia trait due to a novel insertion. Proceedings of the Thalassaemia Meeting, Nice, France.

Kagimoto, T, Morino, Y, and Kishimoto, S. (1978). A new hemoglobin variant. Hb Yarsushiro Alpha^A2 Beta^602 Val replaced by Leu. *Biochim. Biophys. Acta* 532: 195.

Kazazian, HHJ, Orkin, SH, Boehm, CD et al (1986). Characterisation of a spontaneous mutation to a β-thalassaemia allele. *Am. J. Hum. Genet.* 38: 860–867.

Kazazian, HHJ, Dowling, CE, Hurwitz, M et al. (1992). Dominant thalassemia-like phenotypes associated with mutations in exon 3 of the β-globin gene. *Blood* 79: 3014–3018.

Kobayashi, Y, Fukumaki, Y, Komatsu, N et al. (1987). A novel globin structural mutant, Showa-Yakushiji (β110 Leu-Pro) causing a β-thalassemia phenotype. *Blood* 70: 1688–1691.

Landin, B and Rudolphi, O. (1996). A novel mutation in exon 3 of the β-globin gene associated with β-thalassaemia. *Br. J. Haematol.* 93: 24.

Lang, A, Lehmann, H, and King-Lewis, PA. (1974). Hb K Woolwich the cause of a thalassaemia. *Nature* 249: 467–469.

Maquat, LE. (1995). When cells stop making sense: Effects of nonsense codons on RNA metabolism in vertebrate cells. *RNA* 1: 453–465.

Maquat, LE. (1996). Defects in RNA splicing and the consequence of shortened translational reading frames. *Am. J. Hum. Genet.* 59: 279–286.

Murru, S, Loudianos, G, Deiana, M et al. (1991). Molecular characterization of β-thalassemia intermedia in patients of Italian descent and identification of three novel β-thalassemia mutations. *Blood* 77: 1342–1347.

Nagy, E and Maquat, LE. (1998). A rule for termination-codon position within intron-containing genes: When nonsense affects RNA abundance. *Trends Biol. Sci.* 23: 198–199.

Ohba, Y, Hattori, Y, Harano, T et al. (1997). β-thalassemia mutations in Japanese and Koreans. *Hemoglobin* 21: 191–200.

Öner, R, Öner, C, Wilson, JB et al. (1991). Dominant β-thalassaemia trait in a Portuguese family is caused by a deletion of (G)TGGCTGGTGT(G) and an insertion of (G)GCAG(G) in codons 134, 135, 136 and 137 of the β-globin gene. *Br. J. Haematol.* 79: 306.

Park, SS, Barnetson, R, Kim, SW et al. (1991). A spontaneous deletion of β33/34 Val in exon 2 of the β globin gene (Hb Korea) produces the phenotype of dominant β thalassaemia. *Br. J. Haematol.* 78: 581.

Podda, A, Galanello, R, Maccioni, L et al. (1991). Hemoglobin Cagliari (β60[E4] VAL→Glu): A novel unstable thalassemic hemoglobinopathy. *Blood* 77: 371–375.

Ristaldi, MS, Pirastu, M, Murru, S et al. (1990). A spontaneous mutation produced a novel elongated β-globin chain structural variant (Hb Agnana) with a thalassemia-like phenotype. *Blood* 75: 1378–1380.

Sansone, G, Carrell, RW, and Lehmann, H. (1967). Haemoglobin Genova: β28(B10) Leucine → Proline. *Nature* 214: 877–879.

Smith, CM III, Hedlund, B, Cich, JA et al. (1983). Hemoglobin North Shore: A variant hemoglobin associated with the phenotype of β-thalassemia. *Blood* 61: 378–383.

Stamatoyannopoulos, G, Woodson, R, Papayannopoulou, T et al. Inclusion-body β-thalassemia trait. A form of β thalassemia producing clinical manifestation in simple heterozygotes. *N. Engl. J. Med.* 290: 939–943.

Streisinger, G, Okada, Y, Emrich, J et al. (1966). Frame shift mutations and the genetic code. Cold Spring Harbor Symposium on Quantitative Biology, p. 77.

Thein, SL. (1993). β-thalassaemia. In Higgs, DR and Weatherall, DJ, editors. *Baillière's Clinical Haematology. International Practice and Research: The Haemoglobinopathies.* London: Baillière Tindall. pp. 171–176.

Thein, SL, Hesketh, C, Taylor, P et al. (1990). Molecular basis for dominantly inherited inclusion body β-thalassemia. *Proc. Natl. Acad. Sci. U.S.A.* 87: 3924–3928.

Thein, SL, Best, S, Sharpe, J et al. (1991). Hemoglobin Chesterfield (β28 Leu→Arg) produces the phenotype of inclusion body β thalassemia. *Blood* 77: 2791–2793.

Thermann, R, Neu-Yilik, G, Deters, A et al. (1998). Binary specification of nonsense codons by splicing and cytoplasmic translation. *EMBO J.* 17: 3484–3494.

Thillet, J, Cohen-Solal, M, Seligmann, M, and Rosa, J. (1976). Functional and physicochemical studies of hemoglobin St. Louis β28(B10) Leu→Gln. A variant with ferric β heme iron. *J. Clin. Invest.* 58: 1098–1106.

Vetter, B, Neu-Yilik, G, Kohne, E et al. (2000). Dominant β-thalassaemia: a highly unstable haemoglobin is caused by a novel 6 bp deletion of the β-globin gene. *Brit. J. Haemat.* 108: 176–181.

Waye, JS, Eng, B, Francombe, WH et al. (1995). Novel seventeen basepair deletion in exon 3 of the β-globin gene. *Human Mutation* 6: 252–253.

Weatherall, DJ, Clegg, JB, Knox-Macaulay, HHM et al. (1973). A genetically determined disorder with features both of thalassaemia and congenital dyserythropoietic anaemia. *Br. J. Haematol.* 24: 681–702.

Williamson, D, Brennan, SO, Muir, H, and Carrell, RW. (1983). Hemoglobin Collingwood β60(E4) Val→Ala, a new unstable hemoglobin. *Hemoglobin* 7: 511.

Williamson, D, Brown, KP, Langdown, JV et al. (1997). Mild thalassemia intermedia resulting from a new insertion/frameshift mutation in the β-globin gene. *Hemoglobin* 21: 485–493.

Zhang, J, Sun, X, Qian, Y et al. (1998a). At least one intron is required for the nonsense-mediated decay of triosephosphate isomerase mRNA: A possible link between nuclear splicing and cytoplasmic translation. *Mol. Cell. Biol.* 18: 5272–5283.

Zhang, J, Sun, X, Qian, Y, and Maquat, LE. (1998b). Intron function in the nonsense-mediated decay of β-globin mRNA: Indications that pre-mRNA splicing in the nucleus can influence mRNA translation in the cytoplasm. *RNA* 4: 801–815.

15

Hereditary Persistence of Fetal Hemoglobin and δβ Thalassemia

W. G. WOOD

INTRODUCTION

Hereditary persistence of fetal hemoglobin (HPFH) and δβ thalassemia are descriptive terms used for a range of hemoglobin disorders that are characterized by decreased or absent β-chain synthesis and a variable compensatory increase in γ-chain synthesis. HPFH was first observed in two healthy West African individuals who appeared to have sickle cell anemia with only sickle (HbS) and fetal hemoglobin (HbF) (Edington and Lehmann, 1955). Each produced a child with HbA and with a high level of HbF and it was considered that this might be an interaction of HbS with an unusual form of thalassemia. Additional cases were reported from East Africa with a similar mild sickling disorder; it was shown that the carriers of the high HbF condition did not have thalassemic features and the term HPFH was introduced (Jacob and Raper, 1958). Further cases were discovered in the West Indies and the United States, and the first homozygote was found (Wheeler and Krevans, 1961). He was clinically normal and had 100 percent HbF, indicating a complete absence of δ- and β-chain production. It soon became established that the gene responsible for this condition was allelic to the β-globin gene (Conley et al., 1963).

The first type of δβ thalassemia to be described was Hb Lepore (Gerald and Diamond, 1958). This abnormal hemoglobin was shown to contain a fusion δβ-globin chain produced by a crossover between the δ- and β-globin genes (Baglioni, 1962). As the δβ-fusion chain was inefficiently produced and there was no synthesis of normal δ- or β-globin chains it resulted in a thalassemic condition (see Chapter 12). Soon afterwards, a form of thalassemia with normal HbA$_2$ and unusually high levels of HbF was described in several racial groups (Fessas et al., 1961; Zuelzer et al., 1961). When the first homozygote for this condition was observed (Brancati and Baglioni, 1966), with a thalassemic disorder and 100 percent HbF, it was clear that no δ- or β-globin chains were produced in this condition and hence it became known as δβ thalassemia.

Further heterogeneity in these conditions was demonstrated after it was discovered that there are two types of γ-globin chains (Schroeder et al., 1968). While the HbF in many HPFHs and δβ thalassemias contained both $^G\gamma$- and $^A\gamma$-globin chains, other cases had only one or the other.

Once the β-like globin genes had been cloned, these conditions were analyzed at the molecular level and it became clear that deletions within the β-globin gene cluster underlie most cases of δβ thalassemia and many cases of HPFH. Different deletions were observed that removed both the δ- and β-globin genes. The size and positions of the deletions bore no obvious relationship to the underlying phenotypes but these studies demonstrated that HPFH and δβ thalassemia were closely related conditions. The discovery that some HPFH conditions were not due to deletions demonstrated that there was even further heterogeneity within these disorders.

CLASSIFICATION

HPFH and δβ thalassemia were originally distinguished on what appeared to be clear-cut hematologic and clinical grounds. Heterozygous δβ thalassemia had a similar red cell picture to β thalassemia, with hypochromic and microcytic erythrocytes, but a normal level of HbA$_2$ (<3.0 percent) (see Chapter 10). In addition, there was a raised level of HbF (5 percent to 15 percent) that had a heterogeneous intercellular distribution. Homozygotes or compound heterozygotes with β thalassemia had a clinical picture of thalassemia intermedia or major. In contrast, HPFH heterozygotes had essentially normal red cell indices, a normal level of HbA$_2$, and even higher levels of HbF (15 percent to 30 percent) with a more homogeneous, pancellular distribution of HbF. HPFH homozygotes were clinically normal, albeit with reduced mean corpuscular volume (MCV) and mean corpuscular hemo-

Martin H. Steinberg, Bernard G. Forget, Douglas R. Higgs, and Ronald L. Nagel, editors. *Disorders of Hemoglobin: Genetics, Pathophysiology, and Clinical Management.* © 2001 Cambridge University Press. All rights reserved.

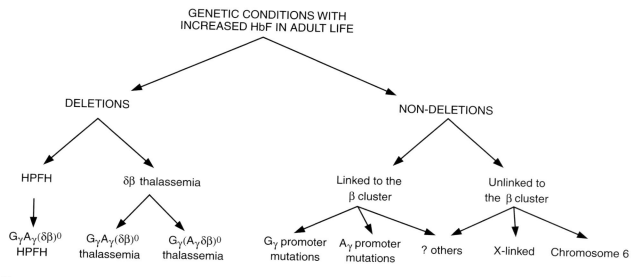

Figure 15.1. Classification of the genetic disorders associated with persistent fetal hemoglobin in adult life.

globin (MCH), while compound heterozygotes with β thalassemia were clinically very mild. However, as more cases with different molecular types of the two conditions were described, these differences became blurred and it is now clear that there is considerable overlap in many of the parameters that were initially used to differentiate them (see below).

The current classification of these conditions is listed in Figure 15.1. The conditions due to gene deletions are classified as HPFH or δβ thalassemia largely on the basis of the level of HbF in heterozygotes and the clinical severity in homozygotes or compound heterozygotes with β thalassemia, where this is known. Included within the HPFH conditions is Hb Kenya, in which production of a hybrid $^A\gamma\beta$ chain is accompanied by increased $^G\gamma$ chain synthesis. The δβ thalassemias are subdivided into those that produce both $^G\gamma$- and $^A\gamma$-globin chains, the $^G\gamma$ $^A\gamma$ $(\delta\beta)^0$ thalassemias (including Hb Lepore), and those that produce only $^G\gamma$ chains, the $^G\gamma(^A\gamma\delta\beta)^0$ thalassemias. Within each of these three groups, there are several different deletions that share a similar clinical and hematologic phenotype; they are usually named after the geographic region in which they were first described.

Conditions associated with increased HbF in adult life that are not due to deletions in the β-globin cluster can also be subclassified (see below). Those in which there is an increase of only the $^G\gamma$- or $^A\gamma$-globin chains are usually due to mutations in the respective promoter, resulting in a variable level of persistent HbF. Several other conditions are due to genes that increase γ-globin gene expression but are not linked to the β-globin complex. These include one localized to chro-

mosome 6 and another to the X chromosome. Additional genes are known to occur but have yet to be localized.

The broad classification of the deletion conditions into three groups, although useful, is rather arbitrary. When the mean levels of HbF and red cell indices are plotted out for each individual deletion it becomes apparent that there is a continuum between δβ thalassemia and the HPFHs and not two distinct groups (Fig. 15.2). Not all conditions fit neatly into one of the groups. For instance, the condition referred to as Indian HPFH or HPFH 3 has 20 percent to 25 percent HbF in heterozygotes, consistent with an HPFH condition but it produces a relatively severe disease when inherited together with β thalassemia, a feature usually associated with δβ thalassemia. The two common types of HPFH of African origin are asymptomatic in homozygotes and appear to be mild in combination with β thalassemia. However, the most common Black β-thalassemia alleles are themselves mild, and it is possible that if these HPFHs were coupled with a severe β-thalassemia allele, a more severe clinical picture might emerge. Indeed, in an early report of a compound heterozygote involving a β^0-thalassemia allele, a more severe interaction was observed (Fogarty et al., 1974). Among the $^G\gamma(^A\gamma\delta\beta)^0$ thalassemias, the Thai type has unusually high levels of HbF [it has been referred to as HPFH 6 (Kosteas et al., 1997)] but from a structural point of view it clearly belongs in the $^G\gamma(^A\gamma\delta\beta)^0$ thalassemias.

Deletions that remove only the β-globin gene and hence produce a β-thalassemia phenotype with a raised HbA_2, also tend to produce increased HbF levels compared to nondeletion β thalassemias. The levels in some individuals overlap with those seen in δβ thalassemia (Fig. 15.2). There are grounds, therefore, for abandoning the classification shown in Figure 15.2

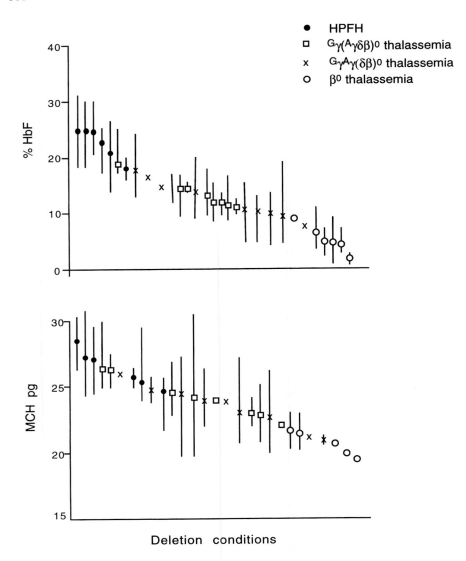

Figure 15.2. The percentage of HbF and of MCH in heterozygotes for HPFH, $^{G}\gamma(^{A}\gamma\delta\beta)^{0}$ thalassemia, $^{G}\gamma^{A}\gamma(\delta\beta)^{0}$ thalassemia, and β^{0} thalassemias due to large deletions. The data are presented as mean and range for each of the defined molecular types for which sufficient information is available

and combining all the deletion conditions into one group. However, as we do not fully understand the mechanisms responsible for the increased HbF in these conditions, this might be premature. When we do, a different classification might naturally emerge. In the meantime, therefore, we have retained the scheme with which most people are conversant.

Deletions Resulting in HPFH or δβ Thalassemia

The structure of the β-globin gene cluster and the surrounding area is illustrated in Figure 15.3. A major regulatory region marked by four erythroid-specific DNase I hypersensitive sites, the locus control region (LCR), lies 5′ to the ε-globin gene. Loss of the LCR, which occurs in the (ε$^{G}\gamma^{A}\gamma\delta\beta)^{0}$ thalassemias, results in inactivation of any remaining β-globin genes (see Chapter 6). The LCR and two other erythroid-specific DNase I hypersensitive sites that have been mapped around the cluster are shown by arrows on the map. Additional regulatory regions include sequences that have enhancer-like activity in transient transfection assays. These have been identified 3′ to the $^{A}\gamma$-globin gene, within IVS 2 of the β-globin gene, 3′ to the β-globin gene, and at three sites in the downstream region, immediately beyond the breakpoints of HPFH-1, HPFH-5, and the Southeast Asian $^{G}\gamma(^{A}\gamma\delta\beta)^{0}$ thalassemia. Several olfactory receptor genes or pseudogenes have been localized in the vicinity of the cluster, three 5′ to the LCR and two 3′ to the β gene (Bulger et al 1999). The area is also rich in repetitive sequences, particularly *Alu* and L1 repeats.

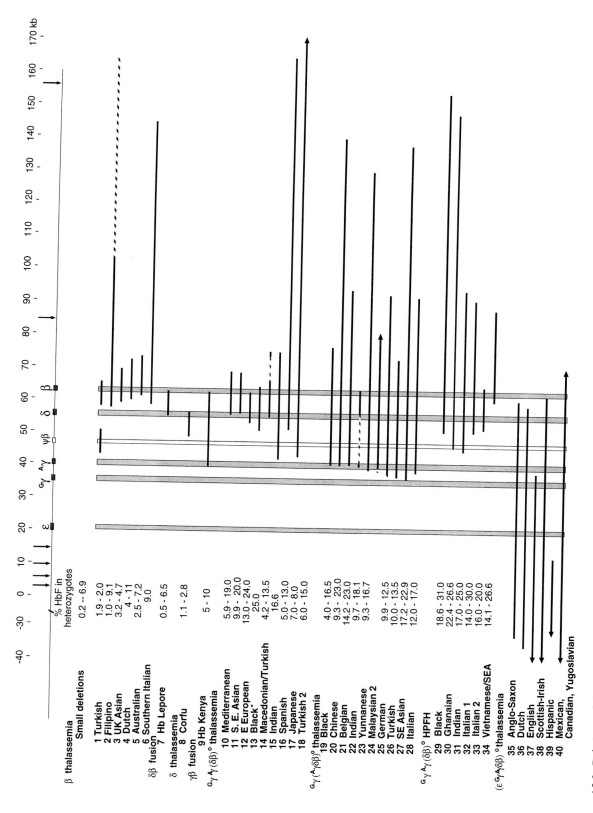

Figure 15.3. Deletions of the β-globin gene cluster causing HPFH, $^G\gamma(^A\gamma\delta\beta)^0$ thalassemia, and $^G\gamma^A\gamma(\delta\beta)^0$ thalassemia; additional large deletions causing β thalassemia and those responsible for $(\epsilon^G\gamma^A\gamma\delta\beta)^0$ thalassemia are provided for comparison. Arrows indicate DNase hypersensitive sites and the four arrows to the left (5') of the ε-globin gene define the LCR. The inverted region in the two double-deletion/inversion cases are shown as a dotted line; for an explanation of the dashed line in the Filipino β thalassemia, see the legend to Table 15.1. * This deletion has only been observed in *trans* to HbS. For references see Wood (1993) and the text.

The deletions resulting in HPFH or δβ thalassemia that have been characterized to date are listed in Table 15.1 and illustrated in Figure 15.3. For comparison, the larger deletions that remove the β-globin gene but spare the δ-globin gene and hence produce a β-thalassemia phenotype are also shown. Deletions of the whole cluster or those that remove its 5' end (including the LCR) and inactivate the remaining genes [(εGγAγδβ)⁰ thalassemias] are also included. The hematologic and clinical aspects of these conditions will be dealt with in a later section.

In both the GγAγ(δβ)⁰ HPFHs and the GγAγ(δβ)⁰ thalassemias, deletions include the δ- and the β-globin gene and extend to a variable degree 3' to the cluster, in some cases for over 100 kb. In the Gγ(Aγδβ)⁰ thalassemias, however, the 5' end of the deletion partially or totally removes the Aγ-globin gene as well.

HPFHs

Hb Kenya. The abnormal β chain in Hb Kenya is a hybrid with a 5' end derived from the γ chain and a 3' end from the β chain (Huisman et al., 1972; Kendall et

Table 15.1. Deletion Breakpoints in δβ Thalassemia, HPFH, and Selected β-Thalassemia Conditions

Condition	Type	5' breakpoint	3' breakpoint	Deletion size (kb)
β thalassemia	Turkish	~43000	~50600	~7.6
	Turkish	~58000	~65600	~7.6
	Filipino	57878	(~103) >165*	(45) >108*
	UK Asian	59127	69456	10.329
	Dutch	59661	72283	12.622
	Australian	61301	73324	12.023
	Italian	58501	~145000	~87
δβ fusion	Hb Lepore	54874–55238	62483–63572	7.398
δ thalassemia	Corfu	48841	56051	7.201
γβ fusion	Hb Kenya	39846–39869	62521–62543	22.675
GγAγ(δβ)⁰ HPFH	Black	51085	~15400	~106
	Ghanaian	46495	~148500	~105
	Indian	45027	~94000	~48.5
	Italian	50375	~91000	~40
	Sicilian	51504	64414	12.910
	SE Asian	60150	~88000	~28
GγAγ (δβ)⁰ thalassemia	Mediterranean	55942	69320	13.378
	SE Asian	55989	68573	12.584
	E European	53177	62301	9.124
	Black	52285	64052	11.767
	Macedonian/Turkish	54686	66151	11.465
	Macedonian/Turkish	73795	75388	1.593
	Indian	42132	74753	32.621
	Spanish	51985	~166000	114
	Japanese	43120	>170000	>130
	Turkish	~43000	~73000	~30
Gγ(Aγδβ)⁰ thalassemia	Black	40680	76487	35.807
	Chinese	40453	~140000	~100
	Indian	40054	40887	0.834
	Indian	56174	63634	7.460
	Italian	39758	~92000	~52
	Belgian	40712	~94000	50
	Yunnanese	39297	~127000	~88
	German	~38000	~90000	~52
	Turkish	37056	73269	36.213
	SE Asian	37233	~138000	~101
	Malay 2	~40000	>80000	>40

* This deletion was originally believed to remove 45 kb (Motum et al., 1993a; Eng et al., 1993; Waye et al., 1994b); analysis of a further family with an identical 5' breakpoint indicated that it extends for >110 kb (Dimovski et al., 1996).

Note: Values are given according to the December 1996 edition of the Genbank β-globin gene cluster sequence and may vary slightly in other editions.

al., 1973), the result of a crossover between the $^A\gamma$ gene and the β gene and deletion of the sequences between (Ojwang et al., 1983). The frequency of Hb Kenya is unknown but relatively rare, and most cases appear to originate from East Africa.

HPFH-1 (or black HPFH). The deletion in this condition begins about 3.75 kb upstream of the δ-globin gene (Fritsch et al., 1979; Tuan et al., 1979, 1983) in an *Alu* repetitive sequence (Jagadeeswaran et al., 1982) and extends for approximately 105 kb (Collins et al., 1987). The breakpoint has been cloned and the newly apposed sequence at the 3′ end characterized (Feingold and Forget, 1989). There is no sequence homology between the 5′ and 3′ ends and additional 5 "orphan" nucleotides have been inserted between the breakpoints.

HPFH-2 (or Ghanaian HPFH). The HPFH-2 deletion begins about 5 kb upstream of the HPFH-1 deletion (Bernards and Flavell, 1980; Tuan et al., 1980, 1983). The 3′ end of the deletion is also shifted about 5 kb to the 5′ side of the HPFH-1 3′ breakpoint (Tuan et al., 1983; Vanin et al., 1983) such that the overall size of these deletions is almost the same. From pulsed field gel electrophoresis, the HPFH-1 and 2 deletions have been estimated to be about 106 and 105 kb, respectively (Collins et al., 1987).

The breakpoint of the HPFH-2 deletion has been cloned and sequenced (Mager et al., 1985; Henthorn et al., 1990). It starts within IVS 2 of the ψβ-globin gene and ends within an L1 repeat element, with three homologous base pairs at the junction itself and no orphan nucleotides.

HPFH-3 (or Indian HPFH). Six Indian HPFH families (Schroeder et al., 1973; Wainscoat et al., 1984) have been studied at the molecular level and shown to have the same deletion (Kutlar et al., 1984; Wainscoat et al., 1984). The 5′ end of the HPFH-3 deletion lies upstream of the ψβ-globin gene, about 1 kb upstream of the HPFH-2 5′ breakpoint in an *Alu* repeat. The deletion extends for 48.5 kb, much shorter than those of the HPFH-1 and HPFH-2 deletions, and ends within a perfect 160 bp palindrome that lies between an L1 repeat on one side and a set of 41 bp repeats on the other side (Henthorn et al., 1986).

HPFH-4 (or Italian HPFH). Three families with HPFH from southern Italy all had the same deletion removing the δ- and β-globin genes (Saglio et al., 1986). The 5′ breakpoint lay between the ψβ-globin gene and the δ-globin gene, close to that of the HPFH-1 deletion. The deletion extends for 40 kb, with the 3′ end lying about 2 kb upstream of the HPFH-3 dele-

tion. Sequence analysis of the breakpoint region has not been reported.

HPFH-5 (or Sicilian HPFH). Two Sicilian brothers with an HPFH phenotype were shown to have a deletion of only about 13 kb (Camaschella et al., 1990). The 5′ end lay within an *Alu* repeat while the 3′ breakpoint was located 692 to 695 bp downstream of the β-gene poly A addition site. The breakpoints shared a 4 bp homology with 5 orphan nucleotides inserted. The deletion ended within the enhancer immediately 3′ to the β gene, removing one of the four GATA-1 sites contained in this element (Camaschella et al., 1990) but the functional significance of that remains unknown.

Southeast Asian HPFH. Motum and co-workers (1993a) described two unrelated Vietnamese patients with HPFH and a novel 30 kb deletion. An apparently identical deletion was subsequently described in families from Vietnam, Cambodia, and China (Dimovski et al., 1994), suggesting that the mutation may be spread throughout Southeastern Asia. This HPFH is the only one described in which the δ-globin gene remains intact. The deletion starts 2 kb upstream of the β-globin gene and extends for about 30 kb, its 3′ end lying within 5 kb of the 3′ ends of the HPFH-3 and -4 deletions.

δβ Thalassemias
Hb Lepore. The Lepore globin chain is a hybrid δβ chain produced by misaligned crossing over between the δ- and the β-globin genes (see Chapter 12 and Fig. 12-4). Three different types of Hb Lepore have been distinguished depending on the position of the crossover: Lepore Washington/Boston, δ87-β116; Lepore Baltimore, δ50-β86; and Lepore Hollandia, δ22-β50. Hb Lepore Washington/Boston is the most common; it and Hb Lepore Baltimore have been found in people of Mediterranean and African origin. Hb Lepore Hollandia has been found in people from Papua, New Guinea, and Bangladesh.

Mediterranean $^G\gamma^A\gamma(\delta\beta)^0$ Thalassemia (Sicilian, Southern Italian δβ Thalassemia). δβ thalassemia is frequently encountered among the thalassemic populations of the Mediterranean and may comprise up to 5 percent of all β thalassemias in some regions. Early gene mapping studies by restriction enzyme analysis had demonstrated the presence of a deletion that gave abnormal sized bands with a probe from IVS 2 of the δ-globin gene (Bernards et al., 1979; Fritsch et al., 1979; Ottolenghi et al., 1982; Tuan et al., 1983). The deletion extended beyond the β-globin gene and encompassed about 13 kb. Cloning and sequencing of the breakpoint demonstrated that the deletion began within δ IVS 2, 188 bp upstream of exon 3 and ended within an L1 repeat (Henthorn et al., 1990).

Southeast Asian $^G\gamma^A\gamma(\delta\beta)^0$ Thalassemia (Thai, Laotian, Vietnamese δβ Thalassemia).

Three independent reports of δβ thalassemia cases from Southeast Asia have been described with a 12.5 kb deletion that is similar to, but clearly different from, the Mediterranean δβ thalassemia. The deletion starts in IVS 2 of the δ-globin gene and ends in the same L1 repeat as the Mediterranean deletion. Restriction enzyme analysis of the Thai (Trent et al., 1988) and Laotian (Zhang et al., 1988) cases are indistinguishable at that level of resolution but sequence analysis was not reported. Craig and co-workers (1994) sequenced the breakpoints of a Vietnamese case and showed that the deletion lies within that of the Mediterranean type, being 47 or 48 bp shorter at the 5′ end and 747 or 748 bp shorter at the 3′ end. It is not entirely clear whether this is identical to the Laotian case, in which fine mapping suggested that the 5′ breakpoint lay 18 to 24 bp downstream of that sequenced in the Vietnamese case. It is possible that closely related but subtly different recombinations between the δ IVS 2 and L1 regions have produced similar deletions and, not surprisingly, similar phenotypes.

Eastern European $^G\gamma^A\gamma(\delta\beta)^0$ Thalassemia.

A 9.1 kb deletion resulting in δβ thalassemia was characterized in a single family of Eastern European origin. The deletion breakpoint was cloned and sequenced and shown to extend from 1.6 kb 5′ to the δ-globin gene cap site into IVS I of the β-globin gene (Palena et al., 1994).

Black $^G\gamma^A\gamma(\delta\beta)^0$ Thalassemia.

A deletion of 12.5 kb that removed the δ- and the β-globin genes was mapped in an American black woman who was a compound heterozygote for the β^S-globin gene (Anagnou et al., 1985). No simple heterozygote for this condition was found but normal MCH, balanced chain synthesis, and a pancellular distribution of the HbF suggested an HPFH phenotype. Restriction mapping data of the 5′ and 3′ breakpoints suggested that this deletion is similar to, but differs from, HPFH-5. A similar deletion was described in a second black family (Waye et al., 19940a) where, in the absence of HbS, a phenotype of δβ thalassemia was observed; interaction with β thalassemia resulted in a clinical picture of thalassemia intermedia. Sequencing of the breakpoints showed that these two deletions were identical and differed slightly in position from that of HPFH-5 (Anagnou, personal communication).

Turkish/Macedonian $^G\gamma^A\gamma(\delta\beta)^0$ Thalassemia.

δβ thalassemia was described in two families from Macedonia by Efremov et al. (1975). Gene mapping demonstrated a deletion extending from 18 to 23 kb 5′ to the δ-globin gene to past the β-globin gene (Efremov et al., 1986). However, some inconsistencies in expected band sizes were observed. Subsequently, Kulozik et al. (1992) described a Turkish family with δβ thalassemia where there were two deletions, with inversion of the sequences between them. Sequencing demonstrated that the 5′ deletion began 53 bp 5′ to the δ-globin gene cap site and ended 11.5 kb downstream, beyond the β-globin gene and just 5′ to the L1 repeat. The second deletion of 1.6 kb began beyond the inverted L1 repeat. The restriction map of this complex rearrangement was similar to that described for the Macedonian cases, suggesting that the two could be the same.

Craig et al. (1994), using a polymerase chain reaction (PCR) approach to identify deletion mutations, described further cases of this inversion-deletion in two Italian and one Greek family. Using the same technique to reanalyze the original Macedonian cases, they demonstrated that the Macedonian and Turkish cases were identical (Craig et al., 1995).

Indian $^G\gamma^A\gamma(\delta\beta)^0$ Thalassemia.

A unique deletion causing δβ thalassemia was found in someone of Indian origin. Cloning and sequencing of the breakpoints demonstrated that the deletion began about 1 kb 3′ of the $^A\gamma$-globin gene and terminated in an L1 repeat, about 11 kb 3′ to the β-globin gene, encompassing 32.6 kb in total (Mishima et al., 1989; Gilman et al., 1992).

Spanish $^G\gamma^A\gamma(\delta\beta)^0$ Thalassemia.

Cases of δβ thalassemia from Spain, including homozygotes, were first reported in 1979 (Gimferrer et al., 1979) and may be a relatively frequent type of thalassemia in that area. The 5′ end of the deletion was mapped to an *Alu* repeat upstream of the δ-globin gene (Ottolenghi et al., 1982). The 3′ breakpoint was shown to lie 8.5 to 9.0 kb beyond the HPFH-1 deletion and the breakpoint has been cloned and sequenced (Camaschelia et al., 1987).

Japanese $^G\gamma^A\gamma(\delta\beta)^0$ Thalassemia.

A Japanese δβ-thalassemia homozygote, the product of a consanguineous marriage, was shown to have a deletion that started about 2 kb 3′ to the $^A\gamma$-globin gene and extended beyond the β-globin gene (Matsunaga et al., 1985). Cloning and sequencing of the breakpoint demonstrated that the deletion ended further downstream than any of the others characterized, including the Spanish δβ-thalassemia deletion (Shiokawa et al., 1988).

Turkish $^G\gamma^A\gamma(\delta\beta)^0$ Thalassemia.

A deletion resulting in $^G\gamma^A\gamma(\delta\beta)^0$ thalassemia was found in a Turkish family (Öner et al., 1996). Starting downstream of the $^A\gamma$-globin gene close to the 5′ ends of the Indian and Japanese type deletions, it extended for about 30 kb, ending in an L1 repeat 3′ to the β-globin gene. Sequencing of the breakpoints will be necessary to demonstrate that this deletion differs from the Indian Gγ Aγ(δβ)⁰ thalassaemia deletion.

Gγ(Aγδβ)⁰ Thalassemia

Black Gγ(Aγδβ)⁰ Thalassemia. Numerous African Americans with high HbF and synthesizing only Gγ-globin chains have been described, some originally as Gγ HPFH, others as Gγ δβ thalassemia (Altay et al., 1977). Molecular analysis of ten families demonstrated that they all had the same deletion of about 34 kb beginning within the 3′ end of the Aγ-globin gene (Henthorn et al., 1985). Cloning and sequencing of the deletion junction showed that its 5′ end was within IVS 2 of the Aγ-globin gene, 87 bp from exon 3 while the 3′ end was located within an L1 repeat 3′ of the β-globin gene.

Chinese Gγ(Aγδβ)⁰ Thalassemia. The first report of a Chinese family with Gγ(Aγδβ)⁰ thalassemia was by Mann et al. (1972). Genomic mapping showed that the 5′ breakpoint of the deletion lay within the Aγ-globin gene (Jones et al., 1981b). When the deletion junction was cloned and sequenced, the 5′ end was shown to be in IVS 2 of the Aγ-globin gene while the 3′ end was about 100 kb away, approximately 11 kb to the 5′ side of the HPFH-2 deletion (Mager et al., 1985). An insert of 36 to 41 bp from an L1 repeat lay between the two junctions. Additional families with the same deletion were described by Trent et al. (1984) and Craig et al. (1994).

Belgian Gγ(Aγδβ)⁰ Thalassemia. A third Aγ-globin gene deletion that started within 30 bp of the Black Gγ(Aγδβ)⁰-thalassemia deletion was described in a Belgian family (Losekoot et al., 1991). The deletion extended for about 50 kb, terminating just 4 bp upstream from the 3′ end of the HPFH-3 deletion and just 1 bp from the midpoint of the 160 bp palindrome that lies in this region (Fodde et al., 1990).

Italian Gγ(Aγδβ)⁰ Thalassemia. An Italian case of Gγ(Aγδβ)⁰ thalassemia has recently been characterized and shown to have a deletion beginning in exon 2 of the Aγ-globin gene and extending for about 52 kb. The 3′ breakpoint of this deletion is close to that of the Indian HPFH (HPFH-3) and the Belgian Gγ(Aγδβ)⁰ thalassemia, in the region of an L1 repeat and a 160 bp palindrome (De Angioletti et al., 1997).

Indian Gγ(Aγδβ)⁰ Thalassemia. A complex double-deletion/inversion rearrangement has been reported in

several Indian families with Gγ(Aγδβ)⁰ thalassemia (Jones et al., 1981a) with similarities to that found in the Macedonian/Turkish Gγ Aγ(δβ)⁰ thalassemia described above. There is a loss of 834 bp from IVS 2 and exon 3 of the Aγ-globin gene and a deletion of 7.46 kb between exon 3 of the δ-globin gene and the 3′ untranslated region of the β-globin gene (Jennings et al., 1985). Additional families with this deletion have been described from India (Matthews et al., 1981; Trent et al., 1984), Kuwait (Amin et al., 1979), and Iran (Craig et al., 1994), suggesting that it may be widespread across the Middle East and the Indian subcontinent.

Yunnanese Gγ(Aγδβ)⁰ Thalassemia. A family from Yunnan province of China was described with several heterozygotes and a homozygote (from a consanguineous mating) with a large deletion starting just upstream of the Aγ-globin gene (Zhang et al., 1993). The 5′ breakpoint was 116 or 117 bp upstream of the Aγ cap site and the deletion extended about 66 kb, terminating in an L1 repeat about 13 kb upstream of the 3′ breakpoint of the Chinese Gγ(Aγδβ)⁰ thalassemia (Zhang and Zhang, 1998).

Malaysian 2 Gγ(Aγδβ)⁰ Thalassemia. George and co-workers (1986) described a Gγ(Aγδβ)⁰-thalassemia homozygote whose relatives were unavailable for study. Beginning within 200 to 400 bp of the Aγ-globin gene cap site the deletion extended an unknown distance beyond the β-globin gene. The size of the abnormal fragments hybridizing with a γ-globin gene probe demonstrated that the deletion differed from the Yunnanese type deletion even though the two 5′ breakpoints were close.

German Gγ(Aγδβ)⁰ Thalassemia. A three-generation German family with Gγ(Aγδβ)⁰ thalassemia was described by Anagnou et al. (1988). The deletion started about 2 kb 3′ to the Gγ-globin gene and ended about 27 kb 3′ to the β-globin gene, close to the 3′ breakpoints of the HPFH-3 and HPFH-4 deletions and the Belgian Gγ(Aγδβ)⁰-thalassemia deletion (Kosteas et al., 1997). Sequence data demonstrated that the 3′ end of the deletion lies 120 bp downstream of the breakpoint in HPFH-4 (Anagnou, personal communication).

Turkish Gγ(Aγδβ)⁰ Thalassemia. A Turkish family with Gγ(Aγδβ)⁰ thalassemia, including a homozygote, has been reported (Reyes et al., 1978; Dincol et al., 1981) and gene mapping demonstrated a large deletion beginning between the Gγ- and Aγ-globin gene (Fritsch et al., 1979; Orkin et al., 1979). Sequencing of the breakpoints demonstrated that the 5′ site lay 1 kb 3′ to the Gγ-globin gene and extended for 36 kb, terminating 48 bp beyond the L1 repeat 3′ to the β-globin gene (Henthorn et al., 1990).

Southeast Asian (Malay-1, Thai, Cantonese) $^{G}\gamma(^{A}\gamma\delta\beta)^{0}$ Thalassemia.

A deletion with a 5′ breakpoint close to that of the Turkish case was described in a Malaysian family by Trent and co-workers (1984). Direct comparison of the two samples demonstrated that they were different deletions but the 3′ extent of the deletion was not determined. A second family with the same 5′ restriction map was described by Fucharoen and co-workers (1987).

Another deletion beginning close to the 3′ end of the $^{G}\gamma$-globin gene was described in a family from Canton [family C (Zeng et al., 1985)]; the extent of the deletion was not ascertained. There were similarities in several abnormal restriction fragment sizes between the Cantonese and Malay-1 deletions, with some apparent differences in weaker bands. Sequencing of the breakpoint junctions will be necessary to confirm the reasonable assumption that the Malay and Cantonese deletions are identical.

Winichagoon and co-workers (1990) described a Thai family with a large deletion starting close to the 3′ end of the $^{G}\gamma$-globin gene. The deletion extended for about 100 kb, ending just short of the Chinese $^{G}\gamma(^{A}\gamma\delta\beta)^{0}$-thalassemia deletion. The abnormal restriction fragments identified with a γ-globin gene probe were similar to those of the Malay-1 deletion. The identity of the Malay and Thai cases was demonstrated by direct comparison with the Malay sample of Fucharoen et al. (1987).

HbF levels are higher in the Malay, Cantonese, and Thai deletion families than in the other forms of $^{G}\gamma(^{A}\gamma\delta\beta)^{0}$ thalassemias, again consistent with these being identical. There is a pancellular distribution of HbF (Trent et al., 1984; Winichagoon et al., 1990) leading to some descriptions of this condition as HPFH-6 (Kosteas et al., 1997). An enhancer-like sequence has been identified in the region between the endpoint of the SE Asian and Chinese $^{G}\gamma(^{A}\gamma\delta\beta)^{0}$ thalassemias.

Other Conditions Related to δβ Thalassemia

$(\varepsilon^{G}\gamma^{A}\gamma\delta\beta)^{0}$ Thalassemia. A number of deletions include the whole β-like globin gene cluster (Fearon et al., 1983; Pirastu et al., 1983; Diaz-Chico et al., 1988; Fortina et al., 1991; Abels et al., 1996). Other deletions remove the 5′ end of the cluster, extending into the β-globin gene in one case (Orkin et al., 1981) but sparing the β-globin gene in two others (Curtin et al., 1985; Taramelli et al., 1986). In these latter two cases, the β-globin gene, although intact, was inactivated. Follow-up studies of the Dutch $(\varepsilon^{G}\gamma^{A}\gamma\delta\beta)^{0}$ thalassemia led to the discovery of the LCR (Grosveld et al., 1987) (see Chapter 6). The importance of the LCR was demonstrated by a deletion that removed the upstream hypersensitive sites but spared HS1 and all of the genes, which, nevertheless, were inactive (Driscoll et al., 1989). Recent studies have shown more extensive conservation of sequences 5′ to the LCR than previously suspected. In mice with a deletion of all structures homologous to the human LCR, DNase sensitivity and developmental regulation of the β-globin gene locus remained intact and mRNA, although reduced in quantity, was present (Bender et al., 2000; Epner et al., 1999). This work suggests that it may be deletion of these sequences 5′ to the LCR that inactivates the β-globin gene in the $(\varepsilon^{G}\gamma^{A}\gamma\delta\beta)^{0}$ thalassemias.

The phenotype of the heterozygous $(\varepsilon^{G}\gamma^{A}\gamma\delta\beta)^{0}$ thalassemias is a normal HbA_2-thalassemia trait. Neonatal hemolytic anemia is present in many, but not all, cases; it spontaneously remits as β-globin chain production replaces γ-globin chain synthesis in the first year of life (Kan et al., 1972; Trent et al., 1990), possibly indicating that fetal and neonatal red cells are more sensitive to the effects of globin chain imbalance than adult cells.

Corfu δ Thalassemia.

A 7.2 kb deletion extending into the δ-globin gene results in a low HbA_2 but has no effect on γ- or β-globin gene expression (Galanello et al., 1990). This deletion has also been found (Wainscoat et al., 1985; Kulozik et al., 1988) in cis to a severe β+-thalassemia allele (IVS1-5 G→A). Heterozygotes for this $\delta^{0}\beta^{+}$ thalassemia show little or no increase in HbF but homozygotes, who have only a trace of HbA, have a mild form of thalassemia intermedia rather than thalassemia major due to their relatively high level of HbF (Traeger-Synodinos et al., 1991). This suggests that the deletion may enhance γ-globin chain production, at least under conditions of erythroid stress.

Nondeletion δβ Thalassemia.

Two Chinese families have been described with the phenotype of δβ thalassemia (hypochromia, microcytosis, normal HbA_2, and HbF of about 22 percent) without a detectable deletion (Zeng et al., 1985; Atweh et al., 1986). In one of these cases it was subsequently shown that the β-globin gene carried the −29 A → G mutation, a mild β+-thalassemia allele (Atweh et al., 1987). Furthermore, there was a nonpolymorphic base substitution in the enhancer 3′ to the $^{A}\gamma$-globin gene (Balta et al., 1994) that could be involved in the increased HbF levels but this awaits experimental confirmation.

Hematology Results and Hemoglobin Analysis

Hematologic findings and the results of hemoglobin analyses on the globin gene deletions discussed above are listed in Tables 15.2 to 15.5. In these analyses, only cases for which the molecular basis has been determined have been included.

Hb Kenya. Hb Kenya carriers have near normal hematologic findings. Hemoglobin analysis reveals low normal levels of HbA_2 (1.4 percent to 1.8 percent) and raised levels of HbF (7 percent to 12 percent), Hb Kenya, and HbA. The proportion of Hb Kenya is more variable, with levels ranging from 5 percent to 23 percent and some suggestion of bimodality, with peaks around 10 percent and 20 percent. The HbF contains only $^G\gamma$-globin gene chains. On interaction with HbS, higher levels of Hb Kenya (17 percent to 19 percent) are observed than in HbA/Kenya cases, while the HbF level (6.6 percent to 11 percent) remains unchanged (Kendall et al., 1973).

$^G\gamma^A\gamma(\delta\beta)^0$ HPFH. Heterozygotes are characterized by normal HbA_2 levels and HbF levels of 15 percent to 30 percent. There are only minor reductions in the red cell indices that are frequently within the normal range. In many of the reported cases, α thalassemia was not excluded and this may explain some instances with reduced MCV and MCH.

Homozygotes have been described for both HPFH-1 (Wheeler and Krevans, 1961; Forget et al., 1976; Orkin et al., 1978; Fritsch et al., 1979) and HPFH-2 (Ringelhann et al., 1970; Acquaye et al., 1977; Tuan et al., 1980; Huisman, 1981; Kutlar et al., 1984) and they are indistinguishable; their hemoglobin consists entirely of HbF (Table 15.5). They are clinically unaffected and have normal or high hemoglobin levels (15 to 18 g/dL), presumably as a result of the higher oxygen affinity of HbF (see Chapter 10). They have microcytic, hypochromic red cells and globin chain synthesis imbalance can be demonstrated, with α/γ-globin ratios of about 2.0 indicating that the output of γ-globin chains does not fully compensate for the lack of β-globin chains.

Compound heterozygotes with β thalassemia are usually clinically silent and have similar hematologic indices to β-thalassemia heterozygotes. Most cases were reported before characterization of the β-thalassemia alleles was feasible and presumably involved mild β-thalassemia mutations that are common in blacks. HbF levels usually fall within the range of 60 percent to 75 percent.

Compound heterozygotes for HPFH and HbS are generally healthy and have a mild sickling disorder (see Chapter 28). They are not usually anemic and there is little evidence of hemolysis. This is ascribed to their high level of HbF and its inhibition of HbS polymerization.

Hematologic indices and hemoglobin analysis of the Indian HPFH heterozygotes are very similar to the two black types (Table 16.2). No homozygotes have been reported but in four families compound heterozygotes with β thalassemia have been observed. Patients were anemic with hemoglobin concentrations of 5.5 to 9.0 g/dL and were classified clinically as thalassemia intermedia. One required splenectomy at age 5 years. In the two Italian types of HPFH, only heterozygotes have been observed and their hematologic and hemoglobin analyses were indistinguishable from HPFH types cited above.

Southeast Asian deletions differ from all the other HPFHs in that the δ-globin gene is intact. Phenotypically they are similar to the other HPFH types except that the HbA_2 level is raised because the δ-globin gene is present.

There are significant differences in the $^G\gamma/^A\gamma$ ratios of the HbF produced in the various deletions that result in HPFH (Fig. 15.4). Heterozygotes for the black HPFH-1 deletion have equal amounts of both chains ($^G\gamma = 50.7 \pm 4.3$ percent). The proportion of $^G\gamma$-globin chain is significantly lower in the Ghanaian HPFH (32.3 ± 4.8 percent) and significantly higher in the Indian type (70.9 ± 2.9 percent); the narrow distributions among these ranges mean that there is little or no overlap between these groups (Kutlar et al., 1984). The Italian type ($^G\gamma = 35.0 \pm 3.2$ percent) overlaps the Ghanaian, while the Sicilian (with only two cases reported) has the lowest $^G\gamma$ level (15 percent and 17 percent) and the Southeast Asian values (61.6 ± 1.7 percent) lie between the black and Indian types. There appears to be no correlation between the HbF concentration and the percent $^G\gamma$-globin chain either within or between the various types of HPFH (Fig. 15.4). Furthermore, the differences between heterozygotes for HPFH-1 and 2 are not maintained in the homozygotes (Table 15.4) and the proportion of $^G\gamma$-globin chains is increased in compound heterozygotes with HPFH and HbS or β thalassemia.

The significance of these observations is not clear. Differences in ratios between the different HPFH types could reflect a direct effect on γ-globin gene expression of the individual deletions; alternatively they may result from differences in polymorphic sequences in and around these genes, like the −158 C or T polymorphism, that differ on the chromosomes where the deletions arose.

Hb Lepore. The hematologic picture in heterozygous Hb Lepore is almost identical to that of β-thalassemia trait. Hemoglobin analysis shows normal levels of HbA_2 together with 5 percent to 15 percent Hb Lepore; Hb Lepore levels do not vary between the different types. HbF levels are usually raised but in most cases do not exceed 5 percent. Direct comparisons within the same laboratory between Hb Lepore and β-thalassemia heterozygotes demonstrate a small but significantly higher

Table 15.2. Summary of Hematologic Data (Mean ± SD) of Deletion HPFH Heterozygotes Sefined by Molecular Analysis

Condition	No. of families/ individuals*	Hb* (g/dL)	MCV† (fl)	MCH† (pg)	HbA₂* (%)	HbF* (%)	Gγ* (%)	α/Non-α synthesis*	Distribution
Black HPFH-1	40/53	12.4 ± 2.2	83.7 ± 4.8	27.1 ± 3.6	1.7 ± 0.4	24.8 ± 3.1	50.7 ± 4.3		Pancellular
Ghanaian HPFH-2	35/64	13.8 ± 1.3	80.3 ± 5.0	25.7 ± 1.6	2.3 ± 0.3	24.5 ± 2.8	32.3 ± 4.8	1.23 ± 0.25	Pancellular
Indian HPFH-3	5/8	14.1 ± 1.1	90.7 ± 5.6	28.5 ± 1.6	1.8 ± 0.3	22.5 ± 2.6	70.9 ± 2.9	1.2	Pancellular
Italian HPFH-4	4/9	13.4 ± 1.6	81.8 ± 5.9	27.2 ± 2.7	1.8 ± 0.1	24.7 ± 5.5	35.0 ± 3.2	1.12 ± 0.05	Pancellular
Sicilian HPFH-5	1/2	13.8 ± 0.3	79.5 ± 2.9	26.0	3.6 ± 0.3	18.0 ± 2.8	16.0 ± 1.4	1.15	Pancellular
SE Asian	4/13	13.2 ± 1.8	85.0 ± 7.9	24.6 ± 1.6	3.8 ± 0.6	20.7 ± 3.8	61.6 ± 1.7	1.46	Pancellular

* Data not necessarily complete for all individuals; extreme outliers are omitted.

† α Thalassemia is not excluded in all cases; some results were obtained after sample had been in transit.

Table 15.3. Summary of Hematologic Data (Mean ± SD) of $^{G}\gamma^{A}\gamma(\delta\beta)^0$ Thalassemia Heterozygotes Defined by Molecular Analysis

Condition	No. of families/ individuals*	Hb (g/dL)	MCV[†] (fl)	MCH[†] (pg)	HbA*$_2$ (%)	HbF* (%)	G$_\gamma$* (%)	α/Non-α* synthesis	Distribution/ % F-cells
Mediterranean	20/24	12.3 ± 1.5	68.2 ± 4.0	22.7 ± 1.8	2.7 ± 0.2	9.6 ± 3.5	43.4 ± 8.2	1.5 ± 0.2	Heterocellular
SE Asian	3/3	13.0 ± 1.1	73.7 ± 2.5	23.9 ± 1.8	2.7 ± 0.3	13.8 ± 5.4	60		Heterocellular/52%
E. European	1/5	13.7 ± 0.9	75.7 ± 1.9	24.8 ± 0.8	2.1 ± 0.3	17.7 ± 4.8	71.5 ± 3.5		Heterocellular/67%
Black	1/1	11.6	70.9		1.9	14.7	50		Heterocellular/50%
Macedonian/Turkish	6/20	12.0 ± 1.0	65.5 ± 6.8	24.5 ± 3.6	2.6 ± 0.4	9.7 ± 2.7	45.6 ± 6.9		Heterocellular
Indian	1/1	11.5	78	26	2.3	16.6	79		Heterocellular
Spanish	?/?	13.1 ± 1.0	69.0 ± 4.6	23.1 ± 3.0	2.3 ± 0.5	10.1 ± 3.9	35.2 ± 7.1	1.46	Heterocellular
Japanese	1/1	12.8	67	21.2	2.9	7.5	49.3		Heterocellular
Turkish	1/2	11.0	64.3 ± 1.8	20.9 ± 0.3	2.5 ± 0.6	10.5 ± 6.3	60	1.37	Heterocellular

* Data not necessarily complete for all individuals; extreme outliers were omitted.
[†] α Thalassemia is not excluded in all cases; some results were obtained after sample had been in transit.

Table 15.4. Summary of Hematologic Data (Mean ± SD) of $G\gamma(A\gamma\delta\beta)^0$ Thalassemia Heterozygotes Defined by Molecular Analysis

Condition	No. of families/individuals*	Hb (g/dL)	MCV† (fl)	MCH† (pg)	HbA$_2$ (%)	HbF (%)	Gγ (%)	α/Non-α synthesis	Distribution/F-cells
Black	20/24	12.6 ± 1.6	74.3 ± 7.4	24.1 ± 2.8	2.4 ± 0.5	11.2 ± 3.4	93.2 ± 4.1	1.43 ± 0.34	Heterocellular
Chinese	5/12	13.9 ± 0.7	72.8 ± 3.8	22.7 ± 1.1	2.5 ± 0.5	11.8 ± 2.1	97.0 ± 2.8	1.38 ± 0.04	Heterocellular/75–90%
Indian	5/16	13.1 ± 1.4	77.1 ± 5.4	24.6 ± 1.3	2.3 ± 0.4	12.9 ± 2.1	99.5 ± 0.5	1.82 ± 0.45	Pancellular
Italian	1/2		68.0 ± 6.2			14.5 ± 3.5			
Belgian	1/3	13.8 ± 2.5	73.5 ± 2.1	26.3 ± 0.6	2.6 ± 0.2	14.5 ± 0.2	82.8 ± 8.8	1.68 ± 0.63	Heterocellular/61–94%
Yunnanese	1/6	13.1 ± 1.0	71.3 ± 4.2	22.9 ± 1.0	1.6 ± 0.1	14.5 ± 3.5	84		Pancellular
German	1/3		72.0 ± 2.8	24.0	2.5 ± 0.1	11.1 ± 1.8	100		Heterocellular/54–77%
Turkish	2/2	12.5 ± 2.1			2.5 ± 0	11.8 ± 2.5		1.96 ± 0.06	Heterocellular/40%
SE Asian	4/9	12.8 ± 1.5	80.0 ± 2.9	26.4 ± 0.9	2.2 ± 0.5	18.8 ± 2.3	96.4 ± 3.6		Pancellular

* Data are not necessarily complete for all individuals; extreme outliers were omitted.

† α Thalassemia is not excluded in all cases; some results were obtained after sample had been in transit.

Table 15.5. Summary of Hematologic Data (Mean ± SD) of δβ Thalassemia and HPFH Homozygotes of Defined Molecular Types

	No of individuals	Hb (g/dL)	MCV (fl)	MCH (pg)	$^{G}\gamma$ (%)	α/γ ratio
HPFH						
Black	3	15.8 ± 1.0	70.0 ± 2.8	24.9 ± 0.2	60.0 ± 1.4	1.7 ± 0.3
Ghanaian	5	17.0 ± 1.2	73.0 ± 5.6	24.2 ± 1.6	58.0 ± 7.0	2.0 ± 0.9
$^{G}\gamma^{A}\gamma(\delta\beta)^{0}$ thalassemia						
Mediterranean	11	10.1 ± 1.6	79.0 ± 4.4	24.2 ± 2.5	53.0 ± 6.4	2.4 ± 1.5
Spanish	10	11.4 ± 1.4	79.3 ± 5.6		~50	4.9 ± 2.9
Turk/Maced	3	11.9 ± 1.2	73.7 ± 3.5	24.0 ± 0.1	53.0 ± 2.8	3.7
Japanese	1	12.0	76	24.7	61.1	2.3
$^{G}\gamma(^{A}\gamma\delta\beta)^{0}$ thalassemia						
Indian	6	10.5 ± 1.2	70.3 ± 5.6	20.8 ± 1.0	100	3.8 ± 1.2
Yunnanese	1	10.7	67	21.3	100	
Malay 2	1	11.8	67	23.7	100	
Turkish	1	9.0	85	25	100	4.9

HbF level in the Hb Lepore heterozygotes. HbF levels are higher in the Baltimore type (mean of 11 cases 4.9 percent, range 2.7 to 11 percent) than in the Washington/Boston cases (mean of 12 cases 2.75 percent, range 0.8 to 5.4 percent) (Ribeiro et al., 1997). This difference is probably due to the different base at position −158 of the $^{G}\gamma$-globin gene (C → T) as shown by the higher proportion of $^{G}\gamma$-globin chains in the Baltimore type (65.9 percent vs. 34.8 percent).

Homozygotes for Hb Lepore contain HbF together with 10 percent to 30 percent Hb Lepore. Their clinical manifestations are variable, ranging from transfusion-dependent thalassemia major to a much milder thalassemia intermedia. A variable clinical picture is also observed in compound heterozygotes with β thalassemia, the severity being, at least in part, dependent on the nature of the β-thalassemia allele.

$^{G}\gamma^{A}\gamma(\delta\beta)^{0}$ Thalassemias. The hematologic findings in the various $^{G}\gamma^{A}\gamma(\delta\beta)^{0}$ thalassemias are similar, with red cell morphology and indices in heterozygotes somewhat milder than those seen in β-thalassemia trait (Table 15.3). HbA$_2$ levels are normal and HbF levels are generally 5 percent to 15 percent. Rather higher levels of HbF are found in the Eastern European and Indian types (although only single families have been studied) but in both cases the red cell indices are reduced. The distribution of HbF in these conditions is heterocellular by the acid elution technique and usually by immunofluorescence. There are no clear-cut differences in the $^{G}\gamma/^{A}\gamma$ ratios between the different $^{G}\gamma^{A}\gamma(\delta\beta)^{0}$ thalassemias, with the possible exceptions that the Eastern European and Indian types have a higher proportion of $^{G}\gamma$-globin chains. In the $^{G}\gamma^{A}\gamma(\delta\beta)^{0}$ thalassemias, in contrast to the HPFH conditions, there appears to be a positive correlation between percent HbF and percent $^{G}\gamma$ chains (Fig. 15.4).

Homozygotes for the Mediterranean, Spanish, Macedonian, and Japanese types of $^{G}\gamma^{A}\gamma(\delta\beta)^{0}$ have been described (Table 15.5). They all have a similar mild form of thalassemia intermedia, with hemoglobin concentrations of 10 to 13 g/dL and only mild hepatosplenomegaly. They may develop more severe anemia during intercurrent infections. Red cell morphology is more severely abnormal than in β-thalassemia trait and the hemoglobin consists of 100 percent HbF, containing both $^{G}\gamma$- and $^{A}\gamma$-globin chains. Compound heterozygotes with β thalassemia show a more variable clinical course, ranging from mild to severe thalassemia intermedia that presumably is dependent on the nature of the β-thalassemia allele. Too few cases have been reported in which both the δβ- and β-thalassemia mutations have been characterized to determine the precise genotype-phenotype relationship.

$^{G}\gamma(^{A}\gamma\delta\beta)^{0}$ Thalassemias. Red cells from $^{G}\gamma(^{A}\gamma\delta\beta)^{0}$-thalassemia heterozygotes, like those from δβ-thalassemia heterozygotes, are characterized by microcytosis and hypochromia (Table 15.4). They show the same pattern of normal HbA$_2$ levels and increased HbF with a heterocellular distribution, as the $^{G}\gamma^{A}\gamma(\delta\beta)^{0}$ thalassemias. The two conditions are distinguished by the γ-globin chain composition of the HbF, which contains nearly all $^{G}\gamma$-globin chains in $^{G}\gamma(^{A}\gamma\delta\beta)^{0}$ thalassemia; the small amounts of $^{A}\gamma$-globin chains present are derived from the normal chromosome in *trans*. The level of HbF is very similar in all the different forms (mean values lie between 11.1 percent and 14.5 percent) except the Southeast Asian type, where they average about 19 percent.

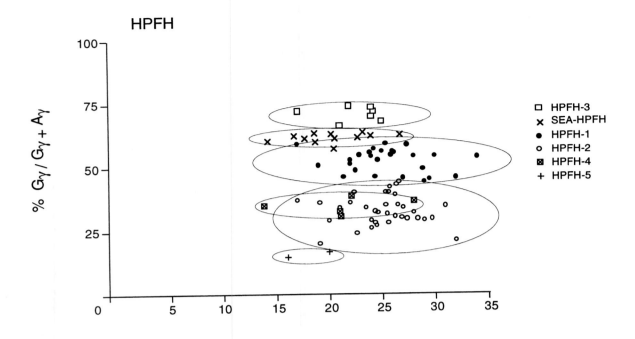

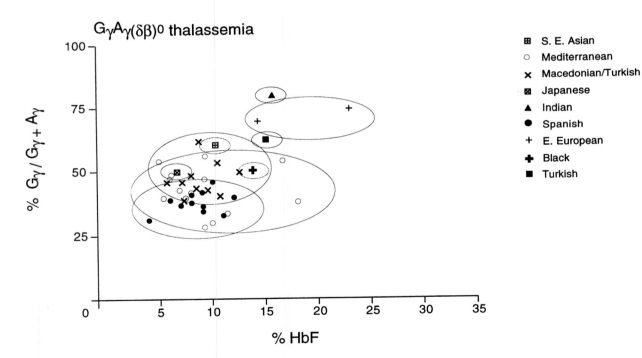

Figure 15.4. A comparison of $^{G}\gamma/^{G}\gamma + {}^{A}\gamma$ ratios versus %HbF in HPFH and $^{G}\gamma^{A}\gamma(\delta\beta)^{0}$-thalassemia heterozygotes.

Homozygotes have been described for the Indian, Yunnanese, Turkish, and Malay-2 types of $^{G}\gamma(^{A}\gamma\delta\beta)^{0}$ thalassemia. Homozygotes appear to be slightly more severely affected than $^{G}\gamma^{A}\gamma(\delta\beta)^{0}$-thalassemia homozygotes, with hemoglobin levels of 7 to 11 g/dL (Table 15.5) and more often have hepatospleno-megaly. The hemoglobin consists of 100 percent HbF containing only $^{G}\gamma$-globin chains. Compound heterozygotes with β thalassemia have a similarly variable clinical course to patients with $^{G}\gamma^{A}\gamma(\delta\beta)^{0}$ thalassemia.

The Intercellular Distribution of HbF in HPFH and δβ Thalassemia

A major feature of the δβ thalassemia and HPFH that is not well understood is the intercellular distribution of HbF. In δβ thalassemia where the HbF level is below 10 percent, the distribution is clearly heterocellular and even a sensitive immunofluorescence technique detects a proportion of cells devoid of HbF (see Chapter 10). In deletion HPFH, where the HbF level is above 20 percent, all of the cells contain detectable HbF and its distribution is said to be pancellular, but the amount of HbF varies from cell to cell. Examination of centrifuged cells from δβ-thalassemia heterozygotes shows that the concentration of HbF is greater in older cells (Wood et al., 1977), whereas there is no such trend in HPFH heterozygotes (Wood et al., 1982). This suggests that there is selective cell survival in δβ thalassemia, with cells producing the most γ chains having the least chain imbalance and the longest life span.

Overall, therefore, there is a correlation between the percentage HbF and the number of HbF-containing cells; however, there is no study published in which the HbF level and the intercellular distribution have been examined across a broad range of conditions using the same techniques in the same laboratory. It is certainly the case that individuals with β thalassemia and an unknown nondeletion HPFH condition (see below) may retain a heterocellular HbF distribution despite an HbF level of 23 percent while an HPFH-2 heterozygote with a relatively low HbF of 14 percent has a pancellular distribution (Craig and Thein, personal communication). This implies that the nature of the underlying molecular defect as well as the level of γ-globin gene expression may determine the distribution level of HbF.

As the same molecular defect is present in all the cells, why should there be this cellular heterogeneity in γ-globin chain production? One explanation is that this is an example of position effect variegation brought about by the altered chromosomal environment that surrounds the globin genes as a result of the deletion. For instance, the enhancer that normally lies about 100 kb from the γ-globin genes is brought closer to them in the HPFH-1 and 2 deletions (see below). While this element has enhancer properties, its effect on the γ-globin gene promoters may not produce as stable an interaction as with its normal target, resulting in reduced gene expression. Its effect may be to increase the probability of γ-globin gene expression in a stochastic way, resulting in variability from cell to cell. If similar but even less effective elements are active in other deletions, one could envisage that many cells may not produce any γ-globin chains, as in the δβ thalassemias. Additional epigenetic effects could also be at work as a result of the altered chromatin structure brought about by the deletion.

PATHOPHYSIOLOGY OF HPFH AND δβ THALASSEMIA

The hematologic and clinical consequences of the disorders resulting from the deletion of the δ- and the β-globin gene is determined by the degree of compensatory γ-globin chain production. With greater production of the γ chain, there is less globin-chain imbalance, the red cells have more hemoglobin, and red cell survival is closer to normal (see Chapter 11). (δβ)^0-thalassemia heterozygotes have less chain imbalance than β-thalassemia heterozygotes while the imbalance is reduced to almost undetectable levels in HPFH heterozygotes. Similarly, the MCH is higher in heterozygotes for δβ thalassemia than in β thalassemia and again is close to normal in HPFH. The amount of γ-globin chain production does not fully compensate for the lack of β-globin chains in HPFH, even in those conditions with the highest HbF levels, since in the homozygous state the cells are microcytic and hypochromic and the α/γ-globin chain synthesis ratio is about 2. Nevertheless, this is sufficient to prevent clinical problems.

δβ-thalassemia homozygotes have thalassemia intermedia of variable severity as the level of γ-globin gene expression is generally lower than in HPFH, but this condition is still milder than homozygous β^0 thalassemia where there is little compensatory γ-globin chain production. Too few cases have been characterized to determine whether the variability in clinical severity among δβ-thalassemia homozygotes is directly related to the underlying molecular defect. It is likely that in homozygous δβ thalassemia as in homozygous β thalassemia there is significant differential red cell survival. The intercellular distribution of HbF is heterogeneous and those cells with the most γ-globin chains—and least chain imbalance—survive longest. Even in heterozygotes, cells with higher amounts of HbF survive longer (Zelkowitz et al., 1972; Wood et al., 1977).

Given that the pathophysiology of the δβ thalassemia is dependent on the level of HbF produced, it is not surprising that there is little difference hematologically between heterozygotes for $^G\gamma^A\gamma(\delta\beta)^0$ thalassemia and $^G\gamma(^A\gamma\delta\beta)^0$ thalassemia. Although both γ-globin genes are active in one case and only one γ-globin gene in the other, similar HbF levels are found in the heterozygotes. $^G\gamma(^A\gamma\delta\beta)^0$-thalassemia homozygotes may have a somewhat more severe clinical course reflecting the inability to increase γ-globin chain production under the added stress of anemia.

Clinical Aspects and Treatment

HPFH is not usually associated with clinical problems, and several homozygotes have been detected by chance rather than by hematologic presentation. However, the numbers reported are small and long-term follow-up to determine whether there are late sequelae to maintaining a high hemoglobin level is lacking. Compound heterozygotes with β thalassemia are also usually unaffected clinically, although a combination with β^0 thalassemia might lead to a more severe phenotype.

Compound heterozygotes for HPFH and HbS may be confused with sickle cell anemia or HbS-β^0 thalassemia because only HbS and HbF are present (see Chapter 28). However, the level of HbF is sufficiently high, with a pancellular distribution, that intracellular polymerization of the HbS molecules is inhibited in the vast majority of cells and the resulting condition is almost uniformly mild.

The increased production of HbF in δβ thalassemia is in general not sufficient to compensate for the lack of β-globin chain production, and in homozygotes or compound heterozygotes with β thalassemia the clinical picture is one of thalassemia intermedia of variable severity. At the more severe end, patients may require regular transfusions and iron chelation therapy, while in other cases transfusions may only be necessary following acute disturbances such as infections. A detailed description of the treatment of thalassemia intermedia is given in Chapters 13 and 37.

Mechanisms Producing Deletions That Result in δβ Thalassemia and HPFH

The fusion globins Lepore and Kenya presumably arose by misalignment followed by crossing over between two nonhomologous genes, with loss of the sequences between them. A similar mechanism has been invoked to explain the two small deletions flanking an inverted region in Indian $^G\gamma(^A\gamma\delta\beta)^0$ thalassemia. A complex folding of the cluster, possibly stabilized by inverted repeat sequences, may have resulted in misalignment of the $^A\gamma$-, δ-, and β-globin genes, with two crossovers producing the final rearrangement (Jones et al., 1981a; Jennings et al., 1985). A similar double deletion/inversion rearrangement occurs in the Macedonian/Turkish $^G\gamma^A\gamma(\delta\beta)^0$ thalassemia; in this case the second deletion lies 3' to the β-globin gene and a complex mechanism must be involved (Kulozik et al., 1992).

The majority of the deletions are due to illegitimate recombination and there is only minimal homology of a few nucleotides at the breakpoints. Most show clean breakage and reunion, although in some cases a few "orphan" nucleotides of unknown origin have been inserted. Several of the deletions start or end within repetitive sequence elements (*Alu* or LINES) but given their frequency within the cluster, this occurs no more often than would be expected by chance. Breakpoints within the genes themselves do seem to occur more often than would be expected, but this is possibly due to ascertainment bias (Henthorn et al., 1990).

It was noted that the HPFH-1 and HPFH-2 deletions were of a similar size overall (about 100 kb) and that the 5' and 3' breakpoints were staggered by about 5 kb. The Anglo-Saxon and Dutch types of $(\varepsilon^G\gamma^A\gamma\delta\beta)^0$ thalassemia where all the genes are deleted or inactivated, are also of similar length and with staggered ends but at the 5' end of the complex. These observations led Vanin et al. (1983) to speculate that this could arise if the β-globin gene cluster was normally maintained as a single chromosomal loop with a length of about 100 kb. Loss of the loop through recombination between the anchorage points could produce deletions of the observed size. The variation in positions of the deletions implied movement of the loop through the anchorage points, perhaps during replication. Additional deletions of this size have been characterized since Filipino β thalassemia, Spanish $^G\gamma^A\gamma(\delta\beta)^0$ thalassemia, and Thai $^G\gamma(^A\gamma\delta\beta)^0$ thalassemia, consistent with the loop hypothesis. However, there are clusters of deletions of other sizes; four are about 50 kb long and seven are between 11.5 and 13.5 kb. (Table 15.1). As more and more deletions are mapped, the lengths are tending toward a continuum, making the concept of fixed-size loops less convincing.

How Do the Deletions Cause Raised HbF in Adults?

Table 15.1 lists the details of the different δβ thalassemia and HPFH deletions that have been characterized. The extent of these deletions are shown in Figure 15.3, together with deletions within the cluster that do not lead to significant increases in HbF in adults, for comparison. Part or all of the δ- and β-globin genes are deleted in almost all of the δβ thalassemias and HPFHs, while part or all of the $^A\gamma$-globin gene is also lost in the $^G\gamma(^A\gamma\delta\beta)^0$ thalassemia, explaining the lack of production of $^A\gamma$-globin chains.

It is clear from Figure 15.3 that neither the size nor the position of the deletions distinguishes the δβ thalassemia from the HPFH. While some deletions are confined to the β-globin gene cluster itself, others extend a considerable distance (> 100 kb) 3' to the β-globin gene. Although it was originally hoped that defining the molecular basis of δβ thalassemias and HPFH would provide an explanation for the persistent HbF production, as more and more deletions have been characterized it has become increasingly difficult to provide a simple, unifying explanation. Several hypotheses have been proposed.

Loss of Regulatory Regions. Because the δβ and $^A\gamma\beta$ fusion chains are associated with gene deletions and the former but not the latter resulted in significantly greater levels of HbF in adults, Huisman et al. (1974) suggested that a regulatory region responsible for repressing γ-globin gene expression in adult life might lie between the ^Aγ- and the δ-globin genes. When further data made this proposal untenable, it was modified to suggest that there were two mutually exclusive domains within the cluster, one fetal and one adult, marked by boundaries (Bernards and Flavell, 1980). Loss of parts of the adult domain would make it defective and shift the equilibrium toward γ-globin gene expression. With the addition of many more deletions, it is now clear that no simple domain boundary exists between the fetal and adult genes and that the loss of no single element can explain the various phenotypes.

The evidence against a single regulatory element is obtained from a comparison of the areas deleted in those conditions that do not result in such high HbF levels. Overlapping deletions in Turkish β thalassemia, Corfu δ thalassemia, Hb Lepore, and UK Asian β thalassemia cover the area from 2 kb 3' of the ^Aγ-globin gene to 5 kb beyond the β-globin gene. All of these disorders have average HbF levels of less than 4 percent. β-globin cluster constructs, with and without the region between the ^Aγ- and δ-globin genes, have been studied in transgenic mice. The γ-globin genes are more or less completely switched off in adults containing the whole complex (Gaensler et al., 1993) and no increase in γ-globin gene expression was observed in the mice with the deleted ^Aγ-δ region (Zhang et al., 1997; Calzolari et al. 1999).

Australian, Dutch, Filipino, and Italian β-thalassemia deletions extend further in the 3' direction than the Turkish and UK Asian deletions and several of these cases have levels of HbF, up to 11 percent, which could implicate a regulatory element in the 3' region of the gene cluster. However, these conditions have only been described in single families and the influence of other factors such as the sequence at ^Gγ −158 (see below) or unlinked heterocellular HPFH genes has not been excluded. Furthermore, most of the 3' sequences lost in these deletions are retained in the HPFH-5 deletion. In the case of the Italian β thalassemia, the 3' end of the deletion is close to the enhancer sequence that has been identified at the end of the HPFH-1 and HPFH-2 deletions (see below) and expression of the γ genes may be influenced by this element.

The Eastern European ^Gγ^Aγ(δβ)^0-thalassemia deletion (about 18 percent HbF) differs from Hb Lepore (about 3 percent HbF) only by removal of 1.5 kb immediately upstream of the δ-globin gene, including its promoter. In contrast, the Mediterranean (about 10 percent HbF) and Southeast Asian ^Gγ^Aγ(δβ)^0-thalassemia deletions (about 10 percent HbF) differ from Hb Lepore only by the deletion of sequences 3' to the β-globin gene. When sequences both 5' to δ and 3' to β are deleted, much higher levels of HbF are found in adults (Italian 2 HPFH with about 20 percent HbF and Black ^Gγ^Aγ(δβ)^0 thalassemia with about 20 percent HbF). It is possible, therefore, that there are two or more regions around the δ- and β-globin gene that act in combination and are involved in keeping the γ-globin gene switched off in adults.

Competition between ^Gγ^Aγ and δβ. As globin gene expression appears to involve interaction of the LCR with gene promoters, it was suggested that the γ-globin genes may be in competition with the δ- and the β-globin gene for expression during adult life (see Chapter 7). In normal circumstances, this competition would favor the δ- and the β-globin gene as a result of the chromatin conformation, stage-specific *trans*-acting factors, or both. However, when both the δ- and the β-globin gene promoters are deleted, the γ-globin gene promoters may be free to interact with the LCR, albeit at submaximal levels, resulting in the persistent HbF (Wood, 1989; Townes and Behringer, 1990). This suggestion was strengthened by analyses of nondeletion HPFH (see below) in which there is evidence for competition in *cis* between β- and γ-globin genes.

Evidence for promoter competition within the β-globin gene cluster is provided by the extremely high levels of HbA_2 in heterozygotes for β-thalassemia alleles involving deletion of a β-globin gene promoter (see Chapters 10 and 12). The increased HbA_2 synthesis occurs in *cis* and appears to be the result of increased transcription of the δ-globin gene. It also appears that such patients have slightly higher levels of HbF compared to those with alleles that leave the promoter intact. In most of the HPFH and δβ-thalassemia deletions both δ- and β-globin gene promoters are missing; however, the Southeast Asian HPFH is a clear exception as the δ-globin gene remains intact and yet HbF levels of more than 20 percent are found in heterozygotes. Furthermore, in three of the ^Gγ^Aγ(δβ)^0-thalassemia deletions (Mediterranean, Southeast Asian, Macedonian/Turkish), the 5' end of the deletion lies within the body of the δ-globin gene, leaving the promoter intact.

Competition between β- and γ-globin genes could not, on its own, explain the phenotypic differences between the ^Gγ^Aγ(δβ)^0 thalassemias and HPFH. It also contradicts data from transgenic mouse studies that show autonomous regulation and switching off of γ-globin gene expression during development in constructs lacking the β-globin gene (Dillon and Grosveld, 1991; Peterson et al., 1995; Arcasoy et al., 1997). However, given that the mouse does not have a fetal hemoglobin and that the human γ-globin gene in mice is expressed largely in embryos, it is not clear whether this model reflects all aspects of human globin gene regulation.

Newly Apposed Enhancer Sequences. An alternative explanation for the persistent γ-gene expression is that there is a positive influence of the sequences translocated to the 3′ end of the complex (Tuan et al., 1983; Feingold and Forget, 1989). It was proposed, for instance, that when the ${}^{A}\gamma$- and β-globin genes are fused (Hb Kenya), the β IVS 2 and 3′ enhancers can activate both the fusion gene promoter and the ${}^{G}\gamma$-globin gene.

Analysis of the sequences immediately 3′ to the large HPFH-1 deletion showed that this region, marked by an erythroid specific DNase I hypersensitive site extending from 1.1 to 1.4 kb 3′ to the HPFH-1 breakpoint (Elder et al., 1990), has enhancer activity in a classical transient transcription assay (Feingold and Forget, 1989). Furthermore, this site is no longer hypersensitive on a chromosome from which the LCR has been deleted, suggesting that it is influenced by LCR activity even though it lies more than 150 kb away (Forrester et al., 1990). As a result of the HPFH-1 and 2 deletions, this sequence is brought to within 10 to 15 kb of the γ-globin genes.

As enhancers detected in transient transfection assays do not always show the same activity when they are incorporated into a chromosome, particularly if they come under the influence of strong regulatory elements such as the LCR, it was important to test this element in vivo. Arcasoy et al. (1997) produced mice with human HPFH-deletion transgenes that contained in various combinations LCR core elements, the two γ-globin genes, and the enhancer 3′ to the HPFH-1 and -2 deletions (Fig. 15.5). Only mice containing all three elements showed significant amounts of γ-globin gene expression as adults, demonstrating that the enhancer is essential for activating γ-globin genes in the mouse

model and strongly suggesting that it is in deletion HPFH patients as well.

A 0.7 kb region with similar enhancer activity in transiently transfected erythroid cells has been identified immediately 3′ to the HPFH-3 3′ breakpoint (Anagnou et al., 1995). This element has sequences homologous to the simian virus 40 enhancer as well as to the human ${}^{A}\gamma$-gene and chick β-gene enhancers. Its activity was restricted to the γ and ε promoters, having no effect on the δ- or β-gene enhancers. The HPFH-3 deletion moves this sequence element to within –5 kb of the ${}^{A}\gamma$-globin gene, and a similar proximity would occur in the Sicilian and Southeast Asian HPFHs and the Belgian and Turkish and Italian ${}^{G}\gamma({}^{A}\gamma\delta\beta)^{0}$-thalassemia deletions.

A third region with enhancer activity in a transient system lies between the breakpoints of the Thai and Chinese ${}^{G}\gamma({}^{A}\gamma\delta\beta)^{0}$-thalassemia deletions, but is deleted in the latter (Kosteas et al., 1997). In ten Chinese ${}^{G}\gamma({}^{A}\gamma\delta\beta)^{0}$-thalassemia cases from five families, HbF ranged from 9 percent to 23 percent (mean 13 percent HbF). HbF levels in the three members of the Thai family ranged from 17 percent to 23 percent (mean 20 percent). While the difference in HbF levels between the two conditions is consistent with a positive effect of this enhancer element, additional families with the Thai

Figure 15.5. The role of the enhancer element (shaded box) found 3′ to the HPFH-1 and HPFH-2 deletions (open boxes) in producing the HPFH phenotype in transgenic mice. Only a construct containing the LCR, the γ-globin genes, and this enhancer resulted in mice with persistent γ-gene expression in adult life.

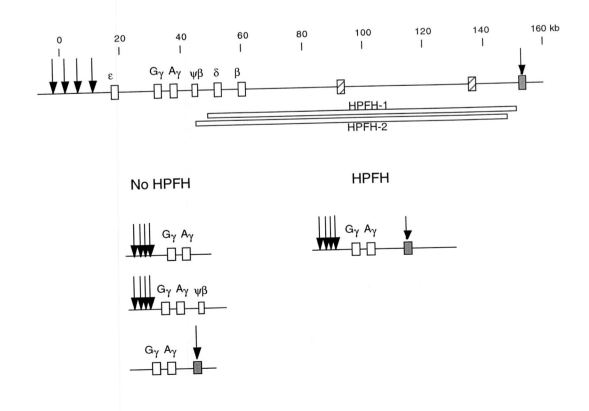

defect are needed to ensure that the high HbF levels are always associated with this $^{G}\gamma(^{A}\gamma\delta\beta)^{0}$ deletion. An open reading frame in the enhancer sequence shares 36 percent homology with the open reading frame in the HPFH-1 enhancer and both appear to be related to an olfactory receptor gene (Kosteas et al., 1996; Forget, 1998; Bulger et al., 1999; Feingold et al., 1999). Furthermore, the element appears to enhance only γ-globin genes and not ε- or β-globin genes in transient transfection assays. To date, the other two distant 3′ elements have not been tested for activity in vivo in a transgenic mouse assay that also includes the LCR.

If an enhancer element brought into the proximity of the γ-globin genes can activate them, could the mechanism be operative in all cases of δβ thalassemia and HPFH? It is difficult to answer this question at present since the region beyond the β-globin gene has not been systematically searched for such elements. Furthermore, the distance over which each enhancer can exert its effect and whether the phenomenon is sequence dependent are unknown. It may be that there is no simple explanation for persistent γ-globin gene expression in the deletion HPFH conditions. While there may be a unifying mechanism linking them all, it seems equally likely that all of the above mechanisms may play a role, with the relative importance of each varying from deletion to deletion. Given the large number of elements that regulate expression—positively and negatively—within the β-globin cluster, it is not surprising that still other regulatory elements reside downstream from the cluster. The balance between regulatory sequences that tend to increase the interaction of the LCR with the γ-globin gene promoters and those that tend to decrease it may ultimately determine the amount of HbF in the red cells, and hence the degree of compensation for the lack of β-globin chain production.

Nondeletion HPFH

Persistent HbF production in the absence of deletions within the β-globin gene cluster is usually due to a mutation in a promoter of one of the two γ-globin genes that causes an increase in the expression of that gene (Fig. 15.1). Other mutations within the β-globin gene cluster may also cause increased HbF production, and genes not linked to the β-globin gene cluster clearly influence HbF levels as well.

Mutations of the γ-Globin Gene Promoters

A form of HPFH with lower HbF levels than reported for African-Americans was recognized as relatively common in Greece (Fessas et al., 1961; Fessas and Stamatoyannopoulos, 1964), and the HbF contained only $^{A}\gamma$-globin chains (Huisman et al., 1970). Several compound heterozygotes with β thalassemia were described, all of whom had more than 50 percent HbA even though severe β+ thalassemia and β0 thalassemia genes are the most common in Greece. This led to the suggestion that the β-globin chain gene was in cis to the HPFH determinant.

Huisman et al. (1975) described a family in whom the propositus had a hemoglobin pattern of approximately 50 percent HbS, 25 percent HbA, and 25 percent HbF, with a low level of HbA₂. The β^{S}-globin gene was inherited from a parent with normal HbF levels while the other parent had HbA but with a high HbF level. This implied that the genes for the β^{A}- and γ-globin chains were on the same chromosome. Furthermore, the case was unusual in that the γ-globin chains were almost entirely $^{G}\gamma$ and the case was characterized as $^{G}\gamma$ β+HPFH. A British HPFH family was described with HbF levels of about 8 percent that only contained $^{A}\gamma$-globin gene chains. In this family were three homozygotes with about 20 percent HbF, normal levels of HbA₂, and the remainder of the hemoglobin, HbA, clearly demonstrating that the γ-, δ-, and β-globin genes must be active on the same chromosome (Weatherall et al., 1975).

Reports on a number of other conditions in which the HbF contained only $^{G}\gamma$- or $^{A}\gamma$-globin chains soon followed. When it became possible to analyze the β-globin gene cluster at the molecular level, it became clear that these types of HPFH were not due to gene deletions (Bernards and Flavell, 1980; Tuan et al., 1980; Jones et al., 1982). The molecular basis of the first of these conditions was elucidated by Collins et al. (1984), who showed that the $^{G}\gamma$-globin gene from the $^{G}\gamma$ β+ HPFH chromosome carried a C→G mutation at position −202. At the time of these studies there was no direct evidence that this base substitution was directly responsible for the condition but similar reports followed rapidly. Giglioni et al. (1984) demonstrated a C→T substitution at −196 in the $^{A}\gamma$-globin gene of an Italian HPFH patient; Greek HPFH was shown to have a G→A substitution at $^{A}\gamma$ −117 (Collins et al., 1985; Gelinas et al., 1985); and the British HPFH had a T→C substitution at −198 in the $^{A}\gamma$-globin gene (Tate et al., 1986). These rare mutations were always associated with high levels of HbF (Waber et al., 1986; Metherall et al., 1988). Furthermore, the same mutations turned up in different racial groups in individuals with similar phenotypes, suggesting independent origins (Gelinas et al., 1986). Finally, direct evidence that the substitutions were responsible for persistent γ-globin gene expression was provided in transgenic mice (Berry et al., 1992; Starck et al., 1994; Peterson et al., 1995).

The mutations in the γ-globin gene promoters that have been described to date are listed in Table 15.6 and shown in Figure 15.6. Homozygotes have been described in the Greek and Tunisian nondeletion types of HPFH in addition to the British HPFH.

Table 15.6. Summary of Hematologic Data (Mean ± SD) of Nondeletional HPFH Heterozygotes Defined by Molecular Analysis

Condition	Mutation	No. of families/ individuals*	Hb (g/dL)	MCV† (fl)	MCH† (pg)	HbA₂ (%)	HbF (%)	Gγ or Aγ (%)	α/Non-α synthesis	Xmn l at −158 in cis	Distribution
Gγ mutations											
Black	−202 C→G	1/5	13.3 ± 1.3	82.0 ± 6.5	27.7 ± 2.0	1.7 ± 0.4	15.6 ± 1.2	99.0 ± 0.5	0.87 ± 0.02	−	Pancellular
Tunisian	−200 +C	1/5	13.1 ± 0.9	95.9 ± 1.8	31.9 ± 0.4	1.5 ± 0.3	25.2 ± 4.1	100 ± 0		+	Pancellular
Black/Sardinian/ British	−175 T→C	2/3	12.7 ± 1.1	85.2 ± 3.1	28.4 ± 1.8	1.3 ± 0.2	20.3 ± 2.8	94.0 ± 5.2	0.97 ± 0.17	−	
Japanese	−114 C→T	1/2					12.5 ± 2.1	89.0 ± 4.2		+	
Australian	−114 C→G	1/1	14.2	92		2.3	8.6	90		−	
Aγ mutations											
Black	−202 C→T	1/5	12.9 ± 0.9	84.4 ± 5.9	30.0 ± 2.3	2.7 ± 1.0	2.5 ± 0.9	92.8 ± 2.8	1.05 ± 0.13	−	Heterocellular
British	−1.98 T→C	3/22	14.2 ± 1.2	83.1 ± 3.3	29.0 ± 1.0	2.5 ± 0.4	6.9 ± 2.2	92.2 ± 1.8	1.06 ± 0.05	−	Heterocellular
Italian/Chinese	−196 C→T	4/8	normal	normal	30.0 ± 0.9	1.8 ± 0.6	13.7 ± 2.0	95.0 ± 0.2		−	
Brazilian	−195 C→G	1/3	normal	normal	normal	2.1	5.4 ± 1.4	89.0 ± 2.5			
Black	−175 T→C	3/7	normal	normal	normal	1.5 ± 0.2	37.4 ± 1.0	78.0 ± 5.5		+	Pancellular
Greek/Black	−117 G→A	64/144	14.2 ± 1.1	85.9 ± 4.5	28.4 ± 2.4	2.0 ± 0.3	12.1 ± 2.8	93.4 ± 4.7	0.95 ± 0.10	−	Pancellular
Black‡	−114 to −102 del	2/2	11.4 ± 2.9	75.5 ± 2.1	26.8 ± 0.3	2.1 ± 0.0	31.0 ± 1.2	85.7 ± 5.7		−	
Georgia	−114 C→T	1/2	normal	normal	normal	2.5 ± 0.4	3.8 ± 1.3	90.9 ± 0.8		−	

* Data are not necessarily complete for all individuals; extreme outliers omitted.

† α Thalassemia not excluded in all cases; some results were obtained after sample had been in transit.

‡ Only described in combination with HbS.

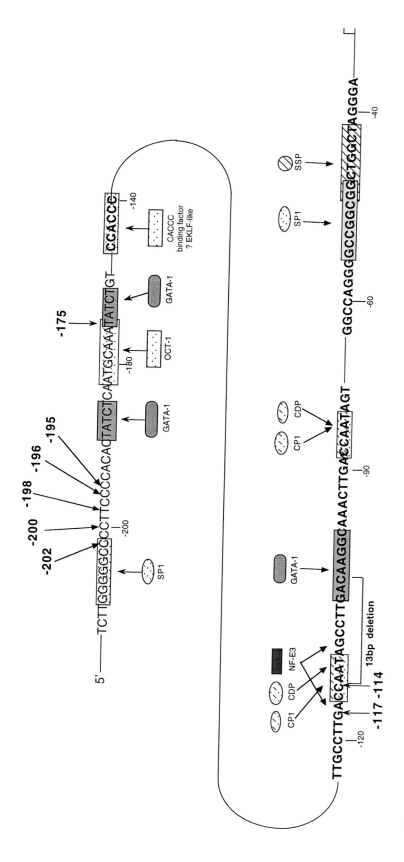

Figure 15.6. Transcription factor binding sites in the promoter of the γ-globin genes. Both genes have identical sequences in this region; mutations that result in nondeletion HPFH are indicated.

$^{G}\gamma \beta^{+}$ HPFH

Black −202 C→G. This condition has been observed in several African-American families (Huisman et al., 1975; Collins et al., 1984), including the original family described by Huisman et al. (Yang et al., 1988). HbF levels vary from 16 percent to 21 percent with a pancellular distribution. In combination with HbS there is no anemia and a very mild disorder results.

Tunisian −200 +C. A single family has been reported with an additional nucleotide inserted at position −200 of the γ-globin gene promoter. Heterozygotes had 18 percent to 27 percent HbF while levels of 48 percent and 49 percent HbF were found in two homozygotes (Pissard et al., 1996).

Black −175 T→C. This condition was originally described in an African-American family by Friedman et al. (1976) and was further characterized by Surrey et al. (1988). It was subsequently found in a Sardinian (Ottolenghi et al., 1988) and a British (Craig et al., 1993) family. In heterozygotes, the HbF level is about 20 percent, rising to about 30 percent if inherited with HbS, a combination that is not associated with any clinical problems (see Chapter 28). This HPFH has also been observed in combination with β⁰ thalassemia, without any clinical consequences (Pistidda et al., 1997). The compound heterozygote had 64 percent HbF, 2.5 percent HbA₂, and the remainder HbA. Interestingly, the HbF still only contained $^{G}\gamma$-globin gene chains, suggesting that it was derived solely from the HPFH chromosome.

Japanese −114 C→T. The single family described with this condition has heterozygotes with HbF levels of 11 percent and 14 percent (Fucharoen et al., 1990), which are significantly higher than the levels in heterozygotes with the same mutation in the $^{A}\gamma$-globin gene.

Australian −114 C→G. A single individual with normal hematologic findings and 8.6 percent HbF has been described with this condition (Motum et al., 1994).

$^{A}\gamma \beta^{+}$ HPFH

Black −202 C→T. This mutation was found in a single black family. It is associated with much lower levels of HbF (1.6 percent to 3.9 percent) than the C→G substitution at the same site in the $^{G}\gamma$-globin gene. (Hattori et al., 1986; Gilman et al., 1988a).

British −198 T→C. Several families with this condition have been described, all of North European origin (Weatherall et al., 1975; Donald et al., 1988; Yang et al., 1988; Craig et al., 1994). HbF levels in heterozygotes range from 3 percent to 10 percent, with 18 percent to 20 percent in homozygotes. The HbF has a heterocellular distribution, and is positively correlated with the proportion of F-cells. In cord blood, the percentage HbF and the ratio of $^{G}\gamma$- to $^{A}\gamma$-globin chains are normal, suggesting that the mutation has little effect when the γ-globin genes are maximally expressed in fetal life (Wood et al., 1982).

Italian/Chinese −196 C→T. This substitution has been reported in several Italian (Giglioni et al. 1984) and Chinese (Farquhar et al., 1983; Gelinas et al., 1986; Yang et al. 1988) families. It produces HbF levels of 12 percent to 16 percent in heterozygotes, rising to about 23 percent in individuals with a β-thalassemia gene in *trans*. This mutation has also been found in *cis* to the common β⁰-thalassemia allele (CAG→TAG) in Sardinia (Ottolenghi et al., 1982, 1987).

Brazilian −195 C→G. A single Brazilian family of European origin, with HbF levels of 4.5 percent to 7.0 percent, has been described with this mutation (Costa et al., 1990).

Black −175 T→C. This condition has been described in two African-American families and leads to extremely high HbF levels of 30 percent to 40 percent (Stoming et al., 1989; Coleman et al., 1993). Individuals with HbS or HbC in trans are clinically and hematologically normal. Although this is a mutation of the $^{A}\gamma$-globin gene promoter, there are significantly higher levels of $^{G}\gamma$-globin chains (18 percent to 38 percent) than in any of the other $^{A}\gamma$-globin gene promoter mutations, suggesting that the presence of the −158 C→T mutation in the $^{G}\gamma$-globin gene promoter in cis may cause this anomaly.

Cretan −158 C→T. This mutation was observed in three individuals from Crete and is the $^{A}\gamma$-globin gene equivalent of the C/T polymorphism in the $^{G}\gamma$-globin gene promoter (Patrinos et al., 1998). It occurs in cis to the $^{G}\gamma$-globin gene −158 C→T mutation, and both changes together cause only a small increase in HbF, with both types of γ-globin gene chains produced. It appears to have arisen twice by different gene conversion events.

Greek −117 G→A. Greek HPFH was originally characterized in the Greek population (Fessas and Stamatoyannopoulos, 1964; Sofroniadou et al., 1975; Clegg et al., 1979) but is found throughout the Southern Mediterranean (Ottolenghi et al., 1988; Camaschella et al., 1989) and has been observed as a new mutation in a black family (Huang et al., 1987). The mean HbF level in heterozygotes is 12 percent with a pancellular distribution. Homozygotes have twice as much HbF (Camaschella et al., 1989) while compound heterozygotes with β thalassemia have HbF levels of about 30 percent. They are mildly anemic but this combination does not usually cause a symptomatic clinical disorder.

Black –114–102 Deleted. Two individuals with this condition in association with HbS have been described, having about 30 percent HbF (Gilman et al., 1988b).

Georgia – 114 C→T. A 3 percent to 5 percent increase in HbF levels was reported in two brothers with this substitution (Öner et al., 1991).

The mechanism of Increased HbF Production in the γ-Globin Gene Promoter Mutants. It seems probable that the nondeletion HPFH mutations alter the binding of various transcription factors to the γ-globin gene promoter (see Chapter 7). For instance, if adult red cells contain factors that bind to the promoter and repress its expression, a mutation might decrease the avidity of the factor for its recognition sequence, hence partially relieving the repression. Alternatively, the change may allow the binding of a positively acting factor present in adult red cells that normally would not bind. Attempts have been made to analyze the proteins that bind to this region and to document the changes that occur with the mutant sequences. They have demonstrated the complexity of the region, in which binding sites for different proteins frequently overlap (Fig. 15.6).

These γ-globin gene promoter lesions cluster in three regions. One, around positions –114 to –117, involves the distal CCAAT box while a second at –175 may involve an overlapping Oct-1/GATA-1 site. The third group, from –195 to –202, does not directly involve a known protein binding site but may disrupt binding to a neighboring G-rich box. The distal CCAAT box can bind at least two CCAAT binding proteins, CP1 and CDP. Binding of both proteins is increased by the $^A\gamma$ –117 mutation (Gumucio et al., 1988; Mantovani et al., 1988; Superti-Furga et al., 1988). This mutation also decreases the binding of GATA-1 to the 3′ side of the CCAAT box as well as the binding of NF-E3, an uncharacterized protein (Mantovani et al., 1988; Superti-Furga et al., 1988). CP1 binding is abolished in the $^G\gamma$ –114 C→T mutation (Fucharoen et al., 1990) while CP1, CDP, and NF-E3, but not GATA-1, binding is lost in the 13 bp deletion of this region (Mantovani et al., 1989).

The –175 mutation abolishes the binding of the Oct-1 protein and alters the binding of GATA-1, which also includes this residue in its binding site. Different reports suggest that the GATA-1 binding is either slightly increased (Mantovani et al., 1988), somewhat decreased (Martin et al., 1989), or unaffected (Gumucio et al., 1988), Altered binding of Sp1 to the G-rich area upstream of the –195 to –202 region has been reported in gel-shift assays comparing normal and mutant oligonucleotides. However, binding increased in the $^G\gamma$

–202 C→G (Sykes and Kaufman, 1990) and $^A\gamma$ –198 mutations (Ronchi et al., 1989; Fischer and Nowock, 1990; Gumucio et al., 1991) but decreased in the $^A\gamma$ –202 C→T (Sykes and Kaufman, 1990) and $^A\gamma$ –196 mutants (Ronchi et al., 1989; Gumucio et al., 1991). The $^G\gamma$ –202 C→G mutation also creates a new binding site for the stage selector protein (Jane et al., 1993). It has been suggested that mutations in this region disrupt an intramolecular triplex that may be the binding site for a repressor (Ulrich et al., 1992; Bacolla et al., 1995). No consistent themes run through these binding studies and as with the deletion forms of HPFH, different mechanisms may operate for each mutation. The results of these in vitro studies may not truly reflect the pattern of binding in vivo, when the DNA is in chromatin. The results are not always reproducible from laboratory to laboratory, reflecting the use of different oligonucleotide probes, and differences in nuclear protein extraction procedures.

Several of these mutants have also been studied in transient transfection assays or in vitro transcription assays, usually involving a comparison of the normal and mutant promoter to drive transcription of a reporter gene such as the chloramphenicol acetyl transferase gene (CAT). The results of these studies have been variable, with either little or no difference seen or a three- to eight-fold increase in expression (Rixon and Gelinas, 1988; Lanclos et al., 1989; Lloyd et al., 1989; Nicolis et al., 1989; Fischer and Nowock, 1990; Gumucio et al., 1990; Ulrich and Ley, 1990; Motum et al., 1993c). The increased expression of 50- to 100-fold seen in vivo has not been reproduced, again reflecting the inadequacies of these expression systems.

Several of these γ-globin gene promoter mutants have been tested in transgenic mice. Using an LCR –γβ gene construct, Berry et al. (1992) showed suppression of the normal γ-globin gene in adult mice, while the same construct carrying the γ^{-117} HPFH mutation showed high levels of γ-globin mRNA in adult life. Subsequent studies (Peterson et al., 1995; Ronchi et al., 1996) demonstrated a γ/γ + β ratio of about 25 percent. The persistence in adults was dependent on the proximal CCAAT box whereas expression of the γ-globin gene in earlier stages of development was much less sensitive to mutations to either CCAAT box. Other mutations that specifically eliminated the binding of GATA-1, NF-E3, or both factors—in effect mimicking the –117 mutation—did not result in increased HbF in adult life, implying that silencing is a multifactorial phenomenon.

Smaller increases in adult γ-globin gene expression were seen in mice carrying a HS2- $^G\gamma^A\gamma$ –117 δβ construct, with γ/γ + β ratios of 4.7 percent to 6.1 percent, compared to 0.6 percent to 1.5 percent in HS2- $^G\gamma^A\gamma$ δβ-construct-bearing mice with a normal γ-globin gene (Roberts et al., 1997). In the absence of the LCR, the

HPFH phenotype was not reproduced in HS2-$^{G}\gamma^{A}\gamma$ $^{-117}$ δβ transgenic mice, although in the $^{G}\gamma^{-202}$ γδβ mice, a low level of $^{G}\gamma$-globin expression persisted in adults (Starck et al., 1994). An intact LCR may be necessary, therefore, to obtain high HbF levels in adult mice but other factors, such as the proximity of the LCR to the promoters, may also cause the differences in expression between the constructs.

An $^{A}\gamma$-globin gene -114 C→T mutation that leads to HbF levels of 3 percent to 5 percent in adults has also been tested in an LCR γβ construct in transgenic mice and the modest increase in γ-globin gene expression was reproduced (Ronchi et al., 1996).

Competition between γ- and β-Globin Genes in Nondeletion HPFH. Individuals with γ-globin gene promoter mutations have balanced globin chain synthesis and a normal MCH (Table 15.6). When combined with an HbS or HbC gene in *trans*, the hemoglobin composition in the $^{G}\gamma$−200 and −175 mutations and the $^{A}\gamma$−175 mutations and −114 to −102 deletions, is approximately 25 percent HbF, 25 percent HbA, and 50 percent HbS or HbC. This indicates that the combined output from the γ- and the $β^A$-globin genes on the affected chromosome is approximately normal (see Chapter 7). The mild anemia seen in compound heterozygotes for β thalassemia and the $^{A}\gamma$−196 and −117 mutations may indicate that the total γ- + β-globin mRNA output from the HPFH chromosome in these cases is slightly less than normal. Nevertheless, it appears that the increase in γ-globin chain production is matched by a decrease in β-globin chain production, and that this reciprocity only occurs in *cis*. This reciprocal relationship could be explained if there were competition between these two genes for access to the LCR. Altered binding of transcription factors to the γ-globin gene promoter as a result of the base substitutions, might well alter the balance of association with the LCR, resulting in a more stable binding than would normally occur in adult red cells. It is known that during the normal developmental switch from γ- to β-globin gene expression, both genes are transcriptionally active in the same cell and that there is continual alternation of activation of the two genes (Wijgerde et al., 1995). Decreased binding of a repressor protein or increased binding of an activator to the γ-globin gene promoter could, therefore, increase the gene's competitiveness. Different mutants would result in different probabilities of a productive interaction with the LCR; hence the variability in the amount of HbF produced (see Chapter 7).

The Intercellular Distribution of HbF in the Nondeletion HPFHs. The distribution of HbF in γ-globin gene promoter mutants tends to be heterocellular when the levels are low and pancellular when they are high (Boyer et al., 1977). Among the British $^{A}\gamma$ HPFH heterozygotes, the HbF concentration was 3.5 percent to 14 percent and correlated well ($r = 0.94$) with the proportion of F-cells (32 percent to 69 percent); among the homozygotes, HbF concentration was about 20 percent and had a pancellular distribution (Wood et al., 1982). Mutations in the promoter might increase the probability of γ-globin gene expression, but via unstable interactions with regulatory elements. Stochastic variability would again produce intercellular heterogeneity, with the proportion of F-cells and the amount of HbF/F-cell dependent on the strength of transcription factor binding.

HPFH Unlinked to the β-Globin Gene Cluster. A number of families, most with thalassemia or sickle cell disease, have been reported to have HPFH that segregates independently of the β-like globin gene cluster (Gianni et al., 1983; Giampaolo et al., 1984; Martinez et al., 1989; Thein and Weatherall, 1989; Oppenheim et al., 1990; Seltzer et al., 1992; Craig et al., 1996; Craig et al., 1997). Analysis is made difficult by the possibility of genetic heterogeneity and incomplete penetrance. Furthermore, the distribution of HbF levels in these families may be continuous, making phenotypic identification of normal and affected individuals difficult. Thus the pattern of inheritance is rarely clear in these families and examples of autosomal or sex-linked dominant, codominant, or recessive patterns have all been reported.

X-Linked. Analysis of HbF levels in healthy Japanese adults led Miyoshi et al. (1988) to suggest that an X-linked gene was involved in increasing HbF levels with a frequency of 11 percent of males affected and 21 percent of females being carriers (see Chapter 10). Support for that suggestion came from analysis of F-reticulocytes and F-cells in sickle cell disease patients, including sib pairs (Dover et al., 1992). The study showed that codominant high and low F-cell production alleles resided at Xp22.2-22.3. Furthermore, it was proposed that this locus accounts for 40 percent of the variability of HbF levels in sickle cell anemia, an effect of much greater magnitude than β-globin gene cluster haplotype, age, sex, or α-globin gene number, which together could account for only about 10 percent of the variability (Chang et al., 1995).

Chromosome 6-Linked. The value of a single large family in the study of unlinked HPFH has been dramatically demonstrated (Thein and Weatherall, 1989). Starting from a patient with homozygous $β^0$ thalassemia who had an extremely mild course, with 10 to 12 g/dL HbF, a family study was carried out that showed clear-cut evidence for an HPFH-like gene not linked to the β-globin gene cluster. The family study was extended until nearly 200 members were accumulated. The pattern of inheritance in this family was initially unclear and assignments of phenotypes made difficult by not only the interacting β thalassemia but also α thalassemia. Nevertheless, by using statistical analysis to take account of the influence of thalassemia, the −158 C→T polymorphism, age and sex, it was possible by multiple regression analysis to demonstrate the presence of a major gene affecting F-cell levels in this family (Thein et al., 1994). By using polymorphic markers covering the whole genome it proved possible to localize this gene to a small area of chromosome 6, 6q22.3-q24 (Craig et al., 1996).

How either the chromosome 6 or X chromosome-linked genes affect HbF levels and F-cells remains unknown. It is possible that these loci code for *trans*-acting factors that bind within the β-globin gene cluster and directly affect gene transcription. It is equally plausible that there are genes that act much more indirectly, perhaps by altering the kinetics of erythropoiesis and mimicking the increased HbF seen in stress erythropoiesis.

Other Sequence Differences Within the β-Globin Gene Cluster Affecting HbF Production. Within the β-globin gene cluster there are numerous polymorphisms affecting either single nucleotides or oligonucleotide motifs. Associations have been noted between some of these polymorphisms and higher HbF levels, usually under conditions of erythroid expansion such as in sickle cell disease or thalassemia. The best known of these is the C→T polymorphism at position −158 of the γ-globin gene, creating an *XmnI* restriction site (Gilman and Huisman, 1985; Labie et al., 1985a, 1985b). Normal individuals homozygous for T at −158 may have a slight increase in F-cells and those with a $^{G}\gamma$-$^{G}\gamma$ gene arrangement—a result of gene conversion—where both genes have the T at −158 have HbF levels of 2 percent to 6 percent (Gilman and Huisman, 1984). Sickle cell disease and β-thalassemia patients with the −158 C→T mutation tend to have higher HbF levels and a higher proportion of $^{G}\gamma$-globin chains. Additional differences within the cluster—some linked to haplotype—also influence HbF levels in these patients. These motifs have been postulated to modulate the phenotype of sickle cell anemia via their effects on HbF levels and they are discussed in more detail in Chapter 26. Other polymorphic regions within the cluster associated with variability in HbF levels in sickle cell and β thalassemia include an $(AT)_x (T)_y$ polymorphism upstream of the β-globin gene promoter (Elion et al., 1992), substitutions upstream of the $^{G}\gamma$-globin gene and in $^{G}\gamma$ IVS 2 (Lanclos et al., 1991; Pissard and Beuzard, 1994), and a $(AT)_x N_{12} (AT)_y$ polymorphism within the HS 2 element of the LCR (Beris et al., 1992; Öner et al., 1992; Merghoub et al., 1996). In none of these cases is there direct evidence from functional studies that different alleles at these sites are responsible for altering γ-globin gene expression and the possibility remains that they are markers in linkage disequilibrium with as yet unidentified elements.

CONCLUSIONS

The discovery that HPFH homozygotes with 100 percent HbF are clinically unaffected promoted the idea that reactivation of HbF production in adult life would be an effective therapeutic strategy for the severe β-globin gene disorders. It was hoped that an understanding of the natural mutations that cause HPFH might provide sufficient insight into the regulation of the γ- and the β-globin genes to allow manipulation of the hemoglobin switching process. While considerable progress has been made in identifying the molecular basis of many of the HPFH conditions, a complete understanding of how these lead to persistent fetal hemoglobin production still eludes us. Among the deletion conditions it seems clear that it is the influence of the newly apposed enhancer elements that is responsible for maintaining the γ-globin gene in an active state in some cases; the nature and mode of action of those elements are under active investigation. We do not know, however, whether this is the mechanism in all the deletion cases and, if not, what other mechanisms are active.

Many of the nondeletion conditions are due to base substitutions in the promoters of the γ-globin gene, altering the binding of transcription factors and preventing suppression of these genes in adult life. The lack of any consistent pattern to these protein binding site changes suggests that the developmental regulation of these genes is a complex multifactorial process and additional investigations are required to provide a more detailed understanding of the way these disruptions enable the mutant γ-globin genes to compete with the β-globin genes in adult erythroid cells.

Our understanding of γ- and β-globin gene regulation may be limited because we are unaware of important contributors in the process; for instance, stage-specific transcription factors. One way in which such factors might be identified is by identifying the genes that influence adult HbF levels but are not linked to the β-globin gene. Positional cloning has localized at least two such genes and further work should result in their identification, as well as the localization of other genes that act similarly. To date, the knowledge we have gained about the molecular basis of HPFH and δβ-thalassemia mutations has considerably increased our understanding of the regulation of the globin genes. Continued progress may ultimately allow us to manipulate the expression of these genes for the benefit of patients with severe hemoglobinopathies.

References

Abels, J, Michiels, JJ, Giordano, PC et al. (1996). A *de novo* deletion causing εγδβ-thalassemia in a Dutch patient. *Acta Haematol.* 96: 108–109.

Acquaye, CTA, Oldham, JH, and Konotey-Ahulu, FID. (1977). Blood donor homozygous for hereditary persistence of fetal haemoglobin. *Lancet* 1: 796–797.

Altay, C, Schroeder, WA, and Huisman, THJ. (1977). The $^{G}\gamma$ $\delta\beta$ thalassaemia and $^{G}\gamma$-β^0-HPFH conditions in combination with β thalassaemia and HbS. *Am. J. Hematol.* 3: 1–14.

Amin, AB, Pandya, NL, Diwin, PP et al. (1979). A comparison of the homozygous states for $^{G}\gamma$ and $^{G}\gamma^{A}\gamma$ $\delta\beta$ thalassaemia. *Br. J. Haematol.* 43: 537–548.

Anagnou, NP, Papayannopoulou, T, Stamatoyannopoulos, G, and Nienhuis, AW. (1985). Structurally diverse molecular deletions in the β-globin gene cluster exhibit an identical phenotype on interaction with the β^S-gene. *Blood* 65: 1245–1251.

Anagnou, NP, Papayannopoulou, T, Nienhuis, AW, and Stamatoyannopoulos, G. (1988). Molecular characterization of a novel form of $(^{A}\gamma\delta\beta)^0$-thalassemia deletion with a 3′ breakpoint close to those of HPFH-3 and HPFH-4: Insights for a common regulatory mechanism. *Nucl. Acids Res.* 16: 6057–6066.

Anagnou, NP, Perez-Stable, C, Gelinas, R et al. (1995). Sequences located 3′ to the breakpoint of the hereditary persistence of fetal hemoglobin-3 deletion exhibit enhancer activity and can modify the developmental expression of the human fetal $^{A}\gamma$-globin gene in transgenic mice. *J. Biol. Chem.* 270: 10256–10263.

Arcasoy, MO, Romana, M, Fabry, ME et al. (1997). High levels of human γ-globin gene expression in adult mice carrying a transgene of deletion-type hereditary persistence of fetal hemoglobin. *Mol. Cell. Biol.* 17: 2076–2089.

Atweh, GF, Zhu, D-e, and Forget, BG. (1986). A novel basis for $\delta\beta$-thalassaemia in a Chinese family. *Blood* 68: 1108–1113.

Atweh, GF, Zhu, X-X, Brickner, HE et al. (1987). The β-globin gene on the Chinese $\delta\beta$-thalassaemia chromosome carries a promoter mutation. *Blood* 70: 1470–1474.

Bacolla, A, Ulrich, MJ, Larson, JE et al. (1995). An intramolecular triplex in the human galla-globin 5′-flanking region is altered by point mutations associated with hereditary persistence of fetal hemoglobin. *J. Biol. Chem.* 270: 24556–24563.

Baglioni, C. (1962). The fusion of two peptide chains in hemoglobin Lepore and its interpretation as a genetic deletion. *Proc. Nat. Acad. Sci. U.S.A.* 48: 1880–1886.

Balta, G, Brickner, HE, Takegawa, S Jr et al. (1994) Increased expression of the $^{G}\gamma$ and $^{A}\gamma$ globin genes associated with a mutation in the $^{A}\gamma$ enhancer. *Blood* 83: 3727–3737.

Bender, MA, Bulger, M, Close, J, and Groudine, M. (2000). β-globin gene switching and DNase I sensitivity of the endogenous β-globin locus in mice do not require the locus control region. *Mol. Cell.* 5: 387–393.

Beris, P, Kitundu, MN, Baysal, E et al. (1992). Black β-thalassemia homozygotes with specific sequence variations in the 5′ hypersensitive site-2 of the locus control region have high levels of fetal hemoglobin. *Am. J. Hematol.* 41: 97–101.

Bernards, R and Flavell, RA. (1980). Physical mapping of the globin gene deletion in hereditary persistence of foetal haemoglobin. *Nucl. Acids Res.* 8: 1521–1534.

Bernards, R, Kooter, JM, and Flavell, RA. (1979). Physical mapping of the globin gene deletion in $(\delta\beta)^0$ thalassaemia. *Gene* 6: 265–280.

Berry, M, Grosveld, F, and Dillon, N. (1992). A single point mutation is the cause of the Greek form of hereditary persistence of fetal haemoglobin. *Nature* 358: 499–502.

Boyer, SH, Margolet, L, Boyer, ML et al. (1977). Inheritance of F cell frequency in heterocellular hereditary persistence of fetal hemoglobin: An example of allelic exclusion. *Am. J. Hum. Genet.* 29: 256–271.

Brancati, C and Baglioni, C. (1966). Homozygous $\beta\delta$ thalassaemia ($\beta\delta$-microcythaemia). *Nature* 212: 262–264.

Bulger, M, von Doorninck, JH, Saitoh, N et al. (1999). Conservation of sequence and structure flanking the mouse and human β-globin loci: the β-globin genes are embedded within an array of odorant receptor genes. *Proc. Natl. Acad. Sci. U.S.A.* 96: 5129–5134.

Calzolari, R, McMorrow, T, Yannoutsos, N et al. (1999). Deletion of a region that is a candidate for the difference between the deletion forms of hereditary persistence of fetal hemoglobin and $\delta\beta$-thalassaemia affects β- but not γ-globin gene expression. *EMBO J.* 18: 949–958.

Camaschella, C, Serra, A, Saglio, G et al. (1987). The 3′ ends of the deletions of Spanish $\delta\beta^0$-thalassaemia and Black HPFH 1 and 2 lie within 17 kilobases. *Blood* 70: 593–596.

Camaschella, C, Oggiano, L, Sampietro, M et al. (1989). The homozygous state of G to A −117$^{A}\gamma$ hereditary persistence of fetal hemoglobin. *Blood* 73: 1999–2002.

Camaschella, C, Serra, A, Gottardi, E et al. (1990). A new hereditary persistence of fetal hemoglobin deletion has the breakpoint within the 3′ β-globin gene enhancer. *Blood* 75: 1000–1005.

Chang, YC, Smith, KD, Moore, RD et al. (1995). An analysis of fetal hemoglobin variation in sickle cell disease: The relative contributions of the X-linked factor, β-globin haplotypes, α-globin gene number, gender and age. *Blood* 85: 1111–1117.

Clegg, JB, Metaxatou-Mavromati, A, Kattamis, C et al. (1979). Occurrence of $^{G}\gamma$ Hb F in Greek HPFH: Analysis of heterozygotes and compound heterozygotes with β thalassaemia. *Br. J. Haematol.* 43: 521–536.

Coleman, MB, Adams, JGI, Steinberg, MH et al. (1993). $^{G}\gamma^{A}\gamma$ (β^+) hereditary persistence of fetal hemoglobin: The G gamma −158 C→T mutation in cis to the −175 T→C mutation of the $^{A}\gamma$-globin gene results in increased $^{G}\gamma$-globin synthesis. *Am. J. Hematol.* 42: 186–190.

Collins, FS, Stoeckert, CJ, Serjeant, GR et al. (1984). $^{G}\gamma\beta^+$ hereditary persistence of fetal hemoglobin: Cosmid cloning and identification of a specific mutation 5′ to the $^{G}\gamma$ gene. *Proc. Natl. Acad. Sci. U.S.A.* 81: 4894–4898.

Collins, FS, Metherall, JE, Yamakawa, M et al. (1985). A point mutation in the $^{A}\gamma$-globin gene promoter in Greek hereditary persistence of fetal haemoglobin. *Nature* 313: 325–326.

Collins, FS, Cole, JL, Lockwood, WK, and Iannuzzi, MC. (1987). The deletion in both common types of hereditary persistence of fetal hemoglobin is approximately 105 kilobases. *Blood* 70: 1797–1803.

Conley, CL, Weatherall, DJ, Richardson, SN et al. (1963). Hereditary persistence of fetal hemoglobin: A study of 79 affected persons in 15 Negro families in Baltimore. *Blood* 21: 261–281.

Costa, FF, Zago, MA, Cheng, G et al. (1990). The Brazilian type of nondeletional ^Aγ-fetal hemoglobin has a C→G substitution at nucleotide –195 of the ^Aγ-globin gene. *Blood* 75: 1896–1897.

Craig, JE, O'Hea, AM, Bametson, R, and Thein, SL. (1993). The molecular basis of HPFH in a British family identified by heteroduplex formation. *Br. J. Haematol.* 84: 106–110.

Craig, JE, Barnetson, RA, Prior, J et al. (1994). Rapid detection of deletions causing δβ thalassemia and hereditary persistence of fetal hemoglobin by enzymatic amplification. *Blood* 83: 1673–1682.

Craig, JE, Efremov, GD, Fisher, C, and Thein, SL. (1995). Macedonian (δβ⁰) thalassemia has the same molecular basis as Turkish inversion-deletion (δβ⁰) thalassemia. *Blood* 85: 1146–1147.

Craig, JE, Rochette, J, Fisher, CA et al. (1996). Dissecting the loci controlling fetal haemoglobin production on chromosomes 11p and 6q by the regressive approach. *Nat. Genet.* 12: 58–64.

Craig, JE, Rochette, J, Sampietro, M et al. (1997). Genetic heterogeneity in heterocellular hereditary persistence of fetal hemoglobin. *Blood* 90: 428–434.

Curtin, P, Pirastu, M, Kan, YW et al. (1985). A distant gene deletion affects β-globin gene function in an atypical γδβ-thalassemia. *J. Clin. Invest.* 76: 1554–1558.

De Angioletti, M, Lacerra, G, and Carestia, C. (1997). Breakpoint characterization of the Italian (AγδβΒ)⁰ thalassemia showing 3′ breakpoint clustering with those of Indian HPFH and Belgian (Aγδβ)⁰ thalassemia. 8th International Conference on Thalassemia, Malta, p. 146.

Diaz-Chico, JC, Huang, JH, Juncic, D et al. (1988). Two new large deletions resulting in εγδβ-thalassemia. *Acta Haematol.* 80: 79–84.

Dillon, N and Grosveld, F. (1991). Human γ-globin genes silenced independently of other genes in β-globin locus. *Nature* 350: 252–254.

Dimovski, AJ, Divoky, V, Adekile, AD et al. (1994). A novel deletion of ~27 kb including the β-globin gene and the locus control region 3′HS-1 regulatory sequence: β⁰-thalassemia or hereditary persistence of fetal hemoglobin? *Blood* 83: 822–827.

Dimovski, AJ, Baysal, E, Efremov, DG et al. (1996). A large β-thalassemia deletion in a family of Indonesian-Malay descent. *Hemoglobin* 20: 377–392.

Dinçol, G, Altay, C, Aksoy, M et al. (1981). Clinical and hematological evaluation of two δ⁰ β⁰-thalassemia homozygotes. *Hemoglobin* 5: 153–164.

Donald, JA, Lammi, A, and Trent, RJ. (1988). Hemoglobin F production in heterocellular hereditary persistence of fetal hemoglobin and its linkage to the beta globin gene complex. *Hum. Genet.* 80: 69–74.

Dover, GJ, Smith, KD, Chang, YC et al. (1992). Fetal hemoglobin levels in sickle cell disease and normal individuals are partially controlled by an X-linked gene located at Xp22.2. *Blood* 80: 816–824.

Driscoll, MC, Dobkin, CS, and Alter, BP. (1989). γδβ-thalassemia due to a *de novo* mutation deleting the 5′ β-glo-

bin gene activation-region hypersensitive sites. *Proc. Natl. Acad. Sci. U.S.A.* 86: 7470–7474.

Edington, GM and Lehmann, H. (1955). Expression of the sickle-cell gene in Africa. *Br. Med. J.* 1: 1308–1311.

Efremov, GD, Nikolov, N, Duma, H et al. (1975). δβ-thalassaemia in two Yugoslavian families. *Scand. J. Haematol.* 14: 226–232.

Efremov, GD, Nikolov, N, Hattori, Y et al. (1986). The 18- to 23-kb deletion of the Macedonian δβ-thalassemia includes the entire δ and β globin genes. *Blood* 68: 971–974.

Elder, JT, Forrester, WC, Thompson, C et al. (1990). Translocation of an erythroid-specific hypersensitive site in deletion-type hereditary persistence of fetal hemoglobin. *Mol. Cell. Biol.* 10: 1382–1389.

Elion, J, Berg, PE, Lapoumeroulie, C et al. (1992). DNA sequence variation in a negative control region 5′ to the β-globin gene correlates with the phenotypic expression of the βˢ mutation. *Blood* 79: 787–792.

Eng, B, Chui, DHK, Saunderson, J et al. (1993). Identification of two novel β⁰-thalassemia mutations in a Filipino family: Frameshift codon 67 (–TG) and a β-globin gene deletion. *Hum. Mutation* 2: 375–379.

Epner, E, Reik, A, Cimbora, D et al. (1999). The beta-globin LCR is not necessary for an open chromatin structure or developmentally regulated transcription of the native mouse beta globin locus. *Mol. Cell. Biol.* 2: 447–455.

Farquhar, M, Gelinas, R, Tatsis, B et al. (1983). Restriction endonuclease mapping of γ-δ-β-globin region in ^Gγ(β)⁺ HPFH and a Chinese ^Aγ HPFH variant. *Am. J. Hum. Genet.* 35: 611–620.

Fearon, ER, Kazazian, HH Jr, Waber, PG et al. (1983). The entire β-globin gene cluster is deleted in a form of γδβ-thalassemia. *Blood* 61: 1273–1278.

Feingold, EA and Forget, BG. (1989). The breakpoint of a large deletion causing hereditary persistence of fetal hemoglobin occurs within an erythroid DNA domain remote from the β-globin gene cluster. *Blood* 74: 2178–2186.

Feingold, EA, Penny, LA, Nienhuis, AW, and Forget, BG. (1999). An olfactory receptor gene is located in the extended human β-globin gene cluster and is expressed in erythroid cells. *Genomics* 61: 15–23.

Fessas, P and Stamatoyannopoulos, G. (1964). Hereditary persistence of fetal hemoglobin in Greece: A study and a comparison. *Blood* 24: 223–240.

Fessas, P, Stamatoyannopoulos, G, and Karaklis, A. (1961). Hereditary persistence of foetal haemoglobin and its combination with alpha and beta-thalassaemia. *8th Congress of the European Society of Haematology*. Vienna: Karger, Basel, p. 302.

Fischer, KD, and Nowock, J. (1990). The T→C substitution at –198 of the ^Aγ-globin gene associated with the British form of HPFH generates overlapping recognition sites for two DNA-binding proteins. *Nucl. Acids Res.* 18: 5685–5693.

Fodde, R, Losekoot, M, Casula, L, and Bernini, LF. (1990). Nucleotide sequence of the Belgian ^Gγ⁺(^Aγδβ)⁰-thalassemia deletion breakpoint suggests a common mechanism for a number of such recombination events. *Genomics* 8: 732–735.

Fogarty, WM Jr, Vedvick, TS, and Itano, HA. (1974). Absence of haemoglobin A in an individual simultaneously heterozygous in the genes for hereditary persistence of foetal haemoglobin and beta-thalassemia. *Br. J. Haematol.* 26: 527–533.

Forget, BG. (1998). Molecular basis of hereditary persistence of fetal hemoglobin. *Ann. N. Y. Acad. Sci.* 850: 38–44.

Forget, BG, Hillman, DG, Lazarus, H et al. (1976). Absence of messenger RNA and gene DNA for β-globin chains in hereditary persistence of fetal hemoglobin. *Cell* 7: 323–329.

Forrester, WC, Epner, E, Driscoll, MC et al. (1990). A deletion of the human β-globin locus activation region causes a major alteration in chromatin structure and replication across the entire β-globin locus. *Genes Dev.* 4: 1637–1649.

Fortina, P, Delgrosso, K, Werner, E et al. (1991). A >200 kb deletion removing the entire β-like globin gene cluster in a family of Irish descent. *Hemoglobin* 15: 23–41.

Friedman, S, Schwartz, E, Ahem, E, and Ahern, V. (1976). Variations in globin chain synthesis in hereditary persistence of fetal haemoglobin. *Br. J. Haematol.* 32: 357–364.

Fritsch, EF, Lawn, RM, and Maniatis, T. (1979). Characterisation of deletions which affect the expression of fetal globin genes in man. *Nature* 279: 598–603.

Fucharoen, S, Winichagoon, P, Chaicharoen, S, and Wasi, P. (1987). Different molecular defects of $^G\gamma$ $(^A\gamma\delta\beta)^0$-thalassaemia in Thailand. *Eur. J. Haematol.* 39: 154–160.

Fucharoen, S, Shimizu, K, and Fukumaki, Y. (1990). A novel C-T transition within the distal CCAAT motif of the Gγ-globin gene in the Japanese HPFH: Implication of factor binding in elevated fetal globin expression. *Nucl. Acids Res.* 18: 5245–5253.

Gaensler, KML, Kitamura, M, and Kan, YW. (1993). Germ-line transmission and developmental regulation of a 150 kb yeast artificial chromosome containing the human β-globin locus in transgenic mice. *Proc. Natl. Acad. Sci. U.S.A.* 90: 11381–11385.

Galanello, R, Melis, MA, Podda, A et al. (1990). Deletion δ-thalassemia: The 7.2 kb deletion of Corfu δβ-thalassemia in a non-β-thalassemia chromosome. *Blood* 75: 1747–1749.

Gelinas, R, Endlich, B, Pfeiffer, C et al. (1985). G to A substitution in the distal CCAAT box of the $^A\gamma$ globin gene in Greek hereditary persistence of fetal haemoglobin. *Nature* 313: 323–325.

Gelinas, R, Bender, M, Lotshaw, C et al. (1986). Chinese $^A\gamma$ fetal hemoglobin: C to T substitution at position −196 of the $^A\gamma$ gene promoter. *Blood* 67: 1777–1779.

George, E, Faridah, K, Trent, RJ et al. (1986). Homozygosity for a new type of $^G\gamma$ $(^A\gamma\delta\beta)^0$-thalassaemia in a Malaysian male. *Hemoglobin* 10: 353–363.

Gerald, PS and Diamond, LK. (1958). The diagnosis of thalassemia trait by starch block electrophoresis of the hemoglobin. *Blood* 13: 61–69.

Giampaolo, A, Mavilio, F, Sposi, NM, Care, A et al. (1984). Heterocellular HPFH: Molecular mechanisms of abnormal γ gene expression in association with β thalassemia and linkage relationship with the β globin gene cluster. *Hum. Genet.* 66: 151–156.

Gianni, AM, Bregni, M, and Cappellini, MD. (1983). A gene controlling fetal hemoglobin expression in adults is not linked to the non-α globin cluster. *EMBO J.* 2: 921–925.

Giglioni, B, Casini, C, Mantovani, R et al. (1984). A molecular study of a family with Greek hereditary persistence of fetal hemoglobin and β-thalassemia. *EMBO J.* 3: 2641–2645.

Gilman, JG and Huisman, THJ. (1984). Two independent genetic factors in the β-globin gene cluster are associated with high $^G\gamma$-levels in the HbF of SS patients. *Blood* 64: 452–457.

Gilman, JG and Huisman, THJ. (1985). DNA sequence variation associated with elevated fetal $^G\gamma$ globin production. *Blood* 66: 783–787.

Gilman, JG, Mishima, N, Wen, XJ, Kutlar, F et al. (1988a). Upstream promoter mutation associated with a modest elevation of fetal hemoglobin expression in human adults. *Blood* 72: 78–81.

Gilman, JG, Mishima, N, Wen, XJ, Stoming, TA et al. (1988b). Distal CCAAT box deletion in the $^A\gamma$ globin gene of two black adolescents with elevated fetal $^A\gamma$ globin. *Nucl. Acids Res.* 16: 10635–10642.

Gilman, JG, Brinson, EC, and Mishima, N. (1992). The 32.6 kb Indian δβ-thalassaemia deletion ends in a 3.4 kb L1 element downstream of the β-globin gene. *Br. J. Haematol.* 82: 417–421.

Gimferrer, E, Baiget, M, and Rutllant, MI. (1979). Homozygous δβ-thalassaemia in a Spanish woman. *Acta Haematol.* 61: 226–229.

Grosveld, F, Blom van Assendelft, G, Greaves, DR, and Kollias, G. (1987). Position-independent, high-level expression of the human β-globin gene in transgenic mice. *Cell* 51: 975–985.

Gumucio, DL, Rood, KL, Gray, TA et al. (1988). Nuclear proteins that bind the human γ-globin gene promoter: Alterations in binding produced by point mutations associated with hereditary persistence of fetal hemoglobin. *Mol. Cell. Biol.* 8: 5310–5322.

Gumucio, DL, Lockwood, WK, Weber, JL et al. (1990). The −175 T-C mutation increases promoter strength in erythroid cells: Correlaion with evolutionary conservation of binding sites for two *trans*-acting factors. *Blood* 75: 756–761.

Gumucio, DL, Rood, KL, Blanchard-McQuate, KL, Gray, TA et al. (1991). Interaction of Sp1 with the human γ globin promoter: Binding and transactivation of normal and mutant promoters. *Blood* 78: 1853–1863.

Hattori, Y, Kutlar, F, Mosley, CJ et al. (1986). Association of the level of $^G\gamma$ chain in the fetal hemoglobin of normal adults with specific haplotypes. *Hemoglobin* 10: 185–204.

Henthorn, PS, Smithies, O, and Nakatsuji, T. (1985). $(^A\gamma\delta\beta)^0$-thalassaemia in blacks is due to a deletion of 34 kbp of DNA. *Br. J. Haematol.* 59: 343–356.

Henthorn, PS, Mager, DK, Huisman, THJ, and Smithies, O. (1986). A gene deletion ending within a complex array of repeated sequences 3′ to the human beta-globin gene cluster. *Proc. Natl. Acad. Sci. U.S.A.* 83: 5194–5198.

Henthorn, PS, Smithies, O, and Mager, DL. (1990). Molecular analysis of deletions in the human β-globin cluster: Deletion junctions and locations of breakpoints. *Genomics* 6: 226–237.

Huang, HJ, Stoming, TA, Harris, HF et al. (1987). The Greek $^{A}\gamma\,\beta^{+}$-HPFH observed in a large black family. *Am. J. Hematol.* 25: 401–408.

Huisman, TH. (1981). The first homozygote for the hereditary persistence of fetal hemoglobin observed in the southeastern United States. *Hemoglobin* 5: 411–416.

Huisman, THJ, Schroeder, WA, Stamatoyannopoulos, G et al. (1970). Nature of fetal hemoglobin in the Greek type of hereditary persistence of fetal hemoglobin with and without concurrent β-thalassemia. *J. Clin. Invest.* 49: 1035–1040.

Huisman, THJ, Wrightstone, RN, Wilson, JB et al. (1972). Hemoglobin Kenya, the product of fusion of γ and β polypeptide chains. *Arch. Biochem. Biophy.* 153: 850–853.

Huisman, THJ, Schroeder, WA, and Efremov, GD. (1974). The present status of the heterogeneity of fetal hemoglobin in β-thalassaemia: An attempt to unify some observations on thalassemia and related conditions. *Ann. N. Y. Acad. Sci.* 232: 107–124.

Huisman, THJ, Miller, A, and Schroeder, WA. (1975). A $^{G}\gamma$ type of hereditary persistence of fetal hemoglobin with β chain production *in cis. Am. J. Hum. Genet.* 27: 765–777.

Jacob, GF and Raper, AB. (1958). Hereditary persistence of foetal haemoglobin production, and its interaction with the sickle-cell trait. *Br. J. Haematol.* 4: 138–149.

Jagadeeswaran, P, Tuan, D, Forget, BG, and Weissman, SM. (1982). A gene deletion ending at the midpoint of a repetitive DNA sequence in one form of hereditary persistence of fetal haemoglobin. *Nature* 296: 469–470.

Jane, SM, Gumucio, DL, Ney, PA et al. (1993). Methylation-enhanced binding of Sp1 to the stage selector element of the human γ-globin gene promoter may regulate developmental specificity of expression. *Mol. Cell. Biol.* 13: 3272–3281.

Jennings, MW, Jones, RW, Wood, WG, and Weatherall, DJ. (1985). Analysis of an inversion within the human beta globin gene cluster. *Nucl. Acids Res.* 13: 2897–2906.

Jones, RW, Old, JM, Trent, RJ et al. (1981a). Major rearrangement in the human β-globin gene cluster. *Nature* 291: 39–44.

Jones, RW, Old, JM, Trent, RJ et al. (1981b). Restriction mapping of a new deletion responsible for $^{G}\gamma$ (δβ)^{0} thalassemia. *Nucl. Acids Res.* 9: 6813–6825.

Jones, RW, Old, JM, Wood, WG et al. (1982). Restriction endonuclease maps of the β-like globin gene cluster in the British and Greek forms of HPFH, and for one example of $^{G}\gamma\beta^{+}$ HPFH. *Br. J. Haematol.* 50: 415–422.

Kan, YW, Forget, BG, and Nathan, DG. (1972). Gamma-beta thalassemia: A cause of hemolytic disease of the newborn. *N. Engl. J. Med.* 286: 129–134.

Kendall, AG, Ojwang, PJ, Schroeder, WA, and Huisman, THJ. (1973). Hemoglobin-Kenya, the product of a γ-β fusion gene: Studies of the family. *Am. J. Hum. Genet.* 25: 548–563.

Kosteas, T, Pavlou, O, Palena, A et al. (1996). Complete sequencing and functional analysis of the HPFH-6 enhancer: Detection of multiple motifs for transcription factors and identification of an open reading frame. *Blood* 88: 150a.

Kosteas, T, Palena, A, and Anagnou, NP. (1997). Molecular cloning of the breakpoints of the hereditary persistence of fetal hemoglobin type-6 (HPFH-6) deletion and sequence analysis of the novel juxtaposed region from the 3′ end of the β-globin gene cluster. *Hum. Genet.* 100: 441–445.

Kulozik, A, Yarwood, N, and Jones, RW. (1988). The Corfu δβ^{0} thalassemia: A small deletion acts at a distance to selectively abolish β globin gene expression. *Blood* 71: 457–462.

Kulozik, AE, Bellan-Koch, A, Kohne, E, and Kleihauer, E. (1992). A deletion/inversion rearrangement of the β-globin gene cluster in a Turkish family with δβ^{0}-thalassemia intermedia. *Blood* 79: 2455–2459.

Kutlar, A, Gardiner, MB, Headlee, MG et al. (1984). Heterogeneity in the molecular basis of three types of hereditary persistence of fetal hemoglobin and the relative synthesis of the $^{G}\gamma$ and $^{A}\gamma$ types of γ chain. *Biochem. Genet.* 22: 21–35.

Labie, D, Dunda-Belkhodja, O, Rouabhi, F et al. (1985a). The −158 site 5′ to the $^{G}\gamma$ gene and $^{G}\gamma$ expression. *Blood* 66: 1463–1465.

Labie, D, Pagnier, J, Lapoumeroulie, C et al. (1985b). Common haplotype dependency of high $^{G}\gamma$-globin gene expression and high HbF levels in β-thalassemia and sickle cell anemia patients. *Proc. Natl. Acad. Sci. U.S.A.* 82: 2111–2114.

Lanclos, KD, Michael, SK, Gu, TC et al. (1989). Transient chloramphenicol acetyltransferase expression of the $^{G}\gamma$ globin gene 5′-flanking regions containing substitutions of C→T at position −158, G→A at position −161, and T→A at position −175 in K562 cells. *Biochim. Biophys. Acta* 1008: 109–112.

Lanclos, KD, Oner, C, Dimovski, AJ et al. (1991). Sequence variations in the 5′ flanking and IVS-ll regions of the $^{G}\gamma$ and $^{A}\gamma$ globin genes of β^{S} chromosomes with five different haplotypes. *Blood* 77: 2488–2496.

Lloyd, JA, Lee, RF, and Lingrel, JB. (1989). Mutations in two regions upstream of the $^{A}\gamma$ globin gene canonical promoter affect gene expression. *Nucl. Acids Res.* 17: 4339–4352.

Losekoot, M, Fodde, R, Gerritsen, EJA et al. (1991). Interaction of two different disorders in the β-globin gene cluster associated with an increased hemoglobin F production: A novel deletion type of $^{G}\gamma + (^{A}\gamma\delta\beta)^{0}$-thalassemia and a δ^{0}-hereditary persistence of fetal hemoglobin determinant. *Blood* 77: 861–867.

Mager, DL, Henthorn, PS, and Smithies, O. (1985). A Chinese $^{G}\gamma+(^{A}\gamma\delta\beta)^{0}$ thalassemia deletion: Comparison to other deletions in the human β-globin gene cluster and sequence analysis of the breakpoints. *Nucl. Acids Res.* 13: 6559–6575.

Mann, JR, MacNeish, AS, Bannister, D et al. (1972). δβ-thalassaemia in a Chinese family. *Br. J. Haematol.* 23: 393–402.

Mantovani, R, Malgaretti, N, Nicolis, S et al. (1988). The effects of HPFH mutations in the human γ-globin promoter on binding of ubiquitous and erythroid specific nuclear factors. *Nucl. Acids Res.* 16: 7783–7797.

Mantovani, R, Superti-Furga, G, Gilman, J, and Ottolenghi, S. (1989). The deletion of the distal CCAAT box region of the $^{A}\gamma$-globin gene in black HPFH abolishes the binding of the erythroid specific protein NFE3 and of the CCAAT displacement protein. *Nucl. Acids Res.* 17: 6681–6691.

Martin, DK, Tsai, SF, and Orkin, SH. (1989). Increased γ-globin expression in a nondeletion HPFH mediated by an erythroid-specific DNA-binding factor. *Nature* 338: 435–438.

Martinez, G, Novelletto, A, Di Rienzo, A et al. (1989). A case of hereditary persistence of fetal hemoglobin caused by a gene not linked to the β-globin cluster. *Hum. Genet.* 82: 335–337.

Matsunaga, E, Kimura, A, Yamada, H et al. (1985). A novel deletion in δβ-thalassemia found in Japan. *Biochem. Biophys. Res. Commun.* 126: 185–191.

Matthews, JH, Rowlands, D, Wood, JK, and Wood, WG. (1981). Homozygous $^G\gamma\delta\beta$ thalassaemia. *Clin. Lab. Haematol.* 3: 121–127.

Merghoub, T, Perichon, B, Maier-Redesperger, M, Labie, D et al. (1996). Variation of fetal hemoglobin and F-cell number with the LCR-HS2 polymorphism in nonanemic individuals. *Blood* 87: 2607–2609.

Metherall, JE, Gillespie, FP, and Forget, BG. (1988). Analyses of linked β-globin genes suggest that nondeletion forms of hereditary persistence of fetal hemoglobin are bona fide switching mutants. *Am. J. Hum. Genet.* 42: 476–481.

Mishima, N, Landman, H, Huisman, THJ, and Gilman, JG. (1989). The DNA deletion in an Indian δβ-thalassaemia begins one kilobase from the $^A\gamma$ globin gene and ends in an L1 repetitive sequence. *Br. J. Haematol.* 73: 375–379.

Miyoshi, K, Kaneto, Y, Kawai, H et al. (1988). X-linked dominant control of F-cells in normal adult life: Characterization of the Swiss type as hereditary persistence of fetal hemoglobin regulated dominantly by gene(s) on X chromosome. *Blood* 72: 1854–1860.

Motum, PI, Hamilton, TJ, Lindeman, R et al. (1993a). Molecular characterisation of Vietnamese HPFH. *Hum. Mutat.* 2: 179–184.

Motum, PI, Kearney, A, Hamilton, TJ, and Trent, RJ. (1993b). Filipino β⁰ thalassaemia: A high Hb A₂ β⁰ thalassaemia resulting from a large deletion of the 5′ β globin gene region. *J. Med. Genet.* 30: 240–244.

Motum, PI, Lindeman, R, Harvey, MP, and Trent, RJ. (1993c). Comparative studies of nondeletional HPFH γ-globin gene promoters. *Exp. Hematol.* 121: 852–858.

Motum, P, Deng, Z-M, Huong, L, and Trent, RJ. (1994). The Australian type of nondeletional $^G\gamma$-HPFH has a C→G substitution at nucleotide −114 of the $^G\gamma$ gene. *Br. J. Haematol.* 86: 219–221.

Nicolis, S, Ronchi, A, Malgaretti, N et al. (1989). Increased erythroid-specific expression of a mutated HPFH γ globin promoter requires the erythroid factor NFE-1. *Nucl. Acids Res.* 17: 5509–5516.

Ojwang, PJ, Nakatsuji, T, Gardiner, MB et al. (1983). Gene deletion as the molecular basis for the Kenya-$^G\gamma$-HPFH condition. *Hemoglobin* 7: 115–123.

Öner, R, Kutlar, F, Gu, L-H, and Huisman, THJ. (1991). The Georgia type of nondeletional hereditary persistence of fetal hemoglobin has a C→T mutation at nucleotide −114 of the $^A\gamma$-globin gene. *Blood* 77: 1124–1128.

Öner, C, Dimovski, AJ, Altay, C et al. (1992). Sequence variations in the 5′ hypersensitive site-2 of the locus control region of β^S chromosomes are associated with different

levels of fetal globin in hemoglobin S homozygotes. *Blood* 79: 813–819.

Öner, R, Öner, C, Erdem, G et al. (1996). A novel (δβ)⁰-thalassemia due to an approximately 30-kb deletion observed in a Turkish family. *Acta Haematol.* 96: 232–236.

Oppenheim, A, Yaari, A, Rund, D et al. (1990). Intrinsic potential for high fetal hemoglobin production in a Druz family with β-thalassemia is due to an unlinked genetic determinant. *Hum. Genet.* 86: 175–180.

Orkin, SH, Alter, BP, Altay, C et al. (1978). Application of endonuclease mapping to the analysis and prenatal diagnosis of thalassemias caused by globin-gene deletion. *N. Engl. J. Med.* 299: 166–172.

Orkin, SH, Alter, BP, and Altay, C. (1979). Deletion of the $^A\gamma$ globin gene in $^G\gamma$ δβ-thalassemia. *J. Clin. Invest.* 64: 866.

Orkin, SH, Goff, SC, and Nathan, DG. (1981). Heterogeneity of DNA deletion in γδβ-thalassemia. *J. Clin. Invest.* 67: 878–884.

Ottolenghi, S, Giglioni, B, Taramelli, R et al. (1982). Molecular comparison of δβ-thalassemia and hereditary persistence of fetal hemoglobin DNAs: Evidence of a regulatory area? *Proc. Natl. Acad. Sci. U.S.A.* 79: 2347–2351.

Ottolenghi, S, Giglioni, B, Pulazzini, A et al. (1987). Sardinian δβ⁰-thalassemia: A further example of a C to T substitution at position −196 of the $^A\gamma$ globin gene promoter. *Blood* 69: 1058–1061.

Ottolenghi, S, Camaschella, C, Comi, P et al. (1988). A frequent $^A\gamma$-hereditary persistence of fetal hemoglobin in northern Sardinia: Its molecular basis and hematologic phenotype in heterozygotes and compound heterozygotes with β-thalassemia. *Hum. Genet.* 79: 13–17.

Palena, A, Blau, A, Stamatoyannopoulos, G, and Anagnou, NP. (1994). Eastern European (δβ)⁰ thalassemia: Molecular characterization of a novel 9.1 kb deletion resulting in high levels of fetal hemoglobin in the adult. *Blood* 83: 3738–3745.

Patrinos, GP, Kollia, P, Loutradi-Anagnostou A et al. (1998). The Cretan type of non-deletional hereditary persistence of fetal hemoglobin [Aγ −158 C to T] results from two independent gene conversion events. *Hum. Genet.* 102: 629–634.

Peterson, KR, Li, QL, Clegg, CH et al. (1995). Use of yeast artificial chromosomes (YACs) in studies of mammalian development: Production of β-globin locus YAC mice carrying human globin developmental mutants. *Proc. Natl. Acad. Sci. U.S.A.* 92: 5655–5659.

Pirastu, M, Kan, YW, Lin, CC et al. (1983). Hemolytic disease of the newborn caused by a new deletion of the entire β-globin cluster. *J. Clin. Invest.* 72: 602–609.

Pissard, S and Beuzard, Y. (1994). A potential regulatory region for the expression of fetal hemoglobin in sickle cell disease. *Blood* 84: 331–338.

Pissard, S, M'rad, A, Beuzard, Y, and Roméo, P-H. (1996). A new type of hereditary persistence of fetal haemoglobin (HPFH): HPFH Tunisia β⁺ (+C-200)$^G\gamma$. *Br. J. Haematol.* 95: 67–72.

Pistidda, P, Frogheri, L, Guiso, L et al. (1997). Maximal γ-globin expression in the compound heterozygous state for −175 $^G\gamma$ HPFH and β⁰39 nonsense thalassaemia: A case study. *Eur. J. Haematol.* 58: 320–325.

Reyes, GR, Pina-Camara, A, Felice, AE et al. (1978). δβ thalassemia in a Mexican family: Clinical differences among homozygotes. *Hemoglobin* 2: 513–529.

Ribeiro, ML, Cunha, E, Goncalves, P et al. (1997). Hb Lepore-Baltimore (δ^{68Leu}-β^{84Thr}) and Hb Lepore-Washington-Boston (δ^{87Gin}-$\beta^{IVS-II-8}$) in Central Portugal and Spanish Alta Extremadura. *Hum. Genet.* 99: 669–673.

Ringelhann, B, Konotey-Ahulu, FID, Lehmann, H, and Lorkin, PA. (1970). A Ghanaian adult, homozygous for hereditary persistence of foetal haemoglobin and heterozygous for elliptocytosis. *Acta Haematol.* 43: 100–110.

Rixon, MW and Gelinas, RE. (1988). A fetal globin gene mutation in $^A\gamma$ nondeletion HPFH increases promoter strength in a non-erythroid cell. *Mol. Cell. Biol.* 8: 713–721.

Roberts, NA, Sloane-Stanley, JA, Sharpe, JA et al. (1997). Globin gene switching in transgenic mice carrying HS2-globin gene constructs. *Blood* 89: 713–723.

Ronchi, A, Nicolis, S, Santoro, C, and Ottolenghi, S. (1989). Increased Sp 1 binding mediates erythroid-specific overexpression of a mutated (HPFH) γ-globulin promoter. *Nucl. Acids Res.* 17: 10231–10241.

Ronchi, A, Berry, M, Raguz, S et al. (1996). Role of the duplicated CCAAT box region in γ-globin gene regulation and hereditary persistence of fetal haemoglobin. *EMBO J.* 15: 143–149.

Saglio, G, Camaschella, C, Serra, A et al. (1986). Italian type of deletional hereditary persistence of fetal hemoglobin. *Blood* 68: 646–651.

Schroeder, WA, Huisman, THJ, Shelton, JR et al. (1968). Evidence for multiple structural genes for the γ-chain of human fetal hemoglobin. *Proc. Natl. Acad. Sci. U.S.A.* 60: 537–544.

Schroeder, WA, Huisman, THJ, and Sukumaran, PK. (1973). A second type of hereditary persistence of fetal hemoglobin in India. *Br. J. Haematol.* 25: 131–135.

Seltzer, WK, Abshire, TC, Lane, PA et al. (1992). Molecular genetic studies in black families with sickle cell anemia and unusually high levels of fetal hemoglobin. *Hemoglobin* 16: 363–377.

Shiokawa, S, Yamada, H, Takihara, Y et al. (1988). Molecular analysis of Japanese δβ-thalassemia. *Blood* 72: 1771–1776.

Sofroniadou, K, Wood, WG, Nute, PE, and Stamatoyannopoulos, G. (1975). Globin chain synthesis in Greek type ($^A\gamma$) of hereditary persistence of fetal haemoglobin. *Br. J. Haematol.* 29: 137–148.

Starck, J, Sarkar, R, Romana, M et al. (1994). Developmental regulation of human γ- and β-globin genes in the absence of the locus control region. *Blood* 84: 1656–1665.

Stoming, TA, Stoming, GS, Lanclos, KD et al. (1989). An $^A\gamma$ type of non-deletional hereditary persistence of fetal hemoglobin with a T→C mutation at position −175 to the cap site of the $^A\gamma$ globin gene. *Blood* 73: 329–333.

Superti-Furga, G, Barberis, A, Schaffner, G, and Busslinger, M. (1988). The −117 mutation in Greek HPFH affects the binding of three nuclear factors to the CCAAT region of the γ-globin gene. *EMBO J.* 7: 3099–3107.

Surrey, S, Delgrosso, K, Malladi, P, and Schwartz, E. (1988). A single-base change at position −175 in the 5′-flanking region of the $^G\gamma$-globin gene from a black with $^G\gamma$-β^+ HPFH. *Blood* 71: 807–810.

Sykes, K and Kaufman, R. (1990). A naturally occurring gamma globin gene mutation enhances SP1 binding activity. *Mol. Cell. Biol.* 10: 95–102.

Taramelli, R, Kioussis, D, Vanin, E et al. (1986). γδβ-thalassaemias 1 and 2 are the result of a 100 kbp deletion in the human β-globin cluster. *Nucl. Acids Res.* 14: 7017–7029.

Tate, VE, Wood, WG, and Weatherall, DJ. (1986). The British form of hereditary persistence of fetal haemoglobin results from a single base mutation adjacent to an S1 hypersensitive site 5′ to the $^A\gamma$ globin gene. *Blood* 68: 1389–1393.

Thein, SL, Sampietro, M, Rohde, K et al. (1994). Detection of a major gene for heterocellular hereditary persistence of fetal hemoglobin after accounting for genetic modifiers. *Am. J. Hum. Genet.* 54: 214–228.

Thein, SL and Weatherall, DJ. (1989). A non-deletion hereditary persistence of fetal hemoglobin (HPFH) determinant not linked to the β-globin gene complex. In *Hemoglobin Switching, Part B: Cellular and Molecular Mechanisms.* Stamatoyannopoulos, G and Nierhuis, AW, editors. New York: Alan R Liss, pp. 97–111.

Townes, TM and Behringer, RR. (1990). Human globin locus activation region (LAR): Role in temporal control. *Trends Genet.* 6: 219–223.

Traeger-Synodinos, J, Tzetis, M, Kanavakis, E, Metaxotou-Mavromati, A et al. (1991). The Corfu δβ thalassaemia mutation in Greece: Haematological phenotype and prevalence. *Br. J. Haematol.* 79: 302–305.

Trent, RJ, Jones, RW, Clegg, JB et al. (1984). ($^A\gamma\delta\beta$)⁰ thalassaemia: Similarity of phenotype in four different molecular defects, including one newly described. *Br. J. Haematol.* 57: 279–289.

Trent, RJ, Svirklys, L, and Jones, P. (1988). Thai (δβ)⁰-thalassemia and its interaction with γ-thalassemia. *Hemoglobin* 12: 101–114.

Trent, RJ, Williams, BG, Kearney, A et al. (1990). Molecular and hematologic characterization of Scottish-Irish type (εγδβ)⁰ thalassemia. *Blood* 76: 2132–2138.

Tuan, D, Biro, PA, de Riel, JK et al. (1979). Restriction endonuclease mapping of the human gamma globin gene loci. *Nucl. Acids Res.* 6: 2519–2544.

Tuan, D, Murnane, MJ, de Riel, JK, and Forget, BG. (1980). Heterogeneity in the molecular basis of hereditary persistence of fetal haemoglobin. *Nature* 285: 335–337.

Tuan, D, Feingold, E, Newman, M et al. (1983). Different 3′ end points of deletions causing δβ-thalassaemia and hereditary persistence of fetal hemoglobin: Implications for the control of γ-globin gene expression in man. *Proc. Natl. Acad. Sci. U.S.A.* 80: 6937–6941.

Ulrich, MJ, Gray, WJ, and Ley, TJ. (1992). An intramolecular DNA triplex is disrupted by point mutations associated with hereditary persistence of fetal hemoglobin. *J. Biol. Chem.* 267: 18649–18658.

Ulrich, MJ and Ley, TJ. (1990). Function of normal and mutated γ-globin gene promoters in electrophorated K562 erythroleukemia cells. *Blood* 75: 990–999.

Vanin, EF, Henthorn, PS, and Kioussis, D. (1983). Unexpected relationships between four large deletions in the human β-globin gene cluster. *Cell* 35: 701–709.

Waber, PG, Bender, MA, Gelinas, RE et al. (1986). Concordance of a point mutation 5′ to the $^A\gamma$ globin gene in $^A\gamma\beta^+$ HPFH in Greeks. *Blood* 67: 551–554.

Wainscoat, JS, Old, JM, and Wood, WG. (1984). Characterization of an Indian $(\delta\beta)^0$ thalassemia. *Br. J. Haematol.* 58: 353–360.

Wainscoat, JS, Thein, SL, Wood, WG et al. (1985). A novel deletion in the β globin gene complex. *Ann. N. Y. Acad. Sci.* 445: 20–27.

Waye, JS, Eng, B, Coleman, MB et al. (1994a). δβ-thalassemia in an African-American: Identification of the deletion endpoints and PCR-based diagnosis. *Hemoglobin* 18: 389–399.

Waye, JS, Eng, B, Hunt, JA, and Chui, DHK. (1994b). Filipino β-thalassemia due to a large deletion: Identification of the deletion endpoints and polymerase chain reaction (PCR)-based diagnosis. *Hum. Genet.* 94: 530–532.

Weatherall, DJ, Cartner, R, and Wood, WG. (1975). A form of hereditary persistence of fetal haemoglobin characterized by uneven cellular distribution of haemoglobin F and the production of haemoglobins A and A_1 in homozygotes. *Br. J. Haematol.* 29: 205–220.

Wheeler, JT, and Krevans, JR. (1961). The homozygous state of persistent fetal hemoglobin and the interaction of persistent fetal hemoglobin with thalassemia. *Bull. Johns Hopkins Hosp.* 109: 217–233.

Wijgerde, M, Grosveld, F, and Fraser, P. (1995). Transcription complex stability and chromatin dynamics in vivo. *Nature* 377: 209–213.

Winichagoon, S, Fucharoen, S, Thonglairoam, V, and Wasi, P. (1990). Thai $^G\gamma$ $(^A\gamma\delta\beta)^0$-thalassemia and its interaction with a single γ-globin gene on a chromosome carrying β^0-thalassemia. *Hemoglobin* 14: 185–197.

Wood, WG. (1989). HbF production in adult life. Stamatoyannopoulos, G, Nienhuis, AW, editors. *In Hemoglobin switching, Part B: Cellular and molecular mechanisms.* New York: Alan R, Liss. pp. 251–267.

Wood, WG, (1993). Increased HbF in adult life. In Higgs, DR, and Weatherall, DJ, editors. *Baillière's clinical haematology: The haemoglobinopathies.* London: Baillière Tindall. pp. 177–214.

Wood, WG, Clegg, JB, Weatherall, DJ et al. (1977). $^G\gamma$ $\delta\beta$ thalassaemia and $^G\gamma$ HPFH (Hb Kenya type) comparison of 2 new cases. *J. Med. Genet.* 14: 237–244.

Wood, WG, MacRae, IA, Darbre, PD, Clegg, JB et al. (1982). The British type of non-deletion HPFH: Characterization of developmental changes *in vivo* and erythroid growth *in vitro. Br. J. Haematol.* 50: 401–414.

Yang, KG, Stoming, TA, Fei, YJ et al. (1988). Identification of base substitutions in the promoter regions of the $^A\gamma$- and $^G\gamma$-globin genes in $^A\gamma$- (or $^G\gamma$-) β^+-HPFH heterozygotes using the DNA-amplification-synthetic oligonucleotide procedure. *Blood* 71: 1414–1417.

Zelkowitz, L, Torres, C, Bhoopalan, N et al. (1972). Double heterozygous βδ-thalassemia in Negroes. *Arch. Intern. Med.* 129: 975–979.

Zeng, Y-T, Huang, S-Z, Chen, B et al. (1985). Hereditary persistence of fetal hemoglobin or $(\delta\beta)^0$-thalassemia: Three types observed in South-Chinese families. *Blood* 66: 1430–1435.

Zhang, J-W, Stamatoyannopoulos, G, and Anagnou, NP. (1988) Laotian $(\delta\beta)^0$-thalassemia: Molecular characterization of a novel deletion associated with increased production of fetal hemoglobin. *Blood* 72: 983–988.

Zhang, J-W, Song, W-F, Zhao, Y-J et al. (1993). Molecular characterization of a novel form of $(^A\gamma\delta\beta)^0$ thalassemia deletion in a Chinese family. *Blood* 81: 1624–1629.

Zhang, X-Q and Zhang, J-W. (1998). The 3′ breakpoint of the Yunnanese $(^A\gamma\delta\beta)^0$-thalassemia deletion lies in an L1 family sequence: Implications for the mechanism of deletion and the reactivation of the $^G\gamma$-globin gene. *Hum. Genet.* 103: 90–95.

Zhang, Z, Lin, C, Wang, S, and Gaensler, KML. (1997). Globin gene switching in β-globin YAC transgenic with a 12.5 kb deletion of the region between the $^A\gamma$ and δ genes. *Blood* 90: 129a.

Zuelzer, WW, Robinson, AR, and Booker, CR. (1961). Reciprocal relationship of hemoglobins A_2 and F in beta chain thalassemias, a key to the genetic control of hemoglobin F. *Blood* 17: 393–408.

SECTION III

α THALASSEMIA

DOUGLAS R. HIGGS

At all stages of development, human hemoglobin is made up of two α-like and two β-like globin chains. In embryonic life the ζ and ε genes are fully active producing embryonic hemoglobin ($\zeta_2\varepsilon_2$). Between 6 and 8 weeks of gestation there is a switch in expression so that the α- and γ-globin genes become fully expressed producing fetal hemoglobin ($\alpha_2\gamma_2$). Finally, at around the time of birth, there is a further switch from γ- to β-globin gene expression so that in adult red cells HbA ($\alpha_2\beta_2$) predominates.

In α thalassemia, the synthesis of α-globin chains is downregulated so that in fetal life there is anemia and the excess γ-globin chains form soluble tetramers (γ_4) called Hb Bart's. In adult life, α thalassemia also causes anemia but, because by this time the γ to β switch is complete, the excess non-α chains assemble into β_4 tetramers, called HbH. The degree of anemia and the amounts of the abnormal hemoglobins (Bart's and H) produced broadly reflect the degree to which α-globin synthesis has been downregulated.

We now know that normal individuals have four α-globin genes, arranged as linked pairs of genes at the tip of each copy of chromosome 16, written in shorthand as αα/αα. α Thalassemia most commonly results from the deletion of one (−α) or both (−−) α genes from chromosome 16. Carriers of α thalassemia (−α/αα and −−/αα) have a mild hypochromic microcytic anemia and may produce detectable amounts of Hb Bart's at birth. In addition, occasional cells containing HbH may be detected in adults with the −−/αα genotype, although hemoglobin electrophoresis is unremarkable. In all other respects, carriers of α thalassemia are entirely normal and the most important consideration, from a clinical and hematologic point of view, is to ensure that such patients do not become misdiagnosed and inappropriately treated for "iron deficiency" anemia.

α Thalassemia is probably the most common disease-causing mutation affecting mankind. There is good circumstantial evidence that α thalassemia has attained such high frequencies by virtue of its selective advantage in areas where falciparum malaria is or has been endemic. In tropical and subtropical regions of the world, the carrier frequency of the mildest type of α thalassemia (−α) is very high and may be present in more than 90 percent of individuals in such populations. In Southeast Asia and the Mediterranean basin, the more severe defect (−−) is also present at high frequencies (up to 10 percent). In these areas, various combinations of alleles are seen. Homozygotes for the −α/ haplotype (−α/−α) have a mild hypochromic microcytic anemia. Compound heterozygotes (−−/−α) have a hemolytic anemia producing large amounts of Hb Bart's at birth and similar levels of HbH in adult life, a condition known as HbH disease. Homozygotes for the −−/ haplotype (−−/−−) have a lethal condition referred to as the Hb Bart's hydrops fetalis syndrome. As predicted from the distribution of the −−/ haplotype, HbH disease and the Hb Bart's hydrops fetalis syndrome are mainly found in individuals of Southeast Asian and Mediterranean origins.

Within the "malaria belt", there has been selection for a very wide range of hemoglobin variants and different types of α and β thalassemia. The major hemoglobinopathies include the HbS mutation and HbE. Co-inheritance of α thalassemia has an important influence on the hematology and clinical manifestations of these common β-chain abnormalities and β thalassemia.

The molecular basis of α thalassemia is now understood in great detail. Normally, the α-like genes are arranged along chromosome 16 in the order in which they are expressed in development (telomere-ζ2-α2-α1-centromere). Furthermore, we now know that the cluster lies in a telomeric, gene-rich region of the genome, surrounded by widely expressed genes. Full expression of the α-like genes is critically dependent on the presence of a regulatory element (called HS −40), which lies 40 kb upstream of the cluster (toward the telomere). As many as 36 deletions removing one

Martin H. Steinberg, Bernard G. Forget, Douglas R. Higgs, and Ronald L. Nagel, editors. *Disorders of Hemoglobin: Genetics, Pathophysiology, and Clinical Management.* © 2001 Cambridge University Press. All rights reserved.

($-\alpha/$) or both genes have been characterized and of these, six ($-\alpha^{3.7}/$, $-\alpha^{4.2}/$, $--^{SEA}/$, $--^{MED}/$, $-(\alpha)^{20.5}/$, and $--^{FIL}/$) represent by far the most common causes of α thalassemia worldwide. In addition, many different point mutations affecting the structural genes have been identified; these cause the less common nondeletional forms of α thalassemia ($\alpha^T\alpha/$). This information has allowed researchers and hematologists to establish logical and robust screening programs for identifying patients with α thalassemia. This, in turn, allows clinicians to provide accurate genetic counseling and prenatal diagnosis for the severe syndromes of α thalassemia, including Hb Bart's hydrops fetalis and transfusion-dependent forms of HbH disease.

In addition to these common forms of α thalassemia, there are many rare and unusual molecular defects that have been identified. These are important because they provide an explanation for patients with hitherto undiagnosed anemia, but they also help us to understand how the α cluster is normally regulated in vivo. Rarely, α thalassemia is caused by deletions that remove the α-globin regulatory element (HS-40). In general these mutations have been observed outside of the "malaria belt", indicating that they are sporadic genetic events that have not been selected during evolution. These natural deletions first indicated the existence of this unexpected form of long-range control of α-globin gene expression.

There are also two rare forms of α thalassemia that are found in association with a variety of developmental abnormalities and, in particular, with mental retardation [so-called α thalassemia with mental retardation, (ATR) syndromes]. The first group of patients have large (>1 Mb) deletions from the tip of chromosome 16 including the α-globin genes (ATR-16). These usually result from chromosome truncations or translocations and, in fact, this syndrome provided the first examples in human genetics of subcytogenetic chromosomal translocations, which are now known to underlie many cases of unexplained mental retardation. The second group of patients are now known to have mutations in a trans-acting factor (called ATRX) encoded on the X-chromosome (ATR-X syndrome). These patients have α thalassemia with profound mental retardation, facial abnormalities, and urogenital anomalies. In this case, it is thought that the X-encoded factor regulates expression of many genes, the α genes being but one target.

Finally, there is a rare and unexplained form of α thalassemia that is seen as an acquired mutation in patients with myelodysplasia, hence called the ATMDS syndrome. These patients inherit a normal complement of α genes ($\alpha\alpha/\alpha\alpha$), but later in life develop myelodysplasia and presumably acquire a clonal genetic abnormality during the course of their disease. It is interesting that the majority of these patients are elderly males who at some stage of their disease have abnormal erythropoiesis. It will be fascinating to solve the molecular basis of this unusual form of α thalassemia in the years to come.

In the following chapters, we review in detail the epidemiology, molecular pathology, pathophysiology, and clinical syndromes of α thalassemia.

16

Pathophysiology of α Thalassemia

STEPHEN A. LIEBHABER
STANLEY L. SCHRIER

The pathophysiology of α thalassemia is a direct consequence of a deficiency in α-globin chain synthesis. One or more mutations diminishing α-globin synthesis result in accumulation of uncomplexed β-globin chains. This in turn leads to red cell damage, the consequent shortening of erythrocyte life span in the peripheral circulation and to a lesser extent to ineffective erythropoiesis. A reduction of α-globin chain synthesis reflects not only the number of α-globin genes affected by mutation(s), but also which of the two α-globin loci (α1 versus α2) is affected, whether the mutation involved is deletional or non-deletional, and whether the nondeletional mutation(s) partially or fully blocks gene expression (Chapter 17).

Erythrocyte damage caused by the excess α-globin chains is primarily due to a multifaceted membrane toxicity. Defects in β-globin chain synthesis (β thalassemia) can ameliorate α thalassemia by rebalancing the α/β chain synthesis ratio. Thus, understanding the basis for the broad spectrum of clinical severity (phenotypes) in individual patients with α thalassemia demands a detailed knowledge of the underlying genetic defect(s) and the impact of that defect on overall levels and balance of globin chain synthesis. This chapter describes the pathophysiologic consequences of defects in this system. Detailed molecular descriptions of the α-globin gene cluster,

the individual α-globin gene mutations, and an extensive catalog of genetic defects affecting the α-globin gene cluster are discussed in Chapter 17 and the clinical and laboratory features of α thalassemia are covered in Chapter 18.

STRUCTURE AND FUNCTION OF THE HUMAN α-GLOBIN GENE CLUSTER

Located at the telomere of chromosome 16, the human α-globin gene cluster, shown in a simplified form in Figure 16.1, contains a single embryonic ζ-globin gene and two co-expressed fetal/adult α-globin genes, (Deisseroth et al., 1977; Fischel-Ghodsian et al., 1987; Higgs et al., 1989) (Chapter 17). ζ-Globin gene expression is restricted to the primitive erythroblasts in the blood islands of the extraembryonic yolk sac (5 to 7 weeks of gestation) (Heuhns and Beaven, 1971; Peschle et al., 1985; Albitar et al., 1989). Both α-globin loci are also transcribed during this period (Albitar et al., 1992a). As erythropoiesis switches from the yolk sac to the definitive lineage in the fetal liver, the ζ-globin gene is silenced and α-globin gene expression is reciprocally enhanced (Peschle et al., 1985; Albitar et al., 1989; Albitar et al., 1992b). Of interest, the long held assumption that ζ- and α-globin genes have unique and essential developmental roles in erythroid development has been brought into question by the recent finding that normal development and viability in the mouse can be entirely supported by the expression of either gene alone (Leder et al., 1997; Russell and Liebhaber, 1998).

The two α-globin genes encode an identical α-globin protein. These two genes have maintained remarkable homology during evolution via multiple rounds of gene conversion (Liebhaber et al., 1980; Michelson and Orkin, 1980; Liebhaber et al., 1981; Orkin and Goff, 1981; Higgs et al., 1984). Both α-globin genes have identical promoters for 633 bp 5′ to the transcription start site (Michelson and Orkin, 1983). Their transcribed regions became divergent via two base substitutions and a 7bp insertion/deletion in intron 2 and via eighteen base substitutions and a single-base deletion in the 113-base 3′ untranslated region (UTR) (Liebhaber et al., 1980; Michelson and Orkin, 1980; Liebhaber et al., 1981; Orkin and Goff, 1981). Thus the fully processed α1- and α2-globin mRNAs have identical coding regions and can be distinguished only on the basis of their 3′ UTR structures (Liebhaber and Kan, 1981; Orkin and Goff, 1981; Hunt et al., 1982).

Martin H. Steinberg, Bernard G. Forget, Douglas R. Higgs, and Ronald L. Nagel, editors. *Disorders of Hemoglobin: Genetics, Pathophysiology, and Clinical Management.* © 2001 Cambridge University Press. All rights reserved.

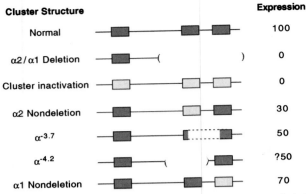

Figure 16.1. Categories of α thalassemia mutations and their impact on α-globin chain synthesis.

UNEQUAL EXPRESSION OF THE TWO α-GLOBIN GENES

Although the two α-globin mRNAs encode an identical α-globin chain, they are not equally expressed. Assays based on the 3′ UTR structural divergence have been used to quantify the relative expression of the two α-globin mRNAs (Liebhaber and Kan, 1981; Orkin and Goff, 1981; Hunt et al., 1982, Kropp et al., 1989; Molchanova and Huisman, 1996). These assays reveal that the α2 locus, that is 5′ to the α1 locus, produces approximately 2.6-fold more mRNA (Liebhaber and Kan, 1981; Liebhaber et al., 1985; Liebhaber et al., 1986; Molchanova and Huisman, 1996; Smetanina et al., 1996). This dominance of the α2 locus is specific to the definitive (fetal/adult) red cell series; expression of the two α-globin loci is equal in the primitive erythroblasts (Albitar et al., 1992a). The molecular basis for the higher expression of the α2-globin gene in definitive erythroblasts is not firmly established. Since the α2/α1 globin mRNA ratio of 2.6 is the same in transcriptionally active bone marrow as it is in transcriptionally silent reticulocytes, one can deduce that the stability of these two mRNAs is equivalent (Liebhaber and Kan, 1981; Orkin and Goff, 1981). Unequal expression— and the dominance of the α2-globin gene—appears rather to reflect the positioning of the two α-globin genes within the cluster (Liebhaber et al., 1985; Vestri et al., 1994).

The predominance of the α2-globin gene in the synthesis of α-globin mRNA would predict a corresponding dominant role of this gene in α-globin chain synthesis. Although there is some difference in the literature as to the full extent of such a difference (Liebhaber et al., 1986, Molchanova et al., 1996), a number of lines of evidence support this dominant role. First, the α1- and α2-globin mRNAs are translated with equal efficiency (Shakin and Liebhaber, 1986). This implies that the higher rate of transcrip-

tion of the α2-globin gene is paralleled by a correspondingly higher level of α2-globin synthesis. A second line of evidence is based on direct monitoring of protein synthesis from the two α-globin loci. Since the two α-globin genes normally encode an identical protein, differential monitoring of protein expression was approached by measuring expression of mutated α-globin genes that encoded mutant α-globin proteins (Liebhaber et al., 1986). These data demonstrate that α-globin structural mutants encoded at the α2 locus are expressed at two to three times the level of those encoded at the α1 locus. Thus these data confirm the dominant role of the α2-globin locus in α-globin chain synthesis and predict that loss of the α2 locus results in a more severe α thalassemia phenotype than loss of the α1 locus (detailed later and in Chapter 17).

RELATIONSHIP OF α-GLOBIN GENE MUTATION TO LOSS OF α-GLOBIN SYNTHESIS

Mutations in the α-globin gene cluster can inactivate either of the two α-globin loci (-α, $\alpha^T\alpha$, $\alpha\alpha^T$) or can result in the loss of both loci (- -) (Higgs et al., 1989; Liebhaber, 1989; Russell and Liebhaber, 1992; also see Chapter 17). In the case of mutation of a single gene, the net loss of α-globin synthesis reflects several variables: (1) whether the mutation is deletional (-α) or nondeletional ($\alpha^T\alpha$ or $\alpha\alpha^T$); (2) whether loss of gene expression is partial or complete; (3) whether the nondeletion mutation inactivates the α1 ($\alpha\alpha^T$) or α2 ($\alpha^T\alpha$) locus; and (4) whether there are compensating changes in the expression of the remaining α-globin locus (Russell and Liebhaber, 1992). These issues are discussed in detail in Chapters 17 and 18.

In general, the α thalassemia determinants can be arranged in the order of their severity (from (αα) to (- -) (see Figs 17.1 through 17.4). The phenotypes resulting from their interactions become increasingly severe (from α thalassemia trait to hydrops fetails) as the resulting level of α-globin synthesis decreases (see Table 18.1.) Categorizing α thalassemias and their corresponding underlying genetic defects is only a general guide for phenotype/genotype correlations. In reality, these clinical syndromes can overlap with each other, and the clinical severity within each of the categories can vary significantly (see Chapter 18). Thus, it is possible to predict with only reasonable accuracy the severity of the α-thalassemia phenotype based on a detailed description of the underlying genotypes.

Loss of a single α-globin gene by the $-\alpha^{3.7}$ deletion is by far the most common molecular defect in α thalassemia. This deletion is generated by a crossover at the most extensive repeat within the α-globin gene complex, the Z-homology box (see Chapter 17 for details) (Orkin et al., 1979; Michelson and Orkin, 1983; Higgs et al., 1984). This unequal crossover generates a single functional α-globin gene that encodes an mRNA that is identical to the α1-globin mRNA and contains the α1-globin mRNA 3′ UTR sequence (Fig. 16.1). Of central importance to the phenotypic impact of this deletion is the fact that the resultant "α1"-globin gene formed by the crossover is expressed at a level midway between that of the native (minor) α1- and (major) α2-globin genes (Liebhaber et al., 1985). Thus the loss of the α2 gene by $-\alpha^{3.7}$ is offset by a doubling in expression of the remaining locus (Liebhaber et al., 1985).

The second most common single α-globin gene deletion, the $-\alpha^{4.2}$ (Embury et al., 1980), is generated by unequal exchange mediated by different repeated units within the X-box (Fig. 16.1) (Embury et al., 1980; Higgs et al., 1984). In this case there is no conclusive evidence for a "compensatory" increase in the expression of the remaining α-globin locus in the affected cluster.

NONDELETION α THALASSEMIA MUTATIONS

A full spectrum of nondeletion mutations has been identified in α thalassemia. These mutations individually impact on gene transcription, transcript processing, translational efficiency, mRNA stability, or protein stability (Russell and Liebhaber, 1992; also see Chapter 17 for detailed catalog and analysis).

Correlating disease severity with specific nondeletion mutations has supported the major role of the α2-globin locus in α-globin expression (Kattamis et al., 1988). Specific supporting data include the following: Mutation of the AUG translation initiation codon at the α2-globin locus results in a higher morbidity than the same mutation at the α1-globin gene locus (Pirastu et al., 1984; Liebhaber et al., 1986; Paglietti et al., 1986; Moi et al., 1987; Ayala et al., 1996; Oner et al., 1997). Individuals with loss of a single gene by nondeletional inactivation of the α2 locus ($\alpha^T\alpha/\alpha\alpha$) can have hematologic parameters more in line with loss of two genes as occurs in α thalassemia trait (-α/-α) (Bianco et al., 1997). Nondeletion defects at the α2 locus in *trans* to a single gene deletion ($\alpha^T\alpha/-\alpha$) can result in HbH disease rather than the α thalassemia trait usually associated with loss of two α-globin genes (Merritt et al., 1997). Nondeletion mutations at the α2 locus in *trans* to a double deletion ($\alpha^T\alpha/-$ -) can result in HbH disease that is more severe than seen with the corresponding nondeletion mutations at the α1 locus ($\alpha\alpha^T/-$ -) (Curuk et al., 1993) or the deletion muta-

tion (-α/- -) (Pressley et al., 1980; Chan et al., 1985; Kattamis et al., 1988; Chan et al., 1997) Finally, homozygosity for a nondeletional mutation at the α2-globin locus ($\alpha^T\alpha/\alpha^T\alpha$), including the frequent Hb Constant Spring mutation (α^{CS}/α^{CS}), can result in HbH disease instead of the α thalassemia trait seen with (-α/-α) (Winichagoon et al., 1980; Pootrakul et al., 1981; Morle et al., 1985; Paglietti et al., 1986; Fucharoen et al., 1988).

This description of single gene defects predicts a rank order of severity (Fig. 16.1). Based on their contributions to α-globin gene expression, the native α2- and α1-globin genes can be assigned relative expression levels of 2.6 and 1.0 "units" of α-globin expression respectively. Thus, the normal cluster encodes 3.6 "units" of α globin. A nondeletion defect at the α2 locus would yield a net residual synthesis of 1.0 units (from the remaining α1 locus); loss of the α2 gene by the $-\alpha^{3.7}$ deletion would yield a residual 2.0 "units" (from the upregulated recombinant α1 locus), and nondeletional mutation of the α1 gene would yield a residual 2.6 "units." Therefore, the rank order of severity of single gene loss is nondeletion α2 mutation ($\alpha^T\alpha$)>-$\alpha^{3.7}$> nondeletion α1 mutation ($\alpha\alpha^T$).

A final category of nondeletion mutations that can result in loss of α-globin synthesis is that of missense mutations that lead to highly unstable globin chains. The first example in this category was the α2 globin chain mutant Hb Quong Sze (α125 leu→pro). (Liebhaber and Kan, 1983). Such mutant globins would be expected to be rapidly cleared from the cell with the net loss of protein expressed by the affected locus equivalent to that seen with other nondeletion mutations. If, however, the unstable mutant interferes in some way with functional hemoglobin tetramer assembly or combines with other globin chains and targets them for destabilization and destruction, they may manifest as "dominant" thalassemia mutations (Chapter 14). Production of unstable structural mutants can also increase the severity of the thalassemic phenotype by "exhausting" the proteolytic system and thus accentuating membrane toxicity caused by the unpaired globin chains (see later).

LOSS OF BOTH α-GLOBIN LOCI

The impact of large deletions (- -) encompassing both α-globin loci on α-globin gene expression is straightforward. Simple heterozygosity for the double deletion (- -/αα) results in α thalassemia trait clinically equivalent to homozygosity for the single gene deletion (-α/-α). There is no evidence for a compensatory increase in the expression of the remaining α-globin genes on the opposite chromosome. It is of interest, however, to note that several of the most common large mutations, and in particular the 20.5 kb Southeast Asia deletion (Ottolenghi et al., 1974; Taylor et al., 1974; Winchagoon et al., 1984) (see also Chapter 17), can derepress the adjacent ζ-globin gene (Randhawa et al., 1984; Chui et al., 1986; Tang et al., 1992; Ireland et al., 1993; Chui and Wayne, 1998). Mechanism(s) for this derepression of the linked ζ-globin gene are undefined.

MECHANISMS LEADING TO ANEMIA IN INDIVIDUALS WITH α THALASSEMIA

Several related components contribute to anemia in individuals with α thalassemia. As outlined previously and in Chapters 17 and 18, the primary abnormality is underproduction of α-globin chains. Important secondary effects occur because of the continued production of excess γ-globin chains in fetal life, which associate to form Hb Bart's, the γ_4 tetramer, and excess β-globin chains in adult life forming the β_4 tetramer, HbH. By mechanisms discussed later, these excess, unmatched non-α-globin chains damage the developing erythroid precursor, giving rise to intramedullary hemolysis or ineffective erythropoeisis. Also, the presence of Hb Bart's and HbH causes premature destruction of mature red cells, which gives rise to the predominant aspect of α thalassemia, intracorpuscular, extravascular hemolysis.

The effects of α-globin chain insufficiency have been most extensively studied in patients with the deletional form of HbH disease (- -/-α), HbH disease with Hb Constant Spring (- -/α^CS α) and homozygotes for Hb Constant Spring (Pootrakul et al., 1981). Each aspect of the pathophysiology is dealt with in the following discussion.

Many aspects of the pathophysiology of α thalassemia were described more than 40 years ago. Two groups of investigators virtually simultaneously described the syndrome of HbH disease (Rigas et al., 1956; Gouttas et al., 1955). Affected patients had a hypochromic microcytic anemia of variable severity, target cells on peripheral smear, reticulocytosis, and inclusions in a few erythrocytes, many more of which could be produced by incubating blood with mild oxidant dyes such as Brilliant Cresyl Blue (BCB). Red cells were resistant to hypotonic solutions in the osmotic fragility test and signs of hemolysis, including a short ^{51}Cr red cell survival, splenomegaly, and elevated indirect reacting bilirubin, were present. A key finding was an abnormal hemoglobin, accounting for up to 40 percent of the total hemoglobin which had more rapid electrophoretic mobility at pH 8.6 than HbA. When this hemoglobin, now called HbH, was allowed to

stand, it turned brown and precipitated forming aggregates that looked somewhat like the red cell inclusions. This conversion was accentuated by the addition of mild oxidants.

Subsequent studies (Dance et al., 1963) identified the disorder as a moderately severe form of α thalassemia, with the deletion or inactivation of 3 α-globin genes leading to a clinically significant unbalance in α-globin chain synthesis. The α/β synthesis ratio was 0.3 to 0.6 instead of 1.0 (Wood and Stamatoyannopoulos, 1976), and the defect in synthesis of α-globin chains led to an accumulation of otherwise normal β-globin chains in adults and γ-globin chains in the fetus. Instead of forming normal α:β dimers, which then tetramerize, excessive β-globin chains assemble into HbH tetramers (Gabuzda, 1966; Nathan and Gunn, 1966). In the neonatal period, before β-globin chain synthesis reaches adult levels, excess unmatched γ-globin chains accumulate and form the γ_4 tetramers of Hb Bart's (Lehmann, 1970). These homotetramers are susceptible to oxidant injury (Rigas and Koler, 1961; Gabuzda, 1966) and are functionally useless as oxygen delivery pigments because their affinity for oxygen is at least ten times greater than HbA, they demonstrate no Bohr effect, and the oxyhemoglobin dissociation curve is not sigmoidal, as there is no heme-heme interaction. In fact, the curve resembles that of myoglobin, a compound that holds but cannot deliver oxygen (Benesch and Benesch, 1964).

A critical factor underlying the pathophysiologic differences between α and β thalassemia is that in the α thalassemias, the excess β- or γ-globin chains can form partially soluble but physiologically ineffective hemoglobin homotetramers that do not precipitate extensively until they are exposed to damaging effects—mostly oxidant in nature—in the circulation. In contrast, in the β thalassemias, the excess unmatched α-globin chains that accumulate cannot form soluble tetramers, but produce insoluble aggregates of α-chain monomers even in very early marrow erythroid precursors. These aggregates affect membrane assembly and accelerate programmed cell death (Chapter 11).

HEMOLYSIS IN α THALASSEMIA

Hemolysis is the major cause of anemia in patients with α thalassemia. ^{51}Cr-labeled α thalassemic red cells have a short half-life in the circulation (Rigas et al., 1956; Rigas and Koler, 1961; Pearson and McFarland, 1962; Gabuzda et al., 1965; Nathan and Gunn, 1966). [51]Cr red cell survival in patients with HbH disease was 12 to 19 days (normal, > 26 days) (Rigas and Koler, 1961; Pearson and McFarland,

1962; Malamos et al., 1962). HbH bound more ^{51}Cr than did HbA and had a higher fractional turnover, which impaired the reliability of ^{51}Cr red cell labeling (Pearson and McFarland, 1962; Gabuzda et al., 1965). However careful studies using glycine-2-^{14}C incorporation into hemoglobin showed that in HbH disease, red cell survival was one-third normal (Gabuzda et al., 1965). External counting revealed splenic sequestration (Malamos et al., 1962). Other signs of uncompensated hemolysis were present. Patients with HbH disease are mildly jaundiced with indirect reacting hyperbilirubinemia, reticulocytosis of 2.5 to 16 percent (Malamos et al., 1962), and usually palpable splenomegaly. An intracorpuscular abnormality causes inadequate synthesis of normal α-globin chains, leading to extravascular erythrocyte destruction by macrophages of the reticuloendothelial system.

Marrow erythroid hyperplasia and reticulocytosis are the response to hemolysis (Gouttas et al., 1955; Rigas et al., 1956). Serum erythropoietin levels are increased as are levels of soluble transferrin receptor (sTfR), an indicator of erythroid activity (Papassotiriou et al., 1998; Rees et al., 1998). These increases are directly related to the HbH concentration, which in turn reflects the globin chain imbalance (Papassotiriou et al., 1998).

These original observations raise two important questions. First, how does decreased α-globin chain synthesis produce abnormalities of the affected erythrocytes that are recognized in the microvasculature and reticuloendothelial organs leading to removal of these cells? Second, why are patients with HbH disease anemic, since a rate of hemolysis three times normal falls easily within the ability of normal bone marrow to increase red blood cell (RBC) production fivefold to sevenfold? Ferrokinetic studies show an increase in erythropoiesis up to six times normal (Malamos et al., 1962) in some but not all patients with HbH disease. More recent data addressing factors contributing to hemolysis are considered next.

RBC Shape

Unbalanced globin chain synthesis leads to a deficiency in the amount of hemoglobin per cell (low mean cell hemoglobin, MCH), and because hemoglobin accounts for 30 to 35 percent of the red cell content, mean cell volume (MCV) is low, producing the hypochromic target cells and microcytosis. However, in addition to these well-characterized morphologic findings, there are frequently fragmented or bizarrely shaped erythrocytes.

Sophisticated modern technology such as the Technicon Bayer H* Analyzer (Chapter 34) has

allowed more precise identification of erythrocyte indices. MCH tracings show that as a consequence of time in the circulation, there is red cell fragmentation (Fig. 16.2) in HbH disease and HbH/Hb[CS] disease, producing populations of tiny hemoglobin-containing fragments. These fragments likely have short survival time. Cell fragments with much decreased surface area volume ratio have great difficulty undergoing the elongated elliptical deformation that normally allows 8 μm diameter red cells to pass through 3μm diameter capillaries and 2 μm slits in reticuloendothelial sinusoids (see Chapters 21 and 22).

Several studies noted that while both α- and β-thalassemic erythrocytes had decreased MCH and MCV, the decrease in mean cell hemoglobin concentration (MCHC) was greater in the α thalassemias with α[CS], observations that led to studies on red cell hydration (Gabuzda et al., 1965).

RBC Hydration

One approach to assessing the extent of erythrocyte hydration is by examining the density of peripheral blood on density gradients. In patients with severe α thalassemia, all erythrocytes, not only the reticulocytes and young red cells, are uniformly light and are found at the top of a discontinuous Stractan gradient (see Fig. 10.9) and are therefore hyperhydrated (Schrier et al., 1989). This contrasts with erythrocytes of comparably anemic patients with β thalassemia where a few of the younger red cells are light, but other erythrocytes found throughout the gradient may be as dense and dehydrated as those in sickle cell anemia with an MCHC >45 (Schrier et al., 1989) (Chapter 22).

Using the Technicon Bayer H*3 Analyzer, a quantitative assessment of erythrocyte hydration is possible. About 50 percent of red cells from patients with HbH disease have MCHC levels <28 (they are definitely hypochromic) whereas 70 percent of patients with HbH/Hb[CS] and 20 percent of patients with homozygous Hb[CS] have hypochromia of this degree (Bunyaratvej et al., 1983; Bunyaratvej et al., 1992) (Chapter 18). Reticulocytes, as they left the marrow (see colored area in Fig. 16.2), were already well hydrated, with an increased MCV and decreased MCHC.

Why the α thalassemia red cell is hyperhydrated is not clear. The K-Cl co-transporter is a pH- and volume-activated transporter that functions in the normal remodeling of reticulocytes to mature red cells where it controls the loss of K-Cl and water, leading to a reduction in the MCV (see Chapters 11 and 22). This transporter closes down in normal red cells but stays open in β thalassemia and sickle erythrocytes, where it is

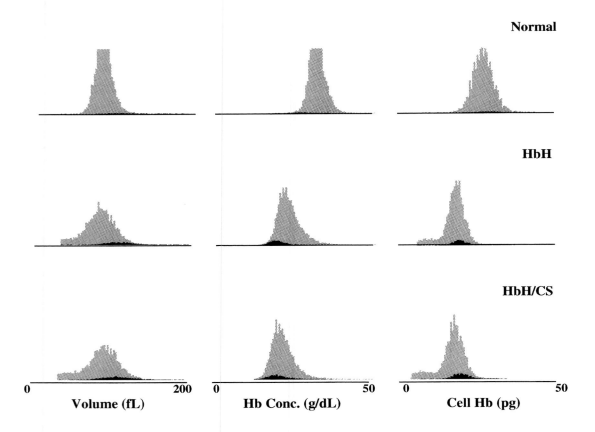

Figure 16.2. Technicon analyses of HbH and HbH/Hb^CS. Technicon-Bayer H* analyses of red cells from a normal subject (top row) a patient with HbH disease (middle row), and a patient with HbH/Hb^CS (bottom row). The dark tracing represents the overall red cell population and the colored area at the bottom of the tracing identifies the reticulocytes. Note the "tail" in the plots of hemoglobin content for the two patients, identifying a population of hemoglobin-containing red cell fragments. (*Blood*, 89, 1762, 1997, Figure 2 p. 1765, with permission)

partly responsible for the cell dehydration (see Chapters 11, 20, and 22). It is an unproven hypothesis that in α thalassemia, the K-Cl co-transporter closes down early, preventing the usual loss of K-Cl and water that is part of the remodeling process.

ROLE OF THE SPLEEN AND MACROPHAGES IN RBC REMOVAL

In the final common pathway of extravascular destruction, abnormalities of red cell deformability (Chapter 22) slow the passage of affected cells in the microvasculature. Macrophages in the reticuloendothelial organs scrutinize these cells and detect any cell surface signals that could alert the macrophages to retard, bind, and engulf the defective erythrocyte. Cellular abnormalities that could

contribute to splenic and macrophagic phagocytosis are discussed next.

Red Cell Deformability

Normally 8-μm diameter erythrocytes must undergo a remarkable elliptical elongation to allow passage through 3-μm diameter capillaries and even smaller slits in the sinusoids of the reticuloendothelial system. Any increase in rigidity will hold up passage through the microvascular bed and delay transit through reticuloendothelial system organs (see Chapters 20 through 22). Deformability measurements made by osmotic gradient ektacytometry (Schrier et al., 1989) showed that HbH erythrocytes were very rigid. This was a surprise because there are three major factors that control red cell deformability: the ratio of surface area/volume, MCHC, and membrane features (Chapter 22). Older measurements of osmotic fragility, which are in fact an index of surface area volume, showed distinct resistance to osmotic lysis (Rigas et al. 1956), thereby indicating that the surface area/volume was increased. The MCHC (reflecting cell hydration) is very low in HbH disease, indicating that intracellular viscosity resulting from elevated hemoglobin concentrations would not contribute to reduced red cell deformability (Schrier et al., 1989). Thus two of the three factors that determine red cell deformability (surface area volume and

MCHC) would be expected to increase cell deformability as they themselves increase. In fact, the opposite occurs. Increased red cell rigidity was even more apparent when populations of defined MCHC were compared in normal and HbH cells. The ektacytometric curves suggest an unexplained interaction of the normal HbA present in HbH erythrocytes with the cytosolic face of the membrane producing extreme rigidity (Schrier et al., 1989). Erythrocytes in HbH/HbCS are even more rigid than in gene deletion HbH disease (Bunyaratvej et al., 1983) and are most rigid in homozygous Hb Constant Spring cells (Schrier et al., 1997). Extreme rigidity could lead to the observed red cell fragmentation in parts of the vasculature where there is elevated shear stress. Rigid fragments are subjected to rapid removal, as rigidity impairs passage through the sinusoids of the reticuloendothelial system.

Red Cell Membrane Deformability and Stability

Isolated red cell membranes from patients with HbH disease were studied because analysis of the extreme rigidity of intact cells indicated that the abnormal membrane was likely to contribute to this defect. Isolated membranes from patients with HbH disease were 2.2 to 3 times more rigid than normal (Schrier et al., 1989, 1997). Membranes from patients with HbH/HbCS were even more rigid, and the least deformable membranes came from patients with homozygous Hb Constant Spring (Schrier et al., 1997). These measurements confirmed that a membrane abnormality contributed to the erythrocyte rigidity.

Membrane stability describes the ability of isolated erythrocyte membranes to resist fragmentation under the impetus of an intense elliptically deforming shear stress (Schrier et al., 1989) (Chapter 21). Membrane stability is generally thought to be a function of the membrane skeleton, and the interaction of the skeleton with the major transmembrane protein, band 3 HbH membranes, were more stable than normal (Schrier et al., 1989). Membranes are even more stable in HbH/HbCS and maximally stable in HbCS/HbCS (Schrier et al., 1997). This contrasts with the findings in β thalassemia membranes, which are unstable (Chapter 11). Erythrocyte and perhaps membrane rigidity are likely to flow slowly in the vasculature of the reticuloendothelial organs, giving macrophages ample opportunity to look for engulfment signals, which include bound IgG and complement components or altered membrane phospholipid bilayer asymmetry.

Red Cell Inclusions

HbH disease inclusions occurred spontaneously in some RBC, were more common in splenectomized subjects, and could be induced by incubating red cells with mild oxidants such as Brilliant Cresyl Blue (BCB) or new methylene blue (Gouttas et al., 1955; Rigas et al., 1956; Rigas and Koler 1961; Bunyaratvej et al., 1983). Inclusion-rich red cells can be found in the spleen after splenectomy (Rigas and Koler, 1961), explaining the increase of inclusion-containing cells in HbH patients after splenectomy. When red cells from patients with HbH disease were separated by density into young, middle-aged, and old cells, the level of soluble HbH was highest in young cells where the number of inclusion-containing cells was lowest. As the cells aged and became denser, the level of soluble HbH decreased, and the proportion of inclusions increased. This led to the interpretation that after about 45 days of in vivo aging, HbH began to precipitate, forming inclusions that damaged the cell and led to at least partial removal in the spleen (Rigas and Koler, 1961). By electron microscopy, inclusions are seen in 67 ± 8.7 percent of deletion HbH erythrocytes and in 81 ± 8.7 percent of HbH/HbCS cells (Bunyaratvej et al., 1983). Cytosolic levels of HbH are different in these two variants of HbH disease, with the deletion type red cells having mean levels of 9.3 percent HbH and 15.3 percent HbH/HbCS cells, levels directly proportional to the number of inclusions (Winichagoon et al., 1980). This may account for the increase in hematological severity observed in patients with HbH/HbCS (see previously).

Proof that red cell inclusions in HbH disease consisted of β-globin chain tetramers was obtained by combining electron microscopy with monoclonal antibodies against β globin (Wickramasinghe et al., 1996). Membrane-bound inclusions interfere with the ability of the cell to undergo the requisite tank treading motion down the microvasculature and contribute to slowing of their passage (Chapter 21). As these aggregates contain heme, it is likely that they will enhance local oxidative damage. Because this heme has already been converted to hemichromes, it remains attached to the β_4 tetramer and has already undergone oxidative alteration (Rachmilewitz et al., 1969).

Lipid Signaling

How does the α-globin chain synthetic defect lead to erythrocyte membrane alterations that are recognized by macrophages? One hypothesis is that the denatured HbH inclusions adjacent to the membrane cause damage by oxidant mechanisms, which alters the normal pattern of phospholipid bilayer asymmetry (Chapter 22). Macrophages recognize surface phosphatidylserine (PS) translocated to the outer membrane leaflet of the phospholipid bilayer of erythrocytes fated for removal. It is possible to determine the number of red cells that have PS exposure using the label Annexin V complexed to fluorescein isothiocyanate (FITC). Deletion HbH disease, Hb Constant Spring homozygotes, and HbH/HbCS have a progressive increase in the number of red cells with translocated PS (Table 16.1), although the absolute number of such cells is small (Kuypers et al., 1998). However, one can imagine that the number of PS-exposing cells is low because they are effectively removed by the macrophages in the spleen and other reticuloendothelial organs.

Membrane Immunoglobulin G (IgG) and Complement Components

Macrophages target red cells with IgG on the outer surface for removal by identifying the Fc domains of IgG. Increases in membrane IgG and complement components are a likely cause of the increased phagocytosis seen in α thalassemia (Chinprasertsuk et al., 1997) (Chapters 11 and 20). Nonsplenectomized patients with deletion HbH disease have erythrocyte IgG levels that are normal; however, after splenectomy the IgG levels are increased. HbH/HbCS cells, even from nonsplenectomized subjects, have more membrane-associated IgG than either normal or deletion HbH disease cells (Wiener et al., 1991; Chinprasertsuk et al., 1997). This finding is consistent with the splenic sequestration of ^{51}Cr-labeled red cells (see previously) and would support the idea that splenic macrophages are active in removing HbH disease cells that have increased levels of surface IgG. Splenectomy permits these erythrocyte to remain in the circulation.

Table 16.1. Phosphatidal Serine Exposure in Normal and Thalassemic Red Cells

Mutation	AV binding (%)	± SD	n
Normal control	0.26	0.20	42
HbH	0.53	0.60	17
HbH/HbCS	1.00	1.66	16
HbH/HbCS splenectomized	1.11	–	1
HbCS/HbCS	0.85	0.61	5
HbE-β thalassemia	0.45	0.37	10
HbE-β thalassemia splenectomized	9.5	7.5	4
β thalassemia intermedia	0.07	–	1
β thalassemia intermedia splenectomized	3.4	3.7	2
All thalassemic cells	1.42	1.01	56

From Kuypers et al., 1998, with permission.

Role of Macrophages

Serum macrophage colony-stimulating factor (M-CSF) levels are elevated in HbH disease and correlate inversely with the patient's hemoglobin levels. It is proposed that such raised M-CSF levels enhance the extent of macrophage attack on HbH cells and contribute to the severity of the anemia (Wiener et al., 1996).

BIOCHEMICAL/CELLULAR OBSERVATIONS THAT UNDERLIE THE ALTERATIONS LEADING TO HEMOLYSIS

A challenge remains to discover how an impairment in synthesis of α-globin chains leads to the cellular alterations that result in hemolysis. Several biochemical studies provide a partial explanation.

Membrane Skeletal-Bound β Globin

In HbH disease, there is a prominent globin band on sodium dodecyl sulfate-polyacrylamide gel electrophoresis (SDS-PAGE) of red cell membranes (Fig. 16.3) (Advani et al., 1992). A variable amount of this globin consists of HbA, probably in the form of αβ dimers. However, when one isolates membrane skeletons (Chapter 22), only β globin is present, likely the excess unmatched β-globin chains, now firmly attached to the membrane skeleton, a mirror image of the finding in severe β thalassemia (Advani et al., 1992) (Fig. 16.4). Thiol disulfide exchange chromatography revealed that this skeletal bound β globin was depleted of thiols and thus had become partially oxidized (Advani et al., 1992). It was hypothesized that skeletal bound, partially oxidized β globin accounted for much of the observed membrane pathophysiology in α thalassemia. Damage produced by the accumulation of β-globin chains may be reduced by proteases which directly attack and occasionally destroy excess β-globin chains (Sancar et al., 1981).

Hb Constant Spring variants provided opportunity for further exploring the pathophysiology of the α thalassemias. As noted previously, HbH/HbCS usually produces a more severe anemia than deletional forms of HbH disease, and there are very few kinetic studies to indicate whether there is more hemolysis, more ineffective erythropoeisis, or less red cell production to account for the difference. However, cellular studies have shown (Pootrakul et al., 1981, Bunyaratvej et al., 1994) that these red cells are hyperhydrated and have more inclusions. Furthermore, they are poorly deformable, and their membranes are very rigid and hyperstable (Schrier et al., 1997). Biochemically these changes represent

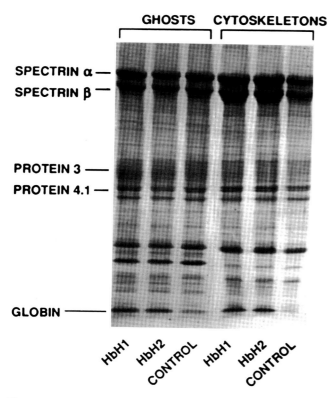

Figure 16.3. Polyacrylamide gel (SDS-PAGE) analysis of red cell membranes (ghosts) and membrane skeletons from a normal subject and two patients with HbH disease. The skeletons are prepared by extracting intact ghosts with Triton, leaving skeletons consisting primarily of spectrin, actin, and band 4.1. Note that in the two HbH samples there are dense bands in the globin position in both the ghosts and skeletons. (*Blood,* 79, 1058, 1992, Figure 2, p. 1060, with permission.)

the presence on the red cell membrane skeleton of partially oxidized α^{CS} chains, in addition to the partially oxidized β globin. In Hb^{CS}/Hb^{CS} there are deposits of partially oxidized β globin and α^{CS} chains on the membrane skeleton. It is likely that their combined presence accounts for the differences in cellular pathophysiology (Schrier et al., 1997).

Oxidant Injury

Membrane skeletal-associated globin with attached hemes, hemichromes (Rachmilewitz et al., 1969), and iron causes local oxidant damage to the membrane. The earliest reports of HbH disease noted the presence of inclusions whose numbers could be increased by incubation with mild oxidants such as methylene blue and BCB (Gouttas et al., 1955; Rigas, 1956). Erythrocytes of patients with HbH disease can undergo further hemolysis when exposed in vivo to oxidant drugs such as the sulfonamides (Rigas and Koler, 1961).

In experiments designed to model oxidant damage, normal erythrocytes were incubated with phenylhydrazine and methylhydrazine (Chapter 11).

Figure 16.4. The globin composition of red cell membranes (ghosts) and membrane skeletons analyzed by Triton-acid-urea-gel electrophoresis, which resolves hemoglobins into the component globin chains. Note that in the HbH ghosts there were mixtures of α and β globin, but in the skeletons there were only β-globin chains. (*Blood,* 79, 1058 1992, Figure 3, p. 1060, with permission.)

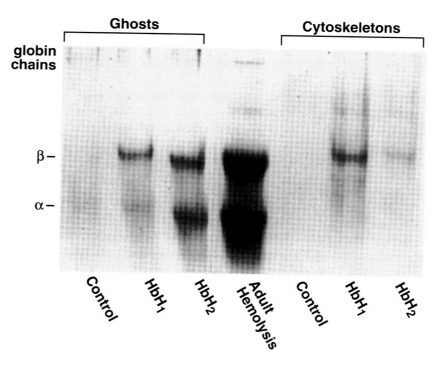

Phenylhydrazine induced the binding of oxidized α-globin chains to the membrane skeleton, and the resulting membranes were unstable as measured in the ektacytometer, findings seen in the erythrocytes of severe β thalassemia (Chapter 10). Conversely, methylhydrazine induced the binding of oxidized β globin to the membrane skeleton, and the membranes were hyperstable, exactly as in severe α thalassemia. These experiments supported the distinct pathophysiologic roles of excess, oxidized globin chains (Schrier and Mohandas, 1992). When isolated and purified α- and β-globin chains were resealed within normal erythrocytes, similar changes occurred, supporting the hypothesis that the specific oxidized excess globin chains are responsible for the cellular pathophysiology (Scott et al., 1992).

Hexosemonophosphate shunt activity was decreased in young red cells of HbH disease (Nathan et al., 1969). This metabolic pathway controls the return of oxidized glutathione to the reduced form and the generation of the reducing agent NADPH. Furthermore, superoxide dismutase, GSH peroxidase, and catalase were increased in HbH disease cells and superoxide dismutase and GSH peroxidase activities were further increased in HbH/Hb^{CS} (Prasartkaew et al., 1986). Curiously, catalase activity, rather than altering in concert with the other two antioxidant enzymes, increased more in HbH than in Hb H/Hb^{CS} (Prasartkaew et al., 1986). Together, these measurements suggest that the α thalassemia erythrocyte is under oxidant stress and that the antioxidant systems are, perhaps, struggling to control the damage.

Other Evidence of RBC Membrane Damage

Several studies have sought to further explain membrane damage in α thalassemia. Spectrin binding to inside-out membrane vesicles prepared from HbH disease erythrocytes is reduced by half (Shinar et al., 1989). This effect could be reproduced by adding heme-containing β-globin chains to normal red cell membranes (Shalev et al., 1996). This observation is consistent with the study showing that the assembly of the membrane skeleton in α thalassemia is probably defective. Free spectrin, actin, and band-4.1 are present in the supernatant wash medium in the course of preparing of α thalassemia red cell membranes by stepwise hypotonic lysis (Yuan et al., 1995). These findings suggest that the membrane skeleton in α thalassemia is deficient or defective and thus likely to be unstable. In fact, the converse occurs; α-thalassemia membranes are hyperstable as discussed previously (Schrier et al., 1989). Therefore, the pathophysiologic interpretation of these results remains elusive.

INEFFECTIVE ERYTHROPOIESIS IN α THALASSEMIA

Ferrokinetics

Ferrokinetic studies in HbH disease showed that ^{59}Fe red cell utilization at 14 days was 62 percent, with a normal rate of more than 85 percent (Pearson and McFarland, 1962). Another study (Malamos et al., 1962) of six patients with HbH disease showed that whereas erythropoiesis was increased up to six times normal, red cell ^{59}Fe utilization varied from 53 to 70 percent, with a mean of 62.6 percent. This rate signifies moderate to mild ineffective erythropoeisis, explaining in part the inability of apparently increased marrow erythropoiesis to compensate for the modest degree of hemolysis. Comparable ferrokinetic data on HbH/^{CS} and Hb^{CS}/Hb^{CS} are not yet available.

Soluble Transferrin Receptor

Two groups studying soluble transferrin receptor levels and also erythropoietin and reticulocyte levels proposed that the discrepancy between the level of reticulocytes and soluble transferrin receptor indicates a degree of ineffective erythropoeisis (Rees et al., 1998; Papassoptiriou et al., 1998).

Morphologic Data

Although most descriptions of HbH inclusions indicate that they occur primarily in circulating red cells as they age (Rigas and Koler, 1961), there is evidence that the excess β-globin chains begin to accumulate and precipitate in marrow erythroid precursors (Fessas and Yataghavas, 1968; Wickramasinghe et al., 1984). Such deposition of insoluble β globin could provide the basis for oxidant or other sorts of cellular injury, leading to intramedullary erythroid precursor death.

Apoptosis (Programmed Cell Death)

If ineffective erythropoiesis can be correlated with marrow erythroblast apoptosis, as has been reported for severe β thalassemia (Chapter 11), then there should be increased apoptosis in severe α thalassemia. Preliminary studies showed that in marrow erythroid precursors from patients with HbH disease, the extent of apoptosis is approximately twice normal (Pootrakul, 1997). This finding is in sharp contrast to the five times normal apoptosis rate in the same cells seen in severe forms of β thalassemia, but is consistent with the much more severe degree of ineffective erythropoiesis in β thalassemia (Pootrakul, 1997) (Chapter 11). A consequence and hallmark of apoptosis is the movement of PS from the inner to the outer leaflet of the membrane bilayer. As discussed, macrophages recognize cells bearing PS on their outer surface, perhaps via the CD36 receptor, and remove such cells efficiently as part of the apoptotic process (Chapter 11).

Other Mechanisms Causing Ineffective Erythropoiesis

An additional mechanism for the enhanced removal of α thalassemia erythroid precursors from the marrow may be their excessive surface IgG (Wiener et al., 1991). In HbH disease these marked cells may be attacked and removed by marrow macrophages with Fc receptors.

PATHOPHYSIOLOGY OF THE Hb BART'S HYDROPS FETALIS SYNDROME

Hb Bart's hydrops fetalis is the most severe form of α thalassemia, and α-globin chains are not produced (Chapter 18). Because α-globin chains are normally made throughout fetal life, no functional hemoglobins can be synthesized in affected fetuses. Tetramers of γ-globin chains accumulate and form Hb Bart's, but this homotetramer binds oxygen with high affinity and cannot release it to tissues. Unlike HbH, Hb Bart's has little propensity to precipitate and form inclusions (Chui and Wayne, 1998). If the molecular defect causing α thalassemia allows the fetus to synthesize ζ-globin chains, this embryonic α-like globin can form functional Hb Portland (ζ2γ2), which allows in utero survival until the third trimester (Chapter 18). Hydropic fetuses are profoundly anemic, even though the measured hemoglobin level may be as high as 10 g/dL owing to the presence of Hb Bart's and embryonic hemoglobins. Their erythrocytes are hypochromic and microcytic, and erythropoiesis is vastly expanded to compensate for the tissue hypoxia. Extramedullary erythropoiesis is found in liver and spleen, and nucleated red cells circulate. Severe anemia causes congestive heart failure with anasarca and capillary leak—the "hydrops" of hydrops fetalis. Presumably, the anemia during early development and organogenesis causes many other congenital defects, including a massively enlarged placenta. For reasons still unclear, there are severe maternal complications, including hypertension and polyhydramnios. The clinical and hematologic features of Hb Bart's hydrops fetalis syndrome are described in detail in Chapter 18.

CONCLUSIONS

The pathophysiology of the α-thalassemia syndromes is directly related to the accumulation of excess unmatched β-globin chains. When these non-α-globin chains accumulate in the erythrocyte, as in

HbH disease, under the impetus of oxidant injury they precipitate, forming inclusions that damage the red cell membrane and lead to abnormal shapes, red cell rigidity, and fragmentation. These cells have difficulty traversing the microvasculature, particularly of reticuloendothelial organs such as the spleen. Further injury alters membrane phospholipid bilayer asymmetry and leads to membrane deposition of IgG and complement components. These provide signals for macrophages to remove affected cells from the circulation. Accumulation and deposition of excess β-globin chains also occur during marrow erythropoiesis. Kinetic data, supported by measurements of increased erythroid apoptosis, indicate that some increase in ineffective erythropoiesis occurs in HbH disease.

References

Adirojnanon, P and Wasi, P. (1980). Levels of haemoglobin H and proportions of red cells with inclusion bodies in two types of haemoglobin H disease. *Br. J. Haematol.* 46: 507–509.

Advani, R, Sorenson, S, Shinar, E et al. (1992). Characterization and comparison of the red blood cell membrane damage in severe human α and β thalassemia. *Blood* 79: 1058–1063.

Albitar, M, Peschle, C, and Liebhaber, SA. (1989). Theta, zeta, and epsilon globin messenger RNAs are expressed in adults. *Blood* 74: 629–637.

Albitar, M, Peschle, C, and Liebhaber, SA. (1992a). Developmental switch in the relative expression of the α1- and α2-globin genes in humans and in transgenic mice. *Blood* 79: 2471–2474.

Albitar, M, Care, A, Peschle, C, and Liebhaber, SA. (1992b). Developmental switching of mRNA expression from the human α-globin cluster: Fetal/adult pattern of (α-globin gene expression. *Blood* 80: 1586–1591.

Ayala, S, Colomer, D, Aymerich, M et al. (1996). Nondeletional α-thalassemia: First description of α^{Hph}α and α^{Nco}α mutations in a Spanish population. *Amer. J. Hematol.* 52: 144–149.

Beaudry, MA, Ferguson, DJ, Pearse, K et al. (1986). Survival of a hydropic infant with homozygous α-thalassemia-1. *J. Pediatr.* 108: 713–716.

Benesch, R and Benesch, RE. (1964). Properties of haemoglobin H and their significance in relation to function of haemoglobin. *Nature* 202: 773–775.

Bianco, I, Cappabianca, MP, Foglietta, E et al. (1997). Silent thalassemias: Genotypes and phenotypes. *Haematologica* 82: 269–280.

Bunyaratvej, A, Sahaphong, S, Bhamarapravati, N, and Wasi, P. (1983). Different patterns of intraerythrocytic inclusion body distribution in the two types of haemoglobin H disease. *Acta Haematol.* 69: 314–318.

Bunyaratvej, A, Butthep, P, Fucharoen, S, and Saw, D. (1992). Erythrocyte volume and haemoglobin concentration in haemoglobin H disease: Discrimination between the two genotypes. *Acta Haematol* 87: 1–5.

Chan, V, Chan, TK, Liang, ST et al. (1985). Hydrops Fetails due to an unusual form of Hb H Disease. *Blood* 66: 224–228.

Chan, V, Chan, VW-Y, Tang, M et al. (1997). Molecular defects in HbH hydrops fetalis. *Br. J. Haematol.* 96: 224–228.

Chinprasertsuk, S, Wanachiwanawin, W, Pattanapanyasat, K et al. (1997). Relation of haemolytic anaemia and erythrocyte-bound IgG in α- and β-thalassemic syndromes. *Eur. J. Haematol.* 58: 86–91.

Chui, DH, Wong, SC, Chung, S-W et al. (1986). Embryonic ζ-globin chains in adults: A marker for α-thalassemia-1 haplotype due to a >17.5 kb deletion. *N. Engl. J. Med.* 314: 76–79.

Chui, DH and Wayne, JS. (1998). Hydrops fetalis caused by α-Thalassemia: An emerging health care problem. *Blood* 91: 2213–2222.

Clegg, JB, Weatherall, DJ, and Milner, PF. (1971). Constant Spring—an α-chain termination mutant? *Nature* 234: 337–371.

Curuk, MA, Dimovski, AJ, Baysal, E et al. (1993). Hb Adana or α2[59Gly]β2, a severely unstable α1-globin variant, observed in combination with the (α) 20.5 kb α-thal-1 deletion in two Turkish patients. *Am. J. Hematolo.* 44: 270–275.

Dance, N, Huehns, ER, and Beaven, GH. (1963). The abnormal haemoglobins in haemoglobin-H disease. *Biochem. J.* 87: 240–248.

Deisseroth, A, Neinhuis, A, Turner, P et al. (1977). Localization of the human α-globin structural gene chromosome 16 in somatic cell hybrids by molecular hybridization assay. *Cell* 12: 205–218.

Embury, SH, Miller, JA, Dozy, AM et al. (1980). Two different molecular organizations account for the single α-globin gene of the α-thalassemia-2 genotype. *J. Clin. Invest.* 66: 1319–1325.

Fessas, P and Yataghanas, X. (1968). Intraerythroblastic instability of Hemoglobin B (HgbH). *Blood* 31: 323–331.

Fischel-Ghodsian, N, Nocholls, RD, and Higgs, DR. (1987). Long range genome structure around the human α-globin complex analyzed by PFGE. *Nucl. Acids. Res.* 15: 6197–6207.

Fucharoen, S, Thongliruam, V, and Winichagoon, P. (1988). Hematologic changes in α-thalassemia. *Am. J. Clin. Pathol.* 89: 193–196.

Gabuzda, TG, Nathan DG, and Gardner, FH. (1965). The metabolism of the individual C[14]-labeled hemoglobins in patients with HbH-thalassemia, with observations on radiochromate binding to the hemoglobins during red cell survival. *J. Clin Invest.* 44: 315–325.

Gabuzda, TG. (1966). Hemoglobin H and the red cell. *Blood* 27: 568–579.

Gouttas, A, Fessas, PH, Tsevrenis, H, and Xefteri, ME. (1955). Description diune nouvelle variète dianèmie hèmolytique congènitale. *Sang* 26: 911–915.

Huehns, ER and Beaven, GH. (1971). Developmental changes in human hemoglobins. *Clin. Dev. Med.* 37: 175.

Higgs, DR, Hill, AVS, Bowden, DK et al. (1984). Independent recombination events between the duplicated human α-globin genes: Implications for their concerted evolution. *Nucl. Acids Res.* 12: 6965–6977.

Higg, DR, Vickers, MA, Wilkie, AOM et al. (1989). A review of the molecular genetics of the human α-globin gene cluster. *Blood* 73: 1081–1104.

Hunt, DM, Higg, DR, Winichagoon, P et al. (1982). Haemoglobin Constant Spring has an unstable chain messenger RNA. *Br. J. Haematol.* 51: 405–413.

Ireland, JH, Luo, HY, Chui, DH et al. (1993). Detection of the (—SEA) double α-globin gene deletion by a simple immunologic assay for embryonic zeta-globin chains. *Am. J. Hematol.* 44: 22–28.

Kattamis, C, Tzotzos, S, Kanavakis, E et al. (1988). Correlation of clinical phenotype to genotype in haemoglobin H disease. *Lancet* 1: 442–444.

Kropp, GL, Fucharoen, S, and Embury, SH. (1989). Selective enzymatic amplification of α2-globin DNA for detection of the hemoglobin Constant Spring mutation. *Blood* 15: 1987–1992.

Kuypers, FA, Yuan, J, Lewis, RA et al. (1998). Membrane phospholipid asymmetry in human thalassemia. *Blood* 91: 3044–3051.

Leder, A, Daugherty, C, Whitney, B and Leder P. (1997). Mouse zeta- and alpha-globin genes: Embryonic survival, alpha-thalassemia, and genetic background effects. *Blood* 90: 1275–1282.

Lehmann, H. (1970). Different types of alpha-thalassemia and significance of haemoglobin Bartis in neonates. *Lancet* 11: 78.

Liebhaber, SA, Goosens, M, and Kan, YW. (1980). Cloning and complete nucleotide sequence of human 5′ alpha-globin gene. *Proc. Natl. Acad. Sci. U.S.A.* 77: 7054–7058.

Liebhaber, SA, Goossens, M, and Kan, YW. (1981). Homology and concerted evolution at the alpha1- and alpha2 loci of human alpha-globin. *Nature* 290: 26–29.

Liebhaber, SA and Kan, YW. (1981). Differentiation of the mRNA transcripts origination from alpha1- and alpha2-globin loci in normals and alpha-thalassemics. *J. Clin. Invest.* 68: 439–446.

Liebhaber, SA and Kan, YW. (1983). Alpha-thalassemia caused by an unstable α-globin mutant. *J. Clin Invest.* 71: 461–466.

Liebhaber, SA, Cash, FE, and Main, D. (1985). Compensatory increase in alpha-1 globin gene expression in individuals heterozygous for the alpha-thalassemia-2 deletion. *J. Clin Invest.* 76: 1057–1064.

Liebhaber, SA, Cash, FE, and Ballas, SK. (1986). Human α-globin gene expression: The dominant role of the α2-locus in mRNA and protein synthesis. *J. Biol. Chem.* 261: 15327–15333.

Liebhaber, SA. (1989). α-Thalassemia: A review. *Hemoglobin* 13: 685–731.

Liebhaber, SA, Griese, EU, Weiss, I et al. (1990). Inactivation of human α-globin gene expression by a de novo deletion located upstream of the α-globin gene cluster. *Proc. Natl. Acad. Sci. U.S.A.* 87: 9431–9435.

Liebhaber, SA, Wang, Z, Cash, F et al. (1996). Developmental silencing of the embryonic zeta-globin gene: Synergistic action of promoter and 3′ flanking region combined with stage-specific silencing by the transcribed segment. *Mol. Cell. Biol.* 6: 2637–2646.

Malamos, B, Gyftaki, E, Binopoulos, D, and Kesse, M. (1962). Studies of haemoglobin synthesis and red cell survival in haemoglobinopathy H. *Acta Haematol.* 28: 124.

Merritt, D, Jones, RT, Head, C et al. (1997). Hb Seal Rock [(alpha 2)142 term→Glu, codon 142 TAA→GAA]: An extended alpha chain variant associated with anemia, microcytosis, and alpha-thalassemia-2 (– 3.7 Kb). *Hemoglobin* 21: 331–344.

Michelson, AM and Orkin, SH. (1980). The 3′ untranslated regions of the duplicated human alpha-globin genes are unexpectedly divergent. *Cell* 22: 371–377.

Michelson, AM and Orkin, SH. (1983). Boundaries of gene conversion within the duplicated human α-globin genes. *J. Biol. Chem.* 258: 15245–15254.

Moi, P, Cash, FE, Liebhaber, SA et al. (1987). An initiation codon mutation (AUG→GUG) of the human α1-globin gene: Structural characterization and evidence for a mild thalassemic phenotype. *J. Clin. Invest.* 80: 1416–1421.

Molchanova, TP and Huisman, THJ. (1996). The importance of the 3′ untranslated region for the expression of the α-globin genes. *Hemoglobin* 20: 41–54.

Morle, F, Lopez, B, Henni, T, and Godet, J. (1985). α-Thalassemia associated with the deletion of two nucleotides at position –2 and –3 preceding the AUG codon. *EMBO J.* 4: 1245–1250.

Nathan, DG and Gunn, RB. (1966). Thalassemia: The consequences of unbalanced hemoglobin synthesis. *Am. J. Med.* 41: 815–830.

Nathan, DG, Stossel, TB, Gunn, RB et al. (1969). Influence of hemoglobin precipitation on erythrocyte metabolism in α and β thalassemia. *J. Clin Invest.* 48: 33–41.

Oner, C, Gurgey, A, Oner, R et al. (1997). The molecular basis of HB H disease in Turkey. *Hemoglobin* 21: 41–51.

Orkin, SH, Old, J, Lazarus, H et al. (1979). The molecular basis of α-thalassemias: frequent occurrence of dysfunctional α-loci among non-Asians with Hb H disease. *Cell* 17: 33–42.

Orkin, SH and Goff, SC. (1981). The duplicated human alpha-globin genes: Their relative expression as measured by RNA analysis. *Cell* 24: 345–351.

Ottolenghi, S, Lanyon, WG, Paul, J et al. (1974). Gene deletion as the cause of α-thalassemia. *Nature* 251: 389–392.

Paglietti, E, Galanello, R, Moi, P et al. (1986). Molecular pathology of haemoglobin H disease in Sardinians. *Br. J. Haematol.* 63: 485–496.

Papassotiriou, I, Traeger-Synodinos, J, Kanavakis, E et al. (1998). Erythroid marrow activity and hemoglobin H levels in hemoglobin H disease. *J. Pediatr. Hematol. Oncol.* 20: 539–544.

Pearson, HA and McFarland, W. (1962). Erythrokinetics in thalassemia. Studies in Lepore trait and hemoglobin H disease. *J. Lab. Clin. Med.* 59: 147.

Peschle, C, Mavilio, F, Care, A et al. (1985). Haemoglobin switching in human embryos: Asynchrony of zeta—alpha and epsilon—gamma-globin switches in primitive and definite erythropoietic lineage. *Nature* 313: 235–238.

Pirastu, M, Saglio, G, Chang, JC et al. (1984). Initiation codon mutation as a cause of α-thalassemia. *J. Biol. Chem.* 259: 12315–12317.

Pootrakul, P, Winichagoon, P, Fucharoen, S, et al. (1981). Homozygous haemoglobin Constant Spring: A need for revision of concept. *Hum. Genet.* 59: 250–255.

Prasartkaew, S, Bunyaratvei, A, Fucharoen, S, and Wasi, P. (1986). Comparison of erythrocyte antioxidative enzyme activities between two types of haemoglobin H disease. *J. Clin. Pathol.* 39: 1299–1303.

Pressley, L, Higgs, DR, Clegg JB et al. (1980). *N. Engl. J. Med.* 24: 1383–1388.

Rachmilewitz, EA, Peisach, J, Bradley, TB Jr, and Blumberg, WE. (1969). Role of haemichromes in the formation of inclusion bodies in haemoglobin H disease. *Nature* 222: 248–250.

Randhawa, ZI, Jones, RT, and Lie-Injo, LE. (1984). Human hemoglobin Portland II (ζ2β2). *J. Biol. Chem.* 259: 7325–7330.

Rees, DC, Williams, TN, Maitland, K et al. (1998). Alpha thalassaemia is associated with increased soluble transferrin receptor levels. *Br. J. Haematol.* 103: 362–369.

Rigas, DA, Koler, RD, and Osgood, EE. (1956). Hemoglobin H: Clinical, laboratory, and genetic studies of a family with a previously undescribed hemoglobin. *J. Lab. Clin. Med.* 47: 51–64.

Rigas, DA and Koler, RD. (1961). Decreased erythrocyte survival in hemoglobin H disease as a result of the abnormal properties of hemoglobin H: The benefit of splenectomy. *Blood* 18: 1–17.

Russell, JE and Liebhaber, SA. (1992). Molecular genetics of thalassemia. In R. S. Verma *Advances in genome biology*, Vol. 2. Greenwich, CT: JAI Press Inc.

Russell, JE and Liebhaber, SA. (1998). Reversal of α and β thalassemia in adult mice by expression of human embryonic globins. *Blood* 92: 3057–3063.

Sancar, GB, Cedeno, MM, and Rieder, RF. (1981). Rapid destruction of newly synthesized excess α-globin chains in Hb H disease. *Blood* 57: 967–971.

Schrier, SL, Rachmilewitz, E, and Mohandas, N. (1989). Cellular and membrane properties of alpha and beta thalassemic erythrocytes are different: Implication for differences in clinical manifestations. *Blood* 74: 2194–2202.

Schrier, SL and Mohandas, N. (1992). Globin-chain specificity of oxidation-induced changes in red blood cell membrane properties. *Blood* 79: 1586–1592.

Schrier, SL, Bunyaratvej, A, Khuhapinant, A et al. (1997). The usual pathobiology of hemoglobin constant spring red blood cells. *Blood* 89: 1762–1769.

Scott, MD, Rouyer-Fessard, P, Soda, BM et al. (1992). α- and β-haemoglobin chain induced changes in normal erythrocyte deformability: Comparison to thalassemia intermedia and Hb H disease. *Br. J. Haematol.* 80: 519–526.

Shakin, SH and Liebhaber, SA. (1986). Translational profiles of α1, α2, and β-globin mRNAs in human reticulocytes. *J. Clin Invest.* 78: 1125–1129.

Shalev, O, Shinar, E, and Lux, SE. (1996). Isolated beta-globin chains reproduce, in normal red cell membranes, the defective binding of spectrin to alpha-thalassemic membranes. *Br. J. Haematol.* 94: 273–278.

Shinar, E, Rachmilewitz, EA, and Lux, SE. (1989). Differing erythrocyte membrane skeletal protein defects in alpha and beta thalassemia. *J. Clin Invest.* 83: 404–410.

Smetanina, NS, Oner, C, Baysal, E et al. (1996). The relative levels of $\alpha 2$-, and $\alpha 1$- and ζ-mRNA in HB H patients with different deletional and nondeletional α-thalassemia determinants. *Biochim. Biophys. Acta* 1316: 176–182.

Tang, W, Luo, H-Y, Albitar, M et al. (1992). Human embryonic zeta-globin chain expression in deletional alpha-thalassemias. *Blood* 80: 517–522.

Taylor, JM, Dozy, A, Kan, YW et al. (1974). Genetic lesion in homozygous α thalassemia (hydrops fetalis). *Nature* 251: 392–393.

Vestri, R, Pieragostini, E, and Ristaldi, MS. (1994). Expression gradient in sheep $\alpha\alpha$ and $\alpha\alpha\alpha$ globin gene haplotypes: mRNA levels. *Blood* 83: 2317–2322.

Wickramasinghe, SN, Lee, MJ, Furukawa, T et al. (1996). Composition of the intra-erythroblastic precipitates in thalassemia and congenital dyserythropoietic anaemia (CDA): Identification of a new type of CDA with intra-erythroblastic precipitates not reacting with monoclonal antibodies to alpha- and beta-globin chains. *Br. J. Haematol.* 93: 576–585.

Wickramasinghe, SN, Hughes, M, Fucharoen, S, and Wasi, P. (1984). The fate of excess α globin chains within erythropoietic cells in α thalassaemia 2 trait, α thalassaemia 1 trait, haemoglobin H disease and haemoglobin Q-H disease: An electron microscope study. *Br. J. Haematol.* 56: 473–482.

Wiener, E, Wanachiwanawin, W, Kotipan, K et al. (1991). Erythroblast- and erythrocyte-bound antibodies in alpha- and beta- thalassemia syndromes. *Transfusion Med.* 1: 229–238.

Wiener, E, Wanachiwanawin, W, Chinprasertsuk, S et al. (1996). Increased serum levels of macrophage colony-stimulating factor (M-CSF) in alpha- and beta-thalassemia syndromes: Correlation with anaemia and monocyte activation. *Eur. J. Haematol.* 57: 364–369.

Wood, WG and Stamatoyannopoulos, G. (1976). Globin synthesis erythroid cell maturation in alpha thalassemia. *Hemoglobin* 1: 135–151.

Yuan, J, Bunyaratvej, A, Fucharoen, S et al. (1995). The instability of the membrane skeleton in thalassemic red blood cells. *Blood* 86: 3945–3950.

17

Molecular Mechanisms of α Thalassemia

DOUGLAS R. HIGGS

INTRODUCTION

Before describing the various ways in which α-globin gene expression may be downregulated in patients with α thalassemia, it is worth briefly reviewing how the genes within the α-globin gene cluster are normally regulated.

Following activation of the α and β loci toward the end of the third week of gestation there is a transition during development from the production of embryonic hemoglobin (Hb Portland, $\alpha_2\gamma_2$; Hb Gower-I $\zeta_2\varepsilon_2$; Hb Gower-II, $\alpha_2\varepsilon_2$) to fetal hemoglobin (HbF, $\alpha_2\gamma_2$), to the major (HbA, $\alpha_2\beta_2$) and minor (HbA$_2$, $\alpha_2\delta_2$) adult hemoglobins (see Chapters 3 through 7).

Whereas both α- and ζ-globin chains are synthesized in primitive erythroblasts in the yolk sac (up to 6 to 7 weeks of gestation), definitive line erythroblasts in the liver almost exclusively synthesize α-globin (from 6 weeks onwards) (Peschle et al., 1985). Using more sensitive mRNA assays, θ-transcripts are detected in yolk sac, fetal liver (Leung et al., 1987), adult blood (Albitar et al., 1989), and bone marrow (Ley et al., 1989). Very small amounts of ζ-globin mRNA are also present throughout fetal life (for example, see Hill et al., 1985) and ζ-globin (as Hb Portland) can be detected in the cord bloods of non-thalassemic newborns (for example, see Chui et al., 1989) (see Chapter 10).

Although the protein products of the α2- and α1-globin genes are identical, two methods exploiting the sequence divergence in their 3′ noncoding regions have enabled the relative amounts of α2- and α1-globin mRNA to be determined in reticulocytes (Liebhaber and Kan, 1981; Orkin and Goff, 1981). In fetal and adult life the steady-state level of α2-mRNA predominates over α1-mRNA by approximately 3:1, probably from differences at the level of transcription of the two genes. More recently, these findings have also been confirmed using quantitative reverse transcriptase polymerase chain reaction (RT-PCR) analyses (Molchanova et al., 1994). Does this mean that the protein synthesis directed by the α2-globin gene in vivo similarly outweighs that from α1-globin gene? Unfortunately, the answer to this important question is still unclear.

Assessment of the ribosome loading of α2- and α1 mRNA has shown that they have identical translational profiles and therefore should be translated with equal efficiencies, predicting a dominant role for the α2-globin locus (Shakin and Liebhaber, 1986). It follows that, in heterozygotes, naturally occurring structural mutations of the α2-globin gene should represent about 37 percent of the peripheral blood hemoglobin and α1 mutants about 13 percent. However, two studies addressing this point come to different conclusions. In the first (Liebhaber et al., 1986), it was found that α2 variants represented 24 percent to 40 percent whereas α1 variants represented 11 percent to 23 percent, suggesting a predominant role for the α2-globin gene at both mRNA and protein levels. In contrast, a more extensive survey of α-globin gene variants by Molchanova et al. (1994) found that in heterozygotes the average proportion of stable variants resulting from α2 mutations (23.5 percent) was only slightly higher than from α1 mutations (19.7 percent), suggesting a less efficient translation of the α2 mRNA and a more equal contribution from the two genes at the protein level. Further work will be needed to resolve this issue since this is clearly important for understanding the pathophysiology of the nondeletional forms of α thalassemia (see below).

The mechanisms by which tissue-specific, developmental control of globin gene expression is achieved is currently under intense investigation and the details are discussed more fully in Chapters 3 through 8. Besides sequences in and around the structural genes, expression of the α-like globin genes is also critically dependent on a remote regulatory sequence (called HS-40) found 40 kb upstream of the ζ2-globin gene (Higgs et al., 1990; Jarman et al., 1991; and see Fig. 17.1).

Martin H. Steinberg, Bernard G. Forget, Douglas R. Higgs, and Ronald L. Nagel, editors. *Disorders of Hemoglobin: Genetics, Pathophysiology, and Clinical Management.* © 2001 Cambridge University Press. All rights reserved.

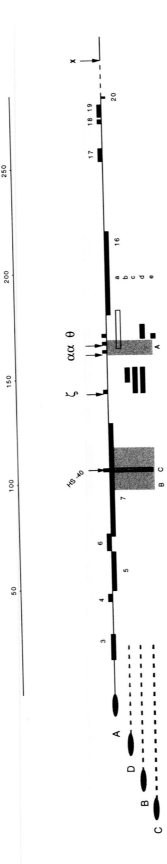

Figure 17.1. The normal α-globin gene cluster and its variants. The major polymorphic, telomeric variants (**A–D**) of 16p as described in the text are indicated with dotted lines (not to scale). Beyond the subtelomeric region the diagram shows the α-globin gene cluster located at the tip of 16p, surrounded by nonglobin genes including the IL9-receptor pseudogene (3); genes of unknown function (4, 5, 6, 16, 17); a DNA repair enzyme MPG (6); RhoGDIγ (18) an inhibitor of the dissociation of GDP from Rho; and PDI (19) a protein disulfide isomerase (further details are given in Flint et al., 1997). Genes illustrated above the line are transcribed toward the centromere and those below, toward the telomere. The ψζ1, ψα2, and ψα1 pseudogenes within the α cluster are not shown. Previously described erythroid-specific DNase I hypersensitive sites (Higgs et al., 1990) are shown as arrows above the line. X denotes the position of chromosomal translocations (summarized in Table 17.1). Shown as shaded boxes are the shortest region of overlap for α-globin deletions (**A**) and natural deletions of the regulatory element (HS-40) (**B**). The area removed in the knockout experiment described in the text is indicated (**C**). The α-ZF deletion (see page 417) is marked as (a) and four rearrangements that do not perturb α-globin gene expression are indicated (b–e; summarized in Higgs et al., 1989, and b is described in Fei et al., 1989). The scale is in kilobase pairs and coordinate 1 is the first nucleotide in the sequence described by Flint et al. (1997).

VARIANTS OF THE α-GLOBIN GENE CLUSTER THAT DO NOT CAUSE α THALASSEMIA

Some mutations of the α-globin gene cluster are common and provide useful genetic markers for the α-globin gene cluster and the 16p telomere. These mutations do not cause α thalassemia and will be reviewed before discussing α thalassemia-causing mutations. In addition they illustrate some of the chromosomal rearrangements and DNA sequence changes that have taken place during the evolution of this multigene family. Furthermore, some mutants help to differentiate between those regions of the gene cluster that are important for expression in vivo and those that may be irrelevant.

Chromosomal Rearrangements Involving 16p13.3

Rarely, chromosomal translocations involving 16p13.3 place the α-globin locus at the tip of another chromosome as seen, for example, in some parents of patients with the ATR-16 syndrome (see Chapter 19). To date we know of 15 individuals (Table 17.1) with such balanced translocations and none of them has α

Table 17.1. Hematologic Findings in Patients with Translocations Involving 16p13.3

Code	Age	Sex	Cytogenetics	Approximate distance of breakpoint from the α-globin genes (Mb)	Hb (g/dL)	MCV (fl)	MCH (pg)	α/β globin synthesis	Reference(s)
AOD	30	F	46, XX t(1;16)(p36;p13.3)	~2	13.3	86	29	0.9	Lamb et al., 1989; Wilkie et al., 1990
LGR	36	F	46, XX t(10;16) (q26.13;p13.3)	~1.2	12.9	89	28	ND	Buckle et al., 1988; Wilkie et al., 1990; Daniels et al., in preparation
KG	AD	F	46, XX t(21;16) ? not visible	~1.8	13.5	88	28	1.0	Daniels et al., in preparation
EW	50	F	46, XX t(16;20) (p13.3;q13.3)	~1.2	11.5	87	28	ND	Daniels et al., in preparation
DJW	75	F	46, XX t(16;20) (p13.3;q13.3)	~1.2	11.0	94	32	ND	Daniels et al., in preparation
JM	51	M	46, XY t(5;16) (q31.1–31.1;p13.3)	~1.7	15.0	88	30	1.2	Harris and Higgs, 1993
PT	32	M	46, XY t(16;17) (p13.3;q24.2)	~1.5	15.3	89	30	1.1	Harris and Higgs, 1993
AMW	33	F	46, XX t(7;16)(q32;p13.3)	>2	12.6	93	30	ND	Germino et al., 1990
HM	33	F	46, XX t(3;16) (q23;p13.13)	ND	13.1	89	31	ND	Unpublished
DF	26	F	46, XX t(X;16) (p11.4;16p13.3)	~1.75	14.1	88	29	ND	KM May, personal communication
RP	34	F	46, XX t(5;16) (p15.3;p13.13)	>2	12.8	88	30	ND	Daniels et al., in preparation
DL	30	F	46, XX t(10;16) (q26.13;p13.3)	~1.2	12.1	94	30	ND	Daniels et al., in preparation
ATA	17	F	46, XX t(16;22) (p13.3;q11.21)	>2	13.5	94	29	ND	European Polycystic Kidney Disease Consortium, 1994, and unpublished
AbA	48	F	46, XX t(16;22) (p13.3;q11.21)	>2	13.0	98	30.3	ND	European Polycystic Kidney Disease Consortium, 1994; and unpublished
GD	36	M	46, XY t(16;11)	>1.5	13.6	80	27	ND	Daniels et al., in preparation

thalassemia. Since the centromeric breakpoints of these chromosomal translocations lie 1 to 2 Mb from the α-globin genes, these findings demonstrate that the *cis*-acting sequences required for full α-globin gene regulation are not perturbed by rearrangements on this scale. In two individuals with unbalanced translocations, and three copies of 16p13.3, the α/β-globin chain synthesis ratios were 1.5 and 1.6 (Wainscoat et al., 1981; Buckle et al., 1988; and unpublished data), again showing that the additional, misplaced copy of the α-globin gene complex is expressed even though its genomic position has been altered. Ultimately, it will be of great interest to know exactly where these breakpoints lie with respect to the α-globin genes and how close other breakpoints would have to be to affect α-globin gene expression.

Variation at the 16p Telomere

The α-globin gene locus lies very close to the telomere of the short arm of chromosome 16 (Fig. 17.1). Four alleles of the α-globin genes lie 170 kb (A), 245 kb (D), 350 kb (B), or 430 kb (C) from the 16p telomeric repeats (Wilkie et al., 1991; Higgs et al., 1993; and see Fig.17.1). Detailed analysis has shown that these polymorphic, subtelomeric alleles are structurally quite different. For example, beyond the region of divergence the A and B alleles are more closely related to nonhomologous chromosomes than to each other. The A allele is related to the subtelomeric regions of Xqter and Yqter, whereas the B allele is more like 9qter, 10pter, and 18pter. Despite these major structural differences at the 16p telomere, the hematologic indices of individuals with A and B alleles are indistinguishable.

Variation in the Number of Globin Genes

As a result of unequal genetic exchange (see below), phenotypically normal individuals may have 4, 5, or 6 α-globin genes (Goossens et al., 1980; Higgs et al., 1980b; Galanello et al., 1983; Gu et al., 1987) and 3, 4, 5, or 6 ζ-like genes (Winichagoon et al., 1982; Felice et al., 1986; Trent et al., 1986a; Titus et al., 1988). A curiously high frequency of the ααα chromosome (gene frequency about 0.01 to 0.08) is found in most populations that have been studied. Why this occurs is not yet clear although it is possible that there is some selective advantage associated with the ααα chromosome. Although there appears to be an excess of α-globin mRNA (Higgs et al., 1980b; Liebhaber and Kan, 1981) and α-globin (Higgs et al., 1980b; Sampietro et al., 1983; Higgs et al., 1984a; Henni et al., 1986; Camaschella et al., 1987; Kulozik et al., 1987) produced from the ααα arrangement, homozygotes (αααα/αααα)

seem to be hematologically normal (Galanello et al., 1983; Trent et al., 1985).

Several members of a recently described family have an unusual, complex rearrangement in which three α-globin gene clusters (αα:αα:αα) are present on one copy of chromosome 16 (Fichera et al., 1994). Provisional data suggest that at least two and possibly all three clusters are fully active. A carrier for this abnormal chromosome (αα:αα:αα/αα) has an α/β-globin chain synthesis ratio of 2.7. Patients who co-inherit the αα:αα:αα chromosome with a mild form of β thalassemia produce sufficient excess α-globin chains to have β thalassemia intermedia (Fichera et al., 1994).

Chromosomes bearing a single ζ-globin gene (ζ2 rather than the normal ζ2-ψζ1 arrangement, see Fig. 17.3) are relatively common (gene frequency about 0.05) in West Africans (Winichagoon et al., 1982; Rappaport et al., 1984; Felice et al., 1986; Higgs et al., 1986; and unpublished data) and occur sporadically in other populations. There is no discernible phenotype associated with the genotype (Winichagoon et al., 1982; Felice et al., 1986; Trent et al., 1986a; and unpublished data) and, to date, only one homozygote has been identified who appears hematologically normal.

A triplicated ζ-globin gene arrangement has the structure ζ2-ψζ1-ψζ1 (Hill et al., 1985) and was originally identified in Southeast Asia where its frequency is 0.09 to 0.20 (Winichagoon et al., 1982; Chan et al., 1986; Higgs et al., 1986); it is also particularly common throughout Melanesia, Micronesia, and Polynesia, where phenotypically normal homozygotes (ζζζ/ζζζ) have been described (Higgs et al., 1986; Trent et al., 1986a; Hill et al., 1987a). Elsewhere, the triplicated ζ-globin gene is uncommon. Structural analysis of this arrangement shows that it has arisen by an unusual interchromosomal recombination event (Hill et al., 1985, 1987a) between Ia and IId haplotypes (see Chapter 32 for a description of α-globin gene haplotypes). All of the ζζζ chromosomes studied from Southeast Asia and the Pacific have this unusual structure (Hill et al., 1987a) suggesting that they have a common, single origin. Some of these chromosomes appear to have been subsequently modified, as shown by the presence of a *Bgl* II polymorphism in 8 percent to 15 percent of cases (Hill et al., 1987a) and the occasional presence of the Hb Constant Spring mutation on the linked α2-globin gene (Winichagoon et al., 1982). A very rare example of a chromosome with four ζζζζ genes was described by Titus et al. (1988).

Gene Conversion in the α-Globin Gene Cluster

DNA strand exchanges involved in misaligned but reciprocal recombination (mentioned above) may also resolve with nonreciprocal genetic exchange (known also as gene conversions; reviewed in Strachan and Read, 1996). During the process of gene conversion, genetic information may be exchanged between allelic or nonallelic homologous sequences without any crossovers or chromosomal rearrangements occurring. Gene conversion events between both the α1/α2 pair and the ζ2/ψζ1 pair may occur quite frequently. DNA sequence analysis suggests that gene conversion events have taken place between α1 and α2 (Michelson and Orkin, 1983) and ζ2 and ψζ1 genes (Proudfoot et al., 1982; Hill et al., 1985) throughout evolution. A likely example of such a conversion between α2 and α1 has been documented in individuals expressing an unexpectedly high level of HbI, an α-globin gene variant ($\alpha^{16\ Lys\rightarrow Glu}$), in whom the same mutation is present on both in cis (Liebhaber et al., 1984) (see Chapter 45). Further possible examples of nonreciprocal exchange have recently been described by Molchanova et al. (1994), who observed identical sequence mutations affecting the α1 and α2 genes on independent chromosomes; one possibility is that these arise by conversion from one gene to another.

Analysis of the downstream ζ-like gene in several populations has shown that it exists in two distinct forms (Hill et al., 1985). In one its structure is clearly that of a pseudogene (ψζ1) and in the other (ζ1) the ψζ1 gene has undergone a gene conversion by the ζ2 gene such that it becomes more similar to the functional ζ-globin gene although it still appears not to be expressed in vivo. The frequency of the ζ2-ζ1 chromosome varies from one population to another (0.14 to 0.57), and phenotypically normal individuals homozygous for either ζ2-ψζ1 or ζ2-ζ1 chromosomes have been observed (Hill et al., 1985). Conversions of the ζ2 gene by ψζ1 have not yet been described although several candidate chromosomes have been identified.

In addition to these examples of gene conversion it seems likely that, as in other mammalian multigene families (Collier et al., 1993) short segmental conversions may also be responsible for transferring thalassemic and nonthalassemic variants within and between different chromosomal backgrounds.

Deletions and Insertions Within the α-Globin Gene Complex

Two uncommon deletions involving the θ1 gene remove either 1.8 kb or 6.0 kb from between the intact α1-globin gene and the α-globin 3′ hypervariable region (HVR) (Fei et al., 1988) (Fig. 17.1). Neither variant was associated with any phenotypic abnormalities in the neonatal period, and an adult heterozygous for the 1.8-kb deletion also appears normal. An individual with the 6.0-kb deletion also had a −ζ chromo-

some (Fei et al., 1988). Another individual apparently has the same 6.0-kb deletion; in this case the arrangement was present in cis to the θ1 deletion (Higgs et al., 1989). Similarly, Ballas, Fei, and Huisman, THJ (personal communication) found that both of these rearrangements may exist on the same chromosome. Thus these individuals have deletions at both the 5′ (10 kb) and 3′ (6 kb) ends of the cluster with no discernible effect on α-gene expression. Finally, in a large survey of newborn babies (Fei et al., 1989), a small (2.5 kb) deletion (see Fig. 17.1) between the ζ- and ψζ-globin genes was observed in two hematologically normal babies from Sardinia.

Phenotypically silent insertions are also recognized in the α-globin gene complex. An insertion of 0.5 to 0.7 kb between the α2 and α1 genes was identified in the nonthalassemic chromosome of a Chinese individual (Nakatsuji et al., 1986). This most probably arose from a reciprocal crossover between a normal chromosome (αα) and the common α-thalassemia determinant (−α³·⁷, see below). In addition, an insertion/deletion polymorphism in the 5′ flanking region of the α-globin gene complex that appears to involve members of the Alu family of repeats has been observed (Higgs et al., 1989).

Restriction Site Polymorphisms

On average 1 in 80 bp of the α-globin gene cluster varies between individuals (Higgs et al., 1986). Some of these changes have been identified as restriction fragment length polymorphisms (RFLP) within and flanking the α-globin gene cluster (Higgs et al., 1986). They can be divided into common (the frequency of the rarer allele in most populations being 0.05 to 0.50) and uncommon (less than 0.05) variants; the latter are frequently race or population specific. Analysis of nine common polymorphisms (including the ψζ1-ζ1 polymorphism and the inter-zeta hypervariable region, IZHVR) showed that linkage disequilibrium exists between these genetic markers and some common α-globin gene cluster haplotypes (nonrandom linkage groups) could be derived. Although a large number of haplotypes are recognized, in each population only one or two are common and several others are present at low frequencies. The α-globin gene haplotypes are described in more detail in Chapter 32. There is no evidence that α-globin gene expression differs between the common α-globin gene cluster haplotypes.

Recently DNA sequence analysis has revealed six minor variants of the HS-40 regulatory element (Harteveld et al., submitted). Again, these polymorphic haplotypes are found in normal, nonthalassemic individuals and provide informative examples of in vivo mutagenesis that allows one to relate the structure of this important regulatory region to its function.

Variable Number of Tandem Repeats (VNTRs)

Preliminary Southern blot analysis identified several VNTRs in and around the α-globin gene locus. The number of repeats in these arrays may be altered at mitosis or meiosis producing highly polymorphic segments of the cluster. Recently DNA sequence analysis of the terminal 300-kb region of 16p (Flint et al., 1997) identified at least 10 VNTRs in this region consistent with the view that such sequences tend to cluster at the ends of human chromosomes (Royle et al., 1988). In the α-globin gene complex there appears to be no relationship between the structure of such regions and the associated phenotype. Whatever their function, if any, they are of great value as genetic markers throughout the genome and have been used to produce individual-specific genetic fingerprints (Jeffreys, 1987; Fowler et al., 1988).

VARIANTS THAT CAUSE α THALASSEMIA

Analysis of the human α-globin gene cluster has revealed a remarkable degree of polymorphism due to point mutations, deletions, and insertions of DNA. These polymorphisms are found in all populations. Variants that cause α thalassemia are largely limited to tropical and subtropical regions of the world where malaria is, or has been, endemic (see Chapters 30 and 32). However, some rare and very informative mutations have been found in individuals outside of these regions. In contrast to β thalassemia, in which mutations are frequently due to point mutations in the structural genes (Chapter 12), α thalassemia is most often due to deletions involving one or both of the α-globin genes. Less frequently, deletions removing the α-globin regulatory element (HS-40) are seen. This difference in molecular pathology—deletions rather than point mutations—represents another contrast between the α- and β-like globin gene clusters, which may also reflect their different chromosomal environments (see Chapter 5).

α⁺-Thalassemia Due to Gene Deletions

Heteroduplex and DNA sequence analysis has shown that the α-globin genes are embedded within two highly homologous, 4-kb duplication units whose sequence identity has been maintained throughout evolution by gene conversion and unequal crossover events (Lauer et al., 1980; Zimmer et al., 1980; Michelson and Orkin, 1983; Hess et al., 1984). These regions are divided into homologous subsegments (X, Y, and Z) by nonhomologous elements (I, II, and III; Fig. 17.2A). Reciprocal recombination between Z segments (Fig. 17.2B), which are 3.7 kb apart, produces chromosomes with only one α gene, the $-\alpha^{3.7}$ rightward deletion (Embury et al.,

1980), that cause α thalassemia and others with three α-globin genes ($\alpha\alpha\alpha^{anti3.7}$) (Goossens et al., 1980; Higgs et al., 1980b). These events can be further subdivided, depending on exactly where within the Z box the crossover took place, into $-\alpha^{3.7I}$, $-\alpha^{3.7II}$, and $-\alpha^{3-7III}$ (Higgs et al., 1984b). These subregions are defined by sequence differences in the $Z\alpha2$ and $Z\alpha1$ boxes that can be detected by Southern blot hybridization.

Recombination between homologous X boxes, which are 4.2 kb apart, also gives rise to an α-thalassemia determinant, the $-\alpha^{4.2}$ (leftward deletion) (Embury et al., 1980) and an $\alpha\alpha\alpha^{anti4.2}$ chromosome (Trent et al., 1981). Further recombination events between the resulting chromosomes (α, αα, ααα) give rise to quadruplicated α-globin genes ($\alpha\alpha\alpha\alpha^{anti3.7}$ and $\alpha\alpha\alpha\alpha^{anti4.2}$) (Trent et al., 1981; De Angioletti et al., 1992) or other unusual rearrangements.

Three rare deletions that produce α⁺ thalassemia have been described (Fig. 17.2A). One removes the entire α1 gene and its flanking DNA ($-\alpha^{3.5}$) has been observed in two Asian Indian patients (Kulozik et al., 1988). Its breakpoints have not yet been examined in detail and thus it is not clear whether this represents a nonhomologous recombination event (see later) or whether further sequences homologous to the Z box lie downstream of the α1-globin gene. A second deletion, referred to as $(\alpha)\alpha^{5.3}$, was observed in a family from Italy (Lacerra et al., 1991). It removed the 5′ end of the α2-globin gene; the 5′ breakpoint lies 822 bp upstream of the mRNA cap site of the ψα1 gene; the 3′ breakpoint is in IVS1 of the α2 gene. Sequence analysis suggests that this deletion has arisen by an illegitimate recombination event. A third rare α⁺-thalassemia deletion was described in a Chinese patient with HbH disease (Zhao et al., 1991). This 2.7-kb deletion removed the α1-globin gene but since the breakpoints have not been sequenced the mechanism by which it occurred is unknown.

The variety of independent recombination events giving rise to −α and ααα chromosomes identified in human populations suggest that recombination between the homologous X and Z boxes is relatively frequent and several indirect observations also support this notion. Both −α and ααα chromosomes are present in most population groups. Moreover, the −α determinant is associated with many different hemoglobin variants (e.g., see Higgs et al., 1989 and Table 17.2), HVR alleles and α-globin gene haplotypes (Goodbourn et al., 1983; Winichagoon et al., 1984; Flint et al., 1986). Furthermore, in population isolates such as Papua New Guinea and Vanuatu the −α determinants are only found on the common α-globin gene haplotypes for that population, suggesting that they have arisen de novo in each population group (Flint et al., 1986) rather than having been "imported" from other populations and selected. Moreover, some α-glo-

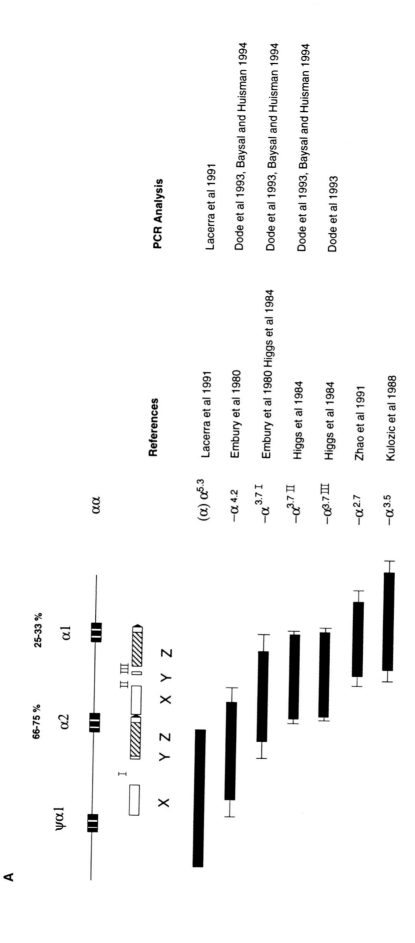

Figure 17.2. (A) Deletions that cause α⁺ thalassemia. Above, the α-globin genes are shown with duplication units divided into X, Y, and Z boxes and regions of nonhomology as I, II, III. Below, the extent of each deletion is represented by a black bar. The thin bars at the end of each thick bar denote the regions of uncertainty for the deletion breakpoints. Primary references for the characterization and examples of PCR analysis of these deletions are shown on the right-hand side of the diagram.

412

B

RIGHTWARD CROSSOVER(Z BOX):-

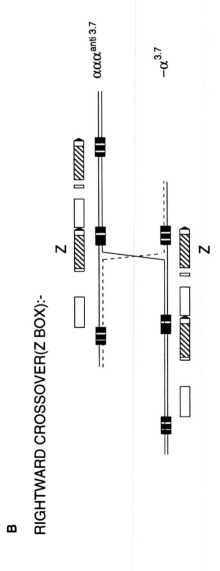

LEFTWARD CROSSOVER(X BOX):-

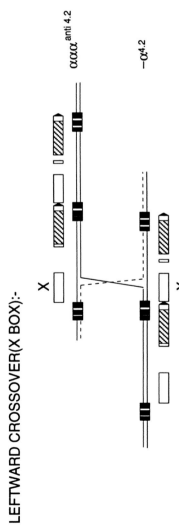

Figure 17.2. (B) The mechanism by which the common deletions underlying α thalassemia occur. Crossovers between misaligned Z boxes give rise to the $-\alpha^{3.7}$ and $\alpha\alpha\alpha^{\text{anti}3.7}$ chromosomes. Crossovers between misaligned X boxes give rise to $-\alpha^{4.2}$ and $\alpha\alpha\alpha^{\text{anti}4.2}$ chromosomes.

Table 17.2. α-Globin Variants Associated with Deletional Forms of α Thalassemia

	Variant	Haplotype	Population(s)	Reference(s)
Hb Evanston	α^{14} Trp→Arg	$-\alpha^{3.7}$	black	Moo-Penn et al., 1978; Honig et al., 1984
Hb Hasharon	α^{47} Asp→His	$-\alpha^{3.7}$ and $\alpha\alpha$	Mediterranean, Ashkenazi Jews	Pich et al., 1973; Del Senno et al., 1980; Giglioni et al., 1980; Mavilio et al., 1980; Liebhaber and Cash, 1985; Liebhaber et al., 1986
Hb G Philadelphia	α^{68} Asn→Lys	$-\alpha^{3.7}$ and $\alpha\alpha$	Algerian, Mediterranean, Black, Melanesian	Sancar et al., 1980; Surrey et al., 1980; Bruzdzinski et al., 1984; Sciarratta et al., 1984; Liebhaber and Cash, 1985; Hill, 1985; Liebhaber et al., 1986
Hb Q (Mahidol)	α^{74} Asp→His	$-\alpha^{4.2}$	Southeast Asian	Lie-Injo et al., 1979; Higgs et al., 1980a
Hb Duan	α^{75} Asp→Ala	$-\alpha^{4.2}$	Chinese	Liang et al., 1988
Hb Stanleyville II	α^{78} Asn→Lys	$-\alpha^{3.7}$	black	Costa et al., 1990
Hb Nigeria	α^{81} Ser→Lys	Not determined	black	Honig et al., 1980
Hb J Capetown	α^{92} Arg→Gln	$-\alpha^{3.7I}$	South African	Lambridis et al., 1986
Hb J Tongariki	α^{115} Ala→Asp	$-\alpha^{3.7III}$	Melanesian	Old et al., 1978; Higgs et al., 1984b

bin gene variants (e.g., HbG Philadelphia, α^{68} Asn→Lys see Chapter 45) are found on both normal $\alpha\alpha$ chromosomes and chromosomes bearing an α-thalassemia determinant ($-\alpha$), suggesting a connection between the two through recombination or gene conversion (Strachan and Read, 1996). Similar observations have been made for the poly(A) signal mutation found in Saudi Arabia, which is present on both $\alpha\alpha$ and $\alpha\alpha\alpha$ chromosomes (Thein et al., 1988). It is interesting that the relative frequencies of the various types of α thalassemia observed throughout the world correlate with the length of the homologous segments that serve as target areas for the crossovers involved [$-\alpha^{3.7I}$ (1436 bp) > $-\alpha^{4.2}$ (1339 bp) > $-\alpha^{3.7II}$ (171 bp) > $-\alpha^{3.7III}$ (46 bp)]. Correlations between frequency of recombination and target size have been noted in other systems (Jinks-Robertson et al., 1993); however, since the α-thalassemia determinants are highly selected for in many areas (Flint et al., 1986), these observations may not truly reflect recombination rates. Direct evidence for a high rate of recombination between the duplicated α-globin genes has recently been obtained using sperm typing by PCR (Lamb and Clegg, 1996). Analysis of DNA extracted from the spermatozoa of a Caucasian donor indicated a recombination frequency of about 1.7×10^{-4}.

Expression From the α+ Chromosomes

Although the relative expression of mRNA from the α2- and α1-globin genes on a normal chromosome is approximately 3:1, there are several lines of evidence which show that the α gene in the various $-\alpha$ chromosomes behaves like neither an α1- nor α2-globin gene.

For example, homozygotes for the $-\alpha^{4.2}$ determinant who essentially have two α1-globin genes ($-\alpha^{4.2}/-\alpha^{4.2}$) appear to express more α globin than the predicted 25 percent of normal (Bowden et al., 1987), and homozygotes for $-\alpha^{3.7III}$ with the equivalent of two α2-globin genes ($-\alpha^{3.7}/-\alpha^{3.7}$) express less than the predicted 75 percent of normal (Bowden et al., 1987). Direct measurements of α-globin mRNA levels in patients with the $-\alpha^{3.7}$ determinant also suggest that the remaining α-globin gene is expressed at a level roughly halfway between that of a normal α2- and normal α1-gene (Liebhaber et al., 1985). Because the transcriptional units of all the recombined genes ($-\alpha^{3.7I}$, $-\alpha^{3.7II}$, $-\alpha^{3.7III}$, $-\alpha^{4.2}$) are virtually identical to either the native α1- or α2-globin gene, the alteration in expression most likely results from a change in the rate of transcription of the gene. Assuming that this is a *cis* effect, it could be brought about by the new combinations of flanking sequences, possibly a release of transcriptional interference from the upstream gene (Proudfoot, 1986) or by the change in chromosome conformation as a result of the deletions.

Another possibility is that the promoters of the α2- and α1-globin genes compete for interaction with the single HS-40 regulatory element in a similar way to which the γ- and β-globin genes are thought to compete for the β-globin gene cluster locus control region (LCR) (see Chapters 7 and 15). In this case a single promoter in the $-\alpha$ chromosome would have continuous access to HS-40 and might consequently be expressed more efficiently.

Although there is no a priori reason to anticipate changes in ζ-globin gene expression in patients with the $-\alpha$ haplotype, it is useful to know that none of the

−α mutations is associated with any significant change in ζ-globin expression (Chui et al., 1986).

α⁰ Thalassemia Due to Deletions of the Structural α-Globin Genes

All of the deletions described in this section either completely or partially [−(α)^{5.2} and (α)^{20.5}] delete both α-globin genes (Figs. 17.3 and 17.4), and therefore no α-chain synthesis is directed by these chromosomes in vivo. Homozygotes for such chromosomes have the Hb Bart's hydrops fetalis syndrome (see Chapter 18). Several deletions remove both α- and ζ-globin genes (Felice et al., 1984; Chan et al., 1985; Di Rienzo et al., 1986; Fischel-Ghodsian et al., 1988; Fortina et al., 1988, 1991; Vickers and Higgs, 1989; Waye et al., 1992); although heterozygotes for these variants survive and appear to develop normally, it appears that homozygotes do not survive even the early stages of gestation because neither embryonic nor fetal hemoglobin can be made (see Chapter 18).

Some, but not all, heterozygotes for deletions in which the embryonic gene remains intact have continued expression of very small amounts of ζ-globin chain in both fetal (Chui et al., 1989) and adult life (Kutlar et al., 1989; Tang et al., 1992). This may be analogous to the persistent γ-globin chain production documented in patients with similar downstream deletions of the β-globin gene complex (see Chapter 15). However, the amount of ζ globin present in adults with these types of α thalassemia is much less than the level of γ-globin chain present in individuals with comparable deletions of the β-globin gene complex. It seems that this increase of embryonic globin expression is not simply due to the increased erythropoiesis since, in one study no ε- or ζ-globin gene transcripts were detected in several patients with erythroid hyperplasia (Ley et al., 1989).

At the 3′ end of the α-globin gene complex most of these deletions include the θ1 gene whose function is not yet known. In one individual, homozygous for the −−^{SEA} deletion, who was treated with blood transfusion, both θ1 genes are deleted and yet the child appears to have developed normally (Fischel-Ghodsian et al., 1987).

Recently all of the DNA stretching for 300 kb from the 16p telomere was cloned, characterized, and sequenced (Flint et al., 1997). This enabled a definition of the full extent of several deletions that include the ζ-, α-, and θ-globin genes. These deletions extend from 100 kb to over 250 kb (Fig. 17.4) and remove other genes that flank the α-globin gene cluster including a DNA repair enzyme (methyl adenine DNA glycosylase), an inhibitor of GDP dissociation from Rho (RhoGDIγ), a protein disulfide isomerase (PDI-R), and several anonymous housekeeping genes. Despite this, such patients appear phenotypically normal apart from having α-thalassemia trait (−−/αα) or HbH disease (−−/−α) In patients with more extensive deletions from 16p 13.3, α thalassemia is associated with developmental abnormalities and mental retardation (see Chapter 19).

Detailed analysis of several determinants of α⁰ thalassemia indicates that they often result from illegitimate or nonhomologous recombination events (Nicholls et al., 1987). Such events may involve short regions of partial sequence homology at the breakpoints of the molecules that are rejoined but they do not involve the extensive sequence-matching required for homologous recombination as described previously.

Sequence analysis has shown that members of the dispersed family of *Alu* repeats are frequently found at or near the breakpoints of these deletions. *Alu*-family repeats occur frequently in the genome (3×10^5 copies) and seem to be particularly common in and around the α-globin gene cluster, where they make up about 25 percent of the entire sequence (Flint et al., 1997). *Alu* repeats may provide partially homologous sequences that promote DNA-strand exchanges during replication, or possibly a subset of *Alu* sequences may be more actively involved in the process. To date, at least eight deletions causing α thalassemia have been shown to have one or both breakpoints lying in Alu sequences. It is interesting that similar illegitimate recombination events in the β-globin gene locus less frequently involve *Alu* sequences, suggesting that this type of recombination may be, to some extent, locus specific (Henthorn et al., 1990).

Detailed sequence analysis of the junctions of the α-globin gene deletions has revealed a number of interesting features including palindromes, direct repeats, regions of weak homology, and frequent occurrence of the motif GAGG. One of the deletions (−−^{MED}) also involves a more complex rearrangement that introduces a new piece of DNA bridging the two breakpoints of the deletion. This inserted DNA originates from upstream of the α-globin gene cluster and appears to have been incorporated into the junction in a manner that suggests that the upstream segment lies close to the breakpoint regions during replication (Nicholls et al., 1987).

At least two of the largest deletions (−−^{HW} and −−^{BR}, Fig. 17.4) result from chromosomal breaks in the 16p telomeric region that have been "healed" by the direct addition of telomeric repeats (TTAGGG)_n. This mechanism is described in further detail below.

α Thalassemia Due to Deletions of the α-Globin Regulatory Element

Expression of the α-globin genes is critically dependent on a segment of DNA that lies 40 kb upstream of

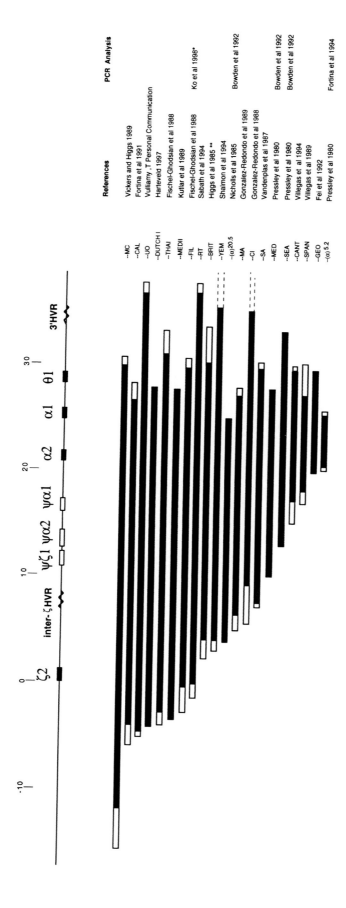

Figure 17.3. Deletions that cause α⁰ thalassemia. Above, the α-globin gene complex is shown (scale in kilobases; 0 indicates the ζ2 globin mRNA cap site). Below, the extent of each deletion is shown by a black bar. Regions of uncertainty for each breakpoint are shown by white boxes. To the right, are the shorthand notations, primary references for the characterization, and examples of PCR analysis for each deletion.

*Although Ko et al. (1998) originally reported that their primers amplified the - -THAI deletion, it has subsequently been shown that, in fact, these primers inadvertently characterized the - -FIL mutation (S. Chong et al., 2000).

**The - -BRIT deletion may be the same as a rare α-thalassemia defect described in a black patient (Steinberg et al., 1986).

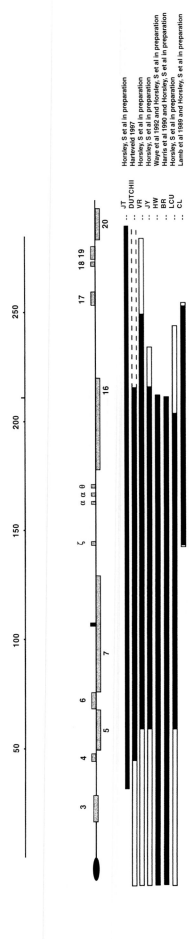

Figure 17.4. Rare, large deletions that cause α thalassemia but no other associated abnormalities. Above, the terminal 300 kb of chromosome 16p as described in the legend to Figure 17.1 (scale in kilobases). Below, black bars indicate the extent of each deletion. Regions of uncertainty for the breakpoints are shown by white boxes. The dashed lines in the α - -DUTCH II mutation indicate that the 3′ end of this deletion has not yet been investigated. To the right, are the shorthand notations and primary references for each deletion.

the α2-globin gene (Higgs et al., 1990). This region is associated with an erythroid-specific DNase I hypersensitive site and is referred to as HS-40. Detailed analysis of HS-40 has shown that it contains multiple binding sites for the erythroid-restricted *trans*-acting factors GATA-1 and NF-E2 (Jarman et al., 1991; Strauss et al., 1992).

The first indication that such a remote regulatory sequence might exist came from observations on a patient with α thalassemia (Hatton et al., 1990). Analysis of the abnormal chromosome (αα)^RA from this patient showed a 62-kb deletion from upstream of the α-globin gene complex (Fig. 17.5), which includes HS-40. Although both α-globin genes on this chromosome were intact and entirely normal they appeared to be nonfunctional. Since this observation, ten more patients with α thalassemia due to a deletion of HS40 and a variable amount of the flanking DNA have been described (see Fig.17.5 for references). A 20 to −24 kb segment of DNA containing HS-40 is deleted in all of these chromosomes and all of these mutations give rise to the phenotype associated with α⁰ thalassemia: Some patients have α thalassemia trait [αα/(αα)] while others have HbH disease [-α/(αα)].

Interspecific hybrids each containing an abnormal copy of chromosome 16 from such patients have been made by fusing Epstein-Barr virus transformed cell lines with mouse erythroleukemia cells (MEL). In contrast to normal copies of chromosome 16, the abnormal chromosomes produce less than 1 percent human α-globin mRNA, suggesting that deletions removing HS-40 severely downregulate expression of the α-globin genes and are responsible for the associated α thalassemia. More recently a specific knockout of HS-40 (Bernet et al., 1994) from such a chromosome, together with many experiments in transgenic mice (Higgs et al., 1998), has confirmed that HS-40 is the major active element deleted by these arrangements.

The mechanisms by which these mutations have arisen are quite diverse. In the (αα)^RA chromosome, the deletion resulted from a recombination event between partially homologous *Alu* repeats that are normally 62 kb apart (Hatton et al., 1990).

In the (αα)^MB chromosome (Flint et al., 1996), the deletion arose via a subtelomeric rearrangement. The chromosomal breakpoint was found in an *Alu* element located about 105 kb from the 16p subtelomeric region. A new telomere acquired by recombination between this *Alu* element and a subtelomeric *Alu* repeat associated with the newly acquired chromosome end stabilized the broken chromosome.

In five cases, (αα)^CMO, (αα)^IdF, (αα)^TAT, (αα)^IC, and (αα)^TI, the chromosomes appear to have been broken and then stabilized by the direct addition of telomeric repeats to nontelomeric DNA (Flint et al., 1994).

Sequence analysis suggests that these chromosomes are "healed" via the action of telomerase, an enzyme that is normally involved in maintaining the integrity of telomeres (Blackburn, 1992; Flint et al., 1994).

Three remaining examples, (αα)^IJ, (αα)^MCK, and (αα)^SN (Fig. 17.5), have undefined mechanisms. However, it is interesting that in both (αα)^IJ and (αα)^MCK, the deletions appear to have arisen de novo, since neither parent has the abnormal chromosome.

α Thalassemia Due to a Deletion Extending Downstream of the α-Globin Gene Cluster

During a study to identify thalassemia in families from the Czech Republic, Indrak et al. (1993) reported a novel deletion (more than 18 kb) involving the α1- and θ-globin genes, α-^ZF (Fig. 17.1). Heterozygotes for this deletion have a mild hypochromic microcytic anemia (hemoglobin concentration, 12.6 g/dL, MCH 22 pg, MCV 68 fl) with a reduced α/β-globin chain biosynthesis ratio of 0.62 to 0.66, and HbH inclusions. These findings suggest that although the α2 gene appears intact it has been inactivated by the novel deletion.

Further analysis of this interesting case (Higgs et al., 1998; Barbour et al., 2000) has confirmed that the remaining α2 gene on the α-^ZF chromosome is structurally intact, including all critical *cis*-acting sequences, and has no inactivating point mutations. Nevertheless, functional studies in which the abnormal chromosome was isolated as an interspecific hybrid with MEL cells, confirmed that the α2 gene has been inactivated by the deletion; such hybrids produce no human α-globin mRNA.

Detailed in vivo analysis of this mutation has shown that the α-globin gene and its promoter have been made inaccessible to DNase I and other endonucleases. Furthermore, the CpG island associated with the gene, which spans the α-globin gene promoter, has become fully methylated whereas normally this region is unmethylated. At present the mechanism by which this occurred is not clear but it is of interest that the region of the chromosome abutted to the α2 gene by the deletion corresponds to an *Alu*-dense, methylated region that contains no DNase I hypersensitive sites (Flint et al., 1997). Perhaps the simplest explanation is that the juxtaposition of the α2 gene next to a piece of relatively inert chromatin has induced a "chromosomal position effect." In such situations it is thought that a repressive chromatin structure spreads over a gene that is normally active and prevents its expression (Shaffer et al., 1993). Further studies will be needed to test this hypothesis.

It is not clear whether this mutation has simply identified an unimportant block of "heterochromatin"

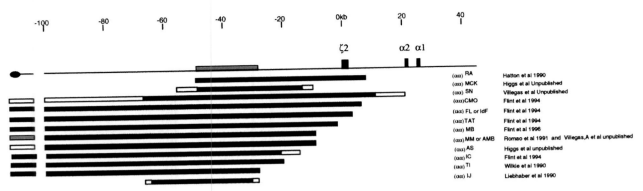

Figure 17.5. Deletions extending upstream of the α-globin gene cluster that cause α thalassemia by removing the α-globin gene regulatory element, HS-40. Above, the α cluster (scale in kilobases; 0 indicates the ζ2 globin mRNA cap site). The stippled box represents the shortest region of overlap among all deletions that includes HS-40. The oval represents the 16p telomere. The extent of each deletion is indicated by black bars and the uncertainty of breakpoints is shown by white boxes. Primary references and shorthand notations are shown on the right.

or if this region normally plays an important role in regulating the α-globin gene cluster. Studies in transgenic mice have shown that although this region contains no positive regulatory sequences, α-globin mRNA expression from a large construct containing this region is expressed at higher levels and in a more stable manner than those that do not span this area (Higgs et al., 1998). Further studies are under way to assess the role of this fascinating area of the α-globin gene cluster.

Nondeletion Types of α Thalassemia

In all surveys reported so far, α thalassemia is much more frequently due to gene deletions than to single point mutations or oligonucleotide insertions and deletions involving the canonical sequences that control gene expression (so-called nondeletion variants, in which the affected gene is denoted α^T). This is in contrast to the situation in β thalassemia where point mutations affecting almost every stage of gene expression are known (see Chapter 12) and deletions are less frequent.

Nondeletion types of α thalassemia were first described in 1977 (Kan et al., 1977) and shown to result from a variety of mechanisms (Higgs et al., 1981). At present we know of 41 well-defined causes of nondeletion α thalassemia (Table 17.3). Twenty-five of these occur in the α2 gene, seven in the α1 gene, and six occur on a –α chromosome. In three cases the mutation has not yet been assigned to an α-globin gene.

As a group, the nondeletion α-thalassemia determinants (α^T, α, and $\alpha\alpha^T$) appear to have a more severe effect on α-globin gene expression and hematologic phenotype than simple deletions that remove one or

another of the α-globin genes (see Chapter 18). This may be explained by the majority of mutations affecting the α2 gene, whose expression may predominate over the α1 gene (see above); this may also lead to a bias in ascertainment. In addition, unlike when one α-globin gene is deleted (see above), there appears to be no compensatory increase in expression of the remaining functional α gene when the other is inactivated by a point mutation. Furthermore, some highly unstable variants may have multiple secondary effects on red cell interactions that produce a more severe phenotype than predicted from the anticipated decrease in α-globin gene expression (compare with similar β globin mutations described in Chapter 14). At present these general assertions are based on a small number of observations and further evaluation of the pathophysiology of each mutation will be needed in the future.

Mutants That Affect mRNA Splicing. Three nondeletion α-thalassemia variants affect RNA splicing. One ($\alpha^{\text{IVS I; 5 bp del}}\alpha$) results from a pentanucleotide deletion at the 5' donor site of IVS1 of the α2-globin gene (Orkin et al., 1981; Felbar et al., 1982). This mutation affects the invariant GT sequence and eliminates splicing from the normal donor site while activating a cryptic donor consensus that lies in exon I. Aberrantly spliced mRNA was detected in a transient expression system and in bone marrow from an affected patient. By contrast, in peripheral blood very little, if any, mRNA from the mutated α2-globin gene was detected, suggesting that the aberrantly spliced mRNA is unstable. Heterozygotes for this mutation have the phenotype of α-thalassemia trait and homozygotes have a correspondingly more severe form of α-thalassemia trait.

A mutation of the acceptor site of IVS1 of the α2-globin gene ($\alpha^{\text{IVS1; 116(A}\rightarrow\text{G)}}\alpha$) was recently described by Harteveld et al. (1996c). Abnormal splicing leads to the retention of IVS1, which introduces a premature stop at codon 31. Low levels of abnormal mRNA in reticulocytes are thought to be due to posttranscriptional mRNA instability. Although all eleven carriers for this mutation have reduced α/β-globin chain synthesis ratios

Table 17.3. Nondeletion Mutants that Cause α Thalassemia

Affected gene	Affected sequence	Location§	Mutation	Alternative notation	Identification	Distribution	Reference(s)
mRNA Processing							
α2	IVS 1 (donor)	163008–163012	IVS 1;5 bp del	$\alpha^{Hph}\alpha$	R: Hph I	Mediterranean	Orkin et al., 1981
α2	IVS1–116 (acceptor)	163122	IVS 1; 116 (A→G)		C:Sac II	Dutch Caucasian	Harteveld et al., 1996c
α1	IVS-1-117 (acceptor)	166927	IVS 1; 117 (G→A)		R: Fok I	Asian Indian	Çürük et al., 1993a
α2	Poly(A) signal	163673–163688	PA; 16 bp del		R: Hae III	Arab	Tamary et al., 1997
α2*	Poly(A) signal	163693	PA; 6 A→G	$\alpha^{TSaudi}\alpha$		Middle East, Mediterranean	Higgs et al., 1983
α2	Poly(A) signal	163691	PA; 4 A→G			Mediterranean	Yüregir et al. 1992
α2	Poly(A) signal	163692–163693	PA; 2 bp del			Asian Indian	Hall et al., 1994;
mRNA Translation†							
-α	Initiation codon	163912	IN; A→G		R: Nco I	Black	Harteveld et al., 1994
-α$^{3.7II}$	Initiation codon	162909–162910	IN; 2 bp del			North African, Mediterranean	Olivieri et al., 1987; Morlé et al., 1985;
α2	Initiation codon	162913	IN; T→C		R: Nco I	Mediterranean	Morlé et al., 1986
α1	Initiation codon	166716	IN; A→G		R: Nco I	Mediterranean	Pirastu et al. 1984
α2	Initiation codon	162913	IN; 1 bp del			Mediterranean	Paglietti et al., 1986; Moi et al., 1987
-α	Exon I	163005–163006	Cd 30/31; 2 bp del		R: Nco I	Vietnam	Waye et al., 1996
α2	Exon II	163146–163154	Cd 39/41; del/ins			Black	Safaya and Rieder, 1988
α1	Exon II	166986–167000	Cd 51–55; 13 bp del			Yemenite-Jewish	Oron-Karni et al., 1997
α2	Exon III	163509–163520	Cd 113–116; 12 bp del		R: Bst NI	Spain	Ayala et al., 1997
α2	Exon III	163519	Cd 116; G→T		C: Bfa I	Spanish	Ayala et al., 1996
α2	Termination codon	163597	TER; T→C (Constant Spring)	$\alpha^{CS}\alpha$	R: Mse I	Southeast Asian	Liebhaber et al., 1987; Clegg et al., 1971
α2	Termination codon	164597	TER; T→A (Icaria)	$\alpha^{Ic}\alpha$	R: Mse I	Mediterranean	Clegg et al., 1974; Efremov et al., 1990
α2	Termination codon	163598	TER; A→C (Koya Dora)	$\alpha^{KD}\alpha$	R: Mse I	Indian	De Jong et al. 1975
α2	Termination codon	163597	TER; T→G (Seal Rock)	$\alpha^{SR}\alpha$	R: Mse I	Black	Bradley et al., 1975; Merritt et al., 1997
α2	Termination codon	163599	TER; A→T (Paksé)		R: Mse I	Laotian	Waye et al., 1994
Posttranslational							
-α	Exon I	162954	Cd 14; T→G (Evanston) {W→R}			Black	Honig et al., 1984
α2	Exon I	163000	Cd 29; T→C (Argrinio) {L→P}			Mediterranean	Hall et al., 1993

(continued)

Table 17.3 (continued)

	Affected gene	Affected sequence	Location§	Mutation	Alternative notation	Identification	Distribution	Reference(s)
Posttranslational (con't)	α2	Exon I	163002–163004	Cd 30; 3 bp del {ΔE}			China	Chan et al., 1997
	α1	Exon II	163143–163145	Cd 38/39; 3 bp del; (Taybe) {ΔT}			Arabia	Pobedimskaya et al., 1994
	α1	Exon II	167011	Cd 59; G→A (Adana) {G→D}			Turkey	Çürük et al., 1993b
	α2	Exon II	163207	Cd 59; G→A (Adana) {G→D}			China	Chan et al., 1997
	α1	Exon II	167013–167018	Cd 60/61; 3 bp del (Clinic) {ΔK}		C: Dde I	Spain	Ayala et al., 1998
	α2	Exon II	163215–163217	Cd 62; 3 bp del			Greece	Harteveld, 1998
	α2	Exon III	163484	Cd 104; G→A (Sallanches) {C→Y}		C: Bsp MI	French	Morié et al., 1995
	α2	Exon III	163499	Cd 109; T→G (Suan Dok) {L→R}	$\alpha^{SD}\alpha$	C: Sma I	Southeast Asia	Sanguansermsri et al., 1979
	α	Exon III	(163502)	Cd 110; C→A (Petah Tikva) {A→D}	$\alpha^{PT}\alpha$		Middle East	Honig et al., 1981
	α2	Exon III	163547	Cd 125; T→C (Quong Sze) {L→P}	$\alpha^{QS}\alpha$	C: Msp I	Southeast Asia	Goossens et al., 1982
	$-\alpha^{3.7}$	Exon III	163547	Cd 125; T→A {L→Q}			Israel	Oran Kani (personal communication)
	α1	Exon III	167370	Cd 129; T→C (Tunis-Bizerte) {L→P}		C: Nci I	Tunisa	Darbellay et al., 1995
	α2	Exon III	163559	Cd 129; T→C (Utrecht) {L→P}		C: Hpa II	Netherlands	Harteveld et al., 1996a
	α2	Exon III	163561	Cd 130; G→C (Sun Prarie) {A→P}			Asian Indian	Harkness et al., 1990
	α2	Exon III	163564	Cd 131; T→C (Questembert) {S→P}			Yugoslavia	Rochette et al., 1995
	α2	Exon III	163580	Cd 136; T→C (Hb Bibba) {L→P}			Caucasian	Prchal et al., 1995
Uncharacterized	α	Unknown	Unknown	Not determined			Black	Mathew et al., 1983
	α	Unknown	Unknown	Not determined			Greek‡	Trent et al., 1986b
	α	Unknown	Unknown	Not determined			Pacific	Hill et al., 1987b

Abbreviations: R, removes; C, creates.

* This mutation has been found in both α2-like genes on an $\alpha\alpha\alpha^{anti3.7}$ chromosome present in Saudi Arabian individuals.
† The elongated α chains associated with Hb Wayne, which results from a frameshift (deletion of either C at α 138 or A at α 139 of the α2-globin gene) and Hb Grady, which results from a crossover in phase (with insertion of three residues at α 118) are not known to be associated with α thalassemia although the critical interactions that would clearly reveal this have not been described.
‡ Its interaction with α⁰-thalassemia determinants to produce the Hb Bart's hydrops fetalis syndrome suggests that both α-globin genes may be affected.
§ These numbers refer to the sequence published in Flint et al., (1997). Location in parentheses assumes α2 defect.

(0.78 to 0.85), their hematologic indices appear remarkably normal (Harteveld et al., 1996c). It remains to be seen if this applies to all carriers of the mutation.

A third splicing defect is caused by mutation of IVS1-117 of the α1-globin gene (α $^{IVS1\ 117;\ G \rightarrow A}$α) (Çürük et al., 1993a). In this case, the nature of the abnormal splicing has not been established. Furthermore, the evidence that this mutation causes α thalassemia is based solely on its consistent effect of lowering the level of HbS in individuals with sickle cell trait. In the future it will be interesting to document the full hematologic effect of this mutation in normal individuals.

Mutations Affecting the poly(A) Addition Signal. The highly conserved sequence motif AATAAA is present 10 to 30 bp upstream of most poly(A) addition sites and forms part of the signal for mRNA cleavage and polyadenylation of primary transcripts (see Chapter 6). This sequence is required for transcriptional termination and some evidence suggests that, when mutated, transcription may proceed into neighboring genes and "interfere" with their expression.

Presently there are four known mutations of the α2-gene polyadenylation signal (Table 17.3). The first to be identified (AATAAA→AATAAG) was found in the Saudi Arabian population. Heterozygotes have the hematologic phenotype of severe carriers of α-thalassemia trait but homozygotes have HbH disease with 5 percent to 15 percent HbH in their peripheral blood (Pressley et al., 1980b; Zhao, personal communication; and unpublished). The mechanisms by which this mutation causes such a severe phenotype are not fully understood.

Homozygotes for other nondeletion mutations that inactivate the α2 gene do not always have HbH disease and when present it is often mild with low levels of HbH (see below). By contrast homozygotes for the α$^{PA6;A \rightarrow G}$α haplotype always have HbH disease with high levels of HbH. It is interesting that in these individuals α2 mRNA is reduced but not absent and therefore, if the α1 gene were fully active, one would expect to see a severe form of α-thalassemia trait rather than HbH disease. The implication of these findings is that the poly(A) site mutation downregulates both α-globin genes on the same chromosome. In some rare individuals, the α$^{PA6;A \rightarrow G}$ mutation is duplicated producing a chromosome with three α-globin genes, α$^{PA6;A \rightarrow G}$ α$^{PA6;A \rightarrow G}$α, which still interacts with the α$^{PA6;A \rightarrow G}$α chromosome to produce HbH disease (Thein et al., 1988).

Analysis of the α$^{PA6;A \rightarrow G}$ mutation has shown that it has at least two effects. It reduces the amount of α2, mRNA that accumulates and, in a transient assay, readthrough transcripts extending beyond the mutated poly(A) addition site are detected. Recently, extended transcripts were also detected in reticulocytes of patients with this defect using RT-PCR (Molchanova et al., 1995). It seems possible that transcription extending through the normal termination point could run on and interfere with expression of the linked α1-globin gene.

Given the reduction in α-globin chain synthesis associated with the α$^{PA6;A \rightarrow G}$α haplotype, it is somewhat surprising that compound heterozygotes for this mutation and a common α^0-thalassemia determinant are not more severely affected (Zhao, personal communication).

Since the original description of the α$^{PA6;A \rightarrow G}$α allele, three other poly(A) signal mutations have been described (Table 17.3). At present there are insufficient data to know whether these mutations downregulate expression in a similar way. In particular, no homozygotes for these mutations have been identified. Compound heterozygotes for these mutations and α^0 thalassemia have HbH disease as expected (Fei et al., 1992; Yüregir et al., 1992; and unpublished).

Mutations Affecting Initiation of mRNA Translation. Several nondeletion mutations affect mRNA translation and five of them disrupt the initiation consensus sequence CCRCCATG (Table 17.3). Two mutations occur on chromosomes with a single α-globin gene. In one (−α$^{IN;\ A \rightarrow G}$), the mutation abolishes translation of mRNA from the gene. It was identified via its interaction with a second α-thalassemia chromosome, −α$^{IN;\ A}$/−α; affected patients had the typical hematologic features of HbH disease with 2.4 percent and 7.2 percent HbH (Olivieri et al., 1987). In the other case (−α$^{IN;2bp\ del}$) a 2-bp deletion from the consensus sequence reduces the level of mRNA translation by 30 percent to 50 percent (Morlé et al., 1985, 1986). This mutation produces HbH disease in homozygotes (−α$^{IN;2bp\ del}$/−α$^{IN;2bp\ del}$) who have a mild hypochromic microcytic anemia (hemoglobin level, 9.7 to 9.9, MCV 63 fl, MCH 18 to 20 pg) with 4.5 percent to 5.6 percent HbH (Tabone et al., 1981).

Two mutations (α$^{IN;\ T \rightarrow C}$ and α$^{IN;\ 1bp\ del}$) abolish translation of mRNA from the α2 gene. Six of seven homozygotes for the α$^{IN;\ T \rightarrow C}$α haplotype have a severe form of α-thalassemia trait but one had a mild form of HbH disease with 2.6 percent HbH (Cao et al., 1991; Galanello et al., 1991; Galanello et al., 1992; and unpublished). Compound heterozygotes for this mutation with common α^0-thalassemia defects have HbH disease with between 8 percent and 24 percent HbH in the blood.

One mutation (αα$^{IN;\ A \rightarrow G}$) abolishes translation of mRNA from the α1-globin gene (Moi et al., 1987). In the single family reported with this mutation, compound heterozygotes (- -/αα$^{IN;\ A \rightarrow G}$) had relatively low levels of HbH (1.5 percent and 3 percent), suggesting that mutation of the α1 gene causes a less severe degree of α-globin chain deficit than a similar mutation of the α2 gene. This mutation adds weight to the argument that the α2 gene is expressed at a higher level than the α1 gene.

In-frame Deletions, Frameshifts, and Nonsense Mutations.

In 1988, Safaya and Rieder (1988) described a black American with HbH disease and HbG Philadelphia ($-\alpha^{68\ \text{Asn}\rightarrow\text{Lys}}$) who synthesized only α^G and no α^A chains. The patient was shown to have the genotype $-\alpha/-\alpha^G$ and they therefore concluded that the $-\alpha$ chromosome was inactivated by a further mutation. Sequence analysis showed that this single α-globin gene has a dinucleotide deletion from one or other of the Glu (GAG) or Arg (AGG) codons (30 and 31). A loss of two nucleotides leads to a frameshift and a novel protein sequence in exon2 from codons 31–54 followed by a new, in-phase termination codon (TAA) at position 55. Hence the $-\alpha^{\text{Cd}30/31;2\text{bp del}}$ haplotype is an inactive α^0-thalassemia determinant.

Mutations affecting the α-globin translational reading frame have also been noted on chromosomes with two α-globin genes. Three affect the α2-globin gene. In one ($\alpha\alpha^{\text{Cd}39/41\text{del/ins}}\alpha$) there is a deletion of 9 bp (codons 39 to 41) replaced by an 8 nucleotide insertion that duplicates the adjacent downstream sequence. The mutation changes the mRNA reading frame, introducing a new termination signal (TGA) 10 codons downstream.

In another patient, a 12-bp deletion of the α2 gene results in the loss of four amino acids (codons 113–116) from the α-globin chain, which is reduced from its normal length of 141 amino acids to 137. It is thought that this produces an unstable α chain, which is rapidly broken down and unable to form a hemoglobin tetramer, like some mutants described below. In a heterozygote, this mutation produced the phenotype of α-thalassemia trait.

The third mutation in this group has a single base change ($\alpha^{\text{Cd}116;\ G\rightarrow T}$), which results in a premature termination codon and inactivation of the α2 gene. Again carriers for this mutation have α-thalassemia trait.

A single Spanish family with a frameshift mutation in the α1-globin gene has been described by Ayala et al. (1997). Two affected individuals ($\alpha\alpha^{\text{Cd}51-55;13\text{bp del}}/\alpha\alpha$) have α-thalassemia trait. Direct sequence analysis of the α1 gene revealed a 13-bp deletion, between codons 51 and 55. This mutation results in an mRNA reading frameshift that introduces a new stop signal at codon 62.

Chain Termination Mutants

Potentially nine single nucleotide variants of the natural termination codon (TAA) of the α2-globin gene can exist. Two (TGA and TAG) encode stop (nonsense) mutations; the others encode amino acids (Fig. 17.6).

When mutations change the stop codon to one of these amino acids they allow mRNA translation to continue to the next in-phase termination codon (UAA) located within the polyadenylation signal (AAUAAA), in each case extending the α-globin chain by 31 amino acids from the natural C-terminal arginine (codon 141). Of the six predicted α2-globin gene termination codon variants, five have been described, each with a unique amino acid at α142. These are Hb Constant Spring (α 142 Gln), Hb Icaria (α 142 Lys), Hb Koya Dora (α 142 Ser), Hb Seal Rock (α 142 Glu), and Hb Paksé (α 142 Tyr) (Table 17.3). An extended α-globin gene variant with leucine at position 142 is predicted but has not yet been described.

How chain termination mutants cause α thalassemia has been difficult to elucidate although there are now sufficient observations to provide a plausible explanation. Nevertheless, we still do not fully understand how the unusual hematologic phenotype associated with these mutations arises. Heterozygotes clearly have α thalassemia, but the MCV is higher than normally seen (for examples see Weatherall and Clegg, 1975; Schrier et al., 1997). Homozygotes have an unexpectedly severe form of thalassemia considering that only two of the four α-globin genes are inactive (Lie-Injo et al., 1974; Pootrakul et al., 1981) and compound heterozygotes have an unusually severe form of HbH disease (for example, see Fucharoen et al., 1988; and Chapter 18).

Hb Constant Spring is the most extensively studied of this group. Heterozygotes for the mutation $\alpha^{\text{TER};\ T\rightarrow C}\alpha/\alpha\alpha$ have about 1 percent Hb Constant Spring in their red cells rather than the 25 percent variant usually found in carriers of other point mutations (Weatherall and Clegg, 1975). It seems likely that the α2 gene containing this mutation is transcribed normally, although this has not been formally demonstrated. Substantial amounts of the abnormal α^{CS} mRNA are found in erythroid precursors from the bone marrow but the level decreases during erythroid maturation and is virtually absent from reticulocytes (Liebhaber and Kan, 1981; Hunt et al., 1982). The synthesis of α^{CS}-globin chains follows the same pattern, decreasing from bone marrow to reticulocytes (Kan et al., 1974; Weatherall and Clegg, 1975). From these findings it was suggested that α^{CS} mRNA is unstable, possibly due to disruption of a sequence in the 3′ noncoding region that is translated inappropriately as a result of the chain termination mutant (Hunt et al., 1982). There are now experimental data to support this interpretation. Weiss and Liebhaber (1994) showed that translational readthrough disrupts a putative RNA/protein complex associated with the α2 globin 3′UTR, which is required for mRNA stability in erythroid cells.

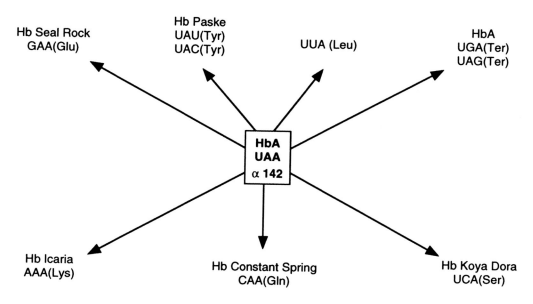

Figure 17.6. The potential and actual α-globin chain termination mutant hemoglobins that can be produced by a single base change in the α-globin gene termination codon α 142 UAA (redrawn from Weatherall and Clegg, 1975).

Unstable α-Globin Chain Variants Associated with α Thalassemia

Some globin variants alter the tertiary structure of the hemoglobin molecule, making the αβ dimer or tetramer unstable (see Chapters 14 and 44). Such molecules may precipitate within the red cell forming insoluble inclusions (Heinz bodies) that damage the red cell membrane. This situation classically causes a chronic hemolytic anemia with equal loss of α- and β-like globin chains from the red cell (see Chapter 44).

Over the past few years it has become apparent that some α-globin chain variants are so unstable that they undergo very rapid, postsynthetic degradation. In this case, since the α chains probably do not form dimers or tetramers, there is no associated loss of normal β-globin chains that remain, in excess within the red cell: Such patients, by definition, have α thalassemia. Many of these α-globin chain variants are so unstable that they cannot be detected by conventional protein analysis. Therefore, affected patients often present with nondeletional α thalassemia that can only be explained when the mutation is identified by DNA sequence analysis.

Such patients have complex hematologic findings because the defects may involve the α1- or α2-globin gene, may cause different degrees of instability, and may be greatly influenced by interacting alleles. For example, some mutants may be fully or temporarily stabilized when incorporated into a dimer or tetramer; the co-inheritance of α thalassemia will reduce the normal pool of free α-globin chains and drive abnormal α chains into dimers or tetramers. In this case, subsequent instability may cause loss of both α-like and β-like chains, changing the pathophysiology from α thalassemia to a hemolytic anemia. This is discussed further in Chapter 18. The easiest way to look at the effect of these mutations is to consider simple heterozygotes who usually have the phenotype of α-thalassemia trait with low or undetectable amounts of the α-globin variant. This contrasts with similar classes of mutations in the β-globin gene where simple heterozygotes have β thalassemia intermedia or the phenotype of Cooley's anemia (see Chapter 14).

To date, seventeen unstable α-globin gene variants have been shown to produce this phenotype to a greater or lesser extent (Table 17.3). Mutations affecting the heme pocket, internal hydrophobic regions of the molecule that normally maintain its conformation or hydrophobic residues involved in the formation of α1β1 contacts are most frequent (see Chapters 9 and 44).

MOLECULAR DIAGNOSIS OF α THALASSEMIA

Patients with well-defined phenotypes of α thalassemia (see Chapter 18) have inherited one or more of the determinants described in this chapter. Most common deletional forms of α thalassemia can be diagnosed by analyzing both α-globin-specific BamH I fragments and α-globin-specific Bgl II fragments using conventional Southern blot analyses (Old and Higgs, 1983). However, when both the α- and ζ-globin gene have been deleted (e.g., - -FIL, - -THAI; Fig. 17.3), breakpoints can only be identified using probes located outside of the α-globin gene complex.

Over the past few years several PCR-based analyses have been developed to diagnose the common forms of α^+ and α^0 thalassemia (see Figs. 17.2 and 17.3 and Table 17.3). Now that the entire sequence of the human α-globin gene cluster has been published (Flint et al., 1997) it is a simple matter to design primers to amplify any of the currently known α-globin deletions that have been described. However, one should bear in mind that although PCR-based assays will identify the deletions for which they are designed, they will not necessarily identify unexpected mutations that can often be suspected and confirmed by Southern blot analysis.

It is more difficult to screen for the nondeletional forms of α thalassemia. However, because the $\alpha1$ and $\alpha2$ genes can be amplified independently, those that cause a restriction site change can be readily identified (see Table 17.3). In the remaining cases for which one strongly suspects a nondeletion mutation, the simplest procedure is to screen with single strand conformation analysis, denaturing gradient gel electrophoresis, and/or DNA sequence analysis (for example, see Harteveld et al., 1996b).

CONCLUSIONS

This chapter has reviewed all of the natural sequence and structural variants that have been observed in and around the human α-globin gene cluster. These mutations have been of great value in pointing to regions of the chromosome that are important in the regulation of α-globin gene expression. Equally, some have ruled out other segments of the cluster as being important in this respect. From a clinical and hematologic point of view it is important to remember that the mutations which cause α thalassemia are among the most frequently encountered human genetic abnormalities (see Chapter 32) and in some areas of the world give rise to severe genetic diseases (see Chapter 18). The careful definition of these mutants has therefore underpinned the development of logical and comprehensive screening programs (see Chapters 18, 32, 35, and 36) to prevent the most severe forms of α thalassemia.

References

Albitar, M, Peschle, C, and Liebhaber, SA. (1989). Theta, zeta and epsilon globin messenger RNAs are expressed in adults. *Blood* 74: 629–637.

Ayala, S, Colomer, D, Pujades, A et al. (1996). Haemoglobin Lleida: A new α_2-globin variant (12 bp deletion) with mild thalassaemic phenotype. *Br. J. Haematol.* 94: 639–644.

Ayala, S, Colomer, D, Aymerich, M, Abella, E, and Vives Corrons, JL. (1997). First description of a frameshift mutation in the α_1-globin gene associated with α-thalassaemia. *Br. J. Haematol.* 98: 47–50.

Ayala, S, Colomer, D, Gelpi, JL, and Vives Corrons, JL. (1998). α-Thalassaemia due to a single codon deletion in the α_1-globin gene. Computational structural analysis of the new α-chain variant. Hum Mutat *11*, 412

Barbour, VM, Tufarelli, C, Sharpe JA et al. (2000). α-Thalassemia resulting from a negative chromosomal position effect. *Blood* (in press).

Baysal, E and Huisman, THJ. (1994). Detection of common deletional α-thalassaemia-2 determinants by PCR. *Am. J. Hematol.* 46: 208–213.

Bernet, A, Sabatier, S, Picketts, DJ et al. (1994). Targeted inactivation of the major positive regulatory element (HS –40) of the human α-globin gene locus. *Blood* 86: 1202–1211.

Blackburn, EH. (1992). Telomerases. *Ann. Rev. Biochem.* 61: 113–129.

Bowden, DK, Hill, AVS, Higgs, DR et al. (1987). Different hematologic phenotypes are associated with leftward ($-\alpha^{4.2}$) and rightward ($-\alpha^{3.7}$) α^+-thalassemia deletions. *J. Clin. Invest.* 79: 39–43.

Bowden, DK, Vickers, MA, and Higgs, DR. (1992). A PCR-based strategy to detect the common severe determinants of α thalassaemia. *Br. J. Haematol.* 81: 104–108.

Bradley, TB, Wohl, RC, and Smith, GJ. (1975). Elongation of the α-globin chain in a black family: Interaction with HbG Philadelphia. *Clin. Res.* 23: 1314.

Bruzdzinski, CJ, Sisco, KL, Ferrucci, SJ, and Rucknagel, DL. (1984). The occurrence of the $\alpha^{\text{G-Philadelphia}}$-globin allele on a double-locus chromosome. *Am. J. Hum. Genet.* 36: 101–109.

Buckle, VJ, Higgs, DR, Wilkie, AOM et al. (1988). Localisation of human α globin to 16p13.3-pter. *J. Med. Genet.* 25: 847–849.

Camaschella, C, Bertero, MT, Serra, A et al. (1987). A benign form of thalassaemia intermedia may be determined by the interaction of triplicated α locus and heterozygous β thalassaemia. *Br. J. Haematol.* 66: 103–107.

Cao, A, Rosatelli, C, Pirastu, M, and Galanello, R. (1991). Thalassemias in Sardinia: Molecular pathology, phenotype-genotype correlation and prevention. *Am. J. Pediatr. Hematol. Oncol.* 13: 179–188.

Chan, V, Chan, TK, Liang, ST et al. (1985). Hydrops fetalis due to an unusual form of HbH disease. *Blood* 66: 224–228.

Chan, V, Chan, TK, Cheng, MY et al. (1986). Organization of the ζ-α genes in Chinese. *Bri. J. Haematol.* 64: 97–105.

Chan, V, Chan, VWY, Tang, M et al. (1997). Molecular defects in HbH hydrops fetalis. *Br. J. Haematol.* 96: 224–228.

Chong, SS, Boehm, CD, Higgs, DR, and Cutting, GR. (2000). Single-tube multiplex-PCR screen for common deletional determinants of α-thalassemia. *Blood* 95: 360–362.

Chui, DHK, Wong, SC, Chung, SW et al. (1986). Embryonic ζ-globin chains in adults: A marker for α-thalassemia-1 haplotype due to a >17.5 kb deletion. *N. Engl. J. Med.* 314: 76–79.

Chui, DHK, Mentzer, WC, Patterson, M et al. (1989). Human embryonic ζ-globin chains in fetal and newborn blood. *Blood* 74: 1409–1414.

Clegg, JB, Weatherall, DJ, and Milner, PG. (1971). Haemoglobin Constant Spring—a chain termination mutant? *Nature* 234: 337–340.

Clegg, JB, Weatherall, DJ, Contopoulos-Griva, I, Caroutsos, K et al. (1974). Haemoglobin Icaria, a new chain termination mutant which causes α-thalassaemia. *Nature* 251: 245–247.

Collier, S, Tassabehji, M, and Strachan, T. (1993). A *de novo* pathological point mutation at the 21-hydroxylase locus: Implications for gene conversion in the human genome. *Nat. Genet.* 3: 260–265.

Costa, FF, Sonati, MF, and Zago, MA. (1990). Hemoglobin Stanleyville II (α78 Asn→Lys) is associated with a 3.7 kb α gene deletion. *Hum. Genet.* 86: 319–320.

Çürük, MA, Baysal, E, Gupta, RB, and Huisman, THJ. (1993a). An IVS-I-117 (G→A) acceptor splice site mutation in the α1-globin gene is a nondeletional α-thalassaemia-2 determinant in an Indian population. *Br. J. Haematol.* 85: 148–152.

Çürük, MA, Dimovski, AJ, Baysal, E et al. (1993b). Hb Adana or $α_2 59(E8)Gly→Aspβ_2$, a severely unstable $α_1$-globin variant, observed in combination with the $-(α)20.5$ kb α-thal-1 deletion in two Turkish patients. *Am. J. Hematol.* 44: 270–275.

Darbellay, R, Mach-Pascual, S, Rose, K et al. (1995). Haemoglobin Tunis-Bizerte: A new $α_1$ globin 129 Leu→Pro unstable variant with thalassaemic phenotype. *Br. J. Haematol.* 90: 71–76.

De Angioletti, M, Lacerra, G, Castaldo, C et al. (1992). $αααα^{anti3.7\ type\ II}$: A new α-globin gene rearrangement suggesting that the α-globin gene duplication could be caused by intrachromosomal recombination. *Hum. Genet.* 89: 37–41.

De Jong, WW, Khan, PM, and Bernini, LF. (1975). Hemoglobin Koya Dora: High frequency of a chain termination mutant. *Am. J. Hum. Genet.* 27: 81–90.

Del Senno, L, Bernardi, F, Marchetti, G et al. (1980). Organisation of α-globin genes and mRNA translation in subjects carrying haemoglobin Hasharon (α47 Asp-His) from the Ferrara region (Northern Italy). *Eur. J. Biochem.* 111: 125–130.

Di Rienzo, A, Novelletto, A, Aliquo, MC et al. (1986). Molecular basis for HbH disease in Italy: Geographical distribution of deletional and non-deletional α-thalassaemia haplotypes. *Am. J. Hum. Genet.* 39: 631–639.

Dodé, C, Krishnamoorthy, R, Lamb, J, and Rochette, J. (1993). Rapid analysis of $-α^{3.7}$ thalassaemia and $ααα^{3.7}$ triplication by enzymatic amplification analysis. *Br. J. Haematol.* 83: 105–111.

Efremov, GD, Josifovska, O, Nikolov, N et al. (1990). Hb Icaria-HbH disease: Identification of the Hb Icaria mutation through analysis of amplified DNA. *Br. J. Haematol.* 75: 250–253.

Embury, SH, Miller, JA, Dozy, AM et al. (1980). Two different molecular organizations account for the single α-globin gene of the α-thalassaemia-2 genotype. *J. Clin. Invest.* 66: 1319–1325.

European Polycystic Kidney Disease Consortium. (1994). The polycystic kidney disease 1 gene encodes a 14 kb transcript and lies within a duplicated region on chromosome 16. *Cell* 77: 881–894.

Fei, YJ, Fujita, S, and Huisman, THJ. (1988). Two different theta (θ)-globin gene deletions observed among black newborn babies. *Br. J. Haematol.* 68: 249–254.

Fei, YJ, Kutlar, F, Harris, HF et al. (1989). A search for anomalies in the ζ, α, β, and γ globin gene arrangements in normal Black, Italian, Turkish and Spanish newborns. *Hemoglobin* 13: 45–65.

Fei, YJ, Liu, JC, Walker, ELDI, and Huisman, THJ. (1992). A new gene deletion involving the α2-, α1-, and θ1-globin genes in a Black family with HbH disease. *Am. J. Hematol.* 39: 299–303.

Felbar, BK, Orkin, SH, and Hamer, DH. (1982). Abnormal RNA splicing causes one form of α-thalassaemia. *Cell* 29: 895–902.

Felice, AE, Cleek, MP, McKie, K et al. (1984). The rare α-thalassaemia-1 of Blacks is a ζα-thalassaemia-1 associated with deletion of all α- and ζ-globin genes. *Blood* 63: 1253–1257.

Felice, AE, Cleek, MP, Marino, EM et al. (1986). Different ζ-globin gene deletions among black Americans. *Hum. Genet.* 73: 221–224.

Fichera, M, Rappazzo, G, Spalletta, A et al. (1994). Triplicated α-globin gene locus with translocation of the whole telomeric end in association with β-thalassaemia trait, results in a severe syndrome. *Blood* 84: 260a.

Fischel-Ghodsian, N, Higgs, DR, and Beyer, EC. (1987). Function of a new globin gene. *Nature* 329: 397.

Fischel-Ghodsian, N, Vickers, MA, Seip, M et al. (1988). Characterization of two deletions that remove the entire human ζ-α globin gene complex (- -^{Thai} and - -^{Fil}). *Br. J. Haematol.* 70: 233–238.

Flint, J, Hill, AVS, Bowden, DK, Oppenheimer, SJ et al. (1986). High frequencies of α thalassaemia are the result of natural selection by malaria. *Nature* 321: 744–749.

Flint, J, Craddock, CF, Villegas, A et al. (1994). Healing of broken human chromosomes by the addition of telomeric repeats. *Am. J. Hum. Genet.* 55: 505–512.

Flint, J, Rochette, J, Craddock, CF et al. (1996). Chromosomal stabilisation by a subtelomeric rearrangement involving two closely related *Alu* elements. *Hum. Mol. Genet.* 5: 1163–1169.

Flint, J, Thomas, K, Micklem, G et al. (1997). The relationship between chromosome structure and function at a human telomeric region. *Nat. Genet.* 15: 252–257.

Fortina, P, Delgrosso, K, Rappaport, E et al. (1988). A large deletion encompassing the entire α-like globin gene cluster in a family of Northern European extraction. *Nucl. Acids Res.* 16: 11223–11235.

Fortina, P, Dianzani, I, Serra, A et al. (1991). A newly-characterized α-thalassaemia-1 deletion removes the entire α-like globin gene cluster in an Italian family. *Br. J. Haematol* 78: 529–534.

Fortina, P, Parrella, T, Sartore, M et al. (1994). Interaction of a rare illegitimate recombination event and a poly A addition site mutation resulting in a severe form of α thalassaemia. *Blood* 83: 3356–3362.

Fowler, SJ, Gill, P, Werrett, DJ, and Higgs, DR. (1988). Individual specific DNA fingerprints from a hypervariable region probe: α-globin 3′HVR. *Hum. Genet.* 79: 142–146.

Fucharoen, S, Winichagoon, P, Pootrakul, P et al. (1988). Differences between two types of HbH disease, α-thalassemia 1/α-thalassemia 2 and α-thalassemia 1/Hb Constant Spring. *Birth Defects: Original Articles Series* 23: 309–315.

Galanello, R, Aru, B, Dessì, C et al. (1992). HbH disease in Sardinia: Molecular, haematological and clinical aspects. *Acta Haematol. (Basel)* 88: 1–6.

Galanello, R, Monne MI, Paderi, L et al. (1991). Homozygous non-deletion α 2 globin gene mutation (initiation codon mutation): clinical and haematological phenotype. *Brit. J. Haematol.* 79: 117–119.

Galanello, R, Ruggeri, R, Paglietti, E et al. (1983). A family with segregating triplicated alpha globin loci and beta thalassemia. *Blood* 62: 1035–1040.

Germino, GG, Barton, NJ, Lamb, J et al. (1990). Identification of a locus which shows no genetic recombination with the autosomal dominant polycystic kidney disease gene on chromosome 16. *Am. J. Hum. Genet.* 46: 925–933.

Giglioni, B, Comi, P, Taramelli, R et al. (1980). Organization of α-globin genes in Hb Hasharon (α47 asp-his) carriers. *Blood* 56: 1145–1149.

Gonzalez-Redondo, JM, Diaz-Chico, JC. Malcorra-Azpiazu, JJ et al. (1988). Characterization of a newly discovered α-thalassaemia-1 in two Spanish patients with HbH disease. *Br. J. Haematol.* 70: 459–463.

Gonzalez-Redondo, JM, Gilsanz, F, and Ricard, P. (1989). Characterization of a new α-thalassemia-1 deletion in a Spanish family. *Hemoglobin* 13: 103–116.

Goodbourn, SEY, Higgs, DR, Clegg, JB, and Weatherall, DJ. (1983). Molecular basis of length polymorphism in the human ζ-globin gene complex. *Proc. Nat. Acad. Sci. U.S.A.* 80: 5022–5026.

Goossens, M, Dozy, AM, Embury, SH et al. (1980). Triplicated α-globin loci in humans. *Proc. Natl. Acad. Sci. U.S.A.* 77: 518–521.

Goossens, M, Lee, KY, Liebhaber, SA, and Kan, YW. (1982). Globin structural mutant $\alpha^{125Leu-Pro}$ is a novel cause of α-thalassaemia. *Nature* 296: 864–865.

Gu, YC, Landman, H, and Huisman, THJ. (1987). Two different quadruplicated α-globin gene arrangements. *Br. J. Haematol.* 66: 245–250.

Hall, GW, Thein, SL, Newland, AC et al. (1993). A base substitution (T→C) in codon 29 of the α2-globin gene causes α thalassaemia. *Br. J. Haematol.* 85: 546–552.

Hall, GW, Higgs, DR, Murphy, A et al. (1994). A mutation in the polyadenylation signal of the α2 globin gene (AATAAA → AATA- -) as a cause of α thalassaemia in Asian Indians. *Br. J. Haematol.* 88: 225–227.

Harkness, M, Harkness, DR, Kutlar, F et al. (1990). Hb Sun Prairie or α-2130 (H13)Ala→Pro-β—2: A new unstable variant occurring in low quantities. *Hemoglobin* 14: 479–490.

Harris, PC, Barton, NJ, Higgs, DR et al. (1990). A long range restriction map between the α-globin complex and a marker closely linked to the polycystic kidney disease I (PKDI) locus. *Genomics* 7: 195–206.

Harris, PC, and Higgs, DR. (1993). Structure of the terminal region of the short arm of chromosome 16. In Davies, KE, and Tilghman, SM, editors. *Genome analysis.* Cold Spring Harbor Laboratory Press. pp. 107–134.

Harteveld, CL, Losekoot, M, Haak, H et al. (1994). A novel polyadenylation signal mutation in the α2-globin gene causing α thalassaemia. *Br. J. Haematol.* 87: 139–143.

Harteveld, CL, Giordano, PC, Losekoot, M et al. (1996a). Hb Utrecht [α2 129(H12)Leu→Pro] a new unstable α2-chain variant in *cis* to a ζ-gene triplication and associated with a mild α-thalassemic phenotype. *Br. J. Haematol.* 94: 483–485.

Harteveld, CL, Heister, JG, Giordano, PC et al. (1996b). Rapid detection of point mutations and polymorphisms of the α-globin genes by DGGE and SSCA. *Hum. Mutat.* 7: 114–122.

Harteveld, CL, Heister, JG, Giordano, PC et al. (1996c). An IVS-1-116 (A→G) acceptor splice site mutation in the α2-globin gene causing α+-thalassaemia in two Dutch families. *Br. J. Haematol.* 95: 461–466.

Harteveld, CL, Losekoot, M, Fodde, R et al. (1997). The involvement of Alu repeats in recombination events at the α-globin gene cluster: Characterization of two α0-thalassemia deletion breakpoints. *Hum. Genet.* 99: 528–534.

Harteveld, CL. (1998). The molecular genetics of α-thalassemia: Structure and expression of the α-globin gene cluster. Thesis. Ridderprint, Ridderkerk, The Netherlands.

Harteveld, CL, Muglia, M, Passarino, G et al. (Submitted). Genetic polymorphism of the major regulatory element upstream of the human α-globin gene cluster.

Hatton, C, Wilkie, AOM, Drysdale, HC et al. (1990). Alpha thalassemia caused by a large (62 kb) deletion upstream of the human α globin gene cluster. *Blood* 76: 221–227.

Henni, T, Belhani, M, Morle, F et al. (1986). α-Globin gene triplication in severe heterozygous β-thalassemia. *Acta Haematol.* 74: 236–239.

Henthorn, PS, Smithies, O, and Mager, DL. (1990). Molecular analysis of deletions in the human β-globin gene cluster: Deletion junctions and locations of breakpoints. *Genomics* 6: 226–237.

Hess, JF, Schmid, CW, and Shen, C-KJ. (1984). A gradient of sequence divergence in the human adult α-globin duplication units. *Science* 226: 67–70.

Higgs, DR, Hunt, DM, Drysdale, HC, Clegg, JB et al. (1980a). The genetic basis of Hb Q-H disease. *Br. J. Haematol.* 46: 387–400.

Higgs, DR, Old, JM, Pressley, L et al. (1980b). A novel α-globin gene arrangement in man. *Nature* 284: 632–635.

Higgs, DR, Pressley, L, Aldridge, B et al. (1981). Genetic and molecular diversity in nondeletion HbH disease. *Proc. Natl. Acad. Sci. U.S.A.* 78: 5833–5837.

Higgs, DR, Goodbourn, SEY, Lamb, J et al. (1983). α-Thalassaemia caused by a polyadenylation signal mutation. *Nature* 306: 398–400.

Higgs, DR, Clegg, JB, Weatherall, DJ et al (1984a). Interaction of the ααα-globin gene haplotype and sickle haemoglobin. *Br. J. Haematol.* 58: 671–678.

Higgs, DR, Hill, AVS, Bowden, DK et al. (1984b). Independent recombination events between duplicated human α-globin genes: Implications for their concerted evolution. *Nucl. Acids Res.* 12: 6965–6977.

Higgs, DR, Ayyub, H, Clegg, JB, Hill, AVS et al. (1985). α-Thalassaemia in British people. *Br. Med. J.* 290: 1303–1306.

Higgs, DR, Wainscoat, JS, Flint, J et al. (1986). Analysis of the human α-globin gene cluster reveals a highly informative genetic locus. *Proc. Natl. Acad. Sci. U.S.A.* 83: 5165–5169.

Higgs, DR, Vickers, MA, Wilkie, AOM et al. (1989). A review of the molecular genetics of the human α-globin gene cluster. *Blood* 73: 1081–1104.

Higgs, DR, Wood, WG, Jarman, AP et al. (1990). A major positive regulatory region located far upstream of the human α-globin gene locus. *Genes Dev.* 4: 1588–1601.

Higgs, DR, Wilkie, AOM, Vyas, P et al. (1993). Characterisation of the telomeric region of human chromosome 16p. *Chromosomes Today* 11: 35–47.

Higgs, DR, Sharpe, JA, and Wood, WG. (1998). Understanding α globin gene expression: A step towards effective gene therapy. *Sem. Hematol.* 35: 93–104.

Hill, AVS. (1985). The distribution and molecular basis of thalassemia in Oceania. PhD Thesis, Oxford University.

Hill, AVS, Nicholls, RD, Thein, SL, and Higgs, DR. (1985). Recombination within the human embryonic ζ-globin locus: A common ζ-ζ chromosome produced by gene conversion of the Ψζ gene. *Cell* 42: 809–819.

Hill, AVS, Gentile, B, Bonnardot, JM et al. (1987a). Polynesian origins and affinities: Globin gene variants in Eastern Polynesia. *Am. J. Hum. Genet.* 40: 453–463.

Hill, AVS, Thein, SL, Mavo, B et al. (1987b). Non-deletion haemoglobin H disease in Papua New Guinea. *J. Med. Genet.* 24: 767–771.

Honig, GR, Shamsuddin, M, Mason, RG et al. (1980). Hemoglobin Nigeria (α-81 Ser→Cys): A new variant associated with α-thalassemia. *Blood* 55: 131–137.

Honig, GR, Shamsuddin, M, Zaizov, R, St et al. (1981). Hemoglobin Peta Tikvah (α110 Ala-Asp): A new unstable variant with α-thalassemia-like expression. *Blood* 57: 705–711.

Honig, GR, Shamsuddin, M, Vida, LN et al. (1984). Hemoglobin Evanston (α14 Trp→Arg): An unstable α-chain variant expressed as α-thalassemia. *J. Clin. Invest.* 73: 1740–1749.

Hunt, DM, Higgs, DR, Winichagoon, P et al (1982). Haemoglobin Constant Spring has an unstable α chain messenger RNA. *Br. J. Haematol.* 51: 405–413.

Indrak, K, Gu, Y-C, Novotny, J, and Huisman, THJ. (1993). A new α-thalassemia-2 deletion resulting in microcytosis and hypochromia and *in vitro* chain imbalance in the heterozygote. *Am. J. Hematol.* 43: 144–145.

Jarman, AP, Wood WG, Sharpe, JA et al. (1991). Characterization of the major regulatory element upstream of the human α-globin gene cluster. *Mol. Cell. Biol.* 11: 4679–4689.

Jeffreys, AJ. (1987). Highly variable minisatellites and DNA fingerprints. *Biochem. Soc. Trans.* 15: 309–317.

Jinks-Robertson, S, Michelitch, M, and Ramcharan, S. (1993). Substrate length requirements for efficient mitotic recombination in *Saccharomyces cerevisiae*. *Mol. Cell. Biol.* 13: 3937–3950.

Kan, YW, Todd, D, and Dozy, AM. (1974). Haemoglobin Constant Spring synthesis in red cell precursors. *Br. J. Haematol.* 28: 103–107.

Kan, YW, Dozy, AM, Trecartin, R, and Todd, D. (1977). Identification of a nondeletion defect in α-thalassemia. *N. Engl. J. Med.* 297: 1081–1084.

Ko, T-M, Tseng, L-H, Kao, C-H et al. (1998). Molecular characterization and PCR diagnosis of Thailand deletion of α-globin gene cluster. *Am. J. Hematol.* 57: 124–130.

Kulozik, AE, Thein, SL, Wainscoat, JS et al. (1987). Thalassaemia intermedia; interaction of the triple α-globin gene arrangement and heterozygous β-thalassaemia. *Br. J. Haematol.* 66: 109–112.

Kulozik, A, Kar, BC, Serjeant, BE et al. (1988). α-thalassemia in India: Its interaction with sickle cell disease. *Blood* 71: 467–472.

Kutlar, F, Gonzalez-Redondo, JM, Kutlar, A et al. (1989). The levels of ζ, γ, and δ chains in patients with HbH disease. *Hum. Genet.* 82: 179–186.

Lacerra, G, Fioretti, G, De Angioletti, M et al. (1991). (α)α$^{5.3}$: A novel α$^+$-thalassemia deletion with the breakpoints in the α2-globin gene and in close proximity to an Alu family repeat between the Ψα2- and Ψα1-globin genes. *Blood* 78: 2740–2746.

Lamb, J and Clegg, JB. (1996). Measurement of aberrant recombination between duplicated globin genes in normal human sperm. *Am. J. Hum. Genet.* 59: A306.

Lamb, J, Wilkie, AOM, Harris, PC et al. (1989). Detection of breakpoints in submicroscopic chromosomal translocation, illustrating an important mechanism for genetic disease. *Lancet* 2: 819–824.

Lamb, J, Harris, PC, Wilkie, AOM et al. (1993). De novo truncation of chromosome 16p and healing with (TTAGGG)$_n$ in the α-thalassemia/mental retardation syndrome (ATR-16). *Am. J. Hum. Genet.* 52: 668–676.

Lambridis, AJ, Ramsay, M, and Jenkins, T. (1986). The haematological puzzle of Hb J Cape Town is partly solved. *Br. J. Haematol.* 63: 363–368.

Lauer, J, Shen, C-KJ, and Maniatis, T. (1980). The chromosomal arrangement of human α-like globin genes: Sequence homology and α-globin gene deletions. *Cell* 20: 119–130.

Leung, S-O, Proudfoot, NJ, and Whitelaw, E. (1987). The gene for θ-globin is transcribed in human fetal erythroid tissues. *Nature* 329: 551–554.

Ley, TJ, Maloney, KA, Gordon, JI, and Schwartz, AL. (1989). Globin gene expression in erythroid human fetal liver cells. *J. Clin. Invest.* 83: 1032–1038.

Liang, S, Tang, Z, Su, C et al. (1988). Hb Duan [α75(EF4)ASP→ALA], Hb Westmead [α122(H5)HIS→GLN], and α-thalassemia-2 (–4.2 kb deletion) in a Chinese family. *Hemoglobin* 12: 13–22.

Lie-Injo, LE, Ganesan, J, Clegg, JB, and Weatherall, DJ. (1974). Homozygous state for Hb Constant Spring (slow moving Hb X components). *Blood* 43: 251–259.

Lie-Injo, LE, Dozy, AM, Kan, YW, Lopes, M et al. (1979). The α-globin gene adjacent to the gene for HbQ-α 74 Asp-His is deleted, but not that adjacent to the gene for HbG-α 30 Glu Gln; three fourths of the α-globin genes are deleted in HbQ-α-thalassemia. *Blood* 54: 1407–1416.

Liebhaber, SA and Kan, YW. (1981). Differentiation of the mRNA transcripts originating from the α1- and α2-globin loci in normals and α-thalassemics. *J. Clin. Invest.* 68: 439–446.

Liebhaber, SA and Cash, FE. (1985). Locus assignment of α-globin structural mutations by hybrid-selected translation. *J. Clin. Invest.* 75: 64–70.

Liebhaber, SA, Rappaport, FE, Cash, FE et al. (1984). Hemoglobin I mutation encoded at both α-globin loci on the same chromosome: Concerted evolution in the human genome. *Science* 226: 1449–1451.

Liebhaber, SA, Cash, FE, and Main, DM. (1985). Compensatory increase in α1-globin gene expression in individuals heterozygous for the α-thalassemia-2 deletion. *J. Clin. Invest.* 76: 1057–1064.

Liebhaber, SA, Cash, FE, and Ballas, SK. (1986). Human α-globin gene expression. The dominant role of the α2-locus in mRNA and protein synthesis. *J. Biol. Chem.* 261: 15327–15333.

Liebhaber, SA, Coleman, MB, Adams, JGI et al. (1987). Molecular basis for non-deletion α-thalassemia in American blacks α2[116GAG->UAG]. *J. Clin. Invest.* 80: 154–159.

Liebhaber, SA, Griese, E-U, Weiss, I et al. (1990). Inactivation of human α-globin gene expression by a *de novo* deletion located upstream of the α-globin gene cluster. *Proc. Natl. Acad. Sci. U.S.A.* 81: 9431–9435.

Mathew, CGP, Rousseau, J, Rees, JS, and Harley, EH. (1983). The molecular basis of α-thalassaemia in a South African population. *Br. J. Haematol.* 55: 103–111.

Mavilio, F, Marinucci, M, Massa, A et al. (1980). Hemoglobin Hasharon (α2 47(CD5) Asp-His β2) linked to α-thalassemia in Northern Italian carriers. *Acta Haematol.* 63: 305–311.

Merritt, D, Jones, RT, Head, C et al. (1997). Hb Seal Rock [(α2) 142 Term→Glu, codon 142 TAA→GAA]: An extended α chain variant associated with anemia, microcytosis, and α-thalassemia-2 (–3.7 kb). *Hemoglobin* 21: 331–334.

Michelson, AM and Orkin, SH. (1983). Boundaries of gene conversion within the duplicated human α-globin genes. Concerted evolution by segmental recombination. *J. Biol. Chem.* 258: 15245–15254.

Moi, P, Cash, FE, Liebhaber, SA et al. (1987). An initiation codon mutation (AUG→GUG) of the human α1-globin gene: Structural characterization and evidence for a mild thalassemia phenotype. *J. Clin. Invest.* 80: 1416–1421.

Molchanova, TP, Pobedimskaya, DD, and Huisman, THJ. (1994). The differences in quantities of α2- and α1-globin gene variants in heterozygotes. *Br. J. Haematol.* 88: 300–306.

Molchanova, TP, Smetanina, NS, and Huisman, THJ. (1995). A second, elongated, α2-globin mRNA is present in reticulocytes from normal persons and subjects with terminating codon or poly A mutations. *Biochem. Biophys. Res. Commun.* 214: 1184–1190.

Moo-Penn, WF, Jue, DL, and Baine, RM. (1978). Hemoglobin J Rovigo (α53 Ala→Asp) in association with β-thalassemia. *Hemoglobin* 2: 443–445.

Morlé, F, Lopez, B, Henni, T, and Godet, J. (1985). α-Thalassaemia associated with the deletion of two nucleotides at position –2 and –3 preceding the AUG codon. *EMBO J.* 4: 1245–1250.

Morlé, F, Starck, J, and Godet, J. (1986). α-Thalassemia due to the deletion of nucleotides –2 and –3 preceding the AUG initiation codon affects translation efficiency both in vitro and in vivo. *Nucl. Acids Res.* 14: 3279–3292.

Morlé, F, Francina, A, Ducrocq, R et al. (1995). A new α chain variant Hb Sallanches [α2 104(G11) Cys→Tyr] associated with HbH disease in one homozygous patient. *Br. J. Haematol.* 91: 608–611.

Nakatsuji, T, Landman, H, and Huisman, THJ. (1986). An elongated segment of DNA observed between two human α-globin genes. *Hum. Genet.* 74: 368–371.

Nicholls, RD, Higgs, DR, Clegg, JB, and Weatherall, DJ. (1985). α0-Thalassemia due to recombination between the α1-globin gene and an *Alu*I repeat. *Blood* 65: 1434–1438.

Nicholls, RD, Fischel-Ghodsian, N, and Higgs, DR. (1987). Recombination at the human α-globin gene cluster: Sequence features and topological constraints. *Cell* 49: 369–378.

Old, JM, and Higgs, DR. (1983). Gene analysis. In Weatherall, DJ, editor. *The thalassemias, methods in hematology.* Edinburgh: Churchill Livingstone. pp. 74–102.

Old, JM, Clegg, JB, Weatherall, DJ, and Booth, PB. (1978). Haemoglobin J. Tongariki is associated with α thalassaemia. *Nature* 273: 319–320.

Olivieri, NF, Chang, LS, Poon, AO et al. (1987). An α-globin gene initiation codon mutation in a Black family with HbH disease. *Blood* 70: 729–732.

Orkin, SH and Goff, SC. (1981). The duplicated human α-globin genes: Their relative expression as measured by RNA analysis. *Cell* 24: 345–351.

Orkin, SH, Goff, SC, and Hechtman, RL. (1981). Mutation in an intervening sequence splice junction in man. *Proc. Natl. Acad. Sci. U.S.A.* 78: 5041–5045.

Oron-Karni, V, Filon, D, Rund, D, and Oppenheim, A. (1997). A novel mechanism generating short deletion/insertions following slippage is suggested by a mutation in the human α2-globin gene. *Hum. Mol. Genet.* 6: 881–885.

Paglietti, E, Galanello, R, Moi, P et al. (1986). Molecular pathology of haemoglobin H disease in Sardinians. *Br. J. Haematol.* 63: 485–496.

Peschle, C, Mavilio, F, Care, A et al. (1985). Haemoglobin switching in human embryos: Asynchrony of ζ-α and ε-γ-globin switches in primitive and definite erythropoietic lineage. *Nature* 313: 235–238.

Pich, PG, Gallo, E, Mazza, U, and Ricco, G. (1973). Study on a case of double heterogosis between Hb C and beta-thalassaemia. *Boll. Soc. Ital. Biol. Sper.* 49: 507–512.

Pirastu, M, Saglio G, Chang, JC et al. (1984). Initiation codon mutation as a cause of α-thalassemia. *J. Biol. Chem.* 259: 12315–12317.

Pobedimskaya, DD, Molchanova, TP, Streichman, S, and Huisman, THJ. (1994). Compound heterozygosity for two α-globin gene defects Hb Taybe (α1; 38 or 39 minus Thr) and a poly A mutation (α2; AATAAA→AATAAG), results in a severe hemolytic anemia. *Am. J. Hematol.* 47: 198–202.

Pootrakul, P, Winichagoon, P, Fucharoen, S, Pravatmuang, P et al. (1981). Homozygous haemoglobin Constant Spring: A need for revision of concept. *Hum. Genet.* 59: 250–255.

Prchal, JT, Adler, B, Wilson, JB et al. (1995). Hb Bibba or α-2 136(H19)Leu→Pro-β-2 in a caucasian family from Alabama. *Hemoglobin* 19: 151–164.

Pressley, L, Higgs, DR, Aldridge, B et al. (1980a). Characterisation of a new thalassaemia 1 defect due to a partial deletion of the α globin gene complex. *Nucl. Acids Res.* 8: 4889–4898.

Pressley, L, Higgs, DR, Clegg, JB et al. (1980b). A new genetic basis for hemoglobin-H disease. *N. Engl. J. Med.* 303: 1383–1388.

Pressley, L, Higgs, DR, Clegg, JB, and Weatherall, DJ. (1980c). Gene deletions in α thalassaemia prove that the 5′ ζ locus is functional. *Proce. Na. Acad. Sci. U.S.A.* 77: 3586–3589.

Proudfoot, NJ, Gil, A, and Maniatis, T. (1982). The structure of the human ζ-globin gene and a closely linked, nearly identical pseudogene. *Cell* 31: 553–563.

Proudfoot, NJ (1986). Transcriptional interference and termination between duplicated α-globin gene constructs suggests a novel mechanism for gene regulation. *Nature* 322: 562–565.

Rappaport, EF, Schwartz, E, Poncz, M, and Surrey, S. (1984). Frequent occurrence of a ζ-globin region deletion in American Blacks accounts for a previously-described restriction site polymorphism. *Biochem. Biophys. Res. Communic.* 125, 817–823.

Rochette, J, Barnetson, R, Varet, B et al. (1995). Hb Questembert is due to a base substitution (T → C) in codon 131 of the α2-globin gene and has an α-thalassemia biosynthetic ratio. *Am. J. Hematol.* 48: 289–290.

Royle, NJ, Clarkson, RE, Wong, Z, and Jeffreys, AJ. (1988). Clustering of hypervariable minisatellites in the proterminal regions of human autosomes. *Genomics* 3: 352–360.

Sabath, DE, Detter, JC, and Tait, JF. (1994). A novel deletion of the entire α globin locus causing α-thalassemia-1 in a Northern European family. *Hematopathology* 102: 650–654.

Safaya, S and Rieder, RF. (1988). Dysfunctional α-globin gene in hemoglobin H disease in blacks. *J. Biol. Chem.* 263: 4328–4332.

Sampietro, M, Cazzola, M, Cappellini, MD, and Fiorelli, G. (1983). The triplicated alpha-gene locus and heterozygous beta thalassaemia: A case of thalassaemia intermedia. *Br. J. Haematol.* 55: 709–710.

Sancar, GB, Tatsis, B, Cedeno, MM, and Rieder, RF. (1980). Proportion of hemoglobin G Philadelphia ($\alpha_2^{68Asn-Lys}\beta_2$) in heterozygotes is determined by α-globin gene deletions. *Proc. Natl. Acad. Sci. U.S.A.* 77: 6874–6878.

Sanguansermsri, T, Matragoon, S, Changloah, L, and Flatz, G. (1979). Hemoglobin Suan-Dok ($\alpha_2^{109(G16)Leu-Arg}\beta_2$): An unstable variant associated with α-thalassemia. *Hemoglobin* 3: 161–174.

Schrier, SL, Bunyaratvej, A, Khukapinant, A et al. (1997). The unusual pathobiology of hemoglobin Constant Spring red blood cells. *Blood* 89: 1762–1769.

Sciarratta, GV, Sansone, G, Ivaldi, G et al. (1984). Alternate organisation of alpha G-Philadelphia globin genes among US black and Italian Caucasian heterozygotes. *Hemoglobin* 8: 537–548.

Shaffer, CD, Wallrath, LL, and Elgin, SCR. (1993). Regulating genes by packaging domains: Bits of heterochromatin in euchromatin? *Trends Genet.* 9: 35–37.

Shakin, SH and Liebhaber, SA. (1986). Translational profiles of α1-, α2-, and β-globin messenger ribonucleic acids in human reticulocytes. *J. Clin. Invest.* 78: 1125–1129.

Shalmon, L, Kirschmann, C, and Zaizov, R. (1994). A new deletional α-thalassemia detected in Yemenites with hemoglobin H disease. *Am. J. Hematol.* 45: 201–204.

Steinberg, MH, Coleman, MB, Adams, JG III et al. (1986). A new gene deletion in the alpha-like globin gene cluster as the molecular basis for the rare α-thalassemia-1 (- -/αα) in blacks: HbH disease in sickle cell trait. *Blood* 67: 469–473.

Strachan, T and Read, AP. (1996). *Human Molecular Genetics.* Oxford: BIOS Scientific Publishers Ltd.

Strauss, EC, Andrews, NC, Higgs, DR, and Orkin, SH. (1992). In vivo footprinting of the human α-globin locus upstream regulatory element by guanine/adenine ligation-mediated PCR. *Mol. Cell. Biol.* 12: 2135–2142.

Surrey, S, Ohene-Frempong, K, Rappaport, E et al. (1980). Linkage of $\alpha^{G-Philadelphia}$ to α-thalassemia in African-Americans. *Proc. Natl. Acad. Sci. U.S.A.* 77: 4885–4889.

Tabone, P, Henni, T, Belhani, M et al. (1981). Hemoglobin H disease from Algeria: Genetic and molecular characterisation. *Acta Haematol. (Basel),* 65: 26–31.

Tamary, H, Klinger, G, Shalmon, L et al. (1997). α-Thalassemia caused by a 16 nt deletion in the 3′ untranslated region of the α2-globin gene including the first nucleotide of the poly A signal sequence. *Hemoglobin* 21: 121–130.

Tang, W, Luo, H-y, Albitar, M et al. (1992). Human embryonic ζ-globin expression in deletional α-thalassemias. *Blood* 80: 517–522.

Thein, SL, Wallace, RB, Pressley, L et al. (1988). The polyadenylation site mutation in the α-globin gene cluster. *Blood* 71: 313–319.

Titus, EAB, Hsia, YE, and Hunt, JA. (1988). α-Thalassemia screening reveals quadruple ζ-globin genes in a Laotian family. *Hemoglobin* 12: 539–550.

Trent, RJ, Higgs, DR, Clegg, JB, and Weatherall, DJ. (1981). A new triplicated α-globin gene arrangement in man. *Br. J. Haematol.* 49: 149–152.

Trent, RJ, Mickleson, KNP, Wilkinson, T et al. (1985). α Globin gene rearrangements in Polynesians are not associated with malaria. *Am. J. Hematol.* 18: 431–433.

Trent, RJ, Mickleson, KNP, Wilkinson, T et al. (1986a). Globin genes in Polynesians have many rearrangements including a recently described γγγγ/. *Am. J. Hum. Genet.* 39: 350–360.

Trent, RJ, Wilkinson, T, Yakas, J et al. (1986b). Molecular defects in 2 examples of severe HbH disease. *Scandi. J. Haematol.* 36: 272–279.

Vandenplas, S, Higgs, DR, Nicholls, RD et al. (1987). Characterization of a new α^0 thalassaemia defect in the South African population. *Br. J. Haematol.* 66: 539–542.

Vickers, MA and Higgs, DR. (1989). A novel deletion of the entire α-globin gene cluster in a British individual. *Br. J. Haematol.* 72: 471–473.

Villegas, A, Calero, F, Vickers, MA et al. (1989). α Thalassaemia in two Spanish families. *Eur. J. Haematol.* 44: 109–114.

Villegas, A, Sanchez, J, Ricard, P et al. (1994). Characterization of a new α-thalassemia-1 mutation in a Spanish family. *Hemoglobin* 18: 29–37.

Wainscoat, JS, Kanavakis, E, Weatherall, D et al. (1981). Regional localisation of the human α-globin genes. *Lancet* 2: 301–302.

Waye, JS, Eng, B, and Chui, DHK. (1992). Identification of an extensive ζ-α globin gene deletion in a Chinese individual. *Br. J. Haematol.* 80: 378–380.

Waye, JS, Eng, B, Patterson, M, and Chui, DHK. (1994). Identification of a novel termination codon mutation (TAA → TAT, Term → Tyr) in the α2 globin gene of a Laotian girl with hemoglobin H disease. *Blood* 83: 3418–3420.

Waye, JS, Eng, B, Patterson, M et al. (1996). Novel mutation of the α2-globin gene initiation codon (ATG→A-G) in a Vietnamese girl with HbH disease. *Blood* 88: 28b.

Weatherall, DJ and Clegg, JB. (1975). The α chain termination mutants and their relationship to thalassaemia. *Philos. Trans. R. Soc. London (B)* 271: 411–455.

Weiss, IM and Liebhaber, SA. (1994). Erythroid cell-specific determinants of α-globin mRNA stability. *Mol. Cell. Biol.* 14: 8123–8132.

Wilkie, AOM, Buckle, VJ, Harris, PC et al. (1990). Clinical features and molecular analysis of the α thalassaemia/mental retardation syndromes. I. Cases due to deletions involving chromosome band 16p 13.3. *Am. J. Hum. Genet.* 46: 1112–1126.

Wilkie, AOM, Higgs, DR, Rack, KA et al. (1991). Stable length polymorphism of up to 260 kb at the tip of the short arm of human chromosome 16. *Cell* 64: 595–606.

Winichagoon, P, Higgs, DR, Goodbourn, SEY et al. (1982). Multiple arrangements of the human embryonic ζ-globin genes. *Nucl. Acids Res.* 10: 5853–5867.

Winichagoon, P, Higgs, DR, Goodbourn, SEY et al. (1984). The molecular basis of α-thalassaemia in Thailand. *EMBO J.* 3: 1813–1818.

Yüregir, GT, Aksoy, K, Curuk, MA et al. (1992). HbH disease in a Turkish family resulting from the interaction of a deletional α-thalassaemia-1 and a newly discovered poly A mutation. *Br. J. Haematol.* 80: 527–532.

Zhao, J-B, Zhao, L, Fei, Y-J et al. (1991). A novel α-thalassemia-2 (−2.7 kb) observed in a Chinese patient with HbH disease. *Am. J. Hematol.* 38: 248–249.

Zimmer, EA, Martin, SL, Beverley, SM et al. (1980). Rapid duplication and loss of genes coding for the α chains of hemoglobin. *Proc. Natl. Acad. Sci. U.S.A.* 77: 2158–2162.

18

Clinical and Laboratory Features of the α-Thalassemia Syndromes

DOUGLAS R. HIGGS
DONALD K. BOWDEN

INTRODUCTION

As discussed in Chapter 17 we currently know of about fifty mutations associated with α^+ thalassemia (chromosomes in which α-globin chain synthesis is reduced) and about forty that cause α^0 thalassemia (chromosomes in which α-globin chain synthesis is abolished). There are potentially several hundred different interactions that could take place between the large number of α-thalassemia determinants described. Phenotypically, these interactions result in one of three broad categories: α-thalassemia trait, in which there are mild hematologic changes but no major clinical abnormalities; HbH disease; and the Hb Bart's hydrops fetalis syndrome. We consider each of these in this chapter.

The information in Chapter 17 suggests that the α-thalassemia determinants could be arranged in the order of the severity (from αα to - -) as shown in Table 18.1. In general the phenotypes resulting from their interactions correlate well with the reduction in α-chain synthesis predicted for each mutation. Although this scheme accurately predicts the outcome of interactions between α^0 thalassemia and α^+ thalassemia caused by a simple deletion, the pathophysiology (see Chapter 16) and consequent hematologic effects appear more complex and less predictable when nondeletional defects are involved. One might expect that nondeletional defects affecting the α2 gene would cause a greater reduction in α-globin synthesis than those affecting the α1 gene (see Chapters 6 and 17) and in general this appears to be so. However, aberrantly processed mRNA or structurally abnormal globin chains may have additional deleterious effects on erythropoiesis and red cell metabolism, producing a more severe effect on phenotype than would be predicted simply from the associated reduction in normal α-globin chain synthesis.

α-THALASSEMIA TRAIT

The term α-thalassemia trait describes a spectrum of phenotypes spanning the clinical and hematologic gap between normal individuals and those with HbH disease (see below). People with α thalassemia usually originate from tropical or subtropical regions of the world (see Chapter 32) and have a hypochromic, microcytic blood picture with a normal or slightly reduced level of HbF and HbA_2. The main differential diagnosis is from iron deficiency, the anemia of chronic disorders, the low HbA_2 types of β-thalassemia trait (see Chapter 12), and, rarely, sideroblastic anemia. In addition to the hypochromic microcytic red cell indices (Pornpatkul et al., 1969), characteristic, diagnostic features of α-thalassemia trait include a raised level of Hb Bart's (γ^4) at birth (Hunt and Lehmann, 1959; Weatherall, 1963), the presence of HbH (β^4) inclusions in adults (originally observed by McNiel, 1968 and Pornpatkul et al., 1978), and the demonstration of a reduced α/β-globin chain synthesis ratio (Kan et al., 1968). Unfortunately, these diagnostic parameters fail to identify a significant proportion of carriers for α thalassemia and discriminate poorly between carriers with different molecular defects. Before the application of molecular biology to this problem (around 1980) these "blunt" diagnostic tools produced a huge amount of confusing literature on the distribution, frequency, and genetics of α thalassemia (reviewed in Weatherall and Clegg, 1981).

The geographic distribution and frequency of α thalassemia is now well documented (Chapter 32), and we know that α-thalassemia trait most frequently results from interactions between a normal α-globin complement and one of the α^0 or α^+ thalassemia defects (Higgs et al., 1989). However, α-thalassemia trait also occurs in some homozygotes and compound heterozygotes for α^+ thalassemia (e.g., $-\alpha/-\alpha$, $-\alpha/\alpha^T\alpha$, and some $\alpha^T\alpha/\alpha^T\alpha$).

Martin H. Steinberg, Bernard G. Forget, Douglas R. Higgs, and Ronald L. Nagel, editors. *Disorders of Hemoglobin: Genetics, Pathophysiology, and Clinical Management.* © 2001 Cambridge University Press. All rights reserved.

Table 18.1. Interactions Producing the Phenotype of α Thalassemia

			αα	ααᵀ	−α	αᵀα	−αᵀ	(αα)	− −
						α⁺		**α⁰**	
α⁰	− − (αα)	T T		H H	H H	H,Hy			Hy
α⁺	−αᵀ αᵀα −α ααᵀ αα	T T T N			H T T	T H	H		

Abbreviations: N, nonthalassemic; T, α-thalassemia trait; H, HbH disease; Hy, Bart's hydrops fetalis syndrome.

α/β-Globin mRNA and Globin Synthesis Ratios in α-Thalassemia Trait

Heterologous cell free assays consistently show that mRNA from the reticulocytes of patients with α thalassemia direct the synthesis of less α than β globin (Benz et al., 1973; Grossbard et al., 1973; Gambino et al., 1974; Pritchard et al., 1974), which is due to underrepresentation of α-globin mRNA (Housman et al., 1973; Kacian et al., 1973; Kan et al., 1974; Natta et al., 1976). Hunt et al. (1980) were the first to analyze the α/β-globin mRNA ratios in carriers of α thalassemia, and although the precise genotypes of the patients studied were not known, they demonstrated clear differences between normal individuals and carriers of α thalassemia (Fig. 18.1).

Subsequently studies using reverse transcription polymerase chain reaction (RT-PCR)-based quantitation of α- and β-globin mRNA in erythrocytes of patients with known genotypes have confirmed those observations (Lin et al., 1994; Smetanina et al., 1996). Although Hunt et al. (1980) showed no overlap in the α/β-globin mRNA ratios of normal individuals and those with α-thalassemia trait, more recent studies demonstrated wider variation (Lin et al., 1994; Smetanina et al., 1996). Nevertheless, Smetanina et al. (1996) confirmed that the α/β-globin mRNA ratios of patients with two functional α genes (−α/−α and - -/αα) are quite distinct from those of nonthalassemic individuals.

The α/β-globin chain ratios in erythrocytes from patients with well-defined α-globin genotypes, measured by in vitro hemoglobin synthesis (Clegg and Weatherall, 1967; Kan et al., 1968; Weatherall et al., 1970; Pootrakul et al., 1975) broadly reflect the α/β-globin mRNA ratios. Data accumulated from the current literature are summarized in Table 18.2 and Figure 18.2. Again the α/β-globin chain ratios in carriers of α thalassemia with two functional α genes can be clearly distinguished from those in normal individuals.

It is interesting that the same trends in mRNA, globin synthesis, and hematologic indices (see below) are seen when comparing individuals with four, three, or two functional α-globin genes. In each case, individuals with two α genes can be clearly distinguished from those with four genes. The values in those with three genes (−α/αα) overlap the two groups but are more closely related to those with four genes (αα/αα).

Figure 18.1. α/β-globin specific RNA ratios determined by cDNA hybridization with total RNA prepared from the peripheral blood of nonthalassemic individuals or obligate carriers with mild (α thalassemia 2) or severe (α thalassemia 1) α-thalassemia trait or HbH disease. The data are redrawn from Hunt et al. (1980).

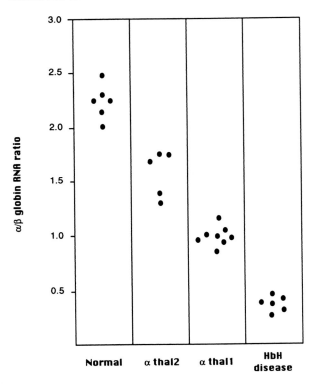

Table 18.2. Hematologic Data for Mendelian α Thalassemia

α-globin genotype	Age (y)		Hemoglobin (g/dL)		RBC ($\times 10^{12}$/L)		MCV (fl)	MCH (pg)	%HbH (%)	α/β ratio
			M	F	M	F				
αα/αα	1–4	N	–		–		–	–	–	
		μ	12.6		4.55		79	27.5	0	
		SD	0.8		0.35		4	2.0	–	
	5–9	N	–		–		–	–	–	
		μ	13.2		4.6		81.5	28.5	0	
		SD	0.8		0.3		4	2.0	–	
	10–15	N	–		–		–	–	–	
		μ	13.9		4.7		84	29.5	0	
		SD	1.0		0.3		4.5	2.0	–	
	≥16	N	–	–	–	–	–	–	–	27
		μ	15.5	14.0	5.2	4.6	90	30	0	1.06
		SD	1.0	1.0	0.35	0.3	5	2.0	–	0.11
–α/αα	1–4	N	55		52		55	52	–	
		μ	10.9		4.74		73.0	23.2	0	
		SD	1.2		0.53		6.4	2.5	–	
	5–9	N	49		49		49	49	–	
		μ	11.8		4.87		76.4	24.5	0	
		SD	0.86		0.50		5.6	2.2	–	
	10–15	N	42		42		42	42	–	
		μ	12.5		5.00		80.2	25.2	0	
		SD	1.2		0.48		6.1	1.8	–	
	≥16	N	81	106	77	102	191	184	–	29
		μ	14.3	12.6	5.42	4.88	81.2	26.2	0	0.87
		SD	1.4	1.2	0.58	0.53	6.9	2.3	–	0.12
$\alpha^T\alpha/\alpha\alpha$	10–15	N	4		4		4	4	–	
		μ	12.8		5.3		71.7	24.2	0	
		SD	0.2		0.26		2.4	1.3	–	
	≥16	N	22	17	21	17	39	38	–	12
		μ	14.5	12.5	5.76	5.21	75.5	24.8	0	0.75
		SD	0.9	0.6	0.49	0.50	4.68	1.7	–	0.12
–α/–α	1–4	N	10		10		10	10	–	
		μ	10.1		5.08		63.0	19.9	0	
		SD	1.7		0.30		6.1	6.1	–	
	5–9	N	7		7		7	7	–	
		μ	10.8		5.0		66.2	21.5	0	
		SD	1.4		0.5		3.0	0.9	–	
	10–15	N	14		14		14	14	–	
		μ	12.0		5.47		72.1	22.1	0	
		SD	0.9		0.49		8.7	2.3	–	
	≥16	N	31	45	30	45	77	75	–	8
		μ	13.9	12.0	5.98	5.30	71.6	22.9	0	0.72
		SD	1.7	1.0	0.81	0.49	4.1	1.3	–	0.12
––/αα	1–4	N	6		5		6	5	–	
		μ	11.2		5.79		60.7	19.6	0	
		SD	0.6		0.58		4.9	1.2	–	
	5–9	N	8		7		8	7	–	
		μ	11.0		5.47		62.5	20.3	0	
		SD	0.8		0.48		3.4	0.8	–	
	10–15	N	13		14		14	13	–	
		μ	12.2		5.83		67.5	21.4	0	
		SD	1.0		0.70		3.4	1.8	–	
	≥16	N	63	83	54	71	145	130	–	31.
		μ	13.7	12.1	6.28	5.65	69.1	21.7	0	0.65
		SD	1.1	1.1	0.63	0.49	4.4	1.7	–	0.12

(continued)

Table 18.2 (continued)

α-globin genotype	Age (y)		Hemoglobin (g/dL) M	Hemoglobin (g/dL) F	RBC (× 10¹²/L) M	RBC (× 10¹²/L) F	MCV (fl)	MCH (pg)	%HbH (%)	α/β ratio
$\alpha^T\alpha/-\alpha$	1–4	N	1		1		1	1	–	
		μ	10.8		5.78		59	18.7	0	
		SD	–		–		–	–	–	
	5–9	N	1		1		1	1	–	
		μ	11.4		5.79		60.2	19.7	0	
		SD	–		–		–	–	–	
	≥16	N	6	6	5	6	12	12	–	4
		μ	12.3	10.6	5.78	5.10	66.1	21.0	0	0.8
		SD	1.05	0.65	0.80	0.37	3.3	1.5	–	0.06
$\alpha^T\alpha/\alpha^T\alpha$	1–4	N	2		2		2	2	2	
		μ	7.9		4.25		63.3	18.9	14.2	
		SD	3.2		2.30		2.9	2.8	5.3	
	5–9	N	1		1		1	1	1	
		μ	6.9		3.5		68	19.7	8.4	
		SD	–		–		–	–	–	
	10–15	N	3		3		3	3	3	
		μ	10.7		5.97		58.3	17.8	7.6	
		SD	2.8		0.82		5.7	2.8	8.0	
	≥16	N	2	3	2	3	6	6	5	5
		μ	11.2	9.9	5.82	5.21	60.5	18.9	10.5	0.47
		SD	0.5	1.4	0.35	0.56	4.77	1.2	7.6	0.18
$-\alpha/--$	1–4	N	17		16		17	16	13	
		μ	9.6		5.77		57.7	17.0	5.7	
		SD	0.8		0.66		8.5	2.2	3.4	
	5–9	N	11		11		11	11	10	
		μ	9.6		5.52		58.7	17.7	4.8	
		SD	0.8		0.86		6.4	2.5	4.0	
	10–15	N	19		18		19	18	15	
		μ	9.5		5.47		59.3	17.7	5.1	
		SD	0.8		0.76		5.6	1.3	2.4	
	≥16	N	28	59	24	58	121	120	110	32
		μ	11.1	9.4	6.10	5.14	64.8	19.1	7.0	0.44
		SD	1.1	1.2	0.82	0.78	7.2	2.3	4.8	0.20
$\alpha^T\alpha/--$	1–4	N	4		3		4	3	3	
		μ	7.8		5.16		67.4	16.6	19.6	
		SD	1.4		1.13		16.7	5.3	2.1	
	5–9	N	8		8		8	8	8	
		μ	8.8		4.69		66.6	19.3	13.4	
		SD	1.9		1.23		7.7	2.5	7.2	
	10–15	N	8		8		8	8	8	
		μ	9.2		5.03		66.1	17.8	22.8	
		SD	0.9		0.49		3.4	1.5	3.5	
	≥16	N	6	5	3	5	14	14	13	17
		μ	10.5	8.5	5.10	4.68	68.0	18.7	22.3	0.32
		SD	1.0	0.7	0.31	0.66	5.9	1.5	6.5	0.15

Note: The number of samples *(N)*, mean (μ), and unbiased estimate of the standard deviation (SD) are shown for the nine possible combinations of the αα, –α, $\alpha^T\alpha$, and - - genotypes (excluding - -/- -), in increasing order of severity, for the age groups (years) 1–4, 5–9, 10–15, and ≥ 16 (adult). The normal data are derived from Dallman (1977); Dallman and Siimes, (1979); Lubin (1987); the principal sources for the α-thalassemia data are described in the text. In addition to the unpublished data sets acknowledged in Higgs et al. (1989), further valuable series were contributed by C.C. Thompson (Hamilton, Ontario) and T. Sophocleous (Nicosia). Because of significant sex differences, the hemoglobin and RBC count are tabulated separately for men and women; although both MCV and MCH tend to be slightly higher in men than women, the relative differences are much smaller (~1 fl and ~0.5 pg, respectively), so these data are pooled, as are the α/β-globin chain synthesis ratios for all ages.

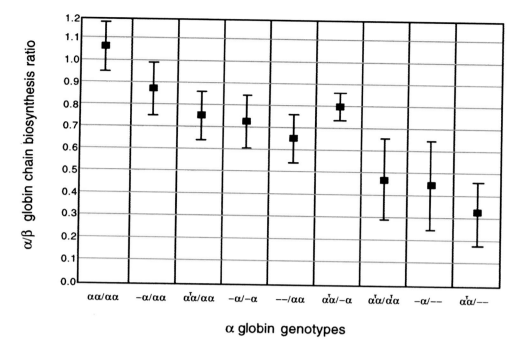

Figure 18.2. The α/β-globin chain biosynthesis ratios in individuals with well-defined α-globin genotypes. The data are derived from the references in the note in Table 18.2.

At present mRNA and globin synthesis ratios have been evaluated in relatively few patients with nondeletional determinants of α thalassemia. Nevertheless, one would predict that α/β mRNA ratios might be a poor way to evaluate such patients since, in some instances, the red cell precursors will contain nonfunctional mRNA and in many cases structurally abnormal mRNA and globin chains may be metabolized in quite complex ways during erythroid maturation. All of these observations highlight the absolute necessity for accurate genotype analysis when counseling or evaluating individuals with α-thalassemia trait.

Red Cell Indices and Hematologic Findings in α-Thalassemia Trait

In the following discussion we first consider the effect of α-globin deletions on red cell indices, comparing normal individuals and those with α-thalassemia trait. Like Ganczakowski et al. (1995) and Williams et al. (1996), we make no distinction between the $-\alpha^{3.7}$ and $-\alpha^{4.2}$ defects. Although the hematologic effects of such deletions will be illustrated by reference to specific studies, it is important to remember that these measurements can vary from one normal population to another (Owen and Yanochik-Owen, 1977), and, in practice, slight variations may be obtained even in healthy, nonthalassemic individuals (Ross et al., 1988). In general, individuals

with α thalassemia trait due to simple gene deletions ($-\alpha/\alpha\alpha$, $-\alpha/-\alpha$, and $--/\alpha\alpha$) have lower total hemoglobin levels, mean corpuscular hemoglobin concentration (MCHC), mean corpuscular volume (MCV) and mean corpuscular hemoglobin (MCH) but higher red blood cell (RBC) counts than nonthalassemic individuals (see Table 18.2 and Fig. 18.3).

The degree of abnormality varies among parameters. The greatest differences are seen in MCH (Table 18.2 and Figs. 18.3 and 18.4); individuals with α thalassemia clearly make less hemoglobin per cell than normal individuals. Nevertheless, patients with α-thalassemia trait maintain adequate hemoglobin levels (within ~1.0–1.5 g/dL of normal) at all stages of development (Table 18.2, Figs. 18.3 and 18.4). It appears that the main compensatory mechanism for the underproduction of hemoglobin in each red cell occurs via an increase in the concentration of red cells (RBC count) maintained in the peripheral blood.

Developmental changes in the hematologic indices of individuals with α-thalassemia trait follow the same patterns as those of normal individuals. Hemoglobin concentration, PCV, MCH, and MCV fall rapidly after birth and begin to rise slowly in the second year. The red blood cell count is relatively low at birth and then rises slowly. Throughout development one can clearly distinguish the hematologic indices found in people with the αα/αα, $-\alpha/\alpha\alpha$, and $-\alpha/-\alpha$ genotypes. For all parameters there is a greater difference between those with the $-\alpha/-\alpha$ and $-\alpha/\alpha\alpha$ genotypes than between those with the $-\alpha/\alpha\alpha$ and αα/αα genotypes. The smaller data set for individuals with the $--/\alpha\alpha$ genotype most closely resembles those with $-\alpha/-\alpha$ geno-

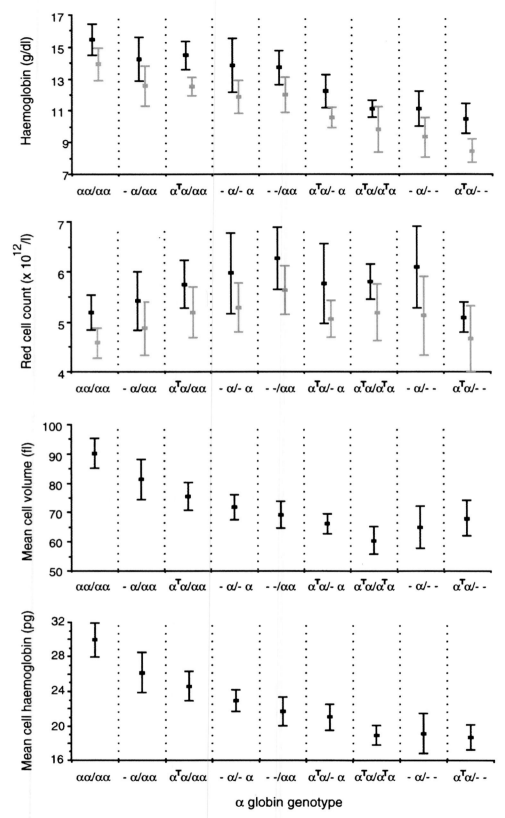

Figure 18.3. The red blood cell indices in patients with various genotypes associated with α-thalassemia. For each set of data the mean and 1 standard deviation are shown. For the level of hemoglobin and estimates of red cell count, differences between males (solid lines) and females (gray lines) are shown. These data are from Wilkie (1991).

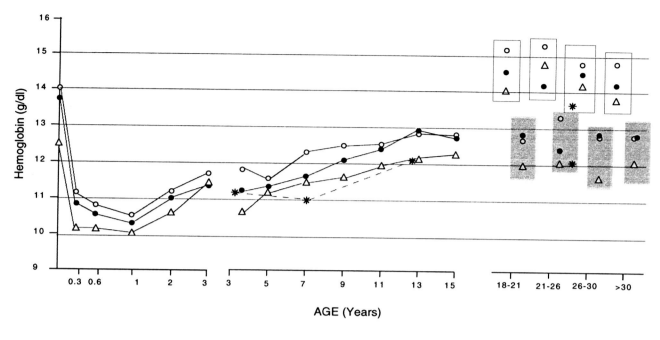

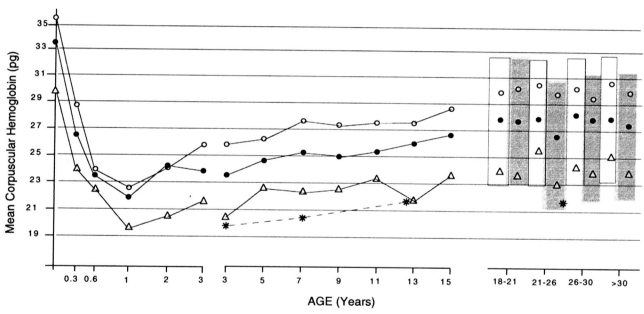

Figure 18.4. Developmental changes in the level of hemoglobin (above) and MCH (below) in individuals with the αα/αα (○), -α/αα (●), -α/-α (△), and - -/αα (*) genotypes. Beyond the age of 15 years results are grouped into males (hatched surround) and females (stippled background).

type. Few differences are seen between males and females prior to puberty, after which there are significant sex-dependent differences in both hemoglobin and RBC count in all genotypes (Fig. 18.4).

At present there are insufficient developmental data to extend these conclusions to all determinants of α thalassemia. However, there is now adequate information to compare hematologic indices in adults with various interactions that produce α-thalassemia trait (Table 18.2 and Fig. 18.3). Although there is a good correlation between the predicted reduction in α-chain synthesis and hemoglobin concentration, MCV, and MCH there is considerable overlap. Therefore, these indices are of only limited value in distinguishing one genotype from another. However, it is clear that with the exception of the −α/αα genotype most carriers of deletional types of α thalassemia can be distin-

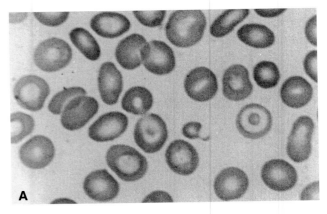

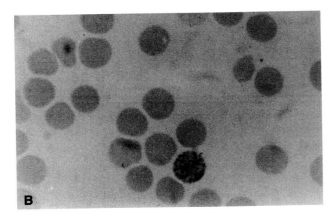

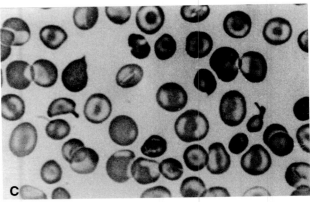

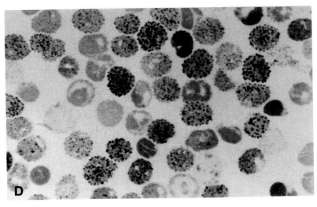

Figure 18.5. Typical hematologic findings in patients with α-thalassemia trait (**A**) and HbH disease (**C**). Rare HbH inclusions may be found in patients with α-thalassemia trait (**B**) whereas they are commonly found in patients with HbH disease (**D**).

guished from normal individuals on the basis of their MCH, which is usually less than 26 pg and always below 27 pg (Higgs et al., 1989; Higgs, 1993; and Table 18.2)

The peripheral blood film in patients with α-thalassemia trait varies from one genotype to another but often shows hypochromasia, with occasional poikilocytes and target cells (Fig. 18.5). The reticulocyte count is usually raised to 2 percent to 3 percent in patients with the severe forms of α-thalassemia trait. Red cell survival and erythrokinetic studies have not usually been carried out. The red cell ^{51}Cr half-life estimates in two cases of α-thalassemia trait reported by Wasi et al. (1974) were 25 days and 29.5 days (normal range 25 to 30 days).

Hemoglobin Analysis in α-Thalassemia Trait

The patterns of hemoglobin seen in adult individuals with α-thalassemia trait are indistinguishable from those seen in normal individuals, although as a group they may have slightly lower levels of HbA$_2$. In a small survey (Maude et al., 1985), throughout development there appeared to be no significant differences in the levels of HbA$_2$ and HbF between individuals with the αα/αα, –α/αα, and –α/–α genotypes (Fig. 18.6a).

Prior to the application of molecular genetic methods to the diagnosis of α thalassemia there was good evidence that a raised level of Hb Bart's in the neonatal period (Fig. 18.7) indicated the presence of α thalassemia (Weatherall, 1963, and reviewed in Wasi et al., 1974). However, it was not clear if normal individuals produced Hb Bart's at birth or if only individuals with α thalassemia had a raised level of Hb Bart's at birth. Furthermore, the relationship between the amount of Hb Bart's and the underlying molecular defect was not known. These issues have now been evaluated in many surveys correlating the level of Hb Bart's with the α-globin genotype. Most surveys using assays that detect 0.5 percent to 1 percent Hb Bart's in cord blood detect a large proportion of neonates with α thalassemia but not all cases of the –α/αα genotype (e.g., see Higgs et al., 1980). Therefore, surveys based solely on the presence of Hb Bart's in cord blood consistently underestimate the frequency of α thalassemia. Furthermore, although the levels of Hb Bart's are generally related to the degree of α-chain deficit they do not accurately distinguish the various α-thalassemia genotypes.

During the first 6 months after birth, the level of Hb Bart's in individuals with α thalassemia declines

(a)

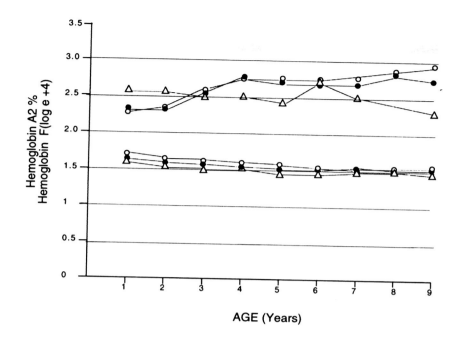

(b)

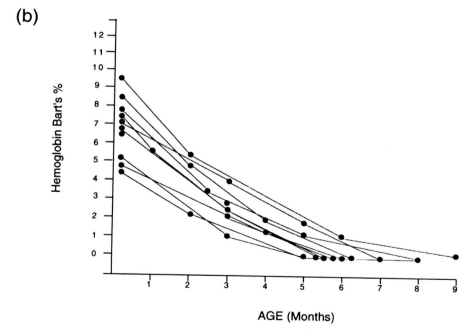

Figure 18.6. Above, developmental changes in the levels of HbA₂ (above in **a**) and HbF (below in **a**) in patients with the αα/αα (○), -α/αα (●), and -α/-α (△) genotypes (data from Maude et al., 1985). Below, developmental changes in the level of Hb Bart's in individuals with α thalassemia during the first few months of life. (Redrawn from Weatherall, 1963.)

(Fig. 18.6b) and eventually becomes undetectable by conventional assays (Weatherall, 1963) although minute amounts may be detected immunologically (Wasi et al., 1979). Similarly small amounts of embryonic ζ-globin chains can be detected in some adults with α thalassemia (Chui et al., 1986) and it has been suggested that these assays can be used as a simple way of detecting carriers of α thalassemia

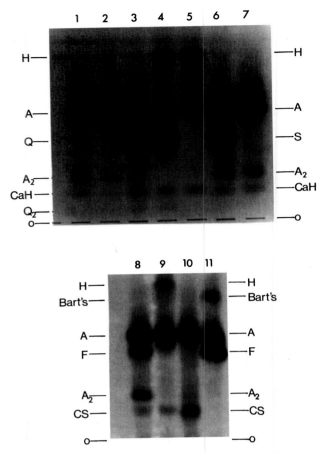

Figure 18.7. Hemoglobin electrophoresis (stained with commassie blue) in normal individuals (1, 2, and 7), a heterozygote for HbQ (3), HbQ-H disease (4), HbH disease (5 and 9), a heterozygote for HbS (6), a homozygote for Hb Constant Spring (CS) (10), and a cord blood with an elevated level of Hb Bart's (11). ○ denotes the origin and CaH indicates the position of carbonic anhydrase.

(Ausavarungnirun et al., 1998). At present, neither is commonly used. Unfortunately, from a diagnostic point of view, Hb Bart's is not replaced by an equivalent amount of HbH in adults; however, occasional cells containing HbH can be detected (Fig. 18.5) in up to 65 percent of individuals with α-thalassemia trait (Galanello et al., 1984). In our experience using the standard HbH preparations (Gibbons et al., 1991), inclusions are usually found in individuals with α-thalassemia trait due to the - -/αα, $\alpha^T\alpha$/αα, –α/α^T, $\alpha^T\alpha$/$\alpha^T\alpha$, and (αα)/αα genotypes but very rarely in those with the –α/αα and –α/–α genotypes. Various modifications of the standard HbH preparation may significantly increase the sensitivity of this assay (Maungsapaya et al., 1985; Kuptamethi et al., 1988).

α-Thalassemia commonly occurs in areas where β-globin variants (e.g., HbS, HbC, and HbE) are also common. The presence of α thalassemia can alter the proportion of variant hemoglobin found in the peripheral blood and therefore, where α thalassemia coexists with β variants, the proportion of hemoglobin variant can be a sensitive guide to the presence of α thalassemia (see Chapters 27 to 29 and 43).

Management and Genetic Counseling of People with α-Thalassemia Trait

Individuals with α-thalassemia trait are clinically normal and require no treatment. Nevertheless, it is important to recognize this condition to avoid unnecessary investigation of the hypochromic microcytic indices and to ensure that the patient does not receive inappropriate treatment with iron and folic acid, which may be harmful.

A diagnosis of α-thalassemia trait should be considered in any individual from tropical or subtropical areas of the world (see Chapter 32) who has a reduced MCH but a normal level of HbA_2 (<3.5 percent) and a normal iron status; such patients with MCH of 26 pg or less almost always have α-thalassemia trait. In some patients there may be a family history of HbH disease or Hb Bart's hydrops fetalis (see below). In most patients with α^0 thalassemia and some with α^+ thalassemia, the diagnosis can be confirmed by demonstrating HbH inclusions in the peripheral blood. In most clinical situations there is no need to pursue investigations beyond this stage since a definitive diagnosis can only be made by DNA analysis.

The main indication for further investigation occurs when a potential carrier of α thalassemia requires genetic counseling to avoid bearing children with the Hb Bart's hydrops fetalis syndrome or, rarely, severe transfusion-dependent forms of HbH disease (see below). Ideally, one should identify all Southeast Asian women with an MCH of 26 pg or less before or soon after they become pregnant (most carriers of the common α^0-thalassemia defects will have an MCH of between 20 and 26 pg). The partners of such individuals should be screened and if they too have α-thalassemia trait, with an MCH of 26 pg or less, the couple should be offered counseling and genotype analysis (see below). If resources are available this approach should be extended to individuals of Mediterranean or mixed origins who are much less commonly at risk (Chapter 36).

α-Thalassemia Trait and Pregnancy

The physiologic changes of pregnancy result in an increase in plasma volume (~40 percent to 45 percent) and red cell mass (20 percent to 30 percent), which by the third trimester results in a variable fall

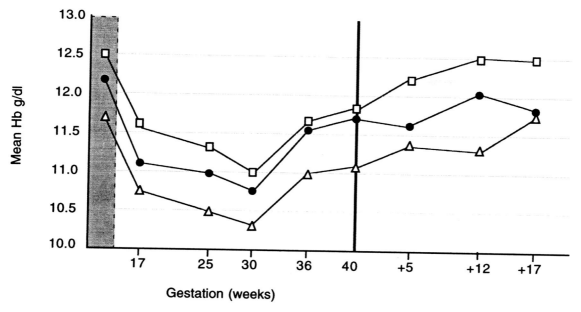

Figure 18.8. Changes in the level of hemoglobin in pregnant women with the αα/αα (□), -α/αα (●), and -α/-α (△) genotypes. Results in shaded area indicate normal values prior to pregnancy. The thick black vertical line denotes the usual time of birth. (Redrawn from Ganczakowski et al., in preparation.)

in hemoglobin concentration (10.5 to 14.5 g/dL) even in normal women (Letsky and Redman, 1987). In addition increased maternal and fetal demands for hematinics may lead to a further drop in hemoglobin if there is no supplementation. It is not surprising, therefore, that pregnant women with HbH disease, and to a lesser extent α-thalassemia trait, may become anemic.

Ganczakowski et al. (in preparation) studied 515 pregnant women with the αα/αα (53 percent), -α/αα (34 percent), and -α/-α (13 percent) genotypes. The changes in hemoglobin (Fig. 18.8) and red cell indices were similar in all three groups with the greatest fall in hemoglobin (~1.4 g/dL) occurring around 30 weeks of pregnancy. Only a small proportion (6 percent) of women with the -α/-α genotype developed a hemoglobin of less than 9 g/dL, which was not significantly different from those in the αα/αα group, of whom 5 percent developed a hemoglobin below 9 g/dL. The red cell indices (MCV and MCH) showed a small increase (5 percent to 7 percent of nonpregnant value) in pregnant women with α thalassemia (-α/αα and -α/-α).

α-Thalassemia Causing a Mild Hemolytic Anemia

Carriers for both deletional and nondeletional forms of α-thalassemia trait have hypochromic microcytic red cell indices but are asymptomatic. Homozygotes for some nondeletional mutations have more severely affected red cell indices (Paglietti et al., 1986) but nevertheless have the phenotype of α-thalassemia trait. Homozygotes for other nondeletional mutations (e.g., $\alpha^{T\ Saudi}\alpha/\alpha^{T\ Saudi}\alpha$) may have HbH disease (see Table 17.1 and below), and those with still others have an intermediate phenotype with a mild hemolytic anemia; this situation has been particularly well documented in patients homozygous for the Hb Constant Spring mutation ($\alpha^{CS}\alpha/\alpha^{CS}\alpha$).

The homozygous state for Hb Constant Spring was first described by Lie-Injo et al. (1974). Since that time several homozygotes have been described (Lie-Injo et al., 1975; Pongsamart et al., 1975) with a survey of 22 patients presented by Pootrakul et al. (1981). In this report, all of the patients had mild anemia (hemoglobin 10.3 ± 1.4 g/dL) and the majority of cases had mild jaundice with total serum bilirubin levels elevated in 8 of 14 cases examined. Splenomegaly was detectable in most cases and mild hepatomegaly in about half.

The hematologic indices were very unusual for patients with α thalassemia. The RBC count was low ($3.9 \pm 0.9 \times 10^{12}$/L) with a normal MCV (88 ± 6 fl) and only slightly reduced MCH (26 ± 3 pg). The peripheral blood films showed mild anisocytosis and hypochromia with a few fragmented cells. Approximately 6 percent of the cells showed basophilic stippling and reticulocyte counts were consistently raised (6.0 ± 3.3 percent). ^{51}Cr RBC survival was reduced (17.3 and 20.5 days) in the two patients studied. In 6 of 15 patients studied transferrin iron saturation was greater than 50 percent. All of these findings suggest that these patients have a mild hemolytic anemia.

Starch gel electrophoresis (e.g., see Fig. 18.7) provided conclusive evidence that these patients have α thalassemia. One newborn infant had 14.2 percent Hb Bart's, which fell to 4.6 percent at 8 months (Lie-Injo et al., 1975). In the study of Pootrakul et al. (1981) seven adults had raised levels (1.8 percent to 3.6 percent) of Hb Bart's and similarly raised levels have been seen in adults in other studies. The levels of Hb Constant Spring varied from 2.6 percent to 11.6 percent.

Another surprising aspect of this condition is that prolonged incubation of reticulocytes revealed an α/β-globin synthesis ratio of 1.5 ± 0.16 rather than a reduced ratio as one would expect. This appears to result from the fact that globin synthesis only remains linear in the cells of $\alpha^{CS}\alpha/\alpha^{CS}$ α homozygotes for approximately 30 minutes, an unexpectedly short time for samples with such a high reticulocyte count. This, together with the rapid removal of excess β-globin chains, accounts for the high α/β ratios observed in 2- to 3-hour incubations (Derry et al., 1984). It remains to be seen if other patients, homozygous for some nondeletional forms of α thalassemia, yield similar findings to those with Hb Constant Spring.

HbH DISEASE

Interactions between the many determinants of α thalassemia (Table 18.1) lead to a spectrum of clinical and hematologic phenotypes ranging from normal individuals to infants with the lethal, Hb Bart's hydrops fetalis syndrome. Young children (>6 to 12 months) and adults with sufficient globin chain imbalance to produce readily detectable levels of HbH (>1 percent to 2 percent) in the peripheral blood on routine hemoglobin electrophoresis (Fig. 18.7) are said to have HbH disease. HbH inclusions are always detectable in the peripheral blood of such individuals (Fig. 18.5).

Not surprisingly, patients defined in this way span a wide range of clinical and hematologic phenotypes. The majority are clinically well and in these the epithet HbH "disease" is inappropriate. Some have thalassemia intermedia. The most severe forms of HbH disease may be lethal late in gestation or in the perinatal period, causing a condition referred to as HbH hydrops fetalis (see below).

Extensive surveys have demonstrated that most cases of HbH disease occur in patients from Southeast Asia, the Mediterranean basin, and the Middle East (see Chapter 32). This geographic distribution is easily explained now that we understand the molecular basis of this disorder (Table 18.1). HbH disease most commonly results from the interaction of α^0 and α^+ thalassemia. Although α thalassemia is common throughout all tropical and subtropical regions, α^0

determinants (and hence HbH disease) are predominantly found in the Mediterranean and Southeast Asia. In Southeast Asia the most common genotype associated with HbH disease is $-^{SEA}/-\alpha$, whereas in the Mediterranean, $-^{MED}/-\alpha$ and $-(\alpha)^{20.5}/-\alpha$ are the most frequent. Less often HbH disease results from the interaction of α^0 thalassemia with nondeletional forms of α^+ thalassemia (genotype $--/\alpha^T\alpha$). HbH disease can also occur in homozygotes for some nondeletional forms of α^{p1} thalassemia (genotype $\alpha^T\alpha/\alpha^T\alpha$). Again these molecular defects are most frequently seen in Southeast Asia and the Mediterranean but also occur at high frequencies in some areas of the Middle East (see Chapter 32). Despite these useful geographic "rules of thumb," one should be aware that patients with α thalassemia trait and HbH disease have been described in almost every racial group. On detailed investigation, patients originating from regions where α thalassemia is otherwise rare are often found to have unusual and biologically interesting molecular defects.

α/β mRNA and Globin Synthesis Ratios in Patients With HbH Disease

As one would expect from the studies of α/β mRNA ratios in carriers of α thalassemia (see above), the red cell precursors of patients with HbH disease contain about one-half to one-quarter of the amount of α-globin mRNA present in normal red cell precursors (Benz et al., 1973; Kacian et al., 1973; Lin et al., 1977; Hunt et al., 1980; Smetanina et al., 1996) as demonstrated in Figure 18.1. Again this is generally reflected in the α/β-globin chain synthesis ratios of patients with the deletional forms of HbH disease (average of 0.44, SD 0.2; see Table 18.2 and Fig. 18.2). Excess β-globin chains synthesized during erythroid maturation mainly form β^4 tetramers but in addition supply a small intracellular pool of β chains that combine with newly synthesized α chains as they become available. Nevertheless, HbH is not present in the peripheral blood in amounts reflecting the rate at which it is synthesized, indicating that it must be lost from the red cells while they are in the circulation (see Chapter 16 for further details).

Red Cell Indices and Hematologic Findings in HbH Disease

As before, we first consider the effect of α-globin deletions on red cell indices, comparing individuals with one functional α gene ($--/-\alpha$) with normal individuals. Those who inherit only a single α gene have lower levels of total hemoglobin, MCH, and MCV but higher red cell counts than nonthalassemic individuals (Table 18.2 and Fig. 18.3). These differences in hematologic indices are seen at all stages of development (see Table 18.2) although there are no substantial data on infants with HbH disease in the perinatal period or during the early months of life. Perhaps the most important hematologic finding is that, using data accumulated from a variety of surveys (see Table 18.2), patients with HbH disease are anemic with, on average, approximately 3 g/dL less hemoglobin than age-and sex-matched normal individuals. It has been noted in some surveys that there may be striking fluctuations in the level of hemoglobin measured sequentially in the same individual over the course of 1 to 2 years (Wasi et al., 1974; Piankijagum et al., 1978), although in our experience this is not common. The wide fluctuations in hemoglobin observed in Wasi's series may have been partly due to concomitant iron and folate deficiencies.

The peripheral blood film shows hypochromia and polychromasia with variable anisopoikilocytosis and target cells (Fig. 18.5). The reticulocyte count is usually raised to around 3 percent to 6 percent although higher counts may be observed. Nucleated red cells and basophilic stippling may be present (Wasi et al., 1974) but in our more limited experience this is quite rare.

The red cell survival, as estimated by ^{51}Cr studies, is reduced in patients with HbH disease, with reported figures ranging from 8 to 17 days (Rigas and Koler, 1961; Pearson and McFarland, 1962; Woodrow et al., 1964; Knox-Macaulay et al., 1972) (normal range 25 to 32 days). External scanning indicates that most of the red cell destruction occurs in the spleen (Rigas and Koler, 1961; Woodrow et al., 1964). Srichaikul et al. (1984) performed full erythrokinetic studies on nine nonsplenectomized patients with HbH disease. They demonstrated a reduced red cell volume, increased plasma volume, and a reduced red cell survival of 6 to 19.5 days with sequestration of ^{51}Cr labeled red cells in the liver and spleen. In addition they showed that patients with HbH disease have a rapid clearance of ^{59}Fe with relatively good ^{59}Fe incorporation into red cells, compared to patients with β thalassemia. They also found that the patient's PCV was correlated to the red cell survival. Together these findings suggest that both hemolysis and ineffective erythropoiesis contribute to anemia in HbH disease but the predominant mechanism is hemolysis.

Although bone marrow examination is rarely necessary in the investigation of patients with HbH disease, when conducted it shows erythroid hyperplasia with only slight or absent deposition of hemosiderin (Wasi et al., 1974).

Over the past 10 to 15 years the precise genotype of many patients with HbH disease has been established. In addition to the common deletional forms (- -/–α)

discussed above, HbH disease may also result from interactions involving nondeletional determinants (- -/α^{T}α and α^{T}α/α^{T}α). Data from several studies (Table 18.2, Fig. 18.3) show that patients with nondeletional HbH disease and the α^{T}α/α^{T}α genotype have hematologic indices that are similar to those with the deletional type of HbH disease, whereas those with the deletional type of HbH disease (- -/α^{T}α) are slightly more anemic with lower red cell counts and higher MCV. Limited data (Table 18.2) indicate that these differences are present throughout development. A few studies have compared the hematologic findings in patients with deletional forms of HbH disease (- -/–α) and those with specific nondeletional defects including (- -/α^{CS}α) (HbH-Constant Spring) (Fucharoen et al., 1988), (- -/α^{Nco}α), and (- -/α^{Hph}α) (Galanello et al., 1983b, 1992). In all of these nondeletional genotypes one finds lower levels of hemoglobin and RBC counts but higher MCVs than in the pure deletional types of HbH disease.

Hemoglobin Analysis in HbH Disease

Infants who go on to develop HbH disease later in life produce large amounts (19 percent to 27 percent) of Hb Bart's (γ^4) at birth (Pootrakul et al., 1967; Wasi et al., 1969, 1974). During the first few months of life Hb Bart's falls, and by adulthood it is replaced by variable amounts of HbH. The level of Hb Bart's at birth often exceeds that of HbH in adult life. This is consistent with other observations (Rachmilewitz and Harari, 1972), showing that HbH is less stable than Hb Bart's. Adults with HbH disease have 0.8 percent to 40 percent HbH in circulating red blood cells. It has been consistently noted that patients with the nondeletional type of HbH disease produce larger amounts of HbH (Higgs and Weatherall, 1983; Kattamis et al., 1988; Galanello et al., 1992; Baysal et al., 1995). Hb Bart's may still be detected in some adults with HbH disease but HbH usually predominates; occasionally the fetal pattern, with an excess of Hb Bart's, persists (Ramot et al., 1959). The reasons why some patients with HbH disease produce significant amounts of Hb Bart's is not clear. It is possible that some have co-inherited γ-globin genes with mutations that are associated with increased γ-globin synthesis (see Chui et al., 1990 and Chapter 15).

HbH and Hb Bart's are easily detected as fast migrating bands on hemoglobin electrophoresis (Fig. 18.7). In addition, HbH can be precipitated from peripheral blood red cells after incubation for 3 hours at room temperature in the presence of dyes such as brilliant cresyl blue or methyl violet (see Gibbons et al., 1991, for details). These characteristic inclusions are artifacts produced by the redox action of the dye (Fig. 18.5). The proportion of cells containing HbH inclusions is directly related to the level of HbH detected in the peripheral blood. Again, patients with nondeletional α thalassemia have a higher proportion of "HbH cells" than those with the deletional types of HbH disease (Winichagoon et al., 1980). Even after prolonged incubation it is unusual to find inclusions in every cell; the reason for this heterogeneity is not clear. Splenectomized patients have large numbers of pre-formed inclusions in the red cells that can be detected by brilliant cresyl blue or methyl violet staining.

As discussed below, Hb Bart's is not a functional hemoglobin. Similarly HbH shows no heme-heme interaction or Bohr effect and has a much higher oxygen affinity than HbA (Benesch et al., 1961). Therefore, neither of these hemoglobins contribute to O_2 transport and their presence will compound the effects of anemia in patients with HbH disease. Other minor changes in the hemoglobin composition found in patients with HbH disease include a tendency to low levels of HbA_2 (1 percent to 2 percent) probably due to the lower affinity of α chains for δ than γ chains; when the supply of α chains is limited less HbA_2 is formed (Chapter 8 and 10). In addition, other abnormal hemoglobins may be detected in patients with α-chain termination mutations (e.g., see Weatherall and Clegg, 1975) and some unstable mutants associated with α thalassemia (see Chapter 17). Finally, some α-chain variants, such as HbJ Tongariki and HbG Philadelphia, may be linked in *cis* to α-thalassemia variants (see Table 17.2).

Clinical Features of HbH Disease

Although HbH disease is quite a common genetic disorder in the Mediterranean, Middle East, and Southeast Asia, there have been relatively few systematic studies addressing the natural history of this condition or the relationship between genotype and phenotype. Most physicians caring for patients with HbH disease agree that there is a remarkably wide clinical spectrum but often comment on the mild nature of this condition. Even from the biased perspective of hospital-based studies, the majority of patients appear to have little disability (Weatherall and Clegg, 1981; Wasi, 1983; Wong, 1984; Kattamis et al., 1988; George et al., 1989; Galanello et al., 1992). A minority may be severely affected, requiring regular blood transfusion and rare cases may present as hydropic, newborn infants (see below).

The largest clinical experience of HbH disease, including data from 500 adults and 502 children, was summarized by Wasi et al. (1974) and much of the discussion below is based on this description. At birth, infants destined to develop HbH disease were said to have near normal levels of hemoglobin with no hepatosplenomegaly. The clinical features of HbH disease (see below) develop in the first year of life. The age at which patients were first seen in Wasi's study ranged from birth to age 74 years with more than half of the patients being older than age 20 years. Anecdotally, survival into adult life appears to be the rule but there are no actuarial data to quantify this assertion. Patients with HbH disease most frequently come to medical attention either because they are found to have a hypochromic microcytic anemia during routine hematologic investigations for other reasons or because they present with symptoms of acute or chronic anemia (e.g., pallor, fatigue, and breathlessness). Of those with acute anemia, the majority are children. The degree of anemia may fluctuate and hemoglobin levels can fall quite dramatically (Wasi et al., 1974), causing episodes of profound weakness and pallor requiring hospital admission and blood transfusion. The cause of such events is not understood and may vary from one environment to another. They may arise from increased hemolysis associated with intercurrent infection or administration of oxidant drugs such as sulfonamides (Rigas and Koler, 1961), or transient aplasia (Bowden DK, unpublished observation). It is unusual for patients with HbH disease to require regular blood transfusion and even in cases where this has been thought necessary, it is not always clear what criteria have been used to make such a decision.

A much less common presentation occurs when patients develop cholecystitis. Gallstones are quite frequent in patients with HbH disease and in 95 patients followed by Piankijagum et al. (1978) for 2 years, there were four episodes of cholecystitis. Most patients with HbH disease in Wasi's study had enlarged livers (about 70 percent of cases) and spleens (about 80 percent of cases). In our more limited experience significant hepatomegaly is unusual in patients with uncomplicated HbH disease unless they have iron loading. Hypersplenism, which can significantly aggravate the anemia and lead to reduced platelet and white blood cell counts, occurs in about 10 percent of patients (Wasi et al., 1974). Severe liver disease has been reported in patients with HbH disease but it is not clear that this was directly attributable to thalassemia.

About one-third of patients with HbH disease were said to have bone changes associated with thalassemia (Wasi et al., 1969). In general these are mild but may affect the facial features. Only 1 percent of patients have impaired physical development (Wasi et al., 1969). Clinically significant extramedullary hematopoiesis does not occur in HbH disease (Wasi et al., 1974; Weatherall and Clegg, 1981). Other complications of HbH disease include leg ulcers (Daneshmend and Peachey, 1978), which are rare (Wasi et al., 1974) and, possibly, an increased susceptibility to certain infections (Wasi et al., 1974; Piankijagum et al., 1978; Cao et al., 1991).

Can one predict phenotype from genotype? The numbers of patients studied in detail are too small to draw firm conclusions. Nevertheless, several studies agree that patients with nondeletional forms of HbH disease are more anemic and jaundiced, have greater degrees of hepatosplenomegaly, more severe bone changes, and more episodes of infection than patients with deletional forms of HbH disease (Higgs and Weatherall, 1983; Fucharoen et al., 1988; Kattamis et al., 1988; George et al., 1989; Galanello et al., 1992; Higgs, 1993; Baysal et al., 1995; Kanavakis et al., 1996). Some studies suggest that patients with nondeletional HbH disease present earlier in life than those with deletional types of HbH disease (Fucharoen et al., 1988). These findings are consistent with the more severe hematologic phenotype reported in patients with nondeletional HbH disease (see above). Most patients reported as requiring regular blood transfusion have nondeletional HbH disease as do all patients with HbH hydrops fetalis (see below).

HbH Disease and Pregnancy

Detailed hematologic studies are not available for pregnant women with HbH disease; however Wasi et al. (1974) reported that in Thailand some pregnant women with HbH disease (- -/–α and - -/αᵀα) have hemoglobin levels of 4 to 5 g/dL, which return to 8 to 10 g/dL a few months after delivery. Many of the patients were also found to be iron deficient. Galanello et al. (1992) described the outcome of 58 pregnancies in twenty-four women with HbH disease. Seven (12 percent) resulted in miscarriage. In ten cases (16 percent) they noted a hemoglobin <7.5 g/dL and in five cases (8 percent) they found a hemoglobin <6.0 g/dL, for which they considered transfusion necessary. The figures are similar to our experience; we have never observed a hemoglobin of less than 7.2 g/dL in a pregnant woman with HbH disease. Nevertheless, several reports describe the need for occasional transfusion in pregnant patients with HbH disease (summarized in Ong et al., 1977).

Iron Status in Patients with HbH Disease

The clinical manifestations of iron overload frequently encountered in patients with β thalassemia intermedia and major (Chapter 13) are rarely seen as a

result of HbH disease (Weatherall and Clegg, 1981; Wasi, 1983; Tso et al., 1984; Chim et al., 1998). Bone marrow iron stores are usually unremarkable and Sonakul et al. (1978) noticed less tissue hemosiderosis at autopsy in patients with HbH disease than those with homozygous β thalassemia. Ferrokinetic studies have suggested that although iron absorption is increased in HbH disease (Lin et al., 1992) iron utilization appears normal, consistent with this being primarily a hemolytic anemia (Srichaikul et al., 1984; Lin et al., 1992).

Most young patients with HbH disease have normal (Galanello et al., 1983a) or only slightly raised levels of serum ferritin (Anuwatanakulchai et al., 1984; Tso et al., 1984). However, significantly raised levels may be found in older patients (e.g., see Fig. 18.9), those treated with regular blood transfusion, and those given inappropriate medication with iron (Galanello et al., 1983a). In the study of Galanello et al. (1992) no difference in the levels of serum ferritin were seen between patients with deletional and nondeletional HbH disease.

One should be aware that HbH disease may coexist with the common form of hereditary hemochromatosis (Feder et al., 1996), which may account for unex-

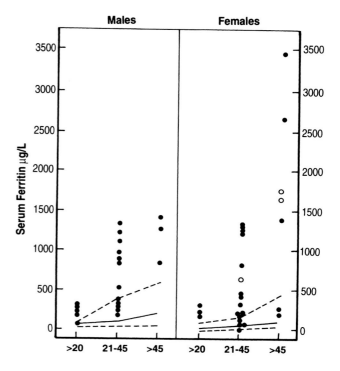

Figure 18.9. Serum ferritin levels of patients with HbH disease according to sex and age group. The solid lines connect the median control values of the different age groups and the dotted ones the upper and lower values of the corresponding control range. Splenectomized subjects are shown as open circles. (Redrawn from Tso et al., 1984.)

plained iron overload in occasional patients with HbH disease (Lin et al., 1990; Galanello et al., 1992).

Treatment Recommendations for Patients with HbH Disease

The overwhelming impression is that most patients with HbH disease are clinically well; they are often unaware of their condition and may go on to have families of their own. Therefore, the major point to make about the management of patients with HbH disease is that no specific treatment other than folic acid supplements should be offered unless there are well-defined reasons for doing so. Oral iron is not required routinely for patients with HbH disease and may be deleterious due to the potential for iron overload (see above). Nevertheless, when appropriate, one should suspect and investigate iron, folate, and B12 deficiency in patients with HbH disease and treat just as for nonthalassemic patients. Most clinicians recommend that all patients with chronic hemolytic anemias should be given regular folic acid supplements (Shojania and Gross, 1964; Nathan and Oski, 1987). Women with HbH disease who are not iron overloaded should be given the same supplements in the management of pregnancy as nonthalassemic women according to local obstetric practices.

Occasional blood transfusions may be required when the level of hemoglobin suddenly dips. Hemolytic episodes occur most commonly in children (Bowden, unpublished observation) who should therefore be examined at least every 12 months to determine steady-state levels of hemoglobin (many adult patients are so well that they neglect to come for review). Occasionally both hemolytic and aplastic episodes can result in rapid falls in the hemoglobin level to the point where transfusion is potentially life saving. Hence, education is a very important part of management. Any episodes of profound weakness and pallor should prompt individuals or families to take the patient to the hospital as a matter of urgency. Aplastic episodes usually last only 1 week or so with rapid recovery and transfusion is not necessarily required. It is important to exclude the coexistence of G-6-PD deficiency in males, which is common in many communities and may cause hemolysis in individuals with HbH disease. Naphthalene, antimalarials, and sulfonamides are the most common causes of hemolytic episodes in G-6-PD deficient children. In many cases the cause of sudden severe anemia in HbH disease remains unknown. Particular care must be taken to monitor pregnant women with HbH disease who may have especially low levels of hemoglobin (see above). In all of these situations it is reasonable to provide temporary support with blood transfusion.

Chronic blood transfusion should be avoided for all but the most carefully considered cases. Once instituted, the patients will require all the long-term care, including iron chelation, used for patients with homozygous β thalassemia (see Chapter 13). The clearest examples in which this should be considered are (1) patients who are unable to maintain normal cardiovascular function with the given level of hemoglobin; (2) patients who would otherwise develop the chronic problems associated with erythroid expansion (thalassemic facies, extramedullary tumors, etc.). In most hematologists' experience these criteria very rarely apply to patients with HbH disease.

Splenomegaly is one of the most common complications of HbH disease and may be accompanied by hypersplenism. Wasi et al. (1969) reported that splenectomy in fifty patients with HbH disease increased the level of hemoglobin by 2 to 3 g/dL (other reports are reviewed in Wagner et al., 1982 and Kanavakis et al., 1986). While splenectomy may be indicated in some cases to ameliorate the problems associated with splenomegaly or hypersplenism, this should be very carefully balanced against the potential complication of venous thrombosis, which has been reported in some patients with HbH disease following splenectomy (Tso et al., 1982; Sonakul and Fucharoen, 1992). Based on the discussion on iron status (see above), ferritin or iron estimations should be carried out at least annually. Iron loading may be caused by regular blood transfusion, inappropriate iron therapy, or abnormal absorption; in many patients several mechanisms contribute. Based on preliminary evaluation it may be necessary to assess iron loading by liver biopsy to determine the need for chelation. Alternatively liver iron storage can be evaluated by noninvasive methods such as dual energy computed tomography (CT) (Chapman et al., 1980) or magnetic resonance imaging (MRI) scanning (Jensen et al., 1994), thus avoiding the need for liver biopsy (the detection of iron overloading is discussed further in Chapter 37). At present we do not know whether iron loading in HbH disease can ever be severe enough to cause cirrhosis and liver failure.

Other complications, such as leg ulcers, have been reported in patients with HbH disease and require the general medical or surgical treatment appropriate for the clinical situation. Gallstones occur commonly and routine ultrasound should be carried out at some stage during late teens. When present, gallstones should be managed conservatively; few patients require cholecystectomy.

Genetic Counseling of Patients with HbH Disease

The presence of HbH disease in one or both partners is not known to impair their ability to have children, although there are no data to evaluate fertility in such individuals. Once a diagnosis has been made in any patient of reproductive age it is important to offer them advice about the potential problems of producing children with the Hb Bart's hydrops fetalis syndrome, and their partner should be tested to see if they are at risk of producing such a pregnancy. Since there are so many potential interactions (see Table 18.1) it will be necessary to obtain a full genotype analysis from both partners to evaluate the relative risks of all possible outcomes.

In each case the primary aim is to avoid pregnancies leading to Hb Bart's hydrops fetalis or the uncommon, severe forms of HbH hydrops fetalis and transfusion-dependent HbH disease.

Hb BART'S HYDROPS FETALIS SYNDROME

The combination of generalized edema, ascites, and pleural and pericardial effusions in a developing fetus (hydrops fetalis) may occur in a wide variety of fetal and maternal disorders (Holzgreve et al., 1984; Nicolaides et al., 1985; Jauniaux et al., 1990; Arcasoy and Gallagher, 1995). The predominant causes vary from one population to another. In the West, rhesus immunization used to be the major cause, but with the widespread introduction of immunoprophylaxis and the decline in rhesus isoimmunization (Clarke and Whitfield, 1977) "nonimmune" causes (intrauterine infection, chromosomal abnormalities, congenital cardiac and renal defects) now account for 75 percent of cases (Machin, 1981; Nicolaides et al., 1985). In Southeast Asia, 60 percent to 90 percent of all cases are caused by α thalassemia, giving rise to the Hb Bart's hydrops fetalis syndrome (Lie-injo, 1959; Thumasathit et al., 1968; Liang et al., 1985; Tan et al., 1989; Ko et al., 1991). Throughout Southeast Asia where the frequency of α-thalassemia trait is high (4.5 percent to 14 percent, see Chapter 32), between 1:200 and 1:2,000 infants inherit no functional α-globin genes from their parents. Since α-globin chains are normally produced throughout development, contributing to embryonic, fetal, and adult hemoglobins, affected fetuses suffer from severe hypochromic anemia *in utero,* which causes hypoxia, heart failure, and consequently hydrops fetalis (Fig. 18.10). Such infants produce large amounts of nonfunctional Hb Bart's and small amounts of functional, embryonic hemoglobin (Hb Portland, $\zeta_2\gamma_2$), which allows sufficient tissue oxygenation for them to survive until the third trimester of pregnancy when they are usually born prematurely and die (see below).

The Hb Bart's hydrops fetalis syndrome nearly always results from the co-inheritance of two α^0-thalassemia defects (Table 18.1). In Southeast Asia, - - ^{SEA}/ - - ^{SEA} is the most common genotype but in areas where the - - ^{FIL} (Fischel-Ghodsian et al., 1988), - - ^{THAI} (Fischel-Ghodsian et al., 1988), and - - ^{HW} (Waye et al., 1992) determinants occur some hydropic babies may be compound heterozygotes (- - ^{FIL}/- - ^{SEA} and - - ^{THAI}/ - - ^{SEA}). These three, less common defects (- - ^{FIL}, - - ^{THAI}, and - - ^{HW}) remove both the fetal/adult and embryonic α-globin-like genes. Since homozygotes do not produce any normal embryonic hemoglobins [Portland, Gower 1 ($\zeta_2\epsilon_2$), and Gower 2 ($\alpha_2\epsilon_2$)] they die very early in gestation and do not produce the classical hydrops fetalis syndrome (Fischel-Ghodsian et al., 1988). α^0 Thalassemia is much less common in other regions of the world. Nevertheless, rare cases of Hb Bart's hydrops fetalis have been reported in individuals of Greek (--^{MED}/- -^{MED}) (Diamond et al., 1965; Sharma et al., 1979; Kattamis et al., 1980; Pressley et al., 1980),

Figure 18.10. **(A)** The typical peripheral blood films of an infant with the Hb Bart's hydrops fetalis syndrome, showing many immature red cell precursors and hypochromic, microcytic, anisopoikilolytic red cells. **(B)** The typical clinical features of a hydropic infant at birth (see text). For full color reproduction, see color plates 18.10A and B. For full color reproduction, see color plate 18.10

A

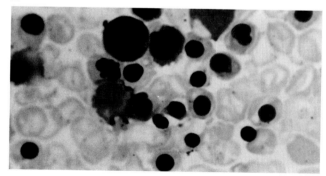

B

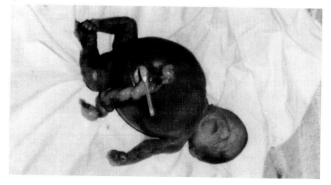

Cypriot (- -^{MED}/- -^{MED}, - -^{MED}/-$\alpha^{20.5}$, -$\alpha^{20.5}$/-$\alpha^{20.5}$) (Sophocleous et al., 1981; Nicholls et al., 1985), Sardinian (- -^{MED}/- -^{MED}) (Galanello et al., 1990), Turkish (-$\alpha^{20.5}$/-$\alpha^{20.5}$) (Gurgey et al., 1989), and Asian Indian (Old et al., in preparation) origins. Many of these cases occur in restricted population groups or, in some cases, result from consanguineous marriages. Given the large number of α-thalassemia mutations that have been described (Chapter 17) one should be aware of potential, rare interactions in such situations. Very rarely, severe fetal anemia with or without overt hydrops fetalis may also result from the co-inheritance of both deletion and nondeletional α thalassemia (Table 18.1), an interaction that normally causes HbH disease (see above). The best examples were described by Chan et al. (1985), who have reported two cases of HbH hydrops fetalis (see below).

mRNA and Globin Synthesis in the Hydrops Fetalis Syndrome

Using complementary cDNA probes Kan et al. (1974) were first to demonstrate that there is no detectable α-globin mRNA in patients with the Hb Bart's hydrops fetalis syndrome. This has subsequently been confirmed in several studies (e.g., see Hunt et al., 1980). Consequently, no α-globin chain synthesis is detected in the peripheral blood of such infants (Weatherall et al., 1970) although β-globin synthesis appears entirely unaffected, underscoring the fact that there appears to be no regulatory feedback at any level between α- and β-globin chain synthesis.

Red Cell Indices and Hematologic Findings in the Hb Bart's Hydrops Fetalis Syndrome

The peripheral blood of infants with the Hb Bart's hydrops fetalis syndrome contains large, hypochromic red cells and shows considerable anisopoikilocytosis (Fig. 18.10). Some elongated cells are said to have the appearance of "sickle cells" (Wasi et al., 1974). The typical hematologic findings in infants with the hydrops fetalis syndrome are summarized in Table 18.3, the most striking abnormality being the severe degree of anemia with a mean hemoglobin of 6.5 g/dL (Vaeusorn et al., 1985). The reticulocyte count is high (Wasi et al., 1974) and the blood contains many nucleated red cells (Fig. 18.10). The bone marrow is hyperplastic and there are many sites (liver, spleen, kidney, and adrenals) of extramedullary hematopoiesis, predominantly erythropoietic, with widespread deposition of hemosiderin. The cause of the anemia is poorly understood and is probably multifactorial, involving underproduction of hemoglobin, hemolysis, and ineffective erythropoiesis. The role of Hb Bart's in the hemolysis and/or ineffective ery-

thropoiesis is not clear; unlike HbH (see above), Hb Bart's is soluble and appears relatively stable. Factors other than anemia (e.g., plasma protein concentration, umbilical blood flow) may contribute to the development of hydrops fetalis (Wasi et al., 1974).

Developmental Changes in Hemoglobin Composition

We now know that the Hb Bart's hydrops fetalis syndrome most commonly results from deletion of all four α-globin genes; α mRNA is undetectable (Kan et al., 1974) and therefore the primary abnormality is an inability to synthesize α-globin chains.

In affected individuals, the embryonic hemoglobins Gower 1 and Portland I are expressed normally, in the first few weeks of life, although there is no Hb Gower 2. Severe anemia probably develops at around 6 to 7 weeks of gestation when the switch from embryonic ζ- and ϵ- to fetal α- and γ-globin gene expression occurs (Peschle et al., 1985). In the absence of α-globin chain synthesis no HbF can be made and excess γ chains form soluble tetramers of Hb Bart's, which makes up to about 90 percent of the total hemoglobin. Toward the end of gestation, as the fetal γ to adult β switch occurs, small amounts of HbH appear in the fetal blood. Neither Hb Bart's nor HbH display any heme-heme interaction (Benesch et al., 1961; Horton et al., 1962), or Bohr effect and both bind oxygen very highly, as in the R state of normal hemoglobin (see Chapter 9). Consequently, oxygen delivery to the fetus is severely impaired throughout most of development and it is remarkable that the fetus survives at all. Viability depends on the persistent synthesis of embryonic ζ-globin chains. In affected individuals Hb Portland I and to a lesser extent Portland II make up about 10 percent to 20 percent of the fetal blood. Hb Portland displays a normal pattern of oxygen dissociation (Tuchinda et al., 1975) and can therefore deliver oxygen to the developing fetus.

The molecular and cellular basis for persistent ζ-globin expression is not understood. A very small increase in ζ-globin chains (Chui et al., 1986, 1989; Kutlar et al., 1989; Tang et al., 1992; Ausavarungnirun et al., 1998) is seen in some carriers of deletions that cause α thalassemia and, superficially, this resembles the persistent γ-globin gene expression that accompanies some deletions that remove the β-globin genes (hereditary persistence of fetal hemoglobin, HPFH, see Chapter 15). However, the levels of ζ globin observed in carriers of α thalassemia (<1 percent) are much lower than levels of γ globin in HPFH. It seems likely that mechanisms other than increased ζ-globin gene transcription (e.g., cell selection or alterations in ζ-globin mRNA stability)

Table 18.3. Hematology in the Normal Developing Fetus and Those with the Hb Bart's Hydrops Fetalis Syndrome

Age (wk)	RBC ($\times 10^{12}$/L)	Hb (g/dL)	PCV (%)	MCV (fl)	MCH (pg)	Reticulocytes (%)	Hb Bart's (%)	Hb Portland (%)	Reference
Nonthalassemic									
30–31	4.79 ± 0.74	19.1 ± 2.2	60 ± 8	127 ± 12.7	38*	5.8 ± 2			Nathan and Oski, 1987
~40	5.14 ± 0.7	19.3 ± 2.2	61 ± 7.4	119 ± 9.4	34*	3.2 ± 1.4	<1		Nathan and Oski, 1987
~40	4.7 ± 0.8	16.5 ±3.0	51 ± 9	108 ± 10	34 ± 3	–			Dallman, 1977
Hydrops fetalis									
28–43	2.2 ± 0.8	6.5 ± 2.3	30.4 ± 13.8	136 ± 23	31.9 ± 9	–	86.9 ± 5.1	13.1 ± 5.8	Vaeusorn et al., 1985
30–40	–	6.7	–	100–190	–	Variable, may be >60%	70–80	–	Wasi et al., 1974
28–38	–	4.9 (3–8.5)	21.3	–	–	–	–	–	Thumasathit et al., 1968

Note: Mean values ± SD.
* Calculated MCH.

must be operating to allow such high levels of Hb Portland to accumulate. However, it is interesting that the embryonic Hb Gower 1 does not persist in this condition, suggesting that the effect specifically acts on ζ-globin expression rather than a general effect on embryonic globin expression.

Clinical and Autopsy Findings

Following a gestation of about 33 weeks (range 23 to 43 weeks) infants with the Hb Bart's hydrops fetalis syndrome usually die *in utero*, during delivery, or within an hour or two of birth (Thumasathit et al., 1968; Liang et al., 1985; Nakayama et al., 1986; Vaeusorn et al., 1985; Chui and Waye, 1998). Occasionally even without specific treatment, some babies survive for a few days (Nakayama et al., 1986; Isarangkura et al., 1987). Typically, affected infants are pale, slightly jaundiced, growth retarded, and edematous with a massive, friable placenta (see Fig. 18.10). The skin may be affected by a "blueberry muffin" rash caused by subcutaneous nodules of extramedullary hematopoiesis (Beutler et al., 1995). In one study the placenta to fetal weight ratio ranged from 0.37 to 1.16 (mean 0.68) compared to the normal ratio of 0.15 to 0.25 (Liang et al., 1985). Sometimes the abdomen is distended with ascites but not all cases are grossly hydropic (e.g., Chui and Waye, 1998). Developmental abnormalities have been reported in up to 17 percent of cases (Guy et al., 1985; Liang et al., 1985; Nakayama et al., 1986). These include hydrocephaly (Liang et al., 1985), microcephaly (Liang et al., 1985), abnormal limb development (Liang et al., 1985; Carr et al., 1995; Harmon et al., 1995; Abuelo et al., 1997; Chitayat et al., 1997), and urogenital abnormalities, including undescended testes, variable degrees of hypospadias, ambiguous genitalia, and even male pseudohermaphroditism (reviewed in Wasi et al., 1969; Wasi et al., 1974; Ongsangkoon et al., 1978; Liang et al., 1985; Isarangkura et al., 1987; Abuelo et al., 1997).

At autopsy, ascites is usually pronounced and there are often pleural and pericardial effusions. Organ weights are usually reported with respect to gestational age, body weight, and body length (Fig. 18.11). The combination of edema and disturbed growth in hydropic babies can severely distort these relationships. With this caveat, enlargement of the heart, liver, and to a

Figure 18.11. The placental weight, body weight, fetal length, and brain weight of a series of infants with the Hb Bart's hydrops fetalis syndrome. The open circles represent the mean values and 95 percent confidence limits. (Redrawn, with permission from S. Fucharoen, from Vaeusorn et al., 1985.)

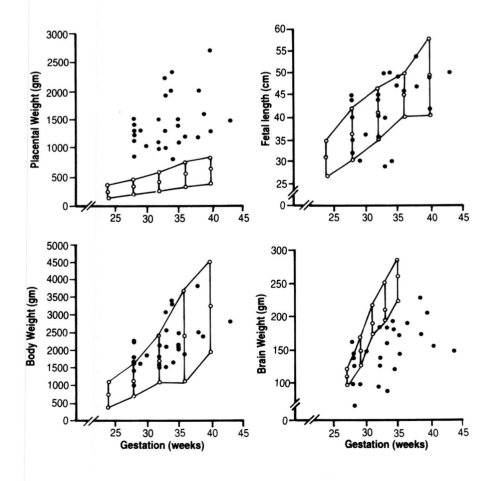

lesser degree the spleen are usually observed, whereas retarded development of the lung, thymus, adrenals, and kidney are often reported (Wasi et al., 1969, 1974; Nakayama et al., 1986; Vaeusorn et al., 1985). Of particular interest there is a progressive decrease in brain weight relative to that expected for gestational age from about 8 weeks of gestation (see Fig.18.11). Again, many congenital abnormalities have been noted at postmortem including cardiac defects (Liang et al., 1985; Vaeusorn et al., 1985), pulmonary hypoplasia (Vaeusorn et al., 1985), and undescended and intraabdominal testes (Nakayama et al., 1986) (reviewed in Abuelo et al., 1997).

Histologically, interstitial edema is noted in all tissues. There are multiple sites of extramedullary erythropoiesis. Up to 60 percent to 70 percent of the liver parenchyma may consist of developing red cells. The placenta is vascular and edematous containing many nucleated red cells. It has been speculated that hematologic changes in this condition may cause occlusion of small blood vessels with subsequent disruption of end organs (e.g., as in abnormal limb development) (Chitayat et al., 1997). It is interesting that, even though the vast majority of infants with hydrops fetalis have an identical genotype there is considerable variation in the pace and extent of abnormal development in each fetus.

Maternal Complications

Mothers of infants with this disorder often give a history of previous stillbirths or neonatal deaths; early miscarriages are probably uncommon. All reports point to an increased incidence of serious maternal complications (see Table 18.4, Liang et al., 1985; Nakayama et al., 1986; Vaeusorn et al., 1985).

In the antenatal period most problems arise in the third trimester when some mothers note a cessation of fetal movements. Common complications include anemia, preeclampsia (hypertension, fluid retention with or without proteinuria), polyhydramnios (excessive accumulation of amniotic fluid), oligohydramnios (decreased amniotic fluid), antepartum hemorrhage, and the premature onset of labor (Table 18.4). Less common general medical and obstetric complications have also been reported (Guy et al., 1985; Liang et al., 1985; Nakayama et al., 1986; Vaeusorn et al., 1985). Labor and delivery may be particularly difficult and assistance (in the form of embryotomy, breech, forceps, and Caesarean section) is required in approximately 50 percent of cases. Postpartum complications include retained placenta, hemorrhage, eclampsia (fits and coma), sepsis, and anemia. It has been suggested that, without medical care, up to 50 percent of women carrying affected fetuses would die as a result of such pregnancies (Vaeusorn et al., 1985). However, to date, there have

Table 18.4. Maternal Complications in the Hb Bart's Hydrops Fetalis Syndrome

	Hydrops (%)			Nonhydrops[‡] (%)
Antepartum				
Anemia	65			17
Preeclampsia	61	78	35	7
Eclampsia	0	1.5		<1
Polyhydramnios	59	3	17.5	<1
Antepartum hemorrhage	6.5	11[†]		3
Placenta previa	4.3			
Abruptio placenta	*		10	
Premature delivery	93	35		5–10
Delivery and postpartum				
Malpresentation	37			<5
Assisted vaginal delivery	35	34		5
Caesarean section	17	14		2–3
Retained placenta	*			*
Postpartum hemorrhage		11[†]		5
Anemia	46			*
Reference	Liang et al., 1985	Vaeusorn et al., 1985	Nakayama et al., 1986	Liang et al., 1985; Llewellyn-Jones 1969

* Recorded but figures are not given.
[†] Includes ante- and postpartum hemorrhage.
[‡] These figures are only a guide since they will vary greatly depending on the population studied and the level of antenatal care provided.

been no retrospective studies of maternal mortality rates in communities where medical assistance is unavailable.

HbH Hydrops Fetalis

Nearly all babies with the Hb Bart's hydrops fetalis syndrome inherit no α-globin genes. However, three reports describe seven rare neonates with severe anemia and various changes associated with hydrops fetalis due to the co-inheritance of α^0 and α^+ thalassemia (Chan et al., 1985; Trent et al., 1986; Ko et al., 1991; Chan et al., 1997). In three well-characterized cases the α^+ thalassemia resulted from mutations in the $\alpha2$ gene associated with highly unstable α-globin variants (Ko et al., 1991; Chan et al., 1997; and Ko, personal communication).

Mothers of these children gave a history of previous neonatal deaths due to anemia. At birth all affected infants were anemic (hemoglobin, 3.4 to 9.7 g/dL) with large amounts of Hb Bart's (31 percent to 65 percent). Five of the seven infants died at birth and two survived following intrauterine blood transfusion but have remained transfusion dependent.

These cases thus represent the transition between severe, transfusion-dependent HbH disease (see above) and Hb Bart's hydrops fetalis. As accurate molecular diagnosis becomes more common we would expect to identify further similar cases. It is not clear why some patients with α^0, α^+ thalassemia interactions should be so severely affected while others with an identical interaction (e.g., see Ko et al., 1991 and Bowden, unpublished) may survive normally.

Long-Term Survival of α^0-Thalassemia Homozygotes

As noted above, there is considerable variability in the clinical course of infants with the Hb Bart's hydrops fetalis syndrome. Although most die *in utero*, during delivery or within 1 or 2 hours of birth others may survive for several days (Isarangkura et al., 1987); in some cases the diagnosis may not be immediately obvious in a newborn infant. It is therefore not surprising that during the past 10 years, as neonatal care has continued to improve, several homozygotes for α^0 thalassemia have survived either as a result of treatment prior to confirmation of the diagnosis or as a result of preplanned intervention. Currently we know of nine such cases (Table 18.5). Most have been delivered prematurely by Caesarean section and transfused soon after birth. Two were transfused *in utero* from 25 weeks onwards. Most infants have a stormy postnatal period with cardiopulmonary problems, and there is disturbingly high frequency of congenital abnormalities including patent ductus arteriosus, limb deformi-

ties, and urogenital abnormalities in male infants. Subsequent development has been abnormal in at least half of the children and all require regular blood transfusion and chelation therapy for survival.

Prevention and Management

Ideally one should screen and identify couples at risk of conceiving a fetus with the Hb Bart's hydrops fetalis syndrome prior to or early in pregnancy, as set out above (see section on management of patients with a thalassemia trait). The majority of these patients will be of Southeast Asian origin but less commonly individuals of Mediterranean or mixed origins may be at risk (Petrou et al., 1992). For accurate prenatal diagnosis, it is essential to determine precisely the parental genotypes by Southern blot or PCR-based strategies (see Chapters 17, 35, and 36). If both parents carry one or other of the known α^0-thalassemia defects there will be a one in four chance that they will conceive a fetus with the Hb Bart's hydrops fetalis syndrome. However, if both parents have α^0-thalassemia haplotypes in which both α and ζ genes are deleted (e.g., - -^{FIL}/- -^{THAI}) then they will not produce hydropic infants since homozygotes (e.g., - -^{FIL}/- -^{FIL}) and compound heterozygotes (e.g., - -^{FIL}/- -^{THAI}) for these defects will be lost soon after conception (Fischel-Ghodsian et al., 1988). Compound heterozygotes for the - -^{SEA}/- -^{FIL} mutations have the common form of hydrops fetalis. If at-risk couples request prenatal testing, fetal DNA can be obtained from chorionic villi sampling (CVS) or fetal cells obtained by amniocentesis. DNA and hemoglobin analysis can be performed on blood samples obtained by cordocentesis in the second trimester of pregnancy. These techniques are discussed in Chapter 35.

Ultrasonography can also be useful in the management of pregnancies at risk for the Hb Bart's hydrops fetalis syndrome (Guy et al., 1985; Ghosh et al., 1987; Saltzman et al., 1989; Kanokpongsakdi et al., 1990; Tongsong et al., 1996). In most cases placental thickness is greater than 2 SD above normal after 12 weeks of gestation; by 18 weeks it is abnormal in all cases (Ghosh et al., 1987, 1994). Similarly the cardiothoracic ratio is increased (> 0.5) in most, if not all, affected fetuses by 13 to 14 weeks gestation (Lam and Tang, 1997). Other features including subcutaneous edema, hepatomegaly, pleural effusion, pericardial effusion, enlarged umbilical vessels, and oligohydramnios and ascites appear with increasing frequency from about 12 weeks onwards (Lam and Tang, 1997) but are not consistently detected by ultrasonography until 22 to 28 weeks of gestation (Tongsong et al. 1996).

These findings can be of help in two situations. First they may alert an obstetrician to the diagnosis if this has not been considered earlier in pregnancy. Second, in

Table 18.5. Summary of Clinical and Hematologic Data for Infants Who Have Survived the Hb Bart's Hydrops Fetalis Syndrome

Case	Sex	Delivery (weeks of gestation)	Method	First transfusion	Neonatal problems	Hb at birth (g/dL)	Wt at birth (g)	Hb Portland (%)	Subsequent development	References
1	M	34	CS	Intrauterine at 25 weeks	Missing one third of foot, syndactyly, hand defects, hypospadias, incompletely descended right teside	Transfused	2,100	Transfused	Psychological testing at 21/12 showed developmental delay ≡16 mo, motor delay at 21/12 ≡ 7–16/12, growth below the third percentile at 21/12	Carr et al., 1995; Abuelo et al., 1997
2	M	32	CS	At birth	Cardiopulmonary convulsions, PDA, hypospadias, cholestatic jaundice, subarachnoid hemorrhage	9.7	2,300	20	At 14 mo = 6–9 mo; at 6 y, delay in speech and hearing. Height at the 10th percentile, weight at the 5th percentile	Beaudry et al., 1986; Jackson et al., 1990
3	F	28	CS	At birth	Respiratory distress, jaundice	(PCV 29.1%)	1,080	19	At 5 y normal development. 50% height, 25% weight	Bianchi et al., 1986; Fischel-Ghodsian et al., 1987; Jackson et al., 1990
4	NR	28	PV (breech)	At birth	NR	NR	NR	7	Gross motor delay 10 mo. height 5%, weight 5%	Jackson et al., 1990
5	F	31	CS	At birth	Jaundice, PDA, heart failure	7.9	1,600	NR	At 27 mo, growth retarded (less than third percentile). Spastic quadriplegia and profound developmental delay	Lam et al., 1992
6	M	33	CS	At birth	Jaundice, metabolic instability, cortical infarcts on CT scan, right inguinal hernia	9.7	1,850	17*	Spastic diplegia at 20 mo. Mild global development delay	S. Howarth, 1996 and C. Cole, 1998 (personal communication)
7	F	32	PV	At birth	PDA, cardiopulmonary, "blueberry muffin" rash	~7.0	1,623	10	Severe growth retardation, asymmetry in hand size. Limited neuropsychiatric assessment appears normal at 5 y	D.K. Bowden, 1992 (unpublished)
8	M	35	PV	At birth	Penoscrotal hypospadias	(PCV 30%)	1,900	22	At 6/12 weight at the 10th percentile, length at the 3rd percentile	C.K. Li (personal communication)
9	NR	37	CS	Intrauterine at 26 weeks	Cardiopulmonary, thrombocytopenia, left portal vein obstruction	NR	NR	NR	Neurologically normal at 3 y	Naqvi et al., 1997

Abbreviations: CS, Caesarean section; PV, pev vaginum; PDA, patent ductus arteriosus; NR, not recorded.
* Not confirmed as Hb Portland.

453

areas where DNA analysis is currently unavailable, it provides a reasonable way to monitor and select at-risk pregnancies for further investigation by hemoglobin electrophoresis of samples obtained by cordocentesis (Lam and Tang, 1997).

At present there is no suitable treatment for the Hb Bart's hydrops fetalis syndrome. Early intervention with intrauterine transfusions (Carr et al., 1995; Abuelo et al., 1997; Naqvi et al., 1997) are difficult to justify because even when successful the child is committed to lifelong blood transfusion and iron chelation. To address this, there have been three unsuccessful attempts to perform *in utero* hematopoietic stem cell transplantation (Diukman and Golbus, 1992; Eddleman, 1996; Westgren et al., 1996). Again, survivors of such unsuccessful procedures (Westgren et al., 1996) require lifelong transfusion. In addition, we do not yet understand when or why other congenital abnormalities occur in this condition; therefore, current attempts to treat this condition are associated with an unknown risk of rescuing infants with multiple, often severe developmental abnormalities. Until these problems have been adequately addressed and solved [e.g., by using the excellent mouse model developed by Pászty et al. (1995; Pászty, 1997); see below and Chapter 34], further human experimentation should be avoided. Given the serious obstetric risk to the mother of an affected fetus it seems most prudent to advise early termination of pregnancy in all cases.

THE ACQUIRED FORM OF α THALASSEMIA ASSOCIATED WITH MYELODYSPLASIA

Very rarely patients with myelodysplasia (MDS) develop an unusual form of HbH disease with a striking hypochromic microcytic anemia, classical HbH inclusions (Fig. 18.12), and detectable levels of HbH in the peripheral blood. Most cases are of North European origin and in all cases where archival data are available there is no evidence of preexisting α thalassemia. The first cases to be reported were diagnosed as having a variety of hematologic malignancies including leukemias, myelofibrosis, myeloproliferative diseases, and acquired sideroblastic anemias. Most of these reports preceded the accurate definition of MDS set out by the French-American-British (FAB) group (Bennett et al., 1982). A recent review of fourteen cases of acquired α thalassemia by Craddock (1994) demonstrated that all of these patients have one or another form of MDS and therefore we now refer to this condition as the α thalassemia/myelodysplasia syndrome (ATMDS).

Table 18.6 summarizes the findings in fifty-four patients with ATMDS including all cases so far described plus twenty-two previously unpublished cases studied in our laboratory. The patients are predominantly male (fifty out of fifty-four) with a mean age of 66 years at presentation. It is of interest that two of the four female patients had an atypical underlying hematologic disease: one had acute lymphoblastic leukemia (Kueh, 1982); another developed MDS after treatment for essential thrombocythemia, whereas most patients with this syndrome have primary MDS. The course of this disease is quite variable. The predominant clinical features are those associated with myelodysplasia; about 30 percent have splenomegaly. Most patients eventually develop acute myeloid leukemia or refractory cytopenias as one would expect in a group of patients with MDS.

α-Globin mRNA and Chain Synthesis Ratios in Patients With ATMDS

The α- to β-globin mRNA ratio has only been studied in three patients with ATMDS but was severely reduced (0.06 to 0.50) in all cases (Higgs et al., 1983). The α/β-globin chain synthesis ratio was similarly reduced (mean 0.28, range 0.05 to 0.67) in all twenty-two patients in which this has been reported. In the most severely affected individuals α-chain synthesis was almost abolished (Fig. 18.13). The α/β-chain synthesis ratio may vary quite considerably during the course of the disease (Higgs et al., 1983).

Red Cell Indices and Hematologic Findings in ATMDS

Patients with ATMDS are always anemic at presentation (mean hemoglobin 8.5 g/dL) with a reduced RBC count (4.3×10^{12}/L) and severe hypochromic (mean MCH 22 pg) and microcytic (mean MCV 75 fl) indices. These abnormalities are even more striking when compared with a control population of patients with MDS (D. Oscier, personal communication) who tend to have slightly higher MCH values (mean MCH 31 pg) than normal at presentation (Fig. 18.14). The red cell diameter width (RDW) was increased in all patients studied. These findings are reflected in the peripheral blood red cell morphology (Fig. 18.12). All patients studied have hypochromic microcytic red cells and in many cases there is marked anisopoikilocytosis. In some cases it appears that there are at least two populations of cells, one quite well hemoglobinized and another consisting of "ghost cells" containing very little hemoglobin (Fig. 18.12).

Hemoglobin Analysis in ATMDS

All patients with ATMDS have detectable amounts of HbH in peripheral red blood cells at some stage in

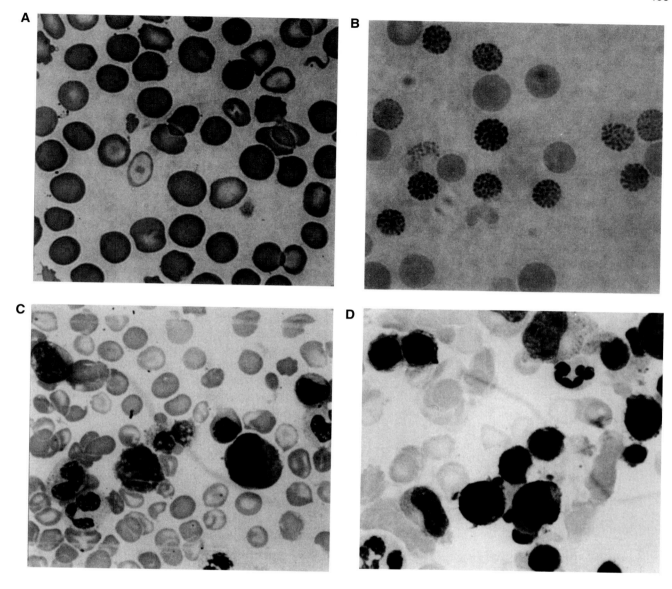

Figure 18.12. Peripheral blood film (**A**) and peripheral blood stained with brilliant cresyl blue (**B**) from a patient with ATMDS and an α/β-globin chain biosynthesis ratio of less than 0.1. Bone marrow samples from the same patient (**C, D**) showing erythroid expansion with dyserythropoietic features including binuclearity and cytoplasmic vacuolation. The neutrophils appear hypogranular. For full color reproduction, see color plates 18.12A–D.

At presentation, the proportion of red cells containing HbH inclusions after incubation with brilliant cresyl blue varies between 0.5 percent and 93 percent (mean 38 percent). Just as the α/β-globin synthesis ratio varies in the course of the disease the proportion of HbH and cells containing HbH inclusions also vary within an individual with ATMDS.

the disease; the recorded levels at presentation range between 1 percent and 57 percent (mean 15 percent). Often it is not possible to obtain accurate estimations of HbH because of prior blood transfusion. In some patients trace amounts of Hb Bart's have been found. In the presence of these high affinity hemoglobins the whole blood oxygen dissociation curve is shifted to the left (Weatherall et al., 1981).

The Molecular and Cellular Basis for ATMDS

The simplest situation to evaluate occurs in patients with less than 10 percent of the normal levels of α-globin mRNA and α-globin synthesis (see Table 18.6 and Fig. 18.13). This level of α-globin synthesis is less than one sees in patients with one functional α-globin gene and implies that all four α-genes are downregulated. Structural analysis of the α-globin genes and

Table 18.6. Hematologic and Clinical Data on Patients with ATMDS

	Age	Sex	Race	Spleno-megaly	Hb (g/dL)	MCV (fl)	MCH (pg)	% BCB	% HbH	α/β RATIO	Karyotype	Diagnosis	Reference
1	60	M	CA		N/A	N/A	N/A	30	N/A	N/A		Erythroleukemia	White et al., 1960
2	46	M	CA		N/A	N/A	N/A	20	N/A	N/A		Erythroleukemia	White et al., 1960
3	49	F	CA		N/A	N/A	N/A	1	N/A	N/A		Erythroleukemia	White et al., 1960
4	72	M			7.8	93	16	N/A	N/A	N/A		Atypical hemolytic anemia	Bergren and Sturgeon, 1960
5	74	M			8.7	74	22	N/A	N/A	N/A		Atypical hemolytic anemia	Bergren and Sturgeon, 1960
6	56	M	CA		N/A	N/A	N/A	N/A	10	N/A		Atypical CML	Beaven et al., 1963
7	76	M			N/A	N/A	N/A	N/A	N/A	N/A		AML	Labie et al., 1968
8	70	M	CA	+	6.1	66	15	93	42	N/A	46 XY	Erythroleukemia	Rosenzweig et al., 1968
9	80	M		−	10.0	97	29	N/A	10	N/A	46 XY	Erythroleukemia	Rosenzweig et al., 1968
10	73	F	CA	+	4.6	63	15	60	20	0.13		Myeloproliferative disorder	Hamilton et al., 1971
11	66	M	CA	+	7.7	N/A	N/A	60	N/A	N/A		Erythroleukemia	Andre et al., 1972
12	72	M	CA		8.6	N/A	N/A	30	15	N/A		Erythroleukemia	Beaven et al., 1978
13	47	M	LE		N/A	71	21	40	20	N/A		Sideroblastic anemia	Boehme et al., 1978
14	65	M	CA	−	N/A	80	N/A	50	18	N/A		Sideroblastic anemia	Boehme et al., 1978
15	81	M	CA	−	11.3	66	16	90	57	0.07	46 XY	Myeloproliferative disorder	Weatherall et al., 1978
16	84	M	CA	−	6.9	69	19	60	18	0.39		Myeloproliferative disorder	Lindsey et al., 1978
17	82	M	SP	+	N/A	N/A	N/A	80	27	N/A		Sideroblastic anemia	Villegas et al., 1979
18	85	M	SP	+	10.7	59	N/A	12	N/A	N/A		Myelodysplasia (RAEB)	Villegas et al., 1979
19	68	M	CA	+	10.6	75	26	80	37	0.05		Myeloproliferative disorder	Veer et al., 1979
20	59	M	OR	+	4.0	N/A	N/A	9	3	0.67		AML	Tanaka et al., 1979
21	30	M	IN	−	4.3	N/A	N/A	1	N/A	N/A		Myelofibrosis	Dash and Dash, 1980
22	42	M	OR	+	N/A	78	N/A	N/A	2	N/A		Myelofibrosis	Nakatsuji et al., 1980
23	63	M	OR	−	N/A	N/A	N/A	66	27	0.1	46 XY	Myeloproliferative disorder	Yoo et al., 1980
24	18	F	OR	+	6.0	66	19	50	N/A	N/A	46 XX	ALL	Kueh, 1982
25	68	M	IT		7.5	97	21	N/A	4	0.43		Sideroblastic anemia	Massa et al., 1987
26	61	M	CA	+	5.9	69	19	4	4	0.09	46 XY	Myelofibrosis	Higgs et al., 1983
27	77	M	CA	−	12.7	89	29	57	20	0.09	46 XY	Myeloproliferative disorder	Higgs, unpublished (JP)
28	78	M	CA	−	9.0	82	28	7	1	0.66		Myeloproliferative disorder	Higgs, unpublished (AC)
29	86	M	CA		8.8	N/A	23	14	10	0.29		Sideroblastic anemia	Higgs, unpublished (RC)
30	76	M	CA		7.9	N/A	23	N/A	4	N/A		Myelodysplasia	Higgs, unpublished

No.	Age	Sex	Race	Spl.							Karyotype	Diagnosis	Reference
31	56	M	CA		8.3	69	N/A	N/A	1	0.53		Sideroblastic anemia	Higgs, unpublished
32	65	M	CA		9.7	84	27	N/A	N/A	N/A	46 XY	Sideroblastic anemia post-AML	Higgs, unpublished
33	68	M	CA	+	10.2	59	16	N/A	37	N/A		Sideroblastic anemia	Higgs, unpublished
34	72	M	OR	-	8.9	78	N/A	N/A	33	0.15	46 XY	Myelodysplasia (RA)	Anagnou et al., 1983
35	29	M	CA	-	8.4	98	N/A	34	2	N/A		Sideroblastic anemia	Tokuda et al., 1984
36	75	M	CA	-	7.3	59	18	70	27	0.18		Myelodysplasia (RAEBT)	Annino et al., 1984
37	64	M	OR	+	9.2	76	22	N/A	1	N/A	46 XY	Myelodysplasia (RA)	Abbondanzo et al., 1988
38	56	M	CA	-	6.0	78	24	N/A	N/A	N/A	46 XY20q-	Refractory anemia	Yoshida et al., 1990
39	74	M	CA		8.2	69	21	64	3	N/A		Erythroleukemia	Bürgi et al., 1992
40	76	M	CA	-	9.3	84	29	1	N/A	0.47		Myelodysplasia	Higgs, unpublished (CS)
41	87	F	CA	-	8.2	80	26	20	N/A	0.62		Essential thrombocythemia	Higgs, unpublished (MG)
42	72	M	CA	+	11.9	59	17	40	17	0.09	46 XY	Myelodysplasia (RA)	Higgs, unpublished (DW)
43	68	M	CA	-	8.9	91	29	6	N/A	0.6	47 XY del20+8	Myelodysplasia (RA)	Higgs, unpublished (CW)
44	63	M	CA	+	5.2	N/A	N/A	20	N/A	N/A	46 XY	Myelodysplasia (RA)	Higgs, unpublished (DB)
45	60	M	CA		5.6	67	10	35	3	0.18	46 XY	Myelodysplasia (RA)	Higgs, unpublished (JP)
46	72	M	CA	-	6.9	80	24	48	9	0.09	46 XY	Myelodysplasia (RA)	Higgs, unpublished (JS)
47	63	M	CA	-	9.0	65	18	8	8	N/A	46 XY	Myelodysplasia (CMML)	Higgs, unpublished (WW)
48	73	M	CA	+	8.9	67	N/A	N/A	3	N/A		Myelodysplasia	Higgs, unpublished (EP)
49	57	M	CA	-	9.7	76	23	25	1	N/A		Myelodysplasia (RA)	Higgs, unpublished (GL)
50	78	M	CA	-	12.2	85	29	30	23	N/A		Myelodysplasia (RA)	Higgs, unpublished (AS)
51	60	M	CA	-	10.3	70	23	4	2	N/A		Myelodysplasia (RA)	Higgs, unpublished (LF)
52	78	M	CA	-	11.9	79	23	25	15	0.13		Myelodysplasia (RAEB)	Higgs, unpublished (HW)
53	75	M	CA	-	7.9	73	23	42	15	N/A		Myelodysplasia (RAEB)	Higgs, unpublished (FC)
54	83	M	CA	-	11.0	69	19	75	38	0.09		Myelodysplasia (RAEB)	Higgs, unpublished (AK)
Average	66				8.5	75	22	38	15	0.28			
S.D.	14				2.15	11	5	27	14	0.22			

Abbreviations: CA, Caucasian; LE, Lebanese; SP, Spanish; OR, Oriental; IN, Asian Indian; IT, Italian; N/A, not available. Splenomegaly was either present (+), absent (–), or not recorded. These data were compiled by C.F. Craddock (Craddock, 1994).

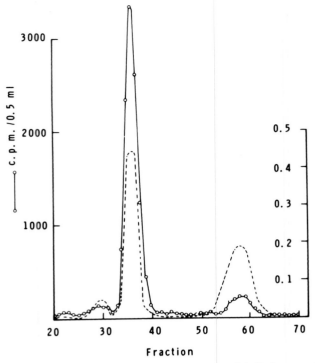

Figure 18.13. Separation of radioactively labelled α- and β-globin chains (○-○) from a patient with ATMDS. The OD²⁸⁰ profile is shown as a dashed line. The profile reveals a severely reduced level of α-globin chain synthesis (α-globin peak is around fraction 58).

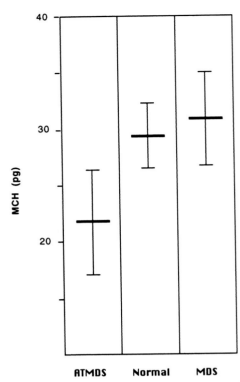

Figure 18.14. The MCH values in patients with ATMDS, normal individuals, and a group of patients with myelodysplasia (MDS). The mean is shown as a thick horizontal bar. 1 SD (ATMDS and MDS) or 2 SD (normal) values are shown as thin vertical lines.

–130 kb of their flanking regions on chromosome 16p has revealed no abnormalities in such severely affected patients (Higgs et al., 1983; Craddock, 1994). Furthermore, provisional analysis of the pattern of methylation appears normal (Anagnou et al., 1983; Craddock, 1994). Although we have not excluded small rearrangements or single nucleotide changes, two cis-acting mutations seems a very unlikely basis for ATMDS. It seems more plausible, therefore, that the α genes are downregulated by a trans-acting mutation either in a factor that normally controls α-gene expression or in a gene that exerts a dominant negative effect.

It seems possible that in the ATMDS clone there is trans-acting defect that completely abolishes α-gene expression. The very low levels of α mRNA and α-globin chain synthesis (Fig. 18.13) might be the product of a small number of normal hematopoietic clone(s) or MDS clone(s) unaffected by the α-thalassemia mutation. Clonal evolution in this situation would explain the variations in HbH and α/β-globin chain synthesis observed during the course of the disease. Alternatively, the ATMDS mutation might cause variable downregulation of α-globin expression in all cells within a single MDS clone. This could provide a less satisfactory explanation for changes in HbH and globin synthesis during progres-

sion of the disease. At present we are unable to distinguish between these two possibilities.

This issue is of importance in designing further experiments to analyze ATMDS. For example, Helder and Deisseroth (1987) made interspecific hybrids between bone marrow from ATMDS patients and APRT deficient mouse erythroleukemia (MEL) cells. After selection, such hybrids retained human chromosome 16 derived from the ATMDS patient and this chromosome directed normal levels of human α-globin synthesis. While this might provide strong evidence that ATMDS results from a trans-acting mutation the interpretation critically depends on whether the human cell that originally fused with the MEL cell could have been from an unaffected clone.

The problem now is to localize and ultimately identify the acquired trans-acting abnormality in ATMDS. This would be of great importance to our understanding of α gene regulation and might also elucidate the molecular pathway to clonal evolution in MDS. Are there any clues to help this search? One of the most striking features of ATMDS is the marked sex bias (>90 percent of the patients are male) not seen in previous studies of MDS (Juneja et al., 1983; Noël et al., 1993). Superficially this might suggest involvement of the X chromosome with only one somatic mutation required to create a null mutation in XY males. However, this argument also applies to females because in each hematopoietic stem cell one X chromosome is inactivated by Lyonization. It is interesting that another acquired clonal hematopoietic disorder (paroxysmal nocturnal hemoglobinuria, PNH) results from mutations in an X-linked gene and this occurs with equal frequency in males and females. The X-chromosome hypothesis might apply to a gene that escapes X inactivation (so that females have two active copies) and is not present on the Y chromosome or if there were a high frequency of Y chromosome loss in the MDS clones. In the absence of such a clue we are left to search for nonrandom chromosome abnormalities. To date no consistent chromosome abnormalities have been found in the four ATMDS patients studied in this way.

Finally, are there any candidate genes? One would expect the general erythroid transcription factors (GATA-1, NF-E2, etc.) to affect α- and β-globin expression equally. However, the ATRX gene (see Chapter 19) encodes a putative transcriptional regulator that specifically affects α-globin gene expression. To date, provisional analysis of this gene in several patients has detected no abnormality.

INTERACTIONS BETWEEN α THALASSEMIA AND STRUCTURAL GLOBIN VARIANTS

Historically, interactions between α thalassemia and structural variants of the α- and β-globin chains were of considerable importance in developing our understanding of the genetics of hemoglobin synthesis (see Chapter 6). Now that we have a more detailed knowledge, one of the main reasons for considering these interactions is to provide a framework for interpreting the many different patterns they produce on routine hemoglobin electrophoresis. The co-inheritance of α thalassemia with some clinically important hemoglobinopathies is discussed in Chapters 27 to 29 and 43.

Interactions between α Thalassemia and α-Globin Structural Variants

When a patient inherits an entirely normal β-globin genotype and a full complement of α-globin genes with one containing a mutation for an α-globin structural variant, the amount of variant hemoglobin produced will depend on the rate at which it is synthesized, its stability, its affinity for β-globin chains (see below), and on whether the mutation affects the α_2- or α_1-globin gene. As discussed in Chapters 6, 8, and 17, although the ratio of α_2:α_1 mRNA is 3:1 there is still some disagreement about the relative contributions of the two genes to hemoglobin synthesis. In addition there is con-

siderable methodologic variation in the quantitation of hemoglobin variants. Not surprisingly the reported proportions of α-globin variants range from 0 (e.g., Hb Quong Sze) to 35 percent (e.g., Hb J Toronto) with an average value of about 25 percent (Chapter 45). Even if one excludes highly unstable α-globin gene mutants there is still considerable variation but, in general, mutations affecting the α_2 gene are present at higher levels than those affecting the α_1 gene (Huisman et al., 1996, and available via http://globin.cse.psu.edu). Hematologically most α-globin variants are quite innocuous although some give rise to high oxygen affinity (e.g., Hb Luton), congenital cyanosis (e.g., Hb M Boston), or hemolytic anemias (Chapter 44). Some heterozygotes for highly unstable mutants (e.g., Hb Quong Sze) may have the phenotype of α-thalassemia trait and these are best considered as determinants of nondeletional α thalassemia (see Chapter 17 and above). The effect of co-inheriting α thalassemia with α globin variants is to increase the proportion of the variant and to reinforce any associated clinical phenotype (Table 18.7). This principle is best demonstrated by the variant HbG-Philadelphia (α68) asn→lys (Chapter 45). Individuals with HbG-Philadelphia may have a full complement of four α genes and 20 percent to 25 percent of the variant hemoglobin with no hematologic abnormality (Bruzdzinski et al., 1984; Molchanova et al., 1994). In some individuals the HbG Philadelphia

---

Table 18.7 Interactions between α-Globin Variants and α Thalassemia

		Predicted* % of variant Hb	Hematologic phenotype
αα/α^{v}α	β^A/β^A	25[†]–37.5[‡]	Normal
αα/αα^v	β^A/β^A	12.5[†]–25[‡]	Normal
αα/α^{v}α^v	β^A/β^A	50	Normal
–α/α^{v}α	β^A/β^A	30[†]–50[‡]	α-thalassemia trait
–α/αα^v	β^A/β^A	16.6[‡]–30[†]	α-thalassemia trait
-α/α^{v}α^v	β^A/β^A	66	α-thalassemia trait
- -/αα^v	β^A/β^A	30[†]–50[‡]	α-thalassemia trait
–α^v/αα	β^A/β^A	50	α-thalassemia trait
–α^v/-α	β^A/β^A	50	α-thalassemia trait
- -/α^{v}α	β^A/β^A	50[†]–70[‡]	α-thalassemia trait
–α^v/-α^v	β^A/β^A	100	α-thalassemia trait
- -α^v/-α^v	β^A/β^A	100	HbH disease

Note: By reference to Huisman et al. (1996) all of these assumptions almost never apply to any known variant and estimated values often differ greatly from these predicted values.

* Assuming that the α^v variant is synthesized efficiently, completely stable, and associates with β^A chains with the same kinetics as α^A chains.

† Assuming that the relative contribution of α2 and α1 is 1:1.

‡ Assuming that the contribution of α2 and α1 is 3:1.

variant is present on an $-\alpha^{3.7}$ haplotype giving rise to genotypes $-\alpha^G/\alpha\alpha$, $-\alpha^G/-\alpha$, $-\alpha^G/-\alpha^G$ that produce 30 percent to 35 percent, about 45 percent, and 100 percent HbG Philadelphia, respectively (Milner and Huisman, 1976; Sancar et al., 1980; Pardoll et al., 1982); such patients have the hematologic phenotype of α-thalassemia trait. Rarely the $-\alpha^{3.7}$ haplotype may interact with α^0 thalassemia to produce HbH disease ($- -/-\alpha^G$). Such patients produce only HbH and HbG and have the classical clinical and hematologic phenotypes associated with HbH disease. The condition is referred to as HbG-H disease (Rieder et al., 1976; Sancar et al., 1980). A list of all mutations directly linked to an α-thalassemia determinant is given in Table 17.2; their interactions with other α-globin haplotypes are very similar to those described above for HbG Philadelphia (also see Table 18.7).

The interaction between HbI ($\alpha^{16 \, lys \to glu}$) and α thalassemia was initially very puzzling (Schwartz and Atwater, 1972). Most often this variant accounts for 24 percent to 28 percent of the total hemoglobin (Huisman et al., 1996). However, in one family, who also had α thalassemia, the level was about 70 percent. It is now known that rarely the HbI mutation may occur on both the α_2- and α_1-globin genes on the same chromosome, presumably as a result of gene conversion (Liebhaber et al., 1984) (see Chapter 45 and Table 18.7).

The interactions between α thalassemia and highly unstable α-globin variants are described above and in Chapter 17. In general, the genotypes in these cases give rise to α-thalassemia trait and the $- -/\alpha^T\alpha$ genotype is associated with HbH disease. There is a tendency for such individuals to fall at the severe end of the clinical spectrum of patients with HbH disease, including patients with HbH hydrops (see above).

Interactions between α Thalassemia and β-Globin Structural Variants

When a patient inherits an entirely normal α-globin genotype and two β-globin genes, one of which encodes a structural variant, the amount of variant hemoglobin produced will depend on its rate of synthesis, its stability, and the pattern of subunit assembly to form αβ dimers (Bunn and McDonald, 1983; Bunn, 1987). Ideally one would predict that equal amounts of HbA and variant hemoglobin would be present in the red cell, but in reality, as for α-globin mutants (see above), considerable variation is observed (Huisman et al., 1996). Some β-globin variants (e.g., HbE and Hb Knossos) are synthesized less efficiently than HbA and represent less than 50 percent of the hemoglobin in heterozygotes. Others (e.g., Hb Köln) are unstable and may represent 30 percent or less of the hemoglobin. The third factor, differences in the rates of αβ-sub-

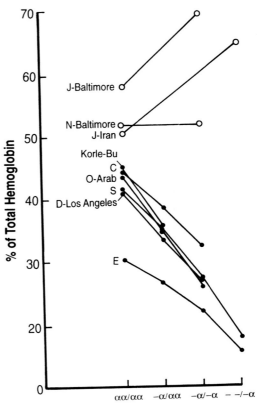

Figure 18.15. Effect of α thalassemia on the proportion of negatively charged (○) and positively charged (●) β-globin variants in heterozygotes. In all cases HbA constitutes the great majority of the remaining Hb. In three-gene deletion α thalassemia, a small amount of HbH (β_4) is present. (Redrawn from Bunn, 1987.)

unit assembly, may influence the accumulated levels of many stable hemoglobin variants.

The formation of αβ dimers is a rate-limiting step in the assembly of hemoglobin. This process is thought to be facilitated by the electrostatic attraction between positively charged α-globin subunits and negatively charged β-globin subunits. Many commonly encountered β-globin variants acquire positive charge (e.g., HbS and HbC) thereby reducing their ability to compete with β^A chains for hemoglobin assembly. In such cases less variant hemoglobin accumulates than HbA. The opposite is seen with negatively charged β-globin variants (Fig. 18.15). These observations are supported by in vitro subunit competition assays using mixtures of normal and variant β-globin subunits (Bunn and McDonald, 1983; Bunn, 1987). In the presence of α thalassemia, in which limiting amounts of α chains are synthesized in the red cell, these effects are exaggerated. The accumulated levels of positively charged β-globin gene variants are further decreased in proportion to the deficit in α-globin chains (Bunn and McDonald, 1983; Bunn, 1987). By contrast the levels of negatively charged variants may increase (Fig. 18.15). This is a good rule of thumb although there are exceptions (e.g., HbN Baltimore) and the situation becomes complex when more than one β variant is involved (e.g., HbS and HbC) or if α-globin variants are also present (see Chapter 8).

The presence of α thalassemia may influence the levels of HbA₂ in the presence of globin variants (see Chapter 10). The δ-globin subunit is considerably more positively charged than the β-globin subunit. In α thalassemia one would therefore expect the amount of HbA₂ to decrease, and, in general, this is what one sees (Wasi et al., 1969, 1974). However, in the presence of a variant, positively charged β subunit, which has less affinity for α subunits, there may be sufficient free α chains to interact with all δ subunits, thereby increasing the level of HbA₂. Such increases have been observed in individuals with sickle cell trait (Whitten and Rucknagel, 1981) and sickle cell disease although whether or not HbA₂ levels are truly increased in these conditions is open to question (see Chapter 34) (see below).

The presence of α thalassemia may also influence the levels of HbF and Hb Bart's in some interactions. Several observations suggest that αγ dimers form less readily than αβ dimers. As discussed before (see above) there is more Hb Bart's in newborns with α thalassemia than HbH in adults with the same genotype. There is some preliminary evidence that the proportion of HbF in newborns is lower in infants with α thalassemia than those with four α genes (Stallings et al., 1983). Evidence also comes from the study of Chui et al. (1990), who described an Italian boy who co-inherited HbH disease and the −117 $^A\gamma$-globin HPFH mutation. They found that approximately 90 percent of the α chains combined with β-globin chains to form HbA (about 78 percent) and 10 percent of the α chains associated with γ-globin chains to form HbF (9.5 percent). Although there were sufficient free γ chains to produce approximately 11 percent Hb Bart's, there were insufficient free β chains remaining to detect HbH on electrophoresis although HbH inclusions were detected. Taken together these findings support the hypothesis that α globin has a higher affinity for β than γ globin. However, the interpretation of these complex interactions is by no means certain, since there are other patients with similar interactions who produce different patterns of hemoglobin expression (e.g., see Rombos et al., 1989).

Hematologic Phenotype of Patients with α Thalassemia and β-Globin Variants

The hematologic phenotype of patients with α thalassemia and stable β-globin gene variants is usually determined by the β-globin mutant and the type of α thalassemia present (see Table 18.8; Chapters 28, 29,

Table 18.8. Proportion of Hemoglobin Variant and Hematologic Phenotypes in Patients with Positively Charged β Globin Variants

		Predicted level of variant	Hemoglobin hematologic phenotype
αα/αα	β^A/β^V	50%*	Normal
−α/αα	β^A/β^V	↓	α-thalassemia trait
−α/−α	β^A/β^V	↓↓	α-thalassemia trait
− −/αα	β^A/β^V	↓↓↓	α-thalassemia trait
− −/−α	β^A/β^V	↓↓↓↓	HbH disease

* Assuming that the variant is synthesized efficiently, completely stable, and associated with α^A chains with the same kinetics as β^A chains.

and 43). Interactions between nondeletional forms of α thalassemia and β-globin variants follow these same principles.

When a patient inherits only one functional α gene (or its equivalent) and a β-globin variant they usually have the clinical and hematologic phenotype of HbH disease. Splenomegaly is particularly prominent in some patients (Giordano et al., 1996). Such interactions have been described with HbC (Giordano et al., 1996), HbE (Thonglairuam et al., 1989), HbS (Matthay et al., 1979), and Hb Hope (DK, Bowden, unpublished). Hemoglobin analysis usually demonstrates HbA with a very reduced amount (10 percent to 20 percent) of the variant hemoglobin. The reported levels of HbH are quite variable in this interaction and sometimes undetectable by routine hemoglobin electrophoresis. Nevertheless, HbH inclusions can usually be demonstrated following incubation with brilliant cresyl blue. Hb Bart's may be detectable in some patients and is characteristically present (1 percent to 6 percent) in carriers for HbE with HbH disease, a condition referred to as HbAE-Bart's disease (Thonglairuam et al., 1989) (see Chapter 43).

Rare interactions between HbH disease and β-globin variants support the electrostatic model for hemoglobin subunit assembly. Su et al. (1992) reported HbH disease in a Chinese patient with the benign β-globin gene mutant Hb Hamilton, which has the same charge as β^A, and it appeared that the level of this mutant was not significantly reduced. Rahbar and Bunn (1987) described an Iranian female with HbH disease and HbJ-Iran (β77 his→asp), a negatively charged subunit. In this case the interaction with α thalassemia produced an increased level (65 percent) of the variant hemoglobin. Finally, Chan et al. (1987) described a Chinese female with a severe transfusion-dependent hemolytic anemia (hemoglobin 3.4 to 6.8 g/dL) resulting from the interaction of HbH disease with Hb New York (β113 val→glu), an unstable negatively charged β-globin variant. In this case the co-inheritance of α thalassemia increased the formation of Hb New York and thus exacerbated the hemolytic anemia.

α Thalassemia in Homozygotes and Compound Heterozygotes for β-Chain Abnormalities

α-Thalassemia is common wherever β thalassemia occurs (see Chapters 31 and 32). Similarly α thalassemia is found wherever HbS and HbE reach polymorphic frequencies (see Chapters 31 & 43). Consequently, there are many potential interactions between the determinants of α thalassemia and these β-globin chain abnormalities. In some cases, the co-inheritance of α thalassemia may significantly alter the phenotype of patients with β-chain hemoglobinopathies. The interactions between α thalassemia and β thalassemia are discussed in Chapter 13. Interactions between α thalassemia and homozygotes for HbE are presented in Chapter 43, and interactions with homozygotes for HbS in Chapter 28.

MOUSE MODELS OF α THALASSEMIA

In the late 1970s, mice mutagenized by radiation (352HB and 27HB) or chemical induction (Hba^{th-J}), were shown to have large (>30 kb) deletions spanning the entire α-globin gene cluster. These deletions also included an undetermined amount of the 5′ and 3′ flanking DNA. Heterozygotes have the typical findings of α-thalassemia trait with a reduced α/β-globin mRNA ratio, reduced α/β-globin chain synthesis ratio (Martinell et al., 1981; Wickramasinghe et al., 1986), and a mild hypochromic microcytic anemia with reticulocytosis (Anderson et al., 1982). Further characterization of Hba^{th-J} mice by Wickramasinghe et al. (1986) showed that differences in the red cell indices between normal and thalassemic mice only became apparent after 4 weeks of age. Hemoglobin analysis of 352HB heterozygotes (Popp et al., 1981) showed that

they produce substantial amounts of a tetramer of the embryonic β-like chain ε^{γ} throughout development. Using electron microscopy, Wickramasinghe et al. (1986) also found intracellular inclusions, thought to be precipitated HbH, in the reticulocytes and mature red cells of neonatal and adult Hba^{th-J} heterozygotes.

Embryos homozygous for these large deletions die approximately 2 days after implantation, long before the differentiation of hematopoietic tissues. This early lethality may be due to removal of critical genes flanking the mouse α-globin gene cluster. Therefore these mutant mice do not provide a model for the Hb Bart's hydrops fetalis syndrome. To develop more appropriate models, gene targeting was recently used to specifically inactivate one (Chang et al., 1996) or both (Pászty et al., 1995) mouse α-globin genes. Heterozygotes with the *α/αα genotype have the phenotype of α-thalassemia trait with a mild hypochromic, microcytic anemia (Table 18.9). Homozygotes (*α/*α) have a more severe anemia with an elevated reticulocyte count and 15 percent HbH. Thus, *α/*α homozygotes are more severely affected than - -/αα heterozygotes. It could be that the targeted 5′ mouse gene is normally expressed at higher levels than the 3′ gene and therefore the output of the affected chromosome is reduced to less than 50 percent of normal. Alternatively, the targeting in this case (Chang et al., 1996) left a neo gene in the cluster (*α) that may affect expression of the remaining α gene. Whatever the mechanism, homozygotes for this mutation (*α/*α) provide a model for HbH disease (Table 18.9). A severe, lethal form of HbH disease was seen in compound heterozygotes for the targeted chromosome and the Hba^{th-J} mutation (- -/*α).

In the targeted knockout made by Pászty et al. (1995) both adult α genes were removed as part of a 16-kb deletion. The targeting event was designed to leave the embryonic α gene (also called x in mouse) intact and functional. Heterozygotes (- -/α) have α-thalassemia trait with a mild hypochromic microcytic anemia and

---

Table 18.9 The Hematologic Data on Mice with Various Forms of α Thalassemia

Genotype	Hemoglobin (g/dL)	MCV (fl)	MCH (pg)	Reticulocytes (%)	HbH	HbH (%)
αα/αα	14.7 ± 1.3	56.7 ± 1.0	16.9 ± 0.4	2.6 ± 0.8		
αα/αα		135.6 ± 1.0*	34.4 ± 0.5*			
*α/αα	13.7 ± 0.8	51.0 ± 1.9	15.1 ± 0.6	2.3 ± 1.5		
*α/*α	13.2 ± 0.7	45.0 ± 1.2	12.2 ± 0.5	11.3 ± 0.6		15
- -/αα (Hba^{th-J})	12.8 ± 1.8	46.1 ± 2.5	13.5 ± 1.2	5.0 ± 0.8	+	ND
- -/*α		(Embryonic lethal)				55–65
- -/αα		122.4 ± 1.0*	33.3 ± 0.3*			Inclusions
- -/- - (βLCRα)		Phenotype of HbH disease			++	
- -/- -		103.8 ± 3.1*	29.6 ± 1.1*		+++	Inclusions

Note: Based on data from Wickramasinghe et al., 1986; Pászty et al., 1995; Chang et al., 1996.

* Values at 14.5 days gestation.

HbH-like inclusions detectable in peripheral red cells incubated with brilliant cresyl blue. Homozygotes for this deletion have no functional α-globin genes and die late in gestation—between 14.5 and 16.5 days of what is normally a 20-day gestation period. Affected fetuses are hydropic and their erythrocytes contain the murine equivalents of Hb Bart's and HbH. In all respects these findings are remarkably similar to what is found for infants with the Hb Bart's hydrops fetalis syndrome. Therefore, these mice represent a valid model of the Bart's hydrops fetalis syndrome. It is of interest that affected mice can be made viable using the human α-globin gene linked to the β-globin locus control region; rescued mice have the phenotype of mild HbH disease (Pászty et al., 1995). In the future these mice with α thalassemia may provide good models for understanding the pathophysiology of HbH disease and the Hb Bart's hydrops fetalis syndrome. However, it is important to note that the preliminary studies of Wickramasinghe et al. (1986) using Hba[th-J] mice suggest that the pathophysiology of HbH disease in mouse and humans may be somewhat different. Finally, these models provide an excellent test bed for approaches to gene therapy prior to any further human experimentation (see above). In addition, together with the recently developed mouse model of sickle cell disease (Pászty, 1997; Pászty et al., 1997; Ryan et al., 1997) (see Chapter 34) they may allow further analysis of the interaction between α thalassemia and sickle cell disease.

CONCLUSIONS

Over the past 20 years we have obtained a comprehensive understanding of the molecular basis of α thalassemia and we now know that a substantial proportion of the world's population have one or another of the genetic conditions summarized in this chapter. Because α thalassemia is so common, the chance finding of a hypochromic, microcytic anemia is often the cause of inappropriate investigation and concern for unaware or inexperienced physicians. Fortunately, once the diagnosis has been made only a small proportion, albeit large numbers, of patients need further attention. Most patients with HbH disease are clinically well whereas a few will have thalassemia intermedia. There is a real need to document more carefully the natural history of HbH disease and to establish more fully the correlation between genotype and phenotype to improve our ability to predict clinical severity. Ultimately, this would enable more precise prenatal counseling and would allow us to develop the best strategies for managing the relatively few patients who will be severely affected by this disorder.

The most important task for the future is to establish inexpensive, effective screening programs to avoid pregnancies leading to the lethal Hb Bart's hydrops fetalis and the rare HbH hydrops fetalis syndromes, which also impose considerable risk to the mother. At-risk couples may still not be routinely identified, even in countries with advanced medical services. The hematology is often a good guide to the underlying molecular defect but genotype analysis is essential for accurate diagnosis and appropriate genetic counseling. At present, attempts to correct the severe forms of α thalassemia by in utero transplantation seem inappropriate since the condition is naturally self-limiting and there is a very serious risk of partial success leading to infants that require lifelong transfusion and may have additional congenital abnormalities. Nevertheless, the establishment of mouse models of these diseases should enable progress to be made in testing appropriate strategies prior to the development of further protocols in humans. Current observations on the clinical and hematologic interactions of α thalassemia with β thalassemia (Chapter 13) and β-chain abnormalities such as that found in sickle cell disease suggest that reducing α-globin synthesis may offer another therapeutic approach to the amelioration of these conditions. Such approaches should arise out of our continued attempts to understand more completely the normal mechanisms by which the α-globin genes are regulated.

ACKNOWLEDGMENTS

We are grateful to Liz Rose for excellent secretarial assistance in the preparation of this chapter and to Dr. W.G. Wood for his comments and revisions. This chapter is substantially based on Chapter 11 by D.R. Higgs, in *The Thalassaemia Syndromes* (4th edition), edited by D.J. Weatherall (in preparation).

References

Abbondanzo, SL, Anagnou, NP, and Sacher, RA. (1988). Myelodysplastic syndrome with acquired hemoglobin H disease. *Am. J. Clin. Pathol.* 89: 401–406.

Abuelo, DN, Forman, EN, and Rubin, LP. (1997). Limb defects and congenital anomalies of the genitalia in an infant with homozygous α-thalassemia. *Am. J. Med. Genet.* 68: 158–161.

Anagnou, NP, Ley, TJ, Chesbro, B et al. (1983). Acquired α-thalassemia in preleukemia is due to decreased expression of all four α-globin genes. *Proc. Natl. Acad. Sci. U.S.A.* 80: 6051–6055.

Anderson, WF, Martinell, J, Whitney, JB III et al. (1982). Mouse models of human thalassaemia. In *Animal models of inherited metabolic diseases*. New York: Alan R. Liss. pp. 11–26.

Andre, R, Najman, A, Duhamel, G et al. (1972). Erythroleucemie avec hemoglobine H acquise et anomalies des antigenes erythrocytaires. *Nouv. Rev. Fr. Hematol.* 12: 29–42.

Annino, L, Di Giovanni, S, Tentori, L Jr et al. (1984). Acquired hemoglobin H disease in a case of refractory anemia with excess of blasts (RAEB) evolving into acute nonlymphoid leukemia. *Acta Haematol.* 72: 41–44.

Anuwatanakulchai, M, Pootrakul, P, Thuvasethakul, P, and Wasi, P. (1984). Non-transferrin plasma iron in β-thalassaemia/Hb E and haemoglobin H diseases. *Scand. J. Haematol.* 32: 153–158.

Arcasoy, MO and Gallagher, PG. (1995). Hematologic disorders and nonimmune hydrops fetalis. *Sem. Perinatol.* 19: 502–515.

Ausavarungnirun, R, Winichagoon, P, Fucharoen, S et al. (1998). Detection of ζ-globin chains in the cord blood by ELISA (enzyme-linked immunosorbent assay): Rapid screening for α-thalassemia-1 (Southeast Asian type). *Am. J. Hematol.* 57: 283–286.

Baysal, E, Kleanthous, M, Bozkurt, G et al. (1995). α-Thalassaemia in the population of Cyprus. *Br. J. Haematol.* 89: 496–499.

Beaudry, MA, Ferguson, DJ, Pearse, K et al. (1986). Survival of a hydropic infant with homozygous α-thalassemia-1. *J. Pediatr.* 108: 713–715.

Beaven, GH, Stevens, BL, Dance, N, and White, JC. (1963). Occurrence of haemoglobin H in leukaemia. *Nature* 199: 1297–1298.

Beaven, GH, Coleman, PN, and White, JC. (1978). Occurrence of haemoglobin H in leukaemia: A further case of erythroleukaemia. *Acta Haematol.* 59: 37–44.

Benesch, RE, Ranney, HM, Benesch, R, and Smith, GM. (1961). The chemistry of the Bohr effect. II. Some properties of hemoglobin H. *J. Biol. Chem.* 236: 2926–2929.

Bennett, JM, Catovsky, D, Daniel, MT et al. (1982). Proposals for the classification of the myelodysplastic syndromes. *Br. J. Haematol.* 51: 189–199.

Benz, EJ, Swerdlow, PS, and Forget, BG. (1973). Globin messenger RNA in hemoglobin H disease. *Blood* 42: 825–833.

Bergren, WR and Sturgeon, PH. (1960). Hemoglobin H: Some additional findings. In *Proceedings of the 7th International Congress in Hematology.* New York, p. 488.

Beutler, E, Lichtman, MA, Coller BS, and Kipps, TJ. (1995). *Williams Hematology.* 5th ed. New York: McGraw-Hill.

Bianchi, DW, Beyer, EC, Stark, AR et al. (1986). Normal long-term survival with α-thalassemia. *J. Pediatr.* 108: 716–718.

Boehme, WM, Piira, TA, Kurnick, JE, and Bethlenfalvay, NC. (1978). Acquired hemoglobin H in refractory sideroblastic anemia. *Arch. Intern. Med.* 138: 603–606.

Bruzdzinski, CJ, Sisco, KL, Ferrucci, SJ, and Rucknagel, DL. (1984). The occurrence of the α$^{G\text{-Philadelphia}}$-globin allele on a double-locus chromosome. *Am. J. Hum. Genet.* 36: 101–109.

Bunn, HF. (1987). Subunit assembly of hemoglobin: An important determinant of hematologic phenotype. *Blood* 69: 1–6.

Bunn, HF and McDonald, MJ. (1983). Electrostatic interactions in the assembly of haemoglobin. *Nature* 306: 498–500.

Bürgi, W, Schlup, P, Deubelbeiss, KA, Fischer, S, and Killer, D. (1992). Erworbene hämoglobin H-krankheit im frühstadium einer erythroleukämie. *Schweiz. Med. Woohenschr.* 122: 348–350.

Cao, A, Rosatelli, C, Pirastu, M, and Galanello, R. (1991). Thalassemias in Sardinia: Molecular pathology, phenotype-genotype correlation and prevention. *Am. J. Pediatr. Hematol. Oncol.* 13: 179–188.

Carr, S, Rubin, L, Dixon, D et al. (1995). Intrauterine therapy for homozygous α-thalassemia. *Obstet. Gynecol.* 85: 876–879.

Chan, V, Chan, TK, Liang, ST et al. (1985). Hydrops fetalis due to an unusual form of HbH disease. *Blood* 66: 224–228.

Chan, V, Chan, TK, Tso, SC, and Todd, D. (1987). Combination of three α-globin gene loci deletions and hemoglobin New York results in a severe hemoglobin H syndrome. *Am. J. Hematol.* 24: 301–306.

Chan, V, Chan, VWY, Tang, M et al. (1997). Molecular defects in Hb H hydrops fetalis. *Br. J. Haematol.* 96: 224–228.

Chang, J, Lu, RH, Xu, S-M et al. (1996). Inactivation of mouse α-globin gene by homologous recombination: Mouse model of hemoglobin H disease. *Blood* 88: 1846–1851.

Chapman, RW, Williams, G, Bydder, G et al. (1980). Computed tomography for determining liver iron content in primary haemochromatosis. *Br. Med. J.* 28: 440–442.

Chim, CS, Chan, V, and Todd, D. (1998). Hemosiderosis with diabetes mellitus in untransfused hemoglobin H disease. *Am. J. Hematol.* 57: 160–163.

Chitayat, D, Silver, MM, O'Brien, K et al. (1997). Limb defects in homozygous α-thalassemia: Report of three cases. *Am. J. Med. Genet.* 68: 162–167.

Chui, DHK, Wong, SC, Chung, S-W et al. (1986). Embryonic ζ-globin chains in adults: A marker for α-thalassemia-1 haplotype due to a >17.5 kb deletion. *N. Engl. J. Med.* 314: 76–79.

Chui, DHK, Mentzer, WC, Patterson, M et al. (1989). Human embryonic ζ-globin chains in fetal and newborn blood. *Blood* 74: 1409–1414.

Chui, DHK, Patterson, M, Dowling, CE, Jr et al. (1990). Hemoglobin Bart's disease in an Italian boy. *N. Engl. J. Med.* 323: 179–182.

Chui, DHK and Waye, JS. (1998). Hydrops fetalis caused by α-thalassemia: An emerging health care problem. *Blood* 91: 2213–2222.

Clarke, C and Whitfield, AGW. (1977). Deaths from rhesus haemolytic disease in England and Wales 1977; accuracy of records and assessment of anti D prophylaxis. *Br. Med. J.* 1, 1665–1669.

Clegg, JB and Weatherall, DJ. (1967). Haemoglobin synthesis in alpha-thalassaemia (haemoglobin H disease). *Nature* 215: 1241–1243.

Craddock, CF. (1994). Normal and abnormal regulation of human α globin expression. D. Phil., University of Oxford.

Dallman, PR. (1977). The red cell. In Dallman, PR, editor. *Blood and blood-forming tissues.* New York: Appleton-Century-Crofts. pp. 1109–1113.

Dallman, PR and Siimes, MA. (1979). Percentile curves for hemoglobin and red cell volume in infancy and childhood. *J. Pediatr.* 94: 26–31.

Daneshmend, TK and Peachey, RD. (1978). Leg ulcers in α thalassaemia (haemoglobin H disease). *Br. J. Dermatol.* 98: 233–235.

Dash, S and Dash, RJ. (1980). Idiopathic myelofibrosis without splenomegaly and with an acquired haemoglobin disorder. *Ind. J. Cancer* 17: 193–195.

Derry, S, Wood, WG, Pippard, M et al. (1984). Hematologic and biosynthetic studies in homozygous hemoglobin Constant Spring. *J. Clin. Invest.* 73: 1673–1682.

Diamond, MP, Cotgreve, I and Parker, A. (1965). Case of intrauterine death due to α-thalassemia. *Br. Med. J.* 2: 278–280.

Diukman, R and Golbus, MS. (1992). In utero stem cell therapy. *J. Reprod. Med.* 37: 515–520.

Eddleman, K. (1996). In utero transfusion and transplantation in α-thalassaemia. In Migliaccio, AR, editor. *Stem cell therapy of inherited disorders.* Rome, Italy.

Feder, JN, Gnirke, A, Thomas, W et al. (1996). A novel MHC class I-like gene is mutated in patients with hereditary haemochromatosis. *Nat. Genet.* 13: 399–408.

Fischel-Ghodsian, N, Higgs, DR, and Beyer, EC. (1987). Function of a new globin gene. *Nature* 329: 397.

Fischel-Ghodsian, N, Vickers, MA, Seip, M et al. (1988). Characterization of two deletions that remove the entire human ζ-α globin gene complex (- -^Thai and - -^Fil). *Br. J. Haematol.* 70: 233–238.

Fucharoen, S, Winichagoon, P, Pootrakul, P, P et al. (1988). Differences between two types of HbH disease, α-thalassemia 1/α-thalassemia 2 and α-thalassemia 1/Hb Constant Spring. *Birth Defects: Original Articles Series* 23: 309–315.

Galanello, R, Melis, MA, Paglietti, E et al. (1983a). Serum ferritin levels in hemoglobin H disease. *Acta Haematol. (Basel)* 69: 56–58.

Galanello, R, Pirastu, M, Melis, MA et al. (1983b). Phenotype-genotype correlation in haemoglobin H disease in childhood. *J. Med. Genet.* 20: 425–429.

Galanello, R, Paglietti, E, Melis, MA et al. (1984). Hemoglobin inclusions in heterozygous α-thalassemia according to their α-globin genotype. *Acta Haematol. (Basel)* 72: 34–36.

Galanello, R, Sanna, MA, Maccioni, L et al. (1990). Fetal hydrops in Sardinia: Implications for genetic counselling. *Clin. Genet.* 38: 327–331.

Galanello, R, Aru, B, Dessì, C et al. (1992). HbH disease in Sardinia: Molecular, haematological and clinical aspects. *Acta Haematol. (Basel),* 88: 1–6.

Gambino, R, Kacian, DL, Ramirez, F et al. (1974). Decreased globin messenger RNA in thalassemia by hybridisation and biologic activity assays. *Ann. N. Y. Acad. Sci.* 232: 6–14.

Ganczakowski, M, Bowden, DK, Maitland, K et al. (1995). Thalassaemia. In Vanuatu, SW Pacific: Frequency and haematological phenotypes of young children. *Br. J. Haematol.* 89: 485–495.

George, E, Ferguson, V, Yakas, J et al. (1989). A molecular marker associated with mild hemoglobin H disease. *Pathology* 21: 27–30.

Ghosh, A, Tang, MHY, Liang, ST, and Ma, HK. (1987). Ultrasound evaluation of pregnancies at risk for homozygous α-thalassaemia-1. *Prenat. Diagn.* 7: 307–313.

Ghosh, A, Tang, MHY, Lam, YH, F et al. (1994). Ultrasound measurement of placental thickness to detect pregnancies affected by homozygous α-thalassaemia-1. *Lancet* 344: 988–989.

Gibbons, RJ, Wilkie, AOM, Weatherall, DJ, and Higgs, DR. (1991). A newly defined X linked mental retardation syndrome associated with α thalassaemia. *J. Med. Genet.* 28: 729–733.

Giordano, PC, Harteveld, CL, Michiels, JJ et al. (1996). Atypical HbH disease in a Surinam patient resulting from a combination of the SEA^{-18.8} and RW^{-3.7} deletions with HbC heterozygosity. *Br. J. Haematol.* 96: 801–805.

Grossbard, E, Terada, M, Dow, LW, and Bank, A. (1973). Decreased globin messenger RNA activity with polysomes in α thalassaemia. *Nat. New Biol.* 241: 209–211.

Gurgey, A, Altay, C, Beksac, MS et al. (1989). Hydrops fetalis due to homozygosity for α-thalassaemia-1, −(α)−20.5 kb: The first observation in a Turkish family. *Acta Haematol. (Scand.)* 81: 169–171.

Guy, G, Coady, DJ, Jansen, V et al. (1985). α-Thalassemia hydrops fetalis: Clinical and ultrasonographic considerations. *Am. J. Obstet. Gynecol.* 153: 500–504.

Hamilton, RW, Schwartz, E, Atwater, J, and Erslev, AJ. (1971). Acquired hemoglobin H disease. *N. Engl. J. Med.* 285: 1217–1221.

Harmon, JV, Osathanondh, R, and Holmes, LB. (1995). Symmetrical terminal transverse limb defects: Report of twenty-week fetus. *Teratology* 51: 237–242.

Helder, J and Deisseroth, A. (1987). S1 nuclease analysis of α-globin gene expression in preleukemic patients with acquired hemoglobin H disease after transfer to mouse erythroleukemia cells. *Proc. Natl. Acad. Sci. U.S.A.* 84: 2387–2390.

Higgs, DR, Pressley, L, Clegg, JB et al. (1980). Detection of α-thalassaemia in Negro infants. *Br. J. Haematol.* 46: 39–46.

Higgs, DR, and Weatherall, DJ. (1983). α-Thalassemia. In Piomelli, S and Yachin, S, editors. *Current topics in hematology.* New York: A.R. Liss. p. 37.

Higgs, DR, Wood, WG, Barton, C, and Weatherall, DJ. (1983). Clinical features and molecular analysis of acquired HbH disease. *Am. J. Med.* 75: 181–191.

Higgs, DR, Vickers, MA, Wilkie, AOM, et al. (1989). A review of the molecular genetics of the human α-globin gene cluster. *Blood* 73: 1081–1104.

Higgs, DR. (1993). α-Thalassaemia. In Higgs, DR and Weatherall, DJ, editors. *Baillière's clinical haematology. International practice and research: The haemoglobinopathies.* London: Baillière Tindall. pp. 117–150.

Holzgreve, W, Curry, CJR, Golbus, MS et al. (1984). Investigation of nonimmune hydrops fetalis. *Am. J. Obstet. Gynecol.* 150: 805–812.

Horton, BF, Thompson, RB, Dozy, AM et al. (1962). Inhomogeneity of hemoglobin VI. The minor hemoglobin components of cord blood. *Blood* 20: 302–313.

Housman, D, Forget, BG, Skoultchi, A, and Benz, EJ. (1973). Quantitative deficiency of chain specific messenger ribonucleic acids in the thalassemia syndromes. *Proc. Natl. Acad. Sci. U.S.A.* 70: 1809–1813.

Huisman, THJ, Carver, MFH, and Efremov, GD. (1996). *A Syllabus of Human Hemoglobin Variants.* Augusta, GA: The Sickle Cell Anemia Foundation.

Hunt, JA and Lehmann, H. (1959). Abnormal human haemoglobins. Haemoglobin 'Bart's': A foetal haemoglobin without α chains. *Nature* 184: 872–873.

Hunt, DM, Higgs, DR, Old, JM et al. (1980). Determination of alpha thalassaemia phenotypes by messenger RNA analysis. *Br. J. Haematol.* 45: 53–64.

Isarangkura, P, Siripoonya, P, Fucharoen, S, and Hathirat, P. (1987). Hemoglobin Barts disease without hydrops manifestation. *Birth Defects: Original Articles Series* 23: 333–342.

Jackson, DN, Strauss, AA, Groncy, PK et al. (1990). Outcome of neonatal survivors with homozygous α-thalassemia. *Pediatr. Res.* 27: 266A.

Jauniaux, E, Van Maldergem, L, De Munter, C et al. (1990). Nonimmune hydrops fetalis associated with genetic abnormalities. *Obstet. Gynecol.* 75: 568–572.

Jensen, PD, Jensen, FT, and Ellegaard, J. (1994). Non-invasive assessment of tissue iron overload in the liver by magnetic resonance imaging. *Br. J. Haematol.* 87: 171–184.

Juneja, SK, Imbert, M, Joualt, H et al. (1983). Haematological feature of primary myelodysplastic syndromes (PMDS) at initial presentation: A study of 118 cases. *J. Clin. Pathol.* 36: 1129–1135.

Kacian, DL, Gambino, R, Dow, LW et al. (1973). Decreased globin messenger RNA in thalassemia detected by molecular hybridization. *Proc. Natl. Acad. Sci. U.S.A.* 70: 1886–1890.

Kan, YW, Schwartz, E, and Nathan, DG. (1968). Globin chain synthesis in alpha thalassemia syndromes. *J. Clin. Invest.* 47: 2515–2522.

Kan, YW, Todd, D, Holland, J, and Dozy, A. (1974). Absence of α globin mRNA in homozygous α-thalassemia. *J. Clin. Invest.* 53: 37a.

Kanavakis, E, Traeger-Synodinos, J, Papasotiriou, I, Vrettou, C et al. (1996). The interaction of α⁰ thalassaemia with Hb Icaria: Three unusual cases of haemoglobinopathy H. *Br. J. Haematol.* 92: 332–335.

Kanavakis, E, Tzotzos, S, Liapaki, A et al. (1986). Frequency of α-thalassemia in Greece. *Am. J. Hematol.* 22: 225–232.

Kanokpongsakdi, S, Fucharoen, S, Vatanasiri, C et al. (1990). Ultrasonographic method for detection of haemoglobin Bart's hydrops fetalis in the second trimester of pregnancy. *Prenat. Diag.* 10: 809–813.

Kattamis, C, Metaxotou-Mavromati, A, Tsiarta, E et al. (1980). Haemoglobin Bart's hydrops syndrome in Greece. *Br. Med. J.* 269: 268–269.

Kattamis, C, Tzotzos, S, Kanavakis, E et al. (1988). Correlation of clinical phenotype to genotype in haemoglobin H disease. *Lancet* 1: 442–444.

Knox-Macaulay, HHM, Weatherall, DJ, Clegg et al. (1972). The clinical and biosynthetic characterization of αβ-thalassaemia. *Br. J. Haematol.* 22: 497–512.

Ko, T, Hsieh, F-J, Hsu, PM, and Lee, TY. (1991). Molecular characterisation of severe α-thalassemias causing hydrops fetalis in Taiwan. *Am. J. Med. Genet.* 39: 317–320.

Kueh, YK. (1982). Acute lymphoblastic leukemia with brilliant cresyl blue erythrocytic inclusions — acquired hemoglobin H? *N. Eng. J. Med.* 307: 193–194.

Kuptamethi, S, Pravatmuang, P, Fucharoen, S et al. (1988). Modified technique for detecting red cells containing inclusion bodies in α-thalassemia trait. *Birth Defects: Original Articles Series* 23: 213–221.

Kutlar, F, Gonzalez-Redondo, JM, Kutlar, A et al. (1989). The levels of ζ, γ, and δ chains in patients with HbH disease. *Hum. Genet.* 82: 179–186.

Labie, D, Rosa, J, and Tanzer, J. (1968). Evidence for β4 and γ4 hemoglobins associated with an acute myeloblastic leukemia. In *Proceedings of the XIIth International Congress in Hematology.* New York. p. 3.

Lam, T-K, Chan, V, Fok, TF, Li, C-K et al. (1992). Long-term survival of a baby with homozygous alpha-thalassemia-1. *Acta Haematol.* 88: 198–200.

Lam, YH and Tang, MHY. (1997). Prenatal diagnosis of haemoglobin Bart's disease by cordocentesis at 12–14 weeks' gestation. *Prenat. Diagn.* 17: 501–504.

Letsky, EA and Redman, CWG. (1987). Blood disorders in pregnancy. In Weatherall, DJ, Leadingham, JGG, and Warrell, DA, editors. *Oxford textbook of medicine.* Oxford: Oxford University Press, pp. 11.31–11.35.

Liang, ST, Wong, VCW, So, WWK et al. (1985). Homozygous α-thalassaemia: Clinical presentation, diagnosis and management. A review of 46 cases. *Br. J. Obstet. Gynaecol.* 92: 680–684.

Lie-Injo, LE. (1959). Haemoglobin of newborn infants in Indonesia. *Nature* 183: 1125–1126.

Lie-Injo, LE, Ganesan, J, Clegg, JB, and Weatherall, DJ. (1974). Homozygous state for Hb Constant Spring (slow moving Hb X components). *Blood* 43: 251–259.

Lie-Injo, LE, Ganesan, J, and Lopez, CG. (1975). The clinical, haematological and biochemical expression of hemoglobin Constant Spring and its distribution. In Schmidt, RM, editor. *Abnormal haemoglobins and thalassaemia — diagnostic aspects.* New York: Academic Press.

Liebhaber, SA, Rappaport, EF, Cash, FE et al. (1984). Hemoglobin I mutation encoded at both α-globin loci on the same chromosome: Concerted evolution in the human genome. *Science* 226: 1449–1451.

Lin, CK, Peng, HW, Ho, CH, and Yung, CH. (1990). Iron overload in untransfused patients with hemoglobin H disease. *Acta Haematol. (Basel)* 83: 137–139.

Lin, C-K, Lin, J-S, and Jiang, M-L. (1992). Iron absorption is increased in hemoglobin H disease. *Am. J. Hematol.* 40: 74–75.

Lin, K-S, Liu, C-H, Lee, T-C et al. (1977). Alpha chain thalassemia in Taiwan. *Clin. Pediatr.* 16: 71–75.

Lin, S-F, Liu, T-C, Chen, T-P et al. (1994). Diagnosis of thalassemia by non-isotope detection of α/β and ζ/α mRNA ratios. *Br. J. Haematol.* 87: 133–138.

Lindsey, RJ, Jackson, JM, and Raven, JL. (1978). Acquired haemoglobin H disease, complicating a myeloproliferative syndrome: A case report. *Pathology* 10: 329–334.

Llewellyn-Jones, D. (1969). *Fundamentals of Obstetrics and Gynaecology.* Vol. 1. London: Faber and Faber Ltd.

Lubin, B.H. (1987). Reference values in infancy and childhood. In Nathan, DG and Oski, FA, editors. *Hematology of infancy and childhood.* Philadelphia: WB Saunders. pp. 1677–1697.

Machin, GA. (1981). Differential diagnosis of hydrops fetalis. *Am. J. Med. Genet.* 9: 341–350.

Martinell, J, Whitney, JB III, Popp, RA et al. (1981). Three mouse models of human thalassemia. *Proc. Natl. Acad. Sci. U.S.A.* 78: 5056–5060.

Massa, A, Tannoia, N, Cerquozzi, S et al. (1987). Molecular characterization of α-thalassemia in Puglia. In Sirchia, G and Zanella, A, editors. *Thalassemia today: The Mediterranean experience.* Milano: Centro Trasfusionale Ospedale Maggiore Policlinico Di Milano Editore, pp. 459–464.

Matthay, KK, Mentzer, WC Jr, Dozy, AM et al. (1979). Modification of hemoglobin H disease by sickle trait. *J. Clin. Invest.* 64: 1024–1032.

Maude, GH, Higgs, DR, Beckford, M et al. (1985). Alpha thalassaemia and the haematology of normal Jamaican children. *Clin. Lab. Haematol.* 7: 289–295.

Maungsapaya, W, Winichagoon, P, Fucharoen, S et al. (1985). Improved technique for detecting intraerythrocytic inclusion bodies in α thalassemia trait. *J. Med. Assoc. Thai.* 68: 43–45.

McNiel, JR. (1968). The inheritance of hemoglobin H disease. Abstracts of the Simultaneous Sessions. XII Congress International and National Society of Hematology. New York, p. 52.

Milner, PF, and Huisman, THJ. (1976). Studies on the proportion and synthesis of haemoglobin G Philadelphia in red cells of heterozygotes, a homozygote, and a heterozygote for both haemoglobin G and α thalassaemia. *Br. J. Haematol.* 34: 207–220.

Molchanova, TP, Pobedimskaya, DD, Ye, Z, and Huisman, THJ. (1994). Two different mutations in codon 68 are observed in Hb G-Philadelphia heterozygotes. *Am. J. Hematol.* 45: 345–346.

Nakatsuji, T, Matsumoto, N, Miwa, S et al. (1980). Acquired hemoglobin H disease associated with idiopathic myelofibrosis and hereditary adenosine deaminase deficiency. *Acta Haematol. J.* 43: 92–98.

Nakayama, R, Yamada, D, Steinmiller, V et al. (1986). Hydrops fetalis secondary to Bart hemoglobinopathy. *Obstet. Gynecol.* 67: 176–180.

Naqvi, A, Waye, JS, Morrow, R et al. (1997). Normal development of an infant with homozygous α-thalassemia. *Blood* 90: 132A.

Nathan, DG and Oski, FA. (1987). *Hematology of Infancy and Childhood.* 3rd ed. Philadelphia: WB Saunders.

Natta, CL, Ramirez, F, Wolff, JA, and Bank, A. (1976). Decreased alpha globin mRNA in nucleated red cell precursors in alpha thalassemia. *Blood* 47: 899–907.

Nicholls, RD, Higgs, DR, Clegg, JB, and Weatherall, DJ. (1985). α⁰-Thalassemia due to recombination between the α1-globin gene and an *Alu*I repeat. *Blood* 65: 1434–1438.

Nicolaides, KH, Rodeck, CH, Lange I et al. (1985). Fetoscopy in the assessment of unexplained fetal hydrops. *Br. J. Obstet. Gynaecol.* 92: 671–679.

Noël, P, Tefferi, A, Pierre, RV et al. (1993). Karyotypic analysis in primary myelodysplastic syndromes. *Blood Rev.* 7: 10–18.

Ong, HC, White, JC, and Sinnathuray, TA. (1977). Haemoglobin H disease and pregnancy in a Malaysian woman. *Acta Haematol. (Basel)* 58: 229–233.

Ongsangkoon, T, Vawesorn, O, and Pootakul, S-n. (1978). Pathology of hemoglobin Bart's hydrops fetalis. 1. Gross autopsy findings. *J. Med. Assoc. Thai.* 61: 71.

Owen, GM and Yanochik-Owen, A. (1977). Should there be a different definition of anemia in Black and White children? *Am. J. Public Health* 67: 865–866.

Paglietti, E, Galanello, R, Moi, P et al. (1986). Molecular pathology of haemoglobin H disease in Sardinians. *Br. J. Haematol.* 63: 485–496.

Pardoll, DM, Charache, S, Hjelle, BL et al. (1982). Homozygous α thalassemia/Hb G Philadelphia. *Hemoglobin* 6: 503–515.

Pászty, C. (1997). Transgenic and gene knock-out mouse models of sickle cell anemia and the thalassemias. *Curr. Opin. Hematol.* 4: 88–93.

Pászty, C, Mohandas, N, Stevens, ME et al. (1995). Lethal alpha-thalassaemia created by gene targeting in mice and its genetic rescue. *Nat. Genet.* 11: 33–39.

Pászty, C, Brion, CM, Manci, E et al. (1997). Transgenic knockout mice with exclusively human sickle hemoglobin and sickle cell disease. *Science* 278: 876–878.

Pearson, HA and McFarland, W. (1962). Erythrokinetics in thalassemia. II. Studies in Lepore trait and hemoglobin H disease. *J. Lab. Clin. Med.* 59: 147–157.

Peschle, C, Mavilio, F, Care, A et al. (1985). Haemoglobin switching in human embryos: Asynchrony of ζ-α and ε-γ globin switches in primitive and definite erythropoietic lineage. *Nature* 313: 235–238.

Petrou, M, Brugiatelli, M, Old, J et al. (1992). Alpha thalassaemia hydrops fetalis in the UK: The importance of screening pregnant women of Chinese, other South East Asian and Mediterranean extraction for alpha thalassaemia trait. *Br. J. Obst. Gynaecol.* 99: 985–989.

Piankijagum, A, Palungwachira, P, and Lohkoomgunpai, A. (1978). Beta thalassemia, hemoglobin E and hemoglobin H disease. Clinical analysis 1964–1966. *J. Med. Assoc. Thai.* 61: 50.

Pongsamart, S, Pootrakul, S, Wasi, P, and Na-Nakorn, S. (1975). Hemoglobin Constant Spring: Hemoglobin synthesis in heterozygous and homozygous states. *Biochem. Biophys. Res. Commun.* 64: 681–686.

Pootrakul, S, Wasi, P, and Na-Nakorn, S. (1967). Studies on haemoglobin Bart's (Hb-γ4) in Thailand: The incidence and the mechanism of occurrence in cord blood. *Ann. Hum. Genet. (Lond.)* 31: 149–166.

Pootrakul, S, Sapprapa, S, Wasi, P et al. (1975). Hemoglobin synthesis in 28 obligatory cases for alpha-thalassemia traits. *Humangenetik* 29: 121–126.

Pootrakul, P, Winichagoon, P, Fucharoen, S et al. (1981). Homozygous haemoglobin Constant Spring: A need for revision of concept. *Hum. Genet.* 59: 250–255.

Popp, RA, Marsh, CL, and Skow, LC. (1981). Expression of embryonic hemoglobin genes in mice heterozygous for α-thalassemia or β-duplication traits and in mice heterozygous for both traits. *Dev. Biol.* 85: 123–128.

Pornpatkul, M, Wasi, P, and Na-Nakorn, S. (1969). Hematologic parameters in obligatory alpha-thalassemia. *J. Med. Assoc. Thai.* 52: 801–811.

Pornpatkul, M, Pootrakul, S-n, Muangsrup, W, and Wasi, P. (1978). Intraerythrocytic inclusion bodies in obligatory alpha thalassemia traits. *J. Med. Assoc. Thai.* 61: 63.

Pressley, L, Higgs, DR, Clegg, JB, and Weatherall, DJ. (1980). Gene deletions in α thalassaemia prove that the 5′ ζ locus is functional. *Proc. Natl. Acad. Sci. U.S.A.* 77: 3586–3589.

Pritchard, J, Clegg, JB, Weatherall, DJ, and Longley, J. (1974). The translation of human globin messenger RNA in heterologous assay systems. *Br. J. Haematol.* 28: 141–142.

Rachmilewitz, EA, and Harari, E. (1972). Slow rate of haemichrome formation from oxidized haemoglobin Bart's (γ4): A possible explanation for the unequal quantities of haemoglobins H (β4) and Bart's in alpha-thalassaemia. *Br. J. Haematol.* 22: 357–364.

Rahbar, S and Bunn, HF. (1987). Association of hemoglobin H disease with Hb J-Iran (β77 His → Asp): Impact on subunit assembly. *Blood* 70: 1790–1791.

Ramot, B, Sheba, C, Fisher, S, Ager, JAM et al. (1959). Haemoglobin H disease with persistent haemoglobin "Bart's" in an oriental Jewess and her daughter. *Br. Med. J.* 2: 1228–1230.

Rieder, RF, Woodbury, DH, and Rucknagel, DL. (1976). The interaction of α-thalassaemia and haemoglobin G Philadelphia. *Br. J. Haematol.* 32: 159–165.

Rigas, DA, and Koler, RD. (1961). Decreased erythrocyte survival in hemoglobin H disease as a result of the abnormal properties of hemoglobin H: The benefit of splenectomy. *Blood* 18: 1–17.

Rombos, J, Voskaridou, E, Vayenas, C et al. (1989). Hemoglobin H in association with the Greek type of HPFH. International Congress on Thalassemia, Sardinia. p. 19.

Rosenzweig, AI, Heywood, JD, Motulsky. AG, and Finch, CA. (1968). Hemoglobin H as an acquired defect of alpha-chain synthesis. *Acta Haematol.* 39: 91–101.

Ross, DW, Ayscue, LH, Watson, J, and Bentley, SA. (1988). Stability of hematologic parameters in healthy subjects. *Am. J. Clin. Pathol.* 90: 262–267.

Ryan, TM, Ciavatta, DJ, and Townes, TM. (1997). Knockout-transgenic mouse model of sickle cell disease. *Science* 278: 873–876.

Saltzman, DH, Frigoletto, FD, Harlow, BL et al. (1989). Sonographic evaluation of hydrops fetalis. *Obstet. Gynecol.* 74: 106–111.

Sancar, GB, Tatsis, B, Cedeno, MM, and Rieder, RF. (1980). Proportion of hemoglobin G Philadelphia (α2 68Asn-Lys β2) in heterozygotes is determined by α-globin gene deletions. *Proc. Natl. Acad. Sci. U.S.A.* 77: 6874–6878.

Schwartz, E, and Atwater, J. (1972). α-Thalassemia in the American Negro. *J. Clin. Invest.* 51: 412–418.

Sharma, RS, Yu, V, and Walters, WAW. (1979). Haemoglobin Bart's hydrops fetalis syndrome in an infant of Greek origin and prenatal diagnosis of alpha-thalassemia. *Med. J. Austra.* 2: 404, 433–434.

Shojania, AM, and Gross, S. (1964). Haemolytic anaemias and folic acid deficiency in children. *Am. J. Dis. Child.* 108: 53–61.

Smetanina, NS, Leonova, JY, Levy, N, and Huisman, THJ. (1996). The α/β and α2/α1-globin mRNA ratios in different forms of α-thalassaemia. *Biochim. Biophys. Acta* 1315: 188–192.

Sonakul, D, and Fucharoen, S. (1992). Pulmonary thromboembolism in thalassemic patients. *Southeast Asian J. Trop. Med. Public Health* 23: 25–28.

Sonakul, D, Sook-aneak, M, and Pacharee, P. (1978). Pathology of thalassemic diseases in Thailand. *J. Med. Assoc. Thai.* 61: 72.

Sophocleous, T, Higgs, DR, Aldridge, B et al. (1981). The molecular basis for the haemoglobin Bart's hydrops fetalis syndrome in Cyprus. *Br. J. Haematol.* 47: 153–156.

Srichaikul, T, Tipayasakda, J, Atichartakarn, V et al. (1984). Ferrokinetic and erythrokinetic studies in alpha and beta thalassaemia. *Clin. Lab. Haematol.* 6: 133–140.

Stallings, M, Abraham, A, and Abraham, EC. (1983). α-Thalassemia influences the levels of fetal hemoglobin components in new born infants. *Blood* 62: 75a.

Su, CW, Liang, S, Liang, R et al. (1992). HbH disease in association with the silent β chain variant Hb Hamilton or α2β211 (A8) Val→Ile. *Hemoglobin* 16: 403–408.

Tan, SL, Tseng, AMP, and Thong, P-W. (1989). Bart's hydrops fetalis — clinical presentation and management — an analysis of 25 cases. *Aust. N. Z. J. Obstet. Gynaecol.* 3: 233–237.

Tanaka, M, Fujiwara, Y, and Hirota, Y. (1979). Globin chain synthesis in acquired hemoglobin H disease. *Acta Haematol. Jpn.* 42: 9–15.

Tang, W, Luo, H-y, Albitar, M et al. (1992). Human embryonic ζ-globin expression in deletional α-thalassemias. *Blood* 80: 517–522.

Thonglairuam, V, Winichagoon, P, Fucharoen, S, and Wasi, P. (1989). The molecular basis of AE-Bart's disease. *Hemoglobin* 13: 117–124.

Thumasathit, B, Nondasuta, A, Silpisornkosol, S et al. (1968). Hydrops fetalis associated with Bart's hemoglobin in northern Thailand. *J. Pediatr.* 73: 132–138.

Tokuda, K, Kyoshoin, K, Kitajima, K et al. (1984). A case of sideroblastic anemia associated with acquired hemoglobin H. *Acta Haematol. (Jpn.)* 47: 1396–1400.

Tongsong, T, Wanapirak, C, Srisomboon, J et al. (1996). Antenatal sonographic features of 100 alpha-thalassemia hydrops fetalis fetuses. *J. Clin. Ultrasound* 24: 73–77.

Trent, RJ, Wilkinson, T, Yakas, J et al. (1986). Molecular defects in 2 examples of severe HbH disease. *Scand. J. Haematol.* 36: 272–279.

Tso, SC, Chan, TK, and Todd, D. (1982). Venous thrombosis in haemoglobin H disease after splenectomy. *Aust. N. Z. J. Med.* 12: 635–638.

Tso, SC, Loh, TT, and Todd, D. (1984). Iron overload in patients with haemoglobin H disease. *Scand. J. Haematol.* 32: 391–394.

Tuchinda, S, Nagai, K, and Lehmann, H. (1975). Oxygen dissociation curve of haemoglobin Portland. *FEBS Lett.* 49: 390–391.

Vaeusorn, O, Fucharoen, S, Ruangpiroj, T et al. (1985). Fetal pathology and maternal morbidity in hemoglobin Bart's hydrops fetalis: An analysis of 65 cases. Abstract presented at the First International Conference on Thalassemia, Bangkok.

Veer, A, Kosciolek, BA, Bauman, AW, and Rowley, PT. (1979). Acquired hemoglobin H disease in idiopathic myelofibrosis. *Am. J. Hematol.* 6: 199–206.

Villegas, A, Perez Gutierrez, A, Diaz Mediavilla, J, and Espinos, D. (1979). Observaciones de alfa-talasemia y de hemoglobina H en espanoles. *Sangre* 24: 1088–1102.

Wagner, GM, Liebhaber, SA, Cutting, HO, and Embury, SH. (1982). Hematologic improvement following splenectomy for hemoglobin-H disease. *West. J. Med.* 137: 325–328.

Wasi, P. (1983). Hemoglobinopathies in Southeast Asia. In Bowman, JE, editor. *Distribution and evolution of hemoglobin and globin loci.* New York: Elsevier. pp. 179–208.

Wasi, P, Na-Nakorn, S, Pootrakul, S et al. (1969). Alpha- and beta-thalassemia in Thailand. *Ann. N. Y. Acad. Sci.* 165: 60–82.

Wasi, P, Na-Nakorn, S, and Pootrakul, S. (1974). The α thalassaemias. *Clin. Haematol.* 3: 383–410.

Wasi, P, Pravatmuang, P, and Winichagoon, P. (1979). Immunologic diagnosis of α-thalassemia traits. *Hemoglobin* 3: 21.

Waye, JS, Eng, B, and Chui, DHK. (1992). Identification of an extensive ζ-α globin gene deletion in a Chinese individual. *Br. J. Haematol.* 80: 378–380.

Weatherall, DJ. (1963). Abnormal haemoglobins in the neonatal period and their relationship to thalassaemia. *Br. J. Haematol.* 9: 265–277.

Weatherall, DJ and Clegg, JB. (1975). The α chain termination mutants and their relationship to thalassaemia. *Phil. Trans. R. Soc. London (B)* 271: 411–455.

Weatherall, DJ and Clegg, JB. (1981). *The Thalassaemia Syndromes.* 3rd ed. Oxford: Blackwell Scientific Publications.

Weatherall, DJ, Clegg, JB, and Boon, WH. (1970). The haemoglobin constitution of infants with the haemoglobin Bart's hydrops foetalis syndrome. *Br. J. Haematol.* 18: 357–367.

Weatherall, DJ, Old, J, Longley, J et al. (1978). Acquired haemoglobin H disease in leukaemia: Pathophysiology and molecular basis. *Br. J. Haematol.* 38: 305–322.

Weatherall, DJ, Higgs, DR, Bunch, C et al. (1981). Hemoglobin H disease and mental retardation. A new syndrome or a remarkable coincidence? *N. Engl. J. Med.* 305: 607–612.

Westgren, M, Ringden, O, Eik-Nes, S et al. (1996). Lack of evidence of permanent engraftment after in utero fetal stem cell transplantation in congenital hemoglobinopathies. *Transplantation* 61: 1176–1179.

White, JC, Ellis, M, Coleman, PN et al. (1960). An unstable haemoglobin associated with some cases of leukaemia. *Br. J. Haematol.* 6: 171–177.

Whitten, WJ and Rucknagel, DL. (1981). The proportion of HbA$_2$ is higher in sickle cell trait than in normal homozygotes. *Hemoglobin* 5: 371–378.

Wickramasinghe, SN, Rayfield, LS, and Brent, L. (1986). Red cell volume distribution curves and intracellular globin chain precipitation in the α-thalassaemic mouse, Hba^{th-J}. *Br. J. Exp. Pathol.* 67: 73–83.

Wilkie, AOM. (1991). The α thalassaemia/mental retardation syndromes: Model systems for studying the genetic contribution to mental handicap. Doctor of Medicine, University of Oxford.

Williams, TN, Maitland, K, Ganczakowski, M et al. (1996). Red cell phenotypes in the α$^+$ thalassaemias from early childhood to maturity. *Br. J. Haematol.* 95: 266–272.

Winichagoon, P,[1] Adirojnanon, P, and Wasi, P. (1980). Levels of haemoglobin H and proportions of red cells with inclusion bodies in the two types of haemoglobin H disease. *Br. J. Haematol.* 46: 507–509.

Wong, HB. (1984). Thalassemias in Singapore. *J. Singapore Paediatr Soc.* 26: 1–14.

Woodrow, JC, Noble, RL, and Martindale, JH. (1964). Haemoglobin H disease in an English family. *Br. Med. J.* 1: 36–38.

Yoo, D, Schechter, GP, Amigable, AN, and Nienhuis, AW. (1980). Myeloproliferative syndrome with sideroblastic anemia and acquired hemoglobin H disease. *Cancer* 45: 78–83.

Yoshida, N, Horikoshi, A, Kanemaru, M et al. (1990). An erythremia with acquired HbH disease and chromosomal abnormality. *Rinsho Ketsueki* 31: 963–968.

---

[1] Reference cited as Winichagoon et al., but is mistakenly published as Adirojnanon and Wasi.

19

The Alpha Thalassemia/Mental Retardation Syndromes

RICHARD J. GIBBONS
DOUGLAS R. HIGGS

The rare association between α thalassemia and mental retardation might easily have been dismissed as the chance occurrence of two common conditions. However, when Weatherall and colleagues (Weatherall et al., 1981) described three mentally retarded children with α thalassemia and a variety of developmental abnormalities, interest was stimulated by the unusual nature of the α thalassemia.

The children were of North European origin, where α thalassemia is uncommon (Chapter 32), and although one would have expected to find clear signs of this inherited anemia in their parents, it appeared to have arisen de novo in the affected offspring. It was concluded that the combination of α thalassemia, mental retardation (ATR), and the associated developmental abnormalities represented a new syndrome and that a common genetic defect might be responsible for the diverse clinical manifestations.

We now know that these original suspicions were correct, although it subsequently became clear that there are two distinct syndromes in which α thalassemia is associated with mental retardation (Wilkie et al., 1990a, 1990b). In the first (ATR-16) we have found large (1 to 2 Mb) chromosomal rearrangements that delete many genes from the short arm of chromosome 16; it is an example of a contiguous gene syndrome. In the second syndrome (ATR-X) a complex phenotype, including α thalassemia, results from

mutations in an X-encoded factor, which is a putative regulator of gene expression. Mutations in this gene downregulate α gene expression and also perturb the expression of other, as yet unidentified, genes.

THE ATR-16 SYNDROME

To date, seventeen individuals have been identified with the ATR-16 syndrome (Table 19.1). Often one is alerted to this condition by observing the unusual association of α thalassemia and mental retardation in individuals originating from outside of the areas where thalassemia commonly occurs (Chapter 32). There are two common patterns of inheritance. In eleven cases neither parent had α thalassemia (αα/αα × αα/αα) and the affected offspring had the phenotype of severe α thalassemia trait (genotype - -/αα). In five cases one parent had the phenotype of mild α thalassemia trait; the other parent was nonthalassemic (-α/αα × αα/αα) and the child had HbH disease (genotype - -/-α). In all such cases initial molecular genetic analyses have shown that affected children fail to inherit the entire ζ-α globin cluster from one parent or the other of the parents.

Chromosomal Abnormalities in ATR-16 Patients

In some cases conventional cytogenetic analysis may immediately demonstrate the underlying genetic abnormality. Because the α-globin complex lies close to the 16p telomere (Fig. 19.1), any chromosomal abnormality affecting this region may give rise to α thalassemia (Wilkie et al., 1990a). In some ATR-16 patients gross chromosomal abnormalities resulting in deletions (Wilkie et al., 1990a), formation of ring chromosomes (e.g., Neidengard and Sparkes, 1981; Quintana et al., 1983; Callen et al., 1989), or translocations (e.g., Buckle et al., 1988) have been observed. Although such abnormalities may arise as de novo genetic events, often one parent carries a balanced translocation that the child inherits in an unbalanced fashion (see Figs. 19.2 and 19.3 for examples) resulting in monosomy for 16p and loss of the α cluster.

In many cases of ATR-16, initial high resolution cytogenetic analysis detects no abnormality. However, even chromosomal rearrangements involving large fragments of DNA (5 to 10 Mb) may not be detected by routine cytogenetics. In this situation the pattern of inheritance of variable numbers of tandem repeats (VNTRs) within the α cluster may reveal the underlying molecular defect. In Figure 19.3 (originally described by Lamb et al., (1989), the parental 16p alleles can be distinguished from each other. The mother in this family carried an

Martin H. Steinberg, Bernard G. Forget, Douglas R. Higgs, and Ronald L. Nagel, editors. *Disorders of Hemoglobin: Genetics, Pathophysiology, and Clinical Management.* © 2001 Cambridge University Press. All rights reserved.

Table 19.1 Cytogenetic and Hematologic Data and Origin of ATR-16 Mutations

Case	Sex	MR	Phenotype	Genotype	Conventional cytogenetics	Chromosomal abnormality	Parental origin	Mechanism	Reference
OD	M	Moderate	HbH	-/-α	Normal	46,XY −16, +der(16)t(1;16)(p36;p13.3)	Maternal	Inherit 16:1 unbal trans	Lamb et al., 1989; Wilkie et al., 1990
DA	M	Mild	Trait	-/-αα	Abnormal	45,XY −15, −16 +der (16)t(15;16)(q13.1;p13.3)	Paternal	de novo	Wilkie et al., 1990
CU	M	Mild	Trait	-/-αα	Abnormal	46,XY −16 +der(16)t(9;16)(21.2;p13.3)	Maternal	de novo	Wilkie et al., 1990; Rack et al., 1993.
MR	F	Mild	Trait	-/-αα	Abnormal	46,XX −16, +der(16)t(9;16)(21.2;13.3)	Paternal	de novo	Rack et al., 1993
Aa	F	Borderline	Trait	-/-αα	Abnormal	46,XX −16, +der(16)t(10;16)(q26.13;p13.3)	Maternal	Inherit 16:10 Unbal trans	Buckle et al., 1988; Wilkie et al., 1990
BO	M	Mild	HbH	-/-α	Normal	46,XY del(16)(p13.3)	Paternal	de novo truncation	Wilkie et al., 1990; Lamb et al., 1993
DO	F	Mild	HbH	-/-α	Normal*	46,XY del(16)(p13.3) +?	Maternal	Unknown	Wilkie et al., 1990
HA	M	Borderline	HbH	-/-α	Normal	46,XY del(16)(p 13.3) +?	Paternal	Unknown	Wilkie et al., 1990
WI	M	Borderline	Trait	-/-αα	Normal	46,XY del(16)(p13.3) +?	Paternal	Unknown	Wilkie et al., 1990
LF	M	Unknown	NR	NA	Abnormal	46,XY −16 +der(16)t(X;16)(p11.4;p13.3)	Maternal	Inherit unbal trans	K. May (personal communication)
CH(BE)	F	NA	Trait	-/-αα	Normal	46,XX +der(16)t(16;16)(q24;p13.3)	Unknown	Inversion/deletion	Rönich and Kleihauer, 1967 and unpublished
W(BE)	M	NA	Trait	-/-αα	Normal	46,XX +der(16)t(16;16)(q24;p13.3)	Unknown	Inversion/deletion	Rönich and Kleihauer, 1967 and unpublished
C(WA)	F	Borderline	Trait	-/-αα	Normal	46,XX −16, +der(16)t(16;20)(p13.3;q13.3)	Maternal	Inherit unbal trans	Unpublished
M(GR)	M	Borderline	Trait	-/-αα	Normal	46,XY del(16)(p13.3) +?	Maternal	Inherit 16:21 unbal trans	Unpublished
J(GR)	F	Borderline	Trait	-/-αα	Normal	46,XY del(16)(p13.3) +?	Maternal	Inherit 16:21 unbal trans	Unpublished
C(BE)	F	MR+	HbH	-/-α	Normal	46,XX +der(16)t(16;16)(q24;p13.3)	Maternal	Inversion/deletion	Rönich and Kleihauer, 1967 and unpublished
GE	M	Severe	Trait	-/-αα	NA	45,XY −16−22 +der(16)(16qter−16p13.3::22q11.21−22qter)	Maternal	Inherit unbal trans	European Polycystic Kidney Disease Consortium, 1994

* At low resolution.

Abbreviations: Unbal, unbalanced; trans, translocation; MR+, mental retardation not qualified; NA, not available.

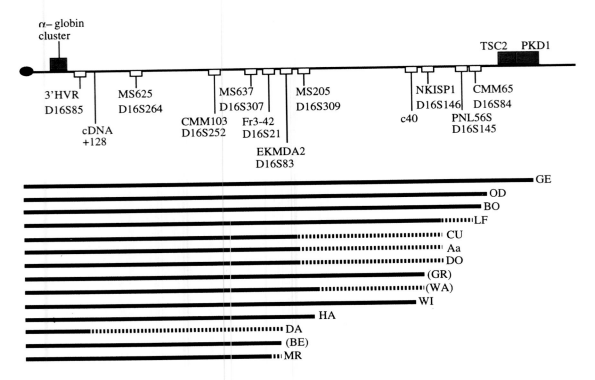

Figure 19.1. Summary of known ATR-16 deletions (S. Horsley et al., unpublished data and R. Daniels et al., unpublished data). Above the 16p telomere is shown as a black oval and the positions of the α-globin cluster, the gene-encoding tuberous sclerosis (TSC2), and the adult form of polycystic kidney disease (PKD1) are shown. The positions of other "anchor" markers are also shown. Below, the extent of each deletion is shown with the patient code alongside (see Table 19.1). Deletions known to result from chromosomal translocations are shown in red; those for which the mechanism is unknown or due to chromosomal truncation are blue. Solid bars indicate regions known to be deleted, and broken lines indicate the region of uncertainty of the breakpoints. The yellow bar below represents the maximum extent of deletions that cause α thalassemia with no associated abnormalities (see Chapter 16). For full color reproduction, see color plate 19.1

unbalanced (16:1) translocation, which both of her children inherited in an imbalanced fashion. Her son OD (Table 19.1) was monosomic for 16p, and therefore had α thalassemia (in this case HbH disease), whereas her daughter was trisomic for 16p. Both children had mental retardation, dysmorphic facies, and a variety of associated developmental abnormalities.

VNTRs are not always informative; therefore more recently, fluorescence in situ hybridization (FISH) studies have been used to analyze ATR-16 families. In this type of study, large segments (~40 kb) of chromosome 16 in cosmid vectors are used as probes to show the presence or absence of the corresponding sequences in the 16p telomeric region with fluorescence microscopy (Buckle and Kearney, 1994). By analyzing the chromosomes of both parents and the affected child, it is possible to

Figure 19.2. High resolution cytogenetic analysis in an individual with ART-16 syndrome demonstrating a translocation between chromosomes 9 and 16. The normal (→) and abnormal (▶) copies of chromosome 16 are indicated with arrows.

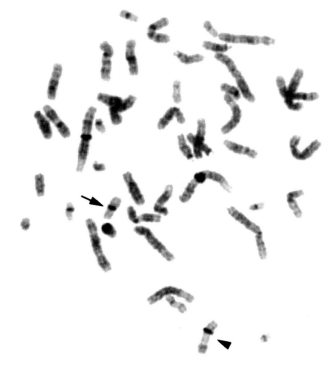

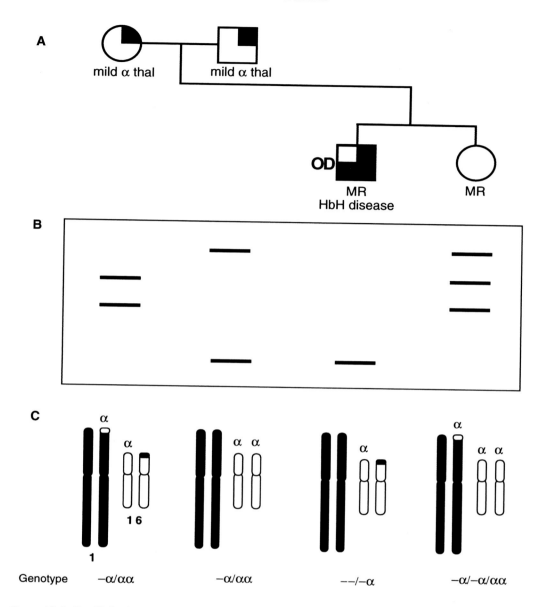

Figure 19.3. Familial subcytogenetic translocation (from Lamb et al., 1989). (A) Pedigree indicating parents with mild α thalassemia only; son (OD) with mental retardation and severe α-thalassemia (HbH disease) and daughter with mental retardation. (B) Schematic representation of restriction fragment length polymorphism analysis using a fully informative marker closely linked to the α-globin cluster. Each track corresponds to the individual shown above. (C) Segregation of 1:16 translocation and α-globin complex (α) in each family member. The resulting genotype is shown. Note that both children have inherited the paternal chromosome carrying the (-α) allele. It has not been determined whether the mother's normal or translated chromosome 16 bears her (-α) allele.

define the extent of 16p monosomy and the mechanism by which it has arisen. In the example shown in Figure 19.4A, FISH analysis showed that the mother of children with the ATR-16 syndrome carries a 5:16 translo-

cation (unpublished observation) that was inherited in an unbalanced fashion (as in Fig. 19.3) by her offspring. In the second example (case HA in Wilkie et al., 1990a), both parents were normal, but FISH analysis demonstrated a de novo loss of material from the end of chromosome 16 (Fig. 19.4B) in their child HA (Table 19.1). These types of chromosomal abnormality, which can be detected only by FISH or molecular analyses, are referred to as *cryptic*.

Using a combination of conventional cytogenetics, FISH, and molecular analysis, at least three types of chromosomal rearrangements (inherited or de novo translocation, inversion/deletion, and truncation) have now been found in ATR-16 patients (Fig. 19.1 and Table 19.1). At present none of the breakpoints associated with the 16p translocations has been sequenced. Similarly, the inversion/deletion event

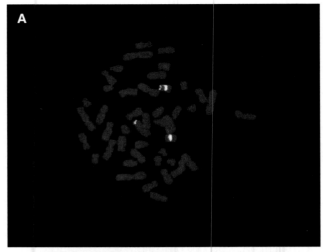

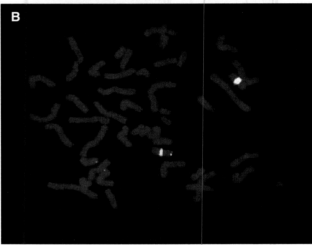

Figure 19.4. (A) An example of an unbalanced translocation in a parent of a child with the ATR-16 syndrome. (B) Loss of 16p material in an individual with the ART-16 syndrome. For full color reproduction, see color plate 19.4

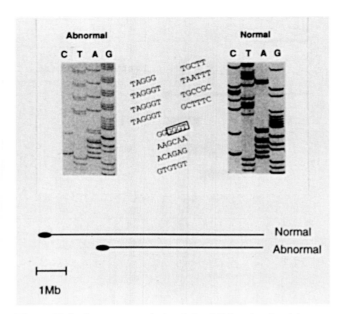

Figure 19.5. Sequence analysis of the BO breakpoint (also see Fig. 19.1). The chromosome has broken and been "healed" directly by the addition of telomeric (TTAGGG) repeats (see Lamb et al., 1993).

(CHBE, WBE, CBE) has only been partially characterized. The telomeric truncation seen in BO (Table 19.1) has been fully analyzed (Lamb et al., 1993). In this important case it appears that the chromosome was broken, truncated, and "healed" by the direct addition of telomeric repeats $(TTAGGG)_n$ (Fig. 19.5) as described for some less extensive 16p deletions in Chapter 17.

A review of the literature has also identified other less well-characterized chromosomal abnormalities that may cause the ATR-16 syndrome. For example, Pawlowitzki et al. (1979) described a child with the unbalanced karyotype 46,XX,−16, +der(16), t(16;20)(p13;q11) who, at the age of 9 months, had severe hypochromia (MCH was 17.6 pg). It is likely that this child had α thalassemia, but this was not investigated. There are a number of other reports of possible chromosome 16p

deletions, including ring (16), associated with mental retardation, but hematologic results were either not mentioned (Pergament et al., 1970; Bauknecht et al., 1976; Golden et al., 1981; Nielsen et al., 1983; Quintana et al., 1983; Anneren and Gustavson, 1984; Nazarenko et al., 1987; Chodirker et al., 1988) or reported as equivocal (Neidengard and Sparkes, 1981; Emanuel et al., 1982). Further analysis of DNA from the ring (16) patient of Neidengard and Sparkes (1981) indicated that the α-globin complex had indeed been deleted from the ring chromosome (Callen et al., 1989), the breakpoint lying between EKMDA2 and NIKSP1 (see Fig. 19.1; unpublished results), and the ring (16) patient of Quintana et al. (1983) is also missing the α-globin complex from the involved chromosome (Callen et al., 1989). Although such cases of α thalassemia and mental retardation have doubtless been overlooked, it is likely that the syndrome is rare, because each case has been the result of a unique and independent chromosome mutation.

How Do Chromosomal Abnormalities Give Rise to the ATR-16 Syndrome?

In the light of these observations, it is clear that individuals with ATR-16 may have quite variable degrees of chromosomal imbalance, and consequently there is considerable variation in the associated phenotypes (Table 19.2). The degree of 16p monosomy varies from ~1 to 2 Mb (Fig. 19.1), but at least eleven patients have additional

Table 19.2. Clinical Findings in Patients with ATR-16 Syndrome

Case	MR	Normal BW	Neonatal problems	Microcephaly	Short stature	Facial dysmorphism	Genital abnormalities	Skeletal abnormalities	Miscellaneous abnormalities
OD	Moderate	+	+	-	-	+	+	-	CAL
DA	Mild	+	+	-	-	+	+	+	SPC, HT
CU	Mild	+	-	-	-	+	-	+	SPC
MR	Mild	+	-	-	+	+	-	+	SPC
Aa	Borderline	+	+	-	-	+	-	-	UG, HPN
BO	Mild	+	-	+	-	+	+	+	IC, P
DO	Mild	+	+	-	-	+	-	-	IC
HA	Borderline	+	+	-	+	+	-	+	E
WI	Borderline	+	-	-	-	+	-	+	AN, IC
LF	U	NA	NA	NA	NA	+	+	NA	T, CS, CHD, H
CH(BE)	NA	NA	NA	NA	NA	+	NA	NA	NA
W(BE)	NA	NA	NA	NA	NA	+	NA	NA	NA
C(BE)	+*	-	+	-	NA	+	-	NA	S
C(WA)	Borderline	+	+	-	+	+	-	+	S, PVC, LFW, SD, NW
M(GR)	Borderline	+	+	-	-	+	-	+	
J(GR)	Borderline	+	+	+	-	+	-	+	CHD
GE	Severe	NA	-	-	-	-	-	-	TS, RC, E

* Mental retardation not classified. NA, data not available; U, unable to assess at time of death; CAL, café au lait patches; SPC, single palmar crease; HT, hypoplastic enamel of teeth; UG, unsteady gait; HPN, high placed nipples; IC, impaired coordination; P, ptosis; E, epilepsy; AN, accessory nipple; T, tracheobronchomalacia; CS, choanal stenosis; CHD, congenital heart disease; H, hydrocephalus; S, strabismus; PVC, paralyzed vocal cord (unilateral); LFW, left facial weakness; SD, sacral dimple; NW, neck webbing; M, myopia; TS, tuberous sclerosis; RC, renal cysts; PL, pigmented lesions (hypo and hyper).

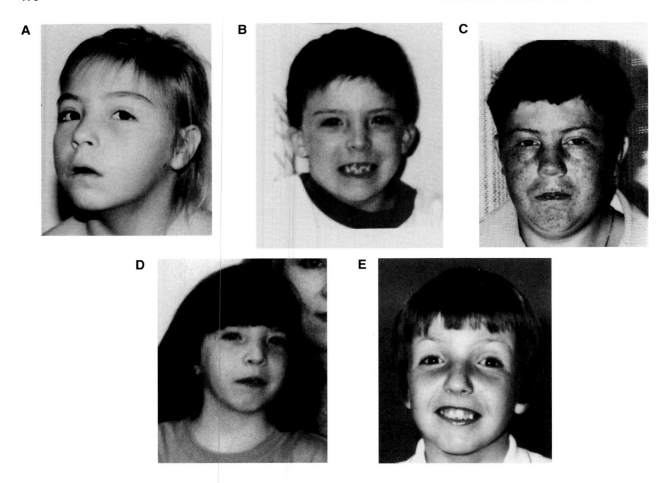

Figure 19.6. The facial appearance of patients with the ATR-16 syndrome. Common features include relative hypertelorism, a small chin and mouth, a "beaked" nose, downslanting palpebral fissures, and crowded teeth.

chromosomal aneuploidy. In some cases imbalance of the non-16 material may dominate the clinical picture. For example, in DA (Table 19.1), loss of material from chromosome 15 while forming the abnormal derivative t(15:16) chromosome produced the striking phenotype associated with the Prader-Willi syndrome.

In only one patient (BO) can all of the clinical features be attributed solely to loss of material from 16p (Lamb et al., 1993). In two other patients (DO and WI, see Fig. 19.1 and Table 19.1), however, current data suggest that the predominant abnormality may similarly result from 16p monosomy. Several of these patients have a similar facial appearance, similar degrees of mild mental retardation, and some associated developmental abnormalities in common (Fig. 19.6 and Table 19.2).

By studying such a group of patients, one might hope to gain insight into how 16p monosomy gives rise to developmental abnormalities. Initially it

seemed possible that hemizygosity for the embryonic ζ globin gene might give rise to neonatal hypoxia and consequent developmental abnormalities. However, we now know that many patients with relatively small (up to 200 kb) deletions (Chapter 17 and Fig. 19.1), including the entire ζ-α cluster, may be developmentally normal. Another possibility is that deletion of a large number of genes from one copy of chromosome 16 may unmask mutations in its homolog; the more genes that are deleted the greater the probability of this occurrence. However, this is unlikely to be the explanation for most ATR-16 cases because it is estimated that normal individuals carry only a few harmful mutations of this type in the entire genome (Vogel and Motulsky, 1986). A further possibility is that some genes in 16p are imprinted (Hall, 1990) so that deletions could remove the only active copy of the gene. At present there is no evidence for imprinting of the 16p region (reviewed in Schneider et al., 1996), and in the few ATR-16 cases analyzed, there appears to be no major clinical differences between patients with deletions of the maternally or paternally derived chromosomes (Table 19.1). It seems more likely, therefore, that some genes in the 16p region encode proteins whose effect is critically determined by the amount produced, so-called dosage-sensitive genes (see Fisher and Scambler, 1994). Examples of such genes include those encoding proteins that form heterodimers, those required at a critical level for a rate-determining step of a regulatory pathway, and tumor suppressor genes (e.g., TSC2, see later). Removal of such critical, dosage-sensitive genes might account for many of the clinical effects seen in ATR-16 patients.

Some of these points can be addressed from currently available data. It is clear that removal of up to ~250 kb of 16p, including an estimated 20 genes (Horsley et al., unpublished), has little or no effect on phenotype other than producing α thalassemia (see Chapter 17 and Fig. 19.1 for summary). Furthermore, patients with deletions of up to 1 Mb of 16p may be quite mildly affected (Daniels et al, unpublished). However, the single patient with 16p monosomy for the terminal 2 Mb of 16p (BO) is more severely affected (IQ53). One patient (GE) whose deletion extends just beyond the BO breakpoint had the phenotype of severe mental retardation, tuberous sclerosis, and polycystic kidney disease (European Polycystic Kidney Disease Consortium, 1994). Subsequently, patients with even quite small interstitial deletions (3 to 6 kb) around the TSC2 and PKD1 loci have been shown to have the variable but often severe syndrome of tuberous sclerosis (European Chromosome 16 Tuberous Sclerosis Consortium, 1993 and J. Sampson, personal communication), thus providing clear examples where removal of a critical gene from the terminal region of 16p can account for most, if not all, of the clinical features.

These findings suggest that the accumulated loss of many genes from chromosome 16p may have a relatively mild effect. However, this region may contain fewer critical genes that exert a severe effect when only one copy is deleted. Characterization of further patients with 16p monosomy and identification of all expressed sequences within 16p13.3 will help in localizing such critical genes in this area.

The ATR-16 syndrome has been an important model for improving general understanding of the molecular basis for mental retardation. It provided the first examples of mental retardation resulting from a cryptic chromosomal translocation and truncation. Further work has shown that such telomeric rearrangements may underlie a significant proportion of cases of unexplained mental retardation (Flint et al., 1995). The current challenge is to understand in detail the mechanisms by which monosomy causes developmental abnormalities; the ATR-16 syndrome provides an excellent model for addressing this issue.

THE ATR-X SYNDROME

As additional patients with α thalassemia and mental retardation were identified throughout the 1980s, it became clear that a distinct group of affected individuals existed in whom no structural abnormalities of the α cluster or 16p could be found. In contrast to the ATR-16 syndrome, patients in this "nondeletional" group were phenotypically uniform; they were male and had severe mental retardation with a remarkably similar facial appearance (Wilkie et al., 1990b; Gibbons et al., 1991). That this group had a distinct and recognizable dysmorphism was underscored when additional cases were identified on the basis of their facial features alone (Wilkie et al., 1991). Ultimately, it was shown that this unusual syndrome of a thalassemia with severe mental retardation results from an X-linked abnormality (see later) and the condition is now referred to as the ATR-X syndrome.

The Clinical and Hematologic Features of the ATR-X Syndrome

More than 100 cases of the ATR-X syndrome from more than 70 families have now been characterized, and a definite phenotype is emerging (Table 19.3). In the great majority of cases, the children have profound and global developmental delay. They have marked hypotonia as neonates and in early childhood, all milestones are delayed. Many do not walk until later in childhood, and some never do. Almost all have no speech, frequently have only situational understand-

Table 19.3. Summary of the Major Clinical Manifestations of the ATR-X Syndrome

Clinical feature	Total	Percentage
Severe mental retardation*	108/110	98
Normal birth weight	65/72	90
Neonatal hypotonia	59/68	87
Seizures	36/104	35
Characteristic face	86/96	90
Microcephaly	67/88	76
Genital abnormalities	83/94	88
Skeletal abnormalities	83/91	91
Cardiac defects	21/98	21
Renal/urinary abnormalities	16/98	16
Gut dysmotility	66/86	77
Short stature	51/74	69

Total represents number of patients on whom appropriate information is available and includes patients who do not have thalassemia but in whom ATR-X mutations have been identified.
* Two patients too young (< 1 year) to assess degree of mental retardation.

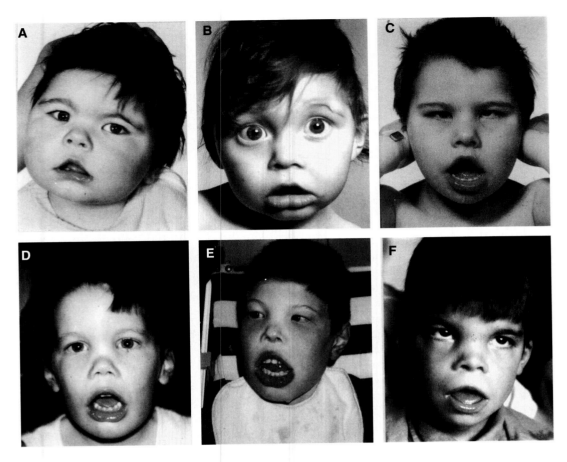

Figure 19.7. The facial appearance of patients with the ATR-X syndrome as described in the text.

ing, and are dependent for almost all activities of daily living. However, in one family with four affected male cousins, one had profound mental retardation, whereas the others had IQs of 41, 56, and 58 (Guerrini et al., 2000). The basis for this marked variation is unknown but indicates that mutations in the ATR-X gene may be responsible for a wider spectrum of intellectual handicap than previously thought.

In early childhood the distinctive facial features are most readily recognized (Fig. 19.7): upswept, frontal hair, telecanthus, epicanthic folds, flat nasal bridge and mid-face hypoplasia, and a small triangular upturned nose with the alar nasae extending below the columella and septum. The upper lip is tented and the lower lip full and everted, giving the mouth a "carplike" appearance. The frontal incisors are frequently widely spaced, the tongue protrudes, and there is prodigious dribbling. A wide spectrum of associated abnormalities affect many systems (Table 19.4). The most intriguing defects are the genital abnormalities seen in almost all children (Gibbons et al., 1995a). These may be very mild as in undescended testes, but the spectrum of abnormality extends through hypospadias, micropenis, to external female genitalia with the affected children being defined as male pseudohermaphrodites. Of particular interest is that these abnormalities breed true within families (McPherson et al., 1995). Recurrent vomiting or regurgitation, sometimes treated by fundoplication, is a common feature and seems likely to be a manifestation of a more generalized dysmotility of the gut (Table 19.4). An apparent reluctance to swallow probably reflects the discoordinated swallowing that has been observed. The tendency to aspirate is commonly implicated as a cause of death in early childhood. Computed tomography or magnetic resonance brain imaging frequently shows no abnormality, although mild cerebral atrophy may be seen. In two cases partial or complete agenesis of the corpus callosum has been reported.

The hematology is often surprisingly normal considering the presence of α thalassemia. Neither the hemoglobin concentration nor mean cell hemoglobin is as severely affected as in the classic forms of α thalassemia (Fig. 19.8), perhaps reflecting the different pathophysiology of the conditions. Where there is more than one affected member in a family, there is frequently marked variation in the frequency of cells with HbH inclusions. In one French family (Lefort

Table 19.4. Clinical Manifestations of the ATR-X Syndrome

Manifestation	Description
Genital abnormalities	Small/soft testes, cryptorchidism, gonadal dysgenesis, inguinal hernia, micropenis, hypospadias, deficient prepuce, shawl scrotum, hypoplastic scrotum, ambiguous genitalia, female external genitalia.
Skeletal abnormalities	Delayed bone age, tapering fingers, drumstick distal phalanges, brachydactyly, clinodactyly, bifid thumb, fixed flexion deformities of joints, overriding toes, varus or valgus deformities of feet, scoliosis, kyphosis, hemivertebra, segmentation defects of the vertebrae, spina bifida, coxa valga, chest wall deformity.
Renal/urinary abnormalities	Renal agenesis, hydronephrosis, small kidneys, vesicoureteric reflux, pelvoureteric junction obstruction, exstrophy of bladder, urethral diverticulum, urethral stricture.
Cardiac defects	Atrial septal defect, ventricular septal defect, patent ductus arteriosus, tetralogy of Fallot, transposition of the great arteries, dextracardia with situs solitus, aortic stenosis, pulmonary stenosis.
Gut dysmotility	Discoordinated swallowing, eructation, gastroesophageal reflux, vomiting, hiatus hernia, recurrent ileus/small bowel obstruction, volvulus, intermittent diarrhea, severe constipation.
Miscellaneous	Apneic episodes, cold/blue extremities, blepharitis, conjunctivitis, entropion, cleft palate, pneumonia, umbilical hernia, encephalitis, optic atrophy, blindness, sensorineural deafness, prolonged periods of screaming/laughing, self-injury.

et al., 1993), two third-degree relatives had 30 and 13 percent of cells with HbH inclusions, respectively, whereas an affected fifth-degree relative had less than 0.001 percent cells with inclusions. This suggests that the hematologic picture is complicated by other, possibly genetic, variables.

Evidence That the ATR-X Syndrome is An X-Linked condition

The five original "nondeletion" cases described by Wilkie et al. (1990b) were sporadic and, apart from male gender, there were no immediate clues to the genetic etiology. Somatic cell hybrids composed of mouse erythroleukemia call lines containing each copy of chromosome 16 from an affected boy produced human α globin in a manner distinguishable from similar hybrids containing chromosome 16 from normal individuals. It seemed likely that the defect in globin synthesis lay in *trans* to the α-globin cluster. This was confirmed in a family with four affected sibs in whom the condition segregated independently of the α-globin cluster (Donnai et al., 1991).

Preliminary observations indicated that the syndrome mapped to the X chromosome, and hence it was named the ATR-X syndrome. Subsequent linkage analysis of 16 families localized the disease to the region Xq13.1–q21.1, confirming that the associated α thalassemia results from a *trans*-acting mutation (Gibbons et al., 1992).

The ATR-X syndrome behaves as an X-linked recessive disorder; only boys are affected. Female carriers have a normal appearance and intellect, although approximately one in four carriers has subtle signs of α thalassemia with very rare cells containing HbH inclusions (Gibbons et al., 1992). Almost all carriers have a highly skewed pattern of X inactivation in leukocytes (derived from mesoderm), hair roots (ectoderm), and buccal cells (endoderm). In each case the disease-bearing X chromosome is preferentially inactivated. In one exception a developmentally normal 3-year-old female carrier had a balanced pattern of X inactivation and almost as many HbH inclusions as her affected brother (Gibbons et al., 1992).

Identification of the ATR-X Disease Gene

Initial analysis of unrelated ATR-X cases revealed no cytogenetic abnormalities involving Xq. Nevertheless, it seemed possible that a gene deletion or rearrangement might be found in some cases, and DNA samples from a panel of ATR-X patients were therefore screened. At first, no abnormalities were found within the disease interval using a combination of polymerase chain reaction, conventional Southern analysis, and pulsed field gel electrophoresis.

The isolation of cDNA fragments mapping to this interval provided the opportunity to study candidate genes for ATR-X (Gecz et al., 1993). cDNAs (from M. Fontes and colleagues) isolated by direct selection using yeast artificial chromosomes (YACs) mapping to this region were screened by hybridization to DNA samples from a panel of patients. Using an 84 bp cDNA frag-

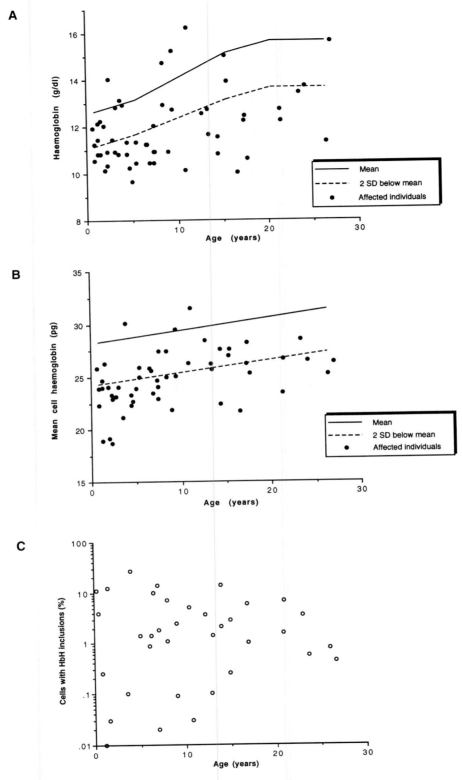

Figure 19.8. (A) Hemoglobin levels and (B) mean cell hemoglobins in subjects with ATR-X syndrome at various ages. Solid line indicated the mean and dashed line 2 standard deviations below the mean (Dallman, 1977). For any subject only one result within each consecutive 5-year period is given. (C) Proportion of red cells with HbH inclusions in subjects with ATR-X syndrome after 1 percent brilliant cresyl blue incubation at room temperature. Only one result is given for each subject. The percentage of positive cells is plotted on a logarithmic scale.

ment, the hybridization signal was absent in one individual. Further mapping with genomic probes isolated with the cDNA probe indicated that this patient had a 2.0 kb deletion, of which approximately 1.6 kb was subsequently shown to encode mRNA. The cDNA fragment was used to isolate further cDNA clones (Gibbons et al., 1995b) and eventually a contig spanning a substantial portion of the cDNA was isolated.

Using cDNA fragments from this putative ATR-X gene to probe Northern blots, two closely migrating transcripts of approximately 10 kb were observed in mRNA from the Epstein–Barr Virus (EBV)-transformed lymphocytes of normal individuals. However, expression of the gene was virtually absent in the patient with the 2 kb deletion. ATR-X mRNA was detected in all other ATR-X patients, but in some there was a marked alteration in the relative intensities of the two transcripts. Furthermore, the ratio was identically altered in other affected members of the same family providing circumstantial evidence that mRNA expression from this gene was perturbed in other ATR-X individuals.

Single-strand conformation polymorphism analysis was carried out on a panel of ATR-X patients using cDNA covering the majority of the known protein coding sequence. Mutations in nine additional pedigrees were detected of which seven were missense mutations and two were premature inphase stop mutations (see later). Taken together, these findings showed beyond reasonable doubt that mutations in the proposed ATR-X gene (initially known as *XH2*

but now designated ATRX) were responsible for the syndrome (Gibbons et al., 1995b).

Characterization of the ATRX Gene and Its Potential Role in Gene Expression

We now know that the ATRX gene spans about 300 kb of genomic DNA and contains 36 exons (Picketts et al., 1996). It encodes at least two alternatively spliced ~10.5 kb mRNA transcripts, which differ at their 5′ ends and are predicted to give rise to slightly different proteins of 265 and 280 kD, respectively (Fig. 19.9). The proteins can be broadly divided into three regions (Fig.

Figure 19.9. Schematic diagram of the complete ATRX cDNA (upper figure). The boxes represent the 36 exons, thin horizontal lines represent the introns (not to scale). The largest open reading frame is shown as an open box (lower figure) with the 5′ and 3′ UTR sequences as black lines with the poly(A) tail denoted (An). The positions of the mutations are shown by circles; open circles indicate mutations that would cause protein truncation. The alternate splicing that resuls in transcripts lacking exons 6 and 7 or lacking exon 7 only is shown by inverted Vs. The alternate initiation codons are labeled M1 and M2. The principal domains, the N-terminal hydrophilic domain, the central domain containing the highly conserved helicase motifs, and the C-terminal domain are indicated. Additional domains are shown as black boxes and include the zinc finger motif (ZEFM), the potential coiled coil (CC), a stretch of 21 glutamic acid residues (E), the P box (P), and a glutamine rich region (Q). In the lower part of the figure is a graphical representation of the amino acid similarity between human and mouse ATRX proteins.

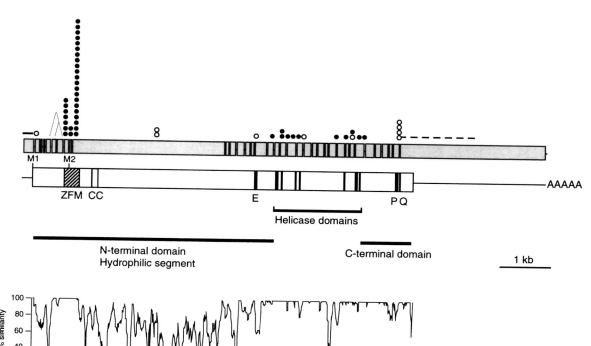

19.9): an N-terminal hydrophilic segment (~1640 amino acids), a central region containing alternating hydrophilic and hydrophobic stretches (~855 amino acids), and a C-terminal domain (~135 amino acids). Within the N-terminal region lies a complex cysteine rich segment (ZFM, Fig. 19.9) part of which shows striking similarity to a PHD finger domain (Gibbons et al., 1997). The PHD finger is a putative zinc-binding domain Cys_4-His-Cys_3) 50 to 80 amino acids long that has been identified in a growing number of proteins, many of which are thought to be involved in chromatin-mediated transcriptional regulation (Aasland et al., 1995). The functional significance of this segment is shown by the high degree of conservation between human and mouse (97 of 98 amino acids) and the fact that it represents a major site of mutations in patients with ATR-X syndrome containing more than 60 percent of all mutations (Fig. 19.9 and see later). Also within the N-terminal region is a segment of protein that has a high probability of forming a coiled coil, a structure implicated in protein-protein interactions. Although this structure resides in an evolutionarily less conserved region, a similar coiled coil is predicted in the mouse protein (Picketts et al., 1998). Two reports of proteins that interact with ATRX involve this region (Le Douarin et al., 1996; Ohsawa et al., 1996). Using the yeast two-hybrid approach to identify proteins that interact with the mouse chromatin associated protein mHP1α, Le Douarin and colleagues identified a partial mouse ATRX sequence corresponding to this region. Cardoso et al. (1998) explored the protein interactions of this region further in a yeast system and showed binding to the SET domain of the polycomb-like protein EZH2.

The central and C-terminal regions show the greatest conservation between mouse and human sequences (94 percent) (Picketts et al., 1998). The central portion of the molecule contains motifs that identify ATRX as a novel member of the SNF2 subgroup of a superfamily of proteins with similar adenotriphosphatase and helicase motifs. Other members of this subfamily are involved in a wide variety of cellular functions including the regulation of transcription (SNF2, MOT1 and brahma), control of the cell cycle (NPS1), DNA repair (RAD16, RAD54 and ERCC6), and mitotic chromosome segregation (lodestar). An interaction with chromatin has been shown for SNF2 and brahma and may be a common theme for all this group (reviewed in Carlson and Laurent, 1994). The helicase domains may be interchanged between members of the same group without substantially changing the specific function of the protein, indicating that regions outside of this central domain may be responsible for the individual properties of these proteins (Carlson and Laurent, 1994 and references therein). The ATRX protein, although showing marginally higher sequence homology to RAD54 than other members of this group, does not obviously fall into a particular functional category by virtue of homology in these flanking segments. There is no clinical evidence for ultraviolet sensitivity or the premature development of malignancy in the ATR-X syndrome that might point to it being the result of a defect in DNA repair mechanisms. Furthermore, cytogenetic analysis has not shown any evidence of abnormal chromosome breakage or segregation. Rather, the consistent association of ATR-X with α thalassemia suggests that the protein normally exerts its effect at one or more of the many stages involved in gene expression.

The extreme C-terminus of ATRX encodes two additional domains of potential functional importance that are highly conserved in the mouse. The P-box (Fig. 19.9) is an element conserved among other SNF-2 like family members involved in transcriptional regulation, and a stretch of glutamine residues (Q-box) represents a potential protein interaction domain.

ATRX mutations appear to downregulate expression of the α- rather than the closely related β-globin genes. Activation of the α- and β-globin genes involves a common group of lineage-restricted (GATA-1 and NF-E2) and ubiquitous (CACC box) DNA-binding factors (reviewed in Chapter 4). A key difference, however, is that the α-globin genes lie in a region of constitutively "open", transcriptionally active chromatin, and their expression is regulated by a remote tissue-specific enhancer. The β-globin genes lie within a segment of chromatin that is "closed" in nonerythroid cells but which "opens" in a tissue-specific manner under the influence of a remote locus control region (Vyas et al., 1992; Craddock et al., 1995). It is conceivable that the ATRX protein acts to derepress or activate the α-globin genes by interaction with chromatin, whereas these functions are subserved by alternative mechanisms in the β-globin cluster. The analysis of α-globin regulation and its perturbation by ATRX mutations offer a unique opportunity to understand exactly how the protein regulates gene expression.

As patients with the ATR-X syndrome have multiple associated congenital abnormalities, it seems likely that ATRX mutations exert pleiotropic effects. By analogy with SNF2, for example, ATRX may regulate expression of a restricted class of genes; perturbation in expression of these "target" genes could affect development of many different systems, including the central nervous system.

ATRX is a candidate for playing an important part in the development of the central nervous system. It is a widely expressed gene with relatively high levels in brain, heart, and skeletal muscle compared with lung and liver. Its murine homolog *Mxnp* is expressed in the early primitive streak (7.0 days postcoitum), which represents the earliest stage of mouse development at which Mxnp expression has yet been studied (Stayton et al., 1994). Although its expression is widespread, there are considerable changes in the levels of expression in different cell types during development.

Recently we have developed a panel of antibodies to the N-terminal region of the ATRX protein (McDowell et al., 1999). In interphase it appears that the protein is found entirely within the nucleus where it is found in discrete regions associated with pericentromeric heterochromatin. In metaphase, ATRX is similarly found close to the centromeres of many chromosomes but, in addition, is found at the stalks of acrocentric chromosomes, where the ribosomal (rDNA) genes are located. These physical locations have provided important clues to another potential role of ATRX protein in the establishment and/or maintenance of methylation in the genome (see below).

Mutations of the ATRX Gene

Now that the ATRX gene has been fully characterized (Gibbons et al., 1995b; Picketts et al., 1996), it will be important to establish the full range of disease causing mutations to facilitate genetic counseling and to elucidate functionally important aspects of the protein. Thirty-three different mutations have been documented (Table 19.5 and Fig. 19.9) including twenty missense mutations, four nonsense mutations, one three base pair insertion, and six splicing defects, of which four cause frameshifts and protein truncation and two cause deletions. The missense mutations in particular are clustered in two regions, the zinc finger motif and the helicase domain. Analysis of the mutations and their resulting phenotypes leads to important conclusions. A number of mutations predicted to cause protein truncation are scattered throughout the gene (Fig. 19.9). Where this leads to the loss of critical domains it would be expected to cause loss of function. Using the monoclonal antibodies against ATRX and Western blot analysis, the levels of ATRX protein were found to be significantly reduced in patients with diverse mutations and in some the protein was virtually undetectable (McDowell et al., 1999). Nevertheless, these mutations are not lethal. Furthermore the resulting phenotype is similar for diverse mutations, which is consistent with the view that the common final pathway of these mutations is a decrease in normal ATRX activity. In some of the splicing mutants, including some presented here, the levels of normal ATRX mRNA range from less than 1 to 30 percent (Villard et al., 1996c). That key features of the ATRX syndrome are found in the presence of substantial amounts of normal ATRX mRNA suggests that the target pathways are sensitive to the dosage of this protein. One reason for such sensitivity could be that, like the related SNF2 protein (Peterson and Herskowitz, 1992; Wilson et al., 1996), ATRX may be required in carefully controlled stoichiometric amounts for the formation of multiprotein complexes.

Recently, an important new finding points to a role for the ATRX protein in establishing or maintaining the pattern of methylation in the human genome. Mutations of ATRX cause consistent changes in the pattern of methylation of rDNA (where the protein has been shown to bind, see above), Y-specific repeats, and subtelomeric repeats. One possibility is that ATRX alters access of the de novo methylase to its binding sites. Alternatively, ATRX (like Mi-2) might be a member of a protein complex (so called histone deacetylase/methylbinding domain protein complexes) involved in establishing or maintaining the pattern of methylation in the genome (Gibbons et al., 2000).

Since the discovery of the ATRX gene, most new cases are defined on the basis of severe mental retardation with the typical facial appearance associated with a mutation in the ATRX gene. This allows a less biased evaluation of the effect of ATRX mutations on the commonly associated clinical features.

Six different mutations are associated with the most severe urogenital abnormalities (Table 19.5). In four, the protein is truncated resulting in the loss of the C-terminal domain, including a conserved element (P in Fig. 19.8) and polyglutamine tract (Q in Fig. 19.9). These mutations therefore may have the greatest potential to disrupt ATRX function. The available data indicate that in the absence of significant ATRX function, particularly that of the C-terminal domain, severe urogenital abnormalities are inevitable. Consistent with this finding, in families with such mutations, severe urogenital abnormalities breed true (McPherson et al., 1995) and an identical, independently arising nonsense mutation (Peds 17 and 38) gives rise to a similar phenotype. In one family with a splicing defect that produces variable amounts of normal ATRX mRNA (Mutation 23 in Table 19.5), urogenital abnormalities were only seen in the patient with the least amount of normal ATRX mRNA (Lefort et al., 1993; Villard et al., 1996c).

The relationship between ATRX mutations and α thalassemia is less clear. Since the presence of excess β chains (HbH inclusions) was originally used to define the ATR-X syndrome, current observations are inevitably biased. Nevertheless, there is considerable variability in the degree to which α globin synthesis is affected by these mutations. Some patients do not have HbH inclusions (Villard et al., 1996a, 1996b, 1996c), although this does not rule out downregulation of α-globin expression because inclusions may not appear until there is 30 to 40 percent reduction in chain synthesis (Higgs et al., 1989). There appears to be no con-

Table 19.5. Summary of ATRX Mutations

Mutation no.	Case	Nucleotide	Amino acid	Mutation*	De novo†	Genital‡ abnormality	HbH inc cells %	Reference
1	Ped N1, DL	1–213		D		++	0	Unpublished
	Ped N1, ML	1–213		D		++	nd	Unpublished
	Ped N1, JP	1–213		D		++	0	Unpublished
2	Ped 59, III-M	324	37	N; C>T; Arg > stop		normal	0.006	Guerrini et al., 2000
	Ped 59 II-F	324	37	N; C>T; Arg > stop		normal	0.003	Guerrini et al., 2000
	Ped 59 II-S	324	37	N; C>T; Arg > stop		normal	0	Guerrini et al., 2000
	Ped 59 III-A	324	37	N; C>T; Arg > stop		normal	0	Guerrini et al., 2000
3	Ped 29, GH	866	177	I; CAA; Q		+	0.12	Gibbons et al., 1997
	Ped 29, JH	866	177	I; CAA; Q		+	0.003	Gibbons et al., 1997
	Ped 29, GC	866	177	I; CAA; Q		+	nd	Gibbons et al., 1997
4	Ped 12, case 3	869–931	178–198	S; deletion 63bp; in frame A873G	+	+	0.1	Picketts et al., 1996
	Ped N17	869–931	178–198	S; deletion 63bp; in frame A873G	+	+	0	Picketts et al., 1996
	Ped 46	869–931	178–198	S; deletion 63bp; in frame A873G		++	0.4	Gibbons et al., 1997
	Ped 49	869–931	178–198	S; deletion 63bp; in frame A873G	+	normal	1.5	Gibbons et al., 1997
5	Ped 51	905	190	M; C > G; Pro > Ala		++	4.8	Gibbons et al., 1997
6	Ped 39	913	192	M; G > C; Leu > Phe		normal	<0.01	Gibbons et al., 1997
7	Ped 35	936	200	M; G > C; Cys > Ser	+	++	31.5	Gibbons et al., 1997
8	Ped 32	995	220	M; T > C; Cys > Arg		++	0.01	Gibbons et al., 1997
9	Ped 50	1002	222	M; G > C; Trp > Ser		++	0.003	Gibbons et al., 1997
10	Ped 30, 232	1054	239	M; C > A, Phe > Leu		nd	2	Unpublished
11	Ped 19	1056	240	M; G > T; Cys > Phe	+ GS	++	6	Gibbons et al., 1997
12	Ped 9, case 1	1073	246	M; C > T; Arg > Cys		++	1.4	Gibbons et al., 1997
	Ped 9, case 2	1073	246	M; C > T; Arg > Cys		++	0.8	Gibbons et al., 1997
	Ped 4	1073	246	M; C > T; Arg > Cys	+	++	5.2	Gibbons et al., 1997
	Ped 7	1073	246	M; C > T; Arg > Cys		++	14	Gibbons et al., 1997
	Ped 8, RH	1073	246	M; C > T; Arg > Cys		++	14	Gibbons et al., 1997
	Ped 8, MC	1073	246	M; C > T; Arg > Cys		+	3.5	Gibbons et al., 1997
	Ped 16	1073	246	M; C > T; Arg > Cys		++	1	Gibbons et al., 1997
	Ped 18	1073	246	M; C > T; Arg > Cys		++	1.8	Gibbons et al., 1997
	Ped 6	1073	246	M; C > T; Arg > Cys		+	6.8	Gibbons et al., 1997
	Ped 24	1073	246	M; C > T; Arg > Cys	+	+	0.05	Gibbons et al., 1997
	Ped 24	1073	246	M; C > T; Arg > Cys	+	+	0.1	Gibbons et al., 1997
	Ped 25, SG	1073	246	M; C > T; Arg > Cys		+	0.01	Gibbons et al., 1997
	Ped 25, JL	1073	246	M; C > T; Arg > Cys		++	0.25	Gibbons et al., 1997
	Ped 31	1073	246	M; C > T; Arg > Cys		nd	3	Gibbons et al., 1997
	Ped 33	1073	246	M; C > T; Arg > Cys		++	0.006	Gibbons et al., 1997
	Ped 34	1073	246	M; C > T; Arg > Cys	+	nd	nd	Gibbons et al., 1997
	Ped 43	1073	246	M; C > T; Arg > Cys		++	2.2	Gibbons et al., 1997
	Ped 48	1073	246	M; C > T; Arg > Cys		+	0.4	Gibbons et al., 1997
	Ped 55	1073	246	M; C > T; Arg > Cys		nd	4.2	Gibbons et al., 1997

#	Pedigree / case	Position	Position	Mutation*	†	‡ Genital abnormality		Reference
	Ped 62 IV:1	1073	246	M; C > T; Arg > Cys		++	+	Unpublished
	Ped 62 IV:7	1073	246	M; C > T; Arg > Cys		+	+	Unpublished
13	Ped 36	1076	247	M; A > G; Asn > Asp		++	+	Unpublished
14	Ped 11, case 1	1083	249	M; G > A; Gly > Asp	+ GL	++	2.5	Gibbons et al., 1997
	Ped 11, case 2	1083	249	M; G > A; Gly > Asp	+ GL	nd	3.9	Gibbons et al., 1997
15	Ped 10, case 1	2064	576	N; C > A; Ser > stop		+++	2.8	Unpublished
	Ped 10, case 2	2064	576	N; C > A; Ser > stop		+	2.1	Unpublished
	Ped 10, case 3	2064	576	N; C > A; Ser > stop		++	10	Unpublished
	Ped 10, case 4	2064	576	N; C > A; Ser > stop		++	1.4	Unpublished
	Ped 58, CB	2064	576	N; C > A; Ser > stop		++	2.2	Unpublished
	Ped 58, MR	2064	576	N; C > A; Ser > stop		normal	nd	Unpublished
16	Ped 20, case 11	4654		S; G>A; insertion 53bp; frameshift		+++	3.6	Picketts et al., 1996
	Ped 20, case 12	4654		S;G>A; insertion 53bp; frameshift		++	0.9	Picketts et al., 1996
17	Ped 22, case 15	4950	1538	M; T>G; Val>Gly¶		+++	11	Picketts et al., 1996
18	Ped 14, case 5	5163	1609	M; A>G; His>Arg		+++	1.6	Gibbons et al., 1995
19	Ped 5, NE	5177	1614	M; T>C; Cys>Arg		++++	>5	Gibbons et al., 1995
20	Ped 21, case 13	5287	1650	M; G>T; Lys>Asn		normal	0.4	Gibbons et al., 1995
	Ped 21, case 14	5287	1650	M; G>T; Lys>Asn		normal	0.6	Gibbons et al., 1995
21	Ped 37	5376	1680	M; T>C; Ile>Thr		++++	+	Unpublished
22	III-1	5474	1713	M; C>T; Pro>Ser		normal	0	Villard et al., 1996b
23	IV-10	5610–5785		S; deletion 176bp; frameshift		+++	30	Villard et al., 1996c
	IV-9	5610–5785		S; deletion 176bp; frameshift		normal	13	Villard et al., 1996c
	IV-16	5610–5785		S; deletion 176bp; frameshift		normal	<0.001	Villard et al., 1996c
24	Ped 54	6294–6359		S; deletion 66bp; in frame		+	+	Unpublished
25	Ped 23, MEF	6441	2035	M; A>T; Asp>Val		+++	7	Gibbons et al., 1995
	Ped 23, MF	6441	2035	M; A>T; Asp>Val		+++	27	Gibbons et al., 1995
26	Ped 15, case 6	6554		S; insertion 124bp; frameshift	+	++	1.4	Picketts et al., 1996
27	Ped 3, SW	6587	2084	M; T>C; Tyr>His		++	>5	Gibbons et al., 1995
28	JM3,4, IV-1	6729	2131	M; G>A; Arg>Gin		+++	nd	Villard et al., 1996a
29	Ped 13, case 4	6825	2163	M; A>G; Tyr>Cys	+	+	12	Gibbons et al., 1995
30	Ped 17, case 8	7493	2386	N; C>T; Arg>stop	+	++++	0.02	Gibbons et al., 1995
	Ped 17, III-1	7493	2386	N; C>T; Arg>stop	+	++++	nd	Gibbons et al., 1995
	Ped 38	7493	2386	N; C>T; Arg>stop		++++	v.rare	Unpublished
31	Ped 27, case 1	7499	2388	N; G>T; Glu>stop		++++	0.03	Gibbons et al., 1995
	Ped 27, case 2	7499	2388	N; G>T; Glu>stop		++++	nd	Gibbons et al., 1995
32	IV-18	7538–7545		S; deletion 8bp; frameshift		++++	0§	Ion et al., 1996
33	Ped 26, case 1	7538–9126		D		++++	1.1	Gibbons et al., 1995
	Ped 26, case 2	7538–9126		D		++++	0.03	Gibbons et al., 1995
	Ped 26, case 3	7538–9126		D		++++	0.09	Gibbons et al., 1995

* Mutation; D, deletion; M, missense; N, nonsense; S, splice site.

† + = mutation demonstrated to have arisen de novo within family; GS, gonosomal mosaicism; GL, germline mosaicism.

‡ Genital abnormality range from normal: + very mild = high lying testes to ++++ = ambiguous genitalia or male pseudohermaphrodite.

¶ This previously unpublished, relatively conservative amino acid change in a nonconserved location may represent a polymorphism rather than a disease-causing mutation.

§ 0/5000 red cells had HbH inclusions but α/β globin chain ratio = 0.85, 15 percent below control samples.

nd, not determined.

sistent relationship between the degree of α thalassemia and the predicted severity of the ATRX mutations and therefore no correlation with abnormal sexual differentiation.

Patients with identical mutations may have different, albeit stable, degrees of α thalassemia, suggesting that the effect of ATRX protein on α-globin expression may be modified by other genetic factors. This is most clearly illustrated by comparing the hematology of cases with identical mutations (Table 19.5). In the 3′ splicing mutation (Mutation 4, Table 19.5), whereas cases in pedigrees 12, 46, and 49 have α thalassemia, in the affected individual in pedigree N17 no HbH inclusions could be detected. Furthermore, comparison of the twenty-one pedigrees with the common C1073T mutation (Mutation 12, Table 19.5) shows a variation in frequency of HbH inclusions of more than four orders of magnitude. This variation may be analogous to mutations of other members of the SNF2 family whose effects are modified by a variation in many genes encoding proteins that interact with SNF2-like proteins (Hirschhorn et al., 1992; Carlson and Laurent, 1994).

Recently it has been shown that phenotypic variability extends to the degree of intellectual handicap (see previously). A nonsense mutation in exon 2 (Mutation 2, Table 19.5) has been identified in an ATR-X pedigree in which the degree of mental retardation in four affected individuals varies from mild to severe. The basis for this variation is not understood, but it suggests that the clinical spectrum for ATRX mutations may be considerably broader than previously defined. Mutation in the ATRX gene has been identified in a case of Juberg-Marsidi syndrome (severe mental retardation, variable degree of sensorineural deafness, hypogenitalism, and short stature: Mutation 28, Table 19.5) and in a number of other cases in which α thalassemia appears not to be present. However, given that these features are seen within the spectrum of abnormalities associated with a single mutation, the case for phenotype splitting is not persuasive. Systematic mutation analysis of a broad population of patients with learning difficulties should help determine the extent of the phenotypic spectrum associated with ATRX mutations and their prevalence.

CONCLUSIONS

From the initial simple clinical observations made almost 20 years ago in patients with unusual forms of thalassemia, two important genetic mechanisms by which mental retardation may arise have been elucidated. Further analysis of the ATR-16 syndrome will provide some answers to how chromosomal imbalance may give rise to developmental abnormalities. Understanding the ATR-X syndrome has raised many new questions. It seems likely that mutations in this class of genes, which appear to regulate many other genes, may be a common cause of syndromal mental retardation. By using information gathered from the ATR-X syndrome it may be possible to identify other similar conditions. At the same time it will be important to identify the "target" genes that are regulated by ATRX. Finally, having established that ATRX is almost certainly involved in the normal regulation of α globin gene expression, we will want to understand exactly what role it plays in this process.

ACKNOWLEDGMENTS

We thank Liz Rose for excellent secretarial help in the preparation of this chapter. The content is substantially based on Chapter 12 by Higgs, D.R. and Gibbons, R.J. in The Thalassaemia Syndromes (4th Edition), edited by Weatherall, D.J. (in preparation).

References

Aasland, R, Gibson, TJ, and Stewart, AF. (1995). The PHD finger: Implications for chromatin-mediated transcriptional regulation. Trends Biol. Sci. 20: 56–59.

Anneren, G and Gustavson, K-H. (1984). Partial trisomy 3q (3q25→qter) syndrome in two siblings. Acta Paediatr. Scand. 73: 281–284.

Bauknecht, T, Betteken, F, and Vogel, W. (1976). Trisomy 4p due to a paternal t(4p–; 16p+) translocation. Hum. Genet. 34: 227–230.

Buckle, VJ, Higgs, DR, Wilkie, AOM. (1988). Localisation of human α globin to 16p13.3-pter. J. Med. Genet. 25: 847–849.

Buckle, VJ and Kearney, L. (1994). New methods in cytogenetics. Curr. Opin. Genet. Dev. 4: 374–382.

Callen, DF, Hyland, VJ, Baker, EG et al. (1989). Mapping the short arm of human chromosome 16. Genomics 4: 348–354.

Cardoso, C, Timsit, S, Villard, L et al. (1998). Specific interaction between the XNP/ATR-X gene product and the SET domain of the human EZH2 protein. Hum. Mol. Genet. 7: 679–684.

Carlson, M and Laurent, BC. (1994). The SNF/SWI family of global transcriptional activators. Curr. Opin. Cell Biol. 6: 396–402.

Chodirker, BN, Ray, M, McAlpine, PJ et al. (1988). Developmental delay, short stature and minor facial anomalies in a child with ring chromosome 16. Am. J. Med. Genet. 31: 145–151.

Craddock, CF, Vyas, P, Sharpe, JA et al. (1995). Contrasting effects of α and β globin regulatory elements on chromatin structure may be related to their different chromosomal environments. EMBO J. 14: 1718–1726.

Dallman, PR. (1977). The red cell. In Dallman, PR, editor. *Blood and blood-forming tissues*. New York: Appleton-Century-Crofts.

Donnai, D, Clayton-Smith, J, Gibbons, RJ, and Higgs, DR. (1991). α thalassaemia/mental retardation syndrome (non-deletion type): Report of a family supporting X linked inheritance. *J. Med. Genet.* 28: 734–737.

Emanuel, B, Zackai, E, Cryer, D, and Rappaport, E. (1982). Deletion mapping of chromosome 16: Phenotypic manifestations and molecular studies of the α-globin complex. *Am. J. Hum. Genet.* 34: A124.

European Chromosome 16 Tuberous Sclerosis Consortium. (1993). Identification and characterization of the tuberous sclerosis gene on chromosome 16. *Cell* 75: 1305–1315.

European Polycystic Kidney Disease Consortium. (1994). The polycystic kidney disease 1 gene encodes a 14 kb transcript and lies within a duplicated region on chromosome 16. *Cell* 77: 881–894.

Fisher, E and Scambler, P. (1994). Human haploinsufficiency — one for sorrow, two for joy. *Nat. Genet.* 7: 5–7.

Flint, J, Wilkie, AOM, Buckle, VJ et al. (1995). The detection of subtelomeric chromosomal rearrangements in idiopathic mental retardation. *Nat. Genet.* 9: 132–140.

Gecz, J, Villard, L, Lossi, AM et al. (1993). Physical and transcriptional mapping of DXS56-PGK1 1 Mb region: identification of three new transcripts. *Hum. Mol. Genet.* 2: 1389–1396.

Gibbons, RJ, Bachoo, S, Picketts, DJ et al. (1997). Mutations in a transcriptional regulator (hATRX) establish the functional significance of a PHD-like domain. *Nat. Genet.* 17: 146–148.

Gibbons, RJ, Brueton, L, Buckle, VJ et al. (1995a). The clinical and hematological features of the X-linked α thalassemia/mental retardation syndrome (ATR-X). *Am. J. Med. Genet.* 55: 288–299.

Gibbons, RJ, McDowell, TL, Raman, S et al. (2000). Mutations in the human SWI/SNF-like protein ATRX cause widespread changes in the pattern of DNA methylation. *Nature Genet.* (in press).

Gibbons, RJ, Picketts, DJ, Villard, L, and Higgs, DR. (1995b). Mutations in a putative global transcriptional regulator cause X-linked mental retardation with α-thalassemia (ATR-X syndrome). *Cell* 80: 837–845.

Gibbons, RJ, Suthers, GK, Wilkie, AOM et al. (1992). X-linked α thalassemia/mental retardation (ATR-X) syndrome: Localisation to Xq12–21.31 by X-inactivation and linkage analysis. *Am. J. Hum. Genet.* 51: 1136–1149.

Gibbons, RJ, Wilkie, AOM, Weatherall, DJ, and Higgs, DR. (1991). A newly defined X linked mental retardation syndrome associated with α thalassaemia. *J. Med. Genet.* 28: 729–733.

Golden, NL, Bilenker, R, Johnson, WE, and Tischfield, JA. (1981). Abnormality of chromosome 16 and its phenotypic expression. *Clin. Genet.* 19: 41–45.

Guerrini, R., Shanahan, JL, Carrozzo, R et al. (2000). A nonsense mutation of the *ATRX* gene causing mild mental retardation and epilepsy. *Ann. Neurol.* 47: 117–121

Hall, JG. (1990). Genomic imprinting: review and relevance to human diseases. *Am. J. Hum. Genet.* 46: 857–873.

Higgs, DR, Vickers, MA, Wilkie, AOM et al. (1989). A review of the molecular genetics of the human α-globin gene cluster. *Blood* 73: 1081–1104.

Hirschhorn, JN, Brown, SA, Clark, CD, and Winston, F. (1992). Evidence that SNF2/SWI2 and SNF5 activate transcription in yeast by altering chromatin structure. *Genes Dev.* 6: 2288–2298.

Ion, A, Telvi, L, Chaussain, JL et al. (1996). A novel mutation in the putative DNA Helicase *XH2* is responsible for male-to-female sex reversal associated with an atypical form of the ATR-X syndrome. *Am. J. Hum. Genet.* 58: 1185–1191.

Lamb, J, Harris, PC, Wilkie, AOM. et al. (1993). De novo truncation of chromosome 16p and healing with (TTAGGG)$_n$ in the α-thalassemia/mental retardation syndrome (ATR-16). *Am. J. Hum. Genet.* 52: 668–676.

Lamb, J, Wilkie, AOM, Harris, PC et al. (1989). Detection of breakpoints in submicroscopic chromosomal translocation, illustrating an important mechanism for genetic disease. *Lancet* ii: 819–824.

Le Douarin, B, Nielsen, AL, Garnier, J-M et al. (1996). A possible involvement of TIF1α and TIF1β in the epigenetic control of transcription by nuclear receptors. *EMBO J.* 15: 6701–6715.

Lefort, G, Taib, J, Toutain, A et al. (1993). X-linked α-thalassemia/mental retardation (ATR-X) syndrome. Report of three male patients in a large French family. *Ann. Genet.* 36: 200–205.

McDowell, TL, Gibbons, RJ, Sutherland, H et al. (1999). Localization of a putative transcriptional regulator (ATRX) at pericentromeric heterochromatin and the short arms of acrocentric chromosomes. *PNAS* 96: 13983–13988

McPherson, E, Clemens, M, Gibbons, RJ, and Higgs, DR. (1995). X-linked alpha thalassemia/mental retardation (ATR-X) syndrome. A new kindred with severe genital anomalies and mild hematologic expression. *Am. J. Med. Genet.* 55: 302–306.

Nazarenko, SA, Nazarenko, LP, and Baranova, VA. (1987). Distal 15q trisomy caused by familial balanced translocation t(15;16) (q24;p13) and an unusual mosaicism in the proband's mother. *Tsitol. Genet.* 21: 434–437.

Neidengard, L and Sparkes, RS. (1981). Ring chromosome 16. *Hum. Genet.* 59: 175–177.

Nielsen, KB, Dyggve, HVK, and Olsen, J. (1983). A chromosomal survey of an institution for the mentally retarded. *Dan. Med. Bull.* 30: 5–13.

Ohsawa, K, Imai, Y, Ito, D, and Kohsaka, S. (1996). Molecular cloning and characterization of annexin V-binding proteins with highly hydrophilic peptide structure. *J. Neurochem.* 67: 89–97.

Pawlowitzki, IH, Grobe, H, and Holzgreve, W. (1979). Trisomy 20q due to maternal t(16;20) translocation: first case. *Clin. Genet.* 15: 167–170.

Pergament, E, Pietra, MGC, Kadotani T et al. (1970). A ring chromosome no. 16 in an infant with primary hypoparathyroidism. *J. Pediatr.* 76: 745–751.

Peterson, CL and Herskowitz, I. (1992). Characterisation of the yeast *SWI1, SWI2* and *SWI3* genes, which encode a global activator of transcription. *Cell* 68: 573–583.

Picketts, DJ, Higgs, DR, Bachoo, S et al. (1996). *ATRX* encodes a novel member of the SNF2 family of proteins: mutations point to a common mechanism underlying the ATR-X syndrome. *Hum. Mol. Genet.* 5: 1899–1907.

Picketts, DJ, Tastan, AO, Higgs, DR, and Gibbons, RJ. (1998). Comparison of the human and murine ATRX gene identifies highly conserved, functionally important domains. *Mamm. Genome* 9: 400–403.

Quintana, A, Sordo, MT, Estevez, C et al. (1983). 16 Ring chromosome. *Clin. Genet.* 23: 243.

Rack, KA, Harris, PC, MacCarthy, AB et al. (1993). Characterization of three de novo derivative chromosomes 16 by 'reverse chromosome painting' and molecular analysis. *Am. J. Hum. Genet.* 52: 987–997.

Rönich, P and Kleihauer, E. (1967). Alpha-thalassämie mit HbH und Hb Bart's in einer deutschen Familie. *Klin. Wochenschrift* 45: S1193–1200.

Schneider, AS, Bischoff, FZ, McCaskill, C et al. (1996). Comprehensive 4-year follow-up on a case of maternal heterdisomy for chromosome 16. *Am. J. Med. Genet.* 66: 204–208.

Stayton, CL, Dabovic, B, Gulisano, M et al. (1994). Cloning and characterisation of a new human Xq13 gene, encoding a putative helicase. *Hum. Mol. Genet.* 3: 1957–1964.

Villard, L, Gecz, J, Mattéi, JF et al. (1996a). XNP mutation in a large family with Juberg-Marsidi syndrome. *Nat. Genet.* 12: 359–360.

Villard, L, Lacombe, D, and Fontés, M. (1996b). A point mutation in the XNP gene, associated with an ATR-X phenotype without α-thalassemia. *Eur. J. Hum. Genet.* 4: 316–320.

Villard, L, Toutain, A, Lossi, A-M et al. (1996c). Splicing mutation in the ATR-X gene can lead to a dysmorphic mental retardation phenotype without α-thalassemia. *Am. J. Hum. Genet.* 58: 499–505.

Vogel, F. & Motulsky, A.G. (1986) Human Genetics. Problems and approaches (2nd ed.). Springer-Verlag, Berlin.

Vyas, P, Vickers, MA, Simmons, DL et al. (1992). Cis-acting sequences regulating expression of the human α globin cluster lie within constitutively open chromatin. *Cell* 69: 781–793.

Weatherall, DJ, Higgs, DR, Bunch, C et al. (1981). Hemoglobin H disease and mental retardation. A new syndrome or a remarkable coincidence? *N. Engl. J. Med.* 305: 607–612.

Wilkie, AOM, Buckle, VJ, Harris, PC et al. (1990a) Clinical features and molecular analysis of the α thalassaemia/mental retardation syndromes. I. Cases due to deletions involving chromosome band 16p13.3. *Am. J. Hum. Genet.* 46: 1112–1126.

Wilkie, AOM, Zeitlin, HC, Lindenbaum, RH et al. (1990b) Clinical features and molecular analysis of the α thalassemia/mental retardation syndromes. II. Cases without detectable abnormality of the α globin complex. *Am. J. Hum. Genet.* 46: 1127–1140.

Wilkie, AOM, Pembrey, ME, Gibbons, RJ et al. (1991). The non-deletion type of α thalassaemia/mental retardation: a recognisable dysmorphic syndrome with X-linked inheritance. *J. Med. Genet.* 28: 724.

Wilson, CJ, Chao, DM, Imbalzano, AN et al. (1996). DNA polymerase II homoenzyme contains SWI/SNF regulators involved in chromatin remodeling. *Cell* 84: 235–244.

SECTION IV

SICKLE CELL DISEASE

MARTIN H. STEINBERG
RONALD L. NAGEL

GENETICS AND PATHOPHYSIOLOGY

A mutation in the gene for β globin, a subunit of adult hemoglobin A (HbA), is the proximate cause of sickle cell disease. An adenine (A) to thymine (T) substitution in codon 6 (GAG→GTG) of the β-globin gene specifies the insertion of valine in place of glutamic acid in the β-globin chain (β^s; $\beta^{6glu \rightarrow val}$). Sickle hemoglobin (HbS, $\alpha_2\beta_2^s$) has the unique property of polymerizing when deoxygenated. When the polymer is present in sufficient quantity, it injures the erythrocyte and evokes the sickle cell disease phenotype. The sickle mutation had four distinct origins in Africa about 3,000 years ago and one in the Indo-European world, probably earlier. Its high prevalence in blacks and selected other ethnic groups results from the survival advantage of the heterozygote under the selective pressure of falciparum malaria infestation that blossomed several thousand years ago.

Sickle cell disease is the product of the various effects that follow red cell sickling. It is typified by acute, recurrent, and chronic complications affecting many organs and tissues. Unique among hemolytic anemias is the vasculopathy of sickle cell disease. Sickle cells interact with other blood cells and with the vascular endothelium, causing vascular injury, tempering vascular tone, and occluding small and sometimes large blood vessels. Vasoocclusion within the microcirculation and at times in larger vessels can occur almost anywhere blood flows and is responsible for most of the severe complications of the disease.

A summary of the pathophysiology of sickle cell disease is shown in Figure 1 and illustrates how the presence of sickle polymer can be involved in the cause of the many abnormalities described in sickle cell disease and lead to vasoocclusion and organ damage. Additional mutations in the sickle β-globin gene and the co-inheritance of other hemoglobin variants affect the relative amount of sickle polymer. Compound heterozygous conditions can result in phenotypes resembling sickle cell anemia (HbS-D Los Angeles, HbS-O-Arab) or sickle cell trait (HbSE, HbS-Hb Korle Bu). Fetal hemoglobin (HbF) is not incorporated into polymer; thus it not only reduces HbS concentration but also inhibits its polymerization. Combined heterozygotes with HbS and hereditary persistence of HbF—where 20 percent to 30 percent of the hemoglobin in each red cell is HbF—are nearly normal. This relationship between polymerization and the clinical phenotype argues for the primacy of polymerization in the pathophysiology of sickle cell disease.

Polymerization of HbS is dependent on temperature, pH, small hemoglobin binding molecules such as 2,3 bisphosphoglyceric acid (BPG), and oxygen. Fully oxygenated HbS cannot enter the polymer phase whereas partially or fully deoxygenated HbS can. If HbF is mixed with HbS, neither the HbF tetramer ($\alpha_2\gamma_2$) nor the $\alpha_2\beta^s\gamma$ hybrid tetramer enters the polymer phase. When a polymer-free solution of HbS is deoxygenated, a delay occurs before any polymer is detected. Polymer then rapidly accumulates. This observation is accounted for by the double-nucleation hypothesis that considers an initial homogeneous nucleation of polymer in solution and the subsequent explosive heterogeneous nucleation on the template of already formed polymers. Most important for understanding the pathophysiology of the disease, the delay time is inversely dependent on HbS concentration to the 30th to 50th power. A spectrum of cells with a range of densities and HbS concentrations exist in each affected individual. They have a broad span of delay times and this variability predicts different fates for different sickle erythrocytes. The initiation of vasoocclusion is likely to depend on features intrinsic to the sickle erythrocyte, such as its polymer content, delay time, and membrane damage, and also local factors extrinsic to this cell, such as the condition of the endothelium, balance of vasodilators and vasoconstrictors, and activation of leukocytes and platelets.

Martin H. Steinberg, Bernard G. Forget, Douglas R. Higgs, and Ronald L. Nagel, editors. *Disorders of Hemoglobin: Genetics, Pathophysiology, and Clinical Management.* © 2001 Cambridge University Press. All rights reserved.

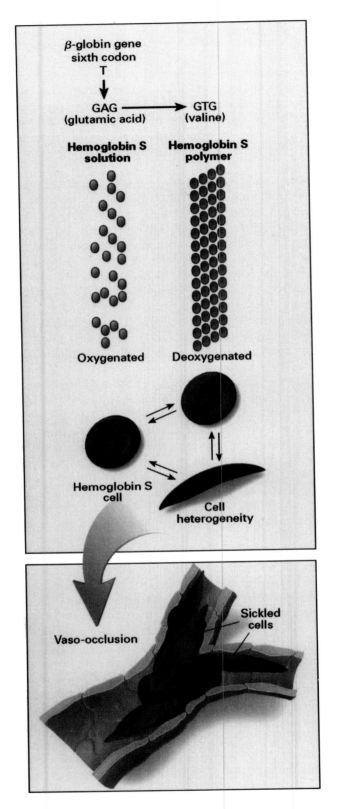

Because of cellular heterogeneity, sickle erythrocytes do not survive equally. Survival is most dependent on the level of HbF and the amount of membrane damage. Most hemolysis in sickle cell disease occurs extravascularly in the reticuloendothelial system. Some sickle cells entrapped in the microvasculature may be fated for early destruction. Linking hemolysis to the vasoocclusive process is the fall in dense cell numbers during the first stages of the painful episode followed by reticulocytosis, a response to increased hemolysis. Reticulocytes contain adhesive ligands and actively regulate their volume. Their rebound late in a painful episode might help explain the tendency of episodes to come in clusters. Increased hemolysis is rarely a cause of clinically significant worsening of the anemia of sickle cell disease.

Conceptually simple, the process by which normal tissue perfusion is interrupted by sickle cells is complex and not fully understood. Available data suggest that the obstruction occurs first in the small postcapillary venules by a combination of erythrocyte adhesion to the vascular endothelium and obstruction by dense cells. Nevertheless, it is not clear if this is the mechanism of vasoocclusion in all tissues. Large arteries—especially to the brain and lungs—can also become occluded. Obstruction by sickle cells might cause obstruction in the lungs but the mechanism might not always involve red cell adhesion.

Experimental evidence suggests that many different elements in the sickle cell, on the sickle cell, on endothelial cells, dissolved in the plasma, suspended in the plasma, intrinsic to the vascular wall, and extrinsic to the patient, provoke and mediate vasoocclusion.

Sickle hemoglobin polymer—perhaps also high concentrations of unpolymerized oxidized HbS—may cause secondary damage to cell contents and membrane. Cation homeostasis is impaired in some sickle cells and cell density is increased. The reduced capacity of these cells to maintain their normal K^+ gradients is mediated by activation of cation transporters by deoxygenation, acidification, cell swelling, Ca^{++} influx, and sickling. Membrane lipids may be asymmetrically distributed, with the procoagulant aminophospholipids translocated to the outer leaflet of the membrane lipid bilayer.

Section 4. Pathophysiology of sickle cell disease. The nucleotide and amino acid substitution of HbS—a GAG to GTG substitution in the sixth codon of the β-globin gene leading to the replacement of a glutamic acid residue by a valine residue—are shown at the top. Upon deoxygenation, after a delay time, HbS polymer forms, causing cell sickling and damage to the membrane. Red cells are heterogeneous with a range of cell densities, membrane injury and HbF content. Some cells adhere to the endothelium and lead to vasoocclusion. (From Steinberg M H., 1999.) Management of sickle cell disease. *New England Journal of Medicine*, 340, 1021–1030). For full color reproduction, see color plate numbered section 4.

Cellular damage enables adhesive interactions between sickle cells and endothelial cells. By assorted attachment mechanisms, the association of sickle and endothelial cells is postulated to delay cellular passage so that polymerization, sickling, and vasoocclusion occur during microvasculature transit. Mature sickle cells circulate in the company of leukocytes, platelets, and "stress" reticulocytes. Stress reticulocytes are found in individuals with hemolytic disease and display adhesive ligands that facilitate erythrocyte–endothelial interactions.

Finally, sickle cell disease patients vary in phenotype. The variability is in part due to environmental influences but is largely genetic. It represents the activity of polymorphic modifier (epistatic) genes. Three epistatic effectors are known—α thalassemia, β-globin gene cluster haplotypes, and genes linked and unlinked to the β-globin gene cluster that influence HbF levels. Other polymorphic epistatic genes will also probably be defined, and promising candidates include those that code for erythrocyte ion transport proteins, proteins that modify red cell interactions with the vasculature, and proteins that influence vascular reactivity. One hope for the next decade is that our understanding of the genetic basis of disease variability will be improved; that would provide invaluable prognostic information.

DIAGNOSIS

The cornerstone of diagnosis is the detection and quantification of HbS by various means. Blood films show sickled cells, Howell-Jolly bodies, and Pappenheimer bodies in most patients with sickle cell anemia; in HbSC disease, target cells, folded cells, and HbC-type crystals may be present; in HbS-β thalassemia, hypochromia, microcytosis, and target cells are found.

Imprecision defining sickle hemoglobinopathies has permeated the medical literature and the hospital charts of affected patients. Sickle cell disease is a phenotype with distinctive clinical and hematologic features, where at least half of the hemoglobin is HbS. Sickle cell trait is not considered a type of sickle cell disease because of its clinically benign features due to the low concentration of HbS. Among the genotypes that determine the sickle cell disease phenotype are homozygosity for the HbS mutation (sickle cell anemia), compound heterozygosity for HbS and HbC, or HbSC disease, compound heterozygosity for HbS and β thalassemia, or HbS-β thalassemia, and other compound heterozygous sickling disorders. Whenever possible, a diagnosis of sickle cell disease should be assigned by its genotype since this designation allows the best assessment of prognosis and only a genotypic diagnosis permits accurate genetic counseling.

CLINICAL FEATURES

Sickle cell trait is asymptomatic and characterized by about 60 percent HbA and 40 percent HbS in the blood. Because of the low concentrations of HbS, carriers have none of the hemolytic or vasoocclusive events typical of the severe sickling disorders. Their sole clinical complication is hematuria, which is usually mild and self-limiting. Hyposthenuria is usually present but is clinically unimportant. Both of these renal abnormalities result from sickling in the hypertonic, hypoxic, acidotic environment that typifies the normal renal medulla. There is no valid reason to restrict the activities or occupation of normal individuals with sickle cell trait.

Hemolytic Anemia

In sickle cell anemia, HbSC disease, and in the HbS-β thalassemias, a variety of abnormalities linked to hemolytic anemia and the vasoocclusive process are present. A major cause of hemolysis is the short life span of the irreversibly sickled cell (ISC). Most patients tolerate chronic hemoglobin levels of 5 to 7 g/dL well. Hemoglobin level remains quite constant over time unless erythropoiesis is depressed. Bacterial infection may transiently reduce erythropoiesis. Dramatic but transient falls in hemoglobin level can occur in association with infection by the human B19 parvovirus. Children with sickle cell anemia and splenomegaly, and less often adults with HbSC disease or HbS-β thalassemia, may have splenic sequestration crisis—a sudden pooling of red cells in a damaged spleen. The spleen rapidly enlarges as the hemoglobin level plummets, and transfusion may be lifesaving. Persistent hyperbilirubinemia, a consequence of hemolysis, is associated with a high prevalence of gallstones. Stones may appear at remarkably young ages and are present in the majority of adults.

Vasoocclusive Events

Vasoocclusive events of the sickling disorders can occur acutely, producing dramatic clinical findings, or be chronic, nonpainful, but nevertheless disabling. Painful episodes are the most common acute clinical event. Limb pain is usually bilateral, raising the possibility that the triggering event for painful episodes is not vasoocclusion.

The most common deficiency in pain treatment is infrequently given and inadequate doses of analgesics. Painful episodes are sometimes triggered by an infection, temperature extremes, or physical or emotional stress. Often they begin with little warning. For severe pain, parenteral opiates are required, given at frequent fixed intervals, not "as-needed," until the pain has diminished and they can be tapered, stopped, and oral analgesics instituted. Some patients prefer patient-controlled analgesia. In a given year, nearly 40 percent of patients with sickle cell anemia will not have a severe painful episode. A small minority of patients are nearly always in severe pain. The cause of this is complex, management is extremely difficult, and expert advice on treatment is warranted. Most patients with acute pain episodes are neither drug addicts nor seekers. Reliable individuals can be given oral drugs such as acetaminophen with codeine to take for pain they feel is manageable at home. Rapid institution of narcotic analgesics in sufficient amounts and frequency to relieve pain and frequent monitoring of the effects of treatment with adjustments as needed are the foundation of pain treatment.

The acute chest syndrome, characterized by fever, chest pain, cough, and lung infiltrates, affects one-third of all sickle cell anemia patients. The etiology varies. Chest syndrome is most common but least severe in young children, where it is often secondary to infection. In adults, pain often precedes this event and mortality is higher than in children. Fat embolism is a common cause of the most severe events during which hemoglobin and platelet levels fall and the leukocyte count increases.

More common in HbSC disease than in sickle cell anemia, the pathology of sickle retinopathy includes the distinctive "black sea fan," "black sunburst," and salmon patches with hemorrhagic, infarctive, proliferative, and resolving lesions. Conjoint effects of a higher PCV, increased cell density, and greater blood viscosity in HbSC disease may account for the higher prevalence of retinopathy in HbSC disease than in sickle cell anemia; it is also possible that the lower HbF levels of HbSC disease play a role. Paradoxically, the high prevalence of proliferative retinopathy in HbSC disease may be an expression of the benignity of this genotype relative to sickle cell anemia, where peripheral retinal vessels are occluded early in the course of disease so that further damage and proliferative lesions cannot develop. The enhanced circulatory competence of the HbSC disease cell preserves this retinal circulation, permitting the later development of proliferative lesions.

Pregnancy in sickle cell disease is associated with a high rate of obstetrical complications. Spontaneous abortion has a 1 percent to 20 percent incidence even with the best management.

Priapism in sickle cell anemia may have a nocturnal onset, occur spontaneously, or be an unwanted response to erotic stimulation. Regardless of the initial stimulus, the normal process of detumescence fails. In sickle cell anemia, this failure almost always results from impaired venous outflow. Recurrent attacks of stuttering priapism can last for several hours and be self-limited. They usually have a nocturnal onset. Erectile function is mostly preserved between these attacks that can recur over years. Major episodes of priapism often follow a history of stuttering attacks, last for days, and can be excruciatingly painful. They usually result in impotence by causing irreversible damage to the corpora.

Liver disease is the most prevalent and serious complication of sickle cell anemia that affects the digestive system. Hepatomegaly is found in 80 percent to 100 percent of patients. Often a melange of diverse pathologies, sickle cell liver disease may be contributed to by intra- and extrahepatic cholestasis, viral hepatitis, cirrhosis, hypoxia and infarction, erythrocyte sequestration, iron overload, and drug reactions.

Two major abnormalities characterize the renal lesions associated with sickle cell disease. Medullary disease is found in nearly all individuals with sickle cell anemia and in most with sickle cell trait. Glomerulopathy, not present in sickle cell trait, begins very early in life but becomes clinically important as patients age. It often culminates in renal failure with severe anemia.

The heart is usually enlarged and systolic murmurs are common. Contractility is normal and overt congestive heart failure is uncommon.

Children with sickle cell disease may develop "hand-foot" syndrome—a sickling–induced periostitis of metacarpal and metatarsal bones that mimics acute rheumatoid arthritis. Osteonecrosis of the hips and shoulders is painful and often disabling, and by 30 years of age, half of all individuals with sickle cell anemia have this abnormality.

The first appearance of a leg ulcer usually signifies the high likelihood of recurrence over a period of many years. Usually appearing on the lower leg, most small and superficial ulcers heal spontaneously with rest and careful local hygiene. At times leg ulcers are deep, huge and circumferential, exceedingly painful, disabling, and defy all simple and many complex therapeutic measures.

Compared to individuals with β thalassemia with similar hemoglobin concentrations, the blood pressure of patients with sickle cell anemia is higher, suggesting the possibility that they have "relative" hypertension. Survival decreases and the risk of stroke increases as blood pressure rises even though the blood pressure at which these risks increase is below the level defining early hypertension in the normal population. This suggests that "relative" hypertension is pathogenetically important and should be carefully evaluated with early treatment provided.

Infection is the major cause of death in children in the first years of life, and the most common offending agent is *Streptococcus pneumoniae*. During the course of sickle cell anemia, and to a lesser extent in HbSC and HbS-β thalassemia, splenic function decreases and is ultimately lost, because of repetitive infarction. Early in life the spleen may be large but hypofunctional. It then atrophies and seems to disappear although it has been known to regenerate after bone marrow transplantation. Hyposplenic patients are susceptible to infection with encapsulated bacteria. Sepsis, pneumonia, meningitis, and otitis are common infections in children and can progress with devastating rapidity.

Sepsis is the major cause of death in children. Causes of death in adults are more varied. About 20 percent are related to organ failure, but often death is unexpected and occurs in the midst of an acute event like a pain episode. In the United States, the median age of death is about 45 years in sickle cell anemia and about 65 years in HbSC disease. Survival past childhood is still unusual in underdeveloped countries.

TREATMENT

Sickle cell disease is a chronic disorder, and attention should be given to good nutrition, immunizations, and avoidance of extremes of temperature, dehydration, and activity. Vaccination against *S. pneumoniae* using the 23-valent vaccine is recommended for children beginning at age 2 years with booster doses at age 5 years. Prophylactic penicillin should be started at 3 to 4 months of age. Children less than age 3 years should receive 125 mg of an oral penicillin twice a day, and older children, 250 mg orally twice a day. This treatment has reduced the incidence of pneumococcal sepsis and death. Even children vaccinated against *S. pneumoniae* who are on penicillin prophylaxis die of pneumococcal sepsis, perhaps because they do not take their medication faithfully. If severe pneumococcal disease has not occurred, and if the patient is enrolled in a comprehensive care program, prophylactic penicillin can be safely discontinued at age 5 years.

Many events can provoke right upper quadrant pain in sickle cell disease, often making a firm diagnosis of cholecystitis difficult. When stones are asymptomatic or symptoms and laboratory findings are equivocal, it is probably best not to recommend cholecystectomy.

The pain of osteonecrosis is sometimes relieved by nonsteroidal antiinflammatory agents. But, as destruction progresses, pain becomes severe and function is lost, the effected joint—most often the hip—needs replacement. Leg ulcers usually heal spontaneously with rest and careful local hygiene. Large ulcers heal slowly.

Treatment for sickle cell disease is evolving. In couples at risk, the probabilities of having children with sickle cell disease and the feasibility of preimplantation and antenatal diagnosis should be clearly presented. Neonatal screening can identify infants with sickle cell disease and direct their parents toward comprehensive care programs. Early in parenthood, counseling on the dangers of infection and fever, acute anemic episodes, recommended immunizations, and prophylactic penicillin can be lifesaving. Periodic physician visits should concentrate on parent and patient education, health maintenance, and careful control of blood pressure.

A general feature of sickle cell disease is its clinical heterogeneity. Some patients have very mild disease and others suffer many complications. We still do not fully understand the reasons for this phenotypic diversity but it is likely that genetic and environmental modulators both contribute.

The ten chapters that follow examine the pathophysiology of sickle cell disease, dissecting the causes of hemolysis, sickle vasoocclusion, effects of HbS on the erythrocyte membrane, and the interactions of sickle cells with the vascular endothelium. Included in this section is an exploration of the genetic variability of sickle cell anemia. Clinical aspects of sickle cell disease and sickle cell trait are discussed with special emphasis on the nature and treatment of the painful episodes that typify this disorder.

Much has been learned about the pathophysiology of sickle cell disease in recent years. Most important, advances in treatment are now being translated into improved quality of life and longevity.

20

General Pathophysiology of Sickle Cell Anemia

RONALD L. NAGEL
ORAH S. PLATT

INTRODUCTION

Diggs and Ching (1934) first proposed the linkage of polymerization, vasoocclusion, and the clinical manifestations of sickle cell disease:

The elongated and spiked cells interlock and pass with more difficulty through narrow spaces than do normal cells. Since the distortion is increased under conditions of anoxemia, it is reasonable to assume that it will be greatest in tissue where there is stasis. The sudden pains experienced by patients with sickle cell anemia, which often disappear as mysteriously as they come, may in part be explained by this capillary blockade.

Their hypothesis emphasized the role of the irreversibly sickled cell (ISC) in physically initiating stasis, hypoxemia, and vasoocclusion. Although the ISC is the most obviously abnormal cell seen in the peripheral blood, it is becoming increasingly clear that the more normal looking and abundant reversibly sickled cells, and even the reticulocyte, are critical for initiating and maintaining vasoocclusion. One of the unusual features of sickle erythrocytes is their tendency to adhere to vascular endothelial cells, a tendency that has obvious pathophysiologic implications (see Chapter 21). Polymerization and sickling take time (Hofrichter et al., 1974). Passage through the microcirculation also takes time. Under most physiologic situations, the 1 second it takes a red cell to traverse the microcirculation is shorter than it takes for it

to sickle (Mozzarelli et al., 1987) and no vasoocclusion occurs. The more the movement of cells is retarded by endothelial adherence, the more likely it is that sickling and vasoocclusion will occur. One of the attractive aspects of the adherence/occlusion hypothesis is that it provides another approach to designing therapeutic interventions and for examining the possible genetic modifiers of clinical severity. In addition, while it has been assumed that obstruction in sickle cell anemia occurred primarily in the capillaries, this phenomenon has been documented only in the retina. Direct observation of other circulatory beds have detected obstruction at the level of precapillary sphincters or postcapillary venules, with capillary obstruction occurring as retrograde phenomena. Anemia and rheologic and hemodynamic aspects of sickle cell disease must be considered as part of its pathogenesis.

ANEMIA

Anemia in sickle cell disease is primarily the consequence of the dramatically shortened survival of some sickle erythrocytes but the precise level of circulating hemoglobin is the product of a complex set of factors. Understanding the mechanism of anemia in sickle cell disease has obvious and not so obvious implications. Among the latter, for example, is that high total hemoglobin levels in sickle cell anemia are a risk factor for avascular bone necrosis and retinopathy, for painful episodes and acute chest syndrome (Serjeant et al., 1996). Hence, the anemia has both adverse consequences and compensatory functions. Factors known to determine the level of anemia are (1) intravascular and extravascular (including ineffective erythropoiesis) red cell destruction; modulators of hemolysis are the numbers of circulating dense cells (including ISCs), characterized by very short survival and F-cells that when endowed with sufficient HbF per cell, have a particularly long survival; (2) the adequacy of red cell production by the marrow aided by the production of growth factors; (3) hemodilution or hemoconcentration; (4) the extent of the right shift of the hemoglobin-oxygen equilibrium curve, modulated by levels of HbS, HbF, 2,3 BPG, serum phosphate, mean corpuscular hemoglobin concentration (MCHC), and the numbers of dense cells.

Hematologic Characteristics of the Anemia

Hematologic Parameters. In the first weeks of life infants with sickle cell anemia have lower hemoglobin levels than normal children (Serjeant et al., 1981; Hayes et al., 1985). As in normals, hemoglobin levels

Martin H. Steinberg, Bernard G. Forget, Douglas R. Higgs, and Ronald L. Nagel, editors. *Disorders of Hemoglobin: Genetics, Pathophysiology, and Clinical Management.* © 2001 Cambridge University Press. All rights reserved.

fall during the next few months but patient values are consistently below those of controls (Fig. 20.1). A nadir of about 8 g/dL is reached at about 1 year of age and maintained until midadolescence. During childhood, girls have somewhat higher hemoglobin levels than boys, but differences barely reach statistical significance. During the 3rd decade (ages 20 to 24 years) that relationship is reversed (Hayes et al., 1985) and thereafter, men have higher mean levels than women. In Jamaican adults 25 to 40 years of age, the 5th to 95th percentiles for hemoglobin concentration are approximately 6 to 11.6 g/dL for men and 5.9 to 10.2 g/dL for women. It is generally believed that the gender difference is due to production of androgens in males after onset of puberty; the delay in onset of the difference when compared to normals is almost certainly related to the delayed onset of puberty in the patients (Platt et al., 1984).

When cross-sectional analysis of clinic populations is used to assess age-related changes in hemoglobin level, there is a decline in later years of life. This is probably related to a decreased renal function, with a consequent decrease in erythropoietin production (Sherwood et al., 1986). Patients with overt renal disease were excluded from this study (Fig. 20.2), but subclinical abnormalities of renal function may very well have been present. Although the steady-state hemoglobin concentration of an individual patient tends to remain constant over time—barring the onset of a complicating chronic disorder (Odenheimer et al., 1984)—marked variations in hemoglobin level can occur during acute illnesses, secondary to fluctuations in hemolytic rates and erythropoiesis activity and due to changes in plasma volume related to dehydration and fluid replacement therapy.

Usually, changes in PCV follow those in hemoglobin concentration, but values are much less reliable because of the abnormal physical properties of sickle cells. Even when oxygenated, sickle cells are stiff (Chien, 1977; Kaul et al., 1983a), and they neither pack normally during centrifugation (although prolonged centrifugation or use of microhematocrit tubes can considerably improve the situation), nor flow normally through the orifice of impedance counters. Automatic counters based on sphering and scattering offer a more accurate calculated PCV. The red cell count does not suffer from these limitations and shows changes similar to those observed for hemoglobin concentration.

Because of their abnormal physical properties, the mean corpuscular volume (MCV) of sickle cells, like the PCV, cannot be accurately measured. Despite that

Figure 20.1. Total hemoglobin concentration (mean ± 1 SD) versus age. Closed circles, sickle cell anemia; open circles, normal control. From age 0 to 6 years. (From Serjeant et al., 1981, with permission.)

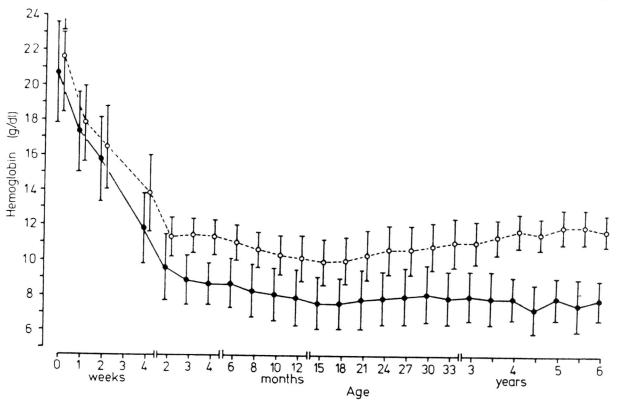

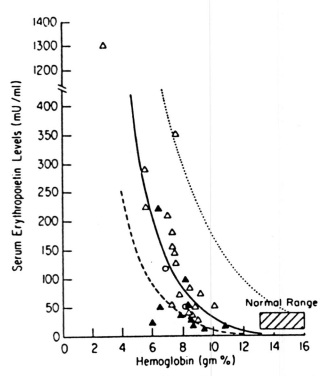

Figure 20.2. Erythropoietin levels in sickle cell anemia for eighteen pediatric (△) and ten adult (▲) patients; two children with Sβ⁺-thal disease (○) are also shown. The regression equation log (SIE − 10) = 8.91 − 0.54 (Hb) − 0.04 (age) is shown for the mean of the two age groups. Regression line of erythropoietin levels in nonhemoglobinopathy anemias for thirteen patients with nonhemolytic and four patients with autoimmune hemolytic.

disadvantage, results from impedance counters provide useful clinical information. During the first months of life, the MCV falls, as it does in normal persons, but then begins to rise at about age 6 months. The average MCV of normal controls continues to fall for several more months; it then begins to rise, but remains significantly lower than that of patients (Serjeant et al., 1981) (Fig. 20.3).

Some of the macrocytosis of sickle cell anemia is related to the presence of increased numbers of reticulocytes, with their increased volume, but this explanation is insufficient in most cases so other factors must be involved. Patients with higher levels of HbF have higher MCVs (Milner et al., 1986); it is likely that both abnormalities reflect abnormal red cell maturation, because both changes are markedly exaggerated during therapy with hydroxyurea (see Chapter 38). The MCV falls with iron deficiency and in both α and β thalassemia. It rises with folate deficiency; changes in either direction from a patient's usual value may provide the first evidence of nutritional deficiency or bleeding. Changes in mean corpuscular hemoglobin parallel those in the MCV.

MCHC cannot be measured accurately by impedance counters and reflects only the most gross changes in red cell morphology (Fig. 20.4). Two techniques can provide useful information on this very important determinant of sickling: density gradient centrifugation and laser light scattering. In the first, red cells are separated according to density fractions, which in turn can be related to the MCHC of normal red cells of the same density (Fabry and Nagel, 1983). Laser light scattering can be used to measure MCHC directly on a cell-by-cell basis (Mohandas et al., 1980), if cells are sphered by appropriate reagents. The Technicon H-series uses isovolumetric sphering of erythrocytes and

Figure 20.3. Mean corpuscular volume (MCV) (mean ± 1 SD) in SS (●) and AA control (○) from ages 0 to 6 years. (From Serjeant et al., 1981, with permission.)

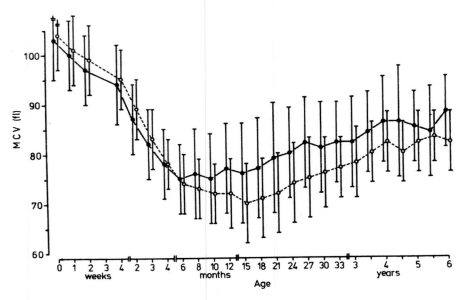

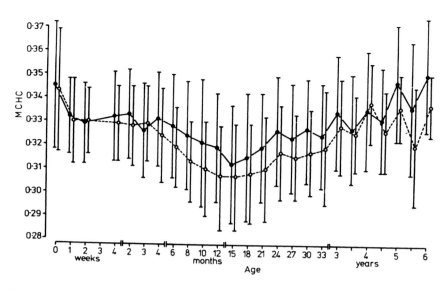

Figure 20.4. Mean corpuscular hemoglobin concentration (MCHC). SS disease (●) and AA controls (○) from age 0 to 6 years. (From Serjeant et al., 1981, with permission.)

Figure 20.5. Isopycnic gradient of ten sickle cell anemia (SS) and one normal (AA) whole blood. The gradients are made of Percoll-Stractan mixtures and centrifuged at 37°C. On the top of the gradient are reticulocytes and on the bottom, in the case of normal blood, the oldest cells; in the case of SS, some red cells have normal density and many cells are moderately dehydrated or very dehydrated (bottom of the range of distribution). Among the very dehydrated are the ISCs. Also depicted are the mean MCHC per fraction and the average density across the gradient. Notice that there is considerable interindividual variation as to the amount of light red cells and very dense red cells among sickle cell anemia patients. Some have a lot of very dense cells, some have very little. In addition, the intermediate density fraction varies as well as the extent of low-density red cells. Two modifier genes (epistatic effects) affect this distribution: the copresence of α-thalassemia trait and high expression of HbF. For full color reproduction, see color plate 20.5.

reduces the error considerably, but not entirely, since some ISCs do not sphere.

When MCHC data are calculated from the centrifuged microhematocrit, they are less affected by artifact, but still reflect only averages. Nevertheless, with this type of MCHC measurement small differences between sickle erythrocyte and normal MCHCs are detected in children, which might well be related to differences in iron deficiency between the two groups (Serjeant et al., 1981). Coexisting α thalassemia has an effect on average red cell indices when the effect of reticulocytosis is taken into account (Embury et al., 1984). Isopycnic gradient centrifugation is a more powerful tool to study and detect these changes than the use of routine blood cell counters, but this is a research tool (Fig. 20.5).

Reticulocytosis is universally present but levels more than 25 percent should suggest a coexisting complication. Reticulocytes are observed mostly in the lighter

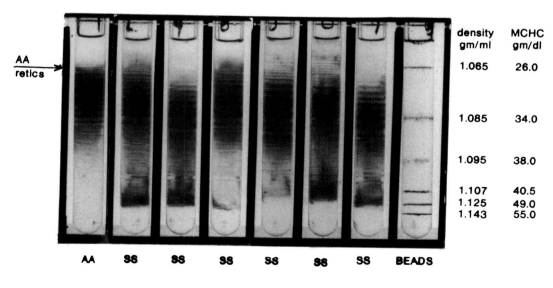

density gm/ml	MCHC gm/dl
1.065	26.0
1.085	34.0
1.095	38.0
1.107	40.5
1.125	49.0
1.143	55.0

AA retics

AA   SS   SS   SS   SS   SS   SS   BEADS

A

TYPES OF RETICULOCYTES

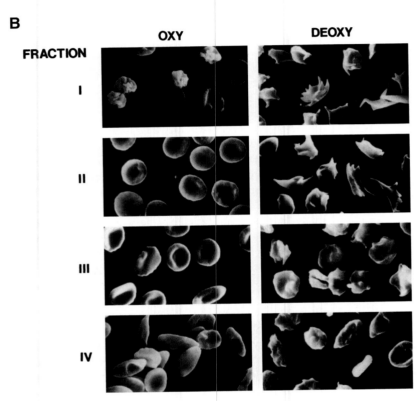

Figure 20.6. Stress reticulocytes. (A) Classification of reticulocytes, between 1 and 4 types according to the number of intracellular vital stained inclusions (that correlate with the age of the reticulocyte). 1 and 2 are definitive "stress" reticulocytes. (B) Scanning microscopy of stress reticulocytes on top fraction and different shape (oxy and deoxy) in denser sickle red cells.

fractions of density separated sickle red cells (Kaul et al., 1983a), but they can be also found in the other fractions including the dense ISC class. Among the reticulocytes stained with supravital stains, there are a considerable proportion of "stress" reticulocytes (Fig. 20.6). These have rather tightly packed stained dots in the form of pseudonuclei and their surface is characteristically bumpy (as a "sack of potatoes") under scanning electron microscopy. Stress reticulocytes are not present nor-mally in peripheral blood and are evidence of enhanced erythropoiesis.

The red cells of patients with sickle cell anemia characteristically appear normochromic and anisocytic in blood smears. The abnormal shape of red cells led, as discussed before, to the discovery and naming of sickle cell anemia, and the abnormalities seen on blood smears from such patients are among the most impressive changes one shows a beginning medical student (Chapter 24, Figs. 1 and 2). ISCs, dense banana-shaped forms, are virtually pathognomonic; their genesis and significance are discussed in Chapter 22. They are oblong or boatlike in shape, sometimes very elongated, but generally have only two sharp points. Cells with that appearance are generally truly ISCs because they do not change shape when reoxygenated. Nevertheless, some of the less elongated ISCs turn out not to be irreversibly sickled because when venous blood—usually used to make blood films—is oxygenated, a decrease of about 10 percent of the ISC count is common. Most ISCs are dehydrated (Fig. 20.5), but some are dehydrated and look "plump" on the smear, and are detectable in normal or light density fractions of sickle blood instead of the usual densest fraction.

Target cells, observed in variable but generally low numbers, reflect a disproportion between cell membrane area and intracellular volume, while polychromasia provides an index of marrow activity. Increased numbers of white cells and platelets are typical, even during intercritical periods; to some extent those changes also reflect splenic hypofunction, but neutrophil kinetics is also abnormal (see Chapter 24).

Rarely done today, with the advent of rapid solubility tests for HbS, the sickle cell preparation provides morphologists with such descriptors as "holly leaf" and "filamentous" forms (Fig. 20.7), which reflect rapid or slow polymerization of HbS. Nucleated red cells can be observed, but if the number is more than 10 percent, extramedullary hematopoiesis, recovery from aplastic anemia, or other unusual conditions should be suspected. Nucleated red cells can interfere with the white cell and reticulocyte counts in automatic counters.

Extramedullary hematopoiesis is found among patients with sickle cell anemia, but is usually less striking than in thalassemia. The incidence of macroscopic lesions in one series was 7 percent (Seidler and Becker, 1968). As in β thalassemia major, intrathoracic hematopoiesis is generally characterized as unilateral or bilateral, smooth, sharply delineated, often lobulated paraspinal masses, but without erosion of the vertebrae or the ribs. Sometimes these paraspinal masses are associated with similar subpleural and paracostal masses (Gumbbs et al., 1987). Generally, they do not produce symptoms, and although they may initially grow rapidly, they attain a steady state in which no further growth is observed. This complication of the disease is worthwhile to remember since it does not require intervention and misdiagnosis might lead to unnecessary thoracotomy.

Erythrocytic ecdysis (the shedding of long filamentous processes from red cells) (Fig. 20.7) detectable in the blood film is a rare phenomenon observed in some complicated cases of sickle cell anemia: patients have congestive heart failure, acute viral syndromes, pneumonia, malignancy, and syndromes of red cell agglutination (Rao and Patel, 1987). Most of the cases reported have considerable hepatomegaly. Although the processes are in all likelihood spectrin-free spicules

released by sickled cells on reoxygenation (Rao and Patel, 1987), the reason for their appearance only in cases with complications is unknown. In vitro they can be produced by repeated cycles of oxygenation and deoxygenation (Westerman et al., 1984), and have been related to the "hypercoagulability state" in sickle cell anemia (Chapter 22).

Bits and pieces of red cells and spherocytes reflect both intravascular fragmentation and loss of splenic function due to infarction. Howell-Jolly bodies, siderotic granules, and "pocks" seen with Nomarski optics—pitted red cells are actually red cell inclusions that have not been plucked out by the spleen—are further evidence of splenic hypofunction (Chapter 24). As in other hemolytic anemias, serum lactic dehydrogenase (LDH) levels are increased. Many patients exhibit values above 500 IU/L and levels correlate with the number of dense cells (Billet et al., 1988a). Moreover, one of the LDH isoenzyme has been reported to be a "marker" for vasoocclusive crises, but has not been widely used (Miller et al., 1980). Haptoglobin, a specific binder of hemoglobin (Bourantas et al., 1998) and hemopexin, a specific binder of hemin (Muller-Eberhard, 1968) are greatly decreased.

Bone Marrow Expansion. Sickle cell anemia patients have greatly expanded red bone marrow, replacing the fatty marrow space of the long bones (Fig. 20.8). This well-established fact has been dramatically confirmed by magnetic resonance imaging (MRI). Nevertheless, there is an intriguing feature of this marrow expansion: Although data derived from other hemolytic anemias or model systems demonstrate that the marrow has the capacity to expand its erythropoietic activity 6 to 10 times (Crosby and Akeroyd, 1952), sickle cell anemia patients expand their marrow activity to only 3 to 6 times. The difference might be due to the low oxygen affinity of blood in sickle cell anemia. The moderately severe anemia in sickle cell disease may not produce sufficiently intense hypoxia, due to the increased oxygen release at the tissue level (see below).

Bone marrow aspirates typically show increased erythroid activity. Marrow necrosis can be seen even in the absence of symptoms. A mild degree of nuclear/cytoplasmatic dissociation may be present, but frank megaloblastic changes suggest folate deficiency. Bone marrow biopsies demonstrate hypercellularity with erythroid hyperplasia.

Modulation of Anemia

Extent of Red Cell Destruction: Red Cell Survival Measurements. McCurdy and Sherman (1978) showed that sickle cell anemia patients have a red cell survival

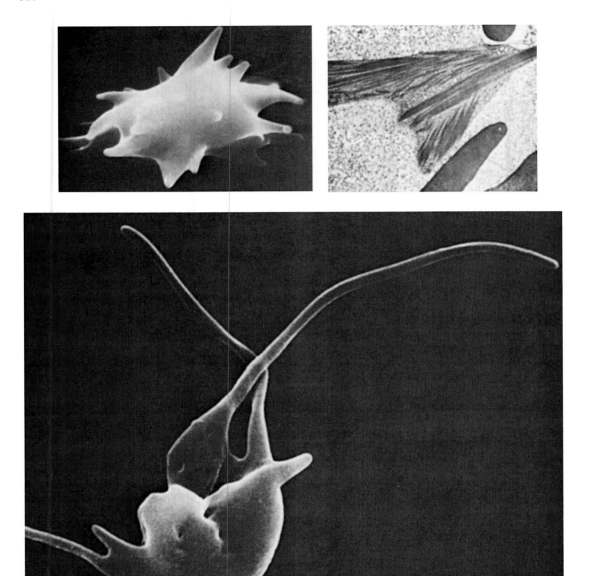

Figure 20.7. The shape and features of sickled cells. Upper diagram shows a "holly leaf" shape of deoxygenated SS cells by scanning electron microscopy (12,000 ×). To the right is an electron microscopy plate of a section of sickled cells demonstrating that the digital protuberances in the sickle cells are generated by fascicles of fibers (polymerized deoxyHbS). The lower diagram shows that, under certain conditions, the digital protuberances can be quite long and cells grossly deformed (ecdysis). It is not surprising that sickled cells of this type lose spicules during circulation.

sity in sickle cell anemia blood is not related principally to red cell aging. In normal blood, the densest cells are considered the oldest. In contrast, in sickle cell anemia, cells that survive the shortest period of time are the ISCs, which are the most dense cells. ISC counts are correlated with hemolysis (Serjeant et al., 1969). Patients with hypersplenism may have ^{59}Cr red cell half-lives of 1 day (Rossi et al., 1964).

Differential Survival of F-Cells. Dover and coworkers (1978) showed that F-cells survive longer than other sickle cells (see Chapter 10). Nevertheless, there may be a discrepancy between the proportion of newly formed F-cells and the final level of HbF. In general, the number of F-cells correctly predicts 70 percent to

that is 15 percent of normal. In nonhypersplenic Jamaican patients with sickle cell anemia (Serjeant et al., 1969) the range is reported to be 2 to 21 days with an average of 10 days for T_{50} Cr or chromium "half-life."

Although the red cell survival rate differs among red cell density classes (Serjeant et al., 1969), cell den-

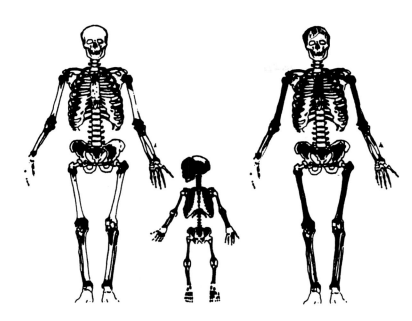

Figure 20.8. Red marrow distribution in the skeleton normal adult (left), normal child (middle), and patient with sickle cell anemia (right).

80 percent of the peripheral level of HbF. In other words, about 25 percent of patients have higher HbF—presumably through preferential survival of the F-cells or effects of other epistatic genes—than predicted by the F-reticulocyte numbers.

Progenitors, Growth Factors, and Anemia.

1. *Erythropoietin.* Serum erythropoietin levels are abnormally low for the extent of the anemia. Sherwood et al. (1986) demonstrated that erythropoietin levels, measured immunologically, increased less as a function of decreasing hemoglobin level in sickle cell anemia than in other anemias, including non-hemoglobinopathic hemolytic anemias (Fig. 20.3). This phenomenon was particularly apparent among patients more than age 10 years. Erslev et al. (1987) using a less sensitive erythropoietin assay did not find this difference.

The reduced erythropoietin response could be the consequence, in part, of the right-shifted oxygen equilibrium curve characteristic of sickle cells. Rightward displacement of the oxygen equilibrium curve is accompanied by an increase in the volume of O_2 per gram of hemoglobin unloaded at the tissue level, and the increase in delivery of O_2 decreases the stimulus for erythropoietin production. An alternative or complementary explanation is that a progressive reduction in renal erythropoietin synthesis is due to progressive renal damage that commonly occurs with aging in sickle cell anemia and is accompanied by increasing anemia (Chapter 24).

2. *Erythroid burst-forming units (BFU-e) and erythroid colony-forming unit s(CFU-e) in sickle cell anemia.* BFU-e and CFU-e are increased in some patients with sickle cell anemia (Pannathur-Das et al., 1984; Croizat and Nagel, 1999) and have increased sensitivity to erythropoietin. BFU-e numbers in sickle cell anemia are inversely correlated with the percentage of HbF and are higher in patients with HbF less than 9 percent. While most circulating BFU-e are not cycling in normal individuals, in sickle cell anemia, ^{3}H-dT suicide studies indicate that these progenitors are in cycle. A significant correlation exists between percentage of BFU-e in cycle and HbF. In contrast, BFU-e is not in cycle in patients with normal numbers of circulating BFU-e, who have more than 9 percent HbF. (Croizat and Nagel, 1993). It must be noted that cycling in these studies was not defined by very stringent criteria, as they are now. No data exist on bone marrow BFU-e in sickle cell anemia.

3. *Other growth factors.* A burst-promoting activity (BPA) was found in sickle cell anemia patients with low HbF levels and actively cycling BFU-es, but not in patients whose BFU-es are not cycling (Croizat, 1994a). This activity was traced to accessory or adherent cells (Croizat et al., 1990;). This BPA-like factor is inhibited by anti-rhGM-CSF, suggesting that GM-CSF is important in sickle cell anemia patients with low HbF (Croizat et al., 1990; Croizat and Nagel, 1999). GM-CSF is constitutively increased in the plasma of the most anemic patients with sickle cell anemia, particularly those with low HbF levels (Croizat, 1994a). In patients with high HbF and less anemia, interleukin (IL)-3 and an inhibitory factor from adherent cells play more of a regulatory role (Croizat et al., 1990).

Stem cell factor (SCF) and transforming growth factor (TGF)-β have been identified as regulatory factors specifically affected by the genotype of sickle cell diseases and disease severity. The plasma concentrations of SCF and TGF-β are significantly different when sickle cell anemia patients are compared to controls, and levels of each cytokine tend to vary inversely with the level of HbF. The highest levels of SCF, up to 7,000 pg/mL, are detected in patients with low HbF levels and is accompanied by an increase in the number of SCF+ CD[34] enriched circulating cells. High HbF sickle cell anemia patients have lower levels of SCF factor and an increased concentration of TGF-β, suggesting a regulatory role of TGF-β on either SCF release or c-kit expression on progenitor cells. Occasional elevations of G-CSF, IL-7, and MIP-1α in sickle cell anemia plasma appeared to be nonspecific and were unrelated to HbF concentration. LIF is always undetectable in plasma of these patients (Croizat and Nagel, 1999).

Interestingly, a correlation is present between the extent of erythropoiesis—measured by the levels of soluble transferrin receptors (sTfR)—and SCF and TGF-β in sickle cell anemia patients and controls. sTfR concentrations are significantly increased in all sickle cell anemia samples and sTfR levels are negatively correlated with the percentage HbF. Levels of sTfR are higher in low HbF than in high HbF patients. Erythropoietin levels are increased in low HbF patients (34 to 215 ml U/mL), while in high HbF patients they are in the normal range (3 to 20 mL U/mL). While erythropoiesis is generally increased in sickle cell anemia, the subclass of low HbF sickle patients exhibits a particularly high erythropoietin response, perhaps because they are more anemic. Based on the correlation between sTfR levels and HbF, this determinant accounts for only one-third of the variance, suggesting that other genetic determinants of marrow response to anemia and the extent of hemolysis in sickle cell anemia are present.

4. Long-term culture-initiating cells (LTC-ICs). Mobilization of the early stem and progenitor cells and formation of a large pool of circulating stem cells appear to be a feature of sickle cell anemia. Nevertheless, the permanent stress of anemia and continuous progenitor cell recruitment may result in the decrease or exhaustion of circulating stem and/or progenitor cells regardless of increased levels of growth factors. What is the size of the stem cell pool and the cycling status of circulating stem and progenitor cells in sickle cell anemia?

Primitive hematopoietic stem cells are present in human bone marrow and blood, and in the presence of supportive fibroblasts, give rise to LTC-ICs (Sutherland et al., 1989, 1990). LTC-ICs are in present in normal human blood in small numbers and are primarily quiescent (Ponchio et al., 1995). LTC-ICs and multilineage clonogenic forming cells (CFC) derived from LTC-ICs, were found to be increased about 10 times in sickle cell anemia, particularly in individuals with low HbF levels (Croizat et al., in press). This observation appears consistent with the higher number of circulating CD[34+] cells detected in low HbF patients (Croizat and Raventos-Suarez, 1993), since LTC-ICs express CD[34] antigen (Sutherland et al., 1989). In each patient, the numbers of LTC-ICs are not stable but vary over time. Follow-up studies in individual patients demonstrated that all progenitors fluctuated markedly over time but in a correlated fashion (Croizat et al., in press).

The fact that the number of progenitor cells in blood is higher than the LTC-IC level is not surprising, since mobilized peripheral blood is enriched in CFC,

rather than early stem cells (Sherwood et al., 1986). Sickle cell anemia patients have an individualized degree of mobilization of stem and progenitor cells of both erythroid and granulocytic lineage. A majority of circulating LTC-ICs were found to be quiescent but were rapidly recruited into a cycle resembling mobilized progenitors in cancer patients undergoing chemotherapy and given high doses of growth factors (Ponchio et al., 1995).

To summarize, sickle cell anemia is associated with overall increases in circulating stem cells and progenitor cells, not restricted to the erythroid lineage, but involving also granulocytic progenitors and primitive stem cells. Their numbers vary considerably from individual to individual and over time in an individual and exhibit properties of mobilized progenitors. There is no evidence of LTC-IC or CFC exhaustion. Constitutively mobilized circulating stem cells may be a good target for gene therapy (Chapter 41).

Factors That Can Influence Anemia

Coexisting G-6-PD deficiency appears not to affect the density distribution of sickle erythrocyte, the level of the steady-state hemoglobin concentration, or the clinical status of the patient with sickle cell anemia (Gibbs et al., 1981). While acute hemolytic episodes in sickle cell anemia have been attributed to the coexistence of this enzymatic defect, this must be uncommon (Beutler et al., 1974; Steinberg et al., 1988) (see Chapter 24).

Patients with sickle cell anemia vary considerably in their hemoglobin concentrations and some of the factors responsible for that variation include HbF level and concomitant α thalassemia (see Chapters 24, 26 to 28). α Thalassemia inhibits HbS polymerization by lowering MCHC (see Chapter 28); sickle cell anemia patients with three α-globin genes have higher hemoglobin levels that those with four α-globin genes and those with two α-globin gene have even higher levels. Both high HbF and α thalassemia prolong red cell survival and their effects are independent. β[S]-Globin gene cluster haplotypes are partial predictors of anemia in adults (see Chapter 26). The Senegal and Arab-India haplotypes are associated with the least anemia. Folic acid deficiency and iron deficiency can complicate the course of sickle cell anemia, and are discussed in Chapter 24.

Erythrophagocytosis by Macrophages and Monocytes.

Erythrophagocytosis designates the ingestion of whole red cells by circulating monocytes or neutrophils, or by fixed macrophages of the spleen or liver (Solanki, 1985). Hemolysis in sickle cell anemia is greatly influenced by the presence of dense cells and ISCs (see Chapter 22). Since adult patients are usually asplenic, but continue to have hemolytic anemia, in these patients destruction of red cells must occur elsewhere. One mechanism of extrasplenic red cell destruction is erythrophagocytosis.

Solanki (1985) found erythrophagocytosis—mostly by monocytes and to a lesser degree neutrophils—in 38 percent of 27 patients with sickle cell disease and this was not present in splenectomized individuals. Erythrophagocytosis was inversely related to PCV. Ten percent of circulating monocytes and 0.1 percent to 0.6 percent of all white cells had intracytoplasmic erythrocytes. Kuppfer cells are commonly engorged with erythrophagocytized cells. Marrow and tissue macrophages ingest more sickle than normal red cells in vitro (Hebbel and Miller, 1984).

Two possible mechanisms for erythrophagocytosis, both linked to surface IgG accumulation, exist: an immune mechanism where sickle cells are phagocytized via the Fc receptor because of surface-bound IgG, and a mechanism where the membrane surface is damaged by oxidative stress (Hebbel and Miller, 1984) with increased amounts of denatured HbS deposited on its inner surface and surface IgG accumulation (see Chapter 22). Petz et al. (1984) found that over 60 percent of sickle cell disease patients had red cells with increased numbers of membrane bound IgG molecules. Confirmed by other laboratories, IgG deposition mainly affects dense cells (Green et al., 1985) and the IgG specificity seems to be directed to the membrane α-galactosyl residues (Galili et al., 1985, 1987). Membrane IgG colocalizes with clustered band 3, the anion transporter, that becomes altered in the dense sickle erythrocyte. Macrophages, with receptors for the Fc fragment of immunoglobulins, bind sickle cells in preference to normal cells; they favor cells with the greatest density and the highest amounts of IgG. The intensity of hemolysis is related to the amount of IgG on the erythrocyte surface and cell density. The interplay and relative significance of these mechanisms in the hemolysis of sickle erythrocytes remains to be established and both mechanisms could be similar to those involved in the senescence of normal red cells (Galili, 1988).

Hemodilution. Plasma volume in sickle cell anemia increased beyond that observed in other hemolytic anemias and averaged 55 ± 7.6 mL/kg in 14 adults with sickle cell anemia (Steinberg et al., 1977). Children had plasma volumes about 10 percent higher. Elevated plasma volume makes it difficult to predict red cell mass that is underestimated by the hemoglobin level or PCV. The origin of this abnormality is unknown.

Hemoconcentration. Since patients with sickle cell anemia are particularly prone to dehydration, many ill patients have hemoconcentration. Rehydration is accompanied by a decrease in PCV. The extent of this decrease is difficult to assess in the face of the considerable blood extraction for laboratory tests but usually the hemoglobin concentration after a night of intravenous fluids is more representative of a patient's usual value than the initial test.

Viscosity of Sickle Blood and Its Relation to Anemia

Blood, a viscoelastic material, has characteristics akin to fluids but also to solids (see Chapter 21). As a viscoelastic liquid, its fluid characteristics are dominant (Matrai et al., 1987). Blood viscosity is defined by the proportionality between shear stress and shear strain rate, or how much stress has to be exercised to produce a certain level of strain per unit of time. Shear rate is similar to flow rate, but also depends on the size of the tube through which flow takes place; shear rates are very high in small diameter capillaries. A liquid is particularly viscous when more force is needed to obtain the same flow.

Newtonian fluids have a linear relationship between shear stress and shear rate; non-Newtonian fluids have a nonlinear relationship. Plots of viscosity versus shear rate are flat for Newtonian fluids and have a descending curve for non-Newtonian fluids. Blood is non-Newtonian, so viscosity decreases as the shear rate increases (Fig. 20.9). Increased viscosity at low shear rates is caused by the aggregation of blood cells, which is influenced by plasma factors. Decreased

Figure 20.9. The relation between shear rate and viscosity in a logarithmic plot, for normal blood at 45 hematocrit and 37°C. Since the line is not horizontal and flat, the relation is characteristic of non-Newtonian fluid. The graphic insert on the upper left corner indicates red cells are aggregating at this level of shear rate while the diagram in the lower right corner depicts the red cell deforming at that particular shear rate regimen. (From Chien et al., 1987, with permission.)

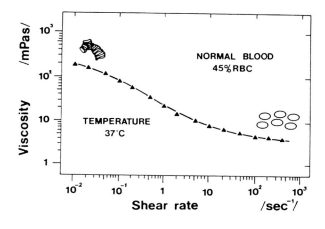

viscosity at high shear rates—assuming nonturbulent flow—is the consequence of red cell deformation. Blood viscosity is normally determined by the PCV, red cell deformability, red cell aggregation, and plasma viscosity.

Bulk viscosity of oxygenated sickle cell disease blood—as contrasted to the deformability or viscosity of individual cells—at the native PCV is lower than normal (Chien, 1977) because the PCV in sickle cell anemia is lower than normal. Aggregation of sickle red cells is diminished, probably because of their abnormal shapes, yet their rigidity is moderately increased. Plasma viscosity is slightly, but significantly, increased, presumably from increases in gamma globulins and fibrinogen. At low shear rates the bulk viscosity of sickle cell disease blood is very low compared to normal blood. The decrease in cell aggregation, and the only moderate influence of cell rigidity at these shear rates, accounts for these results. In contrast, at high shear rates, the bulk viscosity of sickle cell blood is only slightly lower than normal. Here, no effects on cell aggregation are present and viscosity is dominated by decreased erythrocyte deformability or increased rigidity.

Deoxygenation changes blood viscosity in sickle cell anemia considerably (Chien, 1977). While red cell concentration and plasma viscosity remain the same, red cell rigidity increases dramatically because of intracellular HbS polymer. In addition, there are dramatic decreases in red cell aggregation, presumably because of red cell shape changes. As a result, there is a sizable increase in viscosity at all shear rates, but at low shear rates the increased viscosity is still below normal due to the overwhelming effect of a low PCV. At high shear rates, viscosity increased because of decreased red cell deformability. Anemia is in effect adaptive or compensatory in the overall pathophysiology of sickle cell anemia. When the PCV in sickle cell disease is increased by transfusion or pharmacologic treatment with erythropoietin or HbF-increasing drugs, caution is indicated since the increase in PCV and viscosity has the potential to promote vasoocclusive episodes unless there is a corresponding increase in red cell deformability (Schmaltzer et al., 1987).

Clinical Manifestations of Anemia (See also Chapter 24)

Most children and young adults have few clinical manifestations of anemia alone, aside from fatigue and dyspnea on strenuous exertion; occasional patients with hemoglobin concentrations of 4 to 5 g/dL go about their business as usual and are surprised at physician's anxiety over their condition. Still, severe anemia is a risk factor for certain events such as stroke

(see Chapter 24). Despite adaptation, some young children die of congestive heart failure. Those who survive to adult life have large muscular hearts, presumably due to work hypertrophy. As patients enter the 5th to 6th decade, coronary arteries get narrower, hemoglobin levels get lower, and some patients develop angina and get fatigued at tasks that they previously could manage.

Some of the adaptations responsible for such a paucity of symptoms include increased cardiac output, decreased oxygen affinity of the blood, increased blood volume, and probably, increased numbers of open capillaries and general vasodilation of the microcirculation (Lonsdorfer et al., 1983).

HEMODYNAMIC ASPECTS OF SICKLE CELLS

Normal Hemodynamics

Blood circulation involves four functional compartments with considerable overlap and without fixed morphologic delimitations (Fig. 20.10).

1. A high pressure compartment includes conduit vessels such as the aorta and its major branches. Changes in the physiologic state of these vessels generally do not change blood distribution among organs, nor do they contribute considerably to flow resistance. They do contribute to reduction of the pulsatile character of blood circulation, as they attenuate the ejection wave by elastic deformation.

2. A control compartment is formed by arterioles whose contraction can affect flow and distribution and define the postarteriolar capillary pressure. This compartment has high wall shear stresses (5 to 15 Pa) and shear rates (100 to 200 sec^{-1}) and the bulk viscosity is shear dependent.

3. An exchange compartment with the highest surface to volume ratio in the circulatory system, formed largely by capillaries and postcapillary venules. Capillary diameters can be smaller than the red cell diameter and erythrocyte deformation is required for cell passage (Fig. 20.11).

4. A low pressure compartment formed by medium and large veins contains, at any given time, 80 percent of the total blood volume. Flow is slow and sometimes stagnant, and wall shear stresses are low (less than 1 Pa).

Blood Flow and Vessel Size

Blood flow has different characteristics in different sized vessels. In vessels with diameters over 300 μm flow has the characteristic of in vitro bulk viscosity at moderately low shear rates and red cell aggregation or interaction is a significant factor.

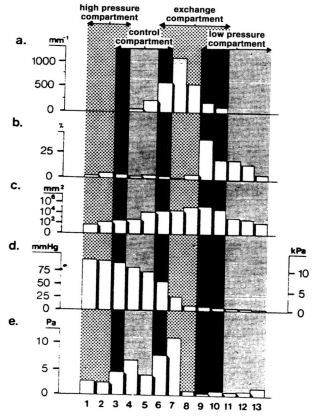

a. – Surface area / volume
b. – % of total volume
c. – Cross-sectional area
d. – Intriluminal pressure
e. – Wall shear stress

Figure 20.10. Distribution of morphologic and hemodynamic parameters in the circulatory system and based in morphometric measurements. The assumptions in this graph include: (1) vessels of equal diameter are assumed belonging to the same cross-section of the vascular tree; (2) temporal variation of diameter and vessel recruitment are ignored; (3) blood rheology is assumed independent of geometric and hemodynamic flow conditions. (From Chien et al., 1987, with permission.)

Single-file flow is characteristic of capillaries. Under these conditions, flow is determined by the deformation of red cells and the red cell/wall interaction. Important features of red cell flow in this type of vessel are their transformation into "parachute shape" (nonaxisymmetric) deformation with stable orientation during flow (Fig. 20.12) and tank-treading where the red cell membrane moves over the cytosol, dissipating energy. In transitional flow, which occurs in vessels between 8 and 300 μm, the number of red cells per section of vessel is much less than in the bulk flow cases and the distribution of the concentration of red cells (and red cell velocities) across the vessel cross-section becomes important. A Newtonian fluid will flow in a tube of these diameters as a parabola of velocities with the highest velocity in the center of the tube and parabolic decreases toward the periphery. Since blood is non-Newtonian, the distribution of red cell velocities across the section has a "blunted" parabola shape (Fig. 20.13). The low velocity near the wall is derived from the increased resistance where the shear is maximal. The non-Newtonian feature of the "blunted center" is the consequence of the increase of viscosity with decreasing shear, which robs those cells traveling in the center of the flow from their legitimate increased velocity. A parabolic velocity profile also implies a gradient of concentration of red cells across the section of the vessel. Fewer are in the periphery, and more in the center. This also means that more plasma travels near the wall and less near the center. All of this, in turn, means that red cells are traveling faster than plasma. Hence, as Fahraeus (1928) predicted, the hematocrits of transitional vessels should be lower than the hematocrit measured in collected blood. This concept is called the "Fahraeus effect," and decreases in the "apparent" viscosity in the transitional-type vessels the "Fahraeus-Linqvist effect" (Fahraeus and Lindqvist, 1929).

Figure 20.11. Frequency distribution of capillary diameters in the human microcirculation. Notice that the diameters are smaller than most red cells, the diameters of which are between 7.5 and 8.5 μm. (From Gaechtgens et al., 1987, with permission.)

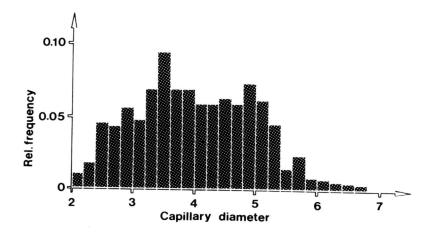

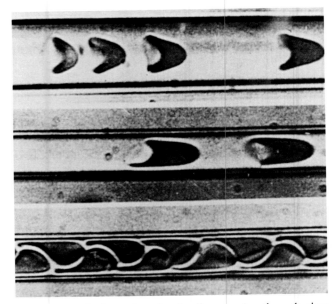

Figure 20.12. Deformation of red cells traversing through glass capillaries between 6 and 12 μm. Notice the "parachute" shape of the single-file flow in the top two capillaries; in the bottom capillary multifile flow has a "zipper" aspect. In vivo observations have confirmed these findings. (From Chien, 1987, with permission.)

Hemodynamics of Blood in Sickle Cell Disease

Vascular Resistance to Sickle Blood. In an isolated "ex vivo" vasculature preparation (Fig. 20.14), the infusion of oxygenated blood from sickle cell anemia patients produces higher vascular resistance and increased transit time when compared to normal red cells (Kaul et al., 1981; Vargas and Blackshear, 1982). Abnormal rheology of oxygenated sickle cell anemia blood may be secondary to the presence of rigid ISCs.

Measurement of microhemodynamic parameters in single unbranched arterioles and in arteriovenous (A-V) networks revealed increased flow resistance to sickle cells. In the cremaster muscle preparation, flow resistance doubled in the A-V network following a bolus infusion of sickle cell anemia blood via the femoral artery (Lipowsky et al., 1982). An initial decrease in resistance suggested that compensatory arteriolar dilation might occur early but prolonged exposure to sickle cells resulted in the deterioration of microvascular flow due to progressive capillary occlusion.

Progressive deoxygenation of sickle cells results in HbS polymerization and loss of red cell deformability. Reduction in the local PO_2 from 40 to 7 mm Hg caused a fourfold increase in the apparent viscosity in single arterioles (Lipowsky et al., 1982). LaCelle (1977), using a similar approach in the cremaster muscle of mice, reported a significant decline in sickle red cell velocity in capillaries when the muscle PO_2 was reduced below 40 mm Hg. In the isolated mesocecum

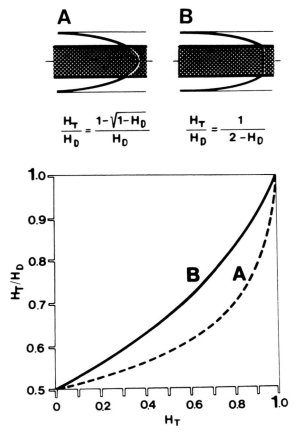

Figure 20.13. Hematocrit dependence of the Fahraeus effect in small vessel flow. A, parabolic flow of the central core of red cells; B, blunted profile of the central core; HT, tube hematocrit; HD, hematocrit of discharge. The central point of the Fahraeus effect is that HT (for small vessels) is lower that HD. The ratio between HT and HD has a different dependency to HD if the flow is parabolic or blunted (see upper diagram formulas). In the lower part of the diagram it is clear that the hematocrit in the tube (or vessel) is lower compared to the discharge hematocrit (that in the collection tube) when the flow is parabolic than when it is blunted. We must remember that due to the abnormal shapes and lower deformability of sickle cells, sickle blood will tend to a blunted flow and a higher small vessel hematocrit than the Fahraeus effect would predict for a normal parabolic flow. (From Chien et al., 1987, with permission.)

preparation, arteriolar red cell velocities fell when the PO_2 of perfusate containing sickle cells was reduced to 60 mm Hg, suggesting a decrease in sickle cell deformability at relatively high PO_2. This result is similar to that observed in vitro (Kaul et al., 1983b).

The obstructive behavior of deoxy as well as oxy sickle cells is highly dependent on the arterial perfusion pressure (Chien, 1977; Kaul et al., 1981). In the isolated mesocecum microvasculature, the arteriolar velocities of oxy sickle red cells are always lower than those of normal human red cells at applied arterial pressure between 100 and 30 mm Hg, and some

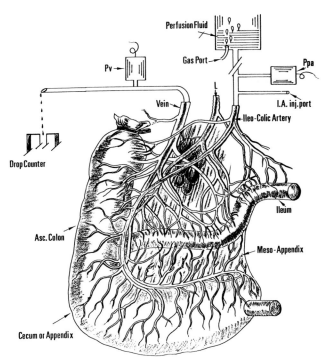

Figure 20.14. Diagramatic sketch of artificially perfused mesocecum (also called mesoappendix) ex vivo preparation of the rat. Pps, arterial perfusion pressure; Pv, venous outflow pressure.

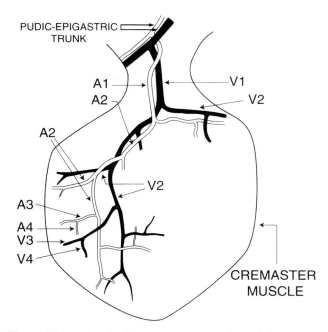

Figure 20.15. "In vivo" cremaster preparation of the mouse. This preparation allow for the observation of the microcirculation in a muscle without detaching the microcirculatory bed from its nerve and vascular connections.

microvascular obstruction is observed when oxygenated sickle cells are infused at 30 mm Hg. Partial deoxygenation of sickle cells (PO_2 of 40 mm Hg) induces sufficient cellular rigidity to produce a drastic reduction in arteriolar velocity and wall shear rates (Fig. 20.15), and about a threefold increase in pressure, even at a perfusion pressure of 100 mm Hg.

The pronounced pressure-dependent ability of partially deoxygenated sickle cells to obstruct the microvasculature suggests that variations in the pressure gradient resulting from changes in vascular dimensions and capillary entry conditions may contribute to stasis and obstruction by sickle cells.

Flow Behavior of Density-Defined Sickle Red Cell Classes. Sickle cells are heterogeneous and their hemodynamic effects are complex since different classes of sickle cells are unequally represented in a given patient and the distribution pattern varies among patients (Fabry and Nagel, 1982). Kaul et al. (1983) have shown that the viscosity of all density cell classes was nearly doubled and the difference between the deoxygenated and oxygenated viscosities remained constant. In contrast, peripheral resistance in the isolated vasculature resulting from infusion of deoxygenated cells was dramatically dependent on cell density, as was the difference in resistance during perfusion of oxygenated or deoxygenated cells (see Chapter 21).

Differences between the viscosity and hemodynamic measurements are most probably due to the different sensitivity of the two methods to the extent of intracellular polymerization of HbS. This difference could be based on the importance of dynamic rigidities in gaining entrance to the microcirculation, which are not represented in bulk viscosity.

Classes of dense cells, such as dense discocytes and ISCs, undergo minimal morphologic (shape) changes following deoxygenation, but are likely to have the most abnormal dynamic rigidities (Nash et al., 1986). In support of this interpretation is the fact that ISCs are mainly observed obstructing the junction of precapillary arterioles and true capillaries (Kaul et al., 1989) (Fig. 20.15). While the roles of ISCs and reversibly sickled cells in the genesis of vasoocclusion have been promoted (Klug and Lessin, 1977; LaCelle, 1977) ISC-induced obstruction is very random, and its occurrence cannot be predicted in a given microvascular bed. Interestingly, ISCs might not pose a problem for capillary flow since they tend to orient themselves along the vessel axis, thereby posing a reduced hazard to flow. Although ISCs could initiate vasoocclusion they are not its sole cause (see Chapter 21).

The role of dense discocytes (MCHC, 39 to 46 g/dL), cells described by Kaul and co-workers (1983a), in microvascular obstruction, has not yet been defined. Due to their moderately high MCHC, dense discocytes may gain access to the capillary beds because they might not contain HbS polymer on the arteriolar side, but will be among the first cells to undergo HbS polymerization upon deoxygenation in the postarteriolar capillaries, and so are likely to obstruct the lumen of these small vessels. Cells with lower MCHC will have already traversed the capillaries before polymerized HbS would have increased their intracellular viscosity sufficiently to cause obstruction.

The Role of Vascular Tone in Blood Flow. How vascular tone and reactivity affect the flow behavior of sickle cells through the microcirculation is not fully understood. The primary cause of vasoocclusion might be a derangement in the microcirculatory control mechanisms, which then secondarily generate stasis and the conditions for vasoocclusion. Microcirculatory blood flow is modulated by periodic vasomotion of the precapillary sphincters and terminal arterioles (Nicoll and Webb, 1955), in response to local metabolic needs. Schmid-Schonbein et al. (1981) have suggested that during vasomotion, periodic partial occlusion of an arteriole tends to increase the fluidity of blood during the slow portion of the cycle, and provides the pressure gradient necessary to propel hemoconcentrated blood during rapid flow period (vasodilation). Abnormal rheologic characteristics are likely to have significant hemodynamic consequences unless appropriate vasomotor adjustments are made. Klug and Lessin (1977) noted that ISCs and sickle cell-induced capillary obstructions in the mesenteric bed of transfused rats could be dislodged by norepinephrine-induced vasomotion.

Using noninvasive laser-Doppler velocimetry, microcirculatory flow in the forearm skin of sickle cell patients has been reported to include the synchronization of periodic flow (termed oscillatory flow) in large groups of contiguous capillaries (Rodgers et al., 1984). The observation of similar patterns in normal and other nonsickle hemoglobinopathies makes the interpretation of this finding less clear.

Using transgenic sickle mice ($\alpha^H\beta^S\beta^{S\text{-Antilles}}$ [β^{MDD}]) (see Chapter 34), in vivo microcirculatory studies of the cremaster muscle preparation (Fig. 20.16) showed adhesion of sickle red cells, restricted to postcapillary venules. Electron microscopy revealed distinct contacts between the red cell membrane and the endothelium surface and sickled red cells were regularly observed in the venular outflow (Kaul et al., 1995). Surprisingly, while under resting conditions (PO$_2$, 15 to 20 mm Hg) there were no differences in the cremaster microvascular diameters of control and transgenic mice; the transgenic mice showed a drastic reduction in microvascular red cell velocities (Vrbc) with the maximal Vrbc decrease (>60 percent) occurring in venules, the sites of red cell adhesion and sickling. Local, transient hyperoxia (PO$_2$, 150 mm Hg) resulted

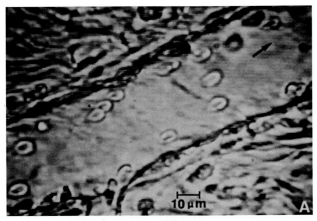

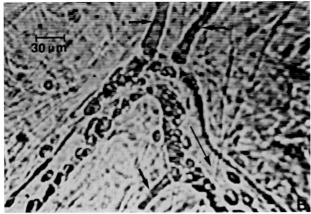

Figure 20.16. Adhesion of sickle red cells in venules. (**A**) Adherent sickle cells of discocytic morphology are seen tethered to the endothelial wall of a venule and are aligned in the direction of the flow (arrow). (**B**) Adhesion of sickle cells at venular bending and at junctions of smaller diameter postcapillary venules. In this instance the postcapillary vessels (small arrows) are totally blocked. Large arrow indicates flow direction. (From Kaul et al., 1981, with permission.)

in striking differences between control and transgenic mice. In controls, oxygen caused a 69 percent arteriolar constriction, accompanied by 75 percent reduction in Vrbc. In contrast, in transgenic mice, hyperoxia resulted in only an 8 percent decrease in the arteriolar diameter and in a 68 percent increase in Vrbc, the latter probably due to an improved flow behavior of red cells as a consequence of unsickling. In effect, the high expression of HbS in the mouse results in not only intravascular sickling but also red cell–endothelium interaction (Kaul et al., 1995a). Blood flow in the mucosal-intestinal microvessels of normal mice was compared with that in transgenic knockout sickle cell mice whose erythrocytes have only HbS and HbF. These animals, in addition to blood flow abnormalities such as sludging in all microvessels, had decreased Vrbc in venules of all diameters. As in the studies of the $\alpha^H\beta^S\beta^{S\text{-Antilles}}$[$\beta^{MDD}$] mice, flow in controls slowed or halted in response to hyperoxia but markedly increased in sickle cell mice (Embury et al., 1999).

VASCULAR OBSTRUCTION IN THE SICKLE SYNDROMES

Vasoocclusion in sickle cell disease involves several components: initiation, extension, damage, and repair. Initiation might involve perfusion pressure changes, vasomotor and humoral factors, anatomic peculiarities, and variable tendency of blood cells to adhere to the endothelium. These events—simultaneously or in succession—may be the dominant modulating factors determining if a circulating sickle erythrocyte can produce obstruction. Nevertheless, initial obstruction need not lead to a clinically significant and extended vasoocclusive event. Changes in perfusion pressure or vessel diameter, for example, have been demonstrated to be capable of reopening an initially obstructed microcirculatory bed (Klug and Lessin, 1977). The possibility of frequent but resolving microvascular occlusion in sickle cell anemia deserves additional scrutiny. The precise role of platelets and white cells, and other hemostatic factors have not been fully elucidated, but their participation in the initial stages of vasoocclusion seems likely. Activated neutrophils may adhere to endothelium, an effect increased by hypoxia. Sickle neutrophils may have increased rigidity and adhere also to sickle erythrocytes. Sickle monocytes can activate endothelial monolayers (NIH Workshop on the Role of Polymorphonuclear Leukocyte in Sickle Cell Disease, Bethesda, MD, May 28, 1999).

That changes in the microcirculation can induce or initiate vasoocclusion by themselves is demonstrated by the induction of dactylitis by ice water exposure of the extremities (Marsden and Shah, 1964). Initiation of a vasoocclusive episode may well be a consequence of alterations in the vascular tone, possibly resulting from changes in metabolic and/or neurohormonal feedback control mechanisms, potentially induced by infection or inflammation, that would abolish the compensatory hemodynamic adjustments required for sickle cell flow. The challenge of the next years will be to define these phenomena. Extension of vasoocclusive events, both contiguously as well as distally, repair and the failure of repair, and tissue damage are other components that also need to be considered.

Sickle cell disease is characterized by recurring episodes of painful vasoocclusive events (see Chapters 24 and 25). Constant, and many times progressive, vasoocclusive injury to several organs may serve as a backdrop for the punctuated acute events. At first, the pathogenesis of vasoocclusion in sickle cell anemia was ascribed entirely to red cell abnormalities (reviewed in Eaton and Hofrichter, 1987). Previous studies have indeed indicated that reduced red cell deformability was a major determinant of rheologic abnormalities, hemolysis, and reduced red cell life span in this disorder. Nevertheless, pleiotropic effects secondary to the presence of HbS significantly complicate the pathogenesis of vasoocclusion to the point where the polymerization tendency of HbS sickle is indispensable but not sufficient to explain the enormous variability of the phenotype of sickle cell disease (Nagel and Fabry, 1985).

For example, hemolysis and oxygenation and deoxygenation of sickle cells in vivo result not only in red cell destruction but also in erythrocyte membrane loss, membrane/cytoskeleton abnormalities, increase in MCHC, and generation of dense cells. Erythropoietic stress due to hemolytic anemia results in the appearance of immature stress reticulocytes in the peripheral circulation. These cells have membrane properties different from those of mature red cells and enhanced adhesivity. In most patients, discocytes with normal MCHC form the largest component of sickle cell disease blood, although large variations in the proportion of reticulocytes, young cells, and dense cells are found (Kaul et al., 1993).

Some features of the phenotype of sickle cell disease are likely to be modulated by genes besides the β^S-globin gene. Some of these effectors are well known, such as α thalassemia, while others are poorly characterized (see Chapter 26). In one model for sickle vasoocclusion, some events are directly attributable to HbS, the primary element, while pleiotropic and epistatic effectors are secondary but indispensable in the generation of the phenotype. Secondary effectors are the basis for the clinical variability of individuals who have the same primary mutation. Sickle hemoglobin is a single mutation but sickle cell anemia is a multigene disease (Nagel, 1992).

HbS Polymerization, Cell Sickling, and Vasoocclusion

HbS polymerization is discussed in Chapter 23. To summarize, polymerization progresses with the characteristics of a nucleation-initiated reaction that requires a critical nucleus—about 10 tetramers—be formed for the reaction to be initiated. One consequence of this model is that there is a delay time during which there is no HbS polymerization because time is required for tetramers to collide and generate the proper sized nucleus. The delay time is exquisitely dependent on the concentration of deoxyHbS and also pH and temperature. As the concentration of deoxyHbS increases, pH falls, and temperature rises, the delay time shortens. This explains the deleterious effects of hyperosmolarity (which shrinks red cells and increases MCHC), acidosis, and fever. Most sickle red cells do not sickle within the period required for the passage through the microcirculation because of this delay time (Eaton and Hofrichter, 1995).

Following nucleation, polymerization can proceed at many nucleation sites simultaneously—particularly when the MCHC is high or the pH low—producing a sickled cell with multiple polymer domains called granular cells. If polymerization proceeds at one or a few nucleation sites producing large polymers, a variety of erythrocyte shapes result: cells resembling bananas, produced by one polymer domain as in the ISCs; stars, produced by two or three domains; and holly-leaf shapes caused by a few domains. Shape alterations can have hemodynamic consequences. ISCs have been seen obstructing the precapillary arteriole sphincter (LaCelle, 1977; Klug et al., 1982; Lipowsky et al., 1987). Granular cells are likely to arise from dense discocytes and are found obstructing either capillaries or venules bedecked by adhered cells (see below).

How rapidly cells are deoxygenated affects the polymer characteristics and their rheology. Kaul and Xue (1991) have shown that gradual deoxygenation of sickle cell disease blood results in the formation of morphologic cell types based on MCHC differences, as noted above. This is accompanied by a gradual increase in the viscosity of whole blood over a given period of deoxygenation. In contrast, rapid deoxygenation results in the transformation of most cells into granular forms regardless of their MCHC. Rapidly deoxygenated sickle cell suspensions show two time-dependent distinct phases in viscosity: first, an initial rapid rise in viscosity to a peak characterized by the presence of mostly granular forms, and second, a significant time-dependent decrease in the whole blood viscosity. This phase is characterized by the appearance of a large percentage of elongated cells. Transmission electron microscopy shows that cells that develop long processes after prolonged deoxygenation contain regions of aligned polymers in addition to regions of very small polymer domains or hemoglobin aggregates in accord with earlier kinetic, morphologic, and ultrastructural analyses of rapidly deoxygenated sickle cells (Fig. 20.7).

Prolonged deoxygenation would then result in elongated shape caused by the growth of the aligned domains. Decreased viscosity in phase two is probably due to the alignment of elongated cells along the direction of flow reminiscent of the viscosity decrease observed in deoxyHbS solutions following polymer alignment (Kaul and Xue, 1991). Other studies have concluded that it is the polymer fraction, not cell morphology, that determines the filterability of deoxy sickle cells but these studies did not employ different deoxygenation rates to produce distinct polymer domain characteristics (Hiruma et al., 1995).

Adhesion of Sickle Cells to the Endothelium (see also Chapter 21). Abnormal adherence of sickle cells to the vascular endothelium is discussed in detail in Chapter 21. In an ex vivo mesocecum preparation of the rat (Kaul et al., 1989), sickle cell anemia cells adhered (Fig. 20.16) exclusively to the venules in an inverse correlation with venular diameter and adherence dependent on cell density (Fig. 20.17) (Kaul et al., 1989). By controlled modifications of cell density under shear flow conditions, adhesion of different density sickle cells is inversely dependent on cell density rather than changes in their intrinsic adhesion potential (Kaul et al., 1994). The adhesive behavior of a given cell population could be distinctly reversed by controlled dehydration/rehydration. In spite of preferential binding of young and low density cells, all sickle cells could potentially adhere to the vascular endothelium.

Based on experiments in a meso-appendix microcirculatory preparation that used specifically labeled dense cells or young sickle red cells (Fig. 20.18), a model of sickle cell vasoocclusion was proposed where increased adhesion of low-density cells in the immediate postcapillary venules is followed by selective trapping of dense cells, resulting in vasoocclusion (Fig. 20.19) (Kaul et al., 1989). While contributions from the several morphologic types of dense cells were not differentiated, more recent work has demonstrated that dense cells were mainly ISCs (Kaul et al., 1994). This is consonant with the clinical observation that the decrease of dense cells from the peripheral circulation during painful episodes mainly involves selective trap-

Figure 20.17. Relationship between venular diameter and sickle red cell adhesion (unseparated cells) in the venules of mesocecum microvasculature. The regression fits the equation $y = 1.0689X^{-1.1206}$, $r = -0.812$, $r^2 = 0.659$, $p < 1 \times 10^{-5}$. (From Kaul et al., 1989, with permission.)

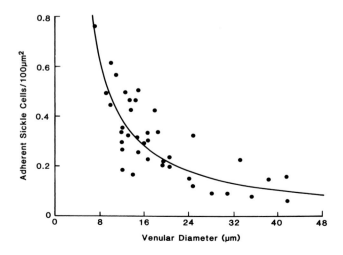

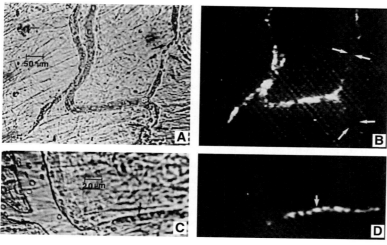

Figure 20.18. Selective trapping of dense cells (fraction SS4) in venular capillary and postcapillary venules and obstruction in a venular capillary following infusion of a mixture of fraction SS2 (discocytes) and FITC-labeled fraction SS4 (ISC and dense unsicklable discocytes) mixes in a ratio of 3:1. (A) Areas of venular obstruction. Arrows indicate *un*obstructed areas with adherent cells. (B) The same area seen under epifluorescence illumination showing localization of FITC-labeled dense fraction SS4 cells trapped in the obstructed venules of various diameters and their absence in areas with adhesion (arrows). (C) A postcapillary venule is seen obstructed with a single file of cells and joins a large diameter venule. The small diameter venule is seen obstructed with a single file of cells and joins a large diameter venule, which shows individual adhered discocytic cells. (D) The same area seen under epifluorescence illumination. Fluorescent dense cells are obstructed along with SS2 cells in the venular capillary. Notice the absence of fluorescence in the individually adherent cells in the larger venule. (From Kaul et al., 1981, with permission.)

Figure 20.19. Proposed model of vasoocclusion in sickle cell anemia in which adhesion occurs first and trapping of rigid sickle cells follows. (Courtesy of D. K. Kaul.).

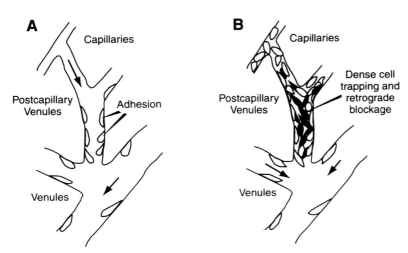

ping of ISCs, presumably following adhesion of deformable cells to the vascular endothelium (see Chapter 25).

Several mechanisms are likely to be involved in the abnormal adherence of sickle red blood cells to vascular endothelium. Red cell age, density, shape, membrane alterations, endothelial pathology, and infection/inflammation may influence these mechanisms. Most sickle red cells are capable of adhesion to the endothelium (Kaul et al., 1994), according to conditions, but the bulk of the phenomenon is driven by young sickle red cells.

Adhesion receptors present only on a subset of sickle reticulocytes, i.e., stress reticulocytes [$\alpha_4\beta_1$ integrin and glycoprotein IV (CD36)] are capable of binding to VCAM-1 expressed on cytokine stimulated endothelial cells and to TSP, respectively (Sugihara et al., 1992; Britain et al, 1993; Swerlick et al., 1993; Joneckis et al., 1993; Gee and Platt, 1995; Natarajan et al., 1996). Induced release of endothelial, large molecular weight von Willebrand factor (vWF) has been shown to enhance overall sickle cell-endothelial interaction in both in vitro and ex vivo systems (Wick et al, 1987; Kaul et al, 1993; Wick et al, 1993; Kaul et al, 1995). Known receptors to vWF (i.e., GPIb and GPIIb/IIIa) are absent in human red cells (Joneckis et al, 1993; Kaul et al, 1993).

The vascular endothelium can release vWF molecules in response to tissue injury and in vivo stimuli, including vasopressin (and its analogue desmopressin), histamine, thrombin, fibrin, and platelet-activating factor (PAF) (Imaizumi et al, 1995). Secondary to inflammation, PAF, which has a myriad of biologic activity, may be released from monocytes. In the isolated mesocecum, PAF induces the release of extra-large vWF and this enhances adhesion (Kaul et al, 1995). Increased vWF levels in the plasma have been reported for sickle cell patients (Richardson et al, 1979; Mackie et al., 1980), although a relationship to disease severity is not clear.

The absence of adhesion receptors for vWF on sickle RBC and the loss of sickle RBC adhesion receptors (e.g., $\alpha_4\beta_1$ and CD36) as the cells mature indicate that other adhesive molecules must be involved. TSP-mediated adhesion may also involve some of the same molecules that bind vWF. For example, both vWF and TSP show binding to the same endothelial ligand, $\alpha_v\beta_3$ (Kaul, 1995; Cheresh, 1987). Other likely candidates are sickle membrane components that are normally present, but are not accessible and then become exposed after repeated sickling, such as modified Band 3 and sulfated glycolipids.

Band 3 is a transmembrane glycoprotein that is involved in anion transport across red cell membrane (Low, 1989). Band 3 has been cloned and sequenced from both mouse (Kopito and Lodish, 1985; Tanner et al., 1988; Lux et al., 1989) and human, showing striking similarities in the two. Band 3 abnormalities in sickle cell anemia include coclustering with hemichromes, which may serve as a signal leading to recognition and removal of senescent red cells by macrophages (Low, 1987). These clusters may also serve as sticky spots to which adhesive proteins may bind readily. Exofacial loops of band 3 have been shown to be involved in cytoadherence of Plasmodium *falciparum*-infected red cells (Crandall et al, 1993) and similar peptides derived from the exofacial loop-3 of band 3 seem to be capable of inhibiting human sickle cell adhesion (Thevine et al, 1995), although this work needs further confirmation. Also, the endothelial molecules involved in this interaction are not known. Sickling-unsickling of sickle cells as well as oxidative processes (Hebbel, 1994) in these cells could result in modifications of exofacial loops of band 3, resulting in vWF binding.

Normally sulfatides are not expressed on the red cell surface but the resulting membrane damage in sickle cells as a consequence of repeated sickling could expose these molecules to the surface. Both vWF and TSP are known to bind sulfated glycolipids in vitro (Roberts et al., 1986). This interaction is effectively inhibited by certain anionic polysaccharides such as high molecular weight dextran sulfate (mol. wt. 500,000) (Ginsburg and Roberts, 1988). Recent studies have shown that sickle cell adhesion to immobilized TSP is also inhibited in the presence of dextran sulfate and chondroitin sulfate A (Joneckis et al., 1996; Hillery et al., 1996). More recently, the effect of inhibitors to this interaction (anionic polysaccharides as high and low molecular weight dextran sulphate) has been explored in HUVEC cultures and mesocecum vasculature, successfully inhibiting adhesion (Barabino et al. [1999]).

The next question is which are the potential adhensive complexes involved in adhesion and expanding the red cell integrins, adhesive proteins, and endothelium receptors? Thus, tripartite adhesive complexes (RBC receptor adhesion protein-endothelial receptor) may contribute to sickle red cell adhesion. Based on known interactions between these components, a number of such complexes may plausibly exist: CD36-TSP-$\alpha_v\beta_3$; sulfatide-TSP-$\alpha_v\beta_3$; sulfatide-vWf-$\alpha_v\beta_3$; sulfatide-laminin-$\alpha_v\beta_3$ (or several potential β_1 integrins). Thus, $\alpha V\beta_3$ could play an important role in sickle red cell adhesion to the endothelium.

In flow systems, peptides and antibodies that inhibit $\alpha_v\beta_3$ function have been shown to inhibit sickle red cell adhesion to endothelium, although the peptides were not absolutely specific for $\alpha_v\beta_3$, and in one study both E-selectin and VCAM-1 also seemed to play important roles. Moreover, cultured endothelial cells were used for these studies, and thus, may differ from the endothelium of intact vessels.

Kaul et al. (2000a) have used monoclonal antibodies (MoAb) directed against $\alpha_v\beta_3$ and GpIIb/IIIa integrins to dissect the role of these integrins in sickle red cell adhesion. The murine MoAb 7E3 inhibits both $\alpha_v\beta_3$ and Gp II/IIIa, whereas MoAb LM609 selectivity inhibits $\alpha_v\beta_3$, and MoAb 10E5 binds only to $\alpha II\beta 3$. Kaul et al. (2000) tested the capacity of these MoAbs to block platelet-activating factor (PAF)-induced sickle red cell adhesion in the ex vivo mesocecum vasculature of the rat. Infusion of washed sickle cells in preparations treated with PAF (200 pg/mL), with or without a control antibody, resulted in extensive adhesion of these cells in venules, accompanied by frequent postcapillary blockage and increased peripheral resistance units (PRU). PAF also caused increased endotheial surface and interendothelial expression of endothelial, expression vWf. Importantly, pretreatment of the vasculature with either MoAb 7E3 F(ab')$_2$ or LM609, but not 10E5 F(ab')$_2$, after PAF almost completely inhibited adhesion in postcapillary venules, the sites of maximal adhesion and frequent blockage. The inhibition of adhesion with 7E3 or LM609 was accompanied by smaller increases in PRU and shorter pressure-flow recovery times. Thus, blockade of $\alpha_v\beta_3$ may constitute a potential therapeutic approach to prevent sickle cell-endothelium interactions under flow conditions.

Hemodynamic Factors and Vasoocclusion in Transgenic Sickle Mouse Models. During steady-state flow in $\alpha^H\beta^S\beta^{S\text{-Antilles}}[\beta^{MDD}]$ mice in vivo adhesion of red cells was restricted to venules. Some sickled cells were regularly observed in the venular outflow. Blood flow was reduced in these animals consistent with intravascular polymer formation. The venular specificity of adhesion is in accord with the finding with human sickle cells in the ex vivo rat mesocecum.

To assess microcirculatory abnormalities in the sickle transgenic mouse, it is important to correlate in vivo arteriovenous hemodynamic profiles with red cell heterogeneity, sickling, and adhesion using defined experimental conditions. Both Vrbc and wall shear rates in the microcirculation are highest in the arterioles but drop steeply as red cells traverse the capillaries to postcapillary venules (Zweifach and Lipowsky, 1984).

The prevailing low wall shear rates in postcapillary venules are expected to provide maximum opportunity for red cell interaction with the vascular endothelium as well as for red cell aggregation. Immediate postcapillary venules are also a part of the exchange compartment along with capillaries and terminal arterioles, and consistent with this, morphologically sickled cells are encountered only in the venular outflow of the transgenic sickle mouse.

Inherent functional differences are present in the endothelial cells of arterioles and venules. Platelet-activating factor (PAF), histamine, and bradykinin induce permeability changes only on the postcapillary side of the circulation by causing separation of intercellular junctions (Fox and Wayland, 1979; Anderson et al., 1984). Increased venular permeability causes hemoconcentration and affects local hemodynamics. Histamine and bradykinin can also affect the arteriolar tone by inducing release of NO (see below).

Red Cell Heterogeneity. Red cell heterogeneity is apparent upon density gradient separation of blood from human sickle cell anemia patients and sickle transgenic mice. Characterized by an increase in both low-density reticulocytes and high-density cells (Clark et al., 1980; Fabry and Nagel, 1982; Kaul et al., 1983a), density fractionated cells have different levels of 2,3 BPG, different oxygen affinity, different shapes, and perhaps different microcirculatory behaviors.

Dense cells are generated by mechanisms discussed in Chapter 22. Membrane oxidation plays a key role in generating the damage observed in integral membrane proteins, cytoskeletal proteins, membrane lipid organization, and ion transport. Cellular dehydration promotes further polymerization and sickling, due to the shortening of the delay time for HbS polymerization. Mechanisms of dehydration involve K:Cl cotransport, the Gardos channel (Ca^{++}-activated K$^+$ loss), and other transport pathways. Membrane damage is particularly severe in dense, dehydrated cells, which exhibit marked reduction in cell deformability and increases in membrane rigidity. Cytoskeletal proteins are altered and rearranged in cells that become irreversibly sickled. Normal lipid asymmetry is also lost and the externalization of phosphatidylcholine renders them most likely to adhere to the endothelium and to monocytes/macrophages.

Nitric Oxide and Other Vasoactive Molecules in Vasoocclusion (see also Chapters 42 and 46). NO is generated from L-arginine and acts on the vascular smooth muscle through guanylate cyclase to produce vasorelaxation (Katisuc and Cosentino, 1994) (see Chapter 42). Both constitutive (cNOS) and inducible (iNOS) forms of nitric oxide synthase (NOS) are expressed in endothelial cells, while only iNOS is present in vascular smooth muscle cells (Katisuc and Cosentino, 1994). cNOS is Ca^{++}-dependent and acts transiently, while iNOS causes longer lasting release of NO (Katusic and Consentino, 1994), perhaps leading to depletion of arginine. L-argi-

nine plasma levels were low in sickle cell anemia and could become rate limiting for NO synthesis. iNOS is inducible after activation of macrophages and other cells by cytokines such as TNF-α or IL-1 (Clark et al., 1991). TNF-α may be elevated in sickle cell anemia. This suggests that arteriolar tone may be modulated by changes in the expression of cNOC with consequences for NO production. Whether this increase in iNOS is accompanied by depleted substrate levels is unknown. Depletion of NO could affect both vascular tone and endothelial function. Induction of NOS in smooth muscle by TNF-α may shorten the half-life for endothelial cNOS mRNA (Yoshizumi et al., 1993).

There is evidence that sickle cells inhibit endothelium-dependent vasorelaxation (Mosseri et al., 1993), probably by inhibition of cNOS gene expression (Phelan et al., 1995). Bank et al. (1996) have shown an increased expression of iNOS in the kidney of $\alpha^H\beta^S\beta^{S-Ant}[\beta^{MDD}]$ mice (Fig. 20.20).

$\alpha^H\beta^S\beta^{S-Ant}[\beta^{MDD}]$ mice showed a significant decrease in the mean arterial blood pressure compared with controls (Kaul et al., 2000a). Lower pressure was associated with significant increase in endothelial NOS (eNOS)

Figure 20.20. Paired immunohistochemistry staining both inducible nitric oxide synthase (iNOS) and nitrotyrosine in individual kidneys of normal and β^S sickle cell mice. Paired photomicrographs are from closely adjacent areas. (From Bank et al., 1996, with permission.) For full color reproduction, see color plate 20.20.

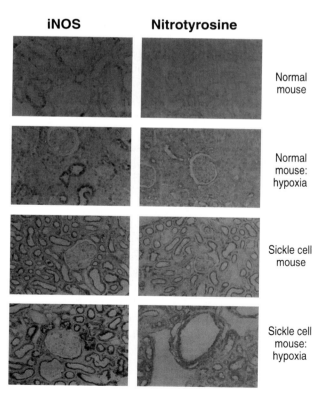

iNOS **Nitrotyrosine**

Normal mouse

Normal mouse: hypoxia

Sickle cell mouse

Sickle cell mouse: hypoxia

expression. Cremaster muscle arterioles in the transgenic mouse showed blunted diameter responses to acetylcholine, an endothelium-dependent vasodilator, and to sodium nitroprusside, an NO-donor. Indomethacin blockade of cyclooxygenase activity did not alter the arteriolar responses to acetylcholine and sodium nitroprusside in control and transgenic mice, or affect blood pressure in transgenic mice.

L-NAME, a nonselective inhibitor of NOS, caused significant increases in blood pressure and decreases in arteriolar diameters in both control and transgenic sickle mice, confirming NOS activity. L-arginine given after L-NAME resulted in a significant recovery of the diameters and blood pressure. Aminoguanidine, an inhibitor of iNOS, did not affect arteriolar diameters or blood pressure in controls or transgenic mice, indicating that iNOS did not contribute to blood pressure and arteriolar responses. Western blotting confirmed the lack of iNOS in the cremaster tissue. A chronic increase in eNOS activity can explain hypotension and altered microvascular responses to NO-mediated vasodilators in transgenic sickle mice. An upregulated NOS/NO activity would maintain microvascular blood flow in the face of red cell rheologic abnormalities in this mouse model and, by extension, in sickle cell disease, providing an important partial compensation to the tendency for vasoocclusion.

NO regulates expression of endothelin-1 (Kourembanas et al., 1991), and endothelium exposed to sickled erythrocytes had a four- to eightfold induction of the endothelin-1 gene (Phelan et al., 1995).

Initiation and Local Extension of the Vasoocclusive Event.

Whatever the mechanisms that precede or lead to vasoocclusion, the next question to be answered is how vasoocclusion becomes established. It is likely that the sickle cell itself is the main factor here, but two different mechanisms of initiation have been observed in animal microcirculatory preparations under direct videomicroscopy: (1) obstruction of the precapillary arteriole sphincter located in the initial portions of the precapillary arteriole by cells that appear to be ISCs; and (2) adhesion of deformable and young nondense sickle cells to the vascular endothelium narrowing the vessel lumen followed by trapping of dense cells, especially ISCs. This mechanism is likely to predominate in the small venules, where adhesion is maximal.

Undefined are the mechanisms for local extension. One hypothesis is that endothelial damage at the site of the initial obstruction could release vasoactive substances downstream, such as prostaglandins and endothelin-1, promoting vasoocclusion.

Distal Extension and Symmetry of Vasoocclusion.

One of the most intriguing features of acute painful episodes (see Chapter 25) is the distal extension of painful sites. Pain many times begins in a single site and in hours or days other painful areas are recruited to the event. Two possibilities for this feature of vasoocclusion are: (1) humoral factors such as cytokines, particularly if they have vasoactive properties or affect the adhesion of sickle cells to the endothelium; (2) the nervous system could respond to the presence of pain by modifying vasoactivity in distal sites.

Serjeant and Chalmers (1990) have proposed that symmetric extensions of pain could be the consequence of a "steal" syndrome. Based on the fact that "cooling" is a major precipitating factor of painful episodes in Jamaica, and that skin cooling in normals leads to cutaneous vasoconstriction with diversion of the blood flow to the bone and muscle circulation (Roddie, 1960), they conjectured that in sickle cell anemia the red marrow is maximally vasodilated and incapable of accommodating an increase in flow. The shift of blood flow would be taken up by the muscle vasculature. This opens the possibility of a decrease in flow to the marrow or blockage due to inability to accommodate increased flow, with the potential of marrow necrosis and the start of a painful episode.

Aseptic Inflammation in Sickle Cell Anemia Painful Episodes.

Acute phase reactants C-reactive protein (CRP), α-1 antitrypsin, and C_3 increase from normal during painful episodes and infections; (Becton et al., 1989; Akinola et al., 1992; Singhal et al., 1993). Akinola et al. (1992) found that CRP, α-1 acid glycoprotein (AGP), and fibrinogen are usually in the normal range during the steady state but with wide fluctuations. About a quarter of sickle cell disease patients had CRP and serum amyloid A levels greater than normal during the steady state of the disease compared to 1 percent of controls (Singhal et al., 1993). Fluctuating subclinical vasoocclusive episodes that elicit acute-phase response may be present in sickle cell anemia.

Endothelial cells can also modulate their surface receptors in response to external stimuli. Infection itself can cause changes in endothelial cells by at least two different mechanisms. Herpes simplex virus 1 (HSV1) can infect endothelial cells and cause them to display Fc receptors. This receptor can increase adherence of sickle red cells by binding to the IgG pathologically found on the surface of sickle red cells (Hebbel et al., 1987). Endothelial cells exposed to parainfluenza 1 or virus-mimicking double-stranded RNA demonstrated increased adherence mediated by an upregulated VCAM1–VLA4 mechanism (Smolinski et al., 1995).

Like parainfluenza 1, TNF-α induced increased adhesion of sickle red blood cells (Vordermeier et al., 1992) through the VCAM1–VLA4 interaction (Swerlick et al., 1993). A more complex reaction to another cytokine, IL-1β was demonstrated when the adherence phenomenon was examined after endothelial cells were exposed to the cytokine for up to 24 hours. Adherence was increased 16-fold over baseline, and at different time points, different endothelial cell receptors were critical: first the vitronectin receptor, then E-selectin, and finally VCAM1 (Natarajan et al., 1996).

Hypoxia itself can induce endothelial cells to become more adhesive to CD36+/VLA4+ sickle reticulocytes. Hypoxic endothelial cells have increased expression of VCAM1 and ICAM1 (intra-cellular adhesion molecule 1), although VCAM1 appears to be the key receptor involved in the increased adherence (Setty and Stuart, 1996). In contrast, exposing endothelial cells to hydroxyurea decreases red blood cell adherence, and changes endothelial cell morphology and cation transport (Adragna et al., 1994).

Evidence That Nonpolymerization-Related-Phenomena Are Major Players in Painful Crises

The fact that polymerization of sickle hemoglobin is the primary event in sickle cell anemia is tautological. Nevertheless, the direct participation of the sickled cell may be of different import in different complications of sickle cell anemia. For example, not all complications of sickle cell anemia correlate with the level of HbF, which is the major, well-understood modulator of disease. Considerable evidence now exists that secondary but relevant events modulate the incidence and pathogenesis of vasoocclusive events in sickle cell anemia.

1. Numbers of dense cells do not correlate at all with the incidence of painful episodes (Billet et al., 1988a; Bailey et al., 1991).
2. Saudi Arabia has two populations of sickle cell anemia patients (see Chapters 26 and 33). Patients with sickle cell anemia linked to the Arab-India β-globin gene haplotype have very high levels of HbF. Patients with sickle cell anemia linked largely to the Benin haplotypes have far lower HbF concentrations. These two groups differ significantly in the prevalence of α thalassemia and MCHC and in the incidence of complications such as dactylitis, acute chest syndrome, and persistence of splenomegaly. Nevertheless, they do not differ in the incidence of painful episodes.
3. α Thalassemia appears to increase the incidence of painful episodes and osteonecrosis (see Chapter 28).
4. HbF levels should have a clear protective effect on painful events if this complication depended predominantly on cell sickling. Yet, two studies (Powars et al., 1980; Baum et al., 1987) have failed to demonstrate the postulated protective effect of HbF on sickle painful episode.
5. High Hbf levels may not protect from stroke (see Chapters 24 and 38).
6. Cyanate, which inhibits polymerization in vitro, failed to modify the incidence of painful episodes (Harkness and Roth, 1975).
7. Although hydroxyurea increased HbF and reduced painful episodes in sickle cell anemia HbF levels did not explain all of the benefit of treatment (see Chapter 38).

These findings strongly suggest that sickle cell painful episode cannot be explained exclusively as the consequence of the capacity of the sickle cell to sickle, either considering the delay time, or with much less likelihood, the extent of polymerization as the relevant factor.

Pathophysiology of Vasoocclusion in the Lung. The lung has two anatomic features that are bound to influence sickle vasoocclusion. Alveolar capillaries do not resemble capillary bends elsewhere and have "sheath" flow where red cells do not march in file but descend as in a waterfall. Precapillary arterioles and postcapillary venules are located in the intersection of alveoli, a structure that changes size and shape when an area of the lung becomes unventilated (atelectasis) (Fig. 20.21). These features make the lung environment especially hazardous for sickle erythrocytes, suggests that atelectasis might be important for producing sickle vasoocclusion, and indicates that combating atelectasis might be an important means of avoiding pulmonary complications of sickle cell anemia.

Mechanisms of lung acute complications are not fully understood but the causes of the acute chest syndrome are expanding (Gladwin et al., 1999; see Chapter 24). Haynes et al. (1993) demonstrated, in a rat lung preparation, that hypoxia and sickle cells synergistically increased the vascular resistance. In this study, the effects of alveolar hypoxia on pulmonary microvascular hemodynamics in sickle red cell–perfused rat lungs were studied under conditions of high and low oxygen tensions and compared with lung perfused with rat and normal human red cell controls. Independent of the PCV of the infused cells, ventilation with the room air gas mixture did not result in any significant differences in the pulmonary arterial pressure, capillary pressure, total pulmonary vascular resistance, or angiotensin II pressor response. Ventilation of lungs perfused with sickle red cells with a hypoxic gas mixture significantly increased the above parameters. No significant accumulation of lung water occurred in sickle cell–perfused lungs compared with controls, judged by capillary filtration coefficient and wet-to-dry lung weight ratio.

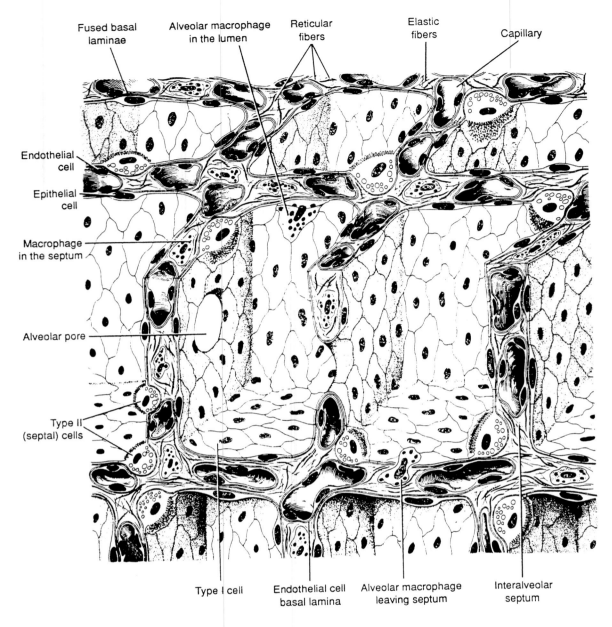

Figure 20.21. Anatomy and vascularization of the alveoli of the lung. Notice that the walls of the alveoli come together in interalveolar spaces that have the capacity of contracting when a portion of the lung suffers atelectasis. Also notice that the capillaries of the walls of the alveoli are wide and the circulation is more in the vein of a thin cascade of cells and in single-file red cells as in the rest of the circulation.

This finding could be the consequence of the retention of sickle cells' due to regional alveolar hypoxia, through a paradoxical vasoconstriction effect in the lung vasculature; this effect is opposite to the effect of hypoxia in the systemic circulation where vasoconstriction can promote the trapping of sickle cells.

To answer this question, Aldrich et al. (1996) used an isolated, perfused rat lung preparation, where each lung was separately ventilated. One lung was exposed to 95 percent O_2, the other to 0 to 21 percent O_2. Lungs were infused with ^{99M}Technicium-labeled sickle cells or normal red cells at a PCV of 30 along with ^{112}Sn-labeled 15 μ microspheres as perfusion markers. After perfusion, lungs were sliced and radioactivity counted. Weight-normalized perfusion was significantly decreased with hypoxia and retention of oxygenated sickle cells averaged 1 percent to 2 percent, a value similar to normal control cells. When sickle cells were perfused in a hypoxic lung their retention was about 30 percent at 2.5 percent O_2 and about 80 percent when lungs were perfused without oxygen. Interestingly, when the hypoxic lung with trapped sickle cells was exposed to O_2, a bolus of dense sickle cells was released (Fig. 20.21). These experiments suggest that sickle cells were entrapped by the induction of sickling and not adhesion, which should have occurred regardless of oxygen tension and might be expected to involve light-density sickle red cells.

In lungs, arteries carry deoxygenated blood and veins carry oxygenated blood. The pulmonary circulation is a highly efficient filter, trapping 99.5 percent of 8 μ microspheres during a single pass. Only 80 percent of similar microspheres are entrapped in the systemic circulation. Pulmonary circulation responds to hypoxia by vasoconstriction, unlike the systemic circulation that vasodilates. This physiology favors entrapment of dense sickle cells. Perhaps the vasculature of the lung has differences in the expression of adhesion molecules or the perfusion pressure might induce wall shear rates that are too high to permit adhesion.

Bovine pulmonary artery endothelial cells (BPAEC) incubated with red blood cells and/or autologous plasma from patients with acute chest syndrome and during steady state, had increased levels of endothelin-1 transcripts and protein in BPAEC supernatants during acute chest syndrome only. Plasma endothelin-1 level was elevated during acute chest syndrome, which decreased during its resolution but not to normal (Hammerman et al., 1997).

In acute chest syndrome caused by bone marrow fat embolism, secretory phospholipase A_2 (sPLA$_2$), an important inflammatory mediator and capable of liberating free fatty acids from fat, is elevated 100-fold compared to normal controls, 35-fold greater than steady-state sickle cell anemia patients, and 5 times greater than patients with pneumonia (Styles et al., 1996). Unknown is whether or not PLA$_2$ generated from fat emboli or fatty acids can impact the generation of sickle cell–mediated microcirculatory obstruction in the lung.

Hemoglobin binding of NO may regulate pulmonary hypoxic vasoconstriction. The lung contains iNOS, cNOS, and eNOS and inhibition of NOS increases pulmonary vascular resistance. It has been suggested that O_2 is the rate-limiting substrate for NO synthesis in lungs and may link oxygenation, NO, and pulmonary vascular tone to maintain an equal ventilation/perfusion (V/Q) ratio (Gladwin et al., 1999). Hypoxic vasoconstriction may be dependent on PCV and during normoxic ventilation anemic animals have increased exhaled NO concentrations and lower pulmonary artery pressures. These observations imply that anemia impairs NO consumption and with hypoxic vasoconstriction causes V/Q mismatch. In sickle cell anemia impaired hypoxic pulmonary vasoconstriction might lead to a fall in hemoglobin-oxygen saturation and HbS polymerization. Transfusion causes very rapid increases in PO$_2$ in some patients with acute chest syndrome, perhaps by restoration of hypoxic pulmonary vasoconstriction and correction of the V/Q ratio.

Pathophysiology of Vasoocclusion in the Retina. Pathologic and clinical aspects of sickle retinopathy are described in Chapter 27; the following discussion is limited to the pathogenesis of vasoocclusion in the retina. Using an adenosine diphosphatase flat-embedding technique that permitted examining retinal vessels en bloc and employing serial sections, the primary site of vasoocclusion in sickle retinopathy was located at the precapillary level (McLeod et al., 1993). An unusual neovascular formation, the hairpin loop, was observed and appeared to result from recanalization of the wall of an occluded vessel. Many autoinfarcted pre-retinal neovascular formations were observed in an older patient with HbSC disease. Small pigmented lesions consisting of retinal pigment epithelial cells ensheathing channels that resembled autoinfarcted vessels were also present. Two patent preretinal formations were studied in detail and their evolution appeared to be influenced by mechanical factors. The vessels appeared to have been extruded from the retina, perhaps owing to hydrostatic pressure secondary to downstream occlusions.

Hemodynamic factors in the retina of sickle retinopathy have also been studied (Roy et al., 1995). Macular blood flow velocity was compared in eighteen patients with sickle cell disease and forty-five normal controls using blue field entoptoscopy, and the relation between macular blood flow velocity and red blood cell density was examined. While there were no significant differences between patients and controls in leukocyte flow velocity, in sickle cell disease patients, leukocyte velocity in the macular capillaries was negatively associated with a greater range of red cell density, suggesting that in sickle red cell density heterogeneity may slow macular capillary blood flow.

Using streptavidin peroxidase immunohistochemistry, Lutty et al. (1994a) investigated changes in distribution and relative levels of components in the fibrinolytic system and growth factors in retina and choroid from two sickle cell disease patients. Antigen localization in the sickle cell patients was compared to localization from two nonsickle cell, nondiabetic control subjects. Tissue plasminogen activator localization and immunoreactivity were comparable in all eyes, but plasminogen activator inhibitor-1 immunoreactivity was elevated within the walls of retinal vessels in the sickle cell tissue. Immunoreactive fibrin was often observed within the lumen of retinal and choroidal vessels and in choroidal neovascularization in sickle cell subjects. Blood vessels containing fibrin generally exhibited elevated plasminogen activator inhibitor-1 immunoreactivity. Von Willebrand's factor and basic fibroblast growth factor immunoreactivity in sickle cell patients were elevated in choriocapillaris and the walls of some retinal vessels. Transforming growth factor-β1 immunoreactivity was significantly lower in sickle cell choriocapillaris than in controls. In chorioretinal pigmented lesions of an HbSC disease patient, basic fibroblast growth factor, TGF-β1, β2, and β3 immunoreactivity were present within migrating retinal pigment epithelial cells. These data suggested that fibrin deposition within retinal and choroidal vessels of sickle cell disease subjects may occur due to elevated plasminogen activator inhibitor-1 activity. Vasoocclusion of choroidal vessels may influence the expression of growth factors in choriocapillaris endothelium, which could stimulate formation of choroidal neovascularization. Fibrosis and gliosis in and near chorioretinal pigmented lesions may be stimulated by migrating retinal pigment epithelial cells and production of basic fibroblast growth factor and TGF-β.

Neovascularization is a common consequence of retina vasoocclusion. Morphometric analysis in postmortem ocular tissue from subjects with sickle hemoglobinopathies (McLeod et al., 1997) demonstrated numerous active and autoinfarcted lesions, representing virtually all stages in preretinal neovascularization. They ranged from single small loops extending from arteries and veins along the retinal surface to the typical complex, elevated sea fan formations. Sea fans developed at hairpin loops and at arteriovenous crossings. There was an average of 5.6 connections between sea fans and retinal vessels; of these, 45 percent were arteriolar, 52.5 percent were venular, and 2.6 percent involved capillaries. Six of eight sea fans were located at arteriovenous crossings. Autoinfarction appeared to occur initially within the sea fan capillaries. The average height of sea fans was 123 μ above the retinal surface. Preretinal neovascularization in sickle cell retinopathy may arise from both the arterial and venous sides of the retinal vasculature and assume a variety of morphologic configurations. Multiple feeding arterioles and draining venules are common, and autoinfarction appears to occur initially at the preretinal capillary level rather than at feeding arterioles. Arteriovenous crossings may be a preferential site for sea fan development.

Vasoocclusion in the retina has been studied in transgenic mice and in a rat animal model. $\alpha^H\beta^S[\beta^{MDD}]$ mice were examined to determine if vascular abnormalities were present in the retina and choroid (Lutty et al., 1994b). One retina from each animal was processed by flat-embedding retinas in glycol methacrylate and the contralateral eye of each animal was embedded whole in glycol methacrylate for histopathologic analysis.

Retinal vascular occlusions resulted in nonperfused areas of retina and arteriovenous anastomoses. Intra- and extraretinal neovascularization was observed adjacent to nonperfused areas. Retinal pigmented lesions were formed by the migration of retinal pigment epithelial cells into sensory retina, often ensheathing choroidal neovascularization. Bilateral chorioretinopathy was present in 30 percent of animals older than age 15 months. These ocular histopathologic changes mimicked many aspects of human proliferative sickle cell retinopathy and permitted the detection of choroid abnormalities not previously characterized. When $\alpha^H\beta^S[\beta^{MDD}]$ mice were given horseradish peroxidase (HRP) intracardially, 42.5 percent of animals without any proliferative retinopathy had retinal blood vessels containing red cell plugs visualized by endogenous peroxidase activity and lacked lumenal HRP-reaction product (Lutty et al., 1998). Besides red cells, fibrin was sometimes present at sites of occlusion. In sections from whole eyes of the same animals, foci of photoreceptor degeneration were associated with areas of choriocapillaris nonperfusion (lumen that lacked HRP-reaction product). In areas with normal photoreceptors, the choriocapillaris appeared perfused and HRP-reaction product was present. In animals with proliferative chorioretinopathy, some neovascular formations lacked luminal HRP-reaction product, suggesting autoinfarction. Nonperfused retinal and choroidal vessels were observed in mice without retinal and choroidal neovascularization, whereas all mice with neovascularization had nonperfused areas. Small foci of HRP loss were associated with areas of nonperfused choriocapillaris. These results suggest that sickle cell–mediated retinal vasoocclusion is an initial event in the chorioretinopathy and outer retinal atrophy that occurs in these sickle transgenic mice.

In a rat model of sickle cell–mediated vasoocclusion in the retina and choroid, dense sickle cells were retained during normoxic conditions but their numbers increased as PO_2 decreased (Lutty et al., 1996) (Fig. 20.22). Neither the reticulocyte-rich sickle cell fraction nor a fraction HbSC disease red cells were retained in significant numbers, an intriguing result since sickle retinopathy is especially common in HbSC disease. Vascular occlusion in the retinal vasculature is the initiating event in sickle cell retinopathy. Red cells from sickle cell anemia patients or HbSC disease patients were separated by density, labeled with fluorescein isothiocyanate (FITC), and infused into ventilated rats. Blood gas levels were altered by changing inspired gas. The retinal vasculature was visualized under dark-field illumination and the FITC-RBCs visualized by fluorescence microscopy. Greater numbers of high-density sickle cells were retained in the normal rat retinal vasculature than normal-density sickle cells. Retention of

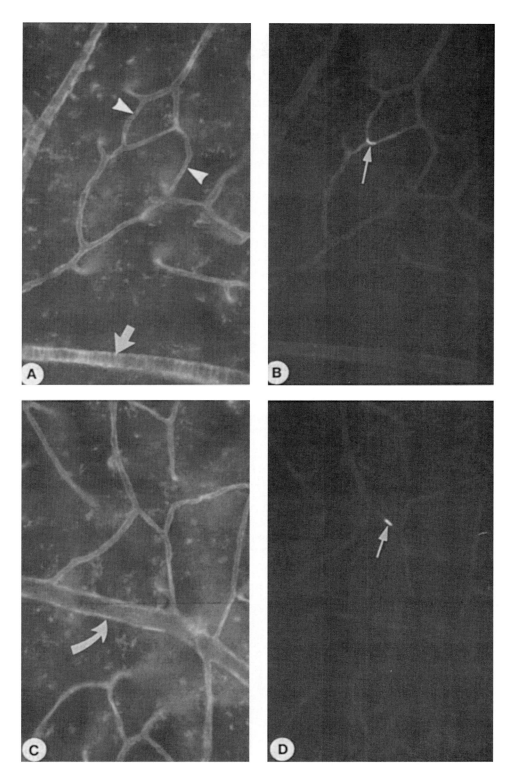

Figure 20.22. Multiple exposure micrograph showing an area in the far peripheral primary capillary network of the rat retina simultaneously demonstrates fluorescent-labeled cells and blood vessels. The SS4 RBCs (arrows) appear to occupy the entire luminal diameter of these capillaries. Magnification 120 ×. (From Lutty et al., 1996, with permission.)

dense sickle cells was inversely dependent on the arterial oxygen tension. Most dense sickle cells were retained in capillaries, but a few were observed within precapillary arterioles. The retained red cell occupied the full luminal diameter of vessels in most cases. In contrast, very few red cells of either normal or high density from

HbSC disease donors were retained in the normal retinal vasculature and retention did not increase significantly with hypoxia. This model demonstrates that high-density sickle cells, which include ISCs, are retained in normal rat retinal vessels and that the number retained is oxygen dependent. Furthermore, it appears that trapping, not adhesion, is responsible for retention of sickle cells in the normal retinal vasculature because there was preferential retention of dense cells, which are known to have lower adherence propensity, and the retained sickle cell blocked the full diameter of the vessel. These results also demonstrate that the mechanism of vascular obstruction by sickle cell anemia and and HbSC disease red cells is different because low retention of HbSC cells was observed.

To see if cytokines influence the retention of sickle erythrocytes in rat retina and if retention could be inhibited by blocking VLA-4 binding to VCAM-1, LPS was administered to rats 20 hours before or TNF-α given 5 hours before administration of density separated and labeled sickle red cells. LPS caused an increase in retention of reticulocyte-enriched fraction while retention of normal control cells was not increased (McLeod et al., 1999). Preincubation of normal-density sickle cells with a peptide that blocks VLA-4 binding to VCAM-1 (TBC-772) inhibited LPS-induced retention, while a control peptide (TBC-1194) had no effect. TNF-α caused a three- to fourfold increase in retention of normal-density cells but did not increase retention of control cells. Preincubation of cells with 200 μM TBC-772 completely inhibited the TNF-α–induced retention. Inhibition of normal-density sickle cell retention was also achieved by administering TBC-772 intravenously before giving the cells but less

inhibition was observed if TBC-772 was administered 8 hours before. It seems that TNF-α and LPS stimulate retention of normal density sickle cells in the retinal vasculature. Since retention can be blocked by VLA-4 antagonists the cells retained after cytokine stimulation may be reticulocytes.

McCally et al. (1999) have recently developed an in vivo noninvasive method to assess the velocity, adherence, and arteriovenous transit time of normal and sickle erythrocytes in retinal and choroidal vessels. FITC-tagged red cells can be observed in the retina of pigmented rats and on the choroid of albino rats. With this technique the authors observed that normal-density sickle cells were transiently retained in retinal vessels, a phenomenon not observed with normal human red cells. Contrary to previous dogma, the red cell flow on choroid was sluggish with even normal human red cells retained in the perimeter of lobules. Sickle red cells were retained in large numbers, in some cases for

Figure 20.23. Difference images of control and transgenic mice (100% O$_2$ vs. room air, 2.5T, TR 1500 msec, TE 40 msec). MRI of mice obtained by comparing the room air image collected while the animal was breathing 100 percent oxygen (B, C, and D). Red and yellow areas indicate positive differences (hypoxic areas) with red indicating the largest change; light and dark blue areas indicate negative differences: gray scale areas had no statistically significant difference. Anatomic image of the α^{H}β^{S}β^{S-Ant}[β^{MDD}] mouse in room air. K, kidney; Li, liver; Lu, lung; S, spleen. (B) Control mouse. Note that there are no *t* statistically significant areas over the kidneys or liver. (C) The same α^{H}β^{S}β^{S-Ant}[β^{MDD}] mouse seen in A. Note that the largest changes are over the liver and the medulla of the upper kidney. (D) An α^{H}β^{S}β^{S-Ant}[β^{MDD}] mouse. Note that the largest changes are over the medulla of the kidney. In this mouse, the spleen also shows changes characteristic of hypoxia. For full color reproduction, see color plate 20.23

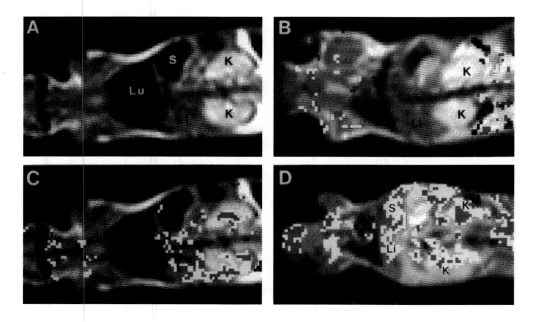

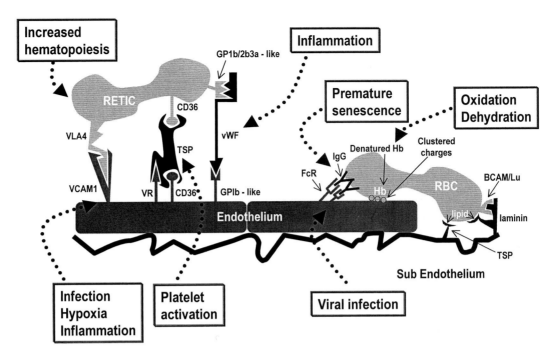

Figure 20.24. An attempt to summarize the pathophysiology of the pleiotropic effects in sickle cell anemia.

extended periods of time. These results suggest that the choroid-capillaris vasoocclusion can play an important role in sickle retinopathy.

Pathophysiology of the Renal Microcirculation. It is clear that the renal microcirculation, particularly in the medulla, is altered to the point that even sickle trait individuals can have renal abnormalities (urine concentration defect, bleeding from the renal papillae) (see Chapter 29). We have previously discussed the evidence that NO is playing an important role (Bank et al., 1998). To this picture has to be added the data from transgenic mice: that with the use of BOLD-MRI significant hypoxia in the blood of the medulla of the kidneys can be detected (Fig. 20.23). This observation establishes that the renal medulla is in constant danger of vasoocclusion, explaining the sickle cell anemia complications of concentration defect (universally), papillary necrosis, and eventual renal insufficiency, both restricted to a subset of patients.

SUMMARY

Central to the pathophysiology of sickle cell anemia is the capacity of HbS to polymerize and produce red cells that have decreased pliability. Still, sickle cell anemia, like many genetic diseases, is associated with multiple pleiotropic effectors (Fig. 20.24) that generate myriad secondary pathogenic events, which contribute to the phenotype of disease. These include (1) the increased capacity of sickle reticulocytes to adhere to the endothelium and to regulate their volume; yet, in some organs such as the lung, sickle cell adhesion might not be a major initiator of vasoocclusion; (2) rheologic/hemodynamic events that cause endothelial damage, alter flow, and cause abnormal vasodilation and an abnormal response to vasoactive substances; (3) a possible cytokine response to increased hematopoiesis and an inflammatory component to vasoocclusive events. Pleiotropic effects are then modified by epistatic effects that are polymorphic among individuals. They most likely include differences in vascular hemodynamics, adhesion, red cell membrane proteins, and cytokine response that account for the interindividual variability of vasoocclusive complications.

References

Adragna, NC, Fonseca, P, and Lauf, PK. (1994). Hydroxyurea affects cell morphology, cation transport, and red blood cell adhesion in cultured vascular endothelial cells. *Blood* 83: 553–560.

Akinola, NO, Stevens, SME, Franklin, IM et al. (1992). Subclinical ischaemic episodes during the steady state of sickle cell anaemia. *J. Clin. Pathol.* 45: 902–906.

Aldrich, TK, Dhuper, SK, Patwa, NS et al. (1996). Pulmonary entrapment of sickle cells: The role of regional alveolar hypoxia. *J. Appl. Physiol.* 80: 531–539.

Anderson, GL, Miller, FN, and Xiu, R-J. (1984). Inhibition of histamine-induced protein leakage in rat skeletal muscle by blockade of prostaglandin synthesis. *Microvasc. Res.* 28: 51–61.

Bailey, S, Higgs, DR, Morris, DR, Serjeant, GR. (1991). Is the painful crisis of sickle cell disease due to sickling? [letter]. *Lancet* 337: 735.

Bank, N, Aynedijan, HS, Qiu, J et al. (1996). Renal nitric oxide synthases in transgenic sickle cell mice. *Kidney International,* 50: 184–189.

Bank, N, Aynedijan, HS, Qiu, J et al. (1996). Renal nitric oxide synthases in transgenic sickle cell mice. *Kidney International,* 50: 184–189.

Barabino, GA, Liu, XD, Ewenstein, BM, and Kaul, DK. (1999). Anionic polysaccharides inhibit adhesion of sickle erythrocytes to the vascular endothelium and result in improved hemodynamic behavior. *Blood* 93, 1422–1429.

Barabino, GA, Wise, RJ, Woodbury, VA et al. (1997). Inhibition of sickle erythrocyte adhesion to immobilized thrombospondin by von Willebrand factor under dynamic flow conditions. *Blood* 89: 2560–2567.

Baum, KF, Dunn, DT, Maude, GH, and Serjeant, GR. (1987). The painful crisis of homozygous sickle cell disease: A study of risk factors. *Arch. Intern. Med.* 147: 1231–1234.

Becton, DL, Raymond, L, Thompson, C, and Berry, DH. (1989). Acute phase reactants in sickle cell anemia. *J. Pediatr.* 115: 99–102.

Beutler, E, Johnson, C, Powars, D, and West, C. (1974). Prevalence of glucose-6-phosphate dehydrogenase deficiency and sickle cell anemia. *N. Engl. J. Med.* 290: 826–828.

Billett, HH, Fabry, ME, and Nagel, RL. (1988b). The hemoglobin distribution width (HDW): A rapid assessment of dense red cells in the steady state and during painful crisis in sickle cell anemia. *J. Lab. Clin. Med.* 112: 339–344.

Billet, HH, Nagel, RL, and Fabry, ME. (1988a). Evolution of laboratory parameters during sickle cell painful crisis: Evidence compatible with dense red cell sequestration without thrombosis. *Am. J. Med. Sci.* 296: 293–8.

Bourantas, KL, Dalekos, GN, Makis, A et al. (1998). Acute phase proteins and interleukins in steady state sickle cell disease. *Eur. J. Haematol.* 61: 49–54.

Brittain, HA, Eckman, JR, Swerlick, RA et al. (1993). Thrombospondin from activated platelets promotes sickle erythrocyte adherence to human microvascular endothelium under physiologic flow: A potential role for platelet activation in sickle cell vaso-occlusion. *Blood* 81: 2137.

Cheresh, DA. (1987). Human endothelial cells synthesize and express an Arg-Gly-Asp-directed adhesion receptor involved in attachment to fibrinogen and von Willebrand factor. *Proc. Natl. Acad. Sci. U.S.A.* 84: 6471–6475.

Chien, S. (1977). Rheology of sickle cells and erythrocytes content. *Blood Cells* 3: 283–303.

Chien, S, Dormandy, J, Matrai, A, eds (1987). *Clinical hemorheology.* Martinus Nijhoff, Dordrecht.

Clark, IA, Rockett, KA, and Cowden, WB. (1991). Proposed link between cytokines, nitric oxide and human cerebral malaria. *Parasitol. Today* 7: 205–207.

Crandall, I, Collins, WE, Gysin, J, and Sherman, I. (1993). Synthetic peptides based on motifs present in human band 3 protein inhibit cytoadherence/sequestration of the malaria parasite *Plasmodium falciparum. Proc. Natl. Acad. Sci. U.S.A.* 90: 4703–4707.

Croizat, H and Nagel, RL. (1988). Circulating BFU-E in sickle cell anemia: Relationship to % HbF and BPA-like activity. *Exp. Hematol.* 16: 946–949.

Croizat, H and Nagel, RL. (1993). Inhomogeneity of the circulating BFU-E regulation in sickle cell anaemia: Accessory cells properties and BFU-E growth factor response pattern. *Br. J. Hematol.* 84: 481–487.

Croizat, HP and Nagel, RL. (1999). Circulating cytokines response and the level of erythropoiesis in sickle cell anemia. *Am. J. Hematol.* 60: 105–115.

Croizat, H, Billett, HH, and Nagel, RL. (1990). Heterogeneity in the properties of burst-forming units of erythroid lineage in sickle cell anemia: DNA synthesis and burst-promoting activity production is related to peripheral hemoglobin F levels. *Blood* 75: 1006–1010.

Croizat, H and Raventos-Suarez, C. (1993). Circulating CD^{34+} cells in sickle cell anemia have distinct properties according to peripheral fetal hemoglobin. *Blood* 82: 34 (abstract).

Croizat, H, Ponchio, L, Nagel, RL, and Eaves, CJ. Characterization of primitive hematopoietic progenitors in the blood of patients with sickle cell anemia. *British J. Hematol.* In press.

Crosby, WH and Akeroyd, JH. (1952). The limit of hemoglobin synthesis in hereditary hemolytic anemia. *Am. J. Med.* 13: 273–283.

DHHS Publication No. (PHS) 83–1682. Washington: US Government Printing Office.

Diggs, LW and Ching, RE. (1934). Pathology of sickle cell anemia. *South. Med. J.* 27: 839–845.

Dover, GJ, Boyer, SH, Charache, S, and Heintzelman, K. (1978). Individual variation in the production and survival of F cells in sickle-cell disease. *N. Engl. J. Med.* 299: 1428–1435.

Eaton, WA and Hofrichter, J. Sickle cell hemoglobin polymerization. *Adv. Protein Chem.* 1990; 40: 63–279.

Embury, SH, Clark, MR, Monroy, G, and Mohandas, N. (1984). Concurrent sickle cell anemia and α-thalassemia: Effect on pathological properties of sickle erythrocytes. *J. Clin. Invest.* 73: 116–123.

Embury, SH, Mohandas, N, Paszty, C, Cooper, P et al. (1999). In vivo blood flow abnormalities in the transgenic knockout sickle cell mouse. *J. Clin. Invest.* 103: 915–920.

Erslev, AJ, Wilson, J, and Caro, J. (1987). Erythropoietin titers in anemic, non-uremic patients. *J. Lab. Clin. Med.* 109: 429–433.

Fabry, ME. (1994). Transgenic animal models. In Embury, SH, Hebbel, RP, Mohandas, N, and Steinberg, MH, editors. *Sickle cell disease—basic principles and clinical practice.* New York: Raven Press, pp. 105–120.

Fabry, ME and Nagel, RL. (1983). The effects of deoxygenation on red cell density: Significance for the pathophysiology of sickle cell anemia. *Blood* 60: 1370.

Fabry, ME, Benjamin, L, Lawrence, C, and Nagel, RL. (1984). An objective sign in painful crisis in sickle cell anemia: The concomitant reduction of high density red cells. *Blood* 64: 559–563.

Fabry, ME, Costantini, F, Pachnis, A et al. (1992a). High expression of human of βˢ and α-globin chains in transgenic mice: Erythrocyte abnormalities, organ damage, and the effect of hypoxia. *Proc. Natl. Acad. Sci. U.S.A.* 89: 12155–12159.

Fabry, ME, Fine, E, Rajanayagam, V et al. (1992b). Demonstration of endothelial adhesion of sickle cells in vivo: A distinct role for deformable sickle cell discocytes. *Blood* 79: 1602–1611.

Fabry, ME, Sengupta, A, Suzuka, SM et al. (1995a). A second generation transgenic mouse model expressing both hemoglobin S (HbS) and HbS-Antilles results in increased phenotypic severity. *Blood* 86: 2419–2428.

Fabry, ME, Suzuka, SM, Rubin, EM et al. (1995b). Strategies for amelioration of sickle cell disease: Use of the transgenic mouse for validation of anti-sickling strategies. In Beuzard, Y, Lubin, B, and Rosa, J, editors. *Sickle cell disease and thalassaemias: New trends in therapy* (proceedings of INSERM Symposium, Paris). Montrouge, France: Colloque INSERM/John Libbey Eurotext. pp. 252–262.

Fahraeus, R. (1928). Die Stromungsverhaltnisse und die Verteilung der Blutzellen im Gefasssystem. *Klin. Wschr.* 7: 100–106.

Fahraeus, R and Lindqvist, T. (1929). The viscosity of blood in narrow capillary tubes. *Am. J. Physiol.* 96: 562–568.

Fox, JR and Wayland, H. (1979). Interstitial diffusion of macromolecules in the rat mesentery. *Microvasc. Res.* 18: 255–276.

Gaehtgens, P, Pries, AR, and Ley, K. (1987). Structural hemodynamic and rheological characteristics of blood flow in the circulation. In Chien, S, Dormandy, J, and Matrai, A, eds. *Clinical hemorheology*. Martinus Nijhoff Dordrecht.

Galili, U. (1988). The natural anti-Gal antibody, the B-like antibody, and human red cell aging. *Blood Cells* 14: 205–228.

Galili, U, Clark, MR, Mohandas, N, Rachmilewitz, E et al. (1985). The natural anti-alpha galactosyl IgG on red cells of sickle cell anemia. *Blood* 64: 48a.

Galili, U, Clark, MR, and Shohet, SB. (1987). Excessive binding of natural anti-alpha-galactosyl immunoglobinG to sickle erythrocytes may contribute to extravascular cell destruction. *J. Clin. Invest.* 77: 27–33.

Gee, BE and Platt, OS. (1995). Sickle erythrocytes adhere to VCAM-1. *Blood* 85: 268–274.

Gibbs, WN, Wardle, J, and Serjeant, GR. (1981). Glucose-6-phosphate dehydrogenase deficiency and homozygous sickle cell disease. *Br. J. Haematol.* 48: 533–543.

Ginsburg, V and Roberts, DD. (1988). Glycoconjugates and cell adhesion: the adhesive proteins laminin, thrombospondin and von Willebrand factor's bind specifically to sulfated glycolipids. *Biochimie* 70: 1651–1659.

Gladwin, MT, Schechter, AN, Shelhammer, JH, and Ognibene, FP. (1999). The acute chest syndrome in sickle cell disease. Possible role of nitric oxide in its pathophysiology and treatment. *Am. J. Crit. Care. Med.* 159: 1368–1376.

Green, GA, Rehn, MM, and Karla, VK. (1985). Cell bound autologous immunoglobulins in erythrocytes subpopulations from patients with sickle cell disease. *Blood* 65: 1127–1133.

Gumbs, RM, Higginbotham-Ford, EA, Teal, JS et al. (1987). Thoracic extramedullary hematopoiesis in sickle cell disease. *A.J.R.* 149: 889–893.

Hammerman, SI, Kourembanas, S, Conca, TJ et al. (1997). Endothelin-1 production during the acute chest syndrome in sickle cell disease. *Am. J. Respir. Crit. Care Med.* 156: 280–285.

Harkness, DR and Roth, S. (1975). Clinical evaluation of cyanate in sickle cell anemia. *Prog. Hematol.* 9: 157–184.

Hayes, RJ, Beckford, M, Grandison, Y et al. (1985). The haematology of steady state homozygous sickle cell disease. 1. Frequency distribution longitudinal observations, effects of age and sex. *Br. J. Haematol.* 59: 369–382.

Haynes, J Jr, Taylor, AE, Dixon, D, and Voelkel, N. (1993). Microvascular hemodynamics in the sickle red blood cell–perfused isolated rat lung. *Am. J. Physiol.* 264: H484–489.

Hebbel, RP and Miller, VB. (1984). Phagocytosis of sickle erythrocytes: Immunological and oxidative determinants of hemolytic anemia. *Blood* 64: 733–741.

Hebbel RP. (1994). Membrane-associated iron. In Embury, SH, Hebbel, RP, Mohandas, N, and Steinberg, MH, eds. *Sickle cell disease-basic principles and clinical practice.* Raven Press, New York, pp. 163–172.

Hebbel, RP, Visser, MR, Goodman, JL et al. (1987). Potentiated adherence of sickle erythrocytes to endothelium infected by virus. *J. Clin. Invest.* 80: 1503–1506.

Hebbel, RP, Yamada, O, Moldow, CF et al. (1980). Abnormal adherence of sickle erythrocytes to cultured vascular endothelium: Possible mechanism for microvascular occlusion in sickle cell disease. *J. Clin. Invest.* 65: 154–160.

Hillery, CA, Ming, MC, Montogomery, RR, and Scott, JP. (1996). Increased adhesion of erythrocytes to components of the extracellular matrix: Isolation and characterization of a red blood cell lipid that binds thrombospondin and laminin. *Blood* 87: 4879–4886.

Hiruma, H, Noguchi, CT, Uyesaka, N et al. (1995). Sickle cell rheology is determined by polymer fraction–not cell morphology *Am. J. Hematol.* 48(1): 19–28.

Hofrichter, J, Ross, PD, and Eaton, WA. (1974). Kinetics and mechanism of deoxyhemoglobin S gelation: A new approach to understanding sickle cell disease. *Proc. Natl. Acad. Sci. U.S.A.* 71: 4864–4868.

Imaizumi, TA, Stafforini, DM, Yamada, Y et al. (1995). Platelet-activating factor: a mediator for clinicians. *J. Int. Med.* 238: 5–20.

Joneckis, CC, Shock, DD, Cunningham, ML et al. (1996). Glycoprotein IV-independent adhesion of sickle red blood cells to immobilized thrombospondin under flow conditions. *Blood* 87: 4862–4870.

Joneckis, CC, Rhonda, RL, Orringer, EP et al. (1993). Integrin α4β1 and glycoprotein IV (CD36) are expressed on circulating reticulocytes in sickle cell anemia. *Blood* 82: 3548–3555.

Katusic, ZS and Cosentino, F. (1994). Nitric oxide synthase: From molecular biology to cerebrovascular physiology. *NIPS* 9: 64–67.

Kaul, DK, Baez, S, and Nagel, RL. (1981). Flow properties of oxygenated HbS and HbC erythrocytes in the isolated microvasculature of the rat. *Clin. Hemorrheol.* 1: 73–79.

Kaul, DK, Chen, D, and Zhan, J. (1994b). Adhesion of sickle cells to vascular endothelium is critically dependent on changes in density and shape of the cells. *Blood* 83: 3006–3017.

Kaul, DK, Fabry, ME, Costantini, F et al. (1995a). In vivo demonstration of red cell-endothelial interaction, sickling and altered microvascular response to oxygen in the sickle transgenic mouse. *J. Clin. Invest.* 96: 2845–2853.

Kaul, DK, Fabry, ME, and Nagel, RL. (1989). Microvascular sites and characteristics of sickle cell adhesion to vascular endothelium in shear flow conditions: Pathophysiological implications. *Proc. Natl. Acad. Sci. U.S.A.* 86: 3356–3360.

Kaul, DK, Fabry, ME, Windisch, P et al. (1983a). Erythrocytes in sickle cell anemia. *Clin. Invest.* 72: 22a.

Kaul, DK, Nagel, RL, and Baez, S. (1983b). Pressure effects on the flow behavior of sickle (HbSS) red cells in isolated (ex-vivo) microvascular system. *Microvasc. Res.* 26: 170–181.

Kaul, DK, Nagel, RL, Chen, D, and Tsai, HM. (1993). Sickle erythrocyte-endothelial interactions in microcirculation: The role of von Willebrand factor and implications for vasoocclusion. *Blood* 81: 2429–2438.

Kaul, DK, Nagel, RL, Llena, JF, and Shear, HL. (1994). Cerebral malaria in mice: Demonstration of cytoadherence of infected red cells and microrheologic correlates. *Am. J. Trop. Med. Hyg.* 50: 512–521.

Kaul, DK, Liu, XD, Fabby, HE, and Nagel, RL (2000a). Impaired nitric-oxide-mediated vasodilation in transgenic sickle mouse *Am J. Physiol* (Heart Circ. Physiol) 270: in press.

Kaul DK, Liu XD, Nagel RL, and Shear, HL. (1998). Microvascular hemodynamics and in vivo evidence for the role of intercellular adhesion molecule-1 in the sequestration of infected red blood cells in a mouse model of lethal malaria. Am. J. Trop. Med. Hyg. 58: 240–247.

Kaul, DK, Tsai, HM, Liu, XD et al. (2000). Monoclonal antibodies to alpha Vbeta3 (7E3 and LM609) inhibit sickle red blood cell-endothelium interactions induced by platelet-activating factor. *Blood* 2000b: 368–374.

Kaul, DK, Tsai, HM, Nagel, RL, and Chen, D. (1995b). Platelet-activating factor enhances adhesion of sickle erythrocytes to vascular endothelium: The role of vascular integrin $\alpha_v\beta_3$ and von Willebrand factor. In Beuzard, Y, Lubin, B, and Rosa, J, eds. *Sickle cell disease and thalassaemias: New trends in therapy* (proceedings of INSERM Symposium, Paris, September 19–22, 1994). Montrouge, France: Colloque INSERM/John Libbey Eurotext. pp. 497–500.

Kaul, DK and Xue, H. (1991). Rate of deoxygenation and rheologic behavior of blood in sickle cell anemia Blood. 77: 1353–1361.

Klug, PP and Lessin, LS. (1977). Microvascular blood flow of sickled erythrocytes. *Blood Cells* 3: 273–282.

Klug, PP, Kay, N, and Jensen, WN. (1982). Endothelial cell and vascular damage in the sickle cell disorders. *Blood Cells* 8: 175–184.

Kopito, RR and Lodish, HF. (1985). Primary structure and transmembrane orientation of the murine anion exchange protein. *Nature* 316: 234–238.

Kourembanas, S, Marsden, PA, McQuillan, LP, and Faller, DV. (1991). Hypoxia induces endothelin gene expression and secretion in cultured human endothelium. *J. Clin. Invest.* 88: 1054–1057.

LaCelle, PL. (1977). Oxygen delivery to muscle cells during capillary occlusion by sickled erythrocytes. *Blood Cells* 3: 273–284.

Lipowsky, HH, Usami, S, and Chien, S. (1982). Human SS red cell rheological behavior in the microcirculation of cremaster muscle. *Blood Cells* 8: 113–126.

Lipowsky, HH, Sheikh, NU, and Katz, DM. (1987). Intravital microscopy of capillary hemodynamics in sickle cell disease. *J. Clin. Invest.* 80: 117–127.

Lonsdorfer, J, Bogui, P, Otayeck, A et al. (1983). Cardiorespiratory adjustments in chronic sickle cell anemia. *Bull. Eur. Physiopath. Resp* 19: 339–344.

Low, PS. (1989). Interaction of native and denatured hemoglobins with band 3: consequences for erythrocyte structure and function. In Agre, P and Parker, JC, eds. Red Blood Cell Membrane, pp. 237–260, Marcel Dekker Inc, New York and Basel, 1989.

Lutty, GA, Merges, C, Crone, S, and McLeod, DS. (1994a). Immunohistochemical insights into sickle cell retinopathy. *Curr. Eye. Res.* 13: 125–138.

Lutty, GA, McLeod, DS, Pachnis, A et al. (1994b). Retinal and choroidal neovascularization in a transgenic mouse model of sickle cell disease. *Am. J. Pathol.* 145: 490–497.

Lutty, GA, Phelan, A, McLeod, DS et al. (1996). A rat model for sickle cell-mediated vaso-occlusion in retina. *Microvasc. Res.* 52: 270–280.

Lutty, GA, Merges, C, McLeod, DS et al. (1998). Nonperfusion of retina and choroid in transgenic mouse models of sicklecell disease. *Curr. Eye. Res.* 17: 438–444.

Lux, SE, John, KM, Kopito, RN, and Lodish, HF. (1989). Cloning and characterization of band 3, the human erythrocyte anion-exchange protein. *Proc. Natl. Acad. Sci. U.S.A.* 86: 9089–9093.

Mackie, I, Bull, H, and Brozovic, M. (1980). Altered factor VIII complexes in sickle cell disease. *Br. J. Hematol.* 46: 499.

Marsden, PD and Shah, KK. (1964). Artificially induced edema in sickle cell anemia. *J. Trop. Med. Hyg.* 67: 31.

Matrai, A, Wittington, RB, and Skalak, R. (1987). Biophysics. In Chein, S, Dormandy, J, and Matrai, A, eds. *Clinical hemorrheology.* Martinus Nijhoff Dordrecht.

McCally, RL, Wajer, SD, Nishiwaki, H et al. (1999). Hemodynamic properties of red blood cells in the retina and choroidal vasculatures and applications to sickle cell disease. *Invest. Ophthalmol. Vis. Sci.* 40 (Suppl): s486.

McCurdy, PR and Sherman, AS. (1978). Irreversibly sickled cells and red cell survival in sickle cell anemia. A study with both DF^{32}P and ^{51}Cr. *Am. J. Med.* 64: 253.

McLeod, DS, Goldberg, MF, and Lutty, GA. (1993). Dual-perspective analysis of vascular formations in sickle cell retinopathy. *Arch. Ophthalmol.* 111: 1234–1245.

McLeod, DS, Merges, C, Fukushima, A, Goldberg, MF et al. (1997). Histopathologic features of neovascularization in sickle cell retinopathy *Am. J. Ophthalmol.* 124: 455–472.

McLeod, DS, Cao, J, Taomoto, M, Vanderslice, P et al. (1999). Antagonist inhibits cytokine-stimulated sickle cell retention in rat retina. *Invest. Ophthalmol Vis. Sci.* 40 (suppl): s707.

Miller, JM, Dickens, AM, Quitiquit, EM, and Davis, DC. (1980). A new isoenzyme of lactate dehydrogenase associated with sickle cell hemoglobin. *J. Natl. Med. Assoc.* 72: 231–236.

Milner, PF, Garbutt, GJ, Nolan-Davis, LV et al. (1986). The effect of HbF and alpha thalassemia on the red cell indices in sickle cell anemia. *Am. J. Hematol.* 21: 383–395.

Mohandas, N, Clark, MR, Kissinger, S et al. (1980). Inaccuracies associated with the automated measurement of mean cell hemoglobin concentration in dehydrated cells. *Blood* 56: 125–128.

Mosseri, M, Bartlett-Pandite, AN, Wenc, K et al. (1993). Inhibition of endothelial-dependent vasorelaxation by sickle erythrocytes. *Am. Heart. J.* 126: 338–346.

Mozzarelli, A, Hofrichter, J, and Eaton, WA. (1987). Delay time of hemoglobin S polymerization prevents most cells from sickling in vivo. *Science* 237: 500–506.

Muller-Eberhard, U, Javid, J, Liem, HH, and Hanstein, HM. (1968). Plasma concentrations of hemopexin, haptoglobin and heme in patients with various hemolytic diseases. *Blood* 32: 811–815.

Nagel, RL. (1994). Lessons from transgenic mouse lines expressing sickle hemoglobin. *Proc. Soc. Exp. Med. Biol.* 205: 274–281.

Nagel, RL and Fabry, ME. (1985). The many pathophysiologies of sickle cell anemia. *Am. J. Hematol.* 20: 195–199.

Nagel, RL, Fabry, MF, Pagnier, J et al. (1985). Hematologically and genetically distinct forms of sickle cell anemia in Africa: The Senegal type and the Benin type. *N. Engl. J. Med.* 312: 880–885.

Nagel RL: Sickle cell anemia is a multigene disease: Sickle Painful Crises, A Case in Point. *Am. J. Hematol.* 42: 96–101, 1992.

Nash, GB, Johnson, CS, and Meiselman, HJ. (1986). Influence of oxygen tension on the viscoelastic behavior of red blood cells in sickle cell disease. *Blood* 67: 110–118.

Natarajan, M, Udden, MM, and McIntire, LV. (1996). Adhesion of sickle red blood cells and damage to interleukin-1β stimulated endothelial cells under flow in vitro. *Blood* 87: 4845–4852.

Nicoll, PA and Webb, RL. (1955). Vascular pattern and active vasomotion as determinants of flow through minute vessels. *Angiology* 6: 291–310.

Odenheimer, DJ, Whitten, CF, Rucknagel, DL, Sarnaik, SA et al. (1984). Stability over time of hematological variables in 197 children with sickle cell anemia. *Am. J. Med. Genet.* 18: 461–470.

Pannathur-Das, R, Alpen, E, Vichinsky, E et al. (1984). Evidence for the presence of CFU-E with increased in vitro sensitivity to erythropoietin in sickle cell anemia. *Blood* 63: 1169–1174.

Petz, LD, Yam, P, Wilkinson, L et al. (1984). Increased IgG molecules bound to the surface of red blood cells of patients with sickle cell anemia. *Blood* 64: 301–304.

Phelan, M, Perrine, SP, Brauer, M, and Faller, DV. (1995). Sickle erythrocytes, after sickling, regulate the expression of the endothelin-1 gene and protein in human endothelial cells in culture. *J. Clin. Invest.* 96: 1145–1151.

Platt, OS, Rosenstock, W, and Espeland, MA. (1984). Influence of sickle hemoglobinopathies on growth and development. *N Engl J Med* 311(1): 7–12.

Ponchio, L, Conneally, E, and Eaves, C. (1995). Quantitate of the quiescent fraction of long-term culture initiating cells in normal human blood and marrow and the kinetics of their growth factor-stimulated entry into S-phase in vitro. *Blood* 86: 3314–3321.

Powars, DR, Schroeder, WA, Weiss, JN et al. (1980). Lack of influence of fetal hemoglobin levels or erythrocyte indices on the severity of sickle cell anemia. *J. Clin. Invest.* 65: 732–740.

Rao, RP and Patel, AR. (1987). Erythrocytic ecdysis in smears of EDTA venous blood in eight patients with sickle cell anemia. *Blood Cells* 12: 543–550.

Roddie, IC. (1960). Circulation to skin and adipose tissue. In *Handbook of physiology*. Vol. III, Section 2. Bethesda, MD. American Physiological Society.

Rodgers, GP, Schechter, AN, Noguchi, CT et al. (1984). Periodic microcirculatory flow in patients with sickle-cell disease. *N. Engl. J. Med.* 311: 1534–1538.

Rhoda, MD, Domenget, C, Vidaud, M, Bardakdjian, M et al. (1988). Mouse alpha chains inhibit polymerization of hemoglobin induced by human β S or beta S-Antilles chains. *Biochim. Biophys. Acta* 952: 208–213.

Richardson, SGN, Matthews, KB, Stuart, J et al. (1979). Serial changes in coagulation and viscosity during sickle-cell crisis. *Brit. J. Hematol.* 41: 95–103.

Roberts, DD, Williams, SB, Gralnick, HR, and Ginsburg, V. (1986). von Willebrand factor binds specifically to sulfated glycolipids. *J. Biol. Chem.* 261: 3306–3309.

Roy, MS, Gascon, P, and Giuliani, D. (1995). Macular blood flow velocity in sickle cell disease: Relation to red cell density. *Br. J. Ophthalmol.* 79: 742–745.

Rossi, EC, Westring, DW, Santos, AS, and Gutierrez, J. (1964). Hypersplenism in sickle cell anemia. *Arch. Intern. Med.* 114: 408–412.

Schmaltzer, EA, Lee, JO, Brown, AK et al. (1987). Viscosity of mixtures of sickle and normal red cells at varying hematocrit levels: Implications for transfusion. *Transfusion* 27: 228–233.

Seidler, RC and Becker, JA. (1968). Intra-thoracic extramedullary hematopoiesis. *Radiology* 83: 1057–1059.

Setty, BN and Stuart, MJ. (1996). Vascular cell adhesion molecule-1 is involved in mediating hypoxia-induced sickle red blood cell adherence to endothelium: potential role in sickle cell disease. *Blood* 1996; 88: 2311–2320.

Serjeant, GR and Chalmers, RM. (1990). Is the painful crisis of sickle cell disease a "steal" syndrome? *J. Clin. Pathol.* 43: 789–791.

Serjeant, GR, Serjeant, BE, and Milner, PF. (1969). The irreversibly sickled cell: A determinant of hemolysis in sickle cell anemia. *Br. J. Haematol.* 17: 527.

Serjeant, GR, Grandison, Y, Lowrie, Y et al. (1981). The development of haematological changes in homozygous sickle cell disease: A cohort study from birth to 6 years. *Br. J. Haematol.* 48: 533–543.

Serjeant, G, Serjeant, B, Stephens, A et al. (1996). Determinant of hemoglobin level in steady state homozygous sickle cell disease. *Br. J. Haematol.* 92: 143–149.

Sherwood, JB, Goldwasser, E, Chilcote, R et al. (1986). Sickle cell anemia patients have low erythropoietin levels for their degree of anemia. *Blood* 67: 46–49.

Singhal, A, Doherty, JF, Raynes, JG et al. (1993). Is there an acute-phase response in steady-state sickle cell disease? *Lancet* 341: 651–653.

Smolinski, PA, Offermann, MK, Eckman, JR, and Wick, TM. (1995). Double-stranded RNA induces sickle erythrocyte adherence to endothelium: A potential role for viral infection in vaso-occlusive pain episodes in sickle cell anemia. *Blood* 85: 2945–2950.

Solanki, DP. (1985). Erythrophagocytosis in vivo in sickle cell anemia. *Am. J. Hematol.* 20: 353–357.

Steinberg, MH, Adams, JG, and Lovell, WJ. (1977). Sickle cell anemia: Erythrokinetics, blood volumes, and a study of possible determinants of severity. *Am. J. Hematol.* 2: 17–23.

Steinberg, MH, West, MS, Gallagher, D, and Mentzer, W. (1988). Effects of glucose-6-phosphate dehydrogenase deficiency upon sickle cell anemia. *Blood* 71: 748–752.

Stuart, J. (1993). Acute phase response and sickle crisis. *Lancet* 341: 664–665.

Styles, LA, Schalkwijk, CG, Aarsman, AJ et al. (1996). Phospholipase A2 levels in acute chest syndrome of sickle cell disease. *Blood* 87: 2573–2578.

Sugihara, K, Sugihara, T, Mohandas, N, and Hebbel, RP. (1992). Thrombospondin mediates CD36+ sickle reticulocytes to endothelial cells. *Blood* 80: 2634–2642.

Sutherland, HJ, Eaves, CJ, Eaves, AC et al. (1989). Characterization and partial purification of human marrow cells capable of initiating long-term hematopoiesis in vitro. *Blood* 74: 1563–1570.

Sutherland, HJ, Lansdorp, PM, Henkelman, DH et al. (1990). Functional characterization of individual human hematopoietic stem cells cultured at limiting dilution on supportive marrow stromal layers. *Proc. Natl. Acad. Sci. U.S.A.* 87: 3584–3588.

Swerlick, RA, Eckman, Jr, Kumar, A, Jeitler, M, and Wick, TM. (1993). α4β1-integrin expression on sickle reticulocytes: vascular cell adhesion molecule-1 dependent binding to endothelium. *Blood* 82: 1891–1899.

Tanner, MJ, Martin, PG, and High, S. (1988). The complete amino acid sequence of the human erythrocyte membrane anion-transport protein deduced from the cDNA sequence. *Biochem J* 256: 703–712.

Thevenin, BJ-M, Rossi ME, Crandall, IW et al. (1995). Inhibition of sickle cell cytoadherence by peptides from exofacially exposed sites of band 3. *J. Invest. Med.* 43: 341A (abstr).

Vargas, FF and Blackshear GI. (1982). Vascular resistance and transit time of sickle red blood cells. *Blood Cells* 8: 139–143.

Vordermeier, S, Singh, S, Biggerstaff, J et al. (1992). Red blood cells from patients with sickle cell disease exhibit an increased adherence to cultured endothelium pretreated with tumour necrosis factor (TNF). *Br. J. Haematol.* 81: 591–597.

Westerman, MP, Cole, ER, and Wu, K. (1984). The effect of spicules obtained from sickle red cells on clotting activity. *Br. J. Haematol.* 56: 557–562.

Wick, TM, Moake, JL, Udden, MM et al. (1987). Unusually large von Willebrand factor multimers increase adhesion of sickle erythrocytes to human endothelial cells under controlled flow. *J. Clin. Invest.* 8: 905–910.

Wick, TM, Moake, JL, Udden, MM, and McIntire, LV. (1993). Unusually large von Willebrand factor multimers preferentially promote young sickle and non sickle erythrocyte adhesion to endothelial cells. *Am. J. Hematol.* 42: 284–292.

Yoshizumi, M, Perrella, MA, Burnett, JC Jr, and Lee, ME. (1993). Tumor necrosis factor downregulates an endothelial nitric oxide synthase mRNA by shortening its half-life. *Circ. Res.* 73: 205–209.

Zweifach, BW and Lipowsky, HH. (1984). Pressure-flow relations in blood and lymph microcirculation. In Renkin, EM and Michen, CC, editors. *Handbook of physiology (Section 2: Cardiovascular system). Volume IV, Microcirculation (Part I).* Bethesda, MD: American Physiological Society, pp. 251–308.

21

Cell Adhesion and Microrheology in Sickle Cell Disease

ROBERT P. HEBBEL
NARLA MOHANDAS

It is likely that numerous red cell abnormalities contribute to the complex pathophysiology of sickle cell disease (Hebbel, 1991; Embury et al., 1994). In this chapter we address two factors that relate to the interaction of sickle red cells with their environment: cellular adhesion and membrane microrheology. These aspects of red cell pathobiology are directly relevant to the cardinal clinical features of sickle cell disease, vasoocclusion, and hemolytic anemia.

RED CELL INTERACTIONS WITH ENDOTHELIUM

Since the seminal observations of sickle cell adhesivity (Hoover et al., 1979; Hebbel et al., 1980b), many studies have confirmed and extended the observation that sickle red cells are abnormally adherent to vascular endothelial cells (tabulated in Hebbel and Mohandas, 1994). This phenomenon has been documented using various sources of endothelium (murine; bovine; rat; human umbilical vein, artery, and microvascular) and differing suspending media (platelet-rich or platelet-poor plasma, serum, culture medium, balanced salt solution, whole blood). Various in vitro methods, including both static adhesion assays (with contact facilitated by gravity or centrifugation or pipettes) and flow models (flow chambers, or perfusion of umbilical cords or rodent microvascular beds) have been used to document increased adherence of sickle cells. Most recently, red cell adhesion to endothelium has been observed in vivo using the sickle transgenic mouse (Kaul et al., 1995).

Tenacity of Adherence

Application of increasing shear force to sickle red cells that are already adherent to endothelial cells results in their progressive removal (Smith and LaCelle, 1986; Barabino et al., 1987a; Rowland et al., 1993), revealing heterogeneity in tenacity of adherence. Under flowing conditions, some sickle red cells actually cease movement, but others exhibit rolling along the endothelium as a result of weaker interactions (Barabino et al., 1987a; Kaul et al., 1989). Thus, the standard use of a thorough prewash period in published flow chamber studies (e.g., Barabino et al., 1987a; Wick et al., 1987; Brittain et al., 1993; Swerlick et al., 1993) excludes from analysis any red cells that are adhering with lower tenacity. This complicates attempts to compare adhesion measured in demanding (i.e., flowing) systems versus that observed in less demanding systems (static adhesion assays).

As measured by micropipette technology (Fig. 21.1A), the force (applied normal to the bovine endothelial surface) necessary to detach adherent human red cells was found to be somewhat greater for sickle than for normal cells: 3.08 ± 1.14 versus $2.19 \pm 1.36 \times 10^{-6}$ dyne (Mohandas and Evans, 1984). However, this report underestimated the actual adhesive force for the sickle cells because the calculations failed to take into account the significantly elevated shear modulus (stiffness) of sickle membranes (Evans et al., 1984). Factoring that in, we estimate that the force needed to detach sickle cells from the endothelial surface actually was 10 to 15 times greater than that required for normal red cells. It is likely that forces at least 100-fold higher than those measured in vitro are needed to detach adherent sickle red cells in vivo, since sickle cells tend to adhere at multiple points of contact (Fig. 21.1B) (Mohandas and Evans, 1984) and since physiologic detaching forces are applied tangential to the endothelial cell surface (Fig. 21.1C). Thus, once sickle cells adhere to the vessel wall, they would be extremely difficult to dislodge under physiologic conditions. In fact, some investigators have observed sickle red cells adhering to endothelial cells at shear stress values ranging from 10 to 55 dyne/cm^2 (Kucukcelebi et al., 1980; Smith and LaCelle, 1986; Grabowski, 1987). On the other hand, sickle red cell adherence virtually disappeared at applied shear stress of 2 dyne/cm^2 in the parallel palate flow chamber (Barabino et al., 1987a),

Martin H. Steinberg, Bernard G. Forget, Douglas R. Higgs, and Ronald L. Nagel, editors. *Disorders of Hemoglobin: Genetics, Pathophysiology, and Clinical Management.* © 2001 Cambridge University Press. All rights reserved.

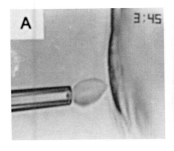
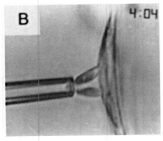
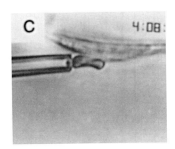

Figure 21.1. Micropipette measurement of red cell adhesivity to endothelium. Individual sickle red cells adherent to bovine endothelial cells (on the surface of microculture beads) were removed by micropipette in the normal direction, and strength of adhesion was calculated (**A**). Some sickle cells exhibit only a single strong contact point (**A**), while others adhere via multiple points of contact (**B**). When red cell removal is attempted in the tangential, physiologic direction (**C**), forces as much as 100 times greater are required. (From Mohandas and Evans, 1985, with permission.)

predicting relevance to only the low shear microvascular beds. Consistent with this, the endothelial adherence of human sickle red cells in the rat microcirculation increases dramatically as venule size diminishes and is maximal in the postcapillary venules (Fig. 21.2) (Kaul et al., 1989). This has been confirmed by observations in the sickle transgenic mouse (Kaul et al., 1995). However, this approach has not resolved whether those cells found immobile in the capillaries have become lodged because they are adherent, poorly deformable, or both.

Adherent Red Cell Subpopulations

Studies attempting to identify the most adherent subpopulation of sickle red cells have provided conflicting results. These can be reconciled, for the most part, by the existence of multiple adherence mechanisms and the fact that various experimental systems demand different tenacities of adhesion to distinguish adherent from nonadherent red cells. Overall, the published data (reviewed in Hebbel and Mohandas, 1994) support the notion that sickle red cells from all density fractions are abnormally adhesive; that is, this is not just a reticulocyte phenomenon. However, the least-dense reticulocyte-rich population is generally found to be the most adhesive subpopulation in studies employing flowing conditions (Barabino et al., 1987a; Wick et al., 1987, 1992; Kaul et al., 1989). In contrast, the most dense fraction—but not its substituent irreversibly sickled cells (ISCs)—tends to be most adhesive in static adhesion assays (Hebbel et al., 1980a, 1980b; Wautier et al., 1985). In studies using micropipette technology (Fig. 21.1), however, adherence seemed to be a feature of irregularly shaped non-ISCs rather than discocytes, regardless of red cell density (Mohandas and Evans, 1985).

Figure 21.2. Adhesion of sickle red cells under flowing conditions. The rat mesocecum was perfused with human sickle red cells. Degree of adhesion increases dramatically as venular diameter decreases (left). The images on the right show that sickle red cells are adherent under flowing conditions in both larger (top) and smaller (bottom) postcapillary venules. The arrow shows the direction of flow. Red cells that are in focus are adherent to endothelium and have ceased flowing. The smaller arrows in the bottom image show that the smallest vessels are completely occluded with sickle red cells. (From Kaul et al., 1989, with permission.)

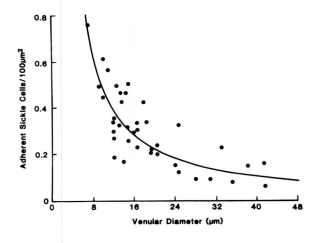
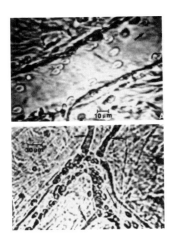

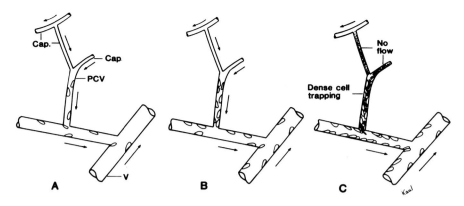

Figure 21.3. Vasoocclusion by secondary trapping of dense (SS4) cells subsequent to adhesion of deformable SS cells. Overall, data are consistent with the idea that accumulation of adherent sickle red cells (left and middle) provides a triggering function and that acute vasoocclusion develops after secondary "log-jamming" by poorly deformable red cells. (From Kaul, 1992, with permission.)

Flow systems are less likely to allow adherence by dense sickle cells because their poor deformability impairs development of the necessary intimacy of endothelial contact that is required for adherence under flowing conditions (Kaul et al., 1994), just as the spiculation that accompanies reversible sickling impairs their ability to attach (Hebbel et al., 1980b). Conversely, cell-cell adhesion in static adhesion assays may be less likely to be impeded by poor deformability. Since the results of in vitro studies thus depend so critically on experimental design, existing data do not allow easy extrapolation to the in vivo situation.

Nevertheless, the basic conclusion from many in vitro experiments is that sickle adhesion is of sufficient tenacity to occur in vivo. Detailed experiments by Kaul and co-workers led them to develop the concept that vasoocclusion is initiated by a two-step process: with abnormal red cell adhesivity comprising a triggering mechanism, and with subsequent "log-jamming" by dehydrated and poorly deformable cells causing propagation (Fig. 21.3). Experimental data in animal models support this hypothesis (Kaul et al., 1989, 1994; Fabry et al., 1992). It is likely that the red cell adherence detected in vitro, or expressed in vivo, will reflect the size and composition of different red cell subpopulations having different mechanisms and tenacities of adhesion. These may vary among patients or temporally for individual patients.

Relevance of Adhesion Affinity

It is reasonable to assume that adhesion mechanisms observable under flowing conditions are high-affinity mechanisms, whereas those observed under static conditions may include low-affinity mechanisms. However, it does not necessarily follow that only the former are of pathophysiologic relevance. As discussed elsewhere (Hebbel, 1997), a stably attached red cell is in mechanical equilibrium, so the forces promoting its detachment—fluid shear force and a peeling torque—must be overcome by the bonding force—the product of bond number and strength per bond. Red cell adhesion that develops under flowing conditions would likely employ higher affinity receptors (only a few of which are necessary) and be rate controlled, with the influence of ligand/receptor on rate being dominant. On the other hand, mechanisms observable in the absence of flowing conditions could involve a low affinity regime where adhesion is equilibrium controlled and time dependent, with the required number of receptors being inversely related to affinity. During interruption of microcirculatory flow, low-affinity mechanisms certainly could participate, especially when limiting vessel diameter allows red cells to establish circumferential contact with endothelium. In that case, a greater number of adhesive contacts is allowed, and the removal tendency conferred by peeling torque could be lost. Thus, we must anticipate that even low-affinity adhesion mechanisms could play a role, depending on the vascular context. Indeed, it may be a critical clue that the described correlation between sickle cell adhesiveness and clinical vasoocclusive severity (Fig. 21.4) (Hebbel et al., 1980a) was identified using an experimental model that probably was measuring one of the low-affinity adhesion mechanisms. In vivo, microvascular blood flow can be intermittent, and red cell passage may be delayed for various reasons (e.g., by activated granulocytes adhering to the inflamed endothelium of the sickle cell disease patient) (Carlos and Harlan, 1994; Hebbel and Vercellotti, 1997; Solovey et al., 1997).

Mechanisms of Sickle Red Cell Adhesion

Both red cell membrane and plasma factors contribute to sickle cell interaction with endothelium (Hebbel et al., 1981; Mohandas and Evans, 1984). The inherent adhesivity of red cells is probably unchanged during acute painful episodes, except as influenced by any changes in red cell subpopulations (see Chapter 25), but plasma obtained during acute

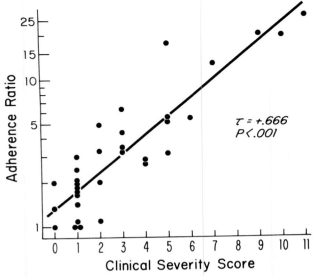

Figure 21.4. Sickle red cell adhesion to endothelial cells corre-lates with clinical vasoocclusive severity. These data were obtained in the absence of plasma proteins other than albumin, so they represent an assessment of inherent (and presumably not receptor-mediated) red cell adhesivity. (From Hebbel et al., 1980a, with permission.)

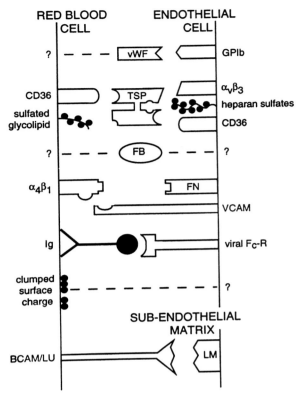

Figure 21.5. Documented mechanisms of sickle red cell adhesiv-ity. FB, fibrinogen; Fc-R, Fc receptor; FN, fibronectin; GPIb, glycoprotein Ib; Ig, immunoglobulin; LM, laminin; TSP, throm-bospondin; VCAM, vascular cell adhesion molecule; vWF, von Willebrand factor.

pain can support greater adherence than plasma obtained during steady state (Hebbel et al., 1981). Studies in vitro have now identified a variety of candi-date mechanisms for sickle red cell adhesion to endothelium in vivo, some of which are based on known receptor structures. Relevant structures on the red cell surface are $\alpha_4\beta_1$ integrins, CD36, basal cell adhesion molecule (BCAM), and sulfatides. Of these, sickle red cells express higher amounts than do their normal counterparts for BCAM (Udahl et al., 1998), CD36 (Browne and Hebbel, 1996), and $\alpha_4\beta_1$ (Joneckis et al., 1993). Corresponding receptors on the endothe-lial surface include GPIb, CD36, $\alpha_4\beta_1$, and VCAM. Considering the probably inflamed nature of sickle endothelium—deduced from studies of circulating endothelial cells (Solovey et al., 1997, 1998)—it is quite possible that the sickle cell disease patient's endothelium differs substantially from that of normal individuals, in ways that are directly relevant to red cell adhesion (Hebbel and Vercellotti, 1997). The following mechanisms have been identified to date (Fig. 21.5).

von Willebrand Factor (vWF). Ultralarge forms of vWF, but not its normal plasma forms, promote sickle red cell adhesion to endothelium (Wick et al., 1987; Brittain et al., 1992; Wick et al., 1992). This occurs under flowing conditions, is greater for least-dense cells, and is much less evident with microvascular than with large vessel endothelial cells. Endothelial cells

express GPIb/V/IX, but investigators have not yet unambiguously identified a specific vWF receptor on sickle red cells, so the mechanism involved is not completely defined. vWF is likely to be most relevant clinically during dehydration, which causes vaso-pressin-induced vWF release, and during endothelial activation when Weibel-Palade bodies can dump their contents. Levels of vWF are increased in sickle cell dis-ease patients even in steady state (Francis and Hebbel, 1994), although multimer composition has not been assessed. Recent data suggest that vWF-mediated adhesion comprises a weaker mechanism than that mediated by either laminin or thrombospondin (Hillery et al., 1996; Joneckis et al., 1996; Barabino et al., 1997).

Thrombospondin (TSP). TSP mediates sickle red cell adhesion in vitro via its ability to bridge CD36 (glyco-protein IV) or perhaps sulfatide expressed on stress reticulocytes and either the vitronectin receptor ($\alpha_v\alpha_3$) or CD36 or perhaps heparan sulfate proteoglycans on the endothelial cell (Sugihara et al., 1992; Brittain et al., 1993; Hillery et al., 1996; Gupta et al., 1999). TSP mediates adherence under both static and flowing conditions and with both microvascular and large-vessel endothelial cells (Sugihara et al., 1992; Brittain et al., 1993). Nonsickle reticulocytes express less CD36 than do sickle reticulocytes (Browne and Hebbel, 1996), and they exhibit little adhesion response to TSP (Sugihara et al., 1992). TSP levels are elevated in some sickle cell disease patients during painful episodes (Browne et al., 1996), most likely due to in vivo platelet activation (Francis and Hebbel, 1994). Thus, the clinical context in which TSP-mediated adhesion is most likely to be relevant is hemostatic perturbation. Based on studies of adhesion to immobilized proteins, it appears that sickle red cell adhesion is stronger to TSP than to vWF (Hillery et al., 1996; Joneckis et al., 1996; Barabino et al., 1997), although it is not yet known if adhesion to immobilized TSP utilizes the same mechanisms as adhesion to soluble TSP.

Fibrinogen (FB). A very modest adhesion-promoting role for FB, probably not mediated by receptors, has been observed in nonflowing experimental systems (Hebbel et al., 1981; Wautier et al., 1983; Smith and LaCelle, 1986; Wick et al., 1987). The existence of weak fibrinogen-dependent adhesive forces was documented by measurements of red cell interaction (Morris et al., 1991, 1992). The relevance of this mechanism perhaps lies in FB's role as an acute phase reactant, increasing in response to concurrent illness and at onset of painful sickle vasoocclusive episodes (Hebbel et al., 1981; Francis, 1991). This mechanism has been tested only under static experimental conditions.

Fibronectin (FN). This protein also has a modest adhesogenic role for sickle red cells under both static and flowing conditions (Wautier et al., 1983; Wick et al., 1987; Kasschau et al., 1996). Removal of collagen-binding plasma proteins—which include but are not limited to FN—diminishes sickle cell adherence in plasma (Mohandas and Evans, 1985). The structures involved in fibronectin-mediated sickle adhesion have not been defined, although known FN receptors are found on both reticulocytes and endothelial cells. Fibronectin levels may fluctuate in sickle patients (Bolarin and Adenuga, 1986).

Immunoglobulin/Fc-Receptors. Because sickle red cells are abnormally gilded with immunoglobulin (Petz et al., 1984; Hebbel and Miller, 1984), they can interact with Fc receptors (Fc-R). The potential relevance of this to red cell/endothelial interaction was established by demonstration that sickle red cells adhere to endothelial cells infected with herpes simplex virus type 1 so they express a glycoprotein having Fc-R function (Hebbel et al., 1987). Whether other, more clinically relevant viruses do this as well has not been examined; but this provides a potential mechanism promoting vasoocclusion in conjunction with viral infection.

$\alpha_4\beta_1$/Vascular Cell Adhesion Molecule-1. Sickle reticulocytes express $\alpha_4\beta_1$ integrin, which can mediate red cell adhesion under flowing conditions through its interaction with endothelial cells, if they have been induced to express vascular cell adhesion molecule-1 (VCAM) by appropriate stimulation [e.g., with tumor necrosis factor (TNF)] (Joneckis et al., 1993; Swerlick et al., 1993; Gee and Platt, 1995). This mechanism nicely illustrates the relevance of endothelial cell surface modulation by cytokines and assorted biological modifiers (Hebbel and Vercellotti, 1997). Interestingly, it has been claimed that stimulation of red cells (presumably reticulocytes) with phorbol has an activating effect on $\alpha_4\beta_1$ (Kumar et al., 1996), although there is lingering concern whether this effect was actually due to contaminating white cells. Involvement of VCAM also seems to be the mechanism by which arachidonate metabolites 15-HETE and 15-HPETE stimulate endothelial cells to be more adhesive for sickle red cells (Setty et al., 1995; Setty and Stuart, 1996).

Laminin (LM). Both soluble and immobilized LM bind to the Lutheran antigen, BCAM/Lu, which is expressed in greater amounts on sickle compared to normal erythrocytes (Udahl et al., 1998). Sickle red cell adhesion to LM has been tested under both flowing and static experimental conditions (Joneckis et al., 1993; Hillery et al., 1996; Barabino et al., 1997; Lee et al., 1998; Udahl et al., 1998). The clinical relevance of this observation may be found in laminin's role as a component of extracellular matrix, which could become important to red cell interaction with the vessel wall should the endothelial barrier be compromised. For example, thrombin-induced endothelial retraction may expose new adhesion molecules (Manodori et al., 1998).

Direct Cell/Cell Adhesion. The original observations of sickle cell adhesion to endothelium were made in the absence of plasma proteins or endothelial stimulation. Under these conditions, adhesion was believed to result from red cell surface charge clustering (Hebbel et al., 1980b). Of interest, sickle cell adhesion can be modulated by manipulation of red cell hydration (Hebbel et al., 1989), which affects the distribution of surface charge on the red cell (Marikovsky et al., 1978). An alternative weak adhesion mechanism may be provided by the altered phospholipid asymmetry of sickle cells (Schlegel et al., 1985) (see Chapter 22). Interestingly, such inherent sickle cell adhesivity was found to be greater for the most dense cells (Hebbel et al., 1980a). Tested only under static experimental conditions, the underlying adhesive force is small, since it apparently cannot overcome gravity (Mohandas and Evans, 1984). Notably, however, it was this mechanism that was tested and found to correlate significantly with clinical vasoocclusive severity (Hebbel et al., 1980a), again suggesting that even low-affinity adhesion mechanisms may be important.

Pathophysiologic Role of Red Cell Adhesion

The hypothesized involvement of endothelial adhesivity in sickle disease pathophysiology provides a mechanism to delay microvascular transit of red cells and, thereby, overcome the delay time required for HbS polymerization. Thus, red cell adhesion to endothelium would be expected to increase the likelihood of sickling in erythrocytes whose transit is arrested by adhesive cells. In fact, several lines of evidence support the notion that red cell adhesion to endothelium may play a role in sickle disease pathophysiology. Among patients with sickle cell anemia, the degree of inherent red cell adhesivity—defined as adherence in absence of plasma—varied over a twentyfold range and correlated with clinical vasoocclusive severity (Hebbel et al., 1980a). Red cell adhesivity was less abnormal for red cells from other genotypes of sickle cell disease that are clinically less severe sickling disorders (Hebbel, 1981). Studies of perfused rat vessels support the hypothesis that vasoocclusion is triggered by adherent deformable red cells, followed by a propagation phase in which less deformable and/or misshapen cells accumulate to complete the vasoocclusion (Fig. 21.3) (Kaul et al., 1989, 1994; Fabry et al., 1992; Kaul, 1992). Interestingly, a positive correlation was observed between vasoocclusive severity and red cell deformability (Ballas et al., 1988; Lande et al., 1988), perhaps revealing a preeminent role for the adhesiveness of the least dense cell subpopulation (as opposed, e.g., to the stiffness of the most dense subpopulation).

The role of red cell adhesion would be influenced by a great variety of factors such as determinants of receptor expression (and affinity) on both red cell and endothelial cell, the concentrations of plasma adhesive proteins that can fluctuate during concurrent illness, and numerous vascular factors such as geometry and flow rates. Thus, the adhesion mechanism that is "most important" may differ from organ to organ, or time to time, or even from patient to patient. Of course, it is possible that a single adhesion occurrence could involve multiple simultaneous mechanisms. As addressed already, it would be misleading to assume that the affinity of each potential mechanism is the preeminent determinant of relevance since even low-affinity mechanisms could

become relevant if multiple contacts are allowed to develop, perhaps circumferentially in a vessel of limiting diameter. To date, no investigation has attempted to define the biophysical principles governing the net effect of simultaneous interactions between adhesive tendency and suboptimal erythrocyte deformability in the context of constraining vascular diameter or variable flow conditions. A hint that this may be important is derived from studies of stroke in the rat perfused with sickle red cells, in which the relevance of NO is demonstrated (French et al., 1997).

We also believe it is likely that adhesive interactions in vivo are influenced by endothelial heterogeneity. In vitro studies showed that the adhesion-promoting effect of vWF was much lower for microvascular compared with large-vessel endothelial cells; conversely, the adhesion-potentiating effect of plasma was markedly greater for microvascular compared with large-vessel endothelium (Fig. 21.6) (Brittain et al., 1992). This undoubtedly reflects the fact that different endothelia express different receptor structures. Most strikingly, CD36 (a TSP receptor) is expressed on microvascular but not large-vessel endothelial cells (Swerlick et al., 1992). The concept of endothelial heterogeneity also extends to temporal considerations whereby endothelial cells can be stimulated by a host of biological modifiers. Thus, sickle red cell adhesion to endothelium increases upon stimulation with TNF (which causes VCAM expression) or IL-1 (which causes expression of various receptors, depending on

Figure 21.6. Endothelial heterogeneity in adhesion response. Sickle red cell adhesion to large vessel endothelium (HUVEC) and microvascular endothelium (MVEC) is markedly different for cells suspended in serum versus ultralarge vWF versus plasma. vWF is the strongest promoter of sickle adhesion to HUVEC, but something else in plasma is the strongest promoter of adhesion to MVEC. (Modified from original data presented elsewhere [Brittain et al., 1992] and reproduced with permission from [Hebbel and Mohandas, 1994].)

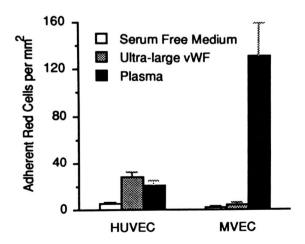

time of exposure) (Vordermeier et al., 1992; Swerlick et al., 1993; Natarajan et al., 1996). In fact, patients are described as having variably elevated levels of major endothelial stimuli such as TNF, platelet activating factor, lipopolysaccharide, hypoxia, thrombin, anti-phospholipid antibodies, L1, homocysteine, and lipoxygenase products (Kucek et al., 1993; Francis and Hebbel, 1994; Setty et al., 1995; Houston et al., 1997; Oh et al., 1997). Since these stimuli also influence receptors for white cells and platelets (Carlos and Harlan, 1994; Frenette et al., 1998), one can speculate that such complex interactions might also be important in the overall process of sickle red cell adhesion.

Studies of circulating endothelial cells recently revealed evidence for abnormal endothelial stimulation in sickle cell disease (Solovey et al., 1997, 1998). Specifically, these studies have revealed abnormal expression of red cell and/or white cell adhesion molecules (ICAM, VCAM, P-selectin, E-selectin) and a procoagulant phenotype (tissue factor expression) on circulating endothelial cells. Ongoing studies are documenting that the phenotype of these circulating endothelial cells reflects that of endothelium remaining in the vessel wall (Hebbel et al., 1999). Thus, it appears that the endothelium is, indeed, abnormally activated (and, therefore, is abnormally pro-adhesive) in the sickle cell disease.

Adherence and the Endothelial Injury Response

As opposed to endothelial stimulation, either physiologic or pathologic, endothelial injury per se is likely to be a component of sickle cell disease (Francis and Hebbel, 1994). In the first place, the intermittent vasoocclusion imposed by sickling (and/or red cell adhesion) would suggest that this disease is an example of "ischemia-reperfusion" physiology. In fact, recent data obtained from the sickle transgenic mouse support this (Osarogiagbon et al., 1997), but pertinent human data have not been collected yet. There are, however, a number of in vitro observations that suggest that sickle adhesion is an endothelial perturbant. Evidence includes elevated numbers of circulating endothelial cells (Sowemimo-Coker et al., 1989; Solovey et al., 1997) and the ability of adherent sickle red cells to inhibit endothelial DNA synthesis (Weinstein et al., 1990), to increase endothelin mRNA (Phelan et al., 1995), to impair NO synthesis (Mosseri et al., 1993), to stimulate arachidonic acid metabolism (Setty et al., 1996), to stimulate prostacyclin release (Wautier et al., 1986; Sowemimo-Coker et al., 1992), and to induce adhesion molecule expression (Sultana et al., 1988). The significance of this perturbation to the vascular pathobiology of sickle disease is not known yet, although numerous aspects of the disease can potentially be ascribed to these effects (Hebbel and Vercellotti, 1997).

Adhesion and Potential Therapies

Several manipulations have been examined in an attempt to diminish sickle adhesivity in vitro. A rationale for a vascular "lubricant" such as FLOCOR™, now in clinical trials, was provided by and observation that it abolished sickle erythrocyte adherence to endothelial cells (Smith et al., 1987). Pentoxifylline (Barabino et al., 1987b) and iloprost (Longenecker et al., 1990) are claimed to impair adhesivity as well. Various peptides and antibodies have been used in identifying mechanisms of adhesion and theoretically could form the basis for antiadhesive therapy. Anionic polysaccharides may prove to be an effective way to impair TSP-mediated adhesion (Hillery et al., 1996; Joneckis et al., 1996; Barabino et al., 1999; Gupta et al., 1999). Intriguingly, the drug hydroxyurea is reported to markedly diminish sickle red cell adhesivity (Bridges et al., 1996), perhaps by downregulating expression of adhesion molecules $\alpha_4\beta_1$ and CD36 (Styles et al., 1997) (see Chapter 38). We can anticipate the development of novel therapeutics based on antiadhesive approaches. One of these may be therapies directed at controlling the expression of adhesion molecules on the endothelial surface (Solovey et al., 1999).

ERYTHROCYTE INTERACTIONS WITH PLATELETS

Little is known about sickle red cell interactions with platelets. Given the variety of receptors on platelets, especially upon their activation, it certainly seems possible that they could participate in conjunction with adhesogenic plasma proteins in the process of red cell binding to endothelium. This has not been studied sufficiently, but sickle cell adhesion is greater in the presence of platelets than in their absence (Antonucci et al., 1990). Increased mixed aggregates of red cells and platelets have been noted in sickle patients (Wun et al., 1997).

ERYTHROCYTE INTERACTIONS WITH MACROPHAGES AND MONOCYTES

Sickle red cells adhere abnormally to peripheral blood monocytes (Schwartz et al., 1985) and macrophages (Hebbel and Miller, 1984) in vitro, which phagocytose them more readily than normal red cells (Hebbel and Miller, 1984; Galili et al., 1986). The most dense red cell subpopulation exhibits the greatest interaction. Comparison of different patients reveals both adherence to macrophages and erythrophagocytosis to be highly variable among patients (Hebbel and Miller, 1984). This interaction presumably explains the fact that macrophages in marrow specimens (Sydenstricker, 1924) or tissues (Bauer et al., 1980) contain ingested red cells.

Mechanisms

Several mechanisms have been implicated. The membrane IgG found on sickle erythrocytes is most strongly implicated (Hebbel and Miller, 1984; Petz et al., 1984; Green et al., 1985; Galili et al., 1986; Schlüter & Drenckhahn, 1986) since adherence and phagocytosis are inhibited by blockade of macrophage Fc receptors or elution of immunoglobulin from the red cells. Red cell membrane epitopes that might be recognized by this Ig include glycolipid with $\alpha1\rightarrow3$Gal (Gallili et al., 1986), modification of the membrane by the peroxidation by-product malondialdehyde (Hebbel and Miller, 1984, 1988), and protein band 3 (Schlüter and Drenckhahn, 1986; Waugh et al., 1986; Turrini et al., 1991). In the latter case, denatured hemoglobin coclusters with band 3 at the cytosol/membrane interface, followed by accumulation of IgG and complement, thereby leading to recognition by macrophage receptors for C3b or Ig (Turrini et al., 1991). Notably, however, macrophages probably can recognize sickle red cells in an immunoglobulin-independent manner due to their disrupted phospholipid asymmetry (Schwartz et al., 1985; McEvoy et al., 1986) and/or their membrane malondialdehyde (Hebbel and Miller, 1984, 1988).

Pathophysiologic Consequences

Indirect evidence supports the hypothesis that abnormal interactions between sickle red cells and macrophages participate in genesis of hemolytic anemia (for a discussion of the pathophysiology of anemia, see Chapter 20). That hemolytic rate probably does not simply correlate with the number of IgG molecules per red cell (Petz et al., 1984) is not surprising since this determination ignores patient-to-patient variability in coating density, IgG type, and proportion of positive cells. On the other hand, hemolytic index does correlate directly with sickle red cell adherence to macrophages in vitro (Hebbel and Miller, 1988). Consistent with this, lower mean PCVs are described for sickle patients having erythrophagocytosis evident in their peripheral blood (Solanki, 1985). Also, blood monocytes from sickle patients are said to show enhanced erythrophagocytic ability during painful episodes (Mendoza et al., 1991). Thus, it is probable that erythrophagocytosis is a significant contributor to the hemolytic component of sickle disease. Abnormal interaction between sickle red cells and macrophages may have other consequences. For example, it probably can adversely affect host defense and contribute to

the infection propensity, since experimental accelerated erythrophagocytosis contributes to macrophage functional blockade (Gill et al., 1966; Hook et al., 1967).

RED CELL RHEOLOGY

The human red cell leaves the bone marrow as a reticulocyte; thereafter, the mature red cell spends its circulatory lifetime of approximately 120 days performing its function of oxygen delivery. To optimally carry out its function, the red cell must repeatedly change its shape and undergo extensive deformation during passage through the microvasculature. The diameter of the human red cell (8 μ) far exceeds that of the capillaries (2 to 3 μ) through which it must pass in the process of delivering oxygen to the tissues. The ability of normal red cells to undergo marked deformations during the passage through capillaries was originally documented in 1675 by van Leeuwenhook, who noted that the blood "globules" underwent deformation into an ellipsoidal shape during passage through the microvasculature but resumed their original shape when they returned to larger vessels. After observing his own blood, van Leeuwenhook noticed with remarkable prescience, that when he was greatly "disordered," globules of his blood appeared hard and rigid, but grew softer and more pliable as his health returned to normal. Since these insightful original observations, elegant studies of Krogh, Branemark and Bagge, Wayland and Frasher, and others who studied red cell deformation in the microvasculature using improved microscopic and microcinematographic techniques have clearly established that the ability of red cells to undergo extensive deformation is essential for its function (Krogh, 1930; Wayland and Frasher, 1973; Branemark and Bagge, 1977). Of particular relevance to the present discussion is the insightful speculation of Ham and Castle about a vicious cycle of erythrostasis due to deoxygenation-induced increased blood viscosity in sickle cell disease (Ham and Castle, 1940).

Cellular deformability is the term generally used to characterize the ability of red cells to undergo deformations. It is a major determinant of microcirculatory flow, since it determines the rate of entry of red cells into capillaries, which in turn influences the pressure drop across small vessels and flow distributions in the vasculature. The deformability of red cells is also an important determinant of bulk viscosity of blood and, as such, plays an indirect but critical role in regulating blood flow in the large blood vessels (see Chapter 20). Two particularly important features to consider in understanding cellular deformability of sickle cells are (1) the marked heterogeneity in the deformability characteristics of individual sickle red cells and (2) the effect of state of cell oxygenation on cell deformability. In comparison to normal red cells, individual sickle red cells exhibit marked heterogeneities in cell density and in various cellular properties. Furthermore, while the state of oxygenation has little or no effect on the rheology of normal red cells, it has a profound influence on the rheologic behavior of sickle red cells. We will summarize our current understanding of rheologic abnormalities of sickle red cells and the mechanistic basis for cell heterogeneity, and indicate how these abnormalities may modulate the pathophysiologic features of sickle cell disease.

Blood Viscosity

Unlike plasma and other Newtonian fluids for which the viscosity is independent of shear rate, the viscosity of a whole blood sample is strongly and inversely dependent on shear rate (see Chapter 20 for additional details). Blood viscosity is determined by PCV, plasma viscosity, red cell aggregation, and red cell deformability (Chien et al., 1982). The viscosity of plasma in sickle cell anemia (1.29 ± 0.02 centipoise [cp]) is slightly higher than that of plasma from normal subjects (1.19 ± 0.01 cp). This increased viscosity is primarily the result of higher total protein concentration of plasma from sickle cell disease individuals. In marked contrast, the bulk viscosity of oxygenated sickle blood is lower than that of normal blood at all shear rates, primarily because of its lower PCV (Fig. 21.7) (Chien et al., 1970, 1982). However, when the PCV of sickle blood is increased to 45 percent by removal of plasma, the viscosity value becomes substantially higher than that of normal blood (Fig. 21.7). While deoxygenation has no effect on the viscosity of normal blood, the viscosity of a sickle blood sample increases with decreased oxygen saturation (Chien et al., 1982; Danish and Harris, 1983). Complete deoxygenation results in a tenfold increase in viscosity at high shear rate values (~200 sec^{-1}). Reduced cellular deformability of sickle red cells is primarily responsible for the increased viscosity of sickle blood.

The physiologic relevance of these findings is that elevated blood viscosity can have detrimental effects on the cardiovascular system and on tissue oxygenation. In this regard, the concept of optimum PCV (defined as the PCV at which hemoglobin flow and hence oxygen delivery is maximized) is worth noting, since it offers insight into the complex relationships among cellular deformability, blood viscosity, and PCV in different red cell disorders (Self et al., 1977; Schmalzer et al., 1987). For patients with red cells of

Figure 21.7. Relationship between viscosity and shear rate for oxygenated sickle blood (PCV of 25 percent) and normal blood (PCV of 45 percent). Also shown is the viscosity of sickle blood at a PCV of 45 percent. (Courtesy of Dr. Shu Chien.)

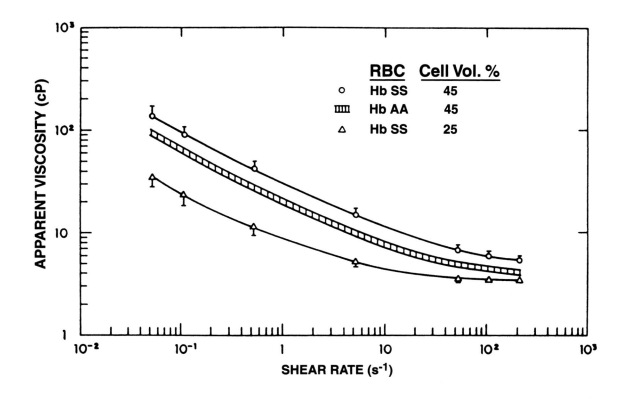

reduced deformability and high whole blood viscosity, lower than normal PCVs are optimal, since at these values hemoglobin flow and oxygen delivery are maximized. Increasing PCV, either by transfusion or by stimulating erythropoiesis, will diminish oxygen delivery because the resultant increase in blood viscosity will reduce blood flow. This concept is particularly relevant for clinical decisionmaking involving transfusions for patients with sickle cell disease (Self et al., 1977; Schmalzer et al., 1987) (see Chapter 37). Increased blood viscosity as a result of elevated PCV could also account for some of the clinical manifestations observed in patients with sickle cell anemia with coexistent α thalassemia or HbS-β^0 thalassemia (Embury et al., 1984a).

Sickle Red Cell Mechanical Fragility

Oxygenated sickle red cells are more susceptible to mechanically induced cell fragmentation than normal red cells. In vitro studies have documented increased sensitivity of sickle red cells to fluid shear stress–induced mechanical fragmentation (Messman et al., 1990), the most dramatic illustration of which is the observation of cell lysis in sickle cell patients undergoing vigorous exercise (Platt, 1982). The most dense sickle red cells are particularly susceptible to mechanical damage. Although the mechanism(s) responsible for increased susceptibility of dense sickle cells have not been unequivocally established, it is interesting to note that the membranes derived from these cells exhibit decreased mechanical stability (Messman et al., 1990). it is likely that weakening of the skeletal protein interactions (spectrin-spectrin or spectrin-actin-protein 4.1) due to accumulated oxidative damage (Hebbel, 1990) is the likely cause of the decreased mechanical stability of these membranes (see Chapter 22).

Deformability of Oxygenated Sickle Cells

Decreased cellular deformability of oxygenated sickle red cells has been documented using a variety of measurement techniques, including viscometry, filtration, ektacytometry, and micropipette aspiration of cells (Chien et al., 1970; Usami et al., 1975; Bessis and Mohandas, 1977; Havell et al., 1978; Clark et al., 1980; Evans et al., 1984; Nash et al., 1984; Schmalzer et al., 1989). In these measurements, reduction in sickle cell deformability is manifested, respectively, by increased viscosity of blood (Chien et al., 1970), decreased filtration rate of dilute cell suspensions through narrow pores (Usami et al., 1975; Schmalzer et al., 1989), decreased ability of cells to undergo deformation in shear fields (Bessis and Mohandas,

1977; Clark et al., 1980), and increased aspiration pressures needed to induce entry of cells into micropipettes (Havell et al., 1978; Evans et al., 1984; Nash et al., 1984). These studies not only documented abnormal rheologic properties of oxygenated sickle blood samples but also showed that there are marked heterogeneities in the degree of rheologic abnormalities of red cells in an individual blood sample and in blood samples from different individuals (Smith et al., 1981; Evans et al., 1984; Nash et al., 1984; Ballas et al., 1988; Lande et al., 1988; Akinola et al., 1992).

The deformation response of an individual red cell to applied fluid force is a complex phenomenon that depends on a number of different cell characteristics, including membrane material properties, cell geometry, and cytoplasmic viscosity (Mohandas et al., 1983; Mohandas and Chasis, 1993). Alterations in each of these cell characteristics have been documented to account for decreased cellular deformability of sickle red cells. By studying cellular deformability of isolated subpopulations of sickle red cells with defined cell densities using ektacytometry, Clark et al. (1980) found that cellular dehydration and the consequent increase in cytoplasmic viscosity are major determinants of the abnormal rheologic behavior of oxygenated sickle red cells (Fig. 21.8). Sickle cell membrane changes also contribute. Studies on resealed ghosts showed that the sickle red cell membrane in isolation exhibits altered material properties, including increased extensional rigidity and decreased membrane mechanical stability (Fortier et al., 1988; Messman et al., 1990). Techniques such as filtration and ektacytometry have proven useful in delineating the cellular basis for the abnormal rheologic behavior of populations of sickle red cells. However, by failing to provide detailed insights into rheologic properties of individual red cells, these measurements have not enabled full definition of physiologic consequences of the abnormal rheology of sickle red cells. To achieve this objective, it is necessary to have detailed information regarding rheologic properties of individual red cells.

Cell Density Heterogeneity

The significance of the rheologic measurements on individual red cells can be put into proper perspective only when viewed in the context of the marked heterogeneity of cell water content of red cells in sickle cell disease and the presence of a large percentage of dehydrated cells (Clark et al., 1982) (see Chapter 22). In normal blood the density of red cells is quite uniform, and there is only limited heterogeneity. In contrast, in sickle cell disease, repeated cycles of sickling and unsickling of mature red cells as well as dehydration of reticulocytes, lead to the generation of dense, dehy-

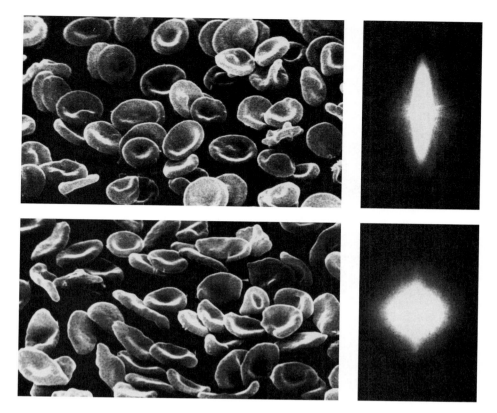

Figure 21.8. Morphology and diffraction patterns of low-density (top left) and high-density (bottom left) oxygenated sickle cells. Discoid morphology is the dominant feature of low-density sickle cells, while irreversibly sickled red cells are enriched in the high-density fraction. Normal cellular deformability of the low-density discoid sickle cells is illustrated by the elliptical diffraction pattern generated by these cells (top right). The diffraction pattern was much more rounded (bottom right) for the undeformable dense dehydrated irreversibly sickled cells.

drated red cells (Fabry and Nagel, 1982). A striking feature of blood samples in sickle cell anemia is the marked heterogeneity in the water content and hence the density of individual red cells (Fig. 21.9). This is evidenced by a broad distribution of the hemoglobin concentration of individual red cells in whole blood samples. In normal blood samples, the hemoglobin concentration of individual red cells ranges between 27 and 38 g/dL, while in sickle cell anemia blood samples it can vary between 23 and 50 g/dL. As a consequence, normal blood contains only a very small fraction of red cells (less than 1 percent) having hemoglobin concentration values greater than 38 g/dL, but sickle cell blood samples contain a substantial fraction of cells (up to 40 percent) with hemoglobin concentrations greater than 38 g/dL.

This increased cell hemoglobin concentration has many deleterious effects on the pathobiology of the sickle red cell. In addition to its marked effect on cellu-

lar deformability of sickle cells, cell dehydration has profound effects on the kinetics and extent of HbS polymer formation upon deoxygenation, and perhaps enhances the tendency of sickle cells to adhere to endothelium. Furthermore, increased cell hemoglobin concentration results in poorly understood events at the cytosol-membrane interface that impact adversely on membrane proteins and lipids, resulting in abnormal rheologic properties of the membrane (Evans et al., 1984; Evans and Mohandas, 1987) and greater susceptibility of the cell to oxidative damage (Hebbel, 1990). Through these effects on the pathobiology of the sickle red cell, cell dehydration plays a major role in various aspects of the pathophysiology of sickle cell disease, including the pathogenesis of hemolytic anemia and vasoocclusive episodes (Embury et al., 1994; Mohandas and Hebbel, 1994).

One important determinant of the number of dense cells in an individual is the level of fetal hemoglobin (HbF). The sickle red cells with the lowest levels of HbF have an increased propensity for cell dehydration (Bertles and Milner, 1968; Horiuchi et al., 1993; Franco et al., 1994, 1998). As there is a marked variation in the amount of HbF among red cells in an individual with sickle cell disease, the number of dense cells is in part determined by the fraction of red cells with low levels of HbF. Strong support for this thesis comes from recent therapeutic studies using hydroxyurea to stimulate HbF production (see Chapter 38).

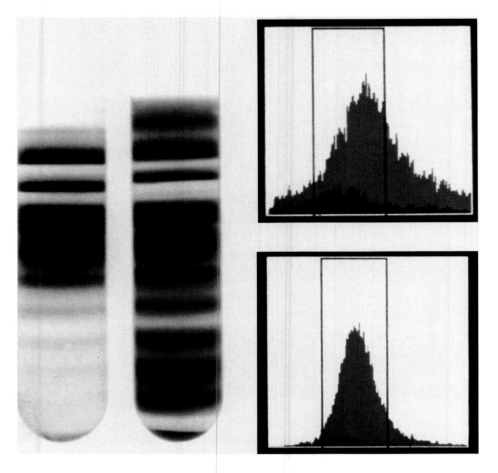

Figure 21.9. High-resolution discontinuous Stractan density gradients of red cells from one normal subject (left) and an individual with sickle cell disease (right). The densities ranged from 1.070 to 1.115 g/mL in approximately 0.004 g/mL increments. Note the marked enrichment of high-density dehydrated cells in the sickle blood sample. Representative example of red cell hemoglobin concentration (cell density) histograms of blood sample from a sickle cell disease patient pre- (top right panel) and posttreatment (bottom right panel) with hydroxyurea is also shown. The histograms of normal blood sample fall within the vertical markers that delineate hemoglobin concentration values of 28 g/dL and 41 g/dL. Note the marked increase in the percentage of red cells (lightly shaded histogram) and reticulocytes (darkly shaded histogram) with hemoglobin concentration >41 g/dL in the sickle blood sample prior to hydroxyurea treatment and the marked decrease in these subpopulations following hydroxyurea treatment.

Following successful stimulation of HbF, there is a marked reduction in numbers of dehydrated red cells in individuals in whom there were large numbers of dense, dehydrated sickle red cells prior to hydroxyurea treatment (Ballas et al., 1989; Mohandas et al., 1991). The normalization of cell density distribution following hydroxyurea treatment is illustrated in Figure 21.9. The reduction in the number of dense red cells appears to be a very good indicator of effective stimu-

lation of HbF in response to hydroxyurea treatment. While it is possible that hydroxyurea treatment by itself may alter red cell water content, the dominant effect appears to be the consequence of stimulation of HbF. Similarly, in individuals who constitutively express high levels of HbF there is a marked reduction in the number of dense sickle red cells. Taken together, these findings demonstrate that the HbF content of the sickle red cell is an important determinant of its state of cell hydration and hence the rheologic properties of sickle cells.

Mechanisms of Cell Dehydration

There is consensus that the membrane permeability changes that accompany repeated cycles of red cell sickling and unsickling play a role in the generation of dense sickle cells. The membrane transport pathways, particularly the calcium-activated potassium efflux (Gardos channel) and KCl cotransport appear to play a major role in the dehydration process and are discussed in detail in the following chapter (Horiuchi et al., 1988; Brugnara, 1995; Franco et al., 1995, 1996, 1997). Particularly relevant to the present discussion is a novel mechanism that has been outlined for the generation of dense sickle cells involving the activation of pH-sensitive KCl cotransporters in reticulocytes (Bookchin et al., 1991; Fabry et al., 1991; Franco et al., 1996). The contribution of reticulocyte dehydration to dense cell formation in sickle cell disease was studied by comparing the density profiles of reticulocytes and mature red cells in a blood sample (Mohandas et al., 1991; Ballas et al., 1992). In individuals with sickle cell anemia, up to 15 percent of reticulocytes had hemoglobin concentrations greater than 38 g/dL compared with less than 1 percent in normal controls. The density profiles of reticulocytes in these blood samples were similar to those of mature sickle red cells (Fig. 21.9); that is, cells recently released from the marrow are rapidly dehydrated. Following treatment with hydroxyurea, there was a profound decrease in the numbers of dense reticulocytes concomitant with decreased numbers of dense mature red cells (Fig. 21.9). These data suggest that reticulocyte dehydration can play a role in the generation of dense sickle cells.

Static and Dynamic Rigidities of Individual Red Cells

Static (time-independent) and dynamic (time-dependent) deformabilities of individual red cells are important determinants of local flow rates and distribution in microvasculature beds (Evans et al., 1984). Abnormal rheology of individual red cells can alter blood flow distribution and, in severe cases, even cause local occlusion of capillaries. When red cells enter small capillaries, they are deformed by extensions and folding. Such deformations cause (1) membrane extension without change in surface area, (2) membrane bending or folding, and (3) shear and displacement of the cytoplasm. The rheologic approximation that has been successfully used to quantitate intrinsic rheologic properties of red cells is based on the view of the cell as a liquid interior encapsulated by a viscoelastic solid membrane shell (Evans and Hochmuth, 1977). In this model, the membrane extension and bending moduli, μ and B, characterize the static rigidities of the cell, and the time constants for recovery from extensional (Te) and bending deformation (Tf), characterize the dynamic rigidities of the cell. To define the contribution of rheologic abnormalities to pathophysiology of sickle cell disease, it is important to have a clear understanding of the changes in these properties for the sickle cells.

The micropipette measurement technique provides the most detailed characterization of the static and dynamic deformabilities of individual red cells (Evans and Hochmuth, 1976; Hochmuth et al., 1979; Evans, 1983; Evans et al., 1984). Membrane extensional modulus (μ) is quantitated by aspirating single red cells into micropipettes with diameters in the range of 1 to 2 μm and determining the relationship between the applied negative pressure and the membrane tongue extension (Fig. 21.10). Higher aspiration pressures required to obtain equivalent tongue extensions indicate increased value for extensional rigidity (i.e., stiffness). Similarly, the bending modulus (B) is determined by measuring the minimum aspiration pressure required to induce folding or buckling of the membrane (Fig. 21.10). To evaluate the dynamic response of the cell to deformation by extension and by folding, the following two procedures are used. First, red cells are extended end to end by diametrically opposed pipettes such that little buckling or curvature change of the membrane surface takes place (Fig. 21.10). Then the cell is quickly released, the length-to-width recovery time course measured, and time constant for extensional recovery (Te) is derived from the best fit of the data using a viscoelastic model for the recovery process. Second, red cells are aspirated by large-caliber (4 μm inner diameter) pipettes such that little extension occurs (Fig. 21.1); the cell simply folds upon entrance into the pipette. The cell is then rapidly expelled from the pipette with a pressure pulse and the time course of unfolding recorded. The time required for the cell width to recover to 1/e of its final width (W∞) is taken as a measure of the time constant for elastic recovery from bending (Tf).

As stated earlier, there is a substantial body of evidence that shows large heterogeneity in the rheologic properties among sickle red cells in a given blood sample and also among different blood samples. This variation in large part is due to different degrees of cell dehydration. Therefore, in assessing rheologic data on sickle red cells it is important to factor into the analysis the contribution of cell density variations. Static and dynamic deformabilities of defined density subpopulations of normal and sickle red cells have been extensively characterized (Evans et al., 1984; Nash et al., 1984). Membrane extensional rigidity is identical in various subpopulations of normal red cells regardless of cell hemoglobin concentration (Fig. 21.11). In contrast, the extensional rigidity of oxygenated sickle cells increases with increasing cell hemoglobin concentration, the extensional rigidity of cells having the highest hemoglobin concentration being eight-fold higher than that of normal cells (Fig. 21.11). Another interesting feature is that sickle cells exhibit persistent deformation more frequently and to a much greater extent than normal cells following mechanical extension (Evans and Mohandas, 1987). Two mechanisms have been identified to account for this abnormal plastic-flow behavior: (1) increased association of sickle hemoglobin with the membrane at elevated hemoglobin concentrations; and (2) altered structural organi-

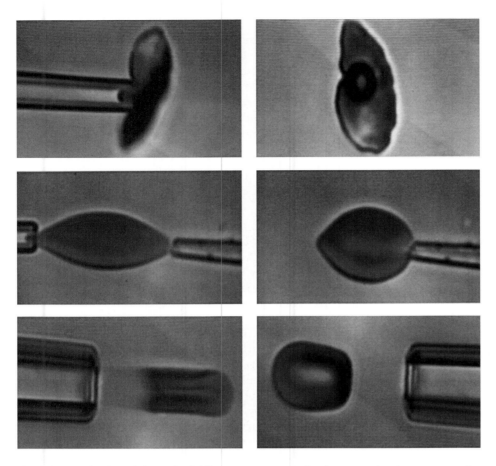

Figure 21.10. Static and dynamic rigidity measurements of red cells by micropipette aspiration. Videomicrograph of pipette aspiration of an irreversibly sickled cell during the course of measurement of membrane extensional rigidity (top left). The pipette inner diameter is 1.5 mm. Bending rigidity of the membrane is measured by determining the minimum pressure at which the membrane begins to wrinkle during the aspiration into the pipette (top right). For this measurement a bent pipette is used so that the cell can be viewed from above to detect accurately the beginning of membrane wrinkling. The time constant for rapid elastic recovery from extensional deformations is determined by end-to-end extension of a red cell by diametrically opposed pipettes (middle left) and following the rate of recovery of the initial shape after release from one of the pipettes (middle right). The time constant from recovery from bending deformations is determined by following the recovery of the unstressed shape after release of a folded cell from a large (4 mm) pipette. Videomicrographs of a red cell just after expulsion from the pipette (bottom left) and during the recovery phase (bottom right) are shown.

zation of the membrane from oxidative damage (Evans and Mohandas, 1987; Hebbel et al., 1990). In contrast to this strong dependence of extensional rigidity on cell hemoglobin concentration, bending rigidity varies little with hemoglobin concentration; for the most dehydrated sickle cells, it increased only by approximately 50 percent (Evans et al., 1984).

The dynamic rigidity of normal cells and oxygenated sickle cells, as reflected by time constants for extensional recovery and recovery from bending, is also strongly dependent on the state of cell hydration (Fig. 21.11). The two time constants (Te and Tf) are the same for normal cells and oxygenated sickle cells at similar cell hemoglobin concentrations and hence similar states of cell hydration. This is in marked contrast with measurements on static extensional rigidity in which the behavior of oxygenated sickle cells is different from that of normal red cells. Furthermore, increases in extensional and folding recovery times with increasing cell hemoglobin concentration are much more pronounced than those seen for static extensional or bending rigidities. The time constant for extensional recovery of a sickle cell increases from 0.125 to 2.5 seconds as the hemoglobin concentration increases from 32 to 48 g/dL (Fig. 21.11). However, the increased recovery times seen at elevated hemoglobin concentrations could be returned to normal values by hydration of the cells (Evans et al., 1984). This implies that increased hemoglobin concentration plays a dominant role in the dynamic behavior of red cells.

The rheologic properties of oxygenated sickle cells are thus strongly influenced by the state of cell hydration and the increased propensity for oxidative dam-

A

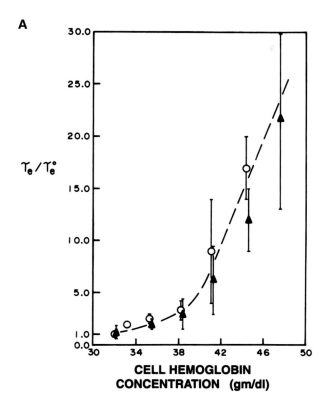

C

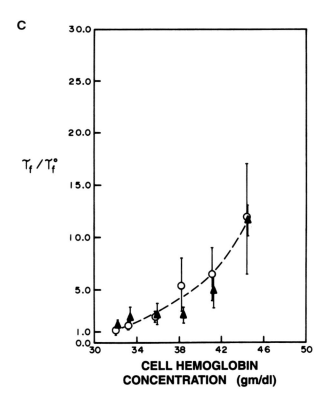

B

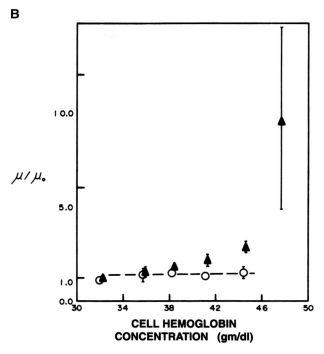

Figure 21.11. Ratio of membrane extensional rigidity measured for cells in specific density fractions (m) to the average value of the extensional rigidity for normal cells in the 32 g/dL fraction (mo) (**B**). Note that while extensional rigidity of sickle red cells increased with increasing cell hemoglobin concentration, the extensional rigidity of normal red cells is independent of cell hemoglobin concentration. Ratio of time constant for rapid elastic recovery from end-to-end extension (**A**) measured for cells in specific density fractions to the average value of the time constant for normal cells in the 32 g/dL fraction (0.12 seconds). Ratio of time constant for recovery from bending deformations (**C**) measured for cells in specific density fractions to the average value of the time constant for normal cells in the 32 g/dL fraction (0.12 seconds). Note that the time constants for recovery from extensional and bending deformations are both strongly dependent on cell hemoglobin concentration. Furthermore, in contrast to extensional rigidity, both normal red cells and sickle red cells show the same dependence on cell hemoglobin concentration for time constants for recovery from extensional and bending deformations. The open circles are the mean values of this ratio for normal red cells and darkened triangles are the mean values for sickle red cells. The standard deviations are shown by brackets about the mean values, and the characteristic behavior of normal red cells is indicated by a dashed line.

age to membranes (Clark et al., 1980; Evans et al., 1984; Clark, 1989; Hebbel et al., 1990).

Temporal Variations in Dense Rheologic Compromised Sickle Cells

Studies have found that the number of ISCs, a morphologically distinct subpopulation of the dense cell fraction, is constant over time and does not fluctuate with vasoocclusive episodes (Serjeant et al., 1969). Recent studies have shown that there are not only substantial differences in the number of dense red cells among individuals with different genotypes of sickle cell disease and among individuals with the same genotype, but also variations in the percentage of dense red cells in individual patients over time (Embury et al., 1984b; Fabry et al., 1984; Ballas et al., 1988; Lande et al., 1988; Akinola et al., 1992; Ballas and Smith., 1992; Mohandas and Ballas, 1994). This variation appears to be particularly striking during the onset and resolution of vasoocclusive episodes (see Chapter 25). It is likely that the "typical" painful event in adults is a dynamic process having two distinct phases: evolution and resolution. During the evolving phase the percentage of dense cells increases above the steady-state value. In addition, anemia worsens slightly as evidenced by a decline in hemoglobin values and a subsequent rise in reticulocyte numbers. During the resolving phase of the episode the percentage of dense cells decreases to below steady-state values but subsequently recovers to the steady-state value over a period of days. Unanswered questions in this regard pertain to the relationship of dense cell sequestration and dense cell generation rates to the observed density changes during these acute episodes. Cell density heterogeneity and hence the extent of rheologic abnormalities of circulating red cells is thus not fixed over time in an individual patient but exhibits dynamic changes that appear to be related to the clinical status of the patient.

Effect of Deoxygenation on Sickle Cell Deformability

An important rheologic feature that distinguishes sickle from normal red cells is the effect of deoxygenation, which has profound influence on deformability and rheology of sickle red cells but has no effect on normal red cells (Danish and Harris, 1983; Nash et al., 1986; Sorette et al., 1987; Keidan et al., 1989; Schmalzer et al., 1989; Mackie and Hochmuth, 1990; Itoh et al., 1992). Measurements using viscometry, filtration, ektacytometry, and micropipette aspiration have shown that the already compromised deformability of oxygenated sickle cells is further dramatically reduced following deoxygenation. This results in increased viscosity of sickle cell disease blood, inability of these cells to traverse narrow pores (causing blockage), loss of ability to manifest dynamic, tank-treading motion in shear fields in the ektacytometer, and dramatic increases in the pressures needed to aspirate sickled cells into micropipettes. The marked increase in the static and dynamic rigidities of sickle red cells following deoxygenation is exemplified by the finding that both static extensional rigidity and the dynamic rigidity increase by two to three orders of magnitude following deoxygenation (Nash et al., 1986; Mackie and Hochmuth, 1990; Itoh et al., 1992).

Just as there is heterogeneity among oxygenated sickle red cells, deoxygenation-induced decreases in cellular deformability also exhibit heterogeneous responses that are cell-density–dependent. During deoxygenation, the critical partial pressure of oxygen (PO_2) at which sickle red cells lose their deformability depends on cell hemoglobin concentration. For example, ektacytometric measurements showed that while loss of cellular deformability of whole sickle blood samples occurred over a broad range of PO_2 values, the loss of deformability for subpopulations of sickle red cells with a narrow range of cell densities occurred over a very small range of PO_2 values (Sorette et al., 1987). The higher the cell hemoglobin concentration, the higher the PO_2 at which the cells lose their ability to deform (Sorette et al., 1987).

This effect of deoxygenation is a direct consequence of increased cytoplasmic viscosity because hemoglobin in the cell interior undergoes a phase transition from a fluid to a solid phase during hemoglobin polymerization. There has been considerable debate concerning the extent of polymer formation necessary to induce altered deformability. Based on filtration studies, it has been suggested that small amounts of polymer formed especially in dense sickle cells can have profound effects on deformability (Green et al., 1988). However, micropipette studies on individual cells at varying PO_2 indicate that loss of deformability is a precipitous event coincident with extensive polymer formation and morphologic sickling (Nash et al., 1986; Itoh et al., 1992). Kinetic studies support the latter view (Mozzarelli et al., 1987). The most convincing evidence to date thus implies that deoxygenation-induced increases in cellular rigidity require a substantial amount of polymer formation and the transition of the hemoglobin from a fluid to a solid phase.

Vascular Tone

The dynamic and shifting balance between stimuli that provoke contraction and relaxation of the vascular tone can also play a significant role in regulating blood flow through the vasculature. In particular, local control of vascular tone by vasoconstrictor or vasodilator substances could be a major regulator of circulatory blood flow. The endothelial cell layer forms the permeability barrier between circulating blood cells and the underlying vascular tissue and as such is in a unique situation to respond to environmental conditions and modulate events in the vasculature via paracrine effects. The first endothelium-derived mediator identified to act on vascular smooth muscle cells was prostacyclin, a vasorelaxing cyclooxygenase product (Weksler et al., 1978). Prostacyclin production can be stimulated by physical perturbations of the endothelial cell membrane. Subsequently, more potent vasodilators have been described, the most potent being NO (Ignarro et al., 1987; Palmer et al., 1987) released by the endothelial cells. Endothelial cells also produce vasoconstrictor substances that include platelet-derived growth factor (PDGF) and endothelin-1 (Berk et al., 1986; Yanagisawa et al., 1988). Particularly relevant to sickle cell disease is the finding that local oxygen tension is a potent environmental modulator of vascular tone, in part through modulating the local release of vasodilators and vasoconstrictors. The vascular response to hypoxia has multiple components that contribute to both the initial responses and the long-term sequelae. The acute response includes the induction of vasoconstriction in pulmonary vasculature and systemic arteries. Chronic hypoxia can lead to remodeling of the vasculature including excess smooth muscle formation. It is likely that imbalances in vascular tone, manifested by local vasospasm or failure of vasodilatory mechanisms, contribute to sickle cell crises and organ damage.

Physiologic Consequences of Altered Red Cell Deformability and Vascular Tone

The marked increase in static and dynamic rigidity of oxygenated sickle cells with elevated hemoglobin concentration has a major influence on the dynamics of their circulation in the microvasculature (Lipowsky et al., 1982, 1987; Kaul et al., 1983, 1986; Kurantsin-Mills et al., 1987, 1988; Dong et al., 1992). This includes a reduced rate of entry of these red cells into capillaries, as well as reductions in flow velocities of these cells during transit through the capillaries. Recent in vivo studies using a transgenic knockout mice model of sickle cell disease lend support to this thesis (Embury et al., 1999). Intravital microscopy was used to compare blood flow in the mucosal-intestinal microvessels of normal mice with that in transgenic knockout sickle mice that have red cells containing only human sickle hemoglobin and that exhibit a degree of hemolytic anemia and pathologic complications similar to the human disease. In sickle mice, in addition to seeing blood flow abnormalities such as sludging in microvessels, decreased blood flow velocity was noted in venules of all diameters. Flow responses to hyperoxia in normal and sickle cell mice were dramatic, but opposite: Hyperoxia promptly slowed blood flow in normal mice but markedly enhanced flow in sickle cell mice, implying that deoxygenation-induced increased rigidity does regulate blood flow in sickle cell disease under normoxic conditions. Increased rigidity can also result in mechanical trapping

of these cells in the microvasculature. These factors can significantly reduce tissue oxygen delivery. Moreover, there is an increased probability of hemoglobin polymerization in these cells as a consequence of longer transit times through regions of low oxygen tension.

The marked increase in static and dynamic rigidity following deoxygenation, in turn, will have additional influences on circulatory dynamics of the sickle cells such as mechanical trapping in the microvasculature and in the reticuloendothelial system. This can lead to blockage of the blood flow, which in turn results in tissue hypoxia and damage. Totally occluded capillaries were indeed observed in the rat mesocecum perfused with sickle red cells (Kaul et al., 1986, 1996). These altered rheologic properties will also contribute to the initiation and propagation of vasoocclusive events. While the effects of rheologic abnormalities of oxygenated sickle cells will be felt throughout the vasculature system, the effects of deoxgenation-induced increases in rigidity will be more restricted, being felt only at sites of low oxygen tension in the vasculature where the cells can undergo sickling. Also, persistence or formation of sickled cells in venous blood can have a major impact on pulmonary circulation. It should be noted that flow disturbances involving deoxygenated cells are likely to be much more pronounced, since the magnitude of the rheologic abnormalities of these cells is much greater.

There is evidence that control of local vascular tone is abnormal not only during sickle cell crises but also in the steady state (Rodgers et al., 1984; Lipowsky et al., 1987; Kennedy et al., 1988). Study of blood flow in nailbed capillary loops showed increased frequency of episodes of stasis or intermittent flow in sickle cell subjects compared to normal subjects (Lipowsky et al., 1987). Large local oscillations in periodic microcirculatory flow have been demonstrated in subjects with sickle cell disease (Rodgers et al., 1984; Kennedy et al., 1988). Synchronization of rhythmic flow occurred in large domains of microvessels in these subjects, perhaps reflecting periodic flow at the level of arterioles rather than in individual capillaries, as seen in normal subjects. While these flow disturbances have been interpreted as due to intermittent occlusion with sickled red cells, it is also possible that local instability of vascular tone and unbalanced regulatory and compensatory mechanisms may also account for these flow disturbances. Existence of an abnormal state of vasodilation and low vascular resistance in sickle cell subjects in the steady state may serve the beneficial effect of producing fast transit times and decrease the likelihood of local cell sickling. During acute painful episodes, however, there could be decreases in vasodilator substances such as prostacyclins and NO and a reciprocal increase in vasoconstrictor substances including endothelin and prostaglandins, leading the balance of vascular tone to be shifted toward vasoconstriction, clearly a maladaptive response. This vasoconstriction would result in the slowing of vascular flow, further obstruction, and more profound deoxygenation of sickle cells.

SUMMARY

Increased adherence to vascular endothelium and rheologic abnormalities are striking features of sickle red cells. Increased or altered surface expression of adhesive molecules on sickle red cells and endothelial cells plays a role in adherence of sickle cells to vascular endothelium. Increased adherence can lead to vessel obstruction and trapping of rheologically compromised red cells. Cellular dehydration and consequent increased cytoplasmic viscosity is a major determinant of the abnormal behavior of sickle red cells. The consequences of these rheologic abnormalities include a reduced rate of entry of these red cells into capillaries, reductions in flow velocities during transit through the capillaries, and mechanical trapping in the microvasculature. There are marked heterogeneities in the extent of adherence and rheologic abnormalities for red cells in individual blood samples and among blood samples from different individuals. The dynamic and shifting balance between stimuli that provoke contraction and relaxation of the vascular tone can also play a significant role in regulating blood flow through the vasculature. The abnormal cell adherence, altered rheology of red cells, and modulation of vascular tone can all contribute significantly to the chronic tissue hypoxia, vasoocclusive episodes, and organ damage that define the vascular pathobiology of sickle disease.

References

Akinola, NO, Stevens, SME, Franklin, IM et al. (1992). Rheological changes in the prodromal and established phases of sickle vaso-occlusive crisis, *Br. J. Haematol.* 81: 598–602.

Antonucci, R Walker, R, Herion, J et al. (1990). Enhancement of sickle erythrocyte adherence to endothelium by autologous platelets. *Am. J. Hematol.* 34: 44–48.

Ballas, SK and Smith, ED. (1992). Red cell changes during the evolution of the sickle cell painful crisis. *Blood* 79: 2154–2163.

Ballas, SK, Larner, J, Smith, ED et al. (1988). Rheologic predictors of the severity of the painful sickle cell crisis. *Blood* 72: 1216–1223.

Ballas, SK, Dover, GJ, and Charache, S. (1989). The effect of hydroxyurea on the rheological properties of sickle erythrocytes in vivo. *Am. J. Hematol.* 32: 104–111.

Ballas, SK, Mohandas, N, Cremins, J et al. (1992). Contribution of reticulocytes and mature erythrocytes to cellular dehydration in various sickle cell syndromes. *Blood* 80 (Suppl 1): 9a (abstract).

Barabino, GA, McIntire, LV, Eskin, SG et al. (1987a). Endothelial cell interactions with sickle cell, sickle trait, mechanically injured, and normal erythrocytes under controlled flow. *Blood* 70: 152–157.

Barabino, GA, McIntire, LV, Eskin, SG, and Udden MM. (1987b). Effect of pentoxifylline on adherence of sickle erythrocytes to vascular endothelial cells. *Clin. Hemorheol.* 7: 339–349.

Barabino, GA, Wise, RJ, Woodbury, VA et al. (1997). Inhibition of sickle erythrocyte adhesion to immobilized thrombospondin by von Willebrand factor under dynamic flow conditions. *Blood* 89: 2560–2567.

Barabino, GA, Liu, XD, Ewenstein, BM et al. (1999). Anionic polysaccharides inhibit adhesion of sickle erythrocytes to the vascular endothelium and result in improved hemodynamic behavior. *Blood* 93: 1422–1429.

Bauer, TW, Moore, W, and Hutchins, GM. (1980). The liver in sickle cell disease, a clinicopathologic study of 70 patients. *Am. J. Med.* 69: 833–837.

Berk, BC, Alexander, RW, Brock, TA et al. (1986). Vasoconstriction: A new activity for platelet-derived growth factor. *Science* 32: 87–89.

Bertles, JF and Milner, PFA. (1968). Irreversibly sickled erythrocytes: A consequence of the heterogeneous distribution of hemoglobin types in sickle cell anemia. *J. Clin. Invest.* 47: 1731–1741.

Bessis, M and Mohandas, N. (1977). Laser diffraction patterns of sickle cells in shear fields. *Blood Cells* 3: 229–239.

Bolarin, DM and Adenuga, AO. (1986). Plasma fibronectin in sickle cell disease. *Acta Haematol.* 75: 209–210.

Bookchin, RM, Ortiz, OE, and Lew, VL. (1991). Evidence for a direct reticulocyte origin of dense red cells in sickle cell anemia. *J. Clin. Invest.* 87: 113–120.

Branemark, PI and Bagge, V. (1977). Intravascular rheology of erythrocytes in man. *Blood Cells* 3: 11–24.

Bridges, KR, Barabino, GD, Brugnara, C et al. (1996). A multiparameter analysis of sickle erythrocytes in patients undergoing hydroxyurea therapy. *Blood* 88: 4701–4710.

Brittain, HA, Eckman, JR, and Wick, TM. (1992). Sickle erythrocyte adherence to large vessel and microvascular endothelium under physiologic flow is qualitatively different. *J. Lab. Clin. Med.* 120: 538–545.

Brittain, HA, Eckman, JR, Swerlick, RA et al. (1993). Thrombospondin from activated platelets promotes sickle erythrocyte adherence to human microvascular endothelium under physiologic flow, a potential role for platelet activation in sickle cell vaso-occlusion. *Blood* 81: 2137–2143.

Browne, PV and Hebbel, RP. (1996). CD36-positive stress reticulocytosis in sickle cell anemia. *J. Lab. Clin. Med.* 127: 340–347.

Browne, PV, Mosher, D, Steinberg, MH, and Hebbel, RP. (1996). Disturbance of plasma and platelet thrombospondin levels in sickle cell disease. *Am. J. Hematol.* 51: 296–301.

Brugnara, C. (1995). Erythrocyte dehydration in pathophysiology and treatment of sickle cell disease. *Curr. Opin. Hematol.* 2: 132–138.

Carlos, TM and Harlan, JM. (1994). Leukocyte-endothelial adhesion molecules. *Blood* 84: 2068–2101.

Chien, S, Usami, S, and Bertles, JF. (1970). Abnormal rheology of oxygenated blood in sickle cell anemia. *J. Clin. Invest.* 49: 623–630.

Chien, S, King, RG, Kaperonis, AA, and Usami, S. (1982). Viscoelastic properties of sickle cells and hemoglobin. *Blood Cells* 8: 53–64.

Clark, MR. (1989). Mean corpuscular hemoglobin concentration and cell deformability. *Ann. N.Y. Acad. Sci.* 565: 284–294.

Clark, MR, Mohandas, N, and Shohet, SB. (1980). Deformability of oxygenated irreversibly sickled cells. *J. Clin. Invest.* 65: 189–196.

Clark, MR, Mohandas, N, Embury, SH et al. (1982). A simple laboratory alternative to irreversibly sickled cell (ISC) counts. *Blood* 60: 659–662.

Danish, EH, and Harris, JW. (1983). Viscosity studies of deoxy hemoglobin S: Evidence for formation of microaggregates during the lag phase. *J. Lab. Clin. Med.* 101: 515–526.

Dong, C, Chadwick, RS, and Schechter, AN. (1992). Influence of sickle hemoglobin polymerization and membrane properties on deformability of sickle erythrocytes in the microcirculation. *Biophys. J.* 63: 774–783.

Embury, SH, Clark, MR, Monroy, G et al. (1984a). Concurrent sickle cell anemia and alpha thalassemia: Effect on pathological properties of sickle erythrocytes. *J. Clin. Invest.* 73: 116–122.

Embury, SH, Garcia, JF, Mohandas, N et al. (1984b). Oxygen inhalation by subjects with sickle cell anemia. Effects on endogenous erythropoietin kinetics, erythropoiesis and pathologic properties of sickle blood. *N. Engl. J. Med.* 31: 291–295.

Embury, SH, Hebbel, RP, Steinberg, MH et al. (1994). Pathogenesis of vasoocclusion. In Embury, SH, Hebbel, RP, Mohandas, N, and Steinberg, MH, editors, *Sickle cell disease: Basic principles and clinical practice.* New York: Raven Press, pp. 311–326.

Embury, SH, Mohandas, N, Paszty, C, Cooper, P et al. (1999). In vivo blood flow abnormalities in the transgenic knockout sickle cell mouse. *J. Clin. Invest.* 103: 915–920.

Evans, EA. (1983). Bending elastic modulus of red cell membrane derived from buckling instability in micropipette aspiration tests. *Biophys. J.* 43: 27–33.

Evans, EA and Hochmuth, RM. (1976). Membrane viscoelasticity. *Biophys. J.* 16: 1–11.

Evans, EA and Hochmuth, RM. (1977). A solid-liquid composite model of the red cell membrane. *J. Membr. Biol.* 30: 351–362.

Evans, EA and Mohandas, N. (1987). Membrane-associated sickle hemoglobin: A major determinant of sickle erythrocyte rigidity. *Blood* 70: 1443–1449.

Evans, E, Mohandas, N, and Leung, A. (1984). Static and dynamic rigidities of normal and sickle erythrocytes: Major influence of cell hemoglobin concentration. *J. Clin. Invest.* 73: 477–488.

Fabry, ME and Nagel, RL. (1982). Heterogeneity of red cells in the sickler: A characteristic with practical clinical and pathophysiologic implications. *Blood Cells* 8: 9–15.

Fabry, ME, Benjamin, L, Lawrence, C, and Nagel RL. (1984). An objective sign in painful crisis in sickle cell anemia: The concomitant reduction of high density red cells. *Blood* 64: 559–564.

Fabry, ME, Romero, JR, Buchanan, ID et al. (1991). Rapid increase in red blood cell density drive by K:Cl contransport in a subset of sickle cell anemia reticulocytes and discocytes. *Blood* 78: 217–225.

Fabry, ME, Fine, E, Rajanayagam, V et al. (1992). Demonstration of endothelial adhesion of sickle cells in vivo, a distinct role for deformable sickle cell discocytes. *Blood* 79: 1602–1611.

Fortier, N, Snyder, LM, Garver, C et al. (1988). The relationship between in vivo generated hemoglobin skeletal protein complex and increased red cell membrane rigidity. *Blood* 71: 1427–1431.

Fox-Robichaud, A, Payne, D, Hassan, SU et al. (1998). Inhaled NO as a viable antiadhesive therapy for ischemia/reperfusion injury of distal microvascular beds. *J. Clin. Invest.* 101: 2497–2505.

Francis, RB Jr. (1991). Platelets, coagulation, and fibrinolysis in sickle cell disease, their possible role in vascular occlusion. *Blood Coag. Fibrinol.* 2: 341–353.

Francis, RB Jr and Hebbel, RP. (1994). Hemostasis. In Embury, SH, Hebbel, RP, Mohandas, N, and Steinberg MH, editors. *Sickle cell disease: Basic principles and clinical practice.* New York: Raven Press, pp. 299–310.

Franco, RS, Barker-Gear, R, Miller, MA et al. (1994). Fetal hemoglobin and potassium in isolated transferrin receptor-positive dense sickle reticulocytes. *Blood* 6: 2013–2020.

Franco, RS, Palascak, M, Thompson, H, and Joiner, CH. (1995). KCl cotransport activity in light versus dense transferrin receptor-positive sickle reticulocytes. *J. Clin. Invest.* 6: 2573–2580.

Franco, RS, Palascak, M, Thompson, H et al. (1996). Dehydration of transferrin receptor-positive sickle reticulocytes during continuous or cyclic deoxygenation: Role of KCl cotransport and extracellular calcium. *Blood* 11: 4359–4365.

Franco, RS, Thompson, H, and Plascak, M. (1997). The formation of transferrin receptor-positive sickle reticulocytes with intermediate density is not determined by fetal hemoglobin content. *Blood* 31: 3195–3203.

Franco, RS, Lohmann, J, Silberstein, EB et al. (1998). Time-dependent changes in the density and hemoglobin F content of biotin-labeled sickled cells. *J. Clin. Invest.* 12: 2730–2740.

French, JA II, Kenny, D, Scott, JP et al. (1997). Mechanisms of stroke in sickle cell disease: Sickle erythrocytes decrease cerebral blood flow in rats after nitric oxide synthase inhibition. *Blood* 89: 4591–4599.

Frenette, PS, Moyna, C, Hartwell, DW et al. (1998). Platelet-endothelial interactions in inflamed mesenteric venules. *Blood* 91: 1318–1324.

Galili, U, Clark, MR, and Shohet, SB. (1986). Excessive binding of natural anti-alpha-galactosyl immunoglobin G to sickle erythrocytes may contribute to extravascular cell destruction. *J. Clin. Invest.* 77: 27–33.

Gee, BE and Platt, OS. (1995). Sickle reticulocytes adhere to VCAM-1. *Blood* 85: 268–274.

Gill, FA, Kaye, D, and Hook, EW. (1966). The influence of erythrophagocytosis on the interaction of macrophages and Salmonella in vitro. *J. Exp. Med.* 124: 173–183.

Grabowski, EF. (1987). Sickle erythrocytes adhere to endothelial cell monolayers (ECM's) exposed to flowing blood. In Nagel, RL, editor. *Pathophysiological aspects of sickle cell vaso-occlusion.* New York: Alan R. Liss, pp. 167–179.

Green, GA, Rehn, MM, and Kalra, VK. (1985). Cell-bound autologous immunoglobulin in erythrocyte subpopulations from patients with sickle cell disease. *Blood* 65: 1127–1133.

Green, MA, Noguchi, CT, Keidan, AJ et al. (1988). Polymerization of sickle hemoglobin at arterial saturation impairs erythrocyte deformability. *J. Clin. Invest.* 81: 1669–1675.

Gupta, K, Gupta, P, Solovey, A et al. (1999). Mechanism of interaction of thrombospondin with human endothelium and inhibition of sickle erythrocyte adhesion to human endothelial cells by heparin. *Biochim. Biophys. Acta.* 1453: 63–73.

Ham, TH and Castle, WB. (1940). Relationship of increased hypotonic fragility to erythrostasis in certain anemias. *Trans. Assoc. Am. Phys.* 55: 127–132.

Havell, TC, Hillman, D, and Lessin, LS. (1978). Deformability characteristics of sickle cells by microelastimetry. *Am. J. Hematol.* 4: 9–17.

Hebbel, RP. (1990). The sickle erythrocyte in double jeopardy: Autooxidation and iron decompartmentalization. *Semin. Hematol.* 27: 51–60.

Hebbel, RP. (1991). Beyond hemoglobin polymerization: The red blood cell membrane and sickle disease pathophysiology. *Blood* 77: 214–237.

Hebbel, RP. (1997). Adhesive interactions of sickle erythrocytes with endothelium. *J. Clin. Invest.* 99: 2561–2564.

Hebbel, RP and Miller, WJ. (1984). Phagocytosis of sickle erythrocytes, immunologic and oxidative determinants of hemolytic anemia. *Blood* 64: 733–741.

Hebbel, RP and Miller, WJ. (1988). Unique promotion of erythrophagocytosis by malondialdehyde. *Am. J. Hematol.* 29: 222–225.

Hebbel, RP and Mohandas, N. (1994). Sickle cell adherence. In Embury, SH, Hebbel, RP, Mohandas, N, and Steinberg, MH, editors. *Sickle cell disease: Basic principles and clinical practice.* New York: Raven Press, pp. 217–230.

Hebbel, RP and Vercellotti, GM. (1997). The endothelial biology of sickle cell disease. *J. Lab. Clin. Med.* 129: 288–293.

Hebbel, RP, Boogaerts, MAB, Eaton, JW et al. (1980a). Erythrocyte adherence to endothelium in sickle-cell anemia. A possible determinant of disease severity. *N. Engl. J. Med.* 302: 992–995.

Hebbel, RP, Yamada, O, Moldow, CF et al. (1980b). Abnormal adherence of sickle erythrocytes to cultured vascular endothelium. Possible mechanism for microvascular occlusion in sickle cell disease. *J. Clin. Invest.* 65: 154–160.

Hebbel, RP, Moldow, CF, and Steinberg, MH. (1981). Modulation of erythrocyte-endothelial interactions and the vasoocclusive severity of sickling disorders. *Blood* 58: 947–952.

Hebbel, RP, Visser, MR, Goodman, JL et al. (1987). Potentiated adherence of sickle erythrocytes to endothelium infected by virus. *J. Clin. Invest.* 80: 1503–1506.

Hebbel, RP, Ney, PA, and Foker, W. (1989). Autoxidation, dehydration, and adhesivity may be related abnormalities of sickle erythrocytes. *Am. J. Physiol.* 256: C579–C583.

Hebbel, RP, Leung, A, and Mohandas, N. (1990). Oxidation-induced changes in microrheologic properties of the red cell membrane. *Blood* 76: 1015–1020.

Hebbel, RP, Solovey, AA, and Solovey, AN. (1999). Circulating endothelial cells have the same activation phenotype as vessel wall endothelium in sickle transgenic mice. *Experimental Biology '99,* Abstract 828.3.

Hillery, CA, Du, MC, Montgomery, RR et al. (1996). Increased adhesion of erythrocytes to components of the extracellular matrix: Isolation and characterization of a red blood cell lipid that binds thrombospondin and laminin. *Blood* 87: 4879–4886.

Hochmuth, RM, Worthy, PR, and Evans, EA. (1979). Red cell extensional recovery and the determination of membrane viscosity. *Biophys. J.* 26: 101–114.

Hook, EW, Kaye, D, and Gill, FA. (1967). Factors influencing host resistance to Salmonella infection. The effects of hemolysis and erythrophagocytosis. *Trans. Am. Clin. Climatol. Assoc.* 78: 230–241.

Hoover, R, Rubin, R, Wise, G et al. (1979). Adhesion of normal and sickle erythrocytes to endothelial monolayer cultures. *Blood* 54: 872–876.

Horiuchi, K, Ballas, SK, and Asakura, T. (1988). The effect of deoxygenation rate on the formation of irreversibly sickled cells. *Blood* 71: 46–51.

Horiuchi, K, Stephens, MJ, Adachi, K et al. (1993). Image analysis studies of the degree of irreversible deformation of sickle cells in relation to cell density and HbF level. *Br. J. Haematol.* 85: 356–384.

Houston, PE, Rana, S, Sekhsaria, S et al. (1997). Homocysteine in sickle cell disease: Relationship to stroke. *Am. J. Med.* 103: 192–196.

Ignarro, LJ, Byrns, RE, Buga, GM et al. (1987). Endothelium-derived relaxing factor from pulmonary artery and vein possesses pharmacologic and chemical properties identical to those of nitric oxide radical. *Circ. Res.* 61: 866–879.

Itoh, T, Chien, S, and Usami, S. (1992). Deformability measurements on individual sickle cells using a new system with pO2 and temperature control. *Blood* 79: 2141–2147.

Joneckis, CC, Ackley, RL, Orringer, EP et al. (1993). Integrin a4b1 and glycoprotein IV (CD36) are expressed on circulating reticulocytes in sickle cell anemia. *Blood* 82: 3548–3555.

Joneckis, CC, Shock, DD, Cunningham, ML et al. (1996). Glycoprotein IV-independent adhesion of sickle red blood cells to immobilized thrombospondin under flow conditions. *Blood* 11: 4862–4870.

Kasschau, MR, Barabino, GA, Bridges, KR et al. (1996). Adhesion of sickle neutrophils and erythrocytes to fibronectin. *Blood* 87: 771–780.

Kaul, D. (1992). Microvascular flow behavior of red cells in sickle cell anemia. *Clin. Hemorheol.* 12: 191–202.

Kaul, DK, and Hebbel, RP. (1999). Leukocyte-endothelial interactions in transgenic sickle mouse during steady-state and after hypoxia-reoxygenation. *Blood* 94 (Suppl): 676a.

Kaul, DK, Fabry, ME, Windisch, P et al. (1983). Erythrocytes in sickle cell anemia are heterogeneous in their rheological and hemodynamic characteristics. *J. Clin. Invest.* 72: 22–29.

Kaul, DK, Fabry, ME, and Nagel, RL. (1986). Vaso-occlusion by sickle cells: Evidence for selective trapping of dense cells. *Blood* 68: 1162–1168.

Kaul, DK, Fabry, ME, and Nagel, RL. (1989). Microvascular sites and characteristics of sickle cell adhesion to vascular endothelium in shear flow conditions, pathophysiological implications. *Proc. Natl. Acad. Sci. U.S.A.* 86: 3356–3360.

Kaul, D, Chen, D, and Zhan, J. (1994). Adhesion of sickle cells to vascular endothelium is critically dependent on changes in density and shape of the cells. *Blood* 83: 3006–3017.

Kaul, DK, Fabry, ME, Constantini, F et al. (1995). In vivo demonstration of red cell-endothelial interaction, sickling and altered microvascular response to oxygen in the sickle transgenic mouse. *J. Clin. Invest.* 96: 2845–2853.

Kaul, DK, Fabry, ME, and Nagel, RL. (1996). The pathophysiology of vascular obstruction in the sickle syndromes. *Blood* 1: 29–44.

Keidan, AJ, Noguchi, CT, Player, M et al. (1989). Erythrocyte heterogeneity in sickle cell disease: Effect of deoxygenation on intracellular polymer formation and rheology of subpopulations. *Br. J. Haematol.* 72: 254–261.

Kennedy, AP, Williams, B, Meydrech, EF et al. (1988). Regional and temporal variation in oscillatory blood flow in sickle cell disease. *Am. J. Hematol.* 28: 92.

Krogh, A. (1930). *The Anatomy and Physiology of Capillaries.* New York: Hafner.

Kucuk, O, Gilman-Sachs, A, Beaman, K et al. (1993). Antiphospholipid antibodies in sickle cell disease. *Am. J. Hematol.* 42: 380–383.

Kucukcelebi, A, Barmatoski, SP, and Barnhart, MI. (1980). Interactions between vessel wall and perfused sickled erythrocytes: Preliminary observations. *Scanning Electron Microsc.* 3: 243–248.

Kumar, A, Eckman, JR, Swerlick, RA et al. (1996). Phorbol ester stimulation increases sickle erythrocyte adherence to endothelium: A novel pathway involving $\alpha_4\beta_1$ integrin receptors on sickle reticulocytes and fibronectin. *Blood* 88: 4348–4358.

Kurantsin-Mills, J, Jacobs, HM, Klug, PP et al. (1987). Flow dynamics of human sickle erythrocytes in the mesenteric microcirculation of the change-transfused rat. *Microvasc. Res.* 34: 152–165.

Kurantsin-Mills, J, Klug, PP, and Lessin, LS. (1988). Vaso-occlusion in sickle cell disease: Pathophysiology of the microvascular circulation. *Am. J. Pediatr. Hematol. Oncol.* 10: 357–372.

Lande, WM, Andrews, DL, Clark, MR et al. (1988). The incidence of painful crisis in homozygous sickle cell disease, correlation with red cell deformability. *Blood* 72: 2056–2059.

Lee, SP, Cunningham, ML, Hines, PC, Joneckis, CC et al. (1998). Sickle cell adhesion to laminin: Potential role for the α5 chain. *Blood* 92: 2951–2958.

Lipowsky, HH, Usami, S, and Chien, S. (1982). Human SS red cell rheological behavior in the microcirculation of cremaster muscle. *Blood Cells* 8: 113–126.

Lipowsky, HH, Sheikh, NU, and Katz, DM. (1987). Intravital microscopy of capillary hemodynamics in sickle cell disease. *J. Clin. Invest.* 80: 117–129.

Longenecker, GL, Beyers, BJ, and McMullan, E. (1990). Red cell-endothelial cell adhesion, role and modulation in sickle cell disease. In Rubanyi, GM and Vanhoutte, PM, editors. *Endothelium-Derived Relaxing Factors.* Basel: Karger, pp. 281–290.

Mackie, LH and Hochmuth, RM. (1990). The influence of oxygen tension, temperature, and hemoglobin concentration on the rheological properties of sickle erythrocytes. *Blood* 76: 1256–1261.

Manodori, AB, Matsui, NM, Chen, JY et al. (1998). Enhanced adherence of sickle erythrocytes to thrombin-treated endothelial cells involves interendothelial cell gap formation. *Blood* 92: 3445–3454.

Marikovsky, Y, Khodadad, JK, and Weinstein, RS. (1978). Influence of red cell shape on surface charge topography. *Exp. Cell Res.* 116: 191–197.

McEvoy, L, Williamson, P, and Schlegel, RA. (1986). Membrane phospholipid asymmetry as a determinant of erythrocyte recognition by macrophages. *Proc. Natl. Acad. Sci. U.S.A.* 83: 3311–3315.

Mendoza, E, Gutgsell, N, Temple, JD, and Issitt, P. (1991). Monocyte phagocytic activity in sickle cell disease. *Acta Haematol.* 85: 199–201.

Messmann, R, Gannon, S, Sarnaik, S, and Johnson, RM. (1990). Mechanical properties of sickle cell membranes. *Blood* 75: 1711–1717.

Mohandas, N and Chasis, JA. (1993). Red cell deformability, membrane material properties and shape: Regulation by transmembrane, skeletal and cytosolic proteins and lipids. *Semin. Hematol.* 30: 171–192.

Mohandas, N and Ballas, SK. (1994). Erythrocyte density and heterogeneity. In Embury, SH, Hebbel, RP, Mohandas, N, and Steinberg, MH, editors. *Sickle cell disease: Basic principles and clinical practice.* New York: Raven Press, pp. 195–204.

Mohandas, N and Evans, E. (1984). Adherence of sickle erythrocytes to vascular endothelial cells: Requirement for both cell membrane changes and plasma factors. *Blood* 64: 282–287.

Mohandas, N, and Evans, E. (1985) Sickle erythrocyte adherence to vascular endothelium. Morphologic correlates and the requirement for divalent cations and collagen-binding plasma proteins. *J. Clin. Invest.* 76: 1605–1612.

Mohandas, N and Hebbel, RP. (1994). Pathogenesis of hemolytic anemia. In Embury, SH, Hebbel, RP, Mohandas, N, and Steinberg, MH, editors. *Sickle cell disease: Basic principles and clinical practice.* New York: Raven Press, pp. 327–334.

Mohandas N, Chasis, JA, and Shohet SB. (1983). The influence of membrane skeleton on red cell deformability, membrane material properties, and shape. *Semin. Hematol.* 20: 225–242.

Mohandas, N, Colella, GM, Fan, S et al. (1991). Dehydration of reticulocytes: A novel mechanism for the generation of dense sickle red cells. *Blood* 78: (Suppl 1): 253a (abstract).

Morris, CL, Gruppo, RA, Shukla, R et al. (1991). Influence of plasma red cell factors on the rheologic properties of oxygenated sickle blood during clinical steady state. *J. Lab. Clin. Med.* 118: 332–342.

Morris, CL, Rucknagel, DL, and Joiner, CH. (1992). Fibrinogen contributes to increased cell-cell adhesion in sickle cells. *Blood* 80 (Suppl): 390a.

Mosseri, M, Bartlett-Pandite, AN, Wenc, K et al. (1993). Inhibition of endothelium-dependent vasorelaxation by sickle erythrocytes. *Am. Heart J.* 126: 338–346.

Mozzarelli, A, Hofrichter, J, and Eaton, WA. (1987). Delay time of hemoglobin S gelation prevents most cells from sickling in vivo. *Science* 237: 500–506.

Nash, GB, Johnson, CS, and Meiselman, HJ. (1984). Mechanical properties of oxygenated red blood cells in sickle cell (HbSS) disease. *Blood* 63: 73–80.

Nash, GB, Johnson, CS, and Meiselman, H. (1986). Influence of oxygen tension on the viscoelastic behavior of red blood cells in sickle cell disease. *Blood* 67: 110–118.

Natarajan, M, Udden, MM, and McIntire, LV. (1996). Adhesion of sickle red blood cells and damage to interleukin-1b stimulated endothelial cells under flow in vitro. *Blood* 87: 4845–4852.

Oh, SO, Ibe, BO, Johnson, C et al. (1997). Platelet-activating factor in plasma of patients with sickle cell disease in steady state. *J. Lab. Clin. Med.* 130: 191–196.

Osarogiagbon, R, Choong, S, Patton, M et al. (1997). Evidence of reperfusion injury physiology in a transgenic mouse model of sickle cell disease. *Blood* In Press.

Palmer, RM, Ferrige, AG, and Moncada, S. (1987). Nitric oxide release accounts for the biological activity of endothelium-derived relaxing factor. *Nature* 327: 524–526.

Petz, LD, Yam, P, Wilkinson, L et al. (1984). Increased IgG molecules bound to the surface of red blood cells of patients with sickle cell anemia. *Blood* 64: 301–304.

Phelan, M, Perrine, SP, Brauer, M, and Faller, DV. (1995). Sickle erythrocytes, after sickling, regulate the expression of the endothelin-1 gene and protein in human endothelial cells in culture. *J. Clin. Invest.* 96: 1145–1151.

Platt, OS. (1982). Exercise-induced hemolysis in sickle cell anemia: Shear sensitive and erythrocyte dehydration. *Blood* 59: 1055–1060.

Rodgers, GP, Schechter, AN, Noguchi, CT et al. (1984). Periodic microcirculatory flow in patients with sickle-cell disease. *N. Engl. J. Med.* 311: 1534–1538.

Rowland, PG, Nash, GB, Cooke, BM et al. (1993). Comparative study of the adhesion of sickle cells and malarial-parasitized red cells to cultured endothelium. *J. Lab. Clin. Med.* 121: 706–713.

Schlegel, RA, Prendergast, TW, and Williamson, P. (1985). Membrane phospholipid asymmetry as a factor in erythrocyte-endothelial cell interactions. *J. Cell. Physiol.* 123: 215–218.

Schlüter, K and Drenckhahn, D. (1986). Co-clustering of denatured hemoglobin with band 3, its role in binding of autoantibodies against band 3 to abnormal and aged erythrocytes. *Proc. Natl. Acad. Sci. U.S.A.* 83: 6137–6141.

Schmalzer, EA, Lee, JO, Brown, AK et al. (1987). Viscosity of mixtures of sickle and normal red cells at varying hematocrit levels: Implications for transfusion. *Transfusion* 27: 228–233.

Schmalzer, EA, Manning, RS, and Chien, S. (1989). Filtration of sickle cells: Recruitment into a rigid fraction as a function of density and oxygen tension. *J. Lab. Clin. Med.* 113: 727–734.

Schwartz, RS, Tanaka, Y, Fidler, IJ et al. (1985). Increased adherence of sickled and phosphatidylserine-enriched human erythrocytes to cultured human peripheral blood monocytes. *J. Clin. Invest.* 75: 1965–1972.

Self, F, McIntire, LV, and Zanger, B. (1977). Rheologic evaluation of Hb S and Hb C hemoglobinopathies. *J. Lab. Clin. Med.* 89: 488–497.

Serjeant, GR, Serjeant, BE, and Milner, PF. (1969). The irreversibly sickled cell: A determinant of hemolysis in sickle cell anemia. *Br. J. Haematol.* 17: 527–533.

Setty, BN, and Stuart, MJ. (1996). Vascular cell adhesion molecule-1 is involved in mediating hypoxia-induced sickle red blood cell adherence to endothelium: Potential role in sickle cell disease. *Blood* 88: 2311–2320.

Setty, BN, Dampier, CD, and Stuart, MJ. (1995). Arachidonic acid metabolites are involved in mediating red blood cell adherence to endothelium. *J. Lab. Clin. Med.* 125: 608–617.

Setty, BN, Chen, D, and Stuart, MJ. (1996). Sickle red blood cells stimulate endothelial cell production of eicosanoids and diacylglycerol. *J. Lab. Clin. Med.* 128: 313–321.

Smith, BD, and LaCelle, PL. (1986). Erythrocyte-endothelial cell adherence in sickle cell disorders. *Blood* 68: 1050–1054.

Smith, CM, Kuettner, JF, Tukey, DP, B et al. (1981). Variable deformability of irreversibly sickled erythrocytes. *Blood* 58: 71–76.

Smith, CM II, Hebbel, RP, Tukey, DP et al. (1987). Pluronic F-68 reduces the endothelial adherence and improves the rheology of liganded sickle erythrocytes. *Blood* 69: 1631–1636.

Solanki, DL. (1985). Erythrophagocytosis in vivo in sickle cell anemia. *Am. J. Hematol.* 20: 353–357.

Solovey, A, Lin, Y, Browne, P, Choong, S et al. (1997). Circulating activated endothelial cells in sickle cell anemia. *N. Engl. J. Med.* 337: 1584–1590.

Solovey, A, Gui, L, Key, NS et al. (1998). Tissue factor expression by endothelial cells in sickle cell anemia. *J. Clin. Invest.* 101: 1899–1904.

Solovey, AA, Solovey, AN, Harness, J et al. (1999). Therapeutic modulation of vascular endothelial cell activation state as therapy for sickle cell disease: NF-κB inhibition as a strategy. *Blood* 94 (Suppl): 676a.

Sorette, MP, Lavenant, MG, and Clark, MR. (1987). Ektacytometric measurement of sickle cell deformability as a continuous function of oxygen tension. *Blood* 69: 316–322.

Sowemimo-Coker, SO, Meiselman, HJ, and Francis, RB Jr. (1989). Increased circulating endothelial cells in sickle cell crisis. *Am. J. Hematol.* 31: 263–265.

Sowemimo-Coker, SO, Haywood, LJ, Meiselman, HJ et al. (1992). Effects of normal and sickle erythrocytes on prostacyclin release by perfused human umbilical cord veins. *Am. J. Hematol.* 40: 276–282.

Styles, LA, Lubin, B, Vichinsky, E, et al, (1997). Decrease of very late activation antigen-4 and CD36 on reticulocytes in sickle cell patients treated with hydroxyurea. *Blood* 89: 2554–2559.

Sugihara, K, Sugihara, T, Mohandas, N et al. (1992). Thrombospondin mediates adherence of CD36 + sickle reticulocytes to endothelial cells. *Blood* 80: 2634–3642.

Sultana, C, Shen, Y, Rattan, V et al. (1998). Interaction of sickle erythrocytes with endothelial cells in the presence of endothelial cell conditioned medium induces oxidant stress leading to transendothelial migration of monocytes. *Blood* 92: 3924–3935.

Swerlick, RA, Lee, KH, Wick, TM, and Lawley, TJ. (1992). Human dermal microvascular endothelial but not human umbilical vein endothelial cells express CD36 in vivo and in vitro. *J. Immunol.* 148: 78–83.

Swerlick, RA, Eckman, JR, Kumar, A et al. (1993). $\alpha_4\beta_1$-Integrin expression on sickle reticulocytes, vascular cell adhesion molecule-1-dependent binding to endothelium. *Blood* 82: 1891–1899.

Sydenstricker, VP. (1924). Further observations on sickle cell anemia. *J. Am. Med. Assoc.* 83: 12–17.

Turrini, F, Arese, P, Yuan, J, and Low, PS. (1991). Clustering of integral membrane proteins of the human erythrocyte membrane stimulates autologous IgG binding, complement deposition, and phagocytosis. *J. Biol. Chem.* 266: 23611–23617.

Udahl, M, Zen, Q, Cottman, M et al. (1998). Basal cell adhesion molecule/Lutheran protein: The receptor critical for sickle cell adhesion to laminin. *J. Clin. Invest.* 101: 1–9.

Usami, S, Chien, S, and Bertles, JF. (1975). Deformability of sickle cells as studied by microsieving. *J. Lab. Clin. Med.* 86: 274–279.

Vordermeier, S, Singh, S, Biggerstaff, J et al. (1992). Red blood cells from patients with sickle cell disease exhibit an increased adherence to cultured endothelium pretreated with tumour necrosis factor (TNF). *Br. J. Haematol.* 81: 591–597.

Waugh, SM, Willardson, BM, Kannan, R et al. (1986). Heinz bodies induce clustering of band 3, glycophorin, and ankyrin in sickle cell erythrocytes. *J. Clin. Invest.* 78: 1155–1160.

Wautier, JL, Pintigny, D, Wautier, MP et al. (1983). Fibrinogen, a modulator of erythrocyte adhesion to vascular endothelium. *J. Lab. Clin. Med.* 101: 911–920.

Wautier, J-L, Galacteros, F, Wautier, MP et al. (1985). Clinical manifestations and erythrocyte adhesion to endothelium in sickle cell syndrome. *Am. J. Hematol.* 19: 121–130.

Wautier, JL, Pintigny, D, Maclouf, J et al. (1986). Release of prostacyclin after erythrocyte adhesion to cultured vascular endothelium. *J. Lab. Clin. Med.* 107: 210–215.

Wayland, H, and Frasher, WA. (1973). Intravital microscopy on the basis of telescopic principles: Design and application of an intravital microscope for microvascular and neurophysiological studies. In Gross, JF, Kaufman, R, and Welterer, E, (editors) *Modern technology in physiologic sciences.* London: Academic Press, p. 125.

Weinstein, R, Zhou, M-a, Bartlett-Pandite, A et al. (1990). Sickle erythrocytes inhibit human endothelial cell DNA synthesis. *Blood* 76: 2146–2152.

Weksler, BB, Ley, CW, and Jaffe, EA. (1978). Stimulation of endothelial cell prostacyclin production by thrombin, trypsin and the ionophore A23187. *J. Clin. Invest.* 62: 923–930.

Wick, TM, Moake, JL, Udden, MM et al. (1987). Unusually large von Willebrand factor multimers increase adhesion of sickle erythrocytes to human endothelial cells under controlled flow. *J. Clin. Invest.* 80: 905–910.

Wick, TM, Moake, JL, Udden, MM, Mc et al. LV. (1992). Unusually large von Willebrand factor multimers preferentially promote young sickle and nonsickle erythrocyte adhesion to endothelial cells. *Am. J. Hematol.* 42: 284–292.

Wun, T, Paglieroni, T, Tablin, F et al. (1997). Platelet activation and platelet-erythrocyte aggregates in patients with sickle cell anemia. *J. Lab. Clin. Med.* 129: 507–516.

Yanagisawa, M, Kurihara, H, Kimura, S, T et al. (1988). A novel potent vasoconstrictor peptide produced by vascular endothelial cells. *Nature* 332: 411–415.

22

Red Cell Membrane in Sickle Cell Disease

CARLO BRUGNARA

Sickle cell disease is a classic example of a genetic disorder of hemoglobin, but many of its clinical manifestations are mediated by cellular interactions that involve the erythrocyte membrane. The membrane of sickle erythrocytes is one of the principal targets of the secondary damage induced by the intracellular polymerization of HbS and cell sickling. Thus, sickle cell anemia is an example not only of a hemoglobinopathy but also of a membrane disease. The damage or changes imposed on the cell membrane by the presence of the abnormal hemoglobin, HbS, play a major role in the pathophysiology of the disease and the associated acute and chronic organ damage. In addition, study of these membrane phenomena provides opportunities to develop new therapeutic strategies for sickle cell disease.

MECHANISMS OF MEMBRANE DAMAGE IN SICKLE CELL DISEASE

Oxidative Damage

There is convincing evidence that HbS has an enhanced tendency to undergo auto-oxidation and is more unstable than HbA (Asakura et al., 1974; Hebbel et al., 1988; Harrington 1998). HbS has a much greater tendency than HbA to interact with and eventually precipitate on the inner surface of the membrane. This process most likely takes place via formation of insoluble hemichromes, oxidation products of methemoglobin, prompting the formation of reactive oxygen radicals and leading to release of iron from heme in the form of highly reactive free iron. The interaction between HbS and the phosphatidylserine (PS) present on the inner leaflet of the lipid bilayer promotes the formation of methemoglobin, hemichromes, and release of heme into the lipid phase (Marva and Hebbel, 1994). In the presence of peroxidation by-products, this process leads to liberation of free iron and additional lipid peroxidation. In addition, the rate of oxidation of HbS becomes 3.4-fold faster in the presence of lipids, which corresponds to a doubling of the oxidation rate for HbS in solution (1.7-fold greater for HbS vs. HbA) (Marva and Hebbel, 1994).

Hebbel proposed that after an initial electrostatic interaction between HbS and the inner membrane, formation of metHb ensues, followed by Hb denaturation, with formation of hemichromes and release of free heme. The presence of free heme promotes lipid peroxidation, which in turn facilitates the release of free iron from heme and induces further oxidative damage. There is evidence that one of the final products of this process, lipid hydroperoxide, is markedly increased in sickle erythrocytes (Sugihara and Hebbel, 1992).

The precipitation of HbS-derived products on the inner surface of the membrane and the associated oxidative damage leads to the formation of Heinz bodies. Heinz bodies affect not only the inner surface of the membrane but also the function of several integral transmembrane proteins, such as band 3 and ankyrin, which aggregate in clusters. Autologous immunoglobulin G (IgG) has been described to bind to the clustered band 3, eventually leading to the removal of the erythrocyte from the circulation (Waugh et al., 1986; Schlüter and Drenckhahn, 1986; Liu et al., 1996).

Hebbel described four major modalities that lead to the abnormal association of iron with the membrane of sickle erythrocytes (Hebbel, 1991, 1994):

Hemichromes: Denatured hemoglobin is a major component of the Heinz bodylike inclusions of sickle cells. Denatured hemoglobin associates in these inclusions with cytoskeletal and integral transmembrane protein. Among these proteins, band 3, with its cytoplasmic domain, plays a dominant role in binding denatured HbS. Approximately 2 to 2.5 hemichrome tetramers or 4 to 5 hemichrome dimers interact with the cytoplasmic domain of each band 3 molecule (Waugh and Low, 1985; Waugh et al., 1987). The aggregates induced by the interaction of hemichromes with the sickle erythrocyte membrane compose up to 1.3 percent of the total membrane proteins, of which two thirds can be accounted for by globin chains (Kannan et al., 1988). These aggregates are rendered insoluble mostly by cross-linking via disulfide bonds, even though other covalent, nonreducible linkages have been demonstrated (Kannan et al., 1988). Increased binding of hemichromes to the cell membrane has been shown in all density fractions of sickle erythrocytes (Campwala and Desforges, 1982).

A similar process can be demonstrated in the densest and presumably oldest fractions of normal blood, indicating that oxidation, hemichrome precipitation, clustering and binding of IgGs are involved in the removal of old erythrocytes from circulation (Kannan et al., 1991).

The association of hemichromes with the erythrocyte membrane had been initially described for unstable hemoglobins exposed to oxidative stress (Rachmilewitz and Harari, 1972; McPherson et al., 1992) and subsequently for β thalassemia (Kahane et al., 1978; Shinar and Rachmilewitz, 1990; Mannu et al., 1995). These alterations are likely to play an important role in the reduced survival of β-thalassemic erythrocytes (Yuan et al., 1992) (Chapter 10).

Free fatty acids seem to promote formation of hemichromes (Akhrem et al., 1989; Harrington et al., 1993; Rifkind et al., 1994). Hemichrome precipitation on the inner side of the membrane leads to the release of hemin and further destabilization of the cytoskeleton (Jarolim et al., 1990).

Free heme: Approximately 5 percent of the heme associated with the cell membrane of sickle erythrocytes is in the form of free heme (Kuross et al., 1988). The amount of free heme, which is measurable in the cytosol, is also fourfold to fivefold increased in sickle erythrocytes (Liu et al., 1988).

Nonheme, free iron: Free iron has been shown to be present in the membrane of sickle erythrocytes (Kuross and Hebbel, 1988; Hartley and Rice-Evans, 1989). Most of the iron, in the form of Fe^{+3}, accumulates at the interface between membrane and cytosol (Sugihara et al., 1992). The association of iron with the membrane is strong, on the order of 10^{12}, such that only chelators with very high affinity are capable of removing iron from the membrane (Shalev and Hebbel, 1996a). It has been postulated that this free, catalytic iron may play an important role in promoting further oxidation of hemoglobin to methemoglobin and deposition of denatured hemoglobin onto the red cell membrane. Thus, catalytic iron associated

with the membrane and HbS in solution could form a redox couple, with the free, ferric iron being available for valence cycling. Shalev and Hebbel have shown that removal of part of the membrane-associated iron with the iron chelator deferiprone (L1) significantly reduces the formation of methemoglobin from HbS in solution (Shalev and Hebbel, 1996b). This finding is relevant for new potential therapies for sickle cell disease. L1 is effective in removing free iron in vitro from sickle and thalassemic erythrocytes (Shalev et al., 1995). Studies with L1 in patients with thalassemia intermedia have also shown a dose-dependent reduction in membrane-associated free iron, up to values of 79 ± 11 percent (n = 4) for L1 dosages of 75 mg/kg per day (Shalev et al., 1995). L1 therapy was also associated with a significant reduction in the activity of the potassium-chloride (K-Cl) cotransporter, which is abnormally increased as the result of oxidative damage present in homozygous β-thalassemic erythrocytes (De Franceschi et al., 1999). A safe, effective, and high affinity iron chelator would be useful to reduce the membrane damage associated with the deposition of free iron.

Nonheme, ferritin iron: The cytosol of sickle erythrocytes contains increased amounts of ferritin (Bauminger et al., 1979). Presence of iron associated with ferritin has also been described in the membrane of sickle erythrocytes (Hartley and Rice-Evans, 1989; Kuross and Hebbel, 1988).

Other relevant targets of free radicals and oxidants are the cysteine residues of proteins, which undergo modification at their sulfydryl moieties. Sickle erythrocytes have a decreased number of titratable thiol residues carried by membrane proteins such as spectrin, ankyrin, protein 3, and protein 4.1 (Rank et al., 1985). This decrease in free thiols has been associated with the increased tendency of sickle erythrocytes to form and shed membrane vesicles (Rank et al., 1988). Dense irreversibly sickled cells (ISCs) have the greatest reduction in membrane thiols and the greatest tendency to shed membrane vesicles. Treatment of sickle erythrocytes with the reducing agent dithiothreitol (DTT) significantly decreases their tendency to form vesicles (Rank et al., 1988). Thiol oxidation is believed to play an important role in the membrane transport abnormalities of sickle erythrocytes, and especially in the activation of the K-Cl cotransport mechanism (see later).

Abnormalities in antioxidant systems have also been described in sickle cells and may tip the balance toward increased oxidation. Sickle erythrocytes have a decreased content of vitamin E, glutathione, glutathione reductase, and catalase (Chiu and Lubin, 1979; Das and Nair, 1980; Lachant et al., 1983; Wettersroem, et al.,

1984). Glutathione peroxidase was abnormally reduced in one study (Das and Nair, 1980), but this difference disappeared when control subjects with high reticulocyte counts were used (Lachant et al., 1983).

Membrane Loss

Sickle erythrocytes, which undergo sickling via cyclic oxygenation and deoxygenation, shed part of their membrane as vesicles (Allan et al., 1981, 1982; Allan and Raval, 1983). This shedding is probably the ultimate stage in the deformation of the cell membrane induced by sickling. These vesicles most likely derive from the membrane spicules formed during sickling and appear to be completely uncoupled from the underlying cytoskeletal network (Fig. 22.1) (Liu et al., 1991). Vesicles may play a role in the hypercoagulability that has been shown in sickle cell disease, although it is not clear what portion of the vasoocclusive manifestation of sickle cell disease is due to intravascular clotting (Frank et al., 1985). In addition, crucial integral membrane proteins are lost with these vesicles. It has been speculated that the increased susceptibility of sickle erythrocytes to damage by complement is due to the loss of factors that normally prevent its activation on the cell membrane (Test and Woolworth, 1994).

Binding of HbS to the Inner Membrane

Hemoglobin can bind to the inner surface of the red cell membrane (Fischer et al., 1975; Eisinger et al., 1982, 1984). An important determinant of binding is the net charge of hemoglobin. Binding is greater for relatively positively charged HbA and follows the sequence HbC >

HbA2 > HbS > HbA > HbF (Fischer et al., 1975; Friedman, 1981; Reiss et al., 1982). Membrane binding is greater for the deoxyHb than for the oxyHb (Shaklai et al., 1981), although a marked depletion of HbA at the cytosol boundary layer accompanies HbS polymerization, suggesting that deoxyHbS may tend to withdraw from the membrane (Eisinger et al., 1984). An important site of interaction between HbA and the cell membrane is the cytoplasmic domain of the anion transporter protein band 3. It has been estimated that approximately half of the band 3 molecules of an erythrocyte have hemoglobin bound to their cytoplasmic domains (Walder et al., 1984). The cytoplasmic portion of band has been shown to bind preferentially to deoxyhemoglobin (Walder et al., 1984).

In sickle erythrocytes, there is a markedly increased deposition of hemoglobin on the inner surface of the membrane, especially in ISCs (Fischer et al., 1975; Lessin et al., 1978; Shaklai et al., 1981). In vitro formation of ISCs is associated with a significant increase in membrane deposition of HbS (Lessin et al., 1978). The static membrane rigidity of oxygenated sickle erythrocytes depends on association of HbS with the membrane (Evans and Mohandas, 1987). In addition, the binding of HbS to transmembrane proteins such as band 3 reduces their mobility in the membrane and may facilitate clustering and abnormal interactions with the cytoskeleton. There is also evidence that the positively charged hemoglobins, such as HbS and HbC, influence the activity of the K-Cl cotransporter and promote potassium, chloride and water loss from the erythrocyte (see later). Although this effect could be mediated by Hb binding to the membrane, no study has provided conclusive evidence to support this possibility.

Phosphorylation

Several reports have described altered patterns of membrane protein phosphorylation in sickle erythrocytes (Dzandu and Johnson 1980; Johnson and Dzandu, 1982; Johnson et al., 1986; Ramachandran et al., 1987; Apovo et al., 1989). Decreased phosphorylation of spectrin/ankyrin and increased phosphorylation of band 3 proteins 4.1 and 4.9 have been observed. It has also been shown that deoxygenation induces nonspecific dephosphorylation of membrane proteins (Fathallah et al., 1995). This dephosphorylation is prevented by pretreatment of the cells with okadaic acid, an inhibitor of protein phosphatases (Fathallah et al., 1995).

Phosphorylation/dephosphorylation mechanisms are involved in the regulation of the function of both cytoskeletal and integral membrane proteins (Boivin, 1988). These control mechanisms are particularly relevant for the modulation of activity of several trans-

Figure 22.1. Model of the long spicule in the deoxygenated sickled cell shows HbS polymers penetrating the membrane skeleton and the lipid bilayer uncoupling from the skeleton (Reprinted with permission from Liu et al., 1991.)

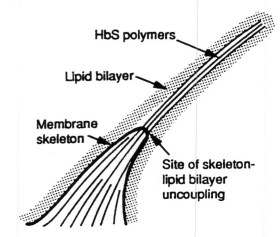

HbS polymers

Lipid bilayer

Membrane skeleton

Site of skeleton-lipid bilayer uncoupling

porters of the cell membrane, including the calcium (Ca) pump, sodium-hydrogen exchanger, band 3, the Ca-activated potassium channel, and K-Cl cotransport (see later). Human erythrocytes possess protein kinase C (PKC) activity (Palfrey and Waseem, 1985), which consists of two major isoforms, the Ca-dependent, phorbol ester-binding isoform PKCa, and the Ca-independent, non-phorbol-ester binding isoform PKCz. The amount of these two isoforms is increased twofold in sickle erythrocytes compared with normal control subjects (Fathallah et al., 1997). Membrane PKC activity is increased approximately sixfold in sickle erythrocytes, whereas the activity of the cytosolic fraction is decreased, especially in dense ISCs (Apovo et al., 1989). Since the activity of several protein kinases is increased in reticulocytes and decreases with cell age/maturation (Jindal et al., 1996), it is not clear how much of this increased PKC activity is specifically due to, or contributes to, the membrane alterations of sickle erythrocytes.

RED CELL MEMBRANE STRUCTURAL ABNORMALITIES IN SICKLE CELL DISEASE

This section reviews the most clinically relevant alterations in membrane structure and function described in sickle erythrocytes, with the exception of their membrane transport properties, which are reviewed separately in the next section.

Altered Cytoskeletal Functions/Interaction

The erythrocyte membrane contains several integral membrane proteins that are embedded into the lipid

bilayer and interact with the underlying cytoskeleton. The functional integrity of the cytoskeleton and its interactions with the integral membrane proteins are crucial for maintaining the mechanical stability of the red cell membrane. The composition of the normal human erythrocyte cytoskeleton is shown in Figure 22.2 (Lux and Palek, 1995).

Several studies have addressed the function of the cytoskeleton and cytoskeleton/integral membrane interactions in sickle cell disease (Platt, 1994). These studies have also attempted to address the issue of the structural basis for the irreversibility of morphologic changes associated with sickling in oxygenated cells, which do not contain appreciable quantities of HbS polymer.

One of the first pieces of evidence for abnormal cytoskeletal function of sickle cells was provided by studies showing that some sickle erythrocytes exposed to oxygen or other factors that reverse HbS polymerization still maintain a deformed shape (Bertles and Döbler, 1969). These cells were defined as ISCs, and subsequent studies showed a defect in the cytoskeleton of ISCs, which is characterized by irreversible deformation of the spectrin-actin lattice (Lux et al., 1976). Ankyrin is functionally abnormal in sickle erythrocytes because it has a markedly decreased binding to spectrin (Platt et al., 1985). Because a similar defect can be found in normal erythrocytes damaged in vitro by exposure to oxidants or in erythrocytes of patients with unstable hemoglobinopathies (Platt and Falcone,

Figure 22.2. Schematic model of the red cell membrane. The relative position of the various proteins is correct, but the proteins and lipids are not drawn to scale. (From Lux and Palek, 1995.)

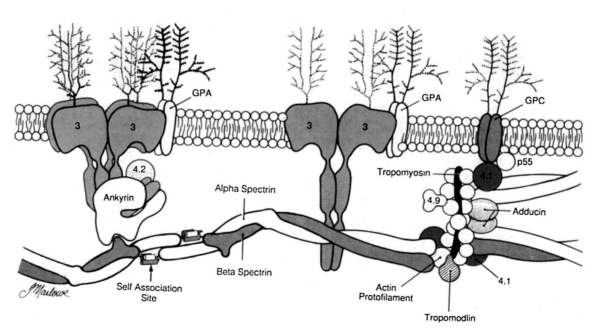

1988), it has been suggested that deposition of denatured hemoglobin on the inner membrane may precipitate these changes in cytoskeletal function. Generation of complexes that include spectrin and hemoglobin on the inner side of the membrane has been associated with increased red cell membrane rigidity in hereditary xerocytosis, heterozygous β thalassemia, and sickle cell disease (Fortier et al., 1988). It has also been proposed that the rigidity of the cytoskeleton of ISCs could be due to an abnormality in β actin, owing to oxidative changes that render two crucial cysteine residues (Cys^{284} and Cys^{373}) unavailable (Shartava et al., 1995). A disulfide bridge is formed between these two cysteine residues in sickle but not normal erythrocytes (Bencsath et al., 1996). The diminished content of reduced glutathione and other crucial antioxidants in ISCs may play a role in facilitating oxidant damage and modification of β actin (Chiu and Lubin, 1979; Das and Nair, 1980; Lachant et al., 1983; Wettersroem et al., 1984). Oxidation induces cross-linking of spectrin and actin with loss of membrane flexibility (Shaklai et al., 1987). (For a detailed description of the increased rigidity and decreased deformability of sickle erythrocytes see Chapter 21.)

Spectrin dimer-dimer association may play a role in the permanent deformation of ISCs (Liu et al., 1993). Evidence for a linkage between the permanent deformation of ISCs and cytoskeletal rearrangement is based on the presence of permanent deformation at 37°C and its absence at 13°C. Because spectrin is free to dissociate and reassociate at 37°C, but not at 13°C, it is possible that spectrin tetramers dissociate into dimers, which may then reassociate into new tetramers in a permanently deformed configuration (Liu et al., 1993).

Protein band 3 can bind to hemoglobin via its cytoplasmic domain. This site may play an important role in facilitating the precipitation of denatured HbS and ultimately inducing the clustering of band 3 with ankyrin, spectrin, protein 4.1, and glycophorin, which is followed by the binding of autologous IgG and the removal of the erythrocyte (Waugh et al., 1986; Schlüter and Drenckhahn, 1986; Kabata and Tichelli, 1994; Liu et al., 1996; Galili et al., 1986). Studies with fluorescence photobleaching recovery and polarized fluorescence depletion have shown abnormal mobility of band 3 (Corbett and Golan, 1993). Some of these changes are dependent on the hydration state of the erythrocytes, but rehydration of sickle erythrocytes could not restore normal mobility for band 3 or glycophorin, indicating the presence of irreversible alterations in the interaction between these two proteins and the underlying cytoskeleton (Corbett and Golan, 1993). More recent studies have provided additional evidence for functional abnormalities of band 3 in

sickle erythrocytes (Platt and Falcone, 1995). Inside-out vesicles (IOV) obtained from sickle erythrocytes showed a marked decrease in the capability of band 3 to bind ankyrin, with normal binding to protein 4.1. Schwartz et al. (1987) reported functional abnormalities in protein 4.1 in sickle erythrocytes, but these results were not confirmed in another study by Platt and Falcone (1995).

Protein band 3 has also been shown to dissociate from the cytoskeleton and be contained in the membrane that comprises the spicule of sickle erythrocytes (Liu et al., 1991). The presence of band 3 can be demonstrated in these spicules by immunofluorescence labeling, whereas immunogold staining for spectrin shows that this protein is limited to the body of the cell and the base of the spicule. This uncoupling of membrane from cytoskeleton is most likely due to the growth of the HbS polymer through gaps in the cytoskeletal network (Fig. 22.1). The detachment of the lipid bilayer containing band 3 and possibly other integral membrane proteins from the cytoskeleton probably facilitates its release from the erythrocyte as membrane vesicles.

Oxidative damage and proteolytic degradation of band 3 have been shown in erythrocytes of normal subjects after acute (20 minutes) hypobaric hypoxia, which simulates an altitude of 4,500 m (Celedon et al., 1998). The human red cells possess specific, membrane-bound proteinases, which are devoted to the proteolytic degradation of oxidatively damaged proteins (Beppu et al., 1994). The function of this proteolytic system in sickle erythrocytes has not been studied.

Altered Membrane Lipid Composition

The normal structure of the lipid bilayer of the red cell membrane exhibits a characteristic asymmetry in the organization of its phospholipids (PL) (Fig. 22.3) (Zwaal and Schroit, 1997). The outer monolayer of the erythrocyte membrane consists of phosphatidylcholine (PC) and sphingomyelin (SM), whereas the inner monolayer consists of the aminophospholipids, phosphatidylethanolamine (PE) and phosphatidylserine (PS). Twenty percent of the PE is found on the outside of the membrane, whereas no PS is seen in the outer leaflet of the membrane of normal erythrocytes. About 70 percent of phosphoinositides are found in the inner monolayer (Kuypers et al., 1994).

The maintenance of this asymmetric PL composition is an active process, which requires adenosine triphosphate (ATP) and is mediated by an ATP-dependent aminophospholipid translocase, which shuttles PS and PE from the outer to the inner leaflets of the bilayer. This translocase is characteristically inhibited by N-ethylmaleimide (NEM) and when intracellular

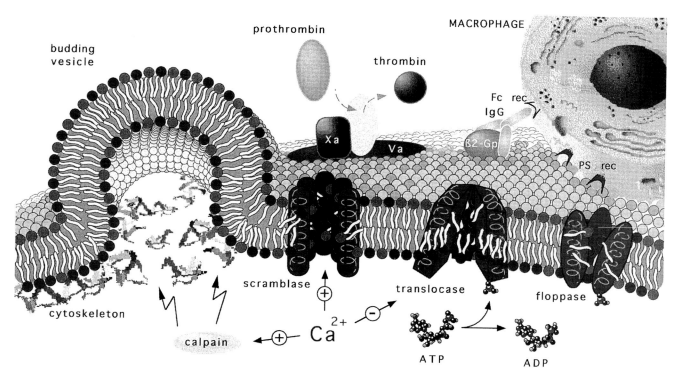

Figure 22.3. The regulation and physiology of membrane phospholipid asymmetry. This model describes how membrane phospholipid asymmetry is generated, maintained, and perturbed as a prerequisite to various phosphatidylserine-related pathophysiologies. Membrane lipid asymmetry is regulated by the cooperative activities of three transporters: (1) the ATP-dependent aminophospholipid-specific translocase, which rapidly transports PS and PE from the cell's outer-to-inner leaflet; (2) the ATP-dependent nonspecific lipid floppase, which slowly transports lipids from the cell's inner-to-outer leaflet; and (3) the Ca^{2+}-dependent nonspecific lipid scramblase, which allows lipids to move randomly between both leaflets. The model predicts that the translocases are targets for Ca^{2+} that directly regulates the transporter's activities. Elevated intracellular Ca^{2+} induces PS randomization across the cell's plasma membrane by providing a stimulus that positively and negatively regulates scramblase and translocase activities, respectively. At physiologic Ca^{2+} concentrations, PS asymmetry is promoted because of an active translocase and floppase but inactive scramblase. Depending on the type of cell, elevated intracellular Ca^{2+} levels can be achieved by cellular activation that generally results in the concomitant influx and accumulation of extracellular Ca^{2+} and by its release from intracellular stores. Increased cytosolic Ca^{2+} can also result in calpain activation, which facilitates membrane blebbing and the release of PS-expressing procoagulant microvesicles. The appearance of PS at the cell's outer leaflet promotes coagulation and thrombosis by providing a catalytic surface for the assembly of the prothrombinase and tenase (not shown) complexes and marks the cell as a pathologic target for elimination by phagocytes. Recognition of the PS-expressing targets can occur by both antibody-dependent and direct receptor-mediated pathways. (Aminophospholipids are shown with red polar headgroups and cholinephospholipids with blue polar headgroups β2-Gp, β2-glycoprotein-1; rec, receptor). (Reprinted with permission from Zwaal and Schroit, 1997.)

Ca reaches micromolar concentrations. An additional system, defined as the nonspecific floppase, transports PS and PE at a much lower rate from the inside to the outside of the bilayer (Zwaal and, Schroit 1997).

The composition of the normal erythrocyte membrane lipid bilayer is shown in Figure 22.3. In response to stimuli such as increased intracellular Ca, or modification of sulfydryl residues, there is a rapid movement of PL between the two layers, which results in the exposure of PS and PE on the outside of the red cell. This movement is mediated by the human plasma membrane phospholipid scramblase; the molecular structure of the scramblase has recently been identified (Zhou et al., 1997). This protein is an ATP-dependent translocase, which is expressed in erythrocytes, platelets, and several other tissues. It is characterized by a very high content of proline (12 percent) and the presence of at least one identifiable protein kinase C phosphorylation site. Most of the protein resides on the cytoplasmic side of the membrane, and only the last nine aminoacids (310 to 318) are predicted to be on the outside of the cell membrane (Zhou et al., 1997). A single Ca-binding site has been identified on the cytoplasmic side, close to the transmembrane domain (Stout et al., 1998), with an apparent affinity for Ca around 40 µmol/L (Zhou et al., 1997). The activity of the PL scramblase is variable among different cells lines, and the levels of expression of this protein is directly related to the capability of each cell line to lose the membrane PL asymmetry in response to an increase in cell Ca (Zhao et al., 1998). Platelets contain approximately ten times more PL scramblase than erythrocytes (Zhao et al., 1998).

Several alterations of membrane lipid structure/function have been described in sickle erythrocytes. The most significant alterations have been reported in the ISC fraction. These cells have fewer membrane lipids per cell, owing to loss of membrane surface area, probably by vesiculation (Allan and Raval 1983).

Loss of lipid asymmetry and exposure of PE and PS in the outside layer of the membrane can occur in vitro when erythrocytes are deoxygenated and sickled (Lubin et al., 1981, 1989; Chiu et al., 1981; Choe et al., 1986). The areas of the membrane subjected to the most extensive rearrangements in PL composition are those of the spicule formed by the membrane protrusions of the polymerized HbS fibers (Frank et al., 1985; Choe et al., 1986). There has never been definitive proof that the cytoskeleton plays a significant role in maintaining the membrane PL asymmetry of normal erythrocytes. However, the portion of membrane that uncouples from the cytoskeleton and forms the spicule of sickled cells (Liu et al., 1991) could be more susceptible to scrambling of PL and appearance on the outer surface of PS.

The reduced PL asymmetry of the cell membrane of deoxygenated sickle cells has been shown to be due to the following (Blumenfeld et al., 1991):

- A twofold decrease in PS uptake (outer to inner layer) by the translocase, and a 50 percent increase in the inner to outer layer translocation.
- A twofold increase in the rate of the outward movement of PE via the translocase, with an unchanged inward transport rate.
- A threefold increase in the passive movement of PC.

All these changes in PL transport are reversible when cells are reoxygenated. Dense ISCs show a slight loss of asymmetry under oxy conditions, with an increased exposure of PE with deoxygenation. Cells in the light fraction (reticulocytes and younger cells) show the largest changes in PL distribution with deoxygenation (Blumenfeld et al., 1991).

Although there are differences among the various reports, deoxygenation seems to increase the outer leaflet content of PE from 12 to 40 percent and that of PS from 0 to 20 percent of the total membrane PE and PS, respectively (Wang et al., 1993; Blumenfeld et al., 1991).

A useful tool in assessing membrane lipid asymmetry is annexin V, a phospholipid binding protein, which has high affinity for PS. I^{125}-labeled annexin V has been used to show increased binding of this probe to sickle cells (Tait and Gibson, 1994). The use of a fluorescence-labeled Annexin V has allowed detailed studies on the loss of PL asymmetry that takes place in sickle erythrocytes (Kuypers et al., 1996). These studies have shown that the fraction of cells that have lost PL asymmetry is variable from patient to patient and averages 2.2 ± 1.2 percent (n = 13). This is at least ten times higher than that observed in normal subjects (Kuypers et al., 1996).

PS and PC are sequestered within the erythrocyte at sites where Heinz bodies are present and are an integral part of the Heinz body together with band 3, protein 4.1, ankyrin, and spectrin (Liu et al., 1996). Sequestration of membrane PL within the Heinz body may be an important factor in the reduced membrane surface area of cells containing Heinz bodies. Therefore, in addition to vesiculation, sequestration of PL within the Heinz body is another possible mechanism that leads to the reduced membrane surface area of ISCs. In addition, it has been shown that PS potentiates by twofold the rate of oxidation of HbS, favoring the formation of methemoglobin, hemichromes, and release of heme into the lipid phase (Marva and Hebbel, 1994).

Dense sickle cells that have PS exposed on the outer membrane contain a lower amount of HbF than PS-negative dense cells. However, PS externalization is not exclusively limited to non-F cells and can be shown in some F cells as well (Yasin et al., 1998). Reinfusion of biotin-labeled dense sickle cell fraction into patients has shown that the circulation half-life of these cells varies from 2 to 7 days, but the percentage of cells with exposed PS did not seem to change over time but rather remained constant as cells aged (Franco et al., 1998b).

The loss of PL asymmetry and the exposure of PE and PS on the outer leaflet of the membrane have several important pathophysiologic implications for sickle cell disease (Fig. 22.3).

Procoagulant Activity

Clotting cascade activation is crucially dependent on the presence of negatively charged phospholipids (Zwaal et al., 1977, 1978). Sickle erythrocytes can accelerate an in vitro coagulation assay (Russel viper venom clotting time) (Chiu et al., 1981). Based on the increased plasma levels of $F_{\cdot 1+2'}$ an indicator of intravascular activation of prothrombin and of D-dimer, an indicator of the intravascular degradation of cross-linked fibrin, there is evidence of activation of the coagulation system in sickle cell disease (Kuypers et al., 1992; Devine et al., 1986; Francis, 1989). Tissue factor procoagulant activity is also elevated in patients with sickle cell disease (Key et al., 1998). However, it is not clear how much of the vascular complications of sickle cell disease can be attributed to hypercoagulability. The vesicles lost from the membrane of sickle cells may also play a role in the generation of this hypercoagulable state (Frank et al., 1985).

Increased Adherence to Monocytes/Macrophages

There have been reports that sickle erythrocytes are abnormally adherent to macrophages/monocytes (Hebbel, 1991; Schwartz et al., 1985). This is due probably to a combination of factors, which include the presence of IgG on the outside membrane, but also the presence of PS on the outside of the cell (Takana and Schroit, 1983; Schlegel and Williamson, 1987).

Increased Adherence to Endothelial Cells

In vitro oxidation of normal human erythrocytes increases their adhesion to cultured bovine endothelial cells (Wali et al., 1987). Normal erythrocyte ghosts adhere strongly to endothelium if they have lost the asymmetry in membrane phospholipid arrangement (Schlegel et al., 1985).

Activation of the Complement Pathway

The alternative complement pathway can be activated by the loss of PL asymmetry associated with deoxygenation (Wang et al., 1993), by exposure to liposomes containing PS and PE, which are normally present only in the inner leaflet of the cell membrane (Tomasko and Chudwin, 1988), or by inducing lipid scrambling with the Ca-ionophore A23187 in intact erythrocytes (Test and Mitsuyoshi, 1997). In vivo activation of complement during painful crises may occur as shown by the increased plasma levels of factor Bb, a by-product of the activation of the alternative pathway C3 convertase (Wang et al., 1993). Activation of the alternative pathway could promote opsonization and clearance of damaged sickle erythrocytes. Mechanisms that normally limit the activation of complement on erythrocytes may be defective in sickle erythrocytes (Test and Woolworth, 1994). Sickle cells and especially dense ISCs are particularly susceptible to hemolysis mediated by the C5b-9 membrane attack complex (MAC). Dense ISCs seem to have an increased binding of MAC to the membrane, but the reason for this behavior has not been clarified. In addition, the binding of the terminal component of the complement cascade, C9, is markedly increased in dense ISCs (Test and Woolworth, 1994). This may indicate a defect in either the homologous restriction factor (HRF) or the membrane inhibitor of reactive lysis (MIRL) mechanisms.

The abnormalities in membrane cytoskeleton and lipid composition are important determinants of the reduced survival of sickle cells (Chapter 20). Decreased deformability and increased rigidity of sickle cells (Chapter 21) and the presence of irreversible deformation and cell dehydration (see the next section) promote the premature removal of erythrocytes from the circulation. The abnormalities in lipid composition of sickle erythrocytes also promote interactions with endothelial cells (also favored by deformation and dehydration, Chapter 21), which result ultimately in vasoocclusion and acute and chronic organ damage. These vascular complications are worsened by the procoagulant activity of these altered erythrocytes and the vesicles they release. Abnormal interactions with mononuclear cells and the complement system also favor the premature removal of sickle erythrocytes from the circulation.

RED CELL MEMBRANE TRANSPORT ABNORMALITIES IN SICKLE CELL DISEASE

Several transport systems control composition, volume, and hydration state of the erythrocytes by transporting cations (Na^+, K^+, and Ca^{+2}) and/or anions (Cl^-, HCO_3^-). The hydration state of the cell is an important factor in the pathogenesis of sickle cell disease, because the polymerization of HbS is so uniquely dependent on the cellular concentration of HbS (Chapter 23) (Eaton and Hofrichter, 1987, 1990). Erythrocyte dehydration leads to increased cellular hemoglobin concentration, which markedly enhances the tendency of the cells to form polymer and sickle. A distinguishing feature of sickle cell disease is the heterogeneity in the volume and water content of erythrocytes (Fabry and Nagel, 1982). In addition to cells with increased volume and normal or low mean cell hemoglobin concentration (MCHC) (representing reticulocytes and very young cells), the blood of patients with sickle cell disease contains dense, dehydrated erythrocytes and reticulocytes. The number of dense, dehydrated high MCHC cells can be estimated with flow cytometry, as the number or percent of cells with MCHC > 38 g/dL, or with density > 1.1009 (Fabry et al., 1984b; Mohandas et al., 1986a; Mohandas et al., 1989; Mohandas and Ballas, 1994). The fraction of dense, dehydrated cells varies with time in each patient and from patient to patient, ranging from 0 to 40 percent. Sickle cell anemia with coincident α thalassemia is associated with reduced numbers of dense cells and with milder hemolytic disease, although there is no reliable correlation between proportion of dense cells and frequency of vasoocclusive crises (Embury et al., 1984; Fabry et al., 1984b; Noguchi et al., 1985; Ballas,

1991). Paradoxically, individuals with the greatest numbers of dense cells appear to have the fewest painful events (Lande et al., 1988). The number of dense cells has been shown to decrease concomitantly with crisis (Fabry et al., 1984a; Lawrence et al., 1985; Lawrence and Fabry, 1987) or to increase in the initial phase of a crisis and subsequently decrease (Ballas and Smith, 1992). The increased cellular concentration of HbS in the dense fractions of sickle cell anemia blood results in several deleterious consequences that play an important role in the pathogenesis of the disease:

- Increased polymerization of HbS, with a reduced delay time for polymerization and presence of polymer even in the oxygenated state (Eaton and Hofrichter, 1987, 1990; Noguchi et al., 1989) (Chapter 22).
- Increased adhesion to endothelium, with resulting endothelial damage and vasoocclusion. (Experimental evidence for high endothelial adhesion of dense cells is extremely dependent on the assay conditions, especially presence or absence of flow (Hebbel et al., 1985; Kaul et al., 1989; Morris et al., 1993; Kaul et al., 1994). For a detailed review of the various studies on adhesion of dense sickle erythrocytes, see Chapter 21).
- Reduced deformability and abnormal rheology (Dong et al., 1992; Hasegawa et al., 1995; Hiruma et al., 1995a; 1995b) (Chapter 21).

Dehydration of sickle erythrocytes can take place by different mechanisms whose identification is relevant for possible new therapeutic approaches to the disease. It has been estimated that a 1 to 4 g/dL decrease in the intracellular HbS concentration (MCHC) could reduce polymerization in sickle cell anemia to the levels seen in the much less clinically severe HbS-β^+thalassemia (Sunshine et al., 1978). Several studies have shown that it is possible to block or reduce cell dehydration in vitro and in vivo by using specific inhibitors for some of the ion transport pathways involved (Brugnara et al., 1996; De Franceschi, Bachir et al., 1997a, 2000) (Chapter 42).

Cell dehydration in sickle erythrocytes is due to loss of potassium. This loss is extreme in ISCs, which exhibit a dramatic reduction in cell potassium content, and an associated marked increase in cell sodium content (Clark et al., 1978b). The magnitude of the potassium loss is much greater than the sodium gain, and consequently ISCs exhibit marked cell dehydration and remarkably increased MCHC.

In the last two decades, there has been great interest in identifying the ion transport pathways that mediate dehydration of sickle erythrocytes. This research was preceded by the seminal work of Tosteson et al. (1952, 1955), which showed for the first time alteration of ion content and transport in sickle erythrocytes (Tosteson et al., 1952; Tosteson et al., 1955; Tosteson, 1955). These reports provided the first evidence that deoxygenation and sickling could induce a decrease in potassium content and an increase in sodium content of sickle erythrocytes and that there were specific changes in cation permeability associated with cell sickling (Fig. 22.4). During the last two decades, research in this area has been focused on identifying different pathways that can lead to dehydration of sickle erythrocytes and on identification of specific inhibitors that could be used safely to prevent dehydration in vivo (Joiner, 1993).

Four major mechanisms have been implicated in the dehydration of sickle erythrocytes.

K-Cl Cotransport, Cell Dehydration, and Cell Magnesium in Sickle Erythrocytes

Erythrocyte K-Cl cotransport is mediated by a member of the chloride-cation contransporter (CCC) family. These transporters use the concentration gradients generated by the active transport via sodium-potassium ATPase to couple the transport of monovalent cations (sodium and/or potassium) with that of monovalent anions (chloride). Members of the CCC family are the thiazide-sensitive Na-Cl cotransporter, the bumetanide-

Figure 22.4. Changes in cell sodium and potassium contents induced by deoxygenation in normal and sickle erythrocytes. (Reprinted with permission from Tosteson et al., 1952.)

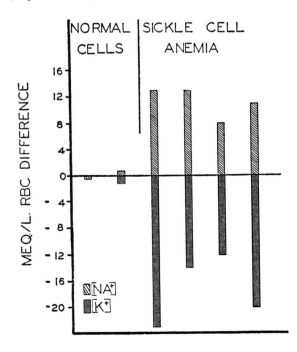

sensitive Na-K-Cl cotransporter and the volume-sensitive K-Cl cotransporter (Lauf et al., 1992; Hass, 1994; Hass and Forbush, 1998).

The prototype of the K-Cl cotransporter has been recently cloned (Gillen et al., 1996). This molecule has been called KCCl and has been shown to correspond to the form expressed in erythroid cells. Human erythrocyte KCCl can be activated by several stimuli or conditions. Some of these are applicable only to in vitro conditions, whereas others may play a role in the dehydration and reduced survival of sickle erythrocytes in vivo. In normal cells, there is no convincing evidence linking dehydration via K-Cl cotransport (or any other pathway) with reduced cell survival.

Cell swelling: Via a still unknown mechanism, swelling of erythrocytes induces activation of K-Cl cotransport with potassium, chloride, and water loss and volume regulatory decrease (Brugnara et al., 1985; Brugnara et al., 1986; Canessa et al., 1986; Brugnara, 1989; Kaji, 1989). Because this process is blocked by phosphatase inhibitors such as okadaic acid and calyculin A, it is likely that the sensitivity of this transporter to volume changes is mediated by a phosphorylation/dephosphorylation mechanism (Jennings and Al-Rohil, 1990; Jennings and Schulz, 1991; Kaji and Tsukitani, 1991). The active form of the transporter is dephosphorylated probably via membrane-associated protein phosphatases (PP1 and PP2A), whereas a still unidentified kinase is responsible for turning off the system.

Acidic pH (with optimum pH around 6.7–7.2): Exposure of erythrocytes to a pH lower than 7.40 leads to marked activation of K-Cl cotransport (Fig. 22.5) (Brugnara et al., 1986). Changes in intracellular pH have been shown to modulate K-Cl cotransport activity (Lauf et al., 1992). Cell dehydration via K-Cl cotransport occurs when sickle erythrocytes are exposed to acidic conditions (Fig. 22.6). (Canessa et al. 1987a; Brugnara et al., 1989; Vitoux et al., 1989; Ellory et al., 1991). It is likely that every time sickle erythrocytes are exposed to an acidic environment, such as in the spleen, kidney, or conditions of slow flow and vasoocclusion, activation of K-Cl cotransport would occur with potassium loss and dehydration.

Removal of intracellular magnesium: The activity of K-Cl cotransport is markedly affected by the cytoplasmic concentration of divalent cations. Mg negatively regulates K-Cl cotransport (Brugnara and Tosteson, 1987; Canessa et al., 1987b). The regulation of erythrocyte magnesium content and the relevance of this mechanism for the pathophysiology of sickle cell disease are discussed later. The inhibition of K-Cl cotransport by increased cell magnesium content has provided a new potential opportunity for preventing dehydration in thalassemic red cells

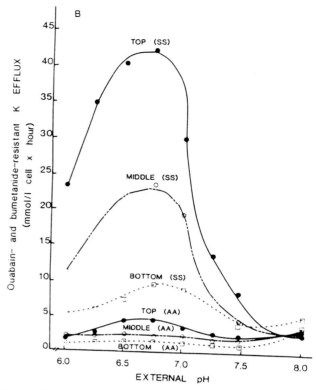

Figure 22.5. Activation of K-Cl cotransport by pH in density separated sickle and normal erythrocytes. Cells were pretreated with carbon monoxide and then nystatin to ensure comparable volume and potassium content. Potassium efflux was measured in isotonic saline media. (Reprinted with permission, from Brugnara et al., 1986.)

(De Franceschi et al., 1997b, 1998) and sickle cell disease (De Franceschi et al., 1997, 2000) (Chapter 42).

Hydrostatic pressure: Increased hydrostatic pressure stimulates a pH- and chloride-dependent potassium permeability in normal human red cells, which is sensitive to magnesium and phosphatase inhibitors (Godart and Ellory, 1996).

Urea and oxidation: Urea is a powerful activator of K-Cl cotransport (Kaji and Gasson, 1995; Culliford et al., 1998). The underlying mechanism has not been clarified, but it probably involves a shift induced by urea from an inactive to a partially activated state of some of the regulatory kinases or phosphatases (Kaji and Gasson, 1995). Deoxygenation also prevents the stimulation of K-Cl cotransport by urea in normal but not in sickle erythrocytes (Gibson et al., 1998). Oxidative damage to the cell membrane activates a potassium permeability pathway that leads to net potassium loss and dehydration (Sheerin et al., 1989). Subsequent work has shown that the K-Cl cotransport activity is markedly increased by oxidative damage of the red cell membrane (Olivieri et al., 1993). Oxidative damage-induced activation of K-Cl cotransport is

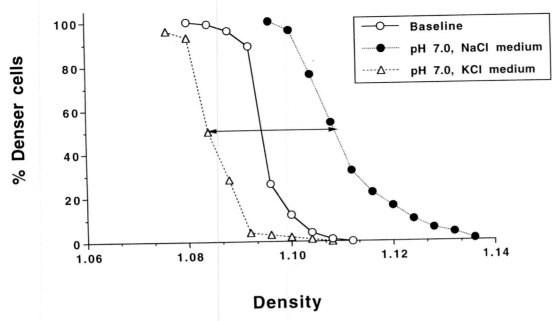

Figure 22.6. Acid pH induces dehydration of the least dense fraction of oxygenated, carbon monoxide-treated, sickle erythrocytes. This process is mediated by K-Cl cotransport and is abolished in a high potassium medium.

believed to play a significant role in the dehydration of β thalassemia erythrocytes (Olivieri et al., 1994). The hemolytic anemia associated with dapsone or ribavirin therapy involves oxidative damage to the cell membrane and activation of K-Cl cotransport (Haas and Harrison, 1989; De Franceschi et al., 1998b).

N-ethylmaeimide (NEM): Exposure of normal human or sheep erythrocytes to this agent results in increased potassium movement via K-Cl cotransport (Lauf et al., 1992). It is not clear if the effect of this agent is mediated via sulfhydryl moieties of the transporter itself or via some of its regulatory mechanisms. The response to NEM is greatly increased in sickle erythrocytes (Canessa et al., 1986).

The activity of K-Cl cotransport is maximal in normal reticulocytes and young cells and is progressively reduced to negligible values in mature and dense normal cells (Hall and Ellory, 1986; Brugnara and Tosteson, 1987; Canessa et al., 1987a,b; Ellory et al., 1990).

Activation of K-Cl cotransport leads to loss of potassium, chloride, and water with cell dehydration and increased intracellular hemoglobin concentration. There have been multiple reports of activation of K-Cl cotransport in sickle erythrocytes (Brugnara et al., 1986; Canessa et al., 1986; Joiner, 1993). When sickle cells are isosmotically swollen or are exposed to acid pH, K-Cl cotransport promotes potassium and chloride loss and cell dehydration (Brugnara et al., 1989). The K-Cl cotransport is most active in the least dense

fraction, which contains most of the reticulocytes and is least active in the densest fractions (Brugnara et al., 1986; Canessa et al., 1987a). K-Cl cotransport is almost completely suppressed at pH 7.40 in isosmotic conditions and a substantial potassium loss is observed only when external pH is lowered below 7.40 (Fig. 22.6). (Dihydroindenyl)oxy-alkanoic acid (DIOA), a relatively specific inhibitor of the K-Cl cotransport, reduces potassium loss in sickle cells (Vitoux et al., 1989). The increased K-Cl cotransport of sickle erythrocytes is almost completely inhibited when the intracellular magnesium concentration is increased (Brugnara and Tosteson, 1987; Canessa et al., 1987b).

Cell heterogeneity is one of the distinguishing characteristics of sickle cell disease (Fabry and Nagel, 1982; Fabry et al., 1984). The activity of K-Cl cotransport is highest in the least dense, reticulocyte-rich fractions of sickle blood (Brugnara et al., 1986; Canessa et al., 1987a). However, even within the reticulocyte-rich fraction of sickle blood, considerable differences exist concerning the function of K-Cl cotransport (Fabry et al., 1991). Etzion et al. (1996) have shown that within the fraction containing most of the sickle reticulocytes, a pool of cells shows an enhanced capability to dehydrate via K-Cl cotransport, and probably accounts for the fast-track dehydration, which had been hypothesized by Lew et al. (1991). Fabry et al. (1991) identified a similar fraction of reticulocytes/young cells and showed that they also have decreased F-cell numbers.

The relationship between fast-track dehydration mediated by K-Cl cotransport and cellular content of HbF (expressed as F cells or F reticulocytes) is not straightforward. Studies in transferrin receptor-positive (TfR) reticulocytes have shown that dense TfR+ cells have a low content of HbF that seems to be a prerequisite for the formation of dense cells at an early reticulocyte stage (Franco et al., 1994). However, since not all non-F cells become dense at an early stage, other factors must play a role in this process. Subsequent studies have shown that these dense, TfR+ reticulocytes have a much greater K-Cl cotransport activity compared with lighter reticulocytes (Franco et al., 1995). It is also possible that TfR+ cells could reach a state of intermediate dehydration via K-Cl cotransport, with the subsequent dehydration being mediated by HbS polymerization, sickling, and activation of the Gardos channel (Franco et al., 1997). This calcium-dependent dehydration would be affected by the cellular content of HbF and be reduced in F cells (Bookchin et al., 1991; Schwartz et al., 1998).

Sickle erythrocytes maturation can be followed using biotin-labeled erythrocytes (Franco et al., 1998a). The life span of non-F erythrocytes is about 2 weeks compared with 6 to 8 weeks for F cells. When labeled cells are reinfused, they exhibit increased density and dehydration within the first week, indicating the presence a fast-track dehydration process.

A different model for "fast-track" dehydration was originally proposed by Lew et al. (1991). In this model, there is an initial dehydration via sickling-induced activation of the Gardos channel, which results in a slight intracellular acidification, which in turn activates K-Cl cotransport in susceptible cells. This mechanism does not seem to exclude F cells among light sickle cells that become denser at pH 7 (without deoxygenation) and therefore does not support the notion that increased HbF may inhibit K-Cl cotransport (Bookchin et al., 1991).

At the present time, no unifying model exists for the fast-track dehydration of light sickle cells. Differences in experimental protocols do not allow reconciliation of different findings by different groups of investigators. Data collected from patients or transgenic sickle mice treated with specific transport inhibitors may be helpful to assess the in vivo relevance of the proposed mechanisms.

Because deoxygenation is associated with an increase in free cytoplasmic magnesium, one would expect that K-Cl cotransport would be decreased by deoxygenation. The sensitivity of K-Cl cotransport to oxygen has been studied in normal and sickle erythrocytes (Gibson et al., 1998). In normal erythrocytes, deoxygenation inactivates K-Cl cotransport and renders it refractory to stimulation by acidification, urea, or cell swelling (Gibson et al., 1998). There was no appreciable inhibition of K-Cl cotransport by deoxygenation in sickle erythrocytes and urea stimulated K-Cl cotransport independently of oxygen tension

(Culliford et al., 1998). When deoxygenation is performed at a relatively acid pH, there is a significant increase in the component of potassium transport that can be attributed to K-Cl cotransport (30 percent at pH 7.40 and 70 percent at pH 7.0, based on DIOA sensitivity) (Olivieri et al., 1991). More recent studies have provided convincing evidence for a stimulation of K-Cl cotransport during deoxygenation (Joiner et al., 1998). This stimulation has been linked to a generalized dephosphorylation of erythrocyte membrane proteins, which is also observed during deoxygenation (Fathallah et al., 1995).

Activation of K-Cl cotransport is not an exclusive property of sickle erythrocytes and has been observed in other hemoglobinopathies, such as homozygous HbC disease (Chapter 27) (Brugnara et al., 1985; Canessa et al., 1986; Brugnara, 1989). A common feature of all hemoglobin variants associated with K-Cl cotransport activation is their relative positive charge. Studies of other positively charged variants have indicated that mutations in the $\beta6$ or $\beta7$ position are strongly associated with increased K-Cl cotransport (Olivieri et al., 1992). The activation of K-Cl cotransport observed in these variants cannot be attributed simply to the presence of younger cells, as some of the hemoglobinopathies studied exhibit mild or no reticulocytosis. We had originally postulated that binding of the positively charged hemoglobin to the inner site of the cell membrane could be involved in K-Cl cotransport activation (Brugnara et al., 1985). Subsequent studies have provided evidence for an abnormal regulation of K-Cl cotransport in HbC disease erythrocytes, which cannot be explained by reticulocytosis (Brugnara, 1989; Canessa et al., 1994). Recent studies have used a transgenic mouse model expressing human HbC to show that the presence of this positively charged variant was associated with K-Cl cotransport activation and dehydration (Fabry et al., 1998).

The activation of K-Cl cotransport by positively charged hemoglobin variants is particularly relevant in the pathogenesis of some of the compound heterozygous sickle hemoglobinopathies. In HbSC disease (Chapter 27), there is a characteristic erythrocyte dehydration that differs from that in sickle cell trait or HbC trait erythrocytes (Fabry et al., 1982). Cell dehydration plays a crucial role in the pathophysiology of HbSC disease, because it allows for the intracellular HbS to reach concentrations that induce clinically significant polymerization and sickling (Fabry et al., 1982). K-Cl cotransport is highly expressed in HbSC erythrocytes and determines their characteristic microcytosis and dehydration (Canessa et al., 1986; Lawrence et al., 1991).

HbS-Oman is a positively charged hemoglobin variant ($\beta6$ Glu-> Val and β 121 Glu->Lys) that further illustrates the importance of hemoglobin charge in the pathogenesis of some sickle hemoglobinopathies (Chapter 28). HbS-Oman accounts for approximately 20 percent of the total hemoglobin in heterozygous patients (Nagel et al., 1998). These low levels, however, are associated with clinically significant disease. The increased polymerization tendency of HbS-Oman cannot account, by itself, for the clinical severity of the disease. It has been shown that HbS-Oman heterozygote erythrocytes have increased K-Cl cotransport, increased reticulocyte density, and increased hemoglobin binding to the cell membrane (Nagel et al., 1998). It seems reasonable to conclude that the interaction of positively charged HbS-Oman with the cell membrane leads to activation of K-Cl cotransport. It is not clear whether this is a direct effect or is mediated via the phosphatases/kinases known to modulate the functional state of the transporter.

Oxidative damage of sickle hemoglobin-containing cells is an additional relevant determinant of the activity and the regulation of K-Cl cotransport. Evidence suggests that erythrocyte K-Cl cotransport is enhanced by oxidative damage in vitro (Sheerin et al., 1989; Olivieri et al., 1993) and in vivo, as seen in thalassemias (Olivieri et al., 1994) with dapsone therapy (Haas and Harrison, 1989; De Franceschi et al., 1998b), and in sickle transgenic mice (De Franceschi et al., 1995).

Magnesium content in sickle erythrocytes: K-Cl cotransport may be regulated by intracellular magnesium and sickle erythrocytes have a reduced magnesium content (Olukoga et al., 1990; Ortiz et al., 1990; De Franceschi et al., 1997). Although total erythrocyte magnesium content is reduced, especially in dense sickle cells, during deoxygenation there is a marked reduction in the 2,3-BPG/hemoglobin ratio, leading to a large increase in the free magnesium concentration of dense sickle cells. Deoxygenation-induced sickling increases membrane permeability to magnesium; the presence of a transient outwardly directed magnesium gradient during deoxygenation provides a possible explanation for the reduced total magnesium content of sickle erythrocytes (Ortiz et al., 1990). Human red cells also possess a specific sodium/magnesium exchange system, whose activity leads to a slow loss of magnesium from the erythrocyte (Feray and Garay, 1986). Sickle erythrocytes exhibit a markedly increased activity of the sodium/magnesium exchanger, which could, in principle, contribute to their reduced total magnesium content; (De Franceschi et al., 2000). As discussed in Chapter 42, oral magnesium supplementation corrects the deficit in intracellular magnesium of sickle erythrocytes, inhibits K-Cl cotransport, and reduces cell dehydration (De Franceschi et al., 1997, 2000). Interestingly, the activity of the sodium/magnesium exchanger is also reduced by oral magnesium supplements (De Franceschi et al., 2000).

Ca-Activated Potassium Channel (Gardos Pathway) and Cell Calcium in Sickle Erythrocytes

Human red cells possess a specific type of potassium channel, which is activated by an increase in cytoplasmic calcium. Because the presence of this channel was first demonstrated by Gardos (1958), this channel is also known as the Gardos channel. This channel belongs to the family of intermediate conductance Ca-gated potassium channels (ISK) (Ishii et al., 1997), and its molecular structure in mouse erythrocytes is known (Vandorpe et al., 1998). The peptide toxin charybdotoxin (ChTX) is a specific inhibitor of the human red cell Gardos channel (Wolff et al., 1988; Brugnara et al., 1995a). Using ^{125}I-ChTX, normal human erythrocytes were found to possess approximately 150 of these channels per cell (Brugnara et al., 1993a).

Glader and Nathan (1978) showed that generation of ISCs under conditions of ATP depletion was dependent on the presence of external calcium and an outwardly directed potassium gradient. When sickle erythrocytes are deoxygenated in the absence of ATP depletion, Ca-dependent formation of dense, dehydrated cells has been observed (Ohnishi et al., 1986; Horiuchi and Asakura, 1987; Horiuchi et al., 1988; Ohnishi et al., 1989; Brugnara et al., 1993b). Gardos channel-mediated generation of dehydrated cells, in vitro and in vivo has also been found in transgenic mouse models of sickle cell disease (Reilly et al., 1994; De Franceschi et al., 1994). The integrated red cell model developed by Lew and Bookchin (1986) has examined the different modalities of dehydration for reticulocytes (Lew et al., 1991) and provided theoretical and experimental evidence for a Ca-dependent process based on transient activation of the Gardos channel (Bookchin et al., 1991). Using rapid deoxygenation/oxygenation cycles which mimic in vivo conditions, the Gardos channel was shown to be the most important mediator of sickle cell dehydration (McGoron, Joiner et al. 2000).

Activation of the Gardos pathway and cell dehydration during deoxygenation are stochastic processes (Lew et al., 1997), and a relatively constant fraction (10 to 45 percent) of cells dehydrate in a Ca-dependent fashion during each deoxygenation cycle. These results were obtained in isolated sickle discocytes with relatively normal density. This cell fraction does not contain an identifiable subpopulation of cells susceptible to dehydration via the Gardos pathway, and the dehydration occurs randomly. Deoxygenation-induced cell dehydration is a probabilistic event; the cells that have the greatest increase in intracellular calcium and activation of the Gardos channel will undergo dehydration (Lew et al., 1997). Clearly, denser cell fractions are a subpopulation with increased susceptibility to sickling and Gardos activation; F cells have decreased susceptibility.

Deoxygenation of sickle erythrocytes leads to a nonspecific dephosphorylation of membrane proteins, which can be prevented by inhibiting protein phosphatases with okadaic acid or stimulating protein kinase C (PKC) with phorbol 12-myristate 13-acetate (PMA) (Fathallah et al., 1995). PKC may regulate the calcium pump and Gardos channel activity in deoxygenated sickle cells (Fathallah et al., 1997).

In vitro, 22-hour exposure to cyclic deoxygenation at pH 6.8 generates both intermediate-density and high-density cells. K-Cl cotransport seems to be mediating formation of intermediate density cells, whereas the Gardos channel mediates formation of high density cells (Schwartz et al., 1998). Because these experiments were carried out using prolonged incubation times, it is not clear whether they are physiologically relevant. However, they seem to reinforce the notion that different modalities of dehydration exist for sickle erythrocytes and may involve K-Cl cotransport and the Gardos channel, either separately or in combination.

There is convincing experimental evidence for increased entry of calcium during cell sickling (Rhoda et al., 1990; Bookchin et al., 1991; Etzion et al., 1993). In sickle discocytes, deoxygenation increases free intracellular calcium two to three times the normal range of 9.4 to 11.4 nmol/L to a range of 21.8 to 31.7 nmol/L (Etzion et al., 1993). These values are close to the threshold for Gardos channel activation, which has been estimated at around 40 nmol/L free calcium in normal cells (Tiffert et al., 1988). It has also been proposed that this calcium permeabilization could be localized to specific areas of the cell membrane that experience the greatest degree of deformation (Mohandas et al., 1986b). These calcium transients lead to activation of the Gardos channel and dehydration. Until recently, no other modalities of activation of the Gardos channel were known, which could be relevant for sickle cell disease. PGE_2 has been found to be a potent stimulator of the Gardos channel to levels capable of inducing erythrocyte dehydration (Li et al., 1996). It has been speculated that the elevated plasma levels of endothelin and PGE_2 observed in sickle cell disease may play an important role in the vasoconstriction/inflammation associated with vasoocclusive episodes and with an increased susceptibility to infections, respectively (Graido-Gonzalez et al., 1998).

Endothelin-1 (ET-1) and ET-3 are potent activators of the Gardos channel in mouse and human erythro-cytes (Rivera et al., 1999; Rivera and Brugnara, 1998). Erythrocytes possess specific receptors for endothelins, which are functionally coupled to the Gardos channel. When ET-1 or ET-3 binds to the receptors, it elicits signaling via a PKC-dependent pathway, which leads to opening of the Gardos channel and dehydration. This new potential modality of cell dehydration is particularly relevant for sickle cell disease, because endothelin levels are abnormally elevated in patients with sickle cell disease in a "steady-state" (Werdehoff et al., 1998; Rybicki and Benjamin, 1998) and increase even further with acute chest syndrome or vasoocclusive crisis (Hammerman et al., 1997). Sickled cells can induce production of endothelin from endothelial cells, potentially promoting a vicious cycle of vasoocclusion and endothelial damage (Phelan et al., 1995). It is possible that local levels of ET-1 and/or PGE_2 become high enough in areas affected by sickling and vasoocclusion to induce activation of the Gardos channel and dehydration. Cell dehydration induced by activation of the Gardos channel would further contribute to the vasoocclusion and endothelial damage/hypoxia. This new pathway for sickle cell dehydration could be exploited pharmacologically, as several specific blockers of endothelin receptors could be used clinically.

The imidazole antimycotic clotrimazole is also a specific inhibitor of the human red cell Gardos channel (Fig. 22.7) (Alvarez et al., 1992; Brugnara et al., 1993b). It most likely acts on the external pore of the channel, because it can displace ^{125}I-ChTX from its binding site on normal erythrocytes (Brugnara et al., 1993). Therefore, the mode of action of clotrimazole on the Gardos channel is not related to inhibition of cytochrome P450, the mechanism of its antifungal effect. Studies in normal human volunteers have shown that oral clotrimazole administration induces ex vivo inhibition of the erythrocyte Gardos channel (Rifai et al., 1995). The inhibition of the Gardos channel by oral clotrimazole is due to the presence in plasma of both the parent compound and several metabolites, which have lost the imidazole ring and are inactive as cytochrome P450 inhibitors (Brugnara et al., 1995). Studies in a transgenic sickle mouse model (SAD mouse) (Trudel et al., 1991; Trudel et al., 1994) have shown that oral clotrimazole induces blockade of the Gardos channel and reduces red cell dehydration in vivo (De Franceschi et al., 1994). Studies in patients with sickle cell disease have also shown inhibition of the Gardos channel and reduction in cell dehydration (Chapter 42) (Brugnara et al., 1996).

Cell calcium and calcium pump activity in sickle erythrocytes: Normal total erythrocyte calcium content varies between 0.9 and 2.8 μmol/L cells (Engelmann and Duhm, 1987). Initial studies on sickle erythrocytes reported increased total cell calcium, with

CYCLIC DEOXYGENATION

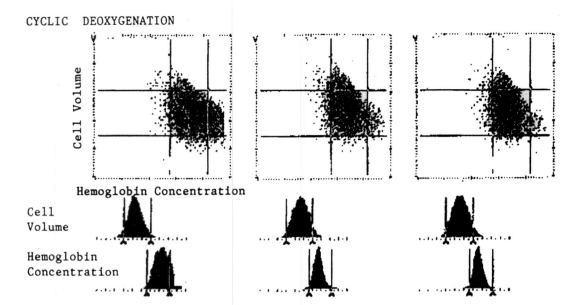

Figure 22.7. Cyclic deoxygenation induces formation of dense sickle erythrocytes, which is blocked by removal of external calcium or by the presence of 10 μmol/L clotrimazole. (Reprinted with permission from Brugnara et al., 1993b.)

values ranging from 110 to 300 μmol/L cells (Eaton et al., 1973; Palek, 1977). Lew and colleagues (1982) provided the first demonstration of free ionized cytoplasmic calcium levels in normal cells using a calcium-chelator loaded intracellularly and ^{45}Ca. Free cytoplasmic calcium was estimated to vary between 11 and 28 nmol/L in normal cells. With the same method, similar estimates of free calcium levels in oxygenated sickle cells were first provided by Bookchin et al. (1985). Studies using the calcium-sensitive dye, fura-2, have estimated free cytoplasmic calcium levels of 18 to 30 nmol/L cells for sickle erythrocytes, levels similar to those of normal controls (Rhoda et al., 1990). Nuclear magnetic resonance studies of normal and sickle erythrocytes have also yielded similar values in the two cell types for ionized cytoplasmic calcium (21 ± 2 versus 18 ± 2 nmol/L) (Murphy et al., 1987).

Elevated total calcium of sickle erythrocytes is the result of a compartmentalization into cytoplasmic vesicles, as first shown by electron probe x-ray analysis of cryosections (Lew et al., 1985) and subsequently confirmed by the use of chlortetracycline as a calcium-sensitive probe (Rubin et al., 1986). These vesicles, derived from the plasma membrane, contain integral membrane proteins, including the Ca-ATPase, in an inside-out configuration. The Ca-ATPase pumps calcium from the cytoplasm into the vesicle and creates a very high internal calcium concentration (Lew et al., 1985; Williamson et al., 1992). Most of the calcium contained in sickle erythrocytes is sequestered into

vesicles and abnormally high free cytoplasmic calcium does not result. It is possible that calcium could leak out of these vesicles into the cytoplasm, especially when the Ca-ATPase is inhibited by severe ATP depletion. This exit of calcium from the vesicles could involve dihydropyridine-sensitive calcium channels (Williamson et al., 1992). However, it is unlikely that such a severe ATP depletion could occur in vivo.

Conflicting reports have been published on the function of the Ca-ATPase in sickle erythrocytes. The activity of this transporter was reported as either reduced, normal, or increased (Carafoli, 1986). The oxidative damage of the sickle red cell membrane could result in a reduced functional capacity of the Ca pump, as a similar defect can be shown in normal erythrocytes exposed to thiol oxidizing reagents and cross-linkers, such as malondialdehyde (Hebbel et al., 1986; Leclerc et al., 1987). However, more recent studies have provided solid evidence for a normal calcium pump activity in oxygenated sickle erythrocytes (Etzion et al., 1993).

Because the free cytoplasmic calcium levels in sickle erythrocytes are not significantly different from those of normal cells, any potential abnormality in calcium pump activity does not seem to be severe enough to affect intracellular calcium under steady state conditions. It remains to be seen if it could become significant during erythrocyte sickling.

Studies in sickle cell trait cells have indicated that calcium entry increases during deoxygenation and returns to normal on reoxygenation (Bookchin and Lew, 1981). Measurements of ^{45}Ca uptake during deoxygenation in sickle erythrocytes loaded with a calcium chelator indicated a marked increase of calcium entry (Bookchin et al., 1985). Calcium entry was partially reduced by the calcium channel blocker nifedipine and by DIDS (30 to 40 percent and 50 percent, respectively) (Rhoda et al., 1990). During deoxygenation, there is a twofold to threefold increase in free cytoplasmic calcium, which results from both a fivefold increase in calcium permeability and a 35 percent inhibition of the calcium pump (Etzion et al., 1993). These changes are larger in sickle cell anemia reticulocytes, but are also present in discocytes.

Several reports have been published on the inhibition of calcium-dependent dehydration of sickle erythrocytes by L-type calcium channel blockers such as nifedipine and nitrendipine (Ellory et al., 1994; Stuart et al., 1994; Ellory et al., 1992a, 1992b). The possible mechanism of action for these compounds is not clear. They could affect calcium entry, at least for the portion that seems to take place via dihydropyridine-sensitive calcium channels and also inhibit directly the Gardos channel. However, the potency of these drugs to inhibit erythrocyte dehydration is relatively low, and near toxic plasma levels would be required to block dehydration. In vitro experiments have shown a potential benefit in combining these agents with other antisickling compounds (Stuart et al., 1994).

Cation Permeability Pathways Induced by Oxidation and Shear Stress in Sickle Erythrocytes

Membrane oxidative damage induced by oxygen free radicals induces a specific increase in potassium loss from erythrocytes (Maridonneau et al., 1983). Measurement of lipid peroxidation products in fresh sickle erythrocytes shows accumulation of thiobarbituric acid reactive substances and increased membrane lipid hydroperoxide, signs of oxidative damage similar to those seen in normal cells after in vitro oxidation (Sugihara et al., 1992).

Mild peroxidative damage induces a deformation-induced leak pathway (Ney et al., 1990; Hebbel and Mohandas, 1991; Sugihara et al., 1991; Sugihara and Hebbel, 1992). A lower degree of cell deformation is required to induce this pathway when oxidative damage is present. This leak pathway is reversible, independent of external calcium and/or chloride, and characterized by a balanced movement of sodium and potassium (potassium loss = sodium gain) (Ney et al., 1990; Sugihara and Hebbel, 1992). When external pH falls below 7, a new component appears, which produces net potassium loss and is not due to enhanced K-Cl cotransport (Sugihara and Hebbel, 1992). When osmolarity decreases, in the presence of deformation, there is a net potassium loss, which is inhibited by DIDS (75 percent) and bromide (50 percent). Because the deoxygenation-induced potassium loss is also reduced by bromide, it is possible that deformation of mildly peroxidated normal red cells in hypotonic medium induces a leak pathway that mimics the increased sodium and potassium leaks observed during deoxygenation (Sugihara, et al., 1994). The multiple effects of even mild oxidative damage on membrane permeability, K-Cl cotransport, and deformation-induced leak suggest that oxidation is an important determinant of cell dehydration in sickle cell disease.

Marked mechanical deformation of normal cells increases cation permeability, which has been attributed to increased membrane tension rather than deformation (Johnson, 1994). Mechanical stress of erythrocytes induces a large increase in potassium permeability, which seems to be mediated, at least in part, by the Gardos channel (Johnson and Tang, 1992). The permeability for chloride seems to be an essential component of this deformation-induced potassium leak, because this potassium movement can be blocked by DIDS (Johnson and Tang, 1993). It has been speculated that deformation-induced permeability could serve as a model for the deoxygenation-induced permeability of sickle erythrocytes, owing to the presence of several common functional features (Johnson and Gannon, 1990).

Deoxygenation Induced Cation Leak, Sodium-Potassium ATPase, Cell Sodium, and Sodium/Hydrogen Exchange in Sickle Erythrocytes

Tosteson et al. (1952) showed that deoxygenation of sickle cells was associated with potassium loss and sodium gain (Fig. 22.4) and that increased permeability was accompanied by stimulation of the sodium-potassium pump and took place through a diffusional pathway (Tosteson, 1955; Tosteson et al., 1955).

Deoxygenation-induced transport of sodium and potassium has been studied by Joiner and colleagues, who found that inward transport of sodium and outward transport of potassium are balanced and do not lead to cell dehydration (Berkowitz and Orringer, 1985; Joiner, 1987; Joiner et al., 1988; Joiner, 1990; Joiner et al., 1993; Joiner et al., 1995). Ion flux is dependent on external (and internal) pH, reaching a maximum value at pH 7.4 to 7.5, with inhibition at pH <7 and >8. Deoxy sodium and potassium flux is activated when oxygen drops below 40 to 50 torr and is chloride independent (Fig. 27.8) (Joiner et al., 1988). The deoxygenation-induced sodium and potassium fluxes are reduced by the anion exchange inhibitor DIDS, and the morphologic sickling is unaffected by DIDS (Joiner, 1990). However, if anion transport via the anion exchanger is inhibited by other

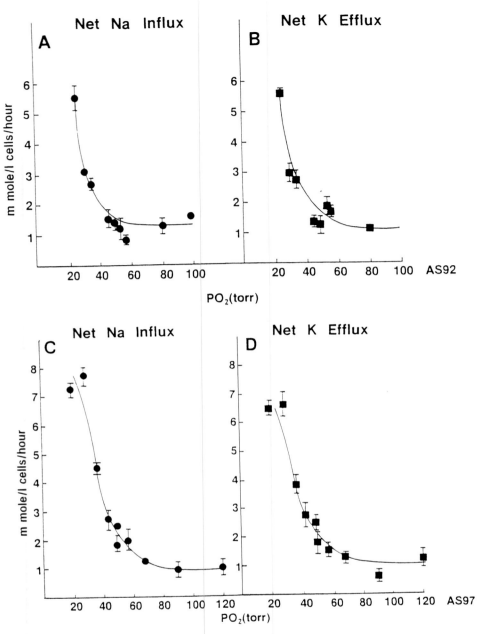

Figure 22.8. Dependence of net cation fluxes in sickle cells on oxygen tension. Cells were equilibrated with mixtures of air and N₂; PO₂ was measured in each sample and was stable over the incubation period. Error bars represent SEM; curves drawn by eye. (Reprinted with permission from Joiner et al., 1988.)

means, the deoxygenation-induced sodium and potassium fluxes are unaffected. Deoxy-ion fluxes are not associated with increased permeability to erythrol, arabinose, or mannitol, indicating that the increased membrane permeability is limited to alkali metal cations (Clark and Rossi, 1990). This deoxygenation-induced pathway is not selective for lithium, sodium, potassium, rubidium, or cesium is linearly dependent on the concentration of sodium or potassium; and is sensitive to changes in membrane potential (Joiner et al., 1993). These properties are suggestive of ion movement via diffusion, with a restriction to monovalent or divalent cations.

The presence of external calcium during deoxygenation inhibits sodium influx more than potassium efflux, resulting in an imbalance between the two fluxes and a net potassium loss (Bookchin et al., 1991; Joiner et al., 1995). This effect is not exclusive for calcium but is present with other divalent cations. Furthermore, no evidence of Gardos channel activation was found in these experiments, indicating that the net potassium loss was indeed mediated by the deoxygenation-induced pathway (Joiner, 1993). Therefore, in the presence of calcium, activation of the deoxygenation-induced pathway leads to cell dehydration.

The sodium-potassium pump may also play a role in cell dehydration. Earlier work in normal human red cells has indicated that activation of the pump in conditions with high sodium content leads to cell dehydration (Clark et al., 1981). In vitro evidence for erythrocyte dehydration mediated by the activation of the sodium-potassium pump has been provided for sickle cells and in hereditary xerocytosis (Joiner et al., 1986). In sickle erythrocytes, deoxygenation would increase cell sodium, which would activate the sodium-potassium pump, with cell dehydration due to the 3 Na_{out}/2 K_{in} stoichiometry of the transporter. However, the reduction in potassium content far exceeds the observed increase in cell sodium, and the integrated red cell model developed by Lew and Bookchin (1986) predicts that this mechanism can account for only a small fraction of the dehydration of sickle cells (Lew et al., 1991).

One important determinant of the deoxygenation-induced sodium and potassium movements is the deformation of the red cell induced by HbS polymerization and cell sickling. Slow, progressive deoxygenation induces the greatest degree of sickling (Asakura and Mayberry, 1984; Horiuchi et al., 1988). Conditions leading to marked morphologic changes are associated with the largest increase in sodium and potassium permeability, suggesting that the deformation induced by the polymer spicule plays a role in the activation of this pathway (Mohandas et al., 1986b).

Cell sodium content in sickle erythrocytes: Sickle erythrocytes of highest density and ISCs have the largest increase in cell sodium that could be due to decreased sodium-potassium pump activity, increased sodium permeability, or both (Clark et al., 1978b; Tosteson and Hoffman, 1960). Potassium transport mediated by the sodium-potassium pump is abnormally decreased in ISCs, whereas the ATPase activity is not (Clark et al., 1978a). This would suggest that there is an abnormal downregulation of the sodium-potassium pump activity in ISCs. The reduced sodium-potassium pump transport activity of dense sickle cells has been attributed to an increased intracellular magnesium/phosphorus ratio. When this ratio is decreased to normal values, the transport activity of the sodium-potassium pump is normalized (Ortiz et al., 1990).

An increased sodium permeability could also contribute to the high cell sodium of dense cells. Increased sodium/hydrogen exchange has been described in reticulocytes of normal and sickle cell anemia subjects (Canessa et al., 1990). However, it has been shown that this system is silent during deoxygenation and that the increase in intracellular calcium associated with deoxygenation is not sufficient to promote translocation of the PKC subunit to the cell membrane and activate the sodium/hydrogen exchanger (Joiner et al., 1998).

These data have outlined a series of mechanisms that ultimately lead to potassium loss and dehydration of sickle reticulocytes and erythrocytes. The relative role of each of these modalities on sickle cell dehydration varies according to the in vitro experimental conditions and may not correspond to events in vivo. Studies in transgenic sickle mice and patients with sickle cell disease have just begun to unravel the complexities of these interactions and assess the in vivo contribution of these mechanisms to erythrocyte dehydration. Several factors play a role in modulating the activity of these pathways and ultimately cell dehydration, and they include cell age (dehydration of reticulocytes and mature cells probably take place through different modalities), cellular content of HbF, and other still undefined factors that may be related to the modulation of the activity of these transport pathways by other receptors or biologically active molecules (PGE_2, endothelin for the Gardos channel, urea, and oxidative damage for K-Cl cotransport).

Rigorous research by many investigators on the transport systems of sickle erythrocytes has provided a basis for the current clinical studies with specific blockers of these pathways. Some of these clinical studies are now addressing issues of clinical efficacy. These new therapeutic approaches are discussed in greater detail in Chapter 42.

INTEGRATION AND SUMMARY

Figure 22.9 summarizes the major mechanisms and alterations in membrane structure and function of sickle erythrocytes. Polymerization of HbS and sickling result in major alterations of structure and function of the erythrocyte membrane. These alterations are present at the levels of membrane lipids, integral membrane proteins, and cytoskeleton. Polymerization of HbS precipitates a series of events that ultimately lead to the premature removal of the cell from the circulation. Membrane oxidation seems to play a key role in generating the damage observed in integral membrane proteins, cytoskeletal proteins, membrane lipid organization, and ion transport. Cellular dehydration plays a key role in promoting further polymerization and sickling, owing to the shortening of the delay time for HbS polymerization. Membrane damage is particularly severe in dense, dehydrated cells, which exhibit marked reduction in cell deformability and marked increase in membrane rigidity. Cytoskeletal proteins are altered and rearranged in these cells in such a way that they remain sickled even in the presence of 100 percent oxygen. Normal lipid asymmetry is also lost in these cells,

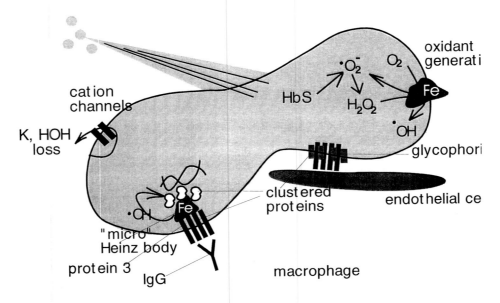

Figure 22.9. Summary of the major mechanisms involved in the structural damage and functional alterations of the membrane of sickle erythrocytes.

and the externalization of phosphatidylcholine renders them most likely to adhere to the endothelium and to monocytes/macrophages. Externalization of phosphatidylcholine promotes coagulation, which is also favored by the release of membrane vesicles from the dense, dehydrated cells. Membrane damage leads to clustering of proteins and formation of hemichromes and Heinz bodies. In these areas, deposition of IgG and complement further enhances the premature removal of the cells from the circulation.

Alterations of the erythrocyte membrane play a major role in the premature removal of erythrocytes from the circulation and in the anemia of sickle cell disease. In addition, they are important determinants in pathogenesis of the vasoocclusion and of the acute and chronic organ damage. They also provide opportunities for the development of new therapies specifically targeted to crucial steps in the pathophysiology of sickle cell membrane damage.

References

Akhrem, AA, Andreyuk, GM, Kisel, MA et al. (1989). Hemoglobin conversion to hemichrome under the influence of fatty acids. *Biochim. Biophys. Acta* 992: 191–194.

Allan, D, Limbrick, AR, Thomas, P et al. (1981). Microvesicles from sickle erythrocytes and their relation to irreversible sickling. *Br. J. Haematol.* 47: 383–390.

Allan, D, Limbrick, AR, Thomas, P et al. (1982). Release of spectrin-free spicules on reoxygenation of sickled erythrocytes. *Nature* 295: 612–613.

Allan, D and Raval, P. (1983). Some morphological consequences of uncoupling the lipid bilayer from the plasma membrane skeleton in intact erythrocytes. *Biomed. Biochim. Acta* 42: 11–12.

Alvarez, J, Montero, M, and Garcia-Sancho, J. (1992). High affinity inhibition of Ca2+-dependent K+ channels by cytochrome P-450 inhibitors. *J. Biol. Chem.* 267: 11789–11793.

Apovo, M, Gascard, P, Rhoda, MD et al. (1989). Alteration in protein kinase C activity and subcellular distribution in sickle erythrocytes. *Biochem. Biophys. Acta* 984: 26–32.

Asakura, T and Mayberry, J. (1984). Relationship between morphologic characteristics of sickle cells and method of deoxygenation. *J. Lab. Clin. Med.* 104: 987–994.

Asakura, T, Onishi, T, Friedman, S et al. (1974). Abnormal precipitation of oxyhemoglobin S by mechanical shaking. *Proc. Natl. Acad. Sci. U.S.A.* 71: 1594–1598.

Ballas, SK. (1991). Sickle cell anemia with few painful crises is characterized by decreased red cell deformability and increased number of dense cells. *Am. J. Hematol.* 36: 122–130.

Ballas, SK and Smith, ED. (1992). Red blood cell changes during the evolution of the sickle cell painful crisis. *Blood* 79: 2154–2163.

Bauminger, ER, Cohen, SG, Ofer, S et al. (1979). Quantitative studies of ferritinlike iron in erythrocytes of thalassemia, sickle-cell anemia, and hemoglobin Hammersmith with Mössbauer spectroscopy. *Proc. Natl. Acad. Sci. U.S.A.* 76: 939–943.

Bencsath, FA, Shartava, A, Monteiro, C et al. (1996). Identification of the disulfide-linked peptide in irreversibly sickled cell beta-actin. *Biochemistry* 35: 4403–4408.

Beppu, M, Inoue, M, Ishikawa, T et al. (1994). Presence of membrane-bound proteinases that preferentially degrade oxidatively damaged erythrocyte membrane proteins as secondary antioxidant defense. *Biochem. Biophys. Acta* 1196: 81–87.

Berkowitz, LR and Orringer, EP. (1985). Passive sodium and potassium movements in sickle erythrocytes. *Am. J. Physiol.* 249: C208–C214.

Bertles, JF and Döbler, J. (1969). Reversible and irreversible sickling: A distinction by electron microscopy. *Blood* 33: 884–898.

Blumenfeld, N, Zachowski, A, Galacteros, F et al. (1991). Transmembrane moobility of phospholipids in sickle erythrocytes: effect of deoxygenation on diffusion and asymmetry. *Blood* 77: 849–854.

Boivin, P. (1988). Role of the phosphorylation of red blood cell membrane proteins. *Biochem. J.* 256: 689–695.

Bookchin, RM and Lew, VL. (1981). Effect of a 'sickling pulse' on calcium and potassium transport in sickle cell trait red cells. *J. Physiol.* 312: 265–280.

Bookchin, RM, Ortiz, OE, and Lew, VL. (1991). Evidence for a direct reticulocyte origin of dense red cells in sickle cell anemia. *J. Clin. Invest.* 87: 113–124.

Bookchin, RM, Ortiz, OE, Somlyo, AV et al. (1985). Calcium-accumulating inside-out vesicles in sickle cell anemia red cells. *Trans. Assoc. Am. Physicians* 98: 10–20.

Brugnara, C. (1989). Characteristics of the volume- and chloride-dependent K transport in human erythrocytes homozygous for hemoglobin C. *J. Membr. Biol.* 111: 69–81.

Brugnara, C, Armsby, CC, De Franceschi, L et al. (1995a). Ca(2+)-activated K+ channels of human and rabbit erythrocytes display distinctive patterns of inhibition by venom peptide toxins. *J. Membr. Biol.* 147: 71–82.

Brugnara, C, Armsby, CC, Sakamoto, M et al. (1995b). Oral administration of clotrimazole and blockade of human erythrocyte Ca(++)-activated K+ channel: The imidazole ring is not required for inhibitory activity. *J. Pharmacol. Exp. Ther.* 273: 266–272.

Brugnara, C, Bunn HF, and Tosteson, DC. (1986). Regulation of erythrocyte cation and water content in sickle cell anemia. *Science* 232: 388–390.

Brugnara, C, De Franceschi, L, and Alper, SL. (1993a). Ca(2+)-activated K+ transport in erythrocytes. Comparison of binding and transport inhibition by scorpion toxins. *J. Biol. Chem.* 268: 8760–8768.

Brugnara, C, de Franceschi, L, and Alper, SL. (1993b). Inhibition of Ca(2+)-dependent K+ transport and cell dehydration in sickle erythrocytes by clotrimazole and other imidazole derivatives [see comments]. *J. Clin. Invest.* 92: 520–526.

Brugnara, C, Gee, B, Armsby, CC et al. (1996). Therapy with oral clotrimazole induces inhibition of the Gardos channel and reduction of erythrocyte dehydration in patients with sickle cell disease [see comments]. *J. Clin. Invest.* 97: 1227–1234.

Brugnara, C, Kopin, AS, Bunn, HF et al. (1985). Regulation of cation content and cell volume in erythrocytes from patients with homozygous hemoglobin C disease. *J. Clin. Invest.* 75: 1608–1617.

Brugnara, C and Tosteson, DC. (1987). Cell volume, K transport, and cell density in human erythrocytes. *Am. J. Physiol.* 252: C269–276.

Brugnara, C and Tosteson, DC. (1987). Inhibition of K transport by divalent cations in sickle erythrocytes. *Blood* 70: 1810–1815.

Brugnara, C, Van Ha, T, and Tosteson, DC. (1989). Acid pH induces formation of dense cells in sickle erythrocytes. *Blood* 74: 487–495.

Campwala, HQ and Desforges, JF. (1982). Membrane-bound hemichrome in density-separated cohorts of normal (AA) and sickled (SS) cells. *J. Lab. Clin. Med.* 99: 25–28.

Canessa, M, Fabry, ME, Blumenfeld, N et al. (1987a). Volume-stimulated, Cl(−)- dependent K+ efflux is highly expressed in young human red cells containing normal hemoglobin or HbS. *J. Membr. Biol.* 97: 97–105.

Canessa, M, Fabry, ME, and Nagel, RL. (1987b). Deoxygenation inhibits the volume-stimulated, Cl(−)-dependent K+ efflux in SS and young AA cells: A cytosolic Mg2+ modulation. *Blood* 70: 1861–1866.

Canessa, M, Fabry, ME, Suzuka, SM et al. (1990). Na+/H+ exchange is increased in sickle cell anemia and young normal red cells. *J. Membr. Biol.* 116: 107–115.

Canessa, M, Romero, JR, Lawrence, C et al. (1994). Rate of activation and deactivation of K:Cl cotransport by changes in cell volume in hemoglobin SS, CC and AA red cells. *J. Membr. Biol.* 142: 349–362.

Canessa, M, Spalvins, A, and Nagel, RL. (1986). Volume-dependent and NEM-stimulated K+, Cl− transport is elevated in oxygenated SS, SC and CC human red cells. *FEBS Lett.* 200: 197–202.

Carafoli, E. (1986). The calcium pump of erythrocytes. Activation and inhibition by natural compounds and by drugs. In Beuzard, Y, Charache, S, and Galacteros, F, editors. *Approaches to the therapy of sickle cell anemia.* Paris: Les editions INSERM. 141: 281–290.

Celedon, G, Gonzalez, G, Sotomayor, CP et al. (1998). Membrane lipid diffusion and band 3 protein changes in human erythrocytes due to acute hyperbaric hypoxia. *Am. J. Physiol.* 275: C1429–C1431.

Chiu, D, Lubin, B, Roelofsen, B et al. (1981). Sickled erythrocytes accelerate clotting in vitro: An effect of abnormal membrane lipid asymmetry. *Blood* 58: 398–401.

Chiu, D and Lubin, BH. (1979). Abnormal vitamin E and glutathione peroxidase levels in sickle cell anemia. *J. Lab. Clin. Med.* 94: 542–548.

Choe, HR, Schlegel, RA, Rubin, E et al. (1986). Alteration of red cell membrane organization in sickle cell anemia. *Br. J. Haematol.* 63: 761–773.

Clark, MR, Guatelli, JC, White, AT et al. (1981). Studies of the dehydrating effect of the red cell Na+/K+ pump in nystain-treated cells with varying Na+ and water content. *Biochim. Biophys. Acta* 646: 422–432.

Clark, MR, Morrison, CE, and Shohet, SB. (1978). Monovalent cation transport in irreversibly sickled cells. *J. Clin. Invest.* 62: 329–337.

Clark, MR and Rossi, ME. (1990). Permeability characteristics of deoxygenated sickle cells. *Blood* 76: 2139–2145.

Clark, MR, Unger, RC, and Shohet, SB. (1978b). Monovalent cation composition and ATP and lipid content of irreversibly sickled cells. *Blood* 51: 1169–1178.

Corbett, JD and Golan, DE. (1993). Band 3 and glycophorin are progressively aggregated in density fractionated sickle and normal red blood cells: Evidence from rotational and lateral mobility studies. *J. Clin. Invest.* 91: 208–217.

Culliford, SJ, Ellory, JC, Gibson, JS et al. (1998). Effects of urea and oxygen tension on K flux in sickle cells. *Pflugers Arch. Eur. J. Physiol.* 435: 740–742.

Das, SK and Nair, RC. (1980). Superoxide dismutase, glutathione peroxidase, catalase and lipid peroxidation of normal and sickled erythrocytes. *Br. J. Haematol.* 44: 87–92.

De Franceschi, L, Bachir, D, Galacteros, F et al. (1997a). Oral magnesium supplements reduce erythrocyte dehydration in patients with sickle cell disease. *J. Clin. Invest.* 100: 1847–1852.

De Franceschi, L, Bachir, D, Galacteros, F et al. (2000). Oral magnesium pidolate: Effects of long-term administration in patients with sickle cell disease. *Br. J. Haematol.* 108: 248–289.

De Franceschi, L, Beuzard, Y, and Brugnara, C. (1995). Sulfhydryl oxidation and activation of red cell K(+)-C1-cotransport in the transgenic SAD mouse. *Am. J. Physiol.* 269: C899–906.

De Franceschi, L, Brugnara, C, and Beuzard, Y. (1997b). Dietary magnesium supplementation ameliorates anemia in a mouse model of beta-thalassemia. *Blood* 90: 1283–1290.

De Franceschi, L, Cappellini, MD, Graziadei, G et al. (1998a). The effect of dietary magnesium supplementation on the cellular abnormalities of erythrocytes in patients with beta thalassemia intermedia. *Haematologica* 83: 118–125.

De Franceschi, L, Saadane, N, Trudel, M et al. (1994). Treatment with oral clotrimazole blocks Ca(2+)-activated K+ transport and reverses erythrocyte dehydration in transgenic SAD mice. A model for therapy of sickle cell disease. *J. Clin. Invest.* 93: 1670–1676.

De Franceschi, L, Shalev, O, Piga, A et al. (1999). Deferiprone therapy in homozygous human β thalassemia removes erythrocyte membrane free iron and reduces K-Cl cotransport activity. *J. Lab. Clin. Med.* 133: 64–69.

De Franceschi, L, Turrini, F, Brugnara, C et al. (1998b). Role of membrane oxidative damage in the pathogenesis of hemolytic anemia induced by ribavirin therapy in patients with chronic hepatitis C infections. *Blood* 92: 10a.

Devine, DV, Kinney, TR, Thomas, PF et al. (1986). Fragment D-dimer levels: An objective marker of vaso-occlusive crisis and other complications of sickle cell disease. *Blood* 68: 317–319.

Dong, C, Chadwick, RS, and Schechter, AN. (1992). Influence of sickle hemoglobin polymerization and membrane properties on deformability of sickle erythrocytes in the microcirculation. *Biophys. J.* 63: 774–783.

Dzandu, JK and Johnson, RM. (1980). Membrane protein phosphorylation in intact normal and sickle cell erythrocytes. *J. Biol. Chem.* 255: 6382–6386.

Eaton, J, Skelton, T, Swofford, H et al. (1973). Elevated erythrocyte calcium in sickle cell disease. *Nature* 246: 105–106.

Eaton, WA and Hofrichter, J. (1987). Hemoglobin S gelation and sickle cell disease. *Blood* 70: 1245–1266.

Eaton, WA and Hofrichter, J. (1990). Sickle cell hemoglobin polymerization. *Adv. Prot. Chem.* 40: 63–279.

Eisinger, J, Flores, J, and Bookchin, RM. (1984). The cytosol-membrane interface of normal and sickle erythro-cytes. Effect of hemoglobin deoxygenation and sickling. *J. Biol. Chem.* 259: 7169–7177.

Eisinger, J, Flores, J, and Salhany, JM. (1982). Association of cytosol hemoglobin with the membrane in intact erythrocytes. *Proc. Natl. Acad. Sci. U.S.A.* 79: 408–412.

Ellory, JC, Culliford, SJ, Smith, PA et al. (1994). Specific inhibition of Ca-activated K channels in red cells by selected dihydropyridine derivatives. *Br. J. Pharmacol.* 111: 903–905.

Ellory, JC, Hall, AC, and Ody, SA. (1990). Factors affecting the activation and inactivation of KCl cotransport in 'young' human red cells. *Biomed. Biochim. Acta* 49: S64–69.

Ellory, JC, Hall, AC, Ody, SA et al. (1991). KCl cotransport in HbAA and HbSS red cells: Activation by intracellular acidity and disappearance during maturation. *Adv. Exp. Med. Biol.* 307: 47–57.

Ellory, JC, Kirk, K, Culliford, SJ et al. (1992a). Nitrendipine is a potent inhibitor of the Ca(2+)-activated K+ channel of human erythrocytes. *FEBS Lett.* 296: 219–221.

Ellory, JC, Nash, GB, Stone, PC et al. (1992b). Mode of action and comparative efficacy of pharmacological agents that inhibit calcium-dependent dehydration of sickle cells. *Br. J. Pharmacol.* 106: 972–977.

Embury, SH, Clark, MR, Monroy, G et al. (1984). Concurrent sickle cell anemia and alpha-thalassemia. Effect on pathological properties of sickle erythrocytes. *J. Clin. Invest.* 73: 116–123.

Engelmann, B and Duhm, J. (1987). Intracellular calcium content of human erythrocytes: relation to sodium transport systems. *J. Membr. Biol.* 98: 79–87.

Etzion, Z, Lew, VL, and Bookchin, RM. (1996). K(86Rb) transport heterogeneity in the low-density fraction of sickle cell anemia red blood cells. *Am. J. Physiol.* 271: C1111–1121.

Etzion, Z, Tiffert, T, Bookchin, RM et al. (1993). Effects of deoxygenation on active and passive Ca2+ transport and on the cytoplasmic Ca2+ levels of sickle cell anemia red cells. *J. Clin. Invest.* 92: 2489–2498.

Evans, EA and Mohandas, N. (1987). Membrane-associated sickle hemoglobin: A major determinant of sickle erythrocyte rigidity. *Blood* 70: 1443–1449.

Fabry, ME, Benjamin, L, Lawrence, C et al. (1984). An objective sign in painful crisis in sickle cell anemia: The concomitant reduction of high density red cells. *Blood* 64: 559–563.

Fabry, ME, Kaul, DK, Raventos-Suarez, C et al. (1982). SC erythrocytes have an abnormally high intracellular hemoglobin concentration. Pathophysiological consequences. *J. Clin. Invest.* 70: 1315–1319.

Fabry, ME, Mears, JG, Patel, P et al. (1984b). Dense cells in sickle cell anemia: The effects of gene interaction. *Blood* 64: 1042–1046.

Fabry, ME and Nagel, RL. (1982). Heterogeneity of red cells in the sickler: A characteristic with practical clinical and pathophysiological implications. *Blood Cells* 8: 9–15.

Fabry, ME, Romero, JR, Buchanan, JD et al. (1991). Rapid increase in red blood cell density driven by K:Cl cotransport in a subset of sickle cell anemia reticulocytes and discocytes. *Blood* 78: 217–225.

Fabry, ME, Romero, JR, Suzuka, SM et al. (1998). Hemoglobin C in transgenic mice with full mouse globin knockouts. *Blood* 92: 330a.

Fathallah, H, Coezy, E, de Neef, RS et al. (1995). Inhibition of deoxygenation-induced membrane protein dephosphorylation and cell dehydration by phorbol esters and okadaic acid in sickle cells. *Blood* 86: 1999–2007.

Fathallah, H, Sauvage, M, Romero, JR et al. (1997). Effects of PKC alpha activation on Ca2+ pump and K(Ca) channel in deoxygenated sickle cells. *Am. J. Physiol.* 273: C1206–1214.

Feray, JC, Beuzard, Y, and Garay, RP. (1988). Na/Mg exchange in sickle cells. *VI International Magnesium Symposium* 22a.

Feray, JC and Garay, R. (1986). A Na-stimulated Mg transport system in human red blood cells. *Biochim. Biophys. Acta* 856: 76–84.

Fischer, S, Nagel, RL, Bookchin, RM et al. (1975). The binding of hemoglobin to membranes of normal and sickle erythrocytes. *Biochim. Biophys. Acta* 375: 422–433.

Fortier, N, Snyder, LM, Garver, F et al. (1988). The relationship between in vivo generated hemoglobin skeletal protein complex and increase red cell membrane rigidity. *Blood* 71: 1427–1431.

Francis, RBJ. (1989). Elevated fibrin D-dimer fragment in sickle cell anemia: Evidence for activation of coagulation during the steady state as well as in painful crisis. *Haemostasis* 19: 105–111.

Franco, RS, Barker-Gear, R, Miller, MA et al. (1994). Fetal hemoglobin and potassium in isolated transferrin receptor-positive dense sickle reticulocytes. *Blood* 84: 2013–2020.

Franco, RS, Lohmann, J, Silberstein, EB et al. (1998a). Time-dependent changes in the density and hemoglobin F content of biotin-labeled sickle cells. *J. Clin. Invest.* 101: 2730–2740.

Franco, RS, Palascak, M, Thompson, H et al. (1995a). KCl cotransport activity in light versus dense transferrin receptor-positive sickle reticulocytes. *J. Clin. Invest.* 95: 2573–2580.

Franco, RS, Thompson, H, Palascak, M et al. (1997). The formation of transferrin receptor-positive sickle reticulocytes with intermediate density is not determined by fetal hemoglobin content. *Blood* 90: 3195–3203.

Franco, RS, Yasin, Z, Lohmann, JM et al. (1998b). The in vivo survival of dense sickle cells: Effects of HbF content and external phosphatidylserine. *Blood* 92: 13a.

Frank, PK, Bevers, EM, Lubin, BH et al. (1985b). Uncoupling of the membrane skeleton from the lipid bilayer. The cause of accelerated phospholipid flip-flop leading to an enhanced procoagulant activity of sickled cells. *J. Clin. Invest.* 75: 183–190.

Friedman, MJ. (1981). Hemoglobin and the red cell membrane: increased binding of polymorphic hemoglobins and measurement of free radicals in the membrane. *The red cell: Fifth Ann Arbor Conference.* New York: Alan R. Liss.

Galili, U, Clark, MR, and Shohet, SB. (1986). Excessive binding of natural anti-alpha-galactosyl immunoglobin G to sickle erythrocytes may contribute to extravascular cell destruction. *J. Clin. Invest.* 77: 27–33.

Gardos, G. (1958). The function of calcium in the potassium permeability of human erythrocytes. *Biochim. Biophys. Acta* 30: 653–654.

Gibson, JS, Speake, PF, and Ellory, JC. (1998). Differential oxygen sensitivity of the K^+-Cl^{1-} cotransporter in normal and sickle human red blood cells. *J. Physiol.* 511.1: 225–234.

Gillen, CM, Brill, SB, Payne, JA et al. (1996). Molecular cloning and functional expression of the K-Cl cotransporter from rabbit, rat and human. A new member of the cation-chloride cotransporter family. *J. Biol. Chem.* 27: 16237–16244.

Glader, BE and Nathan, NG. (1978). Cation permeability alteration during sickling: Relationship to cation composition and cellular dehydration of irreversibly sickled cells. *Blood* 51: 983–989.

Godart, H and Ellory, JC. (1996). KCl cotransport activation in human erythrocytes by high hydrostatic pressure. *J. Physio.* 491: 423–434.

Graido-Gonzalez, E, Doherty, JC, Bergreen, EW et al. (1998). Plasma endothelin-1, cytokine, and prostaglandin E2 levels in sickle cell disease and acute vasoocclusive sickle crisis. *Blood* 92: 2551–2555.

Haas, M. (1994). The Na-K-Cl cotransporters. *Am. J. Physiol.* 267: C869–885.

Haas, M and Forbush, B, 3rd (1998). The Na-K-Cl cotransporters. *J. Bioenerg. Biomembr.* 30: 161–172.

Haas, M and Harrison, JH, Jr. (1989). Stimulation of K-Cl cotransport in rat red cells by a hemolytic anemia-producing metabolite of dapsone. *Am. J. Physiol.* 256: C265–272.

Hall, AC and Ellory, JC. (1986). Evidence for the presence of volume-sensitive KCl transport in 'young' human red cells. *Biochim. Biophys. Acta* 858: 317–320.

Hammerman, SI, Kourembanas, S, Conca, TJ et al. (1997). Endothelin-1 production during the acute chest syndrome in sickle cell disease. *Am. J. Respir. Crit. Care Med.* 156: 280–285.

Harrington, JP. (1998). Alteration of redox stability of hemoglobins A and S by biological buffers. *Compa. Biochem. Physiol. Part B, Biochem. Mol. Biol.* 119: 305–309.

Harrington, JP, Newton, P, Crumpton, T et al. (1993). Induced hemichrome formation of methemoglobins A, S and F by fatty acids, alkyl ureas and urea. *Int. J. Biochem.* 25: 665–670.

Hartley, A and Rice-Evans, C. (1989). Membrane-associated iron species and membrane oxidation in sickle-cell disease. *Biochem. Soc. Trans.* 17: 116–118.

Hasegawa, S, Hiruma, H, Uyesaka, N et al. (1995). Filterability of mixtures of sickle and normal erythrocytes. *Am. J. Hematol.* 50: 91–97.

Hebbel, RP. (1991). Beyond hemoglobin polymerization: The red blood cell membrane and sickle disease pathophysiology. *Blood* 77: 214–237.

Hebbel, RP. (1994). Membrane-associated iron. In Embury, SH, Hebbel, RP, Mohandas, N, and Steinberg, MH, editors. *Sickle cell disease: Basic principles and clinical practice.* New York: Raven Press.

Hebbel, RP and Mohandas, N. (1991). Reversible deformation-dependent erythrocyte cation leak. Extreme sensitivity conferred by minimal peroxidation. *Biophys. J.* 60: 712–715.

Hebbel, RP, Morgan, WT, Eaton, JW et al. (1988). Accelerated autoxidation and heme loss due to instability of sickle hemoglobin. *Proc. Natl. Acad. Sci. U.S.A.* 85: 237–241.

Hebbel, RP, Schwartz, RS, and Mohandas, N. (1985). The adhesive sickle erythrocyte: Cause and consequences of abnormal interactions with endothelium, monocytes/ macrophages, and model membranes. *Clin. Haematol.* 14: 141–161.

Hebbel, RP, Shalev, O, Foker, W et al. (1986). Inhibition of erythrocyte Ca^{2+}-ATPase by activated oxygen through thiol- and lipid-dependent mechanisms. *Biochim. Biophys. Acta* 862: 8–16.

Hiruma, H, Noguchi, CT, Uyesaka, N et al. (1995a). Sickle cell rheology is determined by polymer fraction—not cell morphology. *Am. J. Hematol.* 48: 19–28.

Hiruma, H, Noguchi, CT, Uyesaka, N et al. (1995b). Contributions of sickle hemoglobin polymer and sickle cell membranes to impaired filterability. *Am. J. Physiol.* 268: H2003–2008.

Horiuchi, K and Asakura, T. (1987). Formation of light irreversibly sickled cells during deoxygenation-oxygenation cycles. *J. Lab. Clin. Med.* 110: 653–660.

Horiuchi, K, Ballas, SK, and Asakura, T. (1988). The effect of deoxygenation rate on the formation of irreversibly sickled cells. *Blood* 71: 46–51.

Ishii, TM, Silvia, C, Hirschberg, B et al. (1997). A human intermediate conductance calcium-activated potassium channel. *Proc. Natl. Acad. Sci. U.S.A.* 94: 11651–11656.

Jarolim, P, Lahav, M, Liu, SC et al. (1990). Effect of hemoglobin oxidation products on the stability of red cell membrane skeletons and the associations of skeletal proteins: Correlation with a release of hemin. *Blood* 76: 2125–2131.

Jennings, ML and Al-Rohil, N. (1990). Kinetics of activation and inactivation of swelling stimulated K/Cl transport. The volume sensitive parameter is the rate constant for inactivation. *J. Gen. Physiol.* 95: 1021–1040.

Jennings, ML and Schulz, RK. (1991). Okadaic acid inhibition of K-Cl cotransport. *J. Gen. Physiol.* 97: 799–818.

Jindal, HK, Ai, Z, Gascard, P et al. (1996). Specific loss of protein kinase activities in senescent erythrocytes. *Blood* 88: 1479–1487.

Johnson, R, Dzandu, JK, and Warth, JA. (1986). The phosphoproteins of the sickle erythrocyte membrane. *Arch. Biochem. Biophys.* 244: 202–210.

Johnson, RM. (1994). Membrane stress increases cation permeability in red cells. *Biophys. J.* 67: 1876–1881.

Johnson, RM and Dzandu, JK. (1982). Calcium and ionophore A23187 induce the sickle cell membrane phosphorylation pattern in normal erythrocytes. *Biochim. Biophys. Acta* 692: 218–222.

Johnson, RM and Gannon, SA. (1990). Erythrocyte cation permeability induced by mechanical stress: A model for sickle cell cation loss. *Am. J. Physiol.* 259: C746–751.

Johnson, RM and Tang, K. (1992). Induction of a Ca(2+)-activated K+ channel in human erythrocytes by mechanical stress. *Biochim. Biophys. Acta* 1107: 314–318.

Johnson, RM and Tang, K. (1993). DIDS inhibition of deformation-induced cation flux in human erythrocytes. *Biochim. Biophy. Acta* 1148: 7–14.

Joiner, CH. (1987). Studies on the mechanism of passive cation fluxes activated by deoxygenation of sickle cells. *Prog. Clin. Biol. Res.* 240: 229–235.

Joiner, CH. (1990). Deoxygenation-induced cation fluxes in sickle cells: II. Inhibition by stilbene disulfonates. *Blood* 76: 212–220.

Joiner, CH. (1993). Cation transport and volume regulation in sickle red blood cells. *Am. J. Physiol.* 264: C251–270.

Joiner, CH, Dew, A, and Ge, DL. (1988). Deoxygenation-induced cation fluxes in sickle cells: Relationship between net potassium efflux and net sodium influx. *Blood Cells* 13: 339–358.

Joiner, CH, Jiang, M, Fathallah, H et al. (1998). Deoxygenation of sickle red blood cells stimulates KCl cotransport without affecting Na+/H+ exchange. *Am. J. Physiol.* 274: C1466–1475.

Joiner, CH, Jiang, M, and Franco, RS. (1995). Deoxygenation-induced cation fluxes in sickle cells. IV. Modulation by external calcium. *Am. J. Physiol.* 269: C403–409.

Joiner, CH, Morris, CL, and Cooper, ES. (1993). Deoxygenation-induced cation fluxes in sickle cells. III. Cation selectivity and response to pH and membrane potential. *Am. J. Physiol.* 264: C734–744.

Joiner, CH, Platt, OS, and Lux, SET. (1986). Cation depletion by the sodium pump in red cells with pathologic cation leaks. Sickle cells and xerocytes. *J. Clin. Invest.* 78: 1487–1496.

Kabata, J and Tichelli, A. (1994). Flow cytometric pattern of leukocyte recovery after therapy-induced aplasia. *Acta Haematol. Pol.* 25: 329–342.

Kahane, I, Shifter, A, and Rachmilewitz EA. (1978). Cross-linking of red blood cell membrane proteins induced by oxidative stress in beta thalassemia. *FEBS Lett.* 85: 267–270.

Kaji, DM. (1989). Kinetics of volume-sensitive K transport in human erythrocytes: Evidence for asymmetry. *Am. J. Physiol.* 256: C1214–1223.

Kaji, DM and Gasson, C. (1995). Urea activation of K-Cl transport in human erythrocytes. *Am. J. Physiol.* 268: C1018–1025.

Kaji, DM and Tsukitani, Y. (1991). Role of protein phosphatase in activation of KCl cotransport in human erythrocytes. *Am. J. Physiol.* 260: C176–180.

Kannan, R, Labotka, R, and Low, PS. (1988). Isolation and characterization of the hemichrome-stabilized membrane protein aggregates from sickle erythrocytes. Major site of autologous antibody binding. *J. Biol. Chem.* 263: 13766–13773.

Kannan, R, Yuan, J, and Low, PS. (1991). Isolation and partial characterization of antibody- and globin-enriched complexes from membranes of dense human erythrocytes. *Biochem. J.* 278: 57–62.

Kaul, DK, Chen, D, and Zhan, J. (1994). Adhesion of sickle cells to vascular endothelium is critically dependent on changes in density and shape of the cells. *Blood* 83: 3006–3017.

Kaul, DK, Fabry, ME, and Nagel, RL. (1989). Microvascular sites and characteristics of sickle cell adhesion to vascular endothelium in shear flow conditions: Pathophysiological implications. *Proc. Natl. Acad. Sci. U.S.A.* 86: 3356–3360.

Key, NS, Slungaard, A, Dandelet, L et al. (1998). Whole blood tissue factor procoagulant activity is elevated in patients with sickle cell disease. *Blood* 91: 4216–4223.

Kuross, SA and Hebbel, RP. (1988). Nonheme iron in sickle erythrocyte membranes: Association with phospholipids and potential role in lipid peroxidation. *Blood* 72: 1278–1285.

Kuross, SA, Rank, BH, and Hebbel, RP. (1988). Excess heme in sickle erythrocyte inside-out membranes: possible role in thiol oxidation. *Blood* 71: 876–882.

Kuypers, FA, Lewis, RA, Hua, M et al. (1996). Detection of altered membrane phospholipid asymmetry in subpopulations of human red blood cells using fluorescently labeled Annexin V. *Blood* 87: 1179–1187.

Kuypers, FA, van den Berg, JJM, and Lubin, BH. (1994). Membrane lipids and vesiculation. In Embury, SH, Hebbel, RP, Mohandas, N, and Steinberg, MH, editors. *Sickle cell disease: Basic principles and clinical practice.* New York: Raven Press.

Kuypers, FA, Yee, M, Vichinsky, E et al. (1992). Activation of the prothrombinase complex in sickle cell anemia. *Blood* 80: 75(abstr.).

Lachant, NA, Davidson, WD, and Takanka, KR. (1983). Impaired pentose phosphate shunt function in sickle cell disease: A potential mechanism for increased Heinz body formation and membrane lipid peroxidation. *Am. J. Haematol.* 15: 1–13.

Lauf, PK, Bauer, J, Adragna, NC et al. (1992). Erythrocyte K-Cl cotransport: Properties and regulation. *Am. J. Physiol.* 263: C917–C932.

Lawrence, C and Fabry, ME. (1987). Objective indices of sickle cell painful crisis: Decrease in RDW and percent dense cells and increase in ESR and fibrinogen. *Prog. Clin. Biol. Res.* 240: 329–336.

Lawrence, C, Fabry, ME, and Nagel, RL. (1985). Red cell distribution width parallels dense red cell disappearance during painful crises in sickle cell anemia. *J. Lab. Clin. Med.* 105: 706–710.

Lawrence, C, Fabry, ME, and Nagel, RL. (1991). The unique red cell heterogeneity of SC disease: Crystal formation, dense reticulocytes, and unusual morphology. *Blood* 78: 2104–2112.

Leclerc, L, Girard, F, Galacteros, F et al. (1987). The calmodulin-stimulated ($Ca^{2+}+Mg^{2+}$)-ATPase in hemoglobin S erythrocyte membranes: Effects of sickling and oxidative agents. *Biochim. Biophys. Acta* 897: 33–40.

Lessin, LS, Kurantsin-Mills, J, Wallas, C et al. (1978). Membrane alterations in irreversibly sickled cells: Hemoglobin-membrane interactions. *J. Supramol. Struct.* 9: 537–554.

Lew, VL and Bookchin, RM. (1986). Volume, pH, and ion-content regulation in human red cells: Analysis of transient behavior with an integrated model. *J. Membr. Biol.* 92: 57–74.

Lew, VL, Freeman, CJ, Ortiz, OE et al. (1991). A mathematical model of the volume, pH, and ion content regulation in reticulocytes. Application to the pathophysiology of sickle cell dehydration. *J. Clin. Invest.* 87: 100–112.

Lew, VL, Hockaday, A, Sepulveda, MI et al. (1985). Compartmentalization of sickle-cell calcium in endocytic inside-out vesicles. *Nature* 315: 586–589.

Lew, VL, Ortiz, OE, and Bookchin, RM. (1997). Stochastic nature and red cell population distribution of the sickling-induced Ca2+ permeability. *J. Clin. Invest.* 99: 2727–2735.

Lew, VL, Tsien, RY, Miner, C et al. (1982). Physiological [Ca2+]i level and pump-leak turnover in intact red cells measured using an incorporated Ca chelator. *Nature* 298: 478–481.

Li, Q, Jungmann, V, Kiyatkin, A et al. (1996). Prostaglandin E_2 stimulates a Ca^{2+}-dependent K^+ channel in human erythrocytes and alters cell volume and filterability. *J. Biol. Chem.* 271: 18651–18656.

Liu, SC, Derick, LH, and Palek, J. (1993). Dependence of the permanent deformation of red blood cell membranes on spectrin dimer-tetramer equilibrium: Implication for permanent membrane deformation of irreversibly sickled cells. *Blood* 81: 522–528.

Liu, SC, Derick, LH, Zhai, S et al. (1991). Uncoupling of the spectrin-based skeleton from the lipid bilayer in sickled red cells. *Science* 252: 574–576.

Liu, SC, Scott, JY, Mehta, JR et al. (1996). Red cell membrane remodeling in sickle cell anemia: Sequestration of membrane lipids and proteins in Heinz bodies. *J. Clin. Invest.* 97: 29–36.

Liu, SC, Zhai, S, and Palek, J. (1988). Detection of hemin release during hemoglobin S denaturation. *Blood* 71: 1755–1758.

Lubin, B, Chiu, D, Bastacky, J et al. (1981). Abnormalities in membrane phospholipid organization in sickled erythrocytes. *J. Clin. Invest.* 67: 1643–1649.

Lubin, B, Kuypers, F, and Chiu, D. (1989). Lipid alterations and cellular properties of sickle red cells. *Ann. N.Y. Acad. Sci.* 565: 86–95.

Lux, SE, John, KM, and Karnovsky, MJ. (1976). Irreversible deformation of the spectrin-actin lattice in irreversibly sickled cells. *J. Clin. Invest.* 58: 955–963.

Lux, SE and Palek, J. (1995). Disorders of the red cell membrane. In Handin, RJ, Lux, SE, and Stossel, TP, editors. *Blood: Principles and practice of hematology.* Philadelphia: Lippincott-Raven.

Mannu, F, Arese, P, Cappellini, MD et al. (1995). Role of hemichrome binding to erythrocyte membrane in the generation of band-3 alterations in beta-thalassemia intermedia erythrocytes. *Blood* 86: 2014–2020.

Maridonneau, I, Braquet, P, and Garay, PR. (1983). Na+ and K+ transport damage induced by oxygen free radicals in human red cell membranes. *J. Biol. Chem.* 258: 3107–3113.

Marva, E and Hebbel, RP. (1994). Denaturing interaction between sickle hemoglobin and phosphatidylserine liposomes. *Blood* 83: 242–249.

McGoron, AJ, Joiner, CH, Palascak, MB et al. (2000). Dehydration of mature and immature sickle red blood cells during fast oxygenation/deoxygenation cycles: Role of K-Cl cotransport and extracellular Ca. *Blood* 95: 2164–2168.

McPherson, RA, Sawyer, WH, and Tilley, L. (1992). Rotational diffusion of the erythrocyte integral membrane protein band 3: Effect of hemichrome binding. *Biochemistry* 31: 512–518.

Mohandas, N and Ballas, SK. (1994). Erythrocyte density and heterogeneity. In Embury, SH, Hebbel, RP, Mohandas, N, and Steinberg, MH. editors. *Sickle cell disease: Basic principles and clinical practice.* New York: Raven Press.

Mohandas, N, Johnson, A, Wyatt, J et al. (1989). Automated quantitation of cell density distribution and hyperdense cell fraction in RBC disorders. *Blood* 74: 442–447.

Mohandas, N, Kim, YR, Tycko, DH et al. (1986a). Accurate and independent measurement of volume and hemoglobin concentration of individual red cells by laser light scattering. *Blood* 68: 506–513.

Mohandas, N, Rossi, ME, and Clark, MR. (1986b). Association between morphologic distortion of sickle cells and deoxygenation-induced cation permeability increase. *Blood* 68: 450–454.

Morris, CL, Rucknagel, DL, and Joiner, CH. (1993). Deoxygenation-induced changes in sickle cell-sickle cell adhesion. *Blood* 81: 3138–3145.

Murphy, E, Berkowitz, LR, Orringer, E et al. (1987). Cytosolic free calcium in sickle red blood cells. *Blood* 69: 1469–1474.

Nagel, RL, Daar, S, Romero, JR et al. (1998). HbS-Oman heterozygote: A new dominant sickle syndrome. *Blood* 92: 4375–4382.

Ney, PA, Christopher, MM, and Hebbel, RP. (1990). Synergistic effects of oxidation and deformation on erythrocyte monovalent cation leak. *Blood* 75: 1192–1198.

Noguchi, CT, Dover, GJ, Rodgers, GP et al. (1985). Alpha thalassemia changes erythrocyte heterogeneity in sickle cell disease. *J. Clin. Invest.* 75: 1632–1639.

Noguchi, CT, Rodgers, GP, and Schechter, AN. (1989). Intracellular polymerization. Disease severity and therapeutic predictions. *Ann. N.Y. Acad. Sci.* 565: 75–82.

Ohnishi, ST, Horiuchi, KY, and Horiuchi, K. (1986). The mechanism of in vitro formation of irreversibly sickled cells and modes of action of its inhibitors. *Biochim. Biophys. Acta* 886: 119–129.

Ohnishi, ST, Katagi, H, and Katagi, C. (1989). Inhibition of the in vitro formation of dense cells and of irreversibly sickled cells by charybdotoxin, a specific inhibitor of calcium-activated potassium efflux. *Biochim. Biophys. Acta* 1010: 199–203.

Olivieri, O, Bonollo, M, Friso, S et al. (1993). Activation of K+/Cl-cotransport in human erythrocytes exposed to oxidative agents. *Biochim. Biophys. Acta* 1176: 37–42.

Olivieri, O, De Franceschi, L, Capellini, MD et al. (1994). Oxidative damage and erythrocyte membrane transport abnormalities in thalassemias. *Blood* 84: 315–320.

Olivieri, O, Vitoux, D, Bachir, D et al. (1991). K+ efflux in deoxygenated sickle cells in the presence or absence of DIOA, a specific inhibitor of the [K+, Cl–] cotransport system. *Br. J. Haematol.* 77: 117–120.

Olivieri, O, Vitoux, D, Galacteros, F et al. (1992). Hemoglobin variants and activity of the (K+Cl–) cotransport system in human erythrocytes. *Blood* 79: 793–779.

Olukoga, AO, Adewoye, HO, Erasmus, RT et al. (1990). Erythrocyte and plasma magnesium in sickle-cell anaemia. *East. Afr. Med. J.* 67: 348–354.

Ortiz, OE, Lew, VL, and Bookchin, RM. (1990). Deoxygenation permeabilizes sickle cell anaemia red cells to magnesium and reverses its gradient in the dense cells. *J. Physiol.* 427: 211–226.

Palek, J. (1977). Red cell calcium content and transmembrane calcium movements in sickle cell anemia. *J. Lab. Clin. Med.* 89: 1365–1374.

Palfrey, HC and Waseem, A. (1985). Protein kinase C in the human erythrocyte. Translocation to the plasma membrane and phosphorylation of bands 4.1 and 4.9 and other membrane proteins. *J. Biol. Chem.* 260: 16021–16029.

Phelan, M, Perrine, SP, Brauer, M et al. (1995). Sickle erythrocytes, after sickling, regulate the expression of the endothelin-1 gene and protein in human endothelial cells in culture. *J. Clin. Invest.* 96: 1145–1151.

Platt, OS. (1994). Membrane proteins. In Embury, SH, Hebbel, RP, Mohandas, N, and Steinberg, MH, editors. *Sickle cell disease: Basic principles and clinical practice.* New York: Raven Press.

Platt, OS and Falcone, JF. (1988). Membrane protein lesions in erythrocytes with Heinz bodies. *J. Clin. Invest.* 82: 1051–1058.

Platt, OS and Falcone, JF. (1995). Membrane protein interactions in sickle red blood cells: Evidence of abnormal protein 3 function. *Blood* 86: 1992–1998.

Platt, OS, Falcone, JF, and Lux, SE. (1985). Molecular defect in the sickle erythrocyte skeleton. Abnormal spectrin binding to sickle inside-out vesicles. *J. Clin. Invest.* 75: 266–271.

Rachmilewitz, EA, and Harari, E. (1972). Intermediate hemichrome formation after oxidation of three unstable hemoglobins (Freiburg, Riverdale-Bronx and Koln). *Hamatologie und Bluttransfusion* 10: 241–250.

Ramachandran, M, Nari, CN, and Abraham, EC. (1987). Increased membrane-associated phorbol-12,13 dibutyrate (PDBu) receptor function in sickle red cells. *Biochem. Biophys. Res. Comm.* 147: 56–64.

Rank, BH, Carlsson, J, and Hebbel, RP. (1985). Abnormal redox status of membrane-protein thiols in sickle erythrocytes. *J. Clin. Invest.* 75: 1531–1537.

Rank, BH, Moyer, NL, and Hebbel, RP. (1988). Vesiculation of sickle erythrocytes during thermal stress. *Blood* 72: 1060–1063.

Reilly, MP, Chomo, MJ, Obata, K et al. (1994). Red blood cell membrane and density changes under ambient and hypoxic conditions in transgenic mice producing human sickle hemoglobin. *Exp. Hematol.* 22: 501–509.

Reiss, GH, Ranney, HM, and Shaklai, N. (1982). Association of hemoglobin C with erythrocyte ghosts. *J. Clin. Invest.* 70: 946–952.

Rhoda, MD, Apovo, M, Beuzard, Y et al. (1990). Ca^{2+} permeability in deoxygenated sickle cells. *Blood* 75: 2453–2458.

Rifai, N, Sakamoto, M, Law, T et al. (1995). HPLC measurement, blood distribution, and pharmacokinetics of oral clotrimazole, potentially useful antisickling agent. *Clin. Chem.* 41: 387–391.

Rifkind, JM, Abugo, O, Levy, A et al. (1994). Detection, formation, and relevance of hemichromes and hemochromes. *Methods Enzymol.* 231: 449–480.

Rivera, A and Brugnara, C. (1998). Normal and sickle erythrocytes express an endothelin-1 receptor which is functionally coupled to the Gardos' channel: A new potential pathway for red blood cell dehydration. *Blood* 92: 13a.

Rivera, A, Rotter, A, and Brugnara, C. (1999). Endothelins activate Ca^{2+}-gated K^+ channels via endothelin B receptors in CD-1 mouse erythrocytes. *Am. J. Physiol. (Cell Physiol 46)* 227: C746–C754.

Rubin, E, Schlegel, RA, and Williamson, P. (1986). Endocytosis in sickle erythrocytes: A mechanism for elevated intracellular Ca^{2+} levels. *J. Cell. Physiol.* 126: 53–59.

Rybicki, AC and Benjamin, LJ. (1998). Increased levels of endothelin-1 in plasma of sickle cell anemia patients [letter]. *Blood* 92: 2594–2596.

Schlegel, RA, Prendergast, TW, and Williamson, P. (1985). Membrane phospholipid asymmetry as a factor in erythrocyte-endothelial cell interactions. *J. Cell. Physiol.* 123: 215–218.

Schlegel, RA and Williamson, P. (1987). Membrane phospholipid organization as a determinant of blood cell-reticuloendothelial cell interactions. *J. Cell. Physiol.* 132: 381–384.

Schlüter, K and Drenckhahn, D. (1986). Co-clustering of denatured hemoglobin with band 3: Its role in binding of autoantibodies against band 3 to abnormal and aged erythrocytes. *Proc. Natl. Acad. Sci. U.S.A.* 83: 6137–6141.

Schwartz, RS, Musto, S, Fabry, ME et al. (1998). Two distinct pathways mediate the formation of intermediate density cells and hyperdense cells from normal density sickle red blood cells. *Blood* 92: 4844–4855.

Schwartz, RS, Rybicki, AC, Heath, RH et al. (1987). Protein 4.1 in sickle erythrocytes: evidence for oxidative damage. *J. Biol. Chem.* 262: 15666–15672.

Schwartz, RS, Tanaka, Y, Fidler, IJ et al. (1985). Increased adherence of sickled and phosphatidylserine-enriched human erythrocytes to cultured human peripheral blood monocytes. *J. Clin. Invest.* 75: 1965–1972.

Shaklai, N, Frayman, B, Fortier, N et al. (1987). Crosslinking of isolated cytoskeletal proteins with hemoglobin: A possible damage inflicted to the red cell membrane. *Biochim. Biophys. Acta* 915: 406–414.

Shaklai, N, Sharma, VS, and Ranney, HM. (1981). Interaction of sickle cell hemoglobin with the erythrocyte membrane. *Biochemistry* 78: 65–68.

Shalev, O and Hebbel, RP. (1996). Catalysis of soluble hemoglobin oxidation by free iron on sickle red cell membranes. *Blood* 87: 3948–3952.

Shalev, O and Hebbel, RP. (1996b). Extremely high avidity association of Fe(III) with the sickle red cell membrane. *Blood* 88: 349–352.

Shalev, O, Repka, T, Goldfarb, A et al. (1995). Deferiprone (L1) chelates pathologic iron deposits from membranes of intact thalassemic and sickle red blood cells both in vitro and in vivo. *Blood* 86: 2008–2013.

Shartava, A, Monteiro, CA, Bencsath, FA et al. (1995). A posttranslational modification of β-actin contributes to the slow dissociation of the spectrin-protein 4.1-actin

complex of irreversibly sickled cells. *J. Cell. Biol.* 128: 508–818.

Sheerin, HE, Snyder, LM, and Fairbanks, G. (1989). Cation transport in oxidant-stressed human erythrocytes: heightened N-ethylmaleimide activation of passive K+ influx after mild peroxidation. *Biochim. Biophys. Acta* 983: 67–76.

Shinar, E and Rachmilewitz EA. (1990). Oxidative denaturation of red blood cells in thalassemia. *Semin. Hematol.* 27: 70–82.

Stout, JG, Zhou, Q, Wiedmer, T et al. (1998). Change in conformation of plasma membrane phospholipid scramblase induced by occupancy of its Ca^{2+} binding site. *Biochemistry* 37: 14860–14866.

Stuart, J, Mojiminiyi, FB, Stone, PC et al. (1994). Additive in vitro effects of anti-sickling drugs. *Br. J. Haematol.* 86: 820–823.

Sugihara, T and Hebbel, RP. (1992). Exaggerated cation leak from oxygenated sickle red blood cells during deformation: Evidence for a unique leak pathway. *Blood* 80: 2374–2378.

Sugihara, T, Rawicz, W, Evans, EA et al. (1991). Lipid hydroperoxides permit deformation-dependent leak of monovalent cation from erythrocytes. *Blood* 77: 2757–2763.

Sugihara, T, Repka, T, and Hebbel, RP. (1992). Detection, characterization, and bioavailability of membrane-associated iron in the intact sickle red cell. *J. Clin. Invest.* 90: 2327–2332.

Sugihara, T, Yawata, Y, and Hebbel, RP. (1994). Deformation of swollen erythrocytes provides a model of sickling-induced leak pathways, including a novel bromide-sensitive component. *Blood* 83: 2684–2691.

Sunshine, HR, Hofrichter, J, and Eaton, WA. (1978). Requirements for therapeutic inhibition of sickle hemoglobin gelation. *Nature* 275: 238–240.

Tait, JF and Gibson, D. (1994). Measurement of membrane phospholipid asymmetry in normal and sickle-cell erythrocytes by means of annexin V binding. *J. Lab. Clin. Med.* 123: 741–748.

Tanaka, Y and Schroit, AJ. (1983). Insertion of fluorescent phosphatidylserine into the plasma membrane of red blood cells: recognition by autologous macrophages. *J. Biol. Chem.* 258: 11335–11343.

Test, ST and Mitsuyoshi, J. (1997). Activation of the alternative pathway of complement by calcium-loaded erythrocytes resulting from loss of membrane phospholipid asymmetry. *J. Lab. Clin. Med.* 130: 169–182.

Test, ST and Woolworth, VS. (1994). Defective regulation of complement by the sickle erythrocyte: Evidence for a defect in control of membrane attack complex formation. *Blood* 83: 842–852.

Tiffert, T, Spivak, JL, and Lew, VL. (1988). Magnitude of calcium influx required to induce dehydration of normal human red cells. *Biochim. Biophys. Acta.* 943: 157–165.

Tomasko, MA and Chudwin, DS. (1988). Complement activation in sickle cell disease: A liposome model. *J. Lab. Clin. Med.* 112: 248–253.

Tosteson, DC. (1955). The effects of sickling on ion transport. II. The effect of sickling on sodium and cesium transport. *J. Gen. Physiol.* 39: 55–67.

Tosteson, DC, Carlsen, E, and Dunham, ET. (1955). The effects of sickling on ion transport. I. Effect of sickling on potassium transport. *J. Gen. Physiol.* 39: 31–53.

Tosteson, DC and Hoffman, JF. (1960). Regulation of cell volume by active cation transport in high and low potassium sheep red cells. *J. Gen. Physiol.* 44: 169–194.

Tosteson, DC, Shea, E, and Darling, RC. (1952). Potassium and sodium of red blood cells in sickle cell anemia. *J. Clin. Invest.* 31: 406–411.

Trudel, M, De Paepe, ME, Chretien, N et al. (1994). Sickle cell disease of transgenic SAD mice. *Blood* 84: 3189–3197.

Trudel, M, Saadane, N, Garel, MC et al. (1991). Toward a transgenic mouse model of sickle cell disease: hemoglobin SAD. *EMBO J.* 11: 3157–3165.

Vandorpe, DH, Shmukler, BE, Jiang, L et al. (1998). cDNA cloning and functional characterization of the mouse Ca2+-gated K+ channel, mIK1. Roles in regulatory volume decrease and erythroid differentiation. *J. Biol. Chem.* 273: 21542–21553.

Vitoux, D, Olivieri, O, Garay, RP et al. (1989). Inhibition of K+ efflux and dehydration of sickle cells by [(dihydroindenyl)oxy]alkanoic acid: An inhibitor of the K+ Cl-cotransport system. *Proc. Natl. Acad. Sci. U.S.A.* 86: 4273–4276.

Walder, JA, Chatterjee, R, Steck, TL et al. (1984). The interaction of hemoglobin with the cytoplasmic domain of band 3 of the human erythrocyte membrane. *J. Biol. Chem.* 259: 10238–10246.

Wali, RK, Jaffe, S, Kumar, D et al. (1987). Increased adherence of oxidant-treated human and bovine erythrocytes to cultured endothelial cells. *J. Cell. Physiol.* 133: 25–36.

Wang, RH, Philipps, G, Medof, ME et al. (1993). Activation of the alternative complement pathway by exposure of phosphatidylethanolamine and phosphatidylserine on erythrocytes from sickle cell disease patients. *J. Clin. Invest.* 92: 1326–1335.

Waugh, SM and Low, PS. (1985). Hemichrome binding to band 3: Nucleation of Heinz bodies on the erythrocyte membrane. *Biochemistry* 24: 34–39.

Waugh, SM, Walder, JA, and Low, PS. (1987). Partial characterization of the copolymerization reaction of erythrocyte membrane band 3 with hemichromes. *Biochemistry* 26: 1777–1783.

Waugh, SM, Willardson, BM, Kannan, R et al. (1986). Heinz bodies induce clustering of band 3, glycophorin, and ankyrin in sickle cell erythrocytes. *J. Clin. Invest.* 78: 1155–1160.

Werdehoff, SG, Moore, RB, Hoff, CJ et al. (1998). Elevated plasma endothelin-1 levels in sickle cell anemia: Relationships to oxygen saturation and left ventricular hypertrophy. *Am. J. Hematol.* 58: 195–199.

Wettersroem, N, Brewer, GJ, Warth, JA et al. (1984). Relationship of glutathione levels and Heinz body formation to irreversibly sickled cells in sickle cell anemia. *J. Lab. Clin. Med.* 103: 589–596.

Williamson, P, Puchulu, E, Penniston, JT et al. (1992). Ca2+ accumulation and loss by aberrant endocytic vesicles in sickle erythrocytes. *J. Cell. Physiol.* 152: 1–9.

Wolff, D, Cecchi, X, Spalvins, A et al. (1988). Charybdotoxin blocks with high affinity the Ca-activated K+ channel of Hb A and Hb S red cells: Individual differences in the number of channels. *J. Membr. Biol.* 106: 243–252.

Yasin, Z, Nemeth, TA, Joiner, CH et al. (1998). Phosphatidylserine (PS) externalization in dense sickle cells is not completely prevented by the presence of Hb F. *Blood* 92: 328a.

Yuan, J, Kannan, R, Shinar, E et al. (1992). Isolation, characterization, and immunoprecipitation studies of immune complexes from membranes of beta-thalassemic erythrocytes. *Blood* 79: 3007–3013.

Zhao, J, Zhou, Q, Wiedmer, T et al. (1998). Level of expression of phospholipid scramblase regulates induced movement of phosphatidylserine to the cell surface. *J. Biol. Chem.* 273: 6603–6606.

Zhou, Q, Zhao, J, Stout, JG et al. (1997). Molecular cloning of human plasma membrane phospholipid scramblase: A protein mediating transbilayer movement of plasma membrane phospholipids. *J. Biol. Chem.* 272: 18240–18244.

Zwaal, R. (1978). Membrane and lipid involvement in blood coagulation. *Biochim. Biophys. Acta* 515: 163–205.

Zwaal, RFA, Comfurius, P, and van Deenen, LLM. (1977). Membrane asymmetry and blood coagulation. *Nature* 268: 358–360.

Zwaal, RFA and Schroit, AJ. (1997). Pathophysiologic implications of membrane phospholipid asymmetry in blood cells. *Blood* 89: 1121–1132.

23

Polymer Structure and Polymerization of Deoxyhemoglobin S

FRANK FERRONE
RONALD L. NAGEL

Sickle cell disease originates from a dramatic interplay between structure and function and between thermodynamics and kinetics. A mechanical property, the stiffness of the fiber array formed by deoxyhemoglobin S (deoxyHbS) can have dramatically different consequences depending on the rate of its formation. Of course, the disease is also influenced greatly by the pleiotropic effects stemming from this primary event (Chapters 20 through 22). The pathophysiology of sickle cell disease proceeds from the single site mutation of Glu to Val at position 6 of the β-globin chain. In dilute solution this mutation is largely without consequence, as HbS and HbA display equivalent oxygen-binding thermodynamics (Allen and Wyman, 1954; Gill et al., 1979), response to affinity modifiers (Bunn, 1972), and ligand-binding kinetics (Pennelly and Noble, 1978). Solution structural modifications are limited to subtle effects in the central cavity of the β-globin chains (Hirsch et al., 1999).

This chapter concentrates on the primary event of sickle cell disease: the polymerization of deoxy HbS and its immediate consequences. Before embarking on a detailed description of the various components of this phenomenon, an overview of these intimately linked features is useful.

Consider a sickle red cell in transit through the microcirculation. The cell is densely packed with hemoglobin, so that collisions are frequent between these molecules. As the sickle red cell enters the microcirculation, or perhaps just before, the ambient oxygen tension begins to decrease. As it does, oxygen transport begins to create molecules of deoxyhemoglobin. Because of hemoglobin's cooperative oxygen binding, the dominant tetrameric molecules in the cellular mix will be those carrying four oxygen molecules or no oxygen molecules, with few intermediates.

The deoxygenated molecules abruptly make a small but fatal switch in the packing of the subunits, changing the hemoglobin molecules' quaternary structure. In its new arrangement, the tetrameric molecules, in their inevitable collisions, begin to adhere to each other momentarily. A chance meeting of one or two is still evanescent, but as the size of the cluster grows, the likelihood of falling apart diminishes, until some size—perhaps also a particular structure—is reached at which such a randomly formed cluster is more likely to add members than to lose them. The cluster, now called a homogeneous nucleus, rapidly grows a structured polymer, comprising seven pairs of elementary fibers. Thanks to the structural change that has occurred in the hemoglobin molecule, the hydrophobic mutation site, β6 Val, finds a properly registered hydrophobic receptor in another molecule along the Wishner-Love double strand (see below).

Not all the β6 valines are involved in the stabilization of the polymer, and some of the mutant valines that are not occupied in internal contacts appear at the polymer surface, where they participate in a different type of polymerization. As clusters form and disappear, as described previously, some develop at the surface of the polymer. The extra adhesion provided by the valines at the surface of the fiber endows the nuclear clusters formed there with extra stability, and, as a result, the polymer surface begins to nucleate new fibers. This is called heterogeneous nucleation. In this fashion, an entire network or domain of polymers begins and spreads through the red cell. The fibers themselves bend as they propagate so that the domain widens as it grows, away from the mother fiber, and would completely fan into a radial or spherulitic geometry given enough time and deoxyHbS. If the concentration of hemoglobin in the red cell is high enough, additional homogeneous nuclei may form and develop their own polymer domains.

Fibers within the domain are stable, which makes the array more like a solid than even a highly viscous liquid, and threatens the ability of the red cell to deform while transversing the microcirculation. However, if transit is successful, the return to the lungs is

Martin H. Steinberg, Bernard G. Forget, Douglas R. Higgs, and Ronald L. Nagel, editors. *Disorders of Hemoglobin: Genetics, Pathophysiology, and Clinical Management.* © 2001 Cambridge University Press. All rights reserved.

accompanied by an influx of oxygen and the melting of the polymers back to their monomeric state.

STRUCTURE

The pathophysiology of sickle hemoglobin arises from its ability to form fibers on deoxygenation. The atomic structure of the fibers has not been directly determined but has been inferred from a related crystal structure. Crystals of deoxyHbS contain a planar double strand known as the Wishner-Love structure, which is the assembly unit of the sickle hemoglobin fiber. This has been established by experiments using binary mixtures of HbS and hemoglobin mutants. The overall structure of the polymer has been derived by modeling, based on (1) the crystal structure of a double strand, (2) electron microscopy and image reconstruction of the fiber, (3) model building to conform to the results of (1) and (2), and finally, (4) further mutant analysis to confirm the existence of the putative intradouble strand and interdouble strand contacts in the fiber.

Observations

When deoxy sickle hemoglobin is crystallized, a planar double-stranded structure is formed, with molecules of HbS in each strand offset by a half-stagger relative to the other strand (Wishner et al., 1975). This structure has been studied by x-ray crystallography (Harrington et al., 1997; Padlan and Love, 1985a;

Wishner et al., 1975) with 2.0 Å resolution achieved at present. Higher levels of aggregates have not been successfully reduced to atomic detail other than by model building. In solutions of concentrated HbS, larger fibers of roughly 20 nm diameter are formed, which comprise 14 molecules in cross section (Dykes et al., 1979) (Fig. 23.1). Although the 14-stranded fiber is the smallest fibrillar structure seen in solutions, higher aggregates known as fascicles and macrofibers are also seen (Wellems et al., 1981). Fascicles are bundles of 14-stranded fibers, whereas macrofibers may be collections of twisted strands that are not decomposed solely into 14 strands (because the macrofibers are not multiples of 14) (Fig. 23.2). The proportions of each structure are sensitive to the pH at which the polymerization occurs, with macrofibers and fascicles favored at lower pH (Wellems et al., 1981).

Figure 23.1. (A) Electron micrograph of a fiber. The pitch of the fiber is not fixed, but varies as indicated by the different distances between the minimum diameter points (Bluemke et al., 1988). (B) Fiber model with double strands. The model is built according to the description of Watowich et al. (1989). This 14-strand model (whose end is shown in the inset) was first proposed by Dykes et al. (1978) and is now universally accepted as the basic fiber description. Note the double strands that are a basic structural element of the fiber and are based on a structure determined by crystallography (see Fig. 23.4). The wrapping of the 14 strands leads to a structure that gently varies from narrow to wide along the fiber.

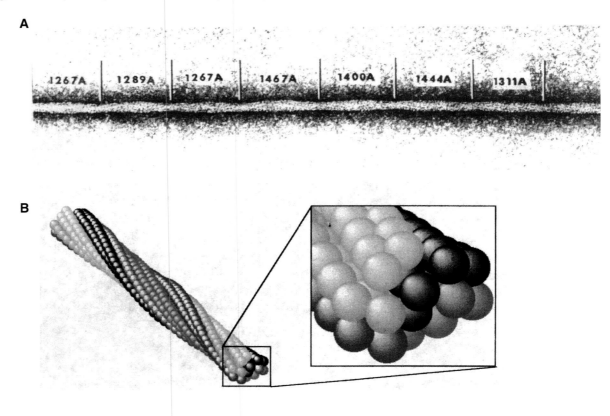

A

1267A   1289A   1267A   1467A   1400A   1444A   1311A

B

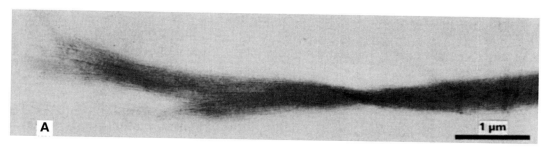

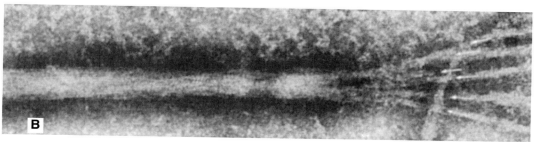

Figure 23.2. Sickle hemoglobin assembly creates structures larger than the fibers shown in Fig. 23.1. (A) Fibers can associate in bundles or fascicles (McDade et al., 1989). Fascicles ultimately form into crystals. The fascicle shown here has a twist, which also appears in crystals. (B) A macrofiber with six fibers extending from the end. Macrofibers are comprised of double strands in antiparallel rows, and such structures appear at low pH (below 6.7 in 0.05 mol/L phosphate buffer). This macrofiber is from the unpublished work of Wellems and Josephs (McDade and Josephs, 1993).

When thin samples are viewed between crossed polarizers on a microscope, the resulting birefringence reveals that polymers will form aligned regions. This alignment is unlike most fibrillar assemblies; it is not the consequence of an alignment transition but a result of the peculiar way in which fibers are formed (see later). Birefringence patterns often show a distinct Maltese cross (Fig. 23.3), which on first inspection appears to signify radial symmetry, as if all fibers came from a common center. On closer study, the fully symmetric crosses are the exception rather than the rule, and time-resolved experiments reveal that these regions initially possess bow-tie geometries, rather than being true spherulites (Basak et al., 1988). The structure producing these areas of alignment flanking an unaligned center is known as a polymer domain. As domains age, they become increasingly spherulitic with the polymers added last possessing the greatest alignment.

Structural Elements

Determining polymer structure for hemoglobin has proved particularly difficult because gelation occurs at high concentrations, complicating the isolation of fibers. Although the structure of the fiber has been described at various times as a hollow tubule or a 16-stranded fiber, the accepted model is now agreed to be a 14-stranded, filled structure, initially identified by Dykes et al. (1978). This fiber is helical and on average 210 Å thick, with an elliptical cross section that leads to a periodic oscillation in the fiber diameter. Modeling is difficult owing to the large number of particles in the cross section, which not only produces complicated patterns, but also diminishes the intensity of any piece of a typical transform. Fiber features are now well established and modeling has proposed atomic contacts within the fiber (Watowich et al., 1989). The atomic scale detail within the fiber is not unambiguous at this time; for example, the precise scale of the separation of the particles in the fiber is still a matter of some dispute (Cretegny and Edelstein, 1993; Watowich et al., 1993) as are certain aspects of the modeling procedure (Mu et al., 1998). An important feature to emerge from the analysis is that the fiber pitch is not fixed, but variable (Fig. 23.1), which will blur straightforward attempts to produce a refined image by correlation. Josephs' group has shown that it can be used for resolution enhancement (Bluemke et al., 1988; Carragher et al., 1988). The proposal that the Wishner-Love double strands were constituents of the 14-stranded structure was strengthened by the observation that some fiber variants were missing external fiber pairs (Dykes et al., 1979). (The mutant Hb Sealy moreover appeared to have a larger structure in which internal pairs are absent (Crepeau et al., 1981). However, the strongest evidence that Wishner-Love double strands make up the polymer came from a set of studies on mutant hemoglobins.

Validation of the Double Strand as a Constituent of the Fiber. The first observation relevant to this issue

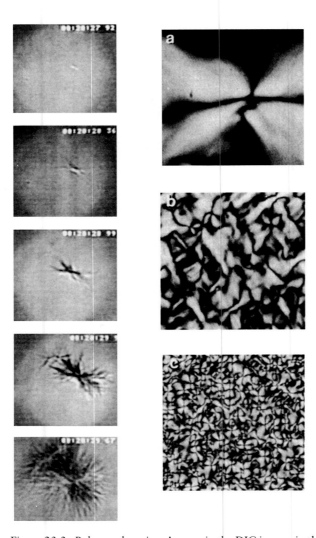

Figure 23.3. Polymer domains. As seen in the DIC images in the left sequence of panels, polymerization produces fibers in attached arrays called domains. In these pictures (Briehl, 1995) laser photolysis (as evidenced by the light-colored circles, of approximately 15 μm diameter) creates deoxyHb, which generates fibers. The attached fibers form twofold symmetric patterns that spread to form larger structures with nearly radial symmetry. These patterns are also visible in birefringence seen as transmission of light when the sample is placed between crossed polarizers and is shown in panels a through c on the right. Each cross or bow-tie defines a polymer domain. Each domain is formed from a single homogeneous nucleation event. The size of the polymer domains is inversely related to the speed of their formation, and speed of formation in turn is related to concentration. The concentrations were 23.4 g/dL, 25.7 g/dL and 27.4 g/dL, respectively. Samples were gelled by temperature jump from 3°C to 23°C (Christoph et al., 1990).

was the discovery of HbC Harlem (Bookchin et al., 1967), a doubly mutated β chain, the sickle mutation and a second mutation that reduced its sickling properties. This observation demonstrated that an additional single amino acid substitution could drastically affect polymerization.

A critical series of experiments that established the identification of the double strands as assembly units of the sickle fiber (Nagel et al., 1980) involved the use of naturally occurring mutants in hybridized copolymerization experiments (binary mixtures), first involving β-globin chain mutants (Bookchin et al., 1970; Nagel and Bookchin, 1975, 1978; Nagel et al., 1980) and later extending to α-globin chain mutants (Benesch et al., 1980).

Underlying these experiments was the idea that hemoglobins with surface mutations but generally without functional abnormalities could be mixed with HbS to establish if they affected polymerization. Because the liganded hemoglobin tetramer will readily split into dimer pairs, the mixture of the hemoglobins would form hybrids and the pure species, according to binomial statistics. The propensity for gelation of the mixtures could be compared with mixtures of HbA and HbS. The use of A/S as a reference was based on experiments described later showing that copolymerization does occur. Of thirty-two β-globin chain variants, eight occur at intermolecular contact sites and all of them affect polymerization. Of the remaining twenty-four variants that do not arise at intermolecular contact sites in the double strand, twenty do not affect polymerization. In addition, it appears that two of the four variants not at intermolecular contact points are adjacent to contacts, and two others occur in the dimer interface, which has been hypothesized as an effect that could alter the copolymerization and thus confound analysis of those particular results. However, the existence of nondouble strand contacts that affect polymerization could arise from particular interactions between double strands and is not as problematic as might first appear. Thus, the mutant studies have predominantly confirmed the double strand hypothesis.

Gelation studies (with a screening method) of deoxygenated binary mixtures of HbS and mutant hemoglobins mentioned before and the extension of this work to the α-globin chains have provided valuable information (Eaton and Hofrichter, 1990) but have not defined the location of all intermolecular contact sites in the HbS polymer because of inherent limitations of experiments based on mixtures of HbS and natural mutants. First, unless the mutation is one of the few that are *cis* to the β^S mutation, the mixtures report only the effect of *trans* mutations (that is, in the β chain not involved in the β6 contact site). Second, the natural mutations provided a restricted repertoire of sites to explore. Third, one needs to assess the possible effects of substitutions on conformation, because the perturbation of a single point mutation could propagate to other regions of the molecule. Fourth, the mutation could involve a substitution that, because of chain length, hydrophobicity, or electrostatic interactions, may not be a good reporter for a particular contact site. The best situation is to have several amino acid substitutions of the same site. Also, if a screening method such as the minimum gelling concentration popular in the 1970s is used to assess gelation, kinetics abnormalities derived from the formation of hybrid tetramers could interfere with the results, particularly if the dimer/dimer interaction is anomalous. Anomalously slow gelation kinetics can affect a scanning method such as minimum gelling concentration, so site-directed mutagenesis, coupled with functional and structural studies of the mutants and an equilibrium method of assessing polymerization (solubility of the deoxy polymer, or c_{Sat}), can provide a greater repertoire of sites and substitutions and more accurate data.

Types of Contacts Within the Fiber

There are two general categories of contacts: those within the double strand and those of the double strands within the fiber. The contacts within the double strand are most precisely determined thanks to the x-ray crystallography. The zigzag nature of the double strand (half stagger) leads to a distinction between the lateral contacts (between adjacent members of the double strand, related by a diagonal displacement) and axial contacts (along an individual strand, related by a vertical displacement). Tables 23.1 and 23.2 list the contacts in the 2 Å resolution double strand structure of Harrington (1997).

The lateral contacts have the most prominence because the mutant β6 appears in one of them and is thus a crucial feature in the polymerization process. (Fig. 23.4) This contact involves burying the β6 in a hydrophobic pocket formed by Leu β88, Phe β85, and several heme atoms. Within the hydrophobic pocket, although the val β6 is buried, it is not fully in van der Waals contacts with the receptor pocket, and this permits a network of water molecules to be located in the contact region and to form bridging hydrogen bonds between the tetramers (Harrington et al., 1997). That the packing of the subunits is not snugly complementary, but allows water, suggests that the variation in pitch may arise as a varying compromise between close packing in the various contact areas.

Table 23.1. Double Strand Lateral Contacts Within 4.0Å Distances in Å

β1	β2									α2	
	Thr4	Pro5	Val6	Ser9	Ala10	Ala13	Lys17	Pro125	Val126	Ser49	His50
Lys66		3.61									
		3.65									
Gly69		3.89									
		3.96									
Ala70		3.83									
		3.88									
Asp73	3.11		3.10								
	3.01		3.92								
Asp79										3.46	2.83
Asn80										3.48	2.88
											3.65
Gly83											3.73
								3.99			
Thr84			3.62					4.10			
Phe85			3.72								
			3.95								
			4.10								
Thr87					4.43	3.65			5.98		
					3.75	4.63			3.83		
Leu88				3.50							
				3.36							
Glu90							5.03				
Lys95							3.49				
							3.93				
							5.78				

Table 23.2. Double Strand Axial Contacts (One Contact within 4.0Å Distances in Å)

	α2					β2			
	Lys16	His20	Glu116	Pro114	Ala115	His116	His117	Phe118	Lys120
α1									
Pro114	3.36 5.85		3.71 3.92						
Ala115	4.81 3.74								
β2									
Gly16									3.08 3.46
Lys17						6.12 3.42	2.86 3.42	3.76 3.91	
Val18									3.21 2.93
Glu22		3.55 4.85							
His117				3.36 3.47	3.37 3.26				
Phe118				3.92 3.55	3.82 3.69				
Gly119					3.78 3.63				
Glu121				3.71 3.79					

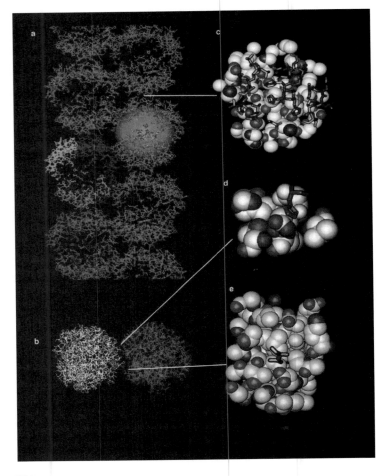

Figure 23.4. (a) The double strand of deoxyHbS, based on the crystal structure of Harrington et al. (1997). The tetramers of HbS have been drawn with the central region excluded for clarity; one tetramer illustrates the exclusion region as a solid green sphere in the center of the molecule. Another tetramer is shown with the four subunits colored differently to differentiate them. Red and purple are β-globin chains; blue and orange are α-globin chains. Contacts along the axis of the double strand (vertical here) are denoted as axial, whereas those that connect diagonally are denoted as lateral. The β6 mutation site is in a lateral contact. Note that both the axial and the lateral contacts are dominated by interactions between the beta chains. (b) An end view of the double strand. The two molecules, with all amino acids now showing, are colored differently to aid the eye. The β6 contact is shown on the bottom (expanded view in (E)), and the salt bridge between αHis50 and βAsp79 is above (expanded view in (d)). (c). The axial contact region in A has been enlarged to allow a better view. Unlike the lateral contact, no single amino acid dominates the geometry. Carbon atoms that are filled to van der Waals radii are yellow, oxygen atoms are red, and nitrogen atoms are blue. (d) The salt bridge between Asp β79 and His α50 in the lateral contact area viewed from the α-globin chain. The His is shown as a green licorice stick drawing in the foreground. (e) The lateral contact region showing the β6 Val (green stick figure, foreground) in the receptor pocket on its complementary chain. (Note that in the crystal there are two distinct such regions.) β88Leu is just forward and above Val; β85Phe is then just below β88 Leu and behind the Val. For full color reproduction, see color plate 23.4.

Axial contacts are dominated by nonpolar contacts between Pro α114 and Ala α115, with His β116, His β117, and Phe β118 (Fig. 23.4). The complementary of these regions involves a far less pronounced bulge and cavity than that seen in the β6 lateral contact. Water is seen again in this interface. Josephs and co-workers have argued that the lowered density of axial contacts at larger fiber diameters limits the fiber size; this presupposes an energetically significant role for the axial contacts (Watowich et al., 1993).

Two salt bridges also appear (cf. Fig 23.4). One is in the lateral contacts, between Asp β79 and His α50. The position of this interaction in the lateral contact at a distance from the β6 interaction restricts what would be a freer rotation of the β6-carrying molecule about the interaction region. In the axial contacts, a salt bridge is found between Glu β22 and His α20. The pH dependence of the polymerization is most likely a consequence of these two His interactions, with possibly offsetting effects from the axial histidines that interact repulsively with Lys 70.

The arrangement of the double strands within the 14-stranded polymer remains the province of model building because atomic structures are lacking. This model building in turn entails the adoption of an accepted 14-strand template from electron microscopy. Within the constraints that any model must exhibit a cross section consistent with the template, the strands can be adjusted to achieve some second target, such as maximal numbers of contacts without steric clash, or maximum agreement with mutant and hybrid studies. The Chicago group (Josephs) (Watowich et al., 1993) and the Geneva group (Edelstein) (Cretegny and Edelstein, 1993) do not agree on the correct density of the template; the Chicago group argues for a less dense cross section to avoid clash. Both models have been criticized based on the failure to retain in the fiber the exact spacing and relative orientation of the molecules in the crystal (Mu et al., 1998).

The Chicago group has produced the most detailed model (Watowich et al., 1989), which has been tested against mutations in a manner similar to that validating the double strand as a fiber constituent. The Watowich-Josephs model has considerable internal space, which is taken up by water. Such regions prevent the unfavorable contacts between strands. In particular only one β6 Val is involved in an intermolecular contact, with the other β6 either solvated within the polymer or facing outward into solution.

However, on further examination, it appears that two of the fourteen molecules in a fiber cross section may utilize *both* β6 contacts within the polymer (Roufberg and Ferrone, in press), although Val in the second contact is slightly displaced from the equivalent position in the primary contact. Such a structure is capable of quantitatively rationalizing the copolymer-

ization studies on HbA-HbS hybrids, which remained problematic within the Watowich-Josephs model, and are discussed in the following sections on thermodynamics. Since only some molecules use both β6 contacts, the many mutant studies would not have readily revealed the presence of the additional sites. One way this might have been revealed is through the identification of mutants that affect polymerization without ostensible contact sites in the Watowich-Josephs model. Very few mutants lack a structural explanation, and of the four known, only one (Hb Sarawa, α6 Asp → Ala) cannot be justified as adjacent to a known contact site. However, this mutant is known to lack hydrogen bonds and thereby loosen the deoxy quaternary structure. In such a case, it is plausible that the more flexible molecule allows the second β6 contacts to be optimized.

Model of the Heterogeneous Nucleus

Besides the fundamental contacts responsible for stabilizing the polymer, another type of contact must be considered. As described previously, and noted in more detail later, the fiber formation process involves the growth of new fibers onto old ones. This process also involves atomic contacts, which have only recently been hypothesized. A survey of the 14-strand polymer surface reveals that four molecules present a β6 mutation site at the polymer surface (Mirchev and Ferrone, 1997). It thus becomes plausible that the same contact partners that appear in the fiber appear on its surface and account for the promotion of new fiber formation on an existing fiber surface. Equally important, the structure of the gel appears to involve cross-links, rather than simply the steric hindrance between solid but featureless fibers.

THERMODYNAMICS

Observations

Polymer formation in sickle hemoglobin creates a mixture of polymers and monomers whose concentration is solely a function of the thermodynamic state of the system, and not of the initial concentration. This final monomer concentration is known as c_{sat} or the solubility, c_s. In contrast, the concentration of hemoglobin in polymers depends on the initial concentration minus the solubility. The solubility is now routinely determined by centrifugation (typically at 140,000 g for 2 hours) of a monomer-polymer mixture so that the polymers may physically be separated from the monomers whose concentration can be assayed spectrophotometrically (Hofrichter et al., 1976; Ross et al., 1977). An older method, the minimum gelling

Figure 23.5. Solubility (c_s or c_{sat}) of sickle hemoglobin in 0.15 mol/L phosphate buffer. (**A**) Temperature dependence of the solubility. Open symbols are measured by determining the concentration of the supernatant after sedimentation (Ross et al., 1977); filled symbols show the concentration determined by measurement of the rate of binding a trace of carbon monoxide, which is set by the concentration of monomers (Liao et al., 1996). (**B**) pH dependence of the solubility is shown measured at 37°C in near physiologic buffer (Poillon and Kim, 1990). The curve is drawn assuming two identical titratable groups per monomer, as found in the double strand structure. The pK of the groups is 7.24 from this curve, which agrees with their identification as histidines.

concentration (MGC), involved the progressive solvent evaporation of a sample to determine the concentration at which gel first formed. Although there are many problematic issues with such a method, the most severe is that polymerization begins with such an infinitesimal polymer formed that the criterion of no polymer is misleading unless unrealistically long times are permitted for equilibration to occur. A third method, which continues to be used with high phosphate buffers, is to conduct kinetic experiments at various initial concentrations and extrapolate the turbidity (typically observed at 700 nm) to zero to determine the minimum concentration (Adachi and Asakura, 1979). More recently, kinetic-based methods have been developed as well (Liao et al., 1996). Figure 23.5 shows the solubility for different temperatures and pH.

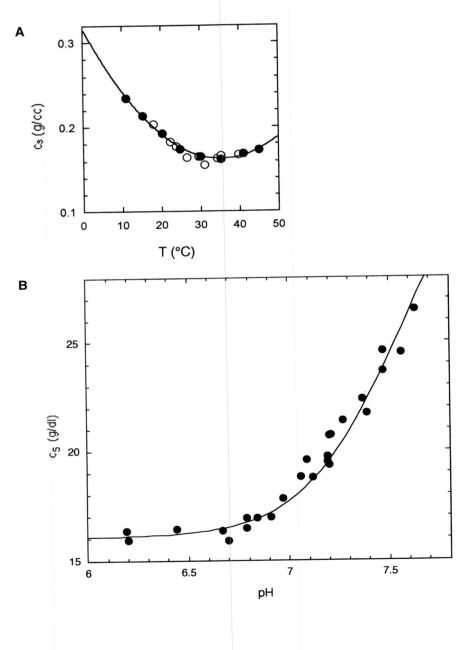

The polymer network that forms does not completely exclude monomers, and it is of interest to know the degree of exclusion and the extent to which monomers may be trapped in the polymer mass. Such issues make it quite difficult to assay the concentration of the packed polymers per se. One way to address this issue is to correlate the measured concentration in the pellet of a centrifuged sample with the monomer concentration of the solution phase. The assumption is that an increase in concentration in the pellet could be attributed to the increase in monomer concentration if the fraction of the gel available to monomers is fixed. This method was used by Sunshine et al. (1979), and from a data set with considerable scatter a value of 0.693 = 0.056 g/mL was deduced. Subsequently a more direct approach using radiolabeled tracers found a smaller value (0.547 ± 0.007) (Bookchin et al., 1994).

Three different types of experiments have probed the polymer network. The simplest involves centrifugation and measurement of the concentration of the pellet produced, as described previously. Another approach used osmotic stress to withdraw water through a permeable membrane and induce gelation and solution packing (Prouty et al., 1985). In a third approach, a small area of HbCO was photolyzed by a focused laser to produce deoxyHbS, which polymerized, and then allowed added hemoglobin to diffuse into the monomer-depleted region (Cho and Ferrone, 1991). This diffusion led to a concentration greater than that of the surroundings. In all these experiments, the maximum observed concentration is about 0.55 g/mL, similar to the concentration deduced by Bookchin as the gel concentration. Thus, there appears to be a question of the extent of trapped hemoglobin in the gel phase.

Both concentrations may be important indicators of different aspects of the gelation process. The polymer itself can have a higher concentration, with little variation, and a value close to that of the crystal. The polymer network can have a lower average concentration, with significant dispersion, based on its particular history. Calculations regarding the formation of the polymer itself require the concentration of that the polymer per se, whereas calculations of monomer interactions with a network or gel, for example, require the lower density value.

Framework for Understanding: The Two-Phase Model

The solubility is related to the equilibrium constant for polymer formation. To understand this equilibrium process more fundamentally, it is helpful to use a two-phase model in which the polymerization is treated analogously to a crystallization (Minton 1975, 1977).

In such a reaction, the chemical potential of monomers in solution, μ_s, is equated to that of monomers in the aggregated phase (crystal or polymer) denoted μ_p. Thus $\mu_s = \mu_p$ and then

$$\mu_s{}^o + RT \ln \gamma c = \mu_p{}^o \qquad (1)$$

Because the solution is crowded, the monomer concentration c is modified by activity coefficients, γ which are a function of c (see later). $\mu_s{}^o$ has contributions from translational and rotational entropy, calculated according to a standard classical statistical mechanics. $\mu_p{}^o$ is the sum of two terms. The first is the chemical potential involved in the contacts (μ_{PC}) by which monomers in the polymer adhere. For example, if the interaction holding monomers in the polymers came entirely from the buried hydrophobic surface of the Val β6, then the standard free energy for burying this residue would be the origin of μ_{PC}. Salt bridges similarly would be included. The second component of $\mu_p{}^o$ is the chemical potential from vibrational entropy, μ_{PV}. The vibrations in this case are those of the molecule about its center of mass while in the polymer. They arise from the width of the potential well in which an attached molecule of HbS finds itself; the broader the well, the greater freedom the molecule possesses to rattle around its mean position in the polymer. It is assumed that there have been no energetically significant internal changes as a result of polymerization. Rewriting equation 1 shows that the solubility is related to a series of chemical potentials:

$$RT \ln \gamma_s c_s = \mu_{PC} + \mu_{PV} - \mu_{ST} - \mu_{SR} \qquad (2)$$

It is worth considering the size of these terms individually. If 1 mol/L (tetramer) is taken as a standard state, then $\mu_{ST} = 19$ kcal/mol and $\mu_{SR} = 18$ kcal/mol, for a total of 37 kcal/mol. On the other hand, $RT \ln \gamma_s C_s = 1.4$ kcal/mol. A large cancellation must be present to overcome the large entropic cost of polymer formation. Fairly good estimates for these values can be obtained by analysis of kinetic experiments. For now, we observe that if the source of the stability of the polymer were entirely due to the burial of the hydrophobic Val β6, one could have as many as four sites (two donor and two acceptors) per HbS tetramer. (Of course, one probably has fewer, but also has salt bridge stabilization. The estimate here is only meant to be a rough one.) Using conventional values for the hydrophobic free energy would give μ_{PC} of about 4 × 1.5 kcal/mol, or about 6.0 kcal/mol of contact stabilization. This leaves almost 30 kcal/mol to be accounted for by vibrations of the monomers in the polymer lattice. Refinements in the nature of the contact energy will still only be a few kcal/mol and will not change the conclusion that the effects of the vibrational term on the polymer stability will be significant.

The enthalpic contributions to the solubility will all arise from μ_{PC}. The enthalpy of association has been determined by vant Hoff analysis of the equilibrium as well as by direct calorimetry (Eaton and Hofrichter, 1990; Ross et al., 1977). There is general but not total agreement. The vant Hoff analysis recaptures the almost linear dependence of the enthalpy on temperature, albeit with a somewhat greater slope. The cause of the discrepancy is not established and may be due to somewhat subtle effects such as nonideality contribution from the polymers.

Since the density of the polymer is less than that of the monomer, it must contain additional water. This is hardly surprising given the structural models of the polymer. This water is not associated in the usual sense, i.e., no bond is made with the polymer. It is, however, different from the remainder of the solution phase in that it contains no monomeric hemoglobin. It is this exclusion that entails a necessary correction for the water associated with polymer formation. The chemical potential accounting for this contribution of approximately 2500 water molecules can be derived using the Gibbs-Duhem equation (cf. Eaton and Hofrichter, 1990) and is given by the expression

$$\mu_w = -RT\int_0^{c_s} \frac{1/c_p - \upsilon}{1 - \upsilon c}\left(1 + \frac{\partial ln\gamma}{\partial ln c}\right)dc \qquad (3)$$

The origin of this effect in the non-ideality corrections is clearly seen by the appearance of the activity coefficient of the monomer (γ) as well as the monomer and polymer specific volumes, υ and ($1/c_p$) respectively. The effect is not large under conditions where c_s is small. For example, at 25°C, μ_w represents about a 5% effect on the free energy of association, and rises to approximately 15% at 10°C, where the solubility is considerably greater. For mixture experiments, where the solubility is larger, this correction is correspondingly more significant. It is also possible, of course, that some water could differ from bulk water, and thereby represent a physical change, which would need to be reckoned in the thermodynamics of assembly. This is a topic of current investigation (see for example, Hentschke and Herzfeld, 1991). It is also interesting that there is no net volume change on polymerization, (i.e., the redistribution of water accounts for no difference in the final volume) (Kahn and Briehl, 1982).

Nonideality

Because the solutions are so crowded, it is necessary to account for the activity of the molecules by multiplying their concentrations by activity coefficients, γ. When concentration is used as a measure of activity, it is assumed that the center-to-center distance accurately represents the likelihood of interaction. In a crowded solution, the edges of the molecules are much closer than their centers, and the likelihood of their interaction rises accordingly. From osmotic pressure data and weight-averaged molecular weight determined by centrifugation, it is possible to determine γ as a function of concentration (Fig. 23.6). These data are well described by a power series,

$$ln\gamma = \sum_{k+1}^6 B_{k+1}c^k \qquad (4)$$

where

$$B_2 = 8V$$
$$B_3 = 15\ V^2$$
$$B_4 = 24.48\ V^3$$
$$B_5 = 35.30\ V^4$$
$$B_6 = 47.4\ V^5$$
$$\text{and } B_7 = 65.9\ V^6$$

Here, V is the volume of a hard sphere and is determined to be 0.79 ± 0.02 cm^3/g, in excellent agreement with the partial specific volume of hemoglobin of 0.75 cm^3/g. (Other functional descriptions are also possible, as discussed by Minton [1998]). In a solution in which a nonpolymerizing species is present that can nonetheless take up significant volume, it is clear that the terms on the right-hand side of Equation 2 are still the same. Therefore c_s will decrease if γ increases. In the

Figure 23.6. Log of activity coefficient, γ, as a function of concentration, as given by Equation 4. Crowding of the solutions under close to physiologic conditions requires significant activity coefficients.

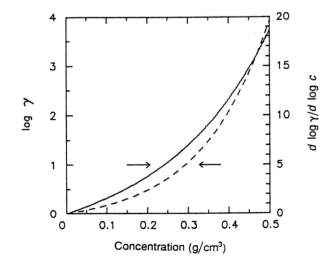

case of molecules with the same volume as hemoglobin that do not copolymerize, such as R-state hemoglobin or HbF, we can simply use Equation 4 for $\ln\gamma$ but use total concentration in the power series.

If a nonpolymerizing species of different volume but the same shape (roughly spherical) is used, it is possible to use scaled particle theory to calculate activities (cf. Minton, 1998). This is useful for explaining the effects of agents such as dextran that reduce the concentration of hemoglobin required for gelation (Bookchin et al., 1999). Theories that can be used for nonsimilar shapes are also known, as reviewed by Minton (1998).

When species copolymerize, the preceding treatment is modified. Because the hemoglobins all have the same volume, the same function for γ is used, but c in Equation 4 is the total hemoglobin concentration. The copolymerizing hemoglobin will have a new μ_{PC} and μ_{PV} (i.e., the contact energy and the potential well in which the contacts sit may both change). The change in these chemical potentials for the ith species are defined as:

$$\Delta\mu^i_P = \mu^i_{PC} + \mu^i_{PV} - (\mu^o_{PC} + \mu^o_{PV}) \qquad (5)$$

in which superscript zero designates the pure HbS polymer. Changes in the vibrational part are specifically included because this is affected by the degree of complementarity of the two sites, and thus changes that alter packing can also alter the vibrations. A copolymerization probability, customarily denoted as e_i can be written as

$$e_i = \exp(-\mu^i_P/RT). \qquad (6)$$

From these the mole fraction of species i in the polymer is

$$f_i = \frac{x_i e_i}{\sum_i x_i e_i} \qquad (7)$$

where x_i is the mole fraction of species i in the solution, and the new solubility becomes

$$\gamma_s C_s = \frac{\gamma^o_s c^o_s}{\sum_i x_i e_i} \qquad (8)$$

where again superscripts indicate the value for pure HbS. For a derivation of these equations the reader is referred to Minton (1975, 1977).

Sickle Hemoglobin Mixture Experiments

By using the preceding analytical tools, it is possible to study the results of hemoglobin mixture experiments. Four hemoglobins have been examined in mixtures with HbS: HbA, HbF, HbC, and HbA$_2$. There are three reasons for investigating the behavior of hemoglobin mixtures. First, the expression of HbS in vivo is often accompanied by the expression of other hemoglobins, and a most promising treatment involves increasing the expression of HbF. Second, gelation in the presence of oxygen necessarily involves species with different solubilities, and therefore necessarily involves understanding mixtures (besides its other facets). Third, analysis of mixture experiments permits inferences about the polymer structure.

A direct approach to determining the detailed polymer composition in a mixture experiment is technically not feasible, and thus the polymer composition must be inferred by using simple models with measurements of the solution phase of the system. This can be done two ways. One involves the measurement of the net solubility (i.e., all hemoglobin in the supernatant after centrifugation). The rise in solubility is the consequence of diminished copolymerization, and from Equation 8, a measurement of solubility can be translated into a copolymerization probability. A second type of experiment consists of determining the composition of the supernatant after gelation and centrifugation. Such compositional analysis has included radiolabeling (Behe and Englander, 1979; Bunn et al., 1982), amino acid analysis (Benesch et al., 1980), and electrophoresis (Benesch et al., 1980; Goldberg et al., 1977). Analyzing the pellet that will contain monomers and polymers after centrifugation of a gel is also possible, although far less common.

In any of the these methods, the results dramatically depend on the procedure used to prepare the mixtures, owing to the dissociation of hemoglobin into its two constituent dimers. Oxyhemoglobin readily dissociates ($K_D = 1$ μmol/L) into two $\alpha\beta$ pairs; deoxyhemoglobin has a dissociation constant about 10^6 lower. The characteristic times for reproportionation of mixtures are thus seconds for ligated species and 1 to 10 hours for deoxygenated hemoglobin. Accordingly, by mixing at least one hemoglobin in the deoxy form, experiments in which reproportionation of the constituent dimers has not occurred is possible. On the other hand, if liganded hemoglobins are mixed before deoxygenation, the outcome will be a mixture of hemoglobin species that include hybrid tetramers with one β^S and one nonsickle β chain and pure HbS and pure additive hemoglobin. A comprehensive review of copolymerization experiments has been compiled by Eaton and Hofrichter (1990) and analyzed for the copolymerization probabilities. That analysis is summarized next (Tables 23.3 and 23.4). The results for nonhybridizing and hybridizing experiments are discussed in turn.

Nonhybridizing mixtures have generally shown virtually no copolymerization within the errors of the

Table 23.3. Copolymerization Probabilities of Unhybridized Hemoglobin Mixtures*

	Determined by solubility	Determined by composition	
S + F		0.14 ± 0.10	Behe and Englander (1979)
	−0.01 ± 0.10	0.16 ± 0.12	Goldberg et al. (1977)
	−0.15 ± 0.10	−0.14 ± 0.10	Benesch et al. (1980)
		0.08 ± 0.10	Benesch et al. (1980)
Average	−0.08 ± 0.07	0.05 ± 0.05	
S + A		0.12 ± 0.10	Behe and Englander (1979)
	−0.05 ± 0.10	0.38 ± 0.22	Goldberg et al. (1977)
	−0.01 ± 0.10	0.20 ± 0.12	Benesch et al. (1980)
		0.24 ± 0.10	Benesch et al. (1980)
Average	−0.03 ± 0.07	0.20 ± 0.06	
S + A$_2$	−0.17 ± 0.12	−0.10 ± 0.13	Benesch et al. (1980)
		0.14 ± 0.10	Benesch et al. (1980)
Average	−0.17 ± 0.12	0.05 ± 0.08	

* Based on compilation by Eaton and Hofrichter (1990) modified to place a base uncertainty of 0.10 on all measurements. More than one entry is given for Benesch et al. (1980) who analyzed the composition of the polymer phase as well as the solution phase. Other entries reflect composition analysis of solution phase alone.

Table 23.4. Copolymerization Probabilities of Hybridized Hemoglobin Mixtures*

	Determined by solubility	Determined by composition	
S + F		0.11 ± 0.10	Behe and Englander (1979)
	0.00 ± 0.10	0.16 ± 0.12	Sunshine et al. (1979)
	0.00 ± 0.10	−0.14 ± 0.10	Sunshine et al. (1979)
	0.06 ± 0.10		Goldberg et al. (1977)
	0.03 ± 0.10		Sunshine et al. (1979)
	0.05 ± 0.10	0.44 ± 0.64	Benesch et al. (1980)
		0.34 ± 0.44	Benesch et al. (1980)
	0.15 ± 0.10		Benesch et al. (1980)
Average	0.05 ± 0.04	0.13 ± 0.10	
S + A		0.55 ± 0.10	Behe and Englander (1979)
	0.38 ± 0.10		Sunshine et al. (1979)
	0.27 ± 0.10		Goldberg et al. (1977)
	0.34 ± 0.10	0.38 ± 0.42	Benesch et al. (1980)
		0.66 ± 0.74	Benesch et al. (1980)
	0.35 ± 0.10	0.24 ± 0.10	Bunn et al. (1982)
	0.46 ± 0.21		Cheetham et al. (1979)
Average	0.34 ± 0.05	0.40 ± 0.07	
S + A$_2$	0.04 ± 0.10	0.26 ± 0.35	Benesch et al. (1980)
		0.43 ± 0.34	Benesch et al. (1980)
	0.07 ± 0.10		Cheetham et al. (1979)
Average	0.06 ± 0.07	0.35 ± 0.24	
S + C	0.40 ± 0.10		Bunn et al. (1982)
	0.40 ± 0.10	0.33 ± 0.11	Bunn et al. (1982)
	0.63 ± 0.24		Cheetham et al. (1979)
Average	0.42 ± 0.07	0.33 ± 0.11	

* Copolymerization calculated with the assumption (see Table 23.3) that the nonhybridized species does not copolymerize at all. More than one entry may be given for a given reference if the measurements were done at different temperatures or by different methods. In particular, Benesch et al. (1980) analyzed the composition of the polymer phase as well as the solution phase. Most entries reflect composition analysis of the solution phase alone. For further detail the reader is referred to Eaton and Hofrichter (1990) on whose analysis this table is based, with the added modification that the uncertainty in copolymerization probability is no less than 0.10.

measurements. For HbF and HbA$_2$, this is the case for both solubility and composition measurement, with small negative values that can be interpreted as equivalent to zero copolymerization. The similarities of the results obtained by the two approaches (solubility and composition) help to validate their conceptual basis, including the use of large activity coefficients. For HbA, solubility measurements also give small, nominally negative values (thus consistent with zero), whereas compositional analysis exhibited a 20 ± 6 percent copolymerization probability. (All averages cited have been error weighted, with the lowest error weight taken as 0.1. The rationale for averaging the results of different experiments is simply to arrive at a consensus among the many studies conducted, with error estimates to suggest the range of results.)

To analyze hybridized mixtures it is necessary to know the copolymerization probability for the unhybridized molecules and the distribution of species. The copolymerization probability follows from the results quoted previously, and the distribution can be assumed to be binomial. That is, if the fraction of non-HbS molecules in the initial mixture is X, then there will be X^2 non-HbS molecules after reproportionation, $(1-X)^2$ HbS molecules, and $2X(1-X)$ molecules that are hybrids. An essentially binomial distribution has been observed and occurs when the free energy of dissociation of the hybrid is simply the mean of the free energies of dissociation of the constituents (Perella et al., 1990). (Thus it is not necessary that the dissociation constants be equal, and indeed they are not [Manning et al., 1996]).

Data for S/F hybrids show no copolymerization, again for both compositional and solubility analysis. S/A and S/C hybrids, however, clearly show extensive copolymerization, and their joint average is 37 ± 3 percent. Agreement is again good between the solubility and compositional analysis. S/A$_2$ hybrids show no copolymerization by solubility analysis, and 35 ± 24 percent copolymerization by composition. Hybrids have also been generated by cross-linking, with varied results that agree as follows: HbS cross-linked with HbF or HbA$_2$ shows no copolymerization, whereas S/A cross-linked molecules exhibit 30 percent copolymerization, consistent with the preceding values.

Why is there no copolymerization of S/A$_2$ or S/F hybrids? HbA$_2$ differs from HbA in only twelve amino acids (Chapter 9). From a study of binary mixtures of HbS with the crossover hemoglobin variants, Hb Lepore Boston-Washington and Hb Lepore Hollandia (Chapters 11 and 14), Nagel and co-workers identified δ22 and δ87 as responsible for the inhibitory effects (Nagel et al., 1979). In an elegant experiment, Adachi and co-workers created a mutant HbA$_2$ in which the δ6 position was replaced by a Val and the δ87 position

altered from Gln to Thr as in HbS or HbA (Adachi et al., 1996b). This double mutant in high phosphate buffers exhibited the same solubility, tenth time, exponential growth, and concentration dependence of kinetics as seen in HbS polymerization. Thus it is extremely likely that the δ87 Gln provides the inhibition seen in the failure of the S/A$_2$ hybrids to copolymerize. By extension, the other eleven amino acid changes (β9, 10, 12, 22, 50, 51, 86, 116, 117, 125, and 126) have no effect. Of particular note are positions 116 and 117, which are His in HbS and are Arg and Asn, respectively, in HbA$_2$. The positive and polar groups can clearly stand in for the somewhat positive charge on His near neutral pH, and not disturb the axial contacts.

Nagel et al. (1979) also have identified γ80 (Asp instead of β80 Asn) and γ87 (Gln instead of β80 Thr) as the most likely source of inhibition of HbF copolymerization, with the contribution of γ22 (Asp instead of β22 Glu) and γ50 (Ser in place of β50 Thr) not conclusively eliminated. When γ87 is mutated from Gln to Thr as well as γ6 mutated to Val, the doubly mutated HbF does not polymerize like HbS (Adachi et al., 1996a), showing that this site cannot be the sole contributor to the inhibitory properties of HbF. Still, mixtures of the doubly modified HbF with HbS showed faster kinetics than seen with HbF/HbS mixtures alone, suggesting at least partial contribution from the 87Gln. Although Asnβ80 makes a contact in the double strand with His α50, there may also be a salt bridge at the neighboring Aspβ79 to the αHis50. Thus, it is hard to be certain how the inhibitory effect of β80Asn→γ80Asp would be produced, although the mutation would clearly be disruptive of the contact arrangement established in HbS. The steric effects at γ22 and γ50 are both subtle changes of one carbon difference. Nevertheless, experimental evidence is needed to exclude them conclusively. Other more subtle influences may also be at work. HbF does not bind 2,3 BPG, for example, and has an altered Bohr effect. If these functional changes have even small correlated structural changes, the ability of HbF to copolymerize may be compromised despite differences in the primary structure. In short, although the amino acids responsible for the lack of copolymerization of HbF have likely been identified, their mode of action has not been rationalized, and, correspondingly, more exotic means of creating the inhibition cannot be conclusively eliminated.

The effects of HbA and HbC may be the consequence of the charged group at β6. HbA and HbC only differ from HbS in the negatively charged Glu or positively charged Lys at β6. Both HbA and HbC would suffer a significant energetic penalty to withdraw the charged group from solution, and thus the copolymerization probability gives a fairly good indication of the fraction of sites internal to the polymer that remain solvated. (Because HbA and HbC have oppositely charged groups but the same copolymerization probability, it is unlikely that the charged group participates in an internal salt bridge.) The double strands themselves use only one β6 and thus might be expected to yield a net copolymerization probability of 0.5, which is similar to the experiment value of 0.37 yet well outside the error range of the measurements. The model of Watowich et al. (1989) maintains this value of 0.5. However, a refined version of that model (Roufberg and Ferrone, in press) increases the number of internal contacts to the fiber and gives a predicted value of 0.36. This lies quite close to the analyzed values of 0.37 for HbS/A and HbS/C hybrids, and 0.3 for cross-linked HbSA.

These copolymerization probabilities, although important for the thermodynamic description, do not imply the absolute exclusion of a given species from a polymer. For example, a copolymerization probability of 0.01 for a given species, which is rather small, in fact amounts only to 2.7 kcal/mol of discrimination, and in a 1:1 mixture would allow one molecule of the mixed species every 100 molecules, or one in every seven layers in the fiber. Therefore, the most accurate statement regarding copolymerization of non-S hemoglobins is that these have copolymerization probabilities less than about 0.06 or an energetic discrimination of at least 1.7 kcal/mol at 25°C. Clearly hybrids of HbS with HbA or HbC can extensively copolymerize, and by extension of the preceding argument, will not always have the β^s subunit in the expected orientation.

One additional mixed hemoglobin, R-state hemoglobin, should be considered. Liganded and unliganded hemoglobins have different quaternary structure. Padlan and Love (1985a) showed that the placement of a molecule HbCO within the deoxyHbS structure could retain the axial contacts but would not make the lateral contacts needed for stability, implying that the deoxy quaternary structure is necessary for polymerization. This is confirmed by experiments in which liganded hemoglobin with the quaternary structure changed by inositol hexaphosphate (IHP) or metHb does polymerize. (Briehl and Salhany, 1975). Yet, the solubility of such liganded T-structure hemoglobin is higher than that for deoxyHbS in the same buffers (Briehl and Salhany, 1975), showing that quaternary structure alone is not sufficient to determine solubility.

The Role of Phosphates and Other Solution Components

Because of the high concentrations of hemoglobin involved in experimental studies, means have been sought to lower the demand for protein, such as the use of dextran in the solution. Another approach taken is to use highly concentrated phosphate buffer, in which the solubility dramatically decreases (Fig. 23.7) (Adachi and Asakura, 1979; Poillon and Bertles, 1979). This also simplifies sample handling, although it has raised questions of applicability (Roth et al., 1979).

The origin of the high phosphate effect on sickle hemoglobin polymerization has not been established Three specific modes of interaction are possible: (1) phosphate buffer competes with the hydrophobic regions for water; by assisting the removal of water from the contact it enhances polymerization; (2) phosphate ions screen charge-charge repulsions and enhance polymerization; and (3) phosphate ions, being larger than water, entail a larger exclusion shell around a hemoglobin molecule. That is, the placement of a hemoglobin molecule in phosphate buffer carves out a larger volume than putting the hemoglobin in water because the diameter of the phosphate ions is greater. A polymer, however, excludes fewer molecules of solvent per molecule in the fiber. Hence, phosphate nonideality can favor polymerization.

Although phosphate ions are the most studied, they are not the only added salts that perturb the solubility (Poillon and Bertles, 1979). A detailed analysis of the

Figure 23.7. Solubility of sickle hemoglobin as a function of the molar phosphate concentration [P]. Data from Adachi and Asakura (1979) are shown as open circles; Data from Poillon and Bertles (1979), shown as filled circles. The solubility drops dramatically as phosphate concentration is increased. This has been used to produce gelation at low concentrations of protein.

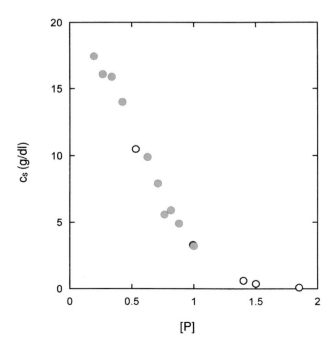

variety of effects shown by the other ions can probably distinguish among the three modes of interaction described previously.

A fourth possibility must also be included, and this is seen in the effects of 2,3 BPG or IHP on polymerization. Although these molecules clearly have direct changes on the solubility, they are also known to modify the affinity of hemoglobin for oxygen and possibly hemoglobin structure. Both IHP and 2,3 BPG (also inorganic phosphates, to a lesser degree) favor the T-quaternary structure in an R-T mixture, and would thus favor the T state by their binding; however, although deoxyHb has fewer than 10^{-4} R state molecules present near neutral pH, the effects persist. It thus seems likely that these allosteric effectors also affect the tertiary structure and that this effect in turn modifies the solubility. Padlan and Love (1985b) point out that the movement of the A helix in deoxyHbS molecules in the double strand is similar to the movement of the A helix induced by the addition of IHP, and thereby provides a structural rationale for the enhanced polymerization in the presence of such allosteric agents.

Oxygen Binding

In dilute solutions, sickle hemoglobin exhibits an oxygen binding curve that is identical to that of HbA (Gill et al., 1979). Concentrated solutions, however, show a right shifted, lower affinity binding curve (Fig. 23.15). From a structural point of view, this qualitative result is readily anticipated since the T structure is required for polymer formation, and the R structure is inhibitory. Consequently, as the equilibrium shifts between R and T in the binding curve, the propensity for forming polymers shifts as well. This in effect adds stability to the T state in a thermodynamic sense (i.e., if the T state favors polymerization, polymerization favors the T state). Thus solutions concentrated enough to gel will naturally be shifted toward the deoxy or T state. The quantitative aspects of this process, however, must be determined by experiments. In structural terms, the question is this: Are all T states equivalent in their propensity to polymerize, or are there further tertiary effects that depend on the number (or nature) of ligands bound?

To answer this question based on a binding curve of solution plus polymers is difficult if possible. An important decomposition of the problem is afforded by the fact that the hemoglobin polymer is optically anisotropic, absorbing more efficiently perpendicular to the polymer axis than along it (Eaton and Hofrichter, 1990) because the hemes act as near perfect planar absorbers, and their planes show a net alignment with respect to the polymer axis. Consequently,

aligned polymers exhibit linear dichroism (difference in absorbance in perpendicular directions). The linear dichroism thus can be used to measure the absorption spectrum and hence oxygen saturation of the polymers per se, rather than inferring the oxygen saturation from a net binding curve.

Such experiments have been carried out for carbon monoxide and oxygen as ligands (Hofrichter, 1979; Sunshine et al., 1982). In carbon monoxide experiments, at 35°C, no binding to the polymer phase was resolved, whereas a small but distinct binding of oxygen was seen at 23.5°C. (Small differences are observed in the binding properties of these two ligands, but differences in the temperature of the experiments may also be sufficient to account for the differences.) These results are consistent with an energetic penalty for ligation within the polymerized T structure. For oxygen, where a quantitative determination is possible, the affinity of the first ligand bound is reduced by a factor of 3.

For the range of oxygenation studied, the binding curve of the polymer also appeared to be noncooperative (Fig. 23.8). The origin of the reduced affinity is not known, but it is fascinating that crystals of HbA

Figure 23.8. Oxygen binding curves of solutions, gels, and polymers of sickle hemoglobin in 0.15 mol/L phosphate buffer. Solution and gel curves (Gill et al., 1980) are measured at pH 7.2 at 25°C, and the polymer curve (Sunshine et al., 1982) is measured at pH 7.0, 23.5°C. The inset shows an expanded view of the polymer binding curve; note that the polymer curve is noncooperative, but with lower affinity than the gel or solution binding curves at low saturation. The solution binding curve has been fit to a MWC curve. The gel binding curve arises from the interplay of the solution and polymer binding curves and the polymerization equilibrium.

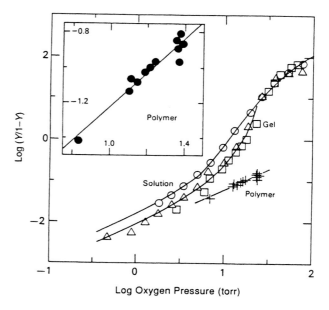

show diminished affinity as well (Mozzarelli et al., 1991). Although the diminution is greater for the crystals (which show affinity about fivefold less than solution T-state affinity, versus threefold for the polymer), about one third of the subunits are exterior in polymers and might thus have fewer constraints than those found in a crystal or the polymer interior. Given a model for ligand binding, such as the familiar Monod-Wyman-Changeux (MWC) model, the binding curve of concentrated solutions can be reconstructed and the agreement, as one might expect, is excellent.

A related experiment is to determine the solubility of partially saturated solutions (Fig. 23.9). As expected, the solubility rises as concentration rises, and nonideality effects make the effect supralinear (Hofrichter, 1979; Sunshine et al., 1982). A quantitative description can be developed by the formalism described previously for mixtures, and the copolymerization probabilities are determined based on the energetic penalties for each ligation state as described previously, coupled with the likelihood of finding the given species as specified by an allosteric model. Agreement between the theory and experiment is very good, suggesting the soundness of equilibrium modeling of polymer formation in the presence of oxygen.

Figure 23.9. Solubility of sickle hemoglobin as a function of solution fractional saturation. Saturation with oxygen is taken from Sunshine et al. (1982) and shown as the filled symbols, whereas saturation with carbon monoxide is taken from Hofrichter (1979) and shown as open symbols. The solid curve shows the solubility determined by using the binding curve data of Figure 23.7 and a correction for associated water. The dashed curve shows the same prediction without the water correction. (For a full description, the reader is referred to Eaton and Hofrichter [1990]).

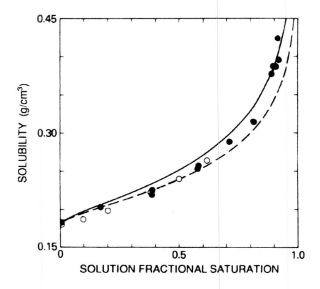

The Bohr Effect and the Sickle Cell

The shift in the oxygen equilibrium of hemoglobin to the right with low pH, first described by Bohr in 1904, facilitates oxygen release from the red cells during their capillary transit through the more acidic environment of metabolizing tissues. Conversely, the Bohr effect facilitates oxygen uptake as the pH of blood passing through the lungs rises.

Oxygen binding properties of HbS are concentration dependent. Although the oxygen binding properties of dilute solutions of HbS were found to be normal (Allen and Wyman, 1954), whole blood from persons with sickle cell anemia had very low affinity for oxygen (Bromberg and Jensen, 1967). Part of the low affinity can be explained by elevated levels of red cell 2,3 BPG, as seen with many anemic states (Charache et al., 1970). Nevertheless, the fundamental reason for this difference is the polymerization of deoxyHbS, which requires a concentration of hemoglobin above that of the c_{SAT} (as is found within the red cells) (Seakins et al., 1973; Bookchin et al., 1976). This was directly verified by Gill et al. (1979), who showed that after partial deoxygenation, a sharp decrease in oxygen affinity coincided with an increase in light scattering indicative of hemoglobin aggregation, in accord with the analysis by Hofrichter (1979) of partially ligated samples.

If polymerization of HbS shifts the oxygen equilibrium curve to the right, and the polymerization reaction occurs at a pH around the intracellular physiologic pH_i 7.2, it follows that the observed Bohr effect (i.e., pH dependence of p^{50}) must be abnormal. Nevertheless, initial reports on the Bohr effect of whole blood on sickle cell anemia red cell suspensions describe it as normal or minimally increased (Rossi-Bernardi et al., 1975; Seakins et al., 1973; Winslow, 1977).

Ueda et al. (1979) exhaustively examined the Bohr effect of whole sickle cell anemia blood at 37°C and constant physiologic carbon dioxide levels (40 mm Hg) (further discussed in Bookchin et al., 1978). The Bohr effect in sickle cell blood was greatly increased, but only between blood pH 7.4 and 7.2 (intracellularly the corresponding pHs are pH 7.2 and 7.0), a pH shift that strongly affects the polymerization of HbS (Fig. 23.10). The dimension of this effect is usually presented as dlog p^{50}/dpH, which is the logarithmic change of p^{50} divided by the logarithmic change of pH, and in effect a measure of the steepness of the slope for this function. In sickle blood α log p^{50}/dpH ranges from –0.92 to –0.99 compared with a normal range of –0.42 to –0.46.

What is the basis of the discrepancy between the early studies and these findings? Some previous work was affected by paucity of data points, but in other instances, methodologic problems conspired against

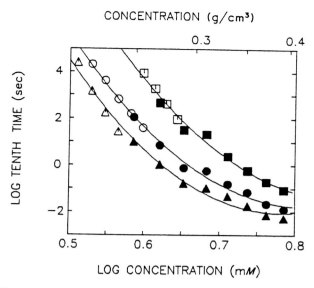

CONCENTRATION (g/cm³)

Figure 23.10. The tenth time (time to reach 10 percent of reaction) for polymerization as a function of initial concentration for three temperatures (15°C, 25°C, and 35°C, squares, circles, and triangles, respectively) (Ferrone et al., 1985b). Filled symbols were collected using a laser photolysis method; the open symbols were collected by a temperature jump method. The concentration dependence is almost fiftieth power at low concentrations but diminishes as concentration increases. The lines have been drawn simply as an aid to the eye.

the correct answer. Winslow (1978) later observed that the method he used to collect oxygen equilibrium data exhibited marked hysteresis (association curve had lower affinity than the association curve), leading to variable results.

This difference in the slope of the Bohr effect in sickle cells suggests that in sickle cell anemia, a drop in blood pH below 7.4 in capillaries causes twice the normal decrease in oxygen affinity and a large release of oxygen from red cells, increasing their risk of sickling. Therefore, even mild transient clinical acidosis with a drop of intracellular pH would be hazardous for patients with sickling disorders. This was shown experimentally when patients with sickle cell anemia infused with low pH isotonic solutions developed painful episodes (Greenberg and Kass, 1958).

KINETICS

The Observations

Because gelation is favored by high temperatures (Fig. 23.4), a convenient method for inducing gelation is to abruptly increase the temperature of a solution prepared at a temperature below solubility. When such an experiment is carried out, the resulting kinetic curves show a dramatic quiescent period

followed by a rapid rise (Hofrichter et al., 1974, 1976). This quiescent period is known as a delay time and is a useful characterization of the kinetic behavior of a given sample. The delay is quite reproducible and is seen in every technique applied to the observation of the reaction, including turbidity, light scattering, birefringence, heat absorption, viscosity, and proton magnetic resonance line width. This delay time is, as described later, an observational effect. The quiescence arises from the failure of the probes to detect a signal, and indeed when more sensitive probes are used, the period of quiescence shortens. With techniques capable of monitoring several decades of signal, the kinetic curve is revealed to be a growing exponential, and the abrupt transition from quiescence to polymerization is seen as the consequence of the exponentially growing process (Eaton and Hofrichter, 1990) (Fig. 23.11).

The delay time is also markedly sensitive to solution conditions, particularly the initial concentration (Hofrichter et al., 1976). For example, delay times in the range of minutes depend inversely on the fortieth power of the initial concentration (Fig. 23.11). To account for this sensitivity, an empirical rule known as the supersaturation equation was formulated, and this rule set the inverse delay time proportional to a high power of the supersaturation, that is, the ratio of initial concentration to solubility. That rule was later modified to include activity, reducing the power law and accounting for nonideality. Unfortunately, the rule does not hold over wide ranges, nor does it follow from the detailed kinetic models that provide a relatively complete description of the kinetics.

In vivo, polymerization is initiated by the removal of oxygen, and in a simulation of that process, carbon monoxide can be removed and kept off indefinitely by steady state laser photolysis (Ferrone et al., 1980, 1985b). This approach has two added virtues: the ability to use very high initial concentrations because HbCO remains soluble up to 50 g/dL, and the ability to repeat the experiment many times because the carbon monoxide will recombine once the laser light is removed. Because the steady state laser can produce significant heating, it is necessary to use a focused spot to maximize the surface/volume ratio and thereby optimize cooling. (Such procedures keep the temperature increases well below 4°C.) Experiments performed under such conditions revealed a new phenomenon. The longest delay times become highly variable under identical conditions (Fig. 23.12), and when the photolyzed areas are inspected, a single domain is invariably observed (Ferrone et al., 1980, 1985b). This stochastic behavior provided the critical key to the mechanism of polymerization.

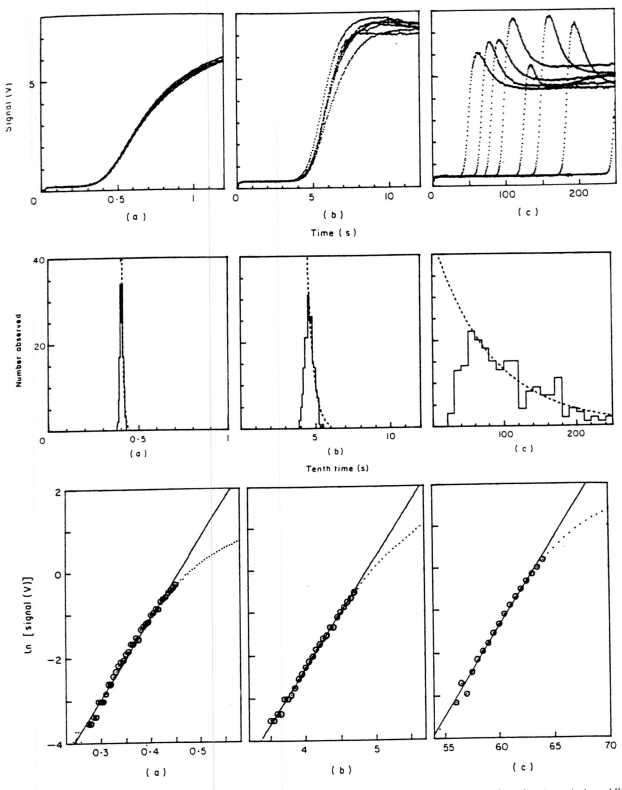

Figure 23.11. Polymerization progress curves for three different temperatures showing the onset of stochastic variation. All experiments were done on a 29 g/dL sample, in a volume of about 10^{-10} cm^3. Left panels show data collected at 29.2°C, center panels show data collected at 18.9°C, and right panels show data for 14.3°C. A total of 150 to 220 curves were collected at each temperature, and representative progress curves are shown in the top row. As the temperature decreases, so does the nucleation rate so that in the right panel, only one nucleus is forming in the sample volume, and the onset of polymerization shows stochastic variation. The central row of panels shows the distribution of the tenth times, which clearly widens. In the third row, representative curves have been plotted semilogarithmically to illustrate the exponential growth process present in *all* the curves (Hofrichter, 1986).

Homogeneous nucleation

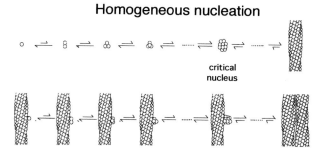

Heterogeneous nucleation

Figure 23.12. The double nucleation mechanism (Ferrone et al., 1980). Polymers may form by homogeneous nucleation or heterogeneous nucleation onto other polymers. In either case, the initial steps are unfavorable, as indicated by the arrows, until a critical nucleus is formed. The critical nucleus is the first aggregate that is equally likely to add monomers or to lose them. No special structure is assumed for the nuclei.

The Mechanism

The high concentration dependence and supersaturation equation suggested that the polymerization process might be nucleation controlled and that the nucleus might simply be given by the exponent in the supersaturation equation. However, a rigorous attempt to use classic theories of nucleation-controlled polymerization produced kinetic curves whose time course was no better than t^2, well below the exponential growth observed (Eaton and Hofrichter, 1978). More rapid growth could be obtained at the expense of nucleation control and thus appeared incompatible with the high concentration dependence. The stochastic variation in delay times suggested a novel mechanism, which has been subsequently verified by differential interference contrast (DIC) microscopy (Samuel et al., 1990). In this double nucleation mechanism, the reaction begins with classic nucleation-controlled polymerization, in a process denoted as homogeneous nucleation. Once a polymer forms, however, the model postulates that new nuclei may form on its surface. Such heterogeneous nucleation will then depend on the amount of material already polymerized, immediately explaining the exponential growth, despite a nucleation-controlled mechanism (Fig. 23.13).

Such a mechanism explains how large time and concentration dependences can be observed simultaneously. It explains why partially melted samples lack a delay time when repolymerized (as there are already an ample number of heterogeneous nucleation sites). It also offers a fascinating explanation for the stochastic variation of delay times seen in small volumes. In those experiments, the stochastic delay arises from the random time involved in the formation of the first poly-

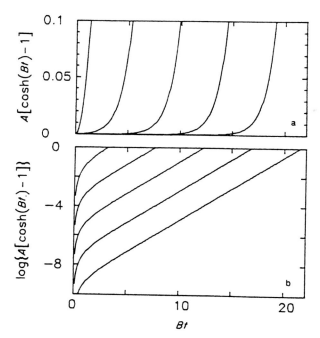

Figure 23.13. Polymerized hemoglobin Δ as a function of time according to the double nucleation mechanism. The mathematical formulation of the double nucleation mechanism of Fig. 23.11 can be solved analytically (Equation 22) for the first 10 percent of the reaction. Δ is the concentration of polymerized monomers, and A and B are constants set by, for example, the initial conditions and the constants that describe polymerization, such as solubility and association rates (Equation 23). For small values of A, the polymerized monomers grow exponentially for most of the initial phase. Because of the exponential growth, the beginning of the reaction is quiescent, giving the illusion that different processes are at work than those once growth is discernible. As the mechanism and its formulation make clear, however, this delay period is observational, and both nucleation and growth are operative during it.

mer, after which the reaction is again deterministic. In that experiment, there is a true delay, not just an observational quiescence. If the reaction were to stop during the stochastic delay, there would be no evidence of the passage of time, unlike that found in delay times on large volumes in which a sparing effect is seen if the reaction is interrupted and resumed. This random behavior has now been seen in DIC microscopy as well as in conventional microscopy in which the location of the first light scattering is spatially resolved.

This mechanism is next described in detail, not only because of its intrinsic interest in describing the nucleation controlled polymerization of HbS, but also because, thanks to its connection with equilibrium thermodynamics, the measurement of kinetics can reveal important features of the basic thermodynamics of HbS assembly. To understand the origin of this connection, it is helpful to follow its development.

The kinetic equations governing this unusual model are straightforward. If the concentration of polymer ends is designated by c_p, and the concentration of monomers in polymers is denoted by Δ, then polymer growth (elongation) is written as

$$\frac{d\Delta}{dt} = k_+ (\gamma c - \gamma_s c_s) c_p \qquad (9)$$

in which k_+ is the monomer addition rate, c the monomer concentration, γ the activity coefficient, and the preceding values are subscripted with s to denote their values at solubility.

The rate of polymer formation by the homogeneous pathway is:

$$\left(\frac{dc_p}{dt} \right)_{\text{hom}} = \frac{k_+ \gamma c \, \gamma_{i^*} \, c_{i^*}}{\gamma_{i^*+1}} \qquad (10)$$

in which k_+ and c are as in Equation 9 and c_{i^*} the concentration of nuclei of size i^*. The γs are activity coefficients for monomers (γ), nuclei (γ_{i^*}) and an activated complex γ_{i^*+1}) taken as the nucleus plus 1. Activity coefficients for the nucleus-plus-1 are calculated assuming an essentially spherical object using scaled particle theory as described previously.

This equation assumes that nucleation is an irreversible step and that the nuclei are in equilibrium with the monomers, a thermodynamic assumption that allows the activity of the nuclei $(\gamma_{i^*} c_{i^*})$ to be computed. Thus, if K_{i^*} is the equilibrium constant for the association of i^* monomers,

$$\gamma_{i^*} c_{i^*} = K_{i^*} (\gamma c)^{i^*} \qquad (11)$$

This is a good assumption as long as growth after nucleation does not substantially deplete the concentration of nuclei (equivalently, does not deplete monomers). We will return to that description presently to show how K_{i^*} and i^* are determined.

The heterogeneous pathway is treated similarly, and one could formally rewrite Equation 10 replacing *het* for *hom*, and *j* for the homogeneous nucleus size *i*, viz.

$$\left(\frac{dc_p}{dt} \right)_{het} = \frac{k_+ \gamma c \gamma'_{j^*} c'_{j^*}}{\gamma'_{j^*+1}} \qquad (12)$$

An important new feature has appeared. The heterogeneous nucleus consists of an aggregate attached to a polymer. The activated complex, therefore, no longer is a spherical object, but one of rather an odd shape, and thus the activated complex activity coefficient has been given a prime to designate that fact. Likewise, the heterogeneous nucleus is an attached aggregate, again written with a prime to distinguish it from an aggregate like the homogeneous nucleus, but simply different in size.

We may formally write an equilibrium for attaching an aggregate of size j^* to polymers as:

$$\gamma'_{j^*} c'^* = K'_{j^*} \gamma_{j^*} c_{j^*} \gamma_p \varphi \Delta \qquad (13)$$

where primes indicate attached aggregates, and unprimed symbols indicate solution aggregates. K_{j^*} is the equilibrium constant for the attachment process, Δ is the concentration of monomers in polymers, φ is the fraction of such polymerized monomers that can accept an aggregate, and γ_p is the activity coefficient of the polymer with no aggregate attached.

Then Equation 12 becomes:

$$\left(\frac{dc_p}{dt} \right)_{het} = \frac{k_+ \gamma c K'_{j^*} \gamma_{j^*} c_{j^*} \gamma_p \varphi \Delta}{\gamma'_{j^*+1}} = k_+ \gamma c K'_{j^*} \gamma_{j^*} c_{j^*} \Gamma \varphi \Delta \qquad (14)$$

in which Γ is the ratio of activity coefficient for a polymer with no aggregate attached to the activity coefficient of a polymer with aggregate size j^*+1 attached (i.e., $\Gamma = \gamma_p/\gamma'_{j^*+1}$. In the initial treatment, Γ was taken as 1 (Ferrone et al., 1985a). The two added parameters are then φ, the fraction of available monomers, and K_{j^*} the equilibrium constant for the attachment process. Initially, these were taken as adjustable parameters to be used in fitting the model to the data. Moreover, K_{j^*} was given a functionally efficient size dependence. Subsequent structural models for heterogeneous nucleation specify these: for example φ is determined from the structural considerations to be 4/14 (Mirchev and Ferrone, 1997).

The kinetic equations for formation of polymers become:

$$\frac{dc_p}{dt} = \left(\frac{dc_p}{dt} \right)_{\text{hom}} + \left(\frac{dc_p}{dt} \right)_{het} \equiv f(c) + g(c)\Delta \qquad (15)$$

and the concentration of monomers in polymers, Δ, grows according to:

$$\frac{d\Delta}{dt} = J(c) c_p \qquad (16)$$

in which

$$J(c) = k_+(\gamma c - \gamma_s c_s) \qquad (17)$$

Analytic solutions for the full set of these equations are not known, and thus an approach was adopted to expand the equations about the initial concentrations, retaining consistent first-order terms in the expansion (Bishop and Ferrone, 1984). The equations after expansion to first-order terms are:

$$\frac{dc_p}{dt} = f(c_0) + \left[g(c_0) - \frac{df(c_0)}{dc_0} \right] \Delta, \qquad (18)$$

$$\frac{d\Delta}{dt} = J_0 c_p \tag{19}$$

From Equations 10, 11, and 14 it is straightforward to show that:

$$f_o = [k_+ K_{i*}/ \gamma_{i*+1}] (\gamma_o c_o)^{i*+1} \tag{20}$$

$$g_o = k_+ \varphi \Gamma K_{j*} K^*_{j*}(\gamma_o c_o)^{j*+1} \tag{21}$$

and the subscript o indicates that the quantities take the values of the initial concentrations. Equations 18 and 19 have a simple, analytic solution, namely:

$$\Delta(t) = A[\cosh(Bt) - 1] = \begin{cases} \frac{1}{2}Ae^{Bt}, & Bt \gg 1 \\ \frac{1}{2}AB^2t^2, & Bt \ll 1 \end{cases} \tag{22}$$

in which the constants A and B are given by

$$A = f_o/[g_o \, df_o/dc]$$
$$B^2 = J_o[g_o \, df_o/dc] \tag{23}$$

and the combination B^2A is uniquely independent of the heterogeneous nucleation process, viz. $B^2A = J_o f_o$. Figure 23.14 shows Equation 22 as the parameters are varied. These equations directly satisfy the requirements that were difficult to reconcile with linear poly-

Figure 23.14. Rate parameters B and B^2A (Equation 22) are shown as a function of initial concentrtion for 15°C, 25°C, and 35°C. (Ferrone et al., 1985a and 1985b). Filled symbols were collected by inducing the reaction by photolysis, the open symbols were collected from temperature jump experiments. B^2A is unaffected by heterogeneous nucleation, and only reflects homogeneous nucleation and growth. B is affected by all parameters, but is dominated by heterogeneous nucleation. Note that the data cannot be fit by a simple straight line, indicating that the nucleus size is variable. The curves through the data arise from fits of the double nucleation mechanism.

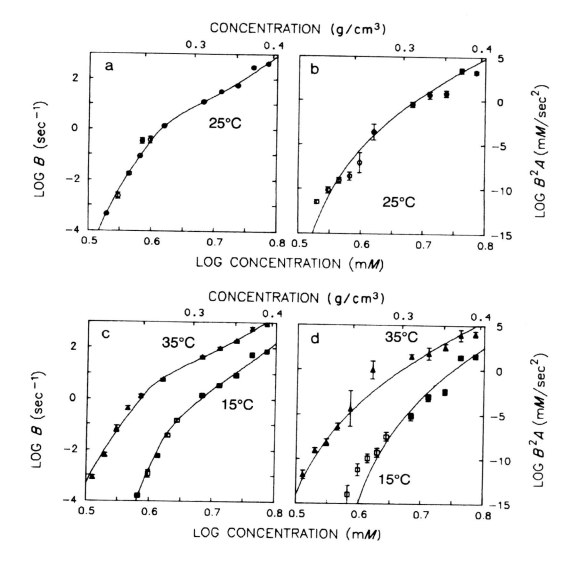

merization, namely an exponential growth rate (Equation 6, when Bt >>1) in which the exponent B is highly concentration dependent (Equation 7). An important further benefit of this formulation is that this solution depends only on the fact that there is a secondary polymer formation pathway that is proportional to the concentration of polymerized monomers. The solutions and decomposition into homogeneous and heterogeneous parts do not depend on the particular details chosen; different expressions of f and g would still give the same solutions. This is important because not all the aspects of the heterogeneous process have been ascertained, so that further evolution of the details is likely. Nonetheless, because of the formulation used, the basic experimental observations already described will continue to be successfully described by the model even as the details evolve. Figure 23.15 shows the values of B and B^2A as a function of concentration as determined from a set of photolysis and temperature jump experiments.

Shear is well known to accelerate the formation of polymers, as the fragmentation of polymers creates new ends to which monomers may add. The previous description of the secondary polymer formation pathway can be easily expanded to include polymer breakage (Bishop and Ferrone, 1984; Eaton and Hofrichter, 1990), as seen in high shear experiments. There is no change in the solution (Equation 6) and only a redefinition of g to include a term for breakage. The concentration dependence of the breakage term is smaller than that of heterogeneous nucleation (although the breakage term may retain some concentration dependence (Samuel et al., 1993). Thus the shape of the polymerization curves will still be exponential, but the concentration dependence of the growth rate (B) and by extension the delay time are expected to be greatly suppressed at high shear, as is in fact observed.

The preceding equations are also readily modified to account for the presence of polymer when the reaction begins, as when there has been incomplete melting of a polymer (Bishop and Ferrone, 1984). If the concentration of polymerized monomers present initially is Δ_{init} then:

$$\Delta = (A + \Delta_{init})\cosh Bt \qquad (24)$$

The effective increase in A means that the reaction will be manifest sooner than usual (i.e., the delay is shortened or effectively abolished because A is typically quite small). The exponential growth process, however, is unchanged, and thus the curves appear simply displaced in time (Fig. 23.16).

It is possible to relate the stochastic variation of the time of onset to the homogeneous nucleation rate, as shown by Szabo (1988). The initial homogeneous nucleation rate is denoted by ζ, and is related to the rate constant for nucleation, f_o, measured in mmol/Ls, by multiplying f_o by the photolyzed volume V and Avogadro's number N_o, with appropriate conversion for mmol/L, that is:

$$\zeta = f_o N_o V. \qquad (25a)$$

Szabo then showed that T(t), the distribution of tenth times t (time to reach 1/10 of final value), is given by:

$$T(t) = \frac{Be^{-\zeta(t)}}{\Gamma(\zeta/B)}(1 - e^{-Bt})^n e^{-\zeta t} \qquad (25b)$$

in which Γ is a gamma function, and n is a parameter that describes the point at which observation of the domain is made, and that is equal to $e^{B(t)}$ with (t) the average tenth time for nonstochastic measurements. The distribution begins small because of the $1-e^{-Bt}$ term. Once t > 1/B, the distribution becomes a decaying exponential, whose decay constant is ζ, the rate of homogeneous nucleation. From Equation 25a, it is evident that small volumes will lead to distributions with long tails. Moreover, the distribution itself can be used as a tool to determine the rate of homogeneous nucle-

Figure 23.15. Distributions of delay times at 20°C for three different initial concentrations (Cao and Ferrone, 1996). Data are collected by simultaneous photolysis of carboxyHbS on many different spots in an array. Because only one homogeneous nucleus forms in each spot (Fig. 23.10), the formations times are random. The distributions are well fit by Szabo's function (Equation 25b) and from that the rate of homogeneous nucleation is determined. Note the high concentration dependence.

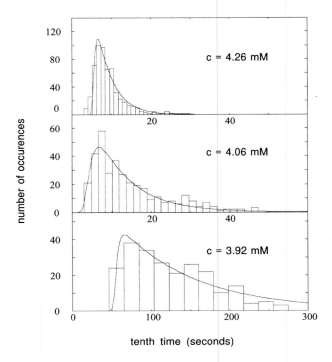

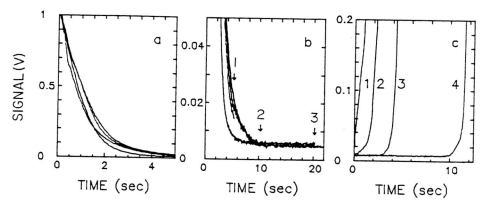

Figure 23.16. Polymerization after incomplete depolymerization from experiments of Mozzarelli et al. (1987). Incompletely melted polymers can seed the formation of new polymers as predicted by the double nucleation mechanism. Panel (**A**) shows a decrease in light scattering, indicating polymer melting, after the decrease in laser intensity in a continuous photolysis experiment. (**B**) The curves seen in (**A**) are shown in an expanded scale. Arrows indicate a point at which laser illumination was increased abruptly to achieve complete photodissociation leading to repolymerization. (**C**) Increase in scattering after photolysis of the incompletely melted samples of (**B**). The greater the amount of polymer remaining, the shorter the delay, as seen in Equation 24, for which the residual polymers gives Δ_{init}.

ation. Figure 23.17 shows distributions at 25°C for three different concentrations.

The stochastic equations are derived from the same double nucleation mechanism as the deterministic equations, so the description of B^2A and the description of the stochastic distribution both yield the homogeneous nucleation rate, or equivalently, knowing one should specify the other. That they do (Cao and Ferrone, 1997) indicates that the model has been correctly formulated.

The concentration dependences of the tenth times (Fig. 23.10) or the parameters B and B^2A (Fig. 23.15) are not only large, but also change with concentration. From the variation in concentration dependence of these figures (i.e., nonlinear log-log plots), one may conclude that the nucleus size is not a constant. This phenomenon has long been observed in droplet condensation and follows from simple thermodynamic descriptions of the nucleation process. This thermodynamic approach yields a new result, namely decomposition of the chemical potential that binds the monomers to the polymer from the vibrational chemical potential that arises from motion of the monomers within a polymer (cf. Equation 2).

The concentration of nuclei may be calculated by equating chemical potentials of i monomers (initially at concentration c_o) to the chemical potential of aggregates of size i. Thus:

$$i(_{RT} + RT \ln \gamma_o c_o) = \mu_{iT} + \mu_{iR} + \mu_{iC} + \mu_{iV} + RT \ln \gamma_i c_i \quad (26)$$

where μ_{RT} is the sum of the rotational and translational chemical potential of the monomer in solution, μ_{iT} and μ_{iR} are the translational and rotation chemical potentials, respectively, of the aggregate and μ_{iC} and μ_{iV} are the contact and vibrational chemical potentials of the monomers in the aggregate. Treating the nuclei as spheres it is easy to show that:

$$\mu_{iT} + \mu_{iR} = \mu_{RT} + 4\, RT \ln i \quad (27)$$

Assuming the nucleus grows as a close packed aggregate, the size dependence of μ_{iC} is obtained by counting contacts between spheres. $\delta(i)$ is a function used to denote the fraction of total contacts made for a given aggregate size. Then:

$$\mu_{iC} = i\delta(i)\, \mu_{PC} = \mu_{PC}(i - \delta, \ln i - \delta_2) \quad (28)$$

where the last equality follows from a fit of an empirical function to experimentally counted spherical contacts in a close packed aggregate (Ferrone et al., 1985a). For the vibrational term, it is assumed that all monomers in the polymer have the same vibrational frequency and thus the same chemical potential. This is equivalent to the Einstein model for solids, and is reasonable to the extent that all modes of vibration are well excited in the polymer. Thus the chemical potential for vibrations in the aggregate is:

$$\mu_{iV} = (i - 1)\, \mu_{PV} \quad (29)$$

in which $i-1$ is used rather than i because the aggregate retains motional freedom. The last two equations (28 and 29) are critical, for they describe a difference in size dependence for the contact and vibrational terms (μ_{PV} and μ_{PC}) that otherwise would remain as an additive pair, as they appear in the solubility equation. Consequently, when Equation 26 is solved for the nucleus size (by setting the concentration derivative of

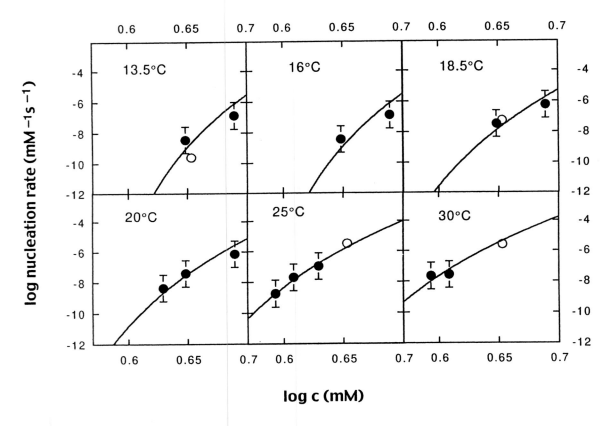

Figure 23.17. Homogeneous nucleation rates for different temperatures and concentrations (Cao and Ferrone, 1997). Rates are determined by collecting distributions of delay times (Fig. 23.15) and fitting Szabo's function (Equation 25b). The fits are shown as the solid lines. The open symbols are taken from the serial experiments of Hofrichter (1986).

the activity to zero), Equation 2 can be used to eliminate μ_{PV}, with the result that the nucleation rate will give μ_{PC} alone. The size of the nucleus is given by

$$i = \xi/\ln S \qquad (30)$$

where we have used the symbol ξ to collect a series of terms, viz:

$$\xi = -4 - \delta_1 \frac{\mu_{pc}}{RT} \qquad (31)$$

and S is the activity supersaturation (i.e., $S = \gamma c/\gamma_s c_s$). The homogeneous nucleation rate can be written as

$$f_0 = qK_+ \frac{\gamma_o c_o \gamma_s c_s}{\gamma_{i^*+1}} \left(\frac{\ln S}{\xi}\right)^\xi e^{1.12\xi} \qquad (32)$$

where

$$q = \frac{\sqrt{8}}{\rho} exp(4(1 - \delta_2)/\delta_1) \qquad (33)$$

and ρ is the ratio of monomer to polymer densities, and δ_1 and δ_2 are the constants from Equation 28. What is remarkable about this equation is that all but two parameters are set by equilibrium measurements: The solubility (and hence the supersaturation S) are known independently. Once the monomer addition rate is measured, as it can be experimentally, only μ_{PC} is a free variable in the nucleation rate equations.

Thus, fits to the homogeneous nucleation rates give values of this contact energy. Such fits are shown in Figure 23.18 (Cao and Ferrone, 1997). The values of the contact energy μ_{PC} generated by such fits are shown in Figure 23.19. At present, the value of μ_{PC} represents the average contact energy, and it remains to decompose it into lateral and axial terms. The value itself is of interest. The cost of burying a Val is known to be approximately 1.5 kcal/mol (Nozaki and Tanford, 1971). A similar cost is attributed to a receptor region. Thus for each monomer there is at least 3 kcal/mol in hydrophobic stabilization. Thus, the hydrophobic effect accounts for a little less than half the net, with the remainder possibly dominated by the salt bridges.

The heterogeneous nucleation pathway is not as thoroughly described as the homogeneous, in part because of the lack, until quite recently, of even a rudimentary structural model for the process. In the initial description, the attachment of the nucleus, K'_{j^*}, was represented by a linear and log term, the coefficients of

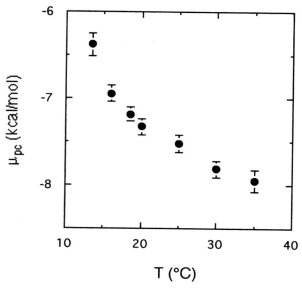

Figure 23.18. Contact energy in the polymer (μ_{PC}) versus T (Cao and Ferrone, 1997). From homogeneous nucleation rates it is possible to deduce the contact chemical potential of the monomers in the polymer. This value differs from the energy of stabilization by the vibrational chemical potential, μ_{PV} and is related to the elementary energetics of stability, such as hydrophobic surface burial and salt bridge formation.

which were treated as adjustable parameters. The fraction of sites available for nucleation, ϕ, was also treated as adjustable. Finally, it was assumed that $\Gamma = 1$. With these assumptions, an excellent description was possible of the heterogeneous nucleation rate, as determined by the exponential growth parameter, B (recall Equation 23). Figure 23.16 shows the comparison of the data and the fit.

There are three aspects to this mechanism, and accordingly, three levels of validation. It is useful to dis-

Figure 23.19. The double nucleation mechanism has been validated by direct observation using differential interference contrast microscopy (Samuel et al., 1990). The pictures are 17 m wide and are taken over 35 seconds. A second polymer is clearly growing along the parent polymer and then splaying off. Sample was 22.2 g/dL, at 21°C.

tinguish this hierarchy because, for example, validation of the conceptual mechanism by direct observation does not itself validate the thermodynamic description of the behavior of nuclei. The most fundamental is the conceptual mechanism as shown in Figure 23.13, involving two types of nucleation-controlled polymerization. The original demonstration of the soundness of the conceptual mechanism arose from the stochastic variation seen in small samples, in which a single molecular event gave rise to many polymers (Ferrone et al., 1980, 1985b). A more direct validation came from the use of DIC microscopy, in which the diffraction shadow of single fibers could be viewed and their growth and morphology observed. There, new fibers were directly observed growing along other fibers (Samuel et al., 1990) (Fig. 23.20). In addition, the DIC observations showed considerable fiber flexibility (so that the tip of the growing fiber danced in brownian motion), as well as cross-linking (observed by adhesion of fibers that had been moving independently). DIC microscopy also provided a fundamental quantitative parameter, k_+, the monomer addition rate constant that was deduced from the rate of polymer elongation.

Given a correct conceptual model, the second aspect is its formulation in terms of rate equations and simplifying approximations. Such approximations include the accuracy of neglecting species other than monomers and polymers, and so forth. The first test of this aspect is to compare the shape of the progress curves with that predicted by Equation 22. The transformation from curves that are close to t^2 (at high concentration) to exponential growth at low concentration supports the expression of the model as shown. Moreover, comparison of stochastic measurements with the measurements of B^2A from well-averaged experiments further validates formulation of the ideas of Figure 23.13 in the equations shown in Equation 22.

Finally, the kinetic model is expressed in thermodynamic terms, because it is constructed around equilibrium nucleation theory. There are three tests of this aspect. The first involves the plausibility of the parameters determined in the fits. Values of μ_{PC} have been discussed previously. A second test involves the enthalpy determined in the reaction. From equation 2,

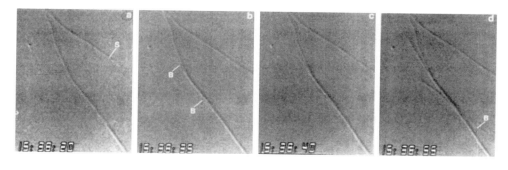

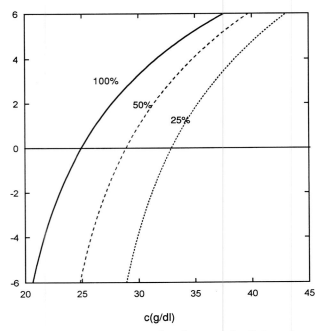

Figure 23.20. Concentration of nuclei in a red cell size volume. From the double nucleation mechanism it is possible to deduce the concentration of nuclei in a volume the size of the red cell after 1-second incubation at fixed saturation conditions. Three different O_2 saturation levels are shown (0, 58, and 80 percent), which yield 100, 50, and 25 percent T-state molecules. R-state molecules are assumed for this calculation to have no possibility of copolymerization. This is only approximately true, but is consistent with the overall accuracy of the calculation.

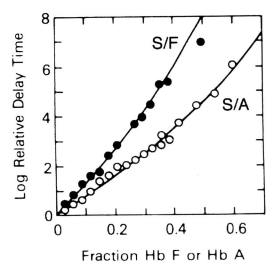

Figure 23.21. Delay times for S/A and S/F mixtures (Sunshine et al., 1979). The presence of non-S hemoglobins such as HbF and HbA causes drastic increases in the delay time. Here, extrapolation of measured data has been used to estimate the relative increase in delay time due to in mixtures. As is apparent, 50 percent AS (effectively sickle cell trait) has a delay time increased sufficiently to be beyond the time for sickling in vivo.

the enthalpy of the log of solubility should arise entirely from the μ_{PC} term, because the μ_{PV} term only contributes 6RT, which exactly balances the enthalphic contributions of μ_{RT}. When the enthalpy from solubility is compared with the enthalpy from μ_{PC}, as determined by nucleation rates, the agreement is excellent (Cao and Ferrone, 1997). The third test involves the nonideality of the nucleus. The nucleation rate depends on the nonideality of the nucleus. This term is surprisingly large and is dependent on the size of the nucleus, which in turn depends on μ_{PC} (see Equations 30 and 31). Thus, the model is highly sensitive to an incorrectly designated nucleus. Tests of the nonideality of the nucleus are presently under way, and preliminary results are encouraging (Ivanova et al., in press).

One consequence of this mechanism and the thermodynamic details of its description is that the concentration of nuclei is predicted to be very small, which frustrates attempts to isolate nuclei by chemical means. Figure 23.21 shows the number of homogeneous nuclei after 1 second, assuming constant nucleation, in a volume of 90 μm^3, which is close to the size of the red cell for a range of hemoglobin concentrations. Calculations are shown for 100, 50, and 25 percent T-state mole-

cules. It is evident that it is possible to have a situation in which a single nucleation event fills an entire cell. It is intriguing that simulations of this process of domain formation display curvature that resembles that seen in slowly deoxygenated cells that sickle (Dou and Ferrone, 1993). Similar domains are seen in DIC microscopy. The sickle morphology thus appears to be the result of the domain structure taken by the polymer. Rapidly deoxygenated cells, on the other hand, can have many domains (if the nucleation rate is greater than 1 in Fig. 23.21) and thus tend to show no gross morphologic changes. The exact point of the changeover from stochastic to deterministic kinetics (i.e., where the number of nuclei becomes > 1) is dependent on many factors that are beyond the scope of this chapter and whose basic features are only superficially known. For example, the rate of deoxygenation may allow the first nucleus to fill the cell before a second nucleation event, or diffusion of oxygen during unloading may mean that the actual volume deoxygenated is less than the whole cell and perhaps confined to a smaller layer near the surface. Such variables will decrease the number of nuclei present.

RECOMBINANT HEMOGLOBINS AND THE POLYMERIZATION OF HbS

Recombinant hemoglobins (Chapter 45) have expanded the number of amino acid substitutions that can be generated at sites not represented by natural mutants or that cannot be produced by chemical procedures. Recombinants provide a means for studying the importance of various amino acids for the thermodynamics and kinetics of polymer formation. Such studies have many specific uses. Recombinants with enhanced polymerization have been used to increase the severity of transgenic mouse models of sickle cell anemia (Li et al., 1997). Mutants expressing modified α- and β-globin chains may be used to increase the antisickling effect for a given degree of expression (Ho et al., 1996). Since HbA copolymerizes, but HbF does not, there has been interest in generating HbA that more closely resembles HbF (McCune et al., 1994).

HbS has been synthesized in *Saccharomyces cerevisiae* (Martin de Llano et al., 1993) and a correctly folded tetramer is produced. This recombinant HbS is identical with naturally occurring, purified HbS as judged by many biochemical and physiologic criteria including its c_{SAT} (Martin de Llano and Manning, 1994). Variant globins can also be expressed in an *Escherichia coli* system, and although misfolding can occur it can be easily repaired (Ho et al., 1996). Because each new mutation carries the potential for altered functional properties in addition to its direct effect on polymerization, it is important to do adequate control experiments on each newly generated mutant. Unless specifically stated, it will be assumed that the properties are not significantly different from HbS. However, the reader is advised to consult the original literature for detailed description, as characterization varies considerably from one laboratory to another.

Because of their novelty, these studies are recounted in somewhat greater detail than other work cited here. Owing to the scarcity of recombinant material, many studies have been carried out in high phosphate buffer, and the applicability of such studies to more physiologic buffer conditions remains a cautionary note (Roth et al., 1979). A final caution is that aggregation of protein is not automatically equivalent to polymer formation, and so observation of, for example, turbidity at 700 nm may not show polymer formation. If light scattering is followed, at least one would expect either a clear delay time, indicative of heterogeneous nucleation, and/or a highly concentration-dependent characteristic time, indicative of nucleation, to suggest similarity of the polymer forms. We now turn to the issues that have been profitably addressed by the recombinant techniques.

Donor Site (β6) Studies

Perhaps the most basic question is how the residue at β6 affects polymer formation. Both β6Leu (Adachi et al., 1991, 1993) and β6Ile (Baudin-Chich et al., 1990) lower the solubility by about half. The similarity

of Leu and Ile in this regard is consistent with the notion that buried surface is responsible, as these two amino acids have similar buried surface and free energy of transfer. The free energy associated with the change $c_s \simeq 0.5\ c_s^o$ (computed as $-RT \ln 2$) is also consistent with the free energy change based on standard hydrophobic energies (Nozaki and Tanford, 1971), as two amino acid changes are needed per molecule. Baudin-Chich (1990) produced a simple steric model of the Ile variant in the acceptor pocket and found a good fit. Hb with Gln also appears to generate polymers (suggested by presence of a delay time, which itself signifies an exponential growth process) (Adachi et al., 1987). The Gln mutant has a solubility 25 to 30 times greater than HbS, which is much less than one would expect based on hydrophobic free energies alone (of course, Gln is hardly a perfect hydrophobe). β6Trp, Phe, Ala, and Glu mutants do not appear to form polymers (Bihoreau et al., 1992), although precipitates form without a delay after a temperature jump (Adachi et al., 1993). Thus one could conclude that polymerization is not only controlled by hydrophobicity but also by stereospecificity. Lesecq et al. (1997) produced a double mutant in which HbS has the added change of β7 Glu $\rightarrow$ Ala. The β7 does not participate in the binding pocket and, not unexpectedly, does not change the solubility or the kinetics of polymerization, although there is evidence the A helix may be destabilized.

Acceptor Site (EF Corner) Studies

The acceptor pocket for the β6Val is formed by Leu β88, Phe β85, and several heme atoms. Replacement of β88 Leu by Ala creates polymers as seen by birefringence (Ferrone, unpublished) and by stochastic kinetics and exponential growth curves (Cao et al., 1997). The mutation leads to an increased solubility, consistent with about 1 kcal/mol of free energy per molecule (Liao et al., 1996; Martin de Llano and Manning, 1994). Similar results are found in both high and low phosphate buffers (Adachi et al., 1994). This result at first seems quite plausible, because Leu is more hydrophobic than Ala, and in fact the magnitude of free energy changes on solvation of Leu versus Ala are even consistent with the magnitude of the difference in energy (Liao et al., 1996). However, when the stereochemistry of the acceptor pocket is studied, it is evident that only part of the Leu is solvent-exposed (Cao et al., 1997). The small bump constituting the Leu surface in the pocket is replaced by a small dimple of the same net surface area when Ala is placed at position β88. Consequently, the contact energy (μ_{PC}) is expected to be the same for the two mutants. Kinetic studies of the homogeneous nucleation rate measure this contact energy and yield this exact unanticipated but reasonable result (Cao et al., 1997). The origin of the difference in solubility must therefore be μ_{PV}, the vibrational chemical potential (recall Equation 2). This is presumably due to the deeper acceptor pocket of the Ala substituted mutant, allowing a fit that is more snug and thus more expensive in loss of entropy. As expected, the kinetics of polymerization are notably slowed by this substitution. When β88 Leu is replaced by Phe, the resulting progress curves fail to demonstrate delay times, and thus the assembly form taken by that mutant remains problematic.

An interesting result arises from the mutation of Lysβ95 to Ile (Himanen et al., 1995). Lysβ95 in the double strands contacts a second Lys (β17) with considerable crystal disorder, as might be expected from the similar charged groups. It has been proposed as a contact between double strands in the fiber, and inspection suggests an ionic interaction with Aspβ94. (In fact, it is possible that such interactions occur within as well as between β chains.) To test this hypothesis a mutant was generated in which Ile replaced Lys. The formation of polymer domains as viewed by birefringence (Ferrone and Liao, unpublished) confirms the formation of aligned polymers. The drastically increased solubility of the mutant (almost 40 g/dla free energy change of 2.8 kcal/mol) suggested that the proposal was correct (i.e., that β95 has a role to play in the formation of polymers) because without its charge partner, Asp β94 would be less solvated in the polymer, particularly with a hydrophobic Ile in close proximity.

An even more striking experimental result was obtained when the foregoing two mutations were combined in a triple mutant (HbS, β88Leu→Ala, β95 Lys→Ile), because the final solubility was the same as that of the β95 mutant alone (Himanen et al., 1996). This result can be nicely reconciled with the previous proposal that the change in β88 Leu→Ala solubility is due to decreased vibrational entropy. If the β95 change also involves a decrease in vibrational freedom within the polymer, the immobilization effected in the β88 Leu→Ala mutation has already occurred, and no further increase in solubility would occur.

Binary mixtures of HbS and a mutant of β87 (HbD Ibadan) had demonstrated that β87 could be inhibitory of the polymerization reaction from a *trans* position with respect to the β chain donating the active β6Val site. Insofar as this is a significant point of difference between HbS and HbF, it is all the more interesting to see how alterations of this amino acid affect polymerization. In high phosphate buffers, β87Leu and Trp mutants of HbS polymerize with characteristic delay times (exponential growth), indicative of polymer formation (Reddy et al., 1997). (Leu mutants also show birefringent domains [Liao and Ferrone, unpublished]).

The Leu mutant has a solubility almost identical to native 87Thr, suggesting that the loss in hydrogen bonds between Ser 9 and Thr 87 (making the polymer less stable) is compensated by increased hydrophobicity (making the polymer more stable.) With β87 Trp, the solubility increases about sixfold, which may be the consequence of steric issues. β87 Gln shows unusually shallow progress curves and very low concentration dependence of the delay time; β87 Asp shows no delay or high concentration dependence. Thus, the polymeric nature of these latter two mutant aggregates remains an open question. Ho et al. (1996) synthesized an HbS variant with β87 Thr → Lys (HbS Ibadan), as well as HbS with both β87 Thr→Lys and α114 Pro→Arg (HbS Ibadan-Chiapas). In the axial contact, 114 interacts with Lys α16, and thus the Arg-Lys repulsion explains the destabilization of the polymer that is observed. McCune et al. (1994) produced an HbS variant with β87 Thr→Gln and the axial β22 Glu→Ala in transgenic mouse lines. Delay time experiments established that this double mutant was a potent inhibitor of gelation. Because β22 Glu forms an axial salt bridge (with α20His), its replacement with the hydrophobe Ala could easily lessen polymer stability.

In an interesting variation of the preceding motif, Adachi and co-workers (1996a) synthesized HbF with γ6Val, which showed aggregation without a delay. When they combined this mutant with HbS, the HbS/Fγ6 hybrids polymerized with a delay time shorter than seen in S/F mixtures under similar (high phosphate) conditions, and with a solubility of about two-thirds that of S/F. When γ87 was mutated to Thr (as found in HbS), the delay time and solubility further decreased for the mixtures to roughly midway between pure HbS and the HbS/Fγ6Val mixture. Finally, a triple modification of HbF was constructed with γ6Val, γ87 Thr, and γ143 Thr and copolymerized with HbA. This polymerized with a clear delay, and high concentration dependence, even though neither of the constituents showed such properties, suggesting an asymmetry in the contacts within the polymer that requires further investigation.

Variants of HbA₂ containing δ6 Val, δ6 Val, δ87 Thr and δ6 Val, δ22 Glu, and δ87 Thr were also produced (Adachi et al., 1996b). With only the Val mutation, aggregates formed without a delay. The double and triple mutants exhibited the same delay time and concentration dependence as HbS in 1.8 mmol/L phosphate buffer, and triple mutants showed the same solubility as HbS, whereas the double mutant appeared to have a solubility almost twice as great. (The latter is hard to reconcile with the identity of the delay times; however, the solubility is obtained from extrapolation of data, and adjustment of the slope of that particular curve to extrapolate to the same solubility might be possible.)

Axial Contacts and Other Multiple Mutants

Besides the work already described, Bihoreau et al. (1992) have synthesized a mutant with an axial change at β23, Val→Ile. This more hydrophilic group would be expected to displace some of the water found in the contact region, and indeed the net effect is to enhance polymerization. This double mutant occurs naturally (as HbS Antilles), and similar enhancement is seen on the β6 Glu→Ile mutant when the β23 is mutated, as the solubility drops to about 60 percent and delay time is halved (Chapter 28).

HbS with the modification Glu β121 Arg has also been produced (Li et al., 1997). This enhances polymerization, as does the natural mutant HbS Oman (β121 Glu→ Lys) and the effects are similar (Chapter 28). The origin of the effect is unclear because the closest axial contact is a Pro (α114). When the preceding axial mutation is coupled with Asp α75 Tyr, the solubility again drops by about half. (Li et al., 1997). A quadruple mutant, with the prior three mutations plus Asp α6→Ala, even further stabilizes the polymer and further decreases the triple mutant solubility by about 40 percent (Li et al., 1997).

KINETICS IN RED CELLS

The small diameter of the capillaries requires cell deformation for passage; erythrocytes have an umbrella shape while in transit (Skalak, 1969). Because a polymer gel has a substantial solid component, intracellular polymer seriously compromises erythrocyte deformability. This was first shown in experiments in which sickled red cells were found incapable of passing through 5 μm pore filters (Jandl et al., 1961). Although solid pores may be an inadequate model for the microcirculation, the experiment established the rigidity of the cell with polymerized hemoglobin. Sickle cells may become trapped in capillaries of the retina (Fabry et al., 1984). In other circulatory beds such as the mesoappendix of the rat or in cremaster preparations in transgenic mice, obstruction by sickle cells has been observed only in the small venules or in the precapillary sphincter (Kaul et al., 1993, 1995). The obstruction in the mesoappendix is a mixture of adhesion of low density sickle cells, which have greater tendency to adhere and are more deformable, and trapping of dense sickle cells, which are less likely to adhere and less deformable. The number of circulating dense cells decreases markedly during a sickle painful episode (Chapter 25). Their increase in the prodromic phase of painful episodes and their scarcity during the episode have been suggested to track an initial event of sickle cell adhesion (increasing initially the number of dense cells) followed by a reduction in dense cells, owing to their trapping in areas bedecked by adherent sickle cells. Studies of the kinetics of sickling in different density classes of sickle cells have not been conducted, apart from some work in sickle transgenic mice. Understanding the different effect of shear stresses on each class of sickle cells and having a complete picture of the impact of the kinetics of polymerization on rheology would fill a significant gap in present understanding.

In red cells, most polymerization occurs in the presence of other, nonpolymerizing components. The kinetics of the gelation of hemoglobin mixtures has been studied in vitro, and, as expected from the sharp sensitivity of the delay time to solution conditions, the delay time of mixtures is strongly sensitive to the fraction of hemoglobin mixtures (Fig. 23.21). This has not yet been successfully analyzed by the double nucleation description in a quantitative way because of the difficulties in assigning nonideality contributions to the heterogeneous part (i.e., the precise value and dependence of Γ in Equation 21). Progress is vital in this area because of the significant effects seen in therapies that augment HbF levels. Similarly, the description of polymerization in the presence of oxygen also depends on having a solid description of the nonideality effects of R-structure molecules unlike the case of mixtures, although there is no database for partially liganded kinetics because such conditions are difficult to characterize and maintain.

Although polymer formation is central to the disease, the relative importance of events following polymer formation is unknown; some of these events are discussed in the preceding three chapters. Polymerization kinetics prevents most cells from sickling that would otherwise do so (Mozzarelli et al., 1987). A red cell takes only a few seconds in the movement from arteries to veins and 15 seconds to reach the lungs. From the range of delay times shown in Figure 23.9, not all cells will have even reached a tenth of the reaction in their passage through the smaller vessels, nor even in the overall transit between successive oxygenation cycles. This argument can be made more quantitatively. Morphologic examination of arterial blood in sickle cell anemia shows that about 10 percent of the circulating cells are sickled, and this is in reasonable agreement with equilibrium analysis that estimates about 5 percent sickle cells. On the other side of the capillaries, the mixed venous return shows about 20 percent sickled cells, in dramatic contrast to the expected equilibrium values of more than 90 percent sickled cells at such pressures (Mozzarelli et al., 1987). Polymer formation kinetics clearly has a pivotal role in determining which cells are eligible for potentially occlusive sickling. Another way of seeing this is to consider the difference between sickle cell trait and sickle cell disease. In a 50:50 mixture of HbA and HbS, the solubility increases by 36 percent to about 24 g/dL, still leaving most of the cells able to sickle (Sunshine et al., 1979). On the other hand, the delay times increase by 10^5 (Fig. 23.21), which is consistent with the asymptomatic nature of sickle cell trait (Chapter 29). A dramatic illustration of the effects of HbF on delay time is provided by hydroxyurea therapy in sickle cell anemia (Chapter 38). In a study of the kinetics of gelation in treated patients, the mean delay time increased nearly fourfold in the first 12 weeks and another twofold in the second 12 weeks of treatment, at which point it was only about twofold shorter than in HbSC disease patients (Bridges et al., 1996).

Because of the profound sensitivity of the kinetics to intracellular concentration, the volume of the erythrocyte is another variable to consider. One hallmark of sickle cell anemia is the heterogeneity of red cell composition and density (Chapters 20 through 22). F cells (Chapter 9) have different HbF concentrations and may have little or no tendency to sickle. Reticulocytes with a low mean cell hemoglobin concentration (MCHC) tend to have less polymer and form single polymer domains. Other sickle cells with normal MCHC tend to sickle with multiple domains. Sickle cells that are biconcave cells with higher density when oxygenated (also known as intermediate high density) tend to have polymer in multiple domains. Finally, the very high density cells, which include irreversibly sickle cells, change very little with deoxygenation, because in spite of abundant polymer, the cell may not deform because the domains are individually too small owing to the extraordinarily high initial concentration.

Chapters 27 and 28 describe the effects of volume changes on HbS polymer associated with HbC and HbS Oman. Individuals with sickle cell trait are well, whereas patients with HbSC disease can be symptomatic. HbC decreases the volume of most HbSC disease red cells, increasing MCHC and the concentration of both HbS and HbC (Bunn et al., 1982). In HbS Oman carriers, levels of this variant are between 11 and 22 percent and the cells are dense, reminiscent of the HbC effect. Individuals with higher expression of HbS Oman were symptomatic and had more dense cells. The c_{SAT} of HbS Oman was 11 g/dL, which establishes a prosickling effect of the second mutation compared with typical values of 16 to 17 g/dL for HbS. Still, the c_{SAT} of HbS Oman is the same as the c_{SAT} of HbS Antilles, and patients heterozygous for HbS Antilles with more than 40 percent of this variant had the same intensity of disease as HbS Oman patients with about half the concentration of variant. The suspicion was then that the second mutation had a further pathogenic effect. Patients homozygous for HbO Arabia, which has the $\beta 121$ Glu$\rightarrow$Lys present in HbS Oman, had red cells with densities similar to homozygotes for HbC. This suggested that patients

with HbS Oman with 22 percent abnormal hemoglobin are sick because the second mutation decreases the c_{SAT} in addition to increasing the MCHC.

The physiological problems arising from sickle hemoglobin polymerization derive in some way from vasoocclusion, itself a consequence, in part, of the rigidity of a polymerized mass of hemoglobin. How do the kinetics of polymer formation or the extent of polymerization affect the cells rigidity? Studies on the viscosity of gels and cell suspensions are available, but key studies are still lacking. The major difficulty is that polymerization generates domains, and sickle cells may be dominated by single domain conditions. It is well known from the rheology of mixtures that the viscosity of an inhomogeneous sample will be dominated by the softer medium. A cell suspension could be dominated by the effects of the cells sliding past each other and be insensitive to the rigidity of individual cells. Similarly, a macroscopic gel could be dominated by interdomain effects that would be different or absent in a single erythrocyte. Until these issues are resolved, trying to reconcile the physiologic effects with rheology studies is difficult. Likewise, there is simply no information by which one might correlate the microstructure of the gel with its deformability. The dramatic differences that are possible can be seen when gels are formed while the solution is stirred. The stirred gel remains fluid, despite being in the same thermodynamic state (i.e., same amount of polymer) as the unstirred gel. Although these cases are extreme, they underscore the dependence of deformability on the manner in which gels are formed.

In contrast to the lack of information on the relationship between the state of oxygenation of sickle cells and their in vivo flow behavior, an extensive body of literature exists on the in vitro characterization of the effect of hemoglobin polymer on the rheology of sickle red cells. Mozzarelli et al. (1987) observed that even small amounts of polymer will cause cells to change their shape, although the rheologic consequences of the small amount of polymers needed for deformation has not been established. On the other hand, Nash et al. (1986) observed an exponential increase in the resistance to aspiration into pipettes as oxygen partial pressure decreased for cells showing morphologic evidence of gelation, most likely due to increasing polymer concentration at greater degrees of deoxygenation. In fractionated cells, Mackie and Hochmuth (1990) observed an increase in rigidity that corresponded well to the concentration of polymerized hemoglobin. Presently, no simple criterion exists with which to calibrate the importance of a given degree of cell rigidity. Nash (1991) noted that immature malarial parasites can continue to circulate despite the significant loss in deformability they cause. Nash argued that therefore substantial changes in deformability are required to compromise circulation, perhaps because of shunting that occurs in the circulation, by passing the capillary bed.

The Red Cell Membrane

Another long-standing question has been the role of the red cell membrane in promoting HbS polymerization. This question was addressed most thoroughly by a set of careful experiments by Bunn and co-workers, who added membrane components to HbS solutions and observed no effects of the membrane on the delay time (Goldberg et al., 1981). It is possible that intact membranes and intact cytoskeleton, not necessarily present in the membrane preparations, might act differently. Sickle cell ghosts, particularly those prepared from dense sickle cells, have globin and hemoglobin attached to the membrane.

However, the greatest weakness of the membrane studies involves the distinction between the homogeneous and heterogeneous process, which was not understood in 1981. The delay time, which was the measured parameter, is most strongly influenced by exponential growth rate B, which in turn contains the heterogeneous nucleation rate. The delay time is more weakly affected by the homogeneous nucleation process. The effects of membrane components would be presumably to overwhelm normal homogeneous nucleation with membrane-induced nucleation from which domains would subsequently grow. (For example, as shown in Figure 23.20, a single nucleation event would outstrip homogeneous nucleation in the low density cells, even though in high density cells the effect would be absent.) Even though homogeneous nucleation might become less significant than membrane-induced nucleation, most polymers would still be formed by heterogeneous nucleation. Therefore, the majority of polymer formation would be unaffected in a bulk experiment, and the stochastic delay could be abolished in a significant number of cases. Consequently, in red cells where the stochastic delay may be much more pronounced, the effects of its abolition might be profound. If the stochastic delay thereby shortens to less than the capillary transit, vasoocclusion could occur.

On the other hand, the single cell experiments of Coletta et al. (1982) show that a population of cells had delay times equivalent to plausible concentration distributions, making it unlikely that there could be many membrane nucleation sites. Still, the effects have not been conclusively eliminated or established. Polymerization may interfere with membrane-mediated processes, such as transport. Hemoglobin denatures at interfaces, and HbS denatures differently than HbA (Hirsch et al., 1980). Perhaps at the water-solid interface in the red cells, polymerization is different from in the rest of the cell. Still, the small surface area involved compared with the bulk cytosolic solution of HbS makes this phenomenon irrelevant for overall polymerization, although it could have consequences for the mechanical and functional properties of the membrane that might indirectly affect red cell volume and polymerization rates.

References

Adachi, K and Asakura, T. (1979). Nucleation-controlled aggregation of deoxyhemoglobin S. Possible difference in the size of nuclei in different phosphate concentrations. *J. Biol. Chem.* 254: 7765–7771.

Adachi, K, Kim, J, Travitz, R et al. (1987). Effect of amino acid at the beta 6 position on surface hydrophobicity, stability, solubility, and the kinetics of polymerization of hemoglobin. Comparisons among Hb A (Glu beta 6), Hb C (Lys beta 6), Hb Machida (Gln beta 6), and Hb S (Val beta 6). *J. Biol. Chem.* 262: 12920–12925.

Adachi, K, Konitzer, P, Kim, J et al. (1993). Effect of β-6 aromatic amino acids on polymerization and solubility of recombinant hemoglobins made in yeast. *J. Biol. Chem.* 268: 21650–21656.

Adachi, K, Konitzer, P, Paulraj, G, and Surrey, S. (1994). Role of Leu-beta88 in the hydrophobic acceptor pocket for Val-beta6 during hemoglobin S polymerization. *J. Biol. Chem.* 269: 17477–17480.

Adachi, K, Pang, J, Konitzer, P, and Surrey, S. (1996a). Polymerization of recombinant hemoglobin F γE6V and hemoglobin F γE6V, γQ87T alone, and in mixtures with hemoglobin S. *Blood* 87: 1617–1624.

Adachi, K, Pang, J, Reddy, LR et al. (1996b). Polymerization of three hemoglobin A_2 variants containing val[86] and inhibition of hemoglobin S polymerization by hemoglobin A_2. *J. Biol. Chem.* 271: 24557–24563.

Adachi, K, Rappaport, E, Eck, H et al. (1991). Polymerization and solubility of recombinant hemoglobins $\alpha_2\beta_2$ (6val) HbS and $\alpha_2\beta_2$(6Leu) (HbLeu). *Hemoglobin* 15: 417–430.

Allen, DW and Wyman, J. (1954). Equilibre de l'hemoglobine de drepanocytose avec l'oxygène. *Rev. Hematol.* 9: 155–157.

Basak, S, Ferrone, FA, and Wang, JT. (1988). Kinetics of domain formation by sickle hemoglobin polymers. *Biophys. J.* 54: 829–843.

Baudin-Chich, V, Pagnier, J, Marden, M et al. (1990). Enhanced polymerization of recombinant human deoxyhemoglobin β6 GluIle. *Proc. Natl. Acad. Sci.* 87: 1845–1849.

Behe, MJ and Englander, SW. (1979). Mixed gelation theory. Kinetics, equilibrium and gel incorporation in sickle hemoglobin mixtures. *J. Mol. Biol.* 133: 137–160.

Benesch, RE, Edalji, R, Benesch, R, and Kwong, S. (1980). Solubilization of hemoglobin S by other hemoglobins. *Proc. Natl. Acad. Sci. U.S.A.* 77: 5130–5134.

Bihoreau, MT, Baudin, V, Marden, M et al. (1992). Steric and hydrophobic determinants of the solubilities of recombinant sickle cell hemoglobins. *Protein Sci.* 1: 145–150.

Bishop, MF and Ferrone, FA. (1984). Kinetics of nucleation controlled polymerization: A perturbation treatment for use with a secondary pathway. *Biophys. J.* 46: 631–644.

Bluemke, DA, Carragher, B, and Josephs, R. (1988). The reconstruction of helical particles with variable pitch. *Ultramicroscopy* 26: 255–270.

Bookchin, RM, Nagel, RL, and Ranney, HM. (1967). Structure and properties of hemoglobin C Harlem: A human hemoglobin variant with amino acid substitution in two residues of the α-polypeptide chain. *J. Biol. Chem.* 242: 248–255.

Bookchin, RM, Nagel, RL, and Ranney, HM. (1970). The effect of α^{73Asn} on the interactions of sickling hemoglobins. *Biochem. Biophys. Acta* 221: 373–380.

Bookchin, RM, Ueda, Y, Nagel, RL, and Landau, LC. (1978). Functional abnormalities of whole blood in sickle cell anemia. In Caughey, WS, editor. *Biochemical and clinical aspects of hemoglobin abnormalities*. New York: Academic Press.

Bookchin, R, Balazs, T, Wang, Z et al. (1999). Polymer structure and solubility of deoxyhemoglobin S in the presence of high concentrations of volume-excluding 70-kDa dextran. *J. Biol. Chem.* 274: 6689–6697.

Bookchin, RM, Balazs, T, and Lew, VL. (1994). Measurement of the hemoglobin concentration in deoxyhemoglobin S polymers and characterization of the polymer water compartment. *J. Mol. Biol.* 244: 100–109.

Bridges, KG, Barabino, G, Brugnara, C et al. (1996). A multiparameter analysis of sickle erythrocytes in patients undergoing hydroxyurea therapy. *Blood* 88: 4701–4710.

Briehl RW. (1995). Nucleation, fiber growth, and melting, and domain formation and structure in sickle cell hemoglobin gels. *J. Mol. Biol.* 245: 710–723.

Briehl, RW and Salhany, JM. (1975). Gelation of sickle hemoglobin. III. Nitrosyl hemoglobin. *J. Mol. Biol.* 96: 733–743.

Bromberg PA and Jensen WN. (1967). Arterial oxygen unsaturation in sickle cell disease. *Am Rev Respir Dis.* 96: 400–407.

Bunn, HF. (1972). The interaction of sickle hemoglobin with DPG, CO_2 and with other hemoglobins: Formation of asymmetrical hybrids. In G. Brewer, ed., *Hemoglobin and red cell structure and function*. New York: Plenum.

Bunn, HF, Noguchi, CT, Hofrichter, J et al. (1982). Molecular and cellular pathogenesis of hemoglobin SC disease. *Proc. Natl. Acad. Sci. U.S.A.* 79: 7527–7531.

Cao, Z and Ferrone, FA. (1996). A 50th order reaction predicted and observed for sickle hemoglobin nucleation. *J. Mol. Biol.* 256: 219–222.

Cao, Z and Ferrone, FA. (1997). Homogeneous nucleation in sickle hemoglobin. Stochastic measurements with a parallel method. *Biophys. J.* 72: 343–352.

Cao, Z, Liao, D, Mirchev, R et al. (1997). Nucleation and polymerization of sickle hemoglobin with Leu β 88 substituted by Ala. *J. Mol. Biol.* 265: 580–589.

Carragher, B, Bluemke, DA, Gabriel, B et al. (1988). Structural analysis of polymers of sickle cell hemoglobin. I. Sickle hemoglobin fibers. *J. Mol. Biol.* 199: 315–331.

Cheethan RC, Huehns ER, and Rosemeyer MA. (1979). Participation of haemoglobins A, F, AZ, and C in polymerisation of haemoglobin. *S. J. Mol. Biol.* 129: 45–61.

Cho, MR and Ferrone, FA. (1991). Monomer diffusion and polymer alignment in domains of sickle hemoglobin. *Biophys. J.* 63: 205–214.

Christoph GW, Hofrichter J, and Eaton WA. (1990). Optical morphology and nucleation of sickle hemoglobin gels. *Biophys J* 57: 237a.

Coletta, M, Hofrichter, J, Ferrone, FA, and Eaton, WA. (1982). Kinetics of sickle haemoglobin polymerization in single red cells. *Nature* 300: 194–197.

Crepeau, RH, Edelstein, SJ, Szalay, M et al. (1981). Sickle cell hemoglobin fiber structure altered by α-chain mutation. *Proc. Natl. Acad. Sci. U.S.A.* 78: 1406–1410.

Cretegny, I and Edelstein, SJ. (1993). Double strand packing in hemoglobin S fibers. *J. Mol. Biol.* 230: 733–738.

Dou, Q and Ferrone, FA. (1993). Simulated formation of polymer domains in sickle hemoglobin. *Biophys. J.* 65: 2068–2077.

Dykes, G, Crepeau, RH, and Edelstein, SJ. (1978). Three dimensional reconstruction of the fibres of sickle cell haemoglobin. *Nature* 272: 506–510.

Dykes, GW, Crepeau, RH, and Edelstein, SJ. (1979). Three dimensional reconstruction of 14-filament fibers of hemoglobin S. *J. Mol. Biol.* 130: 451–472.

Eaton, WA and Hofrichter, J. (1978). Successes and failures of a simple nucleation theory for sickle cell hemoglobin gelation. In W.S. Caughey, ed., pp 443–457 *Biochemical and clinical aspects of hemoglobin abnormalities*. New York: Academic Press.

Eaton, WA and Hofrichter, J. (1990). Sickle cell hemoglobin polymerization. *Adv. Protein Chem.* 40: 63–280.

Fabry, ME, Benjamin, L, Lawrence, C, and Nagel, RL. (1984). An objective sign in painful crisis in sickle cell anemia: The concomitant reduction of high density red cells. *Blood* 64: 559–563.

Ferrone, FA, Hofrichter, J, and Eaton, WA. (1985a). Kinetics of sickle hemoglobin polymerization II: A double nucleation mechanism. *J. Mol. Biol.* 183: 611–631.

Ferrone, FA, Hofrichter, J, and Eaton, WA. (1985b). Kinetics of sickle hemoglobin polymerization. I. Studies using temperature-jump and laser photolysis techniques. *J. Mol. Biol.* 183: 591–610.

Ferrone, FA, Hofrichter, J, Sunshine, H, and Eaton, WA. (1980). Kinetic studies on photolysis-induced gelation of sickle cell hemoglobin suggest a new mechanism. *Biophys. J.* 32: 361–377.

Gill, S, Benedict, RC, Fall, L et al. (1979). Oxygen binding to sickle cell hemoglobin. *J. Mol. Biol.* 130: 175–189.

Gill, S, Spokane, R, Benedict, RC et al. (1980). Ligand-linked phase equilibria of sickle cell hemoglobin. *J. Mol. Biol.* 140: 299–312.

Goldberg, MA, Husson, MA, and Bunn, HF. (1977). Participation of hemoglobins A and F in the polymerization of sickle hemoglobin. *J. Biol. Chem.* 252: 3414–3421.

Goldberg, MA, Lalos, AT, and Bunn, HF. (1981). The effect of erythrocyte membrane perparations on the polymerization of sickle hemoglobin. *J. Biol. Chem.* 256: 193–197.

Greenberg, MS and Kass, EH. (1958). Studies on the destruction of red blood cells: XIII: Observations on the role of pH in the pathogenesis and treatment of painful crisis in sickle cell disease. *Arch. Intern. Med.* 101: 355–363.

Harrington, DL, Adachi, K, and Royer Jr., WE. (1997). The high resolution crystal structure of deoxyhemoglobin S. *J. Mol. Biol.* 272: 398–407.

Hentschke, R and Herzfeld, J. (1991). Theory of nematic order with aggregate dehydration for reversibly assembling proteins in concentrated solutions: Application to sickle-cell hemoglobin polymers. *Phys. Rev.* 43: 7019–7030.

Himanen, J-P, Mirza, UA, Chait, BT et al. (1996). A recombinant sickle hemoglobin triple mutant with independent inhibitory effects on polymerization. *J. Biol. Chem.* 271: 25152–25156.

Himanen, J-P, Schneider, K, Chait, B, and Manning, JM. (1995). Participation and strength of interaction of lysine 95 beta in the polymerization of hemoglobin S as determined by its site-directed substitution by isoleucine. *J. Biol. Chem.* 270: 13885–13891.

Hirsch, RE, Elbaum, D, Brody, SS, and Nagel, RL. (1980). Oxyhemoglobin A and oxyhemoglobin S films at a water/air interface. Absorption spectral studies. *J. Colloid Interface Sci.* 78: 212–216.

Hirsch, RE, Juszczak, LJ, Fataliev, NA et al. (1999). Solution-active structural alterations in liganded hemoglobin C (β6 GluLys) and S (β6 Glu Val). *J. Biol. Chem.* 274: 13777–13782.

Ho, C, Wills, BF, Shen, TJ et al. (1996). Roles of α114 and β87 amino acid residues in the polymerization of hemoglobin S: Implications for gene therapy. *J. Mol. Biol.* 263: 475–485.

Hofrichter J. (1979). Ligand binding and the gelation of sickle cell hemoglobin. *J. Mol. Biol.* 128: 335–369.

Hofrichter, J. (1986). Kinetics of sickle hemoglobin polymerization III. Nucleation rates determined from stochastic fluctuations in polymerization progress curves. *J. Mol. Biol.* 189: 553–571.

Hofrichter, J, Ross, PD, and Eaton, WA. (1974). Kinetics and mechanism of deoxyhemoglobin S gelation: A new approach to understanding sickle cell disease. *Proc. Natl. Acad. Sci. U.S.A.* 71: 4864–4868.

Hofrichter, J, Ross, PD, and Eaton WA. (1976). Supersaturation in sickle cell hemoglobin solutions. *Proc. Natl. Acad. Sci. U.S.A.* 73: 3035–3039.

Jandl, JH, Simmons, RL, and Castle, WB. (1961). Red cell filtration and the pathogenesis of certain hemolytic anemias. *Blood.* 28: 133–148.

Kahn, PC and Briehl, RW. (1982). The absence of volume change in the gelation of hemoglobin-S. *J. Biol. Chem.* 257: 12209–12213.

Kaul, D, Nagel, RL, Chen, D, and Tsai, H-M. (1993). 'Sickle erythrocyte-endothelial interactions in microcirculation: The role of von Willebrand factor and implications for vasoocclusion.' *Blood* 81: 2429–2438.

Kaul, DK, Fabry, ME, Constantini, F et al. (1995). In vivo demonstration of red cell endothelial interaction, sickling and altered microvascular response to oxygen in the sickle transgenic mouse. *J. Clin. Invest.* 96: 2845–2853.

Lesecq, S, Baudin, V, Kister, J et al. (1997). Functional studies and polymerization of recombinant hemoglobin Glu-α2β26(A3)Val/Glu-7(A4) Ala. *J. Biol. Chem.* 271: 17211–17214.

Li, X, Mirza, UA, Chait, BT, and Manning, JM. (1997). Systematic enhancement of polymerization of recombinant sickle hemoglobin mutants: Implications for transgenic mouse model for sickle cell anemia. *Blood* 90: 4620–4627.

Liao, D, Martin de Llano, JJ, Himanen, J-P et al. (1996). Solubility of sickle hemoglobin measured by a kinetic micromethod. *Biophys. J.* 70: 2442–2447.

Mackie, LH and Hochmuth, RM. (1990). The influence of oxygen tesnion, temperature and hemoglobin concentration on the rheologic properties of sickle erythrocytes. *Blood* 76: 1256–1261.

Manning, L, Jenkins, WT, Hess, JR et al. (1996). Subunit dissociations in natural and recombinant hemoglobins. *Protein Sci.* 5: 775–781.

Martin de Llano, JJ and Manning, JM. (1994). Properties of a recombinant human hemoglobin double mutant: Sickle hemoglobin with Leu-88 beta at the primary aggregation site substituted by Ala. *Protein Sci.* 3: 1206–1212.

Martin de Llano, JJ, Schneewind, O, Stetler, G, and Manning, JM. (1993). Recombinant human sickle hemoglobin expressed in yeast. *Proc. Natl. Acad. Sci. U.S.A.* 90: 918–922.

McCune, SL, Reilly, MP, Chomo, MJ et al. (1994). Recombinant human hemoglobins designed for gene therapy of sickle cell disease. *Proc. Natl. Acad. Sci. U.S.A.* 91: 9852–9856.

McDade, WA, Carragher, B, Miller CA, and Josephs, R. (1989). On the assembly of sickle hemoglobin fascicles. *J. Mol. Biol.* 206: 637–649.

McDade, WA and Josephs, R. (1993). On the formation and crystallization of sickle hemoglobin macrofibers. *J. Struct. Biol.* 110: 90–97.

Minton, AP. (1975). Thermodynamic analysis of the chemical inhibition of sickle cell hemoglobin gelation. *J. Mol. Biol.* 95: 289–307.

Minton, AP. (1977). Non-ideality and the thermodynamics of sickle-cell hemoglobin gelation. *J. Mol. Biol.* 100: 519–542.

Minton, AP. (1998). Molecular crowding: Analysis of effects of high concentrations of inert cosolutes on biochemical equilibria and rates in terms of volume exclusion. *Methods Enzymolo.* 295: 127–149.

Mirchev, R and Ferrone, FA. (1997). The structural origin of heterogeneous nucleation and polymer cross linking in sickle hemoglobin. *J. Mol. Biol.* 265: 475–479.

Mozzarelli, A, Hofrichter, J, and Eaton, WA. (1987). Delay time of hemoglobin S polymerization prevents most cells from sickling. *Science* 237: 500–506.

Mozzarelli, A, Rivetti, C, Rossi, GL et al. (1991). Crystals of haemoglobin with the T quarternary structure bind oxygen noncooperatively with no Bohr effect. *Nature* 351: 416–419.

Mu, X-Q, Makowski, L, and Magdoff-Fairchild, B. (1998). Analysis of the stability of hemoglobin S double strands. *Biophys. J.* 74: 655–668.

Nagel, RL and Bookchin, RM. (1975). Mechanism of hemoglobin S gelation. Structural restrictions to supramolecular models of the polymerization of hemoglobin S. In Levere, RD, editor. *Sickle cell anemia and other hemoglobinopathies.* New York: Academic Press.

Nagel, RL and Bookchin, RM. (1977). Studies on the supramolecular structure of the hemoglobin S polymer. In *Molecular interactions of hemoglobin.* INSERM Vol. 70

Nagel, RL and Bookchin, RM. (1978). Areas of interaction in the HbS polymer. In Caughey, WS, editor. *Biochemical and clinical aspects of hemoglobin abnormalities.* New York: Academic Press.

Nagel, R, Bookchin, R, Johnson, J et al. (1979). Structural bases of the inhibitory effects of hemoglobin F and hemoglobin A2 on the polymerization of hemoglobin S. *Proc. Natl. Acad. Sci. U.S.A.* 76: 670–672.

Nagel, RL, Johnson, J, Bookchin, RM et al. (1980). α-Chain contact sites in the hemoglobin S polymer. *Nature* 283: 832–834.

Nash, G, Johnson, CJ, and Meiselman, HJ. (1986). Influence of oxygen tension on the viscoelastic behavior of red blood cells in sickle cell disease. *Blood* 67: 110–118.

Nash, GB. (1991). Red cell mechanics: What changes are needed to adversely affect in vivo circulation? *Biorheology* 28: 231–239.

Nozaki, Y and Tanford, C. (1971). The solubility of amino acids and two glycine peptides in aqueous ethanol and dioxane solutions. *J. Biol. Chem.* 246: 2211–2217.

Padlan, EA and Love, WE. (1985a). Refined crystal structure of deoxyhemoglobin S I. Restrained least squares refinement at 3.0 A resolution. *J. Biol. Chem.* 260: 8272–8279.

Padlan, EA and Love, WE. (1985b). Refined crystal structure of deoxyhemoglobin S. II. Molecular interactions in the crystal. *J. Biol. Chem.* 260: 8280–8291.

Pennelly, RR and Noble, RW. (1978). Functional identity of hemoglobins S and A in the absence of polymerization. In W.S. Caughey, ed, *Biochemical and clinical aspects of hemoglobin abnormalities.* New York: Academic Press, pp. 401–411.

Perella, M, Benazzi, L, Shea MA, and Ackers, GK. (1990). Subunit hybridization studies of partially ligated cyanomethemoglobins using a cryogenic method. *Biophys. Chem.* 35: 97–103.

Poillon, WN and Bertles, JF. (1979). Deoxygenated sickle hemoglobin. *J. Biol. Chem.* 254: 3462–3467.

Poillon, WN and Kim, BC. (1990). 2,3-diphosphoglycerate and intracellular pH as interdependent determinants of the physiologic solubility of deoxyhemoglobin S. *Blood* 76: 1028–1036.

Prouty, MS, Schechter, AN, and Parsegian, VA. (1985). Chemical potential measurements of deoxyhemoglobin S polymerization. *J. Mol. Biol.* 184: 517–528.

Reddy, LR, Reddy, KS, Surrey, S, and Adachi, K. (1997). Role of β87 Thr in the β6 Val acceptor site during deoxy Hb S polymerization. *Biochemistry* 36: 15992–15998.

Ross, PD, Hofrichter, J, and Eaton, WA. (1977). Thermodynamics of gelation of sickle cell deoxyhemoglobin. *J. Mol. Biol.* 115: 111–134.

Rossi-Bernardi L, Luzzana M, Samaja M et al. (1975). The functional properties of sickle cell blood. *FEBS Lett* 59: 15–9

Roth, EFJ, Bookchin, RM, and Nagel, RL. (1979). Deoxyhemoglobin S gelation and insolubility at high ionic strength are distinct phenomena. *J. Lab. Clin. Med.* 93: 867–871.

Samuel, R, Guzman, A, and Briehl, R. (1993). Hemoglobin S polymerization and gelation under shear II. The joint concentration and shear dependence of kinetics. *Blood* 82: 3474–3481.

Samuel, RE, Salmon, ED, and Briehl, RW. (1990). Nucleation and growth of fibres and gel formation in sickle cell haemoglobin. *Nature* 345: 833–835.

Seakins M, Gibbs WN, Milner PF, and Bertles JF. (1973). Erythrocyte Hb-S concentration. An important factor in the low oxygen affinity of blood in sickle cell anemia. J Clin Invest 52: 422–32

Skalak, R. (1969). Deformation of red cells in capillaries. *Science* 164: 717–719.

Sunshine, HR, Hofrichter, J, and Eaton, WA. (1979). Gelation of sickle cell hemoglobin in mixtures with normal adult and fetal hemoglobins. *J. Mol. Biol.* 133: 435–467.

Sunshine, HR, Hofrichter, J, Ferrone, FA, and Eaton, WA. (1982). Oxygen binding by sickle cell hemoglobin polymers. *J. Mol. Biol.* 158: 251–273.

Szabo, A. (1988). Fluctuations in the polymerization of sickle hemoglobin: A simple analytical model. *J. Mol. Biol.* 199: 539–542.

Ueda, Y, Nagel, RL, and Bookchin, RM. (1979). An increased Bohr effect in sickle cell anemia. *Blood* 53: 472–480.

Watowich, SJ, Gross, LJ, and Josephs, R. (1993). Analysis of the intermolecular contacts within sickle hemoglobin fibers: Effect of site-specific substitutions, fiber pitch and double-strand disorder. *J. Struct. Biol.* 111: 161–179.

Watowich, SJ, Gross, LJ, and Josephs, RJ. (1989). Intramolecular contacts within sickle hemoglobin fibers. *J. Mol. Biol.* 209: 821–828.

Wellems, TE, Vassar, RJ, and Josephs, R. (1981). Polymorphic assemblies of double strands of sickle cell hemoglobin. Manifold pathways of deoxyhemoglobin S crystallization. *J. Mol. Biol.* 13: 1011–1026.

Winslow RM. (1997). Blood oxygen equilibrium studies in sickle cell anemia, pp. 235–55. Monograph (PMID: 13105, UI: 77094898).

Winslow RM, Morrissey JM, Berger RL, Smith PD, Gibson CC (1978). Variability of oxygen affinity of normal blood: an automated method of measurement. J Appl Physiol 45: 289–97

Wishner, BC, Ward, KB, Lattman EE, and Lover, WE. (1975). Crystal structure of sickle-cell deoxyhemoglobin at 5 Å resolution. *J. Mol. Biol.* 98: 179–194.

24

Clinical Aspects of Sickle Cell Anemia in Adults and Children

KWAKU OHENE-FREMPONG
MARTIN H. STEINBERG

Sickle-shaped red cells—named by the Chicago physician, J. B. Herrick in 1910 after examining the blood of an anemic dental student from Grenada—were the first hint in Western medical literature for the existence of sickle cell disease (Herrick, 1910). Of course, the inherited nature of sickle cell disease and its symptoms and signs had been recognized in tropical Africa for generations (Konotey-Ahulu, 1974; Ohene-Frempong and Nkrumah, 1994). Herrick withheld publishing his observations for six years as he tried to connect his patients' constellation of signs and symptoms with these peculiar misshapen blood cells and to find additional similar cases. Curiously, although located in the center of Chicago with its burgeoning black population, Herrick, an expert microscopist, never saw another similar case (Savitt and Goldberg, 1989). This may have occurred because of the demographics of his practice and a change in the focus of his interests (Herrick also linked coronary occlusion to myocardial infarction. Sickled cells could arise from "normal" cells as Emmel (1917) reported when he noted that all erythrocytes from an anemic patient sickled in a sealed preparation of fresh blood as did normal-appearing cells of the nonanemic father. Mason (1922) first attached the name *sickle cell anemia* to the clinical and hematologic entity that by now had been reported at least four times in North America. Hahn and Gillespie (1927) confirmed that sickling was oxygen-dependent and reversible and that

almost 10 percent of African Americans had red cells that sickled when deoxygenated. Beet (1949) and Neel (1951) defined the genetics of sickle hemoglobinopathies after Pauling and colleagues (1949) made the electrophoretic identification of HbS and observed that patients with sickle cell anemia had only HbS in their erythrocytes although their parents with sickle cell trait had both normal and sickle hemoglobin. Ingram (1956) found the single amino acid difference that distinguished the sickle β-globin chain from normal. Early historical milestones in the study of sickle cell disease have been summarized by Conley (1980), Serjeant (1992), and Ranney (1994) and are discussed in greater detail in Chapters 1 and 26. Since Ingrams' discovery, progress in understanding the pathophysiology of sickle cell disease and devising an effective treatment has been rapid. But, as discussed elsewhere in this volume, we neither understand completely how HbS leads to the many features of sickle cell disease nor have a simple curative treatment.

Imprecision in defining sickle hemoglobinopathies has permeated the medical literature. Sickle cell disease is a phenotype with distinctive but variable clinical and hematologic features. At least half the hemoglobin present in sickle cell disease is HbS. Sickle cell trait should not be considered a type of sickle cell disease because it is clinically benign (Chapter 29). Among the genotypes that result in sickle cell disease are homozygosity for the HbS mutation, or, sickle cell anemia; compound heterozygosity for HbS and HbC, or, HbSC disease; compound heterozygosity for HbS and β thalassemia, or, Hb S-β thalassemia; and other less common compound heterozygous disorders discussed in Chapter 28. Whenever possible, a diagnosis of sickle cell disease should be assigned by its genotype because this designation allows the best assessment of prognosis, and only a genotypically based diagnosis permits accurate genetic counseling.

"To know syphilis is to know medicine." This popular aphorism of nineteenth century physicians might today be applied to sickle cell disease. The breadth of its clinical and laboratory manifestations and its multitudinous complications present challenges to the pediatrician, internist, general surgeon, obstetrician, orthopedist, ophthalmologist, psychiatrist, and subspecialists in each of these disciplines. This chapter discusses the features of sickle cell anemia from the newborn to the older adult and includes a general approach to diagnosis and treatment.

Just as globin genes switch their expression during development (Chapter 7), the features of sickle cell anemia change as life advances. In the first decade of life, the switch from fetal to adult hemoglobin gene

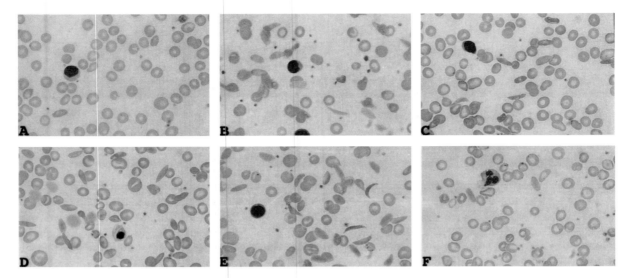

Figure 24.1. Blood films in patients with sickle cell anemia and average or low HbF levels. HbF in these patients are **A**, 0.5 percent; **B**, 1 percent; **C**, 4 percent; **D**, 5 percent; **E**, 7 percent; and **F**, 10 percent. Patients **C** and **F** were taking hydroxyurea. Although some of these patients have more irreversibly sickled cells than patients depicted in Figure 24.2 who have high HbF concentrations, note that patient **A** with the lowest HbF level has very few sickled cells. For full color reproduction, see color plate 24.1

expression underlies the clinical transmutation. Life's first decade is typified by acute problems—high risks of severe life-threatening infection, acute chest syndrome, splenic sequestration, and stroke. Pain is the torment of adolescence. If the worst of childhood and adolescent problems are survived or escaped, young adulthood can be a time of relative clinical quiescence, but vascular damage need not necessarily take a holiday. Chronic organ damage—renal failure, pulmonary deterioration, late effects of previous cerebrovascular disease—becomes paramount in the older adult. Sickle cell anemia is noted for its clinical heterogeneity. Any patient can have nearly all known disease complications; some have almost none but die with a sudden acute problem; some skip one or more phases of the disease but suffer intensely from others. The course of disease can be truncated, lasting two decades or less rather than the five decades now expected in more developed lands, and the spectrum of disease varies throughout the world (Chapter 33).

LABORATORY DIAGNOSIS

Diagnosing sickle cell disease is not difficult; determining the correct genotype can be problematical, especially if family studies and access to molecular diagnostic methods are not available. Examining parents or siblings of affected patients is the least costly

way of establishing the genotype and can be done with simple combinations of blood counts and quantitative studies of hemoglobin fractions. Typical blood counts and hemoglobin studies in different sickle hemoglobinopathies are shown in Tables 28.2 and 28.4.

Blood Counts and Erythrocyte Indices

In sickle cell anemia, the erythrocytes are normocytic or macrocytic, depending on the height of the reticulocyte count and the presence or absence of confounding conditions such as iron or folic acid deficiency. Microcytosis in a suspected case of sickle cell anemia can be seen early in life before erythropoiesis has fully matured, when iron deficiency has developed, or when β thalassemia or α thalassemia is present. HbS-β^0 thalassemia and sickle cell are addressed in Chapter 28. These two conditions are much alike hematologically and clinically, and distinguishing one from the other is difficult. They cannot be separated on the basis of hemoglobin studies or blood counts alone. Hematologic overlap of HbS-β^0 thalassemia and sickle cell anemia-α thalassemia with sickle cell anemia further emphasizes the importance of family studies. Methods of measuring red cell indices and blood counts are considered in Chapter 34.

Blood Films

Sickled cells—the "peculiar" erythrocytes reported by Herrick—are nearly always seen in sickle cell anemia and HbS-β^0 thalassemia but are less common in other forms of sickle cell disease. Typical blood films from patients with sickle cell anemia with high, average, and low HbF concentrations are shown in Figures 24.1 and 24.2. Reflective, in a sense, of the heterogeneity of the disease, some patients have large num-

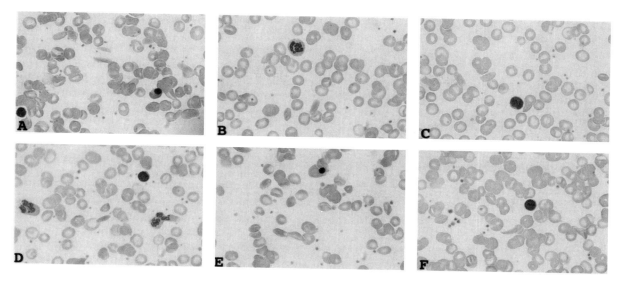

Figure 24.2. Blood films in patients with sickle cell anemia and high HbF levels. HbF in these six patients are A, 19 percent; B, 18 percent; C, 19 percent; D, 21 percent; E, 20 percent; and F, 23 percent. All patients were receiving hydroxyurea. All still have sickled cells in the blood, and these are particularly prominent in patient A. Also note nucleated red cells in A and E. For full color reproduction, see color plate 24.2

bers of irreversibly sickled cells (ISCs), nucleated red cells, Howell-Jolly bodies, and polychromatophilic cells, whereas others display far fewer of these cells. In adults, ISCs remain relatively constant over time, although their percentage does rise early in the course of a painful episode (Ballas and Smith, 1992).

Detecting HbS and Measuring Hemoglobin Fractions

Neonatal diagnosis is discussed in Chapter 36. From neonatal life onwards through early adult life there is a slow but continual decrease in HbF while HbA$_2$ levels increase until ages 1 to 2 years. However, with few exceptions, the hemoglobin fractions present at age 1 year are sufficiently stable so that they can be relied on for diagnosis. In sickle cell anemia unmodified by treatment with hemoglobin "switching" agents (Chapter 38), HbS nearly always forms more than 80 percent of the hemolysate except in infancy when the γ- to β-globin gene switch is incomplete. HbS can be detected by isoelectric focusing, hemoglobin electrophoresis, or high-performance liquid chromatography (HPLC). Hemoglobin fractions may be measured by elution from cellulose acetate strips and spectrophotometric analysis of the eluted fraction, densitometry of stained and cleared cellulose acetate strips, chromatography on "minicolumns," and HPLC (Tan et al., 1993). Densitometry is unreliable for measuring HbA$_2$ and HbF (Schmidt et al., 1974, 1975) (Chapter

9). HPLC is probably the method of choice for quantitation of the major hemoglobins in the newborn and adults. Capillary isoelectric focusing is a recent modification of thin layer isoelectric focusing where hemoglobins are separated in fine capillary tubes. Available commercial systems allow automated data analysis, require small sample size, are rapid and sensitive, conserve expensive reagents, provide quantitative information, and may soon eclipse conventional HPLC (Hempe and Craver, 1994). Hemoglobin electrophoresis at alkaline pH is inexpensive and provides sharp resolution of hemoglobin bands. To confirm the presence of HbS, an additional complementary method, such as citrate agar gel electrophoresis at pH 6.1, is useful. In this method, most hemoglobins move cathodically from their point of origin and with different relative mobilities than is seen with alkaline electrophoresis Figure 24.3 (Robinson et al., 1957; Schedlbauer and Pass, 1989). Sickle hemoglobin can be detected chemically because it is insoluble and precipitates in high molarity phosphate buffer when reduced with sodium dithionite. Sickle solubility tests have no role as the sole means of detecting HbS because they identify only the presence of HbS, are not quantifiable, and cannot reliably distinguish among sickle cell trait, sickle cell anemia, and HbS-β$^+$ thalassemia. Advantages of HPLC are its excellent resolution of various hemoglobins, automation, and ability to quantify hemoglobin fractions. These methods are discussed in greater detail in Chapter 34.

DNA-based methods of detecting HbS have the advantage of specificity but at present are expensive and not widely used clinically. Rapid methodologic advances coupled with price decreases may soon result in greater use of DNA-based techniques for HbS detection. Methods of DNA diagnosis are covered in detail in Chapter 35. DNA-based diagnosis does not provide information on the levels of HbA$_2$ or HbF, which may help define the genotype and prognosis.

GENERAL CLINICAL FEATURES OF SICKLE CELL ANEMIA

One approach to categorizing the pathophysiologic and clinical features of sickling disorders is to separate these features into those that are a consequence of hemolysis of sickle cells and those that follow vasoocclusive episodes caused by sickle cells (Steinberg, 1999) (Chapters 20 and 21). A reduced erythrocyte life span defines all types of hemolytic anemia. Hemolysis is most often identified with benign complications that are amenable to management. Vasoocclusive disease typifies the sickling disorders, and these problems are difficult to manage and are the major cause of morbidity and mortality. This dichotomy is necessarily an oversimplification, and hemolytic anemia and vasoocclusive disease are linked by the presence of "sticky," short-lived sickle cells and reticulocytes, and perhaps many other elements of the disease (Ranney, 1997).

Hemolysis in sickle cell disease—even in sickle cell anemia—is usually only moderate. Symptoms of anemia per se are not the hallmark of this disease. Plasma volume in sickle cell anemia may be expanded 20 to 40 percent, making it difficult to predict the red cell mass from the hemoglobin level. Most patients tolerate chronic hemoglobin levels of 5 to 7 g/dL exceptionally well. Serum erythropoietin levels in sickle cell anemia have been measured and have been considered inappropriately low for the level of hemoglobin (Sherwood et al., 1986). This may be explained by the right-shifted blood hemoglobin-O$_2$ dissociation curve in sickle cell anemia that enhances the delivery of O$_2$ to tissues and the observation that red cell precursor mass appears to be an independent determinant of erythropoietin levels. An expanded erythroid marrow of sickle cell anemia would offset the reduction in peripheral red cell mass, reducing erythropoietin concentrations (Cazzola et al., 1998). Persistent hyperbilirubinemia, a consequence of hemolysis, is associated with a high prevalence of gallstones. Short-lived red cells also place the patient at risk for acutely developing severe anemia when erythropoiesis is temporarily interrupted by B19 parvovirus infection. Pathophysiologic features of the anemia of sickle cell disease are discussed in detail in Chapter 20. Vasoocclusive events of the sickling disorders occur acutely, producing dramatic clinical findings, or can be chronic but nevertheless, over time, disabling. Failure of vital organs is the aftermath of many years of vasoocclusive disease that often is subclinical.

The following sections describe the clinical features of sickle cell anemia grouped by the age where each complication is paramount. Pathophysiologic elements that are distinctive for each organ or complication are included, but the general features of the pathophysiology of sickle cell anemia are presented in Chapters 20 to 22. Painful episodes, the preeminent symptom of sickle cell anemia, and their management are discussed separately in Chapter 25.

Much of our most reliable information on the clinical course and complications of sickle cell disease in developed countries comes from two large observational studies, one in the United States and the other in Jamaica. In the United States, the Cooperative Study of Sickle Cell Disease (Cooperative Study) has followed nearly 4,000 patients, including a newborn cohort of 694 patients, over 20 years (Gill et al., 1995). Patients in Jamaica, all members of a newborn cohort of more than 300 individuals and their matched controls have been followed even longer (Bainbridge et al., 1985). Both studies have the advan-

Figure 24.3. Electrophoretic separation of hemoglobin in normal individuals (2-AA) and patients with sickle cell trait (3-AS), HbS-β$^+$ thalassemia (4-SA), and sickle cell anemia (5-SS), Hb SC disease (6-SC). Control subjects with hemoglobins A, F, S, and C are also shown (lanes 1 and 7). The left panel shows separation by cellulose acetate electrophoresis at pH 8.6; the center panel, citrate agar gel electrophoresis at pH 6.1; and the right panel, isoelectric focusing using pH 4-9 ampholines. For full color reproduction, see color plate 24.3.

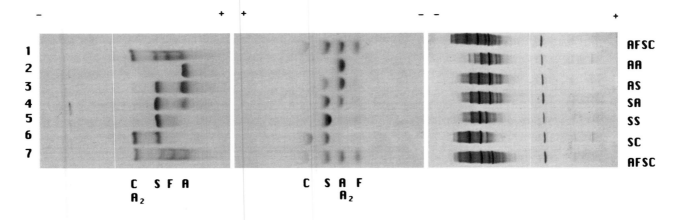

tages of large numbers of patients, contemporaneous controls, longitudinal rather than cross-sectional data, and careful statistical analyses. Cohort studies eliminate the bias of studying only those patients who seek medical care. In the Cooperative Study, in addition to the newborn cohort, a special effort was made to recruit comparatively asymptomatic patients from the community and not to enroll only patients who were regular visitors to the clinic. Neither of these studies were therapeutic trials, although our best studies of the treatment for selected complications of sickle cell anemia grew out of these endeavors. A too common theme that appears continually in the following sections is the lack of controlled clinical trials of treatment in sickle cell anemia. Among the important therapeutic questions that still await answers are these: How should acute chest syndrome be managed—which patients should have exchange transfusion? When will simple transfusion suffice? Can preoperative transfusion sometimes be avoided? Does core decompression of the femoral head retard the advancement of osteonecrosis? Do angiotensin-converting enzyme inhibitors delay sickle nephropathy? Does laser photocoagulation arrest the progression of proliferative retinopathy? When should operative intervention be recommended for priapism? How aggressively should blood pressure be lowered to decrease the chance of stroke (Adams et al., 1992; Styles et al., 1996a; Pegelow et al., 1997; Vichinsky et al., 1997).

Serjeant (1992) and Embury et al. (1994) have provided excellent detailed descriptions of the clinical features of sickle cell disease. It is our intent to summarize recent information about the clinically relevant complications of sickle cell disease and to provide explicit recommendations for treatment. Whenever possible, our recommendations for the management of specific problems are based on the best scientific evidence available. When little or no documentation exists favoring one form of treatment over another, we make this clear and recommend a reasonable way of managing the problem, drawing, if possible, on experience with similar problems in other diseases, data from observational studies, and our knowledge of the pathophysiology of sickle cell disease.

CLINICAL FEATURES OF SICKLE CELL ANEMIA IN DIFFERENT AGE GROUPS

The Neonate

Modern methods make sickle cell disease easily diagnosed in newborns even with their high concentrations of HbF. In the United States and a few other countries, large scale testing of newborns for the pres-

ence of sickle cell disease has been instituted in public health programs (Chapter 36). The prevalence of the various genotypes of sickle cell disease is different in various populations around the world where the disease is common. In the United States, 1 in 400 African-American newborns has some form of sickle cell disease as defined previously. In West and Central Africa, where the disease is most common, approximately 2 percent of all newborns have sickle cell disease. Even with the advent of newborn screening programs for sickle cell disease, most neonates with the disease come to the attention of medical workers only for diagnostic purposes and not because of illness.

At birth and for the first few months of life, children with sickle cell disease usually do not show the typical vasoocclusive complications, probably because of the predominant presence of HbF and F cells. The Cooperative Study reviewed birth outcome and neonatal clinical course of 480 infants with sickle cell disease. Rates of preterm birth (less than 37 weeks), low birth weight (< 2,500 g), and small for gestational age were 9, 10, and 8 percent, respectively, and similar to those in African Americans in general. These figures were similar among the different genotypes of sickle cell disease. However, 59 percent of newborns with sickle cell disease with low birth weight were born at term, compared with 41 percent of all African Americans with low birth weight, a significant difference (Brown et al., 1994).

Although the onset of clinical manifestations of vasoocclusive disease may be delayed, laboratory evidence of the presence of hemolytic disease is present early. Neonatal hyperbilirubinemia has been reported at a higher rate in newborns with sickle cell disease (van Wijgerden, 1983). The prevalence of anemia in newborns with sickle cell disease in the United States is unknown because hemoglobin levels are not measured routinely on term, well-appearing newborns. However, the Jamaican cohort study reported that compared with control neonates, neonates with sickle cell anemia had a lower than normal hemoglobin concentration from as early as age 2 weeks (Serjeant et al., 1981b). In a longitudinal study on the hematologic changes in children with sickle cell disease followed from birth to age 5 years, the Cooperative Study reported that anemia and reticulocytosis were apparent by age 10 weeks in patients with sickle cell anemia (Brown et al., 1994). There are no physical features in a newborn with sickle cell disease that would raise the clinician's suspicion of this diagnosis, which is why screening programs are the most effective way to identify patients before the onset of clinical complications.

Identifying infants who are likely to have severe disease complications would allow more accurate prognosis to be established and distinguish children who might require more intensive treatment and closer observation. Data from the Cooperative Study on 392 infants with sickle cell anemia or HbS-β^0 thalassemia diagnosed before age 6 months with an accumulated 9 years of clinical and laboratory data were analyzed and the analysis validated using data from an additional 115 infants who were observed between ages 6 months and 2 years. Severe outcomes were defined as death, stroke, two or more painful episodes per year for 3 consecutive years, and one or more acute chest events per year for 3 years. Seventeen percent of the newborn cohort were identified as severe. A severe endpoint was achieved at a mean age of 5.6 ± 3.8 years. Several clinical and laboratory parameters were evaluated to determine whether they were associated with severity. Mean steady-state values over the second year of life were used for laboratory parameters. Hemoglobin levels of less than 8 g/dL, leukocyte counts more than 20,000, an episode of dactylitis before age 1 year, and an elevated percentage of pocked red blood cells by age 1 year were significant predictors of adverse outcomes. Combining these risk factors identified a group of forty-one children (10.5 percent of the cohort) with a 0.348 to 0.712 probability of a severe outcome by age 10 years, depending on the number of risk factors present. Application of the severity model to the validation cohort yielded 100 percent positive predictive value and an 88 percent negative predictive value (Miller, 1999). Predictors of severity in sickle cell disease are discussed in greater detail in Chapter 26.

Infants

The Cooperative Study collected data prospectively regarding clinical complications of disease in 694 infants during the first 10 years of life (Gill et al., 1995). Table 24.1 shows the frequency of the most common complications and their prevalence or incidence at different ages in children with sickle cell anemia until age 10 years. There were no gender differences in the occurrence of most of these complications with the exception of acute chest syndrome, which occurred more frequently in boys than in girls (29.1 vs. 20.1 per 100 person-years), and painful events, which had a higher incidence in girls (35.7 vs. 28.9). Constant or episodic scleral icterus and the pattern of recurrent pain in limbs and abdomen often become established in the first year of life. Splenomegaly, another manifestation of sickle cell disease in children, is present before age 6 months in a few infants with sickle cell anemia. The spectrum of complications was the same in children with HbSC disease, but complications occurred at lower rates and at later ages. It is evident from these data that even at the ages when HbF levels are expected to be high, some children with sickle cell disease face increased risk for vasoocclusive complications. The high incidence of pneumococcal bacteremia in infancy is explainable by the documentation of early splenic dysfunction (see later).

In children who are not diagnosed through newborn screening, however, it is difficult for unsuspecting physicians to make the diagnosis on the basis of physical examination alone. The earliest physical sign of the disease is often dactylitis manifested as painful swollen hands and feet ("hand-foot syndrome"). In sickle cell anemia, anemia occurs early, with a mean hemoglobin level of 9.3 g/dL at age 3 months, but remains at about the same level until after age 18 months, when the mean hemoglobin level falls below 9.0 g/dL. During the same period, the mean HbF level

Table 24.1. Incidence of Major Clinical Events in Children with Sickle Cell Anemia in the First 10 Years of Life

Age	Hand-Foot Syndrome	Painful Event	Acute Chest	Cerebrovascular Accident	Acute Anemia		Bacteremia
					Spleen	Other	
< 6 months	14.6	2.9	6.8	0.0	1.0	2.9	1.9
6 to 12 months	31.3	9.5	16.4	0.0	5.5	5.0	9.9
1 year	20.0	24.0	26.8	0.3	6.2	1.7	6.5
2 years	11.0	38.3	26.3	1.3	5.3	3.3	8.7
3 years	3.5	42.4	34.2	0.4	2.0	5.9	4.7
4 years	2.0	49.6	25.5	1.5	1.5	3.9	2.0
5 years	0.0	40.8	22.5	0.7	1.4	2.0	0.0
6 years	0.0	39.2	28.9	2.1	1.0	8.3	4.1
7 years	0.0	41.6	20.8	1.5	0.0	3.0	1.5
8 to 10 years	0.0	37.9	15.2	0.0	0.0	1.9	0.0

Incidence rates, in events per 100 person-years from 427 children with sickle cell anemia observed in the Cooperative Study of Sickle Cell Disease, from October 1978 to October 1988. (Modified from Gill et al., 1995.)

drops from 40.4 to 17.1 percent (Brown et al., 1994). It is unclear why the vast changes in HbF level have so little effect on the degree of anemia, but it may be related to the rise (5.4 to 10.4 percent) in mean reticulocyte count over the same period.

First 10 Years

In the first decade of life the most common sickle cell disease-related clinical events are painful episodes and acute chest syndrome (Gill et al., 1995). Pain, presumed to be caused by vasoocclusive ischemia, often starts as the hand-foot syndrome, where the feet and hands become swollen and tender because of inflammation of the metacarpal and/or metatarsal bones and periosteum (Diggs, 1967; Stevens et al., 1981a). When the hand-foot syndrome is accompanied by fever and persistent localized tenderness and erythema, osteomyelitis should be ruled out. Beyond infancy, the pattern of recurrent pain, typical of sickle cell disease, usually becomes established. The management and pathophysiology of sickle cell disease-related pain are discussed in Chapter 25.

The Spleen in Early Childhood. The spleen undergoes tremendous changes in function and size in the early life of children with severe forms of sickle cell disease. In children with sickle cell anemia and HbS-β^0 thalassemia, splenic dysfunction begins in infancy (Pearson et al., 1969, 1979, 1985). This has been shown in a series of studies by Pearson and others first using technetium-99^M sulfur-colloid liver-spleen scans and later the presence of increased circulating "pocked" or "pitted" red cells as measures of splenic function (Pearson et al., 1969, 1985; Casper et al., 1976; Roogers et al., 1982). Splenic dysfunction is the primary cause of the increased incidence of and mortality from bacterial infection in young children with sickle cell disease. Splenomegaly is a common feature of sickle cell disease early in the life of the patient. The age at onset of splenomegaly and the prevalence of splenomegaly at different ages are different among the major genotypes and among different sickle cell disease populations around the world. In the United States, splenomegaly is seen in children with sickle cell anemia in the first 4 to 5 years of life, but it is rare beyond age 6 years (Powars, 1975). Splenomegaly persists longer in patients with HbS-β^0 thalassemia and in patients with HbSC disease, where it is present over a wider age range (Sears and Udden, 1985; Solanki et al., 1986). In Jamaica, early splenomegaly was associated with increased susceptibility to infection and low HbF concentrations (Stevens et al., 1981b; Roogers et al., 1982). Greek patients with sickle cell anemia had persistent splenomegaly at a higher rate than did

Jamaican patients. (Christakis et al., 1990). Persistent gross splenomegaly is common in patients with sickle cell disease who reside in Africa. This is thought to be related to endemic malaria (Adekile et al., 1988, 1993). The frequency of splenomegaly was higher in a group of Nigerian children with sickle cell anemia than in age-matched patients from the United States (Adeodu and Adekile, 1990). Nigerian children with persistent gross splenomegaly had more frequent episodes of acute anemia, a complication commonly associated with acute attacks of malaria (Adeodu and Adekile, 1990).

Persistent massive splenomegaly is often associated with a hematologic picture of hypersplenism, with lower hemoglobin levels, platelet, and leukocyte counts than expected for age and genotype.

Growth and Development. Delayed growth and sexual development become major issues of concern to the adolescent. Growth delay starts in early childhood but becomes more apparent during adolescence when the growth spurt of normal children separates them from patients with sickle cell disease. Several reports from different population groups in the United States (Platt et al., 1984), Jamaica (Singhal et al., 1994), Italy (Caruso-Nicoletti et al., 1992), and Nigeria (Modebe and Ifenu, 1993; Oyedeji, 1991) have established that children and adolescents with sickle cell disease have impaired growth compared with control children. The growth deficit tends to be greater in weight than in height and is more severe in patients with sickle cell anemia and HbS-β^0 thalassemia than those with HbSC disease and HbS-β^+ thalassemia (Platt et al., 1984). Delayed skeletal maturation and adolescent growth spurt have been reported in sickle cell disease (Singhal et al., 1994). Bone age is often less than chronological age by age 1 year in both boys and girls (Abbasi et al., 1976).

In parallel with delayed growth in weight and height, adolescents with sickle cell disease are delayed in sexual maturation. In general, there is a 1- to 2-year delay in attaining Tanner stages 2 to 5 in both males and females with sickle cell anemia. The age of menorrhea is delayed by 2 to 3 years (Platt et al., 1984; Oyedji, 1995). Fortunately, sexual maturation is eventually achieved and the height, but not the weight, gap is closed by adulthood in most patients. However, size and rate of sexual development are constant measures of comparison among adolescents, and those who are delayed often face severe emotional consequences.

Zinc deficiency has been found in some patients with sickle cell anemia, and treatment with supplemental zinc has been claimed to reverse the sexual immaturity of some patients, promote the healing of leg ulcers, reduce infections, and have some effect on the sickling process (Prasad, 1975). The relationship between zinc deficiency and delayed growth and sexual development in children with sickle cell disease has been confirmed in a recent study (Leonard et al., 1998).

Whether or not zinc deficiency plays an important role in the pathophysiology of well-nourished patients with sickle cell anemia is doubtful, but this has not been the subject of many controlled trials. One trial of 130 patients compared the effects of zinc to placebo in reducing painful episodes. After 18 months of observation, about half as many episodes occurred in the zinc-treated group compared with placebo-treated patients (Gupta and Chanbey, 1995). As zinc deficiency adversely affects helper T cells and cell-mediated immunity, the role of supplemental zinc for preventing infection was studied in thirty-two patients with sickle cell disease, ages 19 to 49 years (Prasad et al., 1999). Twenty-one zinc-deficient patients were divided into two groups: eleven subjects observed for 1 year after which they received 50 to 75 mg of elemental zinc daily, as oral zinc acetate, for 3 years, and ten patients who were observed for 1 year after which they received placebo for 1 year and then switched to zinc supplementation for 2 years. A third group of eleven patients were zinc sufficient and not treated. Zinc supplementation increased in lymphocyte and granulocyte zinc, and increased in interleukin-2 production. Documented bacteriologically positive infections, hospitalizations, and number of vasoocclusive pain episodes were significantly decreased.

Several lines of evidence indicate that tissue zinc deficiency is present in some patients with sickle cell anemia, but there are some inconsistencies in the data. Among the most experienced practitioners, supplemental zinc has not been widely used.

Delayed growth and skeletal and sexual maturation in sickle cell disease may be a result of energy deficiency and chronic malnutrition. Children and adults with sickle cell disease have increased resting energy expenditure (Badaloo et al., 1989; Singhal et al., 1993, 1997; Borel et al., 1998; Kopp-Hoolihan et al., 1999). Resting metabolic rate in twenty patients with sickle cell anemia was 19 percent higher than that in twenty age- and sex-matched control subjects with a normal hemoglobin genotype, and this difference was not accounted for by differences in lean body mass (Singhal et al., 1993). Increased energy expenditure was postulated to reflect the energy expenditure of increased hemolysis and erythropoietic hyperplasia, and its presence may lead to a marginal nutritional state that contributes to abnormal growth.

When basal rates of whole body protein, glucose, and lipid metabolism and resting energy expenditure were measured using stable isotope infusions and indirect calorimetry in eight African-American patients with sickle cell disease and in six control subjects, rest-

ing energy expenditure was 15 percent greater in the patients (Borel et al., 1998b). Whole body protein breakdown and protein synthesis were 32 and 38 percent greater, respectively, in patients than in control subjects; but whole body amino acid oxidation, glucose, and lipid metabolism were not significantly different. Eight children with sickle cell anemia and a mean age of 11.2 years were given a continuous 4-hour infusion of ^{13}C leucine to determine the rate of leucine oxidation, leucine rate of appearance, and nonoxidative leucine disposal, indicators of whole body protein breakdown and synthesis, respectively. Infusion of ^{15}N glutamine was used to assess rates of glutamine utilization. Resting energy expenditure and cardiac output were measured using indirect calorimetry and echocardiography, respectively. Compared with control subjects, patients had a 58 and 65 percent higher rate of leucine appearance and nonoxidative leucine disposal, respectively, a 47 percent higher rate of whole body glutamine utilization, a 19 percent higher resting energy expenditure, and a 66 percent higher cardiac output rate (Salman et al., 1996). These data provide evidence of hypermetabolism with regard to protein, energy, and glutamine utilization and suggest that hemolysis and increased cardiac workload may contribute to excess protein and energy utilization. Additional energy required for the greater rates of whole body protein breakdown and synthesis in these patients contributed significantly to the observed increase in resting energy expenditure, suggesting that dietary energy and protein requirements are enhanced in sickle cell disease.

Voluntary energy intake in sickle cell anemia appears to be similar to that of control subjects, with a normal hemoglobin genotype despite their higher resting metabolic rate. This observation suggests a suboptimal nutritional state. Patients, therefore, may conserve energy by reducing their physical activities. This hypothesis was tested by comparing resting metabolic rate, total daily energy expenditure, and physical activity level in sixteen postpubertal boys with sickle cell disease and sixteen normal matched control subjects. Resting metabolic rate of patients exceeded that of the control subjects, but total energy expenditure was greater in control subjects. Control subjects had nearly 50 percent more physical activity than patients, suggesting that reducing physical activity is a compensatory mechanism for energy deficiency in sickle cell disease (Singhal et al., 1997).

Nearly all studies of energy expenditure in sickle cell disease are flawed by the difficulty of choosing an appropriate control population. Although matching for age and sex is appropriate as far as it goes, controls for hemolysis or anemia are not included. Therefore, results of these studies are not specific for sickle cell disease but compare patients with hemolytic anemia with hematologically normal control subjects. Ideally, to ensure that results reflect the pathophysiology of sickle cell anemia and not hemolytic anemia in general, control subjects should include individuals with other types of chronic hemolytic anemia such as β thalassemia and hereditary spherocytosis. Lacking control subjects with hemolytic anemia, consideration might be given to those with other types of chronic anemia to control for the role of increased cardiac output, but these control subjects may be accompanied by their own set of problems. This lack of appropriate control subjects makes many other studies of sickle cell disease difficult to interpret.

A long-standing and still unanswered question centers about the contribution, if any, of nutritional deficits to the pathophysiology of sickle cell anemia. In developed countries nutritional deficiencies do not seem to be a major factor in the course of disease in most patients. No evidence exists that the many vasoocclusive complications of sickle cell disease or its hemolytic anemia are, except in extreme circumstances, affected by a patient's nutritional status or that nutritional supplementation, with the exception of the rare case of megaloblastic arrest of erythropoiesis resulting from folic acid deficiency, can change the course of disease.

Because of the relationship between plasma homocysteine concentration and folate status, plasma homocysteine concentrations were measured in 120 children with sickle cell anemia who had never received supplemental folic acid (Rodrigues-Cortez et al., 1999). Plasma homocysteine levels in patients with sickle cell anemia and control subjects were similar. In thirty-four children, simultaneous serum folate, red cell folate, and total homocysteine concentrations were measured and their serum folate and red cell folate concentrations were normal. There was no correlation of plasma homocysteine concentration with various clinical or laboratory measures or with red cell folate concentration. These children, who likely had good nutritional status, had normal folate stores in the absence of supplemental folic acid.

Stroke and Neurologic Manifestations. One of the best demonstrations of the vasculopathy of sickle cell disease is the extensive cerebrovascular damage that often leads to stroke and subtle neuropsychological dysfunction. The cause of stroke, often demonstrable by arteriography, is stenosis and/or occlusion of major vessels of the circle of Willis, the internal carotid arteries, and less frequently the vessels of the vertebral-basilar system. At the microscopic level, these large arteries show fragmentation and duplication of the internal elastic lamina, with extensive intimal hyperplasia encroaching on the lumen of the vessel. (Roth-

man et al., 1986; Koshy et al., 1990; Oyesiku et al., 1991). Some vessels also show aneurysmal formation. It is presumed that the vascular damage is initiated by stiff or adherent sickle cells and the high blood flow velocity associated with anemia. Strokes are caused by in situ occlusion or embolism from thrombi formed at the point of vascular damage, or formed at areas of turbulent blood flow created by the vascular damage. (Pavlakis et al., 1989; Koshy et al., 1990; Oyesiku et al., 1991). Stenosis of the major vessels results in increased blood flow velocity, which can be shown by transcranial Doppler ultrasonography (Adams et al., 1988, 1990). Hemorrhagic stroke is thought to be caused often by rupture of aneurysms formed in the vessels of the circle of Willis. Angiographic studies following hemorrhagic stroke have shown the presence of multiple aneurysms, although not all cases of hemorrhage were associated with aneurysm (Koshy et al., 1990; Oyesiku et al., 1991; Overby and Rothman, 1995). Bleeding is commonly subarachnoid but may be intraventricular or parenchymal. Moya Moya disease has been seen in sickle cell patients with stenotic lesions of the major intracranial vessels and may also be a cause of hemorrhage, especially in adults (Seeler et al., 1978; Russel et al., 1984).

The overall prevalence of stroke and incidence of first stroke in patients with sickle cell anemia in the United States are 4.96 percent and 0.61, respectively, per 100 person-years (Ohene-Frempong et al., 1998). Lower rates are found in HbSC disease, 0.84 percent and 0.15 per 100 person-years; in HbS-β+ thalassemia, 1.29 percent and 0.09 per 100 person-years; and in HbS-β⁰ thalassemia, 2.43 percent and 0.08 per 100 person-years. Strokes in sickle cell disease are classified into three clinical types: infarctive, hemorrhagic, and transient ischemic attacks (TIA). Although all types are seen in all age groups, infarctive strokes are more common in children.

Stroke is rare in infants with sickle cell disease: however, beyond age 1 year, its incidence in sickle cell anemia patients is relatively uniform at approximately 0.5 per event 100 patient-years until age 40 years. The exception is a peak of 1.02 events per 100 person-years in patients ages 2 to 5 years and 0.8 events per 100 person-years in patients ages 6 to 9 years. (Ohene-Frempong et al., 1998). However, in thirty-nine children with sickle cell anemia between ages 7 and 48 months without a history of clinical stroke (three had a history of seizures) who were examined with magnetic resonance imaging (MRI) and magnetic resonance angiography (MRA), the overall prevalence of abnormalities in asymptomatic children was 11 percent. One patient had a silent infarct observed on MRI and a stenotic lesion on magnetic resonance angiography; three other patients had stenotic lesions on MRA. Patients with a history of seizures all had lesions consistent with infarcts on MRI. Of the asymptomatic patients who had psychometric testing, one of eighteen was developmentally delayed. One of three patients with a history of seizures had mild developmental delay (Wang et al., 1998). Therefore, very young children with sickle cell anemia without a history of clinical stroke can have infarction in the brain and/or stenosis of major cerebral arteries, similar to those reported in older children. The high incidence in the first decade and the absence of a direct correlation between the incidence of stroke and advancing age suggest that cerebrovascular disease is not likely to be simply the result of cumulative damage caused by sickle cells and abnormal blood flow. Rather, those children experiencing stroke in the first decade may have an additional risk factor, genetic or acquired, which predisposes them to early stroke. However, the risk of stroke persists throughout life for sickle cell disease patients. In sickle cell anemia, the risk of having a first stroke is 11 percent by age 20 years, 15 percent by age 30 years, and 24 percent by age 45 years (Ohene-Frempong et al., 1998).

Compared with the rates of stroke in the United States, the only reliable data on a large number of patients are from the Jamaica cohort study. In their report on stroke in 1992, 5.5 percent of 310 children with sickle cell anemia had a stroke by age 14 years. (Balkaran et al., 1992). This rate seems lower than that of children in the United States where roughly 8 percent of those with sickle cell anemia would have a stroke by this same age (Ohene-Frempong et al., 1998).

Stroke is associated with a high mortality rate in sickle cell disease. In the Cooperative Study, 10 percent of patients with stroke died within 2 weeks after the stroke. All patients who died had sickle cell anemia; almost all had a hemorrhagic stroke, which was associated with a mortality rate of 26 percent. No deaths occurred soon after infarctive stroke. In the Jamaican cohort where stroke is not managed routinely with blood transfusion, six of fifteen children with presumed infarctive stroke died, two immediately after the initial stroke, and four after a recurrent stroke, and one of two patients with a hemorrhagic stroke died.

Several factors were associated with increased risk for stroke. Prior TIA, level of anemia at steady state, rate of acute chest syndrome, acute chest syndrome 2 weeks before the stroke event, and elevated systolic blood pressure, in decreasing order of risk, were associated with infarctive stroke (Ohene-Frempong et al., 1998). Risk factors for hemorrhagic stroke were anemia and elevated leukocyte count at steady state. In this large study, no association was found between stroke and the frequency of painful episodes, priapism, or transfusion therapy within 2 weeks before the stroke event. Increased level of HbF has been reported

in two smaller series to be protective for stroke, an association not noted in the larger Cooperative Study (Powars et al., 1978; Balkaran et al., 1992). There are scant data on the association of stroke in sickle cell disease with either inherited or acquired thrombophilia. However, there has long been a suspicion that other genetic factors may be involved in the predisposition of young children with sickle cell disease to stroke. Moreover, familial aggregation of stroke has been encountered in clinical practice, but a genetic link for stroke in sickle cell disease has not been found. Recently, high homocysteine levels have been associated with stroke in one study, and another study correlated homocysteine levels with acquired folic acid deficiency (Houston et al., 1997; van der Dijs et al., 1998). Correction of the folic acid deficiency led to lower levels of homocysteine. Two recent reports also suggest that additional genetic factors may increase the risk for stroke in sickle cell disease patients. A preliminary report noted that patients with Class II HLA subtypes DRB1 0301 had the highest risk for cerebral infarct, and the lowest risk was in those with DRBI-1501. Within the DQ Class II HLA group, those with DQB1 *0201/02 had a high association with a positive MRI (Hoppe et al., 1999). Systolic hypertension is a risk factor for stroke in sickle cell disease (Peglow et al., 1997; Ohene-Frempong et al., 1998).

An association between specific GT repeat alleles in the angiotensin gene and essential hypertension has been described. This association was tested in a group of children with sickle cell disease. Although those without stroke had the same distribution of the twelve GT alleles as had been reported in African Americans, there was increased frequency of these alleles in the sickle cell disease stroke patients (Tang et al., 1999). It may be useful to obtain a thorough family history of stroke and other thrombotic events and to include evaluation for thrombophilia in laboratory assessment of sickle cell disease patients, particularly those with silent infarcts and stroke. Patients with hemorrhage should also be evaluated for coagulopathy.

α Thalassemia may protect patients with sickle cell anemia from stroke, perhaps because these patients have a higher hemoglobin concentration (Adams, 1994; Ohene-Frempong et al., 1998). Only 20 percent of pediatric patients with sickle cell anemia who had a stroke had α thalassemia, whereas 35 percent of individuals without a history of stroke had α thalassemia (Chapter 28). Other smaller studies have reported similar results. The incidence of infarctive strokes in sickle cell anemia was reduced by more than 50 percent by coincident α thalassemia (Ohene-Frempong et al., 1998). None of 48 patients with homozygous α thalassemia-2 had a stroke. In other studies, α thalassemia was not a deterrent for stroke (Balkaran et al., 1992).

Stroke can be diagnosed by clinical presentation or history. The most common presenting symptoms of infarctive stroke are hemiparesis, aphasia, dysphagia, seizure, and monoparesis (Ohene-Frempong, 1991). The diagnosis is often confirmed or defined further with brain imaging studies that are also done to exclude hemorrhage, which may require surgical intervention. Hemorrhagic stroke often presents as severe headache with vomiting and depressed consciousness. MRI or computed tomography (CT) is able to show parenchymal infarct or hemorrhage, although changes in CT may lag behind the event by several days (Fig. 24.4). Cerebrovascuiar lesions can also be delineated using MRA. Traditional angiography involving catheterization and injection of radiographic dyes is used less frequently, although this method may still be more sensitive and specific than MRA (Kandeel et al., 1996).

Positron emission tomography (PET) added to MRI can improve the detection of cerebral vasculopathy, and PET excels at assessing the functional metabolic state by permitting glucose utilization and microvascular blood flow to be measured. Forty-nine children with sickle cell anemia were studied using PET and MRI, nineteen who had clinically overt stroke, twenty who had life-threatening hypoxic episodes or "soft" neurologic signs, and ten who were normal based on neurologic history and examination. Sixty-one percent of all patients had abnormal MRI findings, 73 percent had abnormal PET findings, and 90 percent showed abnormalities on either the MRI, PET, or both. Eighty-nine percent of patients with overt stroke had an abnormal MRI, 89 percent had abnormal PET, and all had either abnormal MRI, PET, or both. In the twenty subjects with soft neurologic signs, half had abnormal MRI, 65 percent had abnormal PET, and 85 percent had abnormal MRI and/or PET. Sixty percent of the ten neurologically normal subjects had abnormal PET. Eighty-three percent of patients without an overt stroke had imaging abnormalities based on either MRI, PET, or both, suggesting silent ischemia. These imaging abnormalities were associated with lower than average full-scale intelligence quotient whether there was an overt stroke or silent ischemia. Chronic red blood cell transfusion in four patients improved metabolic and perfusion status on repeat PET scans. The use of both PET and MRI identified a much greater proportion of children with sickle cell anemia who had neuroimaging abnormalities, even in the absence of a history of overt neurologic events. In addition, the PET lesions were more extensive and bihemispheric (Powers et al., 1999). These data suggest that PET may be useful as a tool to evaluate metabolic improvement after therapeutic interventions.

Six patients with sickle cell disease and a history of stroke, ages 10 to 28 years, had PET scans using ^{18}F-fluorodeoxyglucose as a tracer. By MRI, two patients had only small vessel disease and four had both large and small vessel disease. In two of four subjects with large vessel disease, PET showed a corresponding metabolic abnormality and also identified an area of hypometabolism extending beyond the anatomic lesion as shown by MRI. PET did not show an abnormality corresponding with small vessel disease. Detailed neuropsychological testing showed cognitive dysfunction in all cases. (Reed et al., 1999). For some patients, PET may add sensitivity in detecting impaired metabolism in the area surrounding a major vessel infarct.

The magnitude of initial brain damage, degree of cerebrovascular disease, age at first stroke, type of stroke, and management determine the long-term outcome of stroke. Children experiencing infarctive stroke often recover motor deficits, but recovery may depend on their age at the time of the first stroke. In one report, only one third of children less than age 5 years old compared to two thirds of those more than 5 years old recovered from motor deficits after initial stroke (Ohene-Frempong, 1991).

In addition to motor deficits, cognitive abnormalities occur in sickle cell disease patients with cerebrovascular disease and stroke. Abnormal neuropsychometric studies are common both in the short- and long-term period after stroke (Wang et al., 1991). Brain MRI and neuropsychological evaluations were conducted to determine whether neuroradiographic evidence of infarct in children with sickle cell disease between 6 and 12 years would result in impairment in cognitive and academic functioning. In 194 children, 135 of whom had sickle cell anemia, MRIs were categorized according to the presence of T_2-weighted, high-intensity images suggestive of infarct and were further categorized on the basis of a clinical history of stroke. An abnormal MRI but no clinical history of cerebrovascular accident was classified as a silent infarct. Neuropsychological evaluations included assessment of both global intellectual functioning and specific academic and neuropsychological functions. Nearly 18 percent of all patients and 22 percent of patients with sickle cell anemia had MRI abnormalities. A clinical history of stroke was found only in children with sickle cell anemia (4.6 percent). Children with a history of stroke performed significantly poorer than children with silent infarcts or no MRI abnormality on most neuropsychological evaluation measures, and individuals with silent infarction performed significantly poorer than children with no MRI abnormality on tests of arithmetic, vocabulary, and visual motor speed and coordination (Armstrong et al., 1996).

Treatment Recommendations: Initial management of infarctive stroke should include stabilization of the patient, judicious intravenous hydration, and transfu-

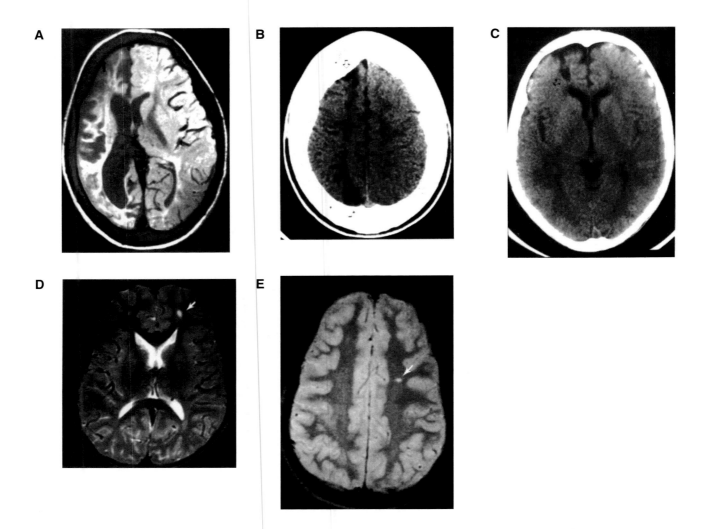

Figure 24.4. MRI and CT scans of cerebral infarction in sickle cell anemia. CT and MRI patterns of cerebrovascular disease. The left side of the photo represents the right side of the brain. (**A**) T_1-weighted MRI from a 12-year-old girl who suffered a right internal carotid artery occlusion 1 year before this study. There is severe loss of cortical and subcortical brain and massive dilation of the ventricular system. The anterior (ACA) and middle cerebral artery (MCA) territories are involved. This is an example of a major vessel occlusion pattern. (**B**) CT showing a linear area (open arrow) of infarction defining the border zone between the MCA and ACA territories. This 10-year-old boy developed mild left hemiparesis. Angiography showed an occluded right internal carotid artery (ICA) with extensive collateral flow from the vertebrobasilar system. (**C**) CT showing another border zone infarction with a wedge-shaped area of infarction extending from the cortical surface to near the frontal pole of the lateral ventricle on the right (open arrow). This 14-year-old boy had a stroke at age 10 years. When the patient was studied at age 14 years after 4 years of chronic transfusion, he had bilateral border zone infarcts (only right side is shown), but both carotid systems were patent on angiography. These lesions are typically seen in cases with large artery, usually the ICA, stenosis or occlusion. In this case the absence of carotid lesions could indicate another mechanism, perhaps repeated bouts of severe anemia, or resolution of lesions after years of transfusion. (**D**) T_2-weighted MRI showing what is also considered by some to be a border zone lesion. The area of

high signal near the frontal pole of the left lateral ventricle (white arrow) is an abnormal area of ischemia in the border zone between the deep and superficial vessels. This area is often abnormal on MRI in sickle cell disease when the CT is normal and the patient may have little if any deficit. This 10-year-old boy was neurologically asymptomatic, but this MRI was done because of abnormal transcranial Doppler studies. (**E**) T_1-weighted MRI from a 13-year-old girl who was neurologically asymptomatic except for headaches. The white arrow shows what has been called an "unidentified bright object." Similar lesions have been noted in asymptomatic elderly patients with vascular risk factors. Although not yet proven by pathologic studies, these small lesions, usually appearing in the subcortical white matter, are likely areas of small infarction caused by microvascular occlusion. Their presence does not imply concomitant large artery stenosis, and the risk of subsequent clinical stroke associated with these lesions is unknown. The patient whose MRI is shown in this panel remained asymptomatic without evidence of stroke 6 years after this study. (From Adams, 1994, with permission.)

sion therapy (Chapter 37). The goal of initial transfusion is to improve oxygenation and reduce the risk of further vasoocclusive and hypoxic damage. Exchange transfusion is preferable to simple transfusion because it allows a rapid decrease in the percentage of sickle cells. Patients with persistent neurologic deficits should be started on rehabilitation therapy as soon as possible. Long-term care involves chronic transfusion therapy to reduce the chance of recurrent stroke and management of iron overload. In untransfused patients the risk of recurrent stroke is as high as 70 percent, whereas it is approximately 10 percent in those maintained at HbS levels of less than 30 percent by chronic transfusion therapy (Powars et al., 1978; Russell et al., 1984; Pegelow et al., 1995). In patients who remain neurologically stable, the HbS level may be allowed to rise to about 50 percent with no added risk of recurrent stroke (Cohen et al., 1992). This reduces the transfusion requirement and the rate of iron accumulation. The duration of chronic transfusion is undetermined. In children, strokes have recurred when transfusion therapy was discontinued after 1 to 2 years or after 5 to 12 years (Wilimas et al., 1980; Wang et al., 1991). The risk of recurrence is not the same in all patients. However, no reliable criteria for safe discontinuation of transfusion have been developed. Children with infarctive stroke have a risk of hemorrhagic stroke later in life (Powers et al., 1990). It is unknown whether continued chronic transfusion therapy will prevent these late outcomes.

Iron overload in sickle cell disease patients on chronic transfusion occurs at rates similar to those in transfusion-dependent thalassemia (Cohen et al., 1991; Brittenham et al., 1993). Iron chelation therapy, when adhered to, is equally effective in reducing iron stores (Cohen et al., 1990). Partial exchange transfusion reduces the rate of iron accumulation and in many cases obviates the need for chelation therapy (Kim et al., 1994). This method of chronic transfusion is applicable to young children as long as they have good venous access required for the procedure and has eliminated iron overload in many patients receiving chronic transfusions. Additional details of transfusion and chelation can be found in Chapter 37.

Stroke in adults may be infarctive or hemorrhagic. In the Cooperative Study, the incidence of stroke in patients ages 20 years and older was 0.59 per 100 person-years. Of the twenty-seven first strokes occurring in, 52 percent were hemorrhagic, 30 percent were infarctive, 11 percent were TIAs, and 7 percent were unclassified. The risk of hemorrhagic stroke was highest in patients ages 20 to 29 years at 0.44 per 100 patient-years. In contrast only five of fifty-two first strokes in sickle cell anemia patients less than 20 years old were hemorrhagic. Although chronic transfusion therapy is effective in decreasing the rate of recurrent infarctive stroke in children, this has not proved to be an effective measure in patients who have their first stroke in adulthood. Moreover, transfusion therapy is often stopped when children make the transition from the pediatric to the adult clinic. Hemorrhagic stroke may be a late sequela of infarctive stroke, suggesting that progressive vascular damage may eventually lead to rupture of abnormal vessels. Such bleeding has occurred even in patients maintained on chronic transfusion therapy.

Management of hemorrhagic stroke includes careful hydration, nimodipine to reduce vasospasm, surgical evacuation of blood, and ligation of accessible aneurysms. Long-term management is unclear. The risk of recurrence is not determined, and the value of chronic transfusion in reducing their recurrence is unproven. A fatality rate of 24 percent within 2 weeks associated with hemorrhagic stroke illustrates the need for ways to prevent this complication. Routine evaluation for aneurysms is not standard practice, although surgical intervention is usually successful in those with aneurysm (Oyesiku et al., 1991).

Because of its ability to increase HbF levels, hydroxyurea (Chapter 38) had been given to some patients with stroke who for different reasons were difficult to transfuse, in whom transfusion was no longer feasible, or who had continued TIA while receiving transfusions (Ware et al., 1995, 1999). Although there has been general success in terms of increased HbF levels, strokes have also recurred in some patients whose HbF was more than 20 percent. In a series of sixteen children treated with hydroxyurea and phlebotomy, stroke recurred in 19 percent (Ware et al., 1999). At this time, using hydroxyurea to prevent recurrent stroke cannot be recommended unless there is no possibility of enrolling the patient in a prophylactic transfusion program.

Stroke Prevention. It is now possible to prevent the first occurrence of stroke in some children with sickle cell anemia. In a series of studies, transcranial Doppler ultrasonography was shown to be capable of selecting children with a high risk of stroke based on blood flow velocity in the major intracranial arteries (Adams et al., 1992a, 1992b, 1997). Transcranial Doppler ultrasonography measures blood flow velocity through intracranial vessels. Blood flow velocity is higher than normal in stenotic vessels. In a study of children with sickle cell anemia and no history of stroke where blood flow velocity of 170 cm/sec or higher in a middle cerebral artery was defined as abnormal, six of twenty-three patients with abnormal transcranial Doppler ultrasonography had a stroke compared with only 1 of 167 with normal transcranial Doppler ultrasonography. In a subsequent multicenter controlled study, 130 children with sickle cell anemia and internal carotid artery or middle cerebral artery blood flow velocity of 200 cm/sec or higher were randomized to chronic transfusion therapy or standard care. After 1 to 26 months of observation, eleven of the patients on standard care had a stroke compared with only one in the transfused group, a reduction of 92 percent in the risk for stroke (Adams et al., 1998).

These important studies raise equally important questions. Should all children with sickle cell anemia be screened, perhaps biannually, for cerebrovascular blood flow by transcranial Doppler ultrasonography? Should those with vascular disease placing them at a high risk of stroke receive transfusions? Most high-risk patients will not have a stroke during a given year, and this must be weighed against the benefits of transfusion. If transfusions are given, how long should they be continued? When transfusions are stopped are patients again at risk for stroke? Methods of transcranial Doppler ultrasonography must be carefully standardized lest some patients receive inappropriate transfusions or fail to receive transfusions at all.

Silent Infarction. MRI studies have identified brain infarcts in 18 to 20 percent of patients who have not had a clinical stroke (Pavlakis et al., 1988; Wiznitzer et al., 1990; Moser et al., 1996). These "silent" infarcts are usually located in the deep white matter in the junctional areas ("borderzones") between the tributaries of the anterior and middle cerebral arteries and the posterior and middle cerebral arteries. Patients with completed strokes usually have infarcts in the cortical regions. The Cooperative Study has recently published its analysis of risk factors for silent infarct among its infant cohort who underwent MRI studies after 5.9 years of age. Eighteen percent of the cohort had a silent infarct. History of seizure, lower rates of painful episodes, and lower hemoglobin level were associated with silent infarcts, as were increased leukocyte count, elevated pocked red cell count, and the number of patients with a Senegal β-globin gene haplotype (Kinney et al., 1999). Silent infarcts are associated with increased neuropsychometric abnormalities. Infants with silent infarcts on MRI performed significantly poorer than children with no MRI abnormality on tests of arithmetic, vocabulary, and visual motor speed and coordination (Armstrong et al., 1996). In this study, children with a history of stroke scored lower than those with silent infarcts or no MRI abnormality on most neuropsychologic evaluation measures.

Although clinicians suspect that "silent" infarcts are associated with increased risk of clinical stroke, this has not been proven conclusively. A broadened definition of stroke that included significant changes in neuropsychometric studies in association with infarcts or vascular changes on brain imaging studies would identify a large number of children with sickle cell disease who may require therapy to prevent further brain damage and overt (motor) stroke. Management of children with sickle cell anemia should include annual transcranial Doppler ultrasonography, starting at age 2 years, to identify those with high risk of stroke for consideration of preventive chronic transfusion therapy. Annual MRI studies may also identify those with "silent" infarcts and cerebrovascular damage.

Neuropathy. Peripheral neuropathies have been described but are not common (Friedlander et al., 1980; Shields et al., 1991; Adams, 1994). Most often they seem to result from adjoining bony disease and nerve entrapment, as when the mental nerve becomes entrapped in the mandibular canal owing to bone infarction, and in spinal radiculopathy, when bone infarction compresses a nerve root. Less often, a mononeuropathy can occur (Shields et al., 1991). One conjecture is that the richly anastamosing arteriolar and capillary network supplying peripheral nerves and the large diameter of these vessels help prevent vasoocclusive damage. Some reports suggest that children with sickle cell anemia who become lead-intoxicated are prone to peripheral neuropathy (Imbus et al., 1978).

Sensorineural hearing loss, particularly in the high frequency range of 2,000 to 8,000 Hz, has been encountered in up to 22 percent of patients with sickle cell disease (Donegan et al., 1982). Sometimes this has been observed in the course of a painful episode, with resolution thereafter. Although the cause of this defect is uncertain, it has been ascribed to vasoocclusive damage to inner and outer hair cells and the stria vascularis. Some patients also have transitory vertigo from apparent labyrinthitis. Although it is not possible to dissociate infectious causes from a vasoocclusive etiology, the latter remains a possibility.

Acute Anemic Episodes. Hemoglobin level remains quite constant over time in sickle cell disease unless erythropoiesis is depressed. Acute anemic episodes describe the episodic lowering of hemoglobin levels below the usual steady-state level in patients with sickle cell disease. Three common causes of acute anemia occur in children with sickle cell disease.

Acute Splenic Sequestration. Initially enlarged, the spleen in sickle cell anemia becomes dysfunctional as early as the first 6 months of life and then begins a slow process of involution that in more than 90 percent of patients culminates in a total loss of functional splenic tissue in late childhood. HbF levels determine, at least partially, the rate of splenic atrophy so that individuals with the highest levels of HbF maintain splenic function longer than those with lower levels. Some individuals with unusually high HbF levels continually have an enlarged functional spleen, and these patients become susceptible to complications of splenomegaly in sickle cell anemia, such as sequestration crisis, splenic infarction, intrasplenic hemorrhage, rupture, and abscess. Acute splenic sequestration, the sudden trapping of red cells in the sinuses of an enlarging spleen accompanied by severe anemia, mild thrombocytopenia, and hypovolemia, has been defined by the Cooperative Study as a decrease of the hemoglobin or packed cell volume (PCV) of at least 20 percent from baseline accompanied by an increase in palpable spleen size of at least 2 cm from baseline. (Jenkins et al., 1960; Gill et al., 1995). Acute splenic sequestration often occurs in association with a febrile upper respiratory illness but its pathophysiology is not clearly understood (Edmond et al., 1985; Seeler and Shwiaki, 1972). Similar to priapism, acute splenic sequestration is another example of trapping or the attenuated exit of sickle cells from a sinusoidal circulatory bed. Sickle cells trapped for any length of time in a hypoxic environment might be expected to hemolyze. Therefore, it may be inaccurate to describe acute splenic sequestration as trapping of sickled cells, as it is neither acute nor followed by increased hemolysis, and plasma is sequestered along with cells. Moreover, the "trapped" red cells are easily released into the general circulation as the acute anemia and hypovolemia are corrected when the spleen shrinks after therapeutic blood transfusion. More likely, blood continues to flow into the sinuses of the spleen but leaves at a much slower rate. A phenomenon causing expansion and subsequent shrinkage of the sinus vascular space within the spleen is a more likely mechanism. This may be due to hypoxic injury to the splenic microvasculature. Splenic sequestration is not always severe, and mild forms with less than 2 cm enlargement of the spleen and less than 2 g/dL drop in hemoglobin level probably predominate.

Rapid enlargement of the liver can also be associated with blood pooling and acute anemia, albeit much less often than splenic sequestration (Hatton et al., 1985; Glader, 1994). Management of both conditions is similar (see later).

Acute splenic sequestration may occur in patients less than age 6 months old. Two cases of acute splenic sequestration, one in a 5-week old and the other in a 2-month old with sickle cell anemia, have been reported. (Bowcock et al., 1988; Pappo and Buchanan, 1989; Airede, 1992). Although rare, acute splenic sequestration can occur in adults with sickle cell anemia and HbSC disease (Bowcock et al., 1988; Orringer et al., 1991; DeCeulaer and Serjeant, 1991). The incidence of acute splenic sequestration in children with

sickle cell anemia was 1.0 per 100 person-years by age 6 months, 6.2 per 100 person-years by age 1 year, 5.3 per 100 person-years by age 2 years, 2.0 per 100 person-years by age 3 years, and 1.0 per 100 person-years by age 6 years (Gill et al., 1995). Acute splenic sequestration is less common in young children with HbSC disease, and its peak incidence of 2.9 per 100 person-years by age 4 years is not reached as early as it is in patients with sickle cell anemia. However, acute splenic sequestration in HbSC disease may occur over a broader age range and is seen in adults and children (Orringer et al., 1991). α Thalassemia may increase the incidence of acute splenic sequestration episodes in children and adults with sickle cell anemia (De Ceulaer and Serjeant 1991). Coincident α thalassemia improves the rheology of sickle erythrocytes and may preserve splenic function into adulthood, setting the stage for acute sequestration episodes at a later age than expected (Chapter 28).

Acute splenic sequestration has a tendency to recur. In the Cooperative Study cohort of newborns, 43 of 694 patients experienced sixty-two episodes of acute splenic sequestration over 10 years (Gill et al., 1995). In addition to acute splenic sequestration, many patients develop episodes of subacute sequestration, with the spleen frequently showing enlargement and reduction in size associated with mild changes in hemoglobin level. In a few patients, there is a chronic hypersplenism with lower hemoglobin level and lower platelet and leukocyte counts than usual (Topley et al., 1981). Sixteen of the forty-three children experiencing acute splenic sequestration underwent splenectomy. Those who had splenectomy were 0.3 to 4.1 years old (median age 1.6 years) at the time of the initial acute splenic sequestration event and were splenectomized at a median age of 2.6 years (range, 0.8 to 5.3 years). None of the splenectomized sickle cell anemia patients developed postsplenectomy-invasive bacterial infection during follow-up evaluation (Gill et al., 1995). Early splenectomy has been used in the management of acute splenic sequestration without apparent increased risk of postsplenectomy bacterial infection (Powell et al., 1992; Wright et al., 1999). The concern that splenectomy may pose additional risk for bacterial infection in young children with sickle cell disease has led some centers to use partial splenectomy (Nouri et al., 1991; Svarch et al., 1996; Idowu and Hayes-Jordan, 1998), although the protective value of this procedure is uncertain, as a case of overwhelming septicemia after partial splenectomy has been reported (Svarch et al., 1999).

Treatment Recommendations: Acute splenic sequestration is a potentially life-threatening complication and should be managed with urgency. Deaths often result from hypovolemic shock and not from anemia. Immediate management of acute splenic sequestration should be directed toward correction of hypovolemia with volume expanders. Transfusion of red cells can follow restoration of blood volume and blood pressure, but this should be performed with caution, because an acutely enlarged spleen tends to release sequestered blood, and hemoglobin levels a few hours after transfusion tend to be higher than expected from the amount of red cells transfused. Red cells should be given in small portions and allowed to equilibrate to avoid hypervolemia. One guide to transfusion for splenic sequestration is that when the observed hemoglobin level is less than 5 g/dL, the initial volume of transfused red cells should be the equal in mL/kg of the observed hemoglobin level. For example, a child with hemoglobin concentration of of 3 g/dL would then receive as an initial transfusion 3 mL/kg of packed red cells. Subsequent transfusion amounts, if clinically indicated, should be estimated based on the hemoglobin level after equilibration of the initial transfusion. The use of diuretics may be advisable in those in whom hypervolemia is imminent or present.

Long-term management for individuals with recurrent acute splenic sequestration or severe hypersplenism includes parental retraining in the palpation of the spleen (this is a part of the initial training of parents of all infants with sickle cell disease), limited term chronic transfusion therapy, or splenectomy. In facing the issue of splenectomy after one or more episodes of acute splenic sequestration, the ease of accessibility of the child to a competent medical facility in the event of an acute event and the functional state of the spleen must be considered. In situations in which it is deemed unlikely that the child can reach a competent medical facility in time, splenectomy should be performed after the first episode of acute splenic sequestration. Where medical access is not a problem, the function of the spleen can be assessed through technetium-99^M sulfur colloid scan or pitted red cell counts. If the spleen is judged functional, it may be prudent to delay splenectomy with chronic transfusion therapy until the child is older than 3 years. Partial splenectomy may be an alternative solution.

Aplastic Crisis. Outside the malaria endemic areas, the most common cause of acute anemia in children with sickle cell disease is the so-called "aplastic crisis": a transient erythroid aplasia or hypoplasia often associated with parvovirus B19 infection. This agent preferentially attacks erythroid precursors—the P antigen of erythocytes is its receptor—so that the bone marrow has few primitive red cells and reticulocytes may be absent. Recovery occurs in 1 to 2 weeks. Not every patient with evidence of B19 parvovirus infection

becomes acutely anemic, and the reason for this is not known. Patients who have been infected with this virus appear to develop lifelong immunity owing to the presence of neutralizing antibodies (Singer et al., 1950; Pattison et al., 1981). In this condition, the transient cessation of red cell production in the marrow coupled with the continued rapid destruction of sickle red cells results in a severe anemia in a few days. The incidence of transient erythroid aplasia has not been determined in many sickle cell disease populations. In the sixty-four acute anemic episodes not resulting from acute splenic sequestration that occurred in thirty-three children 10 years old and younger, the Cooperative Study did not report the specific incidence of erythroid aplasia (Gill et al., 1995). The largest reported series of transient erythroid aplasia comes from the Jamaican cohort study (Serjeant et al., 1993). All ninety-one episodes of "aplastic crisis" occurring in 308 sickle cell anemia patients were associated with parvovirus B19, and the rate of parvovirus B19 infection was the same in both the patients and their normal age-matched control subjects. An additional twenty-three sickle cell anemia patients with parvovirus B19 infection showed mild or no hematologic changes. In one US institution, parvovirus accounted for only 70 percent of the episodes of "aplastic crisis" Rao et al., 1992). Other viruses and bacteria have been associated with transient erythroid aplasia (Serjeant et al., 1981a; Glader, 1994).

The clinical course of transient erythroid aplasia is usually insidious and is often discovered during evaluation of febrile children. Older children may report headache or easy fatigue. The diagnostic hallmark of transient erythroid aplasia is reticulocytopenia (often less than 2 percent) associated with either a minimal or a clinically significant decrease in hemoglobin concentration. Usually, erythropoiesis alone is affected, but concomitant neutropenia and thrombocytopenia have also been reported. Because of its relatively gradual development (acute splenic sequestration develops rapidly), transient erythroid aplasia is often well tolerated. Hemoglobin levels of less than 4 g/dL may be seen in patients whose only complaint may be fever. In patients without evidence of previous parvovirus B19 infection and who do not have increased immunoglobulin G (IgG) for parvovirus B19, it is important to document whether parvovirus B19 is responsible for any episode of reticulocytopenia by obtaining antiparvovirus B19 IgM and IgG levels. Aside from searching for possible bacterial causes of the febrile illness, it is generally not clinically useful to test for other viral infections to establish the etiology of erythroid aplasia. Parvovirus B19 can induce both erythroid aplasia and acute splenic sequestration together (Mallouh and Qudah, 1993).

Transient erythroid hypoplasia may also accompany oxygen treatment in sickle cell disease (Embury et al., 1984). In three patients with sickle cell anemia who inhaled oxygen at a rate of 5 L/min for 5 days, there was a rapid decline in erythropoietin levels that had initially been elevated, a decrease in the number of reticulocytes, and a decrease in the number of ISCs. After cessation of oxygen therapy, erythropoietin levels and the number of ISCs increased promptly, followed by an increase in reticulocytes. In one instance a patient who had a painful episode and who received O_2 treatment developed marrow red cell hypoplasia requiring transfusion (Lane et al., 1988).

Treatment Recommendations: Management of transient erythroid aplasia starts with awareness of whether the patient has had prior infection with parvovirus B19. Routine screening of children with sickle cell disease for parvovirus B19 IgG helps to identify patients who remain at risk and for whom parvovirus B19 infection should be considered whenever they are evaluated for a febrile illness. Patients at risk, or those whose parvovirus B19 status is unknown, should be isolated from pregnant women until the reticulocyte count is determined, because this virus may have untoward effects on the fetus of susceptible women. In the future, patients without B19 parvovirus immunity should be the recipients of parvovirus B19 vaccine. Unlike normal children, children with sickle cell disease are instructed to seek medical attention for all febrile illnesses. This increases the chance that those with parvovirus B19 will be exposed to medical staff. A cluster of parvovirus B19 infections in nurses traced to two sickle cell disease patients hospitalized for transient erythroid aplasia has been reported (Bell et al., 1989).

During the earliest phases of acute illness, antiparvovirus IgM and IgG levels may be negative. It is advisable to repeat these tests 1 week or so later for evidence of recent parvovirus B19 reflected by an increase of IgM antibody. The main therapeutic decision in managing erythroid aplasia is whether transfusion of red cells is required. Patients with a 25 percent or greater decrease in their hemoglobin level from baseline with reticulocyte counts that are declining or are absent, and those who are symptomatic from severe anemia, should be transfused early to shorten the period of acute anemia. In a series of eighty children with strokes at the Children's Hospital of Philadelphia, at least four had a stroke during a period of severe anemia as a result of erythroid aplasia (Ohene-Frempong, 1991). Transfusion should be performed cautiously and in small portions in a manner similar to that described for splenic sequestration to avoid hypervolemia and complications resulting from a sharp rise in blood viscosity (Wayne et al., 1993). Typically, a patient with transient erythroid aplasia begins to show nucleated red cells and reticulocytes within 1 week of the severe reticulocytopenia. In untransfused patients, the reticulocyte counts may rise to dramatic levels during the recovery phase.

Hyperhemolysis. Accelerated hemolysis in conjunction with specific clinical complications of sickle cell disease is a third cause of acute anemia in children with sickle cell disease. Often referred to as "hyperhemolysis," this diagnosis is typified by a reduction in hemoglobin level associated with higher than usual reticulocyte counts. In some reported cases of "hyperhemolysis," the patient may have been examined during the recovery phase of an acute erythroid aplasic episode, and the reticulocytosis does not reflect an increase in hemolysis. Acute chest syndrome is often associated with a 0.5 to 1 g/dL drop in steady state hemoglobin level (Poncz et al., 1985; Vichinsky et al., 1997). Whether this is a result of increased hemolysis is not known. There seems to be little evidence to implicate associated glucose-6-phosphate dehydrogenase (G-6-PD) deficiency in accelerated hemolysis and in the acute anemia of sickle cell disease, although such an association has been reported (Smits et al., 1969; Steinberg et al., 1988). No gender difference in the incidence of acute anemia events is present (Gill et al., 1995). In the absence of malaria, most experts have had difficulty documenting a convincing case of "hyperhemolysis."

Autoimmune hemolytic anemia is found in some patients with sickle cell disease who have undergone transfusion (Chapter 37). It may account for the decrease in hemoglobin concentration from baseline values.

Perhaps the most clinically significant cause of acute hemolysis in sickle cell disease occurs in the context of malaria infection. Acute hemolytic anemia owing to malaria is the leading cause of death in children with sickle cell disease living in malaria-endemic areas of Africa (Fleming, 1989; Gendrel et al., 1992).

Bacterial infection may transiently reduce erythropoiesis and worsen the usual anemia of sickle cell disease. In developed countries, when severe anemia develops, megaloblastic arrest of erythropoiesis may rarely be found. This is usually due to marginal nutrition that causes folic acid deficiency (Glader, 1994).

Treatment Recommendations: Increased hemolysis in a patient with sickle cell disease should be investigated to exclude autoimmune hemolysis that accompanies alloimmunization in patients who have undergone extensive transfusions (Rosse et al., 1998). In these patients, because of the presence of antibodies that are usually panagglutinins, finding blood compatible for transfusion is difficult. Corticosteroids can be used effectively, as for other types of autoimmune hemolytic anemia.

Judicious use of blood transfusion is warranted when anemia is severe. Hemolysis related to malaria infection must be corrected as the infection is treated. It is generally recommended that children with sickle cell disease living in malaria-endemic areas should be protected from malaria. It is unclear, however, whether this protection should be in the form of antimalarial prophylaxis or patient/family education regarding how to respond to febrile illness. The widespread selection of chloroquine resistant *Plasmodium falciparum* in Africa and elsewhere makes that drug unsuitable for routine prophylaxis. It is also unclear whether sulfadoxine-pyrimethamine preparations recommended for malaria prophylaxis during pregnancy is suitable for long-term use in patients with sickle cell disease.

Infection. Infection is the major cause of mortality and morbidity in children in the first years of life, and the most common offending agent is *Streptococcus pneumoniae*. Before the institution of newborn screening for sickle cell disease, pneumococcal vaccination, and penicillin prophylaxis therapy, *S. pneumoniae* bacteremia was the leading cause of death in patients less than age 20 years in the United States (Leikin et al., 1989). Patients with sickle cell disease lose splenic reticuloendothelial function in early life. This was shown by technetium-99^M sulfur colloid liver-spleen scans, which showed absence of splenic uptake in young sickle cell anemia patients even when their spleen was enlarged, an entity called *functional hyposplenism* (Pearson et al., 1979, 1985). The dysfunction of the spleen appears to be unrelated to its size fluctuation in the early years, gradual enlargement until age 3 to 4 years, followed by gradual regression into a contracted fibrotic but possibly revivable organ. Splenic dysfunction is also inferred from the appearance in circulation of red cells containing Howell-Jolly bodies, remnants of nuclear chromatin, normally "culled" from red cells by the spleen, and by the rise in "pocked" (more correctly, pitted) red cells in circulation. The rate of splenic regression is related to the natural reduction in HbF levels that occurs during postnatal development. Ten Saudi Arabs, ages 4 to 26 years, with sickle cell anemia and mean HbF of 20 percent, were found to have splenic abscesses (Al-Salem et al., 1998). Tender, enlarged spleen, abdominal pain, and fever were common presenting features. Six patients had evidence of infection with *Salmonella* species.

Hyposplenic patients are susceptible to infection with encapsulated bacteria such as *S. pneumoniae* and *Haemophillus influenzae*. There is also evidence of abnormal granulocyte function in sickle cell anemia. Circulating neutrophils appear to be activated in the "steady-state" as they have increased activity of phospholipase A_2 (Mollapour et al., 1998). Although these cells might contribute to the initiation of vasoocclusion, they also respond poorly to priming by cytokines and have about half the nicotine adenine dinucleotide phosphate (NADPH) oxidase response of control cells. An impaired response would effect killing of microorganisms, requiring high levels of oxidant radicals for their death, such as *S. pneumoniae* and *H. influenzae*. Sepsis, pneumonia, meningitis, and otitis are the most frequent infections and can progress with devastating rapidity.

The immune defect in sickle cell disease appears to be specific for certain organisms. Primary among these is *S. pneumoniae*. Early studies had shown a defect in opsonization of *S. pneumoniae* antecedent to phagocytosis. This opsonic defect was initially thought to reside in the alternate pathway of complement activation (Johnston et al., 1973). Later, it was shown that the opsonic defect was due to a lack of specific antibodies against pneumococci, perhaps owing to early loss of splenic antibody production function (Bjornson and Lobel, 1979; Bjornson et al., 1985). This opsonic defect is not generalized to all microganisms.

Robinson and Watson (1966) first reported the high frequency of pneumococcal sepsis and meningitis in young children with sickle cell disease. Since then, the relatively high risk of overwhelming pneumococcal infection in patients with sickle cell disease and the associated high rate of mortality have been well documented (Barrett-Connor, 1971; Overturff et al., 1977; Zarkowsky et al., 1986). The incidence of bacteremia in sickle cell disease varies with age and genotype of the disease. Overall, the rate of bacteremia seems to have declined in the United States since the early reports of children with sickle cell disease having bacteremia at 300 to 600 times the rate of normal children (Barrett-Connor, 1971). Factors accounting for the declining rate of bacteremia include the institution of penicillin prophylaxis and the use of pneumococcal and *H. influenzae* type b vaccination. In its cohort of 427 infants with sickle cell anemia followed from 1978 to 1988, the Cooperative Study reported that bacteremia occurred in infants less than 6 months of age. Peak incidence of bacteremia, 9.9 events per 100 person-years, occurred in infants ages 6 to 12 months, declining to less than 5 per 100 person-years after age 3 years (Gill et al., 1995). The second 6 months of life also saw the highest incidence of bacteremia in children with HbSC disease. The Cooperative Study had reported an incidence of bacteremia of 7.98 per 100 person-years for children less than 3 years old with sickle cell anemia; this rate declined to 2.54 per 100 person-years in those ages 3 to 5 years. *S. pneumoniae* was responsible for 67 percent of the cases of bacteremia in those under age 6 years but only 19 percent of cases in individuals older than age 6 years (Zarkowsky et al., 1986). Twenty-four percent of children under age 3 years with sickle cell anemia who had pneumococcal bacteremia died. In 75 percent of the patients who died of sepsis, death occurred within 24 hours after hospitalization (Zarkowsky et al., 1986).

Recent changes in management of febrile illness in young children with sickle cell disease has reduced the rate of mortality (Overturff et al., 1977). In the Cooperative Study infant cohort of 427 children with sickle cell anemia, there were sixty-two cases of *S. pneumoniae* bacteremia with a 14.5 percent mortality after 1,781.4 person-years of observation (Gill et al., 1995).

With increasing age, the cause of bacterial infection in sickle cell disease changes from the pneumococcus to gram-negative organisms such as *Escherichia coli, Klebsiella,* and *Salmonella* species (Wright et al., 1997a; Magnus et al., 1999). Acquisition of natural antibodies, subclinical infection, and in recent years protection offered by pneumococcal vaccination may account for the decline in relative risk of pneumococcal infection despite the permanent loss of splenic function. Until the widespread use of *H. influenzae* type b vaccination, this organism was the second leading cause of sepsis and meningitis in children with sickle cell disease. As the rate of *H. influenzae* infection has declined in the general childhood population, it has also declined in children with sickle cell disease, although it remains higher than in the general population (Overturff et al., 1977; Zarkowsky et al., 1986).

In addition to bacterial sepsis and meningitis, patients with sickle cell disease are at increased risk for osteomyelitis. In the United States, *Salmonella* species are the most common cause of osteomyelitis followed by *Staphylococcus aureus* (Anand and Glatt, 1994; Overturff, 1999). In recent literature from other parts of the world, *Salmonella* species are also reported as the most frequent causes of osteomyelitis in patients with sickle cell disease (Sadat-Ali, 1998; Begue, 1999). However, other gram-negative organisms, such as *Klebsiella* and staphylococcal species, are the leading causes of osteomyelitis in some regions of the world (Aken'Ova et al., 1995).

Eighteen African-American patients with sickle cell disease with human immunodeficiency virus-1 (HIV-1) infection were reported, eleven of whom had quantitative studies of viral load and were under treatment or follow-up monitoring. Although data are scanty, it may be that these HIV-1-infected sickle cell anemia individuals have a lower viral load and higher CD4 cell counts than HIV-1-infected control patients and include more asymptomatic long-term nonprogressors than control subjects. It was hypothesized that asplenia removes an important site for viral replication and accounts for a more indolent disease when HIV-1 and sickle cell anemia coexist (Bagasra et al., 1998).

Treatment Recommendations: Knowledge of the high risk and fatality rate of pneumococcal infection in children with sickle cell disease has resulted in one of the notable successes in the management of this disease. Young children with sickle cell disease who have a febrile illness are managed as if they have pneumococcal sepsis until proven otherwise. This practice mandates that all children with sickle cell disease with significant fever or who simply look or act ill require medical evaluation and prompt antibiotic therapy. Their evaluation should consist at minimum of a physical examination, complete blood count, reticulocyte count (to exclude erythroid aplasia), and blood culture. Lumbar puncture should be done if meningitis is suspected based on the examination or cannot be ruled out because of the young age of the patient. Immediately after the specimens for culture are obtained, broad-spectrum antibiotics should be administered intravenously. A chest x-ray study is advisable in children less than 3 years old, because physical signs of acute chest syndrome may be less obvious in young children and because the presence of acute chest syndrome would alter the course of therapy.

Until the last few years, children less than 6 years old with fever or an ill appearance were admitted and treated with intravenous antibiotics until bacterial cultures were negative (Charache et al., 1989). In recent years, after several reports of successful adoption of this practice, the standard practice has shifted to outpatient management of febrile children with sickle cell disease who are not ill-appearing (Rogers et al., 1990; Bakshi et al., 1991; Wilimas et al., 1993; Charache et al., 1995b). By this practice, the child is given ceftriaxone, a long-acting cephalosporin with excellent antipneumococcal sensitivity, watched for a few hours to ensure the child's continued well-being, and discharged home for outpatient follow-up monitoring. In some institutions, infants are excluded from outpatient management of febrile illness; in others, children are given oral antibiotics for a few days after the intravenous ceftriaxone. This practice change has succeeded largely because in the era of penicillin prophylaxis, pneumococcal vaccination, and comprehensive care, the incidence of pneumococcal sepsis, bacteremia, and meningitis has declined dramatically at major clinical centers. With good follow-up monitoring, outpatients whose cultures grow pathogenic bacteria are returned for further evaluation and appropriate treatment. An unusual fatal hemolytic reaction to ceftriaxone in one child with sickle cell disease has been reported (Bernini et al., 1995). This underscores the need for close follow-up evaluation of those managed as outpatients after receiving ceftriaxone.

Magnus et al. (1999) found that the standardized incidence rates for second and third infections in patients with sickle cell anemia were 4.8 and 15.8 times greater, respectively, than the rate of infection in the sickle cell anemia population at large. This rate implied that the susceptibility to infection is characteristic of a subgroup of patients and that sick patients with previous bacteremia should be investigated early and aggressively for further infection.

Prevention of mortality from pneumococcal infection is the basis for the establishment of newborn screening for sickle cell disease. Twice daily oral penicillin was shown in a double-blind, placebo-controlled trial to effectively reduce the incidence and mortality of pneumococcal bacteremia in children with sickle cell anemia less than age 5 years (Gaston et al., 1986). Since serious infection with pneumococci may start a few weeks after birth, it became imperative to discover children with sickle cell disease early in life, when they are usually asymptomatic, in order to make penicillin prophylaxis available (Consensus Conference, 1987). Forty-four of the fifty states of the United States now include testing for sickle cell disease in their newborn screening programs. In addition to penicillin patients with sickle cell disease should receive pneumococcal vaccination. In the United State, two vaccines are currently available, the 23-valent pneumococcal polysaccharide vaccine (PPV-23) and the recently-licensed 7-valent pneumococcal conjugated vaccine (PCV-7). PCV-7 is available for healthy children as well as those with high risk for invasive pneumococcal infection. There is no contraindication for the use of both vaccines in children or adults although it is recommended that PCV-7 and PPV-23 be given at least two months apart (Vernacchio et al. 1998). The recommended schedule for both vaccines appears below in Table 24.2. Revaccination of children who received the 23-valent

vaccine at age 5 years may have no additional benefit (Bjornson et al., 1996). Some children immunized against pneumococcal infection with the PPV-23 alone have had breakthrough infections (Wong et al., 1992). Even vaccinated children who are prescribed penicillin prophylaxis can die of pneumococcal sepsis, perhaps because they do not take their medication faithfully. How long penicillin prophylaxis should be continued is unclear. A follow-up study to the prophylactic penicillin trial, whose purpose was to determine the efficacy of penicillin prophylaxis in children over age 5 years old with sickle cell anemia, failed to show any significant difference between the penicillin and placebo groups (Falletta et al., 1995). These results do not apply to children with a history of severe pneumococcal infection or splenectomy, as they were excluded from the study. Some clinicians may conclude that penicillin prophylaxis is unnecessary beyond age 5 years. However, splenic dysfunction in sickle cell disease is not restored beyond age 5 years, and older children and adults have died from overwhelming pneumococcal infection. The decision to discontinue penicillin prophylaxis for any child should be carefully considered, taking into account parental understanding of and the ability to respond appropriately to signs of infection and the prior history of pneumococcal infection.

Widespread use of newborn screening for sickle cell disease followed by parental education about infection and administration of penicillin prophylaxis have reduced the high mortality previously seen in young children with sickle cell disease in the United States. Newborn screening programs need to be instituted in other parts of the world where the prevalence of sickle cell disease is high. In Africa, where malaria is a major cause of mortality and morbidity for sickle cell disease patients, prevention of malaria through prophylactic therapy would be useful (Fleming, 1989). However, the increasing prevalence of *Plasmodium falciparum* resistant to chloroquine and other antimalarial agents has made it difficult to select appropriate prophylactic agents.

Table 24.2. Schedule of Pneumococcal Vaccination for Patients with Sickle Cell Disease

Product	Age First Dose	Primary Series	Additional Doses
PCV-7	2–6 m	3 doses, 2 m apart	1 dose at 12–<16 m
	7–11 m	2 doses, 2 m apart	1 dose at 12–<16 m
	12–23 m	2 doses, 2 m apart	—
	≥ 24 m	2 doses, 2 m apart	—
PPV-23	≥ 24 m	1 dose, 2 m after PCV-7	≤10y, 1 dose, 3–5yr later
			≥10y, 1 dose, 5yr later

PCV-7: 7-Valent Pneumococcal Conjugate Vaccine (Prevnar, Wyeth-Ayerst); PPV-23: 23-Valent Pneumococcal Polysaccharide Vaccine.

Increasing penicillin resistance heightens the urgency of an effective vaccine (Chesney et al., 1995; Norris et al., 1996; Woods et al., 1997; Daw et al., 1997). In the United States, surveillance studies of pneumococcal infection in children 18 years old or younger with sickle cell disease have shown that of fifty-six evaluable instances of invasive pneumococcal disease, 21 percent were resistant to penicillin and 24 percent were intermediately susceptible (Adamkiewicz et al., 1999). Sixty-seven percent of individuals taking prophylactic penicillin had resistant strains, a rate twice that of patients not taking prophylaxis. Penicillin prophylaxis does not increase a child's likelihood of nasopharyngeal carriage of penicillin-resistant strains of pneumococcus. However, as the prevalence of penicillin resistance increases, it may become necessary for any local community to alter its antibiotic coverage for children with sickle cell disease suspected of having bacteremia or acute chest syndrome. Even vaccinated children prescribed penicillin prophylaxis die of pneumococcal sepsis, perhaps because they do not take their medication faithfully (Buchanan and Smith, 1986).

Acute Chest Syndrome. Characterized by fever, chest pain, cough, and lung infiltrates, acute chest syndrome, a sometimes lethal complication, affects a third of all patients with sickle cell anemia and is the second most common reason for hospitalization. Acute chest syndrome was defined in the Cooperative Study as "the new appearance of an infiltrate on chest radiograph or, in the presence of pulmonary symptoms and negative chest radiograph, abnormalities on an isotopic scan of the lungs" (Gill et al., 1995; Lisbona et al., 1997). This broad definition attempted to unify a condition characterized by chest pain, varying degrees of respiratory distress, fever, cough, and leukocytosis. In many instances, particularly in young children, the new pulmonary infiltrate is discovered incidentally as part of the evaluation of fever. Acute chest syndrome has its highest incidence in the more severe forms of sickle cell disease, such as sickle cell anemia, sickle cell anemia-α thalassemia, and HbS-β^0 thalassemia.

Acute chest syndrome is a frequent complication of sickle cell disease. In 3,751 patients who were observed for a total of 19,867 person-years, 1,085 (29.2 percent) had at least one episode of acute chest syndrome. Of these individuals, 56 percent had only one episode, and 6 percent had five or more episodes (Castro et al., 1994). Acute chest syndrome occurred more often in sickle cell anemia (12.8 per 100 person-years) and HbS-β^0 thalassemia (9.4 per 100 person-years) than in HbSC disease (5.2 per 100 person-years) and HbS-β^+ thalassemia (3.9 per 100 person-years).

Risk factors for acute chest syndrome in sickle cell anemia patients were low age, low HbF level, high total hemoglobin level, and high steady-state leukocyte count. Children 2 to 4 years old with sickle cell anemia had the highest incidence of acute chest syndrome (25.3 per 100 person-years). The direct relationship between hemoglobin concentration level and acute chest syndrome is unexplained, but it is thought to be related to the higher blood viscosity associated with a high PCV.

The causes of acute chest syndrome are not always clear and may be multifactorial. Its pathogenesis is summarized in Table 24.3. Pulmonary infarction, pulmonary infection, or atelectasis secondary to rib infarction and involuntary splinting, pulmonary embolism, and in situ thrombosis all may eventuate in acute chest syndrome. Newer aspects of its pathophysiology are discussed in Chapter 20. Lungs are particularly vulnerable to vasoocclusive damage in sickle cell disease. Deoxygenated sickle cells that manage to escape trapping in the peripheral microcirculation are returned to the lungs where they are reoxygenated. It is conceivable that cells that become fully sickled by the time they reach the lungs and before they are reoxygenated would be trapped in pulmonary precapillary arterioles, particularly in atelectatic areas, before reoxygenation and unsickling. Large and small branches of pulmonary arteries probably undergo damage similar to that seen in cerebral arteries in sickle cell disease, leading to stenosis and occlusion of the vessels and diminished blood flow to and infarction in some areas of the lung (Koshy et al., 1990). Cumulative microinfarction of the lung is likely to lead to progressive pulmonary dysfunction and chronic lung disease with advancing age (Powars et al., 1988). Sudden vasoocclusion in large vessels is likely to precipitate "pulmonary stroke" manifested as severe acute chest syndrome (Powars et al., 1988). Shunting of deoxygenated and partially oxygenated red cells from the alveolar microcirculation is likely to deposit into the peripheral circulation cells that may sickle readily on further deoxygenation. Partially oxygenated sickle cells have been described in the circulation of patients with sickle cell disease (Asakura et al., 1994).

Isolation of microorganisms in pulmonary secretions or from the blood during the course of acute chest syndrome does not necessarily establish that they are etiologically related to acute chest syndrome, and their presence may represent superinfection in damaged pulmonary tissue. However, it is believed that acute chest syndrome can be triggered by lung infection. It is not surprising that a wide variety of organisms have been associated with acute chest syndrome, and the recovery of these organisms is greatly increased by bronchopulmonary lavage. Infectious

Table 24.3. Pathogenesis of the Acute Chest Syndrome

Mechanism	Evidence
Bone infarction with atelectasis and regional hypoxia	Bone infarctions cause pain with hypoventilation, atelectasis, and subsequent hypoxia. Incentive spirometry reduces radiographic atelectasis in patients with sickle cell anemia and vasoocclusive crisis.
Fat emboli	Bone marrow embolization found in many patients. Lipid-laden alveolar macrophages are recovered from bronchopulmonary lavage fluids in acute chest episodes. Secretory phospholipase A_2 levels elevated and may liberate free fatty acids and promote inflammation.
Infection	Seasonal predilection, pathogenic microorganisms recovered from lung and blood.
Microvascular in situ thrombosis	Increased adherence of erythrocytes to endothelial cells. Pulmonary hypoxia results in entrapment of sickled erythrocytes.
Thromboembolic disease	Pulmonary emboli documented
Vascular injury and inflammation	Endothelin-I levels elevated during acute chest syndrome. Elevated levels of inflammatory mediator. Clinical progression to acute respiratory distress syndrome.

Adapted from Gladwen et al. (1999).

agents include *S. pneumoniae*, *H. influenzae*, *Mycoplasma pneumoniae*, and *Chlamydia pneumoniae* (Miller et al., 1991; Begue, 1999). Parvovirus B19, although typically associated with transient erythroid aplasia, has also been found in acute chest syndrome (Lowenthal et al., 1996). Recent data indicate that about 5 percent of acute chest syndrome episodes are associated with recent B19 parvovirus infection. In many cases of acute chest syndrome, an aggressive search for all possible causes of infections is not carried out. Therefore, many of the published studies on the frequency of infection in acute chest syndrome

may underreport the possibility of such a causative link. A pathogen isolated from blood at the time of acute chest syndrome is often assumed to be its causative agent. Bacteremia was present in only 3.5 percent of the 1,772 episodes of acute chest syndrome reported by the Cooperative Study (Vichinsky et al., 1997). The most frequent organism was *S. pneumoniae* followed by *H. influenzae*, a pathogen much less common now as a cause of serious infection in the United States than in the 1979 to 1988 period of observation in the Cooperative Study report. Children were more likely to have infection-associated acute chest syndrome than were adults. In children less than 2 years old, 14 percent of the episodes of acute chest syndrome was associated with bacteremia, and *S. pneumoniae* was the pathogen in 78 percent of cases. In contrast, only 1.8 percent of patients 10 years or older had bacteremia, and *S. pneumoniae* accounted for only 25 percent of the positive cultures.

Acute chest syndrome is a frequent postoperative complication of sickle cell disease (Vichinsky et al., 1995; Koshy et al., 1995) (see below). It is presumed that this is an extension of the common atelectasis that tends to follow prolonged anesthesia. However, the likelihood that pulmonary infarction is initiated by sickled red cells that were returning to the lungs after slow flow through anesthetized tissue cannot be discounted.

Clinically, the course of acute chest syndrome is variable. Fever, cough, and chest pain are the most common presenting symptoms. Children less than 5 years old present more frequently with fever and cough; older children and adults tend to also have shortness of breath, wheezing, productive cough, chest pain, and chills (Vichinsky et al., 1995). Pain and fever are the most frequent acute events associated with acute chest syndrome. Altogether, 30 percent of the patients with acute chest syndrome had pain, but adults tended to have pain before acute chest syndrome more often than did children. A common scenario is the onset of an acute painful episode followed by acute chest syndrome. Rucknagel et al. (1991) showed that rib infarction was a common precipitating factor of acute chest syndrome. Incentive spirometry was able to reduce the incidence of acute chest syndrome following rib infarction (Bellet et al., 1995).

In other instances, acute chest syndrome may be caused by bone marrow fat embolism (Vichinsky et al., 1994; Castro, et al., 1996). Fat embolism is a common cause of the most severe acute chest events during which hemoglobin and platelet levels fall and the leukocyte count increases. Fat embolism, with its attendant poor prognosis, can be identified by finding lipid within pulmonary macrophages obtained by bronchopulmonary lavage. Fat-laden necrotic bone marrow has been found on autopsy of patients with sickle cell disease who died from severe acute chest syndrome. The detection of fat in circulation and in pulmonary macrophages may help make this diagnosis, which is often overlooked in the management of acute chest syndrome. Elevated levels of phospholipase A_2 have been found in patients with sickle cell disease in association with acute chest syndrome. It has been postulated that free fatty acids released from embolized fat by phospholipase A_2 may cause further damage to lung tissue in this syndrome (Styles et al., 1996).

Treatment Recommendations: Management of acute chest syndrome includes intravenous broad-spectrum antibiotics, careful hydration, and aggressive respiratory therapy with bronchodilators. Antibiotics are usually given, although documented bacterial infection is found in less than 10 percent of cases. The choice of antimicrobial may be predicated on the algorithm for community acquired pneumonia; however, some patients with sickle cell anemia are frequent hospital visitors, and this may modify the choice of a drug. It has become customary to add erythromycin or other agents to cover *Mycoplasma* or *Chlamydia* infection. Oxygen therapy should be given when the patient is hypoxic or tachypneic with signs of respiratory distress. Hydration should be provided carefully to avoid pulmonary edema. Total hydration should not exceed maintenance and replacement of losses. In the context of pain management, often with opioid analgesics and acute chest syndrome, care should be taken to balance the analgesic need and the danger of respiratory suppression.

Simple or exchange transfusion to reduce the percentage of HbS-containing cells and increase the baseline hemoglobin concentration level is useful in hypoxic patients. The timing of transfusion is unclear as is whether exchange transfusion is superior to simple transfusion, although many experts prefer the former. It is the impression of clinicians that patients with infarctive acute chest syndrome, as opposed to infectious acute chest syndrome, have a more rapid recovery in response to blood transfusion, suggesting that early transfusion may prevent progression to severe acute chest syndrome (Mallouh and Asha, 1988). This belief has not been tested in a controlled study. In patients with moderate to severe acute chest syndrome, the goals of transfusion should be to maintain a hemoglobin concentration of 10 g/dL and HbS level of less than 30 percent, levels similar to those used in the management of stroke. Blood less than 5 days old is preferable, as banked blood has low 2,3, BPG levels and a high affinity for oxygen (Festa and Asakura, 1979). Transfusing old blood into a hypoxic sickle cell disease patient could worsen the condition of the patient in the immediate posttransfusion period, as transfused cells have a higher oxygen affinity than nor-

mal until the 24 hours that it takes to restore 2,3, BPG levels elapses.

Prevention of acute chest syndrome should be among the goals of managing sickle cell disease patients in pain, particularly when they are bedridden. The use of incentive spirometry in those with abdominal and chest wall pain for which there may be splinting should be strongly encouraged (Bellet et al., 1995). Routine assessment of oxygen saturation at steady state should be part of general care of sickle cell disease patients. A drop of 3 or more percent oxygen saturation from baseline level at presentation with acute illness is predictive of acute chest syndrome (Rackoff et al., 1993).

Although most children with acute chest syndrome respond well to therapy, a few undergo a rapidly deteriorating course often with disastrous consequences and death. In these cases, patients who may have started with a small infiltrate rapidly develop respiratory distress, increased oxygen requirement, and extensive pulmonary opacification with effusion and edema. Some of these patients require mechanical ventilation and may develop adult respiratory distress syndrome or a syndrome of multiorgan failure. This rapidly deteriorating pulmonary disease is often analogous to pulmonary embolism. Although bone marrow embolism is often a cause of these disastrous episodes, a careful search for fat emboli is infrequently a part of the clinical evaluation. Acute chest syndrome developing in the context of inpatient management of sickle cell disease-related pain has led to the strong, but yet unproven, suspicion that excessive intravenous hydration and use of opiate analgesics may be contributing factors.

Recent studies suggest that nitric oxide (NO) may be involved in the pathogenesis of acute chest syndrome and that inhaled NO may be a useful treatment (summarized in Gladwin et al., 1999). It must be emphasized that although 80 ppm inhaled NO for 15 minutes apparently increases PO_2 and reduces pulmonary artery pressure in acute chest syndrome, there have been no careful clinical trials of this treatment, and it has not yet improved mortality in adult respiratory distress syndrome.

Successful management of severe acute chest syndrome depends to a large degree on the experience of the intensive care unit in managing such patients. Close coordination of intensive care between internists, pulmonologists, hematologists, infectious disease experts, and nursing and respiratory therapists is necessary for achievement of a successful outcome. Response to treatment was recently evaluated in 671 episodes of the acute chest syndrome in 538 patients (Vichinsky et al., 2000). Treatment included phenotypically matched blood transfusions, bronchodilators, and bronchoscopy. Thirteen percent of patients required mechanical ventilation, 3 percent died, and 81 percent recovered. As in prior studies, adults age 20 and above were more severely effected than younger patients. Transfusions improved oxygenation and bronchodilators with a 1 percent rate of alloimmunization. Twenty percent of the patients treated with bronchodilators improved. Eighteen patients died, and the most common causes of death were pulmonary emboli and infectious bronchopneumonia, infection contributing to 56 percent of the deaths.

Long-term outcome of acute chest syndrome is also variable. It is generally believed that repeated episodes of acute chest syndrome lead to restrictive and obstructive lung disease (Powars et al., 1988). In a preliminary report at variance with other studies and accepted wisdom, high resolution CT scans of the chest did not show any difference in the presence of interstitial lung disease in twenty-four adult patients with sickle cell anemia and recurrent acute chest syndrome compared with control patients. (Killic et al., 1998). Pulmonary function abnormalities have been detected in children less than 3 years old with sickle cell anemia (Koumbourlis et al., 1997). A history of acute chest syndrome was associated with lower transcutaneous oxygen saturation in one study (Rackoff et al., 1993). A similar finding was made when children older than age 5 years were compared with younger children. Like the recurrence of stroke in sickle cell disease, acute chest syndrome may be recurrent, and a few patients have repeated severe acute chest syndrome. Such patients and those with chronic hypoxia after surviving severe acute chest syndrome or adult respiratory distress syndrome may benefit from chronic transfusion therapy. Hydroxyurea (Chapter 38) reduced the frequency of acute chest syndrome in adults with sickle cell anemia (Charache et al., 1995). It is unclear whether hydroxyurea alone will prevent recurrent acute chest syndrome or improve hypoxia in patients with pulmonary damage from previous acute chest syndrome.

ADOLESCENCE

Adolescents with sickle cell disease face both the physical limitations associated with sickle cell disease and the psychological impact of a serious chronic disease. While sickle cell disease in older children and adolescents is not fundamentally different, there are a few problems that are more or less common during adolescence. In the second decade of life, patients with sickle cell anemia have a lower incidence of bacteremia, dactylitis, acute splenic sequestration, acute chest syndrome, stroke, and mortality but higher incidence of cholelithiasis and cholecystectomy and severe pain episodes. Although adolescence may be a period of relative stability medically, it is not so psychologically. In fact, much of medical literature dealing with adolescents with sickle cell disease concentrates on psychoso-

cial issues. The management of adolescents with sickle cell disease was reviewed recently by Kinney and Ware (1996). Some of the major issues in adolescents with sickle cell disease include growth and development, management of pain, the psychological impact of and psychosocial adjustment to a chronic disease, and their transition to adult care.

Psychosocial problems reported in adolescents with sickle cell disease include low social adjustment, depression, anxiety, acting out behavior, and negative body image (Morgan and Jackson, 1986). These are not unexpected outcomes from a chronic disease that is associated with severe pain, physical limitations, and an unpredictable course. A series of studies reported by Hurtig et al. (1989) showed that adolescent males are more vulnerable to psychosocial problems than are females and have more difficulty coping with sickle cell disease. Older boys were more likely to be socially withdrawn and were more depressed than younger boys and girls (Hurtig and White, 1989). These findings have been largely substantiated in a more recent study (Barbarin et al., 1994). Kell et al. (1998) reported that family competence was associated with fewer internalizing and externalizing behaviors by the adolescent. Difficulties with medical staff often begin in adolescence and frequently revolve around issues of pain management and inpatient stay. Unpredictable painful episodes may hamper the adolescent's development of a sense of control (Walco and Dampier, 1987).

Psychosocial difficulties of adolescents with sickle cell disease often go unaddressed by pediatric staff who feel unqualified to handle such issues. Those unresolved difficulties become magnified when adolescents are transferred to adult care. Independent of parents, transferred patients may fail to comply with recommended medical therapy and follow-up monitoring. There is growing interest in ensuring that the transition from pediatric to adult care proceed successfully for adolescents with sickle cell disease (Telfair et al., 1994). Professionals in programs caring for adolescents with sickle cell disease need to be aware of these psychosocial issues and to adopt measures to ensure optimal physical and psychological wellness for their patients. A series of guidelines on psychosocial issues drawn by two psychologists, Treadwell and Gil (1994), are recommended for professionals taking care of adolescents and others with sickle cell disease.

YOUNG ADULTHOOD

Pregnancy and Contraception

There is no absolute contraindication to pregnancy in sickle cell anemia, and fertility is probably normal when delayed onset of puberty and the likelihood that initial sexual encounters occur at a later age in sickle cell anemia than in control populations are taken into account (Serjeant 1992; Koshy and Burd, 1994).

The hazards of pregnancy in sickle cell anemia are many, especially for the fetus. Some older medical literature suggests that pregnancy in sickle cell anemia is not worth the risk and that therapeutic abortion and early sterilization is desirable. This is no longer true and modern medical management of pregnancy generally achieves good results, but the rate of obstetrical complications is still higher than in a normal population. In a recent survey of more than 9,300 African-American women delivering at a single maternity center, in fifty women with sickle cell anemia the combined prenatal and perinatal losses per woman were 20 percent compared with 10 percent in women with sickle cell trait or normal hemoglobin (Williams-Murphy et al., 1999). Four percent of women with sickle cell anemia had pyelonephritis compared with 0.3 percent of control women; the incidence of pregnancy-induced hypertension was 20 percent (9.6 percent in control subjects), caesarean sections were necessary in 44 percent of patients (22 percent in control subjects), gestational ages were about 1 week less than in control subjects, and birth weight was 2,700 g versus 3,010 g in control women. Maternal mortality, given access to modern obstetrical care, has been reported to range from less than 0.5 to 2 percent (Powars et al., 1986; Howard et al., 1995; Smith et al., 1996).

It seems logical that placental abnormalities are responsible for the most serious complications of pregnancy in sickle cell anemia and that these abnormalities are a result of anemia and the abnormal characteristics of the sickle erythrocyte. Placental villi may be edematous, infarcted, and fibrotic; and the placenta can be small. Umbilical cord veins showed morphologically abnormal endothelial cells, smooth muscle proliferation, basement membrane thickening, and necrotic areas (Decastel et al., 1999). Oxygen delivery to the fetus is reduced by maternal anemia and a placenta compromised by the effects of sickle cell disease. Patients with sickle cell anemia have about twice the normal rate of multiple pregnancy, placenta previa, abruptio placentae, preterm delivery, fetal distress, and caesarean sections and a fivefold increased occurrence of toxemia (Koshy and Burd, 1994). Infants born to women with sickle cell anemia are more often premature, small, and small for gestational age (Brown et al., 1994).

Few totally convincing randomized controlled studies are available to help the clinician manage the pregnant patient with sickle cell anemia. Although the same can be said about contraceptive methods, here there is far less controversy. Any approved form of contraception is acceptable in sickle cell anemia. The

dangers and the consequences of unwanted pregnancies outweigh the very small risks of contraceptive devices or drugs, and the complications of these methods do not seem to exceed those in the normal population (Serjeant, 1983).

Pregnant patients should be seen by their obstetrician every 1 to 2 weeks and labor closely supervised with continuous fetal monitoring. Sterilization or interruption of pregnancy in women with sickle cell anemia is not medically indicated. Prognostically, women with the highest levels of HbF had a lower rate of fetal perinatal death (Morris et al., 1994). Folic acid and iron supplements should be given if there is evidence of reduced iron stores. Spontaneous abortion has a 1 to 20 percent incidence, even with the best medical management (Koshy and Burd, 1994). Presumably, this is a result of placental insufficiency. When and how to use blood transfusions are the most contentious issues in the management of pregnancy in sickle cell anemia. Some obstetricians believe that transfusions should be used routinely and claim excellent results. Few, if any, controlled trials in the peer-reviewed literature corroborate this claim (Cunningham et al., 1983; Morrison et al., 1991; Howard et al., 1995; El-Shafei et al., 1995). When transfusions are used, there is little, if any, data favoring simple or exchange transfusions. Some evidence shows that where exchange transfusions were believed to be superior, simple transfusions provide the same benefits without as many transfusion-related complications (Chapter 37). Other limited controlled and observational studies suggest that with good prenatal care, fetal loss and other complications are low and transfusions do not improve the outcomes (Milner et al., 1980; Koshy et al., 1988; Smith et al., 1996).

Treatment Recommendations: How should the obstetrician and hematologist manage the pregnant patient with sickle cell anemia given the lack of totally convincing and consistent clinical trials? First, they should establish strong lines of communication so that care can be coordinated. A reasonable plan in the primigravida is to observe the patient carefully and intervene with transfusions only if complications such as toxemia, severe anemia, or worsening symptoms of sickle cell disease ensue. Multiple birth pregnancies also appear to benefit from transfusion (Koshy and Burd, 1991). Multigravidas have their experience with prior pregnancies to help guide the clinician. Uncomplicated previous pregnancies might be managed like those in primigravida, with transfusions reserved for complications. Individuals who have lost previous pregnancies might benefit from the early use of transfusions aimed at keeping the hemoglobin level above 9 g/dL. Sickle cell complications during pregnancy should be managed as they would be if there was no pregnancy, with special attention to avoid potentially teratogenic drugs during the first trimester.

An increasing number of patients have become pregnant or fathered children while taking hydroxyurea. Hydroxyurea is a teratogen in rats, cats, and rhesus monkeys and should not be used if pregnancy is planned. Pregnancy has been reported in at least fourteen women receiving hydroxyurea, usually for myeloproliferative disorders, but in four instances for sickle cell anemia (Steinberg et al., 1998). To date, there have been no adverse outcomes of pregnancy in hydroxyurea-treated women, but it must be emphasized that the study population is quite limited. Developmental defects have not been reported in pregnant patients who took hydroxyurea for other disease. Contraception should be practiced by both women and men receiving hydroxyurea and the uncertain outcome of unplanned pregnancy discussed frankly. If pregnancy occurs while taking hydroxyurea there is little information on which to base a decision for continuation or termination. So far, congenital defects have not been described in pregnancies followed to term. This is no cause for complacency. Hydroxyurea is very likely to be teratogenic in humans and should be avoided when pregnancy is planned. Whether or not previous exposure to hydroxyurea affects fertility and the results of pregnancy is unknown. Complications of hydroxyurea treatment are discussed in more detail in Chapter 38.

Surgery and Anesthesia

Surgery and anesthesia in sickle cell disease are safe, not complication free. For the best outcome, precautions must be observed (Scott-Conner and Brunson, 1994a; Scott-Conner and Brunson, 1994b; Bellet et al., 1995; Halvorson et al., 1997). When the results of more than 700 surgical procedures in sickle cell anemia were analyzed, mortality was about 1 percent, and no deaths occurred in children (Koshy et al., 1995). Nearly 90 percent of patients underwent transfusion preoperatively, but this was not a clinical trial of perioperative management or the effects of transfusion. Patients undergoing moderate risk surgery who underwent transfusion had fewer postoperative acute chest syndromes and painful episodes. Patient who had low risk surgery did not have any acute chest syndromes reported even if they did not undergo transfusion (Koshy et al., 1995).

Whether or not preoperative blood transfusion forestalled intraoperative or postoperative complications had been unanswered until the results of an important clinical trial that partially resolved these questions (Vichinsky et al., 1995). In this trial, discussed in detail in Chapter 37, simple transfusion to a hemoglobin level of about 10 g/dL before surgery

under general anesthesia was equally as effective in preventing postoperative complications as an aggressive regimen that reduced HbS levels to 30 percent or less. Simple transfusion exposed patients to half as much blood, and these individuals had fewer transfusion-related complications. Despite the regimen used, complications, often minor, happened in about one third of surgeries; acute chest syndrome, a major problem, occurred in 10 percent. Still unclear is the complication rate of surgery without routine transfusion.

After tonsillectomy and myringotomy, more than one third of patients had postoperative complications regardless of the method of transfusion, and a history of pulmonary disease was predictive of these complications (Waldron et al., 1999).

Treatment Recommendations: Lacking a randomized direct comparison of preoperative transfusion versus no transfusion in sickle cell anemia, a reasonable approach would be to recommend simple transfusion to a hemoglobin level of 10 g/dL in all patients undergoing intraabdominal and thoracic surgery, tonsillectomy, and other procedures under general anesthesia with moderate or high risk. Incentive spirometry may help prevent acute chest syndrome, the most serious postoperative complication (Bellet et al., 1995). Minor elective procedures in children might be done without preoperative transfusions (Griffin and Buchanan, 1993).

Although common sense suggests that tourniquets be avoided and arterial cross-clamping eschewed, most reports do not indicate problems with these procedures (Stein and Urbaniak, 1980; Vipond and Caldicott, 1998).

Venous Access Devices

Indiscriminate use of intravenous fluid therapy and blood transfusion early in life often culminates in great difficulty finding venous access in teenagers. As the solution to this problem is not simple and is beset with complications, all efforts should be made to use intravenous fluid judiciously (oral rehydration is preferable when feasible). Special attention should be given to avoiding infection and infiltration of intravenous access once it is established, as well as unnecessary blood drawing for laboratory testing.

Implantable central devices such as infusion ports and central venous catheters are associated, by some estimates, with as much as a five to ten times higher risk of complications in sickle cell anemia than when they are used in other diseases (Scott-Conner and Brunson, 1994a; Jeng et al., 1999). These include thrombosis, at times involving large veins and causing superior vena cava syndrome, and sepsis. Some reports found serious complications associated with half the devices implanted. Infections have been estimated to occur at a rate of 5 to 10/1,000 catheter days depending on the indication for catheter placement. Some experts recommend using low doses of warfarin, 2 mg daily, to retard thrombosis of implantable ports and catheters.

Osteonecrosis

Osteonecrosis is painful and often disabling. The age-adjusted incidence rate of osteonecrosis in sickle cell anemia is 2.5 per 100-patient years for both hip and shoulder joints (Milner et al., 1991, 1993). About three fourths of individuals with shoulder disease also have hip involvement (Milner et al., 1993). By age 35 years, half of all individuals with sickle cell anemia have evidence of hip and shoulder osteonecrosis; in childhood, sickle cell disease is the most common cause of this lesion. Because symptoms of hip disease often are present in children and can progress rapidly to disability, management poses a dilemma: to balance the relief of pain and avoidance of loss of joint function with the knowledge that total joint replacement is not yet a permanent "cure" and reoperation, especially of the hip, is likely to be required. This predicament emphasizes the importance of knowing if core decompression in early-stage hip disease, discussed later, is therapeutically beneficial.

Activity-limiting symptoms do not often accompany shoulder disease, which is asymptomatic in 80 percent of patients at the time of its discovery. Hip disease may present acutely and mimic septic arthritis or synovitis. More often, the onset of osteonecrosis is insidious but progressive, and most patients with early-stage disease progress to collapse of the femoral head within 2 years. Hip necrosis is often bilateral, although both hips need not develop disease simultaneously or progress symmetrically. Hip disease can be scored by the system of Ficat, a simplification of an earlier categorization, which classifies by x-ray film and MRI the progressive features of this disorder (Ficat, 1985) (Fig. 24.5 and Table 24.4). The "classic" radiographic lesion, the crescent sign, which is present in Stage III disease, represents an intracapital fracture that begins at the interface of the necrotic lesion and subchondral bone and extends through the area of bone necrosis. Fibrous metaplasia beneath this fracture prevents revascularization and repair, making this lesion irreversible. Many other more or less complicated classification systems have been proposed, some including objective measurements of femoral head involvement and joint destruction (Urbaniak and Jones, 1997). These more elaborate systems may be useful when evaluating and comparing new methods of treatment.

A complete understanding of the pathogenesis of osteonecrosis in sickle cell anemia is lacking, but it may begin with microinfarction of the trabeculae of cancellous bone. Pressure within the marrow of the femoral head is increased when osteonecrosis is recognized clinically or by MRI, but whether this is a cause or a result of osteonecrosis is unclear. It has been reported that in non-sickle cell disease-related osteonecrosis, asymptomatic "normal" hips contralateral to involved hips may have increased pressure. It has been claimed that it is these, rather than "normal" hips with normal pressure, that will ultimately develop clinical disease. PCV, perhaps a surrogate for blood viscosity, is related to the prevalence of osteonecrosis in sickle cell anemia. Patients with higher PCV and with sickle cell anemia-α thalassemia—a genotype associated with an increased PCV compared with sickle cell anemia—have a higher prevalence of osteonecrosis (Steinberg et al., 1984; Milner et al., 1991, 1993; Ballas et al., 1998). In studies of osteonecrosis in patients who did not have sickle cell disease, there has been some association of this lesion with low levels of Protein S and Protein C and hypofibrinolysis and the strong impression that coagulation plays some role in the genesis of this lesion (Urbaniak and Jones, 1997). Recent studies, some reported only in abstract form, have focused on the role of inherited disorders of thrombosis as contributing elements in the pathogenesis of osteonecrosis in sickle cell anemia and have had disparate results. In one report, a C→T mutation at position 677 of the 5, 10 methylenetetrahydofolate reductase gene, which is associated with enzyme thermolability and a putative hypercoagulable state owing to hyperhomocystenemia, was found in 36 percent of forty-five adults with sickle cell disease and osteonecrosis but in only 13 percent of sixty-two patients without osteonecrosis, a significant difference (Kutlar et al., 1998). In other reports, this same mutation was unassociated with vascular complications of sickle cell disease, including osteonecrosis; however, far fewer patients were studied (DeCastro et al., 1998). There was also no relationship between the presence of a mutation in the platelet glycoprotein IIIa gene, a C→T change at position 1565 (a mutation associated with premature coronary artery disease) and osteonecrosis (Zimmerman and Ware, 1998; Zimmerman et al., 1998). Clearly, further work is needed to resolve the role of genetic risk factors for thrombosis, many of which have been examined only in pilot studies or reported in abstract, in the etiology of osteonecrosis. An association has been made between osteonecrosis and the acute chest syndrome (Vichinsky et al., 1994).

Because of pain and loss of joint function, osteonecrosis of the hip can dominate the clinical manifestation of sickle cell anemia. Almost always, it presents with pain in and about the affected joint, at times

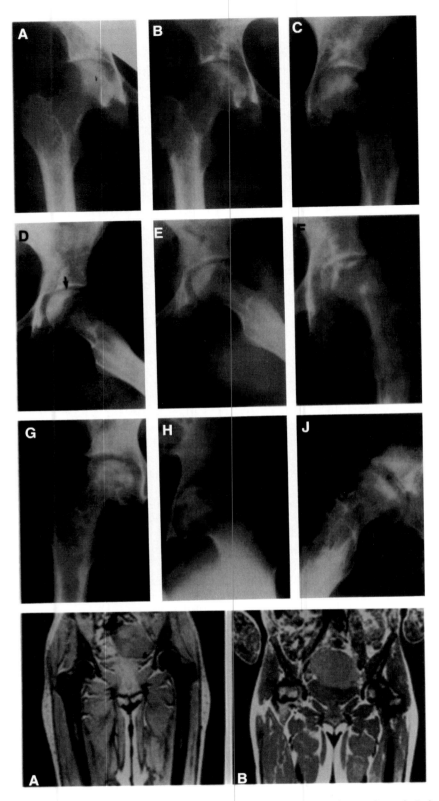

Figure 24.5. Osteonecrosis of the hip in sickle cell disease. In panel (**A**), subpanels A through C, the progression of osteonecrosis in a 19-year-old woman with sickle cell anemia is shown. Although the hip was painful, the x-ray study was initially normal (**A**) but MRI showed osteonecrosis. Core decompression was done (note track) (**B**). In (**C**) the joint space is normal but there is sclerosis. In another patient, a crescent sign appears in a painful hip (**D**). Five weeks later, there is collapse of this segment (**E**). After an additional 15 months, there is extensive joint destruction and total hip replacement was done. Panels (**G**, **H**, and **J**) show advanced degenerative changes in three different patients with sickle cell disease. (**B**) MRI images of the hips in a 30-year-old woman with sickle cell anemia. In subpanel (**A**), the femoral heads are normal. After 1 year, changes of osteonecrosis are evident (**B**). (From Embury et al., 1994, with permission.)

Table 24.4. Modified Ficat System of Grading Osteonecrosis of the Femoral Head

Stage	Imaging Results	Clinical
0	MRI normal (marrow necrosis may be present histologically)	Normal
I	Normal radiograph and CT; abnormal MRI with necrosis (marrow and bone necrosis)	Usually painless
II	Sclerosis and lytic areas on x-ray study; CT and MRI abnormal with necrosis and reactive interface	Pain not always present
III	Femoral head flattening and crescent sign on x-ray study; MRI, crescent sign	Pain present, especially with weight bearing, relieved with rest
IV	Femoral head collapse; joint space narrowing; osteoarthritis	Pain at rest, joint stiffness and weakness; secondary arthritis

From Ficat, 1985; Urbaniak and Jones, 1997.

with spasm of the surrounding musculature. It can be detected early in its evolution by MRI, and only more advanced disease is radiographically visible (Table 24.4). MRI can be used to quantify the extent of damage to the femoral head (Urbaniak and Jones, 1997). The inexorable progress of this complication, once pain and radiographic abnormalities have appeared, has prompted a search for treatment that could stabilize disease progression and relieve pain.

Core decompression is one approach to arresting the progression of osteonecrosis of the hip. Its possible value was discovered serendipitously during measurements of bone marrow pressure and femoral head biopsies when pain decreased after removal of a bone core; controversy has dogged its application. In this method, a core of bone is removed from the femoral neck, stopping well short of the subchondral plate. This procedure has been studied most intensively in osteonecrosis from causes other than sickle cell anemia; results, if variable, have been encouraging. An analysis of more than 1,000 hips from twenty-four different studies, with a 30-month follow-up period showed a clinical and radiographic success rate of 64 percent (Mont et al., 1996). Eighty-five percent of stage I patients had a good result. In comparison, only 23 percent of unoperated patients had a successful outcome. Reports that formed the basis for this syn-

thesis were largely uncontrolled retrospective studies. Treatment of sickle cell osteonecrosis by core decompression decreases pain, restores function, and promotes healing in some patients; but, to date, this method has had limited use (Milner et al., 1994). In a pilot study of thirteen hips (eight patients with sickle cell anemia) followed up for a mean of 42 months, five patients showed one-stage radiologic progression, but pain decreased and mobility increased in eleven hips (Styles and Vichinsky, 1996). Based on these results and the dismal outlook for conservative therapy, a controlled trial of core decompression for hip osteonecrosis in sickle cell disease has been initiated.

Treatment Recommendations: Until now, conservative treatment with bed rest and wheelchair, crutches to reduce the load on weight-bearing joints, nonsteroidal anti-inflammatory drugs, and physical therapy has been the sole means of managing early disease. Pain relief is problematic, consisting of joint protection, rest, heat, hydrotherapy, relaxation techniques, and analgesics. Milder analgesics are often ineffective. If not guarded against, prolonged bed rest can cause flexion contractures. Physical therapy is directed at stretching and strengthening hip adductors and other hip muscles, releasing muscle spasm, training in the proper uses of crutches, quadriceps strengthening, improving upper body strength, and posture retraining. Whether any conservative treatment delays the progression of sickle osteonecrosis is unclear, but the bulk of the evidence suggests that it does not (Washington and Root, 1985; Mankin, 1992). As pain becomes intolerable and joint function is lost, as a final resort, joint replacement is done. Transfusions have not proved useful for pain relief or halting disease progression (Dunsmore et al., 1995).

Pain in osteonecrosis tends to be chronic, and, if possible, narcotic analgesics should be limited. Nevertheless, other analgesics often fail to provide the same measure of comfort that they achieve in degenerative joint disease. As destruction progresses, pain becomes severe and joint function is lost; the affected joint— usually the hip—needs replacement.

Total hip arthroplasty can be successful, but by 4 to 5 years after surgery, about one third of prostheses have failed, and pain can remain a major problem (Milner et al., 1991). Cementless components have been recommended, but their polyethylene surfaces wear and femoral osteolysis may require reoperation (Hickman and Lachiewicz, 1997). Postoperative complications, including infection, fracture, and acute chest syndrome, with persistent pain are common. In different series, the need for revision ranged from 30 to 50 percent, infection occurred in 8 to 30 percent, and failure occurred in about 40 percent of cases monitored for about 5 to 8 years (Urbaniak and Jones, 1997). It seems prudent to delay this type of surgery until symptoms interfere with the activities of daily living. As the results of core decompression for osteonecrosis of the femoral head in sickle cell disease are still being studied, this procedure might best be considered in the context of the ongoing clinical trial. Although the operative management of hip disease is beyond the scope of this discussion, if core decompression is done, great care must be taken to avoid destruction of the femoral head, and postoperative weight bearing must be strictly managed until healing is complete (Urbaniak and Jones, 1997).

When hip disease is too advanced to consider core decompression and total hip arthroplasty is not yet an option, rotational osteotomy has been considered when pain is severe and normal activities impossible (Urbaniak and Jones, 1997). Although some good results have been achieved in patients with sickle cell anemia, adverse outcomes also occur and there are few or no data to recommend when this procedure is indicated or to judge its effectiveness. Expert orthopedic advice should be sought.

Shoulder disease occasionally becomes severely painful. Joint destruction can require total shoulder arthroplasty. There is no published experience with core decompression of the humeral head in osteonecrosis associated with sickle cell anemia, but in uncontrolled studies it has been used with good results in steroid or alcohol-induced disease.

Other Disorders of Bone and Joints

Joint symptoms in addition to hand-foot syndrome and osteonecrosis are commonly encountered. Usually they are minor compared with the other complications of sickle cell anemia. Effusions of large joints may be monoarticular or polyarticular, noninflammatory or inflammatory, and contain sickled cells (Espinoza et al., 1974). Noninflammatory effusions of the knee can be managed successfully by rest and nonsteroidal anti-inflammatory drugs. Acute hematogenous osteomyelitis causes acute pain and swelling and may involve periarticular bone, extending into the joint space and causing effusion. This may be diagnosed by MRI, which is more sensitive than technetium or gallium scanning.

Because of increased production of uric acid and impaired renal function, about one fourth of patients have elevated uric acid levels, and some will have attacks of acute gouty arthritis. Lupus erythematosus is common in African-American women, and the coincidence of lupus and its articular manifestations with sickle cell anemia is not rare. Backaches may often be ascribed to osteoporosis from expanded hematopoiesis and can be treated with physical therapy and mild analgesics.

Myofascial inflammation has also been found and is associated with localized edema, severe pain, inflammatory tissue changes, and myonecrosis (Dorwart and Gabuzda, 1985; Malekgoudarzi and Feffer, 1999).

Bone marrow infarction has been described in sickle cell anemia and other sickle hemoglobinopathies (Charache and Page, 1967). It may be associated with painful episodes involving bone.

Orbital complications are uncommon in sickle cell disease. In one patient with fever, headache, orbital swelling, and optic nerve dysfunction, CT displayed bilateral superior subperiosteal cystic masses, which, during surgical exploration, were bilateral liquefied hematomas (Curran et al., 1997). A review of the literature identified sixteen young patients with sickle cell disease with rapidly developing findings ranging from frontal headache, fever, and eyelid edema to bilateral complete orbital compression syndrome (Curran et al., 1997). Sixty percent had orbital hemorrhage on CT and 80 percent of twelve patients tested had orbital bone marrow infarction. Recovery was complete in 94 percent of cases, 74 percent of whom were treated conservatively, and 11 percent had a recurrence. These unusual events are likely to arise from vasoocclusive disease in the marrow space surrounding the orbits.

Overgrowth of the maxilla and mandible can lead to facial deformity with separation and anterior angulation of the incisors called *sickle gnathopathy*. Rare in developed countries, it has been more characteristic of the disease in Africa, and the deformities can be of a severity to necessitate surgical correction. Diploic spaces of the skull are also widened, giving at times a "hair-on-end" radiographic picture, but these changes are not as prominent as described in patients with poorly treated β thalassemia.

Generalized osteoporosis is commonly present, especially in the spine where vertebrae display a typical "fish mouth" appearance.

Endocrinopathies

Thirty-two men with sickle cell anemia and a mean age of 26.5 years had reduced testosterone and dihydrotestosterone levels and increased luteinizing hormone (LH) and follicle-stimulating hormone (FSH) levels consistent with primary gonadal failure. Zinc levels were decreased in hair and eythrocytes, and their erythrocyte zinc content correlated with serum testosterone. These patients had abnormal secondary sexual characteristics and eunuchoid skeletal proportions (Abbasi et al., 1976). Eighty male and female sickle cell disease patients, ages 4 to 50 years, had gonadal hypofunction with low LH, FSH, cortisol and testosterone levels compared with age- and sex-matched normal control subjects. Semen analysis in twenty-five patients with sickle cell anemia and in twenty-five control subjects showed significantly reduced ejaculate volume, sperm motility, and sperm density in patients in the control population. A significant increase was also observed in the percentage of spermatids and in abnormal spermatozoa, with amorphous and tapered heads in the patients' semen. These abnormalities associated with semen in sickle cell anemia may result from testicular dysfunction and abnormalities in the accessory sex organs, such as the seminal vesicles and the prostate.

To assess the role of the gonads and anterior pituitary gland in the production of poor quality semen of males with sickle cell anemia, FSH, LH, prolactin, and serum testosterone, were assayed radioimmunologically in thirty-three men with sickle cell disease and in twenty-nine age-matched normal control subjects. Individuals with sickle cell disease had significantly lower mean serum testosterone, higher mean FSH, and higher prolactin levels than control subjects. Higher gonadotropins associated with lower testosterone suggested an intact hypothalamic/pituitary axis and a primary testicular defect (Osegbe and Akinyanju, 1987). Hypogonadism in sickle cell anemia may also have a hypothalamic origin (Landefield et al., 1983). In two 19-year-old men with sickle cell anemia and hypogonadism, hypothalamic dysfunction responded to oral clomiphene therapy. Partial hypothalamic hypogonadism was shown by low levels of testosterone, low to low-normal levels of LH and FSH, and a nearly normal rise in gonadotropin levels in response to exogenous gonadotropin-releasing hormone. Treatment with oral clomiphene raised LH, FSH, and testosterone levels to normal, inducing puberty in both patients.

Women with sickle cell disease appeared to be as fertile as control subjects, although they had a 2-year delay in menarche and a 4-year delay for their first pregnancy (Alleyne et al., 1981). The number of infants born to patients with sickle cell disease was less at all ages compared with Jamaican standards, perhaps reflecting lesser fertility after a first pregnancy.

Basal and stimulated cortisol levels and the increment of coritsol at 30, 50, and 120 minutes after adrenocorticotrophic hormone (ACTH) infusion were also similar in patients with sickle cell anemia and control subjects, suggesting normal adrenal function (Saad and Saad, 1992).

Iron overload has been associated with multiple endocrine abnormalities. Three patients with sickle cell disease over 45 years old had received multiple units of transfused red blood cells, had serum ferritin levels of greater than 6,000 ng/mL, and had hypothyroidism (Philips et al., 1992). All patients were diagnosed when they were critically ill, and all died with congestive heart failure shortly after hypothyroidism was found. Postmortem examination in one case showed fibrosis

of the thyroid gland and extensive deposition of iron in the cells lining the thyroid follicles. Males with sickle cell anemia had significantly lower T_3 and higher thyroid-stimulating hormone (TSH) levels than a comparison control group. Stimulation with thyrotropin in ten male sibling pairs showed significant increases in T_3 and TSH in both patients and sibling control subjects, although the increase in TSH was significantly greater in patients with sickle cell anemia. These finding were most consistent with a modest primary thyroid failure (Parshad et al., 1989). However, in another study, T_3 and T_4 levels were similar in patients and controls (el Hazmi et al., 1991).

Reduced height and weight can accompany sickle cell disease. To see whether impaired growth is associated with abnormalities of the growth hormone (GH)/insulin-like growth factor-I (IGF-I)/IGF binding protein-3 (IGFBP-3) axis, twenty-one children with sickle cell disease were examined. Nearly half had a defective GH response to both clonidine and glucagon. Children with an impaired response had slower linear growth velocity, lower circulating concentrations of IGF-I and IGFBP-3, and either partial or complete empty sellae by CT scanning. Dietary intake, body mass index, midarm circumferences, skinfold thickness, serum albumin concentration, and intestinal absorption of D-xylose were similar in the two groups. A single injection of GH produced a smaller increase in circulating IGF-I in children with or without defective GH secretion compared with ten age-matched children with idiopathic short stature and eleven children with isolated GH deficiency, suggesting partial GH resistance in the sickle cell disease group. Defective GH secretion, decreased IGF-I synthesis, and partial resistance to GH in these short children suggest that treatment with IGF-I may be superior to GH therapy for improving their growth (Soliman et al., 1997).

Limited studies of parathyroid function in sickle cell disease have been reported. Concentrations of serum calcium, parathyroid hormone (PTH), 25 hydroxyvitamin D (25 OHD), and 1,25 dihydroxyvitamin D (1,25(OH)2D) were determined in ninety-nine Saudi patients with sickle cell disease and in 104 matching healthy control subjects. Serum calcium and 25 OHD were significantly lower in the patients, and 14 and 12 percent had serum calcium and 25 OHD concentrations, respectively, below the normal range. PTH was significantly higher in the patients; 31 percent had values above normal. There were no significant differences in 1,25(OH)2D levels. These results suggested that patients with sickle cell disease have a tendency toward hypocalcemia associated with high PTH levels, implying impaired intestinal absorption of calcium and vitamin D (Mohammed et al., 1993). In eighteen children with a median age of 8 years with sickle cell anemia living on the tropical island of Curacao, serum calcium concentration was slightly lower than in control children but no individual was hypocalcemic. In contrast to the studies in Saudis, there were no differences in serum concentrations of phosphate, total protein, albumin, PTH, 25 OHD, and 1,25 (OH)2D in patients and control subjects. While possibly contributing to the osteoporosis present in sickle cell disease—a highly conjectural supposition—mineral metabolism in these disorders appears to be very mildly abnormal.

In aggregate, the subtle endocrinologic abnormalities present in sickle cell disease seldom appear to cause clinically apparent problems and infrequently require replacement therapy.

Leg Ulcers

Usually appearing on the lower leg, most small and superficial ulcers heal spontaneously with rest and careful local hygiene. At times leg ulcers are deep, huge and circumferential, exceedingly painful, and disabling. They may defy all simple and many complex therapeutic measures. As expected, there are no trials comparing therapies and only a few controlled trials of any type of ulcer treatment.

In the United States, the Cooperative Study of Sickle Cell Disease found that about 5 percent of patients with sickle cell anemia over age 10 years had leg ulcers on entry into the study. Less than 1 percent of individuals with HbS-β^0 thalassemia had an ulcer, and no ulcers were seen in HbSC disease or HbS-β^+ thalassemia, although they can be found in these genotypes. When incidence rates were examined according to the genotype of sickle cell disease, those 20 years and older with sickle cell anemia had a rate of nearly 20 per 100 patient-years, whereas in sickle cell anemia-α thalassemia, the rate was about 10 per 100 patient-years. In total, about one fourth of patients had a history of or developed a leg ulcer during an observation period that was variable but no more than 8 years. Leg ulcers were uncommon in children—none of 1,700 children younger than 10 years had an ulcer—and began to make their appearance during the early teen years when activities that are most apt to cause trauma to the lower legs become commonplace (Koshy et al., 1989). Beyond age 20 years, the incidence of ulcers increased sharply. Males were more likely to have ulcers than females whether or not they also had α thalassemia. There is a geographic difference in the prevalence of sickle cell leg ulcers. In Jamaica, two thirds of patients may have a history of ulceration (Gueri and Serjeant, 1970). Among 6,302 adults with sickle cell anemia in Nigeria, 7.5 percent had leg ulcers (Durosinmi et al., 1991). How long a population is

observed, where the patients reside, the age of individuals studied, the male/female ratio, and the diligence of inquiring about a history of ulcers all determine the prevalence and incidence of this complication.

The first appearance of a leg ulcer usually signifies the high likelihood of their recurrence over many years. Sometimes an ulcer will appear, disappear with treatment or spontaneously, and never recur. More often they recur after healing but sometimes only after many years. Leg ulcers are most common about the medial and lateral malleoli but can occur on the dorsum of the foot and the anterior or posterior aspects of the leg. They appear bilaterally or unilaterally. It has been said that skin ulceration can occur on the arms and other locations, but if these ulcers have the same cause as the typical sickle cell leg ulcer, they must be quite rare. Ulcers often are first found after trauma to the leg that can seem trivial or appear to be the sequela of an insect bite.

Leg ulcers have been reported in all types of hemolytic anemia, especially the β thalassemias and hereditary spherocytosis, so that they are not a specific complication of sickle cell anemia, although they are far more common in this disorder. Their pathophysiology has not been clearly delineated, but it has been suggested that the poor deformability of the sickle cells and, to a lesser extent, the erythrocytes of β thalassemia and hereditary spherocytosis impair their circulation through the dermal capillaries (Peachey, 1978). Patients with the highest levels of HbF and total hemoglobin are relatively protected from leg ulcers (Gueri and Serjeant, 1970; Koshy et al., 1989) (Fig. 24.6). Individuals with sickle cell anemia-homozygous α thalassemia-2, perhaps because they have higher hemoglobin concentrations and their erythrocytes have greater rheologic competence, have an incidence of ulcers (2.4 per 100 patient-years) less than half that of individuals with sickle cell anemia-heterozygous α thalassemia-2 (Koshy et al., 1989).

Multiple elements are likely to contribute to the development of leg ulcers in sickle cell anemia. These include tropical climate, circulatory dynamics, the "exposed" environment of the leg, anemia, erythrocyte and vascular injury triggered by the polymerization of HbS, and local infection. Both anaerobes and aerobes can be cultured from the base of ulcers more than 50 percent of the time (MacFarlane et al., 1986; Ademiluyi et al., 1988). It is likely that the ulcer flora varies among clinics and regions. Their role in the development and enlargement of ulcers is unknown. Venous pressure measurements and venography in eight patients with leg ulcers were normal, suggesting that venous disease did not contribute to ulceration. Although hemodynamic studies implied venous insufficiency, this was interpreted as the result of peripheral

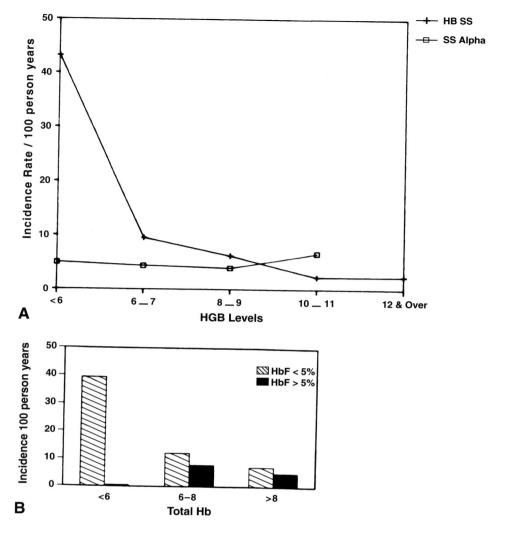

Figure 24.6. Incidence of leg ulcers per 100 patient-years in patients with sickle cell anemia without α thalassemia according to total hemoglobin concentration and HbF level (Koshy et al., 1989).

arteriovenous shunting and the high cardiac output of sickle cell anemia (Billett et al., 1991). Leg ulcers were associated with a higher incidence of HLA-B35 and Cw4 than sickle cell anemia without ulcers, but only nine patients with leg ulcers were examined (Ofosu et al., 1987).

Treatment Recommendations: Perhaps nowhere in the annals of the treatment of sickle cell anemia have more untested remedies been applied than in the therapy of leg ulceration. In the Cooperative Study—a study that did not mandate the choice of treatment—recurrence of ulcers was unaffected by treatment, which included transfusions, the Unna gel dressing, zinc, skin grafts, and topical medications of different types such as antibiotics (Koshy et al., 1989). There are reports touting the use

of erythropoietin, antithrombin III, proprionyl-L-carnitine, perilesional injection of colony-stimulating factors such as GM-CSF, arginine butyrate, pentoxy-fylline, DuoDerm, Solcoseryl, isoxsuprine, zinc sulfate, ozone, oxygen, and hyperbaric oxygen (Phillips et al., 1994; Sher and Olivieri 1994; Pieters et al., 1995; Serjeant et al., 1997; Voskaridou et al., 1999). None of these treatments have been the subject of careful clinical trials. There have been excellent summaries of the treatment of leg ulcers (Table 24.5) (Eckman, 1996). Little that is novel has appeared more recently.

Control of local inflammation and infection ensuring a clean granulating surface for reepithelialization remains the mainstay of treatment. Wet to dry dressings applied several times a day provide debridement. Occasionally surgical debridement is needed to cleanse the ulcer base. Although cultures of the ulcer base are most often positive, topical antibiotics do not uniformly help healing and systemic antimicrobials are usually not indicated. However, when erythema of the ulcer borders and a purulent exudate are present that

Table 24.5. Treatment of Leg Ulcers in Sickle Cell Disease

1. Débridement
    Wet to dry saline dressings
    Hydrocolloid dressings
    Surgical
2. Prevent local edema
    Support hose as needed
    Bed rest and leg elevation as needed
3. Local treatments
    Unna boots (zinc oxide impregnated)
    Hydrocolloid dressings
    Topical antibiotic as needed
    Skin grafting as final alternative
4. Systemic treatments
    Transfusions
    Systemic antibiotic as needed
    Oral zinc sulfate

Adapted from Eckman (1996). All patients should be treated with combinations of treatments listed in 1 to 3. Systemic treatments as listed have not been proven effective, and transfusions may be associated with clinically important complication.

do not rapidly resolve after debridement, topical neomycin-bacitracin-polymyxin ointment and systemic antibiotics, chosen on the basis of culture, can be considered (Baum et al., 1987). A preliminary report suggested that some chronic ulcers resistant to treatment and not complicated by staphylococcal tissue infection, but accompanied by antibodies to staphylolysin and anti-nuclease antibodies, healed after treatment with flucloxacillin (Mangi et al., 1998). Perhaps screening for antistaphylococcal antibodies and treatment of antibody-positive patients with appropriate antibiotics will be useful, but controlled studies must be done before this regimen can be recommended. Dressing the ulcer with an Unna boot protects the involved area and is a reasonable method of conservative management. Even small ulcers can be excruciatingly painful and may require large amounts of narcotic analgesics for relief. Some patients get good analgesic relief from narcotic-containing skin patches. When healing occurs the pain usually disappears. Zinc sulfate, 220 mg orally 3 times a day, has also been recommended (Eckman, 1996).

When healing fails after a trial of conservative treatment that should last 6 to 8 weeks, difficult choices for more radical treatment must be faced. Prolonged bed rest may be helpful but is impractical in most instances. Controlled studies of transfusion have not been reported, but reducing HbS level to less than 30 percent by periodic transfusion can be considered. Hydroxyurea can increase HbF and total hemoglobin level in many individuals with sickle cell anemia and,

on this basis, can be postulated to decrease the recurrence of leg ulcers and to retard their first appearance. No trials have been reported that establish the effectiveness of hydroxyurea as a treatment for sickle cell leg ulcers. Hydroxyurea appears to cause ulcers in patients with myeloproliferative disorders but was not associated with an increase or decrease of leg ulcers in sickle cell anemia (Chapter 38). When leg ulcers cause serious morbidity, a trial of hydroxyurea appears to be reasonable. Surgery is a last resort, as the recurrence rate and chance of graft failure are high. Different procedures have been used including free flaps, myocutaneous flaps, and simple skin grafts. The type of grafting used appears to depend on the size of the ulcer and the experience of the surgeon.

A gel matrix containing the arginine-glycine-aspartic acid (RGD) recognition site of cell surface integrins complexed with sodium hyaluronate was studied in a randomized trial and compared with saline dressings used with the same supportive care (Wethers et al., 1994). Conceptually, this gel was supposed to attract and help anchor cells that would foster healing. RGD gel applied weekly promoted ulcer healing over the 10 weeks of this trial and had an effect even on ulcers that were present for very long times (Fig. 24.7). Whether this treatment will be effective in the long term and prevent recurrence is not known; at this time, the gel product has not been marketed.

All patients, especially those who have had leg ulcers, should be urged to protect their legs with support hose, avoid activities that cause swelling such as prolonged standing, and use local lubricants such as Vanicream, which may prevent excessive skin dryness and cracking.

Priapism

Priapus, the mythological god of procreation and caretaker of vineyards, is personified by an enlarged tumescent phallus, a prerequisite for copulation, that is at times stimulated by excessive quaffing of the grape. This figure is associated with debauchery. Priapism, a prolonged painful erection, undesirable and lasting beyond the period of sexual stimulation, does not provoke sexual profligacy and more often causes impotence. Priapism in sickle cell anemia may have a nocturnal onset, occur spontaneously, or be an unwanted response to erotic stimulation. Regardless of the initial stimulus, the normal process of detumescence fails. In sickle cell anemia, this failure almost always results from impaired venous outflow.

Different mechanisms of priapism and its pathophysiology are best understood by referring to penile anatomy and the normal erectile mechanism (Fig. 24.8). There is no vascular communication between

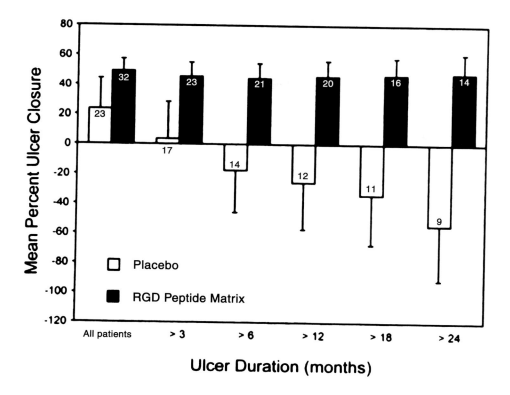

Figure 24.7. Percentage of ulcer healing in patients treated with arginine-glycine-aspartic acid gel and saline control according to the duration of ulcers before treatment (Wethers et al., 1994). In control patients, healing declined with the longer duration of ulcers.

the corpora cavernosa and the corpus spongiosum. Draining the corporal sinusoids are emissary veins that enter progressively larger vessels to form the internal pudendal vein. Sinusoids of the glans drain directly into the deep dorsal veins, allowing, when indicated, shunts to be created that may permit blood to flow from the corpora cavernosa to the corpus spongiosa. Normal erection is initiated by psychogenic, tactile, and neural stimuli that relax arterial vessels and enhance blood delivery to the corporeal bodies. This process is mediated at least partly by reduced α-adrenergic activity. Venous outflow is restricted as draining veins are compressed against the surrounding fascia by distended sinusoids. As the circumference of the penis is limited by the fascial wrapping of the corpora, when the sinusoids become engorged, elongation is paramount. Detumescence reverses this process as α-adrenergic activity increases, feeding arterioles constrict, and venous return is reestablished.

How the blood cells of sickle cell anemia evoke priapism is not known. Conceivably, activated neutrophils and platelets abet sickle erythrocytes in this process by damaging endothelial cells of the vessels draining the corpora cavernosa. NO, or endothelial

Figure 24.8. Anatomy of the penis. Fed by anastomosing branches of the internal pudendal artery, the erectile apparatus consists of two longitudinal cylinders of sinusoidal tissue, the paired corpora cavernosa with their associated arteries. Ventral to the corpora cavernosa is the corpus spongiosum, pierced by the urethra and terminating in the glans penis. A bulbourethral artery feeds the corpus spongiosum. The corporal bodies, except for the glans, are encased in fibrous fascial tunics, the tunica albuginea. There is no vascular communication between the corpora cavernosa and the corpus spongiosum. Draining the corporal sinusoids are emissary veins that enter progressively larger vessels to form the internal pudendal vein. Sinusoids of the glans drain directly into the deep dorsal veins. For full color reproduction, see color plate 24.8

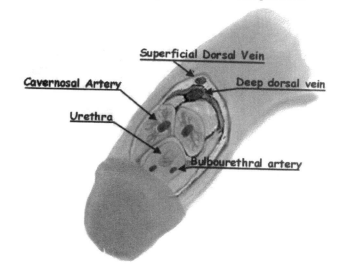

derived relaxing factor, is a potent vasodilator. S-nitrosohemoglobin is formed in the lung, while in tissues, when oxygen is unloaded, NO is transferred to the vessel wall promoting vasodilation (Hofstra et al., 1996). Perhaps HbS increases delivery of NO to the endothelium enhancing vasodilation in the corporal bodies. NO appears to have effects on HbS that differ from HbA, as it increases the O_2 affinity of only HbS; however, this observation has yet to be confirmed (Head et al., 1997).

Where sickle cell anemia is common, it is one of the leading causes of priapism. Less is known about the incidence of priapism in other genotypes of sickle cell disease. Ninety percent of cases of priapism in sickle cell disease are seen in individuals with sickle cell anemia (Sharpsteen et al., 1993). Typically, priapism in sickle cell anemia is said to be bicorporeal—only the corpora cavernosa are affected—and is "low flow"—venous outflow is obstructed rather than arterial flow increased. In children priapism is often associated with normal vascular flow, which perhaps accounts for their better prognosis as a group. Tricorporeal priapism has been described in sickle cell anemia and rarely a "high flow" state, in the absence of penile vascular injury, is present (Sharpsteen et al., 1993; Ramos et al., 1995). With bicorporeal priapism the glans remains soft and urination is normal. A tense glans and impaired urination signal involvement of the spongiosa, which usually implies infarctive damage to the corpora cavernosa.

An alternative construct of priapism in sickle cell anemia holds that prepubertal patients have bicorporeal priapism with high blood flow. Priapic episodes in this population usually last less than 48 hours and tend not to recur; potency is preserved. In contrast, priapism in adults is usually tricorporeal, low flow, recurrent, and long lasting; impotence results in more than half these cases, regardless of treatment (Sharpsteen et al., 1993). These patients have been said to have a higher incidence of stroke, lung disease, renal failure, leg ulcers, and premature death than individuals without priapism.

Recurrent attacks of priapism can last for several hours with tolerable discomfort and be self-limited. These episodes have been termed *stuttering priapism,* and they usually have a nocturnal onset. Erectile function is mostly preserved between these attacks, which can recur over years and number in the dozens. Major episodes of priapism often, but not always, follow a history of stuttering attacks, last for days, and can be excruciatingly painful. They usually destroy sexual function by causing irreversible damage to the corporal bodies. Prolonged or recurrent episodes of priapism cause edema of the vascular septa of the corpora cavernosa, which can lead to fibrosis, destroy the nor-

mal distensible sinusoidal anatomy, and culminate in impotence (Serjeant, 1992).

It has been estimated that nearly 40 percent of adult men with sickle cell anemia have had at least one episode of priapism (Serjeant et al., 1985; Fowler et al., 1991; Serjeant 1992; Hakim et al., 1994). The mean age of onset is 19 years, but it has been reported in children as young as 5 years (Miller et al., 1995). In 400 patients ages 5 to 19 years, only 2 percent were hospitalized with priapism during a 7-year period (Miller et al., 1995). From the literature it is difficult to know the true incidence of priapism in sickle cell anemia. Many different age groups have been studied, most retrospectively; observation periods vary greatly, definitions may be vague, self-reporting may be poor, and the zeal of questioning to determine if priapism has occurred may be suboptimal. High HbF levels may protect against priapism, as they do for other vasoocclusive complications. Priapism has been considered one manifestation of severe vascular disease and has been associated with an increased chance of cerebrovascular accident (Powars and Johnson, 1996; Leong et al., 1997).

One rare complication of priapism is megalophallus (Datta, 1977). In a well-studied case, where penile enlargement followed a prolonged severe priapic event, the proximal two thirds of the penis had a circumference of nearly 20 cm. Using Doppler measurements, penile blood flow was high and MRI showed deoxyHbS in the corpora cavernosa. At least in this instance, corporal fibrosis did not seem to be present and erectile function was preserved. It was hypothesized that sudden loss of elasticity of the tunica albuginea allowed painless penile expansion (Kassim et al., in press).

In the pediatric age group, impotence seems to be a less common result of priapism, and its incidence varies directly with age (Tarry et al., 1987; Chakrabarty et al., 1996). One attack of priapism presages multiple episodes. This may be an indication that sufficient vascular damage is present to alter normal erectile function. It seems reasonable to suspect that subclinical vascular damage precedes overt priapism and to some extent determines the end result of priapic episodes.

Six patients, five with a history of priapism, were studied by nocturnal tumescence testing with polysomnography and MRI of the penis. Nocturnal erections and detumescence times were prolonged and corporeal anatomy varied from normal to intracorporeal fibrosis (Burnett et al., 1995). These studies correlated well with clinical examinations and past history, suggesting to the authors that their routine use was not warranted.

Penile scans using [99m]technetium can be used to distinguish between low and high blood flow states and identify which corporal bodies are affected (Dunn et al., 1995; Miller et al., 1995). They may not be helpful in predicting the clinical course of the event. Intracorporeal pressure and blood gases can be monitored. Doppler flow studies and MRI can also provide information on blood flow and identify which of the corporal bodies are involved. How any of these tests can be used to direct therapy or establish a prognosis is not well understood.

Treatment Recommendations: When should "conservative" treatment—analgesics, hydration, and transfusions—be stopped and operative intervention initiated is the conundrum of managing priapism. Only retrospective studies are available to assist in this decision, and for an individual patient, they do not provide a firm footing on which to base critical treatment options (Chakrabarty et al., 1996). Retrospectively, when the adverse outcome of impotence has occurred after a severe bout of priapism, it is easy to assume that earlier operative intervention would have preserved erectile function. It is entirely possible that the natural history of priapism is unaffected by any treatment, conservative or surgical, and that the ultimate loss of potency is governed by the interplay of intracorporeal and systemic factors.

Most authorities believe that 24 to 48 hours is the maximum time that should elapse before treatment of priapism should be converted from analgesics, hydration, and transfusions to surgical intervention. There are several difficulties with this recommendation. First, there is no agreed upon scale to gauge the severity of the priapic episode or the preceding history of priapism. Conceivably, extreme turgidity with excruciating pain should be managed differently from less degrees of penile engorgement. Most episodes of priapism are preceded by a history of other events, which may be similar, more severe, or less severe, that have resolved satisfactorily, that is, with erectile function preserved. How should this history be incorporated into the treatment plan? Second, there are no published controlled trials comparing different types of treatment of severe acute priapism. It would be valuable to know how hydration, sedation, simple or exchange transfusion, simple aspiration and irrigation, and surgery compare. Whether transfusions are helpful, especially if a major episode has occurred, is not known. If surgery is superior, what type of operation is best? Third, although priapism is a common complication, the experience of any single urologist or hematologist is limited, and the physician's favorite treatment is likely to be based on his or her own fragmented observations. Patients are apt to delay seeking care and be managed by other physicians with different therapies before referral. Because of this uncertainty, the many published schema for managing priapism,

including our own, cannot be taken as a "standard of care" dictating rigid adherence, but are better viewed as general guides formulated on the basis of limited clinical studies, an appreciation of the natural history of this complication, and some understanding of the pathophysiology of priapism in sickle cell anemia.

The following scheme seems to be reasonable for managing acute attacks of major priapism, but it should be taken for what it is, a reasonable suggestion not founded on established facts or etched in granite. Pain should be relieved with narcotic analgesics and adequate fluids provided. If the episode differs from prior episodes of stuttering priapism according to the patient history and physician experience, aspiration and irrigation should be performed within 12 hours from the onset of erection. If this is a typical episode of low flow priapism, a Winter shunt should be placed between the glans penis and corpora cavernosa within 24 hours. If there is tricorporeal involvement, this shunt is unlikely to be effective. This plan requires that crucial decisions be made within 12 hours of onset. Because patients often are reluctant to visit the Emergency Department or clinic based on their prior experience with self-limited priapism, there may be little time for observation.

Invasive treatment for priapism in sickle cell anemia is designed to evacuate stagnant blood within the corpora cavernosa and to prevent immediate recurrence of corporal expansion. The simplest surgical procedure is aspiration of the corporal bodies with irrigation; however, when a major episode of priapism has been present for 24 to 48 hours, aspiration of blood is usually difficult. Most urologists favor creation of shunts between the glans penis and the distal corpora cavernosa with a Tru-cut biopsy needle if corporal irrigation fails. This procedure, popularized by Winter and bearing his name, allows blood from the distended corpora cavernosa to drain into the uninvolved corpus spongiosa. An operative intervention to create larger shunts between the corpora cavernosa and corpus spongiosum can be considered if detumescence is not achieved with the Winter shunt.

Because α-adrenergic activity maintains the vessels feeding the corporal bodies in a constricted state when the penis is flaccid, it was thought that oral and intracavernous administration of α-adrenergic agonists, with or without drainage, may help reverse priapism (Virag et al., 1996, 1997; Bachir et al., 1997). Etilefrine, an α-adrenergic agonist, and other α-adrenergic agents were used in patients with sickle cell anemia and stuttering or acute priapism. When these drugs were used orally in stuttering episodes, recurrence was claimed to be prevented and acute, more severe episodes reversed after intracavernous injection. These observations do not warrant a general recommendation for using these agents because some dangers are associated with α-adrenergic agonists and the reports available do not substitute for well-controlled trials. Vasodilators and even β-adrenergic agents have also been used, but there are no good studies of their usefulness. In one case, "high flow" priapism was treated successfully with bilateral pudendal artery embolization (Ramos et al., 1995).

When impotence results from priapism, implantable penile prostheses have been used with success, although they may be difficult to insert in fibrotic corporal bodies and may be associated with more complications than when used in cases of idiopathic priapism (Monga et al., 1996). Sildenafil (Viagra), a cyclic guanosine monophosphate (cGMP) phosphodiesterase inhibitor is available for treating impotence. It seems unlikely that when the anatomy of the erectile apparatus is permanently damaged, this agent will be effective.

Self-limited attacks of stuttering priapism often resolve after masturbation, cold showers, or exercise. In perhaps the sole double-blinded, placebo-controlled trial of treatment for priapism, stilbestrol reduced attacks of stuttering priapism (Serjeant et al., 1985). Eleven patients with a history of two attacks of priapism weekly were enrolled and after a 2-week baseline period were randomized to receive either 5 mg of stilbestrol daily or placebo. Two individuals stopped having attacks during the baseline period. Five placebo-treated patients continued to have attacks but these subsided when they switched to active drug. Four patients randomized to receive active drug stopped having attacks in 1 to 3 days. A maintenance dose of 2.5 to 5 mg every few days or weekly was usually effective. Stilbestrol can cause gynecomastia, prevent desired erections, and have other undesirable consequences. This was a short-term study of a small and very select group of patients. The general usefulness of this treatment and its ability to stop major episodes of priapism are not known.

Individuals who respond to treatment with hydroxyurea with increases in HbF and other treatment associated changes (Chapter 38) could be less likely to develop priapism. There are no data indicating that this supposition is true, but one brief case report claimed that hydroxyurea abrogated frequent attacks of priapism in a man with sickle cell anemia (Al Jam'a and Al Dabbous, 1998).

Digestive Diseases

Biliary tract disease and parenchymal liver disease are the most prevalent and serious complications of sickle cell anemia that affect the digestive system. Hepatomegaly is found in 80 to 100 percent of patients. Often a mélange of diverse pathologies, liver disease in sickle cell anemia may be contributed to by intrahepatic and extrahepatic cholestasis, viral hepatitis, cirrhosis, hypoxia and infarction, erythrocyte sequestration, iron overload, and drug reactions. Often it is difficult to differentiate among the potential causes of sickle cell liver disease; in a single patient, more than one etiology of liver disease is often present. In common with liver disease in the general population, treatment options are limited.

Abnormal "liver" tests are often present in sickle cell anemia but may not always reflect actual hepatocellular disease or even be related to the hemoglobinopathy (Johnson et al., 1985). Hyperbilirubinemia is usually due to increased levels of unconjugated bilirubin and therefore a manifestation of hemolytic anemia. Bilirubin levels vary considerably among patients, which likely reflects different degrees of liver disease, differing rates of hemolysis, and possibly genetic differences in bilirubin metabolism. Increased levels of alkaline phosphatase, especially in children and adolescents, may reflect growing or injured bones. Protein C and protein S levels are lower in sickle cell anemia compared with healthy individuals, an observation that was accounted for by hepatic dysfunction rather than consumptive coagulopathy (Wright et al., 1997b). There is no evidence that lower levels of these "anticoagulant" proteins play a role in the vasoocclusive process. Hepatic drug metabolism is variously affected in sickle cell disease. Some drugs such as morphine have increased clearance; others such as lidocaine have decreased clearance: still others such as meperidine are unaffected. These differences may exist because of the different routes of drug metabolism, for example, glucuronidation or deethylation (Gremse et al., 1998). In patients with sickle cell disease who have the usual abnormalities of liver tests, insufficient information is available on which to base changes in drug dosing.

An occasional otherwise well patient will have an isolated but striking elevation of unconjugated bilirubin with normal liver tests and no indication of hepatic disease. Perhaps some of these individuals have Gilbert syndrome, now known to be associated with a certain polymorphism in the UDP-glucuronyltransferase (UDPGT1) gene promoter or some related abnormality of bilirubin conjugation. This condition has been described in heterozygous β thalassemia carriers with high bilirubin levels and in neonates with both G-6-PD deficiency and variant genotypes UDPGT1 who have hyperbilirubinemia (Sampietro et al., 1997). UDPGT levels in sickle cell anemia are twofold greater than in control subjects, suggesting that induction of increased enzyme activity may increase bilirubin conjugation (Maddrey et al., 1978).

Results of liver biopsy in sickle cell anemia are highly dependent on the clinical events that prompted the biopsy. Hemosiderosis is often present, a result of chronic transfusions and parenchymal liver disease. Chronic hepatitis and cirrhosis reflect transfusion-transmitted diseases (Comer et al., 1991). When biopsy was done during cholecystectomy, sinusoidal dilation and perisinusoidal fibrosis were the pervasive lesions (Charlotte et al., 1995). Kuppfer cells often contain phagocytized erythrocytes.

As expected in patients who have often received multiple blood transfusions, viral hepatitis is common in sickle cell anemia. Bilirubin levels may be much higher than those found in viral hepatitis uncomplicated by the hemolysis and other liver-related complications of sickle cell anemia (Achord, 1994). Viral hepatitis B (HBV) was often present in transfused patients before it was possible to screen blood for its presence. In Omani children, chronic HBS antigenemia is equally common in pediatric sickle cell anemia and control populations (Soliman et al., 1995). In a North American study, no patient with sickle cell disease who was positive for anti-hepatitis C virus (HCV) was also HBV positive. (Hasan et al., 1996).

Transmission of HCV by transfusions is dependent on the incidence of this disease in the population from which blood donors are recruited. HCV antibodies (anti-HCV) are present in 10 to 20 percent of patients in North America and Saudi Arabia with sickle cell anemia who received blood transfusions (DeVault et al., 1994; Hasan et al., 1996; Al-Fawaz et al., 1996). Of patients receiving more than ten units of blood, 20 to 30 percent were anti-HCV positive, whereas 8 to 9 percent of individuals who received fewer than ten units had anti-HCV antibodies (DeVault et al., 1994; Hasan et al., 1996). When serum alanine aminotransferase levels were persistently elevated, 90 percent of these patients were anti-HCV positive. In Jamaica, 2 to 3 percent of transfused sickle cell anemia patients had anti-HCV (King et al., 1995). HCV infection can be associated with chronic active hepatitis and cirrhosis in about a third of affected individuals (Hasan et al., 1996). Hepatitis E infection has been noted in sickle cell anemia, and as new blood-borne viral hepatitides appear they will undoubtedly be found among patients with sickle cell disease who have undergone transfusion. (Al-Fawaz et al., 1996). With widespread and sensitive tests for HCV, we can expect the incidence of this infection to fall.

Autoimmune hepatitis, diagnosed by biopsy and responsive to immunosuppressive therapy, has been described in patients with sickle cell anemia (El Younis et al., 1996; Chuang et al., 1997).

Sickle hepatopathy, hepatic crisis, and the right upper quadrant syndrome of sickle cell disease have been variously defined (Achord, 1994; Shao and Orringer, 1995). Syndromes of "benign" intrahepatic cholestasis and acute hepatic sequestration, akin to the splenic sequestration syndrome, have been described (see previously). Yet, it is difficult from descriptions in the literature to differentiate among these entities, probably because their causes include viral hepatitis and vasoocclusive disease compounded by hemolysis and cholestasis. A syndrome of increasing hepatomegaly—extreme hyperbilirubinemia with levels approaching 100 mg/dL but only modest increases in transaminase levels, high alkaline phosphatase and γ-glutamyltransferase levels, right upper quadrant pain, increasing anemia, fever, coagulation abnormalities, and differing degrees of hepatic failure—has been recognized. Some patients appear to recover. Others have multiple similar episodes, eventually succumbing to hepatic failure. Many die in the midst of a first acute event.

In the livers of transgenic sickle mice, the inducible isoform of nitric oxide synthase (iNOS) was present in hepatocytes surrounding the central veins, and its activity was increased by hypoxia (Osei et al., 1996). It was hypothesized that NO generation during hypoxia may protect pericentral hepatocytes that are exposed to lower O_2 tensions than periportal cells from ischemic damage. With liver ischemia, pericentral cells are first to display hypoxic damage. Increased NO levels may be protective because of increased blood flow or because they reduce the level of oxidant radicals.

Except for the sequela of some cases of acute viral hepatitis and the frequently devastating consequences of acute right upper quadrant syndrome, the hepatic manifestations of sickle cell anemia do not have a major effect on the course of disease. Liver disease can also be present in HbSC disease and HbS-β^+ thalassemia.

Abdominal pain is a frequent complaint of patients with sickle cell anemia (Scott-Conner and Brunson, 1994a). Whether this pain results from cholelithiasis or cholecystitis, has its roots in intraabdominal vasoocclusive disease, or is related to intraabdominal pathology unrelated to sickle cell anemia is often a difficult question to answer. Some of the causes of abdominal pain in sickle cell anemia are shown in Table 24.6, and one approach to the management of abdominal pain is presented in Figure 24.9. In one series, more than half the episodes of abdominal pain were thought to be due to vasoocclusive episodes, a fourth were due to gallbladder disease or appendicitis, 13 percent had a renal origin, and some were due to pneumonia and gynecologic disease (Scott-Conner and Brunson, 1994a).

Table 24.6. Potential Causes of Abdominal Pain In Sickle Cell Anemia

Enlarged mesenteric and retroperitoneal nodes
Bone and spinal abnormalities
   Marrow hyperplasia
   Bone infarction
      Ribs
      Spine
      Femoral head
   Osteoporosis and vertebral collapse
Nerve root compression
Hepatobiliary disease
   Hepatitis
   Acute hepatic enlargement
      Sequestration
      Intrahepatic cholestasis
   Cholelithiasis
Spleen
   Hemorrhage
   Infarction
   Sequestration
   Abscess
Mesenteric ischemia
Pneumonia
Renal
   Obstructive uropathy
      Stone
      Clot
      Papillary necrosis
Cystitis

Modified from Scott-Conner and Brunson, 1994.

There is little reliable information on other abnormalities of the digestive system in sickle cell anemia. Documented episodes of bowel ischemia are rare, and although pancreatitis has been reported, it is uncommon. Controversy surrounds the incidence of peptic ulcer disease in sickle cell anemia and whether individuals with this disease have reduced acid secretion (Serjeant, 1992).

Treatment Recommendations: The value of interferon for chronic active hepatitis C in sickle cell anemia has not been studied. Its use should be based on the experience in other diseases. Individuals with severe right upper quadrant syndrome can reasonably be offered exchange transfusions. Unless it is unequivocally clear that extrahepatic obstruction is present, surgery should not be recommended.

Gallstones

Cholelithiasis, a consequence of the accelerated bilirubin turnover typical of hemolytic anemia, can appear in the first decade of life and the majority of adults are affected (Krauss et al., 1998). Gallstones were found in about 16 percent of forty-five Kuwaiti children with sickle cell anemia, ages 10.8 ± 5.5 years (Haider et al., 1998). Although HbF concen-

Figure 24.9. An algorithm for the evaluation and management of abdominal pain in sickle cell anemia. (Modified from Scott-Conner and Brunson, 1994.)

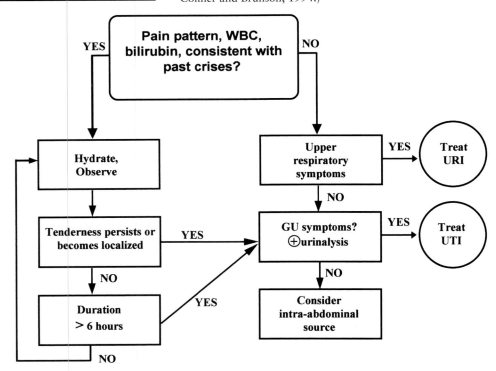

trations were high, consistent with the presence of the Arab-India haplotype, individuals with stones had a lower hemoglobin level and were less likely to have α thalassemia. Perhaps α thalassemia reduces the development of cholelithiasis in adults by reducing hemolysis.

Depending on the degree of calcification, pigmented gallstones in sickle cell anemia may be either radiopaque or radiolucent. Ultrasonography is the preferred means of their detection. Open cholecystectomy accounted for 20 percent of all operations in 717 patients with sickle cell anemia (Koshy et al., 1995). The reported death was a 54-year-old individual with complicated medical problems. Postoperative complications were common but usually minor. In a study of the effects of preoperative transfusion in sickle cell anemia, 211 open cholecystectomies and 153 laparoscopic cholecystectomies were performed (Haberkern et al., 1997). Nineteen percent of these patients had intraoperative, 11 percent transfusion-related, and 10 percent postoperative complications for a total complication rate of 39 percent. Nontransfused patients had the highest rate of postoperative acute chest syndrome and painful episodes. When common duct stones were suspected on the basis of a dilated duct, high alkaline phosphatase levels, and bilirubin that exceeded baseline by 5 mg/dL, the combination of endoscopic retrograde cholangiopancreatography, sphincterotomy, and stone extraction followed by laparoscopic cholecystectomy was an effective approach (Al-Salem and Nourallah 1997).

Treatment Recommendations: Documented episodes of acute cholecystitis are not common, and typical obstructive jaundice is equally infrequent. When stones are asymptomatic or symptoms and laboratory findings are equivocal, it is probably best not to do cholecystectomy. Laparoscopic cholecystectomy patients were hospitalized for a shorter time but had a similar rate of complications as patients who underwent open cholecystectomy.

OLDER ADULTS

Sickle cell anemia, first considered a disease of childhood, can now be found in older adults. Most clinics have seen individuals in their sixth and seventh decades; some patients have a nearly normal life span. Increasing numbers of older adults with sickle cell anemia are probably a result of higher standards of supportive care. In the United States, median ages of death for men and women with sickle cell anemia were 42 and 48 years, respectively, when reported in 1994; these data do not reflect many children who now survive because of prophylactic penicillin and other treatment innovations (Platt et al., 1994). In Jamaica, where more than 3,000 patients with sickle cell anemia were followed, Kaplan-Meir survival curves estimated a life expectancy of 58 years for men and 66 years for women, a reduction of 14 and 10 years, respectively, compared with the general Jamaican population (Wierenga et al., 1999).

Causes of death in adults are varied. About 20 percent of deaths are related to organ failure, but often death is unexpected and occurs in the midst of an acute event such as a pain crisis. In one study of more than 1,000 patients, 17 percent died from sepsis; 15 percent from acute chest syndrome; and 10 percent each from liver failure, stroke, heart failure, and acute anemia. These patients included children and adults, and 35 percent of deaths were in patients 20 years old or younger. In the United States, the median age of death in sickle cell anemia is about 45 years.

Older adults with sickle cell anemia have their own array of complications (Steinberg et al., 1995). We do not understand why some patients with sickle cell anemia survive their peers by decades. It seems unlikely that one or a few laboratory measurements will explain this observation. However, these unusual patients can be examples to others with this disease of the possibility of a long life and should alert physicians that this diagnosis need not be excluded by age alone. Old age in sickle cell anemia does not imply that these are the "golden years." Decades of vascular injury, much of which may be subclinical, begins to result in chronic organ damage and failure. Primarily affected are the lung, heart, bones, and kidneys.

Laboratory and clinical features of a small group of septuagenarians with sickle cell anemia are shown in Table 24.7. In such a small number of cases, generalizations are difficult, but several features of these patients deserve comment. While their life spans were near normal, most of their serious complications became apparent in later life. Curiously, HbF levels, the best predictor of morbidity and mortality, were lower than average (Platt et al., 1991, 1994). However, HbF constantly declines with aging in sickle cell anemia, and there is very little information on HbF in 60- to 80-year-old patients (Rucknagel et al., 1979). Leukocyte counts, also associated with morbidity and mortality in sickle cell anemia, were lower than average (Platt et al., 1994). As both leukocyte counts and HbF decrease with age in sickle cell anemia the levels observed may be an effect—not a cause—of the extended life of these patients (Embury et al., 1994). One other case of a 70-year-old man with sickle cell anemia reported a PCV of 18, HbF of 6.4 percent, and a leukocyte count of 10.3×10^6/L (Shurafa et al., 1982).

Table 24.7. Laboratory Values and Clinical Events in Septuagenarians with Sickle Cell Anemia

Age	Sex	Hb	MCV	Retic	WBC	PLT	HbF	HAPLO	α Genes	Cr	ALT	Bili	Pain	CHF	Leg Ulcer	Acute Chest	ON	CVA	Retina	TX	Other
75	M	5.6	80	13	6.4	249	4.0	BEN/Atyp	3	1.5	23	3.3	0	Y	Y	N	N	N	N	Y	A
71	M	7.8	86	7	6.8	170	5.3	BEN/BEN	3	1.3	27	2.4	10	Y	Y	Y	Y	Y	N	N	D
71	F	7.5	95	14	10.7	433	2.8	BEN/CAR	4	1.5	22	1.7	3	N	Y	N	Y	N	N	N	A
76	M	5.5	96	7	7.6	162	0.2	–	4	4.2	25	2.9	0	Y	Y	N	N	N	N	Y	D
80	M	8.8	84	1.9	11.4	340	5.0	–	–	–	24	0.7	<1	Y	N	N	N	N	N	–	–
73	M	5.5	91	5	11.4	272	–	–	–	1.5	7	4.7	0	Y	N	N	Y	N	N	Y	Y

Hb, hemoglobin level in g/dL; MCV, mean corpuscular volume (fl); Retic, reticulocyte count (percent); WBC, leukocyte count (percent); Retic, reticulocyte count (percent); WBC, leukocyte count (10^9/L); PLT, platelet count (10^9/L); HbF, fetal hemoglobin (percent); HAPLO, β-globin gene cluster haplotype; BEN, Benin; CAR, Central African Republic; Atyp, atypical; α genes, α-globin genotype; Cr, creatinine (mg/dL); ALT, alanine aminotransferase (units); Bili, total bilirubin (mg/dL); Pain, average numbers of pain crises yearly; CHF, congestive heart failure; Y, yes; N, no; Leg Ulcer, presence or history of leg ulcers; Chest, history of acute chest syndrome; ON, osteonecrosis; CVA, history of cerebrovascular accidents; Retina, sickle retinopathy; TX, regular transfusions; A, alive; D, deceased.

Eye Disease

Sickle retinopathy is discussed in detail in Chapter 27 on HbSC disease in which it is most common. Present in about one third to two thirds of adults with HbSC disease, depending on their ages, proliferative sickle retinopathy is far less common in sickle cell anemia. Proliferative retinopathy in HbSC disease may be an expression of the relative benignity of this genotype. In sickle cell anemia, peripheral retinal vessels are occluded early in the course of disease so that further retinal vascular damage and proliferative lesions cannot develop. As hydroxyurea treatment makes sickle cell anemia cells more like HbSC disease cells, the prevalence of proliferative retinopathy may begin to increase in young patients with sickle cell anemia who are treated with this drug.

Some patients with sickle cell anemia have abnormal dark adaptation (Warth et al., 1981). This defect is related to tissue zinc deficiency, a consequence of hyperzincuria in sickle cell anemia, and improves with zinc replacement. Clinical consequences of this laboratory observation have not been reported.

Conjunctival vessels in sickle cell anemia are damaged by vasoocclusion and develop corkscrew and comma-shaped forms, show dropped-out segments, and may become obliterated, ending up with avascular regions of the bulbar conjunctiva. These abnormalities have been considered pathognomonic of sickle cell disease. Their presence is inversely correlated with HbF level and directly related to the numbers of irreversibly sickle cells (Serjeant et al., 1972). Conjuctival abnormalities are less often present in HbSC disease and HbS-β+ thalassemia.

Cardiovascular Complications

Physical work capacity is reduced by about half in adults with sickle cell anemia and 60 to 70 percent in children and is related to the severity of the anemia. Cardiac examinations are rarely normal; the heart is usually enlarged and the precordium hyperactive; systolic murmurs are found in most patients, and premature contractions are often present (Leight et al., 1954). Cardiomegaly and heart murmurs often raise the question of whether congestive heart failure is present. Contractility is normal and overt congestive heart failure is uncommon, especially in children (Covitz, 1994). When heart failure is present, it often can be related to secondary causes such as fluid overload. Hypertension, perhaps becoming more common as the prevalence of renal failure rises, may cause ventricular hypertrophy and heart failure. Cardiac output is increased at rest in individuals with sickle cell anemia and increases further with exercise (Leight et al., 1954). Electrocardiograms often have nonspecific abnormalities and can show signs of ventricular hypertrophy. Cardiac index is increased about twice normal at rest and increases further during exercise. Cardiac index was not related to hemoglobin level or oxygen content, suggesting increased tissue extraction of oxygen. This was postulated to be due to the increased capillary diffusing surface.

Cardiac abnormalities in almost 200 patients ages 13 years and older with sickle cell anemia were studied echocardiographically by investigators of the Cooperative Study of Sickle Cell Disease (Covitz et al., 1995). Compared with normal control subjects, patients had increased left and right ventricular and left atrial chamber dimensions, increased interventricular septal thickness, and normal contractility. These dimensions, except for those of the right ventricle, were inversely related to the hemoglobin level and indicated cardiac dilation. Cardiac dilation was also dependent on age. When homozygous α thalassemia-2 was present, left ventricular dimensions were more normal, but wall thickness was increased (Braden et al., 1996). This difference was postulated to be a result of the higher hemoglobin levels caused by α thalassemia. Nevertheless, the response to exercise was not improved. This failure to improve performance despite a higher hemoglobin level was ascribed to abnormal properties of sickle erythrocytes.

Chest pain, a common entity in sickle cell anemia, often leads to patients being told they have had a "heart attack." In fact, obvious myocardial infarction is unusual but has been reported. Paradoxically, coronary artery occlusion is not common, suggesting that small vessel disease is responsible for the cardiac damage (Covitz, 1994). Gross and microscopic findings consistent with acute (three patients) and healed (four patients) myocardial infarction were found in seven (9.7 percent) of seventy-two consecutive hearts from patients with sickle cell disease studied after autopsy between 1950 and 1982. Gross obstructive and atherosclerotic lesions were absent in all seven patients, whereas microthrombi were present in the arterioles of infarcted tissue in two patients. Anemia, platelet thrombi, coronary vasospasm, and abnormal blood rheology were hypothesized to be etiologically important. Chest pain occurred clinically in six of the seven patients, and electrocardiographic findings typical of infarction were found in two patients. One patient died suddenly. These findings suggest that ischemic heart disease may be present in patients with sickle cell disease and should be considered in all patients with chest pain (Martin et al., 1996).

Sudden unexpected and unexplained death is common in adults with sickle cell anemia (Romero Mestre et al., 1999). In postmortem examinations of the cardiac conduction system and a coronary chemoreceptor from the hearts of two black men who died suddenly, there were abundant foci of old and recent degeneration in the sinus node, atrioventricular node, and His bundle, as well as the coronary chemoreceptor (James et al., 1994). Many capillaries and small arteries were packed with sickled erythrocytes, among which small groups of aggregated platelets were also present. Recent studies have shown platelet-erythrocyte adhesion in sickle cell disease (Wun et al., 1999). Focal fibromuscular dysplasia caused moderate to severe narrowing of many small coronary arteries, including those supplying the conduction system and chemoreceptor. These abnormalities suggest that electrical instability of the heart is at least one component of the lethal terminal events in some individuals. Cardiovascular autonomic function tests were performed in twenty-four patients with sickle cell anemia and thirty-eight healthy white control subjects. Fourteen patients (58.3 percent) were found to have cardiovascular autonomic dysfunction based on abnormal values for at least two cardiovascular autonomic function tests, whereas ten (41.7 percent) had preserved autonomic function. All control subjects had normal cardiac autonomic function. Involvement of autonomic nervous dysfunction may contribute to sudden death in sickle cell anemia.

Pericardial effusions were present in 10 percent of patients and also inversely related to hemoglobin level (Covitz et al., 1995).

Treatment Recommendations: Congestive heart failure in sickle cell anemia should be treated with the usual methods. Severely anemic patients with symptoms of congestive heart failure or angina pectoris may be helped by cautiously increasing their hemoglobin concentration.

Renal Disease

Two major abnormalities characterize the renal lesions associated with sickle cell disease. Medullary disease is present in nearly all individuals with sickle cell anemia and even most carriers of sickle cell trait. Glomerulopathy begins very early in life in sickle cell disease but becomes clinically important as patients age (Powars et al., 1991; Falk and Jennette, 1994). Renal abnormalities in sickle cell anemia are shown in Table 24.8. Acute reversible deterioration of renal function, occasionally severe and requiring dialysis, sometimes develops in hospitalized patients (Sklar et al., 1990a). Deterioration of renal function is often associated with volume contraction, anemia, and infection, and most patients recover with time.

Acidosis, hypoxia, and hyperosmolarity—conditions that favor HbS polymerization—typify the renal

---

Table 24.8. Renal Abnormalities in Sickle Cell Anemia

Distal Nephron
  Impaired urine concentrating ability
  Impaired urine acidification-incomplete renal
    tubular acidosis
  Impaired K^+ excretion
Hematuria
Papillary Necrosis
Proximal Tubule
  Increased phosphate reabsorption
  Increased β_2-microglobulin reabsorption
  Increased uric acid secretion
  Increased creatinine secretion
Hemodynamic changes
  Increased glomerular filtration rate
  Increased renal plasma flow
  Decreased filtration fraction
Glomerular Abnormalities
  Proteinuria
  Nephrotic syndrome with focal glomerular sclerosis
  Chronic renal failure

---

medulla. Even sickle cell trait cells deform in this environment, leading to hyposthenuria and, occasionally, hematuria. In sickle cell anemia, the vasa recta may be severely damaged or lost entirely. Isosthenuria, distal renal tubular acidosis, and impaired potassium excretion are signs of medullary dysfunction. Clinically, the loss of concentrating ability is not important unless access to fluid is restricted. Systemic acidosis is not a clinical problem despite the acidification defect. Hyperkalemia can accompany renal failure and the use of angiotensin-converting-enzyme (ACE) inhibitors and may be worsened by type IV renal tubular acidosis. Hematuria and papillary necrosis are also seen. The former is most always benign, as it is in sickle cell trait.

Proximal renal tubular function is supranormal as creatinine secretion and phosphate reabsorption are increased. This is of no clinical significance but can lead to overestimation of glomerular filtration rate.

An increasing prevalence of renal failure is one hallmark of an aging population of patients with sickle cell anemia. In the United States between 1992 and 1996, there were 345 reported new cases of end-stage renal disease in sickle cell anemia (U.S. Renal Data System 1997 Annual Report, NIDDK, NIH). In one study, patients with a Bantu β-globin gene cluster haplotype (Chapter 26) were more likely to develop renal failure (Powars et al., 1991). This study was a prospective, 25-year longitudinal demographic and clinical cohort study involving 725 patients with sickle cell anemia and 209 patients with HbSC disease. Thirty-six patients developed renal failure, 4.2 percent of patients with sickle cell anemia and 2.4 percent of patients with HbSC disease, with median ages of disease onset of 23.1 and 49.9 years, respectively. Sixty percent of patients older than 40 years had proteinuria, and 30 percent had renal insufficiency. Nephrotic syndrome was found in 40 percent of patients with creatinine levels above 1 mg/dL for children and 1.5 mg/dL for adults. Survival time for patients with sickle cell anemia after the diagnosis of sickle renal failure was 4 years even when they underwent dialysis, and the median age at the time of death was 27 years. Case-control analysis showed that ineffective erythropoiesis with increasingly severe anemia, hypertension, proteinuria, the nephrotic syndrome; and microscopic hematuria was a significant preazotemic predictor of chronic renal failure. Perhaps the lower levels of HbF associated with the Bantu haplotype is responsible for more rapid organ failure. α Thalassemia may prevent or retard sickle glomerulopathy.

In 76 adults with sickle cell anemia, albumin excretion of more than 300 mg/g creatinine was found in 13 percent of patients with heterozygous or homozygous α thalassemia-2 compared with 40 percent of patients with the normal α-globin gene haplotype (Guasch et al., 1999). Unlike the study of Powars, β-globin gene cluster haplotype did not predict the development of renal disease; however, this study population was much smaller and patients were not examined longitudinally.

Years of glomerular hyperfiltration eventuates in renal damage. Important decrements in renal function may be present even when the creatinine is only modestly increased because creatinine is secreted by the proximal tubule. In patients with sickle cell anemia, as in normal individuals, glomerular filtration rate falls with advancing years (Sklar et al., 1990b; West et al., 1992). With renal insufficiency, the prevalence of proteinuria also increases.

Sickle cell nephropathy is a glomerulopathy characterized by glomerular hypertrophy, hypercellularity, mesangial proliferation, and segmental glomerulosclerosis (Falk et al., 1992; Falk, and Jennette, 1994). It is unclear why glomerular hypertrophy occurs, but it may be related to hypoxia, medullary ischemia with increased prostaglandin production, and dilation of efferent glomerular arterioles. Arteriolar dilation may lead to glomerular hypertension, which is ultimately responsible for loss of filtration. Albuminuria and IgG excretion are early hallmarks of glomerular injury (Guasch et al., 1996). Glomerular permeability is increased before renal insufficiency develops and decreases with chronic renal failure (Guasch et al., 1997). Transgenic mice with sickle cell disease (Chapter 34) also have glomerular hyperfiltration and hyposthenuria. These animals excrete increased amounts of stable nitric oxide metabolites and have raised levels of iNOS in their glomeruli (Bank et al., 1996). Perhaps a similar mechanism contributes to glomerular hyperfiltration in patients with sickle cell anemia. Glomerular hypertrophy and hyperfiltration with increased secretion of creatinine explain the very low creatinine levels of children and adolescents with sickle cell anemia and their increased creatinine clearance (Sklar et al., 1990b; Falk et al., 1992; West et al., 1992). Perhaps as a result of glomerular hypertrophy, renal length is increased in sickle cell anemia (Walker et al., 1996).

PCV falls with advancing years, perhaps owing to deteriorating renal function and an increasing incidence of congestive heart failure (West et al., 1992). Acute painful episodes become less of a problem in older adults as their PCV plummets. A low PCV in sickle cell anemia is predictive of less pain (Platt et al., 1991). However, renal failure is a risk factor for early death, with survival reduced by nearly half compared with patients with normal renal function (Powars et al., 1991).

Treatment Recommendations: ACE inhibitors, drugs that can decrease glomerular pressure by dilating the efferent arterioles, can reduce the proteinuria of sickle cell anemia and are being studied as one way of treating sickle nephropathy (Foucan et al., 1998; Falk et al., 1992; Aoki and Saad, 1995). In a randomized double-blind study of twenty-two patients, after 6 months of treatment with 25 mg/day of captopril, there was a 37 percent reduction in microalbuminuria compared with a 17 percent increase in placebo-treated patients (Foucan et al., 1998). There was also a small but significant reduction in diastolic blood pressure in captopril-treated patients. Treating more patients for more extended times will help establish the role of this regimen in the management of nephropathy of sickle cell anemia. ACE inhibitors are renoprotective in other nondiabetic nephropathies, reducing the rate of progression to end-stage renal disease and nephrotic-range proteinuria (Ruggenenti et al., 1999).

Nonsteroidal anti-inflammatory drugs that inhibit the production of prostaglandins can also reduce glomerular filtration rate in sickle cell anemia and might best be avoided in older individuals with signs of incipient renal failure. Dialysis and renal transplantation are used in end-stage sickle cell nephropathy, with outcomes less favorable than in other types of renal failure (Montgomery et al., 1994). If drugs such as hydroxyurea, which increase HbF concentration and attack the vasoocclusive and hemolytic complications of disease, can be used successfully in young children, presumably the glomerulopathy of sickle cell disease can be forestalled or prevented (Chapter 38).

Medullary disease precedes glomerular damage so that drug therapy will need to be started earlier in life to prevent this type of damage; however, these lesions are not as critical as those in the glomerulus.

Concordant with the increase in creatinine, PCV begins to decrease, and, not infrequently, symptoms of severe anemia and congestive heart failure appear and dominate the clinical picture. In sickle cell anemia, erythropoietin levels are lower than predicted, and the judicious use of large doses of erythropoietin can return hemoglobin to the prerenal failure baseline (Fig. 24.10) (Sherwood et al., 1986; Steinberg, 1991). If this approach is chosen, care should be taken not to increase the PCV beyond the level present before the onset of renal disease, as this may have the potential of promoting vasoocclusive episodes.

Hemodialysis can be an effective treatment for end-stage renal failure in sickle cell disease. Renal transplantation has also been advocated. In the most comprehensive examination of the results of renal transplantation in sickle cell disease, the incidence of acute rejection, mean serum creatinine after surgery, and 1-year graft survival in eighty-two patients with end-stage sickle cell nephropathy who underwent renal transplantation after an average dialysis period of 41 months was similar to that for age-matched African-American control subjects. However, the 3-year cadaveric graft survival of 61 percent was poorer than that of control subjects (86 percent). Patient survival at 1 and 3 years posttransplantation was also worse in the sickle cell disease patients. Compared with patients treated with dialysis and wait-listed for transplantation, there was a trend toward improved survival (Ojo et al., 1999). Results from this report differed from those of earlier smaller studies, which concluded that renal transplantation in sickle cell anemia had poor results. This more recent study suggests that the outcome of renal transplantation in sickle cell anemia can be at least as good as dialysis and should be considered for individuals with end-stage renal failure.

Blood Pressure and Hypertension

As a group, patients with anemia have lower than expected blood pressure, and individuals with sickle cell anemia are no exception (Johnson and Giorgio, 1981). In sickle cell anemia, lower than expected blood pressure may be due to renal sodium wasting; however, its cause is not known for certain (Pegelow et al., 1997). Compared with individuals with β thalassemia who had similar hemoglobin concentrations, the blood pressure of patients with sickle cell anemia was higher than expected, suggesting that they may have "relative" hypertension (Rodgers et al., 1993). In this study of eighty-nine patients, there was an association between higher blood pressures and stroke. Figure 24.11 shows blood pressure as a function of age in more than 2,500 African Americans with sickle cell anemia and 800 with HbSC disease (Pegelow et al., 1997). Compared with control subjects, individuals with sickle cell anemia had significantly lower systolic and diastolic blood pressures. Survival decreased and the risk of stroke increased as blood pressure rose (Fig. 24.12), even though the blood pressure at which these risks increased was below the level defining early hypertension in the normal population. This suggests that "relative" hypertension was pathogenetically important. "Relative" hypertension in sickle cell anemia might reflect impaired iNOS activity owing to endothelial cell damage and reduced production of NO that modulates vascular tone.

Blacks in industrialized countries have a high incidence of hypertension, hypertensive nephropathy, and cardiovascular disease. Increasing longevity, a higher prevalence of sickle cell nephropathy, and the consumption of high-calorie, high-salt diets probably all contribute to the rising prevalence of absolute hypertension in patients with sickle cell anemia. When this increased prevalence is considered along with the apparent risks of even "relative" hypertension and the knowledge that reducing blood pressure in people without sickle cell anemia can prevent the consequence of hypertension, it seems reasonable to consider antihypertensive therapy in patients with sickle cell disease who have even borderline hypertension.

Treatment Recommendations: At this time there are no trials of patients with sickle cell anemia that can answer when to begin antihypertensive treatment,

Figure 24.10. Effects of erythropoietin on packed cell volume in sickle cell anemia. Arrows and numbers at the top and bottom of the graph show escalating doses of erythropoietin in units per kilogram given to two patients with sickle cell anemia and renal functional impairment who were treated with injections of erythropoietin three times a week (Steinberg, 1991).

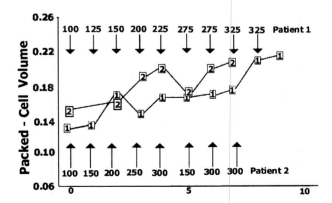

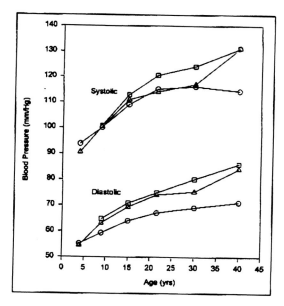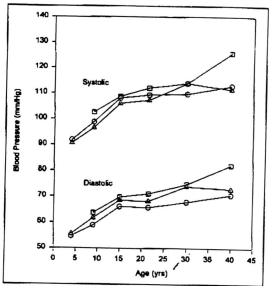

Figure 24.11. Systolic and diastolic blood pressure in male (left panel) and female (right panel) patients with sickle cell anemia (O) and HbSC disease (Δ) and in African-American participants in the NHANES II study (□). In most age categories, both men and women with sickle cell anemia had lower systolic and diastolic blood pressure than NHANES II controls and individuals with HbSC disease. (From Pegalow et al., 1997, with permission.)

what agents are most effective, what the blood pressure goals of treatment should be, and whether blood pressure reduction can reduce the incidence of stroke or prolong life. A reasonable approach, based on experience in the general hypertensive population where the risk of stroke begins well below the "normal" blood pressure of 140/90 mm Hg, is to carefully evaluate the patient and consider beginning antihyperten-

sive treatment when systolic blood pressure rises by 20 mm Hg or the diastolic blood pressure increases by 10 mm Hg. When there is evidence of target organ damage that includes heart disease, nephropathy, and peripheral vascular disease, treatment might be started

Figure 24.12. Survival of male (left panel) and female (right panel) patients with sickle cell anemia classified according to their diastolic blood pressures. High diastolic pressure (H) is the 90th percentile or above, medium diastolic blood pressure (M) the 50th through 89th percentiles, and low (L) diastolic pressure, below the 50th percentile. Mortality is increased for men (P = .007) and women whose diastolic blood pressure is above the 90th percentile, but only the result in males is significant. Blood pressure in the 90th percentile of these sickle cell anemia patients overlaps with "normal" blood pressure. (From Pegalow et al., 1997, with permission.)

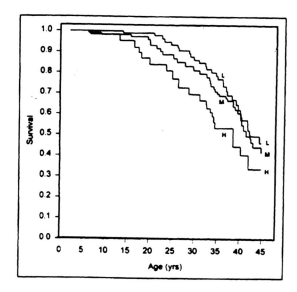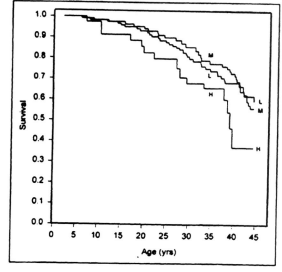

at pressures above 130/85 mm Hg. Treatment at pressures of 120/75 may be indicated when proteinuria is over 1 g/day. ACE inhibitors and calcium antagonists may be especially useful treatments, because the former appear to reduce proteinuria and preserve renal function and the latter may have a higher rate of response in black patients. However, in non-insulin-dependent diabetes and heart failure, some calcium-channel blockers may increase cardiovascular mortality (Estacio et al., 1998). Theoretically, diuretics, by causing hemoconcentration, might predispose to vasoocclusion. In practice, it is not clear if vasoocclusion occurs and the use of diuretics is not contraindicated. Beta-adrenergic-receptor blocking agents can also be used. Renin-dependent hypertension can result from focal area of renal ischemia. Severe blood pressure increases in patients with sickle cell anemia should be evaluated thoroughly to exclude renin-dependent and other forms of secondary hypertension.

Mortality

In the Cooperative Study report on mortality in sickle cell disease patients less than 20 years old who were observed from 1978 to 1988, acute chest syndrome was the second leading cause of death after bacterial sepsis (Leiken et al., 1989). With the recent reductions in deaths from pneumococcal infection in children with sickle cell disease, acute chest syndrome has become the leading cause of mortality at major clinical centers in the United States. Acute chest syndrome was the leading specific cause of death in patients 20 years or older (Platt et al., 1995). There were thirty-two deaths in 1,741 acute chest syndrome events in 949 patients, for an overall death rate of 1.8 percent (Vichinsky et al., 1997). Fourteen of the deaths were in patients less than 20 years old, for a death rate of 1.1 percent, and the death rate in adults was 4.3 percent. Patients with sickle cell anemia and acute chest syndrome had a death rate of 1.9 percent, and in those with HbSC disease, the rate was a similar 1.6 percent. Pulmonary embolism with or without fat embolism, pneumococcal sepsis, extremity pain episode, and respiratory failure within 48 hours of admission were all common in those who died.

HETEROGENEITY OF SICKLE CELL ANEMIA

Epistatic genes that may account for the clinical heterogeneity of sickle cell anemia are discussed in Chapter 26. All genotypes of sickle cell disease display surprising clinical heterogeneity, and knowing the genotype does not predict the resulting phenotype (Embury et al., 1994). Much effort has been devoted to exploring the origins of this heterogene-

ity. Identifying the factors that modulate the course of disease would be useful prognostically, help guide difficult therapeutic decisions, and perhaps provide clues for new methods of treatment. Progress has been made, but the underlying answers are complex. We know most about the roles of HbF and α thalassemia as modulators of the phenotype of sickle cell anemia. In each individual, different genetic and environmental factors are likely to influence the consequences of the sickle mutation.

Clinical diversity in sickle cell anemia is itself an eclectic mixture. Some patients are severely anemic and are dependent on transfusions. Most have only moderate anemia, and a few are barely anemic. Vasoocclusive episodes of many types occur relentlessly in some patients. However, most have episodic events and a few rarely have pain episodes or other vasoocclusive problems. Psychosocial problems may be as crippling as physical events in some instances. Most patients with similarly severe clinical disease cope well and some even flourish. Finally, some patients die very young, whereas others live into the eighth decade. How may we account for these disparities?

In some settings in which sanitation, nutrition, and access to health care are poor, environment influences are paramount. Genetic differences in red cell membrane proteins, leukocytes and platelet function, vascular reactivity, and endothelial cell biology are likely to be pathogenetically important; but their roles in determining disease diversity are not well understood.

GENERAL MEASURES OF TREATMENT

Sickle cell disease is a chronic disorder, and attention should be given to good nutrition, immunizations, and avoidance of extremes of temperature and activity. Nonexertional work should be encouraged. Increased rates of red cell production and inadequate nutrition have led to the routine use of supplemental folic acid, 1 mg/day. Although folic acid levels in children with sickle cell anemia and HbSC disease are similar to those in control populations, there is some evidence that marginally elevated homocysteine levels in sickle cell disease can be reduced by folic acid supplementation, indicating suboptimal levels of folic acid relative to requirements (Van der Dijs et al., 1998). However, some studies suggest that, at least in well-nourished children, folic acid supplementation is unnecessary under usual circumstances (see previously). Pneumococcal sepsis is a leading cause of death in infants with sickle cell anemia. Two preventive measures are used to avert this complication. Vaccination against S. pneumoniae and H. influenzae provide some, if erratic, protection against these organisms. Newer, more immunogenic conjugate vaccines are being tested and appear effective (Ahman

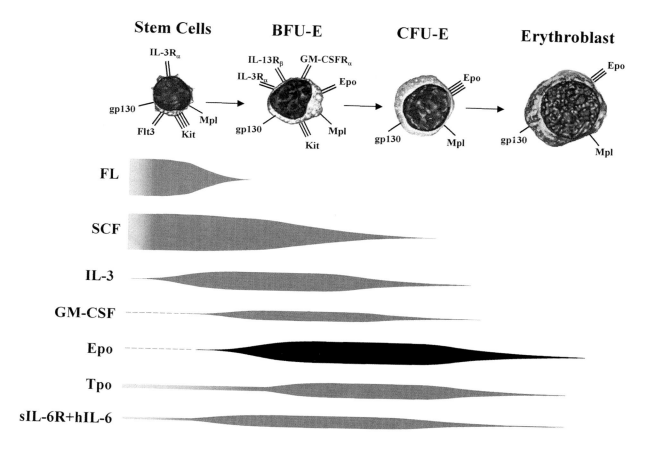

Color Plate 3.1. Diagrammatic scheme of adult erythroid differentiation: Cellular compartments (top panel) and the in vitro influence of growth factors (bottom panel). The level of expression of the corresponding receptors during the cytogeny of erythroid cells is indicated by bars on the cell surface. The growth factors listed influencing proliferation and/or differentiation along the erythroid pathway are: Flt3 ligand and SCF; IL-3 and GM-CSF, EPO and thrombopoietin (TPO). Human stem cells require either SCF or Flt3 ligand to survive and proliferate in culture. Optimal growth of adult erythroid bursts requires the presence of at least three different growth factors: SCF, IL-3 (or, in humans, GM-CSF) and EPO. Formation of erythroid bursts and of CFU-e-derived colonies is influenced by TPO and EPO. TPO also influences the survival of more primitive cells, and in the presence of other factors, induces proliferation of single murine stem cells and of human CD34$^+$ cells in liquid culture. Recently, the combination of IL-6 with its soluble binding receptor (sIL-6R-IL-6) or a fusion molecule called hyper IL-6 has been shown to induce proliferation of stem cells and sustain terminal erythroid differentiation of progenitor cells in the apparent absence of EPO. It should be noted that, although hematopoietic cells do not express the IL-6 receptor, they constitutively express gp130, its signal partner. For a complete list of the factors acting on erythroid differentiation in vitro, see Table 3.2.

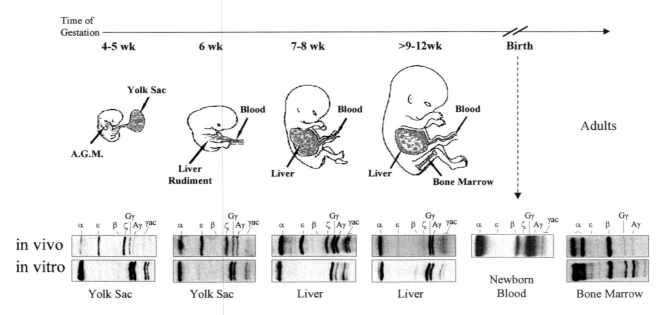

Color Plate 3.2. Erythropoiesis during human ontogeny. Diagram of the anatomic sites (indicated in red) of erythropoiesis and the corresponding globin patterns (bottom) of erythroid cells during development. Globin patterns expressed by erythroid cells in vivo, or by the erythroid progeny of BFU-e in vitro. Note that in yolk sac the in vivo pattern reflects that of primitive erythroblasts, whereas in vitro it is that of the erythroid progeny of definitive lineage BFU-e. In fetal liver stages, the in vivo and in vitro patterns are stable and show minor differences. In the adult stage, the reactivation of fetal globin synthesis under in vitro conditions is shown. The globin pattern expressed by progenitor cells from cord blood is intermediate between those of fetal and adult cells. A tendency for increase in HbA synthesis in vitro has been found, as the in vitro pattern reflects the globin program of progenitors further along in their switch than the red cells present in vivo.

A

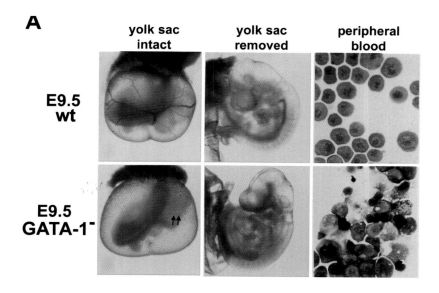

B

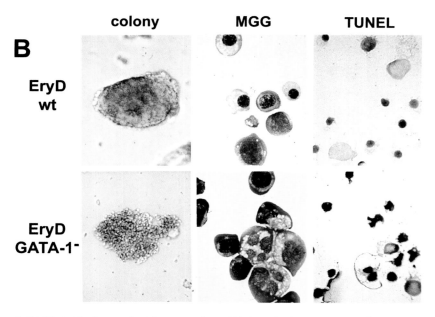

Color Plate 4.3. Loss of GATA-1 blocks erythroid maturation. (**A**) Impaired primitive erythropoiesis in GATA-1⁻ embryos. (**B**) Developmental arrest and apoptosis of cells within definitive erythroid (EryD) colonies generated by in vitro differentiation of GATA-1⁻ ES cells. (Modified from Fujiwara et al., 1996, and Weiss and Orkin 1995b. Copyright 1995 and 1996, National Academy of Sciences, U.S.A. Photographs in panel A provided by Yuko Fujiwara and Stuart Orkin.)

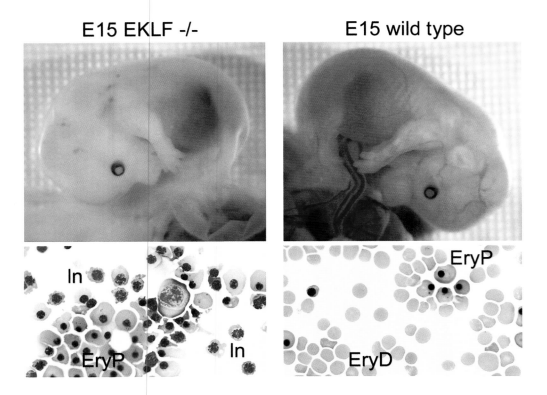

E15 EKLF -/-   **E15 wild type**

Color Plate 4.5. Impaired definitive erythropoiesis in erythroid Krüppel-like factor (ELKF)$^{-/-}$ embryos. Affected embryos are extremely pale, but otherwise structurally normal (top panels). Peripheral blood smears are shown in the bottom panels. In E15 wild-type mice, there are mainly fetal liver-derived enucleated definitive erythrocytes (EryD) and a few yolk sac-derived primitive erythrocytes (EryP). The blood of EKLF$^{-/-}$ littermates contains an increased proportion of normal appearing primitive erythrocytes but few mature definitive erythrocytes. Definitive erythroid cells consist mainly of immature nucleated late normoblasts (In) with irregular, poorly hemoglobinized cytoplasm. Rare circulating enucleated definitive erythrocytes exhibit pallor, microcytosis and poikilocytosis (not shown). (Photographs provided by Andrew Perkins.)

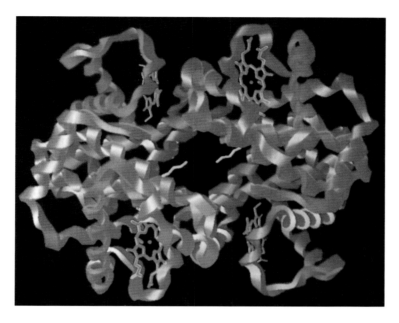

Color Plate 10.13. A GRASP generated figure of Gower II embryonic hemoglobin tetramer. The ε subunits are in green and the α subunits in blue. The two critical ε104Lys residues (whose side chains are in yellow) point to the center of the central cavity from each ε-globin chain.

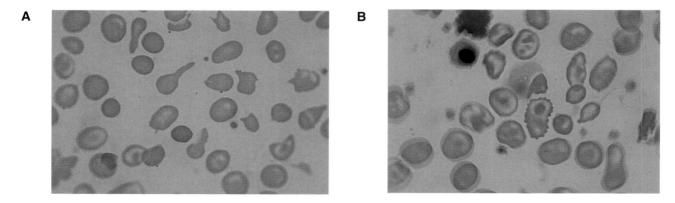

Color Plate 11.1. Peripheral blood smears of patients with β thalassemia intermedia. (A) Nonsplenectomized patient and (B) splenectomized patient.

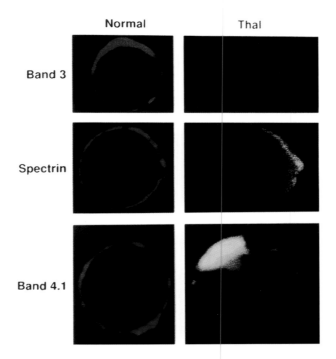

Normal   **Thal**

Band 3

Spectrin

Band 4.1

Color Plate 11.12. Normal and thalassemic marrow erythroid precursors in paired experiments were fixed, permeabilized, and reacted with specific antibodies. The cells were first reacted with Texas Red-labeled rabbit polyclonal antibodies to either band 3, band 4.1, or spectrin, and then with monoclonal FITC-labeled anti-α globin. α-Globin reactivity was never detected in normal erythroid precursors because the antibody detects only denatured or aggregated α-globin. Note smooth rim fluorescence in normals. Overlapping green and red fluorescence produced brilliant yellow fluorescence, indicating colocalization. (From Aljurf et al., 1996, with permission.)

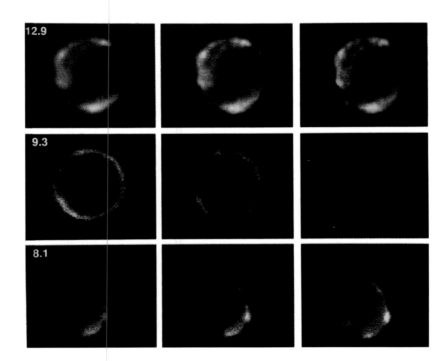

Color Plate 11.13. Incorporation of spectrin into thalassemic erythroid precursors. The middle three cuts at the cell's maximum diameter (equatorial cuts) are shown. The top row shows three sequential images through a proerythroblast of 12.9 μm diameter, the middle row through a polychromatophilic erythroblast of 9.3 μm diameter and the bottom row is through an orthochromic normoblast of 8.1 μm diameter. (From Aljurf et al., 1996, with permission.)

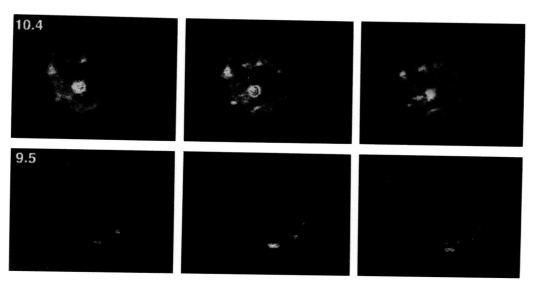

Color Plate 11.14. Incorporation of band 4.1 into two thalassemic polychromatophilic erythroblasts of 10.4 (top row) and 9.5 (bottom row) μm diameter showing three equatorial cuts spaced at 0.5 μm. Note the very abnormal incorporation as well as band 4.1 overlying the nucleus. (From Aljurf et al., 1996, with permission.)

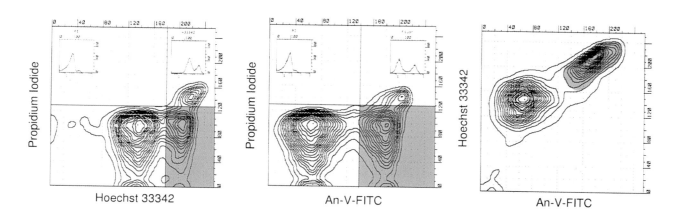

Color Plate 11.16. Fluorescence activated cell sorting. Analysis of isolated and purified marrow erythroid precursors from a patient with β thalassemia major (Cooley's anemia). *Left panel:* The erythroid precursors were incubated with the dye Hoechst 33342 (abscissa), which labels cells dying or undergoing apoptosis, and propidium iodide (ordinate), which under these conditions identifies dead cells. *Middle panel:* Erythroid precursors as above, incubated with propidium iodide (ordinate) and FITC labeled annexin V (abscissa), which binds to apoptotic cells expressing phosphatidylserine on their outer surface. *Right panel:* The cells from the two panels above were FACS analyzed simultaneously for FITC annexin V reactivity (abscissa) and Hoechst 33342 reactivity (ordinate). The colored panels indicate apoptotic cells.

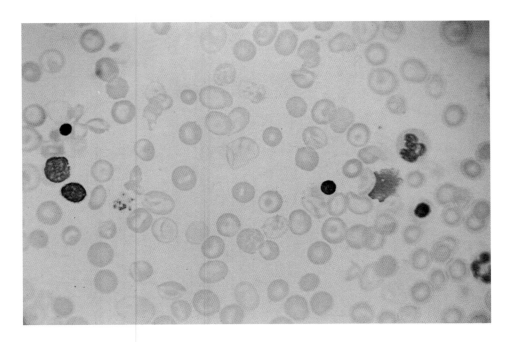

Color Plate 13.8. The blood smear of a patient with thalassemia major showing the typical morphologic changes. (Wright's stain, ×438)

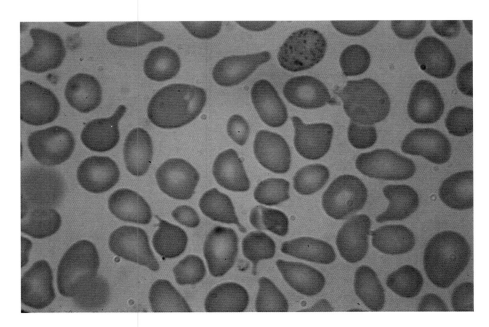

Color Plate 13.11. A peripheral blood smear from the propositus from the first family to be reported with dominantly inherited β thalassemia (Weatherall et al., 1973). Hypochromia is not a major feature but there is a remarkable degree of poikilocytosis and heavy basophilic stippling.

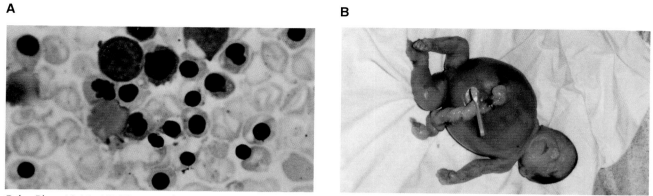

Color Plate 18.10. (**A**) The typical peripheral blood films of an infant with the Hb Bart's hydrops fetalis syndrome, showing many immature red cell precursors and hypochromic, microcytic, anisopoikiolytic red cells. (**B**) The typical clinical features of a hydropic infant at birth (see text).

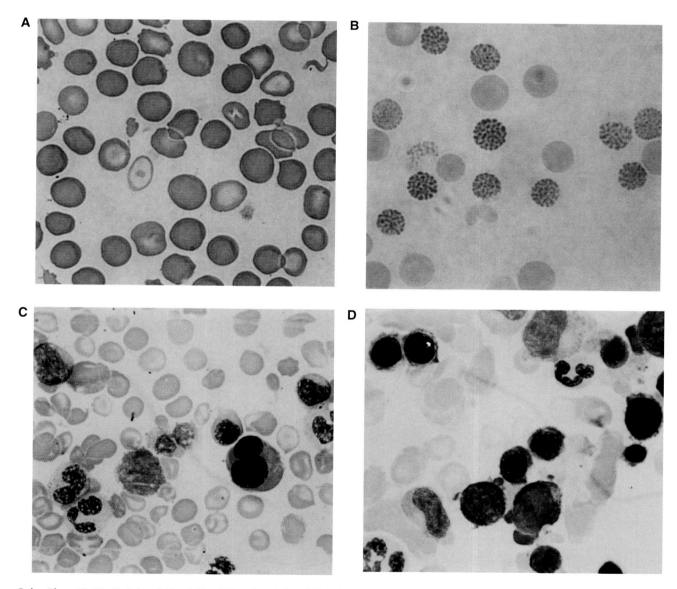

Color Plate 18.12. Peripheral blood film (**A**) and peripheral blood stained with brilliant cresyl blue (**B**) from a patient with ATMDS and an α/β-globin chain biosynthesis ratio of less than 0.1. Bone marrow samples from the same patient (**C, D**) showing erythroid expansion with dyserythropoietic features including binuclearity and cytoplasmic vacuolation. The neutrophils appear hypogranular.

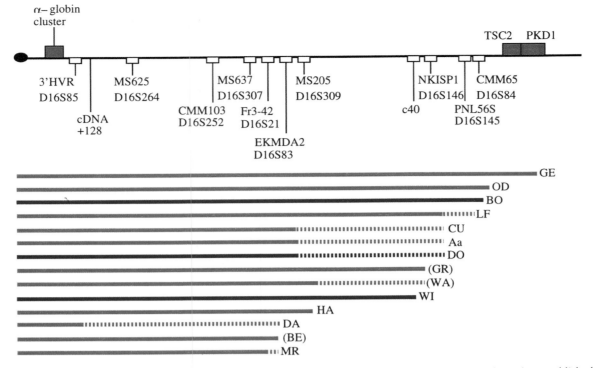

Color Plate 19.1. Summary of known ATR-16 deletions (S. Horsley et al., unpublished data and R. Daniels et al., unpublished data). Above the 16p telomere is shown as a black oval and the positions of the α-globin cluster, the gene-encoding tuberous sclerosis (TSC2), and the adult form of polycystic kidney disease (PKD1) are shown. The positions of other "anchor" markers are also shown. Below, the extent of each deletion is shown with the patient code alongside (see Table 19.1). Deletions known to result from chromosomal translocations are shown in red; those for which the mechanism is unknown or due to chromosomal truncation are blue. Solid bars indicate regions known to be deleted, and broken lines indicate the region of uncertainty of the breakpoints. The yellow bar below represents the maximum extent of deletions that cause α thalassemia with no associated abnormalities (see Chapter 16).

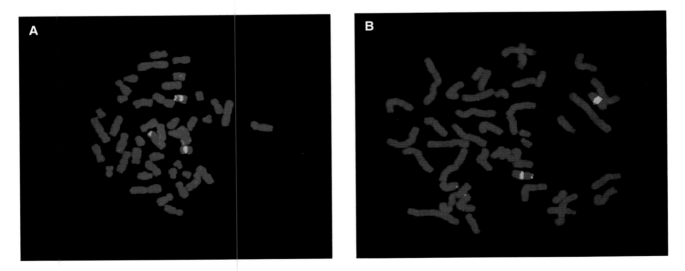

Color Plate 19.4. (A) An example of an unbalanced translocation in a parent of a child with the ATR-16 syndrome. (B) Loss of 16p material in an individual with the ART-16 syndrome.

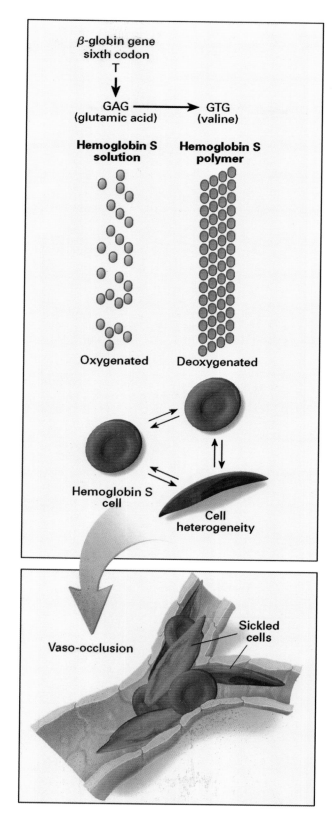

Color Plate Section 4. Pathophysiology of sickle cell disease. The nucleotide and amino acid substitution of HbS—a GAG to GTG substitution in the sixth codon of the β-globin gene leading to the replacement of a glutamic acid residue by a valine residue—are shown at the top. Upon deoxygenation, after a delay time, HbS polymer forms, causing cell sickling and damage to the membrane. Red cells are heterogeneous with a range of cell densities, membrane injury and HbF content. Some cells adhere to the endothelium and lead to vasoocclusion. (From Steinberg M H., 1999.) Management of sickle cell disease. *New England Journal of Medicine*, 340, 1021–1030).

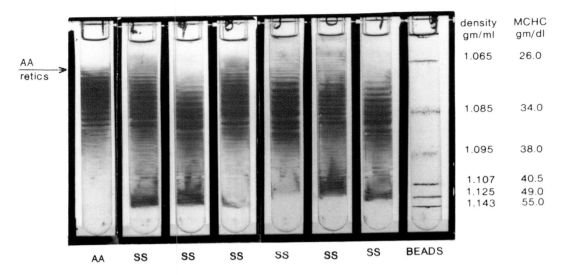

	density gm/ml	MCHC gm/dl
	1.065	26.0
	1.085	34.0
	1.095	38.0
	1.107	40.5
	1.125	49.0
	1.143	55.0

AA   SS   SS   SS   SS   SS   SS   BEADS

Color Plate 20.5. Isopycnic gradient of ten sickle cell anemia (SS) and one normal (AA) whole blood. The gradients are made of Percoll-Stractan mixtures and centrifuged at 37°C. On the top of the gradient are reticulocytes and on the bottom, in the case of normal blood, the oldest cells; in the case of SS, some red cells have normal density and many cells are moderately dehydrated or very dehydrated (bottom of the range of distribution). Among the very dehydrated are the ISCs. Also depicted are the mean MCHC per fraction and the average density across the gradient. Notice that there is considerable interindividual variation as to the amount of light red cells and very dense red cells among sickle cell anemia patients. Some have a lot of very dense cells, some have very little. In addition, the intermediate density fraction varies as well as the extent of low-density red cells. Two modifier genes (epistatic effects) affect this distribution: the copresence of α-thalassemia trait and high expression of HbF.

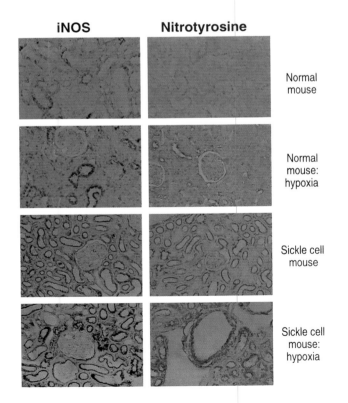

iNOS   Nitrotyrosine

Normal mouse

Normal mouse: hypoxia

Sickle cell mouse

Sickle cell mouse: hypoxia

Color Plate 20.20. Paired immunohistochemistry staining both inducible nitric oxide synthase (iNOS) and nitrotyrosine in individual kidneys of normal and β^S sickle cell mice. Paired photomicrographs are from closely adjacent areas. (From Bank et al., 1996, with permission.)

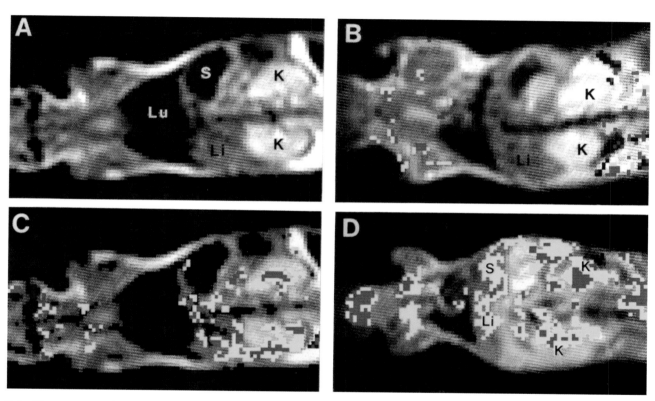

Color Plate 20.23. Difference images of control and transgenic mice (100% O$_2$ vs. room air, 2.5T, TR 1500 msec, TE 40 msec). MRI of mice obtained by comparing the room air image collected while the animal was breathing 100 percent oxygen (**B, C,** and **D**). Red and yellow areas indicate positive differences (hypoxic areas) with red indicating the largest change; light and dark blue areas indicate negative differences: gray scale areas had no statistically significant difference. Anatomic image of the $\alpha^H\beta^S\beta^{S\text{-}Ant}[\beta^{MDD}]$ mouse in room air. *K,* kidney; *Li,* liver; *Lu,* lung; S, spleen. (**B**) Control mouse. Note that there are no *t* statistically significant areas over the kidneys or liver. (**C**) The same $\alpha^H\beta^S\beta^{S\text{-}Ant}[\beta^{MDD}]$ mouse seen in **A**. Note that the largest changes are over the liver and the medulla of the upper kidney. (**D**) An $\alpha^H\beta^S\beta^{S\text{-}Ant}[\beta^{MDD}]$ mouse. Note that the largest changes are over the medulla of the kidney. In this mouse, the spleen also shows changes characteristic of hypoxia.

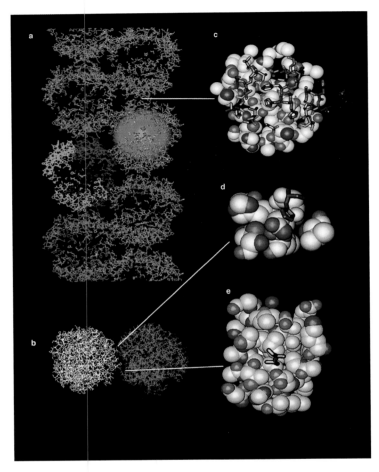

Color Plate 23.4. (a) The double strand of deoxyHbS, based on the crystal structure of Harrington et al. (1997). The tetramers of HbS have been drawn with the central region excluded for clarity; one tetramer illustrates the exclusion region as a solid green sphere in the center of the molecule. Another tetramer is shown with the four subunits colored differently to differentiate them. Red and purple are β-globin chains; blue and orange are α-globin chains. Contacts along the axis of the double strand (vertical here) are denoted as axial, whereas those that connect diagonally are denoted as lateral. The β6 mutation site is in a lateral contact. Note that both the axial and the lateral contacts are dominated by interactions between the beta chains. (b) An end view of the double strand. The two molecules, with all amino acids now showing, are colored differently to aid the eye. The β6 contact is shown on the bottom (expanded view in (e)), and the salt bridge between αHis50 and βAsp79 is above (expanded view in (d)). (c). The axial contact region in a has been enlarged to allow a better view. Unlike the lateral contact, no single amino acid dominates the geometry. Carbon atoms that are filled to van der Waals radii are yellow, oxygen atoms are red, and nitrogen atoms are blue. (d) The salt bridge between Asp β79 and His α50 in the lateral contact area viewed from the α-globin chain. The His is shown as a green licorice stick drawing in the foreground. (e) The lateral contact region showing the β6 Val (green stick figure, foreground) in the receptor pocket on its complementary chain. (Note that in the crystal there are two distinct such regions.) β88Leu is just forward and above Val; β85Phe is then just below β88 Leu and behind the Val.

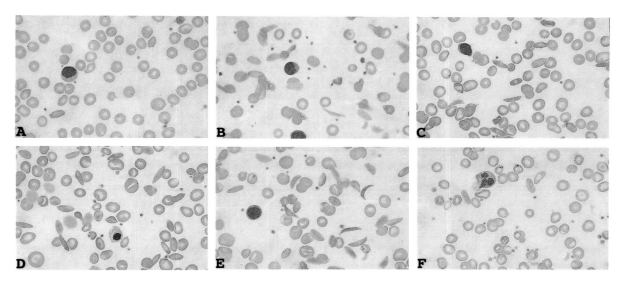

Color Plate 24.1. Blood films in patients with sickle cell anemia and average or low HbF levels. HbF in these patients are **A**, 0.5 percent; **B**, 1 percent; **C**, 4 percent; **D**, 5 percent; **E**, 7 percent; and **F**, 10 percent. Patients **C** and **F** were taking hydroxyurea. Although some of these patients have more irreversibly sickled cells than patients depicted in Figure 24.2 who have high HbF concentrations, note that patient A with the lowest HbF level has very few sickled cells.

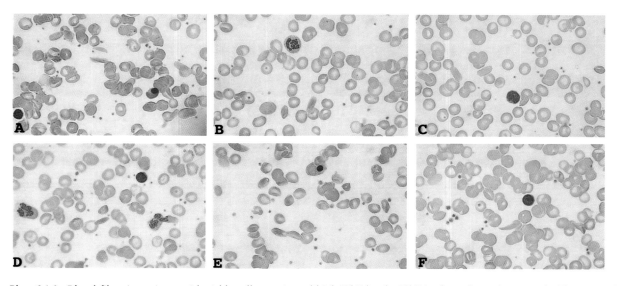

Color Plate 24.2. Blood films in patients with sickle cell anemia and high HbF levels. HbF in these six patients are **A**, 19 percent; **B**, 18 percent; **C**, 19 percent; **D**, 21 percent; **E**, 20 percent; and **F**, 23 percent. All patients were receiving hydroxyurea. All still have sickled cells in the blood, and these are particularly prominent in patient **A**. Also note nucleated red cells in **A** and **E**.

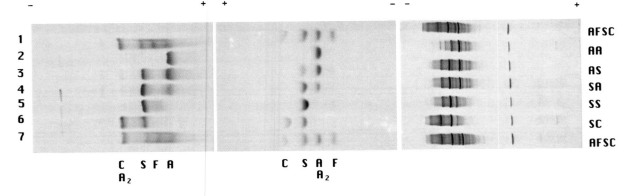

Color Plate 24.3. Electrophoretic separation of hemoglobin in normal individuals (2-AA) and patients with sickle cell trait (3-AS), HbS-β⁺ thalassemia (4-SA), and sickle cell anemia (5-SS), Hb SC disease (6-SC). Control subjects with hemoglobins A, F, S, and C are also shown (lanes 1 and 7). The left panel shows separation by cellulose acetate electrophoresis at pH 8.6; the center panel, citrate agar gel electrophoresis at pH 6.1; and the right panel, isoelectric focusing using pH 4-9 ampholines.

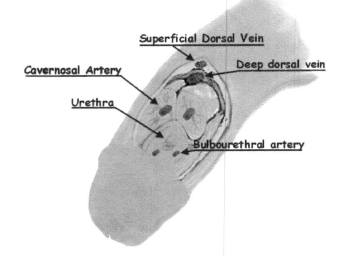

Color Plate 24.8. Anatomy of the penis. Fed by anastomosing branches of the internal pudendal artery, the erectile apparatus consists of two longitudinal cylinders of sinusoidal tissue, the paired corpora cavernosa with their associated arteries. Ventral to the corpora cavernosa is the corpus spongiosum, pierced by the urethra and terminating in the glans penis. A bulbourethral artery feeds the corpus spongiosum. The corporal bodies, except for the glans, are encased in fibrous fascial tunics, the tunica albuginea. There is no vascular communication between the corpora cavernosa and the corpus spongiosum. Draining the corporal sinusoids are emissary veins that enter progressively larger vessels to form the internal pudendal vein. Sinusoids of the glans drain directly into the deep dorsal veins.

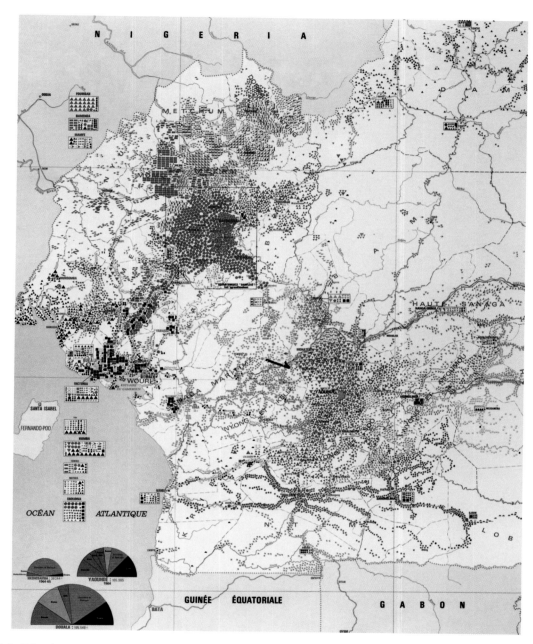

Color Plate 26.8. Ethnologic map of southern Cameroon. Depicted in brown triangle pointing down is the distribution of the Eton people (black arrow). All the symbols in brown are related ethnicities. Of particular interest is the Ewondo people (also carriers of the Camaroon haplotype), depicted by the brown triangle pointing up. (Map from the Service Cartographique de l'ORSTOM. D Laidek, J. Montels, F. Meunier, 1971.)

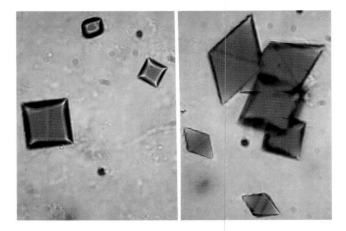

Color Plate 27.2. Crystal forms observed in hemolysates of patients with HbC. (A) Cubic crystals, generated in hemolysates of compound heterozygotes for HbC and Hb Korle-Bu: (B) Tetragonal crystals observed intracellular and in hemolysates of patients homozygous for HbC, with HbSC disease and compound heterozygotes for HbC and HbA and other mutants.

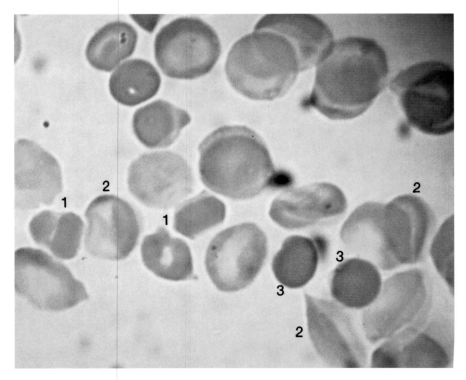

Color Plate 27.7. Erythrocytes in HbSC disease. These cells are characterized by sharp edges, increased red color (particularly in a reticulocyte stained smear), and often by having all the hemoglobin of the cells recruited into the crystal, leaving a ghost of the red cell without cytosolic dissolved hemoglobin. (1) Crystal-containing red cell; (2) "billiard ball" cells; (3) folded cells. (From Lawrence et al., 1991, with permission.)

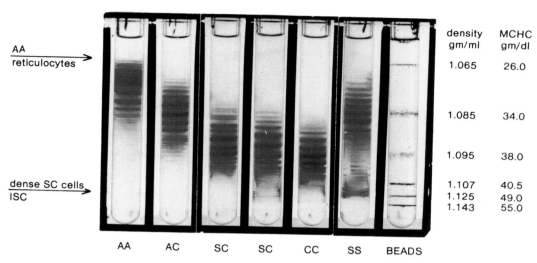

density gm/ml	MCHC gm/dl
1.065	26.0
1.085	34.0
1.095	38.0
1.107	40.5
1.125	49.0
1.143	55.0

AA reticulocytes

dense SC cells
ISC

AA   AC   SC   SC   CC   SS   BEADS

Color Plate 27.11. Percoll-Stractan (Larex) density separation of whole blood from normal hemolysate (AA), HbC trait (AC), and three different HbSC disease individuals and one sickle cell anemia patient (SS). Beads: color-coded density beads to establish the density at different levels of the gradient after centrifugation.

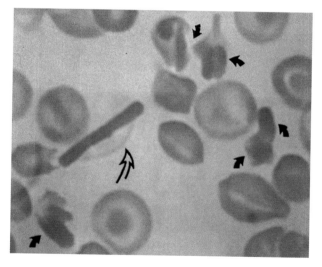

Color Plate 27.13. Blood smear directly from fingerstick blood from a patient with SC$^{\alpha G\text{-Philadelphia}}$ disease. Open arrow depicts a "sugar cane" crystal, a shape not observed in HbC disease or HbSC disease blood. The black arrows depict red cells with more classical forms of HbC-dependent crystals. (From Lawrence et al., 1997 with permission.)

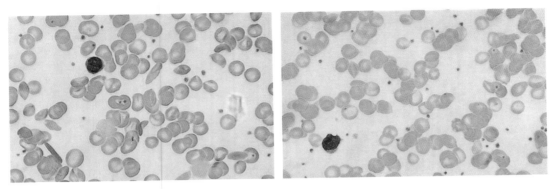

Color Plate 28.1. Blood films in two patients with HbS-β^0 thalassemia. (**Left panel**). The patient has a HbF level of 5 percent. Sickled cells are prominent in addition to microcytosis. In the right panel, with HbF of 2 percent, microcytosis and hypochromia are prominent, and few typical sickled cells are seen.

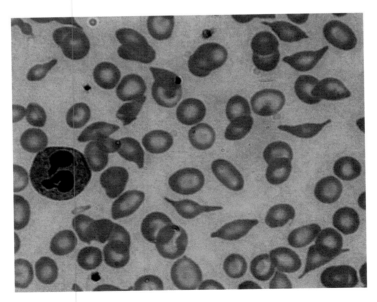

Color Plate 28.6. Erythrocytes in different genotypes of HbS-Oman disease. The peculiar shape of the irreversibly sickled cells has been called "yarn/knitting needle," and it is presumed to result from the polymerization of HbS-Oman in one or two domains.

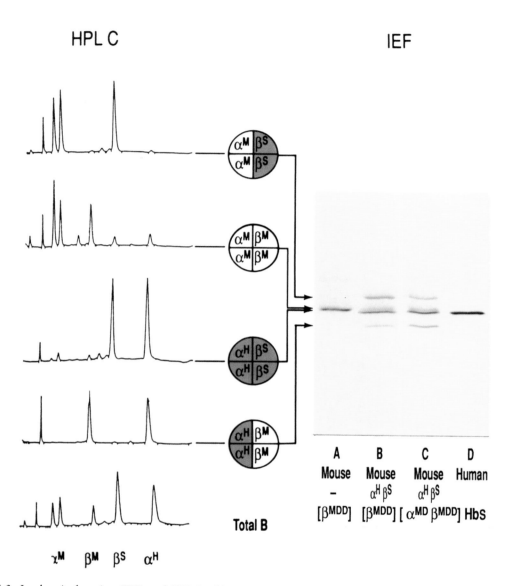

Color Plate 34.3. Isoelectric focusing (IEF) and HPLC of hemoglobins from several transgenic mice expressing human HbS and mouse globins (Fabry et al., 1992a). The bands representing homotetramers composed of dimers of mouse α and human βˢ chains, mouse α and mouse β chains, human α and human βˢ chains, and human α and mouse β chains were separated by isoelectric focusing, isolated from the gel, and separated by denaturing HPLC to allow identification of the tetramers present in the isoelectric focusing gel. (From Fabry et al., 1992, with permission.)

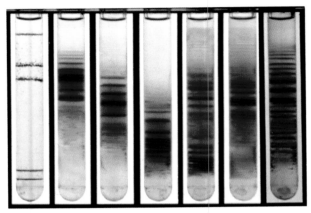

Beads	**AA**	**AC**	**CC**	**SS**	**SOArab**	**HS**

Color Plate 34.5. Percoll®-Larex® continuous density gradient. Red cell density is directly proportional to the mean corpuscular hemoglobin concentration (MCHC). The least dense (lowest MCHC) cells are at the top of the gradient and the highest density cells are at the bottom. This technique provides a method for directly visualizing the distribution of red cell density in a sample of whole blood. The example shows a continuous density gradient with density marker beads and red cells from patients with normal hemoglobin (AA), HbC trait (AC), HbC disease (CC), sickle cell anemia (SS), HbS-O Arabia, and hereditary spherocytosis (HS).

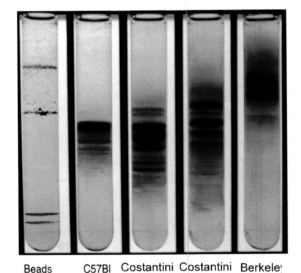

	Beads	C57Bl	Costantini Gilman G1 $\alpha^H \beta^S \gamma$	Costantini Gilman G2 $\alpha^H \beta^S \gamma$	Berkeley $\alpha^H \beta^S$
Knockouts		–	$\alpha^{KK} \beta^{KK}$	$\alpha^{KK} \beta^{KK}$	$\alpha^{KK} \beta^{KK}$
α^H		–	100	100	100
β^S		–	63	93	100
γ		–	27	7	<1
MCH		14.5	14.8	13.1	9.3

Color Plate 34.12. Percoll®-Larex® continuous density gradient of three types of transgenic mice expressing exclusively human hemoglobin. The lightest cells (at the top of the gradient) have low MCHC and are predominantly reticulocytes and the densest cells (at the bottom of the gradient) have high MCHC and are enriched in irreversibly sickled cells. The gradient has physiologic pH and osmolarity and is performed at 37°C. From left to right: density marker beads, C57Bl, Costantini mice with 27 percent γ-globin chains (expressing Gilman G1) at 15 to 30 days, Costantini mice with 7 percent γ globin (expressing Gilman G2) at 15 to 30 days, and the Berkeley mouse. Note the highest density (MCHC) cells in the Costantini G2 mouse and the lowest density (MCHC) cells in the Berkeley mouse.

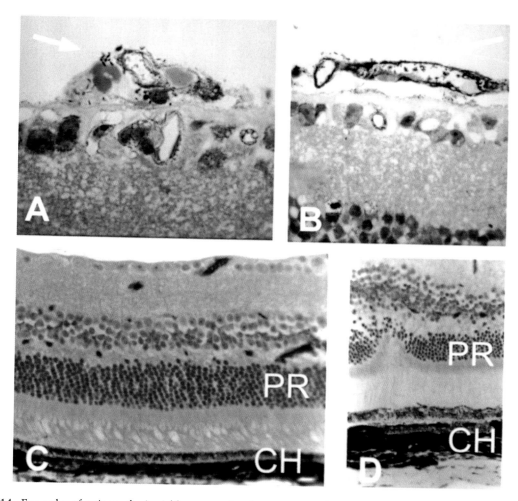

Color Plate 34.14. Examples of retinopathy in sickle transgenic mice expressing the Costantini $\alpha^H\beta^S$ transgene and homozygous for the β^{major} deletion. Panels A and B: pre-retinal neovascularization indicated by arrows. Panel C: a normal retina indicating choroid (CH) and photoreceptor (PR) layers. Panel D: a pathologic retina showing dilated obstructed CH with a disrupted PR layer above it.

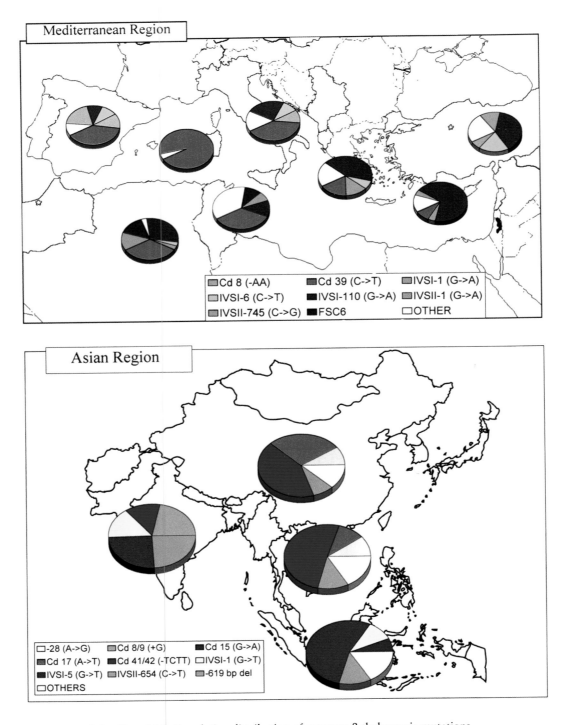

Color Plate 36.2. Population distribution of common β-thalassemia mutations.

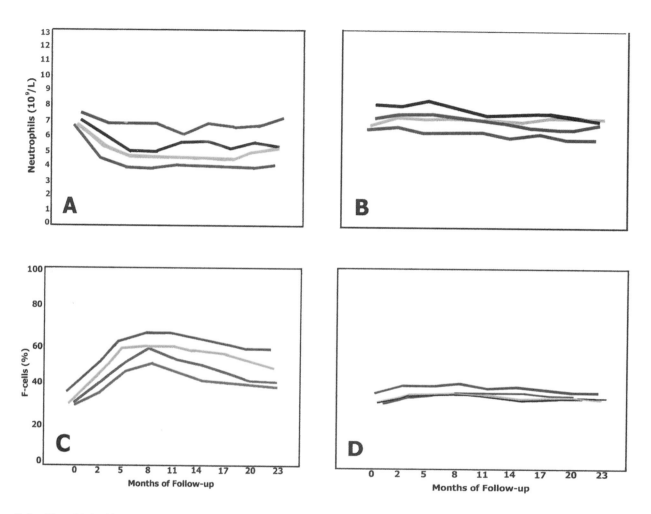

Color Plate 38.4. Changes in neutrophil counts (**A and B**) and F cells (**C and D**) during treatment of sickle cell anemia with hydroxyurea or placebo. Red lines indicate 0 to < 2 pain episodes/year; yellow lines, 2 to <5 episodes/year; blue lines, 5 to < 10 episodes/year; and green lines, ≥ 10 episodes/year. (Panels A and C) Hydroxyurea-treated patients. (Panels B and D) Placebo-treated patients. (Adapted from Charache et al., 1996.)

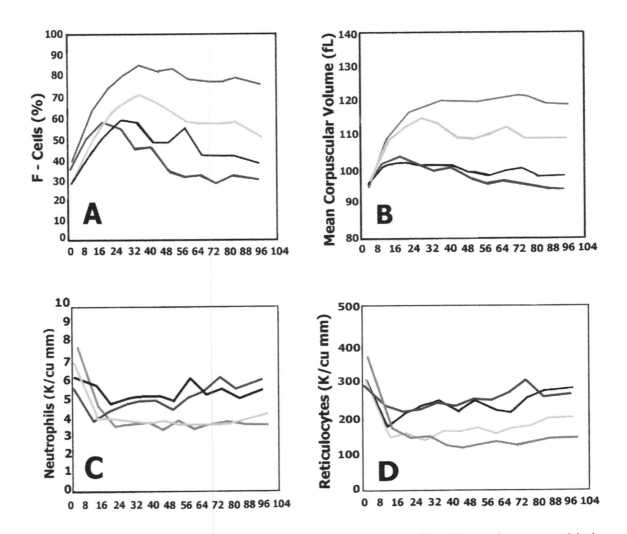

Color Plate 38.5. Variation in F cells, MCV, neutrophil counts, and reticulocyte counts during 2 years of treatment with hydroxyurea. Patients are grouped by the quartile of the final HbF response after two years of treatment (Red-top quartile of HbF response; yellow, third quartile; purple, second quartile; green, lowest [first] quartile). (Adapted from Steinberg et al., 1997a.)

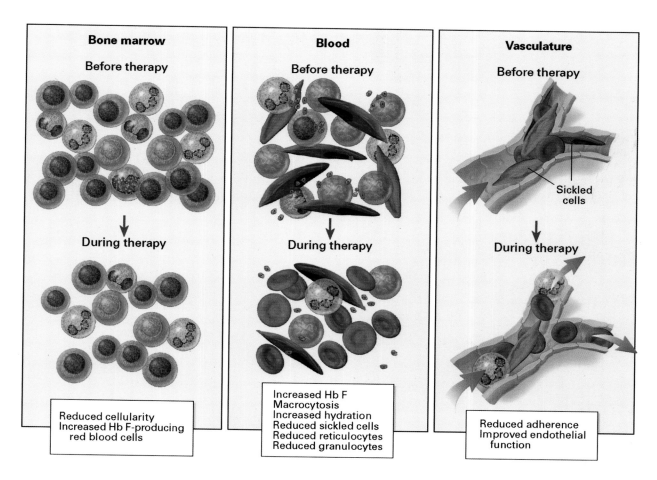

Color Plate 38.7 Mechanisms of action of hydroxyurea. Hydroxyurea acts on the bone marrow and, by its cytotoxic effects, selects a population of erythroblasts that can synthesize increased amounts of HbF. It has no known direct effects on gene expression. Bone marrow cellularity may also be diminished. Higher concentrations of HbF reduce the level of HbS polymer and the numbers of deformed, dense, and damaged erythrocytes. Cells with a high HbF content survive longer, attenuating hemolysis and leading to a reduction in reticulocytes. Circulating granulocytes, monocytes, and platelets are diminished. Fewer dense, poorly adhesive erythrocytes are less apt to adhere to and perturb the endothelium, reducing the likelihood of vasoocclusion. (From Steinberg, 1999 with permission.)

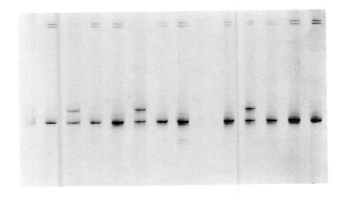

Color Plate 39.7. Evaluation of donor/recipient origin by PCR amplification for the D1S80 minisatellite locus of single BFU-e-derived colonies obtained from a patient with persistent mixed chimerism after BMT for thalassemia.

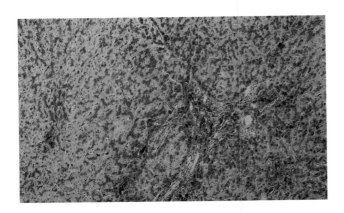

Color Plate 39.8. Pretransplant liver biopsy of a thalassemia patient. The biopsy was prepared by Perls's technique. Hepatic iron concentration was 23 mg/g dry weight.

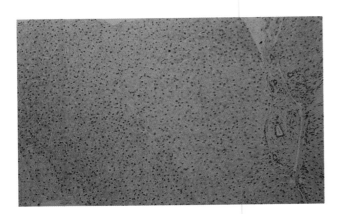

Color Plate 39.9. Liver biopsy (Perls's technique) of the same patient as in Figure 39.8, 8 years after BMT. Hepatic iron concentration was 1.41 mg/g dry weight, normal value <1.6 mg/g (Weinfeld, 1964). The patient had been treated by a course of sequential phlebotomies starting during the third year after transplant.

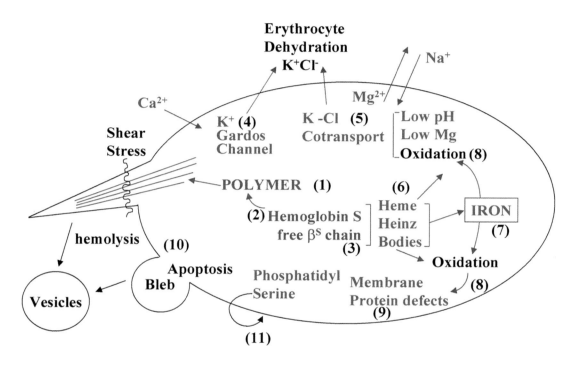

Color Plate 42.1. Sites of red cell physiology that are targets of experimental therapies. Sickle hemoglobin polymer and free β^S-globin chains, primary defects in sickle cell anemia are shown in red, secondary defects are shown in green, and tertiary defects in black.

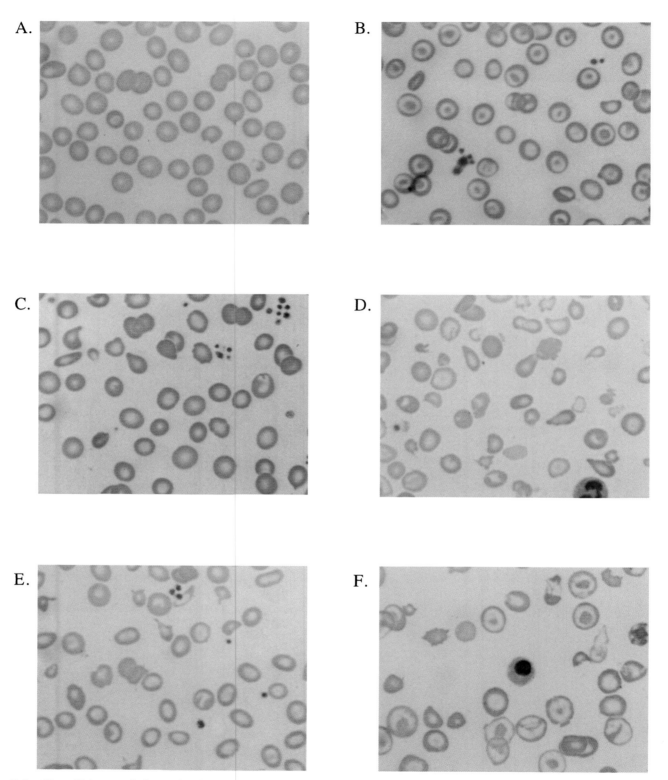

Color Plate 43.3. Morphology of red cells with Wright's staining in various HbE syndromes. (A) HbE heterozygote; (B) HbE homozygote; (C) HbE-α thalassemia-1; (D) Hb E-β thalassemia; (E) AE Bart's disease; (F) EF Bart's disease.

B

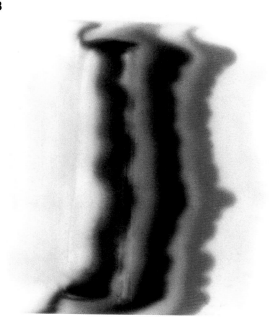

Color Plate 44.7. (**A**) Spectra between 450 and 650 μm of the oxidized form of four M hemoglobins are compared in each case with the normal methemoglobin spectra. In these spectra, the normal chains are met, and the abnormal chains have their own particular spectral properties. (After Shibata et al., 1967.) (**B**) Separation of chains from tetramers of Hb M Boston (α58(E7)His→Tyr), using the P-chloride mercuric benzoate (PCMB) method, and starch block electrophoresis at pH 8.6. Notice that the band to the right has a bright red color and hence the hemes are normal; that is, β chains. The band to the left is dark brown, that is, α^{Boston} chain. The band in the middle is a combination of both colors because it is the undissociated tetramer.

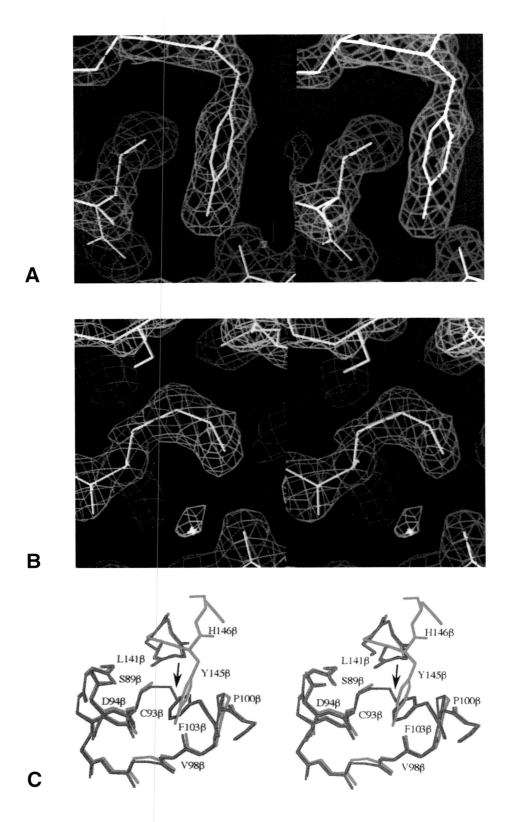

Color Plate 46.4. Stereodiagrams of electron density maps showing the environment of Cys93/β1 for COHbA (**A**) and for SNO-nitrosylHbA (**B**). In (**C**), the environment of Cys93/β1 is shown with side chains, and selected residues and COHbA (red) and SNO-nitrosylHbA (green) have been superimposed. Arrow points to the S-nitroso group.

et al., 1996; Bianco et al., 1997). They should provide far greater protection than currently available products and will soon be available. *H. influenzae* vaccine should also be used in infancy.

Penicillin is given prophylactically, 125 mg twice daily to children younger than 3 years, and 250 mg twice daily to children up to age 5 years (Gaston et al., 1986). Older children do not routinely need continued antibiotic prophylaxis, but the basis for making this decision, as discussed previously, must be carefully considered (Falletta et al., 1995). If severe pneumococcal disease has not occurred, and if the patient is enrolled in a comprehensive care program, prophylactic penicillin can be safely discontinued at age 5 years. Prophylactic penicillin should be started at ages 3 to 4 months. This treatment has reduced the incidence of pneumococcal sepsis and death.

Oxygen

Although oxygen is considered by many a mainstay of treatment, few studies have evaluated its value in normoxic patients with sickle cell anemia. When hypoxia or oxygen desaturation accompanies surgery or an acute chest syndrome, oxygen treatment can reverse these abnormalities. Although the pathophysiology of sickle cell anemia is initiated by the polymerization of deoxyHbS under physiologic conditions, there is no evidence that high concentrations of inhaled oxygen can curtail or prevent this development. Inhaled oxygen can have adverse effects in sickle cell anemia as discussed previously (Embury et al., 1984).

CONCLUSIONS

Treatment for sickle cell anemia is evolving at a gratifying pace, driven by years of laboratory study that have illuminated many features of the pathophysiology of this disease. Better understanding of the use of mainstay treatments such as transfusion and the proper use of opioids coupled with the advent of new treatments such as hydroxyurea and transplantation have typically improved and prolonged life. These modalities include the following:

- Transfusion: Replacement of sickle with normal blood is conceptually the most specific form of treatment. Principles of transfusion therapy in sickle cell anemia are discussed in Chapter 37. Chronic transfusion causes hemosiderosis, alloimmunization, venous access difficulties, and unexpected viral infection, and these hazards should be carefully considered before such a program is undertaken. In most situations, simple transfusions are preferred to exchange transfusions. Anemia alone is rarely an indication for transfusion.

- Hydroxyurea; Hydroxyurea is the first drug treatment that unequivocally improves some symptoms of sickle cell anemia in most patients. Indications for its use and an appropriate drug protocol are discussed in Chapter 38. Children have the greatest petential for benefit, and studies in this population are now under way.

- Transplantation; Stem cell transplantation is currently the only cure for sickle cell anemia (Chapter 40). Its difficulties lie in the lack of suitable marrow donors for about 90 to 95 percent of eligible patients and the 5 to 10 percent mortality rate associated with the current technology of this procedure.

- Experimental therapy: After decades of inactivity, recent years have seen the initiation of many innovative treatments (Chapter 42). Gene therapy, the ultimate goal for cure or reversal of most complications, is still in the early phases of laboratory study (Chapter 41). Many transgenic mouse models of sickle cell disease are available to test the usefulness of newer experimental treatments (Chapter 34).

References

Abbasi, AA, Prasad, AS, Ortega, J et al. (1976). Gonadal function abnormalities in sickle cell anemia: Studies in male patients. *Ann. Intern. Med.* 85: 601–605.

Achord, JL. (1994). Gastroenterologic and hepatobiliary manifestations. In Embury, SH, Hebbel, RP, Mohandas, N, and Steinberg, MH, editors. *Sickle cell disease: Basic principles and clinical practice,* New York: Lippincott-Raven.

Adamkiewicz, TV, Buchanan, GR, Facklam, RR et al. (1999). Invasive *Streptococcus pneumoniae* (Pnc) infections in children with sickle cell disease (SCD): The threat of penicillin resistance. *23rd Annual Meeting of the National Sickle Cell Disease Program.*

Adams, RJ. (1994). Neurologic complications. In Embury, SH, Hebbel, RP, Mohandas, N, and Steinberg, MH, editors. *Sickle cell disease: Basic principles and clinical practice.* New York: Raven Press.

Adams, RJ, McKie, VC, Carl, EM et al. (1997). Long-term stroke risk in children with sickle cell disease screened with transcranial Doppler. *Ann. Neurol.* 42: 699–704.

Adams, RJ, McKie, VC, Hsu, L et al. (1998). Prevention of a first stroke by transfusions in children with sickle cell anemia and abnormal results on transcranial Doppler ultrasonography. *N. Engl. J. Med.* 339: 5–11.

Adams, RJ, Aaslid, R, el Gammal, T et al. (1988). Detection of cerebral vasculopathy in sickle cell disease using transcranial Doppler ultrasonography and magnetic resonance imaging. Case report. *Stroke* 19: 518–520.

Adams, RJ, Nichols, FT 3d, Aasild, R et al. (1990). Cerebral vessel stenosis in sickle cell disease, criteria for detection by transcranial Doppler. *Am. J. Pediatr. Hematol. Oncol.* 12: 277–282.

Adams, RJ, Nichols, FT, Figueroa, R et al. (1992a). Transcranial Doppler correlation with cerebral angiography in sickle cell disease. *Stroke* 23: 1073–1077.

Adams, R, Mckie, V, Nichols, F et al. (1992b). The use of transcranial ultrasonography to predict stroke in sickle cell disease. *N. Engl. J. Med.* 326: 605–610.

Adekile, AD, Mckie, KM, Adeodu, OO et al. (1993). Spleen in sickle cell anemia, comparative studies of Nigerian and U.S. patients. *Am. J. Hematol.* 42: 316–321.

Adekile, AD, Adeodu, OO, Jeje, AA, and Odesanmi, WO. (1988). Persistent gross splenomegaly in Nigerian patients with sickle cell anaemia, relationship to malaria. *Ann. Trop. Paediatr.* 8: 103–107.

Ademiluyi, SA, Rotimi, VO, Coker, AO et al. (1988). The anaerobic and aerobic bacterial flora of leg ulcers in patients with sickle-cell disease. *J. Infect.* 17: 115–120.

Adeodu, OO and Adekile, AD. (1990). Clinical and laboratory features associated with persistent gross splenomegaly in Nigerian children with sickle cell anaemia. *Acta. Paediatr. Scand.* 79: 686–690.

Agbaraji, VO, Scott, RB, Leto, S, and Kingslow, LW. (1988). Fertility studies in sickle cell disease: Semen analysis in adult male patients. *Int. J. Fertil.* 33: 347–352.

Ahman, H, Kayhty, H, Tamminen, P et al. (1996). Pentavalent pneumococcal oligosaccharide conjugate vaccine PncCRM is well-tolerated and able to induce an antibody response in infants. *Pediatric Infect. Dis. J.* 15: 134–139.

Airede A. (1992). Acute splenic sequestration in a five-week-old infant with sickle cell disease [letter]. *J. Pediatr.* 120: 160.

Aken'Ova YA, Bakare, RA, Okunade, MA, and Olaniyi, J. (1995). Bacterial causes of acute osteomyelitis in sickle cell anaemia, changing infection profile. *West Afr. J. Med.* 14: 255–258.

Al-Fawaz, I, Al-Rasheed, A, al-Mugeiren, M et al. (1996). Hepatitis E virus infection in patients from Saudi Arabia with sickle cell anaemia and beta-thalassemia major: Possible transmission by blood transfusion. *J. Viral Hepat.* 3: 203–205.

Alleyne, SI, Rauseo, RD, and Serjeant, GR. (1981). Sexual development and fertility of Jamaican female patients with homozygous sickle cell disease. *Arch. Intern. Med.* 141: 1295–1297.

Al-Salem, AH and Nourallah, H. (1997). Sequential endoscopic/laparoscopic management of cholelithiasis and choledocholithiasis in children who have sickle cell disease. *J. Pediatr. Surg.* 32: 1432–1435.

Al-Salem, AH, Qaisaruddin, S, AIL, Jam'a et al. (1998). Splenic abscess and sickle cell disease. *Am. J. Hematol.* 58: 100–104.

Al Jam'a AH and Al Dabbous, IA. (1998). Hydroxyurea in the treatment of sickle cell associated priapism. *J. Urol.* 159: 1642–1642.

Anand, AJ and Glatt, AE. (1994). Salmonella osteomyelitis and arthritis in sickle cell disease. *Semin. Arthritis Rheum.* 24: 211–221.

Aoki, RY and Saad, STO. (1995). Enalapril reduces the albuminuria of patients with sickle cell disease. *Am. J. Med.* 98: 432–435.

Armstrong, FD, Thompson, RJ Jr, Wang, W et al. (1996). Cognitive functioning and brain magnetic resonance imaging in children with sickle cell disease. Neuropsychology Committee of the Cooperative Study of Sickle Cell Disease. *Pediatrics* 97: 864–870.

Asakura, T, Mattiello, JA, Obata, K et al. (1994). Partially oxygenated sickled cells, sickle-shaped red cells found in circulating blood of patients with sickle cell disease. *Proc. Natl. Acad. Sci. U.S.A.* 91: 12589–12593.

Bachir, D, Virag, R, Lee, K et al. (1997). Prevention and treatment of erectile disorders in sickle cell disease [in French]. *Rev. Med. Interne* 18: 46S–51S.

Badaloo, A, Jackson, AA, and Jahoor, F. (1989). Whole body protein turnover and resting metabolic rate in homozygous sickle cell disease. *Clin. Sci.* 77: 93–97.

Bagasra, O, Steiner, RM, Ballas, SK et al. (1998). Viral burden and disease progression in HIV-1-infected patients with sickle cell anemia. *Am. J. Hematol.* 59: 199–207.

Bainbridge, R, Higgs, DR, Maude, GH, and Serjeant GR. (1985). Clinical presentation of homozygous sickle cell disease. *J. Pediatr.* 106: 881–885.

Bakshi, SS, Grover, R, Cabezon, E, and Wethers, DL. (1991). Febrile episodes in children with sickle cell disease treated on an ambulatory basis. *J. Assoc. Acad. Minor. Phys.* 2: 80–83.

Balkaran, B, Char, G, Morris, JS et al. (1992). Stroke in a cohort of patients with homozygous sickle cell disease. *J. Pediatr.* 120: 360–366.

Ballas, SK and Smith, ED. (1992). Red blood cell changes during the evolution of the sickle cell painful crisis. *Blood* 79: 2154–2163.

Ballas, SK, Talacki, CA, Rao, VN, and Steiner, RM. (1998). The prevalence of avascular necrosis in sickle cell anemia: Correlation with alpha-thalassemia. *Hemoglobin* 13: 649–655.

Bank, N, Aynedjian, HS, Qiu, JH et al. (1996). Renal nitric oxide synthases in transgenic sickle cell mice. *Kidney Int.* 50: 184–189.

Barbarin, OA, Whitten, CF, and Bonds, SM. (1994). Estimating rates of psychosocial problems in urban and poor children with sickle cell anemia. *Health Soc. Work* 19: 112–119.

Barrett-Connor, E. (1971). Bacterial infection and sickle cell anemia. An analysis of 250 infections in 166 patients and a review of the literature. *Medicine (Baltimore)* 50: 97–112.

Baum, KF, MacFarlane, DE, Maude, GH, and Serjeant, GR. (1987). Topical antibiotics in chronic sickle cell leg ulcers. *Trans. R. Soc. Trop. Med. Hygi.* 81: 847–849.

Beet EA. (1949). The genetics of sickle cell trait in a Bantu tribe. *Ann. Eugenics* 14: 279–284.

Begue, P. (1999). Infection and sickle cell anemia. *Pathol. Biol. (Paris)* 47: 19–25.

Bell, LM, Naides, SJ, Stoffman, P et al. (1989). Human parvovirus B19 infection among hospital staff members after contact with infected patients. *N. Engl. J. Med.* 321: 485–491.

Bellet, PS, Kalinyak, KA, Shukla, R et al. (1995). Incentive spirometry to prevent acute pulmonary complications in sickle cell diseases. *N. Engl. J. Med.* 333: 699–703.

Bernini, JC, Mustafa, MM, Sutor, LJ, and Buchanan, GR. (1995). Fatal hemolysis induced by ceftriaxone in a child with sickle cell anemia. *J. Pediatr.* 126: 813–815.

Bianco, I, Cappabianca, MP, Foglietta, E et al. (1997). Silent thalassemias: Genotypes and phenotypes. *Haematologica* 82: 269–280.

Billett, HH, Patel, Y, and Rivers, SP. (1991). Venous insufficiency is not the cause of leg ulcers in sickle cell disease. *Am. J. Hematol.* 37: 133–134.

Bjornson, AB and Lobel, JS. (1979). Direct evidence that decreased serum opsonization of *Streptococcus pneumoniae* via the alternative complement pathway in sickle cell disease is related to antibody deficiency. *J. Clin. Invest.* 79: 388–398.

Bjornson, AB, Lobel, JS, and Harr, KS. (1985). Relation between serum opsonic activity for *Streptococcus pneumoniae* and complement function in sickle cell disease. *J. Infect. Dis.* 152: 701–709.

Bjornson, AB, Falletta, JM, Verter, J et al. (1996). Serotype-specific immunoglobulin G antibody responses to pneumococcal of continued penicillin prophylaxis. *J. Pediatr.* 129: 828–835.

Borel, MJ, Buchowski, MS, Turner, EA et al (1998a). Protein turnover and energy expenditure increase during exogenous nutrient availability in sickle cell disease. *Am. J. Clin. Nutr.* 68: 607–614.

Borel, MJ, Buchowski, MS, Turner, EA et al. (1998b). Alterations in basal nutrient metabolism increase resting energy expenditure in sickle cell disease. *Am. J. Physiol.* 274:E357–364.

Bowcock, SJ, Nwabueze, ED, Cook, AE, and Abound HH. (1988). Fatal splenic sequestration in adult sickle cell disease. *Clin. Lab. Haematol.* 10: 95–99.

Braden, DS, Covitz, W, and Milner, PF. (1996). Cardiovascular function during rest and exercise in patients with sickle-cellanemia and coexisting alpha thalassemia-2. *Am. J. Hematol.* 52: 96–102.

Brittenham, GM, Cohen, AR, McLaren, CE et al. (1993). Hepatic iron stores and plasma ferritin concentration in patients with sickle cell anemia and thalassemia major. *Am. J. Hematol.* 42: 81–85.

Brown, AK, Sleeper, LA, Pegelow, CH et al. (1994). The influence of infant and maternal sickle cell disease on birth outcome and neonatal course. *Arch. Pediatr. Adolesc. Med.* 148: 1156–1162.

Buchanan, GR and Smith, SJ. (1986). Pneumococcal septicemia despite pneumococcal vaccine and prescription of penicillin prophylaxsis in children with sickle cell anemia. *Am. J. Dis. Child.* 140: 428–432.

Burnett, AL, Allen, RP, Tempany, CM et al. (1995). Evaluation of erectile function in men with sickle cell disease. *Urology* 45: 657–663.

Caruso-Nicoletti, M, Mancuso, M, Spadaro, G et al. (1992). Growth and development in white patients with sickle cell diseases. *Am. J. Pediatr. Hematol. Oncol.* 14: 285–288.

Casper, JT, Koethe, S, Rodey, GE, and Thatcher, LG. (1976). A new method for studying splenic reticuloendothelial dysfunction in sickle cell disease patients and its clinical application: A brief report. *Blood* 47: 183–188.

Castro, O. (1996). Systemic fat embolism and pulmonary hypertension in sickle cell disease. *Hematol. Oncol. Clin. North Am.* 10: 1289–1303.

Castro, O, Brambilla, DJ, Thorington, B et al. (1994). The acute chest syndrome in sickle cell disease, incidence and risk factors. The Cooperative Study of Sickle Cell Disease. *Blood* 84: 643–649.

Cazzola, M, Guarnone, R, Cerani, P et al. (1998). Red blood cell precursor mass as an independent determinant of serum erythropoietin level. *Blood* 91: 2139–2145.

Chakrabarty, A, Upadhyay, J, Dhabuwala, CB et al. (1996). Priapism associated with sickle cell hemoglobinopathy in children: Long-term effects on potency. *J. Urol.* 155: 1419–1423.

Charache, S and Page, DL. (1967). Infarction of bone marrow in the sickle cell disorders. *Ann. Intern. Med.* 67: 1195–1200.

Charache, S, Terrin, ML, Moore, RD et al. (1995a). Effect of hydroxyurea on the frequency of painful crises in sickle cell anemia. Investigators of the Multicenter Study of Hydroxyurea in Sickle Cell Anemia. *N. Engl. J. Med.* 332: 1317–1322.

Charache, S, Lubin, B, and Reid CD, editors. (1989). *Management and therapy of sickle cell disease. NIH Publication No. 89–2117.*

Charache, S, Lubin, B, Reid, CD et al. editors. (1995b). *Management and therapy of sickle cell disease. NIH Publication No. 95–2117.*

Charlotte, F, Bachir, D, Nénert, M et al. (1995). Vascular lesions of the liver in sickle cell disease: A clinicopathological study in 26 living patients. *Arch. Pathol. Lab. Med.* 119: 46–52.

Chesney, PJ, Wilimas, JA, Presbury, G et al. (1995). Penicillin- and cephalosporin-resistant strains of *Streptococcus pneumoniae* causing sepsis and meningitis in children with sickle cell disease. *J. Pediatr.* 127: 526–532.

Christakis, J, Vavatsi, N, Hassapopoulou, H et al. (1990). Comparison of homozygous sickle cell disease in northern Greece and Jamaica. *Lancet* 335: 637–640.

Chuang, E, Ruchelli, E, and Mulberg, AE. (1997). Autoimmune liver disease and sickle cell anemia in children: A report of three cases. *J. Pediatr. Hematol. Oncol.* 19: 159–162.

Cohen, A. (1990). Treatment of transfusional iron overload. *Am. J. Pediatr. Hematol. Oncol.* 12: 4–8.

Cohen, AR, Martin, MB, Silber, JH et al. (1992). A modified transfusion program for prevention of stroke in sickle cell disease. *Blood* 79: 1657–1651.

Cohen, AR, Buchanan, GR, Martin, M, and Ohene-Frempong, K. (1991). Increased blood requirements during long-term transfusion therapy for sickle cell disease. *J. Pediatr.* 118: 405–407.

Comer, GM, Ozick, LA, Sachdev, RK et al. (1991). Transfusion-related chronic liver disease in sickle cell anemia. *Am. J. Gastroenterol.* 86: 1232–1234.

Conley, CL. (1980). Sickle-cell anemia—the first molecular disease. In Wintrobe, M, editor. *Blood, pure and eloquent.* New York: McGraw-Hill.

Consensus conference. (1987). Newborn screening for sickle cell disease and other hemoglobinopathies. *JAMA* 258: 1205–1209.

Covitz, W. (1994). Cardiac disease. In Embury, SH, Hebbel, RP, Mohandas, N, and Steinberg, MH, editors. *Sickle cell disease: Basic principles and clinical practice*. New York: Lippincott-Raven.

Covitz, W, Espeland, M, Gallagher, D et al. (1995). The heart in sickle cell anemia: The cooperative study of sickle cell disease (CSSCD). *Chest* 108: 1214–1219.

Cunningham, FG, Pritchard, JA, and Mason, R. (1983). Pregnancy and sickle cell hemoglobinopathies: Results with and without prophylactic transfusions. *Obstet. Gynecol.* 62: 419–424.

Curran, EL, Fleming, JC, Rice, K, and Wang, WC. (1997). Orbital compression syndrome in sickle cell disease. *Ophthalmology* 104: 1610–1615.

Datta, NS. (1977). Megalophallus in sickle cell disease. *J. Urol.* 117: 672–673.

Daw, NC, Wilimas, JA, Wang, WC et al. (1997). Nasopharyngeal carriage of penicillin-resistant *Streptococcus pneumoniae* in children with sickle cell disease. *Pedlatrics* 99: E7.

Decastel, M, Leborgne-Samuel, Y, Alexandre, L et al. (1999). Morphological features of the human umbilical vein in normal, sickle cell trait, and sickle cell disease pregnancies. *Hum. Pathol.* 30: 13–20.

DeCastro, L, Rinder, HM, Howe, JG, and Smith, BR. (1998). Thrombophilic genotypes do not adversely affect the course of sickle cell disease (SCD). *Blood* 92: 161a.

De Ceulaer, K and Serjeant, GR. (1991). Acute splenic sequestration in Jamaican adults with homozygous sickle cell disease, a role of alpha thalassaemia. *Br. J. Haematol.* 77: 563–564.

DeVault, KR, Friedman, LS, Westerberg, S et al. (1994). Hepatitis C in sickle cell anemia. *J. Clin. Gastroenterol.* 18: 206–209.

Diggs, LW (1967). Bone and joint lesions in sickle-cell disease. *Clin. Orthop.* 52: 119–143.

Donegan, JO, Lobel, JS, and Gluckman, JL. (1982). Otolaryngologic manifestations of sickle cell disease. *J. Otolaryngol.* 3: 141–144.

Dorwart, BB and Gabuzda, T. (1985). Symmetric myositis and faciitis: A complication of sickle cell anemia during vasoocclusion. *J. Rheumatol.* 12: 590–595.

Dunn, EK, Miller, ST, Macchia, RJ et al. (1995). Penile scintigraphy for priapism in sickle cell disease. *J. Nucl. Med.* 36: 1404–1407.

Dunsmore, K, Ware, R, Frush, D, and Kinney, T. (1995). Short-term transfusion therapy for avascular necrosis of the hips in children with sickle cell disease. *Int. J. Pediatr. Hematol. Oncol.* 2: 79–83.

Durosinmi, MA, Gevao, SM, and Esan, GJ. (1991). Chronic leg ulcers in sickle cell disease: Experience in Ibadan, Nigeria. *Afr. J. Med. Sci.* 20: 11–14.

Eckman, JR. (1996). Leg ulcers in sickle cell disease. *Hematol. Oncol. Clin. North America* 10: 1333–1344.

Emond, AM, Collis, R, Darvill, D et al. (1985). Acute splenic sequestration in homozygous sickle cell disease, natural history and management. *J. Pediatr.* 107: 201–206.

el-Hazmi, MA, Bahakim, HM, and al-Fawaz, I. (1991). Endocrine functions in sickle cell anaemia patients. *J. Trop. Pediatr.* 38: 307–313.

El-Shafei, AM, Kaur Dhaliwal, J, Kaur Sandhu, A, and Rashid Al-Sharqi, M. (1995). Indications for blood transfusion in pregnancy in sickle cell disease. *Aust. N. Z. J. Obstet. Gynaecol.* 35: 405–408.

El Younis, CM, Min, AD, Fiel, MI et al. (1996). Autoimmune hepatitis in a patient with sickle cell disease. *Am. J. Gastroenterol.* 91: 1016–1018.

Embury, SH, Garcia, JF, Mohandas, N et al. (1984). Effects of oxygen inhalation on endogenous erythropoietin kinetics erythropoiesis and properties of blood cells in sickle cell anemia. *N. Engl. J. Med.* 311: 291–295.

Embury, SH, Hebbel, RP, Mohandas, N, and Steinberg, MH. (1994). *Sickle cell disease: Basic principles and clinical practice*. New York: Lippincott-Raven.

Emmel, VE. (1917). A study of erythrocytes in a case of severe anemia with elongated and sickle-shaped red blood corpuscles. *Arch. Intern. Med.* 20: 586–599.

Espinoza, LR, Spilberg, I, and Osterland, CK. (1974). Joint manifestations of sickle cell disease. *Medicine* 53: 295–305.

Estacio, RO, Jeffers, BW, Hiatt, WR et al. (1998). The effect of nisoldipine as compared with enalapril on cardiovascular outcomes in patients with non-insulin dependent diabetes and hypertension. *N. Engl. J. Med.* 338: 645–652.

Falk, RJ and Jennette, JC. (1994). Renal disease. In Embury, SH, Hebbel, RP, Mohandas, N, and Steinberg, MH, editors. *Sickle cell disease: Basic principles and clinical practice*. New York: Raven-Lippincott.

Falk, RJ, Scheinman, J, Phillips, G et al. (1992). Prevalence and pathologic features of sickle cell nephropathy and response to inhibition of angiotensin-converting enzyme. *N. Engl. J. Med.* 326: 910–915.

Falletta, JM, Woods, GM, Verter, JI et al. (1995). Discontinuing penicillin prophylaxis in children with sickle cell anemia. *J. Pediatr.* 127: 685–690.

Festa, RS, and Asakura, T. (1979). The use of an oxygen dissociation curve analyzer in transfusion therapy. *Transfusion* 19: 107–113.

Ficat, R. (1985). Idiopathic bone necrosis of the femoral head. *J. Bone & Joint surg. Br.* 67: 3–9.

Fleming, AF. (1989). The presentation, management and prevention of crisis in sickle cell disease in Africa. *Blood Rev.* B(I):18–28.

Foucan, L, Bourhis, V, Bangou, J et al. (1998). A randomized trial of captopril for microalbuminuria in normotensive adults with sickle cell anemia. *Am. J. Med.* 104: 339–342.

Fowler, JE Jr, Koshy, M, Strub, M, and Chinn, SK. (1991). Priapism associated with the sickle cell hemoglobinopathies: Prevalence, natural history and sequelae. *J. Urol.* 145: 65–68.

Friedlander, AH, Genser, L, and Swerdloff, M. (1980). Mental nerve neuropathy: A complication of sickle-cell crisis. *Oral Surg.* 49: 15–17.

Gaston, MH, Verter, J, Woods, G et al. (1986). Prophylaxis with oral penicillin in children with sickle cell anemia. *N. Engl. J. Med.* 314: 1593–1599.

Gendrel, D, Kombila, M, Nardou, M et al. (1992). Malaria and hemoglobin S, interactions in African children. *Presse Med.* 21: 887–890.

Gill, FM, Sleeper, LA, Weiner, SJ et al. (1995). Clinical events in the first decade in a cohort of infants with sickle cell disease. *Blood* 86: 776–783.

Glader, BE. (1994) Anemia. In Embury, SH, Hebbel, RP, Mohandas, N, and Steinberg, MH, editors. *Sickle cell disease: Basic principles and clinical practice.* New York: Lippincott-Raven.

Gladwin, MT, Schechter, AN, Shelhammer, JH, and Ognibene, FP. (1999). The acute chest syndrome in sickle cell disease. Possible role of nitric oxide in its pathophysiology and treatment. *Am. J. Crit. Care Med.* 159: 1368–1376.

Gremse, DA, Fillingim, E, Hoff, CJ et al. (1998). Hepatic function as assessed by lidocaine metabolism in sickle cell disease. *J. Pediatr.* 132: 989–993.

Griffin, TC and Buchanan, GR. (1993). Elective surgery in children with sickle cell disease without preoperative blood transfusion. *J. Pediatr. Surg.* 28: 681–685.

Guasch, A, Cua, M, and Mitch, WE. (1996). Early detection and the course of glomerular injury in patients with sickle cell anemia. *Kidney Int.* 49: 786–791.

Guasch, A, Cua, M, You, W, and Mitch, WE. (1997). Sickle cell anemia causes a distinct pattern of glomerular dysfunction. *Kidney Int.* 51: 826–833.

Guasch, A, Zayas, CF, Eckman, JR et al. (1999). Evidence that microdeletions in the alpha globin gene protect against the development of sickle cell glomerulopathy in humans. *J. Am. Soc. Nephrol.* 10: 1014–1019.

Gueri, M and Serjeant, GR. (1970). Leg-ulcers in sickle cell anaemia. *Trop. Geogr. Med.* 22: 155–160.

Gupta, VL and Chaubey, BS. (1995). Efficacy of zinc therapy in prevention of crisis in sickle cell anemia: A double blind randomized controlled clinical trial. *J. Assoc. Physicians India* 43: 467–469.

Haberkern, CM, Neumayr, LD, Orringer, EP et al. (1997). Cholecystectomy in sickle cell anemia patients: Perioperative outcome of 364 cases from the national preoperative transfusion study. *Blood* 89: 1533–1542.

Hahn, EV and Gillespie, EB. (1927). Sickle cell anemia: Report of a case greatly improved by splenectomy. Experimental study of sickle cell formation. *Arch. Intern. Med.* 39: 233–254.

Haider, MZ, Ashebu, S, Aduh, P, and Adekile, AD. (1998). Influence of α-thalassemia on cholelithiasis in SS patients with elevated Hb F. *Acta Haematol.* 100: 147–150.

Hakim, LS, Hashmat, AI, and Macchia, RJ. (1994). Priapism. In Embury, SH, Hebbel, RP, Mohandas, N, Steinberg, MH, editors. *Sickle cell disease: Basic principles and clinical practice.* New York: Lippincott-Raven.

Halvorson, DJ, McKie, V, McKie, K et al. (1997). Sickle cell disease and tonsillectomy: Preoperative management and postoperative complications. *Arch. Otolaryngol. Head Neck Surg.* 123: 689–692.

Hasan, MF, Marsh, F, Posner, G et al. (1996). Chronic hepatitis C in patients with sickle cell disease. *Am. J. Gastroenterol.* 91: 1204–1206.

Hatton, CSR, Bunch, C, and Weatherall, DJ. (1985). Hepatic sequestration in sickle cell anaemia. *Br. Med. J.* 190: 744–745.

Head, CA, Brugnara, C, Martinez-Ruiz, R et al. (1997). Low concentrations of nitric oxide increase oxygen affinity of sickle erythrocytes in vitro and in vivo. *J. Clin. Invest.* 100: 1193–1198.

Hempe, JM and Craver, RD. (1994). Quantification of hemoglobin variants by capillary isoelectric focusing. *Clin. Chem.* 40: 2288–2295.

Herrick, JB. (1910). Peculiar elongated and sickle-shaped red blood corpuscles in a case of severe anemia. *Arch. Intern. Med.* 6: 517–521.

Hickman, JM and Lachiewicz, PF. (1997). Results and complications of total hip arthroplasties in patients with sickle-cell hemoglobinopathies: Role of cementless components. *J. Arthroplasty* 12: 420–425.

Hofstra, TC, Kalra, VK, Meiselman, HJ, and Coates, TD. (1996). Sickle erythrocytes adhere to polymorphonuclear neutrophils and activate the neutrophil respiratory burst. *Blood* 87: 4440–4447.

Hoppe, C, Trachtenberg, E, Klitz, W et al. (1999). HLA type as a predictor of stroke in children with sickle cell disease. *23nd Annual Meeting of the National Sickle Cell Disease Program, San Francisco.*

Houston, PE, Rana, S, Sekhsaria, S et al. (1997). Homocysteine in sickle cell disease, relationship to stroke. *Am. J. Med.* 103: 192–196.

Howard, RJ, Tuck, SM, and Pearson, TC. (1995). Pregnancy in sickle cell disease in the UK: Results of a multicentre survey of the effect of prophylactic blood transfusion on maternal and fetal outcome. *Br. J. Obstet. Gynaecol.* 102: 947–951.

Hurtig, AL and White, LS. (1989). Psychosocial adjustment in children and adolescents with sickle cell disease. *J. Pediatr. Psychol.* 11: 411–427.

Hurtig AL. (1989). Adjustment and coping in adolescents with sickle cell disease. *Ann. N. Y. Acad. Sci.* 565: 172–82.

Hurtig, AL, Koepke, D, and Park, KB. (1989). Relation between severity of chronic illness and adjustment in children and adolescents with sickle cell disease. *J. Pediatr. Psychol.* 14: 117–32.

Idowu, O and Hayes-Jordan, A. (1998). Partial splenectomy in children under 4 years of age with hemoglobinopathy. *J. Pediatr. Surg.* 33: 1251–1253.

Imbus, CE, Warner, J, Smith, E et al. (1978). Peripheral neuropathy in lead-intoxicated sickle cell patients. *Muscle Nerve* 1: 168–171.

Ingram, VM. (1956). A specific chemical difference between the globins of normal human and sickle-cell anaemia haemoglobin. *Nature* 178: 792–794.

James, TN, Riddick, L, and Massing, GK. (1994). Sickle cells and sudden death: Morphologic abnormalities of the cardiac conduction system. *J. Lab. Clin. Med.* 124: 507–520.

Jeng, M, Feusner, J, and Vichinksy, EP. (1999). Risk factors for central venous catheter infections in sickle cell disease. *23rd Annual Meeting of the National Sickle Cell Disease Program.*

Jenkins, ME, Scott, RB, and Baird, RL. (1960). Studies in sickle cell anemia. *J. Pediatr.* 56: 30–38.

Johnson, CS and Giorgio, AJ. (1981). Arterial blood pressure in adults with sickle cell disease. *Arch. Intern. Med.* 141: 891–893.

Johnson, CS, Omata, M, Tong, MJ et al. (1985). Liver involvement in sickle cell disease. *Medicine* 69: 833–837.

Johnston, RB Jr, Newman, SL, and Struth, AG. (1973). An abnormality of the alternate pathway of complement activation in sickle-cell disease. *N. Engl. J. Med.* 288: 803–808.

Kandeel, AY, Zimmerman, RA, and Ohene-Frempong, K. (1996). Comparison of magnetic resonance angiography and conventional angiography in sickle cell disease, clinical significance and reliability. *Neuroradiology* 38: 409–416.

Kassim, CS, Umans, H, Nagel, RL, and Fabry, ME. (in press). Megalophallus as a complication of priapism in sickle-cell anemia: Use of BOLD-MRI. *J. Urol.*

Kell, RS, Kliewer, W, Erickson, MT, and Ohene-Frempong, K. (1998). Psychological adjustment of adolescents with sickle cell disease, relations with demographic, medical, and family competence variables. *J. Pediatr. Psychol.* 23: 301–312.

Killic, S, Grubinic, S, Rayner, C et al. (1998). Sickle cell chronic lung disease: Lack of significant long-term lung damage following recurrent acute chest syndrome. *Blood* 92: 160a.

Kim, HC, Dugan, NP, Silber, JH et al. (1994). Erythrocytapheresis therapy to reduce iron overload in chronically transfused patients with sickle cell disease. *Blood* 83: 1136–1142.

King, SD, Dodd, RY, Haynes, G et al. (1995). Prevalence of antibodies to hepatitis C virus and other markers in Jamaica. *West Indian Med. J.* 44: 55–57.

Kinney, TR and Ware, RE. (1996). The adolescent with sickle cell anemia. *Hematol. Oncol. Clin. North Am.* 10: 1255–1264.

Kinney, TR, Sleeper, LA, Wang, WC et al. (1999). Silent cerebral infarcts in sickle cell anemia, a risk factor analysis. The Cooperative Study of Sickle Cell Disease. *Pediatrics* 103: 640–645.

Konotey-Ahulu, FID. (1974). The sickle cell disease: Clinical manifestations including the "sickle crisis." *Arch. Intern. Med.* 133: 611–619.

Kopp-Hoolihan, LE, van Loan, MD, Mentzer, WC, and Heyman, MB. (1999). Elevated resting energy expenditure in adolescents with sickle cell anemia. *J. Am. Diet. Assoc.* 99: 195–199.

Koshy, M and Burd, L. (1991). Management of pregnancy in sickle cell syndromes. *Hematol./Oncol. Clin. North Am.* 5: 585–596.

Koshy, M and Burd, L. (1994). Obstetric and gynecologic issues. In Embury, SH, Hebbel, RP, Mohandas, N, Steinberg, MH, editors. *Sickle cell disease: Basic principles and clinical practice.* New York: Lippincott-Raven.

Koshy, M, Burd, L, Wallace, D et al. (1988). Prophylactic red-cell transfusions in pregnant patients with sickle cell disease. A randomized cooperative study. *N. Engl. J. Med.* 319: 1447–1452.

Koshy, M, Entsuah, R, Koranda, A et al. (1989). Leg ulcers in patients with sickle cell disease. *Blood* 74: 1403–1408.

Koshy, M, Thomas, C, and Goodwin, J. (1990). Vascular lesions in the central nervous system in sickle cell disease (neuropathology). *J. Assoc. Acad. Minor. Phys.* 1: 71–78.

Koshy, M, Weiner, SJ, Miller, ST et al. (1995). Surgery and anesthesia in sickle cell disease. *Blood* 86: 3676–3684.

Koumbourlis, AC, Hurlet-Jensen, A, and Bye, MR. (1997). Lung function in infants with sickle cell disease. *Pediatr. Pulmonol.* 24: 277–281.

Krauss, JS, Freant, LJ, and Lee, JR. (1998). Gastrointestinal pathology in sickle cell disease. *Ann. Clin. Lab. Sci.* 28: 19–23.

Kutlar, F, Tural, C, Park, D et al. (1998). MTHFR (5, 10-methylenetetrahydrofolate reductase) 677 C→T mutation as a candidate risk factor for avascular necrosis (AVN) in patients with sickle cell disease. *Blood* 92: 695a.

Landefeld, CS, Schambelan, M, Kaplan, SL, and Embury, SH. (1983). Clomiphene-responsive hypogonadism in sickle cell anemia. *Ann. Intern. Med.* 99: 480–483.

Lane, PK, Embury, SH, and Toy, PT. (1988). Oxygen-induced marrow red cell hypoplasia leading to transfusion in sickle painful crisis. *Am. J. Hematol.* 27: 67–68.

Leight, L, Snider, TH, Clifford, GO, and Hellems, HK. (1954). Hemodynamic studies in sickle cell anemia. *Circulation* 10: 653–662.

Leikin, SL, Gallagher, D, Kinney, TR et al. (1989). Mortality in children and adolescents with sickle cell disease. Cooperative Study of Sickle Cell Disease. *Pediatrics* 84: 500–508.

Leonard, MB, Zemel, BS, Kawchak, DA et al. (1998). Plasma zinc status, growth, and maturation in children with sickle cell disease. *J. Pediatr.* 132: 467–471.

Leong, MA, Dampier, C, Varlotta, L, and Allen, JL. (1997). Airway hyperreactivity in children with sickle cell disease. *J. Pediatr.* 131: 278–283.

Lisbona, R, Derbekyan, V, and Novales-Diaz, JA. (1997). Scintigraphic evidence of pulmonary vascular occlusion in sickle cell disease. *J. Nucl. Med.* 38: 1151–1153.

Lowenthal, EA, Wells, A, Emanuel, PD et al. (1996). Sickle cell acute chest syndrome associated with parvovirus B19 infection, case series and review. *Am. J. Hematol.* 51: 207–213.

MacFarlane, DE, Baum, KF, and Serjeant, GR. (1986). Bacteriology of sickle cell leg ulcers. *Trans. R. Soci. Trop. Med. Hyg.* 80: 553–556.

Maddrey, WC, Cukier, JO, Maglalang, AC et al. (1978). Hepatic bilirubin UDP-glucuronyltransferase in patients with sickle cell anemia. *Gastroenterolgy* 74: 193–195.

Magnus, SA, Hambleton, IR, Moosdeen, F, and Serjeant, GR. (1999). Recurrent infections in homozygous sickle cell disease. *Arch. Dis. Child.* 80: 537–541.

Malekgoudarzi, B and Feffer, S. (1999). Myonecrosis in sickle cell anemia. *N. Engl. J. Med.* 340: 483–483.

Mallouh, AA and Asha, M. (1988). Beneficial effect of blood transfusion in children with sickle cell chest syndrome. *Am. J. Dis. Child.* 142: 178–182.

Mallouh, AA and Qudah, A. (1993). Acute splenic sequestration together with aplastic crisis caused by human parvovirus BI 9 in patients with sickle cell disease. *J. Pediatr.* 122: 593–595.

Mangi, MH, Craske, E, Jones, D, and Newland, C. (1998). Incidence of staphylococcal aureus antibodies in resistant chronic sickle cell leg ulcers: Response to antibiotics and role of topical GM-CSF and iodosorb dressing in non-infected patients. *Blood* 92: 527a.

Mankin, H. (1992). Nontraumatic necrosis of bone (osteonecrosis). *N. Engl. J. Med.* 326: 1473–1479.

Martin, CR, Johnson, CS, Cobb, C et al. (1996). Myocardial infarction in sickle cell disease. *J. Natl. Med. Assoc.* 88: 428–432.

Mason, VR. (1922). Sickle cell anemia. *JAMA* 79: 1318–1320.

Miller, ST. (1999). Prediction of clinical severity in children with sickle cell disease: A report from the Cooperative Study (CSSCD). *23rd Annual Meeting of the National Sickle Cell Disease Program.*

Miller, ST, Hammerschlag, MR, Chirgwin, K et al. (1991). Role of *Chlamydia pneumoniae* in acute chest syndrome of sickle cell disease. *J. Pediatr.* 118: 30–33.

Miller, ST, Rao, SP, Dunn, EK, and Glassberg, KI. (1995). Priapism in children with sickle cell disease. *J. Urol.* 154: 844–847.

Milner, PF, Jones, BR, and Dobler, J. (1980). Outcome of pregnancy in sickle cell anemia and sickle cell-hemoglobin C disease. *Am. J. Obstet. Gynecol.* 138: 239–245.

Milner, PF, Kraus, AP, Sebes, JI et al. (1991). Sickle cell disease as a cause of osteonecrosis of the femoral head. *N. Engl. J. Med.* 325: 1476–1481.

Milner, PF, Kraus, AP, Sebes, JI et al. (1993). Osteonecrosis of the humeral head in sickle cell disease. *Clin. Orthop.* 289: 136–143.

Milner, PF, Joe, C, and Burke, GJ, (1994). Bone and joint disease. In Embury, SH, Hebbel, RP, Mohandas, N, and Steinberg, MH, editors. *Sickle cell disease: Basic principles and clinical practice.* New York: Lippincott-Raven.

Modebe, O and Ifenu, SA. (1993). Growth retardation in homozygous sickle cell disease, role of calorie intake and possible gender-related differences. *Am. J. Hematol.* 44: 149–154.

Mohammed, S, Addae, S, Suleiman, S et al. (1993). Serum calcium, parathyroid hormone, and vitamin D status in children and young adults with sickle cell disease. *Ann. Clin. Biochem.* 30: 45–51.

Mollapour, E, Porter, JB, Kaczmarski, R et al. (1998). Raised neutrophil phospholipase A_2 activity and defective priming of NADPH oxidase and phospholipase A_2 in sickle cell disease. *Blood* 91: 3423–3429.

Monga, M, Broderick, GA, and Hellstrom, WJG. (1996). Priapism in sickle cell disease: The case for early implantation of the penile prosthesis. *Eur. Urol.* 30: 54–59.

Mont, MA, Carbone, JJ, and Fairbank, AC. (1996). Core decompression versus nonoperative management for osteonecrosis of the hip. *Clin. Orthop. Relat. Res.* 324: 169–178.

Montgomery, R, Zibari, G, Hill, GS, and Ratner, LE. (1994). Renal transplantation in patients with sickle cell nephropathy. *Transplantation* 58: 618–620.

Morgan, SA and Jackson, J. (1986). Psychological and social concomitants of sickle cell anemia in adolescents. *J. Pediatr. Psychol.* 11: 429–440.

Morris, JS, Dunn, DT, Poddar, D, and Serjeant, GR. (1994). Haematological risk factors for pregnancy outcome in Jamaican women with homozygous sickle cell disease. *Br. J. Obstet. Gynaecol.* 101: 770–773.

Morrison, JC, Morrison, FS, Floyd, RC et al. (1991). Use of continuous flow erythrocytapheresis in pregnant patients with sickle cell disease. *J. Clin. Apheresis* 6: 224–229.

Moser, FG, Miller, ST, Bello, JA et al. (1996). The spectrum of brain MR abnormalities in sickle-cell disease, a report from the Cooperative Study of Sickle Cell Disease. *AJNR Am. J. Neuroradiol.* 17: 965–972.

Neel, JV. (1951). The inheritance of the sickling phenomenon with particular reference to sickle cell disease. *Blood* 6: 389–412.

Norris, CF, Mahannah, SR, Smith-Whitley, K et al. (1996). Pneumococcal colonization in children with sickle cell disease. *J. Pediatr.* 129: 821–827.

Nouri, A, de Montalembert, M, Revillon, Y, and Girot, R. (1991). Partial splenectomy in sickle cell syndromes. *Arch. Dis. Child.* 66: 1070–1072.

Ofosu, MD, Castro, O, and Alarif, L. (1987). Sickle cell leg ulcers are associated with HLA-B35 and Cw4. *Arch. Dermatol.* 123: 482–484.

Ohene-Frempong, K. (1991). Stroke in sickle cell disease, demographic, clinical, and therapeutic considerations. *Semin. Hematol.* 28: 213–219.

Ohene-Frempong, K and Nkrumah, FK. (1994). Sickle cell disease in Africa. In Embury, SH, Hubbel, RP, Mohandas, N, and Steinberg, MH, editors. *Sickle cell disease: Basic principles and clinical practice.* New York: Lippincott-Raven.

Ohene-Frempong, K, Weiner, SJ, Sleeper, LA et al. (1998). Cerebrovascular accidents in sickle cell disease, rates and risk factors. *Blood* 91: 288–294.

Ojo, AO, Govaerts, TC, Schmouder, RL et al. (1999). Renal transplantation in end-stage sickle cell nephropathy. *Transplantation* 67: 291–295.

Orringer, EP, Fowler, VG, Jr, Owens, CM et al. (1991). Case report, splenic infarction and acute splenic sequestration in adults with hemoglobin SC disease. *Am. J. Med. Sci.* 302: 374–379.

Osegbe, DN and Akinyanju, OO. (1987). Testicular dysfunction in men with sickle cell disease. *Postgrad. Med. J.* 63: 95–98.

Osei, SY, Ahima, RS, Fabry, ME et al. (1996). Immuno-histochemical localization of hepatic nitric oxide synthase in normal and transgenic sickle cell mice: The effect of hypoxia. *Blood* 88: 3583–3588.

Overby, MC and Rothman, AS. (1995). Multiple intracranial aneurysms in sickle cell anemia. Report of two cases. *J. Neurosurg.* 62: 430–434.

Overturf, GD. (1999). Infections and immunizations of children with sickle cell disease. *Adv. Pediatr. Infect. Dis.* 14: 191–218.

Overturf, GD, Powars, D, and Baraff, LJ. (1977). Bacterial meningitis and septicemia in sickle cell disease. *Am. J. Dis. Child.* 131: 784–787.

Oyedeji, GA. (1991). The health, growth and educational performance of sickle cell disease children. *East Afr. Med. J.* 68: 181–189.

Oyedeji, GA. (1995). Delayed sexual maturation in sickle cell anaemia patients—observations in one practice. *Ann. Trop. Paediatr.* 15: 197–201.

Oyesiku, NM, Barrow, DL, Eckman, JR et al. (1991). Intracranial aneurysms in sickle-cell anemia, clinical features and pathogenesis. *J. Neurosurg.* 75: 356–363.

Pappo, A and Buchanan, GR. (1989). Acute splenic sequestration in a 2-month-old infant with sickle cell anemia. *Pediatrics* 84: 578–579.

Parshad, O, Stevens, MC, Hudson, C et al. (1989). Abnormal thyroid hormone and thyrotropin levels in homozygous sickle cell disease. *Clin. Lab. Haematol.* 11: 309–315.

Pattison, JR, Jones, SE, Hodgson, J et al. (1981). Parvovirus infections and hypoplastic crisis in sickle-cell anaemia. *Lancet* 1: 664–665.

Pauling, L, Itano, H, Singer, SJ, and Wells, IC. (1949). Sickle cell anemia: A molecular disease. *Science* 110: 543–548.

Pavlakis, SG, Bello, J, Prohovnik, 1 et al. (1988). Brain infarction in sickle cell anemia, magnetic resonance imaging correlates. *Ann. Neurol.* 23: 125–130.

Pavlakis, SG, Prohovnik, I, Piomelli, S, and DeVivo, DC. (1989). Neurologic complications of sickle cell disease. *Adv. Pediatr.* 36: 247–276.

Peachey, RD. (1978). Leg ulceration and haemolytic anaemia: An hypothesis. *Br. J. Dermatol.* 98: 245–249.

Pearson, HA, Spencer, RP, and Cornelius, EA. (1969). Functional asplenia in sickle-cell anemia. *N. Engl. J. Med.* 281: 923–926.

Pearson, HA, McIntosh, S, Ritchey, AK et al. (1979). Developmental aspects of splenic function in sickle cell diseases. *Blood* 53: 358–65.

Pearson, HA, Gallagher, D, Chilcote, R et al. (1985). Developmental pattern of splenic dysfunction in sickle cell disorders. *Pediatrics* 76: 392–397.

Pegelow, CH, Adams, RJ, McKie, V et al. (1995). Risk of recurrent stroke in patients with sickle cell disease treated with erythrocyte transfusions. *J. Pediatr.* 126: 896–899.

Pegelow, CH, Colangelo, L, Steinberg, M et al. (1997). Natural history of blood pressure in sickle cell disease: Risks for stroke and death associated with relative hypertension in sickle cell anemia. *Am. J. Med.* 102: 171–177.

Phillips, G Jr, Becker, B, Keller, VA, and Hartman, J 4th. (1992). Hypothyroidism in adults with sickle cell anemia. *Am. J. Med.* 92: 567–570.

Phillips, G Jr, Eckmam, JR, and Hebbel, RP. (1994). Leg ulcers and myofascial syndromes. In Embury, SH, Hebbel, RP, Mohandas, N, and Steinberg, MH, editors. *Sickle cell disease: Basic principles and clinical practice.* New York: Lippincott-Raven.

Pieters, RC, Rojer, RA, Saleh, AW et al. (1995). Molgramostim to treat SS-sickle cell leg ulcers. *Lancet* 345: 528.

Platt, OS, Rosenstock, W, and Espeland, MA. (1984). Influence of sickle hemoglobinopathies on growth and development. *N. Engl. J. Med.* 311: 7–12.

Platt, OS, Thorington, BD, Brambilla, DJ et al. (1991). Pain in sickle cell disease-rates and risk factors. *N. Engl. J. Med.* 325: 11–16.

Platt, OS, Brambilla, DJ, Rosse, WF et al. (1994). Mortality in sickle cell disease: Life expectancy and risk factors for early death. *N. Engl. J. Med.* 330: 1639–1644.

Poncz, M, Kane, E, and Gill, FM. (1985). Acute chest syndrome in sickle cell disease, etiology and clinical correlates. *J. Pediatr.* 107: 861–866.

Powars, DR. (1975). Natural history of sickle cell disease—the first ten years. *Semin. Hematol.* 12: 267–285.

Powars, DR and Johnson, CS. (1996). Priapism. *Hematol./Oncol. Clin. North Am.* 10: 1363–1372.

Powars, D, Wilson, B, Imbus, C et al. (1978). The natural history of stroke in sickle cell disease. *Am. J. Med.* 65: 461–471.

Powars, D, Weidman, JA, Odom-Maryon, T et al. (1988). Sickle cell chronic lung disease: Prior morbidity and the risk of pulmonary failure. *Medicine (Baltimore)* 67: 66–76.

Powars, D, Adams, RJ, Nichols, FT et al. (1990). Delayed intracranial hemorrhage following cerebral infarction in sickle cell anemia. *J. Assoc. Acad. Minor. Phys.* 1: 79–82.

Powars, DR, Elliott Mills, DD, and Chan, L. (1991). Chronic renal failure in sickle cell disease: Risk factors, clinical course, and mortality. *Ann. Intern. Med.* 115: 614–620.

Powars, DR, Sandhu, M, Nilland-Weiss, J et al. (1986). Pregnancy in sickle cell disease. *Obstet. Gynecol.* 67: 217–228.

Powars, DR, Conti, PS, Wong, WY et al. (1999). Cerebral vasculopathy in sickle cell anemia: Diagnostic contribution of positron emission tomography. *Blood* 93: 71–79.

Powell, RW, Levine, GL, Yang, YM, and Mankad, VN. (1992). Acute splenic sequestration crisis in sickle cell disease, early detection and treatment. *J. Pediatr. Surg.* 27: 215–218.

Prasad, AS, Schoomaker, EB, Ortega, J et al. (1975). Zinc deficiency in sickle cell disease. *Clin. Chem.* 21: 582–587.

Prasad, AS, Beck, FWJ, Kaplan, J et al. (1999). Effect of zinc supplementation on incidence of infections and hospital admissions in sickle cell disease (SCD). *Am. J. Hematol.* 61: 194–202.

Rackoff, WR, Kunkel, N, Silber, JH et al. (1993). Pulse oximetry and factors associated with hemoglobin oxygen desaturation in children with sickle cell disease. *Blood* 81: 3422–3427.

Ramos, CE, Park, JS, Ritchey, ML, and Benson, GS. (1995). High flow priapism associated with sickle cell disease. *J. Urol.* 153: 1619–1621.

Ranney, HM. (1994). Historical milestones. In Embury, SH, Hebbel, RP, Mohandas, N, and Steinberg, MH, editors. *Sickle cell disease: Basic principles and clinical practice.* New York: Lippincott-Raven.

Ranney, HM. (1997). P_{sickle}, the temporary leaky link between sickling and cellular dehydration. *J. Clin. Invest.* 99: 2559–2560.

Rao, SP, Miller, ST, and Cohen, BJ. (1992). Transient aplastic crisis in patients with sickle cell disease, BI 9 parvovirus studies during a 7-year period. *Am. J. Dis. Child.* 146: 1328–1330.

Reed, W, Jagust, W, Al-Mateen, M, and Vichinsky, E. (1999). Role of positron emission tomography in determining the extent of CNS ischemia in patients with sickle cell disease. *Am. J. Hematol.* 60: 268–272.

Robinson, AR, Robson, M, Harrison, AP, and Zuelzer, WW. (1957). A new technique for differentiation of hemoglobin. *J. Lab. Clin. Med.* 50: 745–752.

Robinson, MG and Watson, RJ. (1966). Pneumococcal meningitis in sickle-cell anemia. *N. Engl. J. Med.* 274: 1006–1008.

Rodgers, GP, Walker, EC, and Podgor, MJ. (1993). Is "relative" hypertension a risk factor for vaso-occlusive complications in sickle cell disease? *Am. J. Med. Sci.* 305: 150–156.

Rodriguez-Cortes, HM, Griener, JC, Hyland, K et al. (1999). Plasma homocysteine levels and folate status in children with sickle cell anemia. *J. Pediatr. Hematol. Oncol.* 21: 219–223.

Rogers, DW, Vaidya, S, and Serjeant, GR. (1978). Early splenomegaly in homozygous sickle-cell disease. An indicator of susceptibility to infection. *Lancet* 2: 963–965.

Rogers, DW, Serjeant, BE, and Serjeant, GR. (1982). Early rise in the "pitted" red cell count as a guide to susceptibility to infection in childhood sickle cell anaemia. *Arch. Dis. Child.* 57: 338–342.

Rogers, ZR, Morrison, RA, Vedro, DA, and Buchanan, GR. (1990). Outpatient management of febrile illness in infants and young children with sickle cell anemia. *J. Pediatr.* 117: 736–739.

Romero Mestre, JC, Hernandez, A, Agramonte, O, and Hernandez, P. (199). Cardiovascular autonomic dysfunction in sickle cell anemia: a possible risk factor for sudden death? *Clin. Auton. Res.* 7: 121–125.

Rosse, WF, Telen, M, and Ware, RE. (1998). *Transfusion support for patients with sickle cell disease* Bethesda: AABB Press.

Rothman, SM, Fulling, KH, and Nelson, JS. (1986). Sickle cell anemia and central nervous system infarction, a neuropathological study. *Ann. Neurol.* 20: 684–690.

Rucknagel, DL, Hanash, SH, Sing, CF et al. (1979). Age and sex effects on hemoglobin F in sickle cell anemia. In Stamatoyannopoulos, G and Nienhuis, AW, editors. *Cellular and molecular regulation of hemoglobin switching.* New York: Grune & Stratton.

Rucknagel, DL, Kalinyak, KA, and Gelfand, MJ. (1991). Rib infarcts and acute chest syndrome in sickle cell diseases. *Lancet,* 337: 831–833.

Ruggenenti, P, Perna, A, Gherardi, G et al. (1999). Renoprotective properties of ACE-inhibition in non-diabetic nephropathies with non-nephrotic proteinuria. *Lancet* 354: 359–364.

Russell, MO, Goldberg, HI, Hodson, A et al. (1984). Effect of transfusion therapy on arteriographic abnormalities and on recurrence of stroke in sickle cell disease. *Blood* 63: 162–169.

Saad, ST and Saad, MJ. (1992). Normal cortisol secretion in sickle cell anemia. *Trop. Geogr. Med.* 44: 86–88.

Sadat-Ali, M. (1998). The status of acute osteomyelitis in sickle cell disease. A 15-year review. *Int. Surg.* 83: 84–87.

Salman, EK, Haymond, MW, Bayne, E et al. (1996). Protein and energy metabolism in prepubertal children with sickle cell anemia. *Pediatr. Res.* 40: 34–40.

Sampietro, M, Lupica, L, Perrero, L et al. (1997). The expression of uridine diphosphate glucuronosyltransferase gene is a major determinant of bilirubin level in heterozygous β-thalassaemia and in glucose-6-phosphate dehydrogenase deficiency. *Br. J. Haematol.* 99: 437–439.

Savitt TL and Goldberg, MF. (1989). Herrick's 1910 case report of sickle cell anmia: The rest of the story. *JAMA* 261: 266–271.

Schedlbauer, LM and Pass, KA. (1989). Cellulose acetate/citrate agar electrophoresis of filter paper hemolysates from heel stick. *Pediatrics* 83: 839–842.

Schmidt, RM, Brosious, EM, and Holland, S. (1974). Quantitation of fetal hemoglobin by densitometry. *J. Lab. Clin. Med.* 84: 740–745.

Schmidt, RM, Rucknagel, DL, and Necheles, TF. (1975). Comparison of methodologies for thalassemia screening by Hb A2 quantitation. *J. Lab. Clin. Med.* 86: 873–882.

Scott-Conner, CEH and Brunson, CD. (1994a). Surgery and anesthesia. In Embury, SH, Hebbel, RP, Mohandas, N, and Steinberg, MH, editors. *Sickle cell disease: Basic principles and clinical practice.* New York: Lippincott-Raven.

Scott-Conner, CEH and Brunson, CD. (1994b). The pathophysiology of the sickle hemoglobinopathies and implications for perioperative management. *Am. J. Surg.* 168: 268–274.

Sears, DA and Udden, MM. (1985). Splenic infarction, splenic sequestration, and functional hyposplenism in hemoglobin S-C disease. *Am. J. Hematol.* 18: 261–268.

Seeler, RA and Shwiaki, MZ. (1972). Acute splenic sequestration crises (ASSC) in young children with sickle cell anemia. Clinical observations in 20 episodes in 14 children. *Clin. Pediatr. (Phila)* 11: 701–704.

Seeler, RA, Royal, JE, Powe, L, and Goldberg, HR. (1978). Moya-moya in children with sickle cell anemia and cerebrovascular occlusion. *J. Pediatr.* 93: 808–810.

Serjeant, GR. (1983). Sickle cell hemoglobin and pregnancy. *Br. Med. J.* 287: 628–630.

Serjeant, GR. (1992). *Sickle cell disease.* Oxford: Oxford Medical Publications.

Serjeant, GR, DeCeulaer, K, and Maude, GH. (1985). Stilboestrol and stuttering priapism in homozygous sickle cell disease. *Lancet* 2: 1274–1276.

Serjeant, GR, Serjeant, BE, and Condon, PI. (1972). The conjuctival sign in sickle cell anemia. A relationship with irreversibly sickled cells. *JAMA* 219: 1428–1431.

Serjeant, GR, Topley, JM, Mason, K et al. (1981a). Outbreak of aplastic crises in sickle cell anaemia associated with parvovirus-like agent. *Lancet* 2: 595–597.

Serjeant, GR, Grandison, Y, Lowrie, Y et al. (1981b). The development of haematological changes in homozygous sickle cell disease, a cohort study from birth to 6 years. *Br. Haematol.* 48: 533–543.

Serjeant, GR, Serjeant, BE, Thomas, PW et al. (1993). Human parvovirus infection in homozygous sickle cell disease. *Lancet* 15: 1237–1240.

Serjeant, BE, Harris, J, Thomas, P, and Serjeant, GR. (1997). Propionyl-L-carnitine in chronic leg ulcers of homozygous sickle cell disease: A pilot study. *J. Am. Acad. Dermatol.* 37: 491–493.

Shao, SH and Orringer, EP. (1995). Sickle cell intrahepatic cholestasis: Approach to a difficult problem. *Am. J. Gastroenterol.* 90: 2048–2050.

Sharpsteen, JR Jr, Powars, D, Johnson, C et al. (1993). Multisystem damage associated with tricorporal priapism in sickle cell disease. *Am. J. Med.* 94: 289–295.

Sher, GD and Olivieri, NF. (1994). Rapid healing of chronic leg ulcers during arginine butyrate therapy in patients with sickle cell disease and thalassemia. *Blood* 84: 2378–2380.

Sherwood, JB, Goldwasser, E, Chilcote, R et al. (1986). Sickle cell anemia patients have low erythropoietin levels for their degree of anemia. *Blood* 67: 46–49.

Shields, RW Jr, Harris, JW, and Clark, M. (1991). Mononeuropathy in sickle cell anemia: Anatomical and pathophysiological basis for its rarity. *Muscle Nerve* 14: 370–374.

Shurafa, MS, Prasad, AS, Rucknagel, DL, and Kan, YW. (1982). Long survival in sickle cell anemia. *Am. J. Hematol.* 12: 357–365.

Singer, K, Motulsky, AG, and Wile, SA. (1950). Aplastic crisis in sickle cell anemia. *J. Lab. Clin. Med.* 33: 721–736.

Singhal, A, Davies, P, Sahota, A et al. (1993). Resting metabolic rate in homozygous sickle cell disease. *Am. J. Clin. Nutr.* 57: 32–34.

Singhal, A, Thomas, P, Cook, R et al. (1994). Delayed adolescent growth in homozygous sickle cell disease. *Arch. Dis. Child.* 71: 404–408.

Singhal, A, Davies, P, Wierenga, KJ et al. (1997). Is there an energy deficiency in homozygous sickle cell disease? *Am. J. Clin. Nutr.* 66: 386–390.

Sklar, AH, Perez, JC, Harp, RJ, and Caruana, RJ. (1990a). Acute renal failure in sickle cell anemia. *Int. J. Artif. Organs* 13: 347–351.

Sklar, AH, Campbell, H, Caruana, RJ et al. (1990b). A population study of renal function in sickle cell anemia. *Int. J. Artif. Organs* 13: 231–236.

Smith, JA, Espeland, M, Bellevue, R et al. (1996). Pregnancy in sickle cell disease: Experience of the cooperative study of sickle cell disease. *Obstet. Gynecol.* 87: 199–204.

Smits, HL, Oski, FA, and Brody, JI. (1969). The hemolytic crisis of sickle cell disease, the role of glucose-6-phosphate dehydrogenase deficiency. *J. Pediatr.* 74: 544–551.

Solanki, DL, Kietter, GG, and Castro, O. (1986). Acute splenic sequestration crises in adults with sickle cell disease. *Am. J. Med.* 80: 985–990.

Soliman, AT, Bassiouny, MR, and Elbanna, NA. (1995). Study of hepatic functions and prevalence of hepatitis-B surface antigenaemia in Omani children with sickle cell disease. *J. Trop. Pediatr.* 41: 174–176.

Soliman, AT, el Banna, N, al Salmi, I et al. (1997). Growth hormone secretion and circulating insulin-like growth factor-I (IGF-I) and IGF binding protein-3 concentrations in children with sickle cell disease. *Metabolism* 46: 1241–1245.

Stein, RE and Urbaniak, J. (1980). Use of the tourniquet during surgery in patients with sickle cell hemoglobinpathies. *Clin. Orthop.* 151: 231–233.

Steinberg, MH. (1991). Erythropoietin in anemia of renal failure in sickle cell disease. *N. Engl. J. Med.* 324: 1369–1370.

Steinberg, MH. (1999). Pathophysiology of sickle cell disease. *Bailliere's clinical haematology* 11: 163–184.

Steinberg, MH, Rosenstock, W, Coleman, MB et al. (1984). Effects of thalassemia and microcytosis upon the hematological and vaso-occlusive severity of sickle cell anemia. *Blood* 63: 1353–1360.

Steinberg, MH, West, MS, Gallagher, D et al. (1988). Effects of glucose-6-phosphate dehydrogenase deficiency upon sickle cell anemia. *Blood* 71: 749–752.

Steinberg, MH, Ballas, SK, Brunson, CY, and Bookchin, R. (1995). Sickle cell anemia in septuagenarians. *Blood* 86: 3997–3998.

Steinberg, MH, Castro, O, Ballas, SK et al. (1998). The multicenter study of hydroxyurea in sickle cell anemia (MSH): Mortality at 5–6 years. *Blood* 92: 496a.

Stevens, MC, Padwick, M, and Serjeant, GR. (1981a). Observations on the natural history of dactylitis in homozygous sickle cell disease. *Clin. Pediatr. (Phila.)* 20: 311–317.

Stevens, MC, Hayes, RJ, Vaidya, S, and Serjeant, GR. (1981b). Fetal hemoglobin and clinical severity of homozygous sickle cell disease in early childhood. *J. Pediatr.* 98: 37–41.

Styles, LA and Vichinsky, EP. (1996). Core decompression in avascular necrosis of the hip in sickle-cell disease. *Am. J. Hematol.* 52: 103–107.

Styles, LA, Schalkwijk, CG, Aarsman, AJ et al. (1996a). Phospholipase A2 levels in acute chest syndrome of sickle cell disease. *Blood* 87: 25738.

Svarch, E, Vilorio, P, Nordet, I et al. (1996). Partial splenectomy in children with sickle cell disease and repeated episodes of splenic sequestration. *Hemoglobin* 20: 393–400.

Svarch, E, Nordet, I, and Gonzalez, A. (1999). Overwhelming septicaemia in a patient with sickle cell/beta(O) thalassaemia and partial splenectomy. *Br. J. Haematol.* 104: 930.

Tan, GB, Aw, TC, Dunstan, RA, and Lee, SH. (1993). Evaluation of high performance liquid chromatography for routine estimation of haemoglobins A$_2$ and F. *J. Clin. Pathol.* 46: 852–856.

Tang, DC, Prauner, R, Liu, W et al. (1999). The angiotensin gene GT repeat is associated with strokes in pediatric patients with sickle cell anemia. *23rd Annual Meeting of the National Sickle Cell Disease Program, San Francisco.*

Tarry, WF, Duckett, JW Jr, and Snyder, HMI. (1987). Urological complications of sickle cell disease in a pediatric population. *J. Urol.* 138: 592–594.

Telfair, J, Myers, J, and Drezner, S. (1994). Transfer as a component of the transition of adolescents with sickle cell disease to adult care, adolescent, adult, and parent perspectives. *J. Adolesc. Health* 15: 558–565.

Topley, JM, Rogers, DW, Stevens, MC, and Serjeant, GR. (1981). Acute splenic sequestration and hypersplenism in the first five years in homozygous sickle cell disease. *Arch. Dis. Child.* 56: 765–769.

Treadwell, MJ and Gil, KM. (1994). Psychosocial aspects. In Embury, SH, Hebbel, RP, Mohandas, N, and Steinberg, MH, editors. *Sickle cell disease: Basic principles and clinical practice.* New York: Lippincott-Raven.

Urbaniak, JR and Jones Jr, JP, editors. (1997). *Osteonecrosis: Etiology, diagnosis, and treatment.* Rosemont, IL: American Orthopaedic Association.

van der Dijs, FP, van der Klis, FR, Muskiet, FD, and Muskiet, FA. (1997). Serum calcium and vitamin D status of patients with sickle cell disease in Curacao. *Ann. Clin. Biochem.* 34: 70–72.

van der Dijs, FPL, Schnog, JJB, Brouwer, DAJ et al. (1998). Elevated homocysteine levels indicate suboptimal folate status in pediatric sickle cell patients. *Am. J. Hematol.* 59: 192–198.

van Wijgerden, JA. (1983). Clinical expression of sickle cell anemia in the newborn. *South Med. J.* 76: 477–480.

Vernacchio, L, Neufeld, EJ, MacDonald, K et al. (1998). Combined schedule of 7-valent pneumococcal conjugate vaccine followed by 23-valent pneumococcal vaccine in children and young adults with sickle cell disease. *J. Pediatr.* 133: 275–278.

Vichinsky, E, Williams, R, Das, M et al. (1994). Pulmonary fat embolism: A distinct cause of severe acute chest syndrome in sickle cell anemia. *Blood* 83: 3107–3112.

Vichinsky, EP, Haberkern, CM, Neumayr, L et al. (1995). A comparison of conservative and aggressive transfusion regimens in the perioperative management of sickle cell disease. *N. Engl. J. Med.* 333: 206–213.

Vichinsky, EP, Styles, LA, Colangelo, LH et al. (1997). Acute chest syndrome in sickle cell disease: Clinical presentation and course. *Blood* 89: 1787–1792.

Vipond, AJ and Caldicott, LD. (1998). Major vascular surgery in a patient with sickle cell disease. *Anaesthesia* 53: 1204–1206.

Virag, R, Bachir, D, Lee, K, and Galacteros, F. (1996). Preventive treatment of priapism in sickle cell disease with oral and self-administered intracavernous injection of etilefrine. *Urology* 47: 777–781.

Virag, R, Bachir, D, Floresco, J et al. (1997). Ambulatory treatment and prevention of priapism using alpha-agonists apropos of 172 cases. *Chirurgie* 121: 648–652.

Vichinsky, EP, Neumayr, LD, Earles, AN et al. (2000). Causes and outcomes of the acute chest syndrome in sickle cell disease. *N. Engl. J. Med.* 342: 1855–1865.

Voskaridou, E, Kyrtsonis, MC, Loutradi-Anagnostou, A, and Loukopoulos, D. (1999). Healing of chronic leg ulcers in the hemoglobinopathies with perilesional injections of granulocyte-macrophage colony-stimulating factor. *Blood* 93: 3568–3569.

Walco, GA and Dampier, CD. (1987). Chronic pain in adolescent patients. *J. Pediatr. Psychol.* 12: 215–225.

Waldron, P, Pegelow, C, Neumayr, L et al. (1999). Tonsillectomy, adenoidectomy, and myringotomy in sickle cell disease: Perioperative morbidity. Preoperative Transfusion in Sickle Cell Disease Study Group. *J. Pediatr. Hematol. Oncol.* 21: 129–135.

Walker, TM, Beardsall, K, Thomas, PW, and Serjeant, GR. (1996). Renal length in sickle cell disease: Observations from a cohort study. *Clin. Nephrol.* 46: 384–388.

Wang, WC, Kovnar, EH, Tonkin, IL et al. (1991). High risk of recurrent stroke after discontinuance of five to twelve years of transfusion therapy in patients with sickle cell disease. *J. Pediatr.* 118: 377–382.

Wang, WC, Langston, JW, Steen, RG et al. (1998). Abnormalities of the central nervous system in very young children with sickle cell anemia. *J. Pediatr.* 132: 994–998.

Ware, RE, Zimmerman, SA, O'Branski, EE, and Schultz, WH. (1999). Hydroxyurea as an alternative to blood transfusions for the prevention of recurrent stroke in children with sickle cell disease. *23rd Annual meeting of the National Sickle Cell Disease Program.*

Ware, RE, Steinberg, MH, and Kinney, TR. (1995). Hydroxyurea: An alternative to transfusion therapy for stroke in sickle cell anemia. *Am. J. Hematol.* 50: 140–143.

Warth, JA, Prasad, AS, Zwas, F, and Franke, U. (1981). Abnormal dark adaptation in sickle cell anemia. *J. Labor. Clin. Med.* 98: 189–194.

Washington, E and Root, L. (1985). Conservative treatment of sickle cell avascular necrosis of the femoral head. *J. Pediatr. Orthop.* 5: 192–194.

Wayne, AS, Kevy, SV, and Nathan, DG. (1993). Transfusion management of sickle cell disease. *Blood* 81: 1109–1123.

West, MS, Wethers, D, Smith, J et al. (1992). Laboratory profile of sickle cell disease: A cross-sectional analysis. *J. Clin. Epidemiol.* 45: 893–909.

Wethers, DL, Ramirez, GM, Koshy, M et al. (1994). Accelerated healing of chronic sickle-cell leg ulcers treated with RGD peptide matrix. *Blood* 84: 1775–1779.

Wierenga, KJJ, Hambleton, I, Lewis, N et al. (1999). Life expectancy and risk factors for early death in Jamaican patients with homozygous sickle cell disease. *23rd Annual meeting of the National Sickle Cell Disease Program.*

Wilimas, JA, Flynn, PM, Harris, S et al. (1993). A randomized study of outpatient treatment with ceftriaxone for selected febrile children with sickle cell disease. *N. Engl. J. Med.* 329: 472–476.

Wilimas, J, Goff, JR, Anderson, HR Jr, and Langston, JW. (1980). Efficacy of transfusion therapy for one to two years in patients with sickle cell disease and cerebrovascular accidents. *J. Pediatr.* 96: 205–208.

Williams-Murphy, M, Thorneycroft, I, Little, F, and Hoff, C. (1999). Pregnancy outcome in women with sickle-cell disease in Mobile, Alabama. *J. Invest. Med.* 47: 123a.

Wiznitzer, M, Ruggieri, PM, Masaryk, TJ et al. (1990). Diagnosis of cerebrovascular disease in sickle cell anemia by magnetic resonance angiography. *J. Pediatr.* 117: 551–555.

Wong, WY, Overturf, GD, and Powars, DR. (1992). Infection caused by *Streptococcus pneumoniae* in children with sickle cell disease, epidemiology, immunologic mechanisms, prophylaxis, and vaccination. *Clin. Infect. Dis.* 14: 1124–1136.

Woods, GM, Jorgensen, JH, Waclawiw, MA et al. (1997). Influence of penicillin prophylaxis on antimicrobial resistance in nasopharyngeal *S. pneumoniae* among children with sickle cell anemia. The Ancillary Nasopharyngeal Culture Study of Prophylactic Penicillin Study 11. *J. Pediatr. Hematol. Oncol.* 19: 327–333.

Wright, J, Thomas, P, and Serjeant, GR. (1997a). Septicemia caused by *Salmonella* infection, an overlooked complication of sickle cell disease. *J. Pediatr.* 130: 394–399.

Wright, JG, Malia, R, Cooper, P et al. (1997b). Protein C and protein S in homozygous sickle cell disease: Does hepatic dysfunction contribute to low levels? *Br. J. Haematol.* 98: 627–631.

Wright, JG, Hambleton, IR, Thomas, PW et al. (1999). Post-splenectomy course in homozygous sickle cell disease. *J. Pediatr.* 134: 304–309.

Wun, T, Paglieroni, T, Field, CL et al. (1999). Platelet-erythrocyte adhesion in sickle cell disease. *J. Invest. Med.* 47: 121–127.

Zarkowsky, HS, Gallagher, D, Gill, FM et al. (1986). Bacteremia in sickle hemoglobinopathies. *J. Pediatr.* 109: 579–585.

Zimmerman, SA and Ware, RE. (1998). Inherited DNA mutations contributing to thrombotic complications in patients with sickle cell disease. *Am. J. Hematol.* 59: 267–272.

Zimmerman, RA, Gill, F, Goldberg, HI et al. (1987). MRI of sickle cell cerebral infarction. *Neuroradiology* 29: 232–237.

Zimmerman, SA, Howard, TA, Whorton, MR et al. (1998). The A312G polymorphism in α-fibrinogen is associated with stroke and avascular necrosis in patients with sickle cell anemia. *Blood* 92: 36b.

25

Nature and Treatment of the Acute Painful Episode in Sickle Cell Disease

LENNETTE J. BENJAMIN

INTRODUCTION

The pain of sickle cell disease was recognized in Africa centuries before sickle cell disease was even identified in the Western world (Konotey-Ahulu, 1968). The names for the disease suggested that pain was a prominent if not defining feature of it. In some tribes, it was named onomatopoeically after the crying sounds made by affected children. In Krobo language, it was called *hemkom,* which translates as "body biting" (Konotey-Ahulu, 1991). In other languages, it was called "a state of suffering."

Today, painful episodes are recognized as the hallmark of sickle cell disease (Reid et al., 1995). They are the *bête-noire* of sickle cell patients, the most frequent cause of their visits to the emergency department and hospital admissions, and a strain on caregivers. Advances in diagnosis and treatment, coupled with an expanded understanding of the physiology, pharmacology, and psychology of pain perception, have improved the care of some, but what has been learned has not been universally incorporated into clinical practice (Vichinsky et al., 1982; Foley, 1985; Pasternak et al., 1987; Benjamin, 1989, 1991; Gil et al., 1989, 1994; Payne, 1989, 1997; Shapiro, 1989, 1993; Ballas, 1990, 1995, 1998; Inturrisi, 1990; Shapiro et al., 1990; Ballas and Smith 1992; Benjamin et al., 1994, 1999a; Embury et al., 1994; Gebhart et al., 1994; Koshy et al., 1994; Serjeant et al., 1994;

Charache et al., 1995; Kaul et al., 1996; Cleeland et al., 1997; Wall and Melzack, 1998). Most patients in pain continue to receive inadequate treatment, a situation not solely attributable to an imperfect understanding of pain, pain treatment, or the pathophysiology of sickle cell disease.

In developing countries, and in some parts of the United States, a wide array of agents for treating pain is not available, and regulations further limit choices (Cleeland 1987; International Narcotic Control Board, 1996). In some countries there may not even be access to aspirin (acetylsalicylic acid) or acetaminophen. In others, philosophical or cultural considerations discourage the use of opioids (Cleeland, 1987; Konotey-Ahulu, 1991).

Often, the extent of the pain is not understood by health care providers, who must learn to adjust for their own perceptions of pain and how it is communicated (Armstrong et al., 1995; Turk, 1996a; Shapiro et al., 1997). To manage pain effectively, the health care provider must assess pain in the context of the patient's own beliefs, culture, and problems (Elander and Midence, 1996). A lifetime of unpredictable, sometimes devastating pain that is damaging to the body and complicated by the fear of dying is stressful to sickle cell disease patients as well to their family and their social relations, all of which increases the impact of the pain (Walco and Dampier, 1990; Treadwell and Gil, 1994). Pain interferes with school, work, and the activities of daily living, and it imposes a financial burden (Shapiro et al., 1995).

Historically, the treatment of the acute painful episodes of sickle cell disease has received low priority by both emergency departments and inpatient physicians and nurses, many of whom regard effective relief as unobtainable (Davies, 1990). Because physicians and nurses provide the leadership in the treatment of acute pain, their perceptions and attitudes are critical and may influence care and treatment (Gil et al., 1994). Physicians' and nurses' responses to a patient—empathy, concern, dread, mistrust—influence the patient's pain experience (Murray and May, 1988; Cleeland, 1993; Armstrong et al., 1995). Low expectations can lead to poor results, and many patients unnecessarily accept inadequate pain control (Alleyne and Thomas, 1994; Moore, 1994). Ineffective pain management has broad implications because patients in pain suffer more complications. (Cousins, 1989; Melzack, 1990). Improved analgesia may be associated with less morbidity, lower mortality, shorter hospital stays, and lower costs (Rawal et al., 1984; Foley, 1985; Yeager et al., 1987).

Martin H. Steinberg, Bernard G. Forget, Douglas R. Higgs, and Ronald L. Nagel, editors. *Disorders of Hemoglobin: Genetics, Pathophysiology, and Clinical Management.* © 2001 Cambridge University Press. All rights reserved.

Randomized controlled trials of sickle cell disease pain treatment are sparse (Benjamin, 1990a; Benjamin et al., 1999a, 1999b); in light of the dearth of empirical data, this chapter takes a practical, principle-based approach. Because treatment decisions may be influenced by beliefs about the nature of pain, its mechanisms, and its significance for the patient, this chapter focuses on the nature of acute sickle cell disease pain, how health care providers perceive it, the underlying knowledge needed to choose a course of action, and the practices that are employed in managing the pain. More general reports and extensively detailed reviews may be found elsewhere (Shapiro, 1993; Payne, 1997; Ballas, 1998).

THE NATURE OF ACUTE PAINFUL EPISODES

Definition of Acute Painful Episode

Pain is an unpleasant sensory and emotional experience associated with actual or potential tissue damage, modified by past memories and current beliefs. Pain in sickle cell disease can be acute or chronic. Acute pain can occur alone, be either brief or persistent, can be superimposed on chronic pain, or by frequent recurrence, masquerade as chronic pain (Niv and Davor, 1998). Etiologically, pain can be related to the disease (but it may not be), or to therapy (Foley, 1985). Mechanistically, it can be nociceptive (derived from tissue injury and/or inflammation), neuropathic (derived from nerve injury), or idiopathic (of unknown cause) (Payne, 1997).

Sickle cell anemia pain is said to be worse than postoperative or trauma pain. Bone pain is described as being like a toothache felt through the entire body. It resembles what might be experienced when an extremity is placed in a vise tightened to the extreme, but then is tightened even more—superimposing excruciating pain on unbearable pain. Some women describe the pain of childbirth as paling in comparison to the pain experienced during painful episodes.

The acute painful episode is the most commonly encountered type of sickle cell disease pain in all age groups (Shapiro, 1993; Benjamin et al., 1999a, 2000). It is an episodic, unpredictable, unpleasant sensory and emotional experience for which there is no other explanation, and it can involve any site of the body. Episodes, which last from hours to days, are characterized by exacerbations, migration from one site to another, and a return to the "steady state."

These episodes, which can occur at any time, distinguish sickle cell pain from most other types of pain, such as dental, postoperative, cancer, and obstetrical pain. They can begin in early infancy

(leading to early opioid exposure) and continue throughout life. Moreover, because treatment options for the underlying disease are limited, pain management may be more difficult (Ballas, 1998; Benjamin et al., 1999a, 1999b). Pain management is also complicated by the influence of learned pain behavior, pain memories, and pain therapy-induced pain (Fordyce, 1976; Gil et al., 1993; Basbaum, 1995; Song and Carr, 1999). (Fig. 25.1).

Patients with sickle cell disease may experience innumerable acute pain episodes (Table 25.1) and all kinds of therapies, including surgery. The pathophysiologic mechanisms of the common pain syndromes are variably understood. The most common acute pain events, discussed in detail in Chapter 24, are as follows:

Hand-foot syndrome, or dactylitis, which is a dorsal swelling of the hands and feet that occurs in early childhood (ages 6 months to 4 years) and is often the first manifestation of the disease

Acute inflammation of joints that can accompany dactylitis

Acute chest syndrome

Splenic sequestration in young children and in adults with HbSC disease and HbS-β^+ thalassemia

Intrahepatic sickling or hepatic sequestration in adults

Abdominal pain secondary to bowel infarction and necrosis and cholelithiasis

Priapism due to damage in the corpora cavernosa

PRECIPITATING EVENTS AND THEIR TREATMENT

We do not know what triggers the acute painful episodes of sickle cell anemia. Sickle erythrocyte dehydration, hypoxia, and acidosis promote HbS polymerization in vitro, and it has been presumed that preventing patient exposure to similar circumstances should lessen the likelihood of vasoocclusive episodes (Charache, 1974; Reid et al., 1995).

There is little evidence that painful episodes are initiated by events external to the patient, but some associations have been attributed to changes in weather or psychological stress (Nadel and Portadin 1977). The rainy season in Ghana, West Africa, reportedly produces many sickle pain episodes because the cold water often provokes pain and the cold, wet conditions are linked with some tropical infections. Changes in climate have also been associated with pain (Ibrahim, 1980). Serjeant found exposure to cold in 34 percent of patients presenting with acute painful episodes and proposed a neurovascular etiology with shunting of blood away from the involved regions (Bailey et al., 1991; Serjeant, 1994).

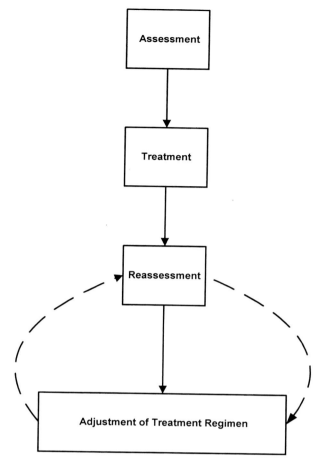

Figure 25.1. Management of pain in sickle cell disease.

Dehydration

Because of hyposthenuria (see Chapters 24 and 29), urinary output in patients with sickle cell anemia may exceed 2 L/d, making them susceptible to dehydration. Because pain is often accompanied by reduced fluid intake and increased water losses, increased fluid intake is essential.

For uncomplicated painful episodes, 5 percent dextrose in water (D5W) and one-quarter to one-half nor-

mal saline can be used for initial fluid replacement. To provide for both urinary water loss and normal daily requirements, the daily fluid intake should be approximately 3 to 5 L for adults and 100 to 150 mL/kg for children (Reid et al., 1995). Needs vary, and hydration should be monitored closely to avoid iatrogenic congestive heart failure or electrolyte imbalance.

Hypoxia

Although deoxygenation induces sickling in vitro, no controlled clinical studies show an association between the painful episode and hypoxia. Studies involving the use of varying concentrations of oxygen and hyperbaric oxygen during sickle cell painful episodes have yielded mixed results. Undesirable effects, such as toxicity related to oxygen therapy (Reinhard et al., 1944) and depression of erythropoiesis during its prolonged use (Embury et al., 1984), have also been reported. Still, the practice of indiscriminately placing patients on oxygen without taking into account the state of oxygenation persists.

Until studies provide evidence to the contrary, oxygen therapy should probably be reserved for those patients who are hypoxic or display acute respiratory distress. Incentive spirometry should be used to open airways and prevent atelectasis.

Infection

Infection has been associated with painful episodes and should always be considered and treated early when present in children (Barrett-Connor, 1968; Buchanan 1994) (See Chapter 24).

Acidosis

Acidosis may be a precipitating event in painful episodes (Reid et al., 1995) and should be managed appropriately (see Chapter 24). Double-blind studies using alkali to abort or relieve a painful episode have not proved effective (McCurdy and Mahmood, 1971).

EPIDEMIOLOGY OF PAIN IN SICKLE CELL DISEASE

Clinicians have long known that patients vary greatly in the number, severity, and frequency of their painful episodes. Recently, the Cooperative Study of Sickle Cell Disease (CSSCD, Chapter 24) has determined specific pain episode rates and risk factors and whether patients with more frequent pain episodes are at greater risk for premature death (Platt et al., 1991, 1994). In this multicenter study, 39 percent of patients had no pain episodes that caused a hospital visit and 1 percent of patients had more than six such episodes per year. Hav-

Table 25.1. Acute Pain Syndromes in Sickle Cell Disease

Acute painful episode
Hand-foot syndrome
Acute chest syndrome
Splenic sequestration or infarction
Hepatic sequestration or intrahepatic sickling
Acute arthritis
Priapism

ing more than three pain episodes per year that required hospitalization was a significant risk factor for disease severity and was associated with increased mortality in patients ages 20 years and older (Platt et al., 1991, 1994). A direct relationship between the incidence of pain episodes and PCV is also found (Serjeant et al., 1984), which may be a consequence of the relationship between PCV and blood viscosity. Lower blood viscosity in more severely anemic individuals may reduce vasoocclusive complications. Fetal hemoglobin (HbF) levels are inversely related to pain frequency.

In a separate CSSCD report on a cohort followed through the first decade of life, painful episodes and acute chest syndrome were the most common disease-related events in sickle cell anemia, HbSC disease, and HbS-β thalassemia patients (Gill et al., 1995). A small study in which patient-kept diaries recorded daily pain showed that patients do not come to the hospital for most of their pain. (Shapiro et al., 1990).

In the CSCCD report, female sickle cell anemia patients had a higher incidence of acute painful episodes than males. (Platt et al., 1991) Half of all sickle cell anemia and HbSC disease children experienced a painful episodes by ages 4.9 and 7.1 years, respectively. One quarter of sickle cell anemia patients in the cohort were taken to medical facilities for pain by age 2.5 years. The rate of painful episode recurrence within 6 months was 32 percent for sickle cell anemia and 19 percent for HbSC disease patients.

Pain and organ damage are influenced by genetic factors such as β-globin gene cluster haplotypes, α thalassemia, HbF level and other, ill-defined factors (Chapter 26). In the CSSCD report (Gill et al., 1995), children with α thalassemia had a higher incidence of painful events and a lower incidence of acute chest syndrome. In general, pain rates for sickle cell diseases vary by genotype and decrease in the following order: sickle cell anemia >HbSC disease> HbS-β+ thalassemia. Substantial variability exists however, even within a genotype (Powars et al., 1990). The genetic basis of the variability is often not clear (Chapter 26), and a better understanding is needed before the risk of pain can be predicted for individuals. A sickle cell anemia patient who has α thalassemia, a Senegal β-globin gene haplotype, and is female has the "best" genetic constitution (Steinberg et al., 1995) The "least" favorable genetic makeup would be a male with four α-globin genes and a Bantu β-globin gene haplotype. Those findings are derived from aggregate data, however, and the genetic markers are insufficient to help in the selection of an individual for more risky therapeutic interventions.

Genetic polymorphism might also play a role in the extent to which pain is perceived. An association, for example, has been reported for deficiency in the cytochrome p450 variant CYP2D and a lower pain threshold (Sindrup et al., 1993). Additional genetic markers, such as polymorphisms for endogenous opioids and opioid and dopamine receptors, might help in determining who is more vulnerable to pain and who has altered opioid responsiveness (Kreek, 1996a, 1996b)

PATHOPHYSIOLOGY OF ACUTE SICKLE PAIN

The pathophysiology of common pain syndromes is poorly understood. While pain in sickle cell anemia is generally attributed to vasoocclusive disease, the disease causes a series of neuropharmacologic and neurophysiologic changes in bone, soft tissue, blood vessels, nerve, and viscera, and those changes are accompanied by neuropsychologic changes. The neuropharmacologic and neurophysiologic changes activate and sensitize nociceptors that respond to chemical stimuli. Vasoocclusion and tissue injury are accompanied by a myriad of reactions that might contribute to acute pain (Francis and Johnson 1991), including vasospasm, inflammation at the site of injury, and elaboration of algesic (pain-producing) chemicals such as histamines, bradykinins, serotonin, prostaglandins, potassium ions, and substance P. Those chemicals can also influence vessel geometry and cellular function (Sinatra, 1993). Kinins circulate in plasma, while histamine, serotonin, prostaglandins, and K+ are found in both plasma and tissues; substance P is found in nerve terminals. The histamine and serotonin that are found in platelets and mast cells may be released by stimuli from tissue injury, heat, and opioid treatment. Neurohumoral alterations invoke persistent sensory responses to the noxious stimuli, and those responses become a form of memory that may determine an individual's reaction to present and future pain (Song and Carr, 1997). The memory of pain often overshadows the primary experience. Thus, acute pain may begin as a vasoocclusive event but be mediated and modulated by various algesic mechanisms and pain memories, and that has implications for combination therapies.

Areas of infarction, necrosis, and blood sequestration can be detected by X-rays, bone scans, magnetic resonance imaging (MRI), computerized tomography, and ultrasonography. Infarctive bone and soft tissue changes revealed by MRI in lower extremities of patients experiencing acute pain episodes (Mankad et al., 1990) and changes in levels of acute phase reactants such as cytokines and coagulation and fibrinolytic proteins support the contribution of ischemia, infarction, and inflammation to the acute painful episode (Benjamin et al., 1994; Ballas, 1998; Devine et al., 1986). Blood oxygen level dependent (BOLD) MRI has been used to assess oxy and deoxyhemoglobin levels in the brain and in painful sites during acute painful episodes and during pain-associated events such as priapism (Kassim et al., in press) and avascular necrosis of the hip (Fabry et al., 1998). Imaging techniques such as positron emission tomography (PET) scans and functional MRI are also under investigation for use in other pain states and have shown promise not only for evaluating pain sites and pain mechanisms but also for providing an objective measure on which to base psychological interventions.

When possible, decisions on how to treat pain should be based on its mechanism. Most acute pain in sickle cell disease is nociceptive. Nociceptive pain involves four electrophysiologic events that occur between the site of tissue damage and the site of pain perception (Farrar, 1999):

1. Tissue injury activates nociceptors.
2. The stimuli are translated into electrical impulses that travel toward the brain.
3. The impulses are modified or modulated at the level of the dorsal horn of the spinal cord by inhibitory actions of endogenous opioid, noradrenergic, and serotonergic systems.
4. Pain is perceived.

Nociceptive pain typically experienced during vasoocclusive episodes results from somatic and/or visceral stimuli. Somatic pain, the most frequent, appears as an intense, localized, sharp or stinging sensation and involves primarily deep structures such as the periosteum, bone marrow, joints, muscles, tendons, ligaments, and arteries. Mediated by fast conducting myelinated fibers of the A (Farrar, 1999) and/or C delta type, these fibers have a high threshold, requiring a strong, usually mechanical, stimulus, and terminate mostly in lamina I. This type of pain can be focal or referred.

Visceral pain is associated with the spleen, liver, lungs, and other organs and is generally vague, poorly localized, diffuse, dull, and often associated with nausea, vomiting, and sweating. It is mediated by unmyelinated fibers, the slower conducting C fibers, and/or by A delta fibers, which are activated by inflammation, ischemia, and rapid distention. C fibers are polymodal, meaning that they mediate mechanical, thermal, and chemical stimuli. They also enter the spinal cord through the dorsal horn and end mostly in the outer layer of lamina II. Some patients have sharper visceral pain that is more localized and felt nearer the site of the injured viscera. This type of visceral pain is frequently associated with muscle spasm, tenderness, and hyperesthesia, and is rarely associated with nausea and vomiting.

The amount of nociceptive activity is influenced by the intensity and duration of the stimuli and the microenvironment of the nociceptors. Besides exciting the nociceptor membrane, chemical messengers work indirectly on the microcirculation contributing to pain at both the injured site and surrounding structures (Cousins, 1989; Sorkin, 1997). As previously noted, chemical messengers and mediators of inflammation elaborated in response to tissue damage can amplify pain.

Neuropathic pain is likely to occur in sickle cell anemia and has not been adequately appreciated (Table 25.2). Neuropathic pain can be epicritic or protopathic. Epicritic pain is associated with A delta fibers and can be lancinating, sharp, or prickly while protopathic pain is usually described as dull, burning, and poorly localized due primarily to involvement of the polymodal C fibers. Maladaptive changes in the peripheral and sensory nervous systems following injury may underlie the symptoms. Neuropathic pain arising from nerve injury is manifested by spontaneous pain, hyperalgesia allodynia (a painful response to a stimulus that is not normally pain producing, e.g., light touch), hyperalgesia (a heightened or exaggerated response to stimuli that is usually painful, e.g., amplification of pain by inflammation), or sensory deficits, or it may have a sympathetic component. Possible sources of neuropathic sickle cell disease pain include nerve ischemia from vasoocclusion, nerve compression from bone infarction or vertebral collapse, nerve injury from noxious substances elaborated at the sites of pain, ill-defined events during acute painful episode, or therapy-induced factors. Neuropathic pain should be considered during acute painful episodes when allodynia, burning, or lancinating pain or electrical or painful paresthesias occur and are only partially relieved by, or are unresponsive to, opioids. Neuropathic pain can persist or recur spontaneously between painful events.

Table 25.2. Possible Neuropathic Pain in Sickle Cell Disease

Pain	Reference
Orbital infarction	Blank and Gill, 1981
Orbital apex syndrome	Al-Rashid, 1979
Mental nerve neuropathy	Konotey-Ahulu, 1972
	Freedlander et al., 1980
	Seelering and Royal, 1982
Mononeuropathy	Shields et al., 1991
Ischemic optic neuropathy	Slavin and Barondes, 1988
Neuropathies, trigeminal neuralgia	Asher, 1980
Spinal cord infarction	Rothman and Nelson, 1980

Pain perception involves not just situational factors, but also mood, psychological state, pain memories, expectations based on experience with similar pain, and coping mechanisms (Gil et al., 1989; McGrath, 1994; Farrar, 1999). After several painful episodes, some sickle cell disease patients fail to readjust; they become fearful and fixed on the possibility of another painful episode or even death. In those instances, organic pain may be amplified or propagated by psychogenic factors, the treatment of which is pivotal to the success of therapy (Fordyce, 1976). Conditioned drug-taking behavior caused by undermedication during acute pain and overmedication during chronic pain may also contribute to pain (Weisman and Haddox, 1989; White and Horoi, 1993; Benjamin et al., 1994; Gil et al., 1994). Psychological factors such as stress can also be the primary factor in precipitating an acute painful episode. The psychophysiology of stress is described as "an integration of the pain experience" (Maier and Watkins, 1998).

Integration of Pain Mechanisms in Persistent Pain

Persistent pain, regardless of the mechanism causing it, results in long-term changes in the spinal cord, brain stem, and thalamus, and at the site of injury. After peripheral trauma, laboratory experiments have shown increased nociceptive transmission and peripheral and central sensitization of nociceptors. Peripheral sensitization is a reduction in the threshold of the afferent peripheral terminal nociceptors. Central hypersensitization is the progressive "wind-up" of dorsal horn neuronal discharge that follows from the expansion of the receptive fields of dorsal horn neurons; it can be caused by afferent input-induced increased excitability of the spinal neurons (Wall and Melzack, 1994). These secondary changes may include structural remodeling of neuronal circuits.

In addition to reducing the pain threshold, persistent pain from tissue injury results in hyperalgesia, a prolongation of the response to noxious stimuli and extension of pain and hypersensitivity to uninjured tissues (secondary hyperalgesia). Such hyperalgesia may occur as a result of the lowered response threshold at the vasoocclusive site or the release and spread of pain- or inflammation-producing substances. These include the peptidergic transmitters, substance P, vasoactive intestinal polypeptide, somatostatin, calcitonin gene-related peptide, and cholecystokinin. The descending pathways seem to involve serotonin, norepinephrine, and endogenous opioids. With secondary hyperalgesia, the hypersensitive state outlasts the injury and increases the sensory and reactive dimensions of pain, making pain control more difficult. Persistent painful stimuli evoke

memory that, in turn, is influenced by peak intensity of previous pain, current pain intensity, emotion, and pain expectation (Kaiko et al., 1989).

MECHANISM-BASED APPROACH TO TREATMENT OF ACUTE PAIN

The ability to control pain with a specific agent may differ in different pain states. Treatment need not be limited to a single agent, however, and analgesics that work by different mechanisms may be additive or synergistic when taken together. When analgesia is balanced, lower doses of each drug can be used and the adverse effects of each are reduced accordingly.

Balanced analgesia can be applied to nociception (Wall and Melzack, 1994) (Fig. 25.2). Nonsteroidal antiinflammatory agents (NSAIDs) affect transduction; opioids, including neuraxial (epidural and subarachnoid) opioids, influence transmission and modulation, and systemic opioids influence perception. Persistent opioid use induces postsynaptic morphologic changes (Basbaum, 1995), and balanced analgesia offers the possibility of preventing such changes, as well as the neuroendocrine response to pain. A combined analgesic regimen can almost eliminate postoperative pain (Dahl and Kehlet, 1993). Because of the benefits of the balanced administration of epidural local anesthetics and opioids (along with NSAIDs), drug combinations are rapidly becoming a standard for postoperative analgesia and may be beneficial in sickle cell disease (Yaster et al., 1994).

Analgesia may relieve pain without abolishing neuroendocrine stress and improving outcomes. Systemic and neuraxial opioids, for example, have little effect on the neuroendocrine stress response. While optimal pharmacologic management is the mainstay in acute pain therapy, patients with pain as a prominent and recurring feature of a chronic disease generally fare best with a combination of acute and chronic pain treatment modalities.

NSAID AND OPIOID THERAPY

The mainstay of medical treatment in managing pain in sickle cell anemia is therapy that includes nonopioid and opioid analgesics and analgesic adjuvants.

Nonopioid Analgesics

The nonopioid analgesic agents are the first line drugs for treatment of pain of mild to moderate intensity (Table 25.3). Although aspirin is the prototypic drug for this group, acetaminophen and NSAIDs are the most frequently used.

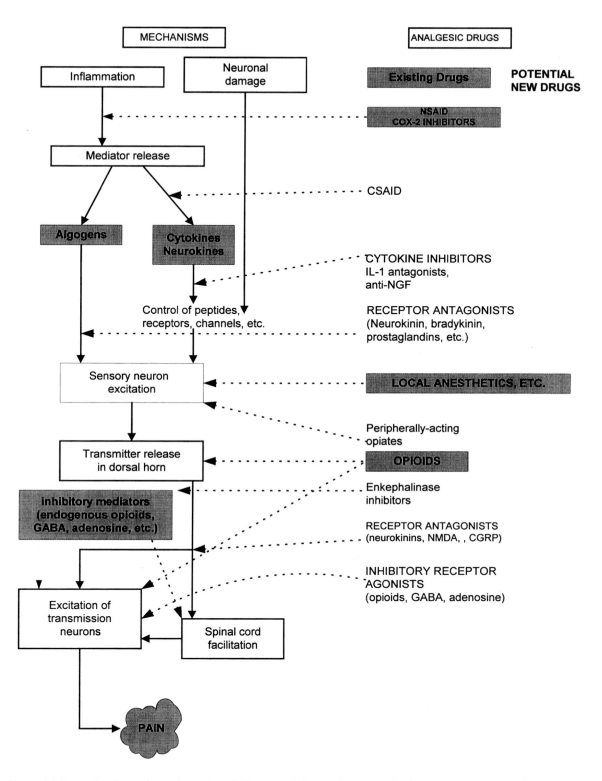

Figure 25.2. Mechanisms of pain in sickle cell disease and classes of drugs useful for treating each type of pain.

Table 25.3. Analgesics Commonly Used Orally for Mild to Moderate Pain: Equianalgesia and Starting Doses

Name	Equianalgesic dose* (mg)	Starting oral dose range (mg)	Comments	Precautions
A. Nonopioids				
Aspirin	650	650	Often used in combination with opioid analgesics	Renal dysfunction; avoid during pregnancy, in hemostatic disorders, and in combination with steroids
Acetaminophen	650	650	Like aspirin but does not affect platelet functions	
Ibuprofen (Motrin®)	ND†	200–400	Higher analgesic potential than aspirin	Like aspirin
Fenoprofen (Nalfon®)	ND	200–400	Like ibuprofen	Like aspirin
Diflunisal (Dolobid®)	ND	500–1000	Longer duration of action than ibuprofen; higher analgesic potential than aspirin	Like aspirin
Naproxen (Naprosyn®)	ND	250–500	Like diflunisal	Like aspirin
Choline magnesium Triasalicylate (Trilisate®)	ND	1,500	Does not affect platelet function	Like aspirin (see also comments)
B. Morphine-like agonists (opioids)				
Codeine	32–65	32–65	Often used in combination with nonopioid analgesics; biotransformed, in part to morphine	Impaired ventilation; bronchial asthma; increased intracranial pressure
Oxycodone	5	5–10	Also in combination with nonopioid analgesics, which limits dose escalation	Like codeine
Meperidine	50	50–100	Biotransformed to normeperidine, a toxic metabolite	Normeperidine accumulates with repetitive dosing causing CNS excitation; not for patients with impaired renal function or receiving monoamine oxidase inhibitors
Propoxyphene HCl (Darvon®) Propoxyphene napsylate (Darvon-N®)	65–130	65–130	Often used in combination with nonopioid analgesics; long half life, biotransformed to potentially toxic metabolite (norpropoxyphene)	Propoxyphene metabolite accumulates with repetitive dosing; overdose complicated by convulsions. Useful as transition drug at home after taper, taking advantage of structural similarity to dolophine and the long life of the metabolite norpropoxyphene
C. Mixed opioid agonist-antagonists				
Pentazocine (Talwin®)	50	50–100	In combination with nonopioid; in combination with naloxone to discourage parenteral abuse	May cause psychotomimetic effects; may precipitate withdrawal in opioid-dependent patients

Abbreviation: ND, not determined.

* For these equianalgesic doses (see also comments) the time of peak analgesia ranges from 1.5 to 2 hours and the duration from 4 to 6 hours. Oxycodone and meperidine are shorter-acting (3 to 5 hours) and diflunisal and naproxen are longer acting (8 to 12 hours).

† These doses are recommended starting from which optimal dose for each patient is determined by titration and the maximal dose limited by adverse effects.

Aspirin is the analgesic for first-line treatment of pain of mild to moderate intensity. For children under age 12 years, acetaminophen or paracetamol is the analgesic of choice because of the association of aspirin with Reye's syndrome.

NSAIDs work by blocking the action of cyclooxygenase (COX), which converts arachidonic acid to prostaglandins. Gastric, renal, and platelet toxicities often limit their use. Cyclooxygenase exists in two isoforms. COX-1, which is constitutive and present throughout the body, mediates the synthesis of prostaglandins that regulate normal physiologic functions. COX-2, which is inducible, mediates the synthesis of prostaglandins that support the inflammatory process and is important in pain production. NSAIDs inhibit both cyclooxygenases, with COX-1 inhibition accounting for the side effects most commonly associated with NSAIDs and COX-2 inhibition accounting for the therapeutic effects. Two agents that selectively inhibit COX-2 have recently been approved by the U.S. Food and Drug Administration, but it is too early to assess their efficacy in the treatment of acute pain.

NSAIDs such as ketorolac tromethamine seem to inhibit not only COX, but also lipooxygenase, which converts arachidonic acid to leukotrienes, important contributors to inflammation and peripheral nociceptor sensitization. Ketorolac has received mixed reviews in studies primarily designed to see if it has an opioid-sparing effect (Wright et al., 1992; Perlin et al., 1994).

Acetaminophen and other para-aminophenol derivatives are similar to aspirin in analgesic and antipyretic properties but have modest antiinflammatory effects. Their mechanism of action is not known although they are thought to act both centrally and peripherally. They are well absorbed when administered orally and have an onset of action of 30 to 60 minutes. The drugs are metabolized in the liver and excreted in the urine. They also differ from NSAIDs in that they do not impair platelet aggregation or produce gastric ulcerations, but patients who have preexisting liver disease are at risk for severe hepatoxicity and those who receive large doses (>4,000 mg/d) over extended periods are vulnerable to nephrotoxicity (American Pain Society, Quality of Care Committee, 1995).

Many preparations contain acetaminophen in combination with codeine and equivalent opioids such as hydrocodone and dextropropoxyphene. While the ceiling effect of acetaminophen limits the amount of the combination that can be prescribed, many patients and some prescribers will escalate the dose to increase the opioid effect without consideration for the potential deleterious effect of acetaminophen. The fact that these preparations contain acetaminophen is often overlooked as well when patients are taking coumadin, and it can lead to an increased risk for bleeding.

Routes of Administration. NSAIDs exist in oral, parenteral, and rectal formulations and short-intermediate- and long-acting preparations so treatment can be tailored to the needs of the patient. Rectal preparations include acetaminophen, aspirin, and indomethacin. Intravenous preparations include indomethacin, which is seldom used because of a high incidence of side effects, and ketorolac, the use of which is restricted to 120 mg/d for 5 days because of potential nephrotoxicity. In Europe and Japan, intravenous lysine acetylsalicylate and diclofenac are available, and there has been one study of the intravenous lysine salt of aspirin in the treatment of an acute painful episode in sickle cell anemia (Benjamin, 1991).

Aspirin and ibuprofen are short acting, with a duration of action of 4 to 6 hours. Naprosyn, ketoprofen, diclofenac, and diflunisal are intermediate with a duration ranging from 6 to 12 hours. Long-acting NSAIDs include sustained-release preparations.

Opioid Analgesics

Opioid analgesics are the first-line drugs for the treatment of painful episodes of moderate to severe intensity. Their effective use requires understanding of their clinical pharmacology and the sites and mechanism of action (Reisine et al., 1995). Important pharmacologic differences between opioids are based on complex interactions with central nervous system receptors. Morphine-like agonist drugs bind to opioid receptors and produce analgesia; opioid antagonists bind to opioid receptors blocking the effects of morphine-like agonists and lack analgesic properties (Raynor et al., 1994) (Table 25.4). Between these extremes are mixed agonist-antagonist drugs that, depending on clinical circumstances, have agonist or antagonist properties.

Few well-controlled studies compare the efficacy and side effects of opioids during repeated dosing, a comparison most relevant to clinical management of sickle cell anemia (Kaiko et al., 1983b). A rationale for and the appropriate use of opioids is based on the knowledge of their pharmacologic properties derived from clinical trials in postoperative, cancer, dental, and trauma patients. Pharmacokinetic studies of the disposition and fate of opioids have started to provide a better understanding of some causes of interpatient variation in their efficacy (Galer et al., 1992; Dampier et al., 1995; Mather et al., 1996; Inturrisi, 1997).

Morphine-Like Agonists

Morphine is the prototype opioid analgesic. Morphine-like agonists share with morphine a similar profile of both desirable and undesirable pharmacodynamic effects (Table 25.5). They differ in relative analgesic

Table 25.4. Different Classification Systems for Opioids

Weak or strong opioids	Opium and its derivatives	Agonists/antagonists
Weak	Natural opium alkaloids	Agonists
Codeine	Phenanthrene derivatives	Alfentanil
Propoxyphene (Darvon)	Morphine	Alphaprodine
Hydrocodone (Vicodin)	Codeine	Codeine
Strong	Semisynthetic derivatives of	Dihydromorphinone
Alfentanil (Alfenta)	opium alkaloids	Dihydrohydroxymorphinone
Alphaprodine (Nisentil)	Morphine derivatives	Fentanyl
Buprenorphine (Buprenex, Temgesic)	Dihydromorphinone	Levorphanol
Butorphanol (Stadol, Dorphanol)	Dihydrohydroxymorphinone	Meperidine
Cholecystokinin	Thebaine derivatives	Methadone
Dihydromorphinone, hydromorphone	Buprenorphine	Morphine
(Dilaudid)	Oxycodone	Oxycodone
Dihydrohydroxymorphinone,	Synthetic compounds	Propoxyphene
oxymorphone (Numorphan)	Morphinans	Sufentanil
Fentanyl (Sublimaze)	Levorphanol	Partial agonists
Levorphanol (Levo-Dromoran)	Nalbuphine	Buprenorphine
Meperidine (Demerol)	Naloxone	Agonist-antagonists
Methadone (Dolophine)	Naltrexone	Butorphanol
Morphine	Phenylheptylamines	Nalbuphine
Nalbuphine (Nubain)	Methadone	Pentazocine
Naloxone (Narcan)	Propoxyphene	Antagonists
Naltrexone (Trexan)	Phenylpiperidine	Cholecystokinin
Oxycodone (Percocet, Tylox, OxyIR,	Alfentanil	Naloxone
Roxicodone)	Alphaprodine	Naltrexone
Pentazocine (Talwin)	Fentanyl	
Sufentanil (Sufenta)	Meperidine	
	Sufentanil	

potency and oral to parenteral analgesic potency, factors critical in dose selection. They also differ in pharmacokinetics and their biotransformation to pharmacologically active metabolites (Foley, 1985; Inturrusi and Hanks, 1993; Mather et al., 1996), factors critical to dose adjustment especially when opioid administration is continued beyond 24 hours. This dosage information is primarily derived from controlled clinical trials employing single-dose relative potency assays comparing other opioids with morphine (Houde et al., 1966).

Morphine. The plasma half-life of 2 to 3 hours is shorter than its 4 to 6 hour duration of analgesia, thereby limiting accumulation. This linearity of pharmacokinetic properties following chronic administration of large doses contributes to its safety. The delayed-release morphine preparations provide analgesia with a duration of 8 to 12 hours for MS Contin® and Roxanol SR® or 24 hours for Kadian®, allowing the sickle cell disease pain patient relative freedom from repetitive dosing, especially at night. The preparations are safe and effective.

Morphine and butorphanol administered by the intramuscular route were equally effective in sickle cell disease (Gonzalez et al., 1988). Morphine by intermittent injection versus patient-controlled analgesia was also equally effective (Gonzalez et al., 1991).

Based on single-dose studies in patients with either acute or chronic pain, the relative potency of intramuscular to oral morphine is 1:6 (Kaiko, 1988). With repeated dosing on a regularly scheduled 24-hour basis, the intramuscular to oral ratio is reduced to 1:3 (Kaiko, 1988). Therefore, in patients with acute pain who are being titrated using a prn schedule, the 1:6 ratio should be used initially with a switch to the 1:3 ratio for continued dosing when a pharmacologic steady state is attained.

Patients should be initially titrated on immediate-release morphine and once stabilized, converted to the delayed-release preparation according to either an 8 or a 12-hour dosing schedule. To manage acute breakthrough pain, "rescue" dosing with immediate-release morphine should be made available to patients receiving delayed-release preparations (Lapin et al., 1989). Various protocols have been proposed for treatment of pain during painful episodes with oral dosing alone (Friedman et al., 1986; Conti et al., 1996).

Table 25.5. Opioid Analgesics Commonly Used for Severe Pain

Name	Equianalgesic dose* (mg)	IM/PO potency	Starting oral dose range (mg)	Comments	Precautions
a. Morphine-like agonists					
Morphine	10	6	30–60[b]	Standard of comparison for opioid analgesics	Lower doses for aged patients; impaired ventilation; bronchial asthma; increased intracranial pressure; liver failure
Hydromorphone (Dilaudid®)	1.5	5	4–8	Slightly shorter acting HP in dosage form for tolerant patients	Like morphine
Methadone (Dolophine®)	10	2	10–20	Good oral potency; long plasma half-life	Like morphine; may accumulate with repetitive dosing causing excessive sedation
Levorphanol (Levo-Dromoran®)	2	2	2–4	Like methadone	Like methadone
Oxymorphone (Numorphan®)	1	– – See comments – –		Not available orally	Like morphine
Meperidine (Demerol®)	75	4	Not recommended	Slightly shorter acting; used orally for less severe pain (see table)	Normeperidine (toxic metabolite) accumulates with repetitive dosing causing CNS excitation; not for patients with impaired renal function or receiving monoamine oxidase inhibitors[c]
Codeine	130	1.5	See comments	Used orally for less severe pain (see table)	Like morphine
b. Mixed agonist-antagonists					
Pentazocine (Talwin®)	60	3	See comments	Use orally for less severe pain; mixed agonist-antagonist; less abuse liability than morphine; included in IV of Controlled Substances Act	May cause psychotomimetic effects; may precipitate withdrawal in opioid-dependent patients; not for myocardial infarction*
Nalbuphine (Nubain®)	10	– – See comments – –		Not available orally; like in pentazocine but not scheduled	Incidence of psychotomimetic effects lower than with pentazocine
Butorphanol (Stadol®)	2	– – See comments – –		Not available orally like in nalbuphine	Like in pentazocine
c. Partial agonists					
Buprenorphine (Buprenex®)	0.4	– – See comments – –		Not available orally; sublingual preparation not yet in U.S.; less abuse liability than morphine; does not produce psychotomimetic effects	May precipitate withdrawal in opioid-dependent patients

Abbreviations: IM, intramuscular; PO, oral.

* For these equianalgesic doses (see also comments) the time of peak analgesia in nontolerant patients ranges from one-half to 1 hour and the duration from 4 to 6 hours. The peak analgesic effect is delayed and the duration prolonged after oral administration.

[a] These doses are recommended starting IM doses from which the optimal dose for each patient is determined by titration and the maximal dose limited by adverse effects.

[b] A value of 3 is used when calculating an oral dosage regimen of 94th around-the-clock.

[c] Irritating to tissues on repeated administration.

681

Morphine-6-glucuronide, an active metabolite of morphine, is primarily responsible for the drug's analgesic properties (Osborne et al., 1990). This metabolite is eliminated by the kidney and accumulates in patients with renal insufficiency. Its accumulation may contribute in part to adverse effects (Peterson et al., 1990; Osborne et al., 1992). An alternative opioid should be considered when a patient receiving morphine experiences a decrease in renal function and an increase in undesirable effects.

Table 25.5 lists morphine-like agonists that may be substituted for morphine. An alternative may be selected based on the need of a particular patient not only to overcome an adverse effect of morphine—vomiting or sedation—but in consideration of the patient's favorable experience with another opioid or even local availability of other morphine-like opioids. No evidence suggests that any opioid has greater analgesic efficacy than morphine or that morphine will be more or less effective in any individual (Galer et al., 1992).

Elevated morphine clearance values have been observed in children and adolescents receiving the drug during painful episodes (Zipursky et al., 1992; Dampier et al., 1995). Morphine clearance values decreased with increasing age or PCV.

Hydromorphone. Hydromorphone is a short half-life opioid used as an alternative to morphine by the oral and parenteral routes. It is more soluble than morphine and available in a 1 mg/mL and a 10 mg/mL concentrated dose form.

Levorphanol. Levorphanol, a long half-life opioid, is also a useful alternative to morphine but must be used cautiously to prevent accumulation. For patients who are unable to tolerate morphine, hydromorphone, or methadone, levorphanol represents a useful medication with an oral to parenteral potency ratio of 1:2.

Oxymorphone. Oxymorphone, a congener of morphine, has had a limited but important role in the management of pain. It is currently most widely used in suppository form, is infrequently used parenterally on a chronic basis, and is not available orally.

Methadone. Methadone has been both advocated and discouraged for pain management. Based on single-dose studies, its oral to parenteral potency ratio is 1:2. Plasma half-life averages 24 hours (range, 13 to 50 hours) but its duration of analgesia is often only 4 to 8 hours. Because of the discrepancy between its plasma half-life and the duration of analgesia, repetitive doses lead to drug accumulation and to sedation and confusion. Even death can occur when patients are not carefully monitored. Methadone can be a useful alternative

to morphine for patients who have developed some degree of tolerance to morphine. Equianalgesic discrepancies exist when switching from high doses of short-acting drugs to methadone (see below). Methadone is the least potent of the common opioid analgesics, requiring larger doses for a similar effect.

Meperidine. Repetitive dosing of meperidine (Demerol®) can lead to accumulation of its toxic metabolite, normeperidine, resulting in central nervous system (CNS) hyperexcitability (Kaiko et al., 1983a). Characterized initially by subtle mood effects and followed by tremors, multifocal myoclonus, and occasionally seizures, CNS hyperexcitability occurs commonly in patients with renal disease, but it can occur following repeated administration in patients with normal renal function (Eisendrath et al., 1987).

The pharmacology of meperidine has been studied more extensively than that of any other opioid in the sickle disease pain patient population (Abbuhl et al., 1986; Pryle et al., 1992; Yang et al., 1995a). The studies suggest decreased serum levels (Abbuhl et al., 1986) and a possible circadian rhythm with poorer pain relief at night (Ristchel et al., 1983). Although peak levels were higher at night, the elimination half-life was much shorter. A more recent study suggested no difference in meperidine pharmacokinetics between adult sickle cell anemia patients studied in a non-crisis condition and normal controls (Yang et al., 1995a). These findings suggest potential pharmacokinetic changes related to physiologic effects produced by a vasoocclusive episode.

Two further studies have examined meperidine serum levels after repeated intramuscular dosing of hospital patients admitted for treatment of painful episodes. The first found that therapeutic levels of meperidine were present for only about 25 percent of hospital days when given in doses ranging from 4 to 20 mg/kg/d (Hunt et al., 1988). For almost 20 percent of hospital days, potentially toxic blood levels of normeperidine were observed. Pain assessment data suggested that pain relief was generally poor. A similar study of both intramuscular and oral dosing suggested an increased risk of seizures at normeperidine serum levels of 1 mg/mL, which was associated with daily doses greater than 25 mg/kg (Pryle et al., 1992). Since 50 mg of meperidine administered orally has the analgesic equivalent of 650 mg of aspirin, it is a poor oral agent, and accumulation of toxic metabolites occurs according to dose whatever the route of administration.

Oxycodone. In the United States, oxycodone is available for oral but not parenteral administration both as immediate-release and continuous-release (8- to 12-hour duration) preparations. It is a suitable alternative opioid for sickle cell disease pain. Information on the use of oxycodone alone for the management of severe pain is increasing as more preparations are available free of the risk of dose-related toxicity from the nonopioid ingredients. Lower doses (e.g., 5 mg) in combination with nonopioids (aspirin, acetaminophen) are frequently used for moderate pain. The fixed dose oxycodone combinations should not be used chronically in large doses for more severe pain because of the risk of dose-related toxicity from the nonopioid ingredients.

Fentanyl. Fentanyl is an opioid agonist that has not been subjected to a definitive relative potency assay and therefore is not listed in Table 25.5. However, fentanyl is estimated to be approximately 80 to 100 times as potent as morphine (Reisine et al., 1995). It is a highly lipophilic drug with shorter duration of action than parenteral morphine. Fentanyl has been evaluated for the management of postoperative pain by intravenous (Andrews and Prys-Robert, 1983) and epidural (Cousins and Mather, 1984) routes of administration. A transdermal patch device is used for chronic pain requiring opioid analgesia (Simmonds et al., 1988)

Codeine. The pharmacokinetics of oral codeine have been compared in sickle cell anemia patients at "baseline" and normal controls (Mohammed et al., 1993a; 1993b). Free plasma codeine concentrations were substantially lower in sickle cell anemia because of a two-fold higher degree of protein binding and a shorter half-life (1.7 vs. 2.4 hours). Drug clearance was higher and the volume of distribution was significantly smaller in sickle cell anemia compared with controls. These data suggest the need for dosage modifications in sickle cell anemia to achieve optimal drug levels for analgesia (Chen et al., 1991). Pharmacogenetic factors could possibly have contributed to failed or lessened analgesia in some of the patients (see Pharmacogenetics section).

Agonist-Antagonist Analgesics. The mixed agonist-antagonist analgesics (Table 25.5) include pentazocine, butorphanol, and nalbuphine. They produce analgesia in the non-tolerant patient but may hasten withdrawal in patients who are tolerant-dependent to morphine-like drugs. Therefore, these analgesics might best be used in patients without a history of chronic opioid exposure and before repeated administration of morphine-like agonists. Mixed agonist-antagonists have a ceiling effect for respiratory depression and are less likely to be abused than the morphine-like drugs. These drugs play a limited role in the management of chronic pain because the incidence and severity of the psychotomimetic effects increase with dose escalation (Inturrisi and Hanks, 1993). Nalbuphine is currently only available for parenteral use, and the oral preparation of pentazocine is

marketed in combination with naloxone. Butorphanol is available for both parenteral and nasal use.

Partial Agonist Analgesics. The partial agonist buprenorphine (Table 25.5) has less abuse liability than the morphine-like drugs, but like the mixed agonist-antagonists, it may also cause withdrawal in patients who have received repeated doses of morphine-like agonists and developed physical dependence. However, it does not produce the psychotomimetic effects seen with the mixed agonist-antagonists and is available in both a sublingual and parenteral form. Only the latter form is available in the United States. Buprenorphine's respiratory depressant effects are reversed only by large doses of naloxone. It is useful for moderate to severe pain requiring an opioid analgesic, but like the agonist-antagonists, it should be used before the morphine-like agonists are introduced (Inturrisi and Hanks, 1993).

Side Effects

Respiratory depression is the most serious, and constipation the most common, adverse effect of opioids. Respiratory depression is usually seen in opioid-naïve patients following acute drug administration and is associated with and often preceded by other signs of central nervous system depression, including sedation and mental clouding. Tolerance develops rapidly to those effects with repeated drug administration, allowing opioid analgesics to be used in the management of persistent acute pain and chronic cancer pain without significant risk of respiratory depression.

Nonetheless, the potential seriousness of this adverse effect must be understood. Morphine-like agonists can cause brain stem respiratory depression to the point of apnea. Death due to morphine-like agonist overdose is nearly always due to respiratory arrest. Therapeutic doses of morphine may depress all phases of respiratory activity (rate, minute volume, and tidal exchange). As CO_2 accumulates, it stimulates central chemoreceptors, resulting in a compensatory increase in respiratory rate which masks the degree of respiratory depression. At equianalgesic doses, the morphine-like agonists produce equivalent degrees of respiratory depression. Individuals with impaired respiratory function or bronchial asthma are at greatest risk of experiencing clinically significant respiratory depression in response to usual doses of the drugs.

If respiratory depression occurs, it can be reversed by the administration of the specific opioid antagonist, naloxone. In patients chronically receiving opioids who develop respiratory depression, naloxone, diluted 1:10, should be titrated carefully to prevent the precipitation of severe withdrawal symptoms. When meperidine is used chronically, naloxone may cause seizures by blocking the depressant action of meperidine and allowing manifestation of the convulsant activity of the active metabolite, normeperidine (Inturrisi and Hanks, 1993). If naloxone is to be used in this situation, diluted doses slowly titrated with appropriate seizure precautions are advised.

Opioid effects on the medullary chemoreceptor trigger zone cause nausea and vomiting, which vary with the drug and the patient. Some advantage may result from switching to an equianalgesic dose of another opioid. Alternatively, an antiemetic may be added to the regimen.

While useful in preanesthesia, sedation from opioids is not a desirable substitute for sleep from the comfort of opioid-induced pain relief. Sedation can limit therapy and may precede respiratory depression, particularly in ambulatory patients. The CNS depressant actions of these drugs can be expected to be at least additive with the sedative and respiratory depressant effects of sedative-hypnotics such as barbiturates and benzodiazepines.

Although it has been suggested that methadone produces more sedation than morphine, this has not been supported by single-dose controlled trials or surveys in hospitalized patients. Methadone's half-life is longer than morphine's and can lead to cumulative CNS depression after repeated doses. Excessive sedation may be prevented or attenuated by a reduction in dose and dosing interval so that a lower dose is given more frequently. Other CNS depressants, including sedative-hypnotics and antianxiety agents, that potentiate the sedative effects of opioids should be avoided. Concurrent administration of dextroamphetamine in 2.5 to 5.0 mg oral doses twice daily or methylphenidate 5 to 10 mg twice daily may reduce the sedative effects of opioids. Tolerance usually develops to the sedative effects of opioid analgesics within several days of administration.

Opioids act at multiple sites in the gastrointestinal tract and spinal cord to produce a decrease in intestinal secretions and peristalsis, resulting in a dry stool. Because tolerance to smooth muscle effects develops very slowly, constipation will persist when the drugs are used for chronic pain. At the same time that the use of opioid analgesics is initiated, provision for a regular bowel regimen, including cathartics and stool softeners, should be started.

Urinary retention is most common in the older patient. Opioid analgesics increase smooth muscle tone and can cause bladder spasm and an increase in sphincter tone. Catheterization may be necessary to manage this transient side effect.

At high doses, all opioid analgesics can produce multifocal myoclonus (Bruera and Pereira, 1997). This complication is most prominent with the repeated administration of large parenteral doses of meperidine

(more than 25 mg/kg/d) due to accumulation of normeperidine.

Route of Administration (Table 25.6)

Oral. Oral opioids differ substantially in their presystemic elimination (i.e., the degree to which they are inactivated as they are absorbed from the gastrointestinal tract and pass through the liver into the systemic circulation). As indicated in Table 25.5, morphine, hydromorphone, meperidine, and oxymorphone have ratios of oral to intramuscular potency of 1:3 to 1:5. Methadone, levorphanol, and oxycodone are subject to less presystemic elimination, resulting in an oral to intramuscular potency ratio of at least 1:2. The failure to recognize these differences often results in a substantial reduction in analgesia when the change from the parenteral to oral administration is attempted without upward dose titration. Orally administered drugs have a longer onset of action and a longer duration of effect, while drugs administered parenterally have a rapid onset of action but a shorter duration of effect (Jacobson et al., 1997).

Intravenous and Intramuscular. Intravenous bolus administration provides the most rapid onset and shortest duration of action. Time to peak effect correlates with the lipid solubility of the opioid, ranging from 2 to 5 minutes for methadone to 10 to 15 minutes for morphine. Intramuscular and subcutaneous routes are commonly used for postoperative pain and have a slower onset (e.g., 30 to 60 minutes) than intravenous and more rapid onset than oral administration. Continuous intravenous infusion is useful for some patients who cannot be maintained on oral opioids (Ives and Guerra 1987; Portenoy and Payne, 1992). This mode of administration allows for complete systemic absorption and can be supplemented with bolus injections to conveniently titrate opioid dosage in patients with rapidly escalating pain.

Table 25.6. Routes of Opioid Administration

Subcutaneous
Oral
Rectal
Transdermal
    Passive drug transfer
    Active drug transfer (iontophoresis)
Intravenous
Intramuscular
Sublingual
Buccal
Inhalatory
Epidural

Subcutaneous. For patients who cannot absorb orally administered opioids because of nausea and vomiting, gastrointestinal intolerance, or obstruction, parenteral routes can be used. A continuous subcutaneous infusion mode of opioid delivery avoids the problems associated with intramuscular or subcutaneous injection, or poor intravenous access. Most opioids available for parenteral use can be administered by continuous subcutaneous infusion, meperidine being the exception. Using subcutaneous infusion often avoids the need to administer large and repeated parenteral bolus doses to the tolerant patient. The features and limitations of this mode of opioid administration have been described (Coyle et al., 1995).

Rectal. Rectal administration is an alternative to the parenteral route for patients unable to take opioid orally. Rectal suppositories containing hydromorphone, oxymorphone, and morphine are available.

Epidural. Epidural analgesia is widely used for the management of acute postoperative and obstetric pain and provides a longer duration of analgesia at doses lower than required by systemic administration (McQuay, 1994). Cross-tolerance to prior systemic opioids and the rapid development of tolerance to epidural opioids seen in some patients may limit the use of this route. Controlled studies in sickle cell disease patients are required to define the indications and the most appropriate opioids for epidural use.

Transdermal. Transdermal systems for fentanyl (TTS-Fentanyl, Duragesic R®) are currently available in four dosage strengths that vary in drug delivery rate from 25 to 100 µg/hr (Christensen et al., 1996). The systems that currently exist are used in the treatment of chronic pain, although relative potency studies of the type that form the basis for the values in Table 25.5 have not yet been reported. As with other modes of opioid administration, individualization of dosage is required. The patch limits fluctuations in drug concentrations in blood over the dosing interval. When it is removed, drug concentrations in blood decline slowly, so that pharmacodynamic effects may not diminish for many hours and adverse effects must be monitored.

Other Modes of Administration. Patient-controlled analgesia (PCA) is a mode of opioid administration in which patients, within limits, can titrate their analgesia requirements (Holbrook, 1990; McPherson et al., 1990; Perlin et al., 1993; Shapiro et al., 1993). PCA has been widely used for postoperative pain and PCA can be used safely and efficaciously in patients with pain due to sickle cell disease. Controlled studies that clarify some of the psychological issues involved with PCA—how

the patients' knowledge that they are controlling analgesic dosing influences their requirement in a particular environment—are required to help determine the real advantages of PCA over more conventional self-administration techniques, such as oral dosing.

MANAGEMENT OF ACUTE SICKLE PAIN

The management of acute pain in patients with sickle cell disease requires a physician-nurse team that develops a trusting collaborative relationship with the patient, takes pain seriously, assesses its nature, and understands the indications and limitations of treatment.

Stages of Pain Management

Four sequential stages typify pain management (Cleeland, 1993) (Fig. 25.1):

1. Assessment: Health care provider's self-appraisal of attitude as well as of the nature of the pain and its significance for the patient. Providers who understand the pain are more likely to consider a biopsychosocial approach that incorporates treatment modalities besides analgesic. They may also be more likely to use other health care providers with complementary expertise.

2. Treatment: Planning and execution of assessment-based management of pain. Some treatments may be directed toward the source and the sensory features of the pain. Others may be directed toward the emotional responses or the experiential meaning of pain for the patient, such as fear, anxiety, hopelessness, or helplessness (Whitten and Fischhoff, 1974; Fordyce, 1976; Keefe et al., 1992). The objective and subjective features coexist, overlap, and dictate the extent that each treatment is integrated into the plan of care. Where availability of analgesics is a major consideration, measures such as massage, heat, imagery, and relaxation must assume a greater role.

3. Reassessment: Evaluation of the effectiveness of treatment and of changes in the patient's condition.

4. Regimen-adjusting processes: Titration, maintenance, rescue, and tapering: a dynamic system dictated and driven by the feedback loops of reassessment.

Principles of Pain Management

Individualized analgesic therapy is fundamental to the appropriate and successful management of acute sickle cell disease pain (Foley, 1985). This involves assessment-based selection of the right analgesic, administered in the right dose, on the right schedule, with timely and appropriate adjustments that maximize pain relief and minimize adverse effects (Inturrisi and Hanks, 1993). New treatments should be added one at

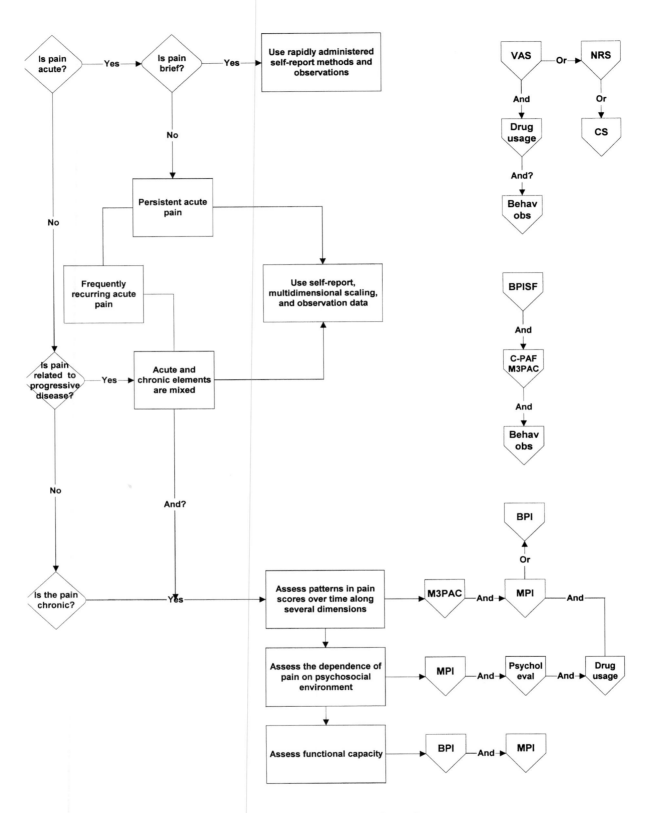

Figure 25.3. Instruments useful for assessing pain in sickle cell disease (from Champan, 1990).

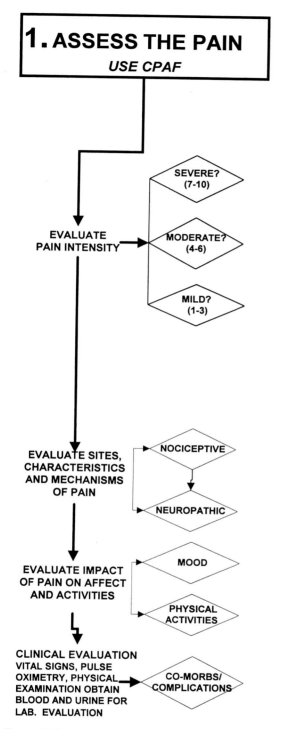

Figure 25.4. Assessment of pain.

a time and reassessed frequently. Adequate time must be allowed for success based on types of treatment.

Pain Assessment Techniques. Sensory and reactive dimensions of pain that will be measured should be specified and instruments should be selected accord-

ingly (Fig. 25.3). Sensory qualities of pain include intensity, location, characteristics, and the underlying physiologic or neurologic mechanisms (Fig. 25.4). Reactive parameters include the interference of pain with physical functioning and distress associated with the patient's emotional suffering due to the combination of the illness and pain.

Acute pain assessment requires that the instruments used for subjective reports:

1. Place a minimal burden on the patient
2. Be easily understood
3. Produce a wide range of scores that show sensitivity to analgesic interventions
4. Demonstrate appropriate reliability and validity (Chapman and Syrjala, 1990; Cleeland and Ryan, 1994).

For pain lasting a few hours, a unidimensional scale (e.g., 10 cm visual analogue or 0 to 10 numerical rating scale of pain intensity) is advocated by many and persistent acute pain (lasting days or weeks) should be evaluated similarly. In the clinical management of persistent acute pain or chronic pain, assessing pain with a multidimensional model that includes self-report, behavioral observations, and functional evaluations is desirable (Fig. 25.3) (Chapman and Syrjala, 1990). The instruments selected should permit evaluation of factors that account for most of the variance in the pain report.

Patients presenting with acute sickle pain should be screened for psychological distress and behavioral manifestations commonly seen in chronic pain syndromes.

The Memorial Pain Assessment Card (MPAC) (Houde 1982) is a simple multidimensional instrument that fits the criteria for use in acute pain settings. It consists of a four-part folding card that assesses: (1) pain intensity on a visual analog scale (VAS); (2) categorical descriptors of pain; (3) relief VAS; and (4) mood VAS. The MPAC requires less than 1 minute to complete and has been validated; the mood scale correlated with more complex multidimensional tools measuring psychologic distress (Fishman et al., 1987). The Montefiore Modification of the Memorial Pain Assessment Card (M₃PAC) replaces the 3 VASs of the MPAC with visual numerical scales (VNS) and adds sedation, where ratings of 0 to 10 are circled (Fig. 25.5). Instead of categorical descriptors, it employs human figure drawings on which painful sites are marked to facilitate delineation of origins.

Categorical pain scales assess pain intensity as none, mild, moderate, or severe (0–3) and relief in response to therapy as none, little, moderate, good, or complete (0–5). Some are critical of this method of assessing pain because there is not linearity among the numbers. Clinically, however, some patients express

DATE ___/__/__ TIME __:__

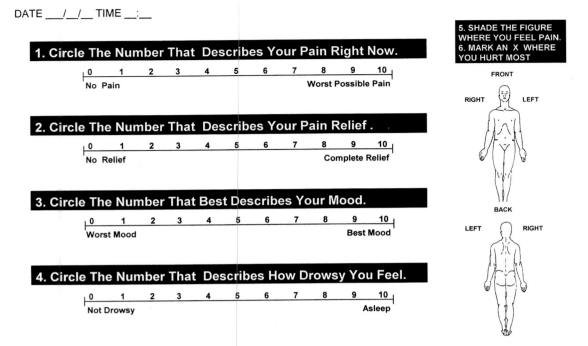

Figure 25.5. The Montefiore Modification of the Memorial Pain Assessment Card (M₃PAC).

Figure 25.6. A pain assessment rating scale.

1. RECORD DATE AND TIME AT EACH ASSESSMENT			
DATE			
TIME (24 HR)			
2. HOW MUCH YOU HURT RIGHT NOW? NO PAIN? = 0 MILD? = 1 MODERATE ? = 2 SEVERE? = 3			
OVERALL			
HEAD			
RIGHT UPPER EXTREMITY			
LEFT UPPER EXTREMITY			
CHEST ANTERIOR			
CHEST POSTERIOR			
RT LOWER EXTREMITY			
LEFT LOWER EXTREMITY			
LOWER BACK			
ABDOMEN			
SUM OF SITES			

their pain and especially their relief with greater certainty with a verbal descriptor scale. Patients will also report that they are consistently "redefining 10" (Benjamin et al., 1999a; 1999b) when the 0 to 10 scale is used as the sole measure. A global (overall) assessment of pain is insufficient, if not inappropriate when pain is persistent because the exacerbations, subsidences, and migration of pain can be missed (Fig. 25.6). Although an assessment including painful sites takes more time, it provides information that helps determine treatment response, and if new pain occurs, allows prompt intervention.

The Brief Pain Inventory Short Form (BPISF) (Benjamin et al., 1996; Cleeland and Ryan, 1994) uses 0 to 10 numerical rating scales to assess present pain intensity (sensory dimension) and pain at its worst, average, and least, as well as pain interference (reactive dimension) with 7 activity and mood related items over the preceding 24 hours. It has been validated in adults with sickle cell disease when used during visits to a Day Hospital (Benjamin et al., 2000). Pain now and least pain are sensitive in measuring response to therapy. Concurrent validity of the M₃PAC and categorical scales for evaluation of acute sickle pain in adults has also been established with the BPISF.

Behavioral observations in adults, alone or as the major modality in pain assessment, can lead to an underestimation of pain, suboptimal treatment, and underestimation of response to treatment. In infants and young children, however, behavioral observation can be very useful (McGrath, 1990). The African-American Oucher Scale, which contains faces of

African-American children, is valid for assessing their pain (Beyer and Knott, 1998).

Bioclinical Pain Assessment. Sickle cell painful episodes are a source of frustration to physicians since objective signs of the pain are lacking. Many providers are uncomfortable with the notion that the patient is the pain authority and the self-report the gold standard. That, coupled with a discomfort prescribing opioids, causes some patient assessments to be totally based on perceived behaviors or disregarded entirely, and the patient to be perceived as faking. While consistency with appropriately selected assessments should eliminate some of these biases, the quest for objective tests for pain and a monitor of response to therapy continues.

Some biologic markers of pain have been defined. Dense sickle erythrocytes decrease during the course of a painful episode (Fabry et al., 1984), and RDW (the coefficient of variation of red cell volume calculated by the Coulter Counter) and hemoglobin distribution width (HDW) (calculated by the Bayer H*3, a measure of the distribution of intracellular hemoglobin concentrations) (Lawrence and Fabry, 1985, Billet et al., 1988a, 1988b) change. The clinical utility of these tests to diagnose and treat painful episodes is being tested. Since dense cells vary with clinical state, reference to a steady-state level is indispensable for interpreting changes during the evolution of pain.

Disappearing dense cells have been reported as secondary to their trapping in the microcirculation, propagating vascular obstruction (Kaul et al., 1996) (Chapter 20). Other studies have noted a lack of relationship between dense cells and number of painful crises (Warth and Rucknagel, 1984) and have shown an inverse relationship between sickle erythrocyte deformability and numbers of irreversible sickled cells and painful event rates. Dense cells not only participate in vasoocclusion, they also have major roles in the pathogenesis of hemolytic anemia. Thus, changes in relative amounts of dense cells could be attributed to one or any combination of independent phenomena that include changes in their rate of formation, changes in their rate of destruction or sequestration, or changes in the relative size of other cell subpopulations (see Chapters 20–22). Nonetheless, there is a potential value in monitoring changes in dense cells that may provide insight into the development and course of painful episodes and be helpful in monitoring therapeutic interventions, like hydroxyurea, that influence cell density.

A complex series of events involving inflammatory mediators also occurs during vasoocclusion. Acute phase reactants like C reactive protein (CRP) and serum amyloid A (SAA) and inflammatory cytokines like IL-6 are increased during painful events (Benjamin et al., 1993). Physiological and psychological adjustments are made by the body and the stress response of the hypothalamic-pituitary-adrenal axis is activated. Some changes or adjustments that can be appreciated clinically include fever, leukocytosis and shift in liver metabolism which results in increased acute phase proteins. Behavioral changes include reduced activity, reduced food and water intake, increased pain sensitivity and reactivity, cognitive alterations and depressed mood. The activity of the sympathetic nervous system and the hypothalamic-pituitary axis is increased. Nitric oxide (NO) levels have also been reported to be altered during painful episodes (Rees et al., 1995). These interrelated mediators of inflammation affect endothelial cells, macrophages, hepatocytes, and neuronal tissue, all of which contain inducible nitric oxide synthase (iNOS). Several clinical features of patients with sickle cell disease suggest endothelial dysfunction and abnormalities in NO synthesis. These include relative hypotension, glomerular hyperfiltration, and priapism. Vascular endothelial cells have been found to have μ3 opioid receptors that, when exposed to opioids, release NO (Stefano et al., 1995). Therapeutic effects can be altered when endothelium is damaged, and exposure to agents like morphine can possibly cause paradoxical vasoconstriction.

Pain is the final common pathway of many processes. While difficult, it may be helpful to identify in individuals which mechanisms are dominant in the pathophysiology of a given painful event.

Analgesic Selection. Initially, pain intensity drives treatment decisions (Fig. 25.7). The World Health Organization (WHO) Analgesic Ladder provides an operational framework for selection of agents according to intensity. Non-opioids or aspirin equivalent analgesics such as acetaminophen or NSAIDS are prescribed for mild pain (Table 25.3); with moderate pain or pain that breaks through treatment with non-opioids alone, an opioid such as codeine or its equivalent is added; with severe pain, morphine or an equivalent opioid is the drug of choice, given either alone or in combination with non-opioids. At all pain levels, adjuvant drugs are added when indicated based upon pain characteristics and side effects as detailed below (Jacox et al., 1994).

Determining a Starting Dose and Treating the Patient Promptly. A starting dose is determined by the intensity of the pain and prior analgesic history. If a patient presents with severe pain and is receiving morphine-equivalent opioid treatment for the first time, 4 to 5 mg IV or 8 to 10 mg of morphine SC or IM could be an appropriate starting dose. In children, the starting dose could be 0.1 to 0.15 mg/kg of morphine (Weisman and Schechter, 1992; Benjamin

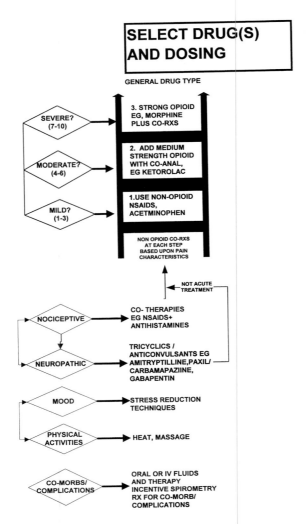

Figure 25.7. Classes of analgesic drugs for different pain severity and co-therapies that may be useful. Initially, pain intensity drives treatment decisions. The World Health Organization (WHO) Analgesic Ladder provides an operational framework for selection of agents according to pain intensity.

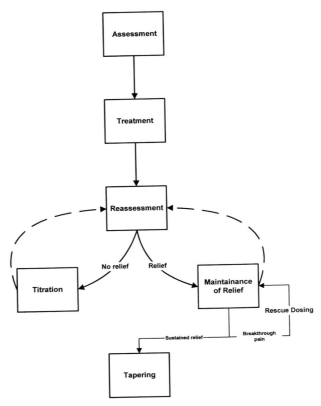

Figure 25.8. Stages in management of the acute painful episode. Treatment adjustment practices include titration, maintenance, rescue dosing, and dose tapering.

et al., 1999a, 1999b). In a patient previously treated with morphine-equivalent opioids, the starting dose would be based on history of the efficacious and safe dosage generally required by the patient for pain of similar intensity.

Rapid Reassessment (Fig. 25.8). Reassessment is based on the efficacy and side effects of the therapy that is administered throughout the treatment course. Given the inability to predict the nature and course of pain or the response to any analgesic selected, a rapidly administered multidimensional tool is preferable to a simplified unidimensional pain intensity scale of 0 to 10 as the sole measure of pain and response to therapy. Global pain intensity difference, pain characteristics, pain relief, and mood are measures that can

be used to gauge efficacy while the sedation scale is used for side effects.

The mood scale also screens for psychological distress and can indicate whether additional interventions are required. Pain memories and expectations and the process by which the individual decides to deal with the pain are also assessed. The use of several pain scales allows for repetitive valid measurement of pain intensity, relief, and mood. Inadequate assessment is a major obstacle to matching treatment to needs and a major factor in undertreatment.

Dose Adjustments. After the initial treatment, dose scheduling is crucial to the effectiveness of any analgesic. Treatment adjustment practices include titration, maintenance, rescue dosing, and dose tapering (Fig. 25.8). Responsiveness to therapy refers to the balance between analgesia and its side effects and indicates that satisfactory relief without intolerable or unmanageable side effects can be accomplished (Fig. 25.9). Labeling individuals resistant or poor responders to treatment or impossible to treat is inappropriate if titration has not been attempted. If pain is controlled with the loading dose, a titration phase might be unnecessary. Then, maintenance and rescue dosing would be instituted. If

TREATMENT ADJUSTMENT DECISIONS

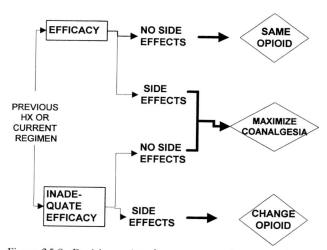

Figure 25.9. Decision points for treatment adjustment of acute pain.

Figure 25.10. Titration of drugs used for pain relief in sickle cell disease.

pain is not adequately relieved with the loading dose, the maintenance medication dose and intervals should be determined following dose titration. When pain relief is sustained, the drug is slowly tapered and discontinued. The WHO Ladder is then employed for remaining or new pain.

Titration. Titration should not be confused with prn dosing, where the patient must request medication after pain returns to a level requiring treatment and the treatment is given only if the request falls within a predetermined time limit. Dose titration, through frequent reassessment of responsiveness to therapy and prompt retreatment at 15 to 30 minutes, permits individualization of care and adjusts for intrapatient pharmacokinetic, pharmacodynamic, and pharmacogenetic differences. Titration can be done by several methods (Fig. 25.10), and frequent reassessments and prompt treatment based on the reassessments are critical. After the initial dose, one method would be to give half the starting dose following each reassessment at intervals as frequent as every 30 minutes, titrating to good pain relief. Vital signs and O_2 saturation should be monitored closely and the patient should be observed for excessive sedation. Usually dose titration is accomplished within 2 to 4 hours. PCA devices can be used for dose titration

DOSE ADJUSTMENT: TITRATION

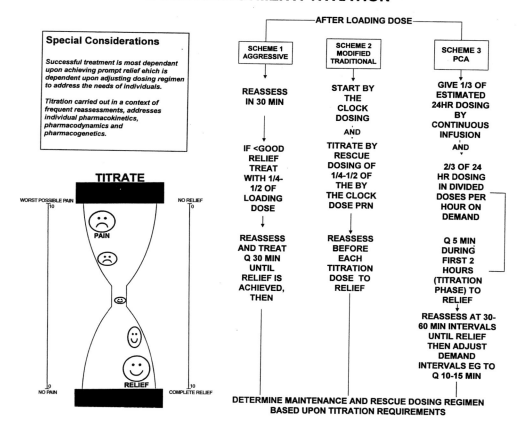

and maintenance or for maintenance therapy following titration with bolus or infusion dosing.

Maintenance Dosing and Rescue Dosing. Maintenance dosing also varies widely. Thus, the dose and intervals selected as maintenance dosing should always be accompanied by rescue dosing that can be employed as needed for additional titration or for breakthrough pain.

A starting maintenance dose can be the medication required in the titration phase divided by the hours treated, or the hourly dose can be set at half of the loading dose divided by the elimination half-life in hours (Max, 1990). The dosing interval can be determined by observing a treated patient until the pain first reappears and prescribing for intervals that fit within that time. An alternative method would be to rely on the history. After determining the appropriate dose and dosing intervals—this could be every 2 to 3 hours—an around-the-clock schedule should be begun. A rescue dose of one-quarter to one-half the maintenance dose prn should be prescribed for breakthrough pain. Deciding whether to arouse a sleeping patient for a maintenance dose is a

matter of clinical judgment but bypassing a scheduled administration of a short half-life medication is probably unwise inasmuch as the pharmacologic objective is to maintain the plasma level of the drug above a minimal effective level. For more prudent management, a long-acting sustained-relief preparation could be prescribed to maintain relief during sleep, or if for some reason oral agents are not tolerated, a transdermal patch, while not a treatment for acute pain, could be tried for continuous delivery of enough opioid to control pain during the night. Alternatively, one-third of the estimated 24-hour dosing could be administered by continuous infusion (Payne, 1989; Benjamin, 1990).

Ideally, once the maintenance and rescue dosing are established, reassessments will dictate continued therapy until the patient's condition permits dose reduction by tapering (Fig. 25.11). More commonly, reassessment will uncover changes in the clinical response to therapy that require modifications in the dosing regimen related to pharmacologic properties of the drugs,

Figure 25.11. Drug dose titration and tapering.

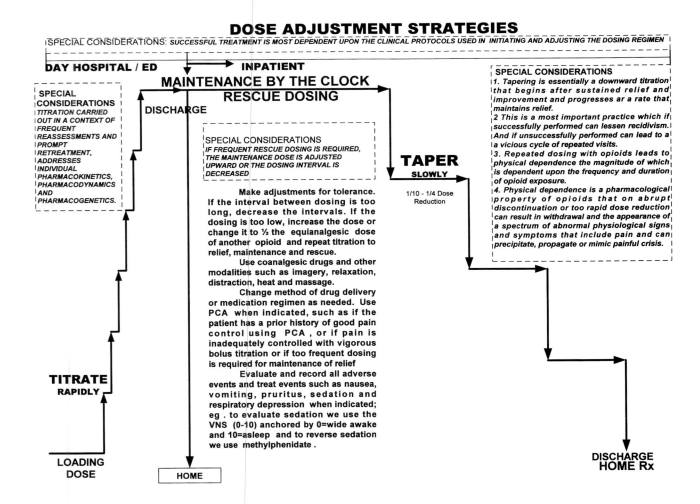

pain mechanisms and host factors. Perhaps disease-induced elements and factors related to suboptimal pain treatment over time can cause physical and behavioral changes that can alter opioid responsiveness.

Development of Tolerance. Tolerance—lowered drug responsiveness requiring adjustments to a higher dose to maintain analgesia—is probably the primary reason for opioid analgesic dose escalation. Tolerance can significantly diminish a favorable balance of analgesia and side effects and limit opioid usage. The initial adjustment is increased dose or decreased intervals. It often results in an increase in the side effects of constipation and sedation and, at higher doses, in adverse effects including myoclonus, grand mal seizures, cognitive impairment, and hallucinations. If side effects occur with pain relief, adjuvant therapies to enhance analgesia and lessen the opioid requirement can be used (Fig. 25.9). If pain relief is not restored and side effects increase, the opioid can be changed.

Changing Drug or Route of Administration. When opioids are switched, often the lack of attention to route-dependent differences in dose accounts for the common reports of undermedication. A table of relative potency provides a framework for a starting point (Table 25.5). If switches are needed for reasons of tolerance, toxicity, or lack of efficacy, the equianalgesic starting dose of the new drug should be decreased by half because of incomplete cross-tolerance, and the dose titrated to the patient's needs.

The relative potency of some opioid analgesics may change with repetitive dosing, particularly opioids with a long plasma halflife such as methadone (Bruera et al., 1996a). The slower onset of analgesia after oral administration often requires some adaptation by a patient who is accustomed to the more rapid parenteral onset. If switching from the parenteral to oral routes presents problems, one solution might be to reduce the parenteral dose slowly and increase the oral dose over a 2 to 3 day period. When parenteral meperidine is used for severe acute pain, its usage beyond a few days can be hazardous. Prescribing oral meperidine for acute and chronic pain is discouraged. (see above)

Altered Opioid Pharmacokinetics. Opioid pharmacokinetics are altered by drug-disease interactions. Clinically, the duration of action depends on the dose, pain intensity, prior opioid experience, and pharmacokinetics and must be assessed in each individual. Several factors could contribute to altered analgesic pharmacokinetics in patients with sickle cell disease. These include increased binding of opioids to acute phase reactants, liver damage that alters drug metabolism, and hyperfiltration and hyposthenuria that increase drug clearance

(Olkkola et al., 1995; Olsen, 1975). The acute phase reactant alpha$_1$ acid glycoprotein has been shown to increase binding of meperidine, decreasing its availability for analgesia (Williams et al., 1985; Kremer et al., 1988). Decreased metabolism may decrease morphine efficacy because a metabolite, morphine-6-glucuronide, accounts for most of the analgesic action. Moreover, increased renal clearance may accelerate the removal of the metabolite, further decreasing the drug's analgesic action. Pharmacokinetic studies are warranted in persons whose management is consistently compromised by lack of efficacy or unacceptable side effects (Portenoy, 1994).

Pharmacogenetic Impact on Altered Opioid Responsiveness. Genetic differences rather than drug-seeking behavior should be considered first as a cause of poor responsiveness to treatment. The cytochrome P450 system plays a crucial role in the metabolism of most drugs, and genetic polymorphisms can be responsible for both the failure of therapeutic agents and their adverse effects. The CYP 2D6 enzyme is one of more than 30 subsets of the CYP system, and it plays a major role in the transformation of drugs to active or inactive forms; it transforms codeine into morphine and hydrocodone into hydromorphone (Mortimer et al., 1990; Quiding et al., 1992) (Table 25.7). CYP 2D6 polymorphisms have been found in approximately 7 percent of people of African and European descent.

When codeine is prescribed for moderate pain, the inborn inability to metabolize it to morphine will reduce the drug's efficacy and increase the side effects attributable to codeine, which will accumulate. In poor metabolizers, meperidine could produce greater efficacy and fewer side effects because of decreased conversion to the toxic metabolite, while morphine could be less effective because of reduced conversion to its active metabolite. Conversely, extensive metabolizers of morphine would convert to more active derivatives with increased efficacy while in such individuals receiving meperidine, toxicity from normeperidine would be increased. Some investigators have suggested that patients deficient in CYP 2D6 may have a lower pain threshold (Sindrup et al., 1991).

Table 25.7. Metabolism of Weak/Moderate Opioid to Strong Opioids

Opioid ⟶	Metabolic fate
Codeine	Morphine
Hydrocodone	Hydromorphone
Oxycodone	Oxymorphone

Table 25.8. Adjuvant Drugs for Pain

Drug	Dosage	Therapeutic effects	Comments
Steroids			
Corticosteroids			
Prednisolone	10 mg tid PO	Potentiates analgesia Elevates mood Improves appetite	Effective for pain caused by compression of nerves or spinal cord or from intracranial pressure; risk of GI bleeding
Dexamethasone	4 mg PO q6h or less	Potentiates analgesia	Side effects: nausea, vomiting, fluid retention → hypertension, edema, cardiac failure
Progestin			
Medroxyprogesterone acetate	2–3 g/d for 10 days; 2 g for 3 weeks; 1 g thereafter		
Antidepressants			
Amitriptyline	Start 10–25 mg hs, increase gradually to 75–100 mg hs	Potentiates opioid analgesia Elevates mood, induces sleep	Effective for deafferentation pain (postherpetic neuralgia)
Doxepin	Start 10–20 mg hs, increase gradually to 75–150 mg		
Imipramine	200 mg hs for severe depression	Antidepressant	High dose to treat severe depression as required
Anxiolytics			
Hydroxyzine	Start with 25 mg tid PO; increase to 50–100 mg q4–6h	Potentiates opioid analgesia Reduces anxiety	
Diazepam	5–10 mg PO, IV, or rectally bid or tid	Relief of acute anxiety and panic; also antiemetic and sedative	More antiemetic and fewer sedative effects than chlorpromazine; risk of orthostatic hypotension and hypotonia
Phenothiazines			
Methotrimeprazine	10–20 mg IM or 20–30 mg PO	Produces moderate analgesia without risk of tolerance or physical dependence	Used as alternative to narcotics if they are contraindicated
Chlorpromazine	10–25 mg q4–8h	Reduces anxiety Produces hypnosis	Risk of orthostatic hypotension; rarely causes jaundice and neurologic reaction
Prochlorperazine	5–10 mg q4–8h	Antiemetic No analgesic effect Reduces anxiety	
Fluphenazine	1–3 mg every day		Combined with an antidepressant, useful in neuropathic pain
		Antiemetic Analgesic	
Haloperidol	Start 1 mg tid PO, increase to 2–4 mg tid PO	Decreases confusion	More potent antiemetic than chlorpromazine
		Antiemetic	
Anticonvulsant			
Carbamazepine	Start 100 mg daily, increase by 100 mg q4 days to 500–800 mg/d	Anticonvulsant	Useful for neuropathic pain; continuous hematologic monitoring required Decreases abnormal CNS neuronal activity

To take clinical advantage of pharmacogenetic differences, tests for polymorphisms must become routine. Then the choice of drugs and dosing regimen could be based on the patient's metabolic profile.

Adjuvant Drugs to Increase Efficacy and Lessen Side Effects (Table 25.8). Maintenance opioid therapy that includes nonopioid drugs can improve a patient's quality of life. Antihistamines, particularly hydroxyzine, are the most common adjuvant medications used in combination with opioids or with opioids plus NSAIDs. They counteract the opioid-induced release of histamines by mast cells, reduce nausea, and have sedating properties.

Pain characteristics can help estimate the possibility of a neuropathic component (Fig. 25.4). While most adjuvant therapies targeting neuropathic pain have a slow onset of action requiring weeks for efficacy, the recognition of this mechanism as a possible component of the pain in the acute setting is important (American Pain Society, Quality of Care Committee, 1995).

Epicritic lancinating, sharp, or prickly pain is variably responsive to anticonvulsants. Agents that suppress neuronal firing rates include carbamazepine, phenytoin, valproate, lamotrigine, gabapentin, benzodiazepines, and barbiturates. Side effects of major concern include drowsiness, dizziness, headache, nausea, vomiting, and diplopia. Idiosyncratic reactions include aplastic anemia and hepatic failure. Protopathic pain is usually described as dull, burning, and poorly localized and it is commonly treated with antidepressants. The tricyclic antidepressants and serotonin reuptake inhibitors have the most analgesic actions. Amitriptyline is favored as a first choice because it exhibits greater balance in its nora-drenergic/serotonin reuptake inhibitor properties. Side effects of tricyclic antidepressants include dry mouth, urinary retention, somnolence, memory impairment, cardiac arrhythmias, orthostatic hypotension, and weight gain. If introduced slowly, tolerance to most of the side effects will develop over time. Besides systemic treatments, topical application of capsaicin has proved useful in some forms of neuropathic pain (Dejgard et al., 1988).

Other adjuvant therapies have a limited but important role in pain treatment (Table 25.8). These include steroids (Bruera et al., 1985), the alpha-2 adrenergic agent clonidine (Max et al., 1990), phenothiazines (Lechin et al., 1989), local anesthetics such as lidocaine or mexiletine (Dejgard et al., 1988), bisphosphonates, and benzodiazepines (Swerdlow, 1984). Only intravenous steroids and epidural lidocaine have received attention in sickle cell disease (Griffin et al., 1994; Yaster et al., 1994). The benefits do not outweigh the risks of causing or exacerbating preexisting osteonecrosis or, in the case of steroids, occult infection. In one study of corticosteroids in acute painful episodes in children, pain was relieved initially but most patients returned to the emergency department with recurring pain within 24 hours (Griffin et al., 1994).

Psychological and Physical Modalities. Although pain intensity and quality are the main criteria for

Figure 25.12. Planning treatment of pain in sickle cell disease. Besides opioid drugs, psychological, cognitive, behavioral, and physical assessment should figure prominently in the treatment plan.

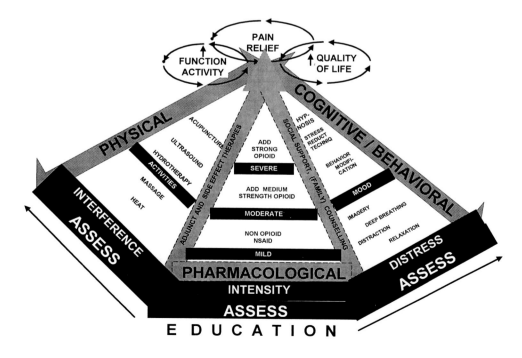

drug selection, psychological, cognitive, behavioral, and physical assessment should figure prominently in the treatment plan (Fig. 25.12). Relaxation, imagery, and stress reduction techniques (Turk, 1996b) can change dysfunctional thinking patterns. The coping strategies used by an individual can be major predictors of pain and adjustment to sickle cell disease in children and adolescents. In one study, active coping strategies were associated with fewer emergency department visits (Gil et al., 1993). Behavioral strategies seek to replace anxiety and distress with more adaptive behaviors.

Medication use is a common measure of pain behavior. Although subject to the bias of self-reporting at home, it can be an objective measure in the hospital. Self-regulation approaches have been evaluated in sickle cell disease with the speculation that the positive effects of this approach could influence not only psychological factors but also cause vasodilation and an increase in skin temperature (Hall et al., 1992), as has been accomplished by biofeedback and hypnosis (Zeltzer et al., 1979; Thomas et al., 1984; Cozzi et al., 1987; Hall et al., 1992). While most patients were amenable to this approach, patients with major psychological factors influencing their pain were generally not motivated to learn self-regulation.

Physical measures that could be employed include heat and massage. Heat has cellular, vascular, and musculoskeletal effects. It increases cellular metabolism, oxygen demand, and arterial flow. Acupuncture (Co et al., 1979), ultrasound, and physical manipulations are best prescribed by physiatrists and performed by skilled physical therapists.

Tapering. Opioid administration leads to physiologic adaptation of the body to opioid presence (physical dependence). To prevent withdrawal, opioid use should be tapered over several days (Fig. 25.12). How tapering will occur should be based on assessments and explained in the collaborative treatment plan. The route and intervals of administration that were used for treatment should be continued at least until the dose has been tapered to half the starting dose without increasing pain. Less anxiety-provoking for the patient, this permits the tapering process to continue with greater confidence in predicting and assessing the response to medication and it does not introduce confounding factors such as wide variations in the bioavailability of oral drugs.

Various tapering schemes are possible, but the pain should be controlled at each step of the taper. One method is to decrease the dose by 25 percent, alternating with the original dose at the onset of tapering (Fig. 25.11). If the patient is receiving 8 mg of morphine every 2 hours, 8 mg alternating with 6 mg every 2 hours for at least 2 cycles of each dose should be given. If both

control pain equally, then 6 mg every 2 hours followed by 6 mg alternating with 4 mg, and so on, can be given until tapering is completed. During this process assessments should continue with the same diligence employed during the titration and maintenance phases. Tapering is essentially downward titration. Each dose must be adequate for maintaining pain control with a reduction in dosing until the patient is both free of significant pain (VAS <4) and free of morphine equivalent opioids or the patient can be discharged home on oral medication. A rush to discharge without adequate drug tapering or a switch to an oral dose that is not equianalgesic can create problems of recidivism and sometimes, the "iatrogenic pseudoaddiction syndrome," a term coined to capture some consequences of undertreatment (see below). Adjuvant therapies such as clonidine (oral or transdermal 0.1 mg daily) to override withdrawal symptoms, antidepressants, education, and self-administered techniques such as imagery, relaxation, and behavior modification could prove vital to the success of achieving and maintaining the results of tapering.

Following the observation of at least 12 but preferably 24 hours with stability or continued resolution of pain, the patient can be discharged. Although this management strategy will lessen early recidivism, strategies centered on switching to morphine-equivalent short half-life oral medication and discharging patients to complete treatment on their own and to self-taper will sometimes work. This practice may be initially successful but backfire when repeated over many episodes.

Economic imperatives forcing early discharge might best be dealt with by emphasizing assessment-based treatment that follows the principles of pain management. Patients experiencing signs of withdrawal should be assessed to find out the extent of symptoms (Table 25.9). These patients, and those who exhibit frequent recidivism, should be provided with early intervention and prevention by more judicious tapering coupled with the use of adjuvant medications and techniques. The economic benefit of shortening a single hospitalization should be weighed against the possibility of frequent future hospitalizations (Yang et al., 1995b; Davis et al., 1997; Woods et al., 1997).

Home Treatment. A graded stepladder approach based on pain intensity is employed when a nonopioid (aspirin equivalent) analgesic alone and a codeine-equivalent opioid analgesic in combination with a nonopioid analgesic are prescribed for home use. When oral morphine-equivalent opioids are also required for home use, the opioid should not be the same as that used for acute severe pain.

Follow-up psychological, cognitive, behavioral, and physical factors should figure prominently in the plan for ongoing pain management (Fig. 25.12). During

Table 25.9. Himmelsbach Scale for Abstinence Assessment

Mild	1. Yawning
	2. Lacrimation
	3. Rhinorrhea
	4. Perspiration
Moderate	5. Muscle tremor
	6. Dilated pupils
	7. Goose flesh
	8. Anorexia
Marked	9. Air hunger
	10. Restlessness
	11. Insomnia
	12. Elevated blood pressure
Severe	13. Emesis
	14. Diarrhea
	15. Weight loss

follow-up outpatient visits, these assessments can be expanded and explored in greater detail as possible precipitants or propagators of pain. Based on these assessments, techniques such as biofeedback, hypnosis, electrical stimulation, heat, and massage should be factored into treatment by a multidisciplinary team.

Unfortunately, a few patients have such frequent visits to emergency departments and hospital admissions for recurring or persistent pain that they do not keep appointments for follow-up and routine health maintenance visits. Their management is generally one of crisis intervention with acute and chronic opioid therapy with little or no attention to psychosocial or experiential factors.

APPROACH TO THE PATIENT WITH FREQUENT PAIN EPISODES

Difficult patients are not just born; they are, in part, created by their passage through the medical system. Not only has this system failed to cure; it may have done unpleasant things to make matters worse. (Hartrick and Pitcher, 1995)

Overview

Recurrent acute painful events superimposed on a background of constant pain present the most perplexing and vexing problem in the care of patients with sickle cell disease. The admission note for persons who are admitted for frequent pain generally reads, "This is one of multiple admissions for this 20-year old male/female well known to...." Actually, these patients in their current predicament are rarely

known, in part because they are only seen in the emergency department or comparable outpatient facility or during an admission where conducting an in-depth assessment is impossible. They are designated negatively by harsh terms such as "drug seeking" or are called addicted to opioids or "frequent flyers."

Owing to the complex manner in which each person arrives at this frequent pain state, which may be influenced by disease progression, comorbidities, psychosocial pathology, and inadequate pain treatment, the relative contributions of each factor have often gone unappreciated. Fragmented care by multiple providers, the lack of stability in subsequent provider/patient relationships, and the instability of a patient whose life has been disrupted by frequent pain and whose pain beliefs derive from experience, present an apparent insurmountable obstacle to treatment.

Some patients have literally fallen into a downward spiral of frequent pain as a by-product of disparate practices in the use of opioids (Fig. 25.13). These practices violate principle-based strategies until the patient is hopelessly entrapped in a behavior that becomes a self-fulfilling prophecy regarding perceived drug-seeking motives. As one person with sickle cell disease stated, "Regarding drug seeking behavior, yes! When I come to the hospital, I am seeking drugs—to relieve my pain."

Caregivers who regard each painful event of most persons who have frequent visits to emergency departments and hospitalizations as drug-seeking behavior will often withhold medication while another well-meaning approach is to "just give them what they want" through liberal prescription writing. Pain medication issues become all consuming and disease-related factors as contributors to pain can be neglected, leading to the labeling of some patients as "addicts." Fixating on drug abuse liability and confusing withdrawal with physical dependence or iatrogenic pseudoaddiction resulting from the endless loop created by unrelieved pain in a disease requiring opioids for pain severely compromises management (Weisman and Haddox, 1989).

As the frequency of admissions for painful events increases, the patient's report of pain is less likely to be believed and undermedication becomes more common (Armstrong et al., 1995). If pain management practices are optimal, then efforts to identify coexisting morbidities and their more intensive treatment with hydroxyurea or blood transfusions, for example, may be indicated.

Consequences of Uncritical Opioid Use

In sickle cell disease as in other painful conditions (Cousins, 1989), a tendency exists to undermedicate patients who require opioids during acute pain because of fear of addiction (Marks and Sacher, 1973)

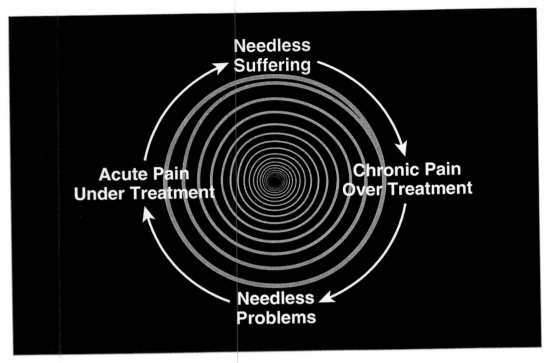

Figure 25.13. Cycle of pain in sickle cell disease.

Figure 25.14. Sequelae of suboptimal pain treatment for the acute painful episode of sickle cell disease. Too little medication results in needless suffering due to unrelieved pain, withdrawal, and altered opioid responsiveness while excessive medication results in needless problems of increased pain—allodynia, hyperalgesia, and side effects.

and to overmedicate them during chronic pain due to insufficient knowledge of clinical pharmacology. Too little medication results in needless suffering due to unrelieved pain, withdrawal, and altered opioid responsiveness (Fig. 25.14). Too much results in needless problems of increased pain—allodynia, hyperalgesia, and side effects.

The utility of a regimen is measured by its good and bad effects and by the dangers of nontreatment. Undertreatment leads to increased pain and longer

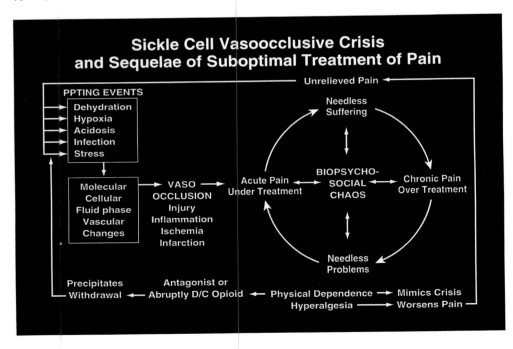

hospitalizations. Respiratory impairment and mental changes can occur with under- or overtreatment. Splinting and atelectasis—consequences of unrelieved pain—are more likely than opioid-induced respiratory depression since tolerance to this side effect generally occurs before tolerance to the analgesic effect. Opioid use and misuse have created a crisis in pain management in sickle cell disease plagued by myth, anecdote, empirical observation, and mistrust, magnified by the failure in provider-patient communication (Weisman and Haddox, 1989; Benjamin et al., 1994). The stages of treatment leading to iatrogenic pseudoaddiction and awareness that this treatment-induced entity is preventable should provide incentive for improving pain management.

Considering the importance of the opioid analgesic agents in the management of acute and chronic pain in sickle cell disease, strategies to improve opioid responsiveness with their use would be valuable. A series of studies has implicated the EAA receptor system in the development and maintenance of morphine tolerance, dependence, and sensitization. Inturrissi (1993) has shown the ability of a competitive (LY274614) and several noncompetitive NMDA receptor antagonists including dextromethorphan, ketamine, and d-methadone to attenuate or reverse the development of tolerance to morphine's antinociceptive (analgesic) effect. Besides reduction of tolerance by, for example, coadministration of NMDA antagonists (Elliot et al., 1995), agents that selectively block excitatory opioid receptor functions, such as calcium channel blockers (Santillan et al., 1994; Mayer et al., 1995) and ultra-low-dose naloxone and naltrexone, are commercially available and could be useful (Crain and Shen, 1995).

Efforts to develop a model approach for optimization of care and destigmatization of individuals experiencing frequently recurring pain and requiring chronic and frequent opioid therapy have suggested the following program (Benjamin et al., 1994).

Improved Functioning and Decreased Hospitalizations for the Patient with Frequent Pain (Fig. 25.15)

Intake/Assessment. A preparatory phase discusses why the individual is a candidate for the protocol—from the patient's and caregivers' perspectives—its purpose, general goals, and steps, and may require several visits. History, physical examination, and initial psychosocial assessment should include a detailed pain and pain management history with an estimate of the average daily requirement of opioids and other analgesics. Records from other facilities are often helpful.

Patient Education and Consent. Terms placing the program in a pain management context should be used. Many persons who find themselves in the frequent pain category are hypersensitive to any suggestion of abuse or addiction. "Opioid" should be used instead of "narcotic," "medication" instead of "drug," "physical dependence" rather than "addiction," and "taper" rather than "detox program." Patients should understand that pain can have different causes. While assessment tools will be used, current suffering is expressed in the narrative; patients must be allowed to tell their story and past, present, and future pain management should be discussed with the available cognitive behavioral strategies (Table 25.10).

Stabilization Phase: Change from a Short to a Long Half-Life Opioid (Table 25.11). The physiological impact of chronic short-acting opioids like morphine is different from the physiological impact of long-acting opioids like methadone. Physiological effects of a short half-life opioid are the net result of the intermittent peaks of opioid actions and side effects, followed by relative withdrawal that occurs approximately 4 times daily. Methadone and other long-acting agents have sustained effects at specific opioid receptors or other sites of action, also dependent upon their pharmacokinetic properties, but with only one daily cycle and no opioid withdrawal. Tolerance to the acute effects of nausea and sedation develops commonly while analgesia tolerance and physical dependence develop variably.

Stabilization of the Hypothalamic-Pituitary-Adrenal Axis. Neuroendocrine alterations accompany pain and vary according to opioid pharmacokinetics. Most sickle cell disease patients require intermittent opioid treatment for acute painful episodes but some require daily opioids. Opioids may change neurotransmitter-neuroendocrine function (Kreek, 1992; Reisine et al., 1995). When administered acutely, both short-acting and long-acting exogenous opioids have similar effects on neuroendocrine function. Chronic administration of short-acting opiates like morphine seems to have the same effects as acute opiate administration. In contrast, chronic administration of a long-acting exogenous opioid like methadone seems to have a different effect and allows normalization of neuroendocrine function (Kreek, 1992). In humans, acute opiate administration causes inhibition of ACTH, luteinizing hormone, and β endorphin release; altered cortisol release; lower blood levels of testosterone and cortisol with flattened diurnal variation of the latter; and increased release of vasopressin and prolactin.(Kreek, 1992). Methadone is very useful in normalizing the hypothalamic-adrenal-pituitary axis (Kreek, 1992; 1996a).

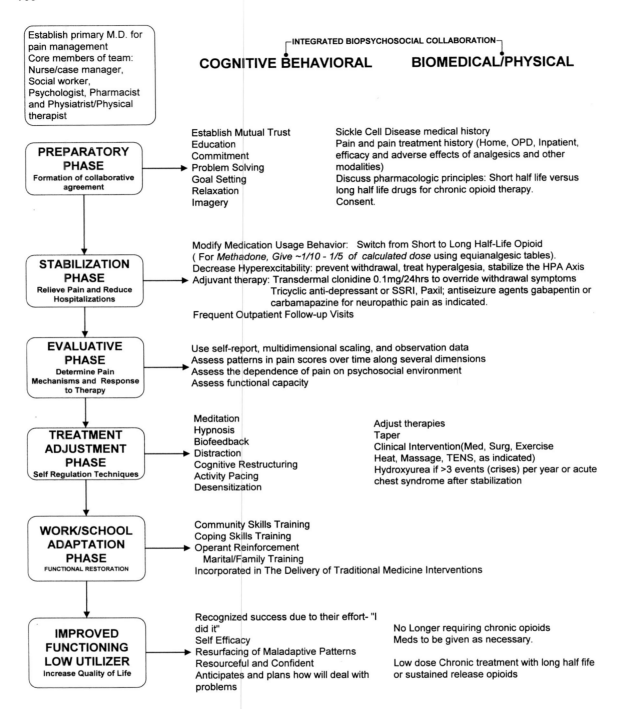

Figure 25.15. Approach to management of the patient with sickle cell disease with frequent attacks of acute pain.

Determine the Equianalgesic Dose of Methadone. The methadone equianalgesic dose can be adjusted by one-fifth to one-tenth depending on the amount and duration of daily dosing. When individuals are treated chronically and with high dose short-acting opioids, the equianalgesic ratios change (Manfredi et al., 1997;

Bruera et al., 1996a; 1996b). One can arrive at a similar dosing ratio by adjusting by half for tolerance, three-fourths for physical dependence, and a factor for tolerance. If the 24-hour dose for an individual is 120 mg parenteral morphine equivalents, an adjustment for tolerance would be 120 mg methadone orally and an adjustment for physical dependence would be 60 mg methadone orally.

Dose and dosing intervals should be calculated according to patient needs (q6 to q12h). Once stability

Table 25.10. Cognitive–Behavioral Objectives

Objectives	Practices	Specify individual issues
Combat demoralization	Reconceptualize patients' view of problem from overwhelming to manageable	
Enhance outcome efficacy	Skills to deal adaptively with problems included in treatment	
Foster self-advocacy	Reconceptualize from passive, reactive, and helpless to active, resourceful and competent	
Break up automatative maladaptive patterns	Monitor thoughts, feelings and behavior and learned interrelationships	
Skills training	Overt and covert behavior, how to respond adaptively to problems	
Attribute success to their efforts	Reiterate	
Facilitate maintenance and generalization	Anticipate and plan for how to deal with problems	

Source: Adapted from Fernandez and Turk, 1989.

is reached the dose should not be increased. Methadone is a racemic mixture. Its dextroisomer has NMDA antagonist properties, which decreases the potential for tolerance (Inturrisi et al., 1990). Other morphine equivalent opioids should not be used concurrently with methadone on an outpatient basis. During acute episodes methadone should be adjusted to approximately one-third of the chronic dose and titrated with short half-life agents. If the patient is hospitalized, the goal of tapering is to discontinue the drug or to change to a low dose long half-life agent.

Table 25.11. Plasma Half-Life Values for Opioids and Their Active Metabolites

Plasma half-life	Hours
Short Half-Life opioids	
Morphine	2–3.5
Hydromorphone	2–3
Codeine	3
Meperidine	3–4
Pentazocine*	2–3
Nalbuphine*	5
Butorphanol*	2.5–3.5
Long Half-Life opioids	
Methadone	24
Levorphanol	12–16
Propoxyphene	12
Norpropoxyphene†	30–40
Normeperidine†	14–21

* Agonist-antagonists.
† Metabolite of propoxyphene with metabolite of meperidine.

Clonidine patches 0.1 mg/24 hrs. can be used to suppress withdrawal symptoms whether converting from short to long-acting medications or tapering to prevent withdrawal. These measures should result in stabilization of the patient, allowing a more extensive evaluation and treatment. Tricyclic antidepressants or serotonin reuptake inhibitors or antiseizure medication may be used for possible neuropathic components or depression.

Evaluative Phase. Frequent visits are essential during the evaluative phase. A biopsychosocial evaluation plan should have been formulated at the beginning of treatment with more extensive biopsychosocial assessments of pain as therapy progresses. (Fig. 25.3) Toxicology screen for methadone, opioids and illicit drugs should be judiciously used but their use for punitive purposes may adversely affect pain management. When patients are screened for illicit substances and for opioids, methadone and other drugs prescribed for pain-related symptoms, compliance with current medications should also be assessed.

Patients report reasons for illicit drug use ranging from easy access to peer pressure to treating unrelieved pain to reduction of withdrawal symptoms. Accordingly, careful questioning allows not only early identification of illicit substance use but also prompt intervention to rectify inadequate treatment.

Treatment Adjustment Phase. Tapering is not always smooth and several attempts may be needed during hospitalizations. Home care may also be adjusted accordingly. Improvement is slow and more than three admissions may be needed before any gains are appreciated. In a small subset of patients, dose titration and opioid tapering are extremely challenging. Most patients with average pain frequency and some frequent pain patients can have their dose tapered with relative ease while others undergoing minor dose reductions experience profound withdrawal symptoms. Perhaps over time, disease-induced elements, pharmacogenetics, and other medication-related factors can cause physical and behavioral changes that alter opioid responsiveness and responsiveness to other medications.

Persistent pain and opioid use cause neuronal plasticity resulting in anatomic, physiologic, and biochemical changes in the brain and spinal cord, altering the response to opioids (Basbaum, 1995). Amplification of the injury may be associated with latent hyperexcitability, tolerance, and physical dependence. Pain management that began in infancy with inadequate or no assessment and escalated to inadequate treatment practices confounded by inattention to the pharmacologic properties of tolerance and physical dependence can perpetuate crises in management.

Tolerance, Physical Dependence, and Addiction Are Not Interchangeable

Confusing addiction and physical dependence and using them interchangeably is common, especially in chronic opioid users. Some behaviors that are iatrogenic effects of chronic opioid exposure—undertreatment, overtreatment, and failure to prevent withdrawal—are erroneously regarded as verification of addiction (Marks and Sacher, 1973; Payne, 1989). Continuous or intermittent chronic opioid treatment can produce tolerance—lowered drug responsiveness requiring adjustment to a higher dose to maintain analgesia. Physical dependence is characterized by withdrawal symptoms occurring from heightened responsiveness to opioid antagonists or too rapid reduction or abrupt discontinuation of the opioid (Portenoy, 1994). However, a decline in analgesia can also occur because of increased activity in nociceptive pathways and psychological processes, leading to the need for escalating doses that, in turn, lead to tolerance (Cox and Werling, 1991; Trujillo, 1991; Cousins, 1994). Mislabeling these pharmacologic properties as addiction can lead to years of compromised care. Addiction connotes a highly aberrant psychological and behavioral syndrome. While studies show that addiction is rare when opioids are given for clinical pain, opioid addiction in sickle cell disease has not been adequately studied and the phenomenon of pseudoaddiction is infrequently recognized and

poorly understood. When a patient escalates his or her drug doses beyond that prescribed, this has been interpreted by some as an addiction rather than a consequence of unrelieved pain (O'Brien, 1996; O'Brien and McLellen, 1996).

A commonality of drugs used in addictive states and for pain treatment contributes to confusion. The language used also influences our attitudes. Both addiction and physical dependence begin with the initiation of narcotic/opioid use. In the addict, drug use is frequently influenced by peer pressure while medication use by the patient for pain relief is influenced by the prescribing practices of the physician (Inturrisi and Hanks, 1993). Continued peer pressure in addictive disease coupled with the perceived desirable aspects of the drugs may lead the new user to persist in chronic opiate use. Persistent pain patients may receive chronic opioids by prescription. Tolerance in either case can occur and implies that increasing amounts of medications will be used to achieve the desired goal, which, for the drug abuser, is usually the euphoria or "high," as contrasted with the pain patient, for whom the desired goal is relief (Foley, 1991; Kreek 1992, 1996a; Reisine et al., 1995).

Physical dependence is a property of the opiate/opioid agents. Differences are present, however, in the withdrawal symptoms of pain patients and persons who have addictive disease. In pain patients who undergo withdrawal, the pain generally occurs in the sites of their clinical pain. The patient is most often unable to distinguish pain of disease from pain of withdrawal. In addictive disease, withdrawal includes abnormal vital signs such as increased heart rate and blood pressure, anomalies in neuroendocrine responsiveness, and behavioral defects as seen in depression (Blasig et al., 1973; Kreek, 1992, 1996a). Although the signs and symptoms of withdrawal after discontinuation of short-acting opioids are most striking during the first 48 to 96 hours after their cessation, a protracted abstinence syndrome, including subtle signs and symptoms of withdrawal, can be present for 6 months or more (Blasig et al., 1973; Cousins, 1994). Failure to understand and consider the possible occurrence of these clinically important events contributes to the perpetuation of pain. For example, sleep disturbance is primarily regarded as a consequence of pain due to disease processes when it may be also a manifestation of protracted abstinence.

Diminishing Symptoms of Withdrawal and Protracted Abstinence Syndrome

Unsettling symptoms such as restlessness, generalized irritability, inability to concentrate on simple intellectual tasks, insomnia, and multiple awakenings characterize the protracted abstinence syndrome (Kreek, 1992; Gardner and Lowinson, 1993). Excessive activity of the noradrenergic system contributes to many acute signs and symptoms of this syndrome. Manipulation of the noradrenergic systems alone, for instance by use of the α-adrenergic receptor agonist, clonidine, can diminish or eliminate some withdrawal symptoms (Aghajanian, 1978; Kimes et al., 1990; Quan et al., 1993). However, other mechanisms must also be involved as sometimes symptoms persist. Frequent pain patients with sickle cell anemia on chronic opioid therapy commonly have sleep disturbance and restlessness that are consistent with the disease or the protracted abstinence syndrome. An overlap between the effects of the disease and medication effects may be present. Overlap between pain pathophysiology (Melzack, 1990), sickle cell disease pathophysiology, and the various inducers of the stress response is likely. Stress is a presumed precipitator of painful episodes (Nadel and Portadin, 1977; Gil et al., 1994; Reid et al., 1995): Unrelieved pain causes hypoxia, dehydration, acidosis, and stress (Wall, 1988; Cousins, 1994) all of which may cause painful vasoocclusive events and could propagate the pain episode (Fig. 25.14). Withdrawal, which can follow rapid drug tapering or when persons on chronic opioid therapy miss a dose of medication—especially short half-life drugs—may precipitate painful events and mimic an acute pain attack. Variable outcomes following opioid exposure may reflect pharmacogenetic differences among patients (Galer et al., 1992).

Functional restoration employs skill training with social workers, psychologists, and physiatrists/physical therapists after which the individual rejoins the work force or returns to school. The person is now prepared for functional enhancement and prevention tactics to recognize and manage problems. The maladaptive patterns and pain memories have to be recognized and the person engaged in an ongoing process of improving the quality of life. Decreased hospital utilization and quality of life enhancement along with the satisfaction that "they did it" have propelled some high utilizers to a different setting that fosters self-advocacy, self-reliance, and self-satisfaction (Benjamin et al., 1994).

SUMMARY

Painful episodes are the chief clinical feature of sickle cell disease. These are acute—often excruciating—bouts of pain in the chest, abdomen, or extremities that often involve multiple areas simultaneously, last days or even weeks, and require opioids for relief. Interestingly, some patients never describe a painful episode. Others have them continuously. These agonizing attacks of acute pain must be separated from more chronic pain of osteoporosis that usually affects the spine, the pain associated with osteonecrosis of hips and shoulders, and the milder aches, pains, and soreness that are frequently present between severe episodes. The day-to-day management of sickle cell disease often equates with the management of acute and chronic pain, a skill that is unfortunately underdeveloped in most physicians.

Patients with sickle cell anemia and HbS-β^0 thalassemia have twice as many pain episodes yearly as individuals with HbSC disease and HbS-β^+ thalassemia; among individuals who have three to ten episodes yearly, about 5 percent of the patients account for more than 30 percent of painful episodes. Nearly 40 percent of individuals with sickle cell anemia do not have a pain episode in a given year. Pain rates are highest during the third and fourth decades of life and mortality is elevated in adults with the most frequent pain episodes.

The pain rate varies directly with PCV and inversely with HbF level. The proportion of dense cells may change as a painful episode evolves. A small decrease in PCV and rise in reticulocytes may occur, but this is insufficient to be diagnostically useful in the individual patient. As pain wanes, dense cell numbers fall and cellular deformability increases. These findings may signify the early trapping and loss of deformable cells—perhaps as they adhere to microvascular endothelium, compromise flow, and initiate ischemia—with the subsequent release of young, deformable, and conceivably more adherent cells. This may presage rapidly recurrent pain attacks; repeat pain episodes are common. Unfortunately, no useful laboratory test can tell if a vasoocclusive pain episode is occurring and the history remains the best clue.

Painful episodes are often stereotypical, affecting individuals in the same manner from episode to episode. Patients usually know if the pain they are experiencing is different from their typical painful episode and the wise physician should heed their advice about the need for hospitalization or likelihood that the pain has an alternative explanation other than "pain crisis." The pain of acute cholecystitis, splenic sequestration crisis, splenic infarction, and right upper quadrant syndrome may sometimes be mistaken for uncomplicated pain episodes. Neither acute, severe anemia nor newly deranged liver function are features of the painful episode. Acute painful episodes are often the heralding events in the acute chest syndrome. Occasional pain episodes end with multiorgan failure. No data allow one to foretell if a "usual" pain episode will have a mortal outcome.

After an assessment of the duration and severity of the pain and the history of response to pain treatment, the decision if hospitalization is needed can be made. Important in this consideration is whether associated complicating factors such as excessive tachycardia, hypotension, fever more than 101°F, marked leukocytosis, a fall in hemoglobin level, or evidence of pneumonia by examination or chest X-ray are present. If the pain episode seems uncomplicated, and after 24 to 36 hours of treatment in the emergency department or day hospital, pain has not diminished to the point where the patient feels that it is manageable at home, hospitalization is warranted.

Most pain episodes do not have an identifiable precipitating cause but this does not mean that one should not be diligently sought. Painful episodes are sometimes triggered by an infection, temperature extremes, or physical and emotional stress. Pneumonia is the most prevalent infection associated with acute pain episodes. Commonly, painful episodes begin with little warning; some patients, however, may sense that a painful episode is soon to occur—they feel that something is not right. Physical examination is usually not helpful for determining if an acute pain episode is in progress but sometimes there is localized swelling and pain over an involved bone. A chest X-ray should be obtained in most patients sufficiently ill to be hospitalized to exclude acute chest syndrome or pneumonia. Low-grade fever can accompany the acute painful episode but higher elevations may point to infection or extensive tissue damage.

References

Abbuhl, S, Jacobson, S, Murphy, JG, and Gibson, G. (1986). Serum concentrations of meperidine in patients with sickle cell crisis. *Ann. Emerg. Med.* 15: 433–438.

Aghajanian, GK. (1978). Tolerance of locus coeruleus neurones to morphine and suppression of withdrawal response by clonidine. *Nature.* 276: 186–187.

Alleyne J, Thomas VJ. (1994). The management of sickle cell crisis pain as experienced by patients and their carers. *J. Adv. Nurs.* 19: 725–732.

Al-Rashid, RA. (1979). Orbital apex syndrome secondary to sickle cell anemia. *J. Pediatr.* 95: 426–427.

American Pain Society, Quality of Care Committee. (1995). Quality improvement guidelines for the treatment of acute pain and cancer pain. *JAMA.* 274: 1874–1880.

Andrews, CJH and Prys-Roberts, C. (1983). Fentanyl: a review. *Clinics Anaesth.* 1: 97–122.

Armstrong ED, Pegelow CH, Gonzalez JC, and Martinez A. (1995). Impact of children's sickle cell history on nurse and physician ratings of pain and medication decisions. *J. Pediatric. Pyschol.* 17: 651–664.

Asher, SW. (1980). Multiple cranial neuropathies, trigeminal neuralgia, and vascular headaches in sickle cell disease, a possible common mechanism. *Neurology.* 30: 210–211.

Bailey, S, Higgs, DR, Morris, J, and Serjeant, GR. (1991). Is the painful crisis of sickle-cell disease due to sickling? *Lancet.* 337: 735.

Ballas, SK. (1990). Treatment of pain in adults with sickle cell disease. *Am. J. Hematol.* 34: 49–54.

Ballas, SK. (1991). Sickle cell anemia with few painful crises is characterized by decreased red cell deformability and increased number of dense cells. *Am. J. Hematol.* 36: 122–30.

Ballas, SK, and Smith, ED. (1992). Red blood cell changes during the evolution of the sickle cell painful crisis. *Blood* 79: 2154–63.

Ballas, SK. (1995). The sickle cell painful crisis in adults: phases and objective signs. *Hemoglobin* 19: 323–333.

Ballas, SK. (1998). Sickle-cell pain. Seattle. *IASP Press.*

Barrett-Conner, E. (1968). Bacterial infection and sickle cell anemia: An analysis of 250 infections in 106 patients and a review of the literature. *Medicine* 50: 97–112.

Basbaum, AI. (1995). Insights into the development of opioid tolerance. *Pain* 61: 349–352.

Benjamin, LJ. (1989). Pain in sickle cell disease. In Foley KM and Payne RM, editors. *Current therapy of pain.* Toronto: BC Decker, pp. 90–104.

Benjamin, LJ. (1990a). Sickle cell pain. In Max, Portenoy, and Laska, editors. *Advances in pain research and therapy, the design of analgesic clinical trials.* New York: Raven Press. pp. 17–331.

Benjamin, LJ. (1990b). Conventional and experimental approaches to the treatment of pain crisis. In Mankad, VN and Moore, RB, editors. *Sickle cell disease: Pathophysiology, diagnosis and treatment.* New York: Praeger Scientific.

Benjamin, LJ. (1991). Sickle cell disease. In Max, Portenoy, Laska, editors. *Advances in pain research and therapy.* New York: Raven Press, pp. 317–331.

Benjamin, LJ, Yatco, E, and Swinson, GI. (1993). *Interleukin-6, Interleukin-1 and Interleukin I Receptor Antagonist (IL-IRA), Mediators and Regulators of the Inflammatory Response Are Altered During Acute Painful Vaso-occlusive Crisis.* Philadelphia, PA: National Sickle Cell Disease Program.

Benjamin, LJ, Swinson GI, Fulchon, C, and McKegney, F. (1994). Frequently recurring pain in sickle cell disease, assessment, treatment and prevention strategies. In Beuzard, Y, Lubin, BH, and Rosa, editor. *Sickle cell disease and thalassaemias: New trends in therapy.* Colloque Inserm, Vol. 234, pp. 433–434.

Benjamin, LJ, Edwards, KR, Swinson, GI, and Cleeland, CS. (1996). *Use of the Brief Pain Inventory Short Form (BPISF) for assessment of acute sickle cell pain.* 21st Annual Meeting of the National Sickle Cell Disease Program 1996, Mobile, AL, p. 84.

Benjamin, LJ, Swinson, G, Fulchon, C, and McKegney, F. (1999a). Frequently recurring pain in sickle cell disease: Assessment, treatment and prevention strategies. In Beuzard Y, Lubin, BH, and Rosa, J, editors. *Sickle cell disease and thalassaemias: New trends in therapy.* Colloque INSERM, John Libbey Eurotext Limited, p. 433.

Benjamin, LJ, Dampier, CD, Jacox, AK, Odesina, V et al. (1999b). *Guideline for the Management of Acute and Chronic Pain in Sickle Cell Disease.* APS Clinical Practice

Guidelines. Series No. 1. Glenview, IL: American Pain Society.

Benjamin, LJ, Swinson, GI, and Nagel, RL. (2000). Sickle cell anemia day hospital: An approach for the management of uncomplicated painful crises. *Blood.* 95: 1130–1137.

Beyer, JE and Knott, CB. (1998). Construct validity estimation for the African American and Hispanic Versions of The Oucher Scale. *J. Pediatr. Nurs.* 13: 20–31.

Billett, HH, Nagel, RL, and Fabry, ME. (1988a). Evolution of laboratory parameters during sickle cell painful crisis: Evidence compatible with dense red cell sequestration without thrombosis. *Am. J. Med. Sci.* 296: 293–298.

Billett, HH, Fabry, ME, and Nagel, RL. (1988b). Hemoglobin distribution width: A rapid assessment of dense red cells in the steady state and during painful crisis in sickle cell anemia. *J. Lab. Clin. Med.* 112: 339–344.

Blank, JP and Gill FM. (1981). Orbital infarction in sickle cell disease. *Pediatr.* 67: 879–881.

Blasig, J, Herz, A, Reinhold, K, and Zieglgansberger, S. (1973). Development of physical dependence on morphine in respect to time and dosage and quantification of the precipitate withdrawal syndrome in rats. *Psychopharmacology* 33: 19–48.

Bruera, E, Roca, E, Cedaro, L, Carraro, S et al. (1985). Action of oral methylprednisolone in terminal cancer patients: A prospective randomized double-blind study. *Cancer Treat. Rep.* 69: 751–754.

Bruera, E, Pereira, J, Watanabe, S, Belzile, M et al. (1996a). Opioid rotation in patients with cancer pain. A retrospective comparison of dose ratios between methadone, hydromorphone and morphine. *Cancer* 78: 852–857.

Bruera, E, Pereira, J, Watanabe S et al. (1996b). Opioid rotation in pain: A retrospective comparison of dose ratios between morphone and morphine. *Cancer* 78: 852–857.

Bruera, E and Pereira, J. (1997). Neuropsychiatric toxicity of opioids. In Jensen, TS, Turner, JA, and Wissenfeld-Hallin, Z, editors. *Proceedings of the 8th World Congress on Pain.* Vol. 8.

Buchanan, GR. (1994). Infection. In Embury, SH, Hebbel, RP, Mohands, N, and Steinberg, MH, editors. *Sickle cell disease: Basic principles and clinical practice.* New York: Raven Press, pp. 567–587.

Chapman, CR and Syrjala, KL. (1990). Measurement of pain. In Bonica, JJ, editor. *The management of pain.* Malvern: Lea & Febiger, pp. 580–594.

Charache, S. (1974). The treatment of sickle cell anemia. *Arch. Intern. Med.* 133: 698–705.

Charache, S, Terrin, ML, Moore, RD et al. (1995). Effect of hydroxyurea on the frequency of painful crises in sickle cell anemia. *N. Engl. J. Med.* 332: 1317–1322.

Chen, ZR, Somogyi, AA, Reynolds, G, and Bochner, F. (1991). Disposition and metabolism of codeine after single and chronic doses in one poor and seven extensive metabolisers. *Br. J. Clin. Pharmacol.* 31: 381–390.

Christensen, ML, Wang, WC, Harris, S et al. (1996). Transdermal fentanyl administration in children and adolescents with sickle cell pain crisis. *J. Pediatr. Hematol. Oncol.* 18: 372–376.

Cleeland, CS. (1987). Barriers to the management of pain. *Oncology* 1(Suppl): 19–26.

Cleeland, CS. (1993). Strategies for improving cancer pain management. *J. Pain Symptom. Manage.* 8: 361–364.

Cleeland, CS, Gonin R, Baez L et al. (1997). Pain and treatment of pain in minority patients with cancer. *Ann. Intern. Med.* 127: 813–816.

Cleeland, CS and Ryan, KM. (1994). Pain assessment: Global use of the Brief Pain Inventory. *Ann. Acad. Med. Singapore* 23: 129–138.

Co, LL, Schmitz, TH, Havdala, H et al. (1979). Acupuncture: An evaluation in the painful crises of sickle cell anaemia. *Pain* 7: 181–185.

Conti, C, Tso, E, and Browne, B. (1996). Oral morphine protocol for sickle cell crisis pain. *Md. Med. J.* 45: 33–35.

Cousins, MJ. (1989). John J. Bonica distinguished lecture. Acute pain and the injury response: Immediate and prolonged effects. *Reg. Anesth.* 14: 162–179.

Cousins, MJ. (1994). Acute postoperative pain. In Wall, PD and Melzack, R, editors. *Textbook of pain.* New York: Churchill Livingstone. pp. 357–385.

Cousins, MJ and Mather, LE. (1984). Intrathecal and epidural administration of opioids. *Anesthesiology* 61: 276–310.

Cox, BM and Werling, LL. (1991). Opioid tolerance and dependence. In Pratt, JA, editor. *The biological bases of drug tolerance and dependence.* New York: Academic Press, pp. 199–229.

Coyle, N, Mauskop, A, Maggard, J, and Foley, KM. (1995). Continuous subcutaneous infusions of opiates in cancer patients with pain. *Oncol. Nurs. Forum.* 13: 53–57.

Cozzi, L, Tryon, WW, and Sedlacek, K. (1987). The effectiveness of biofeedback-assisted relaxation in modifying sickle cell crises. *Biofeedback Self Regul.* 12: 51–61.

Crain, SM and Shen, KF. (1995). Ultra-low concentrations of naloxone selectively antagonize excitatory effects of morphine on sensory neurons, thereby increasing its antinociceptive potency and attenuating tolerance/dependence during chronic cotreatment. *Proc. Natl. Acad. Sci. U.S.A.* 92: 10540–10544.

Dahl, JB and Kehlet, H. (1993). The value of pre-emptive analgesia in the treatment of postoperative pain. *Br. J. Anaesth.* 70: 434–439.

Dampier, CD, Setty, BN, Logan, J et al. (1995). Intravenous morphine pharmacokinetics in pediatric patients with sickle cell disease. *J. Pediatr.* 126: 461–467.

Davies, SC. (1990). The hospital management of patients with sickle cell disease. *Haematologica* 75(Suppl 5): 96–106.

Davis, H, Moore, RM, and Gergen, PJ. (1997). Cost of hospitalizations associated with sickle cell disease in the United States. *Public Health Report* 112(1): 40–43.

Dejgard, A, Peterson, P, and Kastrup, J. (1988). Mexiletine in the treatment of chronic painful diabetic neuropathy. *Lancet,* 1: 9–11.

Devine, DV, Kinney, TR, Thomas, PF et al. (1986). Fragment D-dimer levels: An objective marker of vaso-occlusive crisis and other complications of sickle cell disease. *Blood* 68: 317–319.

Eisendrath, SJ, Goldman, B, Douglas, J et al. (1987). Meperidine-induced delirium. *Am. J. Psychiatr.* 144: 1062–1065.

Elander, J and Midence, K. (1996). A review of evidence about factors affecting quality of pain management in sickle cell disease. *Clin. J. Pain* 12: 180–193.

Elliott, K, Kest, B, and Inturrisi, CE. (1995). NMDA receptors, mu and kappa opioid tolerance and perspectives on new drug development. *Neuropsychopharmacology* 13: 347–356.

Embury, SH, Garcia, J, Mohandas, N et al. (1984). Effects of oxygen inhalation on endogenous erythropoietin kinetics, erythropoiesis, and properties of blood cells in sickle cell anemia. *N. Engl. J. Med.* 2311: 291–295.

Embury, SH, Hebbel, RP, Mohandas, N, and Steinberg, MH. (Eds.). (1994). *Sickle Cell Disease: Basic Principles and Clinical Practice.* New York: Raven Press.

Fabry, ME, Benjamin, L, Lawrence, C, and Nagel, RL. (1984). An objective sign in painful crisis in sickle cell anemia: The concomitant reduction of high density red cells. *Blood* 64: 559–563.

Fabry, ME, Kassim, A, Umans, H, and Nagel, RL. (1998). Clinical application of BOLD-MRI to extremities in sickle cell pain episodes. *Blood* 92: 525a.

Farrar, JT. (1999). Therapeutic use of non-opioid analgesics: Non-steroidals, antidepressants, anticonvulsants, and miscellaneous agents. *Proceedings of the Third Conference on Pain Management and Chemical Dependency* pp. 31–34.

Fernandez, E and Turk, DC. (1989). The utility of cognitive coping strategies for altering pain perception: a meta-analysis. *Pain* 38: 1231–35.

Foley, KM. (1985). The treatment of cancer pain. *N. Engl. J. Med.* 313: 84–95.

Foley, KM. (1991). Clinical tolerance to opioids. In Basbuarn, AJ and Basson, JM, editors. *Towards a new pharmacology of pain.* John Wiley: Chicester, pp. 181–204.

Fordyce, WE. (1976). *Behavioral Methods for Chronic Pain and Illness.* St. Louis: Mosby-Yearbook.

Francis, RB, Jr and Johnson, CS. (1991). Vascular occlusion in sickle cell disease: Current concepts and unanswered questions. *Blood* 77: 1405–1414.

Friedlander, AH, Genser, L, and Swerdloff M. (1980). Mental nerve neuropathy: a complication of sickle-cell crisis. *Oral Surg Oral Med Oral Pathol.* 49: 151–7.

Friedman, EW, Webber, AB, Osborn, HH et al. (1986). Oral analgesia for treatment of painful crisis in sickle cell anemia. *Ann. Emerg. Med.* 7: 787–791.

Galer, BS, Coyle, N, Pasternak, GW, and Portenoy, RK. (1992). Individual variability in the response to different opioids: Report of five cases. *Pain* 49: 87–91.

Gardner, EL and Lowinson, JH. (1993). Drug craving and positive negative hedonic brain substrates activated by addicting drugs. *Neurosciences* 5: 359–368.

Gebhart, GF, Hammond, DL, and Jansen, TS. (1994). *Proceedings of the 7th World Congress on Pain, Progress in Pain Research and Management.* Vol. 2. Seattle: IASP Press.

Gil, KM, Abrams, MR, Phillips, G et al. (1989). Sickle cell disease pain: The relation of coping strategies to adjustment. *J. Consult. Clin. Psychol.* 57: 725–731.

Gil, KM, Thompson, RJ, Jr, Keith, BR et al. (1993). Sickle cell disease pain in children and adolescents: Change in pain frequency and coping strategies over time. *J. Pediatr. Psychol.* 18: 621–637.

Gil, KM, Phillips, G, Edens, J et al. (1994). Observation of pain behaviors during episodes of sickle cell disease pain. *Clin. J. Pain.* 10: 128–132.

Gil, K, Phillips, G, Webster, DK et al. (1995). Experimental pain sensitivity and reports of negative thoughts in adults with sickle cell disease. *Behav. Ther.* 26: 273–293.

Gill, FM, Sleeper, LA, Weiner, SJ et al. (1995). Clinical events in the first decade in a cohort of infants with sickle cell disease. Cooperative Study of Sickle Cell Disease. *Blood* 86: 776–783.

Gonzalez, ER, Ornato, JP, Ware, D et al. (1988). Comparison of intramuscular analgesic activity of butorphanol and morphine in patients with sickle cell disease. *Ann. Emerg. Med.* 17: 788–791.

Gonzalez, ER, Bahal, N, Hansen, LA et al. (1991). Intermittent injection vs patient-controlled analgesia for sickle cell crisis pain. Comparison in patients in the emergency department. *Arch. Intern. Med.* 151: 1373–1378.

Griffin, TC, McIntire, D, and Buchanan, GR. (1994). High-dose intravenous methylprednisolone therapy for pain in children and adolescents with sickle cell disease [see comments]. *N. Engl. J. Med.* 330: 733–737.

Hall, H, Chiarucci, K, and Berman, B. (1992). Self-regulation and assessment approaches for vaso-occlusive pain management for pediatric sickle cell anemia patients. *Int. J. Psychosom.* 39: 28–33.

Hartrick, CT and Pitcher, CE. (1995). Tutorial 17: How to manage a difficult pain patient. *Pain Dig.* 5: 93–97.

Holbrook, CT. (1990). Patient-controlled analgesia pain management for children with sickle cell disease. *J. Assoc. Acad. Minor. Phys.* 1: 93–96.

Houde, RW, Wallenstein, SL, and Beaver, WT. (1966). Evaluation of analgesics in patients with cancer pain. In Lasagna, L, editor. *International encyclopedia of pharmacology and therapeutics. Section 6. Clinical pharmacology.* Vol. 1. New York: Pergamon Press.

Hunt, BJ, Richmond, R, Allen, S, and Davies, SC. (1988). Analgesia in sickle cell crisis. *Br. J. Haematol.* 69: 129.

Ibrahim, AS. (1980). Relationship between meteorological changes and occurrence of painful sickle cell crises in Kuwait. *Trans. R. Soc. Trop. Med. Hyg.* 74: 159–161.

Inturrisi, CE. (1993). Pharmacokinetic-pharmacodynamic (PK-PD) relationship of opioid analgesics. In Chapman, CR and Foley KM, editors. *Current and emerging issues in cancer pain: Research and practice.* New York: Raven Press, p. 1985.

Inturrisi, CE. (1997). Preclinical evidence for a role in glutamatergic systems in opioid tolerance and dependence. *Sarn Neurosci.* 9: 110–119.

Inturrisi, CE, Portenoy, RK, Max, MB et al. (1990). Pharmacokinetic-pharmacodynamic relationships of methadone infusions in patients with cancer pain. *Clin. Pharmacol. Ther.* 47: 565–577.

Inturrisi, CE and Hanks, GWC. (1993). Opioid analgesic therapy. In Doyle, D, Hanks, GWC, and Macdonald, N, editors. *Oxford textbook of palliative medicine*. New York: Oxford University Press. pp. 168–183.

International Narcotics Control Board. (1996). *Availability of Opiates for Medical Needs*. New York: UN.

Ives, TJ and Guerra, MF. (1987). Constant morphine infusion for severe sickle cell crisis pain. *Drug. Intell. Clin. Pharm.* 21: 625–627.

Jacobson, SJ, Kopecky, BA, Joshi, P, and Babul, N. (1997). Randomized trial of oral morphine for painful episodes of sickle-cell disease in children. *Lancet* 350: 1358–1361.

Jacox, A, Carr, DB, and Payne, R. (1994). New clinical-practice guidelines for the management of pain in patients with cancer. *N. Engl. J. Med.* 330: 169–173.

Kaiko, RF, Foley, KM, Grabinski, PY et al. (1983a). Central nervous system excitatory effects of meperidine in cancer patients. *Ann. Neurol.* 13: 180–185.

Kaiko, RF, Wallenstein, SL, Rogers, AG, and Houde RW. (1983b). Sources of variation in analgesic responses in patients with chronic pain receiving morphine. *Pain* 15: 191–200.

Kaiko, RF. (1988). Commentary: Equianalgesic dose ratio of intramuscular/oral morphine, 1:6 versus 1:3. In Foley, KM and Inturrisi, CE, editors. *Advances in pain research and therapy, Vol. 6*. Raven Press. New York: pp. 87–94.

Kaiko, RF, Foley, KM, Grabinski, PY et al. (1989). Central nervous system excitatory effects of meperidine in cancer patients. *Ann. Neurol.* 13: 108–185.

Kassim, CS, Umans, H, Nagel, RL, and Fabry, ME. (in press). Megalophallus as a complication of priapism in sickle-cell anemia: Use of BOLD-MRI. *J.Urol.*

Kaul, DK, Fabry, ME, and Nagel, RL. (1996). The pathophysiology of vascular obstruction in the sickle syndromes. *Blood Rev.* 10: 29–44.

Keefe, FJ, Dunsmore, J, and Burnett, R. (1992). Behavioral and cognitive-behavioral approaches to chronic pain: Recent advances and future directions. *J. Consult. Clin. Psych.* 60: 528–536.

Kimes, AS, Bell, JA, and Londed, ED. (1990). Clonidine attenuates increased brain glucose metabolism during naloxone-precipitated morphine withdrawal. *Neuroscience* 34: 633–644.

Konotey-Ahulu, F. (1972). Mental-nerve neuropathy: a complication of sickle-cell crisis. *Lancet.* 2: 388.

Konotey-Ahulu, FI. (1991). Morphine for painful crises in sickle cell disease [letter; comment]. *Br. Med. J.* 302: 1604.

Koshy, M, Leikin, J, Dorn, L et al. (1994). Evaluation and management of sickle cell disease in the emergency department (an 18-year experience): 1974–1992. *Am. J. Ther.* 1: 309–320.

Kreek, MJ. (1992). Rationale for maintenance pharmacotherapy of opiate dependence. In O'Brien, CP and Jaffee, JH, editors. *Addictive states*. New York: Raven Press, pp. 205–230.

Kreek, MJ. (1996a). Opiates, opioids and addiction. *Mol. Psych.* 1: 232–254.

Kreek, MJ. (1996b). Treatment of addictions: Biological correlates. In Koslow, SH, Murthy, RS, and Coelho, GV, editors. *Decade of the brain: India/USA research in mental health and neurosciences*. pp. 145–159.

Kremer, TM, Wilting, J, and Janssen, LH. (1988). Drug binding to human alpha-1-acid glycoprotein in health and disease. *Pharmacol. Rev.* 40: 1–47.

Lapin, J, Portenoy, RK, Coyle, N et al. (1989). Guidelines for use of controlled-release oral morphine in cancer pain management. *Cancer Nurs.* 12: 202–208.

Lawrence, C, Fabry, ME, and Nagel, RL. (1985). Red cell distribution width parallels dense red cell disappearance during painful crises in sickle cell anemia. *J. Lab. Clin. Med.* 105: 706–710.

Lechin, F, van der Dijs, B, Lechin, ME et al. (1989). Pimozide therapy for trigeminal neuralgia. *Arch. Neurol.* 9: 960–962.

Maier, SF and Watkins, LR. (1998). Cytokines for psychologists: implications of bidirectional immune-to-brain communication for understanding behavior, mood, and cognition. *Psychol Rev* 105: 83–107.

Manfredi, PL, Borsook, D, Chandler, SW, and Payne, R. (1997). Intravenous methadone for cancer pain unrelieved by morphine and hydromorphone: Clinical observations. *Pain* 70: 99–101.

Mankad, VN, Williams, JP, Harpen, MD, Manci, E et al. (1990). Magnetic resonance imaging of bone marrow in sickle cell disease: Clinical, hematologic, and pathologic correlations. *Blood* 75: 274–283.

Marks, RM and Sachar, EJ. (1973). Undertreatment of medical inpatients with narcotic analgesics. *Ann. Intern. Med.* 78: 173–181.

Mather, LE, Denson, DD, and Raj, PP. (1996). Tutorial 22: Pharmacokinetics and pharmacodynamics of analgesic agents. *Pain Dig.* 6: 34–41.

Max, MB. (1990). Improving outcomes of analgesic treatment: Is education enough? *Ann. Intern. Med.* 113: 885–889.

Mayer, DJ, Mao, J, and Price, DD. (1995). The development of morphine tolerance and dependence is associated with translocation of protein kinase C. *Pain* 61: 365–374.

McCurdy, PR, and Mahmood, L. (1971). Intravenous urea treatment of the painful crisis of sickle-cell disease. A preliminary report. *N. Engl. J. Med.* 285: 992–994.

McGrath, PA. (1990). *Pain in Children: Nature, Assessment, Treatment*. New York: Guilford Press.

McGrath, PA. (1994). Alleviating children's pain: A cognitive-behavioral approach. In Wall, PD and Melzack, R, editors. *Textbook of pain*. London: Churchill Livingstone, pp. 1403–1418.

McPherson, E, Perlin, E, Finke, H et al. (1990). Patient-controlled analgesia in patients with sickle cell vaso-occlusive crisis. *Am. J. Med. Sci.* 299: 10–12.

McQuay, HJ. (1994). Epidural analgesics. In: Wall, PD, and Melzack, R, editors. *Textbook of pain*. London: Churchill Livingstone, pp. 1025–1034.

Melzack, R. (1990). The tragedy of needless pain. *Sci. Am.* 262: 27–33.

Mohammed, SS, Ayass, M, Mehta, P et al. (1993a). Codeine disposition in sickle cell patients compared with healthy volunteers. *J. Clin. Pharmacol.* 33: 811–815.

Mohammed, SS, Christopher, MM, Mehta, P et al. (1993b). Increased erythrocyte and protein binding of codeine in patients with sickle cell disease. *J. Pharm. Sci.* 82: 1112–1117.

Moore, D. (1994). Patient/physician model for painful crises. An alternative pathway for care. Presented at the 19th Annual meeting of the National Sickle Cell Disease Program. Pain Symposium. New York, 1994.

Mortimer, O, Persson, K, Ladona, MG et al. (1990). Polymorphic formation of morphine from codeine in poor and extensive metabolizers of dextromethorphan: Relationship to the presence of immunoidentified cytochrome P-450IID1. *Clin. Pharmacol. Ther.* 47: 27–35.

Murray, N and May, A. (1988). Painful crises in sickle cell disease—patients' perspectives. *Br. Med. J.* 297: 452–454.

Nadel, C and Portadin, G. (1977). Sickle cell crises: Psychological factors associated with onset. *N. Y. State J. Med.* 77: 1075–1078.

Niv, D and Davor, M. (1998). Transition from acute to chronic pain. In: *Arnoff*, GM, editor. *Evaluation and treatment of chronic pain.* 3rd ed. Baltimore: Williams & Wilkins.

O'Brien, CP. (1996). Drug addiction and drug abuse. In *Goodman and Gilman's The Pharmacological basis of therapeutics.* 9th ed. New York: McGraw Hill, pp. 557–569.

O'Brien, CP and McLellan, AT. (1996). Myths about the treatment of addiction. *Lancet* 347: 237–240.

Olkkola, KT, Hamunen, K, and Maunuksela, EL. (1995). Clinical pharmacokinetics and pharmacodynamics of opioid analgesics in infants and children. *Clin. Pharmacokinet.* 28: 385–404.

Olsen, GD. (1975). Morphine binding to human plasma proteins. *Clin. Pharmacol. Ther.* 17: 31–35.

Osborne, RJ, Joel, SP, and Slevin, M. (1990). Morphine and metabolite behavior after different routes of morphine administration: Demonstration of the importance of the active metabolite morphine-6-glucuronide. *Clin. Pharmacol. Ther.* 47: 12–19.

Osborne, R, Thompson, P, Joel, S et al. (1992). The analgesic activity of morphine-6-glucuronide. *Br. J. Clin. Pharmacol.* 34: 130–138.

Pasternak, GW, Bodnar, RJ, Clark, JA, and Inturrisi, CE. (1987). Morphine-6-glucuronide, a potent mu agonist. *Life Sci.* 41: 2845–2849.

Pasternak, GW and Inturrisi, CE. (1995). Pharmacological modulation of opioid tolerance. In *Central & peripheral nervous systems.* Ashley Publ. Ltd. pp. 271–281.

Payne, R. (1989). Pain management in sickle cell disease. Rationale and techniques. *Ann. N.Y. Acad. Sci.* 565: 189–206.

Payne, R. (1997). Pain management in sickle cell anemia. *Anesth. Clin. N. Am.* 15: 306–318.

Perlin, E, Finke, H, Castro, O et al. (1993). Infusional/patient-controlled analgesia in sickle-cell vaso-occlusive crises. *Pain Clin.* 6: 119.

Perlin, E, Finke, H, Castro, O et al. (1994). Enhancement of pain control with ketorolac tromethamine in patients with sickle cell vaso-occlusive crisis. *Am. J. Hematol.* 46: 43–47.

Peterson, GM, Randall, CT, and Paterson, J. (1990). Plasma levels of morphine and morphine glucuronides in the treatment of cancer pain: Relationship to renal function and route of administration. *Eur. J. Clin. Pharmacol.* 38: 121–124.

Platt, OS, Thorington, BD, Brambilla, DJ et al. (1991). Pain in sickle cell disease. Rates and risk factors. *N. Engl. J. Med.* 325: 11–16.

Platt, OS, Brambilla, DJ, Rosse, WF et al. (1994). Mortality in sickle cell disease. Life expectancy and risk factors for early death. *N. Engl. J. Med.* 330: 1639–1644.

Portenoy, RK and Payne, R. (1992). Acute and chronic pain. In Lowinson, JH, Ruiz, P, Millman, RB, et al., editors. *Substance abuse: A comprehensive textbook.* Baltimore: Williams & Wilkins. pp. 691–721.

Portenoy, RK. (1994). Opioid tolerance responsiveness: Research findings and clinical observations. In Gebhart, GF, Hammond, DL, and Jensen, TS, editors. *Proceedings of the 7th World Congress on Pain. Progress in Pain Research and Management.* Seattle: IASP Press.

Powars, DR. (1990). Sickle cell anemia and major organ failure. *Hemoglobin* 14: 573–598.

Pryle, BJ, Grech, H, Stoddart, PA et al. (1992). Toxicity of norpethidine in sickle cell crisis. *Br. Med. J.* 304: 1478–1479.

Quan, DB, Wandres, DL, and Schroeder, DJ. (1993). Clonidine in pain management. *Ann. Pharmacother.* 27: 313–315.

Quiding, H, Olsson, GL, Boreus, LO, and Bondesson, U. (1992). Infants and young children metabolise codeine to morphine. A study after single and repeated rectal administration. *Br. J. Clin. Pharmacol.* 33: 45–49.

Rawal, N, Sjöstrand, UH, Christoffersson, E et al. (1984). Comparison of intramuscular and epidural morphine for postoperative analgesia in the grossly obese: Influence on postoperative ambulation and pulmonary function. *Anesth. Analg.* 63: 583–592.

Raynor, K, Kong, H, Chen, Y et al. (1994). Pharmacological characterization of the cloned kappa-, delta-, and mu- opioid receptors. *Mol. Pharmacol.* 45: 330–334.

Rees, DC, Cervi, P, Grimwade, D et al. (1995). The metabolites of nitric oxide in sickle-cell disease. *Br. J. Haematol.* 91: 834–837.

Reid, CD, Charache, S, Lubin, BH et al. (1995). *Management and Therapy of Sickle Cell Disease.* U.S. Department of Health and Human Services, National Institute of Health.

Reinhard, EH, Moore, CV, Dubach, R et al. (1944). Depressant effects of high concentration of inspired oxygen on erythrocytogenesis: Observations on patients with sickle cell anemia with description of observed toxic manifestations of oxygen. *J. Clin. Invest.* 3: 682–698.

Reisine, T, Pasternak, G, Goodman, and Gilman. (1995). Opioid analgesics and antagonists. In *Goodman, Rall, Nies, Taylor,* editors. *The pharmacological basis of therapeutics.* New York: Pergamon Press, pp. 521–555.

Ritschel, WA, Bykadi, G, Ford, DJ et al. (1983). Pilot study on disposition and pain relief after i.m. administration of meperidine during the day or night. *Int. J. Clin. Pharmacol. Ther. Toxicol.* 21: 218–223.

Rothman, SM and Nelson, JS. (1980). Spinal cord infarction in a patient with sickle cell anemia. *Neurology.* 30: 1072–1076.

Santillan, R, Maestre, JM, Hurle, MA, and Florez, J. (1994). Niprodipine, a calcium channel blocker, enhances opiate analgesia in patients with cancer pain tolerant to morphine. Gebhart, GF, Hammond, DL, Jensen, TS, editors. *Progress in pain research and management, Vol. 2.* Seattle: IASP Press.

Seeler, RA and Royal, JE. (1982). Mental nerve neuropathy in a child with sickle cell anemia. *Am. J. Pediatr. Hematol. Oncol.* 4: 212–213.

Serjeant, GR, Ceulaer, CD, Lethbridge, R et al. (1994). The painful crisis of homozygous sickle cell disease: Clinical features. *Br. J. Haematol.* 87: 586–591.

Shapiro, BS. (1989). The management of pain in sickle cell disease. *Pediatr. Clin. North. Am.* 36: 1029–1045.

Shapiro, BS. (1993). Management of painful episodes in sickle cell disease. In Scheaffer, NL, Berde, CB, and Yaster, M, editors. *Pain in infants, children and adolescents.* Baltimore: Williams & Wilkins. pp. 385–410.

Shapiro, BS, Dinges, DF, Orne, EC, Ohene-Frempong, K et al. (1990). Recording of crisis pain in sickle cell disease. In Tyler, DC and Krane, EJ, editors. *Advances in pain research therapy.* New York: Raven Press, pp. 313–321.

Shapiro, BS, Cohen, DE, and Howe, CJ. (1993). Patient-controlled analgesia for sickle-cell-related pain. *J. Pain Symptom Manage.* 8: 22–28.

Shapiro, BS, Dinges, DF, Orne, EC et al. (1995). Home management of sickle cell-related pain in children and adolescents: Natural history and impact on school attendance. *Pain* 61: 139–144.

Shapiro, BS, Benjamin, LJ, Payne, R, and Heidrich, G. (1997). Sickle cell-related pain: Perceptions of medical practitioners. *J. Pain Symp. Manage.* 14: 168–174.

Shields, RW Jr, Harris, JW, and Clark, M. (1991). Mononeuropathy in sickle cell anemia: anatomical and pathophysiological basis for its rarity. *Muscle Nerve.* 14: 370–374.

Simmonds, MA, Blain, C, Richenbacher, J, and Southern, MA. (1988). A new approach to the administration of opiates: TTB (fentanyl). *J. Pain Symp. Manage.* 3: 818.

Sinatra, RS. (1993). Pathophysiology of Acute pain. In Sinatra, RS, Hord, H, Ginsburg, R, and Preble, LM, editors. *Acute pain mechanisms and management.* St. Louis: Mosby Year Book, pp. 44–57.

Sindrup, SH, Grodum, E, Gram, LF et al. (1991). Concentration-response relationship in paroxetine treatment of diabetic neuropathy symptoms: A patient-blinded dose-escalation study. *Ther. Drug Monit.* 13: 408–414.

Sindrup, SH, Poulsen, L, Brosen, K et al. (1993). Are poor metabolisers of sparteine/debrisoquine less pain tolerant than extensive metabolisers? *Pain* 53: 335–349.

Slavin, ML and Barondes, MJ. (1988). Ischemic optic neuropathy in sickle cell disease. *Am J Ophthalmol.* 105: 21221–3.

Song and Carr. (1999). Pain and memory. *Pain clinical updates, International Association for the Study of Pain.* Vol. VII. pp. 1–4.

Sorkin, LS. (1997). Basic pharmacology and physiology of acute pain processing. *Anesth. Clin. North Am.* 15: 235–249.

Stefano, GB, Hartman, A, Bilfinger, TV et al. (1995). Presence of the $\mu 3$ opiate receptor in endothelial cells: Coupling to nitric oxide production and vasodilation. *J. Biol. Chem.* 270: 30290–30294.

Steinberg, MH, Hsu, H, Nagel, RL et al. (1995). Gender and haplotype: Effects upon hematological manifestations of adult sickle cell anemia: Effects of haplotype in sickle cell anemia. *Am. J. Hematol.* 48: 175–181.

Swerdlow, M. (1984). Anticonvulsant drugs and chronic pain. *Clin. Neuropharmacol.* 7: 51–82.

Thomas, JE, Koshy, M, Patterson, L et al. (1984). Management of pain in sickle cell disease using biofeedback therapy: A preliminary study. *Biofeedback Self Regul.* 9: 413–420.

Treadwell, M and Gil, KM. (1994). Psychosocial aspects. In Embury, SJ, Hebbel, RP, Mobandas, N, and Steinberg, MJ, editors. *Sickle cell disease: Basic principles and clinical practice.* New York: Raven Press, pp. 517–529.

Trujillo, KA and Akil, H. (1991). Inhibition of morphine tolerance and dependence by the NMDA receptor antagonist MK-801. *Science* 215: 85–87.

Turk, DC. (1996a). Clinicians' attitudes about prolonged use of opioids and the issue of patient heterogeneity. *J. Pain Symptom. Manage.* 11: 218–230.

Turk, DC. (1996b). Biopsychosocial perspective on chronic pain. In Gatchel, RJ and Turk, DC, editors. *Psychological approaches to pain management: A practitioner's handbook.* New York: Guilford Press.

Vichinsky, EP, Johnson, R, and Lubin, BH. (1982). Multidisciplinary approach to pain management in sickle cell disease. *Am. J. Pediatr. Hematol. Oncol.* 4: 328–333.

Walco, GA and Dampier, CD. (1990). Pain in children and adolescents with sickle cell disease: A descriptive study. *J. Pediatr. Psychol.* 15: 643–658.

Wall, PD. (1988). The prevention of post-operative pain. *Pain* 33: 289–290.

Wall, PD and Melzack, R. (1994). *Textbook of Pain.* New York: Churchill Livingstone.

Warth, JA and Rucknagel, DL. (1984). Density ultracentrifugation of sickle cells during and after pain crisis: Increased dense echinocytes in crisis. *Blood* 64: 507–515.

Weissman, DE and Haddox, JD. (1989). Opioid pseudo-addiction—an iatrogenic syndrome. *Pain* 36: 363–366.

Weisman, SJ and Schechter, NL. (1992). Sickle cell anemia: Pain management. In Sinatra, RS, Hord, AH, Ginsberg, B, and Preble, LM, editors. *Acute pain: Mechanisms and management.* St. Louis: Mosby-Year Book. pp. 508–516.

White, NM and Hiroi, N. (1993). Amphetamine conditioned cue preference and the neurobiology of drug seeking. *Semi. Neurosc.* 5: 329–336.

Whitten, CF and Fischhoff, J. (1974). Psychosocial effects of sickle cell disease. *Arch. Intern. Med.* 133: 681–689.

Williams, D, Chung, H, Turner, E et al. (1985). Protein binding diminishes the efficacy of meperidine. *Blood* 66(Suppl 1): 67a.

Woods, K, Karrison, T, Koshy, M et al. (1997). Hospital utilization patterns and costs for adult sickle cell patients in Illinois. *Public Health Rep.* 112: 44–51.

Wright, SW, Norris, RL, and Mitchell, TR. (1992). Ketorolac for sickle cell vaso-occlusive crisis pain in the emergency department: Lack of a narcotic-sparing effect. *Ann. Emerg. Med.* 21: 925–928.

Yang, YM, Hoff, C, Hamm, C et al. (1995a). Pharmacokinetics of meperidine in sickle cell patients. *Am. J. Hematol.* 49: 357–358.

Yang, YM, Shah, AK, Watson, M, and Mankad, VN. (1995b). Comparison of costs to the health sector of comprehensive and episodic health care for sickle cell disease patients. *Public Health Rep.* 110: 80–86.

Yaster, M, Tobin, JR, Billett, C et al. (1994). Epidural analgesia in the management of severe vaso-occlusive sickle cell crisis. *Pediatrics* 93: 310–315.

Yeager, MP, Glass, DG, Neff. (1987). Epidural anesthesia and analgesia in high-risk surgical patients. *Anesthesiology* 66: 729.

Zeltzer, L, Dash, J, and Holland, JP. (1979). Hypnotically induced pain control in sickle cell anemia. *Pediatrics* 64: 533–536.

Zipursky, A, Robieux, IC, Brown, EJ et al. (1992). Oxygen therapy in sickle cell disease. *Am. J. Pediatr. Hematol. Oncol.* 14: 222–228.

26

Genetics of the β^S Gene: Origins, Genetic Epidemiology, and Epistasis in Sickle Cell Anemia

RONALD L. NAGEL
MARTIN H. STEINBERG

EARLY DISCOVERIES

The discovery of the genetic basis of sickle cell anemia blends with the history of medical genetics. One outcome of studies of sickle cell anemia was substantial advancement of the scientific and medical understanding of genetic diseases. In Western literature, the first efforts to determine the genetic basis of red cell sickling were reported by Emmel, who suggested its heritability after observing sickling in a father and son (Emmel, 1917). Taliaferro and Huck (1923), studying a large kindred, concluded that sickling was a dominant characteristic, which in some members was responsible for severe anemia and in others for only clinically asymptomatic "latent" sickling. A genetic distinction between these two states was not clarified until 1949 when James V. Neel (1949) first suggested that sickle cell anemia was the homozygous state, and sickle cell trait (asymptomatic sickling) was the heterozygous state of an undefined genetic defect. Collection of further pedigree data by Neel (1951) and independently by Beet (1949) lent strong support to this concept.

Pauling and co-workers (1949), based on the observations of I. Sherman (1940), a medical student, that sickle cells were birefringent, provided a powerful insight into the genetic basis of this disease. Events leading to the proposal that sickling was an abnormal-

ity of the hemoglobin molecule were recounted by William Castle to Maurice B. Strauss:

He and I (Castle and Pauling) were both members of a committee that evaluated the publication of the book by Vannevar Bush, "*Science, the Endless Frontier*" that, among other places, met in Denver, I think in 1945. On the overnight train between Denver and Chicago, not long after leaving Denver, I had a conversation with Dr. Pauling about the molecular relation of antibody to antigen, etc., which was very informative to me. I then sketched a little bit of the work that Dr. Ham (Thomas H. Ham) and I had been doing since 1940 on sickle cell disease and mentioned that, as stated by Dr. I.J. Sherman in 1940, when the cells were deoxygenated and sickled they showed birefringence in polarized light. This, I stated, meant to me some type of molecular alignment or orientation, and ventured to suggest that this might be "the kind of thing in which he would be interested." I am equally clear that I did not make the further generalization that it was orientation of the hemoglobin that might be doing this.

A somewhat different account of the events leading to the demonstration of HbS was more recently provided by Pauling (Pauling, 1994). In this account, Pauling recalled a presentation by Castle at a Bush report meeting in Boston that described the twisted shape of the sickled cell in venous blood and its normal shape in arterial blood. He deduced that these differences perhaps lay in different forms of hemoglobin, one lacking oxygen, the other, oxygenated, and reasoned, based on his earlier work, that sickle cell anemia must be due to the alignment of complementary strands of hemoglobin molecules that grow and ultimately deform the red cell, reversing this alignment when oxygen is loaded.

In either case, there is no doubt that Pauling made the critical connection, because only a year later, and on the heels of Neel's paper, he and two of his postdoctoral fellows, Itano and Singer, published a now classic article (1949). The article contained no allusion to Castle's conversation but established that an abnormality of the hemoglobin molecule generated the sickling phenomenon.

Pauling et al. (1949) showed that HbS was chemically different from normal hemoglobin, based on different isoelectric points and faster electrophoretic migration in the free boundary method of Tiselius. He also proposed that these differences were based on a charge difference between the two molecules. Pauling and colleagues reported their failure to show a difference in the number of charged amino acids between the two molecules, and theorized that a neutral substitution could modify the conformation of the polypeptide chain and change the ionization constant of acidic or basic residues. This insightful idea—one that much later was found to apply to other abnormal hemoglobins—turned out not to be applicable to HbS. Pauling's error was a result of the intrinsic difficulty of detecting small changes in the number of amino acids by amino acid analysis when the total number of residues in a polypeptide chain is large. Most important, Pauling et al. (1949) demonstrated that sickle cell trait or "sicklemia" red cells contained both HbA and HbS, whereas sickle cell anemia cells had only HbS. This biochemical finding clearly supported the genetic notion advanced by Neel (1949).

The biochemical definition of HbS had to wait until Ingram (1956) developed a technique capable of probing the primary sequence of a protein. This technique (peptide mapping or "fingerprinting") involved digestion of the protein with trypsin followed by two-dimensional separation of the generated peptides—electrophoresis in one direction and chromatography at right angles to the electrophoresis. This powerful and relatively easy technique changed the history of biochemistry by improving and accelerating the study of proteins. Its first application was the study of HbS: Only one of the peptides in the "fingerprint" of this hemoglobin differed from its counterpart in normal hemoglobin. Sequence analysis of that peptide revealed that the substitution of valine for glutamic acid in position six of the β-globin chain was the physical basis of HbS (Ingram, 1957). That finding explained, among other things, the electrophoretic difference between these two hemoglobins, and it was the first demonstration of a single amino acid substitution in a human protein.

Pauling's groundbreaking idea led to the concept of molecular disease, a physiologic abnormality secondary to a change in a critical protein. For our understanding of genetic diseases, this comes close to the impact that the germ theory of Pasteur and Koch in the previous century had for physicians and scientists.

THE AFRICAN SICKLE GENE AND ITS DISPERSION THROUGHOUT THE WORLD

The Molecular Biology of the β^S Gene

Molecular biological methods allow disease genes to be examined directly. Globin genes were among the first to be located in the human genome. As has happened before, hemoglobinopathies became a model system, this time for the study of disease at the gene level. Goldstein et al. (1963) elucidated the sequence of the β-globin chains of hemoglobin. The DNA sequence of the β-globin gene revealed that the change from glutamic acid to valine in β globin was produced

by substitution of the triplet GTG for GAG in sixth codon of the first exon of the gene. Deisseroth et al. (1975), using hybrid cell lines, finally assigned the β-globin gene to chromosome 11, flanked on its 5′ end by the parathyroid hormone gene, the two γ-globin genes and the δ-globin gene and on its 3′ side by the C-Ha-ras-1 gene and the insulin gene (Chapter 6).

African β^S-Globin Gene Cluster

An important chapter in understanding the genetics of sickle cell anemia began with the discovery by Kan and Dozy (1978) that the β^S-globin gene was in linkage disequilibrium with a polymorphic site located in its 3′ flanking region that was identifiable by an Hpa I restriction endonuclease cleavage site. In 60 percent of African Americans homozygous for the HbS gene, the abnormal gene was linked to the absence of this site (Hpa I negative [–]), whereas in 40 percent, a Hpa I cleavage site was present (Hpa I positive [+]). This result contrasted with a frequency of this site of only 6 percent of black Americans with normal hemoglobin. It was proposed, based on limited data, that linkage to the wild type Hpa I positive site was characteristic of West Africans, whereas a Hpa I negative site was characteristic of East Africans (Kan and Dozy, 1980). These data did not show definitively that the mutation had occurred in two different chromosomal backgrounds, because a secondary mutation at the Hpa I site could have postdated the sickle mutation.

Rapidly thereafter, Mears et al. (1981a, 1981b) showed in samples of human blood from three regions of Africa, each characterized by a high β^S-globin gene frequency, that the distribution of the Hpa I linkage disequilibrium was more complex. Hpa I polymorphism was segregated in Africa in three locations. Atlantic West Africa and Bantu-speaking Central Africa had Hpa I negative-linked β^S genes, whereas Central West Africa had Hpa I positive-linked β^S genes. This observation increased the possibility that the β^S mutation could have been multicentric in origin. Nevertheless, it would still be possible, albeit with diminishing probability, that these mutations occurred after the sickle mutation.

In parallel work, Orkin and co-workers (Orkin et al., 1983; Antonarakis et al., 1985) developed the concept of haplotype based on a series of restriction endonuclease-defined polymorphisms. In these studies, DNA sequence differences in the β-globin gene cluster were detectable by restriction enzymes that fail to cut DNA if the enzyme target sequence is not exactly correct. These authors linked specific thalassemia mutations to particular haplotypes with the hope that haplotypes could serve as diagnostic tools. This approach was not totally successful because it rapidly became evident that more than one thalassemic mutation was linked to the same haplotype and that more than one haplotype was linked to the same mutation. Nevertheless, the effort to understand the relationship between thalassemia and β-like globin gene cluster haplotypes stimulated others to apply this technique to detect the origins of the sickle mutation. A breakthrough came when eleven restriction sites were examined to define haplotypes in sickle cell anemia patients from the three regions in Africa previously studied (Mears et al., 1981a, 1981b; Pagnier et al., 1984) (see below). In addition to these three major haplotypes linked to the β^S-globin gene, a fourth minor African haplotype, the Cameroon (see below), has been found to be a "private" haplotype of the Eton ethnic group indicating a fourth origin of the HbS gene in Africa (Lapoumeroulie et al., 1989). In this group, the Cameroon haplotype reached polymorphic frequencies but expansion beyond the original ethnic group did not occur.

Epidemiology of the β^S-Globin Gene in Africa

Based on their analyses of eleven polymorphic restriction sites, Pagnier et al. (1984) established that the β^S-globin gene was present on three distinctly different chromosomes (Fig. 26.1). Each was identifiable by its specific array of DNA polymorphisms, or haplotypes, and each was largely localized to one of the three separate geographic areas (Atlantic West Africa, Central West Africa, and Bantu-speaking Central and Southern Africa). The β^S gene in Africa is principally distributed around these three main geographic locations, each exhibiting a center of high frequency surrounded by regions of declining frequencies. In Central West Africa the central gene frequency was 0.12 to 0.14 (minimum, 0.02); in the Congo and Zaire the central frequency was 0.12 to 0.14 (minimum, 0.02); around Senegal in Atlantic West Africa the central frequency was 0.08 to 0.10 (minimum, 0.02) (Fig. 26.2). This finding was interpreted as indicating that the β^S gene originated at least three times, with subsequent expansions of the frequency of the abnormal gene, in each of these geographical areas. The strongest argument for this interpretation is the geographic segregation of these distinct haplotypes, one of which is associated with the β^S gene in each of these locales. Atypical haplotypes, haplotypes different from the major haplotypes associated with the β^S gene, are all explainable by crossing-over events around a "hot spot" of recombination 5' to the ψβ-globin gene (Chakravarti et al., 1984). Differences between atypical and typical haplotypes of each geographic area are generally found in the region 5' to this "hot spot" (Srinivas et al., 1988).

Strikingly, of more than twenty haplotypes associated with the β^S-globin gene in Jamaica, whose black population was generated by forced migration from Africa during the eighteenth century (see later), the three haplotypes previously described (Pagnier et al., 1984) comprised more than 95% of the cases (Wainscoat et al., 1983; Antonarakis et al., 1984). This showed that the three geographically segregated haplotypes were the major β^S-linked haplotypes in Africa (Fig. 26.1) and suggested that the rest might represent "private" haplotype linkages generated by fresh mutations, gene conversion, or more classic crossing-over events around the putative "hot spot" 5' to the ψβ-globin gene. Nevertheless, these three major haplotypes and other atypical haplotypes have coexisted in Jamaica only since the eighteenth century, limiting the potential for the suggested crossing-over events (Fig. 26.3).

Further evidence regarding the separate origin of the three major haplotypes linked to the β^S-globin gene came from the studies of Chebloune et al. (1988) on variable repeats of the ATTTT motifs found about 1.5 kb 5' to the β-globin gene and the AT repeats (followed by T runs of different size) found about 0.5 kb 5' to the β-globin gene. Early DNA sequencing in this region (Spritz, 1981; Moschonas et al. 1982) suggested that these repeats were polymorphic. Chebloune and co-workers (1984) used S_1 nuclease digestion and hybridization with single stranded probes (with ATTTT repeated either four or five times with $(AT)_x T_y$ probes having $\times = 7$ or 11 and $Y = 7$ or 3. (Fig. 26.4). Their results were complemented by sequence data from −1080 bp 5' to the cap site of the β-globin gene. It is apparent that the combination of these polymorphic areas is unique for each haplotype, supporting the independent origin of the haplotype region located 3' to the hot spot of recombination.

Time Line for the Appearance and Expansion of the β^S-Globin Gene in Africa

Once the HbS mutation occurred, its increasing frequency was connected with the relative protection the heterozygote (sickle cell trait carrier) had from death owing to *Plasmodium falciparum* malaria. When carriers of sickle cell trait become infected with *P. falciparum*, their mortality is lower than that of noncarriers because increased sickling rates of parasitized cells renders them prone to splenic removal (Chapter 30). Parasitized cells become static and highly deoxygenated because of their adherence to venule endothelium during deep vascular schizogony. Further protection is provided by persistence of high levels of HbF for longer times in some children with sickle cell trait.

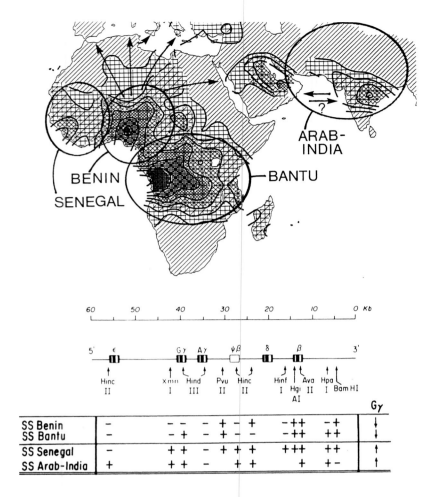

Figure 26.1. (**Upper diagram**) The incidence of HbS in the African continent, the Mediterranean, the Middle East, and the Indian subcontinent according to Bodner and Cavalli-Sforza and the approximate boundaries of the four known major β^S-linked haplotypes. The arrow depicts the possible routes of gene flow involving the Benin haplotypes and their presence in Morocco, Algeria, Turkey, eastern oasis of Saudi Arabia, and by the data presented here, in Sicily. (**Lower diagram**) Haplotypes of the β-globin gene cluster. This cluster corresponds to a 60 kb stretch of DNA that contains the β-globin gene and other highly homologous globin genes. It is generally inherited en bloc but a "hot spot" of recombination has been located around the ψβ-δ region. Depicted by arrows are also the location of the sites recognized by several restriction endonucleases. These sites are polymorphic in human populations, which means that they can be present (+) or absent (–) in different individuals. Haplotypes correspond to the set of + and – sites. Although about twenty different haplotypes are found in different ethnic groups, only five to seven are common. Linkage disequilibrium is present with the β^S gene because 90.7 percent of them are associated with one haplotype (a single change in Hinc II is observed in most of these). In the top of this figure is depicted the β-like gene cluster and indicated by arrows the endonuclease-definable polymorphic sites. The rest of the figure illustrates the haplotypes defined for β^S and β^A in Sicilian populations (n = number of chromosomes found.) (The nomenclature of the Roman numeral haplotypes is according to Orkin et al., 1982.)

An important question is when the β^S mutation expansion occurred. Although the age of the β^S mutation is not known with precision, expansion of the mutation probably occurred coincident with malaria, a strong selective factor, becoming endemic. This coincided with the establishment of significant agriculture that favored large sedentary populations and created a need for irrigation, which by generating still-water ponds, provided good breeding grounds for the *Anopheles* mosquito (Diamond, 1997) (Chapter 30). Accordingly, the expansion of the mutation in Africa occurred about 2,000 to 2,500 years ago and was perhaps further enhanced by the arrival in Africa of the Southeast Asian agricultural complex in the Bantu-speaking portions of Africa about 1,500 years ago (Diamond, 1997). The Bantu haplotype-linked mutation seems to have originated before the Bantu expansion so that it could not have occurred less than 2,000 years ago.

Some calculations put the origin of the β^S gene tens of thousands of years ago (Kurnit, 1979). Based on the mistaken premise that the Hpa I polymorphism followed the β^S mutation, and that in Africa, Hpa I-positive and-negative people coexisted in the same

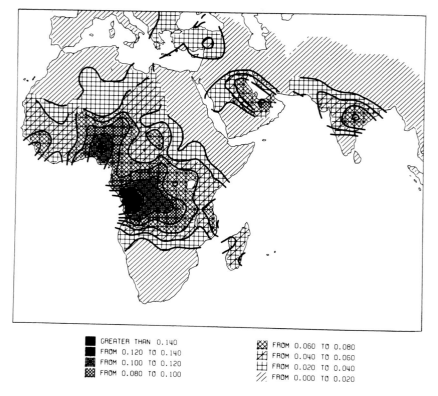

GREATER THAN 0.140
FROM 0.120 TO 0.140
FROM 0.100 TO 0.120
FROM 0.080 TO 0.100

FROM 0.060 TO 0.080
FROM 0.040 TO 0.060
FROM 0.020 TO 0.040
FROM 0.000 TO 0.020

Figure 26.2. Isogenic (equal gene frequencies are corrected) map of the gene frequency of the β^S gene in Africa. Notice three areas of high gene frequency and decreasing concentric lines around each one of these foci. (Bodmer and Cavalli-Sforza)

population, this analysis is likely to be incorrect (Stine et al., 1992). Others have proposed that the mutation could have been "lying around" and that the expansion by malaria should be separated from the origin of the mutation (Bodmer and Solomon, 1979). This last issue deserves further consideration but cannot currently be accepted for lack of supportive evidence. Although β^S mutations could have occurred in Africa and elsewhere before agriculture existed, it is unlikely that without a positive selection, a mutation would remain long in a population, especially when the homozygote has such low fitness. Repeated mutations could have arisen and disappeared over time. The mutations present when malaria became endemic and the number of β^S carriers whose progeny expanded abruptly are critical. We can exclude the possibility of localized coexistence of all or several of the major African haplotypes in any significant number, as all of them would have been expanded simultaneously, although not necessarily with the same intensity, and they would coexist today in the same geographic locations. The geographic segregation of the β^S-globin gene-linked haplotypes is a strong argument that a single mutation was available for expansion in each geographic area.

Genetic and Anthropologic Consequences of the Study of β^S-Linked Haplotypes in Africa

A mutation of the β-globin gene is, by necessity, linked to a particular haplotype of polymorphic DNA sites that exist within 60 kbp of the affected gene (Fig. 26.1). As each new β-globin gene mutation occurs, it has the opportunity of being associated with a different haplotype. Interestingly, the number of β-globin gene cluster haplotypes in all populations is limited to about five to ten, with three to four haplotypes predominant in each population. In different ethnic groups, the nature and frequency of the haplotypes differ. Consequently, if a population exhibits a β-globin gene mutation exclusively associated with a single haplotype, we can assume that the mutational event occurred only once or was unicentric. Three important restrictions to this assumption apply. First, the mutation could have appeared more than once but then disappeared from the population by mechanisms such as genetic drift, gene flow, or selective pressure. Second, the mutation could have appeared more than once, but each time in the same haplotype. The likelihood of these two events occurring depends on the mutational frequency and on the frequency of haplotypes linked to the mutation in the population under study. Third, the strength of the conclusion regarding the unicentricity or multicentricity of a β-globin gene mutation depends on the extent of linkage of the β-globin gene to all the polymorphic sites under consideration. The

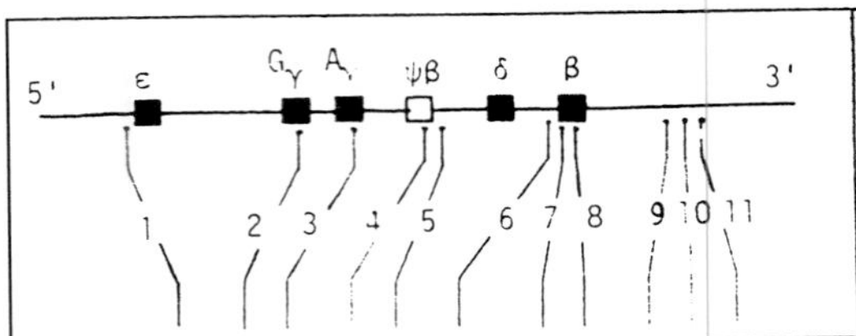

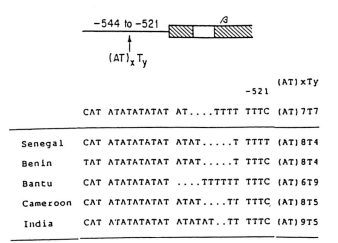

Figure 26.3 table: List of haplotypes of DNA polymorphisms in the β-globin gene cluster. Diagram at top shows sites 5′ — ε — Gγ Aγ — ψβ — δ — β — 3′, with polymorphism sites numbered 1, 2, 3, 4, 5, 6, 7, 8, 9, 10, 11.

	No.	1	2	3	4	5	6	7	8	9	10	11	βA Am.Blacks	βA Jam.Blacks	βA Total	βS Am.Blacks	βS Jam.Blacks	βS Total	βA Meds	βS Meds
	1	+	−	+	−	−	+	+	+			−	1		1	1	2	3	8	
d	2	+	+	−	+	+	+	+	+	+	+	+	1	1	2	5	6	11	1 5	
c	3	−	+	−	+	+	+	+	+	+	+	+	3	3	6					
	4		−		+	+	+	+	−	−	+	+	2		2					
	5	+	−	+	+	+	+	+	•		+	+	1	2	3					
	6	+	−	−	−	+	+	+	+		+	+	1		1					
	7	+	−	+	−	+	−	−		+		+	1		1					
e	8	−	−	−	+	−	+	+	+	+	+	+	2	1	3	1	2	3		
f	9	−	−	−	−	+	−	−	+	−		+	1		1		1	1	12	
	10	+	−	−	+	−	+	+	+	+		+	1		1				1	
	11	−	−	−	+	+	+	+	+	+		+	5		5				42	
	12	−	−	−	+	+	+	+	+	+		+	3	5	8					
	13	+	−	−	+	+	+	+	+	+		+	1	3	4					
	14	+	+	−	−	−	+	−	−	+		+	1		1					
	15	+	−	−	+	+	+	+	+	−		−	1		1					
	16	−	−	+	+	−	+	+	+			−	1		1					
g	17	+	+	−	+	+	+	+	+	+		−	1		1	2		2	2	
h	18	−	−	−	+	−	+	+	+	+		−	1		1	1		1		
A	19	−	−	−	+	−	+	+	−		+	+	1		1	45	63	108		9
B	20	−	+	−	−	−	+	+	+	−	+	+				17	15	32		2
i	21	+	−	−	+	−	+	+	−		+	+				1		1		
j	22	−	−	−	−	−	+	+	+	−		+				1		1		
k	23	+	+	−	−	−	+	+	+	−		+				2		2		
	24	−	−	−	−	+	+	+	+			−		1	1				22	
	25	−	−	−	−	−	−	−	+			+		1	1					
l	26	−	−	−	−	−	+	+	+	E		+		1	1		1	1	1	
m	27	−	−	+	+	+	+	+	−			+					1	1		
n	28	+	−	+	−	−	+	+	+			+					1	1		
o	29	+	−	+	+	−	+	+	+	+		+					1	1	1	
p	30	−	−	−	+	+	+	+	−		+	+					1	1		
	31	+	−	+	+	+	+	+	+			−							5	
	32	+	−	+	+	+	−	−		+		+							4	
	33	+	+	−	+	+	−	−		+		+							4	
	34	+	−	+	+	+	+	+				−							1	
	35	+	−	−	−	+	+	+				+							1	
	36	+	+	−	+		+	+				+							1	
	37	+	+	−	+	−	+	+				−							1	
	38	+	+	−	−	+	+	+				+							1	
	TOTAL:												29	18	47	76	94	170	122	11

Figure 26.3. List of haplotypes of DNA polymorphisms in the β-globin gene cluster associated with various β-globin gene-bearing chromosomes in Jamaica (Antonarakis et al., 1984). Each haplotype is numbered. The haplotypes associated with the βˢ chromosomes are also indicated by letters. The three most common such haplotypes are denoted with the capital letters (A, B, and C). Meds, Mediterranean subjects; Am., American; Jam., Jamaican. The DNA polymorphisms examined are: 1, Hinc II, 5′ to ε-globin gene; 2, Hind III, $^G\gamma$-globin gene IVS-2; 3, Hind III, $^A\gamma$-globin gene IVS-2; 4, Hinc II, ψβ-globin gene; 6, Hinf I, 5′ to β-globin gene; 7, HgiA I, β-globin gene; 8, Ava II, β^{IVS-2}; 9, Hpa I, 3′ to β-globin gene; 10, Hind III, 3′ to β-globin gene; 11, BamH I, 3′ to β-globin gene. In haplotype 26, E in the DNA polymorphism no. 10 column denotes an extra band on the autoradiogram, which represents a polymorphism pattern different from + or − at that site. The asterisk in haplotype 5 in the DNA polymorphism no. 9 column refers to a polymorphism (7.0-kb fragment) different from that designated + or −.

Figure 26.4. The $(AT)_x(T)_y$ repeat motif found in the mid −500 region 5′ to the βˢ gene according to haplotype. The right column summarizes the motif for each haplotype.

−544 to −521 ——— β
$(AT)_x T_y$
−521 ———— $(AT)_x T_y$

					$(AT)_x T_y$
	CAT	ATATATATAT	AT....TTTT	TTTC	(AT)7T7
Senegal	CAT	ATATATATAT	ATAT.....T	TTTT	(AT)8T4
Benin	TAT	ATATATATAT	ATAT.....T	TTTC	(AT)8T4
Bantu	CAT	ATATATATAT	....TTTTTT	TTTC	(AT)6T9
Cameroon	CAT	ATATATATAT	ATAT....TT	TTTC	(AT)8T5
India	CAT	ATATATATAT	ATATAT..TT	TTTC	(AT)9T5

weight of this last issue increases proportionally to the age of the mutation. Chakravarti et al. (1984) provided evidence that not all polymorphic sites usually included in the β-globin gene cluster haplotypes are equally linked to the β-globin gene because there is a "hot spot" of recombination between the ψβ-globin gene and the δ-globin gene. Sequence divergence in the 5′ portion of the haplotype should be expected if the mutation emerged many generations ago. (Fig. 26.5) (see below).

Anthropologic Implications of the Distribution of the β^S-Globin Gene in Africa

Haplotypes are valuable in anthropologic studies involving gene flow because they serve as markers for geographically specific mutations whose migration can be easily traced (Nagel, 1984). Available evidence suggests that about 4,000 years ago, the populations living in sub-Saharan Africa were racially diverse, with three major racial groups predominating: Negroes in West

Africa, Pygmies in Equatorial Africa, and Bushmen (Sen people) in Southern Africa. In contrast, various Semitic and Hamitic groups lived in northern Africa: Cushites, Berbers, Nilo-Saharans, etc. Based on exhaustive linguistic data, Greenberg (1973) postulated, that about 2,000 years ago, the balance of power drastically changed in favor of the Negroes of West Africa.

Domestication of plants expanded agricultural land needs, and the development of effective weapons propelled a massive invasion-migration. Populations living in the margins of the Benue River (Eastern Nigeria) successfully invaded the east and south of Africa, engulfing and later eradicating the indigenous Pygmies and Bushmen. Pygmies were restricted to certain forest regions of equatorial Africa, a limited portion of their historic range. Bushmen, in turn, were chased into the Kalahari desert in Namibia, a significant change from their earlier environment, where they are found today.

Linguistics provides the primary evidence for these events. In West Africa, more than 400 completely unrelated languages are spoken. In equatorial and southern Africa, all the spoken languages have clear interconnections, detectable by the use of similar words, and are regarded collectively as Bantu stock. Since the language closest to that of the Bantu group is spoken in eastern Nigeria, a region contiguous to the Bantu territory, it was concluded that the Bantu expansion originated here. Expertise in agriculture, metallurgy, and fluvial transportation, characteristics

Figure 26.5. The locations of fifteen polymorphic sites are indicated, the numbers below them signifying the distance in kb between adjacent sites. The restriction endonucleases are A, Ava II; B, BamH I; Ha Hpa I; Hc Hinc II; Hd, Hind III; Hf, Hinf I; Hi, HgiA I; R, Rsa I; T, Taq I. The positions of the repeated elements are indicated by *; the location of the chi site is marked by X. The observed and expected recombination rates over the entire cluster are denoted by the lines —— and — —, respectively.

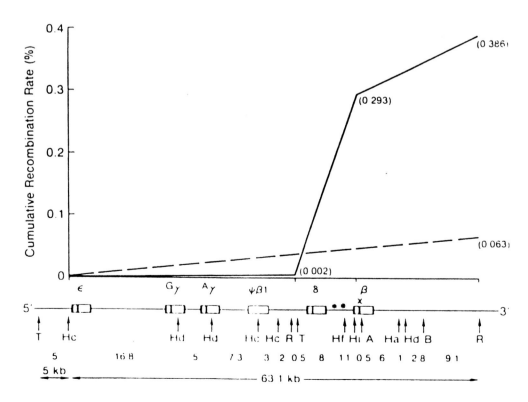

of this group, is consistent with the undertaking of such a monumental territorial conquest.

Sow et al. (1995) have examined the haplotypes of carriers of the β^S-globin gene in the Republic of Guinea, which shares borders with Senegal, Mali, Ivory Coast, and Liberia. The present day Republic of Guinea has a population of more than 7 million and occupies about 250,000 km^2 of the north Atlantic Coast of sub-Saharan Africa. Its major ethnic groups are the Peuhl (about 33 percent), the Malinke (related to the Mandingo and other Mende-speaking ethnic groups, about 31 percent) and the Soussous (about 11 percent). The rest, amounting to 25%, are smaller ethnic groups, some related to the major groups but others entirely independent. Among the latter, the ethnicities with the highest numbers are the Guerze, the Kissi, and the Toma.

Of fifty-six chromosomes bearing the β^S gene linked to the Senegal haplotype, Sow found that all were in subjects of Malinke, Soussou, and Peuhl origin. The only two chromosomes with Benin haplotype were in Malinke individuals, an ethnic group that straddles between Guinea and Mali, where some Malinke subethnic groups have the β^S gene linked to the Benin haplotype (Fig. 26.6A). The extent of Malinke presence in this region is the consequence of the expansion of the Mali Empire between the twelfth and fifteenth centuries that spread Mende-speaking people into Senegal, Gambia, Guinea, Sierra Leone, and western Mali. The Soussou ethnic group, currently living in the coastal region of Guinea and Guinea-Bissau, was probably related to the Ghana Empire (Fig. 26.6B), which was dominant in the tenth-century (Bohannan and Curtin, 1971). The Peuhl (also called Fulani), whose origin is presently disputed, occupy the mountainous central region of Guinea, known as Fouta Djallon. This historical data provide a context for the genetic evidence that in Atlantic West Africa—Senegal, Guinea, Ivory Coast, and Liberia—the β^S gene is in linkage disequilibrium with the Senegal haplotype.

Mitochondrial DNA evidence indicates that individuals living in Senegal and surrounding regions have been separated from ethnic groups in Central West Africa for 40 thousand years (Stine et al., 1992). This isolation has been breaking down in the last centuries, as the Mali-related Malinke groups move into present day Guinea (Bohannan and Curtin, 1971; Stine et al., 1992).

HbS-linked haplotypes in Africa have provided the first biological evidence of the Bantu expansion (Fig. 26.7). The Bantu haplotype linked to the β^S-globin gene exists exclusively in African populations found west of the Benue river, supporting the Greenberg hypothesis. Ojwang et al. (1987), studying sickle cell anemia patients from the Luo and Lubya tribes of Western Kenya, established that fifty-six of fifty-eight cases stud-

ied carried the Bantu haplotype. Moreover, Ramsay and Jenkins (1987), who studied several ethnic groups in the northern portions of South Africa, the southernmost extreme of Bantu-speaking Africa, also found the β^S-globin gene linked to the Bantu haplotype.

Based on the examination of many polymorphic sites and the finding of the same haplotypes in the normal population, it is unlikely that the initially described Hpa I linkage disequilibrium arose a posteriori to the β^S mutation. Rather, the Hpa I polymorphism and these related haplotypes must have preexisted the HbS mutation.

So far we have dealt only with the origins of the HbS mutation. Next, we turn to the issue of how these separate mutations acquired high frequencies in their central foci and why there are genetic clines, or frequency decreases nearly concentrically around their centers of highest frequency. Amplification of the β^S-globin gene frequency is the result of the selective influence of *P. falciparum* malaria. Spread of the HbS gene over large distances and across ethnic barriers occurred through gene flow coupled with the presence of malaria throughout equatorial Africa.

Gene flow could have occurred by two mechanisms. Commerce and industrial contacts almost always involved the exchange of genes, even between unrelated ethnic groups. Slave owners in Africa, unlike those in Europe, freed the children of dead slaves, and the freed children remained with their erstwhile captors, providing the opportunity to spread their genes within the captors' ethnic group.

Genetic clines are a result of reduced gene flow as the distance from the center of origin and expansion increases. With the Cameroon haplotype of the Eton group, polymorphic frequencies were also reached, but did not expand beyond the original ethnic group except for some small spillover into the Ewondo, a contiguous ethnic group in central Cameroon (Fig. 26.8)

Some have postulated that the origin of the major African haplotypes can be explained by recombination (Livingstone, 1989). If so, this should generate at least two different β^S-globin gene associated haplotypes for any given geographic area; this has not been observed. The polymorphic frequencies of the three major haplotypes linked to the β^S gene indicate that haplotypes are selected for as long as they carry the β^S gene. Thus, overwhelming differential survival of one of two β^S-linked haplotypes generated by a hypothetical crossover, to the point where the other is extinguished, is unlikely. The appearance of the Cameroon haplotype in the midst of the Benin haplotype, an observation not explainable by recombination, and the presence of haplotype-specific sequences on both sides of the "hot spot" of recombination, make the recombination theory of the origin of the β^S gene untenable. Flint et al. (1993a) have proposed

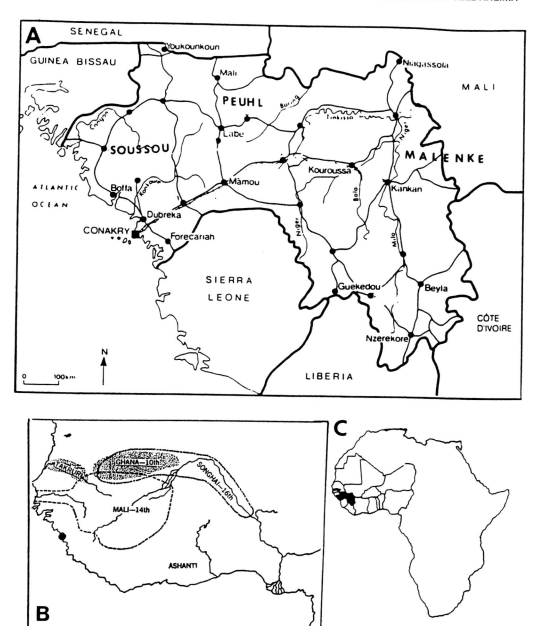

Figure 26.6. (**A**) Map of the Republic of Guinea—south of Senegal and bordering on Mali, Ivory Coast, and Liberia. (**B**) Ghana Empire. (**C**) Present-day Republic of Guinea on the northern Atlantic coast of sub-Sahara Africa.

that gene conversion could be involved in the generation of haplotypes. Gene conversion has occurred between the γ-globin genes. Also, instances of double recombination or gene conversion could explain some rare haplotypes such as those described by Goncalves et al. (1994a). Nevertheless, evidence of gene conversion has not been found in the majority of the major haplotypes linked to the β^S-globin gene. Finally, detailed sequencing of many sections of the β-globin gene cluster beyond the

restriction endonuclease polymorphic sites used to assign a haplotype has shown that in the great majority of cases, each of the major haplotypes linked to HbS shows almost complete fidelity in all regions analyzed (Lanclos et al., 1991).

GENETIC AND ANTHROPOLOGIC STUDIES OF β^S-LINKED HAPLOTYPES IN THE MEDITERRANEAN BASIN

Strong historical evidence of the connection between Sicily and North Africa raised the suspicion that the β^S gene was introduced into **Sicily** by gene flow from Africa (Fig. 26.9). A high prevalence of African red cell

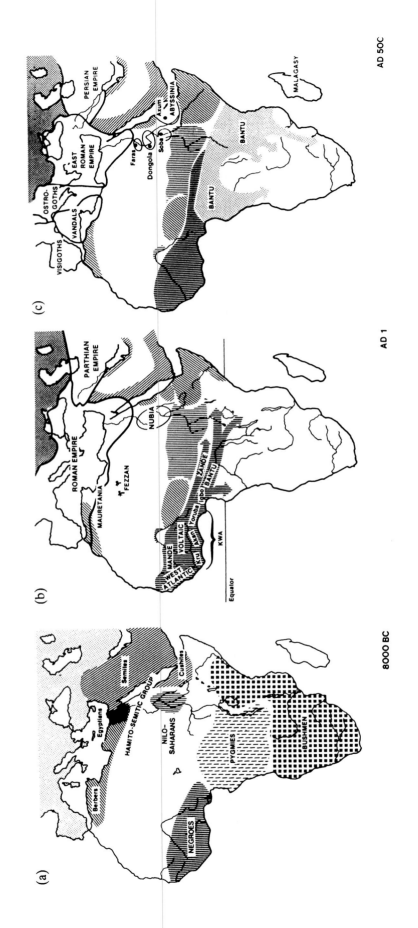

Figure 26.7. Black Africans originally inhabited only western Africa. By AD1 they could be distinguished linguistically. West African language speakers resided in areas where the Senegal β-globin gene is now found, and speakers of the Kwa language resided where the Benin haplotype is present. The Bantu expansion began in eastern Nigeria (see text). The Bantu haplotype distribution is explainable if this haplotype originated at the time of the Bantu expansion.

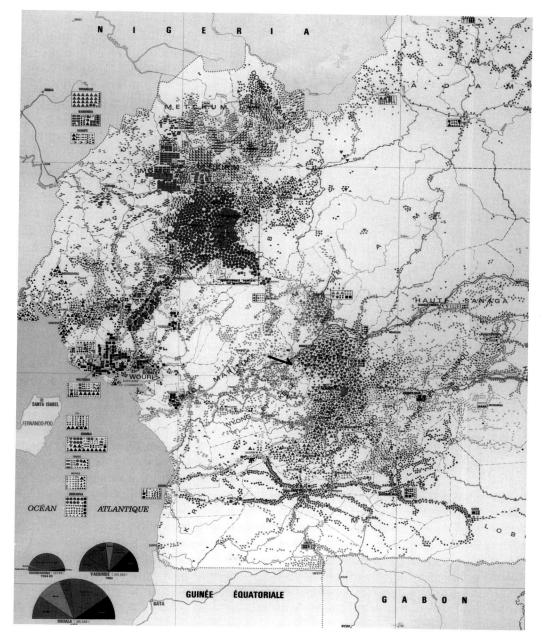

Figure 26.8. Ethnologic map of southern Cameroon. Depicted in brown triangle pointing down is the distribution of the Eton people (black arrow). All the symbols in brown are related ethnicities. Of particular interest is the Ewondo people (also carriers of the Camaroon haplotype), depicted by the brown triangle pointing up. (Map from the Service Cartographique de l'ORSTOM. D Laidek, J. Montels, F. Meunier, 1971.) For full color reproduction, see color plate 26.8.

antigens is present among the Sicilian carriers of the β^S gene (Sadler et al., 1978). Although the HbS of Sicilian sickle cell anemia patients and African Americans was identical, differences in HbF levels and erythrocyte 2,3 biphosphoglycerate concentration appeared to be sig-

nificantly different; however, few subjects were studied (Roth et al., 1980).

Sicilian β^A- and β^S-globin gene-bearing chromosomes show that the β^S gene is in linkage disequilibrium in 100 percent of the cases with the Benin haplotype, which to date has not been found in normal Sicilians (Maggio et al., 1986; Ragusa et al., 1988) (Fig. 26.10). This suggests that the β^S gene was introduced into Sicily from central West Africa, most probably via North Africa (Fig. 26.1). Absence of a Taq I restriction site between the γ-globin genes of all sickle cell anemia chromosomes, a characteristic also shared by the Benin haplotypes in Africa (Ragusa et al., 1988), gives further credence to the African origin of this chromosome, as

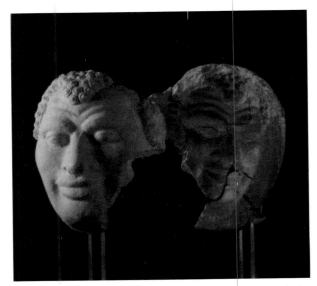

Figure 26.9. A sculpture and its cast of an African male found in Sicily and dated from the Roman era. Arqueological Museum of Siracusa, Sicily, Italy. Along with other evidence such as the mosaic floors of Piazza Armerina, this finding establishes the presence of Africans in Sicily in the Roman era.

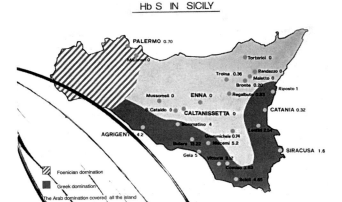

Figure 26.10. Frequency of the β^S-globin gene in several towns in Sicily. The higher frequencies for this gene are the southern coast of the island that faces Africa, which likely facilitated contacts during Roman times. This coast is also the site for the invasion of Italy by Muslims in 700 PE. The Arab invasion also included Sudanese troops, which explains the high incidence of the gene in Butera, site of the Sudanese garrison (see text).

this feature is specific for sub-Saharan Black populations and is absent in Mediterranean and Oriental peoples (Wainscoat et al., 1986).

In some Sicilian towns, the HbS gene has a high frequency. Highest is in Butera, where 12 percent of the population carry this gene. A founder effect is likely because of the strategic position this town occupied during the Arab conquest of Sicily when Butera was headquarters of an Arab military unit containing Sudanese regiments. Still, the question must be asked whether 12 percent of the genes of the population of Butera are truly of African origin. Introduced β^S-globin genes could have been expanded in frequency by malaria, which was rampant in Sicily until it was eradicated by the American Army at the end of World War II. This question was resolved by examining 267 normal chromosomes from 142 people from Butera for β-globin gene markers less likely to be selected for by malaria (Ragusa et al., 1992). The aforementioned Taq I polymorphism (Wainscoat et al., 1986) between the γ-globin genes is especially informative in this regard. Only two instances of the African marker (Taq I negative) were found, showing that the admixture with Africans occurred at a much lower level (less than 1 percent) than previously thought.

A similar approach has detected flow of the β^S gene from central West Africa to North Africa. In **Morocco** and **Algeria** the β^S-globin gene is also linked to the Benin haplotype (Mears et al., 1981b), which most likely traveled through the well-known ancient vertical trans-Saharan routes that are still partially active and commandeered by the Tuareg tribes of Berber origin. DiRienzo et al. (1987) reported that in **Egypt**, all β^S genes were associated with the Benin haplotype. In addition, the Benin haplotype is found in the majority of sickle cell anemia patients in the western portions of **Saudi Arabia**, again suggesting the flow of this gene from central West Africa, perhaps through North Africa, during the Arab slave trade. This observation contrasts with the haplotype associated with the β^S gene in the eastern oases of Saudi Arabia, where it is linked to the Arab-India haplotype, a non-African haplotype, discussed later.

All β^S chromosomes studied in **Greece** and **Albania** were of the Benin haplotype (Kollia et al., 1987; Boletini et al., 1994). Eti-Turk patients with sickle cell anemia and their relatives from Cukurova in southern **Turkey** also had Benin haplotype β^S chromosomes, except for one case where there was linkage to the Arab-India haplotype (Aluoch et al., 1986).

These data establish that the β^S-globin gene found in all of North Africa and the Mediterranean originated entirely from central West Africa.

GENETIC AND ANTHROPOLOGIC STUDIES OF β^S-LINKED HAPLOTYPES IN THE CARIBBEAN

All three major African haplotypes in American populations are associated with the β^S-globin gene and migrated via the eighteenth century British Atlantic slave trade. Slaves originated throughout most of sub-Sahara Africa, reinforcing the use of haplotypes for the study of gene flow to the Americas (Nagel, 1984). Amerindians do not have the HbS gene, so its existence in the

Americas results largely, although not exclusively, from African gene flow. The geographic origins of African slaves varied with time and with the enslaving European power that defined the American port of destination.

In 152 chromosomes from Jamaican patients with sickle cell anemia, 84 percent corresponded to the three major African haplotypes (Wainscoat et al., 1983). Other haplotypes had low individual frequencies and could have arisen as independent mutations or by crossing over, gene conversion, or mutation in the major haplotypes. These minor haplotypes have not had the necessary time to expand, and for gene flow analysis they are irrelevant, except for a few instances of the Arab-India haplotype linked to the β^S gene, which could have been brought to the New World by Indian immigrants (of tribal descent) or by Arab merchants. In a separate study from Jamaica, 90 percent of haplotypes of ninety-four chromosomes from sickle cell anemia patients corresponded to the three major African haplotypes (Antonarakis et al., 1984) (Fig. 26.3).

Based on haplotype and Hpa I restriction site distribution, it can be concluded that the Senegal haplotype is characteristic of populations extending from present-day Senegal to most of the Ivory Coast. A Benin haplotype corresponds to populations from present-day Ghana to Gabon; the Bantu haplotype corresponds to all of Bantu-speaking Africa, including the Central African Republic, Congo, Angola, Mozambique, and other countries of East Africa and southern Africa.

Does the distribution of haplotypes in Jamaica and other regions of the New World reflect the proportion of slaves that came to Jamaica and other countries from different sites in Africa? Before answering this question, a brief analysis of the slave trade is required. The extent of the export of African slaves between the sixteenth- and nineteenth-centuries is not precisely known. The classic analysis by Curtin (1969) estimated that about 10 million Africans were shipped to the new continent (adding some recent corrections to the period 1761 to 1810 and more substantial corrections to the North American trade).

Between 1655 and 1701, the British imported approximately 88,000 slaves to Jamaica; during the eighteenth century, the total importation rose to 662,400 (Curtin, 1969). Approximately 206,200 of these were reexported to other areas within the English sphere of influence, including continental North America. Table 26.1 displays grouping, by port of origin, of the 747,500 slaves imported to Jamaica between 1655 and 1807. The ports of origin coincide fairly well with homogeneous areas in terms of haplotypes (Table 26.2).

To determine composition of a population by origin, haplotype-based percentages would be accurate if the β^S-globin gene frequencies in the areas of origin in Africa

Table 26.1. Slave Imports by Origin into Jamaica (1655–1807): A Comparison of Historical Data with Percentages Calculated on the Basis of HbS-Linked Haplotypes

African ports	Historical import estimates*	Origins calculated by haplotypes†
Atlantic West Africa (Senegambia, Sierra Leone, Windward Coast)	15	1-
Central West Africa (Gold Coast, Bight of Benin, Bight of Biafra)	68	72
Bantu Africa (most of Gabon, Congo, Angola, Namibia)	17	17

In parentheses are the port names used by the English slave traders (Senegambia corresponds to present-day Senegal and Gambia; Sierra Leone encompasses the modern state of Sierra Leone, as well as both Guineas and some of Liberia; Windward Coast corresponds to present-day Ivory Coast and the rest of Liberia; Gold Coast corresponds to modern Ghana; Bight of Benin includes the region from the Volta River to the Benin River, which includes present-day Togo and the Republic of Benin; Bight of Biafra encompasses Nigeria, The Cameroons, and a small portion of Gabon down to Cape Lopez; Central Africa, which includes present day Gabon, the Congo (Brazzaville), Congo (Kinshasa), Angola, and Namibia.
* Curtin, 1969.
† Data of Antonarakis et al., 1984; Wainscoat et al., 1984 corrected for differences in regional HbS gene frequency (see text). A total of 217 HbS-linked chromosomes were studied.

were identical or very similar. In central West Africa and in Bantu-speaking equatorial and southern Africa, the frequency of the HbS gene is similar; but in Senegal, the HbS frequency is about half that of these regions, requiring doubling of the calculated percentage of the Senegal haplotypes for accurate comparisons. Remarkably, these calculations show that the composition by origin of the slave imports is close to the present-day census by haplotype calculation (Curtin, 1969).

β-gene cluster haplotypes in about 150 people, mostly children, with sickle cell disease were studied in Pointe-à-Pitre, **Guadeloupe** (Keclard et al., 1996). Ninety-two percent of all chromosomes belonged to the three major African haplotypes: 73 percent Benin, 11 percent Bantu, and 8 percent Senegal. An ^Aγ^T chain was observed on seven chromosomes, signifying a Cameroon haplotype, and about 5 percent of the β^S chromosomes had atypical haplotypes. Do these numbers fit the historical record of port of origin of the slaves brought into Guadeloupe (Nagel, 1996)?

Table 26.2. Ports of Origin and Homogeneous Haplotype Areas

| African ports | Historical import estimates* | | Origins calculated by haplotypes[†] |
	Virginia (1710–1769)	South Carolina (1733–1807)	
Atlantic West Africa (Senegambia, Sierra Leone, Windward Coast)	27	43	15
Central West Africa (Gold Coast, Bight of Benin, Bight of Biafra)	54	17	62
Bantu Africa (most of Gabon, Congo, Angola, Namibia)	20	40	18

* From Curtin, 1969.
[†] Data of Antonarakis, 1984 based on 76 HbS chromosomes of the Baltimore area.
89 percent of the haplotypes found correspond to the three major forms described (Pagnier et al., 1984).
Corrected for differences in regional HbS gene frequency (see text).

In 1654, 600 Dutch planters and their 300 African slaves arrived in Guadeloupe from Recife (Brazil) to work on sugar plantations. By 1701, the slave numbers had grown to 58,000, imported principally from Mozambique, where the Bantu haplotype predominates. In the eighteenth century, the French Nantes slave trade (Daget, 1976) brought about 240,000 Africans to Guadeloupe. Thirty-five percent came from Angola (Bantu haplotype), about 16 percent from Senegambia and Sierra Leone (Senegal haplotype), and about 45 percent from Benin and Biafra (Benin haplotype) (Curtin, 1969). In the second half of the eighteenth century, the trend was toward a drastic decrease in slaves from the Senegambia and an increase of Beninians and Bantus (Daget, 1976). By the nineteenth century, the British had outlawed the slave trade and enforced their decision by a naval blockade centered around the Senegambia coast. The French responded by building fast ships (Brick Negrieres) capable of outrunning the British cruisers. Shipment of about 100,000 slaves, destined almost entirely for Martinique and Guadeloupe, ran this blockade. Their ports of origin were 80 percent in Bantu-speaking Africa and about 5 percent in Benin, as the rest of Africa had become inaccessible because of the British blockade.

What should the port(s) of origin have been for the present day African-Guadeloupian population? Work conditions at the sugar plantations, called *habitations* by the French slavers, caused such a high death rate that importation of slaves could not keep pace, particularly at the height of the sugar industry. Hence, Africans imported into Guadeloupe at the end of the eighteenth and beginning of the nineteenth centuries had a better chance of contributing their genes to the present-day population. This consideration leads to the conclusion that people of Benin and Bantu origins contributed equally to Guadeloupe, with perhaps a small advantage to the Bantu. Yet the data of Keclard et al. (1996) are not in agreement with the historical record. These investigators found 74 percent Benin haplotypes, 11 percent Bantu haplotypes, and a relatively impressive 8 percent of the Senegal haplotype, which would correspond to about 16 percent importation from Senegambia. An explanation for this discrepancy could increase our knowledge of the effects of haplotype on survival in sickle cell anemia and/or the validity of the historical record.

If the historical record is correct, Senegal and Benin haplotypes are overrepresented. Could this be the consequence of increased survival in the first few years of life of individuals with the Benin and Senegal compared with the Bantu haplotype? A study in Guadeloupe showed that the distribution of haplotypes in sickle cell disease was the same in newborns as in older children, arguing against differential survival as an explanation (Keclard et al., 1997). Thus, the interpretation of the historical record is almost certainly incorrect. Negative population growth might have been overemphasized, or sufficient individuals may have survived, particularly house slaves, who through a high reproductive rate maintained their Bantu genes until the present. Finally, little is known about how slaves were distributed between Martinique and Guadeloupe and how the Nantes slave trade was conducted.

In forty-four **Cuban** children with sickle cell anemia, the haplotype distribution was 43 percent Benin, 38 percent Bantu, and 3 percent Senegal (Muniz et al., 1995); in forty-seven adults, the distribution was 46 percent Benin, 30 percent Bantu, and 9 percent Senegal, a statistically significant difference. When 198 chromosomes from a larger sample of patients with sickle cell anemia, HbSC disease, and HbS-β thalassemia were examined, the HbS gene was linked 51, 41, and 8 percent of the time with the Benin, Bantu, and Senegal haplotypes, respectively. Adjusting for the different frequencies of the HbS gene in Africa, these numbers would predict 16 percent of the ports of origin to be in Atlantic West Africa, 37.3 percent in central West Africa, and 46 percent in Bantu-speaking Africa. Yet the historical record claims a higher percentage from Bantu-speaking Africa (55 percent) and a much lower percentage from Senegal (3.4 percent). These findings suggest a loss of Bantu haplotypes and an excess of Senegal haplotype in sickle cell syndromes in Cuba, particularly among adults, and could reflect the differential survival and severity of the sickle cell disease linked to these haplotypes. In support of this possibility, studies in the United States have shown an association between the Bantu haplotype and more severe disease (Powars, 1991a).

Costa Rica offers yet another challenge for the study of haplotypes linked to the HbS gene. Costa Ricans of African descent are concentrated on the Atlantic and Pacific coasts, and their origin is the result of secondary migration within Central America and the Caribbean. The Atlantic Coast (Puerto Limon) was populated by immigration mostly from Jamaica in the nineteenth century, recruited to work in railroad construction and the banana industry, and reflected the British slave trade in terms of ports of origin. On the Pacific Coast, Guanacaste province is populated by descendants of Africans brought there in the sixteenth century, following the pattern of the Spanish slave trade. In the nineteenth century, an expansion of settlement and agriculture in Guanacaste province was stimulated by immigration from Cuba, because of the exile of the dissident Antonio Maceo. This augmented the number of people of African descent originally generated by the Spanish slave trade (Rodriguez, personal communication). Analysis of haplotypes from a small sample of sickle cell trait carriers revealed that on the Pacific Coast, the Benin haplotype was predominant (68 percent); on the Atlantic Coast, the Bantu haplotype was predominant (52 percent). According to historical records of the slave trade to Jamaica and Cuba collected by Curtin, the main difference in ports of origin between the British and Spanish slave trade in the nineteenth century is the excess of central West

Africans in the former and of Bantu Africans in the latter. Hence, the findings in Costa Rica are in good agreement with the historical record, although they require confirmation in a larger sample.

GENETIC AND ANTHROPOLOGIC STUDIES OF β^S-LINKED HAPLOTYPES IN THE UNITED STATES

Haplotype frequencies in African Americans with HbS offer some surprises. Owing to the bias of the South Carolina slave market, which preferred individuals of Senegalese origin and avoided individuals from the Bight of Biafra, the distribution of haplotypes should depart somewhat from averages predicted by the overall British trade of the eighteenth century, with a higher percentage of individuals from Senegambia and a lesser percentage from central West Africa. Depending on regional differences in the percentages of individuals descended from the South Carolina (Charleston) market or the Virginia (Jamestown) market, the distribution of haplotypes might be expected to vary from region to region.

Such predictions are supported by data of Antonarakis et al. (1984), who examined sickle cell anemia patients from Baltimore, Maryland, who most probably are descendants of slaves imported to Virginia. The finding of lower numbers of Atlantic West African haplotypes, if real, could be derived from a number of sources (Table 26.2). There may be differences between census and imports because of a larger contribution to the present gene pool by slaves imported in the last periods of the slave trade. The proportion of people from different ports of origin varied during the 150 years of the British slave trade and the importation of slaves from Senegambia decreased considerably from 1781 to 1801. If the individuals imported at the end of the slave trade contributed more to the gene pool of present-day African Americans, this may also explain the small discrepancies between the data of Curtin and the calculated results. Differences could also be due to selective reexportation of Senegambia slaves to South Carolina, or an underestimation of the differences in gene frequencies between Atlantic West Africa and the rest of the African Coast. Regardless, the data establish that the frequency of haplotypes linked to the β^S-globin gene varies in different regions of the United States, with more individuals of Senegalese origin in the deep South than in the border states.

Louisiana had a completely different slave trade pattern than the rest of the country. First populated by French immigrants, Louisiana followed initially the French pattern of slave trade, including their importation principally from Senegal (Island of Goree). Later, during the Spanish period, the importation diversified and also included reexportation from other Spanish colonies. When the United States purchased Louisiana, the pattern changed again and an influx of slaves and free slaves form the rest of America followed (Hall, 1992). Two interesting features are unique to Louisiana: First, the Spanish, Portuguese, and to a lesser degree the French had a different policy toward the products of interracial liaisons than did the English. Admixed individuals were classified as mulattos and given an intermediate rank in society. The English considered the mulatto and the black in the same category and discriminated equally against both. The consequence of these divergent policies was a different rate of miscegenation under the two systems, with significant racial mixing reaching into the upper classes in the early history of Louisiana and a retreat from it when the English (ie, Americans of English descent) took over. It would not be surprising to find that whites with sickle cell trait in Louisiana carry the Senegal haplotype linked to the β^S gene. When Louisiana became part of the United States, the English approach prevailed, and laws were approved that classified as Black anyone being 1/64 African. Second, the geography of the delta created conditions by which the slaves could escape and prosper in isolated communities during the French/Spanish period, speaking their own languages and maintaining their own culture. An example is the community of Pointe Coupee (Hall, 1992). It would not be surprising to find that the descendants of the Africans of Pointe Coupee also carry the Senegal haplotype.

GENETIC AND ANTHROPOLOGIC STUDIES OF β^S-LINKED HAPLOTYPES IN IBEROAMERICA

Curtin (1969) presented a comprehensive and thorough census of the Portuguese Atlantic slave trade, and his analysis of historical sources reveals important features of the influx of slaves into **Brazil**. In the second quarter of the sixteenth century, the Dutch seized northeastern Brazil, introduced sugar plantations to the region, and imported African slave labor. Between 1651 and the middle of the nineteenth century, the importation of slaves into Brazil was part of the Portuguese trade. During the second half of the sixteenth century about 50,000 slaves were imported but in the seventeenth century, this number rose to 56,000, being at that time the major component of the slave trade to the Americas. During the beginning of that century the slaves originated primarily from Senegal and surrounding areas. By the middle of the seventeenth century, the main ports of origin had moved to central West Africa (Benin) and by the end of the century to the Bantu-speaking coast (Namibia and Angola). Nevertheless, the dramatically negative population growth documented in that period

makes it unlikely that those forced immigrants made a significant contribution to the present-day Brazilian gene pool.

More interesting is the fact that, according to Goulart (quoted by Curtin [1969]), about 1,800,000 slaves were imported to Brazil in the eighteenth century, including 32 percent from central West Africa and 62 percent from Bantu-speaking Africa. From the beginning of the nineteenth century to the end of the legal trade in 1851, about 1,150,000 individuals were imported.

Through the careful records kept by the Brazilian Foreign Office, we know the ports of origin of a good portion of those introduced specifically to Bahia. About 80 percent of the 50,000 slaves imported between 1817 and 1843 (11 percent of the total Brazilian slave trade for this interval) originated in central West Africa (Benin), and about 20 percent came from Bantu-speaking Africa, a dramatic reversal from the pattern of the eighteenth century. Based on these historical data, one can predict that the percentage of Bantu haplotypes among present-day HbS carriers should be less than the 68 percent characteristic of the eighteenth century trade. The reason for this change was a prosperous bilateral trade between Bahia and Bight of Benin ports (Ouidah, Popo, Apa) involving African slaves and Bahian tobacco. Of forty-seven chromosomes from sickle cell anemia patients examined in Bahia, Brazil, 62 percent were of the Bantu haplotype, and most of the remainder were Benin, numbers in reasonable agreement with the historical record (Curtin, 1986). Sixty-one percent of seventy-four HbS chromosomes from southeastern Brazilian (Sao Paulo) patients were of the Bantu haplotype, whereas from northeastern Brazil, 49 percent of seventy chromosomes were the Bantu type. Almost all of the other chromosomes were the Benin type. These differences, although not statistically significant, may reflect the importation of Nigerian and Ghanaian slaves carrying the Benin haplotype into Bahia (Costa et al., 1994; Goncalves et al., 1994b; Alberto et al., 1998).

A retrospective analysis of all hemoglobinopathy cases diagnosed in a 30-year period in a Buenos Aires Children's Hospital (**Argentina**) revealed that of 140 hemoglobinopathies, HbS was present in 116 cases (Abreu and Penalver, 1992). All of the cases came from the northern and central areas of the country, and African ancestry was found in 20 percent. This African admixture in Argentina is not surprising, as more than 50,000 individuals were imported of slaves into the Rio de la Plata market (Argentina) during the eighteenth century. In the early portion as the century, the ports of origin of the slaves reflected the Spanish slave trade, but in the second half of the century they reflected the French and English slave trade (mostly form Angola, Mozambique, and Namibia) and also reexportation from Brazil, part of the Portuguese slave trade (de Studer, 1984). The prevalence of hemoglobinopathies has been determined in individuals of African descent in two distinct geographic areas in **Ecuador**: in the coastal province of Esmeraldas, particularly the Santiago basin (Rio Cayapas and Rio Onzoles), and in the province of Imbabura, particularly in the intermountain valley, Valle de Chota. In 1,734 samples from Esmeraldas, one fourth carried abnormal hemoglobins, and nearly 20 percent of these had a HbS gene. Of 304 samples from Imbabura, 10 percent had abnormal hemoglobins, largely HbS (Jara et al., 1989).

In **Chile**, the importation of slaves was meager, less than 10,000, and they rapidly disappeared in central and southern Chile as a result of disease—particularly tuberculosis, cold weather, and inhospitable reception by the Amerindian population, mostly Araucanian Indians (Roizen et al., 1973, 1977). In the census of 1812 to 1813, twenty-one central Chilean villages had more than 10 percent of individuals classified as Negroid, but by 1836, there were no more than 1,000 individuals in that category (Roizen et al., 1977). This decrease in the African population has been thought to be a consequence of disease, migration, and involvement in the Chilean war against Peru and Bolivia in 1820 and 1836. In northern Chile, with more favorable climatic conditions and a better reception by the Diaguita Indians, the presence of HbS is detectable in the Elqui and Limari valleys (Etcheverry et al., 1988). In Santiago, Chile's capital, HbS was detected in 1 of 2,084 examined chromosomes (Guzman et al., 1962).

The HbS gene is also present in isolated Indian populations in **Venezuela** (Torres-Guerra et al., 1993). Haplotypes of the βˢ-globin gene have not been reported in Argentina, Ecuador, Venezuela, or Chile.

GENETIC AND ANTHROPOLOGIC STUDIES OF βˢ-LINKED HAPLOTYPES IN THE NEAR EAST

Patients with sickle cell disease from eastern **Saudi Arabia** all have the Arab-India haplotype. In western, haplotypes are more variable but are predominantly Benin (Miller et al., 1986; el-Hazmi, 1990; Padmos et al., 1991). HbS is present in most of the regions of Saudi Arabia, although at variable frequencies (el-Hazmi, 1990). The highest frequency (0.15) was found in Al-Qateef, an eastern province of Saudi Arabia, and the lowest (0.001) in the central region of the country. In some areas, a correlation was evident between malaria endemicity and HbS gene frequency, although a low frequency was encountered in some regions endemic for malaria.

From a hospital-based sample of children with sickle cell anemia in **Kuwait**, the Arab-India haplotype represented 80.4 percent of the chromosomes tested, but African haplotypes were also present, including Benin, 12 percent, and Bantu, 6.5 percent (Adekile and Haider, 1996).

In northern **Oman** there is a multicentric origin of the sickle mutation. Three major haplotypes coexist: 52 percent are Benin (typical and atypical), 26.7 percent are Arab-India (see later), and 21.4 percent are Bantu. These haplotypes arrived in Oman by gene flow, and their distribution is in excellent agreement with the historical record. Ancient contacts between Oman and sub-Sahara West Africa explain the presence of the Benin haplotype; and contacts with Iraq, Iran, present-day Pakistan, and India, account for the Arab-India haplotype. More recent contacts with East Africa (Mombasa), explain the presence of the Bantu haplotype. The pattern of the Arab-India haplotype in the populations of the Arabian peninsula reinforces the hypothesis that the mutation originated in the Harappa culture or in a nearby population and reveals that the Sassanian Empire might have been the vehicle by which this Indo-European sickle mutation migrated to the present-day locations, including Oman (Fig. 26.11) (see later).

MOLECULAR CHARACTERISTICS OF THE INDIVIDUAL AFRICAN βˢ-LINKED HAPLOTYPES

The Benin Haplotype

Extensive sequence analysis of the Benin haplotype has been completed (Lanclos et al., 1991). In the 5′ flanking region of the $^G\gamma$-globin gene of this haplotype, there are two unique sequence changes in positions −369 (C→G) and 309 (C→G) that are linked to the βˢ gene and a novel mutation at −657 (G→T) (Lanclos et al., 1991) (Fig. 26.12). The 5′ flanking region of the $^A\gamma$ gene is more variable. At positions −1315, −1072, −835, and −833, the bases are those found in reference chromosome A (Lanclos et al., 1991), whereas in positions −1121, −611, −604, −603, −588, −369, and +25, the bases are those found in reference chromosome B.

In one kindred where the Benin haplotype was associated with high HbF, the $^G\gamma$-globin gene 5′ flanking region between −472 and the CAP site was identical to the $^A\gamma$-globin gene 5′ flanking region. This indicates a gene conversion, beginning at −472 and ending between the CAP and the beginning of IVS II (Powers and Smithies, 1988; Mishima et al., 1991, 1989).

IVS II sequences appear to be important in γ-globin gene expression in stably transfected K562 cells (Fig. 26.12). This region was examined in the five common haplotypes linked to the βˢ-globin gene (Lanclos et al., 1991). Between nucleotides 500 and 900 of the $^G\gamma$-glo-

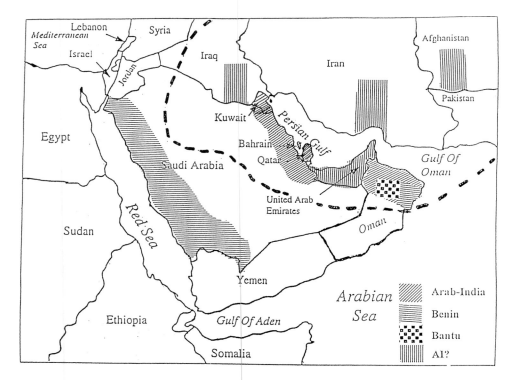

Figure 26.11. Geographic distribution of the haplotype linked to the sickle gene in the Middle East. Broken line: approximate limits of the Sassanian Empire.

bin gene, the first three of four polymorphic sites distinguishing reference chromosomes A and B were type A in the Benin haplotype, but the last one, at position 834, was type B. In addition, the repetitive sequences starting at position 1,062 in the Benin haplotype had some specific mutations; although it was similar to the B chromosome [19(TG) 2(CG) CACG] certain differences were present [9(TC) 19(TG) A 2(TG) 2 (TCG)]. Variability of IVS II of the $^A\gamma$ gene is much greater among haplotypes, and the Benin haplotype contains some singular mutations in that sequence. Between bases 514 and 1,159, a mixture of polymorphic sites corresponding to chromosome A and B is observed; but the four bases following position 743 are unique. Potentially more interesting is the presence of the sequence 10(TG) 4(CG) 7(TG) in the repetitive sequences starting at position 1,062. This pattern is identical to the Bantu but different from the 13(TG) shared by the Senegal and Arab-India haplotypes.

Four unique mutations at positions 1,272, 1,203, 1,207, and 1,208 (TGGG→GCAA) also characterize the Benin haplotype. Repetitive sequences in the $(AT)_x(T)_y$ region 5' to the β-globin gene (Fig. 26.13) are identical between the Senegal and Benin haplotypes but differ in other haplotypes. Surprisingly, few atypical haplotypes have been found in Benin, proba-

bly because 60 percent of the normal population carries the Benin haplotype so that most crossing-over events would be undetectable. Finally, the A→G mutation at position −309 and the C→G mutation at −369 of the $^G\gamma$-globin gene are unique to the Benin haplotype chromosomes linked to the β^S-globin gene (Month et al., 1990). Another example of gene conversion involving the γ-globin genes was found in $^G\gamma$ IVS II in a high HbF-expressing patient with the Benin haplotype. The first half of the $^G\gamma$ IVS II sequence of this patient was indistinguishable from the $^A\gamma$-globin gene (Mishima et al., 1991). The $^A\gamma$ IVS II repetitive region therefore was present in both γ-globin genes in this particular haplotype.

The Senegal Haplotype

In the 5' flanking region of the $^G\gamma$-globin gene of the Senegal haplotype, there are polymorphisms at positions −1280, −1225, −1067, and −807 of the type found in chromosome A, whereas at positions −535 and −534, the polymorphisms are characteristic of chromosome B (Lanclos et al., 1991). This arrangement is found in all haplotypes linked to the β^S-globin gene and is compatible with a short gene conversion in an ancestral African chromosome long before the appearance of the β^S mutation. The thirteen differences between the two reference sequences A and B in the 5' flanking region of the $^A\gamma$ gene (Fig. 26.13) are variably present in the several β^S-globin gene haplotypes, showing more heterogeneity in the $^A\gamma$- than the $^G\gamma$-globin gene.

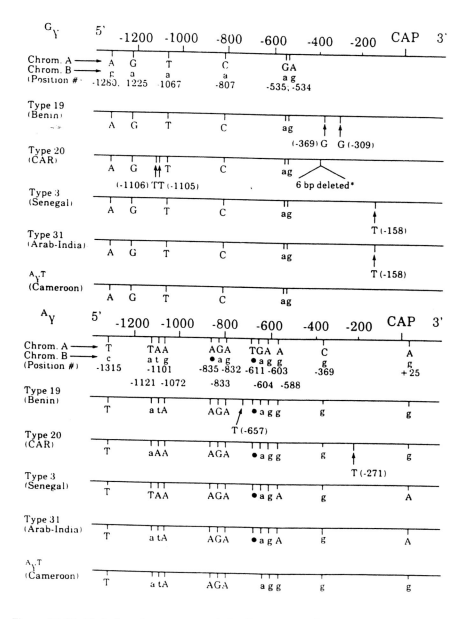

Figure 26.12. Variations in sequences of the ^Gγ (**top**) and ^Aγ (**bottom**) promoter sequences for five sickle cell anemia patients with homozygosity for the five listed β^S-linked haplotypes. Comparison is made to sequences published by Slightom et al. (1980) for the A chromosome; data for the B chromosome were also obtained from Slightom (1990). Capital letters are used for chromosome A and lowercase letters for chromosome B; closed dots indicate that this nucleotide is deleted. Heterozygosity for any of the variations was not observed (Lanclos et al., 1991).

The Bantu Haplotype

Numerous studies have shown the regulatory importance of the regions 5′ to the γ-globin genes (Gilman, 1988) (Chapters 6, 7 and 15). A gene conversion 5′ to the ^Aγ gene of a β^S Bantu haplotype chromosome was found in which ^Gγ-like sequences, starting between bases −306 and −271 (5′ to CAP site of the ^Aγ gene) and extending to between bases 25 and 1,107, have replaced the corresponding ^Aγ sequence (Bouhassira et al., 1989) (Fig. 26.14). The uncertain limits of this gene conversion stem from the extraordinary homology in the sequence of the two γ-globin genes (Powers and Smithies, 1988; Shen et al., 1981). A separate gene conversion in the same region, calculated to have occurred about 1 million years ago, is now fixed in the human population (Slightom et al., 1980). The gene conversion linked to the Bantu haplotype (Bouhassira et al., 1989), seems to be a repeat of this ancient event, showing that this region is prone to rearrangement (Fig. 26.15). This conversion is highly associated with the Bantu haplotype, appears at low or nil frequency in other haplotypes, and does not alter

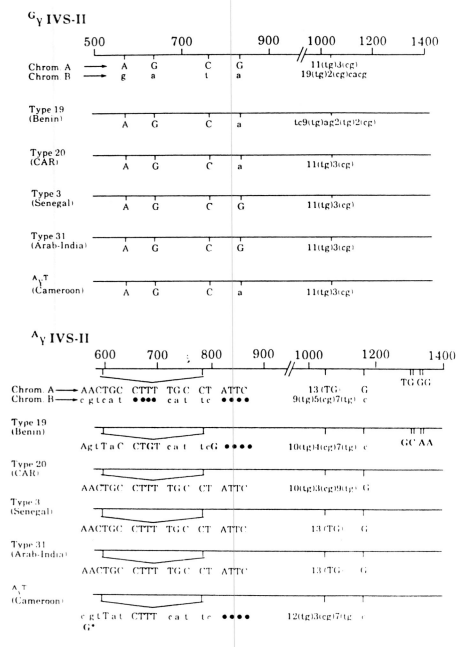

Figure 26.13. Summary of the differences in the sequences of the IVS II ($^G\gamma$ and $^A\gamma$) of the chromosomes from five sickle cell anemia patients with homozygosities for the five different haplotypes. Presentation of the data is similar to that in Fig. 26.3. (**Top**) IVS II of $^G\gamma$; four single-nucleotide differences (at positions + 605, + 669, + 774, + 834) and a difference between the repetitive sequences at position + 1,062 have been observed between the two $^G\gamma$ IVS II segments. The five β^S haplotypes resemble chromosome A, except for position + 834, for the repetitive sequence. (**Bottom**) IVS II of $^A\gamma$; numerous single-nucleotide differences have been found between chromosomes A and B [at positions + 514, + 605, + 670, + 677, + 695, + 741 to + 744 (four- nucleotide deletion), + 753, + 755, + 772, + 780, + 781, + 791 to + 794 (four-nucleotide deletion), and + 1159], and in the repetitive sequences starting at + 1,062. Haplotypes 3 and 31

have sequences identical to that of chromosome A. The sequence of the β^S chromosome with haplotype 19 is unique (T→G at + 743, A→G at + 782, and TGGG→GCAA at + 1,202, + 1,203, + 1,207, and + 1,208); the β^S chromosome with haplotype 20 has a specific repetitive sequence, and the β^S chromosome with haplotype 17 is also different at several positions (Lanclos et al., 1991).

the basic "adult" $^G\gamma$:$^A\gamma$ ratio. These findings strongly suggest that the sequences between −307 and the + 1,062 site of both γ-globin genes are not the sole determinants of differential γ-globin gene expression (Bouhassira et al., 1989).

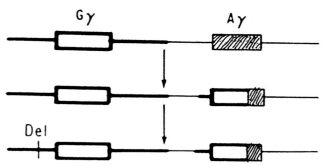

Figure 26.14. The two events detected in the Bantu haplotype. First, a gene conversion in which a 5′ portion of the $^G\gamma$ gene (including a portion of the nontranslated 5′ flanking region) is transposed and replaces the 5′ region of the $^A\gamma$ gene. This leaves the $^A\gamma$ gene with a sequence two thirds of which is of $^G\gamma$ origin. The second event is the appearance of a six-base deletion 5′ to the $^G\gamma$ gene. Three types of β^S chromosomes bearing the Bantu haplotype are shown. The gene cluster at the top represents the expected $^G\gamma$ and $^A\gamma$ arrangement. The bold line represents $^G\gamma$; the thin line represents $^A\gamma$ is replaced by $^G\gamma$. The gene cluster at the bottom represents the appearance of the deletion (Del) in a gene-converted chromosome.

As a majority of Bantu haplotype bearers carry the same gene conversion, the variability of $^G\gamma$ expression among these individuals seems unrelated to sequence changes in this region (Nagel et al., 1987). Undefined sequence changes in other regions could interact with this gene conversion to modify the $^G\gamma$:$^A\gamma$ ratio, and point mutations 5′ to a γ-globin gene can modulate expression of that gene (Collins et al., 1984, 1985; Gelinas et al., 1985; Gilman, 1988) (Chapter 15).

Sequencing of the upstream region of a human $^G\gamma$-globin gene linked to the Bantu haplotype revealed a six base pair deletion between positions −400 and −395 (Fig. 26.1). Further analysis revealed that this mutation was present in 37 percent of sickle cell anemia patients bearing the Bantu haplotype and was

Figure 26.15. The structure of the region where the deletion occurred, 5′ to the $^G\gamma$-globin gene chromosomes bearing the Bantu haplotype. Lowercase letters depict the deleted bases.

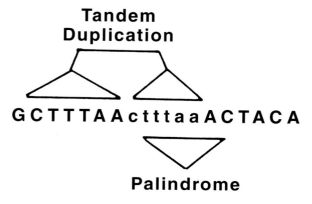

absent in the other haplotypes linked to the β^S-globin gene, as well as in most β^A chromosomes. The most parsimonious interpretation is that the deletion is a very recent event that occurred in the subset of Bantu chromosomes already bearing a gene conversion of the $^A\gamma$ gene by the $^G\gamma$ gene. Its presence in β^S chromosomes is probably the result of a crossing-over between a Bantu β^S chromosome (with deletion and gene conversion) and a β^A chromosome. Bantu chromosomes can be classified into three categories in regard to these features: one displaying the gene conversion and deletion, one displaying only the gene conversion, and a third displaying neither gene conversion nor deletion. The Bantu haplotype, the sole haplotype displaying sequence variability, is also the most heterogeneous in $^G\gamma$-globin gene expression (Nagel et al., 1987).

The presence of the six base pair deletion and gene conversion in the $^G\gamma$-globin gene of some β^A chromosomes having a haplotype different from the Bantu β^S chromosome seems best explained by a presumed crossing-over event between the Bantu β^S haplotype and a β^A chromosome. The chronology of the occurrence of the β^S mutation, the gene conversion, and the 5′ $^G\gamma$ deletion cannot be conclusively defined.

The sequence of the TG repeat region of the Bantu haplotype, starting at position 1,062, is 10(TG) 4(CG) 9(TG), and similar to chromosome B (Lanclos et al., 1991). Since the sequence difference between positions 500 and 900 is similar to $^G\gamma$ rather than $^A\gamma$ and resembles chromosome A, this region might have been involved in yet another gene conversion event.

The Cameroon Haplotype

The Cameroon haplotype is linked to the $^A\gamma^T$ gene (Lapemeroulie et al., 1989; Green et al., 1993) and is identical to haplotype II, which is associated with a subset of β thalassemia in the Mediterranean (Chapter 30). The $^A\gamma^I$ and $^A\gamma^T$ alleles differ at codon 75, which encodes isoleucine or threonine, respectively. Based on protein studies, in the United States $^A\gamma^T$ constituted about 20 percent of Caucasian and 10 percent of African-American β^A chromosomes and was infrequently found linked to a minority (20 percent) of β^S chromosomes of African Americans with sickle cell anemia (Huisman et al., 1985).

The Cameroon haplotype and Mediterranean haplotypes II and VI have in common a high $^G\gamma$:$^A\gamma$ ratio; but lack the −158 C→T mutation characteristic of the Senegal and Arab-India haplotypes (Gilman and Huisman, 1985; Labie et al., 1985a). Haplotype II is linked to β thalassemia and to a four base pair deletion (AGCA) in the region of a GCA repeat, located from −124 to −127 relative to the $^A\gamma$ CAP-site (Gilman et al., 1988). This four base pair deletion has been reported

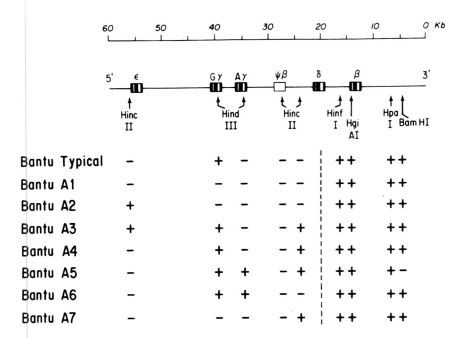

	Hinc II	Hind III		Hinc II		Hinf I / Hgi AI	Hpa I / Bam HI
Bantu Typical	–	+	–	–	–	++	++
Bantu A1	–	–	–	–	–	++	++
Bantu A2	+	–	–	–	–	++	++
Bantu A3	+	+	–	–	+	++	++
Bantu A4	–	+	–	–	+	++	++
Bantu A5	–	+	+	–	+	++	+ –
Bantu A6	–	+	+	–	–	++	++
Bantu A7	–	–	–	–	+	++	++

Figure 26.16. Bantu typical haplotype and seven different atypical haplotypes, all of which, except for BantuA5, can be explained by a simple recombination in the ψβ-δ hot spot.

in the promoters of the $^A\gamma$ alleles on both β^A and β^S chromosomes, but no effect on the expression of the $^A\gamma$-globin gene was noted (Labie et al., 1985a). It was suggested that the four base pair deletion is a common polymorphism linked to the $^A\gamma$ gene (Efstratiadis et al., 1980) (see later).

ATYPICAL HAPLOTYPES

Fewer than 10 percent of Senegalese and Bantu-speaking Africans had their β^S-globin gene linked to an atypical haplotype. Figure 26.16 depicts the atypical haplotypes determined among the twenty-one chromosomes carrying the β^S gene from the central African republic where the Bantu haplotype predominates. Of the eleven atypical haplotypes, four were designated Bantu-A1. In this nomenclature, the name of the typical haplotype is followed by A, if it is atypical, and a correlative number. Two other β^S-globin gene linked haplotypes were designated Bantu-A2. The other five atypical haplotypes (Bantu A3-7) had only one representative each. No homozygote or compound heterozygote for an atypical haplotype was identified.

In ten of the Bantu atypicals, the 3′ portion of the haplotype was identical to the typical Bantu haplotype. 5′ portions of the haplotypes depicted in Fig. 26.16 correspond to those already described in normal haplotypes; 5′ portions of the Bantu-A1 is found in the Mediterranean area in Algeria (Mears et al., 1981b); 5′ portions of Bantu-A2 are identical with haplotypes described in North Africa, Mediterranean haplotype I (Kulozik et al., 1986) and in Senegal (Pagnier et al., 1984); 5′ portions of Bantu-A3 and Bantu-A4 are very similar and differ only in the ε-globin gene site. Since

this site is unstable, as demonstrated among carriers of the Arab-India haplotype in India (Labie et al., 1989), these haplotypes could be related. Haplotype Bantu-A4 is found linked to the β^C-globin gene and is present in normal Africans. The 5′ portion of the Bantu-A6 haplotype is identical with a haplotype common in the Mediterranean. Finally, Bantu-A7 is a combination of 5′ Benin haplotype and 3′ Bantu haplotype. A Benin haplotype is common in β^A chromosomes in Africa, having also been found in the normal population of Benin, in Senegal and Algeria. The haplotype Bantu-A5 is a special case whose origin is still unsettled.

Atypical haplotypes in sickle cell anemia usually result from recombination between haplotypes common in sickle cell anemia and haplotypes rarely associated with the β^S-globin gene. The restriction endonuclease cleavage sites used to assign a haplotype are present in a 63 kb stretch of DNA subdivided into a 34 kb 5′, 19 kb 3′, and 9 kb central domain (Fig. 26.1). Restriction sites within the 5′ and 3′ sectors are nonrandomly associated, whereas the central region is randomly associated with either 5′ or 3′ domains. In the central domain, 5′ to the δ-globin gene is a "hot spot" for recombination (Fig. 26.4). In the United States, more than twenty atypical haplotypes associated with the HbS gene have been identified (Steinberg et al., 1998). This diversity may be explained by the many different genetic backgrounds associated with the β-globin gene in African Americans (Table 26.1). As expected, the distribution of 5′ subhaplotypes mirrored the distribution of haplotypes in African Americans with sickle cell anemia (Antonarakis et al., 1984; Hattori et al., 1986; Schroeder et al., 1989; Rieder et al., 1991; Steinberg et al., 1995b). In African Americans, Senegal and Bantu are less common than Benin haplotypes; thus fewer atypical chromosomes bearing Senegal or Bantu subhaplotypes were found.

One feature of recombination deserves mention. When a 5′ subhaplotype, including the locus control region (LCR), becomes linked to a β^S-globin gene by recombination, there is no assurance that polymorphisms in the LCR, or any other region of the chromosome 5′ to the site of recombination, will be the same as that linked to the β^S-globin gene in the original haplotype. For example, a 5′ Benin subhaplotype from a β^A chromosome may contain polymorphisms distinct from those of the 5′ Benin subhaplotype linked to the β^S-globin gene. The β^S-globin gene has been linked to the 5′ Benin haplotype for only 2,000 to 3,000 years, the approximate age of the HbS gene, whereas 5′ subhaplotypes linked to the β^A-globin gene have evolved for a considerably longer interval. This would allow for many different polymorphisms to be associated with the LCR and other 5′ regions of the β^A chromosome compared with the β^S chromosome, where the sequence of the LCR is relatively monotonous. In some atypical haplotypes of African Americans, the 5′ subhaplotype is likely to be of Caucasian origin, further contributing to genetic diversity and uncoupling the β^S-globin gene from the influence of genetic elements that may have coevolved in the maintenance of high HbF levels.

More recently, Zago et al. (personal communication, 1999) have examined a number of atypical haplotypes in sickle anemia populations from Brazilian and other ethnic groups. Figure 26.17 depicts a number of different ways in which atypical haplotypes can be generated, including single base mutations of endonuclease polymorphic sites and double or triple recombination events. Of course, the recombination at the ψβ-δ hot spot is by far the most common event.

THE INDOEUROPEAN SICKLE GENE

Molecular Biology

Linkage disequilibrium between the β^S-globin gene and a novel haplotype, the Arab-India haplotype, was discovered in sickle cell anemia patients inhabiting the eastern oases of Saudi Arabia (Bakioglu et al., 1985; Wainscoat et al., 1985; Miller et al., 1986) (Fig. 26.1). This haplotype, like the Senegal haplotype, is linked to a XmnI positive restriction site at position −158 5′ to the ^Gγ-globin gene. In the western portions of Saudi Arabia, the β^S gene is linked to the Benin haplotype (Kutlar et al., 1985) (Fig. 26.18).

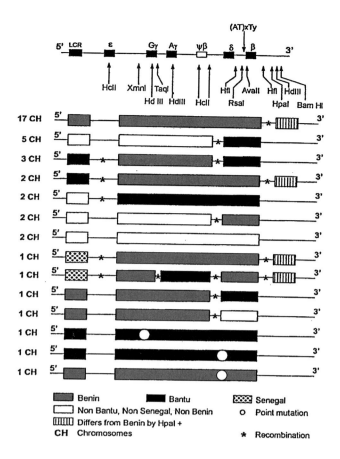

Figure 26.17. Sequence analysis of atypical haplotypes linked to the β^S gene in Brazil.

Kulozik et al. (1986) first described the haplotype linked to the β^S-globin gene in Pan and Kond tribal populations of Orissa, India. In East India there was an 88 percent and in West India a 100 percent association between the HbS gene and this haplotype. The three nontypical haplotypes in individuals from Orissa could have arisen by recombination around the "hot spot" 5′ to the δ-globin gene. As the Bam H1 site 3′ to the β-globin gene is either positive or negative among carriers of these atypical chromosomes, recombination remains a possibility. Among a large number of β^S chromosomes from Orissa, 92 percent were typical Arab-India types, 7 percent differed from the typical types only at the Hinc II site in the ε-globin gene, and 1 percent were atypical (Kulozik et al., 1987).

Labie et al. (1989) have determined the α- and β-globin gene haplotypes of sickle cell anemia, sickle cell trait, and normal individuals belonging to tribes living in malaria-infested areas of northern India (Gujarat, Orissa, and northern Andhra Pradesh) and southern India (Tamil-Nadu). β^S-Globin gene haplotypes in Gujarat, Orissa, and Andhra are characteristic Arab-

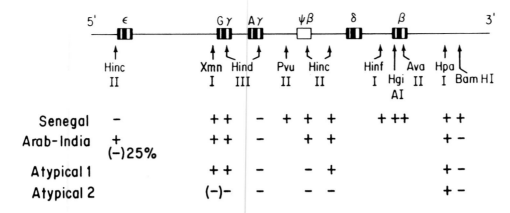

Figure 26.18. Comparison of Senegal and Arab-India haplotype, with the variant haplotype (25 percent) in which the Hinc II is negative. Also two atypical haplotypes that could be the product of recombination.

Indian haplotypes. Of particular interest were the findings in the highland populations of the Nilgieris (Irulas, Kurumbes, Paniyas and Badaga): The majority of the chromosomes bearing the β^S globin gene were of the Indian-Arab type (although almost half the haplotypes lacked the Hinc II site in the ε-globin gene), whereas one was an atypical haplotype. Yet both types of chromosomes were Xmn1-positive and associated with $^G\gamma$-globin gene expression of 67 percent. In addition, another haplotype was found with about 50 percent $^G\gamma$ expression. Surprisingly, the incidence of the $(-\alpha/\alpha\alpha)$ haplotype was found to be 95.2 percent in Gujarat, 42 percent among the Domb and 71.4 percent among Khond in Orissa, and 16.6 percent among the Ganit in Andhra Pradesh. In Irulas and Kurumbes, the frequency of $(-\alpha/\alpha\alpha)$ haplotype was 89.7 percent.

One can conclude that sickle cell anemia in both northern and southern India is associated with at least two haplotypes, but one is predominant. The minor haplotype is possibly related to the typical one by crossing over at the recombination "hot spot," particularly because the endonuclease recognition site is in a microsatellite sequence prone to recombination. Both haplotypes are Xmn1-positive with high $^G\gamma$-globin gene and HbF expression. A third β^S-globin gene haplotype is likely to be independent but is infrequent. High HbF and a high prevalence of α thalassemia predict a mild phenotypical expression of sickle cell anemia among northern and southern Indians (see later).

GENETIC AND ANTHROPOLOGIC IMPLICATIONS OF THE β^S GENE IN INDIA AND THE EASTERN OASIS OF THE ARAB PENINSULA

Lehman and Cutbush (1952) first described HbS in Nilgiris in the present-day state of Tamil-Nadu. Other reports have extended the description of this abnormal hemoglobin to other areas of India, including Orissa, Madhya Pradesh, and Assam, both in tribal groups as well as scheduled Hindu castes. The finding of the same haplotype associated with the β^S gene in tribal populations living in distant regions in India strongly suggests that the mutation arose once, at a time when these tribal populations were in direct contact, and that they were later subjected either to panmixia or gene flow. That is not the situation today, because these populations are isolated from each other geographically and culturally, are endogamic, and are surrounded by mainstream populations that do not bear the β^S-globin gene (Fig. 26.19).

The tribal people recently recognized as "scheduled," a denomination that brings them some status in Indian society, correspond to distinct present-day ethnic groups scattered throughout India and encompass more than 40 million individuals (Vidyarthi and Rai, 1976). Excluded from this analysis are the northeastern and central Himalayan tribes, which are of Oriental or Mongol origin and do not carry the β^S-globin gene. Pertinent to the origins of the HbS gene are the central and southern tribes, which extend from the central-eastern regions of India (Bihar, West Bengal, Orissa, and Madhya Pradesh), to the central-western regions (Rajasthan, Maharashtra, Gujarat, Goa, and Dadra/Nagar Haveli), and to the southern region (Karnataka, Andhra Pradesh, Tamil-Nadu, and Kerala).

Genetic identity of the linked polymorphic structure surrounding the β^S-globin gene in all the tribal peoples studied suggests that this abnormal gene arose unicentrically and at a time when they were in direct contact with each other. Subsequent gene flow is unlikely because they become isolated from each other by the mainstream Indians. Unicentricity implies that the present-day tribals must once have inhabited a geographic location different from today—an ancestral home. Where might this ancestral home be?

The β^S-gene linked to the Arab-India haplotype is found in Saudi Arabia among Shiite Arabs living in the eastern oasis north of the horn of Oman. Sickle cell

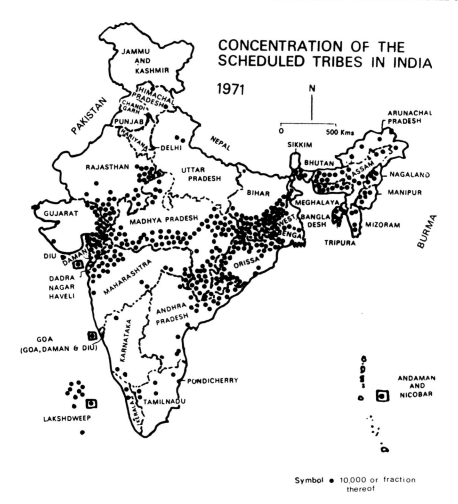

CONCENTRATION OF THE
SCHEDULED TRIBES IN INDIA

1971

Symbol ● 10,000 or fraction
thereof

Figure 26.19. Map of the distribution of scheduled tribes in India. Each dot corresponds to 100,000 individuals or a fraction thereof. The populations reported on in this chapter are encircled.

anemia patients with HbF levels averaging 18 percent who have a benign clinical course has been reported among Iranians (Labie et al., 1989), strongly suggesting the presence of the same Arab-India haplotype. These data would require the ancestral home of the tribal peoples to be in reasonable proximity to the northeast coast of present-day Arabia, to explain the gene flow between these populations.

Time Line of the Origin and Expansion of the Arab-India Sickle Mutation

It has been suggested that the origin of the Indian population preceded the Aryan and Mongol invasions of India and that these populations were part of the original inhabitants of the subcontinent (Basham, 1954; von Furer-Haimendorf, 1968; Bhowmik, 1971; Vidyarthi and Rai, 1976). About 5,000 years ago in Indian history, the Harappa culture flourished in the fertile margins of

the Indus River. This culture reached a high degree of sophistication, developed advanced agricultural techniques with complex grain storage facilities, and had well-designed households and cities (Fig. 26.20) (Fairservis, 1971). The Harappa culture was influenced by contacts with Mesopotamia and the Sumerian civilization (Fariservis, 1971; Kenoyer, 1998).

The present distribution of the Arab-India sickle gene in central and southern Indian tribes and the eastern oasis of Saudi Arabia could have originated in the midst of the Harappan culture. The gene may then have migrated east after the collapse of that civilization and might have been further dispersed and isolated by events not fully understood but which occurred about 2,000 years before the present era (BCE).

During the height of the Harappan civilization, an active agriculture and a high frequency of floods, coupled with a large and concentrated human population, created the proper conditions for the development of pandemic malaria, a necessary condition for the appearance of the β^S-globin gene expansion (Kenoyer, 1998). Skeletal remains of Harappans reveal bone changes that are compatible with, but do not prove, the

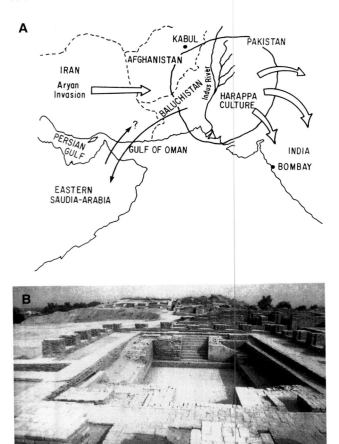

Figure 26.20. (**A**) Hypothesis of the geographic area involved in the origin of the β^S gene in India. Right open arrows depict the dispersion of Harappan culture members after the collapse of this civilization and the Aryan invasion (left open arrow). Black arrows depict the potential gene flow of β^S gene between the Indian subcontinent and the Arabic peninsula (from Labie et al., 1989 with permission of the publishers.) (**B**) Elaborate constructions in Mohanjo Daro. Water bath in the city: One aspect of the enormous development of water engineering in the Harappan culture that sustained an advanced agriculture. The latter is indispensable for the expansion of malaria-selected genes (from Kenoyer, 1998).

presence of sickle cell anemia among these individuals. (Wheeler, 1968; Kennedy, 1981). If tribal dispersion occurred between 2,000 and 4,000 years BCE, the HbS mutation should have arisen between 4,000 and 6,000 years ago. This time frame would make the Indian mutation older than the African one, which arose between 2,000 and 3,000 years ago (Nagel, 1984).

What was the nature of the gene flow that joined Harappans, Saudis, Iraqis, Persians, and Omanis? The period between 200 and 600 CE was characterized by the great influence of Sassanian monarchs from Persia whose religious beliefs included autochthonous paganism, Sassanian Zoroastrianism, and Nestorian

Christianity. The last flourished particularly on the islands between Qatar and Oman. Figure 26.21 shows the limits of the Sassanian empire in this period, which encompassed the region in which the Arab-India haplotype is distributed in the Middle East. An attractive possibility is that flow of this gene occurred during the Sassanian empire, which facilitated contacts between the areas of the world that have a demonstrable or likely presence of the Arab-India haplotype linked to the β^S-globin gene (Hussein et al., 1999).

An alternative explanation would place the origin of the Arab-India haplotype among the Mesopotamian and/or Semitic peoples of the Arab Peninsula, with expansion to India during the British protectorate. This hypothesis seems unlikely on several counts. First, it would be difficult to understand the exclusive distribution of the Arab-India haplotype among the Indian tribals and its absence in other castes. Second, in areas adjacent to Iraq (Syria, Israel, and Jordan) (Rund et al., 1990; el Hazmi, 1990; Flint et al., 1993b; el Hazmi and Warsy, 1997), HbS is linked mainly to the Benin haplotype and not the Arab-India haplotype. Third, Harappan settlements have not been found around Iraq, a region not part of the Sassanian empire.

Figure 26.21. The relationships between α and β haplotypes and clinical features of sickle cell anemia. The clinical features include events such as osteonecrosis, acute chest syndrome, renal failure, and other common disease complications. These associations of haplotype and phenotype in sickle cell anemia are difficult; not all patients exhibit the same complications. Within each haplotype group there is considerable heterogeneity whose cause is yet unknown (from Powars, 1993).

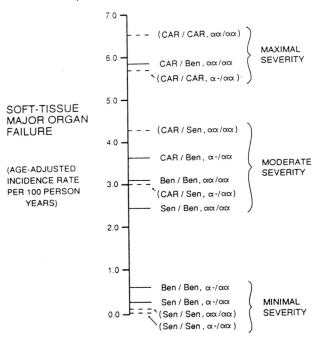

Linkage of the Arab-India haplotype to the β^S-globin gene in Kuwait (Adekile et al., 1996; Adekile, 1997), Bahrain (Al-Arrayed and Haites, 1995), and Oman and the report of a sickle cell anemia patient from Qatar heterozygous for the Arab-India and Benin haplotypes (Bakioglu et al., 1985) strengthen the idea that this Indo-European form of the β^S-globin gene originated in the Indus Valley, migrating by gene flow during the Sassanian Persian empire (224–651 BCE) to the eastern portions of the Arabian Peninsula, including Oman, and to Iraq, Afghanistan, the Indus Valley, and the Caucasus region, when this region was united under Magian Zoroastrianism. Saudi Arabia's western provinces, where this haplotype is very rare (El-Hazmi and Warsy, 1997; Damanhouri, 1997), were outside the Sassanian empire.

High HbF levels in Iranians with sickle cell anemia suggest the possible linkage of the sickle gene to the Arab-India haplotype (Haghshenass et al., 1983).

GENETIC AND ANTHROPOLOGIC IMPLICATIONS OF THE β^S GENE IN THE INDIAN OCEAN

Sickle cell hemoglobin is found at a significant frequency among the inhabitants of Mauritius Island (Kotea et al., 1995). Although the frequency of the β^S gene is higher among individuals of African descent (Creoles), it is also found among the descendants of Indian immigrants. Did all the β^S gene flow come from Africa and reach the descendants of Indian immigrants by admixture, or is the origin of the β^S gene in Mauritius bicentric, that is from Africa but also from the tribal (Adavasi) populations of India? β^S-Globin gene cluster haplotypes were studied in forty-four individuals, members of seventeen families in the Mauritius islands. Of the eighty-eight chromosomes, forty-six were from unrelated individuals, and twenty-nine carried the β^S-globin gene. All β^S carriers of Indian descent had the Arab-Indian haplotype or an atypical Arab-Indian haplotype (two chromosomes), which can be explained by recombination. The other five unrelated individuals carrying the β^S gene were of Creole origin, and all had the Bantu haplotype. The availability of pedigree data made the assignments unambiguous even in sickle trait individuals. These results establish firmly that the origin of the β^S-globin gene among individuals of Indian descent in Mauritius is indeed Indian. In addition, it establishes that Indians of tribal origin were among those who immigrated to the Mauritius islands.

The historical record is informative. British conquest of Mauritius in 1810 barely changed the life of the island because the terms of capitulation left the French with their possessions (including sugar plantations), language, culture, and customs (Addison and Hazareesingh, 1984). The Act of Abolition of the Slave Trade, passed by the British Parliament in 1807, gave hope for emancipation to slaves of African origin, but it took 32 more years for slavery to be abolished in Mauritius. The freed slaves refused to work for pay on the plantations; hence, the sugar industry had to turn to other sources of labor. During his voyage on the HMS Beagle, Darwin was surprised by the planters' apparent lack of concern for their future. He need not have worried since the planters had plans to import indentured Indian labor. This Indian population grew from 24,000 in 1838 to 216,000 in 1870 (Addison and Hazareesingh, 1984; Jha 1986).

There is abundant archival evidence that most of the indentured laborers were "shanghaied"—"recruited" forcefully or under false pretenses—by the British from eastern states of India, such as Bihar, and to a lesser extent, Madras. According to Jha (1986), during the early period of "recruitment" the *arkatis* (recruiters) found the Chotanagpur area of southern Bihar (District of Ranchi) particularly attractive, citing the records for 1836 of the General Department of the Government of India. The tribal populations living there (Oraons, Mundas), fresh from a disastrously unsuccessful rebellion (the Kol insurrection of 1831 to 1832), were "eager to look for greener pastures" and were "easy prey for the *arkatis*." Despite a transient ban on exportation of laborers from India, by 1846, 50,000 of them had reached Mauritius and many, but certainly not all, were tribals (Jha, 1986). Significantly, the main tribal populations living in Chotanagpur, the Oraos, and Mundas (Karan et al., 1978) have today an incidence of sickle trait as high as 8.3 percent, with lower frequencies among the neighboring Desi Bhumij and Ho (Bhatia and Rao 1986). Further immigration from India occurred after 1846, largely of nontribal origins (Addison and Hazareesingh, 1984). These individuals were unlikely bearers of the β^S gene, but instead carried β thalassemia.

The introduction of malaria in the 1860s and its effect on mortality (Addison and Hazareesingh, 1984; Lutz and Wils, 1991) increased the frequency of the β^S gene through selective pressure on heterozygotes. Hence, the β^S gene may be present today at higher frequency in Mauritius than when originally introduced. Because of Indian intermarriage across social barriers in Mauritius, and because of selective pressure, the gene in all likelihood can now be found in families of nontribal ancestry (Bihar, Madras, and Kerala).

Consistent with local history, the second origin of the HbS gene in Mauritius is from Africa. Among three Creole families from Mauritius, the β^S gene was linked exclusively to the Bantu haplotype. The historical record suggests that in the French Colonial period, slaves were imported from Madagascar, Mozambique, and as far north as Zanzibar and Kilwa (Manrakhan, 1990). In populations from those areas of Africa, the β^S-globin gene is linked to the Bantu haplotype, as it is in Creoles in Mauritius.

MOLECULAR CHARACTERISTICS OF THE ARAB-INDIA β^S LINKED HAPLOTYPE

Salient features of the Arab-India haplotype include the presence of the −158 C→T mutation 5′ to the $^G\gamma$-globin gene, which is believed to contribute to the high proportion of $^G\gamma$-globin chains and increased HbF levels in carriers. There is also a unique $(AT)_x(T)_y$ repeat sequence 5′ to the β gene and an unusual sequence in HS-2 of the LCR. In the former case, this motif has the form $(AT)_9T_5$, a structure distinct from the other four typical haplotypes of the β^S chromosome. The tandem repeat motif $(AT)_x(T)_y$ located 5′ to the β-gene CAP-site lies within a negative regulatory region between nucleotides −610 and −490 and binds BP-1, a putative gene repressor (see later). This has been postulated to influence the fractional concentration of HbS in sickle cell trait (Berg et al., 1991; Elion et al., 1992). Although Indians with sickle trait have a lower fractional percentage of HbS than Africans, all Indian populations where sickle cell anemia is prevalent, particularly the Iruleas in the Nilgiris, also have an extremely high incidence of α thalassemia (> 0.85) and in addition have about a 50 percent prevalence of leftward deletions ($-\alpha^{4.2}$). In contrast, African samples have much lower frequencies of α thalassemia, and these are all rightward deletion types ($-\alpha^{3.7}$). In 5′ HS-2 of the Arab-India haplotype, the AT repeat region has the unique form $(AT)_{10}ACACATATACGT(AT)_{12}$ (Adekile et al., 1993). The sequences between 500 to 600 bp and 1400 bp in IVS-II of both γ-globin genes resemble those of reference chromosome A and the Senegal haplotype, but differ from those of other major HbS-associated haplotypes (Lanclos et al., 1991; Adekile et al., 1993). Whether these polymorphisms have a role in causing the higher HbF and $^G\gamma$-globin chain levels in the Arab-India and Senegal haplotypes is not clear.

GENETIC MODULATION OF THE PHENOTYPIC DIVERSITY OF SICKLE CELL ANEMIA

Although sickle cell anemia results from homozygosity of a single, unvarying mutation at position six of the β-hemoglobin locus, phenotypically this disease is remarkably heterogeneous. Some patients are sick all of the time, and some hardly ever (Embury et al., 1994). This clinical heterogeneity of a genetically homogeneous disease has attracted the attention of

clinicians and biomedical scientists who have tried to define the causes of the variability. Geographically linked differences in the phenotype of sickle cell anemia are discussed in Chapter 33. An environmental effect on the course of sickle cell anemia is dramatically apparent in tropical Africa. With good access to medical care, survival to adulthood and a decent quality of life are possible. Lacking that, sickle cell anemia in Africa remains a childhood disease, its course truncated by early death, often from malaria (Ohene-Frempong and Nkrumah, 1994).

In the following sections we discuss the genetic modulation of sickle cell disease, focusing on sickle cell anemia. Although some of the same elements that affect the phenotype of sickle cell anemia are likely to be important in HbSC disease and HbS-β^0 thalassemia, we know less about the modulation of those genotypes. We best understand two general genetic factors that influence the clinical expression of the HbS mutation: those linked to the β-globin gene-like cluster that influence the synthesis of HbF and the α thalassemias. These factors are discussed in the most detail. Perhaps more interesting, as it is possible to explain only a small fraction of the diversity of sickle cell anemia on the basis of β-globin gene or α-globin gene-linked modulation, are candidate genes, epistatic modifiers, which potentially affect the pathogenesis of sickle cell anemia. These genes are likely to act independently of HbS polymerization through which both HbF and α thalassemia work, albeit by different means. We know little about the relationship of these epistatic genes, if any, to the modulation of the vasoocclusive severity of sickle cell anemia. Candidate modifier genes include the following:

- Genes of adhesion-promoting proteins or their receptors (Chapter 21) that could influence interactions among sickle erythrocytes and endothelial cells, platelets, or leukocytes
- Genes coding for proteins that influence thrombosis
- Genes that modulate vasodilation or vasoconstriction
- Genes for proinflammatory or antiinflammatory cytokines
- Modulators of the perception of ischemic tissue damage
- Genes that govern erythroid differentiation
- Genes whose products regulate or modify nitric oxide concentrations in endothelial cells
- Genes that determine the structure of the ion transport channels such as K^+Cl^- cotransport or the Gardos channel, or that regulate ion transport through these channels and affect cell density (Chapter 21).

FETAL HEMOGLOBIN MODULATION OF SICKLE CELL ANEMIA

The β-Globin Gene Cluster and Globin Gene Switching

HbF is the most thoroughly studied genetic modulator of sickle cell anemia, with levels varying more than two orders of magnitude. Most of the known genetic determinants that appear to affect the course of disease influence HbF production. Initially, only very high levels of HbF were considered capable of influencing the phenotype of sickle cell anemia. (Powars et al., 1980, 1984; Noguchi et al., 1988). Further studies have shown that any increment in HbF appears to be clinically and perhaps therapeutically important (Platt et al., 1991, 1994).

Discussed in detail in Chapters 7 and 15, hemoglobin gene switching is the process of sequential globin gene activation and inactivation ending in the near extinction of γ-globin gene expression and its replacement by adult β-globin chain synthesis (Grosveld et al., 1993; Stamatoyannopoulos et al., 1994). Globin gene switching involves the complex interactions of stage-specific transcription factors, chromosomal gene order, gene proximity to the LCR, cis-acting sequences that act positively and negatively in transcriptional regulation, and erythroid-specific and ubiquitous trans-acting factors. Interacting with the promoters of the β-like globin genes, the LCR plays a critical role in their tissue- and developmental-specific expression, and polymorphisms in some of its critical units have been considered vital elements of γ-globin gene regulation in sickle cell anemia. Each hypersensitive site in the LCR contains different combinations of phylogenetically conserved domains for erythroid-specific and ubiquitous DNA-binding proteins. These regulatory elements have redundant functions, and each site may interact preferentially with specific genes of the β-like cluster. For example, HS-1 may interact with the embryonic ε-globin gene, HS-3 with the fetal γ-globin genes, and HS-4 with the adult β-globin gene (Grosveld et al., 1993). Although HS-2 does not appear to have specificity for interaction with the γ-globin genes in transgenic animals, there is some evidence for its association with different HbF levels in sickle cell anemia. The regions of HS-2 that affect globin gene transcription in cell lines and transgenic mice are not completely defined, but they are likely to be transcription factor-binding elements (Caterina et al., 1991; Moon and Ley, 1991; Ellis et al., 1993; Miller et al., 1993). These conserved regions can act synergistically, favoring the hypothesis that the LCR exerts its effects on gene expression as a holocomplex that interacts with only a single promoter at any instant in time (Wijgerde et al., 1995). Studies in transgenic mice using the entire β-globin cluster spanning ~250 kb suggest that most of the sequences required for developmental expression of globin genes are present within this fragment (Peterson et al., 1993). For many years investigators have studied switching, with the goals of learning to reactivate the dormant γ-globin genes therapeutically and of understanding which cis-acting elements and trans-acting factors govern HbF expression.

β-Globin Gene Cluster Haplotypes: Effects on HbF Levels, Hematology, and Clinical Course

Studies of small numbers of African patients with sickle cell anemia and different β-globin gene cluster haplotypes who had distinct hematologic characteristics first suggested that haplotype may be one marker for the phenotypic heterogeneity of sickle cell anemia (Antonarakis et al., 1982; Orkin et al., 1982; Kulozik et al., 1985; Hattori et al., 1986; Kulozik et al., 1987; Nagel et al., 1987; Ragusa et al., 1988; Srinivas et al., 1988; Sharon et al., 1988; Nagel and Labie, 1989; Schroeder et al., 1989; Labie et al., 1989; Month et al., 1990; Ballas et al., 1991; Dimovski et al., 1991; Powars et al., 1991b; Powars et al., 1991b; Öner et al., 1992b; Nagel and Flemming, 1992; Zago et al., 1992). However, most of the detailed and larger studies of the clinical and hematologic effects of haplotype in sickle cell anemia have been in regions were the HbS gene arrived by gene flow. After many years of genetic admixture, patients in such regions are commonly haplotype heterozygotes, complicating interpretation of the potential association of haplotype with phenotype. Reports of the clinical and hematologic effects of haplotype in sickle cell anemia should be interpreted carefully, as often few patients were studied, the patients' ages differed between series—a critical feature because many sickle complications are age dependent—clinical events may not have been sharply defined, and distinctions between haplotype homozygotes and heterozygotes were often not clearly drawn.

Although there are many exceptions, some of the general clinical features of sickle cell anemia found in patients with the common β-gene haplotypes are shown in Figure 26.21. In longitudinal studies from the United States, the Senegal haplotype was associated with fewer hospitalizations and painful episodes (Powars, 1991a, 1991b). An effect of the Senegal haplotype on reducing episodes of acute chest syndrome was of marginal significance. The Bantu haplotype was associated with the highest incidence of organ damage, and renal failure was strongly associated with this haplotype (Powars et al., 1991). Both sex and haplotype affect HbF levels in sickle cell anemia. In 384 patients, hemoglobin concentrations were higher in males with Benin and Bantu haplotypes. In the Senegal haplotype, where the highest HbF levels were present, total hemoglobin concentration was equal in males and females, but HbF concentration was higher in females. Females with the Senegal haplotype and high HbF may have less hemolysis and therefore higher hemoglobin levels (Steinberg et al., 1995b).

In most of Africa, environmental factors, nutrition, and infections make it difficult to distinguish the role of haplotype in modulating the course of disease, but clinical differences have been noted. It appears that Africans with the Senegal haplotype do better than those with other common haplotypes, but there are few clinical data for patients whose haplotype has been determined (Ohene-Frempong and Nkrumah, 1994). Most work suggests that the Arab-India haplotype is also associated with milder disease, although vasoocclusive events do occur (Padmos et al., 1991; El-Hazmi, 1992a, 1992b; Adekile and Haider, 1996).

Although they may be convenient earmarks for genetic regulators of γ-globin gene expression, most of the polymorphic restriction sites used to assign a haplotype have no known role in the differential transcription and temporal regulation of these genes. An exception may be the Xmn I site (−158 C→T), which is 5′ to the $^{G}\gamma$-globin gene in the Senegal and Arab-India haplotypes. This site is associated with high expression of the $^{G}\gamma$ gene compared with the $^{A}\gamma$ gene. In the Saudi population, the −158 C→T mutation is strongly, but imperfectly, correlated with high levels of HbF and $^{G}\gamma$-globin chains in sickle cell anemia (Gilman and Huisman, 1984, 1985; Nagel, 1984; Labie et al., 1985a). In adults and neonates lacking the HbS gene, this polymorphism is also associated with small but significant increases in the synthesis of HbF and $^{G}\gamma$-globin chains (Sampietro et al., 1992; Peri et al., 1997). Individuals with the sickle cell trait, whose β^{S} chromosome carries the Arab-India haplotype, are not anemic and have normal HbF levels. In vitro, erythroid colonies derived from precursor cells obtained from sickle cell trait carriers of the Arab-India haplotype had higher levels of HbF synthesis than did colonies derived from controls (Miller et al., 1987a, 1987b). This system may mimic in some respects perturbed erythropoiesis occurring with hemolysis. With hematopoietic stress it appears that elements in *cis* to the β-globin gene cluster are associated with differences in the levels of HbF (Gilman and Huisman, 1984, 1985; Nagel et al., 1984; Wainscoat et al., 1985; Miller et al., 1987b; Schroeder et al., 1989; Rieder et al., 1991; Green et al., 1993; Chang et al., 1995; Steinberg et al., 1995; Chen et al., 1996; Mrug et al., 1996; Steinberg et al., 1997b; Ofori-Acquah et al., 1999). Even with basal erythropoiesis in people with sickle cell trait and in those with no hemoglobinopathy, these regions may help modulate γ-globin gene expression (Leonov et al., 1996; Merghoub et al., 1996). The −158 C→T mutation may play a permissive role; it may be necessary but insuffi-

cient to promote increased transcription of the $^{G}\gamma$-globin gene. For the γ-globin genes to be expressed at higher than normal levels, expanded erythropoiesis or hemolytic stress must be present. Alternatively, this mutation may represent a polymorphic marker linked to other mutations, for example in HS-2, that are critical for regulating $^{G}\gamma$-globin gene expression. The Cameroon haplotype is also associated with a high $^{G}\gamma{:}^{A}\gamma$ ratio but lacks the −158 C→T mutation characteristic of the Senegal and Arab-India haplotypes. Numerous sequence differences in the 5′ flanking portions and in the large introns of both γ-globin genes appear to be haplotype-specific (Lanclos et al., 1991). Speculation that these polymorphic regions contribute to the variation of HbF in sickle cell anemia has not been supported by functional studies.

The β^{S}-globin gene in the western province of Saudi Arabia is present on the Benin haplotype chromosome and in this portion of the Arabian peninsula, sickle cell anemia resembles the African disease. In Saudi Arabia's eastern province a hematologically milder form of sickle cell anemia is found. Although these patients have high HbF levels, they have vasoocclusive events at a rate similar to their compatriots from the western province (Padmos et al., 1991). More detailed studies are needed to resolve this inconsistency. Attention should be directed to any bias introduced by considering hospital-based patients, who tend to be severely affected. Sickle cell anemia in parts of India and in ethnic Indians in Malaysia is akin to the disease in the eastern province of Saudi Arabia (Brittenham et al., 1979; Lie-Injo et al., 1986), and these individuals also carry the Arab-India haplotype.

Considerable variance in HbF levels exists among individuals with the Senegal and Arab-India haplotypes (Nagel et al., 1984; Kutlar et al., 1985; Wainscoat et al., 1985; Kulozik et al., 1987; Labie et al., 1989). This suggests that elements associated with a haplotype interact with other factors that affect HbF gene expression and HbF levels in blood (Hattori et al., 1986; Schroeder et al., 1989; Nagel et al., 1991; Rieder et al., 1991). Haplotype therefore may serve as a marker for the effects of undefined *cis*- and *trans*-acting factors that temper globin gene expression.

LCR and HbF. Most studies of the influence of the LCR on HbF production have focused on 5′ HS-2, which appears to be the only 5′ hypersensitive site that is polymorphic among HbS-associated haplotypes (Dimovski et al., 1991; Lanclos et al., 1991) (Table 26.3). Because this region probably has some regulatory role in globin gene transcription, it was of interest to see whether polymorphisms of this region were associated with phenotypic variation in sickle cell anemia. In the first study that focused attention on a possible role of

Table 26.3. Sequence Differences in HS-2 of Three βS Chromosomes

Haplotype	−10924 (8580)	−10905 (8598)	−10623–10570 (8883–)	−10390
Reference	T	A	10TA.2CA.2TA.CG.11TA	A
Benin	G	G	8TA.2CA.2TACGTG.7TA	T
Senegal	T	A	9TA.2CA.2TACGTG.7TA	A
Atypical	T	A	9TA.2CA.2TA.CG.10TA	A

The nucleotide positions are given relative to the mRNA capping site of the ε-globin gene (GenBank coordinates). The atypical haplotype was found in a patient homozygous for the Benin haplotype with an unusually high level of HbF. Modified from references (Öner et al., 1992a; Périchon et al., 1993).

HS-2 in determining the level of HbF in sickle cell anemia, HS-2 from a Senegal haplotype homozygote had several sequences that differed from a Benin homozygote in conserved regions of regulatory importance (Öner et al., 1992a). Sharpening this focus was the observation that a sickle cell anemia patient homozygous for the Benin haplotype had 21 percent HbF and 65 percent ᴳγ-chains. In the Benin haplotype, HbF levels are usually much lower, and ᴳγ-chains form about 40 percent of all γ-globin chains. In this patient, the sequence of HS-2 was characteristic of the Senegal type but lacked the −158 Xmn 1 restriction site, suggesting a crossover 5′ to the ᴳγ-globin gene (Öner et al., 1992a). Senegal HS-2 is distinguished by the presence of Sp 1 (−10905) and GATA-binding sites (−10390). Further, the repetitive sequence involving the AT motif forms a sequence similar to that found 5′ in the β gene and the BP 1 binding site (see later). β Thalassemia patients with similar polymorphisms have high HbF levels (Beris et al., 1992). There is little published information beyond this intriguing case to suggest that this portion of HS-2 truly influences γ-globin gene expression in sickle cell anemia. Examining additional exceptional patients who display a discordance between haplotype and HbF levels may help confirm this supposition, and studies of HS-2 polymorphisms in transgenic animals may help to clarify the functional significance of this association.

Mutations in HS-2, such as the A→G transition at position 8,598 in the Benin haplotype, enhance binding of Sp-1, a ubiquitous transcription factor, and a deletion of the Sp-1 binding site decreases β-globin gene expression in transgenic mice (Caterina et al., 1994; Morgan et al., 1996). An A→T transversion at position 9,114 decreases binding of an uncharacterized *trans*-acting factor from nuclear extracts of HEL and HeLa cells (Morgan et al., 1996).

In recent studies, polymorphisms in a tandem repeat of the sequence $(TA)_x N_{10-12}(TA)_y$ which contains a Hox2 binding site, were examined in 100 patients with sickle cell anemia who were 1 to 18 years old (Ofori-Acquah et al., 1999). Fifteen of 200 chromosomes (7.5 percent) had a discordance in the HS-2 tandem repeat that was not characteristic of the haplotype, a higher proportion than reported in other studies (Lu and Steinberg 1996). HbF levels in six Benin haplotype homozygotes with a Senegal-type HS-2 were between 2.6 and 8.5 percent, suggesting that this polymorphism alone did not lead to increased levels of HbF. A region between −1,445 and −1,225 5′ to the promoter of the ᴳγ-globin gene was found by SSCP analysis to vary among haplotypes. In Senegal-Benin chromosomes associated with modest HbF levels, the likely breakpoint for recombination was upstream of −1,500 bp 5′ to ᴳγ-globin gene promoter. On the other hand, when a high HbF was present with the Senegal-Benin chromosome recombination (Öner et al., 1992a), the breakpoint was 3′ to position −369 to −309 in the ᴳγ-globin gene promoter. In carriers of the sickle cell trait with a Benin haplotype, when the normal chromosome had the HS-2 $(AT)_9 N_{12}(AT)_{10}$ structure, HbF (0.9 percent) and F cells (8.3 percent) were about twice as high as in the presence of other configurations for this region (Merghoub et al., 1996). These data suggest that HbF is influenced by elements 3′ to HS-2 and 5′ to the γ-globin gene promoter.

F-cell numbers in nonanemic sickle cell trait carriers where the HbS gene was on a Benin haplotype were more strongly associated with polymorphisms in HS-2 of βᴬ chromosomes, specifically the $(AT)_9N_{12}(AT)_{10}$ configuration, than the −158 C→T change (Merghoub et al., 1997). Because these studies were conducted in the absence of hemolysis or stress erythropoiesis, they are less likely to reflect the effects of differential F-cell survival and more likely to estimate HbF production.

Few chromosomes have been sequenced in limited regions of HS-3, and no variations between the major β-gene haplotypes have been identified (Adekile et al., 1993; Lu and Steinberg, 1996). As HS-3 may be γ-gene specific during development of embryonic and fetal transgenic mice, future studies might examine all phylogenetically conserved sites within HS-III in a larger number of βˢ chromosomes.

β-Globin Gene Silencer

Located −530 bp 5′ to the β-globin gene is an AT-rich region with the core structure, $(AT)_x(T)_y$, which varies polymorphically and is linked to the β-globin gene cluster haplotype (Fig. 26.4). This locus has been proposed to serve as a β-globin gene silencer and may influence the expression of the β-globin gene by binding a putative repressor protein, BP1. The possibility still exists that the area has no functional significance in the regulation of the β-globin gene (Berg et al., 1991; Elion et al., 1992). Depending on the $(AT)_x(T)_y$ composition, BP1 is bound with greater or lesser affinity and may variably inhibit β-globin gene transcription. This region has been proposed as a possible cause of the silent carrier β-thalassemia phenotype (Semenza et al., 1984; Murru et al., 1990).

The Arab-India motif has a higher affinity for BP1 than the Bantu haplotype motif. This may be reflected at the protein level by less HbS in Indian carriers of the $β^S$ gene and a normal α-globin genotype, than in Blacks with sickle cell trait. For example, with the $(AT)_9(T)_5$ motif, HbS levels in sickle cell trait with four α-globin genes were 34 percent compared with about 39 percent with the $(AT)_8(T)_4$ motif, a reduction of nearly 13 percent (Elion et al., 1992). However, nondeletion α thalassemia and iron deficiency, both of which can reduce the percent HbS in sickle cell trait, are also prevalent in this population, and their presence may confound this analysis (Çürük et al., 1993). The −530 area may thus influence the clinical heterogeneity of sickle cell anemia by suppressing $β^S$-globin chain synthesis. As $β^S$ gene transcription declines, a reciprocal increase in γ-globin gene transcription may take place.

The $(AT)_9(T)_5$ motif, together with the −158 C→T polymorphism, may be associated with high HbF in some homozygous β thalassemia patients (Ragusa et al., 1992). In these patients, the $(AT)_9(T)_5$ motif was associated with about 10 g/dL HbF, whereas the $(AT)_7(T)_7$ was accompanied by about 5 g/dL of HbF. Although preliminary, these clinical observations suggest that this motif may have clinically relevant effects on β-globin gene transcription and, perhaps by impairing the production of β globin, increase the synthesis of HbF. As yet no studies in sickle cell anemia relate the composition of the −530 area with HbF levels. If the sequence of the −530 area is always linked to the β-globin gene haplotype, these studies would be redundant; however, if, as noted in the example of the Benin chromosome bearing a Senegal-like HS-2, some form of genetic rearrangement alters the region and affects β- and γ-gene transcription, learning the composition of the −530 $(AT)_x(T)_y$ might be informative.

Four Base Pair Deletion Linked to the $^Aγ$ Gene.

The Cameroon haplotype $β^S$ chromosome invariably accompanied by the $^Aγ^T$ gene is linked to a deletion of 4 bp (AGCA) at −222 to −225 5′ to this allele (Gilman et al., 1988). This is the only β-globin gene haplotype associated with the 4 bp deletion that was present in all racial groups and always linked to the $^Aγ^T$ allele (Coleman et al., 1994). In seventy African-American newborns heterozygous for the $^Aγ^T$-globin chain, this chain was always present at a lower level than the $^Aγ^I$-globin chain. There was no decrease in the percent $^Aγ^T$ compared with $^Gγ$-globin chains in heterozygotes for the 4 bp deletion, but there was a significant decrease in total HbF in newborns with the deletion. The percentage of total $^Aγ$ globin did not differ significantly between the groups with and without the 4 bp deletion. In $^Aγ^I$ homozygotes, HbF averaged 66.5 percent of total hemoglobin, whereas in $^Aγ^I:^Aγ^T$ heterozygotes, HbF averaged 50.2 percent, implying that the 4 bp deletion was associated with decreased expression of not only the $^Aγ^T$-globin gene, but also the $^Gγ$-globin gene in cis. In contrast to other reports, there was no difference in $^Aγ$-globin gene expression relative to the $^Gγ$-globin gene in $^Aγ^T/^Aγ^I$ heterozygotes compared with $^Aγ^I$ homozygotes. Studies in β thalassemia where the 4 bp deletion was present also suggested decreased $^Gγ$ gene expression in cis to the $^Aγ^T$ allele (Manca et al., 1991). Together, these results implicate the region of the 4 bp deletion as a possible cis-acting element that augments the expression of both γ-globin genes when combined with a trans-acting factor. If true, then the 4 bp deletion might modulate the course of sickle cell anemia in individuals with the Cameroon haplotype.

To test the association of the $^Aγ^T$ allele with the 4 bp deletion in $β^A$ chromosomes of sickle cell trait individuals, polymerase chain reaction (PCR) was used to generate a 1.2 kb fragment that included both the $^Aγ$-225 region and codon 75 (Gilman et al., 1993). Direct linkage of the 4 bp deletion to $^Aγ^T$ was shown by Bbv I digestion, which cleaved the normal but not the 4 bp deletion $^Aγ$ promoter, followed by blot hybridization to specific $^Aγ^T$ and $^Aγ^I$ oligonucleotides. In combination with quantitative hemoglobin analysis, these studies confirmed that the 4 bp deletion was associated with low in vivo $^Aγ^T$ expression.

Patients with sickle cell anemia and the Cameroon haplotype (Huisman et al., 1985) had the following γ-globin gene expression ratios. In homozygotes for the Cameroon haplotype the $^Gγ:^Aγ^T:^Aγ^I$ ratios were 45:55:0. Cameroon/Benin haplotype mixed heterozygotes had ratios of 46:21:33; Benin homozygotes had 46:0:54 ratios. All homozygous Cameroon haplotypes were homozygous for the 4 bp deletion, all Cameroon/Benin haplotypes were heterozygous for the deletion, and no Benin homozygotes had the deletion. The coexistence of the $^Aγ^T$ allele with the 4 bp deletion and the low $^Aγ^T:^Aγ^I$ globin ratio in

Cameroon/Benin sickle cell anemia cases is consistent with previous data (Gilman et al., 1988). The $^G\gamma$:$^A\gamma^T$ ratios of 45:55 in homozygous Cameroon haplotypes may indicate a *cis* effect of the 4 bp deletion on $^G\gamma$-globin gene expression, a result also suggested in studies of cord blood samples (Coleman et al., 1994). If the 4 bp deletion decreases both $^A\gamma^T$ and $^G\gamma$ in *cis*, then the $^G\gamma$:$^A\gamma^T$ ratio of Cameroon haplotype homozygotes would remain similar to $^G\gamma$:$^A\gamma^T$ of Benin haplotype homozygotes. Perhaps supporting this possibility, some $^A\gamma$ promoter mutations that increase $^A\gamma$ expression also increase $^G\gamma$ in *cis* (Chapters 6, 7, and 15).

Unfortunately, the number of patients with sickle cell anemia and the Cameroon haplotype for whom clinical data are available is small, making it difficult to gauge what influence this genetic locus may have on HbF levels, and most patients available for study were heterozygous for the haplotype. In one study, patients with a Cameroon haplotype chromosome in *trans* to a Benin, Bantu, or Senegal haplotype chromosome showed no differences in HbF levels, packed cell volume (PCV), or mean cell volume (MCV) (Steinberg et al., 1998) (Table 26.4).

There is additional in vitro evidence for the functional significance of the 4 bp deletion. A *trans*-acting factor was found to bind the 3′ enhancer and the promoter region of the $^A\gamma$-globin gene. Using a series of scanning mutations in gel shift competition assays, the binding site in the promoter was localized to the GCAGCA sequence that included the site of the 4 bp deletion. In a transient expression system, in vitro studies of the promoter containing the 4 bp deletion did not show reduced activity compared to the control sample. However, in this work the construct used lacked the 3′ enhancer previously found to bind the factor, and the site of the 4 bp deletion may facilitate interaction between the promoter and the 3′ enhancer. Preliminary evidence also suggests that the 4 bp dele-

tion creates a new site for the binding of a repressor protein. Finally, the protein product of the homeodomain locus, Hox B2, binds to the promoter and 3′ enhancer of the γ-globin gene in addition to sites in the LCR (Lavelle et al., 1991; Sengupta et al., 1994).

$^G\gamma$ Gene 5′ Regulatory Region

About 1.65 to 1.15 kb 5′ to the $^G\gamma$ gene lies an area of 0.5 kb that has been proposed as yet another region with a potentially regulatory role in γ-globin gene expression (Pissard and Beuzard, 1994). This region, designated the pre-$^G\gamma$ framework, has four polymorphic variants, which, like most other *cis*-acting sequences with possible regulatory roles, are linked to the β-gene cluster haplotype. Interest was drawn to this area because it contained four GATA-1 binding sites, as well as an Sp1 and CRE protein-binding domains. By gel retardation assay, strongest protein binding was associated with the Senegal pre-$^G\gamma$ framework. Functional studies of the polymorphic pre-$^G\gamma$ variants in two erythroid cell lines, measured as the enhancer function of the pre-$^G\gamma$ framework by CAT activity, showed that the Benin haplotype-linked pre-$^G\gamma$ enhancer activity was sevenfold lower than the Bantu and Senegal type pre-$^G\gamma$ framework. Some of these results are difficult to interpret. In patients with sickle cell anemia whose chromosomes formed the basis for this work, the HbF levels of the haplotype homozygotes are different from most results reported. Perhaps they represent transiently elevated HbF in young patients rather than stable adult levels. Whether the pre-$^G\gamma$ framework is one of the important haplotype-linked regulatory regions awaits further study.

When $^G\gamma$-globin gene promoters from Bantu, Senegal, and Benin chromosomes were linked to a CAT reporter gene and to HS-2 sequences from all three haplotypes, the Bantu promoter was associated with decreased CAT expression in K562 cells (human erythroleukemia cells expressing an embryonic-fetal hemoglobin synthesis program), but not MEL cells (murine erythroleukemia cell expressing an "adult" hemoglobin program) (Thomas et al., 1998). Lowest CAT expression was found with the combination of Bantu HS-2 and Bantu $^G\gamma$-globin gene promoter. Although these experiments mirror clinical observations on the effect of the Bantu haplotype on HbF expression and draw additional attention to the γ-globin gene promoter, the physiologic significance of these findings is unclear given the cell lines studied and constructs used.

Table 26.4. Effect of the Cameroon Chromosome in Haplotype Combined Heterozygotes with Benin, CAR, and Senegal Haplotype Chromosomes

Typical haplotype	n	HbF	PCV	MCV
Benin	20	5.9 ± 4.0	24.8 ± 4.0	97 ± 8.9
CAR (Bantu)	7	5.2 ± 3.6	24.4 ± 5.5	92 ± 13.6
Senegal	3	6.2 ± 5.7	23.4 ± 4.6	93 ± 9.9
All	30	5.8 ± 3.7	24.6 ± 5.2	93 ± 10.5

All patients were combined heterozygotes for a Cameroon haplotype chromosome and one of the typical haplotype chromosomes listed in column 1.
PCV, packed cell volume; MCV, mean cell volume.

Non-Gene Deletion Hereditary Persistence of HbF

Mutations in proximal and distal promoters of the $^G\gamma$- and $^A\gamma$-globin genes are likely to be responsible for the phenotype of nondeletional hereditary persistence of fetal hemoglobin (HPFH) (Chapter 15). In these conditions, the HbF level in heterozygotes is 3 to 20 percent, and its distribution among erythrocytes varies according to the HbF level. Either the $^{G}\gamma$ or $^{A}\gamma$ gene is affected, and the β-globin gene in *cis* is expressed (β+). These disorders differ from the first described examples of HPFH caused by large deletions affecting the δ- and β-globin genes, whose phenotype merges with that of δβ thalassemia (Chapter 15). Could this class of mutation be responsible for some instances of sickle cell anemia with very high HbF levels and, therefore, be an additional genetic modulator of disease severity?

In a group of 299 adult patients with sickle cell anemia and a spectrum of HbF concentrations, the γ-globin gene promoters in thirty patients with HbF levels in the highest decile (mean HbF, 12.4 percent) were sequenced and no mutations were encountered. These mutations are rare and are unlikely to account for the high HbF phenotype in most individuals with sickle cell anemia (Lu and Steinberg, 1996). A special case of γ-globin gene promoter mutation is the previously discussed C→T polymorphism at position −158 5′ to the γ-globin gene that is linked to the Senegal and Arab-India haplotypes.

Duplicated, triplicated, or quadruplicated γ-globin loci may also cause high HbF. (Powers et al., 1984; Harano et al., 1985).

Cis-Acting Elements Beyond Hypersensitive Sites of the LCR

Other *cis*-acting elements (for example, in additional phylogenetically conserved regions of the LCR outside the core sequences of its constituent hypersensitive sites) may partake in the regulation of γ-globin gene transcription (Blau and Stamatoyannopoulos 1994; Li and Stamatoyanno-Poulos, 1994; Stamatoyannopoulos et al., 1994; Jackson et al., 1996). Conserved regions of DNA within the LCR, but removed from the core sequences studied previously, were identified by phylogenetic footprinting (Lu and Steinberg, 1996); and patients who were homozygous for the three common haplotypes found in sickle cell anemia, based on extensive examination of other polymorphic regions besides the restriction enzyme sites used to define a haplotype, were studied in a search for differences in phylogenetically conserved sequences among patients with sickle cell anemia and different levels of HbF (Nagel, 1994; Figueiredo et al., 1996a; Lu and Steinberg, 1996). Although differences were present outside the core sequences of HS-2 and HS-3 of the LCR, they were most extensive in regions devoid of identifiable transcription factor binding sites. It seems unlikely that the sequence variations found represented unique changes

that could provide a general explanation for the differential expression of the γ-globin gene in sickle cell anemia. All of the sequence differences that were present were associated with either high or low HbF levels, were present in all or none of the individuals with a specific haplotype, and occurred sporadically among the three haplotypes studied (Plonczynski et al., 1997).

HbF Modulation Unlinked to the β-Globin Gene Cluster

HbF is sequestered in a restricted number of cells called F cells, whose numbers are genetically determined, although the exact genetic elements involved in regulation are unknown (Chapter 7). There are likely genetic determinants of HbF level that are not linked to the β-globin gene cluster that influence HbF concentrations in sickle cell anemia (Miyoshi et al., 1988; Dover et al., 1992) (Chapter 15). One possible "F-cell" production locus is X-chromosome linked and has been localized between DXS143 and DXS16 within Xp22.3–22.2 (Chang et al., 1994). This locus may account, in part, for the higher HbF levels found in females, both healthy ones and those with sickle cell anemia (Miyoshi et al., 1988). Another gene affecting HbF production was localized to chromosome 6q (Thein et al., 1994; Craig et al., 1996). Other *trans*-acting autosomal loci also appear to influence the amounts of HbF in F cells, and collectively these elements have been termed *quantitative trait loci* (Garner et al., 1998a, 1998b). Preliminary studies in monozygotic and dizygotic twins suggest than the Xmn I C→T polymorphism 5′ to the $^{G}\gamma$-globin gene partially explains the variance in HbF levels (Garner et al., 1998a, 1998b; Thein and Craig, 1998). The HbF level in sickle cell anemia is set by the number of F cells, the amount of HbF per F cell, and the differential survival of F and non-F cells (Dover et al., 1978; Dover and Boyer, 1980).

α THALASSEMIA

Interactions of sickle cell anemia and α thalassemia are discussed in detail in Chapters 24 and 28 and are only summarized here. α Thalassemia in Blacks is usually a result of the deletion of one or two α-globin genes. Missing even two of the normal complement of four α-globin genes is not clinically important (Chapters 17 and 18). On average, about a third of blacks carry an α-globin gene deletion, and in some populations this prevalence is even higher so that α thalassemia and sickle cell anemia often coexist (Steinberg and Embury, 1986; Steinberg, 1991). The coexistence of α thalassemia and sickle cell anemia is associated with less hemolysis, higher hemoglobin concentration, lower MCV, and lower reticulocyte count, compared with individuals with normal α-globin gene numbers (Embury et al., 1982; Higgs et al., 1982; Steinberg et al., 1984; De Ceulaer et al., 1983). α Thalassemia does not appear to modify the effect of haplotype on HbF levels in sickle cell anemia. Therefore, it is unlikely that any clinical benefit α thalassemia confers on sickle cell anemia is mediated through its effects on HbF level. α Thalassemia is distributed evenly among all β-globin gene haplotypes in African Americans with sickle cell anemia.

α Thalassemia does have an effect on the phenotype of sickle cell anemia and reduces sickle hemoglobin concentration in red cells. As HbS polymerization depends on hemoglobin concentration, concurrent α thalassemia should diminish the polymerization potential of sickle hemoglobin in sickle cell anemia. Clinically, the outcome of coincident α thalassemia and sickle cell anemia is paradoxical. Vasoocclusive events appear undiminished in sickle cell anemia with α thalassemia, and some types appear to be increased. Fewer dense and poorly deformable cells, as a result of α thalassemia, raise the PCV and because these cells contain HbS, blood viscosity is increased. Raising the number of sickle cells, as occurs with α thalassemia, seems to promote vasoocclusion (Chapters 24 and 28).

Patients with sickle cell anemia and α thalassemia have more episodes of pain and more bone disease than do patients with sickle cell anemia only (Billett et al., 1995). However, more blood may also have beneficial effects in some organs, so that skin ulcers of the leg and retinal vascular disease may be less common in carriers of α thalassemia and sickle cell anemia. In children 2 to 12 years old with sickle cell anemia and high HbF levels who were likely to carry the Arab-India haplotype, gene-deletion or non-gene-deletion types of α thalassemia appeared to preserve splenic function as estimated by ^{99m}Tc colloid scanning (Adekile et al., 1996). Nearly 60 percent of individuals with normally visualized spleens had α thalassemia; when the spleen was not visualized or only partially visualized, α thalassemia was found in only 30 percent of cases. α Thalassemia may also reduce the incidence of stroke in children with sickle cell anemia. Some evidence has suggested that the combination of α thalassemia and sickle cell anemia may promote longevity, but this has not been proven (Mears et al., 1983).

INTERACTIONS OF β-GLOBIN GENE HAPLOTYPE AND α THALASSEMIA

Several studies have examined the way in which α thalassemia interacts with different β-globin gene haplotypes to modify the hematologic and clinical presentation of sickle cell anemia (Rieder et al., 1991; Alfinito et al., 1994; Steinberg et al., 1995; Figueiredo et al., 1996b; Chang et al., 1997; Mukherjee et al., 1997; El-Kalla and Baysal, 1998a, 1998b; Lee et al., 1998; Steinberg et al., 1998) (Table 26.5). In most instances, there is no differential effect of α thalassemia on vasoocclusive complications among carriers of different β-globin gene haplotypes. Regardless of the β-globin gene haplotype, α thalassemia has little effect on HbF concentration beyond that of haplotype alone (Chang et al., 1995). Regardless of the β-globin gene haplotype, α thalassemia reduces MCV by about 8 fl, increases hemoglobin concentration by 0.4 g/dL, and reduces reticulocyte count by 2 percent. There was a substantial effect of sex, however, which confounded the effect of α thalassemia on MCV (Steinberg et al., 1995b).

One notable exception to the usual observation that α thalassemia is an adverse risk factor for vasoocclusive disease was a study of two western Indian populations. Both groups had a HbS gene frequency of over 0.2 and HbF concentrations of 18.5 and 15.5 percent, and were homozygous for the Arab-India haplotype (Shalev et al., 1996). More extensive analysis revealed that both groups had identical polymorphisms within HS-2 and 5' to the β-globin gene. Each group had between 67 and 72 percent F cells. One population, the Valsad tribals, appeared to have a milder clinical course with fewer pain episodes and hospitalizations. Carriers of sickle cell trait in the Valsads had 28 percent HbS versus 36 percent in the nontribal Nagpur population, suggesting the presence of α thalassemia (Chapter 28). The gene frequency of α thalassemia was 0.97 in Valsads, and 76 percent of these patients were homozygous for α thalassemia-2. In contrast, only 24 percent of the more severely affected nontribal Nagpur group had an α thalassemia determinant, and homozygosity was rare. Unfortunately, PCV was not reported in this study. Studies in Saudis and Kuwaitis with the Arab-India haplotype and α thalassemia also suggest that these individuals have a milder disease than those

Table 26.5. Hematologic Features of Sickle Cell Anemia with α Thalassemia

Genotype	Hemoglobin	MCV	Reticulocytes (%)	HbA$_2$ (%)
αα/αα	8.0 ± 1.1	92 ± 7	11 ± 6	2.8 ± 0.4
−α/αα	8.6 ± 1.1	83 ± 7	9 ± 6	3.3 ± 0.6
−α/−α	9.2 ± 1.3	72 ± 4	7 ± 5	3.8 ± 4

Hb, hemoglobin concentration in g/dL; MCV, mean corpuscular volume in femtoliters.

Genotype indicates the number of α-globin genes present in patients with sickle cell anemia.

These data report the average determined from studies of black patients with α thalassemia and sickle cell anemia (from De Ceulaer et al., 1983; Steinberg et al., 1984).

without α thalassemia (Padmos et al., 1991; El-Hazmi, 1992a, 1992b; Adekile and Haider, 1996). α Thalassemia did not affect the hemoglobin concentration in twenty-five patients from the United Arab Emirates who had the Arab-India haplotype but was reported to increase the hemoglobin concentration and the severity of vasoocclusive disease in a small number of patients with Benin and Bantu haplotypes attending the same clinic (El-Kalla and Baysal, 1998a).

Most studies of sickle cell anemia in black patients suggest that α thalassemia increases the likelihood of vasoocclusive complications (Chapter 24). The beneficial effect of α thalassemia on sickle cell anemia with the Arab-Indian haplotype may be explained by the exceptionally high HbF in carriers of this haplotype, which dominates the increased PCV caused by α thalassemia.

HEMOGLOBIN A₂

HbA$_2$, the tetramer of α-and δ-globin chains, impairs the polymerization of HbS to the same extent as the γ-globin chain of HbF (Poillon et al., 1993); δ22 (Ala) and δ87 (Gln) are the residues that inhibit polymerization (Poillon et al., 1993). HbA$_2$ has the advantage of being evenly distributed in all red cells, whereas HbF is sequestered in F cells. The naturally low level of HbA$_2$ makes it an inconsequential contributor to the total hemoglobin concentration, but there are instances when the level of HbA$_2$ is increased far beyond its usual values. Normally, HbA$_2$ is only 2 to 3 percent of the total hemoglobin (Chapter 10). When HbA$_2$ and HbF levels are high, the combination of these two hemoglobins may modulate sickle cell disease and cause a mild phenotype (Waye et al., 1991). HbA$_2$ levels are increased in β thalassemia. Some individuals with β thalassemia trait have HbA$_2$ concentrations that are significantly higher than the usual 5.0 ± 1.1 percent (Steinberg and Adams, 1991). These exceptionally high HbA$_2$ levels are the result of deletions that remove the β-globin gene promoters (Steinberg and Adams, 1991). Elimination of β-globin gene promoters by 5′ deletions may increase the likelihood that the LCR interacts with the δ gene in *cis*.

It is unlikely that variation in HbA$_2$ level affects the phenotype of sickle cell anemia. Although HbA$_2$ is increased in sickle cell anemia with α thalassemia, compared with sickle cell anemia alone, the increase is small, and if any benefit results, it is probably undetectable with our current imprecise means of quantifying phenotypic variation in sickle cell anemia. However, in the rare instances in which β^0 thalassemia is caused by deletions of the 5′ portion of the β-globin gene that cause the HbA$_2$ level to far exceed that

expected, there could be modulation of the compound heterozygote with HbS-β^0 thalassemia. Too few patients with this combination of partial gene deletion β thalassemia and sickle cell anemia have been evaluated to establish the phenotype, which appears to be heterogeneous (Padanilam et al., 1984; Miller et al., 1989; Waye et al., 1991).

ERYTHROCYTE G-6-PD DEFICIENCY

Glucose-6-phosphate dehydrogenase (G-6-PD) deficiency commonly coexists with sickle cell anemia. The effect of G-6-PD deficiency on the disease has been reported to be beneficial, deleterious, or neutral (Piomelli et al., 1972; Beutler et al., 1974; Steinberg and Dreiling, 1974; Bienzle et al., 1975; Gibbs et al., 1980; Al-Nuaim et al., 1997; Bouanga et al., 1998). In 800 males over age 2 years with sickle cell anemia who were analyzed in the United States as part of a multiinstitutional study, G-6-PD deficiency was not associated with differential survival, reduced hemoglobin levels, increased hemolysis, more pain crises, septic episodes, or a higher incidence of acute anemia episodes (Steinberg et al., 1988).

A potential defect in all the studies derives from the difficulty of definitively ascertaining the presence of G-6-PD deficiency in patients with hemolytic anemia who have a young red cell population, although it was unlikely that any errors made substantially confounded the interpretation of the results. Using DNA-based methods to unequivocally detect the GdA$^-$ allele—the gene causing G-6-PD deficiency in the vast majority of African subjects—it was recently reported that the frequencies of GdA$^-$ and of the normal GdB and GdA$^+$ genes were identical in about 200 patients with sickle cell anemia and an equal number of control subjects with only normal hemoglobin (Bouanga et al., 1998). Blood counts were similar in patients with and without G-6-PD deficiency, although the hemoglobin concentration was lower in those with sickle cell anemia and the GdA$^-$ gene. The prevalence of GdA$^-$ did not change according to age. It now seems clear, particularly in males where the expression of this X-linked trait is most apparent, that there is little, if any, modulation of the phenotype of sickle cell anemia by coincident G-6-PD deficiency.

INHERITED DISORDERS OF THROMBOSIS

Because of the possibility that thrombosis and hemostasis play roles in the pathophysiology of sickle cell anemia, coincidental mutations that favor blood coagulation or thrombosis could influence the phenotype of disease (Francis and Hebbel, 1994). Recent studies attempting to relate the presence of mutations in genes for factor V, platelet glycoprotein IIIa, and 5, 10 methylenetetrahydrofolate reductase (MTHFR) to the pathogenesis of specific complications of sickle cell disease have had disparate results.

In one report, a C→T mutation at position 677 of the MTHFR gene, which is associated with enzyme thermolability and a putative hypercoagulable state due to hyperhomocystinemia, was found in 36 percent of forty-five adults with sickle cell disease and osteonecrosis but in only 13 percent of sixty-two patients without osteonecrosis, a significant difference (Kutlar et al., 1998). In other reports, this same mutation was not associated with vascular complications of sickle cell disease, including osteonecrosis and stroke; however, far fewer patients were studied (DeCastro et al., 1998; Zimmerman et al., 1998). For example, the MTHFR mutation was present in 14 percent of fourteen patients with osteonecrosis and 14 percent of patients without osteonecrosis (Zimmerman and Ware 1998). There was also no relationship between osteonecrosis and a mutation in the platelet glycoprotein IIIa gene—C→T at position 1565, which was associated with premature coronary artery disease (Zimmerman and Ware 1998). Factor V Leiden, a common cause of thrombosis in Caucasians, is rare in blacks; and limited studies have not linked this mutation to stroke in sickle cell disease (Kahn et al., 1997; Andrade et al., 1998).

One report of seven children with stroke suggested that, compared with control subjects, protein C levels were reduced in "steady state" or with vasoocclusive crisis (Khanduri et al., 1998). However, these differences, although considered statistically significant, were quite small. To assess the possible role of protein C, protein S, heparin cofactor II, thrombin-antithrombin complexes, five coagulation factors, and resistance to activated protein C in the genesis of cerebral vasculopathy, these factors were measured in children who were being transfused for stroke, children at risk for stroke on the basis of transcranial Doppler flow studies, and untransfused control subjects with sickle cell anemia (Liesner et al., 1998). Most anticoagulant proteins, such as protein C, were reduced in patients with sickle cell anemia. Procoagulant factors such as thrombin-antithrombin complexes were often elevated. Yet there were no differences between patients with sickle cell anemia who had not had transfusions, stroke patients who had transfusions, and individuals at increased risk for stroke. It is difficult to control for the effects of transfusion. Increased flow by transcranial Doppler studies does not equate with cerebrovascular disease (although recent studies with magnetic resonance imaging and position emission tomography scanning suggest that nearly 90 percent of a selected group of children with sickle cell anemia had some ele-

ment of cerebral vasculopathy) (Powars et al., 1999). High levels of antiphospholipid antibodies were found in patients with sickle cell disease and individuals with sickle cell trait, but no relationship to disease complications was noted (Nsiri et al., 1998).

Most of the reports of genetic predisposition to thrombosis in sickle cell anemia are abstracts or of pilot studies. Further work is needed to resolve the role of genetic risk factors for thrombosis in the etiology of osteonecrosis or other complications of sickle cell anemia.

PREDICTION OF PHENOTYPE IN SICKLE CELL ANEMIA

Can the phenotype of sickle cell anemia be predicted on the basis of our knowledge of the genetic modifiers of disease? Finding a reliable method of foretelling disease severity early in life, or perhaps antenatally, becomes increasingly important as new treatments such as bone marrow transplantation, chemotherapeutic manipulation of HbF level, or even gene therapy—all with potentially serious complications—approach clinical use (Platt et al., 1984; Vermylen et al., 1988; Rodgers et al., 1990). Currently, an accurate prediction of disease severity cannot be made on the basis of one or two genetic markers such as α thalassemia or the β-globin gene cluster haplotype, but it could become possible with additional markers. Methods that not only diagnose sickle cell anemia but also determine its prognosis would be of considerable help when hazardous treatments are being considered.

It may be simplistic to expect that even if we could predict the rate of decrease of HbF level in childhood and its steady-state level in adults, we would be able to foretell the course of the disease. Some patients survive many years with few problems even when low HbF levels presage an early and painful demise (Steinberg 1989; 1995a). The distribution of HbF in F cells may be vitally important and not reflected in the measurement of total HbF or F-cell levels. For example, having 10 percent F cells each with nearly 100 percent HbF is not likely to be as advantageous as having 20 percent F cells, each with 50 percent HbF. Factors unrelated to the hemoglobin genes, such as the proteins that influence thrombosis, blood coagulation and anticoagulation, vascular reactivity, erythrocyte membrane structure and function, leukocyte biology, and endothelial cell integrity, may be integral to the pathogenesis of sickle cell anemia (Hebbel, 1991; Embury et al., 1994). When the roles of these determinants are delineated and integrated into a comprehensive model of pathogenesis and environmental influences are controlled, it may then be possible to establish an accurate prognosis for sickle cell disease.

References

Addison, J and Hazareesingh, K. (1984). *A new history of Mauritius*. London and Basingstoke: Macmillan.

Adekile, AD, Dimovski, AJ, Oner, C et al. (1993). Haplotype-specific sequence variations in the locus control region (5′ hypersensitive sites 2, 3, 4) of β^S chromosomes. *Hemoglobin* 17: 475–478.

Adekile, AD, Tuli, M, Haider, MZ et al. (1996). Influence of α-thalassemia trait on spleen function in sickle cell anemia patients with high HbF. *Am. J. Hematol.* 53: 1–5.

Adekile, AD and Haider, MZ. (1996). Morbidity, β^s haplotype and α-globin gene patterns among sickle cell anemia patients in Kuwait. *Acta Haematol.* 96: 150–154.

Adekile, AD. (1997). Historical and anthropological correlates of β^S haplotypes and α and β-thalassemia alleles in the Arabian Peninsula. *Hemoglobin* 21: 281–296.

Al-Arrayed, SS and Haites, N. (1995). Features of sickle cell disease in Bahrain. *La Revue de Sante de la Mediterrannee Oriental* 1: 1.

Al-Nuaim, L, Talib, ZA, El-Hazmi, MAF, and Warsy, AS. (1997). Sickle cell and G-6-PD deficiency gene in cord blood samples: Experience at King Khalid University Hospital, Riyadh. *J. Trop. Pediatr.* 43: 71–74.

Alberto, FL, Arruda, VR, Lima, CSP et al. (1998). Long-term hydroxyurea therapy in thalassemia intermedia and thalassemia major patients. *Blood* 92: 36b.

Alfinito, F, Calabro, V, Cappellini, MD et al. (1994). Glucose 6-phosphate dehydrogenase deficiency and red cell membrane defects: Additive or synergistic interaction in producing chronic haemolytic anaemia. *Br. J. Haematol.* 87: 148–152.

Aluoch, JR, Kilinc, Y, Aksoy, M et al. (1986). Sickle cell anaemia among Eti-Turks: Hematological, clinical and genetic observations. *Br. J. Haematol.* 66: 45–55.

Andrade, FL, Annichino-Bizzacchi, JM, Saad, STO et al. (1998). Prothrombin mutant, factor V Leiden, and thermolabile variant of methylenetetrahydrofolate reductase among patients with sickle cell disease in Brazil. *Am. J. Hematol.* 59: 46–50.

Antonarakis, SE, Boehm, CD, Giardina, PV, and Kazazian, HH. (1982). Nonrandom association of polymorphic restriction sites in the β-globin gene cluster. *Proce. Natl. Acad. Sci. U.S.A.* 79: 137–141.

Antonarakis, SE, Boehm, CD, Serjeant, GR et al. (1984). Origin of the beta S-globin gene in blacks: The contribution of recurrent mutation or gene conversion or both. *Proc. Natl. Acad. Sci. U.S.A.* 81: 853–856.

Antonarakis, SE, Kazazian, HH, and Orkin, SH. (1985). DNA polymorphism and molecular pathology of the human globin gene clusters. *Hum. Genet.* 69: 1–14.

Bakioglu, I, Hattori, Y, Kutlar, A et al. (1985). Five adults with mild sickle cell anaemia share a β^S chromosome with the same haplotype. *Am. J. Hematol.* 20: 297–300.

Ballas, SK, Talacki, CA, Adachi, K et al. (1991). The XMN l site (−158, C→T) 5′ to the ^{G}γ gene: Correlation with the Senegalese haplotype and ^{G}γ globin expression. *Hemoglobin* 15: 393–405.

Basham, AL. (1954). *The wonder that was India*. London: Sidgwick and Jackson.

Beet, EA. (1949). The genetics of the sickle-cell trait in a Bantu tribe. *Ann. Eugenics* 14: 279–284.

Berg, PE, Mittelman, M, Elion, J et al. (1991). Increased protein binding to a −530 mutation of the human β-globin gene associated with decreased b-globin synthesis. *Am. J. Hematol.* 36: 42–47.

Beris, P, Kitundu, MN, Baysal, E et al. (1992). Black b-thalassemia homozygotes with specific sequence variations in the 5′ hypersensitive site-2 of the locus control region have high levels of fetal hemoglobin. *Am. J. Hematol.* 41: 97–101.

Beutler, E, Johnson, C, Powars, D, and West, C. (1974). Prevalence of glucose-6-phosphate dehydrogenase deficiency in sickle cell anemia. *N. Engl. J. Med.* 290: 826–828.

Bhatia, HM and Rao, VR. (1986). *Genetic atlas of Indian tribes*. Parel, Bombay: Institute of Immunohaematology.

Bhowmik, KL. (1971). *Tribal India: A profile in Indian ethnology*. Calcutta: World Press.

Bienzle, U, Sodeinde, O, Effiong, CE, and Luzzatto, L. (1975). Glucose-6-phosphate dehydrogenase deficiency and sickle cell anemia: Frequency and features of the association in an African community. *Blood* 46: 591–597.

Billett, HH, Nagel, RL, and Fabry, ME. (1995). Paradoxical increase of painful crises in sickle cell patients with α-thalassemia. *Blood* 86: 4382–4382.

Blau, CA and Stamatoyannopoulos, G. (1994). Regulation of fetal hemoglobin. In Embury, SH, Hebbel, RP, Mohandas, N, and Steinberg, MH, editors. *Sickle cell disease: Basic principles and clinical practice*. New York: Raven Press.

Bodmer, E and Solomon, WF. (1979). Evolution of sickle variant gene. *Lancet* I: 923.

Bohannan, P and Curtin, P. (1971). *Africa and Africans*. New York: Natural History Press.

Boletini, E, Svobodova, M, Divoky, V et al. (1994). Sickle cell anemia, sickle cell β-thalassemia, and thalassemia major in Albania: Characterization of mutations. *Hum. Genet.* 93: 182–187.

Bouanga, JC, Mouélé, R, Préhu, C et al. (1998). Glucose-6-phosphate dehydrogenase deficiency and homozygous sickle cell disease in Congo. *Hum. Hered.* 48: 192–197.

Bouhassira, EE, Lachman, H, Krishnamoorthy, R et al. (1989). A gene conversion located 5′ to the ^{A}γ gene is in linkage disequilibrium with the Bantu haplotype in sickle cell anemia. *J. Clin. Invest.* 83: 2070–2073.

Brittenham, G, Lozoff, B, Harris, JW et al. (1979). Sickle cell anemia and trait in Southern India: Further studies. *Am. J. Hematol.* 6: 107–123.

Caterina, JJ, Ryan, TM, Pawlik, KM et al. (1991). Human β-globin locus control region: Analysis of the 5′ DNase I hypersensitive site HS 2 in transgenic mice. *Proc. Natl. Acad. Sci. U.S.A.* 88: 1626–1630.

Caterina, JJ, Ciavatta, DJ, Donze, D et al. (1994). Multiple elements in human β-globin locus control region 5′ HS 2 are involved in enhancer activity and position-independent, transgene expression. *Nucleic Acids Res.* 22: 1006–1011.

Chakravarti, A, Buetow, KH, Antonarakis, SE et al. (1984). Nonuniform recombination within the human β-globin gene cluster. *Am. J. Hum. Genet.* 36: 1239–1258.

Chang, YC, Smith, KD, Serjeant, G, and Dover, G. (1994). The X-linked F cell production locus: Genetic mapping and role in fetal hemoglobin production. *Clin. Res.* 42: 237A.

Chang, YC, Smith, KD, Moore, RD et al. (1995). An analysis of fetal hemoglobin variation in sickle cell disease: The relative contributions of the X-linked factor, β-globin haplotypes, α-globin gene number, gender, and age. *Blood* 85: 1111–1117.

Chang, YPC, Maier-Redelsperger, M, Smith, KD et al. (1997). The relative importance of the x-linked FCP locus and β-globin haplotypes in determining haemoglobin F levels: A study of SS patients homozygous for β^S haplotypes. *Br. J. Haematol.* 96: 806–814.

Chebloune, Y, Trabuchet, G, Poncet, D et al. (1984). A new method for detection of small modifications in genomic DNA, applied to the human δβ globin gene cluster. *Eur. J. Biochem.* 142: 473–480.

Chebloune, Y, Pagnier, J, Trabuchet, G et al. (1988). Structural analysis of the 5′ flanking region of the β globin gene in African sickle cell anemia patients. Further evidence for three origins of the sickle cell mutation in Africa. *Proc. Natl. Acad. Sci. U.S.A.* 85: 4431–4435.

Chen, Y, Ruffin, D, and Pace, B. (1996). Mutations in the β globin locus may play an important role in fetal hemoglobin induction by hydroxyurea. *Blood* 88(Suppl 1): 494a.

Coleman, MB, Adams, JG, Steinberg, MH, and Winter, WP. (1994). A four base pair deletion 5′ to the ^Aγ^T gene is associated not only with the decreased expression of the ^Aγ^T-globin gene but also the ^Gγ gene in cis. *Am. J. Hematol.* 47: 307–311.

Collins, FS, Stoeckert, CJ Jr, Serjeant, GR et al. (1984). ^Gγβ+ hereditary persistence of fetal hemoglobin: Cosmid cloning and identification of a specific mutation 5′ to the ^Gγ gene. *Proc. Natl. Acad. Sci. U.S.A.* 81: 4894–4898.

Collins, FS, Metherall, JE, Yamakawa, M et al. (1985). A point mutation in the ^Aγ globin-gene promoter in Greek hereditary persistence of fetal hemoglobin. *Nature* 313: 325–326.

Costa, FF, Arruda, VR, Goncalves, MG et al. (1994). β^S-gene-cluster haplotypes in sickle cell anemia patients from two regions of Brazil. *Am. J. Hematol.* 45: 96–97.

Craig, JE, Rochette, J, Fisher, CA et al. (1996). Dissecting the loci controlling fetal haemoglobin production on chromosomes 11p and 6q by the regressive approach. *Nat. Genet.* 12: 58–64.

Curtin, PD. (1969). *The Atlantic slave trade: A census.* Milwaukee: University of Wisconsin Press.

Çürük, MA, Baysal, E, Gupta, RB et al. (1993). An IVS-I-117 (G→A) acceptor splice site mutation in the a1-globin gene is a nondeletional α-thalassaemia-2 determinant in an Indian population. *Br. J. Haematol.* 85: 148–152.

Daget, S. (1976). In La Traitte des Noirs, Societe Francaise d'Histoire D'Outre-mer, Paris, 1976.

Damanhouri, G. (1997). Sickle cell anaemia haplotypes in the western region of Saudi Arabia. *6th International Conference on Thalassemia and the Haemoglobinopathies,* Abstract #181.

Darwin, C. *The voyage of the HMS Beagle.* London.

DeCastro, L, Rinder, HM, Howe, JG, and Smith, BR. (1998). Thrombophilic genotypes do not adversely affect the course of sickle cell disease (SCD). *Blood* 92: 161a.

De Ceulaer, K, Higgs, DR, Weatherall, DJ et al. (1983). Alpha thalassemia reduces the hemolytic rate in homozygous sickle-cell disease. *N. Engl. J. Med.* 309: 189–190.

Deisseroth, A, Nienhuis, A, Lawrence, J et al. (1975). Chromosomal location of human β globin gene on human chromosome 11 in somatic cell hybrids. *Proc. Natl. Acad. Sci. U.S.A.* 75: 1456–1460.

de Studer, FSE. (1984). *La trata de negros en el Rio de la Plata durante el siglo XVIII.* Buenos Aires, Argentina: Libros de Hispanoamerica.

Diamond, J. (1997). *Guns, germs, and steel. The fates of human societies.* New York: Norton.

DiRienzo, A, Felicetti, A, Terrenato, L. (1987). RFLP's in β^Thal and β^S chromosomes in Egypt. *2nd International Symposium on Thalassemia in Crete.*

Dimovski, AJ, Öner, C, Agarwal, S et al. (1991). Certain mutations observed in the 5′ sequences of the ^Gγ and ^Aγ-globin genes of β^S chromosomes are specific for chromosomes with major haplotypes. *Acta Haematol. (Basel)* 85: 79–87.

Dover, GJ, Boyer, SH, Charache, S, and Heintzelman, K. (1978). Individual variation in the production and survival of F cells in sickle-cell disease. *N. Engl. J. Med.* 299: 1428–1435.

Dover, GJ and Boyer, SH. (1980). Quantitation of hemoglobins within individual red cells: Asynchronous biosynthesis of fetal and adult hemoglobin during erythroid maturation in normal subjects. *Blood* 56: 1082–1091.

Dover, GJ, Smith, KD, Chang, YC, et al. (1992). Fetal hemoglobin levels in sickle cell disease and normal individuals are partially controlled by an X-linked gene located at Xp22.2. *Blood* 80: 816–824.

Efstratiadis, A, Posakony, JW, Maniatis, T et al. (1980). The structure and evolution of the human β globin gene family. *Cell* 21: 653–668.

El-Hazmi, MA. (1990). Beta-globin gene haplotypes in the Saudi sickle cell anaemia patients. *Hum. Hered.* 40: 177–186.

El-Hazmi, MAF. (1992a). Clinical and haematological diversity of sickle cell disease in Saudi children. *J. Trop. Pediatr.* 38: 106–112.

El-Hazmi, MAF. (1992b). Heterogeneity and variation of clinical and haematological expression of haemoglobin S in Saudi Arabs. *Acta Haematol.* 88: 67–71.

El Hazmi, MAF and Warsy, AS. (1997). *Xmn* 1 polymorphism in Yemeni sickle cell disease patients. *Symposium on genetic diseases in Arab population: A wealth of indicative information.*

El-Kalla, S and Baysal, E. (1998a). Genotype-phenotype correlation of sickle cell disease in the United Arab Emirates. *Pediatr. Hematol. Oncol.* 15: 237–242.

El-Kalla, S and Baysal, E. (1998b). α-Thalassemia in the United Arab Emirates. *Acta Haematol.* 100: 49–53.

Elion, J, Berg, PE, Lapouméroulie, C et al. (1992). DNA sequence variation in a negative control region 5′ to the β-globin gene correlates with the phenotypic expression of the β^S mutation. *Blood* 79: 787–792.

Ellis, J, Talbot, D, Dillon, N, and Grosveld, F. (1993). Synthetic human β-globin 5′HS2 constructs function as locus control regions only in multicopy transgene concatamers. *EMBO J.* 12: 127–134.

Embury, SH, Dozy, AM, Miller, J et al. (1982). Concurrent sickle-cell anemia and alpha-thalassemia: Effect on severity of anemia. *N. Engl. J. Med.* 306: 270–274.

Embury, SH, Hebbel, RP, Mohandas, N, and Steinberg, MH. (1994). *Sickle cell disease: Basic principles and clinical practice.* New York: Raven Press.

Emmel, VE. (1917). A study of the erythrocytes in a case of severe anemia with elongated and sickle-shaped red blood corpuscles. *Arch. Intern. Med.* 20: 586–598.

Etcheverry, R, Vacarreza, R, Manuguean, A et al. (1988). Distribution of blood groups and hemoglobin S (sickle) as indices of negroid mixture in Diaguitas Indians of the Elqui and Limari river valleys. *Rev. Med. Chile* 116: 607–611.

Fairservis, WA. (1971). *The roots of ancient India: the archeology of early Indian civilization.* New York: Macmillan Co.

Figueiredo, MS and Steinberg, MH. (1996a). 5′ Hypersensitive site-2 and fetal hemoglobin in Brazilians. *Hemoglobin* 20: 435–438.

Figueiredo, MS, Kerbauy, J, Goncalves, MS et al. (1996b). Effect of α-thalassemia and β-globin gene cluster haplotypes on the hematological and clinical features of sickle-cell anemia in Brazil. *Am. J. Hematol.* 53: 72–76.

Flint, J, Harding, RM, Clegg, JB, and Boyce, AJ. (1993a). Why are some genetic diseases common? Distinguishing selection from other processes by molecular analysis of globin gene variants. *Hum. Genet.* 91: 91–117.

Flint, J, Harding, RM, Boyce, AJ, and Clegg, JB. (1993b). The population genetics of the haemoglobinopathies. In Fleming, AF editor, *Bailliere's clinical haematology.* London: Harcourt Brace Jovanovich.

Francis, RB, Jr and Hebbel, RP. (1994). Hemostasis. In Embury, SH, Hebbel, RP, Mohandas, N, and Steinberg, MH, editors. *Sickle cell disease: Basic principles and clinical practice.* New York: Lippincott-Raven.

Garner, C, Mitchell, J, Hatzis, T et al. (1998a). Haplotype mapping of a major quantitative-trait locus for fetal hemoglobin production, on chromosome 6q23. *Am. J. Hum. Genet.* 62: 1468–1474.

Garner, C, Tatu, T, Reittie, J et al. (1998b) Twins *en route* to QTL mapping for heterocellular HPFH. *Blood* 92: 694a.

Gelinas, R, Endlich, B, Pfeiffer, C et al. (1985). G to A substitution in the distal CCAAT box of the $^A\gamma$-globin gene in Greek hereditary persistence of fetal hemoglobin. *Nature* 313: 323–325.

Gibbs, WN, Wardle, J, and Serjeant, GR. (1980). Glucose-6-phosphate dehydrogenase deficiency and homozygous sickle cell disease in Jamaica. *Br. J. Haematol.* 45: 73–80.

Gilman, JG and Huisman, THJ. (1984). Two independent genetic factors in the β-globin gene cluster are associated with high $^G\gamma$-levels in the HbF of SS patients. *Blood* 64: 452–457.

Gilman, JG and Huisman, THJ. (1985). DNA sequence variation associated with elevated fetal $^G\gamma$ globin production. *Blood* 66: 783–787.

Gilman, JG, Johnson, ME, and Mishima, N. (1988). Four base-pair DNA deletion in human $^A\gamma$ globin gene promoter associated with low $^A\gamma$ expression in adults. *Br. J. Haematol.* 68: 455–458.

Gilman, JG. (1988). Expression of $^G\gamma$ and $^A\gamma$ globin genes in human adults. *Hemoglobin* 1: 707–716.

Gilman, JG, Josifovska, O, Erlingsson, S et al. (1993). Direct demonstration that the A gamma T globin gene is linked to the 4 bp promoter deletion in the beta A chromosome of sickle cell traits. *Am. J. Hematol.* 43: 312–315.

Goldstein, J, Konigsberg, W, and Hill, RJ. (1963). The structure of human hemoglobin. VI. The sequence of amino acids in the tryptic peptides of the beta chain. *J. Biol. Chem.* 238: 2016–2033.

Goncalves, I, Goncalves, J, Perichon, B et al. (1994a). A novel mosaic Bantu/Benin/Bantu β^S haplotype found in several African populations. *Hum. Genet.* 94: 101–103.

Goncalves, MS, Nechtman, JF, Figueiredo, MS et al. (1994b). Sickle cell disease in a Brazilian population from Sao Paulo: A study of the β^S haplotypes. *Hum. Hered.* 44: 322–327.

Green, NS, Fabry, ME, Kaptue-Noche, L, and Nagel, RL. (1993). Senegal haplotype is associated with higher HbF than Benin and Cameroon haplotypes in African children with sickle cell anemia. *Am. J. Hematol.* 44: 145–146.

Greenberg, JH. (1973). In Skinner, EP, editor. *Peoples and culture of Africa.* Garden City, NY: Doubleday, National History Press.

Grosveld, F, Antoniou, M, Berry, M et al. (1993). Regulation of human globin gene switching. *Cold Spring Harb. Symp. Quant. Biol.* 58: 7–13.

Guzman, C, Etcheberry, Regonesi, C et al. (1962). Hemoglobinas anormales en Chile. *Proceedings of the IX Congress of International Hematology,* Mexico, 3: 71–72.

Hall, WM. (1992). *Africans in colonial Louisiana. The development of the Afro-Creole culture in the eighteenth century.* Baton Rouge and London: Louisiana State University Press.

Haghshenass, M, Ismail-Beigi, F, Clegg, JB, and Weatherall, DJ. (1983). Mild sickle-cell anaemia in Iran associated with high levels of fetal haemoglobin. *J. Med. Genet.* 14: 168–171.

Harano, K, Harano, T, Kutlar, F, and Huisman, THJ. (1985). γ-globin gene triplication and quadruplication in Japanese newborns. Evidence for a decreased in vivo expression of the 3′ $^A\gamma$ globin gene. *FEBS Lett.* 190: 45–49.

Hattori, Y, Kutlar, F, Kutlar, A et al. (1986). Haplotypes of beta S chromosomes among patients with sickle cell anemia from Georgia. *Hemoglobin* 10: 623–642.

Hebbel, RP. (1991). Beyond hemoglobin polymerization: The red blood cell membrane and sickle disease pathophysiology. *Blood* 77: 214–237.

Higgs, DR, Aldridge, BE, Lamb, J et al. (1982). The interaction of alpha-thalassemia and homozygous sickle-cell disease. *N. Engl. J. Med.* 306: 1441–1446.

Huisman, THJ, Kutlar, F, Natatsuji, T et al. (1985). The frequency of the γ chain variant $^A\gamma^T$ in different populations, and its use in evaluating γ gene expression in association with thalassemia. *Hum. Genet.* 71: 127–133.

Ingram, VM. (1956). A specific chemical difference between the globins of normal human and sickle-cell haemoglobin. *Nature* 178: 792–794.

Ingram, VM. (1957). Gene mutations in human haemoglobin: The chemical difference between normal and sickle cell haemoglobin. *Nature* 180: 326–328.

Jackson, JD, Petrykowska, H, Philipsen, S et al. (1996). Role of DNA sequences outside the cores of DNase hypersensitive sites (HSs) in functions of the β-globin locus control region. Domain opening and synergism between HS2 and HS3. *J. Biol. Chem.* 271: 11871–11878.

Jara, NO, Guevara Espinoza, A, and Guderian RH. (1989). Abnormal hemoglobins in Negroid Ecuadorian populations. *Sangre (Barc)* 34: 10–13.

Jha, JC. (1993). Early Indian immigration into Mauritius (1834–1842). In Bissoondoyal and Servansing, editors. *Indian labour immigration.*

Kahn, MJ, Scher, C, Rozans, M et al. (1997). Factor V Leiden is not responsible for stroke in patients with sickling disorders and is uncommon in African Americans with sickle cell disease. *Am. J. Hematol.* 54: 12–15.

Kan, YW and Dozy, AM. (1978). Polymorphism of DNA sequence adjacent to the human β-globin structural gene: Relationship to sickle mutation. *Proc. Natl. Acad. Sci. U.S.A.* 75: 5631–5635.

Kan, YW and Dozy, AM. (1980). Evolution of the hemoglobin S and C genes in world populations. *Science* 209: 388–391.

Karan, VK, Prasad, SN, and Prasad, TB. (1978). Sickle cell disorder in Aboriginal tribes of Chotanagpur. *Indian Pediatric.* 14: 287–291.

Keclard, L, Ollendorf, V, Berchel, C et al. (1996). Beta S haplotypes, alpha-globin gene status, and hematological data of sickle cell disease patients in Guadeloupe. *Hemoglobin* 20: 63–74.

Keclard, L, Romana, M, Lavocat, E et al. (1997). Sickle cell disorder, beta-globin gene cluster haplotypes and alpha-thalassemia in neonates and adults from Guadeloupe. *Am. J. Hematol.* 55: 24–27.

Kenoyer, JM. (1998). *Ancient cities of the Indus Valley civilization.* Oxford, New York, Delhi: Oxford University Press.

Kennedy, KAR. (1981). Skeletal biology: When bones tell tales. *Archeology* 34: 17–24.

Khanduri, U, Gravell, D, Christie, BS et al. (1998). Reduced protein C levels—a contributory factor for stroke in sickle cell disease. *Thromb. Heamost.* 79: 879–880.

Kollia, P, Karababa, PH, Sinopoulou, K et al. (1987). Distribution of the β-gene cluster haplotypes in Greece. Feasibility of prenatal diagnosis of thalassemia. *2nd International Symposium on Thalassemia in Crete.*

Kotea, N, Baligadoo, S, Surrun, SK et al. (1995). Bicentric origin of sickle hemoglobin among the inhabitants of Mauritius Island. *Blood* 86: 407–408.

Kulozik, AE, Wainscoat, JS, Serjeant, GR et al. (1986). Geographical survey of the β^S-globin gene haplotypes: Evidence for an independent Asian origin of the sickle-cell mutation. *Am. J. Hum. Genet.* 39: 239–244.

Kulozik, AE, Kar, BC, Satapathy, RK et al. (1987). Fetal hemoglobin levels and β^S globin haplotypes in an Indian population with sickle cell disease. *Blood* 69: 1742–1746.

Kurnit, DM. (1979). Evolution of sickle variant gene. *Lancet* I: 104.

Kutlar, A, Hattori, Y, Bakioglu, I et al. (1985). Hematological observations on Arabian SS patients with a homozygosity or heterozygosity for a β^S chromosome with haplotype 31. *Hemoglobin* 9: 545–557.

Kutlar, F, Tural, C, Park, D et al. (1998). MTHFR (5, 10-methylenetetrahydrofolate reductase) 677 C→T muta-

tion as a candidate risk factor for avascular necrosis (AVN) in patients with sickle cell disease. *Blood* 92: 695a.

Labie, D, Dunda-Belkhodja, O, Rouabhi, F et al. (1985a). The −158 site 5′ to the ^{G}γ gene and ^{G}γ expression. *Blood* 66: 1463–1465.

Labie, D, Pagnier, J, Lapoumeroulie, C et al. (1985b). Common haplotype dependency of high ^{G}γ-globin gene expression and high HbF levels in β-thalassemia and sickle cell anemia patients. *Proc. Natl. Acad. Sci. U.S.A.* 82: 2111–2114.

Labie, D, Srinivas, R, Dunda, O et al. (1989). Haplotypes in tribal Indians bearing the sickle gene: Evidence for the unicentric origin of the beta S mutation and the unicentric origin of the tribal populations of India. *Hum. Biol.* 61: 479–491.

Lanclos, KD, Öner, C, Dimovski, AJ et al. (1991). Sequence variations in the 5′ flanking and IVS-II regions of the ^{G}γ and ^{A}γ-globin genes of b^S chromosomes with five different haplotypes. *Blood* 77: 2488–2496.

Lapoumeroulie, C, Dunda, O, Ducrocq, R et al. (1989). A novel sickle gene of yet another origin in Africa: The Cameroon type. *Hum. Genet.* 89: 333–337.

Lavelle, D, Ducksworth, J, Eves, E et al. (1991). A homeodomain protein binds to gamma-globin gene regulatory sequences. *Proc. Natl. Acad. Sci. U.S.A.* 88: 7318–7322.

Lee, K, Préhu, C, Mérault, G et al. (1998). Genetic and hematological studies in a group of 114 adult patients with SC sickle cell disease. *Am. J. Hematol.* 59: 15–21.

Lehman, H and Cutbush, M. (1952). Sickle cell-trait in Southern India. *Br. Med. J.* i: 289–290.

Leonov, JY, Kazanetz, EG, Smetanina, NS et al. (1996). Variability in the fetal hemoglobin level of the normal adult. *Am. J. Hematol.* 53: 59–65.

Li, Q and Stamatoyannopoulos, JA. (1994). Position independence and proper developmental control of gamma-globin gene expression require both a 5′ locus control region and a downstream sequence element. *Mol. Cell. Biol.* 14: 6087–6096.

Lie-Injo, LE, Hassan, K, Joishy, SK, and Lim, ML. (1986). Sickle cell anemia associated with alpha-thalassemia in Malaysian Indians. *Am. J. Hematol.* 22: 265–274.

Liesner, R, Mackie, I, Cookson, J et al. (1998). Prothrombotic changes in children with sickle cell disease: Relationships to cerebrovascular disease and transfusion. *Br. J. Haematol.* 103: 1037–1044.

Livingstone, FB. (1989). Who gave whom hemoglobin S: The use of restriction site haplotype variation for the interpretation of the evolution of the β^S-globin gene. *Am. J. Hum. Biol.* 1: 289–302.

Lu, ZH and Steinberg, MH. (1996). Fetal hemoglobin in sickle cell anemia: Relation to regulatory sequences cis to the b-globin gene. *Blood* 87: 1604–1611.

Lutz, W and Wils, AB. (1991). The demographic discontinuities of Mauritius. In Lutz and Toth, editors. *Population, economy and environment in Mauritius.* University of Mauritius.

Maggio, A, Acuto, S, LoGioco, P et al. (1986). β^A and β^{thal} DNA haplotypes in Sicily. *Hum. Genet.* 72: 229–230.

Manca, L, Cocco, E, Gallisai, D et al. (1991). Diminished A gamma T fetal globin levels in Sardinian haplotype II beta 0-thalassaemia patients are associated with a four base pair deletion in the A gamma T promoter. *Br. J. Haematol.* 78: 105–107.

Manrakhan, J. (1990). Examination of certain aspects of the slavery-indentured continuum in Mauritius. In Bissoondoyal and Servansing, editors. *Indian labour immigration.* Moka, Mauritius: Mahatma Gandhi Institute.

Mears, JG, Lachman, HM, Cabannes, R et al. (1981a). Sickle gene. Its origin and diffusion from West Africa. *J. Clin. Invest.* 68: 606–610.

Mears, JG, Beldjord, C, Benabadji, M et al. (1981b). The sickle gene polymorphism in North Africa. *Blood* 58: 599–601.

Mears, JG, Lachman, HM, Labie, D, and Nagel, RL. (1983). Alpha thalassemia is related to prolonged survival in sickle cell anemia. *Blood* 62: 286–290.

Merghoub, T, Maier-Redelsperger, M, Labie, D et al. (1996). Variation of fetal hemoglobin and F-cell number with the LCR-HS2 polymorphism in nonanemic individuals. *Blood* 87: 2607–2609.

Merghoub, T, Perichon, B, Maier-Redelsperger, M et al. (1997). Dissection of the association status of two polymorphisms in the β-globin gene cluster with variations in F-cell number in non-anemic individuals. *Am. J. Hematol.* 56: 239–243.

Miller, BA, Salameh, M, Ahmed, M et al. (1986). High fetal hemoglobin production in sickle cell anemia in the eastern province of Saudi Arabia is genetically determined. *Blood* 67: 1404–1410.

Miller, BA, Salameh, M, Ahmed, M et al. (1987a). Analysis of hemoglobin F production in Saudi Arabian families with sickle cell anemia. *Blood* 70: 716–720.

Miller, BA, Olivieri, N, Salameh, M et al. (1987b). Molecular analysis of the high-hemoglobin-F phenotype in Saudi Arabian sickle cell anemia. *N. Engl. J. Med.* 316: 244–250.

Miller, BA, Salameh, M, Ahmed, M et al. (1989). Saudi Arabian sickle cell anemia. A molecular approach. *Ann. N.Y. Acad. Sci.* 565: 143–151.

Miller, JL, Walsh, CE, Ney, PA et al. (1993). Single-copy transduction and expression of human gamma-globin in K562 erythroleukemia cells using recombinant adeno-associated virus vectors: The effect of mutations in NF-E2 and GATA-1 binding motifs within the hypersensitivity site 2 enhancer. *Blood* 82: 1900–1906.

Mishima, N, Brinson, EC, Milner, PF, and Gilman JG. (1991). $^{G}\gamma$ and $^{A}\gamma$ genes are identical from −171 of the promoter midway through γIVSII in a Benin β^{s} haplotype associated with elevated fetal hemoglobins. *Am. J. Hum. Genet.* 48: 1175–1180.

Mishima, N, Gilman, JG, Huey, LO, and Milner, PF. (1989). $^{A}\gamma$ globin gene with $^{G}\gamma$-like promoter in a Benin sickle cell anemia haplotype associated with elevated fetal hemoglobin. In Stamatoyannopouluks G and Nienhuis AW, editors. New York: AR Liss.

Miyoshi, K, Kaneto, Y, Kawai, H et al. (1988). X-linked dominant control of F-cells in normal adult life: Characterization of the Swiss type as hereditary persis-

tence of fetal hemoglobin regulated dominantly by gene(s) on X chromosome. *Blood* 72: 1854–1860.

Month, SR, Wood, RW, Trifillis, PT et al. (1990). Analysis of 5′ flanking regions of the gamma globin genes from major African haplotype backgrounds associated with sickle cell disease. *J. Clin. Invest.* 85: 364–370.

Moon, AM and Ley, TJ. (1991). Functional properties of the β-globin locus control region in K562 erythroleukemia cells. *Blood* 77: 2272–2284.

Morgan, JC, Scott, DF, and Lanclos, KD. (1996). Two mutations in the locus control region hypersensitivity site-2 (5′HS-2) of haplotype 19 β^{s} chromosomes alter binding of *trans*-acting factors. *Am. J. Hematol.* 51: 12–18.

Moschonas, N, deBoer, E, and Flavell, RA. (1982). The DNA sequence of the 5′ flanking region of the human β-globin gene: Evolutionary conservation and polymorphic differences. *Nucleic Acids Res.* 10: 2109–2120.

Mrug, M, Divoky, V, Thornley-Brown, D et al. (1996). Association of a specific β globin gene cluster haplotype with high γ globin expression in non-anemic homozygous β^{0} thalassemia. *Blood* 88(Suppl 1): 149a.

Mukherjee, MB, Lu, CY, Ducrocq, R et al. (1997). Effect of α-thalassemia on sickle-cell anemia linked to the Arab-Indian haplotype in India. *Am. J. Hematol.* 55: 104–109.

Muniz, A, Corral, L, Alaez, C et al. (1995). Sickle cell anemia and beta-gene cluster haplotype in Cuba. *Am. J. Hematol.* 49: 163–164.

Murru, S, Loudianos, G, Cao, A et al. (1990). A β-thalassemia carrier with normal sequence within the β-globin gene. *Blood* 76: 2164–2165.

Nagel, RL, Fabry, ME, Pagnier, J et al. (1984). Hematologically and genetically distinct forms of sickle cell anemia in Africa. The Senegal type and the Benin type. *N. Engl. J. Med.* 312: 880–884.

Nagel, RL. (1984). The origin of the hemoglobin S gene: Clinical, genetic and anthropological consequences. *Einstein Q. J. Biol. Med.* 2: 53–62.

Nagel, RL, Rao, SK, Dunda-Belkhodja, O et al. (1987). The hematologic characteristics of sickle cell anemia bearing the Bantu haplotype: The relationship between G gamma and HbF level. *Blood* 69: 1026–1030.

Nagel, RL and Labie, D. (1989). DNA haplotypes and the β^{s} globin gene. *Progr. Clin. Biol. Res.* 316B: 371–393.

Nagel, RL, Erlingsson, S, Fabry, ME et al. (1991). The Senegal DNA haplotype is associated with the amelioration of anemia in African-American sickle cell anemia patients. *Blood* 77: 1371–1375.

Nagel, RL and Fleming, A. (1992). Epidemiology of the β^{s} gene. *Bailliere's Clin. Haematol.* 5: 331–365.

Nagel, RL. (1994). Origins and dispersion of the sickle gene. In Embury, SH, Hebbel, RP, N Mohandas, N, and Steinberg, MH, editors. *Sickle cell disease: Basic principles and clinical practice.* New York: Raven Press.

Nagel, RL. (1996). The sickle haplotypes in Guadeloupe and the African gene flow. *Hemoglobin* 20: V–VII.

Neel, JV.(1949). The inheritance of sickle cell anemia. *Science* 110: 64–66.

Neel, JV. (1951). The inheritance of the sickling phenomenon with particular reference to sickle cell disease. *Blood* 6: 389–412.

Noguchi, CT, Rodgers, GP, Serjeant, G, and Schechter, AN. (1988). Levels of fetal hemoglobin necessary for treatment of sickle cell disease. *N. Engl. J. Med.* 318: 96–99.

Nsiri, B, Ghazouani, E, Gritli, N et al. (1998). Antiphospholipid antibodies: Lupus anticoagulants anti-cardiolipin and antiphospholipid isotypes in patients with sickle cell disease. *Hematol. Cell. Ther.* 40: 107–112.

Ofori-Acquah, SF, Lalloz, MRA, and Layton, DM. (1999). Localisation of *cis* regulatory elements at the β-globin locus: Analysis of hybrid haplotype chromosomes. *Biochem. Biophys. Res. Commun.* 254: 181–187.

Ohene-Frempong, K and Nkrumah, FK. (1994). Sickle cell disease in Africa. In Embury, SH, Hebbel, RP, and Mohandas, N. *Sickle cell disease: Basic principles and clinical practice.* New York: Raven Press.

Ojwang, PJ, Ogada, T, Beris, P et al. (1987). Haplotypes and alpha globin gene analyses in sickle cell anaemia patients from Kenya. *Br. J. Haematol.* 65: 211–215.

Öner, C, Dimovski, AJ, Altay, C et al. (1992a). Sequence variations in the 5′ hypersensitive site-2 of the locus control region of β^s chromosomes are associated with different levels of fetal globin in hemoglobin S homozygotes. *Blood* 79: 813–819.

Öner, C, Dimovski, AJ, Olivieri, NF et al. (1992b). β^s Haplotypes in various world populations. *Hum. Genet.* 89: 99–104.

Orkin, SH, Kazazian, HH Jr, Antonarakis, SE et al. (1982). Linkage of beta-thalassaemia mutations and beta-globin gene polymorphisms with DNA polymorphisms in human beta-globin gene cluster. *Nature* 296: 627–631.

Padanilam, BJ, Felice, AE, and Huisman, THJ. (1984). Partial deletion of the 5′ β-globin gene region causes β⁰-thalassemia in members of an American black family. *Blood* 64: 941–944.

Padmos, MA, Roberts, GT, Sackey, K et al. (1991). Two different forms of homozygous sickle cell disease occur in Saudi Arabia. *Br. J. Haematol.* 79: 93–98.

Pagnier, J, Mears, JG, Dunda-Belkodja, O et al. (1984). Evidence of the multicentric origin of the hemoglobin S gene in Africa. *Proc. Natl. Acad. Sci. U.S.A.* 81: 1771–1773.

Pauling, L, Itano, HA, Singer, SJ, and Wells, IC. (1949). Sickle cell anemia, a molecular disease. *Science* 110: 543–548.

Pauling, L. (1994). Foreword. In Embury, SH, Hebbel, RP, Mohandas, N, and Steinberg, MH, editors. *Sickle cell disease: Basic principles and clinical practice.* New York: Lippincott-Raven.

Peri, KG, Gagnon, J, Gagnon, C, and Bard, H. (1997). Association of –158(C→T) (*Xmn* I) DNA polymorphism in ^Ggamma- globin promoter with delayed switchover from fetal to adult hemoglobin synthesis. *Pediatr. Res.* 41: 214–217.

Peterson, KR, Clegg, CH, Huxley, C et al. (1993). Transgenic mice containing a 248-kb yeast artificial chromosome carrying the human β-globin locus display proper developmental control of human globin genes. *Proc. Natl. Acad. Sci. U.S.A.* 90: 7593–7597.

Périchon, B, Ragusa, A, Lapouméroulie, C et al. (1993). Inter-ethnic polymorphism of the β-globin gene locus control region (LCR) in sickle-cell anemia patients. *Hum. Genet.* 91: 464–468.

Piomelli, S, Reindorf, C, Arzanian, MT, and Corash, LM. (1972). Clinical and biochemical interactions of glucose-6-phosphate dehydrogenase deficient and sickle-cell anemia. *N. Engl. J. Med.* 287: 213–217.

Pissard, S and Beuzard, Y. (1994). A potential regulatory region for the expression of fetal hemoglobin in sickle cell disease. *Blood* 84: 331–338.

Platt, OS, Orkin, SH, Dover, G et al. (1984). Hydroxyurea enhances fetal hemoglobin production in sickle cell anemia. *J. Clin. Invest.* 74: 652–656.

Platt, OS, Thorington, BD, Brambilla, DJ et al. (1991). Pain in sickle cell disease-rates and risk factors. *N. Engl. J. Med.* 325: 11–16.

Platt, OS, Brambilla, DJ, Rosse, WF et al. (1994). Mortality in sickle cell disease: Life expectancy and risk factors for early death. *N. Engl. J. Med.* 330: 1639–1644.

Plonczynski, M, Figueiredo, MS, and Steinberg, MH. (1997). Fetal hemoglobin in sickle cell anemia: Examination of phylogenetically conserved sequences within the locus control region but outside the cores of hypersensitive sites 2 and 3. *Blood Cells Mol. Dis.* 23: 188–200.

Poillon, WN, Kim, BC, Rodgers, GP et al. (1993). Sparing effect of hemoglobin F and hemoglobin A₂ on the polymerization of hemoglobin S at physiologic ligand saturations. *Proc. Natl. Acad. Sci. U.S.A.* 90: 5039–5043.

Powars, D, Schroeder, WA, Weiss, JN et al. (1980). Lack of influence of fetal hemoglobin levels or erythrocyte indices on the severity of sickle cell anemia. *J. Clin. Invest.* 65: 732–740.

Powars, D, Weiss, JN, Chan, LS, and Schroeder, WA. (1984). Is there a threshold level of fetal hemoglobin that ameliorates morbidity in sickle cell anemia? *Blood* 63: 921–926.

Powars, DR, Elliott Mills, DD, and Chan, L. (1991). Chronic renal failure in sickle cell disease: Risk factors, clinical course, and mortality. *Ann. Intern. Med.* 115: 614–620.

Powars, DR. (1991a). Sickle cell anemia: β^S-Gene-cluster haplotypes as prognostic indicators of vital organ failure. *Semin. Hematol.* 28: 202–208.

Powars, DR. (1991b). β^S-Gene-cluster haplotypes in sickle cell anemia: Clinical and hematologic features. *Hematol. Oncol. Clin. North Am.* 5: 475–493.

Powars, DR, Conti, PS, Wong, WY et al. (1999). Cerebral vasculopathy in sickle cell anemia: Diagnostic contribution of positron emission tomography. *Blood* 93: 71–79.

Powers, PA, Altay, C, Huisman, THJ, and Smithies, O. (1984). Two novel arrangements of the human fetal globin genes: ^Gγ-^Gγ and ^Gγ-^Aγ. *Nucleic Acids Res.* 12: 7023–7034.

Powers, PA and Smithies, O. (1988). Short gene conversion in the human fetal globin gene region: A by-product of chromosome pairing during meiosis. *Genetics* 112: 343–358.

Ragusa, A, Lombardo, M, Sortino, G et al. (1988). Beta S gene in Sicily is in linkage disequilibrium with the Benin haplotype: Implications for gene flow. *Am. J. Hematol.* 27: 139–141.

Ragusa, A, Lombardo, M, Beldjord, C et al. (1992). Genetic epidemiology of β-thalassemia in Sicily: Do sequences 5′ to the Gγ gene and 5′ to the b gene interact to enhance HbF expression in b-thalassemia. Am. J. Hematol. 40: 199–206.

Ramsay, M and Jenkins, T. (1987). Globin gene-associated restriction-fragment-length polymorphisms in Southern African peoples. Am. J. Hum. Genet. 41: 1132–1144.

Rieder, RF, Safaya, S, Gillette, P et al. (1991). Effect of β-globin gene cluster haplotype on the hematological and clinical features of sickle cell anemia. Am. J. Hematol. 36: 184–189.

Rodgers GP, Dover, GJ, Noguchi CT et al. (1990). Hematologic responses of patients with sickle cell disease to treatment with hydroxyurea. N. Engl. J. Med. 322: 1037–1045.

Roizen, Z, Salinas, A, and Rivera, L. (1977). Sickle cell anemia in a Chilean family. Rev. Med. Chile 105: 905–910.

Rona, R, Rozovski, J, and Stekel, A. (1973). Sickle-thalassemia: Study of a Chilean generation. Rev. Med. Chile, 101: 237–239.

Roth, EF, Schiliro, G, Russo, A et al. (1980). Sickle cell disease in Sicily. J. Med. Genetics 17: 34–38.

Rund, D, Kornhendler, N, Shalev, O, and Oppenheim, A. (1990). The origin of sickle cell gene in Israel. Hum. Genet. 85: 521–524.

Sampietro, M, Thein, SL, Contreras, M, and Pazmany, L. (1992). Variation in HbF and F-cell number with the Gγ XmnI (C→T) polymorphisms in normal individuals. Blood 79: 832–833.

Schroeder, WA, Powars, DR, Kay, LM et al. (1989). β-Cluster haplotypes a-gene status and hematological data from SS SC and S-b-thalassemia patients in southern California. Hemoglobin 13: 325–353.

Semenza, GL, Delgrosso, K, Poncz, M et al. (1984). The silent carrier allele: Beta thalassemia without a mutation in the beta-globin gene or its immediate flanking regions. Cell 39: 123–128.

Sengupta, PK, Lavelle, DE, and DeSimone, J. (1994). The 87-kD A gamma-globin enhancer-binding protein is a product of the HOXB2(HOX2H) locus. Blood 83: 1420–1427.

Sharon, B, Poncz, M, Surrey, S, and Schwartz, E. (1988). Non-random association of the Rsa l polymorphic site 5′ to the beta-globin gene with major sickle cell haplotypes. Hemoglobin 12: 115–124.

Shen, SH, Slightom, JL, and Smithies, O. (1981). A history of the human fetal globin gene duplication. Cell 26: 191–203.

Sherman, IJ.(1940). The sickling phenomenon, with special reference to the differentiation of sickle cell anemia from the sickle cell trait. Bull. Johns Hopkins Hosp. 178: 309–324.

Slightom, JL, Blechl, AE, and Smithies, O.(1980). Human fetal Gγ- and Aγ-globin genes: Complete nucleotide sequences suggest that DNA can be exchanged between these duplicated genes. Cell 21: 627–638.

Sow, A, Peterson, E, Josifovska, O et al. (1995). Linkage-disequilibrium of the Senegal haplotype with the βs Gene in the Republic of Guinea. Am. J. Hematol. 50: 301–303.

Spritz, RA. (1981). Duplication/deletion polymorphism 5′ to the human β globin gene. Nucleic Acids Res. 9: 5037–5047.

Srinivas, R, Dunda, O, Krishnamoorthy, R et al. (1988). Atypical haplotypes linked to the βS gene in Africa are likely to be the product of recombination. Am. J. Hematol. 29: 60–62.

Stamatoyannopoulos, G and Nienhuis, AW (1994). Hemoglobin switching. In Stamatoyannopoulos, G, Nienhuis, AW, Majerus, PW, and Varmus, H, editors. The molecular basis of blood diseases. Philadelphia: WB Saunders.

Stamatoyannopoulos, JA, Clegg, C, and Li, Q. (1994). A regulatory element 3′ to the Aγ-globin gene functions in conjuction with an upstream LCR to mediate position-independent γ-globin gene expression. Blood 84: 218a.

Steinberg, MH. (1989). Sickle cell anaemia in a septuagenarian. Br. J. Haematol. 71: 297–298.

Steinberg, MH. (1991). The interactions of α-thalassemia with hemoglobinopathies. Hematol. Oncol. Clin. North Am. 5: 453–473.

Steinberg, MH and Adams, JG III. (1991). Hemoglobin A₂: Origin, evolution, and aftermath. Blood 78: 2165–2177.

Steinberg, MH and Dreiling, BJ. (1974). Glucose-6-phosphate dehydrogenase deficiency in sickle-cell anemia. A study in adults. Ann. Intern. Med. 80: 217–220.

Steinberg, MH and Embury, SH. (1986). Alpha-thalassemia in blacks: Genetic and clinical aspects and interactions with the sickle hemoglobin gene. Blood 68: 985–990.

Steinberg, MH, Ballas, SK, Brunson, CY, and Bookchin, R. (1995a). Sickle cell anemia in septuagenarians. Blood 86: 3997–3998.

Steinberg, MH, Hsu, H, Nagel, RL et al. (1995b). Gender and haplotype effects upon hematological manifestations of adult sickle cell anemia. Am. J. Hematol. 48: 175–181.

Steinberg, MH, Lu, Z-H, Barton, FB et al. (1997). Fetal hemoglobin in sickle cell anemia: Determinants of response to hydroxyurea. Blood 89: 1078–1088.

Steinberg, MH, Lu, ZH, Nagel, RL et al. (1998). Hematological effects of atypical and Cameroon β-globin gene haplotypes in adult sickle cell anemia. Am. J. Hematol. 59: 121–126.

Steinberg, MH, Rosenstock, W, Coleman, MB et al. (1984). Effects of thalassemia and microcytosis upon the hematological and vaso- occlusive severity of sickle cell anemia. Blood 63: 1353–1360.

Steinberg, MH, West, MS, Gallagher, D, and Mentzer, W. (1988). Effects of glucose-6-phosphate dehydrogenase deficiency upon sickle cell anemia. Blood 71: 748–752.

Stine, OC, Dover, GJ, Zhu, D, and Smith, KD. (1992) The evolution of two west African populations. J. Mol. Evol. 34: 336–344.

Taliaferro, WH and Huck, JG. (1923). The inheritance of sickle-cell anemia in man. Genetics 8: 594–598.

Thein, SL and Craig, JE. (1998). Genetics of Hb F/F cell variance in adults and heterocellular hereditary persistence of fetal hemoglobin. Hemoglobin 22: 401–414.

Thein, SL, Sampietro, M, Rohde, K et al. (1994). Detection of a major gene for heterocellular hereditary persistence of fetal hemoglobin after accounting for genetic modifiers. Am. J. Hum. Genet. 54: 214–228.

Thomas, JJ, Kutlar, A, Scott, DF, and Lanclos, KD. (1998). Inhibition of gene expression by the ^{G}Y 5′ flanking region of the Bantu β^S chromosome. *Am. J. Hematol.* 59: 51–56.

Torres-Guerra, E, Torres-Guerra, T, Valbuena, G et al. (1993). Frequency of sickle-cell anemia in the population of "Cuatro Bocas." *Invest. Clin.* 34: 99–105.

Vermylen, C, Robles, EF, Ninane, J, and Cornu, G. (1988). Bone marrow transplantation in five children with sickle cell anaemia. *Lancet* 1: 1427–1428.

Vidyarthi, LP and Rai, BK. (1976). *The tribal culture of India.* New Delhi: Concept Publishing Co.

von Furer-Haimendorf, C. (1968). *Tribes of India: The struggle for survival.* Oxford: Oxford University Press.

Wainscoat, JS, Bell, JI, Thein, SL et al. (1983). Multiple origins of the sickle mutation: Evidence from β^S globin gene cluster polymorphisms. *Mol. Biol. Med.* 1: 191–197.

Wainscoat, JS, Thein, SL, Higgs, DR et al. (1985). A genetic marker for elevated levels of haemoglobin F in homozygous sickle cell disease. *Br. J. Haematol.* 60: 261–268.

Wainscoat, JS, Kulozik, AE, Ramsay, M et al. (1986). A Taq I β-globin DNA polymorphism: An African-specific marker. *Hum Genet.* 74: 90–92.

Waye, JS, Chui, DHK, Eng, B et al. (1991). Hb S/β^o-thalassemia due to the ~1.4-kb deletion is associated with a relatively mild phenotype. *Am. J. Hematol.* 38: 108–112.

Wheeler, Sir M. (1968). *The Indus civilization* (3rd ed.). Cambridge: Cambridge University Press.

Wijgerde, M, Grosveld, F, and Fraser, P. (1995). Transcription complex stability and chromatin dynamics in vivo. *Nature* 377: 209–213.

Zago, MA, Figueiredo, MS, and Ogo, SH. (1992). Bantu β^S cluster haplotype predominates among Brazilian Blacks. *Am. J. Phys. Anthropol.* 88: 295–298.

Zimmerman, SA and Ware, RE. (1998). Inherited DNA mutations contributing to thrombotic complications in patients with sickle cell disease. *Am. J. Hematol.* 59: 267–272.

Zimmerman, SA, Howard, TA, Whorton, MR et al. (1998). The A312G polymorphism in α-fibrinogen is associated with stroke and avascular necrosis in patients with sickle cell anemia. *Blood* 92: 36b.

27

Hemoglobin SC Disease and HbC Disorders

RONALD L. NAGEL
MARTIN H. STEINBERG

HbC ($\beta^{6\ glu \to lys}$), along with HbS and HbE, is one of the three most prevalent abnormal hemoglobins in humans. Its unique features cause erythrocyte dehydration. HbC disease—defined as the homozygous state for the HbC gene—results only in mild hemolytic anemia. In HbSC disease, where equal amounts of HbS and HbC coexist, HbC accentuates the deleterious properties of HbS. This conjunction of variant hemoglobins culminates in both vasoocclusive disease and hemolysis, and makes HbSC disease a clinically significant disorder. Like sickle cell anemia, the hematologic and clinical features of HbSC disease are heterogeneous but all of the complications that make sickle cell anemia notorious can be present.

HbC AND HbC DISEASE

Origins and Distribution of HbC

HbC, the second hemoglobin variant discovered and either the second or third most prevalent abnormal hemoglobin, was initially described by Itano and Neel (1951) and the first homozygous case was reported by Spaet et al. (1953). The β^C-globin gene, generated by a <u>G</u>AG→<u>A</u>AG substitution in codon six of the β-globin gene, converts a glutamic acid residue to lysine. Shortly after its description in African Americans, HbC was found to be common in

Africans. Population studies and genetic evidence showed that the HbC mutation originated on a β^A-globin gene in West Africa and spread throughout the world like the HbS gene (Chapter 27) (Kan and Dozy, 1980; Boehm et al., 1985; Talacki et al., 1990). Based on the population distribution of β-globin gene cluster haplotypes, it has been deduced that the β^S-globin gene found in North Africa arose in West Africa and migrated northward through ancient trans-Saharan trade routes (Mears et al., 1981). Similar data exist for the β^C mutation. Predicated on the identity of their haplotypes, HbC in sub-Saharan Africa and North Africa appears to have had the same origin as in Burkina Faso (previously Upper Volta). Strong gene flow, influenced by the selective pressure of malaria (Olson and Nagel, 1986), has distributed HbC throughout Central West Africa and toward North Africa, particularly Morocco (Labie et al., 1984).

Kan and Dozy first established that the HbC gene was linked to the absence of an Hpa I restriction site 3′ to the β-globin gene (Kan and Dozy, 1980). This simple observation eliminated the possibility that the β^C gene arose from the β^S gene by a second mutation within β-globin gene codon six, a possibility already unlikely because two point mutations are needed to convert the codon for valine (GTG) to one for lysine (AAG).

Most likely, the β^C mutation occurred among ethnic groups in Burkina Faso. Found in Africa in a restricted distribution, HbC reaches its highest frequency in Central West Africa and its gene frequency decreases concentrically outward from this region (Labie et al., 1984; Dack, 1988). Interestingly, HbC is found in Africa almost exclusively in areas where HbS exists. An exception was possibly present in the Dogon area of Mali but more recent data showed that the presence of HbC among the Tanners of the Dogon—a defined endogamic caste—was very low while HbS was absent; however, only a small number of individuals were studied. The Backsmiths caste and the Nobles—coexisting but not mating with the Tanners—had both HbS and HbC. It is therefore possible that the presence of HbC in Tanners could represent a founder effect or genetic drift (Ducrocq et al., 1994). While the possibility of a second origin of the HbC gene in Africa has been raised by the presence of a 3′ β-globin gene Hpa I site in several patients (Feldenzer et al., 1979; Schroeder et al., 1989; Talacki et al., 1990; Steinberg et al., 1996), this site is in the middle of an extensive L1 repeat where a high probability of rearrangement exists (Chakravarti et al., 1984). Two instances of independent origin of the β^C gene have been found in Thailand and in Oman (Daar et al., 1998). In both instances a strong case for independent origin is made by the presence of the mutation in a different chromosomal framework. Evidence that these mutations have expanded by malaria selection and are likely to be recent events is lacking.

Haplotypes of β^C-globin gene-bearing chromosomes were characterized in 25 African Americans by examining eight polymorphic restriction sites within their β-globin gene clusters (Boehm et al., 1985) (Fig. 27.1A). Twenty-two of the 25 chromosomes were identical in all sites, and possessed a haplotype infrequently found among normal African Americans. Three major haplotypes of the β^C-globin gene, termed CI, CII, and CIII, are found. Several minor unusual haplotypes have also been described (Kan and Dozy, 1980; Boehm et al., 1985; Talacki et al., 1990). Of 90 β^C-globin gene chromosomes, 70 percent were CI, 20 percent CII, and 10 percent had other haplotypes that were either CIII or compatible with recombination events (Chakravarti et al., 1984; Talacki et al., 1990; Steinberg et al., 1996). One study of 20 chromosomes showed only 5 percent with the CII haplotype (Schroeder et al., 1989). These characteristics established a typical haplotype in linkage disequilibrium with the β^C-globin gene. Two haplotypes different

from the typical one were observed in three unrelated individuals. These haplotypes were identical to the typical haplotype in the 3′ region and different in the 5′ region of the β-globin gene cluster. Heterogeneity of haplotypes associated with the β^C gene is likely to result from crossovers in the 5′ portion of the β-globin gene cluster, an event that is common and results in atypical haplotypes of the β^S gene (see Chapter 26) (Chakravarti et al., 1984; Nagel and Ranney, 1990).

Trabuchet et al. have studied haplotypes of the β^C-globin gene in areas of Africa where this mutation is prevalent (Trabuchet et al., 1991). In most of 78 β^C chromosomes from individuals living in Burkina Faso

Figure 27.1. β-Globin gene cluster haplotypes associated with the β^C-globin gene. Above each section are depicted the β-like globin genes with approximate size markers in kilobases (kb). (**A**) Haplotypes of β^C-globin gene-bearing chromosomes have determined using eight RFLPs. Shown are the "typical" haplotypes CI, CII, and CIII. Arrows indicate, from left to right, the polymorphic restriction sites, Hind III (2 sites), Hinc II (2 sites), Hinf I, Ava II, Hpa I, and Bam HI. A (+) indicates cleavage, and a (−), lack of cleavage by the designated enzyme. (**B**) Two atypical haplotypes associated with the β^C-globin gene (A$_1$ β^C and A$_2$ β^C). These haplotypes were determined using additional RFLPs as shown. (Modified from Boehm et al., 1985, and Trabuchet et al., 1991).

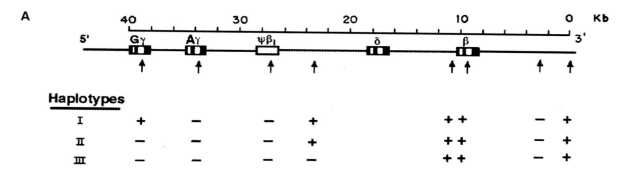

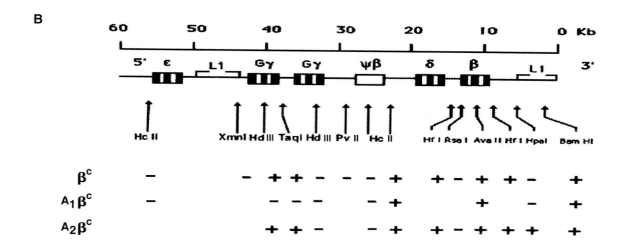

and Benin, the β^C-globin gene was linked to the typical CI haplotype. Additionally, these chromosomes were found to lack the Xmn I site 5' to the β-globin gene cluster and had a Taq I site present between the γ-globin genes. Besides the two atypical haplotypes previously described, a novel haplotype was also found (Fig. 27.1B).

That HbC exists at polymorphic frequencies in parts of Africa suggests that its presence in heterozygotes has some selective advantage. Although the data favoring an advantage for the heterozygous HbC carrier under the selective pressure of *Plasmodium falciparum* are not as strong as those for sickle cell trait, some evidence suggests that HbC trait carriers have less severe parasitemia. HbC also interferes with the lysis of red cells in the late schizont state, impairing the dispersion of merozoites (Olson and Nagel, 1986). Malaria and the red cell is discussed in detail in Chapter 30.

PATHOPHYSIOLOGY OF HbC DISORDERS

Biochemical Features of HbC

HbC was first detected because of its slow migration during cellulose acetate electrophoresis at pH 8.6 (Itano and Neel, 1950). Hunt and Ingram showed that this difference was a consequence of the substitution of lysine acid for glutamic at the β^6 position, which resulted in a net increase of two units of positive charge per molecule (Hunt and Ingram, 1958). Two other mutant hemoglobins, HbE and HbO-Arab, and the normal minor hemoglobin, HbA_2, have the same electrophoretic behavior as HbC on alkaline electrophoresis (see Chapters 10, 43, and 45). However, on citrate agar electrophoresis at pH 6.2, these three hemoglobins migrate similarly to HbA. HbC, because of its interactions with impurities in agar gels, moves slightly anodically under the conditions of agar gel electrophoresis (Winter and Yodh, 1983). Carboxy HbC has decreased solubility in phosphate buffers while deoxy HbC has nearly the same solubility as deoxy HbA (Huisman et al., 1955). In concentrated phosphate buffers, deoxy HbC had even higher solubility than HbA (Itano, 1953). When the viscosity of HbC was compared to that of HbA under oxy conditions and as a function of hemoglobin concentration, both hemoglobins behaved similarly (Condon and Serjeant, 1972). Oxygen affinity of HbC hemolysates "stripped" of 2,3-BPG was normal (Bunn and Briehl, 1970; Murphy, 1976).

HbC Crystallization in Solution. When concentrated solutions of purified hemoglobins are incubated in high molarity phosphate buffer, hemoglobin crystals usually form (Fig. 27.2) (Adachi and Asakura, 1979). In these crystals, hemoglobin can be liganded either as cyanamet, oxy, or CO hemoglobin. Carboxyhemoglobin is preferred for crystallization of ferrous hemoglobin since it inhibits methemoglobin formation that occurs during the long, hot incubation.

Tetragonal HbC crystals form within 25 minutes in a 100 percent HbC solution (Fig. 27.3A). Solutions of HbC containing 0 to 50 percent HbA form a significantly greater number of crystals than similar mixtures with HbF (Hirsch et al., 1988). Ten times fewer crystals were formed with 20 percent HbF compared to 20 percent HbA (Fig. 27.3B). No crystals formed within 2 hours with 30 percent HbF in the mixture but a similar concentration of HbA permitted crystallization. Studies in intact cells in HbC disease showed that cells with crystals isolated from density gradients had very low HbF concentrations. These data suggest that HbF inhibits HbC crystallization in vivo and in vitro (Hirsch et al., 1985).

Forty amino acid differences exist between the β- and γ-globin chains of humans. Of these differences, 21 involve surface or crevice residues and could influence the protein interactions underlying crystal formation (Conley, 1964). To examine which residues could be involved in crystallization, Hirsch et al. studied the potential inhibitory effects of HbA_2, whose δ-globin chains differ from β-globin chains at only 12 sites (Hirsch et al., 1988). HbA_2 inhibited HbC crystallization strongly—slightly surpassing the inhibitory effects of HbF (Fig. 27.3B). Four substitutions are common to δ- and γ-globin chains, but two of them are very conservative changes (position 9 [Ser→Thr or Ala] and

Figure 27.2. Crystal forms observed in hemolysates of patients with HbC. (A) Cubic crystals, generated in hemolysates of compound heterozygotes for HbC and Hb Korle-Bu: (B) Tetragonal crystals observed intracellular and in hemolysates of patients homozygous for HbC, with HbSC disease and compound heterozygotes for HbC and HbA and other mutants. For full color reproduction, see color plate 27.2.

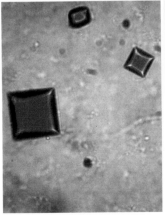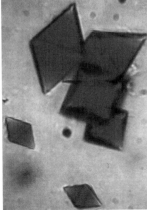

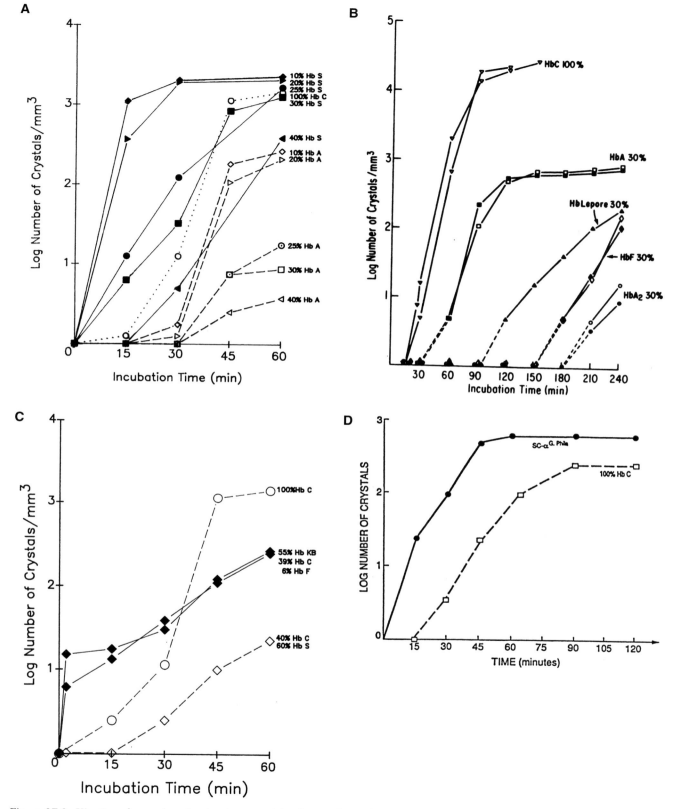

Figure 27.3. Kinetics of crystal nucleation (measured by the numbers of individual crystals generated vs. time) in high phosphate buffer (1.8 mM/L, pH 7.4, 30°C). (A) Hemoglobin mixtures containing HbC and HbA and HbS at different concentrations, demonstrating that HbS accelerates HbC crystallization and that HbA inhibits HbC crystallization. (B) Effect of HbF, HbA$_2$, and Hb Lepore on kinetics of crystallization of HbC. (C) Effect of Hb Korle-Bu in a native hemolysate. (D) Effect of HbG Philadelphia on HbC crystallization in a case of a compound heterozygote for mutations in the β- and α-globin chains. (From Hirsch et al., 1988; Lawrence et al., 1997.)

position 50 [Thr→Ser]) and therefore unlikely to be functionally important. Another site of interest is position 22, where a Glu→Ala difference between β- and δ-globin chains can be contrasted with the very conservative Glu→Asp difference between β- and γ-globin chains. Since both δ- and γ-globin chains are inhibitory, and the former has a negatively charged to neutral mutation while the latter has a conservative mutation, this position is an unlikely candidate for the inhibitory effect. A fourth difference occurs at position 87 where a Thr is replaced by a Gln in both δ- and γ-globin chains. Based on these findings, and the observation that this residue inhibits the polymerization of HbS by HbsF and A_2, γ^{87} Gln may be responsible for the inhibitory effect of HbF and HbA_2 on HbC crystallization (Fig. 27.3B).

To further narrow the assignment of residues in HbF that inhibit HbC crystallization, an examination of the interactions of HbC with Hb Lepore-Boston has proven useful. Hb Lepore-Boston, synthesized by a δβ-globin fusion gene, contains only six of the twelve amino acid differences that distinguish δ and β globin (see Chapters 12 and 15). Hb Lepore-Boston also inhibits HbC crystallization, but less than HbF and HbA_2 (Fig. 27.3B). This reduction in inhibition could arise from the slight difference in hemoglobin conformation that may be surmised by the slight shift of oxygen equilibrium observed in Hb Lepore (Hirsch et al., 1988, 1996). While residue 87 is one site involved in the inhibition of crystallization, other amino acids located between positions 88 and 146 could add to the inhibitory effect of both the γ- and the δ-globin chains. As γ- and δ-globin chains deviate at 13 points between residue 88 and the C-terminal histidine, this could explain the differing effects of HbF and HbA_2 on HbC crystal formation. To date, the available data imply that HbF, HbA_2, and Hb Lepore-Boston inhibit the tendency of HbC to crystallize by an effect mediated, at least in part, by residue 87 of the non-α-globin chain.

Hb Korle-Bu (β73 Asp→Asn) accelerates HbC crystallization and compound heterozygotes with HbC and Hb Korle-Bu have a phenotype with many qualitative characteristics of HbC heterozygotes, made quantitatively more intense by the presence of Hb Korle-Bu (Nagel et al., 1993). The combination of Hb Korle-Bu and HbC produces a mild microcytic hemolytic anemia and in vitro acceleration of crystal formation where precrystal hemoglobin structures convert rapidly into cubic-like crystals (Fig. 27.3C), as opposed to the typical tetragonal crystal structure of homozygous HbC, HbSC disease, and HbC trait. In vitro crystallization studies led to the conclusion that β87 and β73 are contact sites of the oxy crystal (Hirsch et al., 1996).

Hemoglobin $\alpha_2^{G\text{-Philadelphia}}\beta_2^C$ has an increased rate of crystal nucleation compared to $\alpha_2\beta_2^C$ (HbC). This finding implies that position α68, the mutation site of $\alpha_2^{G\text{-Philadelphia}}\beta_2$ (HbG^{Philadelphia}), is a contact site in the crystal of HbC (Lawrence et al., 1997) (Fig. 27.3D).

Mixtures of HbA and HbC crystallize with a different morphology than the classical HbC crystal habit, raising the question of the hemoglobin composition of crystals generated in mixtures of HbC with HbF or HbA_2 (Hirsch et al., 1988). As HbA concentration of the mixture increases, more tetragonal crystals are formed as opposed to typical orthorhombic crystals. HbA alone does not form crystals under these conditions, making it likely that hybrid tetramers ($\alpha_2\beta^C\beta^A$) are incorporated into these crystals and account for their different morphologies. It also suggests strongly that these two hemoglobins co-crystallize. HbS also co-crystallizes with HbC (see below).

Intracellular Crystals in HbC Disease. Are HbC crystals present in vivo? Many early observations of in vivo crystals were made under circumstances where crystal formation could have been induced by the method of cell processing (Diggs et al., 1954; Wheby et al., 1956). When blood from splenectomized HbC disease patients was examined by Percoll-Stractan continuous density gradients, a new, very dense band of cells containing crystals 1 μm or more in size was observed (Fabry et al., 1981). This cell fraction was absent from most HbC disease individuals with intact spleens but present in smaller amounts in some HbC disease patients over age 55 years who could have undergone spontaneous loss of splenic function.

Scanning electron microscopy of cells isolated from density gradients had intracellular HbC crystals (Fig. 27.4). Freeze-fracture preparations, followed by electron microscopy, also showed intracellular crystals (Fig. 27.5). Circulating crystals can be detected in unperturbed wet preparations from individuals with HbC disease but, without splenectomy, they are rare. Together, these observations are consistent with early reports of an increase in intraerythrocytic crystals in HbC disease following splenectomy (Thomas et al., 1955; Jensen et al., 1998).

HbC disease cells, incubated in hypertonic saline, formed crystals rapidly at 56°C but cell lysis occurred; at 4° crystal formation did not occur within 24 hours (Charache et al., 1967) because HbC crystal formation has a negative temperature coefficient—HbC crystals melt at low temperatures. Mutations in other hemoglobins present with HbC as naturally occurring compound heterozygotes can affect in vitro crystallization of HbC. Studies of two HbC compound heterozygotes, HbC/HbN-Baltimore (β95 Lys→Glu) and HbC/Hb Riyadh (β120 Lys→Asn), showed that β120 and β95

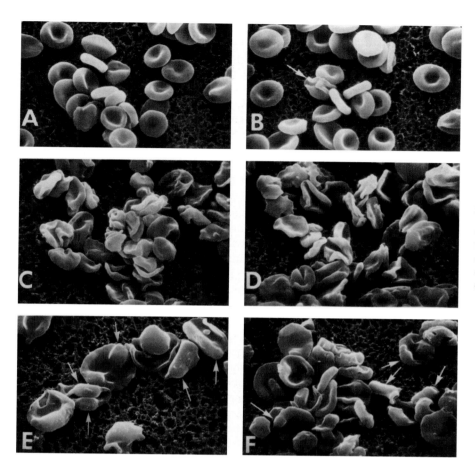

Figure 27.4. Scanning microscopy of HbC disease fractions: (**A and B**) Whole blood; in (**B**) a folded cell. (**C and D**) Middle density red cell fraction. Notice the abundance of folded cells. (**E and F**) The highest density red cell fraction; arrows point to crystal-containing red cells.

are additional contact sites in the crystal. Hb Riyadh (β120 Lys→Asn) inhibited the in vitro crystallization of HbC, explaining the lack of overt pathology, with the exception of microcytosis, in a compound heterozygous infant. In contrast, HbN-Baltimore accelerated the crystallization of HbC, and contributed to abnormal red cell morphology, suggesting strongly that the crystal is sustained by hydrophobic interactions (Hirsch et al., 1997). After a 4-hour incubation at 37 °C the rate of HbC crystallization was not pH dependent, but was accelerated when the cells were dehydrated by incubation in 900 to 1,100 mOsm buffers. Salt concentrations of 1,500 mOsm or higher inhibited crystallization. Deoxygenation with either propane or nitrogen substantially accelerated crystal formation beyond that observed under oxy conditions, but hours were required before crystals appeared so this observation is unlikely to be physiologically relevant.

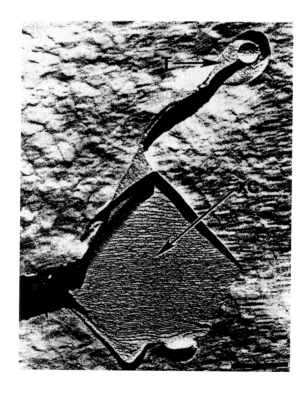

Figure 27.5. Freeze fracture of an HbC disease cell from a splenectomized patient containing a highly ordered crystal (XC) and tail portion (T), that correspond to the membrane of the cell devoid of hemoglobin. This is a negative print (light areas have accumulation of platinum) of a predominantly cross-fractured cell. (From Hirsch et al., 1985, with permission.)

Crystal forms of oxy and deoxy HbC differ (Hirsch et al., 1985). HbC crystals in the red cells of a splenectomized patient homozygous for HbC were found to be in the oxy state and melted after deoxygenation induced either by equilibration with nitrogen or by exposure to dithionite (Hirsch et al., 1985) (Fig. 27.6). When cells from venous and arterial blood were fixed and counted, a small but significant difference in the mean percentage of crystal-containing cells in the arterial circulation versus the venous circulation (1.6 ± 0.22 versus 1.1 ± 0.23 percent) was present. HbC crystals were not observed either in vitro or in vivo in HbC trait (Conley, 1964).

HbC crystals are most likely to form in cells with low HbF content (Hirsch et al., 1985). When the cells of individuals with HbC disease are density fractionated, cells of highest density had the lowest HbF content (Hirsch et al., 1988). In this dense cell fraction, F cells did not contain HbC crystals. HbF inhibition of HbC crystallization might contribute to the potentially beneficial effects of hydroxyurea in HbSC disease in those individuals who have an increase in HbF in response to treatment with this drug (see below).

In HbC disease, HbC crystallizes in its oxy configuration and crystals probably exist in vivo. They are unlikely to play an important role in the pathophysiology of this disorder because they will melt before they enter or as they enter the microcirculation due to the change in their ligand state.

Properties of the HbC Erythrocyte

Morphology. HbC disease erythrocytes are noted for their bizarre morphology. In wet preparations, microcytic and hyperchromic cells are present while in dried stained blood films, target cells, microspherocytes, and cells with crystalline inclusions are found (Conley,

Figure 27.6. Melting of oxy HbC crystal intracellularly by deoxygenation. Time sequence (in seconds) recording of oxy HbC intracellular melting after the addition of isotonic dithionite solution for deoxygenation. Demonstration that the crystal habit of the intracellular crystal is indeed oxy, which is incompatible with the deoxy conformer of HbC. (From Hirsch et al., 1985, with permission.)

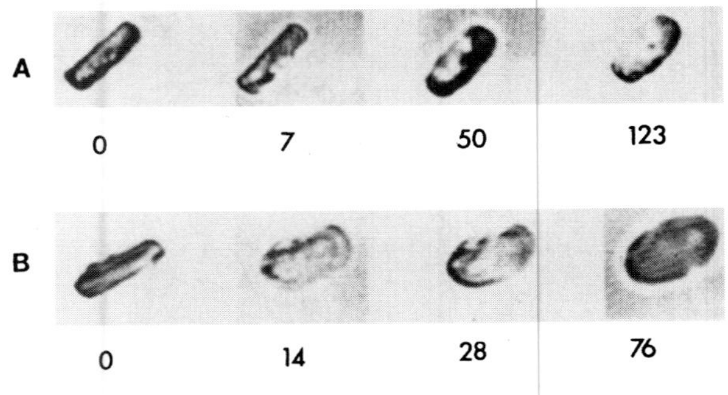

1964). Target cells, a diagnostically useful artifact, are presumably the consequence of the greater surface to volume ratio of HbC disease cells which is, in turn, the consequence of their reduced water content. Incubation of cells containing HbC with 3 percent saline for 4 hours at 37°C reliably induces crystal formation in all cells, a phenomenon regarded as diagnostic of homozygous or heterozygous HbC (Kraus and Diggs, 1956).

Ion Transport and Cation Content. Erythrocytes that contain HbC have a characteristic volume-stimulated K^+ leak. Consequently, intracellular cation and water content of HbC disease cells is strikingly reduced while the cation content of HbC trait and HbSC disease cells is less prominently depleted (see Chapter 22) (Brugnara et al., 1984, 1985). When the cation and water content of HbC disease cells was increased by making the membrane permeable to cations and returning the cells to an isotonic medium, they returned to their original volume by gaining K^+, a behavior that was not observed in control cells. Volume-stimulated K^+ efflux was neither inhibited by ouabain and butamide, nor blocked by inhibitors of Ca^{++}-activated K^+ permeability. A volume-regulated decrease in cell water in HbC disease cells stands in sharp contrast to the usual description of the human red cell as a passive, slightly imperfect osmometer, and probably explained the reduced response of HbC disease cells to changes in the extracellular osmotic pressure. From these observations, it was concluded that HbC disease cells have a potassium transport mechanism that is either absent from, or inactive in, normal cells, and raised the possibility that the presence of the abnormal hemoglobin was responsible for the activity of this transporter (Brugnara et al., 1984, 1985). Volume-stimulated K^+ efflux occurred when osmolarity and pH were both reduced, an effect that was chloride dependent, N-ethylmaleimide (NEM) stimulated, and similar to previously reported K^+Cl^- transporters (Lauf and Theg, 1980; Dunham and Ellory, 1981; Canessa et al., 1986). Transporters of this sort are present in normal and sickle reticulocytes under oxygenated conditions and decrease in activity with cell aging (Canessa et al., 1987). Although red cell life span is shortened to approximately 40 days in HbC disease, this is three times as long as the life span of cells in sickle cell anemia (Prindle and McCurdy, 1970). This suggests that factors beyond the existence of an elevated population of young cells contribute to the high activity of the K^+Cl^- transporter in HbC disease. Ouabain-sensitive flux of the Na/K pump was increased from 5 mmol/L cells/h in normal cells to 12 mmol/L cells/h in HbC disease cells, perhaps due to their reduced Na^+ (Brugnara et al., 1985). Total cellular calcium was elevated in

HbC disease cells as it was in sickle cell anemia and sequestered in endocytic vesicles.

K:Cl contransport is a powerful volume regulator that is found in young red cells. In rabbit erythrocytes, K:Cl cotransport can be described by a two-state system with regulation by dephosphorylation and phosphorylation. When K:Cl contransport is activated and deactivated by stepwise changes in either osmolarity or pH, the time course of K^+ efflux can be calculated and delay times of activation and deactivation measured. The delay time for activation of K^+ efflux in sickle cell anemia cells was 6.2-fold shorter than for HbC disease cells and 5.1-fold shorter than for normal cells. To study the rate of deactivation, cells were first swollen (220 mOsm) to activate the K:Cl cotransport and then shrunk by reestablishing normal osmolarity (300 mOsm). HbC disease cells were deactivated with a delay time 8.1-fold longer than sickle cell anemia cells. When K:Cl cotransport was activated by acidification, similar differences in the delay times for activation and deactivation were observed between HbC disease and sickle cell anemia cells. Moreover, the delay time for activation increased markedly with cell density, but the delay time for deactivation was approximately equal in all density fractions. These studies suggest that K:Cl cotransport is very active in young HbC disease cells but has a longer delay time for deactivation by cell shrinkage than in sickle cell anemia or normal red cells. This implies that a transient activation of K:Cl cotransport in HbC disease reticulocytes, followed by a slow deactivation, may gradually decrease hydration and increase mean corpuscular hemoglobin concentration (MCHC). Implicit in this analysis is that K:Cl contransport regulation by phosphorylation/dephosphorylation might be altered either by a direct effect of HbC and/or by HbC-dependent alteration of enzymes controlling the phosophorylated state.

Oxygen Affinity of HbC Disease Cells. While the oxygen affinity of HbC solutions in the absence of 2,3-BPG was normal (Bunn and Briehl, 1970), the p^{50} of HbC disease cells was increased to 29.5 mm Hg (normal, 26.5 mm Hg) (Murphy, 1976). 2,3-BPG content of HbC disease cells, in micrometer per gram Hb, was equal to that of normal cells while the difference between the intracellular and extracellular pH was increased to -0.280 ± 0.050 for HbC disease cells (normal, -0.195 ± 0.036). Decreased oxygen affinity of HbC disease cells was attributed primarily to reduced intracellular pH, but the "normal" 2,3-BPG content failed to take into account the diminished intracellular water content. When this is considered, the effective 2,3-BPG content is considerably higher than normal and should further decrease oxygen affinity. Decreased oxygen affinity could modulate the anemia of HbC disease by increasing oxygen delivery to tissues (see Chapter 44) and decreasing the stimulus to erythropoietin production (Murphy, 1976).

Osmotic Response and Cellular Dimensions. Cells containing HbC have a diminished osmotic response: Their change in cell volume in response to a change in osmotic pressure is smaller than normal (Charache et al., 1967). Although considered an indication that not all water participates in osmotic equilibrium, this hypothesis is not supported by evidence that all intracellular water acts as a solvent for small molecules and is in rapid exchange with extracellular water (Lee et al., 1984).

Osmotic lysis takes place at a volume of 131 fl in HbC disease cells compared to 151 fl in normal cells, indicating that at the time of lysis, the surface area of the average HbC disease cell is reduced. Mean diameter of HbC disease cells was 6.24 ± 1.25 μm compared to a normal value of 7.81 ± 0.63 μm (Fabry et al., 1981). Erythrocytes of a splenectomized patient with HbC disease had a mean diameter of 6.65 ± 1.15 μm. Reduced osmotic fragility in HbC disease is consistent with an increased surface to volume ratio, an observation consistent with reduced cell volume due to dehydration (Murphy, 1976).

Effect of HbC on Cell Density. High MCHC and low intracellular water content are characteristics of HbC-containing cells (Murphy, 1976; Brugnara et al., 1984, 1985). Red cell density is directly related to the MCHC. Cells in both HbC trait and HbC disease are denser than normal (Fabry et al., 1982). Average MCHC in HbC disease, HbSC disease, HbC trait, and HbA cells were 38, 37, 34, and 33 g/dL, respectively. Cells of all four of these genotypes have a narrow density distribution so that the youngest and lightest cells differ from the oldest and most dense cells by only 3 to 4 g/dL. In contrast, cells of sickle cell anemia have a very wide density distribution. HbC disease, HbSC disease, and HbC trait reticulocytes are denser than normal reticulocytes. This implies either that these cells are denser than normal when they first enter the circulation or that their density changes within their first 24 hours in the circulation when they are still recognizable as reticulocytes.

Increased volume-regulated loss of red cell K^+ and water make the HbC-containing cell dehydrated and more dense than normal. This single feature may be responsible for all of the abnormalities that have been detected in erythrocytes that contain high levels of this hemoglobin.

Binding of HbC to Cell Membranes. HbC, like HbS, interacts more strongly with the erythrocyte membrane than HbA. This interaction has been studied by using changes in the fluorescence intensity of the membrane-imbedded probe, 12-(9-anthroyloxy) stearic acid, whose fluorescence is quenched when it is approached by hemoglobin (Reiss et al., 1982). At pH 6.8, the affinity of HbC for the erythrocyte membrane was about 5 times greater than that of HbA, while the pH dependence of HbC binding is significantly right-shifted from that observed for HbA. Deoxy HbA and HbC were less strongly bound than oxyhemoglobin. These experiments were done at low and nonphysiologic ionic strengths and low hemoglobin concentrations. When the NaCl concentration was increased, HbC was about 90 percent dissociated from the membrane.

At higher hemoglobin concentrations, HbC binding was stronger and higher salt concentrations were required to displace the hemoglobin from the membrane. The cytoplasmic portion of band 3 was implicated as the binding site for both HbA and HbC. HbO-Arab is more strongly bound than HbS and is even more tightly membrane bound than HbC (Ballas et al., 1981). This suggests that both electrostatic charge and the protein conformation in the vicinity of the charged groups play a role in membrane binding. Membrane binding of abnormal hemoglobins may affect those membrane proteins involved in anion or cation movement and play a role in the altered red cell densities observed in cells containing these mutant hemoglobins. Increased density of HbC disease cells may be due to an electrostatic interaction between HbC and components of the red cell membrane (Brugnara et al., 1985). HbE has the same charge as HbC and HbE homozygotes also have microcytic cells, but with a normal MCHC. Factors beyond charge-mediated nonspecific electrostatic interaction may also affect hemoglobin-membrane interactions (Nagel et al., 1981).

Rheologic Properties of HbC Disease Cells.

An ability to pass through 3 μm Millipore filters is one measure of red cell deformability. HbC disease cells were less filterable than normal cells regardless of the osmolarity of the suspending buffer. While the optimum filterability of normal cells occurred at 300 mOsm, HbC disease cells were maximally filterable at 200 mOsm, an observation consistent with the hypothesis that these cells are dehydrated. Using a laser diffraction viscosimeter or ecktactometer that measures cellular elongation in response to a fluid shear stress, cellular deformability was examined as a function of osmolarity of the suspending buffer. HbC disease cells were poorly deformable in isotonic media but deformability improved when osmolarity was reduced to 100 to 200 mOsm (Mohandas et al., 1980). HbC disease cells were more viscous than normal cells when studied by eckacytometry at high PCVs. At the more physiologic

PCV of 30, both oxygenated and deoxygenated HbC disease cells from individuals with intact spleens had similar viscosities that were higher than normal controls (Fabry et al., 1981; Kaul et al., 1981). One splenectomized HbC disease patient was found to have an elevated blood viscosity that was further elevated upon deoxygenation.

In the isolated rat mesoappendix model, HbC disease cells caused a 10 percent to 20 percent increase in peripheral resistance compared to normal controls (Fabry et al., 1981). This minimal circulatory impairment is compatible with the benign clinical course of most HbC disease patients. Adverse affects that might arise because of the high MCHC and reduced deformability of HbC disease cells are probably offset by their small size (Fabry et al., 1981).

Vasoocclusive Disease

Vasoocclusive episodes are not a feature of HbC disease despite the presence of intraerythrocytic HbC crystals. Although poorly deformable, HbC cells are small and rheologically competent. Oxy HbC crystals will tend to melt when HbC cells become lodged in the microcirculation where the pO$_2$ is low (Hirsch et al., 1985). This would restore deformability to the HbC disease red cell and allow any potential vascular obstruction caused by these dense cells to resolve. Vasoocclusion in sickle cell disease is likely to be mediated by complex interactions among altered erythrocyte membranes, vascular endothelial cells—themselves injured by repetitive buffeting from sickle cells—neutrophils, and platelets. There are no data suggesting that these interactions are present in HbC disease.

HbC DISEASE, HbC TRAIT, AND HbC-β THALASSEMIA AND α THALASSEMIA

HbC trait is found in 2 percent of African Americans (Motulsky, 1973). In parts of West Africa, the prevalence of the HbC gene can reach 0.125 (Lehmann and Huntsman, 1974; Labie et al., 1984). In African Americans the prevalence of HbC disease is 1 in 6,000.

Laboratory Features and Diagnosis

Both HbC trait and HbC disease are characterized by target cells in the blood. Individuals with HbC trait are not anemic, have normal mean cell volume (MCV), and normal red cell life span (Prindle and McCurdy, 1970). Their erythrocytes were more dense than normal cells and MCHCs were about 2 g/dL higher than normal and 1 g/dL more than sickle cell trait cells, when this was measured using a Bayer cell counter (Bunn et al., 1982; Hinchliffe et al., 1996).

HbC makes up about 42 percent of the total hemoglobin in HbC trait (Steinberg, 1975). Considering that within this 42 percent resides the 2 percent to 3 percent HbA$_2$ fraction that is not conveniently separated from HbC by electrophoresis, the HbC level in HbC trait is similar to the amount of HbS in sickle cell trait.

Because of its strongly positive charge, HbC can be easily distinguished from HbA, HbS, and HbF by electrophoresis at alkaline and acidic pH and by isoelectric focusing. Different methods of HPLC also can resolve HbC. Other hemoglobin variants such as HbE and HbO-Arab that have a similar positive charge and some hybrid hemoglobin molecules, found when α- and β-globin gene variants are present together, behave like HbC upon alkaline electrophoresis (see Chapter 28). They can usually be distinguished by citrate agar electrophoresis or isoelectric focusing. HbA$_2$ migrates like HbC at alkaline pH but rarely accounts for more than 6 percent and is never more than 12 percent of the total hemoglobin. A band in the position of HbA$_2$ on cellulose acetate that comprises 25 percent to 50 percent of the total hemoglobin is probably HbC or HbE. Many commonly used methods of hemoglobin separation do not distinguish HbA$_2$ from HbC although this is possible to do with some forms of HPLC (see Chapter 34). HbA$_2$ levels cannot usually be used as a guide to the presence of HbC-β^0 thalassemia compound heterozygotes except when HPLC is used for hemoglobin separation. HbC can lead to overestimation of HbA$_1$C concentration when this is measured by immunoassay (Roberts et al., 1998).

α Thalassemia can be present in individuals with HbC trait or in homozygotes with HbC disease. In HbC trait α thalassemia, the concentration of HbC is reduced similarly to HbS levels in sickle cell trait α thalassemia (see Chapters 29). mRNA isolated from individuals with HbC trait, and HbC trait with either homozygous α thalassemia-2 or HbH disease, supported balanced expression of β^C and β^S globin favoring a posttranslational mechanism for the modulation of HbC concentration (Liebhaber et al., 1988). Trimodality in the percentage of HbC in carriers of HbC trait suggested the presence of α thalassemia as a modulatory factor (Huisman, 1977). HbC plus HbA$_2$ concentration was 44 percent, 38 percent, and 32 percent in HbC trait carriers presumed to have four, three, and two α-globin genes, based on globin biosynthesis studies (Huisman, 1977). In other cases where the carrier was presumed to have heterozygous α$^+$ thalassemia, MCV was reduced and HbC and HbA$_2$ together were about 33 percent (Charache et al., 1974; Steinberg, 1975). A case of HbC trait HbH disease, caused by compound heterozygosity for the −α$^{3.7}$ and SEA deletions had splenomegaly, mild anemia, MCV of 59 fl, and 24 percent HbC (Giordano et al., 1997). HbC dis-

ease α thalassemia has been described with a phenotype similar to HbC disease but α-globin gene mapping was not done (Steinberg, 1975).

Compared to the wealth of information on the effects of the interaction of α thalassemia and sickle cell trait, there are little available data on the hematologic and clinical aspects of HbC trait or HbC disease with α thalassemia when α thalassemia was definitively detected by α-globin gene mapping. Since both HbC trait and the −α$^{3.7}$ type of α thalassemia are clinically innocuous there is no reason to believe that their concordance should be any different.

HbC crystals, very prominent target cells, and anemia are present in HbC disease. Mild hemolytic anemia is customary: The PCV is usually 32 percent to 34 percent and hemoglobin concentration between 9 and 12 g/dL, with a moderate reticulocytosis of between 5 percent and 10 percent. Characteristically, the MCV is between 55 and 65 fl (Murphy, 1976). Red cell survival has been studied in only a small number of HbC disease patients. Using DF^{32}P labeled red cells, a mean red cell life span of 38.5 and 35.1 days was found in two individuals with a ^{51}Cr red cell survival of 19 days (Prindle and McCurdy, 1970).

Hemolysis may not be the sole mechanism generating anemia in HbC disease. A reduced oxygen affinity of HbC cells (see above) could account for a portion of the reduction in PCV as these red cells would more readily unload oxygen in the tissues. In turn, erythropoietin production would be stimulated at a lower hemoglobin level than normal. Anemia may therefore appear to be uncompensated because of the decreased oxygen affinity of HbC disease red cells. Dyserythropoietic features, including nuclear disorganization and altered chromatin staining, have been found in erythroblasts of HbC disease but not sickle cell anemia (Wickramasinghe et al., 1982). These findings suggest that ineffective erythropoiesis may account for some of the anemia in this disorder. In children with HbC disease, hemoglobin levels and reticulocyte counts were similar to those in adults and the MCV was between 60 and 80 fl (Olson et al., 1994; Kim et al., 1977).

HbC-β$^+$ thalassemia and β^0 thalassemia have been described, and like HbS-β thalassemia, the observed clinical heterogeneity is a result of a multiplicity of β-thalassemia genes. HbC-β$^+$ thalassemia in Blacks, because of the prominence of the "mild" promoter mutations in this population (see Chapters 12 and 28), has hematologic features of β-thalassemia trait with microcytosis and either no anemia, or very mild anemia. HbC levels are 20 percent to 30 percent, similar to HbS levels in most Blacks with HbS-β$^+$ thalassemia. Like HbS-β$^+$ thalassemia in Mediterranean populations, β$^+$-thalassemia mutations that impair considerably gene expression produce a more severe phenotype approaching that of HbC-β^0 thalassemia.

HbC-β^0 thalassemia can be difficult to distinguish from HbC disease since HbA is absent and HbA$_2$ may not be measured (see above) (Prindle and McCurdy, 1970). Considerable overlap of the hematologic findings in these genotypes makes it impossible to rely on these values and mandates family studies or DNA analysis when it is important to make the distinction between HbC disease and HbC-β^0 thalassemia (Table 27.1). Further complicating the separation of these disorders is the possibility of α thalassemia coincidental with HbC disease, which is likely to cause a phenotype similar to HbC-β^0 thalassemia. HbC trait has been described with gene deletion hereditary persistence of HbF, Hb Lepore, and with $\delta\beta$ thalassemia. All are mild conditions resembling HbC-β^+ thalassemia because of the presence of HbF and Hb Lepore.

Clinical Features of HbC Trait and HbC Disease

HbC trait is not associated with clinical disease. Hematuria and isosthenuria, the best characterized clinical abnormalities of sickle cell trait, are not associated with HbC trait.

Individuals with HbC disease have hematologic and clinical evidence of their hemoglobinopathy but appear to have a normal life span and few signs or symptoms—besides splenomegaly—attributable to their disease. They do not have vasoocclusive events typical of sickle cell disease.

Splenomegaly has been reported in most adult patients with HbC disease and is usually asymptomatic. In the past, splenectomy was frequently recommended with the hope of correcting the anemia; current practice avoids splenectomy in all but very selected cases. Splenectomy is usually followed by a slight, but not clinically important, increase in PCV and by increased numbers of circulating cells containing HbC crystals, that, in spite of their menacing aspect in the smear, seem to have no pathologic consequences. The modest effect of splenectomy on PCV might be expected if the major portion of the anemia were secondary to the elevation of 2,3-BPG, but the postsplenectomy increase in PCV would not be expected if the anemia were largely the consequence of reduced oxygen affinity (Murphy, 1976). Children may have a lower prevalence of splenomegaly (Olson et al., 1994). Spontaneous rupture of the spleen has been described in HbC disease (Lipshutz et al., 1977). Increased density of the HbC-containing erythrocytes does not impair renal concentrating ability (Statius van Eps et al., 1970).

Treatment Recommendations

As HbC disease is clinically asymptomatic and hematologically benign, no special treatment is needed. Iron should be avoided since it will not, in the absence of iron lack, repair anemia or microcytosis. Hemolysis is very mild, so a reasonably nutritious diet should provide sufficient folic acid and supplementation is unnecessary.

Parvovirus B19 can transiently interrupt erythropoiesis but since hemolysis is mild, the sequelae of this infection should not be as serious as in sickle cell anemia, may not reach the threshold of clinical detection, and transfusions should not be needed.

Patients sometimes have aches and pains—we all do—and it is not clear if these can be linked to HbC disease. There is no evidence that HbC disease is accompanied by a reduction in longevity in the Western world, although this might not be true in the harsh environmental conditions of the Sahel (Labie et al., 1984).

HbSC DISEASE

HbSC disease is an altogether different clinical problem than HbC disease because the erythrocytes in this disorder contain equal concentrations of HbC and HbS. Each hemoglobin component exerts its own special pathologic effects that synergistically cause the well-delineated features of HbSC disease.

Cellular Factors Accounting for the Pathophysiology and Severity of HbSC Disease

Sickle cell trait and HbSC disease erythrocytes both have far lower concentrations of HbS than cells of sickle cell anemia. Yet, the expectation that because of low

---

Table 27.1. Hematologic Findings in HbC Disease and HbC-β^0 Thalassemia*

Genotype	Hemoglobin (g/dL)/PCV	MCV (fl)	HbF (%)	Reticulocytes (%)	Spleen
HbC disease	10–15/30–45	60–90	2–4	2–7	↑↑
HbC-β^0 thalassemia	8–12/25–35	55–70	3–10	5–20	↑↑↑

* These data are a composite of many cases reported in the literature. For references, see Bunn and Forget (1986) and Charache et al. (1967).

HbS concentrations polymerization-induced defects will be attenuated or absent is realized only in sickle cell trait. The reasons why sickle cell trait and HbSC disease differ, which elucidate the pathophysiology of HbSC disease, are discussed in the following sections.

Incubation of HbSC disease blood with 3 percent NaCl for 4 hours at 37°C induces the formation of intracellular HbC crystals. These crystals are the most striking and distinctive feature in circulating red cells of patients with HbSC disease, especially when they have a normal complement of α-globin genes. HbC crystals have been noted for decades but have only recently been studied intensively using modern approaches. Crystals are observed in Wright's and vital-dye stained smears and in "wet" preparations from fingerstick blood samples (Fig. 27.7). When α thalassemia is present with HbSC disease, typical crystals are absent in some patients. All HbSC disease patients' red cells exhibit heavily stained conglomerations of hemoglobin that appear marginated with rounded edges in distinction to the straight-edged crystals. Such cells have been called "billiard ball cells."

Figure 27.7. Erythrocytes in HbSC disease. These cells are characterized by sharp edges, increased red color (particularly in a reticulocyte stained smear), and often by having all the hemoglobin of the cells recruited into the crystal, leaving a ghost of the red cell without cytosolic dissolved hemoglobin. (1) Crystal-containing red cell; (2) "billiard ball" cells; (3) folded cells. (From Lawrence et al., 1991, with permission.) For full color reproduction, see color plate 27.7.

Both crystals and "billiard ball cells" are found in the densest fraction of HbSC disease but not sickle cell anemia cells, and represent hemoglobin aggregation distinct from the polymerization of HbS. Regardless of the α-globin gene haplotype, the blood of HbSC disease patients has additional abnormally shaped cells that are strikingly apparent upon scanning electron microscopy (Fig. 27.8). Typical are "folded cells," some with a single fold, and resembling—to the gastronomically inclined—pita bread or a taco. These are most likely the cells that Diggs et al. called "fat cells," since in Wright-stained smears they appear as wide bipointed cells. Other misshapen cells had triconcave shapes, that is, triangular cells with three dimples, very much like those seen in acute alcoholism termed "knizocytes." A remarkable shape was the "triple folded cells" that appeared as two pita breads stuck together (Fig. 27.8). These bizarre shapes are the product of an increased surface to volume ratio. Excessive surface is resolved largely by membrane folding, accounting for the multiplicity of fascinating erythrocyte forms.

Not all cells in HbSC disease contain crystals. An enlarged, infarcted, and perhaps abnormally functioning spleen might fail intermittently in its "pitting" function, allowing hemoglobin crystals and aggregates to remain in the cell. HbS accelerates the crystallization of HbC in vivo as has been demonstrated in vitro (Lin et al., 1989).

HbC shares with HbS the same β⁶ mutation site although HbC contains a new lysine residue and HbS, a valine. HbC crystallizes when oxygenated and HbS

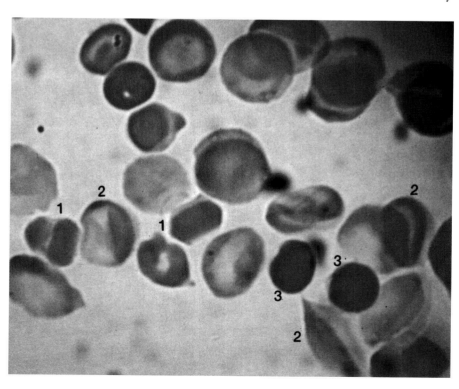

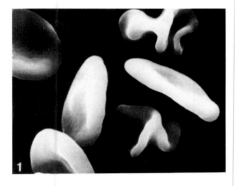

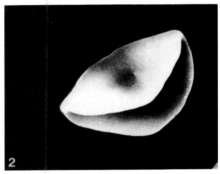

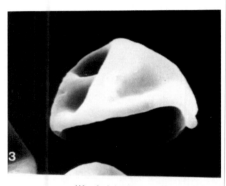

a multi-folded SC cell

Figure 27.8. Several types of red cells found in the blood of HbSC disease patients illustrated by scanning electron microscopy. Folded red cells (top panel), "pita-bread" red cells (middle panel), and highly folded red cell (lower panel) from whole blood of an HbSC disease patient, by scanning electron microscopy.

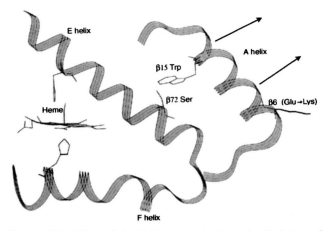

Figure 27.9. View of the F, E, and A helix in the β chains of hemoglobin. Also depicted are the heme, the β15 Trp - β72 Ser bond, and the β6 Lys (the mutation of HbC). The arrows depict the likely movement of the A helix away from the E helix, which is compatible with conformational changes in the central cavity of the tetramer. (From Hirsch et al., 1996, with permission.)

Ratio of HbS to HbC

In HbSC disease, the ratio of HbS to HbC is 50:50. This contrasts with the 40:60 ratio of HbS to HbA in sickle cell trait. Several explanations have been proposed for this difference in HbS level, a difference that may underlie the dissimilar clinical and hematologic features of HbSC disease and sickle cell trait. Charge-related differences in αβ dimer assembly account for the lower proportion of HbS in sickle cell trait and HbC in HbC trait (see Chapters 8 and 29). Although HbC has one additional positive charge compared to HbS, both these abnormal hemoglobins may compete similarly for α-globin chains and because of this, equalize the HbS to HbC ratio.

Just as HbF is unequally distributed among all cells, there is some evidence that HbC is unequally apportioned among all red cells of an individual. Using single-cell electrophoresis, the distribution of HbS in sickle cell trait and HbC in HbC trait was found to vary from cell to cell (Anyaibe et al., 1983). Whether HbS concentration differs among the cells of HbSC disease is unknown. If a difference is present, it could be under genetic control as is HbF, and be one facet of the modulation of the severity of polymerization-related defects in HbSC disease.

HbSC disease is associated with hemolytic anemia and vasoocclusive complications while sickle cell trait is not. It has been proposed that this difference can be largely attributed to the higher proportion and concentration of HbS in HbSC disease (Bunn et al., 1982). While the effects of HbA and HbC on HbS polymerization are equivalent, increasing the percentage HbS from 40 percent to 50 percent—keeping the total

polymerizes when deoxygenated. The mechanism of HbC crystallization is unknown. Hirsch et al. (1996), based on intrinsic fluorescence and ultraviolet Raman spectroscopy data, have demonstrated the weakening of Trpβ15-Serβ72 bond that most likely leads to a displacement of the A helix away from the E helix. More recent data (Hirsch et al., 1999) have extended these studies to demonstrate that the central cavity (between the two β-globin chains) is altered compared to HbA. These features may explain the crystallization tendencies of HbC (Fig. 27.9).

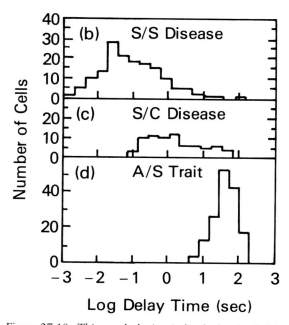

Figure 27.10. This graph depicts individual red cell delay times of polymerization in HbSC disease compared to sickle cell anemias and sickle cell trait. Notice that many HbSC cells behave as sickle trait cells, as far as delay times, but that also some of the cells behave as the slowest sickle cell anemia cells. In effect, delay time of HbSC cells is intermediate between sickle cell anemia and sickle cell trait cells, with overlapping. (From Eaton and Hofrichter, 1990, with permission.)

hemoglobin concentration steady—increased the rate of polymerization nearly 15-fold. This observation is in complete agreement with studies of HbS polymerization in intact red cells (Coletta et al., 1982). The length of the delay time before sickling occurs may play a role in the pathophysiology of HbSC disease, since a long delay may allow a cell to move through hypoxic microvasculature before rigidity and rheologic incompetence ensue, while a shorter delay time may increase a cell's propensity to induce vasoocclusion (Fig. 27.10).

Cation Content

Cation content of HbSC disease red cells is intermediate between normal and HbC disease cells. Oxygenated HbSC disease cells exhibit a volume-stimulated potassium efflux similar to that observed in sickle cell anemia and HbC disease (Brugnara et al., 1985; Canessa et al., 1986). This transporter appears to be chloride dependent and stimulated by N-ethylmaleimide (Canessa et al., 1986). More recently, such a transporter was found in young cells of normal controls and individuals with sickle cell anemia and HbSC disease. It is inhibited by deoxygenation through cytosolic Mg^{++} modulation (Fabry et al., 1982; Canessa et al., 1987b). HbSC disease cells also exhibit a diminished change in cell volume in response to variation of the osmolarity of the suspending medium, which is likely due to volume-regulated K^+ efflux. Volume-regulated K^+ efflux should impact adversely the pathophysiology of disease since any increase of MCHC will aggravate HbS polymerization.

Cell Density and Density-Related Properties

As illustrated in Figure 27.11, HbSC disease cells share the increased red cell density characteristic of all cells containing HbC. Reflecting the increased MCHC,

Figure 27.11. Percoll-Stractan (Larex) density separation of whole blood from normal hemolysate (AA), HbC trait (AC), and three different HbSC disease individuals and one sickle cell anemia patient (SS). Beads: color-coded density beads to establish the density at different levels of the gradient after centrifugation. For full color reproduction, see color plate 27.11.

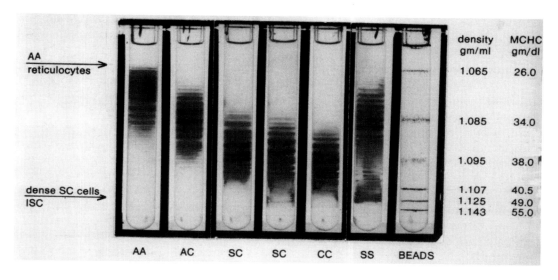

the intracellular HbS concentration is raised to a level where polymerization occurs under physiologic conditions. This contrasts with sickle cell trait cells where polymerization occurs only at high osmolarity and low pH, conditions that, in vivo, are present exclusively in the renal medulla. Reducing the MCHC in HbSC disease to normal levels of 33 g/dL by osmotically swelling HbSC cells resulted in normalization of many of the polymerization-dependent abnormal properties of these cells (Fabry et al., 1982). Among the beneficial effects of cell rehydration are increased hemoglobin oxygen affinity (reduced in HbSC disease), reduction of viscosity of deoxygenated erythrocyte suspensions (increased in HbSC disease), fall in the rate of sickling (similar to that in sickle cell anemia), and reduction in the deoxygenation-induced K^+ leak (greater than that observed in sickle cell anemia). Percoll-Stractan continuous density gradients of the same density profile but different osmolarities were used to determine the osmolarity where the density distribution of HbSC disease cells most nearly matched normal cells. At this osmolarity (240 mOsm), the cells were examined by scanning electron microscopy and were found to be biconcave disks. This is a welcome feature of the rehydration of HbSC disease cells. A discoid shape is indispensable for normal deformation of red cells in the microcirculation and this conformation can be achieved in HbSC disease because these cells have a normal MCH and increased MCHC. In contrast, while some erythrocytes of sickle cell anemia are dehydrated, the majority are normal discocytes with a normal MCH and MCHC. Rehydrating these cells, a maneuver that will also decrease polymerization, will produce cells that are no longer discocytes but that acquire progressively a spheroidal shape. This is an unwelcome feature of rehydrating sickle erythrocytes, since it decreases their deformability. As a therapeutic tool, rehydrating cells in sickle cell anemia makes sense only if the most dense cells can be modified. However, modification of the intracellular hemoglobin concentration is an attractive therapeutic approach for the treatment of HbSC disease.

Analogous to sickle cell anemia, when α thalassemia coexists with HbSC disease fewer dense cells are present (Embury et al., 1984; Fabry et al., 1984). During the course of painful episodes in HbSC disease, dense cells decrease just as they do during pain episodes in sickle cell anemia, suggesting that painful episodes may be accompanied by dense cell sequestration (Fabry et al., 1983; Ballas and Smith, 1992). HbSC disease cells exhibit pathologic properties characteristic of both sickle cell anemia and HbC disease cells and this feature helps explain the greater than anticipated severity of HbSC disease given the cellular content of HbS.

A morphologic analysis of density-separated HbSC disease cells indicated that they became progressively more aberrant in shape as their density increased. The densest fraction of the gradient contained cells with the most abnormal shapes, which were particularly noticeable for their gross pitting and membrane invaginations. Crystal-containing cells are particularly predominant among the highest density fractions. HbSC disease cells destined to become extremely dense are likely also to produce crystals as a by-product of their progressive MCHC increase as the concentration of hemoglobin within crystals is about 68 g/dL. Irreversibly sickled cells are rare in HbSC disease and are found in the densest cell fractions. α Thalassemia is associated with a decrease in the size of the dense cell fraction. In contrast with sickle cell anemia, the highest percentage of reticulocytes is found within a fraction of dense cells, although the youngest, or stress reticulocytes, are predominant in the least dense fraction. While HbC disease cells display similar findings, reticulocytes of normal individuals and patients with other types of hemolytic anemia and sickle cell anemia are the lightest red cells in the blood. This suggests that in HbSC disease reticulocytes exit the marrow as low-density cells and become dense within 24 hours, sinking to the next densest fraction of cells in the blood. Reticulocytes are almost absent from the dense cell fractions that contain the largest proportion of crystal-containing cells. Hyperdense reticulocytes migrate to lower densities if Cl^- is removed from the media, in concordance with a K:Cl contransport-mediated phenomenon. The density distribution of HbSC disease reticulocytes shifts dramatically when Cl^- is removed from the media and replaced by NO_3^- as the percentage of dense cells is reduced and the reticulocyte distribution shifts to lower densities. Since under the conditions of the experiment K:Cl cotransport is abolished, it seems that K:Cl cotransport is responsible for the presence of HbSC disease reticulocytes of unusually high densities. This interpretation is confirmed by direct measurements (Canessa et al., 1987a) in density-defined HbSC disease red cell fractions, where HbSC disease red cells were found to be endowed with an especially active K:Cl cotransport system capable of decreasing volume that was not compensated by Na^+ influx or Na^+/H^+ exchange.

G-6-PD activity in HbSC disease cell fractions, in contrast to normal blood where the distribution of G-6-PD is cell-age dependent, shows similar enzyme activity in all fractions. In conjunction with the peculiar distribution of reticulocytes among HbSC disease cell density fractions and the progressive abnormal shapes with increasing cell density, the data suggest that the mean cell age within different fractions of HbSC disease cells is determined by the admixture of young and old cells.

β-globin Gene Cluster Haplotypes in HbSC Disease

In seventy-three adult patients with HbSC disease a Benin haplotype β^S chromosome was present in 56 percent and Bantu, Senegal, and other haplotype chromosomes present in 25 percent, 6 percent, and 12 percent, respectively (Steinberg et al., 1996). There were no significant differences in the hematologic characteristics of patients with these four β-globin gene haplotypes (Talacki et al., 1990). Haplotypes of the HbC chromosome were consistent with earlier studies (see above). Hematologic features of individuals with HbSC disease who had Benin or Bantu β^S chromosomes were similar whether they had a CI or CII haplotype. β-Globin gene haplotype modulates the hematologic and clinical features of sickle cell anemia via haplotype-linked elements that affect the levels of HbF. HbF levels in HbSC disease are lower than in sickle cell anemia, probably because there is less hemolysis and bone marrow expansion in HbSC disease and possibly because the β^C chromosome may not contain the critical genetic elements that are present in sickle cell anemia and necessary for increased transcription of the γ-globin genes.

Clinical Features of HbSC Disease

HbSC disease has an incidence of about 1:833 live births in African Americans (Motulsky, 1973). In some West African locales such as Northern Ghana, Burkina Faso, and Western Nigeria about one fourth of the population may have HbSC disease (Lehmann and Huntsman, 1974). Slave trading, population migrations, and centuries of conflict have spread the HbS and HbC genes throughout the world, broadening greatly the distribution of the sickle hemoglobinopathies (see Chapter 26). All complications that are found in patients with sickle cell anemia have occurred in individuals with HbSC disease. Yet, most—but not all—of these complications are seen less often and appear at a later time in HbSC disease compared to sickle cell anemia. Hemolysis is less intense so that anemia is milder and the complications of hemolysis—aplastic episode and cholelithiasis—less frequent or severe. Osteonecrosis of bone is nearly as common, proliferative sickle retinopathy is much more prevalent in HbSC disease than in sickle cell anemia, and the mortality of acute chest syndrome may be increased (Embury et al., 1994). Painful episodes occur at about half the frequency as in sickle cell anemia. While longer than in sickle cell anemia, the life span of HbSC disease patients is shortened when compared to control populations. Specific treatments that will prevent complications of this disease are not yet available. In the

following sections, the clinical aspects of HbSC disease that differ most from those of sickle cell anemia are discussed. For details of treatment and many complications, which differ little among the genotype of sickle cell disease, the reader should consult Chapter 24.

Hematology and Laboratory Findings. Hemoglobin electrophoresis, isoelectric focusing, HPLC, and capillary electrophoresis can all accurately determine the relative levels of HbS and HbC. HbS-O Arab and sickle cell anemia/HbG Philadelphia can appear like HbSC disease on alkaline electrophoresis. In the first case, the distinction can be made by agar gel electrophoresis, when HbO separates from HbC. In the example of sickle cell anemia/HbG Philadelphia, the hybrid molecule $\alpha_2{}^G\beta_2{}^S$ migrates like HbC at alkaline pH and only HbS is visualized by citrate agar gel electrophoresis. Both of these disorders have a more severe phenotype than the usual cases of HbSC disease and behave more like typical sickle cell anemia. HbE also migrates like HbC at alkaline pH. HbSE disease is usually a mild disorder with minimal anemia, microcytosis, and few symptoms (Altay et al., 1976; Rey et al., 1991; Schroeder et al., 1998).

Smears of blood from patients with HbSC disease contain target cells, HbC crystals, and a panoply of other deformed cells (see above). Except in the presence of sickle cell–related renal failure or with coincidental medical conditions that can reduce the PCV, patients with HbSC disease do not usually have symptoms of anemia. At any age, PCV in HbSC disease is higher than in sickle cell anemia (West et al., 1992). Median values by age and sex for PCV, MCV, platelet count, and bilirubin are shown in Figure 27.12. PCV rises from 31 to 32 in children ages 2 to 5 years to about 37 in males over age 20 years, a level about five points higher than in females with HbSC disease. Many adult men but fewer adult women have a normal PCV (Serjeant et al., 1973; Bannerman et al., 1979; West et al., 1992). Individuals with high PCV may be at greatest risk for complications such as proliferative retinopathy and osteonecrosis of the femoral head (Condon and Serjeant, 1972; Milner et al., 1991). Leukocyte counts in HbSC disease are normal or only very slightly elevated. Perhaps this is a result of more persistent splenomegaly and less proliferative activity of the bone marrow. Platelet counts are also lower in HbSC disease than in sickle cell anemia, perhaps for similar reasons. Some individuals with HbSC disease have mild thrombocytopenia and this can often be related to an enlarged spleen.

Leukocytosis, thrombocytosis, and reticulocytosis have been linked to the severity of vasoocclusive disease in sickle cell anemia. Mature sickle cells circulate in the company of leukocytes, platelets, and "stress"

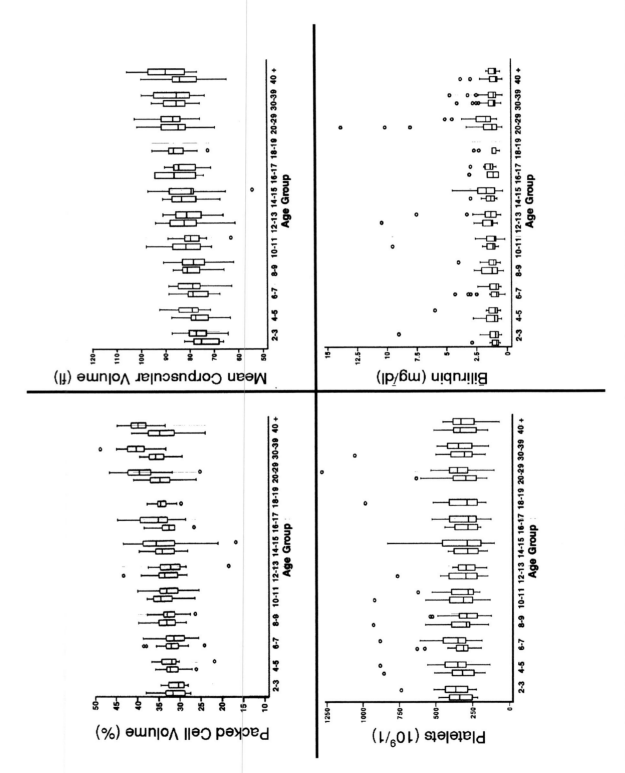

Figure 27.12. PCV, MCV, platelet count, and bilirubin levels in a cross-sectional study of patients with HbSC disease ages 2 years to older than 40 years. PCV, MCV, and reticulocyte counts were available for 586 patients and bilirubin for 467 patients. Box plots show the mean and 25th (bottom of box) and 75th percentile (top of box) of the data (see West et al., 1992, for an explanation of the vertical lines). (Modified from West et al., 1992, with permission.)

reticulocytes. Stress reticulocytes are found in individuals with hemolytic disease and display adhesive ligands that facilitate erythrocyte–endothelial interactions (Sugihara et al., 1992; Brittain et al., 1993; Wick et al., 1993 Gee and Platt, 1995). Increasing evidence points to the complicity of neutrophils in vasoocclusion (see Chapter 20). High granulocyte counts are a risk for mortality in sickle cell anemia (Platt et al., 1994). Neutrophils can interact with sickle cells and with the endothelium, releasing damaging cytokines when activated (Dias-Da-Motta et al., 1996; Hofstra et al., 1996). Activated platelets elaborate thrombospondin that can promote the adherence of sickle erythrocytes to endothelium (Brittain et al., 1993). Perhaps some of the milder features of HbSC disease are accounted for by the lower numbers of these cells in the blood.

Bilirubin is usually normal, reflecting mild hemolytic anemia compared to sickle cell anemia (West et al., 1992). ^{51}Cr survival in thirty-one patients with HbSC disease was 12.6 to 26 days and DF^{32}P mean life span was 29 days (McCurdy et al., 1975; Bannerman et al., 1979). In distinction, by the same method, red cell lifetime for sickle cell anemia patients was between 12 and 24 days (mean, 17.2 days) while the life span of normal cells approached 120 days. Reticulocytes ranged from less than 1 percent to a high of 7 percent, confirming the abatement of hemolysis (Bannerman et al., 1979). As in sickle cell anemia, red cell volume was only modestly reduced while plasma volume was more substantially elevated (McCurdy et al., 1975; Bannerman et al., 1979). Red cell survival, plasma volume, and PCV were unrelated to splenomegaly or splenic function.

Although hemolysis is only modest and within the capacity of a normal bone marrow to counterbalance, compensation is incomplete. Mild anemia in HbSC disease cannot be entirely accounted for by the rate of red cell destruction, since this does not exceed the potential of normal marrow to replace lost cells. In HbSC disease, the PCV and red cell mass average about 80 percent to 85 percent of normal. As conjectured for sickle cell anemia (Steinberg et al., 1977), it was hypothesized that an increased p^{50} and enhanced tissue extraction of O$_2$ blunted erythropoiesis in HbSC disease (Bannerman et al., 1979). While the lack of an appropriate erythropoietic response can probably be traced, at least in part, to low oxygen affinity of the hemoglobin in the red cell (see above), serum erythropoietin levels have not been reported in HbSC disease (Bannerman et al., 1979). Impaired erythropoietin production due to subclinical renal disease or an inappropriate erythroid response intrinsic to the bone marrow could also be involved in the genesis of anemia. Hemoglobin-oxygen affinity of hemoglobin solutions isolated from HbSC disease red cells is normal. However, the red cell density is abnormal in this disorder, which affects the polymerization of the HbS in HbSC disease cells and hemoglobin-oxygen equilibria. HbSC disease cells had a p^{50} of 32 mm Hg when suspended in isotonic media but when osmolality is reduced to 240 mOsm, normalizing the MCHC, the p^{50} was restored to a nearly normal 27.5 mm Hg (Fabry et al., 1982). These results emphasize that the properties of intact cells are most relevant for understanding disease pathophysiology

Even in the presence of erythropoietic stress, the β^C haplotype is associated with a relative low HbF expression compared to most individuals with sickle cell anemia (Table 27.2). HbSC disease patients usually have HbF concentrations less than 2 percent. While hemolysis and bone marrow expansion in HbSC disease is less than in sickle cell anemia, other influences on HbF in HbSC disease may be genetically determined. In parts of Africa where HbC and HbS coexist geographically, the β-globin gene clusters of HbSC disease patients are unavoidably a combination of the typical β^C haplotype and the Benin β^S-globin gene haplotype.

HbSC disease patients usually have low HbF levels but occasionally the HbF in adults is near 10 percent. HbSC disease patients have different combinations of β^C and β^S haplotypes. Individuals with exceptionally high HbF levels might carry recombinations with other β-globin gene cluster haplotypes or non-β-globin gene-linked genetic elements that influence γ-globin gene expression. HbF is unlikely to have a major effect on the hematology or clinical features of HbSC disease because of its low level in the majority of patients (Bannerman et al., 1979). Patients with sickle cell ane-

Table 27.2. Hematologic Features in Different Haplotypes of HbSC Disease

Group-n	Age (y) Gender	Hb (g/dL)	Reticulocytes (%)	MCV (fl)	HbS (%)	HbF (%)
BEN/C-41	32.9/61 F	11 ± 1.4	4.4 ± 3.0	82.6 ± 7.4	51.5 ± 3.4	1.3 ± 1.2
CAR/C-18	33.4/61 F	12 ± 1.5	4.2 ± 1.7	82.1 ± 7.4	53.8 ± 3.4	2.0 ± 2.0
SEN/C-5	30.5/60 F	11 ± 1.2	4.8 ± 0.6	89.3 ± 4.7	53.5 ± 2.7	2.0 ± 1.9
ATYP/C-9	32.5/89 F	12 ± 1.1	4.3 ± 1.5	85.9 ± 8.4	51.3 ± 1.7	1.9 ± 1.6

Adapted from Steinberg et al. (1996), with permission.

mia and a Bantu haplotype have levels of $^G\gamma$-globin chains that are widely dispersed and often far below 50 percent. Individuals with Senegal or Arab-Indian haplotypes have $^G\gamma$-globin chain levels above 50 percent. Individuals with HbSC and HbC disease, regardless of haplotype, have similar $^G\gamma$-globin chain levels despite different degrees of erythropoietic stress.

α Thalassemia, a known modulator of sickle cell anemia (Steinberg and Embury, 1986), does not appear to have a major effect on the hematology of HbSC disease or its clinical course although it is associated with the expected microcytosis (Steinberg et al., 1983; Rodgers et al., 1986).

HbSC/Hb-G Philadelphia Disease.

This genotype has a special phenotype because the hybrid molecule, $\alpha_2{}^{\text{G-Philadelphia}}\,\beta_2{}^C$ increases the rate of crystal nucleation compared to native HbC (Lawrence et al., 1997). HbS enhances this effect in a pathogenetically relevant manner. Heterozygotes for the β^S, β^C, and the $\alpha^{\text{G-Philadelphia}}$ genes (HbSC/Hb-G Philadelphia disease) have abundant circulating intraerythrocytic crystals and increased numbers of folded red cells with a mild clinical course. This phenotype seems to be the result of increased crystallization and decreased polymerization caused by the effects of the $\alpha^{\text{G-Philadelphia}}$ globin chain on the β^C and β^S gene products. Some of the intraerythrocytic crystals in this syndrome, unlike the typical crystal of HbSC disease, are unusually long and thin, resembling sugar cane (Fig. 27.13). A mild clinical course associated with increased crystallization

Figure 27.13. Blood smear directly from fingerstick blood from a patient with SC$^{\alpha\text{G-Philadelphia}}$ disease. Open arrow depicts a "sugar cane" crystal, a shape not observed in HbC disease or HbSC disease blood. The black arrows depict red cells with more classical forms of HbC-dependent crystals. (From Lawrence et al., 1997 with permission.) For full color representation, see color plate 27.13.

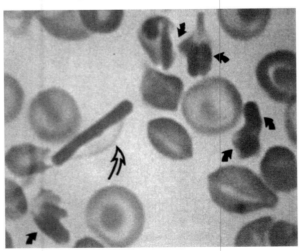

implies that, in HbSC disease, polymerization of HbS is pathogenically more important than the crystallization induced by β^C chains. HbSC/Hb-G Philadelphia disease is an example of nonallelic variant hemoglobins interacting to create a unique phenotype.

Growth and Development.

Growth in HbSC disease is delayed, but less so than in sickle cell anemia. With access to reasonable nutrition, Tanner stages of adult sexual development are achieved at 14 to 16 and 16 to 18 years of age in girls and boys, respectively, 1 to 2 years earlier than in children with sickle cell anemia (Platt et al., 1984). In some studies, HbSC disease does not appear to affect height, weight, and bone age (Stevens et al., 1986). A study of 298 children with sickle cell anemia and 157 children with HbSC disease revealed that, after 5 years, HbSC disease children had normal growth (Stevens et al., 1986).

Mortality.

A 1989 report indicated that 95 percent of patients with HbSC disease in the United States survived to age 20 years (Leikin et al., 1989). These individuals were participants in a university-based Cooperative Study (see Chapter 24) and many attended comprehensive sickle cell centers, making it possible that they had more regular and skilled care than the general population with HbSC disease. Mortality in this series was greatest in children between ages 1 to 3 years and was most often a result of pneumococcal sepsis. Another study, reported in 1990, where 231 individuals with HbSC disease were compared to 785 sickle cell anemia patients, showed an age-specific death rate (per 100 person-years) up to age 30 years of less than one in HbSC disease compared to two to three for sickle cell anemia. Beyond this age, mortality in all patients increased; still, the rate in HbSC disease was less than half that of sickle cell anemia (Powars et al., 1990). In the largest study of mortality from the United States, again from the national Cooperative Study, the median survival in HbSC disease was 60 years for men and 68 years for women; 3 percent, or 27 of 844 individuals, died during the 6-year follow-up (Platt et al., 1994). Survival curves comparing patients with HbSC disease and sickle cell anemia are shown in Figure 27.14. Jamaican children with HbSC disease, diagnosed by cord blood screening and so unlikely to represent a biased sample, had a 95 percent chance of surviving to the age of 2 years (Rogers et al., 1978). It has been theorized that since these reports, the mortality of sickle cell anemia has fallen in developed countries because of the widespread use of prophylactic penicillin and hydroxyurea. Penicillin prophylaxis is not uniformly used in HbSC disease and the indications—if any—for hydroxyurea in HbSC disease are just being defined, so both are unlikely to reduce further mortality. It is con-

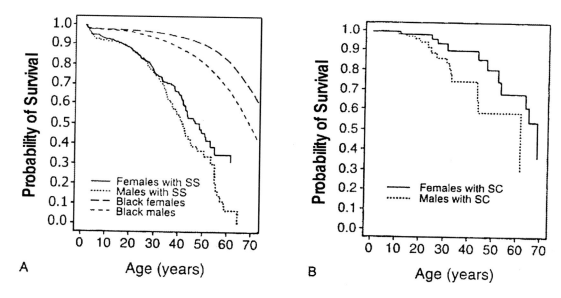

Figure 27.14. Survival curves comparing patients with HbSC disease (SS) and sickle cell anemia. (From Platt et al., 1994, with permission.)

ceivable that, failing major advances in supportive care or in the clinical usefulness of innovative treatments being developed (see Chapters 40 to 42), mortality in HbSC disease will not fall further.

There are few data on risk factors for early death in HbSC disease. Median age of onset for irreversible organ failure—stroke, renal failure, and chronic lung disease—that might contribute to early mortality in HbSC disease is 10 to 35 years later than in sickle cell anemia (Powars et al., 1990). Even in large series of patients, relatively small numbers of deaths occur in HbSC disease, making it difficult to assess the relationship of HbF, leukocyte count, and prior vasoocclusive episodes such as pain and acute chest syndrome to mortality in HbSC disease. HbF levels may not play the key role in morbidity and mortality that they do in sickle cell anemia. It is clear that HbSC disease has a pattern of survival that is different from sickle cell anemia. Increased mortality of HbSC disease is apparent only after age 20 years. Overall prognosis of HbSC disease is therefore better than that for sickle cell anemia.

Vasoocclusive Disease

Patients with HbSC disease can have all of the vasoocclusive problems of sickle cell anemia but usually have a milder clinical course. In a survey of ninety Jamaican patients with HbSC disease, Serjeant found pathology similar to sickle cell anemia, but with generally reduced severity except for retinal vascular disease (Serjeant et al., 1973). He speculated that this latter feature might be related to the higher hemoglobin lev-

els found in HbSC disease. In a pediatric cohort, 50 percent were found to develop symptoms of sickle cell disease by age 5 years but 22 percent remained free of symptoms at age 10 years (Bainbridge et al., 1985). This is consistent with a relatively mild early course of HbSC disease. Many individuals with HbSC disease are active in quite strenuous occupations. Some never have the occasion to seek medical attention for unique events of sickle cell disease and have their diagnosis established incidental to another medical condition (Serjeant et al., 1973). Rarely, the presenting attribute of HbSC disease is calamitous, such as life-threatening acute chest syndrome, sepsis, or splenic sequestration. Therefore, while often mild and needing little medical supervision, HbSC disease should not be neglected. Patients with HbSC disease should be detected by neonatal screening so that they and their families can be enrolled in programs providing education about the potential complications of this disorder and the needed level of continued monitoring.

Proliferative Retinopathy and Eye Disease. Proliferative sickle retinopathy is perhaps the most typical vasoocclusive complication of HbSC disease (Fig. 27.15). More common in this genotype, where it is found in a third of patients as opposed to sickle cell anemia where only 3 percent are affected the pathology of this entity was delineated in detail by Welch and Goldberg in 1966 (Welch and Goldberg, 1966; Fox et al., 1990; Lutty and Goldberg, 1994). Age-adjusted prevalence of proliferative retinopathy in 533 patients with HbSC disease is shown in Table 27.3. The distinctive "black sea fan," "black sunburst," and salmon patches typify this disorder and characterize the hemorrhagic, infarctive, proliferative, and resolving lesions of sickle retinopathy. Conjoint effects of a

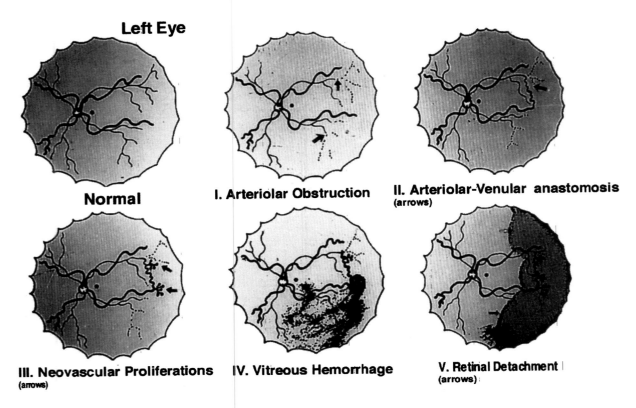

Figure 27.15. Stages of proliferative sickle retinopathy.

higher PCV, increased cell density, and greater blood viscosity in HbSC disease may account for the higher prevalence of retinopathy in HbSC disease than in sickle cell anemia; it is also possible that the lower HbF levels of HbSC disease play a role. A discussion of the pathophysiology of retinopathy in sickle cell disease and the use of transgenic mice to study this condition is presented in Chapter 20.

Paradoxically, the high prevalence of proliferative retinopathy in HbSC disease may be an expression of

the relative benignity of this genotype. A new classification of the peripheral retinal vascular changes in sickle cell disease, based on the appearance of the peripheral retinal vasculature, has been proposed (Penman et al., 1994). Vessels are either "normal" (Type I) or abnormal (Type IIa or IIb) based on qualitative changes such as irregular vascular margins, capillary stumps, hyper- or hypofluorescence, and capillary bed thinning. This classification is based on the observation that proliferative retinopathy develops in response to progressive closure of the vessels of the peripheral retina and the recession centripetally of the margin of retinal perfusion (Talbot et al., 1982, 1996). An abnormal peripheral retinal vasculature is present in about 80 percent of adults with HbSC disease (Kent et al., 1994). By age 17 years, the prevalence of abnormal vascular borders is about 60 percent (Penman et al., 1994). More than 260 patients with sickle cell anemia and 154 with HbSC disease were studied with serial fluorescein angiography and retinal photography, beginning at ages 6 to 12 years (Penman et al., 1994). In the teenage years, each year there is a 6 percent conversion from normal to abnormal vascular border. The occurrence of sickle proliferative retinopathy was always associated with an abnormal vascular border. In sickle cell anemia, peripheral retinal vessels are occluded early in the course of disease so that further retinal vascular damage and proliferative lesions cannot develop. The enhanced circulatory competence of

Table 27.3. Age-Related Prevalence of Proliferative Sickle Retinopathy in HbSC Disease

Age (y)	No. of patients	Percent with retinopathy
0–9	47	0
10–14	77	6
15–19	117	14
20–24	81	27
25–29	67	60
30–39	88	57
>40	56	70
Total	533	32

the HbSC disease cell may preserve this retinal circulation, permitting the later development of proliferative lesions. If this is true, as hydroxyurea treatment makes sickle cell anemia cells more like HbSC disease cells, the prevalence of proliferative retinopathy may begin to increase in young sickle cell anemia patients treated with this drug.

Sickle retinopathy is recognizable by its different stages that include nonproliferative lesions and three stages of proliferative lesions, including neovascularization, vitreous hemorrhage, and retinal detachment. Whether there is an orderly progression from less to more serious stages that precedes retinal detachment and blindness, or if catastrophic changes can arise directly from early stages of proliferative retinopathy, is not well characterized. Characteristically, following vasoocclusion in the peripheral vessels of the retina—the nonproliferative stages of retinopathy—neovascular malformations called "black sea fans" grow from the retinal surface into the vitreous. These fragile new vessels may leak blood into the vitreous, at times in amounts sufficient to reduce vision. Organization of vitreal hemorrhages exerts traction on the inelastic retina, causing tears and allowing vitreal fluid to enter the subretinal space. Retinal detachment, a potential consequence of subretinal fluid invasion, can produce blindness. Of fourteen patients with HbSC disease who were selected for study because they had nonproliferative lesions of peripheral retinal arteriolar occlusion or AV anastomoses, 21 percent developed new sea fans with an average interval of 18 months (range 8 to 36 months). Based on these rather small numbers of patients, the authors estimated that about 14 percent of young adults with HbSC disease develop neovascularization each year (Raichand et al., 1977). Complicating the evaluation of retinopathy in HbSC disease is the propensity for spontaneous regression of proliferative lesions due to autoinfarction (Nagpal et al., 1975). However, these authors caution that withholding treatment in the hopes of a spontaneous regression is dangerous since the incidence of spontaneous vitreal hemorrhage increased from 28 percent to 44 percent in patients observed for 6 to 77 months (Goldberg, 1971; Nagpal et al., 1975).

Twenty-nine patients with HbSC disease, picked randomly from a clinic population, were enrolled and followed with annual or 6-monthly detailed ophthalmologic examinations (Clarkson, 1992). At the initial examination, eleven patients had stage III retinopathy and their average length of followup was 7 months. Twelve patients had normal findings or stage I or II disease and they were followed for 88 months. The lesions that were present are summarized in Table 27.4.

The natural history of proliferative retinopathy in HbSC disease compared with sickle cell anemia, in

Table 27.4. Prevalence of Ocular Lesions in HbSC Disease

Ocular lesion	%
Nonproliferative	
Salmon patch	17
Iridescent spot	28
Black sunburst	62
Proliferative	
Stage III, neovascularization	45
Stage IV, vitreous hemorrhage	21
Stage V, retinal detachment	10

patients who presented with stage III disease, is shown in Table 27.5 (Clarkson, 1992). In the twenty-three patients with HbSC disease, 48 percent had proliferative disease upon initial examination and 74 percent developed stages III to V disease at final examination while there was little change over time in the prevalence of nonproliferative retinopathy in either HbSC disease or sickle cell anemia patients (Clarkson, 1992).

In studies from Jamaica, 115 patients (270 eyes) with HbSC disease were followed sequentially (Condon and Serjeant, 1980a). Efforts were made to ensure that this was a random sample of HbSC disease patients. Proliferative retinopathy was present in 24 percent of patients at the initial examination, arose de novo during the study in 18 percent, and was present at the final examination in 40 percent. The mean age of patients showing progression was 27.7 years. Of forty-three individuals, fifty-eight new lesions were found in eighteen patients less than age 25 years and the highest risk period was age 20 to 24 years. Two-thirds of patients with de novo proliferative lesions were ages 15 to 29 years. About one-third to one-half of patients had autoinfarction during the course of the study. From ages 10 to 39 years, about 7 percent of individuals in each 5-year age bracket developed proliferative retinopathy per 100

Table 27.5. Natural History of Proliferative Retinopathy in Sickle Cell Disease

	Sickle cell anemia	HbSC disease
No. of eyes	17	19
Length of observation (mo)	69	77
Stable disease (%)	59	26
Regression (%)	18	42
Progression (%)	35	58
Vitreous hemorrhage (%)	6	37
Retinal detachment (%)	6	6

Table 27.6. Evolution of Proliferative Retinopathy in HbSC Disease According to Age

Age (y)	Eyes (no.)	Progression (%)	Regression (%)	Stable (%)
10–19	10	40	30	30
20–29	47	60	17	23
30–39	56	43	27	30
>40	24	29	4	67

patient-years of observation (Fox et al., 1990). In further studies of the Jamaican HbSC disease population, the natural history of retinopathy was studied (Fox et al., 1991). These results, summarized in Table 27.6 indicate that progressive disease was most frequent between ages 20 and 39 years. However, visual loss occurred in only 9 percent of patients followed for a mean of 4.5 years (Fox et al., 1991).

Abnormal conjunctival vessels are typical in sickle cell disease but in distinction to proliferative retinopathy, are more common in sickle cell anemia than in HbSC disease. Comma-shaped and corkscrew conjunctival vessels are visible with the ophthalmoscope and typical of sickling hemoglobinopathies. Ophthalmologic abnormalities of sickle cell disease have been comprehensively reviewed (Serjeant, 1992; Embury et al., 1994).

Special problems associated with the treatment of hyphema in carriers of HbS are discussed in Chapter 29.

Treatment Recommendations. Management of sickle proliferative retinopathy is imperfect. Incipient proliferative disease has been treated with focal or pan-retinal section photocoagulation to forestall advancing pathology and impaired vision. Some of the earliest

comparative trials were inconclusive and questioned the role of photocoagulation but different techniques of treatment and new technologies now make these results difficult to interpret. (Condon and Serjeant, 1980b). There are presently no data that conclusively show that prophylactic photocoagulation significantly changes the natural history of retinopathy (Clarkson, 1992). In a randomized trial of argon laser scatter photocoagulation, ninety-nine eyes were treated and seventy-five eyes served as controls, with an average followup of about 45 months (Farber et al., 1991). There was complete or partial regression of sea fans in 81 percent of treated eyes and spontaneous regression in 46 percent of control eyes. New sea fans developed in 34 percent of treated compared to 41 percent of control eyes. The cumulative percentage of treated and control eyes developing either visual loss or vitreous hemorrhage is shown in Figure 27.16.

Using the criteria of visual loss, five control eyes and three treated eyes lost vision during followup, a difference that is not significant and similar to that observed in an observational study, while the incidence of retinal detachment was not clearly reduced (Clarkson, 1992). It was suggested that a controlled trial of patients with HbSC disease, ages 15 to 30 years and with 60 degrees or more of proliferative disease, be undertaken (Clarkson, 1992). Some data suggest that proliferative retinopathy is most prevalent in individuals with higher hemoglobin levels (Condon and Serjeant, 1972). Phlebotomy, to reduce the hemoglobin concentration to 9 to 10 g/dL, has also been advocated as a measure to

Figure 27.16. Survival curves for loss of visual acuity (L) and vitreous hemorrhage (R) in treated (....) and control (- - - - -) eyes. (Modified from Farber et al., 1991, with permission.)

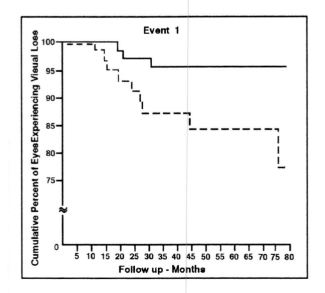

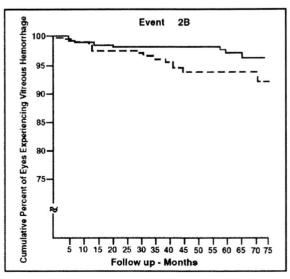

prevent retinopathy or slow its advancement—without evidence of the efficacy of this treatment.

In summary, proliferative retinopathy occurs often in patients with HbSC disease between the ages of 15 and 30 years, is progressive, can culminate in visual loss, and does not have a definitive treatment that can eliminate its most severe endpoints. Averting the costs—monetary and otherwise—of frequent ophthalmologic studies and blindness would be a major adjunct in the management of HbSC disease.

Painful Episodes. In a given year, over one-half of 806 patients with HbSC disease did not have a painful episode, one-third had a single episode of pain, and less than 10 percent had three or more pain episodes (Platt et al., 1991). This rate was about 0.4 episodes per patient-year, less than half the rate in sickle cell anemia. Forty percent of Jamaican patients with HbSC disease had at least one pain episode requiring hospitalization; 17 percent never reported a pain episode. (Serjeant et al., 1973). About 60 percent of HbSC disease patients in Los Angeles reported a least one pain episode (Powars et al., 1990). Treatment of painful episodes is detailed in Chapter 25.

Acute Chest Syndrome. Acute chest syndrome, with its high morbidity, propensity to cause chronic lung disease, and appreciable mortality, is seen in about 30 percent of patients with HbSC disease (Powars et al., 1990). While this incidence is only 50 percent to 75 percent that of sickle cell anemia, progression to chronic lung disease is only 0.1 percent that of sickle cell anemia and the median age of onset is almost one decade later (Powars et al., 1990; Castro et al., 1994). The incidence per 100 patient-years in patients of all ages is 5.2. Typical of this condition, the incidence in children age 5 years is twice that of older individuals (Castro et al., 1994). Only steady-state leukocyte count was a risk factor for acute chest syndrome in HbSC disease. When compared to sickle cell anemia, there were no differences in length of hospitalization or death rate but sickle cell anemia patients were more likely to present with severe pain (Vichinsky et al., 1997).

The Spleen. Splenic function is often preserved in HbSC disease while it is rarely preserved in sickle cell anemia. A positive result of retained splenic function is the reduced incidence of infection with encapsulated bacteria. A negative result is the chance for splenic sequestration crises and splenic infarction to occur in adults. The pathology of the spleen is quite prominent in HbSC disease.

Pocked, or "pitted" red cells are found in increased numbers when splenic function declines and is lost, and can be used as a measure of functional asplenia when splenomegaly is present. When pitted red cell counts were used to evaluate splenic reticuloendothelial function in HbSC disease, there were 4.9 ± 9.1 percent pitted cells in this disorder compared to 11.8 ± 7.0 percent in sickle cell anemia—splenic function was better preserved in HbSC disease. Pitted cells increased with age for the sickle cell anemia group but did not in HbSC disease patients, suggesting they had stabilized splenic function (Fatunde and Scott, 1986). This observation is consistent with the preservation of splenic function to a greater degree and for a longer period in HbSC disease than in sickle cell anemia. However, a discrepancy between pit counting and splenic function tests has been noted in HbC disease (Zago et al., 1986).

Slightly over one-half of all adults with HbSC disease had splenomegaly, 36 percent were asplenic, and 12 percent had normal spleens when evaluated by spleen scanning (Serjeant et al., 1973; Ballas et al., 1982). When "pit" counts were related to spleen scans, no patient with HbSC disease less than age 4 years had functional asplenia while this abnormality was present in 22 percent of individuals ages 4 to 12 years and 45 percent of individuals older than age 12 years (Lane et al., 1995).

Six percent of children with HbSC disease had splenic complications that included acute sequestration crisis, painful infarction, and hemorrhage (Aquino et al., 1997). Similar events can occur in adults with HbSC disease, whereas they are very rare in adult sickle cell anemia (Sear and Udden, 1985). Coexistent hereditary spherocytosis and HbSC disease was deemed responsible for multiple episodes of splenic sequestration crises in one interesting case report. It was hypothesized that increased density and reduced deformability of red cells engendered by both disorders caused increased splenic trapping and sickling (Warkentin et al., 1990).

Infection. The relative risk of bacteremia is less for HbSC disease patients than for sickle cell anemia patients when correction is made for the total nonhospitalized population at risk, but is much larger than that for the normal population; however, the type of systemic infection most commonly found in HbSC disease patients (gram-negative bacteremia) was less life-threatening than the pyogenic bacteremia most commonly found in sickle cell anemia. Normal splenic function, as estimated by "pit" counts in children age 4 years and less with HbSC disease, suggested that prophylactic penicillin need not be used in this age group (Lane et al., 1995). Two adolescents with functional asplenia were reported to die of pneumococcal sepsis. Fatal pneumococcal sepsis has been described in children age 5 years and below, none of whom were receiving penicillin at the time of their terminal illness (Lane et al., 1994). Their splenic function was not known.

Treatment Recommendations. Some authorities question the use of prophylactic penicillin in HbSC disease (Rogers and Buchanan, 1995a, 1995b). A reasonable approach in children who are most susceptible to pneumococcal infection might be to assess splenic function by "pit" counts, the presence of Howell-Jolly bodies, or radionuclide scanning (Yam and Li, 1994). If splenic function is normal, prophylaxis may be withheld. It should be remembered that in sickle cell disease, a large spleen does not always equate with a normally functional spleen. Pneumococcal vaccine should be given at ages 2 and 5 years and parents instructed to seek immediate medical attention for febrile illnesses.

Osteonecrosis. Usually painful and often disabling, the incidence of osteonecrosis in HbSC disease is only slightly lower than in sickle cell anemia, with an age-adjusted incidence rate of 1.9/100 patient-years for the hip joints and 1.7/100 patient-years for shoulders (Milner et al., 1991, 1993). Shoulder disease was uncommon in patients less than age 25 years. In the Cooperative Study of Sickle Cell Disease, osteonecrosis of the femoral heads was almost as prevalent in HbSC disease (8.8 percent) as in sickle cell anemia (10.2 percent), results closely echoed by other studies of large patient groups (Serjeant et al., 1973; Powars et al., 1990; Milner et al., 1991). Median estimated age at diagnosis in HbSC disease was 40 years versus 36 years for sickle cell anemia and 26 years for sickle cell anemia-α thalassemia (Milner et al., 1991).

Renal Disease. The pathophysiology of renal lesions in HbSC disease is similar to that in sickle cell trait and sickle cell anemia. Hematuria is often present and appears to be more frequent than in sickle cell trait (Dacie, 1988). In HbSC disease, renal concentrating ability is lost at a time intermediate between the loss in sickle cell anemia and sickle cell trait (Statius van Eps et al., 1967, 1970; Lesorbe et al., 1978). Maximum concentrating ability in fourteen patients with HbSC diseases, ages 6 to 65 years (mean age 30 years), was 537 mOsm and appeared to decline with age (Statius van Eps et al., 1970). In this study, the two youngest patients, ages 6 and 8 years, had maximally concentrated urines of 640 and 698 mOsm, about 60 percent of normal. In eight children with HbSC disease, ages 10 to 17 years (mean age 11 years), none had an overnight urine concentration greater than 545 mOsm (mean 445 mOsm; normal range 800–1,000 mOsm). Seven of these eight children increased their urine concentration after receiv-

ing dDAVP, although none increased urine concentration to normal (Iyer et al., in press). Renal function deteriorates with age as it does in sickle cell anemia but chronic renal failure is half as common as in sickle cell anemia (2.2 percent) and its median age of onset is 25 years later (Powars et al., 1990, 1991; West et al., 1992). In one study, 73 percent of twenty-seven patients had papillary necrosis based on calyceal blunting by intravenous pyelography (Ballas et al., 1982). In this total patient group, renal function was normal and the clinical significance of this observation is unclear.

Cerebrovascular Disease. Two to three percent of HbSC disease patients had stroke (Powars et al., 1990). This incidence was 3 to 4 times less than in sickle cell anemia. In the Cooperative Study, 0.8 percent of individuals with HbSC disease compared to 4 percent of patients with sickle cell anemia had suffered a stroke at study entry (Ohene-Frempong et al., 1998). The age-adjusted incidence of stroke in HbSC disease was 4 times less than in sickle cell anemia.

Pregnancy. Perinatal mortality in HbSC disease has been reported to vary from 28 percent to nil in the absence of transfusions and from 0 to 9 percent when transfusions were given (Koshy and Burd, 1994). In this heterogeneous collection of patient series with widely different numbers of cases, more recent reports generally had lower mortality. Pregnancy-related complications are higher than in normal controls and not dissimilar to those in sickle cell anemia and the rate of Caesarean sections is similar (Koshy et al., 1988). Although HbSC disease may remain dormant for long periods, stress or pregnancy may result in exacerbation and the pregnant HbSC disease patient may be as severely affected as the sickle cell anemia patient. Pregnancy in sickle cell disease and recommendations for management are discussed in more detail in Chapter 24.

Treatment of HbSC Disease

There are no forms of therapy unique for HbSC disease compared to sickle cell anemia. Vasoocclusive complications, when they occur, are treated the same as in sickle cell anemia. HbSC disease has distinct pathophysiologic features that may provide a future basis for a direct attack on some of the basic mechanisms of disease. These involve reversing the dehydration, increased density, and decreased deformability of HbSC disease erythrocytes (see above). Membrane-active drugs might be especially useful for treatment (Berkowitz and Orringer, 1981; Clark et al., 1982; Benjamin et al., 1986; Wolff et al., 1988; Orringer et al., 1991; Brugnara et al., 1993).

Several drugs block erythrocyte membrane cation-transport channels and can restore toward normal cellular cation content and density (Berkowitz and Orringer, 1981; Clark et al., 1982; Wolff et al., 1988; Orringer et al., 1991; Brugnara et al., 1993) (see Chapter 42). Clotrimazole, an antifungal agent, reduced cellular dehydration in vitro in a transgenic mouse model of sickle cell disease and when given to patients with sickle cell anemia (Brugnara et al., 1993; De Franceschi et al., 1994; Brugnara et al., 1996). Recent studies in sickle cell anemia showed that cell density changes are achievable with well-tolerated doses of this drug (Brugnara et al., 1996). However, the reduction in cell density is modest and less than observed following hydroxyurea treatment of sickle cell anemia. Magnesium salts also interfere with cation transport and cause cell rehydration. Whether these cellular changes will have clinical utility in HbSC disease awaits proof by controlled trials. These types of experimental therapy are discussed in detail in Chapter 42. Hydroxyurea can effect changes in the HbSC disease erythrocyte that may be independent of any change in HbF. Early trials of hydroxyurea in HbSC disease are discussed in Chapter 38.

Transfusions are used in HbSC disease for the same indications as in sickle cell anemia. A recent study has provided much needed information on preoperative transfusion in HbSC disease (Neumayr et al., 1998). Eighteen percent of all patients had some postoperative complication. Postoperative events were compared between the 38 percent of seventy-five patients with HbSC disease who received preoperative transfusions and in the remainder who were not transfused before surgery. This study was not randomized and both simple and exchange transfusions were used. Preoperative hemoglobin level in transfused patients was 12 g/dL with HbA levels between 35 percent and 50 percent. Nine percent of all patients had postoperative acute chest syndrome or painful episodes. Nearly 40 percent of surgery was intraabdominal, and in this group 35 percent of patients who were not transfused had an acute chest syndrome or painful episodes compared to none who were transfused. Based on these observations and the larger study of preoperative transfusion in sickle cell anemia (Vichinsky et al., 1995), it appears prudent to use preoperative transfusion in patients with HbSC disease who face procedures with moderate surgical risk, such as abdominal surgery.

SUMMARY

The positively charged HbC molecule induces changes in the HbC trait and homozygous HbC disease erythrocyte that are a result of cellular dehydration. Although biologically interesting and producing characteristic hematologic features in the HbC-containing cell, the clinical abnormalities associated with HbC trait and HbC disease are trivial. This is not so when HbC is present with HbS. HbSC disease is a clinically important illness with all of the complications of sickle cell anemia, albeit at a reduced rate, and an effective treatment would be a major medical advance.

References

Adachi, H and Asakura, T. (1979). The solubility of sickle and non-sickle hemoglobins in concentrated phosphate buffer. *J. Biol. Chem.* 254: 4079–4084.

Altay, C, Niazi, GA, and Huisman, THJ. (1976). The combination of Hb S and Hb E in a black female. *Hemoglobin* 1: 100–102.

Anyaibe, S, Wilson, P, Scott, R et al. (1983). Relative proportions of human hemoglobins A, S and C in individual erythrocytes of heterozygotes. *Hemoglobin* 7: 227–244.

Aquino, VM, Norvell, JM, and Buchanan, GR. (1997). Acute splenic complications in children with sickle cell hemoglobin C disease. *J. Pediatr.* 130: 961–965.

Bainbridge, R, Higgs, DR, Maude, GH et al. (1985). Clinical presentation of homozygous sickle cell disease. *J. Pediatr.* 106: 881–885.

Ballas, SK, Embi, K, Goshar, D et al. (1981). Binding of β^s, β^c, and $\beta^{O\ Arab}$ globins to the erythrocyte membrane. *Hemoglobin* 5: 501–505.

Ballas, SK, Lewis, CN, Noone, AM et al. (1982). Clinical, hematological and biochemical features of HbSC disease. *Am. J. Hematol.* 13: 37–51.

Ballas, SK, and Smith, ED. (1992). Red blood cell changes during the evolution of the sickle cell painful crisis. *Blood* 79: 2154–2163.

Bannerman, RM, Serjeant, B, Seakins, M et al. (1979). Determinants of haemoglobin level in sickle cell-haemoglobin C disease. *Br. J. Haematol.* 43: 49–56.

Benjamin, LJ, Berkowitz, LR, Orringer, EP et al. (1986). A collaborative, double-blind randomized study of cetiadil citrate in sickle cell crisis. *Blood* 67: 1442–1447.

Berkowitz, LR, and Orringer, EP. (1981). Effect of Cetiadil, an in-vitro anti-sickling agent, on erythrocyte membrane cation permeability. *J. Clin. Invest.* 68: 1215–1220.

Boehm, CD, Dowling, CE, Antonarakis, SE et al. (1985). Evidence supporting a single origin of the $\beta^{(C)}$-globin gene in blacks. *Am. J. Hum. Genet.* 37: 771–777.

Brittain, HA, Eckman, JR, Swerlick, RA et al. (1993). Thrombospondin from activated platelets promotes sickle erythrocyte adherence to human microvascular endothelium under physiologic flow: A potential role for platelet activation in sickle cell vaso-occlusion. *Blood* 81: 2137–2143.

Brugnara, C, Kopin, AS, Bunn, HF et al. (1984). Electrolyte composition and equilibrium in hemoglobin CC red blood cells. *Trans. Assoc. Am. Phys.* 97: 104–112.

Brugnara, C, Kopin, AS, Bunn, HF et al. (1985). Regulation of cation content and cell volume in hemoglobin erythrocytes from patients with homozygous hemoglobin C disease. *J. Clin. Invest.* 75: 1608–1617.

Brugnara, C, De Franceschi, L, and Alper, SL. (1993). Inhibition of Ca²⁺-dependent K⁺ transport and cell dehydration in sickle erythrocytes by clotrimazole and other imidazole derivatives. *J. Clin. Invest.* 92: 520–526.

Brugnara, C, Armsby, CC, Sakamoto M et al. (1995). Oral administration of clotrimazole and blockade of human erythrocyte Ca⁺⁺-activated K⁺ channel: The imidazole ring is not required for inhibitory activity. *J. Pharmacol. Exp. Ther.* 273: 266–272.

Brugnara, C, Armsby, CC, Sakamoto M et al. (1995). Oral administration of clotrimazole and blockade of human erythrocyte Ca⁺⁺-activated K⁺ channel: The imidazole ring is not required for inhibitory activity. *J. Pharmacol. Exp. Ther.* 273: 266–272.

Brugnara, C, Gee, B, Armsby, CC et al. (1996). Therapy with oral clotrimazole induces inhibition of the Gardos channel and reduction of erythrocyte dehydration in patients with sickle cell disease. *J. Clin. Invest.* 97: 1227–1234.

Bunn, HF, and Briehl, RW. (1970). The interaction of 2,3-diphosphoglycerate with various human hemoglobins. *J. Clin. Invest.* 49: 1088.

Bunn, HF, and Forget, BG. (1986). *Hemoglobin: Molecular, Genetic and Clinical Aspects.* Philadelphia: W.B. Saunders.

Bunn, HF, Noguchi, CT, Hofrichter et al. (1982). Molecular and cellular pathogenesis of hemoglobin SC disease. *Proc. Natl. Acad. Sci. U.S.A.* 79: 7527–7531.

Canessa, M, Splavins, A, and Nagel, RL. (1986). Volume-dependent and NEM-stimulated K⁺ Cl⁻ transport is elevated in oxygenated SS SC and CC human cells. *FEBS Lett.* 200: 197–202.

Canessa, M, Fabry, ME, Blumenfeld, N et al. (1987a). A volume-stimulated Cl⁻ dependent K⁺ efflux is highly expressed in young human red cells containing normal hemoglobin or Hb S. *J. Membrane Biol.* 97: 97–105.

Canessa, M, Fabry, ME, and Nagel, RL. (1987b). Deoxygenation inhibits the chloride-dependent volume-stimulated K:Cl cotransport in SS and young AA cells: A modulatory effect of intraerythrocytic Mg²⁺. *Blood* 70: 1861–1866.

Castro, O, Brambilla, DJ, Thorington, B et al. and Coop Study of Sickle Cell Disease (1994). The acute chest syndrome in sickle cell disease: Incidence and risk factors. *Blood* 84, 643–649.

Chakravarti, A, Buetow, KH, Antonarakis, SE et al. (1984). Nonuniform recombination within the human β-globin gene cluster. *American Journal of Human Genetics* 36, 1239–1258.

Charache, S, Conley, CL, Waugh, DF et al. (1967). Pathogenesis of hemolytic anemia in homozygous hemoglobin C disease. *J. Clin. Invest.* 46: 1795–1811.

Charache, S, Conley, CL, Doeblin, TD et al. (1974). Thalassemia in black Americans. *Annals of the New York Academy of Sciences* 232, 125–134.

Clark, MR, Mohandas, N, and Shohet, SB. (1982). Hydration of sickle cells using the sodium ionophore Monesin: A model for therapy. *J. Clin. Invest.* 70: 1074–1080.

Clarkson, JG. (1992). The ocular manifestations of sickle-cell disease: A prevalence and natural history study. *Trans. Am. Ophthalmol. Soc.* 90: 481–504.

Coletta, M, Hofrichter, J, Ferrone, FA et al. (1982). Kinetics of sickle haemoglobin polymerization in single red cells. *Nature* 300: 194–197.

Condon, PI, and Serjeant, GR. (1972). Ocular findings in hemoglobin SC disease in Jamaica. *Am. J. Ophthalmol.* 74: 921–931.

Condon, PI, and Serjeant, GR. (1980a). Behavior of untreated proliferative sickle retinopathy. *Br. J. Ophthalmol.* 64: 404–411.

Condon, PI and Serjeant, GR. (1980b). Photocoagulation in proliferative sickle retinopathy: Results of a 5-year study. *Br. J. Ophthalmol.* 64: 832–840.

Conley, CL. (1964). Pathophysiological effects of some abnormal hemoglobins. *Medicine* 43: 785–787.

Daar, S, Hussain, HM, Nagel, RL et al. (1998). Genetic epidemiology of HbC in Oman: an independent origin for HbC^Oman. *Am. J. Hematol.*

Dacie, J. (1988). *The Haemolytic Anaemias,* 3rd ed. Edinburgh: Churchill Livingstone. pp. 1–588.

De Franceschi, L, Saadane, N, Trudel, M et al. (1994). Treatment with oral clotrimazole blocks Ca²⁺-activated K⁺ transport and reverses erythrocyte dehydration in transgenic SAD mice. A model for therapy of sickle cell disease. *J. Clin. Invest.* 93: 1670–1676.

Dias-Da-Motta, PM, Arruda, VR, Muscará, MN et al. (1996). The release of nitric oxide and superoxide anion by neutrophils and mononuclear cells from patients with sickle cell anaemia. *Br. J. Haematol.* 93: 333–340.

Diggs, LW, Kraus, AP, Morrison, DB et al. (1954). Intraerythrocytic crystals in a white patient with hemoglobin C in the absence of other types of hemoglobin. *Blood* 9: 1172–1184.

Ducrocq, R, Bennani, M, Bellis, G et al. (1994). Hemoglobinopathies in the Dogon country: Presence of β^s, β^c, and δ^A' genes. *Am. J. Hematol.* 46: 245–247.

Dunham, PB, and Ellory, JC. (1981). Passive potassium transport in low potassium sheep red cells: Dependence upon cell volume and chloride. *J. Physiol.* 318: 511–530.

Eaton, WA, and Hofrichter, J. (1990). Sickle cell hemoglobin polymerization. *Adv. Protein Chem.* 40: 6–280.

Embury, SH, Clark, MR, Monroy, GM et al. (1984). Concurrent sickle cell anemia and α thalassemia. *J. Clin. Invest.* 73: 116–123.

Embury, SH, Hebbel, RP, Mohandas, N et al. (1994). *Sickle Cell Disease: Basic Principles and Clinical Practice.* 1st ed. New York: Raven Press.

Fabry, ME, Kaul, DK, Raventos-Suarez, C et al. (1981). Some aspects of the pathophysiology of homozygous hemoglobin C red cells. *J. Clin. Invest.* 67: 1284–1291.

Fabry, ME, Kaul, DK, Raventos-Suarez, C et al. (1982). SC cells have an abnormally high intracellular hemoglobin concentration: Pathophysiological consequences. *J. Clin. Invest.* 70: 1315–1319.

Fabry, ME, Benjamin, L, Lawrence, C et al. (1983). An objective sign of painful crisis in sickle cell anemia. *Blood* 64: 559–563.

Fabry, ME, Mears, JG, Patel, P et al. (1984). Dense cells in sickle cell anemia: The effects of gene interaction. *Blood* 64: 1042–1046.

Farber, MD, Jampol, LM, Fox, P et al. (1991). A randomized clinical trial of scatter photocoagulation of proliferative sickle retinopathy. *Arch. Ophthalmol.* 109: 363–367.

Fatunde, OJ and Scott, RB. (1986). Pitted red cell counts in sickle cell disease: Relationship to age, hemoglobin, genotype and splenic size. *Am. J. Pediatr. Hematol. Oncol.* 8: 329–333.

Feldenzer, J, Mears, JG, Burns, A et al. (1979). Heterogeneity of DNA fragments associated with the sickle-globin gene. *J. Clin. Invest.* 64: 751–755.

Fox, PD, Dunn, DT, Morris, JS et al. (1990). Risk factors for proliferative sickle retinopathy. *Br. J. Ophthalmol* 74: 172–176.

Fox, PD, Vessey, SJR, Forshaw, ML et al. (1991). Influence of genotype on the natural history of untreated proliferative sickle retinopathy—an angiographic study. *Br. J. Opthalmol.* 75: 229–231.

Gee, BE, and Platt, OS. (1995). Sickle reticulocytes adhere to VCAM-1. *Blood* 85: 268–274.

Giordano, PC, Harteveld, CL, Michiels, JJ et al. (1997). Atypical HbH disease in a Surinamese patient resulting from a combination of the -SEA and -$\alpha^{3.7}$ deletions with HbC heterozygosity. *Br. J. Haematol.* 96: 801–805.

Goldberg, MF. (1971). Natural history of untreated proliferative sickle retinopathy. *Arch. Ophthalmol.* 85: 428–437.

Hinchliffe, RF, Norcliffe, D, Farrar, LM et al. (1996). Mean cell haemoglobin concentration in subjects with haemoglobin C, D, E and S traits. *Clin. Lab. Haematol.* 18: 245–248.

Hirsch, RE, Raventos-Suarez, C, Olson, JA et al. (1985). Ligand state of intraerythrocytic circulating Hb C crystals in homozygous CC patients. *Blood* 66: 775–777.

Hirsch, RE, Lin, MJ, and Nagel, RL. (1988). The inhibition of hemoglobin C crystallization by hemoglobin F. *J. Biol. Chem.* 263: 5936–5939.

Hirsch, RE, Lin, MJ, Vidugirus, GVA et al. (1996). Conformational changes in oxyhemoglobin c (Glu$^{\beta6}$→lys) detected by spectroscopic probing. *J. Biol. Chem.* 271: 372–375.

Hirsch, RE, Witkowska, HE, Shafer, F et al. (1997). HbC compound heterozygotes [HbC/Hb Riyadh and HbC/Hb N-Baltimore] with opposing effects upon HbC crystallization. *Br. J. Haematol* 97: 259–265.

Hofstra, TC, Kalra, VK, Meiselman, HJ et al. (1996). Sickle erythrocytes adhere to polymorphonuclear neutrophils and activate the neutrophils' respiratory burst. *Blood* 87: 4440–4447.

Huisman, THJ. (1977). Trimodality in the percentage of β chain variants in heterozygotes: The effect of the number of active HB$_\alpha$ structural loci. *Hemoglobin* 1: 349–382.

Huisman, THJ, van der Schaaf, PC, and van der Sar, A. (1955). Some characteristic properties of Hb C. *Blood* 10: 1079–1091.

Hunt, AJ, and Ingram, VM. (1958). Allelomorphism and the chemical differences of the human hemoglobins A S and C. *Nature* 181: 162–163.

Itano, H. (1953). Solubility of naturally occurring mixtures of human hemoglobins. *Arch. Biochem. Biophys.* 147, 148–159.

Itano, HA, and Neel, JV. (1950). A new inherited abnormality of human hemoglobin. *Proc. Natl. Acad. Sci. U.S.A.* 36: 613–617.

Jensen, WN, Schoefield, RA, and Agner, R. (1998). Clinical and necropsy findings in hemoglobin C disease. *Blood* 12: 74–83.

Kan, YW, and Dozy, AM. (1980). Evolution of the hemoglobin S and C genes in world populations. *Science* 209: 388–391.

Kaul, DK, Baez, S, and Nagel, RL. (1981). Flow properties of oxygenated Hb S and Hb C erythrocytes in the isolated microvasculature of the rat: A contribution to the hemorheology of hemoglobinopathies. *Clin Hemorheol.* 1: 73–86.

Kent, D, Arya, R, Aclimandos, WA et al. (1994). Screening for ophthalmic manifestations of sickle cell disease in the United Kingdom. *Eye* 8: 618–622.

Kim, HC, Weierbach, RG, Friedman, S et al. (1977). Globin biosynthesis in sickle cell, Hb SC, and Hb C diseases. *J. Pediatr.* 91: 13–20.

Koshy, M, and Burd, L. (1994). Obstetric and gynecologic issues. In Embury, SH, Hebbel, RP, Mohandas, N, and Steinberg MH, editors. *Sickle cell disease: Basic principles and clinical practice.* New York: Lippincott-Raven, pp. 689–702.

Koshy, M, Burd, L, Wallace, D et al. (1988). Prophylactic red-cell transfusions in pregnant patients with sickle cell disease. A randomized cooperative study. *N. Engl. J. Med.* 319: 1447–1452.

Kraus, AP and Diggs, LW. (1956). In vitro crystallization of hemoglobin occurring in citrated blood from patients with Hb C. *J. Lab. Clin. Med.* 47: 700–705.

Labie, D, Richin, C, Pagnier, J et al. (1984). Hemoglobins S and C in Upper Volta. *Hum. Genet.* 65: 300–302.

Lane, PA, Rogers, ZR, Woods, GM, Wang, WC et al. (1994). Fatal pneumococcal septicemia in hemoglobin SC disease. *J. Pediatr.* 124: 859–862.

Lane, PA, O'Connell, JL, Lear, JL et al. (1995). Functional asplenia in hemoglobin SC disease. *Blood* 85: 2238–2244.

Lauf, PK and Theg, BE. (1980). A chloride dependent K$^+$ flux induced by N-ethlymaleimide in genetically low K$^+$ sheep and goat erythrocytes. *Biochem. Biophys. Res. Commun.* 92: 1422–1428.

Lawrence, C, Fabry, ME, and Nagel RL. (1991). The unique red cell heterogeneity of SC disease: crystal formation, dense reticulocytes, and unusual morphology. *Blood* 78: 2104–12.

Lawrence, C, Hirsch, RE, Fataliev, NA et al. (1997). Molecular interactions between Hb α-G Philadelphia, HbC, and HbS: Phenotypic implications for SC α-G Philadelphia disease. *Blood* 90: 2819–2825.

Lee, P, Kirk, G, and Hoffman, JF. (1984). Interrelations among Na and K contents, cell volume and buoyant disease. *J. Membrane Biol.* 79: 119–126.

Lehmann, H and Huntsman, RG. (1974). *Man's Haemoglobins.* 2nd ed. Amsterdam: North Holland.

Leikin, SL, Gallagher, D, Kinney, TR et al. (1989). Mortality in children and adolescents with sickle cell disease. *Pediatrics* 84: 500–508.

Lesorbe, B, Pieron, R, Mafart, Y et al. (1978). Defaut de concentration urinaire dans la drepanocytose et l'hemoglobinopathie S-C. Etude de 56 sujets. *Ann. Med. Interne* 129: 289–292.

Liebhaber, SA, Cash, FE, and Cornfield, DB. (1988). Evidence for posttranslational control of Hb C synthesis in an individual with Hb C trait and alpha-thalassemia. *Blood* 71: 502–504.

Lin, MJ, Nagel, RL, and Hirsch, RE. (1989). The acceleration of hemoglobin C crystallization by hemoglobin S. *Blood* 74: 1823–1825.

Lipshutz, M, McQueen, DA, and Rosner, F. (1977). Spontaneous rupture of the spleen in homozygous hemoglobin C disease. *J. Am. Med. Assoc.* 237: 792–793.

Lutty, GA, and Goldberg, MF. (1994). Ophthalmologic complications. In Embury, SH, Hebbel, RP, Mohandas, N, and Steinberg, MH, editors. *Sickle cell disease: Basic principles and clinical practice.* New York: Raven, pp. 703–724.

McCurdy, PR, Mahmood, L, and Sherman, AS. (1975). Red cell life span in sickle cell-hemoglobin C disease with a note about sickle cell-hemoglobin O arab. *Blood* 45: 273–279.

Mears, JG, Lachman, HM, Cabannes, R et al. (1981). Sickle gene. Its origin and diffusion from West Africa. *J. Clin. Invest.* 68: 606–610.

Milner, PF, Kraus, AP, Sebes, JI et al. (1991). Sickle cell disease as a cause of osteonecrosis of the femoral head. *N. Engl. J. Med.* 325: 1476–1481.

Milner, PF, Kraus, AP, Sebes, JI et al. (1993). Osteonecrosis of the humeral head in sickle cell disease. *Clin Orthop.* 289: 136–143.

Mohandas, N, Clark, MR, Jacobs, MS et al. (1980). Analysis of factors regulating erythrocyte deformability. *J. Clin. Invest.* 66: 563–573.

Motulsky, AG. (1973). Frequency of sickling disorders in US blacks. *N. Engl. J. Med.* 288: 31–33.

Murphy, JR. (1976). Hemoglobin CC erythrocytes: Decreased intracellular pH and decreased O_2 affinity anemia. *Semin. Hematol.* 13: 177.

Nagel, RL, and Ranney, HM, (1990). Genetic epidemiology of structural mutations of the β-globin gene. *Semin. Hematol.* 27: 342–359.

Nagel, RL, Raventos-Suarez, C, Fabry, ME et al. (1981). Impairment of the growth of Plasmodium falciparum in HbEE erythrocytes. *J. Clin. Invest.* 68: 303–305.

Nagel, RL, Lin MJ, Witkowska, HE et al. (1993). Compound heterozygosity for hemoglobin C and Korle-Bu: Moderate microcytic hemolytic anemia and acceleration of crystal formation. *Blood* 82: 1907–1912.

Nagpal, KC, Patrianakos, D, Asdourian, GK et al. Spontaneous regression (autoinfarction) of proliferative sickle retinopathy. *Am. J. Ophthalmol.* 80: 885–892.

Neumayr, L, Koshy, M, Haberkern, C et al. and Preoperative Transfusion in Sickle Cell Disease Study Group. (1998). Surgery in patients with hemoglobin SC disease. *Am. J. Hematol.* 57: 101–108.

Ohene-Frempong, K, Weiner, SJ, Sleeper, LA et al. and Cooperative Study of Sickle Cell Disease. (1998). Cerebrovascular accidents in sickle cell disease: Rates and risk factors. *Blood* 91: 288–294.

Olson, JA, and Nagel, RL. (1986). Synchronized cultures of P falciparum in abnormal red cells: The mechanism of the inhibition of growth in HbCC. *Blood* 67: 997–1001.

Olson, JF, Ware, RE, Schultz, WH et al. (1994). Hemoglobin C disease in infancy and childhood. *J. Pediatr.* 125: 745–747.

Orringer, EP, Brockenbrough, JS, Whitney, JA et al. (1991). Okadaic acid inhibits activation of K-Cl cotransport in red blood cells containing hemoglobins S and C. *Am. J. Physiol. Cell Physiol.* 261: C591–C593.

Penman, AD, Talbot, JF, Chuang, EL et al. (1994). New classification of peripheral retinal vascular changes in sickle cell disease. *Br. J. Ophthalmol.* 78: 681–689.

Platt, OS, Rosenstock, WF, and Espeland, M. (1984). Influence of S hemoglobinopathies on growth and development. *N. Engl. J. Med.* 311: 7–12.

Platt, OS, Thorington, BD, Brambilla, DJ et al. (1991). Pain in sickle cell disease—rates and risk factors. *N. Engl. J. Med.* 325: 11–16.

Platt, OS, Brambilla, DJ, Rosse, WF et al. (1994). Mortality in sickle cell disease: Life expectancy and risk factors for early death. *N. Engl. J. Med.* 330: 1639–1644.

Powars, D, Chan, LS, and Schroeder, WA. (1990). The variable expression of sickle cell disease is genetically determined. *Semin. Hematol.* 27: 360–376.

Powars, DR, Elliott Mills, DD, and Chan, L. (1991). Chronic renal failure in sickle cell disease: Risk factors, clinical course, and mortality. *Ann. Intern. Med.* 115: 614–620.

Prindle, KH, and McCurdy, PR. (1970). Red cell life span in hemoglobin C disorders (with special reference to hemoglobin C trait). *Blood* 36: 14–19.

Raichand, M, Goldberg, MF, Nagpal, KC et al. (1977). Evolution of neovascularization in sickle cell retinopathy: A prospective fluorescein angiographic study. *Arch. Ophthalmol.* 95: 1543–1552.

Reiss, GH, Ranney, HM, and Shaklai, N. (1982). Association of hemoglobin C with erythrocytes ghosts. *J. Clin. Invest.* 70: 946–952.

Rey, KS, Unger, CA, Rao, SP, and Miller, ST. (1991). Sickle cell-hemoglobin E disease: Clinical findings and implications. *J. Pediatr.* 119: 949–951.

Roberts, WL, McCraw, M, and Cook, CB. (1998). Effects of sickle cell trait and hemoglobin C trait on determinations of HbA_{1c} by an immunoassay method. *Diabetes Care* 21: 983–986.

Rodgers, GP, Sahovic, EA, Pierce, LE et al. (1986). Hemoglobin SC disease and alpha-thalassemia. Prolonged survival and mild clinical course. *Am. J. Med.* 80: 746–750.

Rogers, DW, Clarke, JM, Cupidore, L et al. (1978). Early deaths in Jamaican children with sickle cell disease. *Br. Med. J.* 1: 1515–1516.

Rogers, ZR, and Buchanan, GR. (1995a). Bacteremia in children with sickle hemoglobin C disease and sickle beta(+)-thalassemia: Is prophylactic penicillin necessary? *J. Pediatr.* 127: 348–354.

Rogers, ZR, and Buchanan, GR. (1995b). Risk of infection in children with hemoglobin S-beta-thalassemia. *J. Pediatr.* 127: 672–672.

Schroeder, WA, Powars, DR, Kay, LM et al. (1989). β-Cluster haplotypes α-gene status and hematological data from SS SC and S-β-thalassemia patients in southern California. *Hemoglobin* 13: 325–353.

Schroeder, WA, Powars, D, Reynolds, RD et al. (1998). Hb-E in combination with Hb-S and Hb-C in a black family. *Hemoglobin* 1: 287–289.

Sear, DA, and Udden, MM. (1985). Splenic infarction, splenic sequestration and functional hyposplenism in hemoglobin S-C disease. *Am. J. Hematol.* 18: 261–268.

Serjeant, GR. (1992). *Sickle Cell Disease.* 2nd ed. Oxford: Oxford Medical Publications.

Serjeant, GR, Ashcroft, MT, and Serjeant, BE. (1973). The clinical features of haemoglobin SC disease in Jamaica. *Br. J. Haematol.* 24: 491–501.

Spaet, TH, Alway, RH, and Ward, G. (1953). Homozygous type "C" hemoglobin. *Pediatrics* 12: 483–490.

Statius van Eps, LW, Schouten, H, La Porte-Wijsman, LW et al. (1967). The influence of red blood cell transfusions on the hyposthenuria and renal hemodynamics of sickle cell anemia. *Clin. Chim. Acta.* 17: 449–461.

Statius van Eps, LW, Schouten, H, Ter Haar Romeny-Wachter, CCh et al. (1970). The relation between age and renal concentrating capacity in sickle cell disease and hemoglobin C disease. *Clin. Chim. Acta.* 27: 501–511.

Steinberg, MH. (1975). Haemoglobin C/alpha thalassaemia: Haematological and biosynthetic studies. *Br. J. Haematol.* 30: 337–342.

Steinberg, MH and Embury, SH. (1986). Alpha-thalassemia in blacks: Genetic and clinical aspects and interactions with the sickle hemoglobin gene. *Blood* 68: 985–990.

Steinberg, MH, Dreiling, BJ, and Lovell, WJ. (1977). Sickle cell anemia: Erythrokinetics, blood volumes, and a study of possible determinants of severity. *Am. J. Hematol.* 2: 17–23.

Steinberg, MH, Coleman, MB, Adams, JG et al. (1983). The effects of alpha-thalassaemia in HbSC disease. *Br. J. Haematol.* 55: 487–492.

Steinberg, MH, Nagel, RL, Lawrence, C et al. (1996). β-globin gene haplotype in Hb SC disease. *Am. J. Hematol.* 52: 189–191.

Stevens, MCG, Maude, GH, Cupidore, LH et al. (1986). Prepubertal growth and skeletal maturation in children with sickle cell disease. *J. Pediatr.* 78: 124–132.

Sugihara, K, Sugihara, T, Mohandas, N et al. (1992). Thrombospondin mediates adherence of CD36⁺ sickle reticulocytes to endothelial cells. *Blood* 80: 2634–2642.

Talacki, CA, Rappaport, E, Schwartz, E et al. (1990). Beta-globin gene cluster haplotype in Hb C heterozygotes. *Hemoglobin* 14: 229–240.

Talbot, JF, Bird, AC, Serjeant, GR et al. (1982). Sickle cell retinopathy in young children in Jamaica. *Br. J. Ophthalmol.* 66: 149–154.

Talbot, JF, Bird, AC, Maude, GH et al. (1996). Sickle cell retinopathy in Jamaican children: Further observations in a cohort study. *Br. J. Ophthalmol.* 72: 727–732.

Thomas, ED, Motulsky, AG, and Walters, DH. (1955). Homozygous hemoglobin C disease: Report of a case with studies on the pathophysiology and neonatal formation of hemoglobin C. *Am. J. Med.* 18: 832–838.

Trabuchet, G, Elion, J, Dunda, O et al. (1991). Nucleotide sequence evidence of the unicentric origin of the β^C mutation in Africa. *Hum. Genet.* 87: 597–601.

Vichinsky, EP, Haberkern, CM, Neumayr, L et al. and Preoperative Transfusion in Sickle Cell Disease Study Group. (1995). A comparison of conservative and aggressive transfusion regimens in the perioperative management of sickle cell disease. *N. Engl. J. Med.* 333: 206–213.

Vichinsky, EP, Styles, LA, Colangelo, LH et al. (1997). Acute chest syndrome in sickle cell disease: Clinical presentation and course. *Blood* 89: 1787–1792.

Warkentin, TE, Barr, RD, Ali, MA et al. (1990). Recurrent acute splenic sequestration crisis due to interacting genetic defects: Hemoglobin SC disease and hereditary spherocytosis. *Blood* 75: 266–270.

Welch, RB, and Goldberg, MF. (1966). Sickle-cell hemoglobin and its relation to fundus abnormality. *Arch. Ophthalmol.* 75: 353–362.

West, MS, Wethers, D, Smith, J, Steinberg, MH and Cooperative Study of Sickle Cell Disease (1992). Laboratory profile of sickle cell disease: A cross-sectional analysis. *J. Clin. Epidemiol.* 45: 893–909.

Wheby, MS, Thorup, OH, and Leavell, BS. (1956). Homozygous hemoglobin C disease in siblings: Further comment on intraerythrocytic crystals. *Blood* 11: 266–272.

Wick, TM, Moake, JL, Udden, MM et al. (1993). Unusually large von Willebrand factor multimers preferentially promote young sickle and nonsickle erythrocyte adhesion to endothelial cells. *Am. J. Hematol.* 42: 284–292.

Wickramasinghe, SN, Akinyanju, OO, and Hughes, M. (1982). Dyserythropoiesis in homozygous haemoglobin C disease. *Clin. Lab. Haematol.* 4: 373–381.

Winter, WP, and Yodh, J. (1983). Interaction of human hemoglobin and its variants with agar. *Science* 221: 175–178.

Wolff, D, Cecchi, X, Spalvins, A, and Canessa, M. (1988). Charybdotoxin blocks with high affinity the Ca⁺⁺ – activated K⁺ channel of Hb A and Hb S red cells: Individual differences in the number of channels. *J. Memberana Biol.* 106: 276–281.

Yam, LT, and Li, CY. (1994). The spleen. Embury, SH, Hebbel, RP, Mohandas, N, and Steinberg, MH, editors. *Sickle cell disease: Basic principles and clinical practice.* New York: Lippencott-Raven, pp. 555–566.

Zago, MA, Costa, FF, Covas, DT et al. (1986). Discrepancy between pit counting and splenic function tests in nutritional anemia and hemoglobinopathy C. *Nouv. Rev. Fr. Hematol.* 28: 84.

28

Compound Heterozygous and Other Sickle Hemoglobinopathies

MARTIN H. STEINBERG

Wherever the sickle hemoglobin (β^S; HbS) gene is widespread, diverse β thalassemia alleles are found as well. Consequently, compound heterozygotes with HbS-β thalassemia are commonplace. Their prevalence depends on the populations' ratio of HbS genes to β thalassemia genes. In the United States and in Africa, where the HbS gene predominates, sickle cell anemia is the prevailing sickle cell disease genotype. Wherever β thalassemia is more frequent than sickle cell trait (eg, Greece, Italy and other Mediterranean countries), HbS-β thalassemia is the prevailing genotype (Chapter 31). Some β thalassemia variants, such as δβ thalassemia, gene deletion hereditary persistence of fetal hemoglobin (HPFH), and Hb Lepore (Chapter 15) also interact with HbS producing different interesting phenotypes. α Thalassemia is present in one third of black patients with sickle cell anemia, and this combination has distinctive hematologic and clinical features.

Compound heterozygotes of HbS with other mutant α- or β-globin genes are also present in populations with a high prevalence of HbS. Depending on the mutation found with HbS, these conditions may resemble sickle cell trait or have a clinical phenotype with hemolytic anemia and vasoocclusive complications. Other hemoglobin variants, often with intriguing phenotypes, have both the sickle mutation and an additional mutation in the same β-globin gene.

In African Americans, HbSC disease (Chapter 27) and the HbS-β thalassemias together are about as common as sickle cell anemia, making the prevalence of sickle cell disease in this population nearly 1 in 300. This chapter examines the molecular, diagnostic, laboratory, and clinical aspects of the compound heterozygous sickle hemoglobinopathies other than HbSC disease. Unless there are special features associated with a genotype discussed in this chapter, the clinical aspects of the associated conditions are discussed in chapters on sickle cell anemia (Chapter 24) and on HbSC disease (Chapter 27) and in chapters focused on the management of and special treatments for those diseases (Chapters 37, 38, 40–42).

Specific approaches to treating the complications of compound heterozygous forms of sickle cell disease do not differ among genotypes. The critical clinical issue is establishing the correct genotypic diagnosis before counseling families, discussing prognosis, or contemplating antenatal diagnosis.

HISTORY

Sickle-β thalassemia was recognized first in Italy, a land where β thalassemia is commonplace (Chapter 31) and where the HbS gene is found in selected subpopulations (Chapter 29) (Silvestroni and Bianco, 1946). Patients with HbS-β thalassemia provided the first clues to the genetic basis of thalassemia (Singer and Fisher, 1952; Sturgeon et al., 1952) Their blood contained less HbA than blood of individuals with sickle cell trait, and their erythrocytes were microcytic and hypochromic. This suggested that the thalassemia gene *interacted* with the HbA gene to reduce the concentration of HbA. Still, some individuals with sickle cell trait and features of thalassemia did not have reduced levels of HbA. In these instances, the thalassemia determinant segregated independently from HbS. This observation generated the hypothesis of noninteracting forms of thalassemia, where the thalassemia gene did not directly affect HbA production, and ultimately led to the concept of β thalassemia and α thalassemia (Ingram and Stretton, 1959). Cases in which a child affected with sickle cell disease did not appear to have inherited the sickle cell gene from both parents first led to the identification of other compound heterozygous types of sickle cell disease (Cooke and Mack, 1934). As mutations of both the β and α-globin genes were delineated with increasing frequency, their interactions with HbS provided additional insights into the polymerization of HbS and the pathophysiology of sickle cell disease.

HbS-β THALASSEMIA AND HbS-β THALASSEMIA-LIKE CONDITIONS

β Thalassemia is classified as β^0 thalassemia and β^+ thalassemia (Chapter 13). In the former, the thalassemia-causing mutation totally abolishes expression of the affected gene; in the latter, the reduction in β-globin gene expression varies with the mutation. HbA is not present in HbS-β^0 thalassemia unless the patient has been transfused, and the hemolysate contains only HbS, fetal hemoglobin (HbF), and 4 to 6 percent HbA_2. Therefore, the phenotype of HbS-β^0 thalassemia mimics that seen in sickle cell anemia and is equally variegated. In HbS-β^+ thalassemia, HbA levels vary from < 5 percent to 45 percent of the hemolysate. Given the primacy of the HbS concentration in determining the phenotype of the resulting disease, individuals with only traces of HbA have a disease resembling sickle cell anemia or HbS-β^0 thalassemia. Most patients with HbA levels of 20 percent or more have a phenotype milder than that of HbSC disease or sickle cell anemia. Classifying HbS-β^+ thalassemia as Types I (HbA, 3 to 6 percent), II (HbA, 8 to 15 percent), or III (HbA, 20 to 25 percent) according to their level of HbA has little current utility given our ability to define exactly the mutation and our appreciation of the relationship of the β-thalassemia mutation to the expression of the β-globin gene.

Because of the confounding influences of genetic modifiers of γ-globin gene expression, α thalassemia, and other more obscure modulators of sickle cell disease (Chapter 26), a rigid genotype-phenotype correlation is difficult to establish in all instances of HbS-β thalassemia. Among the different genotypes of HbS-β^+ thalassemia, higher levels of HbA are usually associated with a milder phenotype and in all types of HbS-β thalassemia, as in sickle cell anemia, higher HbF concentrations temper the disease.

Pathophysiology

β Thalassemia Mutations in HbS-β Thalassemia.
Many different β thalassemia-causing mutations have been described in association with HbS (Table 28.1). In each population where HbS-β thalassemia is found, the molecular basis of β thalassemia reflects the β-thalassemia mutations extant in that population. Because the types of mutations vary among populations, HbS-β thalassemia has a different clinical spectrum in different racial and ethnic groups. HbS-β thalassemia is most common in selected Italian and Greek populations; in Turks, Iranians, and other Middle Eastern nationalities; in tribal groups of the Indian subcontinent; and in blacks of African descent. Table 28.1 lists some β-thalassemia mutations found with the HbS gene in different populations. "Mild"

β-globin gene promoter mutations are prevalent in blacks, accounting for the preponderance of milder forms of HbS-β^+ thalassemia in this racial group.

As with sickle cell disease caused by other genotypes, the pathophysiology of the HbS-β thalassemias is ultimately linked to HbS polymerization and modulated by coincident genetic factors, such as the ability to make large amounts of HbF, and by the cellular concentration of HbS. Two interrelated elements modulate the polymerization tendency of HbS in HbS-β thalassemia: mean corpuscular HbS concentration and the concentration of HbA. In both HbS-β^0 thalassemia and HbS-β^+ thalassemia, reduced β-globin chain accumulation reduces mean corpuscular hemoglobin (MCH) and mean corpuscular volume (MCV). In HbS-β^+ thalassemia, HbA concentration is the major determinant of mean corpuscular HbS concentration.

At its root, the pathophysiology of the sickle-β thalassemias is identical to the pathophysiology of sickle cell anemia (Chapter 20). In HbS-β^+ thalassemia, variable amounts of HbA dilute HbS and inhibit polymerization-induced cellular damage. With HbS-β^0 thalassemia, compared with sickle cell anemia, the effects of thalassemia on sickle erythrocytes—microcytosis, hypochromia, sometimes high levels of HbF—improve the circulatory competence of these cells, marginally reduce hemolysis, and cause a small increase in hemoglobin concentration and packed cell volume (PCV). As in sickle cell anemia-α thalassemia, the increase in PCV is not accompanied by a reduction—there may even be an increase—in painful episodes or other of the vasoocclusive events of sickle cell disease. This may result from increased blood viscosity caused by greater numbers of HbS-containing erythrocytes.

Diagnosis

Microcytosis and elevated concentrations of HbA_2 are typically present in HbS-β thalassemia as they are in heterozygous β thalassemia (Chapter 13). Several caveats must be remembered when considering this diagnosis. In many respects, HbS-β^0 thalassemia resembles sickle cell anemia and in some cases of HbS-β^0 thalassemia, the MCV is near normal, and the HbA_2 is elevated only marginally. Sickle cell anemia-α thalassemia is a nearly exact phenocopy of HbS-β^0 thalassemia. Iron deficiency causes microcytosis in sickle cell anemia, but here the level of HbA_2 is normal or low. When a sickle solubility test is the sole means of diagnosis (it should never be!) or when protein-based methods, such as hemoglobin electrophoresis, are uncritically interpreted, HbS-β^+ thalassemia may be confused with sickle cell trait or even go unsuspected.

Hematologic studies, including the determination of MCV and MCH, and quantification of HbS, HbA_2,

Table 28.1. β Thalassemia Mutations in HbS-β Thalassemia*

β+ thalassemia

Mutation	PCV/hemoglobin	HbA	HbF	MCV	Phenotype
−92 C→T[†]	14.5/	45	1.4	83	Asymptomatic
−88 C→T	10/31	18	15	65–70	Mild
−88 C→T in *cis* to HbS[†]	12/35	90	3	70	Very mild new thal mutation on HbS gene
−29 A→G	11/32	20	11[¶]	65–70	Mild
IVS-1–1 G→C	7.3–11.4/	0	3–9	61–72	Severe Hb Monroe
IVS-1 5 G→C	9/	<5	12	72	Severe Indian, 1 black
IVS-1 5 G→T[†]	8.4/25	8	12	57	
IVS-1 5 G→A		<5			Severe
IVS-1† 6 T→C		35			
IVS-1, 110 G→A	9/	9–11	7	72	Severe
IVS-2 745 C→G		5			Severe
Poly A site AAT→AAC[†]		18			

β⁰ thalassemia

Mutation	PCV/hemoglobin	HbA	HbF	MCV	Phenotype
CD 2/3/4 (−9, + 31 bp)[†]	9/	—	8.5	70–80	
CD 6 −A[†]					
CD 15 TGG→TGA[†]	—	—	—	—	Unknown
CD 25/26 GGT.GAG→G GT.T.GAG[†]	8/	—	14	74	Severe, Tunisians
CD 39 C→T					
CD 44 −C[†]					
CD 106/007 + G[†]					
IVS-1 2 T→C	7/		6	58	Severe
IVS-2 1 G→A					
IVS-2 849 A→G[†]					
IVS-2 849 A→C	10/28		8–35	79	
Frameshift 106/107[†] (+ G)					
−1393 bp	11/32	—	11–19	73	Mild/severe
−530 bp[‡]			30		

* In many instances, few patients or only a single patient were studied so that the values reported may not necessarily be representative of the genotype.

† Examples of HbS-β thalassemia where information is scanty and only one or two cases are reported. Also, patient ages may differ among groups, confounding the interpretation of hemoglobin level, MCV, HbF, and HbA₂. In some instances, no hematologic values are available.

Data reported were assembled from the following references. (Altay et al., 1997; Divoky et al., 1993; Gonzalez-Redondo et al., 1988a, 1988b, 1991; Huisman et al., 1997; Padanilam et al., 1984; Steinberg et al., 1997; Waye et al., 1991a).

‡ One individual, age 9 months, was studied. HbA₂ was 6 percent.

¶ Mean age of patients was about 10 years.

HbF, and when present, HbA levels, form the cornerstone of diagnosis. Blood films from two patients with HbS-β⁰ thalassemia are shown in Figure 28.1. Family studies and the demonstration by DNA analysis of heterozygosity for the sickle β-globin gene and the nature of the β thalassemia mutation are important confirmatory analyses and are critical when antenatal diagnosis and genetic counseling are at issue.

The most confusing diagnostic problem is the differentiation of HbS-β⁰ thalassemia from sickle cell anemia-α thalassemia. Some hematologic distinctions among these phenocopies are shown in Table 28.2 and comparative pedigrees are displayed in Figure 28.2. Most cases of HbS-β thalassemia are accompanied by a reduced MCV and MCH and increased concentration of HbA₂. Depending on the reticulocyte count, HbF level, and nature of the particular β-thalassemia mutation, the MCV may be normal or in the lower range of normality. HbA₂ levels are low in early childhood and cannot be relied on for diagnostic discrimination at this stage of

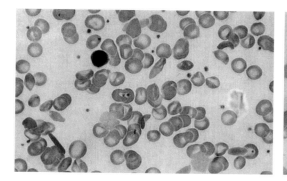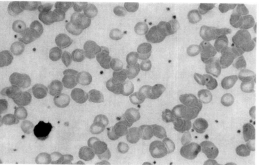

Figure 28.1. Blood films in two patients with HbS-β⁰ thalassemia. (**Left panel**). The patient has a HbF level of 5 percent. Sickled cells are prominent in addition to microcytosis. In the right panel, with HbF of 2 percent, microcytosis and hypochromia are prominent, and few typical sickled cells are seen. For full color reproduction, see color plate 28.1.

life. When the HbF level is very high, HbA_2 levels are often reduced, further compromising the utility of this measurement. Although increased HbA_2 is typical of heterozygous β thalassemia, the increase is in part dependent on how much β-globin chain synthesis is reduced (Chapter 13). HbA_2 is also high when α thalassemia is present with sickle cell anemia. This increase is proportional to the reduction in α-globin chain synthesis and is a result of the differential affinities of non-α-globin chains for α-globin chains, which exist in limited amounts in α thalassemia (Chapters 8, 18, and 29). HbA_2 levels and MCV in sickle cell anemia, HbS-β⁰ thalassemia, and sickle cell anemia-α thalassemia are shown in Figure 28.3. Although HbA_2 levels are highest in HbS-β⁰ thalassemia, lowest in sickle cell anemia, and intermediate in sickle cell anemia-α thalassemia, they have little diagnostic value in an individual.

Microcytosis and the elevated HbA_2 level in sickle cell anemia-α thalassemia cause great confusion with HbS-β⁰ thalassemia. Differentiating between these

genotypes is critical during genetic counseling when antenatal diagnosis is contemplated. Hematologic and electrophoretic studies alone are unable to distinguish between these conditions and family studies and DNA analysis are needed to verify the diagnosis. Although higher on average in HbS-β⁰ thalassemia than in sickle cell anemia, HbF levels span such a broad range that they are diagnostically useless.

In HbS-β⁺ thalassemia, the presence of HbA simplifies the diagnosis. Yet the rare case with very high HbA levels (the highest level reported is 45 percent) might be confused with sickle cell trait, and in instances where HbA is quite low (the lowest levels are less than 5 percent) its presence can be overlooked. Representative hematologic findings in the different genotypes of HbS-β⁺ thalassemia are presented in Table 28.1. During newborn screening for sickle cell disease, small amounts of HbA may be undetected, leading to a false diagnosis of sickle cell anemia and emphasizing the need for confirmatory testing after the initial screening (Strickland et al., 1995) (Chapter 36).

Individuals with HbS-β⁺ thalassemia and very low levels of HbA are often mistakenly diagnosed as having HbS-β⁰ thalassemia. Four β⁺ thalassemia mutations, all producing a severe phenotype, have been described at IVS-1 position 5, and two of these have been associated with severe HbS-β⁺ thalassemia, mas-

Table 28.2. Laboratory Differentiation of Sickle Cell Anemia, Sickle Cell Anemia with α Thalassemia, and HbS-β⁰ Thalassemia*

Diagnosis	Hemoglobin (g/dL)	MCV (fl)	HbA_2 (%)	HbF[†] (%)	α/β[‡]
Sickle cell anemia	7–8	85–95	2.5–3.5	5	0.95
Sickle cell anemia-α thalassemia[§]	8–10	70–85	3.5–4.5	5	1.50
HbS-β⁰ thalassemia	8–10	65–75	4–6	8	0.75

* The laboratory values, except where specified otherwise, reflect ranges found in individuals age 15 and older (Serjeant et al., 1973; Steinberg et al., 1984a).
[†] Average level.
[‡] Ratio of radioactive leucine incorporated into α-and β-globin chains.
[§] α Thalassemia includes both heterozygotes and homozygotes for the $-\alpha^{3.7}$ deletion.

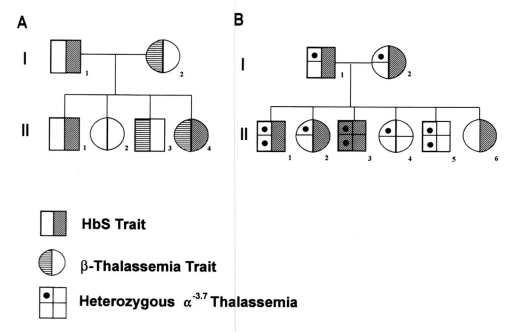

HbS Trait

β-Thalassemia Trait

Heterozygous α⁻³·⁷ Thalassemia

Figure 28.2. Pedigrees of families with HbS-β thalassemia (**A**) and sickle cell anemia with α thalassemia (**B**). II 4 in family A and II 3 in family B have nearly identical hematologic findings with microcytic erythrocytes and increased HbA$_2$ levels. But, A II 4 has HbS-β thalassemia and B II 3 has sickle cell anemia with homozygous α thalassemia-2. The latter individual has inherited a HbS gene from each parent and an α thalassemia gene from each parent. As shown in the pedigree, because the β-globin genes and α-globin genes are on different chromosomes, they are inherited independently, and individuals can have sickle cell trait (or sickle cell anemia) without α thalassemia or with one or two α thalassemia genes. The HbS and β thalassemia genes are allelic.

querading as HbS-β⁰ thalassemia (Huisman et al., 1997; Li et al., 1998). IVS-I position 5 is part of the consensus sequence for the donor splice site of exon 1. When mutated, splicing efficiency is greatly reduced with only a small amount of mRNA correctly spliced.

Hb Monroe (IVS-1 position −1, G→C), initially described in a Tunisian patient and called Hb Kairouan (Vidaud et al., 1998), has been described in several families as a compound heterozygote with HbS. IVS-1 position −1 is between the A and G of β-globin gene codon 30 (AGG), which normally codes for arginine; in Hb Monroe, it is converted to a threonine codon (ACG). The mutation has dual effects; it impairs the use of the normal 5′ splice site by 98 percent, and the threonine residue causes hemoglobin instability. In HbS-Hb Monroe disease, Hb Monroe is not detectable by iso-electric focusing and only in some patients is 0.6 to 1.6 percent Hb Monroe found by high-performance liquid chromatography (HPLC) (Sweeting et al., 1998). Patients with HbS-Hb Monroe appear to have all the clinical and hematologic features of HbS-β⁰ thalassemia.

Two Moroccan adults with sickle cell trait were found to have the −88 C→T β⁺ thalassemia mutation in *cis* to the sickle mutation. Both had a normal α-globin gene haplotype. Reticulocytosis of about 3 percent, mild anemia, and microcytosis (Table 28.1)

Figure 28.3. HbA$_2$ levels and MCV in HbS-β⁰ thalassemia, sickle cell anemia-α thalassemia, and sickle cell anemia. Considerable overlap among these genotypes makes it difficult to rely on HbA$_2$ for diagnostic purposes in an individual case.

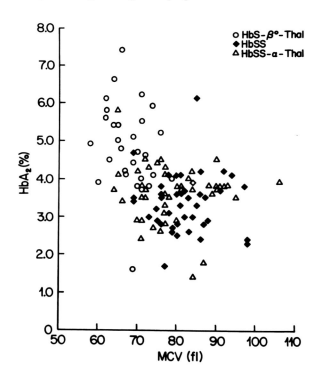

without iron deficiency suggested the presence of mild hemolysis. HbA$_2$ levels were 6 to 7 percent, HbF about 3 percent, and HbS 10 to 11 percent. In one individual, the α/β globin biosynthesis ratio was 1.35 and the ratio of β^S/β^A+β^S was 0.17 (Baklouti, et al., 1987). Further studies of cloned DNA in the patient's family confirmed that the thalassemia mutation was on the same gene as the HbS mutation. Analysis of polymorphisms 5′ to the β^S gene revealed a Benin haplotype chromosome, strongly suggesting that the thalassemia mutation arose anew on the HbS chromosome rather than from a recombination between a β-thalassemia and an HbS chromosome (Baklouti et al., 1989). It was not clear why HbS levels were as low as they were because analysis showed a reduction of β-globin mRNA similar to that found in simple heterozygotes for the −88 C→T mutation. The authors speculated that the reduction in HbS was caused by a posttranslational event and that even without α thalassemia, the β^S chains competed less well than the β^A chains for α-globin chains.

Two Portuguese patients with sickle cell trait had a β-thalassemia determinant that was not linked to the β-globin gene (Fig. 28.4) (Pacheco et al., 1995). Extensive analysis of the β-globin gene DNA failed to find a thalassemia-causing mutation. Carriers had very mild microcytic anemia and increased HbA$_2$ levels; in vitro translation of mRNA showed an α/β ratio of 1.6.

Clinical Features

Both HbS-β^0 thalassemia and HbS-β$^+$ thalassemia with very low levels of HbA, with some exceptions,

have a clinical course and range of complications similar to those present in sickle cell anemia. In HbS-β^0 thalassemia, the average PCV and hemoglobin concentration are higher than in sickle cell anemia, a likely result of the reduction in mean cell HbS concentration and prolonged red cell survival.

In one HbS-β$^+$ thalassemia study, the median PCV was 32 in all patients less than age 10 years. Males, 10 to 19 years old and 20 years and older, had a PCV of 36 and 40, respectively, about 4 to 6 points higher than age-matched females. In all patients, the MCV was 70 to 72 fl compared with about 90 fl in sickle cell anemia. Leukocyte and platelet counts were also reduced compared with sickle cell anemia patients (West et al., 1992). These data were from African-American patients where the preponderance of β$^+$ thalassemia mutations are "mild" (Chapter 12).

A large cooperative study of the clinical course of sickle cell disease in the United States examined clinical differences produced by the common sickle hemoglobinopathies. About 3 percent of patients with HbS-β$^+$ thalassemia died during 6 to 8 years of observation compared with 8 percent of patients with sickle cell anemia, 4 percent with HbS-β^0 thalassemia, and 3 percent with HbSC disease (Platt et al., 1994). Patients with HbS-β$^+$ thalassemia had pain rates about half those observed in HbS-β^0 thalassemia and sickle cell anemia, and similar to that of patients with HbSC dis-

Figure 28.4. Inheritance of sickle cell trait and β thalassemia unlinked to the β-globin gene cluster. The 2 Hinc II/ψβ RFLP are shown with +/−. (From Pacheco et al., 1995.)

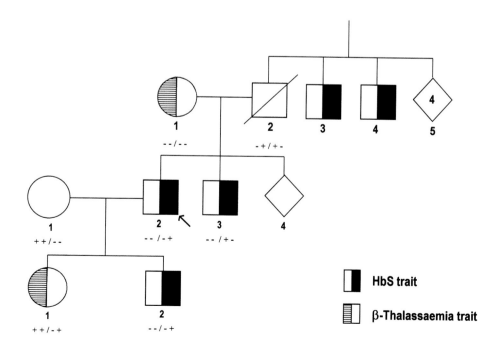

ease (Platt et al., 1991). Osteonecrosis of the femoral head rarely appeared in children with HbS-β^+ thalassemia and was less frequent in adults with this genotype (5.8 percent) than in sickle cell anemia (10.2 percent). In HbS-β^0 thalassemia, osteonecrosis (13.1 percent) was more common than in sickle cell anemia (Milner et al., 1991). Bacteremia was about half as frequent in HbS-β^+ thalassemia and HbS-β^0 thalassemia than in sickle cell anemia and similar to its incidence in HbSC disease. (Zarkowsky et al., 1986). At any age, the incidence of acute chest syndrome in HbS-β^+ thalassemia was less than in sickle cell anemia and HbS-β^0 thalassemia (which did not differ) and similar to that in HbSC disease (Castro et al., 1994). Strokes occur in all genotypes of HbS-β thalassemia but less often than in sickle cell anemia (Ohene-Frempong et al., 1998).

HbS-β^+ thalassemia patients with > 20 percent HbA usually have milder clinical disease than those with sickle cell anemia and HbSC disease, and some can be asymptomatic, the diagnosis established incidentally to other medical problems. Sometimes the mildness of this genotype leads it to be confused with sickle cell trait. Now and then, the presence of HbS is not recognized at all because the patient seems normal hematologically. Nevertheless, microcytosis and reticulocytosis are virtually always present. Failing to recognize mild HbS-β^+ thalassemia can be a serious omission when surgery is planned or pneumonia-like disorders are treated (Kolquist et al., 1996). Individuals with this genotype can encounter severe and devastating problems. Some observations suggest that the mortality of acute chest syndrome is higher in HbS-β^+ thalassemia than in sickle cell anemia (Desselle et al., 1995; Johnson et al., 1994; Kolquist et al., 1996; Zaidi et al., 1996).

Splenic enlargement is more likely to persist into the adult years in HbS-β thalassemia; in some studies it is present in over half the affected patients. As a result, adults may have splenic sequestration episodes. An enlarging spleen in adults can also lead to hypersplenism with falling blood counts and splenic infarction (Serjeant et al., 1973).

In Greek patients with HbS-β thalassemia, detailed studies of renal function showed multiple abnormalities that were similar in all respects to those found in sickle cell anemia.

Some forms of HbS-β^0 thalassemia may have a mild phenotype, which is usually due to very high HbF levels. In rare instances, the β-thalassemia mutation is accompanied by higher than usual levels of HbF and HbA$_2$. Uncommon small gene deletions that affect the 5' portion of the β-globin gene, perhaps because of competition of the transcriptional apparatus for gene promoters (Chapter 12), are typi-

fied by very high HbA$_2$ and HbF levels. Both HbA$_2$ and HbF inhibit the polymerization of HbS. In families with HbS-β^0 thalassemia caused by a -1.4 kb deletion, the combined total of HbF and HbA$_2$ was more than 20 percent of the total hemoglobin and associated with a milder than expected phenotype (Waye et al., 1991b). Other observations suggested that all individuals with this genotype may not be similarly affected (Padanilam et al., 1984). One young child with HbS-β^0 thalassemia caused by a 532 bp deletion in the 5' part of the β-globin gene had 29 percent HbF and 6 percent HbA$_2$, however, this patient's age precluded an assessment of the phenotype (Waye et al., 1991a).

HbS-β THALASSEMIA PLUS α THALASSEMIA

Where more than a few cases are available for analysis, any influence of coexistent α thalassemia on the phenotype of HbS-β^0 thalassemia or β^+ thalassemia is difficult to detect. However, the numbers of observations are still too small to provide a firm conclusion (Kulozik et al., 1991; Steinberg et al., 1984b). Not all reports have ascertained α thalassemia by gene mapping. When the coincidence of these disorders was based on hematologic, electrophoretic, and globin biosynthesis studies, there were no clinical or hematologic differences from patients with HbS-β^0 thalassemia except the presence of balanced globin biosynthesis ratios (Steinberg et al., 1984b). Clinical and hematologic differences were also not observed when heterozygous or homozygous α thalassemia-2 was ascertained by the more reliable method of α-globin gene mapping (Steinberg et al., 1984b).

In summary, although it is true that HbS-β^0 thalassemia is clinically more severe than HbS-β^+ thalassemia, and among people with HbS-β^+ thalassemia, those with more fare better than those with less HbA, rigid, uniformly applicable, genotype-phenotype correlations are difficult to establish because of the many genetic and environmental modulators that influence sickle cell disease (Chapter 26).

HbS-HPFH AND $\delta\beta$ THALASSEMIA

Pathophysiology

Hereditary persistence of HbF (HPFH) connotes the continued expression of HbF into adult life. These conditions, whose molecular basis and clinical spectrum are covered in detail in Chapter 15, are, like all genetic abnormalities of globin, genetically and hematologically heterogeneous. They can be divided into two classes: HPFH caused by extensive deletions within the β-like globin gene complex and HPFH

Table 28.3. HbS with Hereditary Persistence of Fetal Hemoglobin

Nongene deletion

Mutation	Hb/PCV	HbF	$^G\gamma$ (%)	MCV	Phenotype
−202 C→G 5′ $^G\gamma$		20	100		In sickle cell trait, HbA ~30%
−202 C→T 5′ $^A\gamma$	11/30	2.5	32	88	In sickle cell anemia
−175 T→C 5′ $^G\gamma$		30	100		In sickle cell trait, HbS ~40%, HbA ~28%
−175 T→C 5′ $^A\gamma$, 5′ $^G\gamma$ 158 C→T in *cis*	14/42	40	35	85	In sickle cell trait, HbS ~40%, HbA ~17%
13 bp deletion −114 to −102		31	14		HbA 20%
−158 C→T 5′ $^G\gamma$					See discussion of Senegal haplotype in sickle cell anemia (Chapter 26)

Gene deletion HPFH

HPFH-1, ~106 kb	Normal	25	51	70–80	None
HPFH-2 105 kb	Normal	25	32		None

δβ thalassemia

~12 kb§	11/34	25		85	Very mild
~36 kb	9–13/29–45	19–22	90–98	75–91	

From Huisman et al., 1997.

---

caused by point mutations within the promoters of the γ-globin genes. The δβ thalassemias, also caused by large gene deletions, are closely related to gene deletion HPFH (Chapter 15). Compound heterozygotes with HbS-deletion HPFH and δβ thalassemia can be found in black and Mediterranean populations. Mutations described in HbS-HPFH and δβ thalassemia are shown in Table 28.3. This chapter considers mainly the HbS-deletion HPFH and δβ thalassemia syndromes.

Nongene-deletion HPFH occurs with sickle cell anemia, but the elevated HbF level typical of this genotype makes the recognition of this form of HPFH difficult in the absence of family studies, enumeration of F cells, and determination of the HPFH mutation. Nongene-deletion HPFH is more commonly recognized when it is present with sickle cell trait or exists in the absence of an abnormal hemoglobin or β thalassemia. These mutations are discussed in Chapter 15.

Illustrating the role of HbF as a major modulator of sickle cell disease, the level and cellular distribution of HbF in compound heterozygous conditions with HbS determines the phenotype. A pancellular distribution of HbF in HbS-deletion HPFH retards HbS polymerization to the extent that hemolytic and vasoocclusive disease are absent or very minimal. Even though HbS-δβ thalassemia and HbS-deletion HPFH may have nearly equal total HbF levels, in the former condition

all cells are not equally endowed with HbF, so that mild hemolytic anemia is present.

Diagnosis

In blacks, the prevalence of HbS-deletion HPFH is about 0.0001 (Murray et al., 1988). HbF levels are 20 to 30 percent, and the distribution in erythrocytes is nearly equal in all red cells, or pancellular. Anemia and reticulocytosis are absent or mild, irreversibly sickled cells are absent, target cells are present, and HbA$_2$ levels are low or normal because the HPFH chromosome lacks the δ-globin gene. Thirteen unselected patients with HbS-HPFH, diagnosed because the proband had a parent with heterozygous HPFH, but not diagnosed by molecular analysis, were compared with patients with sickle cell anemia and HbS-β^0 thalassemia. In all groups the median age of the patients was between 9 and 12 years, and all individuals had HbF levels greater than 20 percent. Their hematologic findings are summarized in Table 28.4. Differentiating among these genotypes was possible based on the hematologic findings, although the patients with sickle cell anemia and HbS-β^0 thalassemia were selected for this comparison by their high HbF levels. When HbS-deletion HPFH is compared with unselected cases of sickle cell anemia and HbS-β^0 thalassemia that have more ordinary HbF

Table 28.4. Comparisons of HbS-Deletion HPFH with High HbF Sickle Cell Anemia, and HbS-β Thalassemia

Variable	HbS-HPFH	Sickle cell anemia	HbS-β thalassemia
Hemoglobin (g/dL)	13.4	10.2	10.9
HbF (%)	29.2	21.6	24.2
HbA$_2$ (%)	2.0	2.0	3.7
MCV (fl)	78.4	89.2	75
Reticulocytes (%)	1.9	7.3	3.6

Adapted from Murray et al., 1988. Values are means.

levels, the differentiation among these genotypes is even more dramatic.

Hb Kenya is caused by a γβ fusion gene, the product of nonhomologous crossing over between the γ- and β-globin genes. In compound heterozygotes with HbS, there was about 18 percent Hb Kenya, evenly distributed among the red cell population, and HbF averaged about 8 percent. Hb Kenya acted as a deletion HPFH determinant, and vasoocclusive symptoms were not reported. Red cell morphology was normal and anemia absent or minimal (Huisman, 1997; Kendall et al., 1973).

In HbS-δβ thalassemia, the HbF level is 15 to 25 percent. Its cellular distribution is not uniform as it is in HbS-deletion HPFH, but instead HbF is unevenly spread among red cells, or heterocellular. Anemia is mild, with the hemoglobin level averaging 10 to 12 g/dL, reticulocytes are about 2 percent, and the MCV is low-normal. HbA$_2$ levels are normal or low because of the deleted δ-globin gene (Kinney et al., 1978).

Some individuals with sickle cell anemia have very high HbF levels and seem not to have deletion HPFH, δβ thalassemia, or a Senegal haplotype chromosome (Chapter 26). Few of these patients have been carefully studied, but it is likely that some will have a nondeletion HPFH mutation. In a patient with sickle cell anemia who was heterozygous for the Benin and the "MOR" haplotype and lacked the −158 C-T polymorphism, HbF was 24 to 29 percent. The presence of a C→T mutation at −202 5' to the $^Aγ$ globin gene was suspected to cause this marked increase in HbF. Individuals with sickle cell trait who also inherited this mutation had 2 to 4 percent HbF and more than 90 percent $^Aγ$ chains (Gilman et al., 1988).

In some cases of sickle cell anemia with unusually high HbF levels, the increase in HbF may not be linked to the β-globin genelike cluster (Chang et al., 1995, 1997; Craig et al., 1997; Thein et al., 1994). Other instances may be associated with already identified or

still obscure cis-acting elements linked to the β-globin gene that may modulate γ-globin gene expression (Lu and Steinberg, 1996; Ofori-Acquah et al., 1999; Öner et al., 1992; Plonczynski et al., 1997).

Clinical

HbS-deletion HPFH is not associated with hemolytic anemia or acute vasoocclusive disease, although osteonecrosis has been described. The phenotype of HbS-δβ thalassemia also appears to be mild. Vasoocclusive problems can occur, but less often than in sickle cell anemia or HbS-β thalassemia. Splenomegaly is common.

HbS-Hb LEPORE

Hb Lepore, a small collection of hemoglobin variants that result from unequal crossing over between δ- and β-globin genes (Chapter 15), is characterized by the deletion of both these genes from the chromosome and their replacement by a poorly expressed, δβ hybrid, or, Hb Lepore gene. HbS-Lepore was first described in Greece but has since been found in many other geographic areas (Stamatoyannopoulos 1963). Hb Lepore has the same electrophoretic behavior as HbS, but in heterozygotes, accounts for only about 10 percent of the total hemoglobin. It causes a δβ$^+$ thalassemia with levels of Hb Lepore equivalent to the levels of HbA in the IVS-1, 110 G→A HbS-β$^+$ thalassemia. Compound heterozygosity for HbS and Hb Lepore is an uncommon condition, most often described in Mediterranean populations and best diagnosed by family studies that document heterozygous Hb Lepore in a parent or sibling. Failure to note the presence of Hb Lepore by protein-based hemoglobin diagnostic studies can result in the confusion of this genotype with sickle cell anemia or HbS-β^0 thalassemia. It is possible to separate Hb Lepore from HbS by isoelectric focusing. Analysis of DNA can authenticate the presence of the Hb Lepore gene. Because compound heterozygotes with HbS-Hb Lepore have only a single β-globin gene, amplification of the β-globin gene, and allele-specific hybridization or restriction endonuclease cleavage can falsely suggest homozygosity for the HbS gene when in actuality, the patient is hemizygous at the β^6 codon.

Unsurprisingly, reported patients with HbS-Lepore have heterogeneous phenotypes (Fairbanks et al., 1997; Huisman, 1997; Mirabile et al., 1995; Seward et al., 1993; Stamatoyannopoulos and Fessas, 1963; Voskaridou et al., 1995). A typical pedigree, with representative hematologic findings, is shown in Figure 28.5. Compared with sickle cell

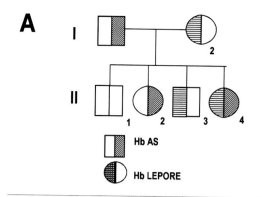

	I₁	I₂	II₄
Hb	15	12	11
MCV	85	70	78
HbS	40	0	75
HbLEPORE	0	10	10
HbA₂	3	2	2
HbF	1	1	10

Hb AS

Hb LEPORE

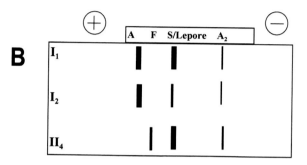

Figure 28.5. Pedigree of a typical family with HbS-Hb Lepore. (A) Hematologic values and the proportions of HbS, HbF, and Hb Lepore are average values taken from most cases reported in the literature. (B) Hemoglobin electrophoresis at pH 8.6 showing the migration of HbA, F, S, and Lepore. HbS and Lepore migrate together making the diagnosis of this compound heterozygous state by electrophoresis difficult. (From Fairbanks et al., 1997; Huisman, 1997; Mirabile et al., 1995; Seward et al., 1993; Stamatoyannopoulos and Fessas, 1963; Voskaridou et al., 1995; Fairbanks et al., 1997.)

anemia and HbS-β⁰ thalassemia, there is milder anemia and a reduction in MCV, HbA₂, and reticulocyte counts. Symptoms can be mild or severe and splenomegaly is common. A paucity of clinical studies of HbS-Lepore disease makes it difficult to define completely its clinical spectrum and compare its severity with that of patients with HbS-β⁺ thalassemia who have low levels of HbA, for example, those with the IVS-1, 110 G→A mutation.

Residues δ22 (ala) and δ87 (gly) inhibit polymerization of HbS (Nagel et al., 1979; Poillon et al., 1993) and, as mentioned, when HbA₂ and HbF levels are high, their combination may cause a mild phenotype (Waye et al., 1991b). Hb Lepore Boston, the type most often reported with HbS, contains the δ87 glycine residue, whereas Hb Lepore Hollandia contains δ22 alanine. It is possible that the presence of Hb Lepore not only reduces the concentration of HbA but also inhibits polymerization, accounting for a milder than expected phenotype.

Treatment Recommendations

With few exceptions, individuals with HbS-β thalassemia-like disorders should be managed like those with sickle cell anemia. Although serious pneumococcal infection is less common in HbS-β⁺ thalassemia with high levels of HbA and may be no more common than in the general population, it does occur (Rogers and Buchanan, 1995b). Little consensus exists on the use of prophylactic penicillin for pneumococcal sepsis in S-β⁺ thalassemia or other "mild" compound heterozygous forms of sickle cell disease discussed in this chapter (Buchanan, 1994; Rogers and Buchanan, 1995a). A rational decision to use prophylactic penicillin in HbS-β thalassemia can be based on an approach similar to that for HbSC disease and is discussed in detail in Chapter 27. In essence, this decision is predicated on an evaluation of splenic function, which, if normal, argues for withholding prophylaxis. Pneumococcal vaccine should be given at age 2 years and parents instructed to seek immediate medical attention for febrile illnesses.

Patients with HbS-β thalassemia and similar disorders have a higher prevalence of proliferative retinopathy than do individuals with sickle cell anemia. They should be monitored like patients with HbSC disease (Chapter 27).

Continued and sometimes advancing splenomegaly predisposes affected individuals to splenic infarction, splenic sequestration episodes, and hypersplenism. These complications raise the issue of splenectomy and its timing during the evolution of the disease. Delaying splenectomy until the first recurrence of an episode of splenic sequestration seems reasonable. Hypersplenism or subacute splenic sequestration may be associated with worsening anemia and the need for transfusion. This may then dictate the need for splenectomy. Splenic infarcts may be painful, recurrent, and associated with intrasplenic hemorrhage. Depending on the severity of symptoms, they may also require splenectomy (Vichinsky et al., 1995).

When the use of general anesthesia is planned, based on observations in HbSC disease and in sickle cell anemia, using preoperative transfusion in patients with HbS-β⁺ thalassemia who face procedures with moderate surgical risk, such as abdominal surgery, appears prudent (Neumayr et al., 1998; Vichinsky et al., 1995). Preoperative transfusions are likely to reduce the incidence of serious complications such as acute chest syndrome.

Sickling Hemoglobins with Two Substitutions in the β-Globin Gene

Six variant hemoglobins have been described with both the β^6 glu→val sickle cell mutation and an addi-tional amino acid substitution in the same β-globin chain (Table 28.5). Most probably, these variants arose from crossing over between chromosomes, with the HbS mutation and chromosomes containing a different mutation. Yet this has never been proven by genetic analysis, and new mutations in a HbS gene or a new HbS mutation in a gene for another abnormal hemoglobin are possible. In four instances (Table 28.5), the hemoglobin variant with the second mutation was characterized before the description of the doubly substituted variant. Hb Korle-Bu and HbO Arab are sufficiently common to suggest that crossing over between these genes and HbS genes are the origin of Hb C-Harlem and S-Oman, respectively.

HbS-Antilles (β6 glu→val; β23 val→ile) was found in a black family from Martinique (Monplaisir et al., 1986). Twenty-four heterozygotes with 40 to 50 percent HbS-Antilles had hemolytic anemia with hemo-globin levels of 11 g/dL, reticulocytes of 4.5 percent, and MCV of 90 fl. Irreversibly sickled cells were pre-sent in the blood film. Heterozygotes for HbS-Antilles had recurrent painful episodes and splenomegaly. Three compound heterozygotes with HbS died with severe anemia, and one child with HbS-Antilles/HbC had severe disease.

Table 28.5. Sickling Hemoglobins with Two Amino Acid Substitutions in the β-Globin Chain

Hb name	Amino acid substitution	Presumed crossover	Presumed mutation*	Phenotype[†]
S-Antilles	β23 val→Ile	HbS(- - -)	GTT→ATT	Migrates ~HbS. Heterozygote affected; compound heterozygote with HbC severely affected
C-Ziguinchor	β58 pro→arg	HbS (Dhofar)	CCT→CGT	Migrates ~HbC. 30–40% in the heterozygote. Normal hematology target cells
C-Harlem	β73asp→asn	HbS (Korle-Bu)	GAT→AAT	Migrates like HbS at alkaline pH and like HbC at acidic pH. Compound heterozygote with HbS~ sickle cell anemia, heterozygote ~40%, normal hematology.
S-Providence	β82 asn→asp	HbS (Providence)	AAG→AAT or AAC	Migrates like HbA. Hematology normal
S-Oman	β121 glu→lys	HbS (O-Arab)	GAA→AAA	Migrates ~HbC. Heterozygote has ~15% HbS-Oman
S-Travis	β142 ala→val	HbS(- - -)	GCC→GTC	Migrates between HbS and HbS at alkaline pH and between HbA and HbS at acidic pH. Unstable, ~15% in heterozygote. Hematology normal.

From Huisman et al., 1997.

Non-HbS mutation and amino acid substitution are shown. All cases are presumed to have the β6 glu→val HbS mutation.

* In no case has the mutation been proven by gene analysis.

[†] Migration refers to cellulose acetate electrophoresis unless noted otherwise.

Like the sickle cell anemia erythrocyte, HbS-Antilles red cells had reduced oxygen affinity, but solutions of HbS-Antilles also had a low p^{50}. This variant had a C_{sat} (a measure of hemoglobin solubility) of 11.9 g/dL compared with 18.4 g/dL for HbS and 24.1 g/dL for an equal mixture of HbS and HbA. HbS-Antilles erythrocytes sickled at physiologic PO_2. Ten to 20 percent of HbS-Antilles erythrocytes had increased density. The percentage of HbS-Antilles cells that sickled at PO_2 between 0 and 70 mm Hg was identical to HbSC disease erythrocytes. At a PO_2 between 40 and 90 mm Hg, the polymer fraction in HbS-Antilles cells was similar to that present in erythrocytes of sickle cell anemia. These findings show that this variant polymerized more readily than HbS at any PO_2. HbS-Antilles polymerizes even when it accounts for only half the cellular hemoglobin, explaining the cellular damage and symptoms of sickle cell disease in heterozygotes and the very severe phenotype in compound heterozygotes with HbS or HbC.

HbS-OMAN

This variant, containing the HbS and HbO-Arab mutation (β121 glu→lys), migrates slower than HbC when electrophoresed at alkaline pH because of an additional positive charge (Langdown et al., 1989). β121 lys appears to stabilize the sickle polymer. C_{sat} was 11 g/dL, nearly identical to that for HbS-Antilles and lower than that for HbS. In all cases described to date, HbS-Oman has been associated with either heterozygous or homozygous α thalassemia-2 (Fig. 28.6).

Figure 28.6. Erythrocytes in different genotypes of HbS-Oman disease. The peculiar shape of the irreversibly sickled cells has been called "yarn/knitting needle," and it is presumed to result from the polymerization of HbS-Oman in one or two domains. For full color reproduction, see color plate 28.6.

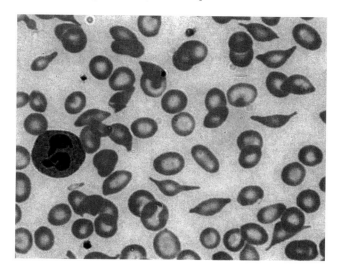

Homozygotes for this variant have not been described but are predicted to have very severe disease, resembling homozygotes with HbS-Antilles, and perhaps made even worse by the presence of α thalassemia. Two different phenotypes appear to exist (Nagel et al., 1998). Patients with HbS-Oman/heterozygous α thalassemia-2, had more than 20 percent of the variant hemoglobin, low hemoglobin levels, MCV about 73 fl, splenomegaly, and vasoocclusive episodes including acute chest syndrome. Their sickle cells had a peculiar morphology described as "yarn/knitting needle," believed to be a consequence of a single domain of HbS-Oman polymerization. Individuals with HbS-Oman/homozygous α thalassemia-2 had about 14 percent variant hemoglobin and further reduction of MCV. They were asymptomatic but had microcytosis. Interaction of this highly charged variant with the membrane—a general feature of hemoglobins with high positive charges, such as HbC and HbA₂—promotes dense cell formation and polymerization even at the relative low concentrations of HbS-Oman found in heterozygous HbS-Oman/heterozygous α thalassemia-2 (Nagel et al., 1998).

Recently, the homozygote state of Hb O_{ARAB} has been studied (Nagel et al., 1999). Density separation of red cells by isopyknic gradients demonstrated that all the homozygous HbO_{ARAB} red cells were denser than normal red cells, similar to homozygous HbC patients. Reticulocytes in homozygotes for HbO_{ARAB} were found in the densest density fraction of whole blood. and cation transport systems in homozygotes for HbO_{ARAB} were abnormal, with K:Cl cotransport activity similar to HbSOman and only somewhat lower than sickle cell anemia red cells. The Gardos channels were indistinguishable from the activity found in HbS, HbC and HbS-Oman cells. These findings support the concept that the erythrocytic pathogenesis of HbO_{ARAB} involves the dehydration of red cells, due, at least in part, to the K:Cl cotransport system. The similarity of the charge and consequences to the red cell of the presence of both HbC and HbO_{ARAB}, the product of two distantly located mutations is intriguing. It raises the possibility that this pathological activity is connected with a charge-dependent interaction of these hemoglobins with the red cell membrane and/or its cytoskeleton and that this abnormality appears early in red cell development. These findings also buttress the interpretation that the O_{ARAB} mutation is indeed responsible for the enhanced phenotype of HbS-Oman.

HbS-HbC HARLEM

A compound heterozygote with HbS and HbS-HbC-Harlem (β6 glu→val; β73 asp→asn) had 50 percent HbS, 43 percent HbC-Harlem, and 7 percent HbF

(Adachi, 1980; Bookchin et al., 1968; Moo-Penn et al., 1975). Hematologic findings were similar to those in sickle cell anemia; there were vasoocclusive episodes, and osteonecrosis of the hips required surgery. Heterozygous HbC-Harlem emulates sickle cell trait. Equal mixtures of HbC-Harlem and HbS had gelling properties identical to 100 percent HbS, predicting that compound heterozygotes would resemble sickle cell anemia. Compound heterozygotes for sickle cell trait and Hb Korle-Bu, however, do not differ from individuals with sickle cell trait alone, indicating that in that variant, the β73 asp→asn substitution does not promote HbS polymerization.

COMPOUND HETEROZYGOTES OF HbS WITH β-GLOBIN CHAIN VARIANTS

Examples without a Clinical Phenotype

Many β-globin chain variants have been described as compound heterozygotes with HbS. In most examples, only one or a few cases have been reported, and gauging the true extent of any hematologic or clinical abnormalities is difficult because confounding genetic and acquired abnormalities are not always excluded. Most of these compound heterozygous combinations are not associated with any clinical disease, and if hematologic abnormalities are present, they are minor. Only when the site and type of amino acid substitution permit participation in the polymerization of HbS, or the variant is unstable or is synthesized in vastly reduced amounts, as with Hb Monroe (see previously), is a clinically apparent phenotype apt to be present. About one third of the β-globin chain variants found with HbS as compound heterozygotes do not separate from HbS by electrophoresis at alkaline pH. Individuals who have these hemoglobins can be mistaken for patients with sickle cell anemia and counseled erroneously or mistreated. Alternative methods of hemoglobin separation and family studies can usually resolve any confusion that may arise. The known compound heterozygotes with HbS that do not have a clinically significant phenotype are listed in Table 28.6.

Examples with a Clinical Phenotype

Some examples of compound heterozygosity for HbS and other β-globin gene variants associated with hematologic or clinical findings are described only once or twice. Their associated phenotype is likely to be incompletely characterized. Often enough, the phenotype is ostensibly the result of the abnormal properties of the variant associated with HbS rather than the polymerization of HbS so that, strictly speaking, these examples may not be a type of sickle cell disease (Table 28.7).

HbO-ARAB

HbO-Arab (β121 glu→lys) is a relatively common variant in blacks and individuals of Arabic descent, and in both populations it has been associated with HbS. Together, the two variants can cause severe sickle cell disease. Because HbO-Arab migrates with HbC when electrophoresed at alkaline pH, HbS-O-Arab disease is confused often with HbSC disease. Patients with unusually severe "HbSC disease" should be carefully evaluated for the presence of HbO-Arab. HbO-Arab can be separated from HbC on electrophoresis at acidic pH and by isoelectric focusing. The β121 residue, also affected in HbD-Los Angeles, is a contact point in the HbS polymer, and substitutions at this residue increase the nucleation rate for polymer formation (Adachi et al., 1988).

Thirty-nine patients with HbS-O-Arab have been reported, allowing an assessment of the clinical phenotype (Zimmerman et al., 1999). Individuals with HbS-O-Arab disease have hematologic and clinical findings indistinguishable from patients with sickle cell anemia (Milner et al., 1970). In thirteen African Americans with HbS-O-Arab disease, ages 3 to 63 years, mean hemoglobin concentration was 8.7 g/dL, reticulocytes 5.8 percent, and HbF 6.7 percent (Zimmerman et al., 1999). Blood films showed target and sickled cells. Acute chest syndrome, stroke, leg ulcers, and painful episodes, along with all of the other complications of sickle cell disease, occurred in all patients. Four patients died, two children from pneumococcal sepsis, a teenager from acute chest syndrome, and an adult from multiorgan failure.

HbD-LOS ANGELES (PUNJAB)

Compound heterozygosity of HbD-Los Angeles (Punjab) β121 glu→gln with HbS, first described in Caucasians, produces hematologic and clinical manifestations similar to those of sickle cell anemia (Sturgeon et al., 1955). The β121 glutamine residue facilitates polymerization of HbS (Adachi et al., 1988). This mutant, widespread throughout the world, is most common in Caucasians of northern India. It is a "typical" HbD, electrophoresing like HbS at alkaline pH, like HbA at acidic pH, and giving a negative sickle solubility test.

HbS-Oman and HbS-O-Arab, where the β 121 substitution is in *cis* or in *trans*, respectively, to the HbS β6 glu→lys substitution, and where both conditions are associated with vasoocclusive disease, illustrate the clinical importance of mutations that stabilize the HbS polymer. In contrast, the β 73 residue, altered in Hb Korle-Bu, does not affect polymerization. Heterozygotes for HbC-Harlem, where the β 73 mutant is in *cis* to the sickle mutation,

Table 28.6. Compound Heterozygotes of HbS with β-Globin Chain Variants That Have No Clinical Phenotype

Name	Substitution	Properties
Hb Deer Lodge	β2 his →arg	Migrates like HbS on alkaline electrophoresis. Compound heterozygotes appear like "sickle cell anemia"
HbG-San Jose	β7 glu →gly	Migrates between HbF and HbS
Hb Saki	β14 leu →arg	Migrates like HbA
HbJ-Baltimore	β16 gly →asp	Migrates faster than HbA at alkaline pH and like HbS at acidic pH
Hb Sinai-Baltimore	β18 val →gly	Migrates~ HbA
HbD-Iran	β22 glu →gln	Migrates~ HbS
Hb Knossos	β27 ala→ser	Migrates like HbA. A "thalassemic" variant. 40% in compound heterozygote with HbS
Hb Muscat	β32 leu→val	Migrates like HbA. 48% in compound heterozygote with HbS
HbG Galveston	β43 glu→ala	Migrates like HbS at alkaline pH, like HbA at acidic pH. Possibly mistaken for sickle cell anemia
Hb Maputo	β47 asp→tyr	Migrates like HbS at alkaline pH, like HbA at acidic pH
Hb Osu-Christiansborg	β52 asp→asn	Migrates like HbS at alkaline pH, like HbA at acidic pH. Possibly mistaken for sickle cell anemia
Hb Ocho Rios	β52 asp→ala	Migrates like HbS at alkaline pH
Hb Korle-Bu	β73 asp→asn	Common variant
Hb Mobile	β73 asp→val	Can be confused electrophoretically with HbS
Hb Pyrgos	β83 gly→asp	Migrates faster than HbA
HbD-Ibadan	β87 thr→lys	Migrates like HbS at alkaline pH, like HbA at acidic pH
Hb Caribbean	β91 leu→arg	Migrates between HbS and HbA
HbN-Baltimore	β95 lys→glu	Migrates much faster than HbA, common in blacks
Hb New Mexico	β100 pro→arg	Migrates like HbS at alkaline pH, between HbS and HbC at acidic pH. High O_2 affinity variant with mild erythrocytosis. 54% with HbS.
Hb Richmond	β102 asn→lys	Migrates as two bands between HbS and HbA
HbP-Galveston	β117 his→arg	Migrates like HbS at alkaline pH
Hb Iowa	β119 gly→ala	Migrates ~HbF at alkaline pH. In a neonate electrophoresis was confused with HbSF pattern and sickle cell anemia was considered
Hb Hofu	β126 val→glu	Migrates faster than HbA. 23% with HbS, mild anemia. This may be due to α thalassemia. No symptoms despite HbS of ~70%.
Hb K-Cameroon	β129 ala→?	Amino acid substitution unclear, ?asp, ?glu
Hb Camden	β131 gln→glu	Migrates faster than HbA at alkaline pH, near HbF at acidic pH
Hb K-Woolwich	β132 lys→gln	Migrates faster than HbA
Hb McKees Rock	β145 tyr→term	Migrates like HbA. High O_2 affinity variant
Hb Rainier	β145 tyr→cys	Migrates like HbA. High O_2 affinity variant

From Hardison et al., 1998; Huisman et al., 1998; Witkowska et al., 1997.

Table 28.7. Compound Heterozygotes of HbS with β-Globin Chain Variants with a Clinical Phenotype

Name	Substitution	Phenotype
Hb Monroe	IVS-1-1 G→C; arg→thr	Severe HbS-$β^0$ thalassemia
HbE	β26 glu→lys	Mild sickle cell disease
Hb Lufkin	β29 gly →asp	Migrates faster than HbA. Mildly unstable. ~45% in compound heterozygote with HbS. Mild hemolysis
Hb 1-Toulouse	β66 lys→glu	Migrates faster than HbS
Hb Quebec-Chori	β87 thr→Ile	Causes sickle cell disease. 60% of hemolysate
Hb San Diego	β109 val→met	Difficult to separate from HbA. High O_2 affinity variant with erythrocytosis
HbD-Los Angeles (Punjab)	β121 glu→gln	Migrates like HbS at alkaline pH and HbA at acidic pH. Fourth most common Hb variant
HbO-Arab	β121 glu→lys	Migrates like HbC
Hb Shelby	β131 gln→lys	Migrates like HbF at alkaline pH and between HbS and HbC at acidic pH
Hb North Shore	β134 val→glu	"Thalassemic" variant causing HbS-$β^+$ thalassemia
Hb Hope	β136 gly→asp	Migrates like HbF at acidic pH and slightly faster than HbA at alkaline pH

From Hardison et al., 1998; Huisman et al., 1998.

resemble heterozygotes for HbS. Only the HbS-HbC-Harlem compound heterozygote has sickle cell disease because of homozygosity for the β 6 glu→val sickle cell mutation, not the β 73 mutation in *trans*.

Hb QUEBEC-CHORI

Hb Quebec-Chori (β87 thr→ile) migrates like HbA on alkaline electrophoresis and by isoelectric focusing, allowing the compound heterozygous state with HbS to be confused with sickle cell trait (Witkowska et al., 1991). Reverse-phase HPLC and electrospray ionization mass spectroscopy separated this variant β-globin chain from β^A. Mixtures of Hb Quebec-Chori with HbS had the same delay time of polymerization as pure HbS. A bulky hydrophobic isoleucine residue substituted at β87 may strengthen the hydrophobic environment in the acceptor pocket for β6 val, stabilize a lateral contact between HbS polymer strands, and accelerate polymerization. Other work has shown the importance of this site in polymer formation (Ho et al., 1996; Reddy et al., 1997) (Chapter 23). Participation of this variant with HbS in the polymerization process caused vasoocclusive symptoms and the hematologic phenotype of sickle cell disease in the compound heterozygote with HbS. Associated with a nonfunctional enlarged spleen, vasoocclusive episodes, mild anemia, reticulocytosis, and sickled cells in the blood, HbS-Hb Quebec-Chori mimics sickle cell anemia and not sickle cell trait. This rare condition, described only once, provides a cautionary note on the evaluation of clinically symptomatic instances of sickle cell trait (Chapter 29).

HbSE DISEASE

Described so far in Turks and in blacks, HbSE disease is usually a mild disorder with minimal anemia, microcytosis (perhaps reflecting the thalassemic nature of the HbE gene or coexistent α thalassemia), and few symptoms (Altay et al., 1976; Rey et al., 1991; Schroeder et al., 1998). However, complications of sickle cell disease can occur, as illustrated by a report of a young woman with HbSE disease who had severe acute chest syndrome associated with B19 parvovirus infection (Eichhorn et al, 1999). HbE and HbA_2 are difficult to separate by electrophoresis, and their combined concentration of 30 to 35 percent is less than the 50 percent HbC present in HbSC disease. Because HbE migrates similarly to HbC on electrophoresis at alkaline pH, their distinction may not be apparent. Although HbE is considered an uncommon genotype in African Americans, the recent influx into the United States of many Asians who carry a HbE gene makes it likely that the prevalence of this disorder will increase in the country. HbSE disease seems milder than HbSC

disease, although it has a higher concentration of HbS. Characterizations of the HbSE phenotype are too sketchy, and insufficient studies of cell density or polymerization in HbSE cells have been done to suggest a reason for this observation; however, this may be due to the thalassemic features of HbE and the differential effects of HbE and HbC on the erythrocyte membrane.

Hb I-TOULOUSE

Hb I-Toulouse (β66 lys→glu) was described in a boy with sickle cell trait splenomegaly, a hemoglobin level of 10.5 g/dL, reticulocytes of 7 percent, and MCV of 110 fl. Similar findings were present in a simple heterozygote for this variant, suggesting that it was the characteristics of this unstable hemoglobin rather than HbS that were responsible for the phenotype (Tejuca et al., 1987).

HB SAN DIEGO

Hb San Diego (β 109 val→met) is a high oxygen affinity variant described in diverse ethnic backgrounds and often results from a new mutation. It has been postulated that the ethnic diversity of this variant is a result of the mutation occurring at a CpG "hot spot" where deamination of methylcytosine leads to a C→T transition (Coleman et al., 1993; Williamson et al., 1995). In a compound heterozygote with HbS, about 70 percent of the hemolysate was Hb San Diego. Mild erythrocytosis with a hemoglobin of 18.8 g/dL and PCV of 58 was caused by the high oxygen affinity variant and not by sickle cell disease.

Hb SHELBY

Hb Shelby (β131 gln→lys), a mildly unstable variant, is associated with hemolytic anemia when present with HbS (Adachi et al., 1993). It appears to interact similarly with HbS and HbA. At age 4 years, the proband with HbS-Hb Shelby had a hemoglobin level of 9.8 g/dL, 14 percent reticulocytes, and an MCV of 70 fl. Hb Shelby formed 43 percent of the hemolysate. Splenomegaly or vasoocclusive symptoms were absent. It is not clear why anemia was present in this compound heterozygote. Based on studies of simple heterozygotes for Hb Shelby, the phenotype of this combination most likely is due to Hb Shelby and not HbS polymerization.

Hb HOPE

Hb Hope (β136 gly→asp) is unstable and when present with HbS, is associated with mild hemolytic anemia but normal reticulocyte counts and no symptoms of vasoocclusive disease (Steinberg et al., 1974). In compound heterozygotes, about half the hemolysate was Hb Hope. ^{51}Cr red cell survival was reduced about 30 percent and Heinz bodies were present in half the red cells. Hb Hope did not appear to affect HbS polymerization because the minimum gelling concentrations of mixtures of Hb Hope and HbS and HbA with HbS were similar. Lack of reticulocytosis was thought to result from the low O_2 affinity of Hb Hope (Steinberg et al., 1976). Again, the phenotype of this combination does not appear to be due to HbS polymerization.

Hb NORTH SHORE

Hb North Shore (β134 val→glu) is associated with the phenotype of mild β thalassemia. A patient with sickle cell trait and Hb North Shore had mild hemolytic anemia, MCV of 71 fl, HbA$_2$ of 4.9 percent, and an α/β synthesis ratio of 3 (Arends et al., 1977). These findings suggested that HbS polymerization did not contribute to the phenotype that was likely to be a reflection of the "thalassemic" properties of this variant (Smith et al., 1983).

SICKLE CELL ANEMIA WITH α THALASSEMIA

Early accounts of the effects of α thalassemia in sickle cell anemia were limited by the inability to detect directly the presence of the common gene deletion type of α thalassemia (Honig et al., 1978; Weatherall et al., 1969). Because of the problems of disease ascertainment and the small number of patients studied, those reports of coexistent α thalassemia and sickle cell anemia were unclear regarding the effect of α thalassemia on the phenotype of sickle cell anemia. Gene mapping and PCR-based methods provided accurate means of detecting of α thalassemia and by the study of substantial groups of patients, have permitted the definition of the phenotype of sickle cell anemia-α thalassemia (Figueiredo et al., 1996; Higgs et al., 1982; Kéclard et al., 1996, 1997; Martinez et al., 1996; Mukherjee et al., 1997; Powars et al., 1990; Steinberg et al., 1995, 1997).

Among blacks with sickle cell anemia, 30 to 40 percent are heterozygous and 2 to 3 percent are homozygous for the common $-\alpha^{3.7}$ kb deletion type of α thalassemia (Higgs et al., 1982; Kéclard et al., 1996, 1997; Steinberg and Embury, 1986; Steinberg et al., 1997). This genotype is also prevalent in Saudi Arabia and India (El-Hazmi and Warsy, 1993; Mukherjee et al., 1997). Some instances of sickle cell anemia with microcytosis, without evidence of β thalassemia or gene deletion α thalassemia, may reflect the presence of nondeletion types of α thalassemia. Although uncommon in blacks, these mutations are not rare on the Arabian peninsula, the Middle East, and in North Africa. Infrequently, the $-\alpha^{4.2}$ kb deletion and HbH disease have been found in individuals with the HbS gene (Adekile and Haider 1996; Embury et al., 1985b; Steinberg et al., 1986). Sickle cell anemia has also been described with triplicated α-globin loci. Few cases have been reported, and although they do not seem to differ from sickle cell anemia, it is not yet possible to know if the phenotype of the disease is affected (Higgs et al., 1984; Kéclard et al., 1996, 1997; Steinberg et al., 1997).

An extensive literature on the interaction of α thalassemia with sickle cell anemia is available and the following seems clearly established. α Thalassemia affects the cellular abnormalities, hematologic values, and clinical features of sickle cell anemia. The extent of this effect depends on the α-globin gene haplotype. In a single patient, the changes produced by α thalassemia may be subtle and difficult to detect, but differences among groups of patients are clear and clinically relevant.

Cellular Effects

α Thalassemia has multiple repercussions in the sickle erythrocyte that culminate in improved cellular survival (Table 28.8). Reduced cellular hemoglobin content, a primary consequence of α thalassemia, is calculated to diminish the polymerization potential of HbS and the cascade of cellular damage that emanates from this phenomenon. Smaller sickle cells may also have rheologic advantages that increase their survival. In sickle cell anemia-α thalassemia, the numbers of dense cells are reduced and fewer irreversibly sickled cells—cells that are least deformable and shortest lived—are present (Billett et al., 1986; Embury et al., 1984; Noguchi et al., 1985). The O_2 affinity of sickle cells,

---

Table 28.8. Cellular and Clinical Effects of α-Thalassemia in Sickle Cell Anemia

Cellular Effects

Reduced HbS polymer
Decreased cation exchange
Decreased erythrocyte density
Increased erythrocyte deformability

Clinical Effects

Increased osteonecrosis
Increased splenic sequestration
Possible increased painful episodes
Fewer leg ulcers
Fewer cerebrovascular accidents

low because of the existence of HbS polymer, may be increased in sickle cell anemia-α thalassemia by the improvement in cellular hydration. Higher O_2 affinity should reduce the fraction of deoxy HbS, further retarding polymerization (Embury and Steinberg, 1994).

Studies using different methods have shown that α thalassemia reduces the density and increases the deformability of oxygenated sickle erythrocytes (Billett et al., 1986; Embury et al., 1984; Noguchi et al., 1985; Serjeant et al., 1983). When sickle cells of equal density were isolated from individuals with four, three, and two α-globin genes, they were equally deformable, showing that the improved deformability associated with α thalassemia is due to the presence of fewer dense cells (Embury et al., 1984). Improved deformability is also probably related to reduced cytoplasmic viscosity caused by a lower mean cell HbS concentration and the advantages of an increased cell surface area to volume ratio. As PCV is the prime determinant of blood viscosity, the rheologic benefit of enhanced deformability of the individual cell is lost when the PCV in sickle cell anemia-α thalassemia cell is increased owing to improved cell survival. Whole blood viscosity in sickle cell anemia-homozygous α thalassemia-2 at a standard PCV of 45 was lower than viscosity of sickle cell anemia blood at the same PCV. When these groups are compared with the patient's original PCV, viscosity was higher in sickle cell anemia-α thalassemia (Serjeant et al., 1983). An additional benefit anticipated from increased cell surface area to volume ratio is protection against deoxygenation-induced K^+ efflux induced by polymerization-provoked membrane distortion (Chapter 22). α Thalassemia protects against deoxygenation-induced cation leak and the rapid dehydration of reticulocytes that generates irreversibly sickled cells (Bookchin et al., 1991; Embury et al., 1985a). Effects of α thalassemia on red cell surface area to volume relationships may explain the lack of effect of α thalassemia on the severity of anemia of young children (Stevens et al., 1986). Persistent splenic function in childhood may condition sickle erythrocytes, a normal function of the spleen, removing excessive membrane.

Hematologic Effects of α Thalassemia

Hematologic manifestations of sickle cell anemia-α thalassemia are a direct consequence of the cellular changes and are summarized in Table 28.9. Black patients with sickle cell anemia-α thalassemia had increased levels of HbA_2, microcytosis, reduced reticulocyte counts, and higher hemoglobin levels. Patients homozygous for the $-\alpha^{3.7}$ kb deletion had more pronounced changes than heterozygotes for this haplotype (Embury et al., 1982; Landin et al., 1995; Schroeder et al., 1989; Steinberg et al., 1984a). It was suggested that the lower mean corpuscular HbS concentration associated with α thalassemia resulted in retarded HbS polymerization and less red cell injury. Higher hemoglobin levels and reduced reticulocyte counts suggested that hemolysis was likely to be reduced and studies of red cell survival in sickle cell anemia-α thalassemia confirmed this notion (De Ceulaer et al., 1983). Children younger than 5 years old do not show similar changes, perhaps because of continued splenic function.

HbA_2 levels are elevated in sickle cell anemia-α thalassemia, an effect that confounds the distinction of this entity from HbS-β^0 thalassemia. It is likely that δ-globin chains compete more effectively than β^S chains for the limited numbers of α-globin chains that are present in α thalassemia and favor the assembly of HbA_2.

Sickle cell anemia-α thalassemia was first thought to be associated with increased HbF levels, but subsequent studies have failed to confirm the observation that was likely to have been the result of the examination of too few patients. Hypothetically, γ-globin chains might compete more favorably than β^S chains for the reduced number of α chains available in sickle cell anemia-α thalassemia and increase HbF levels. Several large studies of sickle cell anemia-α thalassemia found little influence of α thalassemia on HbF concentration in sickle cell anemia, and other

Table 28.9. Effects of α Globin Haplotype on the Hematological Features of Sickle Cell Anemia

Genotype	Number	Hemoglobin (g/dL)	Reticulocytes (%)	MCV (fl)	HbF (%)	HbA_2 (%)
αα/αα	299	8.1	11.4	92	6.2	2.9
−α/αα	152	8.6	9.0	83	5.7	3.3
−α/−α	66	9.2	6.7	72	5.1	3.8

Values reported are averages of three studies that used gene mapping to ascertain the α-globin genotype. The series differed in the mean ages of the patients studied. One series lumped the −α/αα and −α/−α genotype together for hemoglobin, MCV, and HbF levels; only nine −α/−α patients were in this series, and in this table these data were analyzed with the −α/αα genotype. The HbF differences are not significant; however, the patients were not segregated by β haplotype. In patients with α thalassemia and the Senegal haplotype, HbF levels are higher than in the other groups. Other differences are statistically significant.

investigators found that α thalassemia reduced HbF in sickle cell anemia (Dover et al., 1987). It was hypothesized in this latter work that the presence of both α thalassemia and HbF allowed some sickle erythrocyte to survive longer, masking the usual F-cell enrichment characteristic of sickle cell anemia and reducing the total HbF level (Dover et al., 1987). When patients were stratified based on the β-globin gene haplotype, no effect of α thalassemia on HbF was observed (Steinberg et al., 1995, 1997). HbF levels are unaltered by α thalassemia in children with sickle cell anemia and the Arab-India haplotype (Adekile and Haider, 1996). If α thalassemia does modulate HbF in sickle cell anemia, the effects must be quite small.

Clinical Effects

Table 28.8 shows some cellular and clinical effects of coincident α-thalassemia and sickle cell anemia. These observations may be interpreted as follows. An α-thalassemia-induced decrease in mean cell hemoglobin concentration reduces the polymerization tendency of HbS. Cellular damage, a usual consequence of high concentrations of HbS, is reduced, as membrane damage with an increased cation flux and potassium leak is diminished (Embury et al., 1985a). Smaller, less dense, more deformable cells are produced, whose longevity is enhanced. Because of these favorable cellular characteristics, PCV rises. These cellular and hematologic changes produce curious and paradoxical clinical results. Some vasoocclusive complications are increased, others are unaffected, and a few are reduced (Adams et al., 1994; Miller et al., 1988; Milner et al., 1991; Platt et al., 1991).

In sickle cell anemia, blood flow is optimal at the typical PCV found in most patients (Chien et al., 1970, 1982). Presumably, as the PCV rises, flow in some vascular beds is compromised, promoting vasoocclusion. This recalls normal circulatory physiology that links blood flow to the blood viscosity, which is, in turn, fixed primarily by the PCV. The presence of HbS distinguishes sickle cell anemia blood from normal blood. Abnormal intrinsic properties of dense and poorly deformable sickle cells vastly increase blood viscosity at any given PCV.

Clinically, the outcome of coincident α thalassemia and sickle cell anemia is incongruous. Anemia is improved, but vasoocclusive disease generally is not. Some work suggested that α thalassemia increased survival in sickle cell anemia (Martinez et al., 1996; Mears et al., 1983). Yet the largest studies do not confirm that α thalassemia has this effect, and, because of its effects on vasoocclusive crises, α thalassemia is a risk, in some studies, for increased morbidity and mortality (Higgs et al., 1982; Kéclard et al., 1996, 1997;

Powars et al., 1990; Steinberg and Embury, 1986; Thomas et al., 1997).

Vasoocclusive events appear undiminished in sickle cell anemia-α thalassemia (Billett et al., 1986; De Montelembert et al., 1993; Gill et al., 1995; Higgs et al., 1982; Steinberg et al., 1984a). The presence of more HbS-containing red cells, unless HbF levels are simultaneously increased in these cells, seems to promote vasoocclusion (Phillips et al., 1991). Patients with sickle cell anemia-α thalassemia have more episodes of pain and more bone disease than do patients with sickle cell anemia alone, an effect that appears to be due to the higher PCV caused by α thalassemia. In sickle cell anemia-α thalassemia, osteonecrosis of the humeral and femoral heads had an incidence of 4.5 to 4.9 cases per 100 patient-years compared with 2.4 cases for sickle cell anemia without α thalassemia (Milner et al., 1991, 1993).

Cardiovascular function was examined in patients with sickle cell anemia who were homozygous for the common α-thalassemia-2 deletion (Braden et al., 1996). These individuals had increased left ventricular wall thickness, with higher heart rates and blood pressure during exercise compared with patients with sickle cell anemia. The abnormalities noted in sickle cell anemia-α thalassemia suggested that the lower hemoglobin level in sickle cell anemia protects cardiac function.

Nevertheless, more blood and less hemolysis may also have beneficial effects in some organs, so that skin ulcers of the leg and retinal vascular disease may be less common. Twenty percent of pediatric patients with sickle cell anemia who had a stroke (44 patients) and 35 percent without a history of stroke (256 patients) had α thalassemia (Adams et al., 1994). The "no stroke" group also had HbF levels twice as high as the stroke group, but, even when controlling for the effects of HbF, α thalassemia was associated with a lower risk of stroke. Other smaller studies have given similar results (Figueiredo et al., 1996). Recently, the Cooperative Study of Sickle Cell Disease reported that the incidence of infarctive strokes in sickle cell anemia was reduced by more than 50 percent by coincident α thalassemia (Ohene-Frempong et al., 1998). None of forty-eight patients with homozygous α thalassemia-2 had a stroke. In other studies, α thalassemia was not a deterrent for stroke (Balkaran et al., 1992). A protective effect of α thalassemia is related to the associated increase in PCV (Ohene-Frempong et al., 1998).

α Thalassemia may increase the incidence of acute splenic sequestration episodes in children and adults with sickle cell anemia (De Ceulaer and Serjeant, 1991). Improved rheology of sickle erythrocytes in the presence of α thalassemia may preserve splenic function in some adults, setting the stage for acute sequestration episodes at a later age than expected. A positive aspect

804

of α thalassemia-related preserved splenic function, at least in individuals with the Arab-Indian haplotype and high HbF levels, is a reduction in bacterial infection (Adekile and Haider, 1996; Adekile et al., 1996).

Reduced hemolysis in sickle cell anemia-α thalassemia predicts that cholelithiasis should be less common in this genotype, a hypothesis supported by preliminary studies (Adekile and Haider, 1996).

HbS WITH α-GLOBIN CHAIN VARIANTS

Separate inheritance of β- and α-globin genes permits a dizzying array of combinations of sickle cell disease and sickle cell trait with α-globin gene variants and α thalassemia. In this section, the interactions of sickle cell anemia with α-globin gene variants are considered. α-Globin gene variants found with HbS are shown in Table 28.10. Hemoglobin tetramer assembly, discussed in Chapter 8, occurs via the association of αβ dimers. When variants of the α-globin gene are present, hybrid tetramers containing variant α-globin chains and normal α-globin chains are often seen by electrophoresis. In the presence of β-globin chain mutants such as HbS and HbC, additional hybrid tetramers form that can display unique electrophoretic patterns. This often provides a clue for the diagnosis of disorders where both α- and β-globin chain variants are present.

As HbG-Philadelphia (α68 asn→lys) is the most common α-globin gene variant in blacks, many examples of the coincidence of this variant and sickle cell anemia or sickle cell trait have been described (Fig. 28.7) (Charache et al., 1977). An example of the electrophoretic behavior of HbG-Philadelphia found with sickle cell trait and sickle cell anemia is shown in Figure 28.8. In sickle cell anemia, diagnostic confusion can occur because the hybrid molecule, $\alpha^A\alpha^G\beta_2^S$, migrates like HbC on alkaline electrophoresis. Clinically and hematologically, sickle cell anemia-HbG-Philadelphia resembles sickle cell anemia and not HbSC disease.

Sickle cell anemia has also been described with the α-globin gene variants Hb Montgomery (α48 leu→arg) and Hb Chicago (α136 leu→met) (Gu et al., 1993). The phenotype of these individuals resembled that of sickle cell anemia. By hemoglobin electrophoresis and isoelectric focusing, confusing patterns were present that could be resolved by HPLC. An example of isoelectric focusing of these variants is shown in Figure 28.9.

Hb Memphis, α23 glu→gln, is described as migrating with HbS when electrophoresed at both alkaline and acidic pH. This variant was present in older adults with sickle cell anemia and patients had the hematologic features of sickle cell anemia. Red cell survival was 11 days and vasoocclusive episodes and splenomegaly seemed absent. In the best described case, the hemoglobin level was 9.5, reticulocytes 5 to 24 percent, MCV 88 fl, and HbF 6 percent. Many sickled cells were present in the blood. Curiously, in neither the proband nor in three children in the family of the proband who had sickle cell trait and Hb Memphis was there evidence of hybrid molecules such as $\alpha^A\alpha^M\beta_2^S$, $\alpha^A\alpha^M\delta_2$, and $\alpha_2^M\beta_2^S$ that are typical of other α-globin gene variants and might be expected (Cooper et al., 1973). It would be desirable to confirm the diagnosis of Hb Memphis by DNA analysis.

Hb Stanleyville-II α77 pro→arg was described in a boy from Zaïre with findings that were typical of sickle cell anemia with 70 percent HbS and 30 percent Hb Stanleyville-II (Van Ros et al., 1973). A brother with sickle cell anemia had a more severe disease. Individuals with sickle cell trait and Hb Stanleyville-II were well and had the expected distribution of HbA, Hb Stanleyville-II, and hybrid molecules. It was proposed than the mutation to arginine stabilized HbS fiber formation (Rhoda et al., 1983).

Table 28.10. Association of α-Globin Gene Variants with HbS

Variant	Mutation	Phenotype
Hb Memphis	α23 glu→gln	Migrates like HbS at both alkaline and acidic pH
Hb Montgomery	α48 leu→arg	Migrates between HbS and HbA at alkaline pH
Hb Mexico	α54 gln→glu	With sickle cell trait, ~20% Hb Mexico and 50% hybrid hemoglobin
HbG-Philadelphia	α68 asn→lys	Migrates like HbS at alkaline pH and HbA at acidic pH
Hb Stanleyville-II	α77 pro→arg	Migrates like HbS at alkaline pH and HbA at acidic pH
Hb Nigeria	α81 ser→cys	Migrates faster than HbA and hybrid with β^S migrates faster than HbS at alkaline pH
HbG-Georgia	α95 pro→leu	Migrates ~HbS at alkaline pH
Hb Hopkins-II	α112 his→asp	Migrates ~HbA
Hb Chicago	α136 leu→met	Not separated by electrophoresis

From Hardison et al., 1998; Huisman et al., 1998.

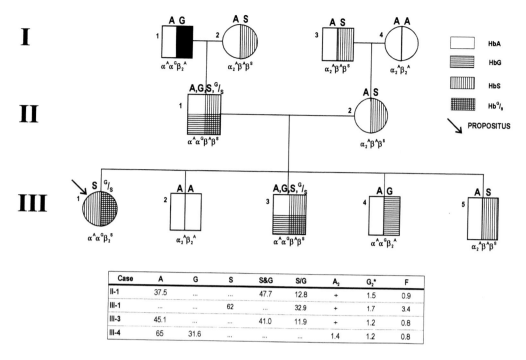

Case	A	G	S	S&G	S/G	A₂	G₂*	F
II-1	37.5	...	...	47.7	12.8	+	1.5	0.9
III-1	...	...	62	...	32.9	+	1.7	3.4
III-3	45.1	...	...	41.0	11.9	+	1.2	0.8
III-4	65	31.6	...	...	...	1.4	1.2	0.8

Figure 28.7. Pedigree of an extended family where HbG-Philadelphia is present with sickle cell trait and sickle cell anemia. Below the pedigree, the percentage of different hemoglobin fractions is shown. (Redrawn from Charache et al., 1977.)

A report of a 3-year-old patient with sickle cell anemia and Hb Hopkins-II (α112 his→asp), a variant with high O_2 affinity, revealed mild anemia and reticulocytosis, no sickled cells in the blood, reduced MCV, and normal splenic function (Witkowska et al., 1997).

Mild sickle cell anemia was reported in a 34-year-old patient homozygous for the HbS gene and heterozygous for Hb Matsue-Oki, α75 asp→asn. This α_2-globin gene variant effects a contact site between deoxy HbS polymer strands. $\alpha^{Matsue-Oki}_2\beta^S_2$ tetramers formed 28 percent

of the hemolysate and migrated on cellulose acetate electrophoresis like HbC. Hb Matsui-Oki migrates like HbS and heterozygotes have between 12 and 24 percent of this variant (Huisman et al., 1998). Although no clinical information was provided in the initial report of this compound heterozygote, it was implied that the phenotype was milder than that of HbSC disease with which it might be confused.

Figure 28.8. Electrophoresis of HbG-Philadelphia present with sickle cell trait and sickle cell anemia. (A) Results of alkaline electrophoresis. (B) Acid agar electrophoresis. Globin chain composition of different hemoglobin bands are shown beneath the electrophoretic separations.

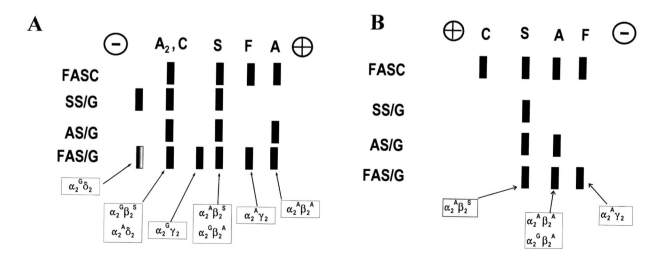

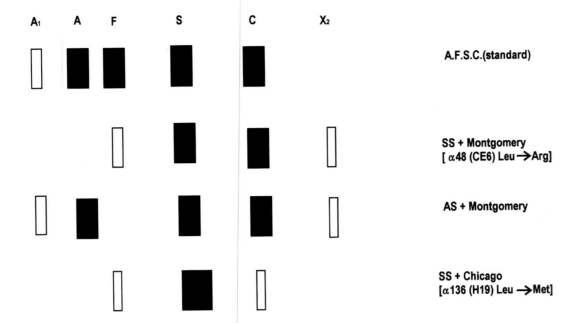

Figure 28.9. Isoelectric focusing of hemolysates from sickle cell trait and sickle cell anemia with Hb Montgomery and sickle cell anemia with Hb Chicago. These α-globin gene variants display confusing patterns by hemoglobin electrophoresis and isoelectric focusing. (Redrawn from Gu et al., 1993.)

HbS WITH OTHER GLOBIN VARIANTS

Variants of the γ-globin chains and the δ-globin chain (Chapter 10) are also found with homozygosity and heterozygosity for the HbS gene. Although they may cause diagnostic confusion, they are not associated with any hematologic or clinical sequela. γ-Globin gene variants are usually detected in infants, where they can form up to 30 percent of the total hemoglobin and similar proportions of the HbF fraction. As γ-globin gene expression diminishes, these variants are reduced to a minor fraction of the small amount of remaining HbF and are usually undetectable.

HbA$_2$′, δ16 gly→sp is the most common δ-globin gene variant in blacks and so is often found in sickle cell anemia and sickle cell trait. It migrates more slowly than HbA$_2$ on electrophoresis at alkaline pH.

Individuals with sickle cell trait have been described with the βδ-globin gene crossover variant Hb P-Nilotic (Congo) (β through residue 22, δ from residue 50). Pedigrees in which the affected but hematologically normal individual had HbS, HbA, and HbP-Nilotic confirm that the chromosome with the fusion gene contains a normal β-globin gene (Dherte et al., 1959; Huisman, 1997). The hemoglobin composition is 40 percent HbS, 35 percent HbA, 22 percent HbP-Nilotic, and 2.3 percent HbA$_2$ (Huisman, 1997).

CONCLUSION

HbS can be present with different forms of α or β thalassemia and dozens of abnormal hemoglobins. Phenotypes associated with these genetic combinations can be pernicious or benign, and the management of clinically significant phenotypes should follow the guidelines proposed for sickle cell anemia or HbSC disease. Most important is the correct delineation of the genotype so that the affected individual can be accurately counseled, especially when antenatal diagnosis is at issue.

References

Adachi, K, Asakura, T, and Schwartz, E. (1980). Aggregation of hemoglobin S and hemoglobin C Harlem with nonsickle hemoglobin in concentrated phosphate buffer. *Blood* 55: 494–500.

Adachi, K, Kim, J, Ballas, S et al. (1988). Facilitation of Hb S polymerization by the substitution of Glu for Gln at beta 121. *J. Biol. Chem.* 263: 5607–5610.

Adachi, K, Surrey, S, Tamary, H et al. (1993). Hb Shelby [β131 (H9)Gln→Lys] in association with Hb S [β6(A3)Glu→Val]: Characterization, stability, and effects on Hb S polymerization. *Hemoglobin* 17: 329–343.

Adams, RJ, Kutlar, A, McKie, V et al. (1994). Alpha thalassemia and stroke risk in sickle cell anemia. *Am. J. Hematol.* 45: 279–282.

Adekile, AD and Haider, MZ. (1996). Morbidity, βs haplotype and α-globin gene patterns among sickle cell anemia patients in Kuwait. *Acta Haematol.* 96: 150–154.

Adekile, AD, Tuli, M, Haider, MZ et al. (1996). Influence of α-thalassemia trait on spleen function in sickle cell anemia patients with high HbF. *Am. J. Hematol.* 53: 1–5.

Altay, C, Niazi, GA, and Huisman, THJ. (1976). The combination of Hb S and Hb E in a black female. *Hemoglobin* 1: 100–102.

Altay, C, Öner, C, Öner, R et al. (1997). Genotype-phenotype analysis in HbS-beta-thalassemia. *Hum. Hered.* 47: 161–164.

Arends, T, Lehmann, H, Plowman, D, and Stathopoulou, R. (1977). Haemoglobin North Shore-Caracas beta 134 (H12) valine replaced by glutamic acid. *FEBS Lett.* 80: 261–265.

Baklouti, F, Francina, A, Dorleac, E et al. (1987). Association in cis of β⁺-thalassemia and hemoglobin S. *Am. J. Hematol.* 26: 237–245.

Baklouti, F, Ouzana, R, Gonnet, C et al. (1989). β⁺ Thalassemia in *cis* of a sickle gene: Occurrence of a promoter mutation on a βˢ chromosome. *Blood* 74: 1818–1822.

Balkaran, B, Char, G, Morris, JS et al. (1992). Stroke in a cohort of patients with homozygous sickle cell disease. *J. Pediatr.* 120: 360–366.

Billett, HH, Kim, K, Fabry, ME, and Nagel, RL. (1986). The percentage of dense cells does not predict sickle cell painful crisis. *Blood* 68: 301–303.

Bookchin, RM, Davis, RP, and Ranney, HM. (1968). Clinical features of Hb C Harlem, a new sickling hemoglobin variant. *Ann. Intern. Med.* 68: 8–18.

Bookchin, RM, Ortiz, OE, and Lew, VL. (1991). Evidence for a direct reticulocyte origin of dense red cells in sickle cell anemia. *J. Clin. Invest.* 87: 113–124.

Braden, DS, Covitz, W, and Milner, PF. (1996). Cardiovascular function during rest and exercise in patients with sickle-cell anemia and coexisting alpha thalassemia-2. *Am. J. Hematol.* 52: 96–102.

Buchanan, GR. (1994). Infection. In Embury, SH, Hebbel, RP, Mohandas, N, and Steinberg, ME, editors. *Sickle cell disease: Basic principles and clinical practice.* New York: Lippincott-Raven, pp. 567–587.

Castro, O, Brambilla, DJ, Thorington, B Levy, PS et al. and Coop Study of Sickle Cell Disease. (1994). The acute chest syndrome in sickle cell disease: Incidence and risk factors. *Blood* 84: 643–649.

Chang, YC, Smith, KD, Moore, RD et al. (1995). An analysis of fetal hemoglobin variation in sickle cell disease: The relative contributions of the X-linked factor, β-globin haplotypes, α-globin gene number, gender, and age. *Blood* 85: 1111–1117.

Chang, YPC, Maier-Redelsperger, M, Smith, KD et al. (1997). The relative importance of the X-linked FCP locus and β-globin haplotypes in determining haemoglobin F levels: A study of SS patients homozygous for βˢ haplotypes. *Br. J. Haematol.* 96: 806–814.

Charache, S, Zinkham, WH, Dickerman, JD et al. (1977). Hemoglobin SC, SS/G_Philadelphia and SO_Arab disease: Diagnostic importance of an integrative analysis of clinical, hematologic and electrophoretic findings. *Am. J. Med.* 62: 439–446.

Chien, S, King, RG, Kaperonis, AA, and Usami, S. (1982). Viscoelastic properties of sickle cells and hemoglobin. *Blood Cells* 8: 53–64.

Chien, S, Usami, S, and Bertles, JF. (1970). Abnormal rheology of oxygenated blood in sickle cell anemia. *J. Clin. Invest.* 49: 623–634.

Coleman, MB, Adams, JG, III, Walker, AM et al. (1993). Hb San Diego [β109(G11)Val→Met] in an Iranian: Further evidence for a mutational hot spot at position 109 of the β-globin gene. *Hemoglobin* 17: 543–545.

Cooke, JV and Mack, JK. (1934). Sickle-cell anemia in a white American family. *J. Pediatr.* 5: 601–607.

Cooper, MR, Kraus, AP, Felts, JH et al. (1973). A third case of hemoglobin Memphis-sickle cell disease. Whole blood viscosity used as a screening test. *Am. J. Med.* 55: 535–541.

Craig, JE, Rochette, J, Sampietro, M et al. (1997). Genetic heterogeneity in heterocellular hereditary persistence of fetal hemoglobin. *Blood* 90: 428–434.

De Ceulaer, K, Higgs, DR, Weatherall, DJ et al. (1983). α-Thalassemia reduces the hemolytic rate in homozygous sickle-cell disease [letter]. *N. Engl. J. Med.* 309: 189–190.

De Ceulaer, K and Serjeant, GR. (1991). Acute splenic sequestration in Jamaican adults with homozygous sickle cell disease: A role of alpha thalassaemia. *Br. J. Haematol.* 77: 563–564.

De Montelembert, M, Maier-Redelsperger, M, Girot, R et al. (1993). β-Globin gene cluster haplotype and α-thalassemia do not correlate with the acute clinical manifestations of sickle cell disease in children. *Blood* 82: 2595–2596.

Desselle, BC, O'Brien, T, Bugnitz, M et al. (1995). Fatal fat embolism in a patient with sickle-beta + thalassemia. *Pediatr. Hematol. Oncol.* 12: 159–162.

Dherte, P, Lehmann H, and Vandepitte, J. (1959). Haemoglobin P in a family in the Belgian Congo. *Nature* 184: 1133–1135.

Divoky, V, Baysal, E, Schiliro, G et al. (1993). A mild type of Hb S-β⁺-thalassemia [−92(C→T)] in a Sicilian family. *Am. J. Hematol.* 42: 225–226.

Dover, GJ, Chang, VT, Boyer, SH et al. (1987). The cellular basis for different fetal hemoglobin levels among sickle cell individuals with two, three, and four alpha-globin genes. *Blood* 69: 341–344.

Eichhorn, RF, Buurke, EJ, Blok, P et al. (1999). Sickle cell-like crisis and bone marrow necrosis associated with parvovirus B19 infection and heterozygosity for haemoglobins S and E. *J. Intern. Med.* 245: 103–106.

El-Hazmi, MAF and Warsy, AS. (1993). On the molecular interactions between α-thalassaemia and sickle cell gene. *Journal of Tropical Pediatrics* 39: 209–213.

Embury, SH, Backer, K, and Glader, BE. (1985a). Monovalent cation changes in sickle erythrocytes: A direct reflection of α-globin gene number. *J. Lab. Clin. Med.* 106: 75–79.

Embury, SH, Clark, MR, Monroy, GM, and Mohandas, N. (1984). Concurrent sickle cell anemia and α thalassemia. *J. Clin. Invest.* 73: 116–123.

Embury, SH, Dozy, AM, Miller, J et al. (1982). Concurrent sickle-cell anemia and alpha-thalassemia: effect on severity of anemia. *N. Engl. J. Med.* 306: 270–274.

Embury, SH, Gholson, MA, Gillette, P, and Rieder, RF. (1985b). The leftward deletion α-thal-2 haplotype in a black subject with sickle cell anemia. *Blood* 65: 169–171.

Embury, SH and Steinberg, MH. (1994). Genetic modulators of disease. In Embury, SH, Hebbel, RP, Mohandas, N, and Steinberg, MH, editors. *Sickle cell disease: Basic principles and clinical practice* New York: Lippincott-Raven, pp. 279–298.

Fairbanks, VF, McCormick, DJ, Kubik, KS et al. (1997). Hb S/Hb Lepore with mild sickling symptoms: A hemoglobin variant with mostly δ-chain sequences ameliorates sickle-cell disease. *Am. J. Hematol.* 54: 164–165.

Figueiredo, MS, Kerbauy, J, Goncalves, MS et al. (1996). Effect of α-thalassemia and β-globin gene cluster haplotypes on the hematological and clinical features of sickle-cell anemia in Brazil. *Am. J. Hematol.* 53: 72–76.

Gill, FM, Sleeper, LA, Weiner, SJ. (1995). Clinical events in the first decade in a cohort of infants with sickle cell disease. *Blood* 86: 776–783.

Gilman, JG, Mishima, N, Wen, XJ et al. (1988). Upstream promoter mutation associated with a modest elevation of fetal hemoglobin expression in human adults. *Blood* 72: 78–81.

Gonzalez-Redondo, JM, Kutlar, A, Kutlar, F et al. (1991). Molecular characterization of Hb S(C) β-thalassemia in American blacks. *Am. J. Hematol.* 38: 9–14.

Gonzalez-Redondo, JM, Kutlar, F, Stoming, TA et al. (1988b). Hb S(C)-β+-thalassaemia: Different mutations are associated with different levels of normal Hb A. *Br. J. Haematol.* 70: 85–89.

Gonzalez-Redondo, JM, Stoming, TA, Lanclos, KD et al. (1988a). Clinical and genetic heterogeneity in black patients with homozygous β-thalassemia from the southeastern United States. *Blood* 72: 1007–1014.

Gu, L-H, Wilson, JB, Molchanova, TP et al. (1993). Three sickle cell anemia patients each with a different α chain variant. Diagnostic complications. *Hemoglobin* 17: 295–301.

Hardison, RC, Chui, DHK, Riemer, CR et al. (1998). Access to a syllabus of human hemoglobin variants (1996) via the World Wide Web. *Hemoglobin* 22: 113–127.

Higgs, DR, Aldridge, BE, Lamb, J et al. (1982). The interaction of alpha-thalassemia and homozygous sickle-cell disease. *N. Eng. J. Med.* 306: 1441–1446.

Higgs, DR, Clegg, JB, Weatherall, DJ et al. (1984). Interaction of the ααα globin gene haplotype and sickle haemoglobin. *Br. J. Haematol.* 57: 671–678.

Ho, C, Willis, BF, Shen, TJ et al. (1996). Roles of α114 and β87 amino acid residues in the polymerization of hemoglobin S: Implications for gene therapy. *J. Mol. Biol.* 263: 475–485.

Honig, GR, Koshy, M, Mason, RG, and Vida, LN. (1978). Sickle cell syndromes. II. The sickle cell anemia-alpha-thalassemia syndrome. *J. Pediatr.* 92: 556–561.

Huisman, THJ, Carver, MFH, and Efremov, GD. (1998). *A syllabus of human hemoglobin variants.* Augusta: Sickle Cell Anemia Foundation.

Huisman, THJ. (1997). Compound heterozygosity for Hb S and the hybrid Hb S Lepore, P-Nilotic, and Kenya: Comparison of hematological and hemoglobin composition data. *Hemoglobin* 21: 249–257.

Huisman, THJ, Carver, MFH, and Baysal, E. (1997). *A syllabus of thalassemia mutations.* Augusta, GA: The Sickle Cell Anemia Foundation. Ingram, VM and Stretton,

AOW. (1959). Genetic basis of the thalassaemia diseases. *Nature* 184: 1903.

Johnson, K, Stastny, JF, and Rucknagel, DL. (1994). Fat embolism syndrome associated with asthma and sickle cell-β+ -thalassemia. *Am. J. Hematol.* 46: 354–357.

Katopodis, MS, Elisaf, HA, Pappas, JC et al. (1997). Renal abnormalities in patients with sickle cell-beta thalassemia. *J. Nephrol.* 10: 163–167, 1997.

Kendall, AG, Ojwang, PJ, Schroeder, WA, and Huisman, THJ. (1973). Hemoglobin Kenya, the product of a gamma-beta fusion gene. *Am. J. Hum. Genet.* 25: 548–563.

Kéclard, L, Ollendorf, V, Berchel, C et al. (1996). βS Haplotypes, α-globin gene status, and hematological data of sickle cell disease patients in Guadeloupe (FWI). *Hemoglobin* 20: 63–74.

Kéclard, L, Romana, M, Lavocat, E et al. (1997). Sickle cell disorder, β-globin gene cluster haplotypes and α-thalassemia in neonates and adults from Guadeloupe. *Am. J. Hematol.* 55: 24–27.

Kinney, T, Friedman, S, Cifuentes, E et al. (1978). Variations in globin synthesis in delta-beta-thalassaemia. *Br. J. Haematol.* 38: 15–22.

Kolquist, KA, Vnencak-Jones, CL, Swift, L et al. (1996). Fatal fat embolism syndrome in a child with undiagnosed hemoglobin S/beta + thalassemia: A complication of acute parvovirus B19 infection. *Pediatr. Pathol. Labor. Med.* 16: 71–82.

Kulozik, AE, Bail, S, Kar, BC et al. (1991). Sickle cell-β+ thalassaemia in Orissa State India. *Br. J. Haematol.* 77: 215–220.

Landin, B, Rudolphi, O, and Ek, B. (1995). Initiation codon mutation (ATG→ATA) of the β-globin gene causing β-thalassemia in a Swedish family. *Am. J. Hematol.* 48: 158–162.

Langdown, JV, Williamson, D, Knight, CB et al. (1989). A new doubly substituted sickling haemoglobin: HbS-Oman. *Br. J. Haematol.* 71: 445–446.

Lu, ZH and Steinberg, MH. (1996). Fetal hemoglobin in sickle cell anemia: Relation to regulatory sequences *cis* to the β-globin gene. *Blood* 87: 1604–1611.

Li, J, Plonczynski, M, Kheradpour, A et al. (1998). Severe Hb S-β+ thalassemia caused by IVS-1 splice site mutations. *Hemoglobin* 22: 383–385.

Martinez, G, Muniz, A, Svarch, E et al. (1996). Age dependence of the gene frequency of α-thalassemia in sickle cell anemia in Cuba. *Blood* 88: 1898–1899.

Mears, JG, Lachman, HM, Labie, D, and Nagel, RL. (1983). Alpha thalassemia is related to prolonged survival in sickle cell anemia. *Blood* 62: 286–290.

Miller, ST, Rieder, RF, Rao, SP, and Brown, AK. (1988). Cerebrovascular accidents in children with sickle-cell disease and alpha-thalassemia. *J. Pediatr.* 118: 847–849.

Milner, PF, Kraus, AP, Sebes, JI et al. (1991). Sickle cell disease as a cause of osteonecrosis of the femoral head. *N. Engl. J. Med.* 325: 1476–1481.

Milner, PF, Miller, C, Grey, R et al. (1970). Hemoglobin O Arab in four negro families and its interaction with hemoglobin S and hemoglobin C. *N. Engl. J. Med.* 283: 1417–1425.

Milner, PF, Kraus, AP, Sebes, JI et al. (1993). Osteonecrosis of the humeral head in sickle cell disease. *Clin. Orthop. Relat. Res.* 289: 136–143.

Mirabile, E, Testa, R, Consalvo, C et al. (1995). Association of Hb S/Hb Lepore and δβ-thalassemia/Hb Lepore in Sicilian patients: Review of the presence of Hb Lepore in Sicily. *Eur. J. Haematol.* 55: 126–130.

Monplaisir, N, Merault, G, Poyart, C et al. (1986). Hb S Antilles (α_2 β_2 6Glu-> Val, 23Val-> #lle): A new variant with lower solubility than Hb S and producing sickle cell disease in heterozygotes. *Proc. Nat. Acad. Sci. U.S.A.* 83: 9363–9367.

Moo-Penn, W, Bechtel, K, Jue, D et al. (1975). The presence of hemoglobin S and C Harlem in an individual in the United States. *Blood* 46: 363–367.

Mukherjee, MB, Colah, RB, Ghosh, K, and Mohanty, D. (1997). Milder clinical course of sickle cell disease in patients with α thalassemia in the Indian subcontinent. *Blood* 89: 732–732.

Murray, N, Serjeant, BE, and Serjeant, GR. (1988). Sickle cell-hereditary persistence of fetal haemoglobin and its differentiation from other sickle cell syndromes. *Br. J. Haematol.* 69: 89–92.

Nagel, RL, Daar, S, Romero, DJ et al. (1998). Hb S-Oman disease: A new dominant sickle syndrome. *Blood* 92: 4375–4382.

Nagel, RL, Bookchin, RM, Labie, D et al. (1979). Structural basis for the inhibitory effects of hemoglobin F and hemoglobin A₂ on the polymerization of hemoglobin S. *Proc. Natal. Acad. Sci. U.S.A.* 76: 670–672.

Nagel, KL, Krishmamoorthy, R, Fattoun, S et al. (1999). The erythrocytic effects of haemoglobin O_{ARAB}. *Br. J. Hematol.* 107: 516–521.

Neumayr, L, Koshy, M, Haberkern, C et al. (1998). Surgery in patients with hemoglobin SC disease. *Am. J. Hematol.* 57: 101–108.

Noguchi, CT, Dover, GJ, Rodgers, GP et al. (1985). Alpha thalassemia changes erythrocyte heterogeneity in sickle cell disease. *J. Clin. Invest.* 75: 1632–1637.

Ofori-Acquah, SF, Lalloz, MRA, and Layton, DM. (1999). Localisation of cis regulatory elements at the beta-globin locus: Analysis of hybrid haplotype chromosomes. *Biochem. Biophys. Res. Commun.* 254: 181–187.

Ohene-Frempong, K, Weiner, SJ, Sleeper, LA et al (1998). Cerebrovascular accidents in sickle cell disease: Rates and risk factors. *Blood* 91: 288–294.

Öner, C, Dimovski, AJ, Altay, C et al. (1992). Sequence variations in the 5′ hypersensitive site-2 of the locus control region of β^s chromosomes are associated with different levels of fetal globin in hemoglobin S homozygotes. *Blood* 79: 813–819.

Pacheco P, Peres MJ, Faustino, P et al. (1995). β-thalassaemia unlinked to the β-globin gene interacts with sickle-cell trait in a Portuguese family. *Br. J. Haematol.* 91: 85–89.

Padanilam, BJ, Felice, AE, and Huisman, THJ. (1984). Partial deletion of the 5′ β-globin gene region causes β^0-thalassemia in members of an American black family. *Blood* 64: 941–944.

Phillips, G Jr, Coffey, B, Tran-Son-Tay, R et al. (1991). Relationship of clinical severity to packed cell rheology in sickle cell anemia. *Blood* 78: 2735–2739.

Platt, OS, Brambilla, DJ, Rosse, WF et al. (1994). Mortality in sickle cell disease: Life expectancy and risk factors for early death. *N. Engl. J. Med.* 330: 1639–1644.

Platt, OS, Thorington, BD, Brambilla, DJ et al. (1991). Pain in sickle cell disease-rates and risk factors. *N. Engl. J. Med.* 325: 11–16.

Plonczynski, M, Figueiredo, MS, and Steinberg, MH. (1997). Fetal hemoglobin in sickle cell anemia: Examination of phylogenetically conserved sequences within the locus control region but outside the cores of hypersensitive sites 2 and 3. *Blood Cells Mol. Dis.* 23: 188–200.

Poillon, WN, Kim, BC, Rodgers, GP et al. (1993). Sparing effect of hemoglobin F and hemoglobin A₂ on the polymerization of hemoglobin S at physiologic ligand saturations. *Proc. Natl. Acad. Sci. U.S.A.* 90: 5039–5043.

Powars, D, Chan, LS, and Schroeder, WA. (1990). The variable expression of sickle cell disease is genetically determined. *Semin. Hematol.* 27: 360–376.

Reddy, LR, Reddy, Ks, Surrey, S, and Adachi, K. (1997). Role of β87 Thr in the β6 Val acceptor site during deoxy Hb S polymerization. *Biochemistry* 36: 15992–15998.

Rey, KS, Unger, CA, Rao, SP, and Miller, ST. (1991). Sickle cell-hemoglobin E disease. Clinical findings and implications. *J. Pediatr.* 119: 949–951.

Rhoda, MD, Martin, J, Blouquit, Y et al. (1983). Sickle cell hemoglobin fiber formation strongly inhibited by the Stanleyville-II mutation (alpha 78 Asw leads to Lys). *Biochem. Biophys. Res. Commun.* 111: 8–13.

Rogers, ZR and Buchanan, GR. (1995b). Bacteremia in children with sickle hemoglobin C disease and sickle beta(+)-thalassemia: Is prophylactic penicillin necessary? *J. Pediatr.* 127: 348–354.

Rogers, ZR and Buchanan, GR. (1995a). Risk of infection in children with hemoglobin S-beta-thalassemia. *J. Pediatr.* 127: 672–672.

Schroeder, WA, Powars, D, Reynolds, RD, and Fisher, JI. (1998). Hb-E in combination with Hb-S and Hb-C in a black family. *Hemoglobin* 1: 287–289.

Schroeder, WA, Powars, DR, Kay, LM et al. (1989). β-Cluster haplotypes α-gene status and hematological data from SS SC and S-β-thalassemia patients in Southern California. *Hemoglobin* 13: 325–353.

Serjeant, BE, Mason, KP, Kenny, MW et al. (1983). Effect of alpha thalassaemia on the rheology of homozygous sickle cell disease. *Br. J. Haematol.* 55: 479–486.

Serjeant, GR, Ashcroft, MT, Serjeant, BE, and Milner, PF. (1973). The clinical features of sickle-cell β thalassaemia in Jamaica. *Br. J. Haematol.* 24: 19–30.

Seward, DP, Ware, RE, and Kinney, TR. (1993). Hemoglobin sickle-Lepore: Report of two siblings and review of the literature. *Am. J. Hematol.* 44: 192–195.

Silvestroni, E and Bianco, I. (1946). Una nova entita nosologgica: La malatia microdrepanocitica. *Haematologica* 29: 455.

Singer, K and Fisher, B. (1952). Studies on abnormal hemoglobins. V. The distribution of type S (sickle cell) hemoglobin and type F (alkali resistant) hemoglobin within the red cell population in sickle cell anemia. *Blood* 7: 1216.

Smith, CM, Hedlund, B, Cich, JA et al. (1983). Hemoglobin North Shore: A variant hemoglobin associated with the phenotype of beta-thalassemia. *Blood* 61: 378–383.

Steinberg, MH, Adams, JG, Thigpen, JT et al. (1974). Hemoglobin Hope (α_2 β_2 136-[gly-asp])-S disease: Clinical and biochemical studies. *J. Lab. Clin. Med.* 84: 632–642.

Steinberg, MH, Coleman, MB, Adams, JG et al. (1986). A new gene deletion in the alpha-like globin gene cluster as the molecular basis for the rare alpha-thalassemia-1 (- -/αα) in blacks: HbH disease in sickle cell trait. *Blood* 67: 469–473.

Steinberg, MH, Coleman, MB, Adams, JG, and Rosenstock, W. (1984b). Interaction between HbS β⁰-thalassemia and α-thalassemia. *Am. J. Med. Sci.* 288: 195–199.

Steinberg, MH and Embury, SH. (1986). Alpha-thalassemia in blacks: Genetic and clinical aspects and interactions with the sickle hemoglobin gene. *Blood* 68: 985–990.

Steinberg, MH, Hsu, H, Nagel, RL et al. (1995). Gender and haplotype effects upon hematological manifestations of adult sickle cell anemia. *Am. J. Hematol.* 48: 175–181.

Steinberg, MH, Lovell, WJ, Wells, S et al. (1976). Hemoglobin Hope: Studies of oxygen equilibrium in heterozygotes, hemoglobin S-Hope disease, and isolated hemoglobin Hope. *J. Lab. Clin. Med.* 88: 125–131.

Steinberg, MH, Lu, Z-H, Barton, FB et al. (1997). Fetal hemoglobin in sickle cell anemia: Determinants of response to hydroxyurea. *Blood* 89: 1078–1088.

Steinberg, MH, Rosenstock, W, Coleman, MB et al. (1984a). Effects of thalassemia and microcytosis upon the hematological and vaso-occlusive severity of sickle cell anemia. *Blood* 63: 1353–1360.

Stevens, MC, Maude, GH, Beckford, M et al. (1986). Alpha thalassemia and the hematology of homozygous sickle cell disease in childhood. *Blood* 67: 411–414.

Strickland, DK, Ware, RE, and Kinney, TR. (1995). Pitfalls in newborn hemoglobinopathy screening: Failure to detect β⁺-thalassemia. *J. Pediatr.* 127: 304–308.

Sturgeon, P, Itano, HA, and Bergren, WR. (1955). Clinical manifestations of inherited abnormal hemoglobin. I The interaction of hemoglobin-S with hemoglobin-D. *Blood* 10: 389–396.

Sturgeon, P, Itano, HA, and Valentine, WN. (1952). Chronic hemolytic anemia associated with thalassemia and sickling trait. *Blood* 7: 350.

Sweeting, I, Serjeant, BE, Serjeant, GR et al. (1998). Hb S-Hb Monroe: A sickle cell β-thalassemia syndrome. *Hemoglobin* 22: 153–156.

Tejuca, M, Martinez, G, Mendez, J et al. (1987). Association of hemoglobin Toulouse with Hb S in a Nicaraguan girl. *Hemoglobin* 11: 43–46.

Thein, SL, Sampietro, M, Rohde, K et al (1994). Detection of a major gene for heterocellular hereditary persistence of fetal hemoglobin after accounting for genetic modifiers. *Am. J. Hum. Genet.* 54: 214–228.

Thomas, PW, Higgs, DR, and Serjeant, GR. (1997). Benign clinical course in homozygous sickle cell disease: A search for predictors. *J. Clin. Epidemiol.* 50: 121–126.

Van, Ros, G, Wiltshire, B, Renoirte Monjoie, A-M et al. (1973). Interaction entre les hémoglobins Stanleyville-II et

S dans une famille du Zäire. Etude de l' hybrid Stanleyvill-II/S (α₂ 78 lys β₂ 6 val). *Biochimie* 55: 1107–1110.

Vichinsky, EP, Haberkern, CM, Neumayr, L et al. (1995). A comparison of conservative and aggressive transfusion regimens in the perioperative management of sickle cell disease. *N. Engl. J. Med.* 333: 206–213.

Vidaud, M, Gattoni R, Stevenin, J et al. (1989). A 5′ splice-region G→C mutation in exon 1 of the human β-globin gene inhibits pre-mRNA slicing: A mechanism for β⁺-thalassemia. *Proc. Natl. Acad. Sci. U.S.A.* 86: 1041–1045.

Voskaridou, E, Konstantopoulos, K, Kollia, P et al. (1995). Hb Lepore (Pylos)/Hb S compounds heterozygosity in two Greek families. *Am. J. Hematol.* 49: 131–134.

Waye, JS, Cai, S-P, Eng, B et al. (1991a). High hemoglobin A₂ β⁰-thalassemia due to a 532-basepair deletion of the 5′ β-globin gene region. *Blood* 77: 1100–1103.

Waye, JS, Chui, DHK, Eng, B et al. (1991b). Hb S/β⁰-thalassemia due to the ~1.4-kb deletion is associated with a relatively mild phenotype. *Am. J. Hematol.* 38: 108–112.

Weatherall, DJ, Clegg, JB, Blankson, J, and McNeil, JR. (1969). A new sickling disorder resulting from interaction of the genes for haemoglobin S and alpha-thalassaemia. *Br. J. Haematol.* 17: 517–526.

West, MS, Wethers, D, Smith, J et al. (1992). Laboratory profile of sickle cell disease: A cross-sectional analysis. *J. Clin. Epidemiol.* 45: 893–909.

Williamson, D, Perry, DJ, Brown, K, and Langdown, JV. (1995). Compound heterozygosity for two β chain variants: Hb S[β6(A3)glu→val] and the high affinity variant Hb San Diego[β 109(G11)val→met]. *Hemoglobin* 19: 27–32.

Witkowska, E, Shackleton, CHL, Medzihradszky, KR et al. (1997). Benign clinical presentation of compound heterozygoyes for Hb S and high oxygen affinity hemoglobin variants. *Blood* 90: 32b.

Witkowska, E, Asakura, T, Tang, D et al. (1998). Compound heterozygote for Hb S and Hb Matsue-Oki α75(EF4)Asp->Asn presents with a mild sickle cell disease phenotype. *Blood* 92:525a.

Witkowska, HE, Lubin, BH, Beuzard, Y et al. (1991). Sickle cell disease in a patient with sickle cell trait and compound heterozygosity for hemoglobin S and hemoglobin Quebec-Chori. *N. Engl. J. Med.* 325: 1150–1154.

Zaidi, Y, Sivakumaran, M, Graham, C, and Hutchinson, RM. (1996). Fatal bone marrow embolism in a patient with sickle cell beta + thalassaemia. *J. Clin. Pathol.* 49: 774–775.

Zarkowsky, HS, Gallagher, D, Gill, FM et al. (1986). Bacteremia in sickle hemoglobinopathies. *J Pediatr* 109: 579–585.

Zimmerman, SA, O'Branski, EE, Rosse, WF, and Ware, RE. (1999). Hemoglobin S/O_ARAB: Thirteen new cases and a review of the literature. *Am. J. Hematol.* 60:279–284.

29

Sickle Cell Trait

MARTIN H. STEINBERG

Nearly 30 years ago, a burst of scientific and political activity was ignited by reports of sudden death in military recruits who had sickle cell trait (Jones et al., 1970). Soon thereafter, screening for sickle cell trait became mandatory; when tests were positive, the opportunity for military service was denied to some carriers, insurance coverage was canceled for others, and an astounding list of complications—retinopathy, retinal artery occlusion, glaucoma, urinary tract infection, low-birth-weight infants, osteonecrosis, bone infarction, hemarthrosis, leg ulcers, strokes of all manner, impaired cognitive function, hypopituitarism, priapism, cardiomyopathy, anesthetic deaths, splenic infarction and hemorrhage, and sundry others—appeared in the sickle cell trait literature. The ubiquity of the trait, coupled with a misunderstanding of its pathogenic potential, led to the interpretation of the coincidental association of the trait with other diseases as evidence of cause and effect. Often ignored was whether the reports reflected a statistically significant association of sickle cell trait with the disorders or merely a random one. One purpose of this chapter is to reviews what is known, what is presumed, and what is false about the clinical features and pathogenicity of sickle cell trait. Another is to review the management of sickle cell trait.

HISTORY

Since antiquity, parents of children with the disease now recognized as sickle cell anemia were rarely noted to be as affected as were their offspring. Moreover, the symptoms were not the same for all affected children in a family. In 1927, 17 years after Herrick's description of sickle cell anemia (Herrick, 1910), Hahn and Gillespie (1927) showed that almost 10 percent of African Americans had red cells that sickled when they were deoxygenated. It required the identification of HbS by Pauling and his colleagues (1949) and their observation that the only hemoglobin in hemolysates of patients with sickle cell anemia was HbS, whereas their parents' hemolysates had both HbS and HbA, for Neel and Beet to characterize the genetics of sickle hemoglobinopathies (Beet, 1949; Neel, 1951).

PATHOGENESIS OF SICKLE CELL TRAIT

Less than half the hemoglobin in the sickle cell trait erythrocyte is HbS. The remainder, mainly HbA, dilutes the HbS. The probability that the mixed hybrid tetramer, $\alpha_2\beta^S\beta^A$, will enter the polymer phase is only half that of the HbS tetramer, $\alpha_2\beta^S_2$ (Poillon et al., 1993) (Fig. 29.1) (Chapter 23). Hemoglobin S polymer concentrations sufficient to injure the red cell are a prerequisite for the expression of the phenotype of sickle cell disease. In sickle cell trait, high concentrations of HbA preclude clinically significant HbS polymer formation at the oxygen saturation and physiologic conditions present in most tissues (Fig. 29.1B) (Chapter 23). HbS polymer appears in sickle cell trait cells only when oxygen saturation falls below 60 percent. Even when sickle cell trait blood is totally deoxygenated, the polymer fraction is only 40 percent of total hemoglobin (Noguchi et al., 1981). Sickle cell trait, therefore, should be clinically benign; with rare exception, clinical and laboratory studies confirm this expectation.

DIAGNOSIS

Clinical indications for detecting sickle cell trait are few. Diagnosis should be sought in the following situations:

- Genetic counseling of couples involved in family planning who are likely to carry a HbS gene
- Surveying populations to establish the prevalence of the HbS gene

Martin H. Steinberg, Bernard G. Forget, Douglas R. Higgs, and Ronald L. Nagel, editors. *Disorders of Hemoglobin: Genetics, Pathophysiology, and Clinical Management.* © 2001 Cambridge University Press. All rights reserved.

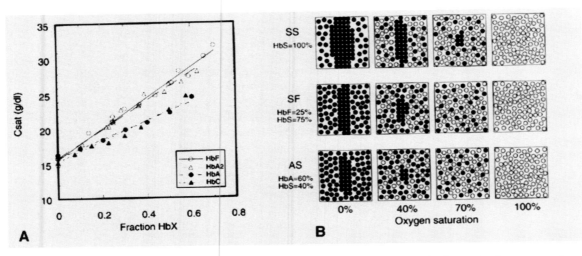

Figure 29.1. (A) Solubility of deoxygenated hemoglobin mixtures. Other hemoglobins prevent HbS polymerization by increasing HbS solubility (Csat). The percent increase in solubility reflects the likelihood of the other hemoglobin type being included in the deoxy HbS polymer. Neither the γ-globin chain of HbF nor the δ-globin chain of HbA_2 is incorporated into the polymer phase, so HbF and HbA_2 inhibit polymerization more than do HbA and HbC. (From Embury et al., 1994, with permission.) (B) Effects of HbA and HbF on HbS polymerization. Closed circles indicate fully deoxygenated hemoglobin and open circles, fully oxygenated hemoglobin. Polymer is indicated by stacked closed circles. (From Embury et al., 1994, with permission.)

- Evaluating hematuria in individuals at risk for sickle cell trait
- Planning treatment of hyphema in individuals at risk for sickle cell trait
- Planning complicated thoracic surgery in individuals at risk for sickle cell trait.

Detecting sickle cell trait requires the demonstration in hemolysate of both HbS and HbA in appropriate proportions. That can be accomplished by isoelectric focusing, hemoglobin electrophoresis, high-performance liquid chromatography (HPLC), and variants of those methods. Alternatively, DNA-based methods can define the condition at the genetic level. Simple HbS heterozygosity cannot be diagnosed by medical history, clinical features, or laboratory testing that does not detect the HbS gene or its abnormal protein product. Several reviews of methods for detecting variant hemoglobins are available in the literature (Adams et al., 1991; Adams, 1994; Dumars et al., 1996; Embury, 1994; Globin Gene Disorder-BCSH Task Force, 1994; Lubin et al., 1991; Steinberg, 1993). Neither hematologic indices measured by electronic cell counting nor peripheral blood film reviews are useful for diagnosis because both are normal in sickle cell trait.

Some of the following methods for detecting HbS can be adapted to measure hemoglobin fraction concentrations, which can be important for distinguishing sickle cell trait from HbS-β⁺ thalassemia and for detecting the coexistence of α thalassemia.

Isoelectric Focusing

In isoelectric focusing, a hemolysate applied to a thin polyacrylamide gel that is placed in an electrical field migrates to the anode or the cathode. HbS tetramers have two more positive charges than HbA tetramers and migrate more slowly toward the anode. Isoelectric focusing uses ampholines to establish ga pH gradient in the polyacrylamide gel (Basset et al., 1978; Drysdale et al., 1971; Galacteros et al., 1980). The electric field then "focuses" the hemoglobin fractions into sharp bands at their isoelectric points. The high resolution of the technique has made it the method of choice for initial screening, especially neonatal screening, in many laboratories. Gels must be evaluated visually, however, and considerable skill is required because many extraneous minor hemoglobin bands are often present. Another problem is that quantitation of hemoglobin fractions is difficult, but just ascertaining that the concentration of HbA is greater than that of HbS may be sufficient for detecting sickle cell trait in adults. Better quantitative information can be obtained by capillary isoelectric focusing, a modification of isoelectric focusing in which hemoglobins are separated in fine capillary tubes. Commercially available systems allow automated data analysis, require small sample size, are rapid and sensitive, and conserve expensive reagents (Hempe and Craver, 1994).

Hemoglobin Electrophoresis

Hemoglobin electrophoresis at alkaline pH is usually done on cellulose acetate membranes that are inexpensive, can be prepared quickly and easily, and provide sharp resolution of hemoglobin bands.

Relative percentages of the major hemoglobin bands can be quantified by densitometry or elution and spectroscopy. Membranes can be fixed and cleared so that the gels can furnish a permanent record of the procedure (Schedlbauer and Pass, 1989). Because HbA and HbS are poorly resolved from HbF with this technique, it is imperative to use an additional, complementary method for newborns. An example is citrate agar electrophoresis, which distinctly separates HbF from HbA and the major common variants. In acid agar electrophoresis, most hemoglobins move cathodically from their point of origin and display different relative mobilities than they do in alkaline electrophoresis (Robinson et al., 1957; Schedlbauer and Pass, 1989). Citrate agar electrophoresis can detect some variants that do not separate from HbA, S, or C by cellulose acetate electrophoresis; when used with cellulose acetate electrophoresis, it can resolve confusion in the identification of many common variants, such as HbG Philadelphia, HbD, and Hb Lepore (Chapter 28).

High-Performance Liquid Chromatography

HPLC offers many advantages including the following: (1) the isolation of many hemoglobins, including HbF; (2) the procedure can usually be automated by a microcomputer interface, which can produce a reliable interpretation of the chromatogram; and (3) the various hemoglobin fractions are quantifiable. HPLC has these disadvantages: (1) it cannot always resolve HbS or HbC from other variants with the same charge; (2) the equipment is expensive to purchase and maintain, and; (3) some systems require great technical skill (Kutlar et al., 1993).

Sickle Solubility Test

When reduced with sodium dithionite, sickle hemoglobin precipitates in high molarity phosphate buffer at neutral pH. That observation forms the basis for the sickle solubility test (Greenberg et al., 1972). With rare exception, the sickle solubility test has no role as a primary screening test or as the sole means of detecting HbS. Because the test indicates only the presence of HbS, and not its quantity, it cannot reliably distinguish between sickle cell trait, sickle cell anemia, and HbS-β^+ thalassemia. Nor is the solubility test useful for neonates who synthesize large amounts of HbF, and it fails to detect the low concentrations of HbS that might be present in some varieties of HbS-β^+ thalassemia or sickle cell trait with α thalassemia (Chapter 28). This test is specific for sickling hemoglobins. It can be useful for distinguishing HbS from variants that may mimic it electrophoretically. Solubility tests sometimes give false-positive results, but rarely with reliable reagents.

DNA-Based Methods

DNA-based methods for detecting HbS have the advantage of being specific and requiring a minimum of material and the disadvantage of costliness and limited availability (they are used primarily in reference laboratories for antenatal diagnosis). A blastocyst, or even a single cell, is sufficient for identifying the HbS mutation, which means that the amount of tissue or blood required for diagnosis is minuscule (Ray et al., 1996). DNA-based methods are covered in detail in Chapter 35. The main method involves amplification of β-globin gene fragments and hybridization with HbS gene-specific oligonucleotide probes.

QUANTITATION OF HBS

Hemoglobins can be quantified after they are isolated by electrophoresis or chromatography. Reliable quantification procedures include spectrophotometric analysis of elusions from cellulose acetate strips, minicolumns, or HPLC, as well as densitometry of stained and cleared cellulose acetate strips (Tan et al., 1993). The cellulose acetate elution method is highly reliable for measuring HbA_2 and variant hemoglobin levels in adults; but because HbF migrates between HbA and HbS, it is not used for newborn samples. Densitometry of cellulose acetate electrophoresis strips is unreliable for measuring HbA_2 and HbF. (Schmidt et al., 1975a, 1975b). While the minicolumn method is reliable, it has been largely supplanted by HPLC (Huisman, 1987), which is the separation technique of choice for quantitation of the major hemoglobins in the newborn. HbS does not perturb the measurement of HbA_1C by HPLC or immunoassay (Roberts et al., 1998).

In uncomplicated, or simple sickle cell trait, HbF levels are usually normal. In individuals with the Senegal or Arab-Indian β-globin gene haplotype, the HbF level may be slightly increased but still within normal range (Kulozik et al., 1996). HbF and F cells (erythrocytes containing HbF) may be increased in individuals with sickle cell trait who have, coincidentally, forms of hereditary persistence of fetal hemoglobin (HPFH) that do not involve gene deletions (Chapter 15).

LEVELS OF HbS IN SICKLE CELL TRAIT

Effects of α-Globin Gene Haplotype

In sickle cell trait carriers who have the normal complement of four α-globin genes, HbS is consistently 40 ± 4 percent of total hemoglobin H. That percentage can be altered by an α-globin gene mutant, additional β globin gene variants in *trans* (or, very rarely, in *cis*), β⁺ thalassemia, iron deficiency anemia, and possibly lead poisoning and megaloblastic anemia. The concentration of a particular hemoglobin type depends on the transcriptional rate of the globin gene, the stability of the globin chain, and the posttranslational assembly and stability of the αβ dimer and hemoglobin tetramer (Chapter 8). Early studies of the proportion of HbS in sickle cell trait (Esan and Adesina, 1974; Nance and Grove, 1972) were unable to detect α thalassemia, the prime modulator of HbS concentration in the condition.

Oxyhemoglobin tetramers rapidly dissociate into αβ dimers. In sickle cell trait, reassociation can occur as the hybrid tetramer $\alpha_2\beta^S\beta^A$. Normal globin biosynthesis provides a slight excess of α chains that are always available to bind non-α chains. As a result, the steady-state accumulation of hemoglobin tetramers in the normal erythrocyte depends predominantly on expression of the non-α-globin genes. Hemoglobin dimers, the basic subunit of the tetramer, are assembled by the electrostatic attraction of α- and β-globin chains (Abraham and Huisman, 1977; Bunn, 1987) (Chapter 8). β^S Globin chains have two more positive charges than β^A chains and therefore bind α chains, which are also positively charged, less avidly. That accounts for HbS levels being 40 percent, rather than the 50 percent level expected on the basis of gene dosage. Mild forms of α thalassemia, however, are extraordinarily common in HbS populations (Chapter 32). Individuals with sickle cell trait who have fewer, or sometimes more, α-globin genes than normal, exhibit altered HbA and HbS ratios.

HbS concentration in sickle cell trait is trimodally distributed, with peaks at 30, 35, and 40 percent (Brittenham, 1977; El-Hazmi, 1986; Embury and Dozy, 1981; Lane and Githens, 1985; Steinberg et al., 1975; Steinberg and Embury, 1986; Wong et al., 1981). Globin biosynthesis studies (DeSimone et al., 1974; Shaeffer et al., 1975) and, more definitively, restriction endonuclease mapping of the α-globin gene cluster show that the trimodal distribution depends on the number of α-globin genes present (Embury and Dozy, 1981; Steinberg and Embury, 1986). The reduction of β^S-globin biosynthesis in sickle cell trait-α thalassemia is shown in Figure 28.2, and the ratios of to α to β globin biosynthesis in three families where there was a proband with that genotype is shown in Figure 28.3. α Thalassemia reduces the number of α chains so that in sickle cell trait, normal β^A and abnormal β^S-globin chains must compete for a smaller α-globin chain pool. Newly synthesized HbS molecules are lost from the cell, perhaps by proteolysis

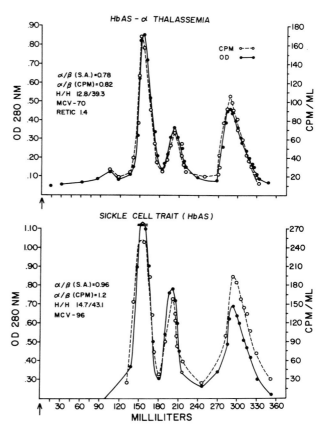

Figure 29.2. Globin biosynthesis in patients with sickle cell trait-α thalassemia (top) and sickle cell trait (bottom). Isotopically labeled globin chains were separated on carboxymethylcellulose columns, and specific activity (S.A.) and total counts (cpm) were measured. The left-most peaks represent the β^A chain, the second peak the β^S chain, and the final peak, the α-globin chain.

Figure 29.3. $\alpha/\beta^A + \beta^S$ biosynthesis in three families where there was a proband with sickle cell trait-α thalassemia. Shown beneath each individual is the $\alpha/\beta^A + \beta^S$ biosynthesis ratio. The normal ratio is 0.85 to 1.25.

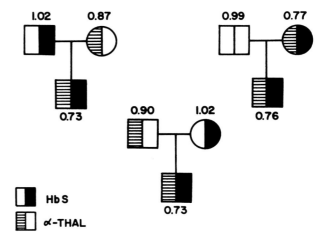

(DeSimone et al., 1977). α Chains dimerize twice as effectively with β^A chains as with β^S chains. Thus, when sickle cell trait and α thalassemia coexist, the level of HbS falls from the usual 40 percent level. Conversely, extra α-globin genes increase the HbS level beyond 40 percent (Higgs DR et al., 1984; Steinberg and Embury, 1986). Table 29.1 shows typical HbS levels in individuals with sickle cell trait who have different numbers of α-globin genes and some hematologic findings in those individuals. Individuals with two α-globin genes have lower HbS levels than those with three α-globin genes, who, in turn, have lower levels that those with the usual complement of four α-globin genes. Individuals with the $-\alpha^{4.2}$ deletion have lower HbS levels than those with the more common $-\alpha^{3.7}$ deletion because of the greater α-globin chain deficit associated with the former type of α thalassemia (Chapters 17 and 18). Rare individuals with sickle cell trait have only a single α-globin gene, or HbH disease (Felice et al., 1984; Matthay et al., 1979; Schwartz and Atwater, 1972; Steinberg et al., 1986). They have HbS levels of about 20 percent, mild anemia, and marked microcytosis, but no detectable HbH. It may be that the presence of only a single normal β-globin gene, the high affinity of α-globin chains for the limited β-globin chains, and the instability of a β^S tetramer preclude HbH (β_4) formation. Heterozygotes for HbC and HbE have similar changes in the level of the variant hemoglobin when α thalassemia is present (Chapters 28 and 43).

Effects of Other Modulators

HbG Philadelphia, an α-globin chain variant (Chapters 18, 45), is occasionally found with sickle cell trait, usually on a chromosome that lacks the α_2-globin gene ($-\alpha^{3.7}$ deletion). Heterozygotes for both HbS and HbG Philadelphia are not anemic and have no evidence of hemolysis. They may have mild microcytosis. Nearly half their hemoglobin is HbS and HbG (Rising et al., 1974). When sickle cell trait or HbC trait (Chapter 27) appear together with HbG Philadelphia, the electrophoretic pattern can be confusing (see Fig. 28.8). Normal α-globin chains combine with β^A, β^S, δ, and in the neonate, γ-globin chains, to make HbA, HbS, HbA_2, and HbF. Similarly, α^G-globin chains combine with the same non-α-globin chains to form HbG and $\alpha^G \beta^S$, α^G δ, and α^G γ hybrids. The electrophoretic mobility of the hybrids depends on their charge, and their proportion hinges on the ease of dimer formation. At alkaline pH, HbS and HbG comigrate and are inseparable. Other α-globin chain variants may be found with sickle cell trait, and, like the example of HbG-Philadelphia, their electrophoretic picture may be puzzling; but they are clinically insignificant. Some of the variants are shown in Table 29.2.

Heterozygotes with β^+ thalassemia and sickle cell trait synthesize more HbS than HbA because of the reduced expression of the β-thalassemia gene in *trans* (Chapter 12). Rarely, a β thalassemia mutation can be *cis* to the β^S-globin gene. A C→T mutation at position

---

Table 29.1. Hematology and Percent HbS in Sickle Cell Trait with α Thalassemia or β Thalassemia

α-Globin genotype	Hemoglobin (g/dL)	MCV (fl)	α/β* Biosynthesis	HbS[†] (%)
ααα/αα	N	N	–	45
αα/αα	N	N	1	40
–α/ααα	N	N	–	40
–α/αα	N-low N	75–85	0.85	35
- -/αα[‡]	?	?	?	?
–α/–α	N-low N	70–75	0.75	30
- -/–α	7–10 g/dL	50–60	0.50	20–25

Sickle cell trait with β^+ Thalassemia in *trans* or in *cis*

β^+ Thalassemia *trans*	8–12	60–70	1.50	70–90
β^+ Thalassemia *cis*	12–13	65	1.50	10

Modified from Steinberg and Embury, 1986.

N signifies normal levels.

* Ratio of radioactivity incorporated into α-globin chains vs. β-globin chains during incubation of reticulocytes with radioisotopes. The normal α/β ratio is 1 ± 0.15. Lower ratios suggest the presence of α thalassemia and higher ratios, β thalassemia.

[†] Remainder of hemoglobin predominantly HbA.

[‡] This genotype has not been reported with sickle cell trait.

Most values represent means from several studies. Although about 50 patients with sickle cell trait and the αα/αα genotype, 40 with the -α/αα genotype and 20 with the -α/-α have been studied, far fewer with the other genotypes have been examined, so the data presented should be interpreted with caution. HbS with β^+ thalassemia assumes a normal α-globin genotype.

Table 29.2. Association of α-Globin Gene Variants with HbS

Variant	Mutation	Phenotype
Hb Memphis	α23 glu→gln	Migrates like HbS at both alkaline and acidic pH
Hb Montgomery	α48 leu→arg	Migrates between HbS and HbA at alkaline pH
Hb Mexico	α54 gln→glu	With sickle cell trait, ~20% Hb Mexico and 50% hybrid hemoglobin
HbG-Philadelphia	α68 asn→lys	Migrates like HbS at alkaline pH and HbA at acidic pH
Hb Stanleyville-II	α77 pro→arg	Migrates like HbS at alkaline pH and HbA at acidic pH
Hb Nigeria	α81 ser→cys	Migrates faster than HbA at alkaline pH, and hybrid with β^S migrates faster than HbS
HbG-Georgia	α95 pro→leu	Migrates like HbS at alkaline pH
Hb Hopkins-II	α112 his→asp	Migrates like HbA

−88 5′ to the β-globin gene was found on a HbS gene on a Benin haplotype chromosome (Baklouti et al., 1989). Affected patients had a normal α-globin genotype with α:β synthesis consistent with β thalassemia trait. They were mildly anemic with microcytosis, high HbA_2, and HbS levels of 10 to 11 percent. The HbS levels were much lower than those associated with HbH disease and sickle cell trait (Felice et al., 1984; Matthay et al., 1979; Schwartz and Atwater, 1972; Steinberg et al., 1986) (Table 29.1) (Chapter 28).

Mutations that produce HPFH (Chapter 15) can be found *cis* and *trans* to the HbS gene in sickle cell trait. They are not associated with a clinical phenotype but can produce confusing electrophoretic findings. Depending on the mutation causing HPFH, there may be minor increases in HbF that usually do not exceed 5 percent or major increases that exceed 20 percent of the total hemoglobin. Individuals with sickle cell trait who inherit the −202 C→T mutation 5′ to the $^A\gamma$ globin gene have 2 to 4 percent HbF and more than 90 percent $^A\gamma$ chains (Gilman et al., 1988). Mutations associated with those conditions are shown in Table 29.3. The compound heterozygous conditions of HbS-deletion HPFH and HbS-δβ thalassemia are discussed in Chapter 28.

Sickle cell trait has been described with the γβ fusion hemoglobin, Hb Kenya (Kendall et al., 1973) (Chapters 15 and 28). Carriers are not anemic but may

have mild microcytosis. The hemolysate contains about 20 percent Hb Kenya and 60 to 70 percent HbS, and the remainder is HbA_2 and HbF.

Iron deficiency selectively inhibits the translation of α-globin mRNA and can produce an acquired form of α thalassemia. Depending on its severity, iron deficiency can mimic sickle cell trait-α thalassemia by depressing HbS levels and causing microcytic erythrocytes. In vitro and perhaps in vivo, lead can do the same (Adams et al., 1974).

Sickle cell trait can coexist with many other β-globin chain variants, including HbD_{Ibadan}, HbD_{Iran}, $HbG_{San\ Jose}$, Hb Osu-Christianbourg, HbE, $HbG_{Galveston}$, Hb Korle Bu, and Hb Richmond (Aksoy and Lehmann, 1957; McCurdy et al., 1974). Resulting phenotypes depend on the pathogenicity of the β-globin variant but usually resemble uncomplicated sickle cell trait (Chapter 28).

Hb Lepore (Chapter 15) is the product of a poorly expressed fusion gene with δ- and β-globin chain components. On electrophoresis, Hb Lepore migrates like HbS at alkaline pH and like HbA at acidic pH. Hb Lepore heterozygotes have about 10 percent of this variant and are associated with the phenotype of β-thalassemia trait. Care should be taken to not confuse heterozygous Hb Lepore with sickle cell trait and HbH disease or the rare instance of sickle cell trait in *cis* to β thalassemia. The anti-Lepore variants HbP Nilotic (HbP Congo) and Hb Lincoln Park exhibit the same electrophoretic behavior as HbS and form about 20 percent of the hemolysate. Unlike Hb Lepore, they do not cause a thalassemia phenotype. Hb Parchman, a possible δβδ-globin chain, migrates like HbS but forms less than 2 percent of the hemolysate (Adams et al., 1982). Hemoglobin variants that could be confused with HbS are listed in Chapter 45.

HbS-Antilles (β6 glu→val; β23 val→Ile) migrates like HbS, giving the electrophoretic appearance of sickle cell trait but producing sickle cell disease in the

Table 29.3. Nongene Deletion Hereditary Persistence of HbF and Sickle Cell Trait

Mutation	HbF	HbA	HbS	$^G\gamma$ (%)
−202 C→G 5′ $^G\gamma$	20	30	50	100
−202 C→T 5′ $^A\gamma$	2–4	60	40	10
−175 T→C 5′ $^G\gamma$	30	30	40	
−175 T→C 5′ $^A\gamma$	40	20	40	85
−158 C→T 5′ $^G\gamma$ in *cis*				

heterozygote. The possibility of its presence should be considered in patients with sickle cell trait who have hemolytic anemia and vasoocclusive disease (Chapter 28). Heterozygotes have 40 to 50 percent HbS-Antilles, and sickling tests are positive. HbS-Antilles can polymerize even when it constitutes only half the hemoglobin, which accounts for the erythrocyte damage and the sickle cell disease symptoms seen in heterozygotes. HbC-Harlem ($\beta6$ glu→val; $\beta73$asp→asn) also migrates like HbS at alkaline pH, is present at a concentration of about 40 percent, and gives a positive test for sickling. It can be separated from HbS at acidic pH. HbC-Harlem heterozygotes do not have abnormal hematology or symptoms.

A unique cause of symptomatic sickle cell trait was found with the coexistence of pyruvate kinase (PK) deficiency in a carrier of the HbS gene. This patient, a 42-year-old Guinean woman, had a HbS level of 44 percent, packed cell volume (PCV) of 25, reticulocytes of 203×10^9/L, cholelithiasis, and a 35-year history of hospitalizations about five times a year for painful crises (Cohen-Solal et al., 1988). Erythrocyte density profiles resembled that seen in HbSC disease (Chapter 27). The p^{50} was 41.5 mm Hg (normal ~25) Severe PK deficiency was documented by a PK level of 1.2U/gHb; 2,3 BPG; of 32.5 μmol/gHb, more than twice normal; adenosine triphosphate (ATP) of 0.76 μmol/gHb, about half normal and confirmed by sequencing the PK gene. High 2,3 BPG levels, a consequence of the metabolic block caused by PK deficiency, increased p^{50}, and decreased hemoglobin oxygen affinity, allowing HbS polymerization. Intraerythrocytic HbS polymer was inferred by hysteresis, different p^{50} values during deoxygenation and reoxygenation studies, of the hemoglobin-oxygen dissociation curves. HbS polymerization under physiologic conditions evidently increased cell density, caused hemolytic anemia, and provoked vasoocclusive episodes. Although it would be useful to know in more detail the clinical details of the vasoocclusive disease in this patient, this case seems to be an exceptional example of a truly symptomatic individual with sickle cell trait. It suggests that metabolic abnormalities can influence the phenotype of sickle cell trait and, by extension, sickle cell disease.

PREVALENCE

In Africa, the frequency of HbS versus HbA is a prime example of balanced genetic polymorphism. In populations where falciparum malaria selected for the mutation, HbS gene frequencies exceed 10 percent (Chapter 30). In some populations, nearly half the members are heterozygous for the sickle cell gene.

In other areas, the prevalence of sickle cell trait depends primarily on the pattern of flow of the HbS

Table 29.4. Prevalence of Sickle Cell Trait in World Populations

Region/country		Prevalence (%)
Africa		
	North Africa	1.3–6.3
	West Africa	13.2–24.4
	Central Africa	5.1–24.5
	East Africa	2–38
	Southern Africa	0.8–20
Middle East		
Central Asia and India	India	20 (in affected tribal populations)
	Transcaucasia	0.5–1
	Turkey	13 (Eti-Turks)
	Iran	
	Saudi Arabia	1–60
Europe		
	Greece	0–32 (mean = 11 in the north)
	Italy (Sicily)	2–4
	Portugal	
United States	United States	8–9 (African Americans)
	Amerindians	Rare
South America	Brazil	4–8
Caribbean		7–14 (excluding Puerto Rico)
Central America		1–20 (dependent on racial origin of population examined)

Data from Africa are summarized from the work of many investigators and adapted from Ohene-Frempong and Nkrumah, 1994.

gene from its origins in Africa, the Middle East, and Asia to Europe and the New World. Also contributory is how long ago the migrations took place and the extent of genetic admixture with the indigenous population (Chapter 26). Table 29.4 shows the prevalence of sickle cell trait in some African locations and in population groups throughout the world. Variations in the prevalence of sickle cell trait from area to area within a country or geographic region are due to the presence or absence of malaria, ancient migrations, isolation, and the extent of miscegenation. In Greece, the highest prevalence is in the northeast, with pockets in the central and western parts of the country (Deliyannis and Tavlarakis, 1955). In Saudi Arabia, the western oasis has a HbS carrier prevalence of about 25 percent compared with 5 percent in the north and east (Gelpi, 1970; Gelpi and King, 1976). In some local populations, likely to be highly inbred, sickle cell trait prevalence may be about 60 percent (El-Hazmi et al., 1996; Winter, 1986). In India, tribal populations predominantly in the east (Orissa, Andhra Pradesh) and south (Nilgiris) have a very high prevalence compared with populations in the north (Brittenham et al., 1977, 1979; Kaur et al., 1997; Nagel, 1994; Ramasamy et al., 1994). Some Caribbean island populations have HbS gene frequencies of more than 5 percent (Serjeant et al., 1986).

Although sickle cell trait is widely distributed in Caucasian populations, it is not the result of selection, but of ancient wars and migrations, the slave trade, and many generations of genetic admixture between the original carriers of the HbS gene and indigenous populations (Chapter 26). In India, Greece, Turkey, Italy, and elsewhere in the Old World, sickle cell trait is found mainly in Caucasians (excluding recent migrants from Africa or the Caribbean). In the United States, the prevalence of sickle cell trait in Caucasians varies according to the population examined, but it is usually less than 0.1 percent (Ewing et al., 1981; Tsevat et al., 1991; Winter, 1986). In Caucasians with sickle cell anemia, the HbS mutation resides on African β-globin gene cluster haplotypes, indicating that the HbS genes in those individuals represent genetic admixture and not new mutations (Rogers et al., 1989).

With rare exceptions, sickle cell trait is not found in Amerindians, North Europeans, and Asians other than certain Indian tribal groups; and when it is present, it is likely to be the result of gene flow and genetic admixture (Livingstone, 1967).

CLINICAL FEATURES

Hematology

Table 29.1 shows hematologic data compiled from various studies of people with sickle cell trait with either a normal α-globin genotype, α thalassemia, or β+ thalassemia. In some studies, the packed cell volume (PCV) in sickle cell trait was slightly reduced but still in normal range; in others, it did not differ from the PCV in control subjects (Ashcroft et al., 1969; Castro and Scott, 1985; Diggs et al., 1933; Polenak and Janerich, 1975; Rana et al., 1993). The disparity may have been due to the differences in methodology and to the use of geographically diverse populations of different sizes and age ranges. Any differences from normal values are small and within normal range, suggesting that they are unlikely to be clinically significant.

Hemolysis is unlikely to occur in uncomplicated sickle cell trait. Reticulocytosis is absent, and isotopic red cell survival studies usually yield normal findings (Barbedo and McCutdy, 1974). α Thalassemia reduces the mean cell volume (MCV) and mean cell hemoglobin (MCH) in sickle cell trait and is sometimes associated with slight, clinically insignificant reductions in hemoglobin concentration.

HbA_2 concentration in sickle cell trait is normal by most measurement techniques, but some yield higher than normal values (Schiliro et al., 1990; Steinberg and Adams, 1991; Whitten and Rucknagel, 1981).

Mortality

Sickle cell trait is not a risk factor for excess mortality in African Americans (Heller et al., 1979). When 65,000 hospitalized African-American men were screened by hemoglobin electrophoresis for hemoglobinopathies, rates of all-cause mortality did not differ between those with sickle cell trait and those with normal hemoglobin. Moreover, both populations were similar in postoperative mortality and risk of death following myocardial infarction. A lack of age-dependent differences in the frequency of sickle cell trait suggested that there was no effect on life span. In 350 men and women, the frequency of sickle cell trait was similar in three age groups: 5 to 20 years, 21 to 49 years, and 50 years and older (Petrakis et al., 1970). Longitudinal studies of 119 carriers of sickle cell trait and control subjects suggested no difference in their mortality (Ashcroft and Desai, 1976). In another study, more than 500 individuals with sickle cell trait and more than 1,000 age- and sex-matched control subjects were monitored for 7 years; there was no difference in mortality rates between the groups (Stark et al., 1980). When more than 30,000 African Americans were screened in a community-based study, the prevalence of sickle cell trait did not vary with age (Castro et al., 1987). The scope of those studies suggests that the results apply to African Americans in general. There is no evidence that sickle cell trait increases mortality in Africans either, but adequate data are not available for analysis (Ohene-Frempong and Nkrumah, 1994). To determine unambiguously whether sickle cell trait increases mortality or morbidity, a very large cohort of affected neonates and matched control subjects would have to be followed for many years, a study which is unlikely to be undertaken and completed.

Reports of sudden death or life-threatening episodes during exercise abound for sickle cell trait, and they have been reviewed extensively (Kark and Ward, 1994). Most of the deaths were attributed to exertional heat illness. Case reports and small clusters of unexpected sudden death in people with sickle cell trait in special situations—military recruits undergoing basic training and athletes engaging in physically stressful sports—raised the possibility that under extremely rigorous conditions, sickle cell trait may be associated with a higher risk of sudden death (Kark and Ward, 1994). That possibility is supported by a study in the military. For 5 years, when 2.1 million recruits underwent basic training in the U.S. Armed Forces, the risk of sudden unexplained death in black recruits with sickle cell trait compared with those without the trait was 27.6 (Kark et al., 1987). Compared with all recruits, blacks without sickle cell trait and whites, the relative risk was 40. (Other sickle cell trait mortality studies suffer from design flaws, principally low power owing to small sample size.) The risk increased progressively with increasing age from a death rate of 12 per 100,000 at ages 17 to 18 years to 136 per 100,000 at ages 31 to 34 years. Perhaps the increasing prevalence of isosthenuria with age in sickle cell trait and the accompanying possibility of dehydration when access to fluids was limited account for the observation. It was not possible to tell if the fractional percent of HbS was associated with sudden death. Individuals with sickle cell trait and coincident α thalassemia have a lower amount of HbS and better preserved urine-concentrating ability than those with trait alone (see later) (Gupta et al., 1991). Work based on using percent HbS used as a surrogate for α thalassemia, and not the determination of α-globin gene haplotype, suggested that α thalassemia was underrepresented in individuals with sudden death (Kark and Ward, 1994). If this is true, it may be because individuals with sickle cell trait-α thalassemia have better preserved urine concentration ability (see below) (Gupta et al., 1991).

In summary, sickle cell trait is not a risk factor for excess mortality in the general population, and restraint during the rigors of conditioning should eliminate any hazard in special groups.

Treatment Recommendations. These observations suggest a prudent course that includes gradual conditioning, liberal fluid intake, and avoidance of overexertion under all conditions, especially when temperatures are high. When that strategy was adopted by the U.S. military in recruit conditioning and training, the death rate in the sickle cell trait population fell to that of the entire recruit population. Its abandonment was associated with a return to increased mortality in carriers of sickle cell trait.

MORBIDITY OF SICKLE CELL TRAIT

Does sickle cell trait interfere with any physical activities? Is it a risk factor for increased morbidity from certain diseases, and do carriers of sickle cell trait show increased mortality from other diseases? The fol-lowing section reviews the effects of sickle cell trait on daily living and selected organ function.

Pregnancy

In Africa, fertility may be increased in women and perhaps men with sickle cell trait (Eaton and Mucha, 1971; Livingstone, 1957). This increased fertility was believed to be one mechanism to explain the high frequency of HbS where malaria is endemic. That concept, however, is not supported by more recent studies (Ezeh and Modebe, 1996; Fleming, 1996; Madrigal, 1989). According to many reports, pregnancy complications are more frequent in sickle cell trait. The risks for bacteriuria, pyelonephritis, and urinary tract infection may be increased as much as twofold (Blattner et al., 1977; Sears, 1978; Walley et al., 1963), and in a well-designed prospective study of 162 pregnancies with sickle cell trait and 1,422 control subjects, the preeclampsia rate was doubled in those with sickle cell trait (Larrabee and Monga, 1997). Also, endometritis occurred more frequently in the women with sickle cell trait, and gestational age and birth weight were reduced in their infants. The effect of maternal age on pregnancy outcome was studied in 157 women with sickle cell trait who were compared with control subjects by age group (14 to 16 and 17 to 28 years old). The pregnancy outcomes were similar, but sickle cell trait mothers had offspring whose mean birth weight was almost 200 g less than that of the control subjects (Hoff, 1983). Retrospective analyses, on the other hand, found no differences in mean birth weight, number of low-birth-weight infants, 5-minute Apgar scores, gestational age, or incidence of delivery complications (Kramer et al., 1978; Polenak and Janerich, 1980). Some studies reporting increased complications of many types, including prematurity and premature rupture of membranes, often lacked appropriate control subjects (Rimer, 1975). Iron supplementation to pregnant African women with sickle cell trait is of little benefit, perhaps because of an increased risk of malaria, but those results are inconclusive (Menedez et al., 1995).

Treatment Recommendations. Sickle cell trait may be associated with increased risks of certain complications of pregnancy, mainly urinary tract infections, but conscientious prenatal care can minimize those risks. Customary means of contraception are safe for women with sickle cell trait.

Growth and Development

Many investigators have questioned whether sickle cell trait influences growth and development. Some have found differences in physical and intellectual growth (McCormack et al., 1975), but the best evidence suggests that there are no such differences between children with sickle cell trait and matched control subjects (Ashcroft et al., 1976, 1978; Kramer et al., 1978; Rehan, 1981). Sickle cell trait is not associated with an increased chance of sudden infant death syndrome (Gozal et al., 1994).

Altitude

In some circumstances, hypoxia at high altitude may affect performance in vigorous exercise and cause changes in the splenic circulation.

Exercise

As discussed previously, risk of sudden death from exertional heat illness is increased during strenuous conditioning regimens in military recruits and athletes with sickle cell trait when optimal hydration is not maintained. What are the physiologic responses to exercise in sickle cell trait? Does this condition impair exercise tolerance and performance? Forty-eight people with sickle cell trait, ages 4 to 21 years, underwent progressive ergometer stress testing at their voluntary maximal performance, and the results were compared with 184 control subjects. Equivocal ischemic changes on electrocardiogram were seen on four from the sickle cell trait group. The maximum workload and heart rate were lower in the sickle cell trait subjects, but there were no complications as a result of the exercise program (Alpert et al., 1982). One study comparing the response to incremental exercise in people with sickle cell trait and control subjects reported no differences in cardiovascular function but did shower lower blood acetate concentrations in sickle cell trait carriers (Bile et al., 1998a). When anaerobic exercise and exercise metabolism after force-velocity tests were compared in sedentary adults with sickle cell trait and closely matched control subjects, there were no differences between the groups (Bile et al., 1996).

Black athletes with sickle cell trait are well represented in elite competitive sports (Murphy, 1973). The percentage of African marathon runners and other competitive athletes with sickle cell trait among the top performers is similar to, or more than, that in the general population (Bile et al., 1998b; Le Gallais et al., 1994). In a recent study, racers in the Cameroon who competed at high altitudes, with some exceptions, had a similar percent of sickle cell trait carriers as the general population. At altitudes of 3,800 to 4,095 meters, the carriers were slower than other competitors (Thiriet et al., 1994). Before and after basic training, a group of individuals with sickle cell trait and control

subjects had similar responses to exercise testing (Weisman et al., 1988c). Acute stressful exercise at an altitude of 1,270 meters and a simulated altitude of 2,300 meters was not associated with differences in cardiopulmonary and gas exchange between subjects with sickle cell trait and control subjects (Weisman et al., 1988a, 1988b). Vigorous arm exercise was associated with sickled cells in effluent venous blood, and the frequency of such cells increased fourfold at simulated altitudes of 4,000 meters (Martin et al., 1989). Performance was unimpaired, and sickled cells were not detected in arterial blood.

Many other studies, summarized elsewhere, show minimal or no adverse effects of sickle cell trait during exercise (Kark and Ward, 1994; Sears, 1978).

Treatment Recommendation. Based on the total body of work on exercise ability and capacity, there is no reason to restrict exercise of any type in persons with sickle cell trait. Restraints need not differ from those used to forestall ill effects of exercise in the general population.

Flying

There are many reports of splenic infarction during flight in unpressurized aircraft at altitudes of 3,000 to 5,000 meters (Sears, 1978). In the early reports, the diagnosis of sickle cell trait was often made by tests for sickling that today would be considered inadequate, and some cases reported may have been instances of HbSC disease or HbS-β^+ thalassemia rather than sickle cell trait. Commercial aircraft are pressurized to 2,500 meters, and splenic infarct and any other complication of HbS polymerization are unlikely to occur under that condition (Green et al., 1971). At present, the U.S. Department of Defense places no restrictions on military aircrew with sickle cell trait (Voge et al., 1991).

Kidney

The kidney medulla is one of the few sites where sickle cell trait erythrocytes are placed in jeopardy. Low PO$_2$, low pH, and high solute concentration provide a milieu where sickling of even the sickle cell trait erythrocyte can occur (Bookchin et al., 1976; Embury et al., 1994; Statius van Eps et al., 1970). Damage to the countercurrent urine-concentrating mechanism and the vasculature of the renal medulla leads to a defect in urine-concentrating ability and hyposthenuria in most adults with sickle cell trait, as well as hematuria in some. Those abnormalities may result from microvascular injury in the vasa recta of the renal medulla. A defect in urine acidification, which in sickle cell anemia is related to the severity of the concentration defect, is not seen in sickle cell trait (Falk and Jennette, 1994; Oster et al., 1976).

The polymerization tendency of HbS may determine the extent of the urine-concentrating defect in sickle cell trait (Gupta et al., 1991). To test this hypothesis, urinary concentrating ability was examined after overnight water deprivation and intranasal arginine vasopressin (dDAVP) in sickle cell trait subjects separated into two groups, one with a normal α-globin complement and one with either heterozygous or homozygous α thalassemia (α thalassemia modulates the HbS concentration in sickle cell trait). The ability to concentrate urine was most impaired in subjects with normal α-globin genotype and least impaired in subjects homozygous for α thalassemia (Gupta et al., 1991). (Urine osmolality was 882 ± 37 mOsm/kg H_2O in α thalassemia homozygotes and 672 ± 38 mOsm/kg H_2O in the heterozygotes.) In all subjects, urinary osmolality correlated linearly and inversely with percentage of HbS. A similar correlation was found between urine-concentrating ability and HbS polymerization tendency at 0.4 oxygen saturation (Fig. 29.4), suggesting that HbS polymer, a function of percent HbS, is responsible for the urine-concentrating defect of sickle cell trait.

Hematuria in sickle cell trait has been reviewed (Sears, 1978). Hematuria occurs episodically in about 5 percent of people with sickle cell trait (Heller et al., 1979). Some studies suggest that hematuria is most common at higher HbS levels (Gupta et al., 1991;

Figure 29.4. Relationship between maximum urine-concentrating ability and polymer fraction at 40 percent oxygen saturation in individuals with sickle cell trait and 4, 3, and 2 α-globin genes. (From Gupta et al., 1991, with permission.)

Kennedy et al., 1986). Bleeding is more frequent in the left kidney, perhaps because of the anatomy of venous drainage system, and men are affected four times more often than women. Although von Willebrand syndrome has been reported in sickle cell trait (Brody et al., 1977; Weinger et al., 1979), no association has been established between any coagulation abnormality and sickle cell trait hematuria.

Papillary necrosis, another cause of hematuria (sometimes with renal colic), may be more frequent in sickle cell trait and is perhaps another consequence of sickling in the renal medulla (Sears, 1978; Zadeii and Lohr, 1997).

Treatment Recommendations. No treatment can stop hematuria in people with sickle cell trait, and radical treatments should be avoided. Although often recurrent, hematuria is usually benign and self-limited, but it could arise from more ominous causes than a damaged renal medulla. Renal and bladder cancer—especially medullary cancer in young patients—stones, glomerulonephritis, and infection should be excluded during an evaluation of a first episode of hematuria.

Renal medullary carcinoma, a rare and aggressive tumor, may be associated with sickle cell trait (Adsay et al., 1998; Coogan et al., 1998; Davidson et al., 1995; Davis et al., 1995; Figenshau et al., 1998; Friedrichs et al, 1997). In a retrospective analysis spanning 20 years, thirty-three black patients, ages 11 to 40 years, who presented with hematuria and pain, had renal medullary carcinoma (Davis et al., 1995). Nine patients had proven sickle cell trait and one had HbSC disease, but all tumor specimens contained sickled cells. The tumors were lobulated with

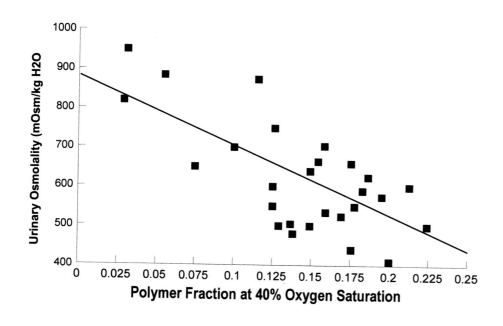

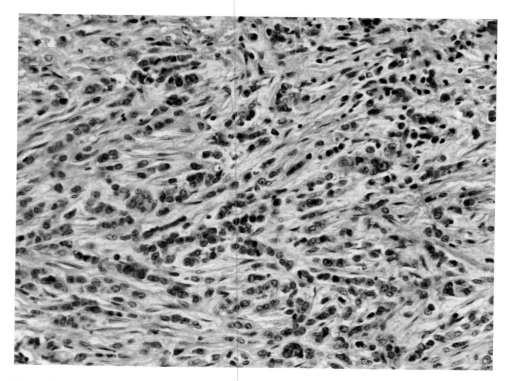

Figure 29.5. Renal medullary carcinoma, showing epithelioid cells and spindle cells in a background of fibrosis and small lymphocytes (400×). (Provided by R. S. Figenshau.) (From Figenshau et al., 1998.)

satellite cortical nodules and widespread metastases. Histologically, the tumors had a reticular, yolk saclike or glandular cystic appearance, with a desmoplastic stroma, hemorrhage, necrosis, neutrophil infiltration, and lymphocyte sheathing (Fig. 29.5). Chemotherapy was uniformly unsuccessful, and survival after diagnosis was about 4 months (Avery et al., 1996).

The diagnosis of sickle cell trait for twenty-three of the patients was based on histologic findings because diagnostic tests documenting sickle cell trait were not reported for them. If sickle cell trait was present in all thirty-three patients, the conclusion that the condition predisposes to this rare tumor seems inescapable. It has been hypothesized that the medullary cancers may originate in terminal collecting ducts, where epithelial cell proliferation has been noted in sickle cell trait. Perhaps rapid cell proliferation and oxygen radicals produced by cell sickling, coupled with preexisting mutations in genes that control cell growth (such as p53), predispose to carcinogenesis.

Other renal or genitourinary system disorders, such as nephrotic syndrome, priapism, pyelonephritis, hypotonic bladder, hypertension, renal failure, renal cortical infarction, and renal vein thrombosis, undoubtedly occur in sickle cell trait; but there is no evidence that they are caused by sickle cell trait. Renal allograft survival in sickle cell trait is equivalent to that in the general population (Chatterjee, 1980).

Spleen

Young black men with sickle cell trait residing at altitudes up to 1,600 meters for many years have normal splenic function as assessed by radionuclide scan and by the number of red cells with "pits" (Nuss et al., 1991). Splenic infarction can occur in individuals with sickle cell trait when they encounter hypobaric conditions. Scuba diving, where divers breathe compressed air, provides an environment with increased PO_2 and poses no risk to carriers of sickle cell trait (Adams, 1984).

Splenic infarcts in African Americans with sickle cell trait are rare, or rarely reported, in the United States. Nor was splenic infarction mentioned in a report of African runners with sickle cell trait who competed at altitudes of up to 4,100 meters (Thiriet et al., 1994). Especially interesting are reports of splenic infarction in Caucasians with sickle cell trait (Gitschier and Thompson, 1989; Lane and Githens, 1985), and Caucasian men are overrepresented in reports of altitude-induced splenic syndrome and splenic infarcts at sea level. In a recent review, twenty of twenty-nine reported cases of splenic syndrome were in white males (Harkness, 1989). Most, but not all, episodes occurred shortly after ascent to about 3,000 meters. This curious observation has led to much speculation (Castro and Finch, 1974; Roth, 1985; Steinberg, 1985;

Steinberg and Embury, 1986). A reasonable supposition is that an African HbS gene, now within the Caucasian gene pool, became isolated from accompanying genes that in Africa evolved along with the HbS gene and modulated its effects. The hypothesized modulating genes may affect the mean corpuscular HbS concentration, which may differ between black and nonblack trait carriers. Some inconclusive evidence suggests that Caucasian carriers with splenic infarction have a higher HbS concentration than black carriers, and that a high mean cell HbS concentration increases the risk of intrasplenic sickling and organ damage. One white splenic infarction patient had a HbS level of 46.5 percent and had five α-globin genes (Shalev et al., 1988). (Table 29.1). In a report in which both father and son had a splenic infarct, the HbS levels were 41 and 45.6 percent, respectively (Goldberg et al., 1985). In another study, however, HbS levels in a small series of nonblack carriers differed little from those in most black carriers of sickle cell trait (Lane and Githens, 1985). If HbS levels are truly higher in Caucasian carriers, it may be a consequence of the absence of α thalassemia and the reduced cation exchange and lower cation content in Caucasians, erythrocytes, a deficit most marked in men (Lasker et al., 1985), or differences in other "protective" genes associated with the HbS gene in blacks.

Rarely, sickle cell trait and hereditary spherocytosis coexist. The dominant phenotype is that of hereditary spherocytosis (Yang et al., 1992). One study reported that two patients with the combination developed acute splenic sequestration crises (Chapter 24), and the postsplenectomy specimens showed erythrostasis and sickling. Perhaps these unusual events (sequestration crises are not a feature of sickle cell trait) were the result of the splenomegaly of hereditary spherocytosis and the high mean cell hemoglobin concentration (MCHC) of HbS-containing hereditary spherocytosis erythrocytes.

Eye

In nonhemoglobinopathic individuals, hyphema (i.e., hemorrhage into the anterior chamber) usually clears uneventfully with topical medical therapy. In sickle cell trait, the naturally low PO_2 in the anterior chamber causes cell sickling and impedes cellular outflow through the trabecular meshwork and Schlemm's canal, raising intraocular pressure. High pressure in the anterior chamber can reduce vascular perfusion pressure elsewhere in the eye, injuring the optic nerve and retina and impairing vision. Anterior segment hypoxia and acidosis set in place the vicious cycle of erythrostasis typical of sickle cell disease. Secondary open-angle glaucoma can result from poorly treated hyphema.

Treatment Recommendations. Black patients and others at risk of carrying the HbS gene who present with hyphema should be screened for the gene without delay. A sickle solubility test is sufficient because it is important to ascertain only whether HbS is present. Management of hyphema in sickle cell trait is beyond the scope of this chapter; it should be supervised by an ophthalmologist who understands the special problems that may arise when the conditions coexist. Intraocular pressure can be controlled medically in perhaps two thirds of the cases. Anterior chamber hypertension of greater than 24 mm Hg for consecutive 24-hour periods and repeated but transient increases greater than 30 mm Hg should be reduced by paracentesis, which can be repeated if necessary. Normal pressure during the first 24 hours of observation suggests, but does not establish, that medical treatment will suffice (Deutsch et al., 1984; Liebmann, 1996).

Many ocular abnormalities, including internuclear ophthalmoplegia, transient monocular blindness, vitreous hemorrhage, and optic atrophy, have been described in sickle cell trait (Finelli, 1976; Leavitt and Butrus, 1994; Sears, 1978); but any association of the disorders with sickle cell trait is likely to be fortuitous. Chronic open-angle glaucoma is no more common in sickle cell trait than in age- and sex-matched control subjects (Steinmann et al., 1983).

Proliferative retinopathy akin to the type known to occur in sickle cell disease has been described in sickle cell trait (Jackson et al., 1995; Nagpal et al., 1977). In all cases, a known cause of proliferative retinopathy such as diabetes or granulomatous disease was present, perhaps predisposing to the development of retinal lesions.

Bones and Joints

Reports of osteonecrosis in sickle cell trait make an unconvincing case for an association between the two common conditions (Sears, 1978; Taylor et al., 1986). Bone infarction has also been described with sickle cell trait, also with no evidence of association beyond coincidence (Lally et al., 1983).

Surgery and Anesthesia

Many hundreds of patients with sickle cell trait have safely undergone anesthesia and surgery (Sears, 1978). In a matched-pair analysis of fifty-six patients with sickle cell trait and control subjects undergoing surgery, the frequency of anesthetic, surgical, and postoperative complications was similar in both groups (Atlas, 1974). The study included few intraabdominal and thoracic procedures, however, and most patients were young.

Treatment Recommendations. Most evidence suggests that anesthetic risk is not increased by sickle cell trait, and the choice of anesthesia need not be limited (Scott-Conner and Brunson, 1994). Thus, there is no rationale for preoperative screening for sickle cell trait (Scott-Conner and Brunson, 1994). With open heart surgery or complicated intrathoracic surgeries, where hypoxia may be intrinsic to the procedure, preoperative transfusion is recommended (Scott-Conner and Brunson, 1994). Screening for sickle cell trait may be prudent under those circumstances, but there are no well-controlled studies on the preoperative management of intrathoracic surgery in sickle cell trait. Not even the use of tourniquets with surgery on extremities has been associated with increased risk in sickle cell trait (Martina et al., 1984; Stein and Urbaniak, 1980).

Malaria

The selection pressure from falciparum malaria is expressed primarily in children, and where malaria is endemic, sickle cell trait children have reduced mortality (Hendrickse et al., 1971). The trait retards the development of cerebral malaria in children less than 5 years old, and it reduces its mortality (Olumese et al., 1997). Although the clinical features, parasite counts, and most laboratory measurements are similar in children with and without sickle cell trait, trait carriers receive transfusions more often. Malaria and the HbS gene are discussed in Chapter 30.

Other Conditions

The grab-bag of other diseases reported in individuals with sickle cell trait in the older literature has been thoroughly reviewed (Sears, 1978). Early reports of impaired pulmonary function in sickle cell trait have been refuted by more carefully controlled studies of (1) diffusing capacity for carbon monoxide and spirometry at simulated altitudes up to 7,500 meters and (2) pulmonary function at rest and after exhaustive exercise in men with sickle cell trait who had been living above 1,600 meters for many years (Dillard et al., 1987; Nuss et al., 1993). Reports of sickle cell disease-like "crises," complicated migraine with occlusion of branches of the middle cerebral artery, venous thrombosis, and retroperitoneal fibrosis could not be linked etiologically to sickle cell trait (Bussone et al., 1984; Humphries and Wheby, 1992). Priapism, a serious complication of sickle cell anemia, also is not associated with sickle cell trait. However, a 39 year old male with sickle cell trait with a past medical history of mild erectile dysfunction (ED) was prescribed sildenafil (Kassim et al, 2000). After taking a dose of

50mg, he had an erection within 15 minutes (a response considerably faster than observed during trials), that was sustained even after ejaculation. His painful erection remained for about 6 hours. Patient subsequently noticed a loss of morning erection followed by gradual worsening of his ED, with complete loss of erection 3 months later. Hemoglobin (Hb) electrophoresis, isoelectric focusing, and globin separation by HPLC were consistent with sickle cell trait. Isopyknic density gradient was also consistent with sickle cell trait. Mass spectroscopy excluded the presence of silent mutations of Hb. While priapism has not been reported in sickle trait individuals, the susceptibility of these individuals to this complication might also depend on inherited modifier genes which have yet to be identified. This case illustrates the possibility that sildenafil can cause priapism in patients with sickle cell trait, although the incidence of this event is unknown.

Leg ulcers have been associated with sickle cell trait in Jamaica. Of 250 patients wisth chromic leg ulcers, 20 percent had sickle cell trait, whereas only 11 percent of the general population carried the HbS gene (Serjeant and Gheri 1970). There are no data to support an increase in leg ulceration in sickle cell trait carriers in less tropical climates.

Erythrocyte glucose-6-phosphate dehydrogenase (G-6-PD) deficiency is common in many populations where sickle cell trait is found. Hemizygotes with the common African type of G-6-PD deficiency rarely encounter clinical difficulties. In a study of more than 65,000 hospitalized African-American men, nearly 1 percent had both sickle cell trait and G-6-PD deficiency. Morbidity from pneumonia and mean age of death were similar for the group with sickle cell trait alone and the group with both sickle cell trait and G-6-PD deficiency (Heller et al., 1979).

Transfusion of Sickle Cell Trait Blood

Minor changes distinguish sickle cell trait from normal blood under storage conditions, but transfused sickle cell trait erythrocytes are equivalent to normal ones in safety, effectiveness (Ahmed et al., 1991; Hipp and Scott, 1974; Ould Amar et al., 1996; Romanoff et al., 1988; Sears, 1978), and survival (Callender et al., 1949). Cryopreserved red cells from individuals with sickle cell trait may hemolyze when deglycerolized (Kelleher and Luban, 1984; Merryman and Hornblower, 1976), but a special deglycerolization protocol can prevent that from happening. Thus, when cryopreservation of rare blood types is undertaken, knowing if the donor has sickle cell trait is useful (Merryman and Hornblower, 1976). Blood from donors with sickle cell trait cannot be consistently leukodepleted with any available filter (Bodensteiner, 1994; Williamson, 1999). While an explanation for this observation has not been found, the low PO_2 and pH of stored blood was invoked as a possible contributor to altered erythrocyte filterability; cell sickling upstream of the filters was not observed. As the standard for transfused blood is rapidly shifting to leuokodepleted units and since sickle cell trait carriers are a large fraction of donors in many locales, loss of units from these donors may seriously reduce blood supplies. Sickle cell trait donors should be avoided when transfusing large amounts of blood into anemic hypoxic neonates (Novak and Brown, 1982).

SCREENING AND COUNSELING

The institution of broad, at times legislatively mandated, population-based screening programs that followed the reports nearly 30 years ago of sudden death in military recruits who had sickle cell trait led to negative consequences in addition to those previously discussed (restricted occupational opportunities and insurance coverage). They also led to feelings of stigmatization and anxiety based on misinformation and to cries of genocide and racism from less temperate voices. More positively, public attention and research dollars were directed to the study and treatment of sickle cell disease, and that effort has yielded notable advances. Many years of sober consideration of the data on sickle cell trait and its complications have quenched the early flames of controversy and directed screening efforts to targeted groups and neonates.

Screening for sickle cell trait is best applied to couples who are planning their family and are likely to carry HbS genes. Before any tests are conducted, however, screening programs should educate clients about sickle cell anemia and sickle cell trait and provide nondirective counseling. Then, when the screening results become available, couples with the HbS gene will understand the implications of having the gene, the chances of having children with sickle cell disease, and their reproductive options (Chapters 35 and 36). As a by-product of neonatal screening for sickle cell disease, many infants with sickle cell trait are now identified. The value of finding sickle cell trait in newborns is questionable; nevertheless, it is reasonable to notify the parents, educate them about the implications of the condition, and offer them further family testing (Anonymous, 1987). Ideally, at-risk, expectant women should be educated before delivery about sickle cell disease and/or sickle cell trait, as appropriate.

Screening at-risk patients is also recommended before major thoracic and cardiovascular surgery and when hyphema is present. The U.S. Armed Forces vary in their approach to sickle cell trait screening by service and even by military installation. While the screening of individuals assigned to flight duty may be prudent, screening the general population for sickle cell trait serves no purpose.

CONCLUSIONS AND RECOMMENDATIONS FOR COUNSELING

When asked about the pathogenicity and the implications of carrying the HbS gene, the physician or counselor should tell an individual who has sickle cell trait that the chances of having offspring with sickle cell disease can be predicted and that antenatal diagnosis of that disorder is available. Clinically significant anemia in sickle cell trait cannot be ascribed to the trait alone. Microcytosis in sickle cell trait is usually a sign of α thalassemia, a clinically insignificant disorder, but it could also be a sign of iron deficiency and therefore should be evaluated. The choice of occupation, except for unusual vocations such as mountaineering, is not limited. Flying in commercial aircraft need not be feared. Unexplained painful events should not be ascribed to sickle cell trait. Hematuria, usually self-limiting and benign, is likely to be due to sickle cell trait but should be evaluated to exclude other causes. Hyposthenuria, clinically irrelevant, is present in most adults. Normal hydration should be maintained; when strenuous exercise is undertaken, fluid intake should match expected losses. If a patient sustains an eye injury, hyphema should be approached with the knowledge that sickle cell trait is present and surgical intervention may be needed. Sickle cell trait-related events are not likely to complicate surgery. Morbidity from most diseases is not increased and, with rare exceptions, length and quality of life are normal.

References

Anonymous. (1987). Newborn screening for sickle cell disease and other hemoglobinopathies. *JAMA* 258: 1205–1209.

Abraham EC and Huisman, THJ. (1977). Differences in affinity of variant β chains for α chains: A possible explanation for the variation in the percentages of β chain variants in heterozygotes. *Hemoglobin* 1: 861–873.

Adams, JG, Baine, R, Eckman, J et al. (1991). *Newborn screening for hemoglobinopathies: Program development and laboratory methods.* Bethesda: NIH.

Adams, JG, De Simone, J, Orbach, H et al. (1974). The effect of lead on the proportion of hemoglobin S in sickle cell trait. *Blood* 44: 944.

Adams, JG, Morrison, WT, and Steinberg, MH. (1982). Hemoglobin Parchman: Double crossover within a single human gene. *Science* 218: 291–293.

Adams, JG III. (1984). Sickle cell trait and scuba diving. *JAMA* 251: 1681–1682.

Adams, JG III. (1994). Clinical laboratory diagnosis. In SH, Embury, RP, Hebbel, Mohandas, N, and Steinberg, MH, editors. *Sickle cell disease: Basic principles and clinical practice* New York: Lippincott-Raven, pp. 457–468.

Adsay, NV, DeRoux, SJ, Sakr, W, and Grignon, D. (1998). Cancer as a marker of genetic medical disease: An unusual case of medullary carcinoma of the kidney. *Am. J. Surg. Pathol.* 22: 260–264.

Ahmed, MA, Al-Ali, AK, al-Idrissi, HY et al. (1991). Sickle cell trait and G6PD deficiency in blood donors in eastern Saudi Arabia. *Vox Sang.* 61: 69–70.

Aksoy, M and Lehmann, H. (1957). The first demonstration of sickle cell haemoglobin E disease. *Nature* 179: 1249–1249.

Alpert, BS, Flood, NL, Strong, WB et al. (1982). Responses to exercise in children with sickle cell trait. *Am. J. Dis. Child.* 136: 1002–1004.

Ashcroft, MT and Desai, P. (1976). Mortality and morbidity in Jamaican adults with sickle-cell trait and with normal haemoglobin followed up for twelve years. *Lancet* 2: 748–786.

Ashcroft, MT, Desai, P, Grell, GA et al. (1978). Heights and weights of West Indian children with the sickle cell trait. *Arch. Dis. Child.* 53: 596–598.

Ashcroft, MT, Desai, P, Richardson, SA, and Serjeant, BE. (1976). Growth, behaviour, and educational achievement of Jamaican children with sickle-cell trait. *Br. Med. J.* 1: 1371–1373.

Ashcroft, MT, Miall, WE, and Milner, PF. (1969). A comparison between characteristics of Jamaican adults with normal hemoglobin and those with sickle cell trait. *Am. J. Epidemiol.* 90: 236–243.

Atlas, SA. (1974). The sickle cell trait and surgical complications. A matched-pair patient analysis. *JAMA* 229: 1078–1080.

Avery, RA, Harris, JE, Davis, CJ Jr et al. (1996). Renal medullary carcinoma: Clinical and therapeutic aspects of a newly described tumor. *Cancer* 78: 128–132.

Baklouti, F, Ouzana, R, Gonnet, C et al. (1989). β+ Thalassemia in *cis* of a sickle gene: occurrence of a promoter mutation on a βS chromosome. *Blood* 74: 1818–1822.

Barbedo, MM and McCurdy, PR. (1974). Red cell life span in sickle cell trait. *Acta Haematolo.* 51: 339–343.

Basset, P, Beuzard, Y, Garel, MC, and Rosa, J. (1978). Isoelectric focusing of human hemoglobin: Its application to screening, to the characterization of 70 variants, and to the study of modified fractions of normal hemoglobins. *Blood* 51: 971–982.

Beet, EA. (1949). The genetics of sickle cell trait in a Bantu tribe. *Ann. Eugenics* 14: 279–284.

Bile, A, Le Gallais, D, Mercier, B et al. (1996). Anaerobic exercise components during the force-velocity test in sickle cell trait. *Int. J. Sports Med.* 17: 254–258.

Bile, A, Le Gallais, D, Mercier, B et al. (1998a). Blood lactate concentrations during incremental exercise in subjects with sickle cell trait. *Med. Sci. Sports Exerci.* 30: 649–654.

Bile, A, Le Gallais, D, Mercier, J et al. (1998b). Sickle cell trait in Ivory Coast athletic throw and jump champions, 1956–1995. *Int. J. Sports Med.* 19: 215–219.

Blattner, P, Dar, H, and Nitowsky, HM. (1977). Pregnancy outcome in women with sickle cell trait. *JAMA* 238: 1392–1394.

Bodensteiner, D. (1994). White cell reduction in blood from donors with sickle cell trait. *Transfusion* 34: 84.

Bookchin, RM, Balazs, T, and Landau, LC. (1976). Determinants of red sickling. Effects of varying pH and of increasing intracellular hemoglobin concentration by osmotic shrinkage. *J. Lab. Clin. Med.* 87: 597–616.

Brittenham, G. (1977). Genetic model for observed distributions of proportions of haemoglobin in sickle-cell trait. *Nature* 268: 635–636.

Brittenham, G, Lozoff, B, Harris, JW et al. (1979). Sickle cell anemia and trait in southern India: Further studies. *Am. J. Hematol.* 6: 107–123.

Brittenham, G, Lozoff, B, Harris, JW et al. (1977). Sickle cell anemia and trait in a population of southern India. *Am. J. Hematol.* 2: 25–32.

Brody, JI, Levison, SP, and Jung, CJ. (1977). Sickle cell trait and hematuria associated with von Willebrand syndromes. *Ann. Intern. Med.* 86: 529–533.

Bunn, HF. (1987). Subunit assembly of hemoglobin: An important determinant of hematologic phenotype. *Blood* 69: 1–6.

Bussone, G, La Mantia, L, Boiardi, A et al. (1984). Complicated migraine in AS hemoglobinopathy. *Eur. Neurol.* 23: 22–25.

Callender, STE, Nickel, JF, and Moore, CV. (1949). Sickle cell disease: Studied by measuring the survival of transfused red blood cells. *J. Lab. Clin. Med.* 34: 90.

Castro, O and Finch, S. (1974). Splenic infarction in sickle cell trait: Are whites more susceptible? *N. Engl. J. Med.* 291: 630–631.

Castro, O, Rana, SR, Bang, KM, and Scott, RB. (1987). Age and prevalence of sickle-cell trait in a large ambulatory population. *Genet. Epidemiol.* 4: 307–311.

Castro, O and Scott, RB. (1985). Red blood cell counts and indices in sickle cell trait in a black American population. *Hemoglobin* 9: 65–67.

Chatterjee, SN. (1980). National study on natural history of renal allografts in sickle cell disease or trait. *Nephron* 25: 199–201.

Cohen-Solal, M, Préhu, C, Wajcman, H et al. (1998). A new sickle cell disease phenotype associating Hb S trait, severe pyruvate kinase deficiency (PK Conakry), and an α2 globin gene variant (Hb Conakry). *Br. J. Haematol.* 103: 950–956.

Coogan, CL, McKiel, CF Jr, Flanagan MJ et al. (1998). Renal medullary carcinoma in patients with sickle cell trait. *Urology* 51: 1049–1050.

Davidson, AJ, Choyke, PL, Hartman, DS, and Davis, CJ Jr. (1995). Renal medullary carcinoma associated with sickle cell trait: Radiologic findings. *Radiology* 195: 83–85.

Davis, CJ Jr, Mostofi, FK, and Sesterhenn, IA. (1995). Renal medullary carcinoma: The seventh sickle cell nephropathy. *Am. J. Surg. Pathol.* 19: 1–11.

Deliyannis, GA and Tavlarakis, N. (1955). Sickling phenomenon in Northern Greece. *Br. Med. J.* 2: 299–301.

DESImone, J, Kleve, LJ, Longley, MA, and Shaeffer, JR. (1974). Unbalanced globin chain synthesis in reticulocytes of sickle cell trait individuals with low concentrations of hemoglobin S. *Biochem. Biophys. Res. Commun.* 59: 564–569.

DeSimone, J, Adams, JG III, and Shaeffer, J. (1977). Evidence for rapid loss of newly synthesized haemoglobin S molecules in sickle cell anaemia and sickle cell trait. *Br. J. Haematol.* 35: 373–385.

Deutsch, TA, Weinreb, RN, and Goldberg, MF. (1984). Indications for surgical management of hyphema in patients with sickle cell trait. *Arch. Ophthalmol.* 102: 566–569.

Diggs, LW, Ahmann, CF, and Bibb J. (1933). The incidence and significance of the sickle cell trait. *Ann. Intern. Med.* 7: 769–778.

Dillard, TA, Kark, JA, Rajagopal, KR et al. (1987). Pulmonary function in sickle cell trait. *Ann. Intern. Med.* 106: 191–196.

Drysdale, JW, Righetti, P, and Bunn, HF. (1971). The separation of human and animal hemoglobins by isoelectric focusing in polyacrylamide gel. *Biochimi. Biophysi. Acta* 229: 42–50.

Dumars, KW, Boehm, C, Eckman, JR et al. (1996). Practical guide to the diagnosis of thalassemia. *Am. J. Med. Genet.* 62: 29–37.

Eaton, JW and Mucha, JI. (1971). Increased fertility in males with the sickle cell trait. *Nature* 231: 456–457.

El-Hazmi, MA. (1986). Studies on sickle cell heterozygotes in Saudi Arabia: Interaction with alpha-thalassaemia. *Acta Haematol.* 75: 100–104.

El-Hazmi, MAF, Warsy, AS, Al-Swailem, AR et al. (1996). Sickle cell gene in the population of Saudi Arabia. *Hemoglobin* 20: 187–198.

Embury, SH. (1994). Prenatal diagnosis. In Embury, SH, Hebbel, RP, Mohandas, N, and Steinberg, MH, editors. *Sickle cell disease: Basic principles and clinical practice.* New York: Lippincott-Raven, pp. 485–503.

Embury, SH and Dozy, A. (1981). The α globin genotypes as a determinant of hematologic parameters in sickle cell trait. In Sigler, PB, editor. *The molecular basis of mutant hemoglobin dysfunction.* New York: Elsevier/North-Holland, pp. 63–67.

Embury, SH, Hebbel, RP, Mohandas, N, and Steinberg, MH. (1994). *Sickle cell disease: Basic principles and clinical practice.* New York: Lippincott-Raven.

Esan, GJ and Adesina, TA. (1974). Phenotypic variation in sickle cell trait. *Scand. J. Haematol.* 13: 370–376.

Ewing, N, Powars, D, Hillburn, J, and Schroeder, WA. (1981). Newborn diagnosis of abnormal hemoglobins from a large municipal hospital in Los Angeles. *Am. J. Public Health* 71: 629–631.

Ezeh, UO and Modebe, O. (1996). Is there increased fertility in adult males with the sickle cell trait? *Hum. Biol.* 68: 555–562.

Falk, RJ and Jennette, JC. (1994). Renal disease. In Embury, SH, Hebbel, RP, Mohandas, N, and Steinberg, MH, editors. *Sickle cell disease: Basic principles and clinical practice.* New York: Lippincott-Raven, pp. 673–680.

Felice, AE, Cleek, MP, McKie, K et al. (1984). The rare alpha-thalassemia-1 of blacks is a zeta alpha-thalassemia-1 associated with deletion of all alpha- and zeta-globin genes. *Blood* 63: 1253–1257.

Figenshau, RS, Basler, JW, Ritter, JH et al. (1998). Renal medullary carcinoma. *J. Urol.* 159: 711–713.

Finelli, PF. (1976). Sickle cell trait and transient monocular blindness. *Am. J. Ophthalmol.* 81: 850–851.

Fleming, AF. (1996). Maternal segregation distortion in sickle-cell trait. *Lancet* 347: 1634–1635.

Friedrichs, P, Lassen, P, Canby, E, and Graham, C. (1997). Renal medullary carcinoma and sickle cell trait. *J. Urol.* 157: 1349–1349.

Galacteros, F, Kleman, K, Caburi-Martin, J et al. (1980). Cord blood screening for hemoglobin abnormalities by thin layer isoelectric focusing. *Blood* 56: 1068–1071.

Gelpi, AP. (1970). Sickle cell disease in Saudi Arabia. *Acta Haematol.* 1970: 89–99.

Gelpi, AP and King, MC. (1976). Screening for abnormal hemoglobins in the middle east: New data on hemoglobin S and the presence of hemoglobin C in Saudi Arabia. *Acta Haematol.* 56: 334–337.

Gilman, JG, Mishima, N, Wen, XJ et al. (1988). Upstream promoter mutation associated with a modest elevation of fetal hemoglobin expression in human adults. *Blood* 72: 78–81.

Gitschier, J and Thompson, CB. (1989). Non-altitude related splenic infarction in a patient with sickle cell trait. *Am. J. Med.* 87: 697–698.

Globin Gene Disorder-BCSH Task Force. (1994). Guidelines for the fetal diagnosis of globin gene disorders. *J. Clin. Pathol.* 47: 199–204.

Goldberg, NM, Dorman, JP, Riley, CA, and Armbruster, EJ Jr. (1985). Altitude-related specific infarction in sickle cell trait—case reports of a father and son. *West. J. Med.* 143: 670–672.

Gozal, D, Lorey, FW, Chandler, D et al. (1994). Incidence of sudden infant death syndrome in infants with sickle cell trait. *J. Pediatr.* 124: 211–214.

Green, RL, Huntsman, RG, and Serjeant, GR. (1971). The sickle-cell and altitude. *Br. Med. J.* 4: 593–595.

Greenberg, MS, Harvey, HA, and Morgan, C. (1972). A simple and inexpensive screening test for sickle hemoglobin. *N. Engl. J. Med.* 286: 1143.

Gupta, AK, Kirchner, KA, Nicholson, R et al. (1991). Effects of α-thalassemia and sickle polymerization tendency on the urine-concentrating defect of individuals with sickle cell trait. *J. Clin. Invest.* 88: 1963–1968.

Hahn, EV and Gillespie, EB. (1927). Sickle cell anemia: Report of a case greatly improved by splenectomy; experimental study of sickle cell formation. *Arch. Intern. Med.* 39: 233–254.

Harkness, DR. (1989). Sickle cell trait revisited. *Am. J. Med.* 87: 30N–34N.

Heller, P, Best, WR, Nelson, RB, and Becktel, J. (1979). Clinical implications of sickle-cell trait and glucose-6-phosphate dehydrogenase deficiency in hospitalized black male patients. *N. Engl. J. Med.* 300: 1001–1005.

Hempe, JM and Craver, RD. (1994). Quantification of hemoglobin variants by capillary isoelectric focusing. *Clin. Chem.* 40: 2288–2295.

Hendrickse, RG, Hasan, AH, Olumide, LO, and Akinkunmi, A. (1971). Malaria in early childhood. An investigation of five hundred seriously ill children in whom a "clinical" diagnosis of malaria was made on admission to the children's emergency room at University College Hospital, Ibadan. *Ann. Trop. Med. Parasitol.* 65: 1–20.

Herrick, JB. (1910). Peculiar elongated and sickle-shaped red blood corpuscles in a case of severe anemia. *Arch. Intern. Med.* 6: 517–521.

Higgs, DR, Clegg, JB, Weatherall, DJ et al. (1984). Interaction of the ααα globin gene haplotype and sickle haemoglobin. *Br. J. Haematol.* 57: 671–678.

Hipp, MJ and Scott, RB. (1974). Altered filterability of CPD-stored sickle trait donor blood. *Transfusion* 14: 447–452.

Hoff, C, Wertelecki, W, Dutt, J et al. (1983). Sickle cell trait maternal age and pregnancy outcome in primiparous woman. *Hum. Biol.* 55: 763–770.

Huisman, THJ. (1987). The separation of hemoglobins and hemoglobin chains by high performance liquid chromatography. In Deyl, Z and Hern, MTW, editors. *Separation of biopolymers and supramolecular structures.* Amsterdam: Elsevier Science, p. 277.

Humphries, JE and Wheby, MS. (1992). Case report: Sickle cell trait and recurrent deep venous thrombosis. *Am. J. Med. Sci.* 303: 112–114.

Jackson, H, Bentley, CR, Hingorani, M et al. (1995). Sickle retinopathy in patients with sickle trait. *Eye* 9: 589–593.

Jones, SR, Binder, RA, and Donowho, EM Jr. (1970). Sudden death in sickle-cell trait. *N. Engl. J. Med.* 282: 323–325.

Kark, JA, Posey, DM, Schumacher HR Jr, and Ruehle, CJ. (1987). Sickle-cell trait as a risk factor for sudden death in physical training. *N. Engl. J. Med.* 317: 781–787.

Kark, JA and Ward, FT. (1994). Exercise and hemoglobin S. *Semin. Hematol.* 31: 181–225.

Kassim, A, Fabry, ME, and Nagel, RL (2000). Acute priapism associated with the use of sildenafil in a patient with sickle cell trait. *Blood* 95: 1878–1879.

Kaur, M, Das, GP, and Verma, IC. (1997). Sickle cell trait and disease among tribal communities in Orissa, Madhya Pradesh and Kerala. *Indian J. Med. Res.* 105: 111–116.

Kelleher, JF Jr and Luban, NL. (1984). Transfusion of frozen erythrocytes from a donor with sickle cell trait. *Transfusion* 24: 167–168.

Kendall, AG, Ojwang, PJ, Schroeder, WA and Huisman, TH. (1973). Hemoglobin Kenya, the product of a gamma-beta fusion gene: Studies of the family. *Am. J. Hum. Genet.* 25: 548–563.

Kennedy, AP, Walsh, DA, Nicholson, R et al. (1986). Influence of HbS levels upon the hematological and clinical characteristics of sickle cell trait. *Am. J. Hematol.* 22: 51–54.

Kramer, MS, Rooks, Y, and Pearson, HA. (1978). Growth and development in children with sickle-cell trait. A prospective study of matched pairs. *N. Engl. J. Med.* 299: 686–689.

Kulozik, AE, Thein, SL, Kar, BC et al. (1996). Raised Hb F levels in sickle cell disease are caused by a determinant linked to the β globin gene cluster. In Stamatoyannopoulos, G and Nienhius, AW, editors. *Developmental control of globin gene expression.* New York: Alan R. Liss, pp. 427–439.

Kutlar, F, Kutlar, A, Nuguid, E et al. (1993). Usefulness of HPLC methodology for the characterization of combinations of the common β chain variants Hbs S, C, and O-Arab, and the α chain variant Hb G-Philadelphia. *Hemoglobin* 17: 55–66.

Lally, EV, Buckley, WM, and Claster, S. (1983). Diaphyseal bone infarctions in a patient with sickle cell trait. *J. Rheumatol.* 10: 813–816.

Lane, PA and Githens, JH. (1985). Splenic syndrome at mountain altitudes in sickle cell trait: Its occurrence in nonblack persons. *JAMA* 253: 2251–2254.

Larrabee, KD and Monga, M. (1997). Women with sickle cell trait are at increased risk for preeclampsia. *Am. J. Obstet. Gynecol.* 177: 425–428.

Lasker, N, Hopp, L, Grossman, S et al. (1985). Race and sex differences in erythrocyte Na$^+$, K$^+$, and Na$^+$-K$^+$-adenosine triphosphatase. *J. Clin. Invest.* 75: 1813–1820.

Le Gallais, D, Prefaut, C, Mercier, J et al. (1994). Sickle cell trait as a limiting factor for high-level performance in a semi-marathon. *Int. J. Sports Med.* 15: 399–402.

Leavitt, JA and Butrus, SI. (1994). Internuclear ophthalmoplegia in sickle cell trait. *J. Neuroophthalmol.* 14: 49–51.

Liebmann, JM. (1996). Management of sickle cell disease and hyphema. *J. Glaucoma* 5: 271–275.

Livingstone, FB. (1967). *Abnormal hemoglobin genes.* Chicago: Aldine.

Livingstone, FB. (1957). Sickling and malaria. *Br. Med. J.* 1: 762–763.

Lubin, BH, Witkowska, HE, and Kleman K. (1991). Laboratory diagnosis of hemoglobinopathies. *Clin. Biochem.* 24: 363–374.

Madrigal, L. (1989). Hemoglobin genotype, fertility, and the malaria hypothesis. *Hum. Biol.* 61: 311–325.

Martin, TW, Weisman, IM, Zeballos, RJ, and Stephson, SR. (1989). Exercise and hypoxia increase sickling in venous blood from an exercising limb in individuals with sickle cell trait. *Am. J. Med.* 87: 48–56.

Martina, WJ, Green, DR, Dougherty, N et al. (1984). Tourniquet use in sickle cell disease patients. *J. Am. Podiatry Assoc.* 74: 291–294.

Matthay, KK, Mentzer, WC Jr, Dozy, AM et al. (1979). Modification of the hemoglobin H disease by sickle trait. *J. Clin. Invest.* 64: 1024–1032.

McCormack, MK, Scarr-Salapatek, S, Polesky, H et al. (1975). A comparison of the physical and intellectual development of black children with and without sickle-cell trait. *Pediatrics* 56: 1021–1025.

McCurdy, PR, Lorkin, PA, Casey, R et al. (1974). Hemoglobin S-G (S-D) syndrome. *Am. J. Med.* 57: 665–670.

Menedez, C, Todd, J, Alonso, PL et al. (1995). The response to iron supplementation of pregnant women with the haemoglobin genotype AA or AS. *Trans. Ro. Soc. Trop. Med. Hygi.* 89: 289–292.

Merryman, HT and Hornblower, M. (1976). Freezing and deglycerolizing sickle-trait red blood cells. *Transfusion* 16: 627–632.

Murphy, JR. (1973). Sickle cell hemoglobin (Hb AS) in black football players. *JAMA* 225: 981–982.

Nagel, RL. (1994). Origins and dispersion of the sickle gene. In Embury, SH, Hebbel, RP, Mohandas, N, and Steinberg MH, editors. *Sickle cell disease: Basic principles and clinical practice.* New York: Lippincott-Raven, pp. 353–380.

Nagpal, KC, Asdourian, GK, Patrianakos, D et al. (1977). Proliferative retinopathy in sickle cell trait. Report of seven cases. *Arch. Intern. Med.* 137: 325–328.

Nance, WE and Grove, J. (1972). Genetic determination of phenotypic variation in sickle cell trait. *Science* 177: 716–720.

Neel, JV. (1951). The inheritance of the sickling phenomenon with particular reference to sickle cell disease. *Blood* 6: 389–412.

Noguchi, CT, Torchia, DA, and Schechter, AN. (1981). Polymerization of hemoglobin in sickle trait erythrocytes and lysates. *J. Biol. Chem.* 256: 4168–4171.

Novak, RW and Brown RE. (1982). Multiple renal and splenic infarctions in a neonate following transfusion with sickle cell trait blood. *Clin Pediatr. (Phila.)* 21: 239–241.

Nuss, R, Feyerabend, AJ, Lear, JL, and Lane, PA. (1991). Splenic function in persons with sickle cell trait at moderately high altitude. *Am. J. Hematol.* 37: 130–132.

Nuss, R, Loehr, JP, Daberkow, E et al. (1993). Cardiopulmonary function in men with sickle cell trait who reside at moderately high altitude. *J. Lab. Clin. Med.* 122: 382–387.

Ohene-Frempong, K and Nkrumah, FK. (1994). Sickle cell disease in Africa. In Embury, SH, Hebbel, RP, and Mohandas, N, editors. *Sickle Cell Disease: Basic Principles and Clinical Practice.* New York: Lippincott-Raven, pp. 423–435.

Olumese, PE, Adeyemo, AA, Ademowo, OG et al. (1997). The clinical manifestations of cerebral malaria among Nigerian children with the sickle cell trait. *Ann. Trop. Paediatr.* 17: 141–145.

Oster, JR, Lee, SM, Lespier, LE et al. (1976). Renal acidification in sickle cell trait. *Arch. Intern. Med.* 136: 30–35.

Ould Amar, AK, Kerob-Bauchet, B, Robert, P et al. (1996). Assessment of qualitative functional parameters of stored red blood cells from donors with sickle cell trait (AS) or with heterozygote(AC) status. *Transfus. Clin. Biol.* 3: 225–233.

Pauling, L, Itano, H, Singer, SJ, and Wells, IC. (1949). Sickle cell anemia: A molecular disease. *Science* 110: 543–548.

Petrakis, NL, Wiesenfeld, SL, Sams, BJ et al. (1970). Prevalence of sickle-cell trait and glucose-6-phosphate dehydrogenase deficiency. *N. Engl. J. Med.* 282: 767–770.

Poillon, WN, Kim, BC, Rodgers, GP et al. (1993). Sparing effect of hemoglobin F and hemoglobin A_2 on the polymerization of hemoglobin S at physiologic ligand saturations. *Proc. Natl. Acad. Sci. U.S.A.* 90: 5039–5043.

Polenak, AP, and Janerich, DT. (1975). Hematocrit among blacks with sickle cell trait. *Hum. Biol.* 47: 493–504.

Polenak, AP, and Janerich, DT. (1980). Birth characteristics of Blacks with sickle cell trait: A case-control study. *Hum. Biol.* 52: 15–21.

Ramasamy, S, Balakrishnan, K, and Pitchappan, RM. (1994). Prevalence of sickle cells in Irula, Kurumba, Paniya and Mullukurumba tribes of Nilgiris (Tamil Nadu, India). *Indian J. Med. Res.* 100: 242–245.

Rana, SR, Sekhsaria, S, and Castro, OL. (1993). Hemoglobin S and C traits: Contributing causes for decreased mean hematocrit in African-American children. *Pediatrics* 91: 800–802.

Ray, PF, Kaeda, JS, Bingham, J et al (1996). Preimplantation genetic diagnosis of β-thalassaemia major. *Lancet* 347: 1696–1696.

Rehan, N. (1981). Growth status of children with and without sickle cell trait. *Clin. Pediatr. (Phila.)* 20: 705–709.

Rimer, BA. (1975). Sickle-cell trait and pregnancy: A review of a community hospital experience. *Am. J. Obstet. Gynecol.* 123: 6–11.

Rising, JA, Sautter, RL, and Spicer, SJ. (1974). Hemoglobin G-Philadelphia-S. A family study of an inherited hybrid hemoglobin. *Am. J. Clin. Pathol.* 61: 92–102.

Roberts, WL, McCraw, M, and Cook, CB. (1998). Effects of sickle cell trait and hemoglobin C trait on determinations of HbA_{1c} by an immunoassay method. *Diabetes Care* 21: 983–986.

Robinson, AR, Robson, M, Harrison, AP, and Zuelzer, WW. (1957). A new technique for differentiation of hemoglobin. *J. Lab. Clin. Med.* 50: 745–752.

Rogers, ZR, Powars, DR, Kinney, TR et al. (1989). Nonblack patients with sickle cell disease have African beta S gene cluster haplotypes. *Jama* 261: 2991–2994.

Romanoff, ME, Woodward, DG, and Bullard, WG. (1998). Autologous blood transfusion in patients with sickle cell trait. *Anesthesiology* 68: 820–821.

Roth, E Jr. (1985). The sickle cell gene in evolution: A solitary wanderer or a nomad in a caravan of interacting genes. *JAMA* 253: 2259–2260.

Schedlbauer, LM and Pass, KA. (1989). Cellulose acetate/citrate agar electrophoresis of filter paper hemolysates from heel stick. *Pediatrics* 83: 839.

Schiliro, G, Comisi, FF, Testa, R et al. (1990). Hematological findings in 375 Sicilians with Hb S trait. *Haematologia* 75: 113–116.

Schmidt, RM, Brosious, EM, and Holland, S. (1975b). Quantitation of fetal hemoglobin by densitometry. *J. Lab. Clin. Med.* 84: 740.

Schmidt, RM, Rucknagel, DL, and Necheles, TF. (1975a). Comparison of methodologies for thalassemia screening by Hb A_2 quantitation. *J. Lab. Clin. Med.* 86: 873–882.

Schwartz, E and Atwater, J. (1972). α-Thalassemia in the American Negro. *J. Clin. Invest.* 51: 412–418.

Scott-Conner, CEH and Brunson, CD. (1994). Surgery and anesthesia. In Embury, SH, Hebbel, RP, Mohandas, N, and Steinberg, MH, editors. *Sickle cell disease: Basic principles and clinical practice.* New York: Lippincott-Raven, pp. 809–827.

Sears, DA. (1978). The morbidity of sickle cell trait: A review of the literature. *Am. J. Med.* 64: 1021–1036.

Serjeant, G and Gueri, M. (1970). Sickle cell trait and leg ulceration. *Br. Med. J.* 1: 820–820.

Serjeant, GR, Serjeant, BE, Forbes, M et al. (1986). Haemoglobin gene frequencies in the Jamaican population: A study in 100,000 newborns. *Br. J. Haematol.* 64: 253–262.

Shaeffer, JR, DESImone, J, and Kleve, LJ. (1975). Hemoglobin syntheis studies of a family with alpha-thalassemia trait and sickle cell trait. *Biochem. Genet.* 13: 11–12.

Shalev, O, Boylen, AL, Levene, C et al. (1988). Sickle cell trait in a white Jewish family presenting as splenic infarction at high altitude. *Am. J. Hematol.* 27: 46–48.

Stark, AD, Janerich, DT, and Jereb, SK. (1980). The incidence and causes of death in a follow-up study of individuals with haemoglobin AS and AA. *Int. J. Epidemiol.* 9: 325–328.

Statius van Eps, LW, Pinedo-Veels, C, Vries, GHD, and Koning, JD. (1970). Nature of concentrating defect in sickle-cell nephropathy. Microradioangiographic studies. *Lancet* 1: 450–452.

Stein, RE and Urbaniak, J. (1980). Use of the tourniquet during surgery in patients with sickle cell hemoglobinpathies. *Clin. Orthop.* 151: 231–233.

Steinberg, MH. (1985). Sickle cell trait and splenic syndrome. *JAMA* 254: 1901–1902.

Steinberg, MH. (1993). DNA diagnosis for the detection of sickle hemoglobinopathies. *Am. J. Hematol.* 43: 110–115.

Steinberg, MH, Adams, JG, and Dreiling, BJ. (1975). Alpha thalassaemia in adults with sickle-cell trait. *Br. J. Haematol.* 30: 31–37.

Steinberg, MH and Adams, JG III. (1991). Hemoglobin A$_2$: Origin, evolution, and aftermath. *Blood* 78: 2165–2177.

Steinberg, MH, Coleman, MB, Adams, JG et al. (1986). A new gene deletion in the α-like globin gene cluster as the molecular basis for the rare α-thalassemia-1 (- -/$\alpha\alpha$) in blacks: HbH disease in sickle cell trait. *Blood* 67: 469–473.

Steinberg, MH and Embury, SH. (1986). Alpha-thalassemia in blacks: Genetic and clinical aspects and interactions with the sickle hemoglobin gene. *Blood* 68: 985–990.

Steinmann, W, Stone, R, Nichols, C et al. (1983). A case-control study of the association of sickle cell trait and chronic open-angle glaucoma. *Am. J. Epidemiol.* 118: 288–293.

Tan, GB, Aw, TC, Dunstan, RA, and Lee, SH. (1993). Evaluation of high performance liquid chromatography for routine estimation of haemoglobins A$_2$ and F. *J. Clin. Pathol.* 46: 852–856.

Taylor, PW, Thorpe, WP, and Trueblood, MC. (1986). Osteonecrosis in sickle cell trait. *J. Rheumatol.* 13: 643–646.

Thiriet, P, Le Hesraan, JY, Wouassi, D et al. (1994). Sickle cell trait performance in a prolonged race at high altitude. *Med. Sci. Sports Exerci.* 26: 914–918.

Tsevat, J, Wong, JB, Pauker, SG, and Steinberg, MH. (1991). Neonatal screening for sickle cell disease: A cost-effectiveness analysis. *J. Pediatr.* 118: 546–554.

Voge, VM, Rosado, NR, and Contiguglia, JJ. (1991). Sickle cell anemia trait in the military aircrew population: A report from the Military Aviation Safety Subcommittee of the Aviation Safety Committee, AsMA. *Aviat. Space Environ. Med.* 62: 1099–1102.

Walley, PJ, Pritchard, JA, and Richards, JR. (1963). Sickle cell trait and pregnancy. *JAMA* 186: 1132–1135.

Weinger, RS, Benson, GS, and Villarreal, S. (1979). Gross hematuria associated with sickle cell trait and von Willebrand's disease. *J. Urol.* 122: 136–137.

Weisman, IM, Zeballos, RJ, and Johnson, BD. (1988b). Cardiopulmonary and gas exchange responses to acute strenuous exercise at 1,270 meters in sickle cell trait. *Am. J. Med.* 84: 377–383.

Weisman, IM, Zeballos, RJ, and Johnson BD. (1988a). Effect of moderate inspiratory hypoxia on exercise performance in sickle cell trait. *Am. J. Med.* 84: 1033–1040.

Weisman, IM, Zeballos, RJ, Martin, TW, and Johnson BD. (1988c). Effect of Army basic training in sickle-cell trait. *Arch. Intern. Med.* 148: 1140–1144.

Williamson LM. (1999). Leukocyte depletion of whole blood and red cells from donors with hemoglobin sickle trait. *Transfusion* 39, Supplement: 108S.

Whitten, WJ and Rucknagel, DL. (1981). The proportion of Hb A$_2$ is higher in sickle cell trait than in normal homozygotes. *Hemoglobin* 5: 371–378.

Winter, WP, editor. (1986). *Hemoglobin variants in human populations.* Boca Raton: CRC Press.

Wong, SC, Ali, MA, and Boyadjian, SE. (1981). Sickle cell traits in Canada. Trimodal distribution of Hb S as a result of interaction with alpha-thalassemia gene. *Acta Haematol.* 65: 157–163.

Yang, Y-M, Donnell, C, Wilborn, W et al. (1992). Splenic sequestration associated with sickle cell trait and hereditary spherocytosis. *Am. J. Hematol.* 40: 110–116.

Zadeii, G and Lohr, JW. (1997). Renal papillary necrosis in a patient with sickle cell trait. *Am. J. Soc. Nephrol.* 8: 1034–1039.

SECTION V

EPIDEMIOLOGY AND GENETIC SELECTION OF HEMOGLOBINOPATHIES AND THALASSEMIA

RONALD L. NAGEL

Malaria is responsible for most common hereditary abnormalities of the human erythrocyte. Genetic resistance to the erythrocytic stage of malaria leads to the selection of red cell genetic defects at gene frequencies that imply positive selective pressure—gene frequencies higher than 0.01. These defects include not only hemoglobin disorders such as HbS, HbC, HbE, and α and β thalassemia—subjects of this book—but also erythrocyte membrane defects such as Southeast Asian ovalocytosis and some forms of elliptocytosis, and metabolic abnormalities such as glucose-6-phosphate dehydrogenase deficiency. *Plasmodium falciparum,* the only lethal variety of malaria, often leads to the death of its victims, particularly before age 5 years, and exercises a very strong selective pressure. Since this age dependency deprives these individuals of reproducing, carriers of innate resistance contribute the variant gene to the next generation more often than nonresistors. In sickle cell anemia or in β thalassemia, the increased reproductive fitness of the heterozygote is compensated, in part, by the decreased fitness of the homozygous state. This is the definition of balanced polymorphism.

In sickle trait, the malaria parasite promotes sickling of the cell permitting the spleen to target parasitized cells for removal. If this mechanism fails to cull parasitized cells from the circulation, parasites fail to prosper in the stage in where their host cells become static and adhere to the endothelium of venules. Still, the actual mecha-nism of parasite growth inhibition or death in sickled erythrocytes is not fully understood. Parasite growth in thalassemic erythrocytes is poor, perhaps because of reduced nutrients and because host oxidative response is increased to a point that parasite viability is reduced. Erythrocytes with high levels of HbF can partially protect the carrier from the parasite, especially in the critical first 5 years of life. HbC seems to interfere with the lysis of red cells in the late schizont state, and the dispersion of merozoites. HbE impairs parasite growth, and oxidative stress might also be increased in HbE erythrocytes. These and many other mechanisms of protection have evolved as adaptations to the great scourge of malaria. In vitro culture of parasites and transgenic mouse technology have increased our understanding of innate resistance to malaria in genetically altered red cells.

Malarial anemia can cause death, particularly in children and pregnant women. Hemolysis can be caused by cell rupture during merozoite release, splenic phagocytosis, increased phagocytosis of infected red cells identified by altered membrane surface or antibody coating, and increased overall phagocytic activity. Reduced erythrocyte production might involve marrow hypoplasia, ineffective erythropoiesis, and inappropriately low erythropoietin levels. Multiple genetic factors also effect the anemia of malaria.

In vitro data clearly indicate that the sickle cell anemia erythrocyte is an inhospitable host for plasmodia—worse than sickle cell trait cells. Yet, patients with sickle cell anemia can die of the infection, not from cerebral or hepatic malaria as in individuals with sickle cell trait or normal hemoglobin, but of the ravages of malaria infection for which they are particularly susceptible—dehydration, acidosis, cytokine release, for example—many of which are prosickling events.

Sickle cell disease and the thalassemias are least common in countries where their biology and treatment are studied most intensively. We have attempted to extend our discussion of hemoglobin disorders beyond the high-technology–driven practice of medicine of developed countries. Present at polymorphic gene frequencies in their regions of origin because of malaria and dispersed throughout much of the world by emigration, war, and slave trading, these disorders differ in their clinical expression according to the genetic background in which they exist and the features of the local environment. In three chapters that follow we discuss the worldwide distribution of sickle cell disease, α thalassemia, and β thalassemia and emphasize the prevalence of these diseases in different populations, the clinical differences that exist, and the segregation of different thalassemia mutations in different populations.

30

Malaria and Hemoglobinopathies

RONALD L. NAGEL

INTRODUCTION

Most red cell genetic defects that occur with high frequency in human populations owe their prevalence to the selective pressure of malaria, the world's most significant, frequent, and devastating disease that even today causes two to four million deaths a year, mostly of children (Kolata, 1984). Malaria arose about 3,000 years ago with the emergence of agriculture (Weisenfeld, 1967). This momentous advance in cultural development, through the establishment of human settlements and irrigation, provided sufficient density of both humans and mosquitos—the two hosts required for the human malarial parasite to complete its life cycle—to render the disease endemic. The Malaysian agricultural complex that arrived in Africa via Madagascar from Southeast Asia, a little over 2,000 years ago, helped increase the population of West and East Africa by the introduction of new crops, but at the same time it increased the spread of malaria.

Humans vary in susceptibility to malaria, and most resistance is either genetic or acquired via immunologic response to prior exposure. Most red cell defects occurring at polymorphic frequencies represent genetic resistance.

Four species of *Plasmodium* cause malaria in humans *(falciparum, ovale, vivax,* and *malariae). P. falciparum* causes the deadly form. The protozoan's life cycle includes a sexual phase, which occurs in the anopheles mosquito, and an asexual phase, which occurs in humans. *P. falciparum* undergoes two developmental stages in humans, one in the liver and one in the erythrocyte (Fig. 30.1). The latter generates gametocytes, which, when ingested by the mosquito, develop into gametes and fuse to form zygotes and the next generation of plasmodia. Although genetic resistance to malaria in humans could involve the hepatic stage, which precedes the erythrocyte stage, there is no information about genetic resistance involving that stage of the cycle.

Genetic resistance involving the erythrocyte stage leads to defects at polymorphic frequencies (higher than 0.01), implying positive selective pressure. These defects include hemoglobin disorders such as HbS, HbC, HbE, and α and β thalassemia; erythrocyte membrane defects such as Southeast Asian ovalocytosis and some forms of elliptocytosis; and metabolic abnormalities such as glucose-6-phosphate dehydrogenase (G-6-PD) deficiency. Genetic resistance to *P. falciparum* may target the following stages of the erythrocytic cycle: (1) merozoite invasion of the red cell; (2) intracellular growth period; and (3) erythocytic lysis that occurs at merozoite maturation and leads to their dispersion (Fig. 30.1).

Although all four types of human malaria can exert selective pressure, *P. falciparum* is the only lethal variety, hence it exerts the strongest pressure. Since *P. falciparum* often kills its human hosts before they reach reproductive age, carriers of innate resistance contribute their genes to the next generation more often than noncarriers, tending to increase frequency of the variant gene. When the variant gene is lethal in the homozygous state (as in sickle cell anemia), those with two copies of it also die prior to reaching reproductive age, tending to decrease the frequency of the variant gene. This results in balanced polymorphism, a concept generated by E. B. Ford (1945), who defined it as "the occurrence together in the same habitat of two or more distinct forms of a species in such proportion that the rarest of them cannot be maintained merely by recurrent mutation." The Ford concept was first applied to hemoglobinopathies by Haldane (1949) (see below), and explains why many of the red cell defects are found in high frequencies in humans.

This chapter analyzes the data available for hemoglobinopathies that afford resistance to *P. falciparum.* Advances in understanding the adhesion of parasitized red cells to the endothelium and the interesting relationships between the HLA system and immunologic-based resistance to malaria are not considered here. However, I have included the red cell membrane

Martin H. Steinberg, Bernard G. Forget, Douglas R. Higgs, and Ronald L. Nagel, editors. *Disorders of Hemoglobin: Genetics, Pathophysiology, and Clinical Management.* © 2001 Cambridge University Press. All rights reserved.

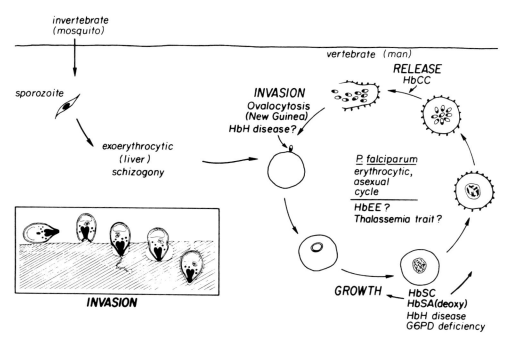

Figure 30.1. Life cycle of *P. falciparum*. Shown are the portions of the cycle principally affected by malaria-resistant red cell abnormalities. Depicted is injection of the malaria sporozoite (which is accomplished by an Anopheles mosquito), followed by invasion into hepatocytes, liver schizogony, and the emergence of merozoites capable of invading red cells. The insert represents stages of invasion: nonspecific adhesion between the merozoite and the red cell, rearrangement of the merozoite to its correct polarity and its specific adhesion, formation of a junction membrane, and invagination of the cell. Between the last two stages flipping of the red cell membrane is observed. The erythrocytic cycle follows, which begins with the ring form, followed by the early and late trophozoites, which are not present in the general circulation followed by schizonts.

defects that are associated in vitro with abnormalities of parasite growth or invasion; those defects might inform our understanding of the membrane alterations associated with the hemoglobinopathies.

METHODOLOGY

In the last two decades, two important methodologies have been introduced in the study of innate resistance to malaria in genetically altered red cells. One is an in vitro method and the other an in vivo method based on transgenic mouse technology.

In Vitro Culture

Pioneering work of Jensen and Trager (1977), just over two decades ago, described the first in vitro culture system for *P. falciparum* and permitted the testing of the relationship between red cell genetic

polymorphisms and the growth of this parasite (Fig. 30.2).

Advantages of the malaria erythrocytic cultures are (1) they largely dispense with the use of humans and monkeys, which are expensive and involve crossing species barriers; (2) the interaction of the red cell with malaria can be studied separately from the role of liver/spleen, antimalarial antibodies, complement, cellular reactions and most cytokines; (3) they avoid the complications derived from the entry into the circulation of stress reticulocytes and leukocytes during the parasite growth phase; (4) mixtures of red cells with different characteristics can be studied; (5) red cells can be modified, and the nutrients individually suppressed or modified in quantity or quality; (6) red cells can be age defined. In essence, most intrinsic properties of the cell membrane, cytoplasm, and hemoglobin can be evaluated.

Nevertheless, the shortcomings of the culture system must also be remembered. Cultures fail to address the role of immunity, the reticuloendothelial system, the complement system, or the splenic/liver filtration system in parasite growth. Culture medium is excessively rich in a variety of nutrients such as glutathione and glucose and the effects of some red cell defects on parasite growth might be apparent only when critical nutrients are in limited supply, for example, β-thalassemia red cells (see below).

Animal Models

More recently, the field has turned to using transgenic mouse models to study the mechanisms of resis-

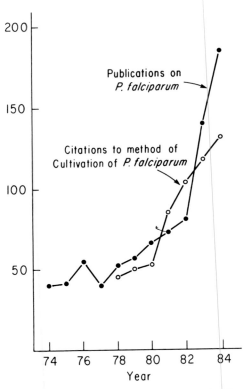

Figure 30.2. Early impact of the discovery by Trager and Jensen of an in vitro culture system for *P. falciparum*, on the number of publications on the subject.

tance by abnormal hemoglobins and other red cell defects (Roth et al., 1988; Shear et al., 1991, 1993; Kaul et al., 1994; Hood et al., 1996). It is possible to test in vivo some of the hypotheses derived from clinical or culture studies. In addition, the models allow the testing of the effect of organs, such as the spleen, in the pathogenic cascade. Finally, the use of transgenic animals with overexpressed or knocked-out genes allows for the assessment of the role of those genes on pathogenesis. This exciting and potentially powerful tool is not devoid of problems such as the study of a different host than humans. Fortunately, we can study these animals with species-appropriate malaria strains but the difference in the anatomy and physiology of some organs needs to be considered when interpreting results in these animal models.

P. FALCIPARUM MALARIA AND HbS

Epidemiologic and clinical studies first suggested that heterozygotes for the β^S gene could acquire *P. falciparum* malaria but were partially protected from dying of the infection (Allison, 1954; Livingston, 1971). In addition, the geographic distribution of the HbS gene and β-thalassemia genes is virtually identical to that of endemic malaria (Livingston, 1971) (Fig. 30.3).

Although the relationship between HbS and malaria has long been known, elucidating the mechanisms of protection is still in progress. Initially, Luzzato et al. (1970) reported that the rate of sickling of parasitized sickle cell trait red cells was 2 to 8 times greater than that of the nonparasitized cells in the same blood. This finding provided the first potential explanation for the protection from malaria conveyed by sickle cell trait erythrocytes: By inducing sickling in cells that normally do not sickle readily, the parasite caused a suicidal infection, since its chances of being removed from the circulation had increased considerably. Yet, there were some problems with this exciting experiment. Deoxygenation of sickle trait cells was done with sodium metabisulfite, which could have introduced artifacts. More important, being an in vitro study done under conditions of total dexoygenation, it did not necessarily demonstrate that this mechanism was relevant to physiologic conditions where zero O_2 saturation is rarely achieved.

Studies of Roth et al. (1978) that followed were the first to use cultured parasitized red cells, an experimental approach made possible by the discovery of the culture conditions needed to propagate *P. falciparum*. Roth's studies (1978) eased the concerns about Luzzatto's experiments, by comparing sickling curves on nonparasitized red cells in culture with those of early and late parasitized red cells, all at physiologic levels of N_2-induced deoxygenation. Accelerated morphologic sickling clearly occurred in sickle cell trait cells containing ring forms of the parasite. Yet, morphologic sickling did not occur in sickle cell trait cells containing trophozoites, a later parasite form, although HbS polymer was nevertheless detectable by electron microscopy. These last results were not surprising based on our present knowledge of the polymerization of HbS (Chapter 23). Since sickle cell trait cells have a low intracellular pH, HbS will polymerize readily, particularly when cells contain late-stage *P. falciparum* trophozoites (see below). This environment will simultaneously produce a great number of nucleation events, preceding polymerization, assuring that none of the nuclei will become large enough to deform the cell and cause morphologic sickling (Chapter 23).

Roth's experiments also demonstrated that, under conditions similar to venous O_2 saturations (about 50 percent), more sickling was detectable in parasitized compared to nonparasitized sickle cell trait erythrocytes. One can reasonably conclude that "suicidal" infection of sickle trait red cells is at least one of the mechanisms by which carriers are protected from lethal infections from *P. falciparum*.

"Suicidal" infection is not the only mechanism involved in the innate resistance of sickle cell trait

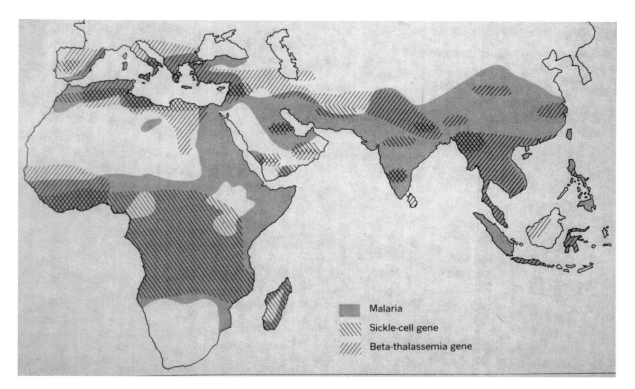

Figure 30.3. Distribution of malaria superimposed with the distribution of the HbS and β-thalassemia genes. (From Scientific American, with permission.)

individuals to malaria. Friedman (1978) demonstrated that sickle cell trait cells, cultured at 17 percent oxygen, sustained the growth of *P. falciparum* normally (Fig. 30.4). After 2 days of normal growth in 17 percent oxygen, the reduction of the oxygen content to 3 percent resulted in parasites not thriving and death in a few days. This deoxygenation effect was even more pronounced in HbSC disease and sickle cell anemia erythrocytes. This finding strongly suggested that parasitized sickle cell trait cells, even if they have survived "suicidal invasion" during their ring form stage, will be seriously hampered during the deep vascular schizogony. In this period, the red cells, whose parasites have reached the early trophozoite stage, proceed to grow "knobs" on their surface (Luse and Miller, 1971) and adhere to the venule endothelium (Raventos-Suarez et al., 1985) (Fig. 30.5). The venules, particularly the smaller ones, become occluded with adherent parasitized cells, becoming partially or totally obstructed due to the secondary trapping of erythrocytes with increased viscosity produced by the presence of parasites (Kaul et al., 1985). This situation causes hypoxia and low pH, although cytokines, such as tumor necrosis factor (TNF)-α, might also have a contributing effect. If the red cell contains β^S globin,

these conditions will favor sickling and reproduce the situation in which the parasite does not thrive (Friedman, 1978).

Still, the actual mechanism of parasite growth inhibition or death in sickled erythrocytes is not fully understood. Friedman et al. (1979a), studying sickle cell trait cells, proposed two possible and not mutually exclusive mechanisms: (1) the loss of K+, which accompanies sickling itself could be detrimental to parasite growth, as had been suggested for *P. lophourea*, an avian malaria parasite (Trager, 1976); (2) the loss of water concomitant with the loss of K+ would progressively increase mean cell HbS concentration and HbS polymerization since this reaction is affected by the 30th power of the initial HbS concentration (Chapter 23). The observation that argues best for the role of either K+ or cell dehydration as the cause of growth inhibition, but does not distinguish between these two possibilities, is the decrease in sickling observed when sickle cell trait cells are suspended in buffers with a high K+ concentration (Olson & Nagel, 1986), a condition that inhibits K+ efflux and concomitant loss of water (Fig. 30.4). Ouabain-treated red cells, enriched in intracellular Na+ but low in K+, sustain the growth of parasites normally (Ginsberg et al., 1986; Tanabe et al., 1986). These studies suggest that it is cell water loss and increased HbS concentration with an increase in the tendency for polymerization of deoxyHbS and not the level of intracellular K+ that is the most likely mechanism of growth inhibition.

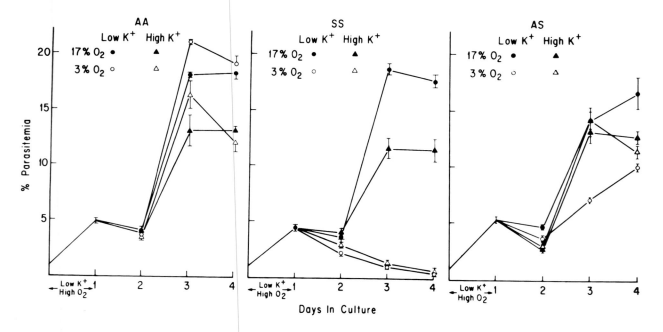

Figure 30.4. Parasitemia time course for synchronized cultures of *P. falciparum* in normal (AA), sickle cell trait (AS), and sickle cell anemia (SS) red cells grown for the first 24 hours in the presence of low and high extracellular K^+ and low (3 percent) or high (17 percent) O_2. Normal cells sustain the growth of *P. falciparum* in high and low oxygen, although they are affected somewhat by the presence of high K^+ in the media. Sickle cell anemia cells fail to sustain the growth of the parasite in low O_2 conditions, while they behave like normal cells in oxygenated conditions. Sickle cell trait cells inhibit normal parasite growth only under conditions of low oxygen and low extracellular K^+. Notice that in the sickle cell anemia cells exposed to low O_2 conditions for 24 hours, the parasitemia decays progressively after invasion (at the end of the first day), due largely to the absence of normal growth during the second day, and leading to a low number of merozoites capable of infecting other cells (which creates the big rise in parasitemia observed between days 2 and 3). Day 3 reports death of parasites, since the parasitemia is lower than in day 2, and parasite death is greater on day 4. Level of extracellular K^+ had no effect in deoxy conditions but some decreased growth is observed, as in the AA cells, in oxygenated conditions with high extracellular K^+ (From Olson and Nagel, 1986, with permission.)

Other work has suggested that sickle polymer is an inappropriate substrate for the proteases of the parasite. Ultrastructural studies of Friedman (1979a) suggested that after 6 hours of deoxygenation, parasitized sickle cell trait cells showed vacuolization that was interpreted as metabolic inhibition. Parasitized sickle cell anemia cells showed disruption of the parasitophorous vacuole and other membranes. This membrane disruption in sickle cell trait erythrocytes might be due to its puncture by spearlike polymers, and suggest that this might account for the cell lysis observed with parasitized

Figure 30.5A. Another depiction of the *P. falciparum* erythrocyte life cycle, emphasizing the deep vascular schizogony. Disappearance of all parasitized red cells from the periphery is due to the attachment of early schizonts to endothelial cells in the venules located, predominantly but not exclusively, in the brain, liver, and to a lesser degree, kidney. This deep vascular schizogony is possible by the appearance of "knobs" in the red cell membrane surface, that with the mediation of adherent proteins (among others, thrombospondin), attach themselves tenaciously to the endothelium of venules. During this period the stage of schizont is reached in which the parasite divides itself into potential merozoites. When these mature, the cell bursts, liberating about fifteen to twenty merozoites, some of which will be successful in infecting other red cells and continuing the life cycle in its erythrocytic stage.

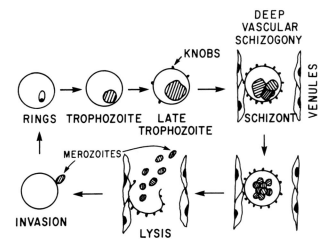

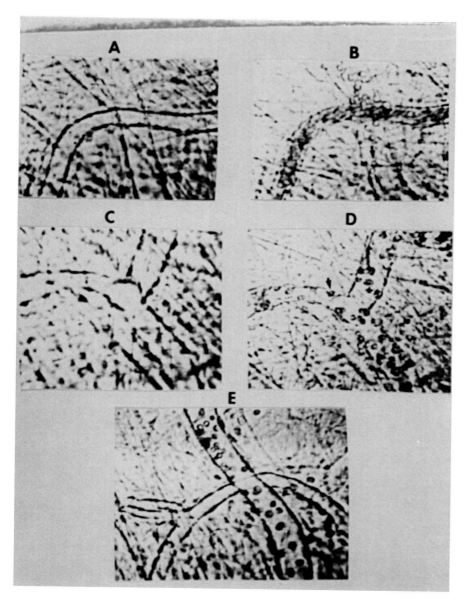

Figure 30.5B. Sequential photographs of the *P. falciparum* parasitized red cells and controls in an ex vivo microcirculatory preparation. (**A**) Perfusion by Ringer's solution. (**B**) Same area as *A*. There are two vessels: One is an arteriole showing the passing bolus of red cells. Another vessel is a venule (vertical) with adhered parasitized red cells. (arrow). (**C**) Another area of the preparation: during Ringer's. (**D**) The same areas as *C* after the bolus has passed and the perfusion continues with Ringer's solution.

erythrocytes in sickle cell anemia. Profound metabolic disruption could produce similar results. Another possibility is that the polymer, with its considerably right-shifted oxygen equilibrium curve, kills the parasite by oxygen toxicity, when it releases O_2 during polymerization. While other studies have confirmed the inhibition of parasite growth in deoxygenated sickle cell trait cells and, in addition, have reported a significant decrease in invasion rate under these conditions (Pasvol et al., 1978; Pasvol, 1980), observations in synchronized cultures, a method that can sensitively detect parasite invasion, refutes this claim (Olson and Nagel, 1986) (Fig. 30.4).

Free protoporphyrin IX was hypothesized to be involved in the death of *P. falciparum* in sickle cell anemia cells and even sickle cell trait erythrocytes but experiments were not performed in parasitized red cells and so there is no direct evidence to support the hypothesis. (Orjih et al., 1981, 1985). Heme toxicity would not readily explain the deoxygenation dependency of the growth inhibition; nevertheless, this mechanism is worth exploring further in sickle cell trait as a potential secondary effect.

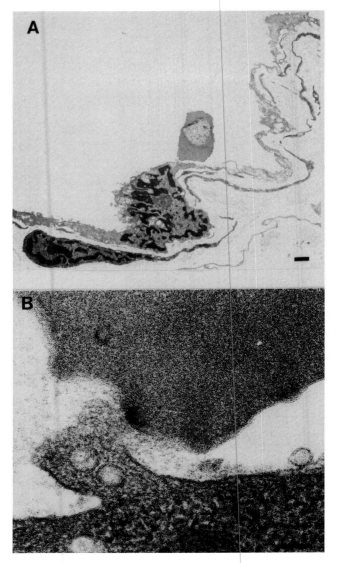

Figure 30.5C. (A) Electron microscopy of single parasitized red cells attached to the membrane. (B) Higher magnification that detects the attachment site. Notice that it involves a knob formation in the parasitized red cell membrane.

In summary, carriers of sickle cell trait are partially protected from *P. falciparum* through at least two mechanisms: (1) a dramatic increase in sickling rates of parasitized sickle cell trait cells makes them prone to be removed from the circulation and is a first line of defense; and (2) parasites that have escaped this defense find themselves incapable of prospering in the stage in which their host cells become static and adhere to the endothelium of venules. This analysis is not contradicted by the higher malaria death rate of patients with sickle cell anemia. In vitro data clearly indicate that the sickle cell anemia erythrocyte is an inhospitable host for plasmodia—worse than sickle cell trait cells. But

patients do die of the infection. They do not die of cerebral or hepatic malaria as do individuals with sickle cell trait or normal hemoglobin, but rather of the ravages of malaria infection for which they are particularly susceptible—dehydration, acidosis, cytokine release, and so on—many of which are directly or indirectly prosickling events.

Mechanisms outlined in this section are compatible with epidemiologic data that suggests that HbS carriers are not innately resistant to acquiring malaria but are less likely to die of it.

A transgenic mouse model of sickle cell disease (reviewed in Nagel, 1994, 1998; Fabry et al., 1992a 1992b) has provided new ways to study the mechanism of malaria protection in vivo, and new data have emerged on Plasmodia species to which rodents are susceptible, and on strains of diverse severity (Shear et al., 1993). Their discovery in Africa, followed by the recreation of their mosquito host habitat in the laboratory, resulted in these murine Plasmodia being used for immunologic and chemotherapeutic studies (Killick-Kendrick, 1978). *P. chabaudi adami* was discovered in the Central African Republic, in the thicket rat, *Thamnomys rutilans*. This Plasmodia preferentially invades mature erythrocytes and causes a self-limited infection in laboratory mice. *Plasmodium berghei*, in contrast, tends to invade reticulocytes and usually causes a lethal infection in laboratory mice. *P. yoelii* 17XNL is related to *P. berghei* and invades reticulocytes but causes a nonlethal infection, although another strain of *P. yoelii*, 17XL, is lethal (see below). *P. vinckei* invades mature erythrocytes and is highly virulent (Landau and Boulard, 1978). In studies of sickle transgenic mice, *P. chabaudi adami*, *P. berghei*, and the *yoelli* strains were used in nonlethal and lethal infections. In these studies, a transgenic mouse line expressing both the β^S gene and the human α-globin genes was used (Fabry et al., 1992b). To increase the relative expression of β^S globin, the transgenic mice, originally produced using the normal inbred strain FvB/N, were bred to homozygosity for a β-thalassemia mutation, Hbb (Skow et al., 1983) on a C57BL/6J background. While these mice did not have anemia they had compensated hemolysis. Thus, they appeared to represent a model intermediate between sickle cell trait and sickle cell anemia.

Sickle transgenic mice and the two parental mouse strains, C57BL/6J and FVB, were injected intraperitoneally with 10^6 *P. chabaudi adami*-infected mouse erythrocytes (Shear et al., 1993). A significant reduction in time of patency (appearance of parasites) and level of parasitemia (Fig. 30.6) was observed in the sickle transgenic mice compared to controls. Sickle transgenic mice and C57BL/6J mice infected with 5×10^5 *P. berghei*-infected-erythrocytes, also were signifi-

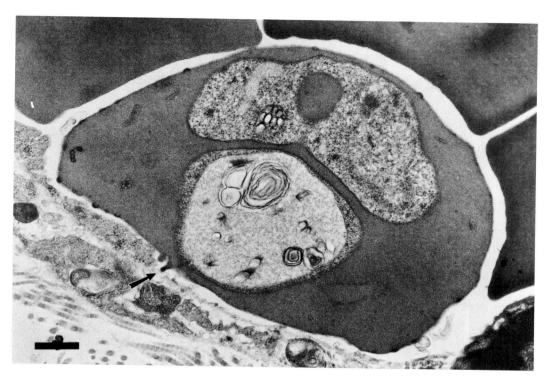

Figure 30.5D. Electron microscopy of vasoocclusion induced by *P. falciparum* parasitized human normal red cells in the rat ex vivo microcirculatory preparation. The venule is obstructed by one parasitized red cell (notice the knobs in the surface) and surrounded by nonparasitized human red cells, recognizable by the absence of knobs (one of the first evidence of rosetting). The parasitized red cell is in direct contact with the endothelium with participation of the knob structure (arrow). (Micrographs by Raventos and Nagel, with permission.)

Figure 30.6. Parasitemia versus time, for *P. chabaudi adami* in transgenic β^S mice and its parental (control) strains.

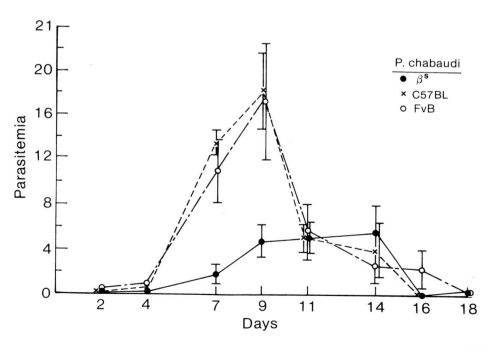

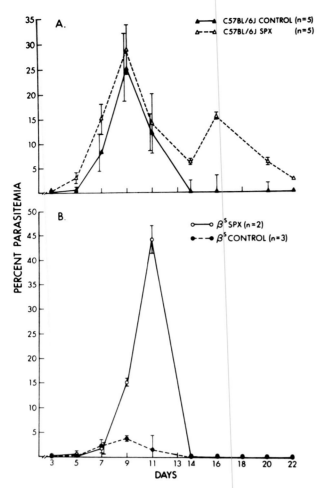

Figure 30.7. Parasitemia versus time in normal and transgenic β^S mice with (control) and without (spx) spleens.

strated that the sickle erythrocytes were fully able to support the growth of *P. chabaudi adami*, suggesting than the protective effect must involve the spleen.

Finally, Hood et al. (1996) challenged three transgenic models, expressing 39 percent, 57 percent, and 75 percent β^S, with *P. yoelli* strain 17XL, which is lethal and appears to cause cerebral malaria (Fig. 30.8). Survival was in direct proportion to the level of expression of the β^S gene: All the low expressors and controls succumbed to the infection by 8 days. Of the intermediate expressors, two of nine animals survived for 6 days, the remainder for more than 15 days. Among the highest β^S expressors, the majority survived for more than 20 days. These results demonstrated that the protection afforded by the β^S gene is particularly active when dealing with lethal forms of malaria, paralleling the human situation.

These studies confirmed and extended previous epidemiologic and in vitro studies indicating that the sickle cell trait phenotype is protective against *P. falciparum* malaria. They also established that the spleen plays a significant role in protecting the sickle transgenic mice from malaria, validating in vivo the Luzzatto hypothesis of "suicidal infection."

MALARIA AND HbC TRAIT AND HbC DISEASE

As discussed in Chapter 27, the frequency of the β^C gene is highest in northern Burkina Faso (formerly

cantly protected, although not to the extent as those injected with *P. chabaudi adami*-infected cells.

These experiments demonstrated in vivo the protective effect of the sickle gene but did not elucidate the mechanisms of this effect. Mechanisms postulated in the culture studies—inability of parasites to grow in HbS-containing cells or host removal of infected cells before the parasites have a chance to mature ("suicidal infection")—were studied first. Diminished parasitemia was consistent with either hypothesis. To investigate the second possibility, transgenic mice were splenectomized prior to infection. Postsurgery, animals were inoculated with 5×10^5 *P. chabaudi adami*-infected erythrocytes. Splenectomized normal mice had a slightly greater parasitemia than nonsplenectomized normal mice, but the most striking difference was between splenectomized and intact sickle transgenic mice. Intact sickle mice had a diminished course of infection whereas in the splenectomized sickle mice, the protective effect was completely abolished (Fig. 30.7). This experiment also demon-

Figure 30.8. Mortality of mice, with different expression levels of β^S, infected with *P. Yoelli* 17XL. Mice with 73 percent and 54 percent expression survived significantly longer than those with 36 percent and 0 percent expression.

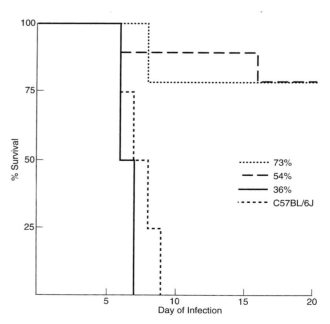

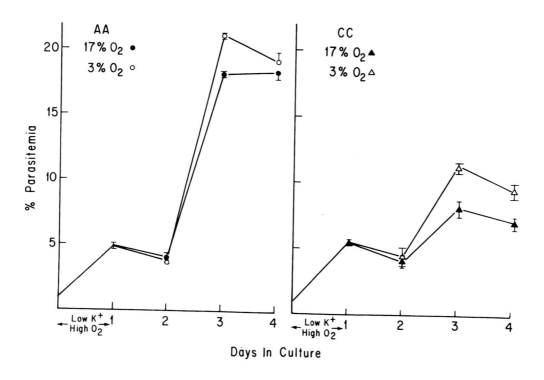

Figure 30.9. The synchronized growth curves of *P. falciparum* in normal (AA) and homozygous HbC (CC) erythrocytes. Red cells have been exposed to different concentrations of K+ [high (abnormal) and low (normal)], during the first 24 hours of culture. HbC cells do not thrive in either condition of extracellular K+, a demonstration that the growth abnormality is not dependent on intracellular K+ level. Notice the similar increase in parasitemia between time 0 and the end of the first 24 hours: The very similar parasitemia at day 1 means that the merozoites from the inoculum were able to invade normal or HbC cells equally well, producing an equivalent increase in the number of the parasitized cells of each type.

Upper Volta) and decreases concentrically in surrounding areas. Our understanding of the interaction between HbC red cells and malaria is less complete than that of the HbS interaction. Friedman et al. (1979b) were the first to document severely decreased growth in vitro of *P. falciparum* in oxygenated HbC disease cells. This finding was confirmed by Olson and Nagel (1986) (Fig. 30.9). Deoxygenation did not significantly modify *P. falciparum* growth in HbC disease cells and, unlike the case with HbS-containing erythrocytes, normal development is not restored when HbC cells are suspended in high extracellular K+ buffer. Parasitized HbC disease cells were very resistant to lysis compared to parasitized normal cells (Fig. 30.10). In synchronized cultures—cultures where all the parasitized forms are at the same stage of development—degenerated schizonts were observed on day 4 (second cycle), an observation compatible with the incapacity

of parasitized HbC-containing cells to complete schizogony. It appears, therefore, that HbC disease cells, due to their dramatically increased osmotic resistance, are incapable of bursting and releasing merozoites in a normal fashion. This interpretation is also compatible with the rather flat growth curve characteristic of HbC cells, in contrast with the down-sloping shape of the growth curves observed with other abnormal red cells.

Not explained is the fact that HbC trait cells in vitro sustain the growth of the parasite as well as normal cells. This is disturbing since the established concept is that the high frequency of HbC in certain

Figure 30.10. Osmotic resistance of parasitized normal and HbC cells. Notice that HbC cells are not completely lysed at 0 Osm.

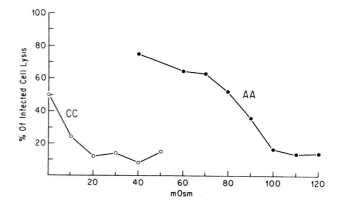

populations is the product of a classical balanced polymorphism. There is no definitive answer to this paradox. One possibility is that the malaria culture system is not sensitive enough to detect the advantages of the HbC trait cells, or that the advantage of these cells pertains to a portion of the malaria cycle not tested by culture, such as endothelial adhesion, interaction with the spleen, or phagocytosis. Alternatively, selection might not favor the HbC carrier at all (see below).

MALARIA AND HbSC DISEASE

In culture, the behavior of HbSC disease cells toward the malaria parasite is distinctive. While the oxygenated HbSC cells are indistinguishable from normal cells as a host for plasmodia, when HbSC cells are partially deoxygenated the parasite rapidly dies; they are almost as inhospitable as sickle cell anemia cells (Friedman et al., 1979b). While the mechanism for this observation is unknown, possibilities include the lowering of intraerythrocyte pH caused by parasite metabolism, inducing more deoxy HbS polymerization in a red cell with high mean corpuscular hemoglobin concentration (MCHC)—a consequence of the presence of HbC (see Chapter 27)—a poor substrate for the parasite. Increased crystallization of HbC induced by the presence of HbS (Lin et al., 1989) could introduce another potentially inadequate substrate for the parasite's proteases. This hypothesis will be possible to test in vivo, since an HbC transgenic mouse has already been produced (Fabry et al., 1998), and an HbSC mouse should not lag far behind.

It has been proposed that selective pressure might operate more on HbSC than on HbC trait individuals (Friedman et al., 1979b). This interpretation, if correct, would be a qualitative extension of balanced polymorphism. Supporting this notion, HbC has been found to coexist with HbS in all geographic locations, although it can be segregated according to caste in the Dogon regions in Mali (Ducrocq et al., 1994) and there is little mortality from HbSC disease before reproductive age, at least in the United States (Leikin et al., 1989). Although this might not be entirely true in the extreme conditions of some parts of sub-Saharan West Africa, it is quite likely that even in that environment, people with HbSC disease have a significantly higher fitness than those with normal HbA (because of the condition's association with resistance to malaria) but an even higher fitness than those with HbC trait, as suggested by the intensity of growth inhibition of HbSC cells in vitro.

A model of this type suggests that there could be an advantage to introducing an additional malaria resistance gene into a population that already has one or more of them: Compound heterozygotes might enhance the resistance mechanisms, rendering a fitter individual in a malarious region. Most of the populations exposed to pandemic malaria exhibit more than one red cell defect that resists the infection. Further work on the state of equilibrium—or lack of it—of HbC gene frequency, and interrelationships of the HbA, HbS, and HbC genes in Africa are needed to test this hypothesis.

MALARIA AND HbE

HbE is the most frequent hemoglobin structural mutation in Southeast Asia and perhaps the world (Flatz et al., 1964; Flatz, 1967) (see Chapter 43). The highest frequency of this gene is observed in the "HbE triangle" where the frontiers of Cambodia, Laos, and Thailand congregate. HbE can be found in other malarious regions such as Bangladesh, the State of Assam in India, Madagascar, South China, Indonesia, and the Philippines. Early epidemiologic studies suggested a connection between this abnormal hemoglobin and malaria (Flatz, 1967). In the central region of Indochina, red cell genetic defects including HbE, α and β thalassemia, and G-6-PD deficiency, are so frequent that Sicard et al. (1979) have calculated that only about 15 percent of the population has "normal" red cells.

The first in vitro study of the relationship between P. falciparum and HbE-containing cells demonstrated a moderate decrease in growth of P. falciparum in HbE disease cells, but normal growth in HbE trait cells (Nagel et al., 1981). A subsequent study appeared to contradict this finding (Santiyanont and Wilairat, 1981), however; the growth curves in HbE disease and HbE trait cells were not generated with the same inoculum. Variability in the number of parasitized cells from one inoculum to another is so great that it may obscure any real difference in effect. This discrepancy was resolved by a third study that confirmed and extended the results of Nagel et al. (1981; Vernes et al., 1986). Diminished growth of parasites in both HbE trait and HbE disease cells, particularly the latter, was observed at 5 percent oxygen and maximized at 20 percent oxygen (Vernes et al., 1986). Vitamin C, an antioxidant, partially inhibited the decrease of growth in the 20 percent oxygen cultures. This possible antioxidant effect is interesting in view of some of the properties of HbE, which is somewhat unstable and capable of generating free radicals and inducing oxidative damage to the red cell membrane (Frischer and Bowman, 1975). Significantly higher levels of antimalarial antibodies and lower parasitemias were present in the carriers of HbE compared to normal individuals from the same areas, an exciting observation that needs confirmation and explanation.

Parasitized HbE disease and HbE trait erythrocytes are phagocytized to a greater extent by normal human monocytes than infected erythrocytes from normal individuals (Bunyaratvej et al., 1986). This phenomenon was particularly prominent in late trophozoites and schizonts, suggesting that the surface of parasitized HbE-containing red cells is modified compared to normal red cells, a situation plausible in view of the potential free radical damage induced by HbE.

Culture-based evidence demonstrated that HbE interferes with the growth of the malaria parasite and this mechanism can render their carriers partially protected from infection. The mechanisms involved are not well understood but oxidative damage to the parasite induced by the instability of HbE is a strong possibility. If confirmed, increased antimalarial antibodies in these individuals might signal frequent but benign infections, conducive to early immunologic resistance and survival through a mechanism of double protection.

NEONATAL RED CELLS AND RED CELLS CONTAINING HbF

P. falciparum growth is reduced in red cells containing HbF in a medium relatively deficient in reduced glutathione. Suggesting that this property is linked to the presence of HbF, and not due to other properties of the host cell, is the fact that all red cells containing HbF retard the growth of plasmodia. Included among these cells are cord blood cells containing a majority of HbF, red cells from infants (F-cells, or cells that contain on average about 20 percent HbF), and red cells from adults homozygous for hereditary persistence of fetal hemoglobin (HPFH), whose red cells contain almost 100 percent HbF (Pasvol et al., 1977). This finding buttresses the notion that this effect is produced directly by HbF and not by the age or morphologic differences that exist among red cell–containing HbF. HbF effects disappeared when parasites were grown in RPMI-1640 and at a PO_2 of 5 percent, a result consistent with the HbF effect being mediated by an increase in intraerythrocytic oxidative stress (Pasvol et al., 1978; Friedman, 1979b). Invasion of *P. falciparum* is increased at least in neonatal cells (Pasvol et al., 1977).

Shear et al. (1998) used transgenic mice expressing human $^A\gamma$- and $^G\gamma$-globin chains who had 40 percent to 60 percent $\alpha^M_2\gamma_2$ hemoglobin to examine the effects of HbF on survival. Animals were infected with three types of rodent malaria, *P. chabaudi adami*, which causes a nonlethal infection mainly in mature red cells, *P. yoelii* 17XNL, which induces a nonlethal infection, invading primarily reticulocytes, and *P. yoelii* 17XL, a lethal variant of *P. yoelii* 17XNL that almost invariably causes death in 1 to 2 weeks. Data indicate that this later strain may cause a syndrome resembling

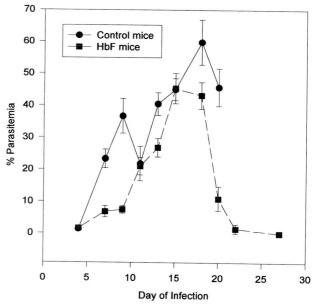

Figure 30.11. Course of *P. yoelli* 17XL (lethal) infection in C57BL/6J controls. (●; *n* = 6) and transgenic mice expressing 40 percent to 60 percent $\alpha^M_2\gamma_2$ hemoglobin (■; *n* = 7). Mice were injected intraperitoneally with 1×10^5 infected erythrocytes on day 0. On the days indicated, smears were prepared from blood taken from the tail vein, stained, and counted. Data are expressed as mean percentage parasitemia ± SEM.

cerebral malaria caused by *P. falciparum* in humans (Kaul et al., 1994). In these transgenic mice infected with *P. chabaudi adami*, the parasitemia rose more quickly, in agreement with previous data (Pasvol et al., 1977), but was cleared more rapidly. Mice infected with *P. yoelii 17XNL* showed a reduction in parasitemia, and splenectomy prior to this infection did not alter this protection. While control mice died between 11 and 23 days, transgenic mice cleared the infection by day 22 and survived (Fig. 30.11); similar results were seen in splenectomized animals. These studies suggest an in vivo protective effect of HbF toward malaria infection not mediated by the spleen.

Light microscopy showed that parasites developed more slowly in HbF-containing than in normal erythrocytes, and electron microscopy showed that hemozoin formation was defective in transgenic sickle mice. Human recombinant plasmepsin II studies demonstrated that HbF is digested only half as well as HbA (Fig. 30.12). It appears that HbF provides protection from *P. falciparum* malaria by the retardation of parasite growth. The mechanism involves resistance to digestion by malarial hemoglobinases based on the data presented and by the well-known properties of HbF as a superstable tetramer (see Chapter 10). Resistance of normal neonates to malaria can now be explained by a double mechanism: Increased malaria

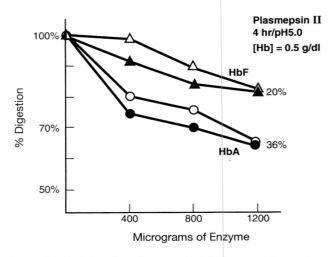

Figure 30.12. Digestion of HbF and HbA by recombinant plasmepsin II. The y-axis represents the percentage digestion; the x-axis represents μg of enzyme (from Shear et al., 1998, with permission.)

invasion rates, reported in neonatal red cells (see above), will direct parasites to fetal cells as well as F-cells, and less to the 20 percent HbA-containing red cells, amplifying the antimalarial effects of HbF.

These findings do not entirely exclude the participation of oxidative stress in this phenomena (see below). HbF is not particularly prone to be a source of free radicals because of its stability; in effect it is resistant to methemoglobin formation as well as heme loss (see Chapter 10).

Impaired growth of *P. falciparum* in HbF-containing cells is important because this effect may explain the decreased parasitemia observed in the first 6 months of life (Pasvol et al., 1978) and might be at least a contributing factor to the advantages of being a carrier of β thalassemia since carriers exhibit a significant retardation of the HbF to HbA switch. This period is critical, as mentioned before, in the resistance toward the infection, since the humoral and cellular defenses are not yet effective.

MALARIA AND β THALASSEMIA

J. B. S. Haldane (1949) first invoked the concept of balanced polymorphism to explain the high frequency of some hemoglobinopathies including β thalassemia. Fewer studies support the selective advantage of β thalassemia compared to other red cell polymorphisms. Early population studies have been summarized (Weatherall and Clegg, 1981; Teo and Wong, 1985). A recent survey in Northern Liberia found an increasing frequency of β-thalassemia trait with increasing age, suggesting that carriers had increased survival (Willcox et al., 1983). Using the criterion of parasite

density with parasitemia greater than $1 \times 10^9/L$ indicative of the probability of lethal infection, a relative risk for lethal infection of 0.45 in children ages 1 to 4 years was calculated, demonstrating clearly the protective effect of β thalassemia toward malaria.

In early culture studies, parasites grew normally in β-thalassemia trait red cells, but parasites were more susceptible to oxidants than were parasites growing in normal cells (Friedman, 1979b). Other studies were also unable to demonstrate inhibited parasite growth in thalassemic red cells under optimal culture conditions (Pasvol and Wilson, 1982; Roth et al., 1983). Yet some workers have shown differences in in vitro parasite growth in β thalassemia red cells by changing the conditions of culture and varying the composition of the culture media (Brockelman et al., 1987). In these studies, replacement of most of the usual culture medium (RPMI 1640) with MEM may have diluted the concentration of amino acids indispensable to the parasites that they obtain normally by digesting hemoglobin. If nutrients are supplied abundantly in the medium the limitations encountered by the parasite in hypochromic red cells would be masked. Many other differences exist between these culture media, illustrating the limitation of interpreting results of single culture conditions.

Anderson et al. (1989) studied 18 β-thalassemia families from the Ferrara region of Italy where the incidence of an inherited low flavin mononucleotide (FMN)-dependent pyridoxine phosphate (PNP) oxidase activity—a sensitive indicator of red cell FMN deficiency—is higher in genetically related family members than in the unrelated spouses, controls, and subjects without family history of thalassemia. There was a markedly higher incidence of red cell flavin adenine dinucleotide deficiency in thalassemia heterozygotes than in their normal relatives. This was indicated by higher stimulation of flavin adenine dinucleotide glutathione reductase activity by flavin adenine dinucleotide and lower glutathione reductase activity per red cell, suggesting an additive effect of thalassemia on red cell flavin adenine dinucleotide deficiency that resulted from the inherited reduction of riboflavin metabolism. There is evidence that diversion of flavin adenine dinucleotide to other flavin adenine dinucleotide enzymes might be an important factor. Any impact of this finding on malaria remains to be investigated.

β-Thalassemia erythrocytes infected with *P. falciparum* have reduced tendency to cytoadhere or to form rosettes (Udomsangpetch et al., 1993). A decrease of parasite antigens is found on the surface of infected β-thalassemia red cells in the trophozoite or schizont stage, but not in the ring forms. Noninhibitory pooled immune serum did not show a difference between parasitized thalassemic red cells and parasitized normal red

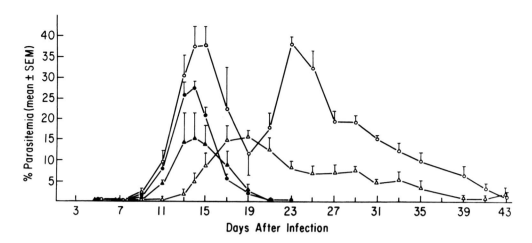

Figure 30.13. Thalassemia mutations project mice from *P. chabaudi* and *P. Chabaudi*, strain 1309 infection. ●-normal mice; ○-splenectomized normal mice; ▲-intact β-thalassemic mice; △-splenectomized β-thalassemic mice.

cells. If confirmed, this finding will suggest another and qualitatively different mechanism of protection by β thalassemia.

Recent studies of the role of oxidant stress in mediating the protection against malaria in β-thalassemia red cells showed red cell age dependency in sensitivity to oxidant stress existed in thalassemia and normal red cells (Senok et al., 1998). Parasite invasion and growth deteriorated with red cell age, particularly in cells with late parasite maturation arrest or abnormal morphology. Although there was a negative correlation between parasite activity and oxidant stress in both normal and thalassemic red cells, the relationship was weak.

Transgenic mice have contributed to the study of β thalassemia and malaria. C57BL/6J mice with a homozygous β-thalassemia syndrome (Skow et al., 1983) and also transgenic thalassemic mice that expressed the human β^A gene were infected with *P. chabaudi adami*, *P. chabaudi* (strain 1309), or *P. berghe*. Thalassemic mice infected with *P. chabaudi adami* had both a delayed and diminished rise in parasitemia compared with both normal C57BL/6J and transgenic thalassemic mice that expressed that β^A transgene (Roth et al., 1988). A 48-hour delay in both detection of parasites and in occurrence of peak parasitemia was observed in the thalassemic mice. Importantly, the level of peak parasitemia in the thalassemic mice was approximately 40 percent of that in the normal and the β^A transgenic mice while normal and β^A transgenic mice were not significantly different from one another. When a more virulent strain of *P. chabaudi* was used, similar delays in patency and peak parasitemia were observed, but the levels of parasitemia were similar to controls (Roth et al., 1988). Thalassemic mice were not protected from *P. berghei*. While parasitemia in the β^A transgenic mice was similar to control mice, parasitemia was greater than in normal mice (Roth et al., 1988). Thalassemic mice may not be protected from *P. berghei* due to the high

level of reticulocytes in these mice. A small but significant increase in parasitemia in the β^A transgenic mice may therefore be due to the slightly elevated reticulocyte count that exists in these animals.

These studies indicate that the thalassemia mutation protects mice from *P. chabaudi adami* and *P. chabaudi*, strain 1309 infection (Fig. 30.13). Correction of the thalassemia phenotype by the β^A transgene abolished this protective effect. It is unlikely that the protection seen with *P. chabaudi* infection is due to reticulocytosis, because the number of mature red cells available for parasite invasion far exceeded the number of infected red blood cells.

In vivo models allow studies of host factors in the protection from malaria. These could involve increased phagocytosis, either because of increased binding of IgG (Luzzi et al, 1991) or intrinsic alteration of the thalassemic erythrocyte (Shinar and Rachmilewitz, 1990). However, splenectomized thalassemic mice had a further delay in the rise of parasitemia, a paradoxical effect needing further study (Roth et al., 1988).

MALARIA AND α THALASSEMIA

Based on the detection of α thalassemia by DNA analysis it was established that the high frequency and distribution of this condition in Melanesia was a result of natural selection by malaria (Flint et al., 1986). α-Thalassemia frequency, but not the frequency of other unlinked DNA polymorphisms, exhibited an altitude- and latitude-dependent distribution that correlated with the presence of malaria endemicity throughout Melanesia. Previous studies in which α thalassemia was detected by hematologic indices were much less sensitive and accurate.

In culture, there was a significant decrease in parasite growth rate in HbH disease red cells or cells from Hb Constant Spring carriers, but normal growth was found in the red cells of persons who lacked only one or two α-globin genes (Ifediba et al., 1985; Yuthavong et al., 1988). Infected α-thalassemia red cells were also found to be more readily phagocytosed than infected normal red cells. These findings underscore the possibility that variant red cells may impair parasite survival by extrinsic mechanisms that could not be detected in culture. For example, variant red cells could offer protection to the host by selective destruction of parasitized red cells in the spleen, an effect undetectable in vitro. Culture data strongly suggest that α-thalassemia red cells are poor hosts for the malaria parasite.

Of particular interest are the findings of Williams et al. (1996) that studied the epidemiology of malaria in Vanuatu, in the northeast Pacific. In a holoendemic region of these islands, they found that the incidence of uncomplicated malaria (*P. falciparum* and *vivax*) as well as splenomegaly (commonly associated with malaria infection) was increased, not decreased, in children less than 5 years of age that carry the $-\alpha/-\alpha$ genotype. No genotype effect was found in children older than 5 years of age. This apparent paradox and contradiction with the above data is resolved by the following hypothesis: α Thalassemia might increase susceptibility to *P. vivax* in young children, and such infection, by cross-reactive cellular and humoral immunity, might afford protection against subsequent, potentially fatal, *P. falciparum*. This ground-breaking hypothesis needs to be examined in more detail but offers the possibility of a final picture in which a mixture of genes and acquired immunity are coparticipants in the protection toward malaria.

MECHANISM OF RED CELL PROTECTION IN THALASSEMIC RED CELLS

Although a definitive mechanism for the inhibition of malarial parasites in β-thalassemia erythrocytes remains elusive, limitation in essential amino acids present in a low MCHC red cell (Allison and Eugui, 1982), increased susceptibility to oxidant stress (Allison and Eugui, 1982), increased vulnerability to cell-mediated damage (phagocytosis) (Allison and Eugui, 1982), and elevation and persistence of HbF in infancy and early childhood (Lehmann, 1972; Weatherall and Clegg, 1981) and associated low pyridoxine-phosphate oxidase activity in thalassemias (Clements et al., 1981) are among the possible causes.

An important player in this phenomenon my be oxidative stress, hence it deserves particular attention. Unfortunately, this phenomenon is complicated and the following assertions have been made: The malaria parasite produces oxidants that can potentially damage the red cell, the red cell hosting the parasite responds with an increased resistance to oxidation, and thalassemic red cells are likely to be already partially damaged by the presence of the red cell defect. The data that support the previous list of events are the following:

1. The malaria-parasitized red cell is under substantial oxidative stress. A strong demonstration of this has been provided by Atamma and Ginsburg (1997), showing that normal red cells and isolated parasites have high reduced glutathione (GSH) over oxidized glutathione (GSSG), and the GSH/GSSG ratio amounts to about 300 in both cases, indicating adequate antioxidant defenses. In the parasited red cell this ratio falls to 30, a tenfold effect, indicating a sizable oxidant challenge.

2. Nevertheless, the red cell mounts a defense against the oxidant, recognizing its danger: increases in its α-tocopherol content (Roth et al., 1984). The depletion of plasma α-tocopherol, retinol, and carotinoids in children with *P. falciparum* (Das et al., 1996), and the previous observation of this in rodent malaria (Roth et al., 1984), suggest that vitamin E is obtained from plasma by the parasitized red cell. In addition, the hexose monophosphate shunt (HMS), which produces NADPH for reductive antioxidant protection, is 78 times higher than normal red cells, and the parasite contributes 82 percent; that of the host cell is increased about 24-fold (Atamma et al., 1994).

3. There is very little doubt that thalassemic red cells are oxidatively damaged and that their red cell membrane has suffered oxidative alteration in addition to the binding of globin chains, mostly in the form of hemichromes (Rachmilewitz et al., 1985; Schrier, 1997).

Hence, a unifying hypothesis of the mechanism of protection will have to involve, among others, a oxidative stress-dependent pathway, of the following sort: The thalassemias, that is, α and β thalassemias, HbE, and Hb Constant Spring protect the carrier from dying of malaria, because the oxidative stress of the parasite invasion of the red cell is added to the intrinsic oxidative stress of the thalassemic red cell condition, producing a red cell with less viability. This allows for the selective destruction and removal of thalassemic parasitized red cells. The details of the mechanisms involved, and the differences between the different thalassemias, will need to be worked out. Nevertheless, the solution of this problem might indicate potential avenues of therapeutic intervention in malaria.

MALARIA AND THE ERYTHROCYTE MEMBRANE

Mutations in Erythrocyte Surface Antigens (Blood Groups)

Duffy System. Defining the role of the Duffy blood group determinants in erythrocyte invasion by *P. vivax* opened a new avenue for understanding red cell resistance to malaria (Miller et al., 1975, 1976). Many Africans and Black Americans are entirely resistant to *P. vivax* malaria (Young et al., 1958). In Gambian individuals 100 percent are Duffy negative (Welch, 1977), a trait also found in Arabs, Oriental Jews, and the Druze, ethnic groups that have admixed with Blacks (Sandler et al., 1979).

The Duffy blood group system is polymorphic and includes five alloantigens, two of which are Mendelian alleles (Fy^a and Fy^b), and map to chromosome 1, since they are syntenic to the Rh loci. Duffy negativity corresponds to a null genotype that lacks the expression of both Fy^a and Fy^b antigens [Fy(a$^-$b$^-$)]. Miller and associates (1976) first demonstrated that Fy(a$^-$b$^-$) erythrocytes were resistant to the invasion of *P. knowlesi*—a Plasmodium akin to *P. vivax,* which normally affects monkeys—merozoites in vitro. As in vitro malaria cultures were not available in early studies, demonstration that carriers of the negative Duffy genotypes were resistant in vivo to *P. vivax* malaria required human volunteers exposed to mosquitos infected with *P. vivax* (Young, 1958). Duffy-negative individuals were resistant to infection while the controls fell sick 11 to 15 days after the exposure. These findings explain the very high frequency of the Duffy null genotype in parts of West Africa and the fact that this haplotype is fixed (100 percent frequency) in some areas of that region. Although *P. vivax* is not life threatening, it can contribute to infant mortality by additive interaction with malnutrition and other infections. Selective pressure mediated by malaria must be operative in this system to explain the high frequency of the Duffy null genotype in populations exposed now or previously to *P. vivax.*

The Duffy system deserves further attention as a model for a receptor involved in the invasion of red cells by plasmodial merozoites because alloantibodies to Fy^a partially block the invasion of *P. knowlesi.* Northern blotting and susceptibility to *Vibrio* cholera neuraminadase demonstrate that both Fy^a and Fy^b reside in a glycoprotein of about 40 kd (Hadley et al., 1984; Tanner et al., 1988; Chaudhuri et al., 1989). The role of the Duffy system as a ligand for merozoite invasion of *P. vivax* has been further studied in a short-term in vitro culture system that allows for significant re-invasion of target erythrocytes by the parasite (Wertheimer & Barnwell, 1989): Study of Duffy-positive and -negative erythrocytes, various primate erythrocytes, enzymatic modification of erythrocytes, and monoclonal antibodies that define a new Duffy determinant, Fy6, provided evidence that the erythrocyte glycoprotein carrying Duffy determinants is required as a ligand for the invasion of human erythrocytes by *P. vivax* merozoites. Blockade of invasion by Fab fragments of the anti-Fy6 monoclonal antibody equal to that of the intact molecule and the correlation of *P. vivax* susceptibility with the presence of the Fy6 determinant suggested that this epitope or a nearby domain may be the active site on the Duffy glycoprotein. However, as for *P. knowlesi,* there is evidence that an alternative pathway for *P. vivax* invasion of simian erythrocytes may exist.

A 135-kd parasite protein from *P. knowlesi,* which binds the Duffy glycoprotein, and a 140-kd parasite protein from *P. vivax* were shown to be homologous to the parasite-binding protein in *P. falciparum* (Wertheimer and Barnwell, 1989; Adams et al., 1992; Sim et al., 1994). Genes for both of these proteins have been cloned (Adams et al., 1992; Fang et al., 1992), and localized to the micronemes, organelles of the apical end of the merozoites (Chitnis and Miller, 1994). The extracellular portion of this Duffy-binding protein can be divided into six domains and the cysteine-rich domain II is the active binding region of the molecule (Chitnis et al., 1996).

Recently, the Duffy antigen has been defined as a novel receptor (DARC) for the chemoattractant cytokine family (Horuk and Peiper, 1996; Horuk et al., 1996; reviewed by Hadley and Peiper, 1997). Chemokines are a superfamily of secreted proteins, molecular weight around 10 kd, that recruit leukocytes to sites of inflammation. They are segregated into two gene clusters, the C-X-C that are chemoattractant to neutrophils and the C-C, chemoattractants for lymphocytes and monocytes (Hadley and Peiper, 1997). Duffy antigen, the DARC receptor, is expressed on endothelial cells of the postcapillary venules throughout the body and littoral cells of the spleen and perhaps endothelial cells of the glomeruli and vasarecta, even when erythrocytes are Duffy negative (Peiper et al., 1995; Chaudhuri et al., 1997). An apparent predilection for the postcapillary venules is intriguing since this is the only site demonstrated for the adhesion of parasitized erythrocytes in microcirculatory preparations and in animal models (Kaul et al., 1994, 1998).

Glycophorins. Receptors for the invasion of *P. falciparum* merozoites are thought to be members of the glycophorin system. Still, the exact role of each of the glycophorins [A(α), B(δ), and C(β)] and the methodology used for implicating them as receptors has been questioned and a role for the anion transporter, band 3, as alternative receptor is also possible.

Although there is some resistance to malarial parasite invasion in red cells carrying polymorphic forms of the glycophorin system, none of the polymorphic forms of the glycophorins that reduce invasion emulate the Duffy system, because this reduction is only partial. Cells showing complete absence of A or α glycophorin [En(a-)] reduce invasion of *P. falciparum* significantly but not completely (Hadley et al., 1988). This is a rare blood group—only about ten individuals in the world are known to carry this genotype—without an apparent effect on erythrocyte function. Higher frequencies of red cells exhibiting the S-s-U- genotype compatible with balanced polymorphism have been found in Equatorial Africa (Pasvol, 1982). Reductions in invasion rates by *P. falciparum* merozoites of 50 percent to 75 percent were observed in these cells. A report that Wr^b- red cells, also polymorphic in Africa, are strongly resistant to invasion has not been confirmed (Pasvol, 1982; Facer and Mitchell, 1984; Yi-qin et al., 1987).

Red cells expressing α-δ hybrid glycophorins generated from the genes specifying A and B glycophorins show 50 percent reduction in invasion rates (Wertheimer and Barnwell, 1989). Tn red cells, which are imperfectly glycosylated exposing a cryptic antigen that can be identified serologically, show considerable resistance to invasion (Dahr et al., 1975).

Studies of the effects of diverse monoclonal antibodies to α-glycophorin (A), showed that all antibodies inhibit invasion of *P. falciparum* and *P. knowlesi* in direct proportion to their effect in decreasing red cell deformability measured by ektacytometry (Pasvol et al., 1989). Parasite invasion and deformability decreased as the antibody recognized epitopes closer to the lipid bilayer. Nearest the bilayer is the site for the Wr^b determinant and antibodies to this site were the most inhibitory. Antibodies against δ-glycophorin (B), Rh, and Kell determinants had no effect. Although this study suggested that deformability may play an important role in parasite invasion and that decreased red cell pliability can impair this important part of its life cycle, this association is not probative. Caution should be exercised in interpreting the effects of antibody on parasite invasion as reagent binding to the red cell surface could itself affect deformability and confound the interpretation of the results (Pasvol et al., 1989).

Gerbich-negative phenotype occurs in about 10 percent of Melanesians living in the malaria-infested northern provinces of Papua New Guinea (Serjeantson et al., 1977). In a survey of 266 individuals, the prevalence of *P. falciparum* and/or *P. vivax* infection in Gerbich-negative subjects was 5.7 percent compared with 18.6 percent in Gerbich-positive individuals (P= .05). *P. malariae* occurred at comparable rates of about 8 percent in Gerbich-negative and Gerbich-positive subjects. These results must be confirmed in further studies.

M^kM^k erythrocytes that lack A and B glycophorins were tested with two *P. falciparum* strains, 7G8 and Camp (Perkins, 1981). These cells were invaded with 50 percent efficiency by 7G8 parasites but only at 20 percent efficiency by the Camp strain. These results raise the possibility of heterogeneity red cell binding determinants among *P. falciparum* malaria variants. Neuraminidase treatment of erythrocytes can inhibit invasion, suggesting the possibility that sialic acid might be involved in the receptor for invasion, but because enzyme treatment could induce conformational changes in the glycosylated protein these findings should be viewed in circumspect. When Tn cells were exposed to Camp, Thai-1, and Thai-2 strains of *P. falciparum*, with and without treatment with neuraminidase, it was concluded that heterogeneity of red cell surface receptors best explained the results (Mitchell et al., 1986).

Partial reduction of parasite invasion rates by all active glycophorin mutants strongly suggests that the receptor site for *P. falciparum* is complex and multivalent with differences in affinity constants among redundant sites. If so, it might be difficult to attack malaria infection by concentrating on blocking invasion receptors. Invasion studies have been carried out using a small number of red cell donors. If in addition to the determinant of interest, these cells also contained other genetic defects that were active but unlinked to the glycophorin mutants, the results might be misinterpreted.

RED CELLS WITH CYTOSKELETON ABNORMALITIES

Southeast Asian Ovalocytosis

Malarial invasion is complex, involving several stages, including initial nonspecific attachment, reorientation of the polarity of the merozoite, red cell membrane flipping, and the zipper-type introjection of the merozoite into the red cell (Miller et al., 1979). Given this complexity, it is not surprising that cytoskeletal proteins could be active participants and that their mutants might generate red cell resistance to *P. falciparum*.

Melanesian, or Southeast Asian, ovalocytosis, is the sole highly polymorphic red cell cytoskeleton abnormality. Present in about 30 percent of the Melanesian population of Papua New Guinea and other aboriginal populations of Southeast Asia, ovalocytosis is characterized by red cells with axial ratios smaller than that of elliptocytes (Lie-Injo et al., 1972; Amato and Booth 1977). Hemolysis is absent. Deformability of these cells is diminished, thermal deformation of these cells is abnormal, and expression of surface blood groups is altered (Booth et al., 1977; Mohandas et al., 1984; Saul et al., 1984).

Epidemiologic evidence suggested that ovalocytosis confers resistance to high levels of parasitemia with *P. falciparum, P. vivax,* and *P. malariae* (Serjeantson et al., 1977). Ovalocytes are highly, but not absolutely, resistant to invasion by *P. falciparum* merozoites (Kidson et al., 1981). These cells are also resistant to the invasion by *P. knowlesi,* which bind a receptor distinct from that used by *P. falciparum* (Hadley et al., 1983).

The phenomena is complicated by the fact that the presence of malaria infection might involve the generation of ovalocytes. In individuals infected with *P. falciparum,* 6.3 ± 8.4 percent of erythrocytes were ovalocytic whereas only 0.46 ± 0.4 percent ovalocytes were seen in controls. Ovalocytes contained significantly fewer parasites than discocytes. These findings could reflect a response of the malarious patient to parasite proliferation in their circulation (Apibal et al., 1989).

In culture studies, hereditary ovalocytosis appeared protective (Bunyaratvej et al., 1997). Interestingly, higher ovalocythemia (75 percent to 100 percent) was found in malarious patients while their ovalocytocytosis parents, without malaria, had 25 percent to 50 percent ovalocythemia. This suggests that the nonovalocytes were being removed from the circulation preferentially. The invasion index was 1.52 ± 0.91 in ovalocytosis while it was 4.45 ± 1.51 in normal individuals. Parents had an infection index of 1.81 ± 0.81, which also indicated significant protection. The same was true for the red cell deformability index. This finding has been interpreted to indicate that it is not red cell shape but decreased deformability that limits parasite invasion.

In contrast to studies mentioned above, in Madang, Papua New Guinea, the prevalence of ovalocytosis did not differ between children with and without acute *P. falciparum* malaria or according to the α-globin gene haplotype (O'Donnell et al., 1998). Two or more linear or irregularly shaped pale regions in the red cells had high sensitivity and specificity (more than 94 percent and 99 percent, respectively) and were considered useful for the morphologic diagnosis of ovalocytosis. In contrast, the presence of ovalocytes had high specificity (100 percent) but low sensitivity (69 percent). In acute malaria, hemoglobin levels and red cells counts were lower in patients with ovalocytosis than normal children. In contradiction with the findings of Bunyaratvej et al., (1997), these authors found that ovalocytosis patients had lower ovalocythemia, suggesting that a selective loss of ovalocytes might contribute to the anemia in the presence of malaria.

Southeast Asian ovalocytosis is due to heterozygosity for an eight amino acid deletion (400 to 408) in erythrocyte band 3. (Liu et al., 1995). This mutant protein is anomalously attached to the membrane cytoskeleton and highly aggregated (oligomerized)

with ankryn, forming stacks containing bands of inter-membrane particles (IMP), which are resistant to alkaline pH and trypsin. Affected cells have a marked decrease in membrane rotational mobility, contributing to their increased rigidity. In effect, these membranes are incapable of cytoskeletal extension, which is indispensable for deformation. Why the merozoite is unable to invade the ovalocytic cell is unknown.

Naturally occurring anti-band 3 autoantibodies bind to erythrocytes infected with the FCR-3 knobby variant of *P. falciparum* (Winograd and Sherman, 1989). These autoantibodies recognized a greater than 240-kd protein in extracts made from surface-iodinated infected erythrocytes. The antigen was present only in erythrocytes infected with a knobby variant, and was removed by trypsin treatment of intact infected cells. Two-dimensional peptide map analysis demonstrated that the antigen was structurally related to band 3. These observations raise the questions of whether band 3 is modified by the infection, whether this is a subclass of Band 3, and whether there are genetic mutants of band 3 that confer innate immunity to malaria. *P. falciparum* invasion and growth in the band 3 variant Memphis (56 Lys→Glu) (Jarolim et al., 1992) was normal (Schulman et al., 1990).

Hereditary Elliptocytosis

Another cytoskeletal defect that has been found to be resistant to invasion by both *P. knowlesi* and *P. falciparum* is elliptocytosis, due to either the absence of glycophorin C or band 4.1 (Hadley and Miller, 1988). These erythrocytes have cytoskeletal abnormalities with reduced interactions that stabilize the anchoring of the cytoskeleton core to the protein imbedded in the bilipid layer and also exhibit alterations in deformability. That invasion is inhibited for two types of plasmodia suggests that this defect alters a stage of invasion later than receptor recognition.

Hereditary elliptocytosis due to protein 4.1 deficiency and structural variants that increase the content of spectrin dimers also exhibit parasite abnormal growth (Schulman et al., 1990), a pattern distinct from that of hereditary spherocytosis (see below).

Hereditary poikilocytosis due to the αI/74 mutant spectrin, was associated with significantly reduced parasitemia. Hereditary elliptocytosis due to the αI/65 variant spectrin also had reduced invasion. Decreased invasion correlated with the percentage of spectrin dimers present within the membrane of variant cells. In contrast, in a partial deficiency of protein 4.1 (HE/4.1 +) that had a normal percentage of spectrin dimers, invasion was unchanged or increased (Facer, 1995). These data suggest that the αI domain variants might interfere with the merozoite/receptor interaction in the surface of the red cell and/or the mechanism of endocytosis. Membrane proteins may become modified during intracellular growth of *P. falciparum*. An 80-kd phosphoprotein associated with the membrane in normal red cells may be a phosophorylated form of 4.1 forming a complex with the MPI antigen of the parasitized red cell or be generated by the intracellular parasite. Erythrocytes of a homozygote for 4.1 (−) hereditary elliptocytosis, whose red cells were completely devoid of protein 4.1, also lacked 80-kd phosphoprotein, demonstrating that this protein is indeed a phosphorylated form of protein 4.1 (Christi et al., 1994). Whether this protein alters the red cell membrane and affects parasite growth and survival remains to be determined. A similar mechanism could operate in other mutations of protein 4.1.

Homozygotes for hereditary elliptocytosis, with protein 4.1 absence and the Leach phenotype due to glycophorin C absence were similarly resistant to parasite invasion, but only the protein 4.1 abnormality had reduction in parasite growth (Christi et al., 1994). Since the p55 protein is deficient in both of these abnormal red cells, the latter protein could be involved in the invasion abnormality but not the parasite growth defect.

Hereditary Spherocytosis

Hereditary spherocytosis has not been reported at polymorphic frequencies in any region of the world. Nevertheless, since the underlying molecular defect is a cytoskeleton protein abnormality it is of great interest to investigate the fate of the *P. falciparum* malaria parasite in these cells and to explore the possibility that red cell membrane proteins are utilized by the parasite, beyond the initial encounter during invasion.

Parasite growth was decreased in direct proportion to the extent of spectrin deficiency in hereditary spherocytosis (Schulman et al., 1990) (Fig. 30.14). This abnormality was unique and characterized by normal growth during the first 2 days followed by abnormal growth with a delay proportional to the decrease of spectrin. In hereditary spherocytes that exhibited a 46 percent decrease in spectrin, abnormal growth was immediate after day 2. Hereditary spherocytosis cells with 23 percent to 32 percent decrease in spectrin had apparent abnormal growth beginning at day 3 or 4. Hereditary spherocytosis cells lacking spectrin deficiency had normal growth. ATP and glutathione levels were normal in infected and noninfected normal cells compared to the infected and noninfected abnormal cells. Preincubation of hereditary spherocytosis cells in culture medium had no effect on the results. It seems unlikely that the hereditary spherocytosis itself is responsible for the abnormal growth. Abnormal inva-

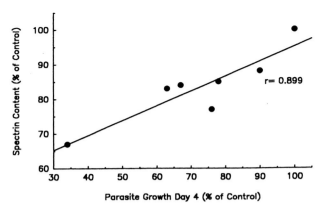

Figure 30.14. Correlation of malarial parasite growth on day 4 in hereditary spherocytosis erythrocytes with cell spectrin content. The line drawn represents the best fit by regression analysis, and r is the correlation coefficient.

sion was excluded as a cause for the growth abnormalities observed. Ankyrin/spectrin deficient mice showed a dramatic decrease in invasion by *P. berghei* and *P. chabaudi* (Shear et al., 1991). These experiments suggest that skeletal membrane proteins may play a role in both invasion and growth, according to the defect that is present and raise questions regarding erythrocyte innate resistance. These include the mechanisms of the growth impairment and delay and the role of host cytoskeleton proteins in the construction of the parasites own set of membranes such as parasitosphorous vacuoles.

In studies of hereditary spherocytosis and elliptocytosis, parsimony suggests that in the absence of invasion defects, spectrin and other interacting proteins, either modified or in the native form, play important roles as constitutive elements of the parasite membranes. Alternatively, the host cytoskeletal proteins may be involved in the events that follow invasion—generation of the parasitosphorous membrane—without direct incorporation into the parasite membranes. Finally, cytoskeleton or membrane proteins could be critical in the insertion of parasite proteins in the red cell surface, and mutations in these proteins could interfere with this adaptive process. No direct evidence for any of these hypotheses exists, and little work has been done in this area. Delauney (1995) has reported higher than 1 percent frequency for band 3 Montefiore in Africa, indicating that the defect is polymorphic.

Mice with abnormalities of erythrocyte membrane spectrin have been utilized to characterize further the roles of spectrin and ankyrin in malaria infection. Homozygous mice expressing the nb mutation synthesize normal amounts of spectrin but no ankyrin. Because of the ankyrin deficiency, only 50 percent of the normal amount of spectrin is bound to the erythrocyte membrane (Bodine et al., 1984). Mice with the sph/spherocytosis mutation synthesize ankyrin but do not synthesize the α chain of spectrin (Barker et al., 1986). Homozygous WBB6F$_1$ (nb/nb), heterozygous (nb/+), and homozygous (+/+) mice were infected with *P. chabaudi*-parasitized erythrocytes. Controls (+/+) displayed a course of nonlethal parasitemia that was patent on day 3, peaked on day 10, and was cleared by day 14 after infection. Heterozygous animals had a lower peak of parasitemia, which cleared by day 17. Strikingly, nb/nb mice did not display a patent parasitemia. The nb/nb mice were also refractory to *P. berghei* (Shear et al., 1991). In contrast, nb/+, +/+, and parental C57BL/6J mice all succumbed to this lethal parasite. Parasites could invade erythrocytes of nb/nb mice, but they did not develop within them. (Shear et al., 1991). Anemic W/W^v mice were completely susceptible to *P. berghei*. Mice carrying the sph/sph mutation synthesize only 20 percent of β chain of spectrin and were not susceptible to infection with *P. chabaudi adami* or *P. berghei*.

DEFORMABILITY OF THE PARASITIZED RED CELL

Deformability of *P. falciparum* infected red cells has been examined by micropipette aspiration techniques (Nash et al., 1989). Erythrocytes containing ring forms exhibited a 50 percent increase in time and critical pressure needed to enter a 3 μ diameter pipette compared with nonparasitized cells. Trophozoite and schizont-containing red cells showed a much greater loss of deformability. This decrease in deformability was attributable to a deficit in cell surface area/volume ratio and slight stiffening of the cell membrane. Shape recovery measurements indicated that the membrane of parasitized cells was not more viscous than normal. The main factor in the drastic loss of deformability of cells containing the trophozoites and schizonts was the presence of the parasite itself.

Deformability of *P. falciparum*-parasitized erythrocytes was unchanged in ring forms of any strain while more mature forms caused increased rigidity that was less in knobless than knobby strains (Paulitschke and Nash, 1993). Strain-dependent differences in rigidity could influence the extent of adherence, vasoocclusion, and parasitized red cell clearance by the reticuloendothelial system.

ANEMIA IN MALARIA

Malarial anemia can cause death, particularly in children and pregnant women. Anemia in *P. falciparum* malaria infected individuals is multifactorial and its prevalence may be underestimated (Phillips and Pasvol, 1992). Two clinical presentations predomi-

nate: (1) severe acute malaria followed by profound anemia; and (2) severe anemia, secondary to repeated attacks of malaria. Children with chronic falciparum malaria in India are apyrexic, moderately to severely anemic, and have hepatosplenomegaly. These patients have more anemia and hemolysis, more neutropenia, atypical lymphocytosis and thrombocytopenia but lesser parasitemia than the acute patients (Sen et al., 1994). Ninety-four percent of 169 patients with cerebral malaria were anemic and one-third required transfusions (Phillips et al., 1986). Anemia was severe in pregnancy and in cases with concomitant bacterial infections and was related to admission parasitemia and serum creatinine. Exchange transfusion might be life-saving in severe malaria, by rapidly reducing parasite load, decreasing intravascular hemolysis, preventing disseminated intravascular coagulation and renal failure, and improving blood rheology and oxygen-carrying capacity (Phillips et al., 1990).

Mechanisms involved in the generation of malaria-associated anemia are hemolysis, decreased red cell production, and associated genetic factors. Hemolysis can be caused by (1) rupture of red cells during merozoites release, (2) splenic phagocytosis, (3) increased phagocytosis of infected red cells detected by altered membrane surface or antibody coating; (4) increased overall phagocytic activity, and (5) hemolysis of uninfected red cells. Reduced erythrocyte production might involve, (1) marrow hypoplasia, (2) dyserythropoeisis that generates ineffective erythropoiesis, and (3) inappropriately low erythropoietin levels. Multiple genetic factors also affect the anemia of malaria.

Hemolysis of Parasitized Red Cells

In *P. falciparum*-infected red cells, parasite development alters the distribution of phosphatidylserine (PS), phosphatidylcholine (PC), and phosphatidylethanolamine (PE) (Schwartz et al., 1987). PE and PS are exposed on the outer layers of the red cell membrane in conjunction with parasite maturation. This phenomenon, which precedes membrane rupture, might affect adhesion and be related to membrane permeability changes.

Following invasion, the parasite produces increased permeability to a variety of solutes. Although permeability is anion selective, there is also a significant increase in cation permeability. Cation permeability increased in the presence of extracellular Cl$^-$ and K$^+$ influx in parasitized red cells (Kirk and Horner, 1995). Cl$^-$-dependent K$^+$ efflux may play a role in volume regulation and hemolysis in parasitized red cells.

Parasitized red cells accumulate Ca^{++} with maturation. Total, exchangeable, and free Ca^{++} are elevated in infected red cells (Kramer and Ginsburg, 1991).

Exchangeable and free Ca^{++} is higher in host cell than in parasite cytosol. This is maintained by the pH gradient across the parasite membrane mediated by the Ca^{++}/H^{+} antiporter. Ca^{++} might contribute to the biochemical, structural, and functional abnormalities of infected red cells.

Individuals from areas of perennial malaria transmission showed a much higher reactivity to band 3 peptides than controls. Loop 3 peptide (of band 3 protein) reactivity was correlated with lower mean parasite count but not with hematocrit, making it unlikely that these antibodies are related to hemolysis (Hogh et al., 1994).

Blood monocytes might affect malaria hemolysis. Activated monocytes caused P. falciparum strain-specific growth inhibition (Mohan et al., 1995). Lipid peroxidation and sensitivity to hemolysis increased with parasite maturity, particularly if infected erythrocytes are exposed to activated monocytes.

During acute P. falciparum malaria, red blood cells were detected that contained ring-infected erythrocyte surface antigen (also known as RESA or Pf155) but no intracellular parasite (Angus et al., 1997). This might indicate the existence of an in vivo mechanism for the removal of intraerythrocytic parasites without red cell destruction and explain the disparity between the fall in hematocrit and decrease in parasite count observed in some hyperparasitemic patients.

A special form of hemolysis in malaria is blackwater fever (fievre bilieuse hemoglobinique) that must be differentiated from hemoglobinuria of other causes (Delacollette et al., 1995). Blackwater fever is sometimes difficult to relate to malaria, because hyperparasitemia can be missed due to an unusual synchronous lysis of infected red cells. Travelers from nonendemic countries into malarious regions can suffer this complication.

Renal failure associated with malaria is a life-threatening complication, frequently accompanied by intense anemia due to brisk hemolysis (Naqvi et al., 1996).

Hemolysis of Cocirculating Uninfected Red Cells

The mean life span of ^{51}Cr-labeled red cells at day 0 of severe P. falciparum malaria was 44 ± 22 days, versus 90 ± 13 days in healthy controls (Looareesuwan et al., 1991). This observation demonstrated that nonparasitized red cells also have reduced life span in P. falciparum malaria. IgM auto-antibodies against red cells could, at least in part, account for this phenomenon (Rosenberg et al., 1973). Similar data exist in mice infected with P. berghei (Lustig et al., 1977).

Before the appearance of parasite-containing red cells in the periphery, red cells of P. yoelli-infected mice have a progressive decrease in cell surface net negative

charge and resistance to linoleic acid-induced lysis. In P. falciparum malaria, a similar decrease in linoleic acid lysis-resistance was observed in uninfected erythrocytes (Sabolovic et al., 1994). This alteration could help the spread of the infection and affect the level of hemolysis. Uninfected red cells in cultures of P. falciparum malaria are susceptible to lysis and peroxidation of the membrane by activated monocytes (Mohan et al., 1995).

In summary, the mechanisms of increased destruction of nonparasitized red cells in a malaria infection are uncertain. Candidate effects are (1) cross-reactivity of autoantibodies, (2) increased phagocytosis because of toxic substances released by the parasitized red cells, (3) cytokines released during infection that alter all red cells, and (4) dyserythropoeisis or hypoxia induced by vasoocclusion within the marrow microcirculation (see below).

Potential Contributions From Host Genetic Factors

Epistatic genes are apt to contribute to the interindividual variability in the response to malaria. Remarkably similar infection rates, morbidity, and antibody responses are found among the Mossi and Rimaibe in the northeast of Ouagadougou (Burkina Faso) (Modiano et al., 1996). In contrast, the Fulani, who live together and are exposed to the same hyperendemic transmission of P. falciparum, have less parasitemia, less morbidity, and a higher antibody response. Mossi and Rimaibe are closely related anthropologically and are of negroid stock with long traditions of sedentary farming. In contrast the Fulani, who have Caucasian physical features, have mysterious origins. They are pastoralists and seminomadic.

A case-control study of malaria in West African children showed that an HLA class I antigen (HLA-Bw53) and a class II haplotype (DRB1 * 1302-DQB1 * 0501), common in West Africa but much less frequent in other populations, are independently associated with protection from P. falciparum severe malaria, with a level of protection similar to that of sickle trait (Hill et al., 1991). This protection may be mediated through class I-restricted cytotoxic T lymphocytes acting against the early liver stage of the infection, since hepatocytes but not red cells carry class I antigens (Hill et al., 1994). The DRB1-1302 locus of the HLA class II haplotype is associated with protection from severe anemia.

A polymorphism of the promotor region of the TNFα-gene (TNF2 allele) seems to be associated with an increased risk of cerebral malaria independent of HLA class I and class II variation (McGuire et al., 1994). This high gene frequency (0.16) of TNF2 indicates a balanced polymorphism and an advantage to this allele that counterbalances the detrimental effect of increasing the risk of cerebral malaria and death of its carriers. This advantage may be mediated through TNF-α parasite cytotoxicity and /or activation of mononuclear cells.

Other epistatic genes may be identified by segregation analysis such as those attempted by Garcia et al. (1998). Sib-pair linkage analysis has also been fruitful. Rihet et al. (1998) has found linkage between blood infection levels and 5q31-q33, a region of the genome that contains numerous candidate genes encoding immunologically active molecules such as IL-4, IL-12, IFN regulatory factor 1, IL-3, CSF-2, IL-9, IL-13, CSF-IR, IL-9, and IL-13.

Marrow Suppression

Abnormalities of Erythroid Progenitors. Erythroid burst-forming units (BFU-e) and erythroid colony-forming units (CFU-e) were reduced in marrow of children with severe *P. falciparum* malaria and greater than 1 percent parasitemia compared to those with less than 1 percent parasitemia, although absolute progenitor deficiency was uncommon (Abdalla and Wickramasinghe, 1988). Bone marrows of twenty-one Thai patients with *P. falciparum* malaria were cultured for CFU-e and BFU-e using AB serum, autologous serum taken during parasitemia, and postparasitemia autologous serum (Jootar et al., 1993). "Parasitemia serum" from uncomplicated cases did not suppress postparasitemia BFU-e but suppressed postparasitemia CFU-e. In complicated cases, "parasitemia serum" suppressed both types of progenitors.

Ineffective Erythropoiesis and Dyserythropoiesis

Iron was present in bone marrow of patients with *P. falciparum* malaria unless iron deficiency preexisted (Phillips et al., 1986). Serum iron rose after treatment. Serum ferritin averaged 1,773 ng/dL. Seventy-three percent of patients had dyserythropoiesis and in 30 percent this was moderate to intense. These findings presented a picture of "chronic disease anemia" marrow with disturbances in iron metabolism.

Erythroblast kinetics were studied using quantitative ^{14}C-autoradiography in acute *P. falciparum* malaria and suggested ineffective erythropoiesis (Dormer et al., 1983). Cell cycle distribution in erythroblasts in chronic *P. falciparum* malaria showed an increased proportion of cells in G2 and arrest during progression through the S phase (Wickramasinghe et al., 1982). Bone marrow aspirates showed increased plasma cells and macrophages, phagocytosis of parasitized red cells, increased eosinophil giant metamyelocytes, and mor-

phologic abnormalities of erythroblasts (Wickramasinghe et al., 1989). Parasitized cells adhered to the endothelium causing microcirculatory obstruction. *P. vivax* malaria marrow showed marked to moderate dyserythropoiesis (Wickramasinghe et al., 1989).

Dyserythropoiesis and ineffective erythropoiesis could not be explained by iron, folic acid, or B12 deficiency. An important difference between *P. vivax* and *P. falciparum* bone marrow was that the microcirculation was not obstructed by parasitized red cells during deep-seated schizogony in *P. vivax* malaria since this parasite does not produce knobs.

Erythropoietin Abnormalities

Marrow suppression could be the consequence of inadequate levels of circulating erythropoietin. Inadequate erythropoietin production was present in almost half of patients with *P. falciparum* malaria at admission, and in close to 70 percent of the patients between days 7 and 15 of the infection, perhaps explaining prolonged anemia (Weatherall et al., 1983; Burgmann et al., 1996). *P. falciparum* produced a rapidly reversible suppression of the marrow response to erythropoietin as estimated by red cell distribution width, a surrogate for young red cells (Kurtzhals et al., 1997).

Spleen and Reticuloendothelial Activity and Hyperactivity

Ultrastructural studies of the spleen in *P. falciparum* malaria showed large numbers of parasitized and nonparasitized erythrocytes in the cytosol of macrophages, littoral, and reticular cells; congestion and abundant parasitized red cells in splenic sinusoids; and cords with rosettes of erythrocytes surrounding immunopresenting cells (Pongponratn et al., 1987). These findings suggest immunologic and nonimmunologic interactions of the spleen with red cells in malaria. Splenic filtration of parasitized red cells is compromised by loss of erythrocyte deformability. Clearance of heat-treated ^{51}Cr-labeled autologous red cells was examined in patients with acute *P. falciparum* malaria and controls (Looareesuwan et al., 1987). With splenomegaly and anemia, clearance was accelerated to 8.4 ± 4.4 minutes versus 63 ± 37 minutes in controls. Clearance was normal in patients without splenomegaly but after treatment the clearance accelerated to levels comparable to those with splenomegaly. Six weeks after infection all patients were normal. These findings suggest that increased splenic filtration in malaria might occur only with palpable splenomegaly during the infection and only after treatment when splenomegaly is absent. Heated red cells might have properties different from parasitized native red cells and the clinical implications of this phenomenon need further study.

Clearance of IgG-coated autologous ^{51}Cr-labeled red cells was studied to assess splenic Fc receptor function in patients with *P. falciparum* malaria (Ho et al., 1990). Clearance half-times were significantly correlated with parasite count and hematocrit. Only half of the patients had half-times significantly shorter than the controls, but these decreased when the parasitemia had disappeared. A failure to increase Fc receptor-mediated red cell clearance in patients with high parasitemia suggests inadequate splenic phagocytic activity when challenged with a considerable antigenic load. Fc receptor function may be important both in the control of the infection and the development of anemia.

The Role of Cytokines

TNF-α. The TNF gene is situated close to the lymphotoxin gene to which it has a 28 percent homology. It is also 70 kb from the D locus of the MHC system, setting the stage for potential linkage disequilibrium between TNF-α and D polymorphisms. Monocytes and activated macrophages are the major TNF-α secreting cells. TNF-α expression can be pathogenic, since it might induce loss of anticoagulant activity of the endothelium, leading to diffuse intravascular coagulation, and increase leukocyte adhesion to endothelium, resulting in a shower of free radicals and tissue damage. TNF-α provides an early defense to infection. TNF-α, originating from macrophages and monocytes, has a dose-dependent effect on erythropoiesis: At high doses it induces anemia in rats while at low doses it induces erythroid hyperplasia (Ulrich et al., 1990).

TNF-α levels measured in Zairian children with *P. falciparum* malaria were 71 pg/mL compared to 10 pg/mL in sick children with other diseases (Shaffer et al., 1991). TNF-α levels correlated strongly with hyperparasitemia and less strongly, but significantly, with anemia. Similar results were obtained in other studies, suggesting that severe malaria is associated with high levels of TNF-α and anemia and that a causal relationship between the two might exist (Grau et al., 1989; Nyakundi et al., 1994).

Monocytes cocultured with *P. falciparum* schizont stage parasitized red cells in the process of rupturing exhibit high levels of TNF-α (Pichyanagkul et al., 1994). Isolated pigment (hemozoin) was found to specifically induce release of TNF-α and IL-1β from monocytes, but pigment digestion with proteases inhibited this response. Pigment in *P. falciparum* malaria is released with endothelium attachment during deep-seated schizogony.

Heat-stable antigens from rodent malaria parasites induced release of TNF-α from mouse macrophages in vivo and in vitro. Similarly, analogous antigens of *P. falciparum* triggered release of TNF-α from monocytes (Taverne et al., 1990). Soluble antigens or insoluble elements such as hemozoin released during merozoite-induced red cell rupture may promote the secretion of TNF-α by monocytes and macrophages.

Interleukins, Interferon γ (INF-γ), and Receptors. Plasma from children with severe malaria contained higher levels of IL-2R than children with mild malaria and the IL-2R level was significantly correlated with parasitemia. In contrast, TNF-α, IL-6, IFN-γ, IL-4 or IL-4R did not differ significantly. A transient increase in IL-3 but not stem cell factor (SCF) was seen early in malaria and in 80 percent of patients that developed anemia (Jacobsen et al., 1994). These cytokines might contribute to the anemia of *P. falciparum* malaria (Burgmann et al., 1997). In patients with severe malaria, elevated levels of TNF-α soluble receptor I and absence of parasite-specific IgG3 carried a bleak prognosis (Sarthou et al., 1997). Elevated levels of IL-6 and INF-γ were be found in most patients with *P. falciparum* before treatment, but in very few with *P. vivax* malaria (Kern et al., 1989). TNF-α and IL-6 correlated with parasite density and complications in the clinical course, but INF-γ levels did not. Low plasma concentrations of IL-10 were found in severe malarial anemia, but not in cerebral malaria or in uncomplicated malaria (Kurtzhals et al., 1998). IL-10 mediates feedback regulation of TNF-α and stimulates bone marrow function in vitro. TNF-α concentrations were significantly higher in cerebral malaria than any of the other group, including patients with severe anemia, and the ratio TNF-α/IL-10 was higher in fully conscious patients with severe anemia than in any other group.

Ninety-one patients of different severity were studied for cytokine expression with and without ex vivo stimulation of whole blood with phytohemagglutinin (PHA). On admission, the patients had elevated TNF-α, IFN-γ, and IL-10 compared to posttreatment values. TNF-α on admission was correlated with disease severity and fever, and PHA stimulation of TNF-α production by lymphocytes was suppressed during the acute phase. High PHA-stimulated TNF-α production was correlated, in turn, with rapid defervescence and parasite clearance (Mordmuller et al., 1997). Exogenous IL-10 inhibits malaria antigen-induced cytokine production by reducing mRNA accumulation, with a maximal effect at the first 2 hours of stimulation (Ho et al., 1998).

These data suggest that IL-10 counterregulates the pro-inflammatory response to *P. falciparum*, mediated by TNF-α. Severe malaria might represent partial failure of this regulatory axis.

Phospholipase A2 (PLA$_2$). PLA$_2$ might be involved in the host response to malaria (Vadas et al., 1993). Levels of PLA$_2$ were measured in Seventy-two children with *P. falciparum* malaria, and a highly significant increase was found in both acute malaria patients as well as convalescents. If the pretreatment level of PLA$_2$ was less than 60,000 units, mortality was about 8 percent, while in those with greater than 60,000 units, mortality was over 33 percent. In addition, PLA$_2$ correlated significantly with TNF-α, density of parasitemia, and anemia. PLA$_2$ has no effect on normal porcine red cells, but its membrane-penetrating capacity is enhanced by attaching a fatty acyl chain to Lys-116 (Mollier et al., 1990). A lauric acid derivative of pig PLA$_2$ is capable of attaching to the infected red cells exclusively, causing their lysis but leaving the noninfected red cells intact. Presumably this effect takes advantage of the increase in membrane permeability observed in red cells infected with mature malaria parasites.

Phospholipase A$_2$, but not A$_1$, activity has been detected in red cells infected with *P. falciparum* trophozoites and schizonts, but not in noninfected cells. Chloroquine, quinine, and artemether, three antimalarial drugs, inhibit the activity of the PLA$_2$. Since the IC50 is within the range of the concentrations found in food vacuoles of the malaria parasite, this inhibition might be relevant to the mechanism of action of these drugs.

Contributions by Preexisting Conditions

Preexisting anemia has an effect on mortality from malarial anemia and other malarial complications. This issue is of great concern in the third world, particularly among children and pregnant women (Cornet et al., 1998). Asymptomatic parasitemia, common in the rainy season in endemic regions, may lead to life-threatening anemia, particularly in those with a poor or inadequate response to drug treatment.

SUMMARY

In the past 15 years, considerable progress has been made in understanding the relationships between hemoglobinopathies and malaria. In sickle trait, the malaria parasite promotes sickling of the cell. This permits the spleen to target parasitized cells for removal from the circulation. If this mechanism fails to cull the invaded cell from the circulation, the parasite cannot grow in the next stage of development where conditions favor the polymerization of HbS. Parasite growth in thalassemic erythrocytes is poor, perhaps because of reduced nutrients (hemoglobin) and because host oxidative response is increased to a point that parasite viability is reduced. Erythrocytes

with high levels of HbF can partially protect the carrier from the parasite, especially in the critical first 5 years of life. HbC seems to interfere with schizont-induced lysis of red cells, and therefore the dispersion of merozoites. HbE impairs parasite growth and oxidative stress might also be increased. These and many other mechanisms of protection have evolved as adaptations to the great scourge of malaria.

The price paid for this innate resistance to malaria is that homozygotes or compound heterozygotes with thalassemia major, sickle cell anemia, HbSC disease, HbE-β thalassemia, and to a far lesser extent, homozygous HbC and HbE, are often seriously ill with decreased survival. In developing countries harboring the highest incidence of these diseases the need for medical care overwhelms its availability.

References

Abdalla, SH and Wickramasinghe, SN. (1988). A study of erythroid progenitors in bone marrow of Gambian children with falciparum malaria. *Clin. Lab. Haematol.* 10: 22–40.

Adams, JH, Sim, BK, Dolan, SA et al. (1992). A family of erythrocyte binding proteins of malaria parasites. *Proc. Natl. Acad. Sci. U.S.A.* 89: 7085–7089.

Allison, AC. (1954). Protection afforded by sickle-cell trait against subtertian malarial infection. *Br. Med. J.* 1: 190–195.

Allison, AC and Eugui, EM. (1982). A radical interpretation of immunity to malaria parasites. *Lancet* 2: 1431–1433.

Amato, D and Booth, PB. (1977). Hereditary ovalocytosis in Melanesians. *Papua New Guinea Med. J.* 20: 26–30.

Anderson, BB, Perry, GM, Clements, JE et al. (1989). Genetic and other influences on red cell flavin enzymes, pyridoxine phosphate oxidase and glutathione reductase in families with beta-thalassaemia. *Eur. J. Haematol.* 42: 354–360.

Anderson, BO, Moore BE, and Banarjee, A. (1994). Phospholipase A2 regulates critical inflammatory mediators of multiple organ failure. *J. Surg. Res.* 56: 199–205.

Angus, BJ, Chotivanich, K, Udomsanpetch, R, and White, NJ. (1997). In vivo removal of malaria parasites from red blood cells without their destruction in acute falciparum malaria. *Blood* 90: 2037–2040.

Apibal, S, Suwannurak, R, Bunyarativej, A et al. (1989). Increased ovalocytic red cells and their low parasitemia in malaria infected subjects. *J. Med. Assoc. Thai.* 72: 129–131.

Atamna, H, Pascarmona, G, and Ginsburg, H. (1994). Hexose-monophosphate shunt activity in intact *Plasmodium falciparum*-infected erythrocytes and in free parasites. *Mol. Biochem. Parasitol.* 67: 79–89.

Atamma, H and Ginsburg, H. (1997). The malaria parasite supplies glutathione to its host cell—investigation of glutathione transport and metabolism in human erythrocytes infected with *Plasmodium falciparum. Eur. J. Biochem.* 250: 670–679.

Barker, JE, Bodine, DM, and Birkenmeier, CS. (1986). Synthesis of spectrin and its assembly into the red blood cell cytoskeleton of normal and mutant mice. In *Membrane skeletons and cytoskeletal-membrane associations*. New York: Alan R. Liss. pp. 313–324.

Barnwell JW. (1999). Malaria. A new escape and evasion tactic. *Nature* 398: 562–563.

Beals, PF. (1997). Anaemia in malaria control: A practical approach. *Ann. Trop. Med. Parasitol.* 91: 713–718.

Berck, HP, Felger, I, Barjer, M et al. (1995). Evidence of HLA class II association with antibody response against the malaria vaccine Spf66 in a naturally exposed population. *Am. J. Trop. Med. Hyg.* 53: 284–288.

Bernstein, S. (1980). Inherited hemolytic disease in mice: A review and update. *Lab. Anim. Sci.* 30: 197–205.

Bodine, DM, Birkenmeier, CS, and Barker, JE. (1984). Spectrin-deficient hemolytic anemia in the mouse: Characterization by spectrin synthesis and mRNA activity in reticulocytes. *Cell* 37: 721–729.

Booth, PB, Serjeantson, S, Woodfield, DG, and Amato D. (1977). Selective depressions of blood group antigens associated with hereditary ovalocytosis among Melanesians. *Vox. Sang.* 32: 99–104.

Brockelman, CR, Tan-ariya, P, Piankijagum, A, and Matangkasombut, P. (1983). An in vitro approach to study innate resistance to *Plasmodium falciparum* infection in folic acid deficient individuals. *Asian Pacific J. Allerg. Immun.* 1: 107–112.

Brockelman, CR, Wongsattayanont, B, Tan-ariya, P, and Fucharoen, S. (1987). Thalassemic erythrocytes inhibit in vitro growth of *Plasmodium falciparum*. *J. Clin. Microbiol.* 25: 56–61.

Bunyaratvej, A, Butthep, P, Yuthavong, Y et al. (1986). Increased phagocytosis of *Plasmodium falciparum*-infected erythrocytes with haemoglobin E by peripheral blood monocytes. *Acta Haematol.* 76: 155–163.

Bunyaratvej, A, Butthep, P, Kaewkettong, P, and Yuthabong, Y. (1997). Malaria protection in hereditary ovalocytosis: Relation to red cell deformability, red cell parameters and degree of ovalocytosis. *Southeast Asian J. Trop. Med. Public. Health* 3: 38–42.

Burgmann, H, Looareessuwan, S, Kapiotis, S et al. (1996). Serum levels of erythropoietin in acute Plasmodium falciparum. *Am. J. Trop. Med. Hyg.* 54: 280–283.

Burgmann, H, Looareeswuwan, S, Weinsinger, EC et al. (1997). Levels of stem cell factor and interleukin-3 in serum in acute *Plasmodium falciparum* malaria. *Clin. Diagn. Lab. Immunol.* 4: 226–228.

Chaudhuri, A, Zbrzezna, V, Johnson, C et al. (1989). Purification and characterization of an erythrocyte membrane protein complex carrying Duffy blood group antigenicity. Possible receptor for *Plasmodium vivax* and *Plasmodium knowlesi* malaria parasite. *J. Biol. Chem.* 264: 13770–13774.

Chaudhuri, A, Nielsen, S, Elkjaer, ML et al. (1997). Detection of Duffy antigen in the plasma membranes and caveolae of vascular endothelial and epithelial cells of nonerythroid organs. *Blood* 89: 701–712.

Chitnis, CE and Miller, LH. (1994). Identification of the erythrocyte binding domains of Plasmodium vivax and Plasmodium knowlesi proteins involved in erythrocyte invasion. *J. Exp. Med.* 180(2): 497–506.

Chitnis, CE, Chaudhuri, A, Horuk, R et al. (1996). The domain on the Duffy blood group antigen for binding Plasmodium vivax and P. knowlesi malarial parasites to erythrocytes. *J. Exp. Med.* 184(4): 1531–1536.

Christi, AH, Maalouf, GJ, Marfalia, S et al. (1994). Phosphorylation of protein 4.1 in *Plasmodium falciparum*-infected human red blood cells. *Blood* 83: 3339–3345.

Clements, JE, Anderson, BB, and Perry GM. (1981). Low red cell activity of pyridoxine phosphate oxidase and glutathione reductase associated with thalassaemia. *Biomedicine* 34: 119–225.

Cornet, M, Le Hesran, JY, Fievet, N et al. (1998). Prevalence of and risk factors for anemia in young children in southern Cameroon. *Am. J. Trop. Med. Hyg.* 58: 606–611.

Dahr, W, Uhlenbruck, G, Gunson, HH, and van der Hart, M. (1975). Molecular basis of Tn-polyglutinability. *Vox Sang.* 29: 36–43.

Delacollette, C, Taelman, H, and Wery, M. (1995). An etiologic study of hemoglobinuria and blackwater fever in the Kivu Mountains, Zaire. *Ann. Soc. Belg. Med. Trop.* 75(1): 51–63.

Delaunay, J. (1995). Genetic disorders of the red cell membrane. *Crit. Rev. Oncol. Hematol.* 19: 79–110.

Dennis, EA. (1994). Diversity of group types, regulation and function of Phospholipase A_2. *J. Mol. Biol.* 268: 13060–13069.

Dormer, P, Dietrich, M, Kern, P, and Horstmann, RD. (1983). Ineffective erythropoiesis in acute human P. falciparum malaria. *Blut* 46: 279–288.

Ducrocq, R, Bennani, M, Bellis, G et al. (1994). Hemoglobinopathies in the Dogon Country: Presence of β^S, β^C, and δ' Genes. *Am. J. Hematol.* 46: 245–247.

Fabry, ME, Nagel, RL, Pachnis, A et al. (1992a). High expression of human β^S and α-globins in transgenic mice: 1) Hemoglobin composition and hematological consequences. *Proc. Natl. Acad. Sci.* 89: 12150–12154.

Fabry, ME, Costantini, FD, Pachnis, A et al. (1992b). High expression of human β^S and α-genes in transgenic mice: II) Red cell abnormalities, organ damage, and the effect of hypoxia. *Proc. Natl. Acad. Sci.* 89: 12155–12159.

Fabry, ME, Romero, JR, Sususka, SM et al. (1998). Hemoglobin C in transgenic mice with full mouse globin knockout. *Blood.* 92: 330a.

Fang, XD, Kaslow, DC, Adams, JH, and Miller, LH. (1991). Cloning of the Plasmodium vivax Duffy receptor. *Mol. Biochem. Parasitol.* 44(1): 125–132.

Facer, CA and Mitchell, GH. (1984). Wr^b negative erythrocytes are susceptible to invasion by malaria parasites. *Lancet* 2: 758–761.

Facer, CA. (1995): Erythrocytes carrying mutations in spectrin and protein 4.1 show differing sensitivities to invasion by Plasmodium falciparum. *Parasitol. Res.* 81(1): 52–7.

Flatz, G, Pik, C, and Sundharagiati, B. (1964). Malaria and haemoglobin E in Thailand. *Lancet* 2: 385–391.

Flatz, G. (1967). Hemoglobin E: Distribution and population dynamics. *Humangenetik* 3: 189–234.

Flint, J, Hill, AV, Bowden, DK et al. (1986). High frequencies of alpha thalassemia are the result of natural selection by malaria. *Nature* 321: 744–747.

Ford, EB. (1945). Polymorphism. *Biol. Rev.* 20: 73–88.

Friedman, MJ. (1978). Erythrocytic mechanism of sickle cell resistance to malaria. *Proc. Natl. Acad. Sci. U.S.A.* 75: 1994–2000.

Friedman, MJ. (1979a). Ultrastructural damage to the malaria parasite in the sickled cell. *Protozoology* 26: 195–199.

Friedman, MJ. (1979b). Oxidant damage mediates variant red cell resistance to malaria. *Nature* 280: 245–249.

Friedman, MJ, Roth, EF, Nagel, RL, and Trager, W. (1979a). *Plasmodium falciparum*: Physiological interactions with the human sickle cell. *Exp. Parasitol.* 4: 73–80.

Friedman, MJ, Roth, EF, Nagel, RL, and Trager, W. (1979b). The role of hemoglobins C, S and N Baltimore in the inhibition of malaria parasite development in vitro. *Am. J. Trop. Med. Hyg.* 28: 777–780.

Frischer, H and Bowman, J. (1975). Hemoglobin E, an oxidatively unstable mutation. *J. Lab. Clin. Med.* 85: 531–538.

Garcia, A, Cot, M, Chipaux, JP et al. (1998). Genetic control of blood infection levels in human malaria: Evidence for a complex genetic model. *Am. J. Trop. Med. Hyg.* 58: 480–488.

Ginsburg, H, Handeli, S, Friedman, S et al. (1986). Effects of red blood cell potassium and hypertonicity on the growth of *Plasmodium falciparum* in culture. *Z. Parasitenkd.* 72: 185–192.

Glaser, KB, Mobilio, D, Chang, JY, and Senko, N. (1993). Phospholipase A2 enzymes: Regulation and inhibition. *Trends Pharmacol. Sci.* 14: 92–98.

Grau, GE, Taylor, TE, Molineaux, ME et al. (1989). Tumor necrosis factor and disease severity in children with falciparum malaria. *N. Engl. J. Med.* 320: 1586–1591.

Gravenor, MB, McLean, AR, and Kwiatkowski, D. (1995). The regulation of malaria parasitemia: Parameter estimates for a population model. *Parasitology* 110: 115–119.

Hadley, TJ and Miller, LH. (1988). Invasion of erythrocytes by malaria parasites: Erythrocyte ligands and parasite receptors. *Prog. Allergy* 41: 49–56.

Hadley, TJ and Peiper, SC. (1997). From malaria to chemokine receptor: Emerging physiological role of the Duffy blood group antigen. *Blood* 89: 3077–3091.

Hadley, TJ, Saul, A, Lamont, G et al. (1983). Resistance of Melanesian elliptocytes (ovalocytes) to invasion by *Plasmodium knowlesi* and *Plasmodium falciparum* malaria parasites *in vitro. J. Clin. Invest.* 71: 780–787.

Hadley, TJ, David, PH, McGinnis, MH, and Miller, LH. (1984). Identification of an erythrocyte component carrying the Duffy blood group F_y^a antigen. *Science* 223: 597–603.

Hadley, TJ, Klotz, FW, Pasvol, G et al. (1987). Falciparum malaria parasites invade erythrocytes that lack glycophorin A and B ($M^k M^k$). *J. Clin. Invest.* 80: 1190–1195.

Haldane, JBS. (1949). The rate of mutation of human genes. Proc VIII Int Cong Genet. Hereditas. 35(supplement): 267–273.

Hill, AVS, Allsopp, CEM, Kwiatkowski, D et al. (1991). Common west African HLA antigens are associated with protection from severe malaria. *Nature* 352: 595–600.

Hill, AVS, Aidoo, M, Allsopp CE et al. (1994). Interactions between *Plasmodium falciparum* and HLA molecules. *Biochem. Soc. Trans.* 2: 282–285.

Ho, M, White, NJ, Looareesuwan, S et al. (1990). *Infect. Dis.* 161: 555–561.

Ho, M, Schollaardt, T, Snape, S et al. (1998). Endogenous interleukin-10 modulates proinflammatory response in *Plasmodium falciparum* malaria. *J. Infect. Dis.* 178: 520–525.

Hogh, B, Petersen, E, Crandall, I et al. (1994). Immune response to band 3 neoantigens on *Plasmodium falciparum*-infected erythrocytes in subjects living in an area of intense malaria transmission are associated with low parasite density and high hematocrit value. *Infect. Immun.* 62: 4362–4366.

Hood, AT, Fabry, ME, Costantini, F et al. (1996). Protection from lethal malaria in transgenic mice expressing sickle hemoglobin. *Blood* 87: 1600–1603.

Horuk, R and Peiper, SC. (1996). The Duffy antigen receptor for chemokines. In Horuk, R, editors. *Chemoattractant ligands and their receptor.* New York: CRC Press.

Horuk, R, Martin, A, Hesselgesser, J et al. (1996). The Duffy antigen receptor for chemokines: Structural analysis and expression in the brain. *J. Leuk. Biol.* 59: 29–35.

Ifediba, TC, Stern, A, Ibrahim, A, and Rieder, RF. (1985). *Plasmodium falciparum* in vitro: Diminished growth in hemoglobin H disease erythrocytes. *Blood* 65: 452–456.

Jacobsen, PH, Morris-Jones, S, Theander, TG et al. (1994). Increased plasma levels of soluble II-2R are associated with severe *Plasmodium falciparum malaria. Clin. Exp. Immunol.* 96: 98–103.

Jarolim, P, Rubin, HI, Zhai, S et al. (1992). Band 3 Memphis: A widespread polymorphism with abnormal electrophoretic mobility of erythrocyte band 3 caused by substitution AAG→GAG(Lys→Glu) in codon 56. *Blood* 80: 1592–1120.

Jensen, JB and Trager, W. (1977). *Plasmodium falciparum* in culture; use of outdated blood and description of the candle jar method. *J. Parasitol.* 63: 833–838.

Jootar S, Chaisiripoomkere W, Pholvicha P et al. (1993). Suppression of erythroid progenitor cells during malarial infection in Thai a caused by serum inhibitor. *Clin. Lab. Haematol.* 15(2): 87–92.

Kaul, DK, Raventos-Suarez, C, Olson, JA, and Nagel, RL. (1985). The role of membrane knobs in microvascular obstruction induced by *Plasmodium falciparum*-infected erythrocytes. *Trans. Assoc. Am. Phys.* XCVIII: 204–214.

Kaul, DK, Nagel, RL, Llena, JF, and Shear, HL. (1994). Cerebral malaria in mice: Demonstration of cytoadherence of infected red cells and microrheologic correlates. *Am. J. Trop. Med. Hyg.* 50: 512–521.

Kaul, DK, Liu, X-D, Nagel, RL, and Shear, HL. (1998). Microvascular hemodynamics and in vivo evidence for the role of intercellular adhesion molecule-1 in the sequestration of infected red blood cells in a mouse model of lethal malaria. *Am. J. Trop. Med. Hyg.* 58: 240–247.

Kern, PF, Hemmer, CJ, Van Damme, J et al. (1989). Elevated tumor necrosis factor alpha and interleukin 6 serum levels as markers for complicated *Plasmodium falciparum. Am. J. Med.* 87: 139–143.

Kidson, C, Lamont, G, Saul, A, and Nurse, GT. (1981). Ovalocytic erythrocytes from Melanesians are resistant to invasion by malaria parasites in culture. *Proc. Natl. Acad. Sci. U.S.A.* 78: 5829–5834.

Killick-Kendrick, R. (1978). Taxonomy, zoogeography and evolution. In Killick-Kendrick, R and Peters, W, editors. *Rodent malaria.* London: Academic Press. pp. 1–52.

Kirk, K and Horner, HA. (1995). Novel anion dependency of induced cation transport in malaria-infected erythrocytes. *J. Biol. Chem.* 270: 24270–24275.

Kolata, G. (1984). The search for a malaria vaccine. *Science* 226: 679–684.

Kramer, R and Ginsburg, H. (1991). Calcium transport and compartment analysis of free and exchangeable calcium in *Plasmodium falciparum*-infected red blood red cells. *J. Protozool.* 38: 594–601.

Kurtzhals, JA, Rodrigues, O, Addae, M et al. (1997). Reversible suppression if bone marrow response to erythropoietin in *Plasmodium falciparum* malaria. *Br. J. Haematol.* 97: 169–174.

Kurtzhals, JA, Adabayeri, V, Goka, BQ et al. (1998). Low plasma concentrations of interleukin 10 in severe malarial anaemia compared with cerebral and uncomplicated malaria. *Lancet* 351: 1768–1772.

Landau, I and Boulard, Y. (1978). Life cycles and morphology. In Killick-Kendrick, R and Peters, W, editors. *Rodent malaria.* London: Academic Press. pp. 53–84.

Lehmann, H. (1972). Abnormal hemoglobins. In Jonxis, JHP and Delafresnaye, JF, editors. Oxford: Oxford University Press. p. 313.

Leikin, SL, Gallagher, D, Kinney, TR et al. (1989). Mortality in children and adolescent with sickle cell disease. Cooperative study of sickle cell disease. *Pediatrics* 84: 500–508.

Lie-Injo, LE, Fix, A, Bolton, JM, and Gilman RH. (1972). Hemoglobin E-hereditary elliptocytosis in Malayan aborigines. *Acta Haematol.* 47: 210–215.

Lin, MJ, Nagel, RL, and Hirsch, RE. (1989). The acceleration of hemoglobin C crystallization by hemoglobin S. *Blood* 74: 1823–1825.

Liu, SC, Palek, J, Yi, SJ et al. (1995). Molecular basis of altered blood cell membrane properties in Southeast Asia ovalocytosis: Role of the mutant band 3 protein in band 3 oligomerization and retention by the membrane skeleton. *Blood* 86: 349–358.

Livingston, FB. (1971). Malaria and human polymorphisms. *Ann. Rev. Genet.* 5: 33–38.

Looareesuwan, S, Ho, M, Wattanagoon, Y et al. (1987). Dynamic alteration in splenic function during acute falciparum malaria. *N. Engl. J. Med.* 317: 675–679.

Looareesuwan, S, Davis, TM, Pukrittayakamee, S et al. (1991). Erythrocyte survival in severe falciparum malaria. *Acta Trop.* 48: 263–270.

Luse, S and Miller, LH. (1971). *Plasmodium falciparum* malaria: Ultrastructure of parasitized erythrocytes in cardiac vessels. *Am. J. Trop. Med. Hyg.* 20: 660–665.

Lustig, HJ, Nussenzweig, V, and Nussenzweig, RS. (1977). Erythrocyte membrane-associated immunoglobulins during malaria infection of mice. *J. Immunol.* 119: 210–216.

Luzzatto, L, Nwachukes-Jarrett, ES, and Reddy, S. (1970). Increased sickling of parasitized erythrocytes as mechanisms of resistance against malaria in sickle cell trait. *Lancet* 1949 1: 319–403.

Luzzi, GA, Merry, AH, Newbold, CI et al. (1991). Surface antigen expression of *Plasmodium falciparum*-infected erythrocytes is modified in α- and β-thalassemia. *J. Exp. Med.* 173: 785–791.

McGuire, W, Hill, AVS, Allsopp, CEM et al. (1994). Variation in the TNF-α promoter region associated with susceptibility to cerebral malaria. *Nature* 371: 508–511.

Migot, F, Chougnet, C, Perichon, B et al. (1995). Lack of correlation between HLA class II alleles and immune responses to Pf155/RESA from *Plasmodium falciparum* in Madagascar. *Am. J. Trop. Med. Hyg.* 52: 252–257.

Mitchell, GH, Hadley, TJ, McGinnies, MH et al. (1986). Invasion of erythrocytes by *Plasmodium falciparum* malaria parasites: Evidence for receptor heterogeneity and two receptors. *Blood* 67: 1519–1523.

Miller, LH, Mason, SJ, Dvorak, JA et al. (1975). Erythrocyte receptors for *Plasmodium knowlesi* malaria: Duffy blood group determinants. *Science* 189: 561–566.

Miller, LH, Mason, SJ, Clyde, DF, and McGinniss, AB. (1976). The resistance factor to *Plasmodium vivax* in Blacks: The Duffy-blood-group genotype, F_yF_y. *N. Engl. J. Med.* 295: 302–306.

Miller, LH, Aikawa, M, Johnson, JG, and Shiroishi, T. (1979). Interaction between cytochalasin B-treated malarial parasites and red cells. Attachment and junction formation. *J. Exp. Med.* 149: 172–177.

Modiano, D, Petrarca, V, Sirima, BS et al. (1996). Different response to *Plasmodium falciparum* malaria in West African sympatric ethnic groups. *Proc. Natl. Acad. Sci. U.S.A.* 93: 11320–13211.

Mohan, K, Dubey, ML, Ganguly, NK, and Mahajan, RC. (1995). *Plasmodium falciparum*: Role of activated blood monocytes in erythrocyte membrane damage and red cell loss during malaria. *Exp. Parasitol.* 80: 54–63.

Mohandas, N, Lie-Injo, LE, Friedman, M, and Mak, JW. (1984). Rigid membranes of Malayan ovalocytes: A likely genetic barrier against malaria. *Blood* 63: 1385–1391.

Mollier, P, Chwetzoff, S, and Menez, A. (1990). A monoclonal antibody recognizing a conserved epitope in a group of phospholipases A2. *Mol. Immunol.* 27(1): 7–15.

Moore, KW, O'Garra, A, de Waal Malefyt, R et al. (1993). Interleukin-10. *Ann. Rev. Immunol.* 11: 165–190.

Mordmuller, BG, Metzger, WG, Juillard, P, Bri et al. (1997). Tumor necrosis factor in *Plasmodium falciparum* malaria: High plasma level is associated with fever, but high production capacity is associated with rapid fever clearance. *Eur. Cytokine Netw.* 8: 29–35.

Nagel, RL. (1994). Lessons from transgenic mouse lines expressing sickle hemoglobin. *Proc. Soc. Exp. Biol. Med.* 205: 274–281.

Nagel, RL. (1998). A knock-out of a mouse: Transgenic mice models for sickle cell anemia. *N. Engl. J. Med.* 339: 194–195.

Nagel, RL and Roth, EF. (1989). Malaria and red cell genetic defects. *Blood* 74: 1213–1221.

Nagel, RL, Raventos-Suarez, C, Fabry, ME et al. (1981). Impairment of the growth of *Plasmodium falciparum* in HBEE erythrocytes. *J. Clin. Invest.* 64: 303–305.

Naqvi, R, Ahmed, E, Akhtar, F et al. (1996). Predictors of outcome of malaria renal failure. *Ren. Fail.* 18: 687–688.

Nash, GB, O'Brien, E, Gordon Smith, EC, and Dormandy, JA. (1989). Abnormalities in the mechanical properties of red blood cells caused by *Plasmodium falciparum*. *Blood* 74: 855–861.

Nichols, ME, Rubinstein, P, Barnwell, J et al. (1987). A new human Duffy blood group specificity defined by a murine monoclonal antibody. Immunogenetics and association with susceptibility to *Plasmodium vivax*. *J. Exp. Med.* 166: 776–780.

Nyakundi, JN, Warn, P, Newton, C et al. (1994). Serum necrosis factor in children suffering from *Plasmodium falciparum* infection in Kilifi district, Kenya. *Trans. R. Soc. Trop. Med. Hyg.* 88: 667–670.

O'Donnell, A, Allen, SJ, Mgone, CS et al. (1998). Red cell morphology and malaria anaemia in children with Southeast Asia ovalocytosis band 3 in Papua New Guinea. *Br. J. Haematol.* 101: 407–412.

Olson, JA and Nagel, RL. (1986). Synchronized cultures of *P. falciparum* in abnormal red cells: The mechanism of the inhibition of growth in HBCC cells. *Blood* 67: 997–1000.

Orjih, AU, Benyal, HS, Chevli, R, and Fitch, CD. (1981). Hemin lyses malaria parasites. *Science* 214: 667–700.

Orjih, AU, Chevli, R, and Fitch, CD. (1985). Toxic heme in sickle cells: An explanation for death of malaria parasites. *Am. J. Trop. Med. Hyg.* 34: 223–227.

Pasvol, G. (1980). The interaction between sickle haemoglobin and the malarial parasite *Plasmodium falciparum*. *Trans. R. Soc. Trop. Med. Hyg.* 74: 701–705.

Pasvol, G and Wilson, RJM. (1982). The interaction of malaria parasites with red blood cells. *Br. Med. Bull.* 38: 133–140.

Pasvol, G, Weatherall, DJ, Wilson, RJM et al. (1976). Fetal haemoglobin and malaria. *Lancet* 1: 1269–1272.

Pasvol, G, Weatherall, DJ, and Wilson, RJM. (1977). Effects of foetal haemoglobin on susceptibility of red cells to *Plasmodium falciparum*. *Nature* 270: 171–173.

Pasvol, G, Weatherall, DJ, and Wilson, RJM. (1978). Cellular mechanism for the protective effect of haemoglobins against P. falciparum malaria. *Nature* 274: 701–703.

Pasvol, G, Chasis, JA, Mohandas, N et al. (1989). Inhibition of malarial parasite invasion by monoclonal antibodies against glycophorin A correlates with reduction in red cell membrane deformability. *Blood* 74: 1836–1843.

Paulitschke, M and Nash, GB. (1993). Membrane rigidity of red blood cells parasitized by different strains of *Plasmodium falciparum*. *J. Lab. Clin. Med.* 122: 581–589.

Peiper, SC, Wang, ZX, Neote, K et al. (1995). The Duffy antigen/receptor for chemokines (DARC) is expressed in endothelial cells of Duffy who lack the erythrocyte receptor. *J. Exp. Med.* 181: 1311–1317.

Perkins, ME. (1981). Inhibitory effects of erythrocyte membrane proteins on the in vitro invasion of the human malarial parasite *(Plasmodium falciparum)* into its host cell. *J. Cell. Biol.* 90: 563–567.

Phillips, RE and Pasvol, G. (1992). Anaemia of *Plasmodium falciparum* malaria. *Baillieres Clin. Haematol.* 5: 315–330.

Phillips, RE, Looareesuwan, S, Warrell DA et al. (1986). The importance of anaemia in cerebral and uncomplicated falciparum malaria: Role of complications, dyserythropoiesis and iron sequestration. *Q. J. Med.* 58: 305–323.

Phillips, RE, Nantel, S, and Benny, WB. (1990). Exchange transfusion as an adjunct to the treatment for severe falciparum malaria: Case report and review. *Rev. Infect. Dis.* 12: 1100–1108.

Pichyanagkul, S, Saengkrai, P, and Webster, HK. (1994). *Plasmodium falciparum* pigment induces monocytes to release high levels of tumor necrosis factor in interleukin 1 beta. *Am. J. Trop. Med. Hyg.* 51: 430–435.

Pongponratn, E, Riganti, M, Bunnag, D, and Harinasuta, T. (1987). Spleen in falciparum malaria: ultrastructural study. *Southeast Asian J Trop Med Public Health* 18: 491–501.

Rachmilewitz, EA, Shinar, E, Shalev, O et al. (1985). Erythrocyte membrane alterations in β-thalassaemia. *Clin. Haematol.* 14: 163–182.

Raventos-Suarez, C, Kaul, DK, Macaluso, F, and Nagel, RL. (1985). Membrane knobs are required for the microcirculatory obstruction induced by *Plasmodium falciparum*-infected erythrocytes. *Proc. Natl. Acad. Sci. U.S.A.* 82: 3829–3833.

Rihet, P, Traore, Y, Abel, L et al. (1998). Malaria in humans: *Plasmodium falciparum* blood infection levels are linked to chromosome 5q31–q33. *Am. J. Hum. Genet.* 63: 498–505.

Rosenberg, EB, Strickland, GT, Yang, S, and Whalen, GE. (1973). IgM antibodies to red cells and autoimmune anemia in patients with malaria. *Am. J. Trop. Med. Hyg.* 22: 146–151.

Roth, EF Jr, Friedman, M, Ueda, Y et al. (1978). Sickling rates of human AS red cells infected in vitro with *Plasmodium falciparum* malaria. *Science* 202: 650–652.

Roth, EF Jr, Raventos-Suarez, C, Rinaldi, A, and Nagel, RL. (1983). Glucose-6-phosphate dehydrogenase deficiency inhibits in vitro growth of *Plasmodium falciparum*. *Proc. Natl. Acad. Sci. U.S.A.* 80: 298–299.

Roth, E, Raventos-Suarez, C, Gilbert, H et al. (1984). Oxidative stress and falciparum malaria: A critical review of the evidence. In *Malaria and the red cell*. New York: Alan R. Liss. pp. 35–43.

Roth, EF Jr, Shear, HL, Costantini, F et al. (1988). Malaria in β-thalassemic mice and the effects of the transgenic human β-globin gene and splenectomy. *J. Lab. Clin. Med.* 111: 35–41.

Sabolovic, D, Bouanga, JC, Danis, M et al. (1994). Alterations in uninfected red blood cells in malaria. *Parasitol. Res.* 80: 70–73.

Sandler, SG, Kravitz, C, Sharon, R et al. (1979). The Duffy blood group system in Israeli Jews and Arabs. *Vox Sang.* 37: 41–44.

Santiyanont, R, and Wilairat, P. (1981). Red cells containing haemoglobin E do not inhibit malaria parasite development in vitro. *Am. J. Trop. Med. Hyg.* 30: 541–544.

Sarthou, JL, Angel, G, Aribot, G et al. (1997). Prognostic value of anti-*Plasmodium falciparum* specific immunoglobin G3, cytokines, and their soluble receptors in West African patients with severe malaria. *Infect. Immun.* 65: 3271–3276.

Saul, A, Lamont, G, Sawyer, W, and Kidson, C. (1984). Decreased membrane deformability in Melanesian ovalocytes from Papua New Guinea. *J. Cell Biol.* 98: 1348–1351.

Schrier, SL. (1997). Pathobiology of thalassemic erythrocytes. *Curr. Opin. Hematol.* 4: 75–78.

Schulman, S, Roth, EF, Jr. Cheng, B et al. (1990). Growth of *Plasmodium falciparum* in human erythrocytes containing abnormal membrane proteins. *Proc. Natl. Acad. Sci. U.S.A.* 87: 7339–7343.

Schwartz, RS, Olson, JA, Raventos-Suarez, C, Y et al. (1987). Altered plasma membrane phospholipid organization in *Plasmodium falciparum*-infected human erythrocytes. *Blood* 69: 401–407.

Sen, R, Tewari, AD, Sehgal, PK, et al. (1994). Clinico-haematological profile in acute and chronic *Plasmodium falciparum* malaria in children. *J. Commun. Dis.* 26: 31–38.

Senok, AC, Li, K, Nelson, EA et al. (1998). Flow cytometric assessment of oxidant stress in age-fractionated thalassaemic trait erythrocytes and its relationship to in vitro growth of *Plasmodium falciparum*. *Parasitology* 116: 1–6.

Serjeantson, S, Bryson, K, Amato, D, and Babona, D. (1977). Malaria and hereditary ovalocytosis. *Hum. Genet.* 37: 161–164.

Shaffer, N, Grau, GE, Dedberg, K et al. (1991). Tumor necrosis factor and severe malaria. *J. Infect. Dis.* 163: 96–101.

Shear, HL, Roth, EF Jr, Ng, C, and Nagel, RL. (1991). Resistance to malaria in ankyrin and spectrin deficient mice. *Br. J. Haematol.* 78: 558–560.

Shear, HL, Roth, EF Jr, Fabry, ME et al. (1993). Transgenic mice expressing human sickle hemoglobin are partially resistant to rodent malaria. *Blood* 81: 222–226.

Shinar, E and Rachmilewitz, EA. (1990). Differences in the pathophysiology of hemolysis of alpha and beta-thalassemia red blood cells. *Ann. N.Y. Acad. Sci.* 612: 118–126.

Sicard, D, Lieurzo, Y, Lapoumeroulie, C, and Labie, D. (1979). High genetic polymorphism of hemoglobin disorders in Laos. *Hum. Genet.* 50: 327–331.

Sim, BKL, Chitnis, CE, Wasniowska, K et al. (1994). Receptor and ligand domains for invasion of erythrocytes by *Plasmodium falciparum* malaria. *Science* 264: 1941–1943.

Skow, LC, Burkhart, BA, Johnson, FM et al. (1983). A mouse model for β-thalassemia. *Cell* 34: 1043–1052.

Tanabe, K, Izumo, A, and Kageyama, K. (1986). Growth of *Plasmodium falciparum* in sodium-enriched human erythrocytes. *Am. J. Trop. Med. Hyg.* 35: 476–481.

Tanner, MJ, Ansteee, DJ, Mallison, G et al. (1988). Effect of endoglycosidase F-peptidyl N-glycosidase F preparations on the surface components of the human erythrocyte. *Carbohydrate Res.* 178: 203–210.

Taverne, J, Bate, CA, Sarkar, DA et al. (1990). Human and murine macrophages produce TNF in response to soluble antigens of *Plasmodium falciparum*. *Parasite Immunol.* 12: 33–43.

Teo, CG and Wong, HB. (1985). The innate resistance of thalassemia to malaria: A review of the evidence and possible mechanisms. *Singapore Med. J.* 26: 504–508.

Trager, W. (1957). The nutrition of an intracellular parasite (avian malaria). *Acta Trop. Med.* 14: 289–393.

Troye-Blomber, M, Olerup, O, Larsson, A et al. (1991). Failure to detect class II associations of the human immune response induced by repeated malaria infections to *Plasmodium falciparum* antigen Pf115/RESA. *Int. Immunol.* 3: 1043–1051.

Udomsangpetch, R, Sueblinvong, T, Pattanapanyasat, K et al. (1993). Alteration in cytoadherence and rosetting of *Plasmodium falciparum*-infected thalassemic red blood cells. *Blood* 82: 3752–3759.

Ulrich, TR, del Castillo, J, and Yin, S. (1990). Tumor necrosis factor exerts dose-dependent effects on erythropoiesis and myelopoiesis in vivo. *Exp. Hematol.* 18: 311–315.

Vadas, P, Taylor, TE, Chimsuku, L et al. (1993). Increased serum phospholipase A2 in Malawian children with falciparum malaria. *Am. J. Trop. Med. Hyg.* 49: 455–459.

Vernes, AJM, Haynes, JD, Tang, DB et al. (1986). Decreased growth of *Plasmodium falciparum* in red cells containing haemoglobin E, a role for oxidative stress, and a sero-epidemiological correlation. *Trans. R. Soc. Trop. Med. Hyg.* 80: 642–648.

Weatherall, DJ and Clegg, JB. (1981). *The Thalaessemia Syndromes*. 3rd ed. Oxford: Blackwell Scientific Publications.

Weatherall, DJ, Abdalla, S, and Pippard, MJ. (1983). The anaemia of *Plasmodium falciparum* malaria. *Ciba Found Symp.* 94: 74–97.

Weisenfeld, SL. (1967). Sickle-cell trait in human biological and cultural evolution. *Science* 157: 1134–1140.

Welch, SG. (1977). The Duffy blood group and malaria prevalence in Gambian West Africans. *Trans. R. Soc. Trop. Med. Hyg.* 71: 295–299.

Wertheimer, SP and Barnwell, JW. (1989). *Plasmodium vivax* interaction with the human Duffy blood group glycoprotein: Identification of a parsite receptor-like protein. *Exp. Parasitol.* 69: 340–348.

Wickramasinghe, SN, Abdalla, S, and Weatherall, DJ. (1982). Cell cycle distribution of erythroblasts in *P. falciparum* malaria. *Scand. J. Haematol.* 29: 83–88.

Wickramsinghe, SN, Looareesuwan, S, Nagachinta, B, and White, NJ. (1989). Dyserythropoiesis and ineffective erythropoiesis in plasmodium vivax malaria. *Br. J. Haematol.* 72: 91–99.

Willcox, M, Bjorkman, A, and Brohult, J. (1983). Falciparum malaria and β-thalassemia trait in northern Liberia. *Ann. Trop. Med. Parasitol.* 77: 335–339.

Williams, TN, Maitland, K, Bennett, S et al. (1996). High incidence of malaria in alpha-thalassaemic children. *Nature* 383: 522–525.

Winograd, E and Sherman, IW. (1989). Naturally occurring anti-band 3 autoantibodies recognize a high molecular weight protein on the surface of *Plasmodium falciparum* infected erythrocytes. *Biochem. Biophys. Res. Commun.* 160: 1357–1363.

Yi-qin, L, Jun-fan, L, Nagel, RL, and Blumenfeld, O. (1987). Erythrocyte membrane glycophorins of Central Africans and some hematological patients. *Chinese Med. J.* 100: 787–794.

Young, MD, Eyles, DE, and Burgess, RW. (1958). Experimental testing of Negroes to *Plasmodium vivax*. *J. Parasitol.* 44: 371–376.

Yuthavong, Y, Butthep, P, Bunyaratvej, A et al. (1988). Impaired parasite growth and increased susceptibility to phagocytosis of *Plasmodium falciparum* infected alpha thalassemia or hemoglobin Constant Spring red cells. *Am. J. Clin. Pathol.* 89: 521–526.

31

Worldwide Distribution of β Thalassemia

DIMITRIS LOUKOPOULOS
PANAGOULA KOLLIA

INTRODUCTION

Originally thought to be confined to the Mediterranean basin, the β thalassemias are now identified in many populations extending in a beltlike fashion over the Near East, the South Caucasus countries, the Indian peninsula, and Southeast Asia. β Thalassemia is also common in people of African descent while extremely rare among Northern Europeans, Japanese, Native Americans, and Australian aborigines. In nations that sustained immigration, the presence of β thalassemia reflects the geographic origin of the immigrant populations. To determine the world distribution of β thalassemia, investigators using a variety of simple techniques and criteria studied thousands of subjects, mostly from 1950 to 1980. Genetic and hematologic data left no doubt that the disease was heterogeneous. Subsequently, application of molecular techniques revealed that (1) the genetic defects underlying the β-thalassemia phenotype are extremely diverse, and (2) within individual populations, a few molecular defects, or even a unique one, could account for most of the cases. The latter finding is of utmost importance not only for its anthropogeographic and historic implications (Flint et al., 1993), but also because it facilitates disease prevention via large-scale carrier identification programs and prenatal diagnosis of at-risk pregnancies (WHO, 1982) (see Chapter 36). Numerous surveys of the distribution of the various molecular defects leading to β thalassemia have accumulated over recent years. In general, even though relatively small numbers of individuals were examined, there are no major disagreements. The present chapter aims to put together the essence of those surveys.

The total number of β-thalassemia patients is difficult to estimate. Sources of information include anecdotes, sporadic case reports from countries where the diagnosis constitutes an interesting finding, and formal registries produced on "representative" population samples in several developing countries with the goal of setting up national prevention programs. How representative the sample populations have actually been is difficult to assess, especially when the surveys cover large territories and do not consider the ethnic origin of those surveyed. Moreover, the fact that the diagnostic criteria used in some large surveys were not standardized or even noted also limits the accuracy of the reported frequencies. The number of surviving homozygous β-thalassemia (thalassemia major) patients depends greatly on the level of the care they received. As a rule, for a given prevalence of heterozygotes, the number of living patients with β thalassemia major varies with the level of medical care. As expected, the balance between prevalence and medical care determines the impact of the disease in each country and dictates the appropriate approach toward its control. A further factor to be considered in the assessment of the total impact of β thalassemia on the public health services of the involved countries often is the frequent co-inheritence of β thalassemia with HbS, HbE, and other hemoglobinopathies.

For the time being, the extensive surveys recorded by Livingstone in 1985 and the WHO registries appear to be the most reliable sources of information. The latter were initially compiled by an *ad hoc* WHO Committee (WHO Reports 1982, 1985, 1989) and are now continually updated by Professor B. Modell in the United Kingdom on behalf of the organization. The extensive data kindly provided by Dr. Modell are summarized in Table 31.1 (Angastiniotis and Modell, 1998; Modell et al., 1998), which shows the incidence of β-thalassemia carriers (and carriers of HbS and HbE) in the main WHO regions along with the expected annual number of births of babies with homozygous β thalassemia or with compound heterozygosity for β thalassemia and a hemoglobinopathy. According to those calculations, about 30,000 infants are born with β thalassemia annually. The number has been dramatically reduced in the few countries where effective prevention programs have been implemented. Assuming a mean survival of 20 years for patients liv-

Table 31.1. Global Distribution and Impact of β-Thalassemia, by WHO Regions (in Rough Approximation)

	Population $\times 10^6$	% carriers of β-thalassemia	Annual number of births $\times 10^6$	Annual number of newborns with β-thalassemia	Total annual number of newborns with any hemoglobinopathy
Europe	850	0.87	13.0	2,100*	4,000†
Nonendemic regions					
Indigenous	260	Almost nil	3.4	0	0
Minority groups	13	Reflects origin	0.27	250*	500
Endemic regions	300	0.2–8.0	5.00	160*	1,800
Greece	10	8.0	0.10	120*	130
Turkey	60	3.0	1.60	350*	500
Italy	55	4.0	0.55	320*	330
Uzbekistan	18	3.0	0.60	320	320
Tajikistan	5	5.0	0.15	180	180
Azerbaijan	8	5.5	0.15	160	180
Eastern Mediterranean Region	400	4.0	15.0	8,450	15,100†
Pakistan	115	5.0	3.50	3,100	3,100
Iran	55	3.0	2.40	1,200	1,200
Iraq	55	3.0	0.85	550	1,500
Sudan	27	4.0	1.20	1,300	2,350
Morocco	27	3.0	0.95	750	1,850
Egypt	55	2.7	2.10	600	800
Afghanistan	15	3.0	1.80	350	350
Tunisia	10	3.5	0.30	150	350
Cyprus	0.7	15.0	0.10	<100*	<100*
Saudi Arabia	14	1.0	0.70	35	280
African Region					
Sub-Saharan Africa	250	0	13.0	A few	200,000‡/**
Nigeria	112	0	5.5	Almost nil	108,000
Zaire	38	0	1.6	Almost nil	28,000
Ghana, Cameroon, Benin, Angola, Ivory Coast, Mali, Congo, Guinea, etc.	80	0	5.0	A few	50,000

North Africa and islands	110	0–2.0	5.0	400	20,000‡/**
Tanzania, Kenya, Uganda	75	0	3.6	Almost nil	18,000
Algeria	26	2.0	0.9	300	700
Mauritius	2	2.0	0.2	<50	<50
Reunion	2.5	2.0	0.2	<50	<50
Southeast Asian Region	1,300	4.0	40.0	15,000	76,800‡
India	850	3.0	25.0	10,000	22,500‡/§
Indonesia	190	3.0	5.3	500	1,500
Bangladesh	120	3.0	5.0	250	3,500
Thailand	60	3.0	1.2	250	24,000‡/§
Myanmar	45	3.0	1.3	250	25,000‡/§
Western Pacific Region	1,550	1.0	32.5	3,500	38,000§
China	1,150	1.7	24.3	3,000	16,000§
Vietnam	68	4.0	2.2	150	3,000§
Philippines	63	1.0	2.1	200	400
Malaysia	18	2.0	0.5	20	1,000§
Cambodia	9	2.8	0.35	<100	1,100§
Laos	5	5.0	0.15	<100	700§
The Americas	730	2.1	17.5	<200	15,000†/§
Caribbean countries	30	1.0	0.8	A few	3,000†/§
United States	250	Reflects % in ethnic minorities	4.1	As high as 200	1,500†/§
Brazil	150	1.0	4.5	100	4,000†/§
Argentina, Colombia, Peru, Venezuela, Chile	200	Reflects % in ethnic minorities	3.5	As high as 200	400†/§

Note: This table is a summary of the detailed tabulation of the global distribution of thalassemia and the hemoglobinopathies assembled and continuously updated by Professor B. Modell (University College, London, UK) on behalf of the World Health Organization.
* Prior to setting up large prevention programs.
† Mostly patients with sickle cell syndromes.
‡ Patients with HbS syndromes.
§ Patients with HbE syndromes.
** Patients with HbC syndromes.

ing where good medical care is available, and a survival of no more than a few years for others, the total number of patients with β thalassemia major should be about 300,000. The annual number of babies born with HbS and HbE disease is much higher.

Micromapping is available for most of the Mediterranean countries, where thalassemia occurs endemically (Siniscalco et al., 1961; Malamos et al., 1965; Tegos et al., 1987; Silvestroni and Bianco, 1975; Cao et al., 1981; Rosatelli et al., 1992). As a rule, most carriers are found at low-altitude fertile areas, where expansion of the thalassemia genes was favored by endogamy and the selective pressure of malaria. In contrast, β-thalassemia genes are almost absent in mountainous areas of the same country or region. Micromapping of the spread of thalassemia across larger countries is impossible because of their size and the differing ethnic origins of their population. On reviewing the relevant literature, an additional cause of uncertainty is the fact that over the years, scientific interest focused more on rare molecular types than on incidence. These reservations apply for all frequencies reported in the tables of this chapter.

MOLECULAR ASPECTS

The development of molecular techniques provided a new perspective in the survey of the global distribution of thalassemia. The recognition that the thalassemic phenotype results from an array of varying mutations and rearrangements of the respective genes has not only offered valuable clues to the mechanistic basis of each condition but has also provided the means for setting up effective prevention programs, which are now expanding because of their relative simplicity and reliability. Within this context, two additional seminal observations are worth mentioning: (1) Most of the common mutations are carried on chromosomes with a specific set of restriction site polymorphisms (the RFLP haplotypes; Kazazian et al., 1984a) (see Chapter 12), and (2) within each population, the number of prevalent β-thalassemia mutations is small, allowing the identification of the great majority of carriers and offspring (Orkin et al., 1982).

More than 175 β-thalassemia mutations have been identified; they are published in several reviews and in this book (see Chapter 12). For the time being, the syllabus published by the Sickle Cell Anemia Foundation in Augusta, Georgia (Huisman et al., 1997; Hardison et al., 1998) and available on the globin gene server at www.globin.psu.edu, constitutes the basic reference. The following paragraphs attempt to provide a concise review of the frequency of the mutations prevailing in various parts of the globe on the basis of the published surveys and the syllabus. The chapter focuses on the frequency of each mutation and its impact on the local control of β thalassemia; some interesting, rare mutations may be omitted. The scientific interest each mutation may present is addressed elsewhere (see Chapter 12). The tables and comments that follow examine the frequency of the β-thalassemia mutations by geographic region, starting with the countries where the recognition of the prevailing thalassemic defects has been successfully applied to prevention programs. The mutations are listed according to the defect they produce, that is, transcriptional mutants, cap site and initiation mutants, RNA processing mutants, truncated proteins following from nonsense and frameshift mutations, 3′ untranslated regions, and polyadenylation site mutations.

SOUTHEAST EUROPE (TABLE 31.2)

Greece

The mean frequency of β thalassemia in Greece (population 10 million) is approximately 8.0 percent and its distribution is heterogeneous (Malamos et al, 1965; Tegos et al., 1987; Table 31.2). The underlying molecular types are extremely diverse (Kattamis et al., 1990; Kollia et al., 1992). The most prevalent is the β^+-IVS1-nt110 (G→A) thalassemia mutation, which occurs in close association with haplotype I. Other common types are β^0-CD39 (C→T) thalassemia, usually carried on haplotype II, β^0-IVS1-nt1 (G→A) thalassemia, usually carried on haplotype V, and the mild β^+-IVS1-nt6 (T→C) mutation, usually carried on haplotype VI. Table 31.2 lists the reported frequencies, while Table 31.3 shows associations between specific mutations and chromosomal haplotypes (Kollia et al., 1992). Assuming that each mutation occurred only once on each haplotype, the fact that the frequency of the β^+-IVS1-nt110 (G→A) mutation is higher on the haplotype I chromosome than the frequency of the normal gene implies that the mutation is very old, the assumption being that it occurred once and then increased in prevalence through endogamy and the selective pressure of malaria, reaching and even exceeding the frequency of the normal haplotype I chromosome. The assumption is supported by the finding of the above mutation almost exclusively on haplotype I, Ava II/ψβ negative chromosomes in clear contrast with the normal β-globin genes, which are found on haplotype I, Ava II/ψβ positive chromosomes (Kollia et al., 1992). Greece harbors also a large variety of rare β-thalassemia mutations as well as several types of δβ thalassemia; of the former, worth mentioning are the very mild −101 C→T and the +6, C→G, 3′ to the termination codon "silent carrier" mutations, which may often escape detection by conventional techniques (Loutradi et al., unpublished

Table 31.2. Distribution of β-Thalassemia in Southeast Europe, Turkey, and Cyprus

Molecular defect*	Greece	Greek/Turkish Cypriots	Turkey	Albania	Bulgaria	Former Yugoslavia
−101 (C→T)	3		6	–	1	–
−87 (C→G)	19		12	–	4	3
−30 (T→A)	1		33	–	1	2
−28 (A→C)			3			
IVS1-1 (G→A)	135	36/40	54	5	49	20
IVS1-5 (G→A, C, T)	5		19	1		
IVS1-6 (T→C)	81	39/35	181	21	30	33
IVS1-110 (G→A)	425	563/309	519	61	101	91
IVS2-1 (G→A)	20		91	3	7	5
IVS2-745 (C→G)	43	36/26	42	1	17	7
CD 29 (C→T)						2
CD 39 (C→T)	193	20/5	48	31	99	7
FSC 5 (−CT)	6		22	2	29	5
FSC 6 (−A)	28	1/–	5		24	7
FSC 8 (−AA)	9	2/–	81		5	7
FSC 8/9 (+G)	1		19		2	
FSC 44 (−C)				4	2	
AATAAA→AATAAG–						
AATAAA→AATGAG–				3	1	4
AATAAA→A - - - - -						
Other	7			1	4	7
Unknown	14	8/13	86	13	32	11
Number of chromosomes	**989**	**705/428**	**1,227**	**146**	**408**	**211**

* *Abbreviations:* CD, codon; FSC, frameshift; IVS, intervening sequence.

observations; Jancovic et al., 1991), the β-thalassemic hemoglobinopathy Hb Knossos, where the substitution of Ser for Ala in codon 27 decreases the amount of the variant mRNA because of defective processing (Orkin et al., 1984a), and Hb Corfu, a 7.2-kb deletion, which removes part of the δ-globin gene and occurs consistently in association with a G→A mutation at position IVS1-nt5 (Wainscoat et al., 1985; Kulozik et al., 1988).

Table 31.3. Association of Molecular Defects with Underlying Haplotypes

Molecular defect*	Haplotypes									
	I	II	III	IV	V	VI	VII	VIII	IX	"New"
IVS1 nt 110	50								1	1
β-39	1	22								1
IVS2 nt 1			3						2	
FSC 8				1						
IVS1 nt 1	1				15					2
IVS1 nt 6						11				
IVS2 nt 745							3			
−87			1						1	
FSC 5					1					
Unknown	1	1	1							
Total	**53**	**23**	**5**	**1**	**16**	**11**	**3**	**–**	**4**	**4**

Polymorphic sites defining the β gene cluster haplotypes. *Hinc* II 5′ to the ε gene; *Hind* III within the $^Gγ$ and $^Aγ$ genes. *Hinc* II within the ψβ and 3′ to the ψβ gene; *Ava* II within the β gene and *Bam* HI 3′ to the β gene; Haplotype I, (+−−−−++); Haplotype II, (−++−+++); Haplotype III, (−+−+++−); Haplotype IV, (−+−++−+); Haplotype V, (+−−−−+−); Haplotype VI, (−++−−−+); Haplotype VII, (+−−−−−+); Haplotype VIII, (−+−+−+−); Haplotype IX, (−+−++++); Haplotype X, (−+−−−−+).

* Abbreviations as in Table 31.2; nt, nucleotide.

Albania, Former Yugoslavia, and Bulgaria

The frequency of β thalassemia in Albania (population 3.2 million) is 7.4 percent. In addition, Albania harbors a 4.5 percent prevalence of HbS carriers (Boletini et al., 1994). β Thalassemia occurs less frequently in the former Yugoslavia (total population 22 million; incidence of carriers 4 percent) (Dimovsky et al., 1990; Efremov, 1992) and nearby Bulgaria (population 10 million; frequency of β thalassemia approximately 3 percent) (Kalaydjieva et al., 1989; Petkov et al., 1990). The distribution of the β-thalassemia gene in the above countries is heterogeneous and the incidence of the various molecular types is almost similar to that of Greece. This is not surprising if one considers the extensive merging of these populations in the past (Table 31.2).

Turkey

β Thalassemia constitutes a major public health problem in the western regions of this large country (population around 55 million) where the frequency of the β-thalassemia trait is reportedly as high as 6.7 percent, exceeding by far the mean frequency over the whole country, which is of the order of 2.0 percent (Dincol et al., 1979). The distribution of the various mutations is similar to that of Greece with most of the defects belonging to the β⁺-IVS1-nt110 (G→A), β⁰-IVS1-nt1 (G→A), and the mild β⁺-IVS1-nt6 (T→C). Other molecular types of β thalassemia occurring in relatively high frequency are the ("Turkish") β⁰-FSC-8 (-AA), the β⁰-IVS2-nt1 (G→A), the β⁺-IVS2-nt745 (C→G), and the β⁰-CD39 (C→T) mutations (Oner et al., 1990; Basak et al., 1992; Tadmouri et al., 1998) (Table 31.2). Of interest also is the occurrence of a β thalassemia whose heterozygotes display an unusually high HbA₂ level resulting from a relatively small (290 bp) deletion that includes the 5′ end of the β-globin gene (reviewed by Thein, 1993).

Cyprus

The extremely high (about 15 percent) frequency of β thalassemia in this small island (population 0.7 million) created a major public health problem until an effective prevention program completely obviated the birth of affected newborns (Angastiniotis and Hadjiminas, 1981). The prevailing β-thalassemia defects are almost similar to those found in the Mediterranean basin, with the β⁺-IVS1-nt110 (G→A) mutation occurring with a significantly higher frequency than in neighboring countries (Table 31.2). It is of interest that Greek Cypriots have the same mutations as their Turkish counterparts (Baysal et al., 1992). Of the rare mutations worth mentioning is the

very mild C→G change in position +33 in the 5′ untranslated region of the β-globin gene, which was recently reported in two individuals of Greek Cypriot origin and results in normal red cell indices and HbA₂ levels in the heterozygotes (Ho et al., 1996).

THE NEAR AND MIDDLE EAST AND THE TRANS-CAUCASUS (TABLE 31.4)

The Lebanese population (3.0 million) is a mixture of individuals of different ethnic origins; the mean incidence of β thalassemia is of the order of 2 percent to 3 percent. The distribution of the mutations resembles that in Cyprus, with the interesting addition of C→T transition at position 29, which results in β⁺ thalassemia and is found in 8 percent of the heterozygotes (Chehab et al., 1987) (Table 31.4). The spectrum of β-thalassemia mutations in the Palestinians in the Gaza strip is similar to the above (Filon et al., 1995). The distribution of β thalassemia in Israel (population around 6 million) is markedly uneven because of the nation's ethnic diversity and intermarriage, which is common in some religious groups. The incidence is highest (up to 20 percent) in Kurdish Jews (no more than 20,000 individuals) and lower in Mediterranean and Arab Jews. The Israeli β-thalassemia alleles include 20 percent of the common Mediterranean mutation β⁺-IVS1-nt110 (G→A), 20 percent of the β⁰-FSC–44 (-C) mutation, and the unique Kurdish mutations β⁺-nt–28 (A→C) and poly(A) nt6 (A→G) (15 percent and 6.5 percent, respectively) (Rund et al., 1990) (Table 31.4). Jordan (population 2.5 million) and Syria (population 15 million) harbor a relatively high frequency of β-thalassemia genes, but accurate numbers are not available. The β⁺-IVS1-nt110 (G→A), β⁰-IVS2-nt1 (G→A), β⁺-IVS2-nt745 (C→G) (Mediterranean), and β⁰-CD37 (G→A) (Saudi Arabian) mutations prevail (Kamel, 1987; Sadiq and Huisman, 1994) (Table 31.4).

β-thalassemia is a major problem in Iran, a large country (population 60 million) with roughly 3.5 percent heterozygotes and a high frequency of consanguineous marriages. The reported mutations are heterogeneous, because of the underlying large ethnic diversity. Of those, β⁰-IVS2-nt1 (G→A), β⁺-IVS1-nt5 (G→C), and β⁺-IVS1-nt110 (G→A) are the most common (Merat et al., 1993; Nozari et al., 1995). Thalassemia is well known also in Iraq, but information regarding its frequency is not available (Kamel, 1987) (Table 31.4).

The Trans-Caucasian countries of the former USSR (Armenia, Georgia, Uzbekistan, Degestan, Tadjikistan, and Azerbaijan) harbor a large number of β-thalassemia genes with frequencies ranging from 1 percent or 2 percent up to 6.5 percent. In the latter

Table 31.4. Distribution of β-thalassemia in the Middle and Near East, the Trans-Caucasus Countries, and the Indian Subcontinent

		Israel								
Molecular defect*	Lebanon	Kurdish Jews	Other Jews	Iran	Azerbaijan	Jordan	Syria	India	Pakistan	Bangladesh
−101 (C→T)		1	4							
−88 (C→T)									2	
−87 (C→G)										
−30 (T→A)			2		2	2		5		
−28 (A→C)		18	1		1					
+1 (A→C)										
IVS1-1 (G→A/T)	2	1	5	128	2	8		141	8	
IVS1-5 (G→A/C/T)	4	1		197	2	5	6	320	4	
IVS1-6 (T→C)	31		47	44	7	8			27	6
IVS1-110 (G→A)	2	9	13	116	20	35	16			
IVS2-1 (G→A)	2	2	11	324	21	21	1			
IVS2-745 (C→G)		1		12		13	6			
CD 15 (G→A)			1					18	13	1
CD 29 (C→T)	4				3					
CD 30 (G→C)		1		17	1					
CD 37 (G→A)			1			8				
CD 39 (C→T)	2	8	7	7	2	2	4			
FSC 5 (−CT)				14		3			16	
FSC 6 (−A)						1				
FSC 8 (−AA)	4				21					
FSC 8/9 (+G)				135	2	3		95	103	1
FSC 16 (−C)									8	
FSC 41/42 (−TTCT)				1				100	18	
FSC 44 (−C)		24	1	49	3					2
25 bp deletion										
619 bp deletion								221	4	
AATAAA→AATAAG		10								
AATAAA→A - - - - -										
Other		3	2	110	12	5				
Unknown		2	5	65		16	3			
Number of chromosomes	51	81	102	1,219	99	130	36	940	221	10

* Abbreviations as in Table 31.2; bp, base pairs.

country (population around 6 million) the annual number of newborns with thalassemia may be as high as 200, because of the high frequency of consanguineous marriages. The Mediterranean β^+-IVS1-nt110 (G→A), β^0-IVS2-nt1 (G→A), and β^+-IVS1-nt6 (T→C) and the Turkish β^0-FSC 8 (-AA) (Kuliev et al., 1994) (Table 31.4), are the most common mutations.

THE INDIAN SUBCONTINENT (TABLE 31.4)

Undoubtedly, β thalassemia major is a common medical problem across India, Pakistan, and Bangladesh, but accurate frequency statistics are not available. This reflects the large and long-lasting heterogeneity of the almost 1 billion inhabitants, who are divided into thousands of caste and tribal units characterized by cultural isolation and high endogamy. The mean reported incidence of β thalassemia in India is around 3 percent to 4 percent, and there are approximately 4,000 affected newborns per year. The distribution of the β-thalassemia trait is heterogeneous with estimates as high as 9.2 percent to 17.0 percent among the Lohanas (Gujarat; northwest; the delta of Indus and other rivers) and the Tamils in Pondicherry (southeast tip of the subcontinent), 7.0 percent in Maharashtra (Bombay area), 3.7 percent in Bengal (Calcutta area; the Ganges delta), and lower than 2.0 percent in Uttar Pradesh (center-north) and Raipur (in Madhya Pradesh) probably in the mountains. Several patients with β thalassemia major have also been recorded in Andhra Pradesh (southeast) and the Bhopal area (Madhya Pradesh; center-north) (reviewed by Brittenham, 1987). The above frequencies are blurred by the inevitable "selection" created by geographic barriers and the highly inbred caste groups, and caution is required when interpreting the reported frequency of the associated molecular defects. From the reports that became available over the last years it appears (1) that the Indian β-thalassemia genes are preferentially carried on specific RFLP haplotypes as in the Mediterranean countries (Kazazian et al., 1984b), and (2) that some of the associated mutations are quite specific for the Indians, such as the β^0 –619 bp deletion at the 3' end of the gene; that mutation occurs in relatively high frequency all over the country, usually in association with haplotype F (VII). Other prevailing mutations are the β^+IVS1-nt5 (G→C) transversion, the β^0-CD 15 (TGG→TAG) transversion, and the β^0-FSC 8/9 (+G) and FSC 41/42 (-TTCT) (Thein et al., 1988; Baysal et al., 1994). The IVS1-nt5 (G→C) mutation appears to occur frequently among the natives of the Maharashtra area, while the Punjabis show a larger diversity of mutations (Garewal et al., 1994). The IVS1-nt5 (G→C) mutation also prevails among the Gond tribal group (Gupta et al., 1991) and

the natives of Uttar Pradesh (Agarwal et al., 1994). The high frequency of the IVS1-nt1 (G→A) mutation reported by Thein et al. (1988) was not confirmed in the other Indian surveys but appears to be common among the Pakistanis (Verma et al., 1997).

Pakistan

As in India, a caste system with high consanguinity, a mean carrier frequency of 5.4 percent, and another 4,000 homozygotes born per year make β thalassemia the most important medical problem in the area. β^0-FSC 8/9 (+G) is relatively frequent in the north (41.3 percent) and β^+-IVS1-nt5 (G→C) in the south (52.2 percent). A few unique mutations are also of interest (Ahmed et al., 1996; Khan and Riazuddin, 1988).

NORTH AFRICA AND THE ARABIC COUNTRIES (TABLE 31.5)

Egypt

The incidence of β thalassemia in this large country (population around 50 million) is low (about 1.2 percent) and would be even lower if not for consanguinity (Kamel, 1987). The mutations β^+-IVS1-nt110(G→A), β^+-IVS1-nt6 (T→C), and β^0-IVS1-nt1 (G→A) comprise almost half of the total, while another quarter remain uncharacterized (Noveletto et al., 1990; Huisman et al., 1997) (Table 31.5).

Morocco, Tunisia, Algeria, and Libya (Total Population Around 50 Million)

These populations are essentially Arabs with a minority of Berbers, whose origin may be Mediterranean. β Thalassemia is unevenly distributed. The mean reported frequency is approximately 2.0 percent and follows from the high frequency of consanguineous marriages. The presence of HbS, especially in the south, creates an additional public health problem (Kamel, 1987). The underlying mutations include a C→T transition at position 39 and β^+-IVS1-nt110 (G→A), β^0-IVS1-nt1 (G→A), and β^0-FCS 6 (-A). An interesting mutation, which appears to be unique in Oran, is IVS1-nt2 (T→C or T→A), which results in β^+ thalassemia (Bouhass et al., 1994).

Saudi Arabia and Neighboring Countries

Thalassemia is a minor problem in this region because of the much greater incidence of sickle cell disease. The prevailing mutations are those found in other Middle East countries and include β^+-IVS1-nt110 (G→A), β^0-IVS2-nt1 (G→A), β^+-IVS1-nt5 (G→C), and

Table 31.5. Distribution of β-Thalassemia in North Africa and the Arab Countries

Molecular defect‡	Egypt	Arab countries*	North Africa†
−30 (T→A)			3
IVS1-1 (G→A, T)	23	20	20
IVS1-5 (G→A, C, T)		318	
IVS1-6 (T→C)	34	16	11
IVS1-110 (G→A)	63	46	47
IVS2-1 (G→A)	8	75	
IVS2-745 (C→G)	13	2	5
CD 15 (TGG→TAG)		12	
CD 22 (A→C)	15		
CD 30 (AGG→ACG)		10	2
CD 30 (AGG→AGC)		1	
CD 37 (TGG→TGA)	1	1	
CD 39 (C→T)	2	51	65
FSC 5 (−CT)	2	17	2
FSC 6 (−A)	3	4	35
FSC 8 (−AA)		33	1
FSC 8/9 (+G)	1	46	
FSC 16 (−C)		9	
FSC 41/42 (−TTCT)		5	
FSC 44 (−C)		11	4
25 bp deletion AATAAA→AATAAG and A - - - - -		4	
Other/Unknown	30	54	45
Number of chromosomes	175	734	241

* Includes Saudi Arabia, Yemen, United Arab Emirates, and Kuwait.

† Includes Tunisia and Algeria (Huisman, Carver and Baysal: *Syllabus of Thalassemia Mutations*, 1997).

‡ Abbreviations as in Table 31.2.

β⁰-CD39 (C→T), as well as some rarer or nonidentified mutations (compiled in Huisman et al., 1997). In one report, the "population-specific" mutation β⁺-IVS1-3′ end −25 bp accounted for 13 percent of the mutations (El-Hazmi et al., 1995), but other studies have not confirmed this.

SOUTHWEST EUROPE (TABLE 31.6)

Italy (Population Around 60 Million)

β Thalassemia is unevenly distributed throughout the country. Reported frequencies of heterozygous carriers vary from 1.5 percent to 2.0 percent in Central Italy, 2.0 percent to 3.0 percent in Northern Italy (as a result of the migration of workers from the south and the high concentration of the gene in the Po valley), 2.6 percent to 12.4 percent in Southern Italy and

Sicily, and 10.5 percent in Sardinia (Silvestroni and Bianco, 1975; Cao et al., 1981; Tentori and Marinucci, 1986; Maggio et al., 1990; Schiliro et al., 1995). The underlying β-thalassemia mutations are also diverse; the frequencies detected in the southern part of Italy closely resemble those of Greece, most probably reflecting the composition of the population of "Magna Grecia" in antiquity, while the β-thalassemia genes of the Po River valley and those of Sardinia are almost exclusively represented by the β⁰ type CD39 (C→T) (Table 31.5). The β-thalassemia types in the big industrial cities of the north (Milano, Torino, etc.) reflect the mutations prevailing in the population groups who came from the south in search of work.

France

As thalassemia does not occur among indigenous French, the identifiable β-thalassemia mutations reflect the origin of the Tunisian, Algerian, and Moroccan populations who immigrated mostly into southern France over the past years. Further north (Parisian area), sickle cell disease, brought in with immigrants from Central Africa and the French Caribbean, constitutes the predominant hemoglobinopathy (Milland et al., 1987).

Spain

β Thalassemia is rare in central Spain, but occurs with relatively high frequency on the island of Minorca and in the south of Spain (2.0 percent to 7.4 percent), where the Moors lived for centuries, and in Galicia, in the northwest corner of the country (5.4 percent), where the condition appears to be a legacy of the ancient Ligures (Baiget and Gimferrer, 1986). The reported incidence of mutations contrast with that of the eastern Mediterranean countries in that the frequency of the IVS1-nt110 (G→A) mutation does not exceed 8.0 percent, while that of the β⁰-CD39 (C→T) and β⁺-IVS1-nt6 (T→C) mutations is significantly increased (6.4 percent and 15.5 percent, respectively) (Table 31.6; Anselem et al., 1988; Ribeiro et al., 1997). Of interest is the "ethnic" mutation CD37 (G→A) occurring in high frequency among the Catalonians in the delta of the Ebro (Galano et al., 1992).

Portugal

The frequency of β thalassemia in this small country of approximately 10 million inhabitants is relatively low (1 percent in the south and 0.5 percent in the north). The β⁰-IVS1-nt1 (G→A), β⁺-IVS1-nt110 (G→A), β⁺-IVS1-nt6 (T→C), and β⁰-CD39 (C→T)

Table 31.6. Distribution of β Thalassemia in Western and Northern Europe

Molecular defect[*]	Italy			Spain	Portugal	France
	South	Po delta	Sardinia			
−101 (C→T)	3	1				
−92 (C→T)	3					
−87 (C→G)	37	3	7			
IVS1-1 (G→A)	184	2	1	103	55	11
IVS1-6 (T→C)	305	2	3	32	57	9
IVS1-110 (G→A)	477	20	15	38	24	27
IVS2-1 (G→A)	48	2	1			1
IVS2-745 (C→G)	112		12	7	1	3
CD 15 (G→A)					33	
CD 39 (C→A)	704	48	2,872	105	96	44
FSC 6 (−A)	28		66	4	11	
FSC 8 (−AA)	1			5		
FSC 76 (−C)	2		20			
Other	49		3	9	3	
Unknown	57			21		10
Number of chromosomes	2,010	78	3,000	324	280	105

[*] Abbreviations as in Table 31.2.

mutations cause 96 percent to 97 percent of the cases (Table 31.6). The interest in these cases in Portugal lies in the fact that the CD39 and the IVS1-1 mutations are carried on more than one haplotype (II, I, and VI for the former; Coutinho Gomes et al., 1988, and III, Va, Vb and IX for the latter; Faustino et al., 1992) indicating either a "hot spot" for recurrent mutations or the very old presence of the defect among the involved population. In addition, two novel mutations were also detected: −90 (C→T) and a 2-bp deletion (AG) within the IVS2 5′ splice site consensus sequence (Tamagnini et al., 1993).

NORTHERN EUROPE

Germany

Thalassemia does not occur among indigenous Germans; the identifiable β-thalassemia mutations reflect the origin of the Turkish, Greek and other workers who migrated into this country over the past years. This statement holds also for the United Kingdom, where the public health problems caused by thalassemia become very pressing because of the large numbers of immigrant Cypriots, Pakistanis, and Indians, who came to the country carrying distinct β-thalassemia genes. However, in 1992 Hall and co-workers reported twenty-three British β-thalassemia carriers whose families did not appear to have had any Mediterranean admixture as far as this could be traced in the past; in seventeen carriers the underlying mutations belonged to common

Mediterranean or Asian types; another three produced a dominant type of β-thalassemia trait (see Chapter 14) and the last three could not be identified. An inherited hypochromic microcytic anemia featuring all hallmarks of β-thalassemia trait and transmitted in an autosomal manner over three generations of an English family independently of the β-globin gene complex may represent another kind of thalassemia (Thein et al., 1993).

Belgium, the Netherlands, Denmark, and the Scandinavian Countries

Thalassemia does not occur among these populations. However, the condition is well known in hospitals where patients from the Mediterranean, Africa, India, and Indonesia are admitted for treatment or bone marrow transplantation. An initiation codon mutation (T→C) reported as a cause of β thalassemia in a Belgian family most probably represents a de novo mutation (Wildmann et al., 1993).

EASTERN EUROPE

Thalassemia does not appear to occur among the inhabitants of the northern part of the former USSR in contrast to the Trans-Caucasus countries, where the condition constitutes a major public health problem (see above). Although extremely rare, a small number of β-thalassemia mutations have been reported in Hungary (Ringelhann et al., 1993) and Czechoslovakia (Indrak et al., 1992). The fact that in almost all cases, they were

Table 31.7. Distribution of β Thalassemia in Southeast Asian Countries

| Molecular defect* | Thailand | Burma | Malaysia and Singapore | | China | | Japan |
			Chinese	Malay	South/West Provinces	Hong-Kong	
−31 (A→G)							45
−28 (A→G)	56	4	8	3	48	7	1
Initiation codon mutations			1				25
+1 (A→C)	1		10	4			
IVS1-1 (G→A/T)	25	34	1	10	8		
IVS1-5 (G→C/C/T)	71	27	2	56			3
IVS2-1 (G→A)							29
IVS2-654 (C→T)	42	2	47	5	22	20	38
CD 17 (A→T)	152	7	14	7	71	9	1
CD 19 (A→G)	54		3	11			
CD 35 (C→A)	10						1
CD 90 (G→T)							44
FSC 41 (−C)	7						
FSC 41/42 (−TTCT)	305	21	83	12	136	45	19
FSC 71/72 (+A)	16		2		11		
FSC 127/128 (−AGG)							11
3.4 kb deletion	17						
Other	18		3	13	16	12	44
Unknown	45	4		12	2		
Number of chromosomes	819	99	174	133	314	93	261

* Abbreviations as in Table 31.2.

those commonly encountered in Central Europe indicates that they were most probably introduced through immigration from the neighboring countries. In addition, there was one novel mutation (FSC 51, -C), which was not further studied, and an initiation codon mutation, which has been reported also in the Japanese but apparently represents a de novo mutation, since it is carried on a different chromosome. Thalassemia major is an important public health problem in Romania, but accurate statistics are not available.

THE FAR EAST (TABLE 31.7)

China

This huge Asian country harbors very few β-thalassemia genes. The mean incidence of β thalassemia among the Hans, who constitute more than 90 percent of the population and reside in the north and northwest provinces is less than 0.5 percent. To the contrary, in the southwest provinces (Guizhou, Sichuan, Guanxi, Guandong), where the inhabitants belong to ethnic groups with large contacts with neighboring Laos, Vietnam, and Cambodia, the incidence of β thalassemia is much higher, ranging from 2.0 percent to 4.0 percent (Antonazakis et al., 1984; Zeng, 1987); this figure holds

also for Taiwan (Liu et al., 1997). In these provinces, the number of patients with β thalassemia major must be high and certainly has a severe impact on the local health authorities; the problem is aggravated by the simultaneous presence of large numbers of α thalassemia and HbE carriers, and effective prevention measures that are vital for reducing the medical impact of these disorders are now being established. The prevailing molecular types include the β^0-FSC 41/42 (-TTCT), the mutation β^+-IVS2-nt 654 (C→T), the β^+ mutation at position −28 (AG), a β^0-CD17 (A→T), another β^0-FSC 71/72 (+A), and other defects (Kazazian et al., 1986; Zhang et al., 1988; Huisman et al., 1997) (Table 31.7).

Thailand, Cambodia, Laos, and Vietnam

These countries are a paradise for the geneticists, because they harbor numerous α- and β-globin gene defects, which give rise to complex genetic diseases and clinical conditions of varying severity. Most defects involve the α-globin genes; they include various types of α thalassemia and the α thalassemia-causing variant Hb Constant Spring (see Chapters 17 and 32). HbE in the homozygous state is a relatively mild disease; HbE thalassemia can be a severe disease (see

Chapter 43). The reported frequencies of β thalassemia in the area vary from 3.0 percent to 9.0 percent (reviewed by Wasi, 1987). In 83 percent of cases β thalassemia is due to β^0-FSC 41/42 (-TTCT), β^0-CD17 (AAG→TAG), and β^+-IVS2-nt654 (C→T) mutations, and the β^+-nt–28 (A→G) mutation upstream of the β-globin gene (Thein et al., 1990) (Table 31.7).

Malaysia

In Malaysia the situation is different from the above, reflecting the different origin of the involved populations. The most frequent defects among Malay patients are the IVS1-nt5 (G→C), followed by the CD19 (A→G) and IVS1-nt1 (G→T) mutations; Indonesians of Chinese origin harbor the Chinese β-thalassemia genes (mostly FSC 41/42) (Yang et al., 1989; George et al., 1992; Table 31.7).

Burma

In Burma six mutations (mainly the IVS1 nt1, the IVS1-nt5, and FSC 41/42 mutations) account for 99 percent of the local β-thalassemia genes (Brown et al., 1992).

Japan

A few years ago, β thalassemia was thought to not occur in Japan. However, this is not the case today, not only because patients with β thalassemia major are occasionally identified under various circumstances, but also because almost half of the underlying molecular defects are unique for the Japanese population. The latter include the A→G mutation at position –31 and a series of mutations in codons 35 (C→A) (Yasunaga et al., 1995), 90 (GAG→TAG) (Hattori et al., 1992), 110 (G→C), and 127/128 (four nucleotides deleted) (Hattori et al., 1989). They also include a new mutation at the initiation codon (ATG→GTG) (Hattori et al., 1991), a FSC insertion (+G) in codon 54 (Fucharoen et al., 1990), and an insertion of a thymidine within or following the TTT sequence of codon 42, which results in a premature stop at codon 43 (transformed into TGA) (Oshima et al., 1996). The other half of the mutations are those usually identified in the Chinese (mostly FSC 41/42; four-nucleotide deletion), but also in the European populations (Yamamoto et al., 1992).

Philippines

The incidence of β thalassemia in the Philippines is relatively low (around 1 percent). The most common (approximately 50 percent) mutation is the "Filipino"

deletion (beginning approximately 4 kb upstream of the β-globin gene and extending beyond it), followed by the codon 67 (-TG) (26 percent) (Waye et al., 1994; Ko et al., 1998).

Korea

The frequency of β thalassemia in Korea is also extremely low, where only a few sporadic cases have been reported; the ATG→ATT mutation at the initiation codon has been described also in China and Japan (Shimizu et al., 1989; Ko et al., 1992).

Melanesia

Surveying the distribution of β thalassemia in Melanesia has provided valuable information because the structure of this population (isolated islands) was not influenced by internal movements or migration from other places over several thousand years. These studies confirmed once again the positive pressure of malaria on the proliferation of the thalassemia defect, given that the average incidence of the thalassemia trait in the coastal, malaria-affected populations was found to be around 5.0 percent with some tribes reaching 20 percent, while in the highlands, where malaria virtually does not exist, the frequency of the trait was only 0.2 percent. The most common molecular defect in the area is the G→C transversion at IVS1-nt5. The fact that this mutation was found on chromosomes bearing a different haplotype also in several Asian Indians and Chinese patients along with the existence of other mutations of the same nucleotide (G→T in the Mediterraneans and G→A in Algeria) suggest that this position may be a "hot" mutational spot (Hill et al., 1988).

AUSTRALIA AND NEW ZEALAND

β Thalassemia has not been reported to occur among the Australian aborigines. However, homozygous β thalassemia is a major problem in Australia, where large numbers of Greek and Italian and other populations harboring a high incidence of the trait have immigrated.

CENTRAL AND SOUTH AFRICA

β Thalassemia is relatively rare among the black African population and may occur with a "patchy" distribution. Kasili's review (1987) contains a few sporadic cases spread out over the countries of East Africa. In West Africa the frequency of β-thalassemia genes varies from 0.8 percent (Nigeria) to 1.3 percent

Table 31.8. Distribution of β Thalassemia in South America, American Blacks, and Blacks from Guadeloupe

Molecular defect[*]	Black Americans	Guadeloupe	Argentina	Brazil
−88 (C→T)	27	4		
−87 (C→A)			2	
−29 (A→G)	76	51		
IVS1-1 (G→T)			8	6
IVS1-5 (G→A)		12		
IVS1-5 (G→C)		15		
IVS1-6 (T→C)			5	13
IVS1-110 (G→A)			19	13
IVS2-1 (G→A)		19	3	
IVS2-745 (C→G)			2	
IVS2-849 (A→G, A→C)	5	7		
CD 6 (−A)	1			
CD 15 (G→A)			1	
CD 24 (T→A)	3	4		
CD 39 (C→T)			40	38
AATAA→AACAAA		9		
Other/Unknown	16	8	5	
Number of chromosomes	**128**	**129**	**85**	**70**

[*] Abbreviations as in Table 31.2.

to 1.7 percent (Ghana) but may go up to 9 percent in some tribes in Liberia (Weatherall and Clegg, 1981). As a rule, β thalassemia runs a mild course in blacks of African descent. This reflects the underlying molecular defects, most of which involve the promoter sequences or the polyadenylation signal, and hence they result in mild curtailment of β-globin gene transcription and a mild β⁺ thalassemia. This information is derived mainly from studies that have been carried out on Africans Americans and are detailed below and in Table 31.8.

THE AMERICAS (TABLE 31.8)

The incidence of β thalassemia in the Americas reflects the structure of the studied population; this also holds true for the underlying molecular defects. As a rule, the β-thalassemia genes in blacks produce mild symptoms. Of these, the −88 (C→T), the −29 (A→G), and the −24 (T→A) substitutions as well as the T→C replacement in the polyadenylation cleavage site occur more frequently. Rarer mutations include: the nt−87 (C→A), IVS2-nt654 (C→T) and the IVS2-nt849 A→G and A→C mutations, all identified in African Americans (Coleman et al., 1992; Antonarakis et al., 1984; Orkin et al., 1984b). The survey of Gonzalez-Redondo et al. (1988) in black patients from the southeastern United States added two new mutations (IVS2-nt848 C→A and CD61 A→T) and reconfirmed two previously reported deletion β thalassemias (a Gγ[Aγδβ]⁰-thalassemia due

to a 34-kb deletion and a 1.35-kb deletion at the 5′ end of the β-globin gene). β Thalassemia is rather frequent in Jamaica, where both the β⁺mild and β⁰ severe varieties occur; this is also valid for the blacks of Guadeloupe who carry in addition to the usual mild β-thalassemia genes the more severe IVS1-nt5 mutations (G→C and G→C) as a result of the admixture of Mediterranean and Indian chromosomes, respectively (Romana et al., 1996). The incidence of β thalassemia in the blacks of Brazil is not expected to be different than that of the other populations of African origin; on the contrary, as both Brazil and Argentina harbor a high incidence of β-thalassemia carriers of Italian and Portuguese origin, the incidence of the various β-thalassemia defects resembles more that of the Mediterranean populations (Sonati et al., 1996; Fonseca et al., 1998). This is also evident with regard to the distribution of β thalassemia across the United States, which is present where the population under study comprises large numbers of Greek and Italian immigrants. The almost complete absence of β thalassemia from Native Americans is a most interesting finding. The explanation offered by Weatherall and Clegg (1981) is that this population migrated form Asia (through the Bering Strait in the last Ice Age) before the genes for β thalassemia or HbE were established in this population, and the absence of malaria in the New World did not favor the expansion of the few β-thalassemia mutations that were carried by the immigrants.

Table 31.9. Diagnostic Criteria and Approach to Carrier Identification

	RBC indices	RBC morphology	HbA_2	HbF	Presence of abnormal hemoglobins	β/α ratio on biosynthesis	Serum iron
High HbA_2 β thalassemia							
	$\Downarrow$	Abnormal	$\Uparrow$	Normal	No	$\Downarrow$	Normal
Super-mild thalassemia genes; "silent" β thalassemia							
	$\downarrow$/Normal	$(\pm)$ normal	$\uparrow$/Normal	Normal	No	$\downarrow$/Normal	Normal
High HbF β thalassemia; $\delta\beta$-thalassemia trait							
	$\Downarrow$	Abnormal	Normal/$\downarrow$	$\Uparrow$	No	$\Downarrow$	Normal
Hb Lepore $\delta\beta$-thalassemia trait							
	$\Downarrow$	Abnormal	Normal/$\downarrow$	Normal	Hb Lepore	$\Downarrow$	Normal
Corfu $\delta\beta$-thalassemia trait							
	$\Downarrow$	Abnormal	Normal/$\downarrow$	Normal	No	$\Downarrow$	Normal
$\gamma\delta\beta$-thalassemia trait							
	$\Downarrow$	Abnormal	Normal/$\downarrow$	Normal	No	$\Downarrow$	Normal
β thalassemia with simultaneous presence of a δ-thalassemia gene (*in cis* or *in trans*)							
	$\Downarrow$	Abnormal	$\downarrow$	Normal	No	$\Downarrow$	Normal
β thalassemia with simultaneous presence of one or more α -thalassemia gene (α^+/α^o -thalassemia)							
	$\Downarrow$	Abnormal*	$\Uparrow$**	Normal	No	$\downarrow$/Normal	Normal
Thalassemic hemoglobinopathy (Hb Knossos etc)							
	$\downarrow$/$\Downarrow$	$(\pm)$ normal	Normal	Normal	Hb Knossos	$\downarrow$/Normal	Normal
Severe chronic iron deficiency							
	$\downarrow$/$\Downarrow$	Abnormal	Normal/low	Normal	No	Normal	$\Downarrow$

*/** Has been reported to be within normal limits.

A STRATEGY TOWARD A COMPREHENSIVE CARRIER IDENTIFICATION: ONGOING AND PLANNED PROGRAMS

Considering the above general rules and their exceptions, the strategy for carrier identification must include a set of screening tests, a set of confirmatory tests, and finally advanced research technology aiming to understand the basis for the detected erythrocyte abnormalities at the molecular level (see Chapter 36). The various flowcharts proposed in the literature take into consideration the prevalence of β thalassemia in the studied populations, the technical feasibilities and competence of the staff, the cost, and the potential benefit. As a rule, the initial detection is based on the red cell indices; simplified osmotic fragility studies and evaluation of red cell morphology can substitute for blood counts in field surveys. This is probably sufficient when surveying large populations with a relatively low prevalence of thalassemia (for example 1 percent to 3 percent) for the purpose of establishing prevention programs. Detection based on erythrocyte indices is confirmed by determination of HbA_2 and HbF; at the same time, a simple hemoglobin electrophoresis will reveal the presence of HbS, HbE, or other variant hemoglobins of potential importance. The sequence of additional testing will depend on the results of the initial tests and include search for red cell inclusion bodies, assessment of the iron status, high-performance liquid chromatography and isoelectric focusing, biosynthetic studies, and identification of thalassemic genes by DNA-based molecular techniques (see Chapters 34 and 35). Basic characteristics of the various β-thalassemia defects along with the approaches suggested for their identification are summarized in Table 31.9. Family studies are often helpful. Within this context, when establishing epidemiologic surveys or population screening programs, a general rule for cost effectiveness is that the complexity of the applied tests should be inversely related to the prevalence of β thalassemia in the population, since the probability of mating between a typical carrier and a silent carrier who may be missed is remote (Fessas et al., 1988).

References

Agarwal, S, Neveed, M, and Gupta, UR. (1994). Characterization of beta-thalassaemia mutations in 57 beta-thalassaemia families seen at Lucknow. *Indian. J. Med. Res.* 100: 106–110.

Ahmed, S, Petrou, M, and Saleem, M. (1996). Molecular genetics of beta-thalassaemia in Pakistan: A basis for prenatal diagnosis. *Br. J. Haematol.* 94: 476–482.

Angastiniotis, M and Hadjiminas, MG. (1981). Prevention of thalassaemia in Cyprus. *Lancet* 1: 369–370.

Angastiniotis, M and Modell, B. (1998). Global epidemiology of hemoglobin disorders. *Ann. N.Y. Acad. Sci.* 850: 251–269.

Anselem, S, Nunes, V, Vidaud, M et al. (1988). Determination of the spectrum of the β-thalassemia genes in Spain by use of dot-blot analysis of amplified β-globin DNA. *Am. J. Hum. Genet.* 43: 95–100.

Antonarakis, S, Orkin, S, Cheng, TC et al. (1984). Beta-thalassemia in American Blacks: Novel mutations in the "TATA" box and an acceptor splice site. *Proc. Nat. Acad. Sci.* 81: 1154–1158.

Antonarakis, S, Kang, J, Lam, VMS et al. (1988). Molecular characterization of β-globin gene mutations in patients with β-thalassaemia intermedia in South China. *Br. J. Haematol.* 70: 357–361.

Baiget, M and Gimferrer, E. (1986). Geographical distribution of hemoglobin variants in Spain. In Winter, WP, editor. *Hemoglobin variants in human populations.* Boca Raton: CRC Press, pp. 141–153.

Basak, AN, Ozcelik, H, Ozer, A et al. (1992). The molecular basis of β-thalassemia in Turkey. *Hum. Genet.* 89: 315–318.

Baysal, E, Indrak, K, Bozkurt, G et al. (1992). The β-thalassemia mutations in the population of Cyprus. *Br. J. Haematol.* 81: 607–609.

Baysal, E, Sharma, S, Wong, SC et al. (1994). Distribution of β-thalassemia mutations in three Asian Indian populations with distant geographical locations. *Hemoglobin* 18: 201–209.

Boletini, E, Svobodova, M, Divoky, V et al. (1994). Sickle cell anemia, sickle cell β-thalassemia, and thalassemia major in Albania: Characterization of mutations. *Hum. Genet.* 93: 182–187.

Bouhass, R, Perrrrin, P, and Trabuchet, G. (1994). The spectrum of β-thalassemia mutations in the Oran region of Algeria. *Hemoglobin* 18: 211–219.

Brittenham, GM. (1987). Globin gene variants and polymorphisms in India. In Winter W, editor. *Hemoglobin variants in human populations.* Vol 2. Boca Raton: CRC Press, pp. 80–109.

Brown, JM, Thein, SL, Weatherall, DJ et al. (1992). The spectrum of beta thalassemia in Burma. *Br. J. Haematol.* 81: 574–578.

Cao, A, Furbetta, M, Galanello, R et al. (1981). Prevention of homozygous β-thalassemia by carrier screening and prenatal diagnosis in Sardinia. *Am. J. Hum. Genet.* 33: 592–605.

Chehab, FF, Der Kaloustian, V, Khouri, FP et al. (1987). The molecular basis of β-thalassemia in Lebanon: Application to prenatal diagnosis. *Blood* 69: 1141–1145.

Coleman, MB, Steinberg, MH, Harrell, AH et al. (1992). The −87 (C→A) β+-thalassemia mutation in a black family. *Hemoglobin* 16: 399–401.

Coutinho Gomes, MP, Gomes da Costa, MG, Braga, LB et al. (1988). β-thalassemia mutations in the Portuguese population. *Hum. Genet.* 78: 13–15.

Dimovski, A, Efremov, DG, Jankovic, L et al. (1990). β-thalassemia in Yugoslavia. *Hemoglobin* 14: 15–24.

Dincol, G, Aksoy, M, and Erdem, S. (1979). Beta thalassaemia with increased haemoglobin A₂ in Turkey. A study of 164 thalassaemic heterozygotes. *Hum. Hered.* 29: 272–278.

El Hazmi, MAF, Warsy AS, and Al-Swailem, AR. (1995). The frequency of 14 β-thalassemia mutations in the Arab populations. *Hemoglobin* 19: 353–360.

Efremov, GD. (1992). Hemoglobinopathies in Yugoslavia: An update. *Hemoglobin* 16: 531–544.

Faustino, P, Osorio-Almeida, L, Barbot, J et al. (1992). Novel promoter and splice junction defects add to the genetic, clinical or geographic heterogeneity of β-thalassemia in the Portuguese population. *Hum. Genet.* 89: 573–576.

Fessas, Ph, Loukopoulos, D, and Kaltsoya-Tassiopoulou, A. (1988). Prevention of thalassemia major and the HbS syndromes in Greece and other countries with high frequency. In Loukopoulos D (editor). *Prenatal diagnosis of thalassemia and the hemoglobinopathies.* Boca Raton: CRC Press, pp. 68–86.

Filon, D, Oron, V, Shawa, R et al. (1995). Spectrum of beta-thalassemia mutations in the Gaza area. *Hum. Mutat.* 5: 351–353.

Flint, J, Harding, RM, Boyce, AJ, and Clegg, JB. (1993). The population genetics of the haemoglobinopathies. *Baillere's Clin. Haematol.* 6: 215–262.

Fonseca, SF, Kerbauy, J, Escrivao, C et al. (1998). Genetic analysis of beta-thalassemia major and beta-thalassemia intermedia in Brazil. *Hemoglobin* 22: 197–207.

Fucharoen, S, Katsube, T, Fucharoen, G et al. (1990). Molecular heterogeneity of beta-thalassaemia in the Japanese: Identification of two novel mutations. *Br. J. Haematol.* 74: 101–107.

Galano, P, Girodon, E, Ghanem, N et al. (1992). High prevalence of the beta-thalassemia nonsense 37 mutation in Catalonians from the Ebro delta. *Br. J. Hematol.* 81: 126–127.

Garewal, G, Fearon, CW, Warren, TC et al. (1994). The molecular basis of β-thalassaemia in Punjabi and Maharashtran Indians includes a multilocus aetiology involving triplicated β-globin loci. *Br. J. Haematol.* 86: 372–376.

George, E, Li, HJ, Fei, YJ, Reese, AL et al. (1992). Types of thalassemia among patients attending a large University Clinic in Kuala Lumpur, Malaysia. *Hemoglobin* 16: 51–66.

Gonzalez-Redondo, JM, Stoming, TA, Lanclos, KD et al. (1988). Clinical and genetic heterogeneity in black patients with homozygous β-thalassemia from the Southeastern United States. *Blood* 72: 1007–1014.

Gupta, RB, Tiwary, RS, Pande, PL et al. (1991). Hemoglobinopathies among the Gond tribal groups of central India; interaction of α- and β-thalassemia with β chain variants. *Hemoglobin* 15: 441–458.

Hall, GW, Barnetson, RA, and Thein, SL. (1992). Beta thalassaemia in the indigenous British population. *Br. J. Haematol.* 82: 584–588.

Hardison, R, Riemer, C, Chui, DHK et al. (1998). Electronic access to sequence alignments; experimental results and human mutations as an aid to studying globin gene regulation. *Genomics* 47: 429–437.

Hattori, Y, Yamane, A, Yamashiro, Y et al. (1989). Characterization of beta-thalassemia mutations among the Japanese. *Hemoglobin* 13: 657–670.

Hattori, Y, Yamashiro, Y, Ohba, Y et al. (1991). A new β-thalassemia mutation (initiation codon A̲TG-G̲TG) found in the Japanese population. *Hemoglobin* 15: 317–325.

Hattori, Y, Yamamoto, K, Yamashiro, Y et al. (1992). Three β-thalassemia mutations in the Japanese: IVS-II-1 (G→A), IVS-II-848 (C→G), and codon 90 (G̲AG→T̲AG). *Hemoglobin* 16: 93–97.

Hill, AVS, Bowden, DK, O'Shaughnessy, DF et al. (1988). β-thalassemia in Melanesia: Association with Malaria and characterization of a common variant (IVS-1 nt 5 G→C). *Blood* 72: 9–14.

Ho, PJ, Rochette, J, Fisher, CA et al. (1996). Moderate reduction of beta-globin transcript by a novel mutation in the 5′ untranslated region: A study of its interaction with other genotypes in two families. *Blood* 87: 1170–1178.

Huisman, THJ, Carver, MFH, and Baysal, E. (1997). *A Syllabus of Thalassemia Mutations.* Augusta, GA: The Sickle Cell Anemia Foundation.

Indrak, K, Brabec, V, Indrakova, J et al. (1992). Molecular characterization of β-thalassemia in Czechoslovakia. *Hum. Genet.* 88: 399–404.

Jankovic, L, Dimovski, AJ, Kollia, P et al. (1991). A CG mutation at nt position 6 3′ to the terminating codon may be the cause of a silent β-thalassemia. *Int. J. Hematol.* 54: 289–293.

Kalaydjieva, L, Eigel, A, and Horst, J. (1989). The molecular basis of β-thalassaemia in Bulgaria. *J. Med. Genet.* 26: 614–618.

Kamel, K. (1987). Hemoglobin variants in the Middle East. In Winter, W, editor. *Hemoglobin variants in human populations.* Vol 2. Boca Raton: CRC Press, pp 45–64.

Kasili, EG (1987). The geographical distribution of some abnormal hemoglobins in Eastern Africa. In Winter, W (editor). *Hemoglobin variants in human populations.* Vol 2. Boca Raton: CRC Press. pp. 30–43.

Kattamis, C, Hu, H, Cheng, G et al. (1990). Molecular characterization of β-thalassemia in 174 Greek patients with thalassemia major. *Br. J. Haematol.* 74: 342–346.

Kazazian, HH, Orkin, SH, Markham, AF et al. (1984a). Quantification of the close association between DNA haplotypes and specific beta-thalassaemia mutations in Mediterraneans. *Nature* 310: 152–154.

Kazazian, HH, Orkin, SH, Antonarakis, SE et al. (1984b). Molecular characterization of seven β-thalassemia mutations in Asian Indians. *EMBO J.* 3: 593–596.

Kazazian, HH, Dowling, CE, Waber, PG et al. (1986). The spectrum of β-thalassemia genes in China and Southeast Asia. *Blood* 68: 964–966.

Khan, SN and Riazuddin, S. (1988). Molecular characterization of beta-thalassemia in Pakistan. *Hemoglobin* 22: 333–345.

Ko, MS, Kim, SI, Cho, HI et al. (1992). A β-thalassemia mutation found in Korea. *Hemoglobin* 16: 313–320.

Ko, TM, Cavilles, AP Jr, Hwa, HL et al. (1998). Prevalence and molecular characterization of beta-thalassemia in Filipinos. *Ann. Hematol.* 77: 257–260.

Kollia, P, Karababa, Ph, Sinopoulou, K et al. (1992). Beta-thalassaemia mutations and the underlying beta gene cluster haplotypes in the Greek population. *Gene Geog.* 6: 59–70.

Kuliev, A, Razulov, IMR, Dadasheva, T et al. (1994). Thalassaemia in Azerbaijan. *J. Med. Gene.* 31: 209–212.

Kulozik, A, Yarwood, N, and Jones, RW. (1988). The Corfu (δβ)⁰-thalassemia; a small deletion acts at a distance to selectively abolish β-globin gene expression. *Blood* 71: 457–462.

Liu, TC, Lib, SF, Yang, TY et al. (1997). Prenatal diagnosis of thalassemia in the Chinese. *Am. J. Hematol.* 55: 65–68.

Livingstone, FA. (1985). *Frequencies of Hemoglobin Variants.* New York: Oxford University Press.

Maggio, A, Di Marzo, R, Giambona, A et al. (1990). Beta-thalassemia mutations in Sicily. *Ann. N. Y. Acad. Sci.* 612: 67–73.

Malamos, B, Fessas, P, and Stamatoyannopoulos, G (1965). Types of thalassemia trait carriers as revealed by study of their incidence in Greece. *Br. J. Haematol.* 8: 5–13.

Merat, A, Haghshenas, M, Mostafavi Pou, Z et al. (1993). β-thalassemia in Southwestern Iran. *Hemoglobin* 17: 427–436.

Milland, M, Berge-Lefranc, JL, Lena, D, and Cartouzou, G. (1987). Oligonucleotide screening of beta thalassemia mutations in the southeast of France. *Hemoglobin* 11: 317–327.

Modell, B, Dazlison, M, and Ingzam, D (1998). APoGI Project. Accessible Publishing of Scientific Information; Information Materials for Haemoglobin Disorders. Department of Primary Care and Population Sciences, and Centre for Health Informatics and Multiprofessional Education, University of London.

Novelletto, A, Hafez, M, Deidda, G et al. (1990). Molecular characterization of thalassemia mutations in Egypt. *Hum. Genet.* 85: 272–274.

Nozari, G, Rahbar, S, Golshiyzan, A, and Rahmanzadeh, S. (1995). Molecular analyses of β-thalassemia in Iran. *Hemoglobin* 19: 425–431.

Oner, R, Altay, C, Gurgey, A, et al. (1990). β-thalassemia in Turkey. *Hemoglobin* 14: 1–13.

Orkin, SH, Kazazian, HH, Antonarakis, SE et al. (1982). Linkage of β-thalassemia mutations and β-globin gene polymorphisms with DNA polymorphisms in human β-globin gene cluster. *Nature* 296: 627–631.

Orkin, SH, Antonarakis, S, and Loukopoulos, D. (1984a). Abnormal processing of β^Knossos RNA. *Blood* 64: 311–313.

Orkin, SH, Antonarakis, SE, and Kazazian, HH Jr. (1984b). Base substitution at position −88 in a beta-thalassemic globin gene. Further evidence for the role of distal promoter element ACACCC. *J. Biol. Chem.* 259: 8679–8681.

Oshima, K, Harano, T, and Harano, K. (1996). Japanese beta zero thalassemia: Molecular characterization of a novel insertion causing a stop codon. *Am. J. Hematol.* 52: 39–41.

Petkov, GH, Efremov, GD, Efremov, DG et al. (1990). β-thalassemia in Bulgaria. *Hemoglobin* 14: 25–33.

Ribeiro, ML, Goncalves, P, Cunha, E et al. (1997). Genetic heterogeneity of beta thalassemia in populations of the Iberian Peninsula. *Hemoglobin* 21: 261–269.

Ringelhann, B, Szelenyi, JG, Horanyi, M et al. (1993). Molecular characterization of beta thalassemia in Hungary. *Hum. Genet.* 92: 385–387.

Romana, M, Keklard, L, Guillemin, G, et al. (1996). Molecular characterization of beta thalassemia mutations in Guadeloupe. *Am. J. Hematol.* 53: 228–233.

Rosatelli, MC, Tuveri, T, Scalas, MT et al. (1992). Molecular screening and fetal diagnosis of β-thalassemia in the Italian population. *Hum. Genet.* 89: 585–589.

Rund, D, Filon, D, Dowling, C et al. (1990). Molecular studies of β-thalassemia in Israel. Mutational analysis and expression studies. *Ann. N. Y. Acad. Sci.* 612: 98–105.

Sadiq, MFG and Huisman, THJ. (1994). Molecular characterization of β-thalassemia in North Jordan. *Hemoglobin* 18: 325–332.

Schiliro, G, Di Gregorio, F, Samperi, P et al. (1995). Genetic heterogeneity of beta-thalassemia in southeast Sicily. *Am. J. Hematol.* 48: 5–11.

Shimizu, K, Park, KS, and Omoto, K. (1989). The DNA polymorphisms of the β-globin gene cluster and the arrangements of the α- and the γ-globin genes in Koreans. *Hemoglobin* 13: 137–146.

Silvestroni, E and Bianco, I. (1975). Screening for microcythemia in Italy; analysis of data collected in the past 30 years. *Am. J. Hum. Genet.* 27: 198–212.

Siniscalco, M, Bernini, L, Latte, B, and Motulsky, A. (1961). Favism and thalassemia in Sardinia and their relationship to malaria. *Nature* 190: 1179–1180.

Sonati, MF, Kimura, EM, Grotto, HZW et al. (1996). Hereditary hemoglobinopathies in a population from Southeast Brazil. *Hemoglobin* 20: 175–179.

Tadmouri, GO, Tuzmen, S, Ozcelik, H et al. (1998). Molecular and population genetic analyses of β-thalassemia in Turkey. *Am. J. Hematol.* 57: 215–220.

Tamagnini, GP, Goncalves, P, Ribeiro, MLS et al. (1993). β-thalassemia mutations in the Portuguese; high frequencies of two alleles in restricted populations. *Hemoglobin* 17: 31–40.

Tegos, C, Voutsadakis, A, Paleologou, N et al. (1987). The incidence and distribution of thalassemias in Greece (a study on 64,814 recruits). *Hellenic Armed Forces Med. Rev.* (in Greek) 21: 27–36.

Tentori, L and Marinucci, M. (1986). Hemoglobin variants and thalassemias in Italy. In Winter, WP, editor. *Hemoglobin variants in human populations.* Vol 1. Boca Raton: CRC Press, pp. 156–164.

Thein, SL. (1993). β-Thalassaemia. *Balliere's Clin. Haematol.* 6: 151–175.

Thein, SL, Hesketh, C, Wallace, RB et al. (1988). The molecular basis of thalassaemia major and thalassaemia intermedia in Asian Indians: Application to prenatal diagnosis. *Br. J. Haematol.* 70: 225–231.

Thein, SL, Winichagoon, P, Hesketh, C et al. (1990). The molecular basis of β-thalassemia in Thailand: Application to prenatal diagnosis. *Am. J. Hum. Genet.* 47: 369–375.

Thein, SL, Wood, WG, Wickramasinghe, SN, and Galvin, MC. (1993). Beta-thalassaemia unlinked to the beta-globin gene in an English family. *Br. J. Haematol.* 82: 961–967.

Verma, IC, Saxena, R, Thomas, E, and Jain, PK. (1997). Regional distribution of beta-thalassemia mutations in India. *Hum. Genet.* 100: 109–113.

Wainscoat, JS, Thein, SL, Wood, WG et al. (1985). A novel deletion in the β-globin gene complex. *Ann. N. Y. Acad. Sci.* 445: 20–27.

Wasi, P. (1987). Geographic distribution of hemoglobin variants in South East Asia. In Winter W (editor). *Hemoglobin variants in human populations.* Vol 2. Boca Raton: CRC Press. pp. 112–127.

Waye, JS, Eng, B, Hunt, JA, and Chui, DHK. (1994). Filipino β-thalassemia due to a large deletion: Identification of the deletion endpoints and polymerase chain reaction (PCR)-based diagnosis. *Hum. Genet.* 94: 530–532.

Weatherall, DJ and Clegg, JB. (1981). *Thalassaemia Syndromes.* 3rd ed. Oxford: Blackwell Scientific Publications.

WHO Working Group Report. (1982). Community control of hereditary anemias. *Bull. WHO* 60: 643–660.

WHO. (1985). Update of the Progress of Hemoglobinopathies Control. Report of the Third and Fourth Annual Meetings of the WHO Working Group for the Community Control of Hereditary Anaemias. Unpublished report of the WHO HMG/WG/ 85.8.

WHO. (1989). Report of the Sixth Annual Meeting of the WHO Working Group on the Feasibility Study on Hereditary Disease Community Control Programs (Hereditary Anaemias). Cagliari, Sardinia, Italy, April 8–9 1989.

Wildmann, C, Laronelle, Y, Vaerman, JL et al. (1993). An initiation codon mutation as a cause of β-thalassemia in a Belgian family. *Hemoglobin* 17: 19–30.

Yamamoto, K, Yamamoto, K, Hattori, Y et al. (1992). Two β-thalassemia mutations in Japan: Codon 121 (GAA-TAA) and IVS-1-130 (G-C). *Hemoglobin* 16: 295–302.

Yang, KG, Kutlar, F, George, E, et al. (1989). Molecular characterization of β-globin gene mutations in Malay patients with Hb E β-thalassaemia and thalassaemia major. *Br. J. Haematol.* 72: 73–80.

Yasunaga, M, Fujiyama, Y, Miyagawa, A et al. (1995). Thalassemia incidentally found by marked erythrocytosis due an ochre mutation at codon 35 in a Japanese man. *Int. Med.* 34: 1198–1200.

Zeng, Y-T. (1987). Hemoglobin variants in China. In Winter W (editor). *Hemoglobin variants in human populations.* Vol 2. Boca Raton: CRC Press. pp. 130–140.

Zhang, J-Z, Cai, S-P, He, X et al. (1988). Molecular basis of β-thalassemia in South China. *Hum. Genet.* 78: 37–40.

32

Geographic Distribution of α Thalassemia

LUIGI F. BERNINI

More than 20 years ago, Weatherall and Clegg (1981) reviewed the world distribution of α thalassemia. That review is still valid for the heterogeneous distribution of α+ and α0 thalassemia determinants, as well as for the regions where HbH (β4) disease and Hb Bart's (γ4) hydrops fetalis have a high prevalence and create public health problems. More recent reviews on the distribution and population genetics of hemoglobinopathies have been published by Livingstone (1985), Hill (1992), and Flint et al. (1998). This chapter summarizes the results of recent investigations dealing with the frequency of α+ and α0 determinants in different countries and ethnic groups. The present contribution does not survey and discuss the changes in the prevalence of α thalassemia brought about by migration. These changes started centuries ago with the displacement of populations, for political and/or economic reasons, from areas at high risk for hemoglobinopathies to other regions and continents in which these inherited disorders were originally unknown or very rare.

Thalassemia phenotypes result from the interactions of wild-type chromosomes with α+ and α0 thalassemia determinants; α+ and α0 refer, respectively, to those forms of α thalassemia in which the production of α-globin chains from a single α-gene cluster is either reduced (α+) or completely abolished (α0). α+Thalassemia involves only one of the two linked α-globin genes and is caused by either gene deletion or nondeletion defects. α0

Thalassemia is usually the result of the deletion of both linked α-globin genes, but it can also be caused by mutations that inactivate the residual α-globin gene left on an α+thalassemia chromosome and, even more rarely, by deletions of the α-globin gene cluster gene Major Regulatory Element (α-MRE) or HS-40. Chapter 17 details the molecular mechanisms of α thalassemia. The segregation in populations of both α+ and α0 alleles accounts for the presence of genotypes with three (shown by the notation –α/αα), two (- -/αα or –α/–α), and one (- -/–α) functional α-globin gene. These genotypes are responsible for the expression of roughly 75, 50, and 25 percent, respectively, of the normal α-globin chain output. The fourth genotype (- -/- -) does not express any α-globin chain and results in a severe fetal anemia, Hb Bart's hydrops fetalis, which is lethal during gestation or soon after birth.

CLINICAL AND HEMATOLOGIC DIAGNOSIS OF THALASSEMIC PHENOTYPES

The diagnosis of HbH disease and the Hb Bart's hydrops fetalis syndrome is usually straightforward. Identification of individuals carrying two or three normal α-globin genes is more difficult. The details of diagnosis are discussed in Chapter 18. α Thalassemia trait can be diagnosed in most cases if iron deficiency and β thalassemia with normal HbA$_2$ levels can be excluded. In contrast, using hematologic indices to identify heterozygotes for α+ thalassemia (silent carriers) is virtually impossible, although when considered as a group, their average hematologic indices and globin biosynthetic ratios are significantly different from individuals with a normal genotype (αα/αα) and α thalassemia trait (- -/αα or –α/–α) (Williams et al., 1996; Bernini and Harteveld, 1998). A particularly useful marker (Weatherall, 1963; Tanpaichitr et al., 1988) that was and still is widely exploited for population screening is a raised level of Hb Bart's in the cord blood of newborn carriers of α+ and α0 thalassemia. Increased amounts of Hb Bart's are detected in nearly all individuals in whom two α-globin genes are deleted or otherwise nonfunctional (Chapter 17) and even in heterozygotes for severe nondeletional mutants of the α2-globin gene. Unfortunately, however, many individuals with the genotype –α/αα are negative for Hb Bart's, which leads to a constant underestimation of α+ thalassemia gene frequencies (Chapter 18).

In a recent survey of abnormal hemoglobins and α thalassemia in Togolese newborns, 15 percent of the infants with a –α/αα genotype did not have any measurable Hb Bart's at birth, whereas 17 percent of the

Martin H. Steinberg, Bernard G. Forget, Douglas R. Higgs, and Ronald L. Nagel, editors. *Disorders of Hemoglobin: Genetics, Pathophysiology, and Clinical Management.* © 2001 Cambridge University Press. All rights reserved.

normal newborns had raised levels (Segbena et al., 1998). In both the αα/αα and -α/αα groups, the only apparent hematologic difference between Hb Bart's positive and Hb Bart's negative infants was that the former had higher HbF levels. Normal newborns positive for Hb Bart's also weighed significantly less than those who were negative for Hb Bart's. These results agree with earlier observations when it was not possible to diagnose α thalassemia in some children positive for Hb Bart's (Folayan-Esan, 1972; Nhonoli et al., 1979). In a survey in Thailand, 13 percent Hb Bart's negative individuals were found among -α/αα genotypes, and no Hb Bart's was seen in normal newborns (Tanphaichitr et al., 1988). Hb Bart's was measured by starch gel electrophoresis, probably the most sensitive method for its detection but not for its quantitation. In Sardinia, 61 percent of the -α/αα genotypes were negative for Hb Bart's (Galanello et al., 1984).

The sensitivity with which Hb Bart's can be identified is influenced by the methodology used. The genetic background of the population investigated and possibly local environmental conditions may also modify the degree of globin chains synthesis imbalance seen in α thalassemia and affect the level of Hb Bart's in cord blood. Also, the bimodal pattern of Hb Bart's values, which is supposed to indicate the deletion or loss of function of either one or two α-globin genes, is likely to be observed in populations in which only the common, deletional α-thalassemia mutations segregate (Higgs et al., 1980a; Segbena et al., 1998). The presence in the population of several α+ thalassemia alleles, deletional and nondeletional, expressing variable amounts of α-globin chains generates many overlapping phenotypes, which can smooth over or obliterate a multimodal distribution. Finally, Hb Bart's disappears rapidly after birth, making the test unsuitable for screening adults. Of the few alternative procedures (Chapter 18), the immunologic quantitation of ζ-globin chains seems the most promising for adult carriers of α⁰ thalassemia (Chui et al., 1988). This test has proved to be highly sensitive and specific in heterozygotes for the - -^{SEA} deletion (Tang et al., 1993; Ausavarungnirun et al., 1998) and might be useful for detecting other common α⁰ thalassemia determinants, such as - -$^{MED\ 1}$ and $-(\alpha)^{20.5}$, where ζ genes remain intact.

MOLECULAR CHARACTERIZATION OF α THALASSEMIA

By the late 1970s, the introduction of Southern blot hybridization and gene mapping allowed the detection of large deletions within the α-globin gene cluster (Dozy et al., 1979; Higgs et al., 1980b, 1981). Ten years later the molecular analysis of α-thalassemia mutations was made much easier by the application of

Polymerase chain reaction (PCR)-based strategies. This approach enabled the amplification and direct sequencing of the α2- and α1-globin genes, fast and nonradioactive diagnosis of the most common large deletions (by gap amplification), the search for common mutants (by allele-specific oligonucleotide [ASO] hybridization), and the complete screening of both genes for unknown mutations (by combined denaturing gradient gel electrophoresis [DGGE], and single strand conformation polymorphism [SSCP] analysis and DNA sequencing) (Dodé et al., 1990; Bowden et al., 1992; Traeger-Synodinos et al., 1993; Harteveld et al., 1996; reviewed by Kattamis et al., 1996). Despite progress in the molecular characterization of α thalassemia, accurate estimations of gene frequency in populations by screening of appropriately sized random samples are infrequent, and reliable data are only available in a few instances.

This probably arises because α thalassemia does not represent a major clinical problem in most regions except for Southeast Asia and southern China. Even in those places, HbH disease is usually well tolerated, although it does represent an important cause of chronic anemia. Similarly, in Oceania, homozygous α+ thalassemia is responsible for mild forms of anemia in a substantial portion of the population (Bowden et al., 1985).

A second reason for the lack of reliable data is that random, large-scale screening procedures are expensive and time-consuming, and not within the reach of most laboratories, although the present technology can provide correct molecular diagnoses. Therefore, the aim of most α thalassemia surveys has been to characterize molecular defects in small numbers of patients with HbH disease, which provides a qualitative picture of the α thalassemia alleles segregating in a given population. Quite often, however, the information cannot be used to deduce the relative frequencies of the different mutations because it may provide biased estimates. For example, HbH disease caused by the interaction of α⁰ determinants with point mutations of α2 genes is usually more severe than HbH disease caused by deletion of either α2 or α1 genes (Chapters 17 and 18). Point mutations may therefore be overrepresented in patients with HbH syndromes. In Southeast Asia (Liu et al., 1994) and in Thailand in particular (Wongchanchailert et al., 1992), Hb Constant Spring is found in about 50 percent of the cases of HbH disease, whereas its gene frequency is lower than that of deletional α+ alleles.

Despite their limitation in the diagnosis of α+ thalassemia, it seems unrealistic to do without the help of hematologic indices for disease detection. A compromise, which can probably provide a reasonably accurate estimate of the frequency of α+ and α⁰ thalassemia, might be to screen for α thalassemia trait (−α/−α and - -/αα) by hematologic analysis in a large population sample and to follow it up by molecular characterization of positive individuals. In addition, screening done at the same time on a modest sample of 200 to 300 random chromosomes by gap PCR and hybridization would detect the frequency of those determinants (single α-globin gene deletions and point mutations) that are difficult or impossible to detect in other ways. The frequency of α^0 and α^+ phenotypes can also be assessed through the complete ascertainment of the prevalence of hydrops fetalis and HbH disease when hospitals and public health records are reliable enough to allow such a calculation (Pirastu et al., 1982; O-Prasertsawat et al., 1990).

WORLD DISTRIBUTION OF α THALASSEMIAS

Tables 32.1 through 32.7 illustrate the distribution of α-thalassemia mutations in different geographic areas. The data have been largely obtained through random population surveys carried out by DNA analysis. Results are given in terms of gene frequencies, indicating the number of chromosomes analyzed and, when the size of the sample allows, the 95 percent confidence limits of the mean. Gene frequencies refer to α^0 thalassemia, deletional α^+ thalassemia, nondeletional α^+thalassemia, and α-globin gene triplications. These kinds of data are the most useful because they allow prediction of the incidence at birth of Hb Bart's hydrops fetalis and HbH disease in each population. α-Globin gene triplications may be an indication of the recombination process that leads to deletion and duplication within the α-globin gene cluster. The frequency of α-globin gene triplication ranges from 0.002 to 0.01 in most populations. It is unclear whether the frequencies are modified by selection or, considering the wide fluctuations, by random genetic drift. They seem much too high to reflect the recombination rate of misaligned α-globin genes.

The interaction of triplicated α-globin genes with heterozygous β thalassemia leads to β thalassemia intermedia in all homozygotes for the α-globin gene triplication and in some heterozygotes (Galanello et al., 1983; Camaschella et al., 1987). The lower section of each table gives the relative proportions of specific α-thalassemia alleles. Sometimes the data on gene frequencies and the distribution of mutations were taken from different sources and combined. Other times, the proportion of mutations characterized by DNA analysis of patients with HbH disease patients were the only data available.

Sub-Saharan Africa

Since the early 1960s, Hb Bart's in the cord blood of African and African-American neonates has been used to screen for α thalassemia (reviewed by Weatherall and Clegg, 1981). When restriction endonuclease analysis of DNA established the presence of two predominant genotypes in α-thalassemic populations, −α/αα and −α/−α, it simultaneously demonstrated that Hb Bart's is a poor predictor of the −α/αα genotype (Higgs et al., 1979, 1980a). The only α thalassemia present in all the African populations investigated was α^+ thalassemia of that genotype (Table 32.1). The deletion is virtually always of the $-\alpha^{3.7}$ type; only in The Gambia about 10 percent of deletions are of the $-\alpha^{4.2}$ type (Hill, 1992). Restriction endonuclease analysis using the enzyme Apa I has revealed in some West Africans that the $-\alpha^{3.7}$ determinant is of subtype I (Dode et al., 1988). The gene frequency of α^+ thalassemia ranges from 0.06 in South Africa to 0.33 to 0.40 in Nigeria; the highest values occur in the equatorial belt from Ivory Coast to Kenya, the lowest (0.05 to 0.08) in North and South Africa. The San hunter-gatherers of the Kalahari desert in Namibia have a very low frequency of α^+ thalassemia, and they show no trace of the sickle β-globin gene (Ramsay and Jenkins, 1984). The investigators suggest that α thalassemia is a vestige of the selective pressure of malaria on the San ancestors before the southward expansion of Bantu people. They further propose that α thalassemia is older than the sickle β-globin gene and is the oldest malaria protective trait in Africa (Chapters 26 and 30). Parts of the screening studies reported in Table 32.1 were carried out in people who were normal and in people who were homozygous for HbS, so that the frequency of α thalassemia in both groups could be compared. If, as suggested (Mears et al., 1983; Kar et al., 1986), the coexistence of α thalassemia does increase the life expectancy of people with sickle cell anemia (Chapter 28), adult HbS homozygotes would have a higher frequency of $-\alpha^{3.7}$ than normal individuals or carriers of the sickle cell trait. Co-occurrence of α thalassemia and sickle cell anemia causes epistatic effects (Chapters 26 and 28), but whether patients with both conditions survive longer than those with sickle cell anemia alone has not been established. Elevated α^+ thalassemia frequencies were found in sickle cell anemia patients in Benin and Upper Volta, but not in Senegal (Pagnier et al., 1984) or in two population samples in Nigeria (Falusi et al., 1987; Adekile et al., 1993). Because the question is unsettled, using caution when interpreting gene frequencies of α thalassemia in sickle cell anemia is prudent. α^0 Thalassemia is not present at detectable levels in sub-Saharan Africa; the rare deletion found in American blacks (Chapter 17) most probably did not originate in Africa. The large deletions detected in North Africa are common in other Mediterranean areas and are probably due to gene flow from there.

Table 32.1. Sub-Saharan Africa

α Thalassemia determinants (gene frequency)	Nigeria (overall) 2N = 1.126	Nigeria (Yoruba)	Nigeria (Ibo)	Nigeria (Hausa)	Nigeria (Fulani)	Sâo Tomé and Principe
α⁰ Thalassemia						
α⁺ Thalassemia (Deletions)	0.26 ± 0.04 (S/S hom.)*	0.25	0.33	0.21	0.04	0.31
	0.24 ± 0.07 (A/A hom.)*					
	0.26 ± 0.06 (A/A + A/S + A/C)*†	0.25	0.27	0.24		
	0.25 ± 0.06 (S/S+S/C)†					
α⁺ Thalassemia (Point Mutations) α-globin gene	0.009*					
	0.005†					
α⁺ (Relative frequencies) −α³·⁷	100%					100%

α Thalassemia determinants (gene frequency)	Gambia 2N = 106	Senegal (overall) 2N = 118	Benin and Upper Volta (overall) 2N = 204	Zambia 2N = 200	Zaire
α⁰ Thalassemia					
α⁺ Thalassemia (Deletions)	0.08 ± 0.05	0.1 ± 0.077 (A/A)	0.16 ± 0.076 (A/A+A/S+A/C+C/C)	0.27 ± 0.06 (3)	0.2
		0.1 ± 0.077 (S/S)	0.28 ± 0.08 (S/S+S/C)		
α⁺ Thalassemia (Point mutations) α-globin gene	0.009	0.02		0.01	
α⁺ (Relative frequencies)					
α 3.7	90%	100%	100%	100%	100%
α 4.2	10%				

α-Thalassemia determinants (gene frequency)	Togo 2N = 340	C.A.R. (overall) 2N = 98	C.A.R. (Pigmies) 2N = 120	Ivory Coast 2N = 468	Kenya	South Africa 2N = 508
α⁰ Thalassemia						
α⁺ Thalassemia (Deletions)	0.26 ± 0.05	0.22 ± 0.11	0.125 ± 0.06*	0.22 ± 0.04	0.19	0.06 (San) − 0.2 (Venda) 0.07 (Sotho-Tswana; Nguni)
		0.25 ± 0.12*				
α⁺ Thalassemia (Point mutations) α-globin gene Triplications	0.012 (1)					0.01 – 0.03
α⁺ (Relative frequencies) −α³·⁷	100 %	100 %	100 %	100 %	100 %	100 %

* (Nigeria) Adekile et al., 1993. (Nigeria) Falusi et al., 1987.

† (Sâo Tomé and Principe) Bento et al. 1997.

(Gambia) Abdalla et al. 1989; (Senegal, Benin, and Upper Volta) Pagnier et al., 1984; (Zambia) Muklwala et al., 1989; (Zaire) Dodé et al., 1988; (Togo) Segbena et al., 1998; (C.A.R.) Pagnier et al., 1984; L. F. Bernini (unpublished)*; (Ivory Coast) Coulibaly (unpublished); (Kenya) reported by Flint et al., 1998; (South Africa) Ramsay and Jenkins, 1987.

Mediterranean Basin

The Mediterranean basin and Southeastern Asia are the only regions of the world where α⁺ and α⁰ thalassemia coexist and where both HbH disease and Hb Bart's hydrops fetalis occur, although the latter is rare in the Mediterranean. The presence of α thalassemia in the coastal countries and on the Mediterranean islands was first recognized in the mid-1950s, when sporadic cases of HbH disease in Greece, continental Italy, Sardinia,

Cyprus, and Israel were identified (Weatherall and Clegg, 1981).

Table 32.2 illustrates the frequency and molecular distribution of α thalassemia in countries within the Mediterranean basin. North Africa is included in this survey, but data from only Algeria and Egypt are included, although α thalassemia is present in Morocco, Tunisia, and Libya (El Hazmi and Warsy, 1996). The highest frequencies of α^+ thalassemia are in Sardinia and Cyprus; the lowest are in Spain. The low frequency of α^0 thalassemia accounts for the rarity of hydrops fetalis, which has been observed only twice in Sardinia (Galanello et al., 1990, and personal communication), once in Turkey, and a few times in Cyprus and Greece (Chapter 18). Deletional α^+ thalassemia is nearly always represented by the $-\alpha^{3.7}$ type I determinant. In one case, however, an initiation codon mutation was linked to a $-\alpha^{3.7\ II}$ deletion. This has also been found in southern Italians and Algerians (Morlé et al., 1985; Di Rienzo et al., 1986).

A remarkable feature of the α thalassemia distribution along the Mediterranean countries is the heterogeneity of mutations and the clustering of the different mutations within regions and provinces of the same country. In Apulia (Italy), for instance, the only α^0 determinant found in HbH disease patients is the $-\alpha^{20.5}$ deletion (Massa et al., 1994). The mutation is also present in other regions of continental Italy, but not in the Mediterranean Islands. The haplotype $-\ -^{MED\ I}$ is present in 100 percent of HbH disease patients who are autochthonous Sardinians (Galanello et al., 1992) and in about 70 percent of Sicilians. In Sicily, the remaining 30 percent of HbH disease is caused by the $-\ -^{CAL}$ determinant, a deletion found originally in a family from Calabria (Fortina et al., 1991) and also reported in a Spanish family (Villegas et al., 1994).

Heterogeneity and clustering are more evident in countries such as Israel, where α thalassemia is prevalent in different ethnic groups such as the Jews of Yemenite, Iraqi, and Kurdish origin and the Israeli Arabs (Rund et al., 1998; Tamary et al., 1998). The major α^+ and α^0 thalassemia determinants, common β thalassemia mutations behave similarly, show a frequency gradient across the major axis of the Mediterranean Basin from Spain to the Middle East. From Portugal and Spain to Turkey, the frequency of deletional α^+ thalassemia decreases as one travels eastward, whereas the frequency of α^+ thalassemia caused by point mutations increases. Although those estimates, inferred from the analysis of HbH disease patients, are not necessarily correct, the conclusion is supported by results obtained by random screens in Latium (Italy) (Foglietta et al., 1995) and by the molecular characterization of HbH disease in Greek and Turkish Cypriots (Baysal et al., 1995).

A similar shift also occurs for α^+ point mutations; $-\alpha2^{\ IVS-1;\ 5bp\ del.}$, $\alpha2^{IN;\ T\to C}$, and $\alpha2^{\ IN:\ A\to G}$ are prevalent in the west Mediterranean from Spain to southern Italy, whereas two mutations of the polyadenylation signal ($\alpha2^{PA;\ 6A\to G}$ and $\alpha2^{PA;\ 4A\to G}$ account for a large proportion of α^+ thalassemia determinants that are prevalent from Greece to Turkey and Israel. The α^0 mutation $-\ -^{MED\ I}$ is ubiquitous throughout the whole area and is followed in frequency by the $-\alpha^{20.5}$ determinant, which has not been found in Sardinia or Sicily.

Two other α^0 haplotypes caused by large deletions are the $-\ -^{CAL}$ and $-\ -^{MED\ II}$. The first, with the exception of a sporadic case in a Spanish family, occurs only in southern Italy and Sicily; the second is found in Turkey and Cyprus and occasionally, probably because of gene flow, in Calabria (Kutlar et al., 1989; Baysal et al., 1995). Gene flow after the Greek westward expansion and colonization of the Mediterranean may similarly explain the distribution of two mutations of the $\alpha2$-globin gene termination codon, Hb Icaria ($\alpha2^{TER;\ T\to A}$) and Hb Constant Spring ($\alpha2^{\ TER;\ T\to C}$). Hb Icaria represents about 4 percent of the α^+ determinants found in Greeks (Traeger-Synodinos et al., 1993), but outside Greece it has been identified only in southern Italy (Lacerra et al., unpublished data) and the Balkans (Efremov, 1992). Hb Constant Spring was reported in Greece (as Hb Athens) and correctly identified later (Fessas et al., 1972). It has recently been found in Greek and Sicilian HbH disease patients (Traeger-Synodinos et al., unpublished data). The haplotype associated with the mutation is identical in Greeks and Sicilians but differs in five of seven markers from the haplotype of the same mutation occurring in Southeast Asia. Therefore, the Mediterranean Hb Constant Spring mutation probably originated independently and migrated, like Hb Icaria, to Southern Italy. Other mutations, such as $-\ -^{YEM}$ (Yemenite community in Israel), have not been found outside the ethnic group in which they were originally identified.

The scenario described previously confirms again the molecular heterogeneity, geographic clustering, and regional specificity of α-thalassemia mutations. These features are only partially attenuated by the effects of the intense population migrations that have occurred throughout the Mediterranean.

Arabian Peninsula

Deletional α^+ thalassemia has a high prevalence throughout the Arabian peninsula (Table 32.3) but is heterogeneously distributed—gene frequencies vary from 0.01 to 0.67—with the highest values being observed in Oman. More than 90 percent of α^+ deletional haplotypes are the $-\alpha^{3.7}$ type and 2 to 5 per-

Table 32.2. Mediterranean Basin

α-Thalassemia determinants (gene frequency)	Sardinia 2N = 868	Sicily 2N = 1276	Calabria 2N = 600	Apullia	Latium
α⁰ Thalassemia	0.002 – 0.003	≤ 0.001			0.007
α⁺ Thalassemia (Deletions)	0.13 ± 0.02(North) 0.18 ± 0.06 (South)	0.05 ± 0.013		≈ 0.03 (alpha 0 + alpha +)	0.048 ± 0.02
α⁺ Thalassemia (Point mutations)	0.02	0.004			0.01
α-globin gene Triplications	0.002	0.004			0.007
α⁺ (Relative frequencies)					
-α³·⁷	83%	84%	76%	82%	80%
-α⁴·²	1.2%	6%			2.8%
α₂ IN; T→C	11%	6%			2.8%
α₂ IVS 1;5 bp del	3.2%	4%		12%	14%
α₁ IN; A→G	1.3%				
(α₂/α₁) T			24%	6%	
α⁰ (Relative frequencies)					
- -MED I	100%	71%	Present		
-(α)20.5			Present		50%
- -CAL			Present	100%	50%
- -MED II		29%			

α-Thalassemia determinants (gene frequency)	Spain 2N = 800	Portugal 2N = 200	Greece 2N = 454	Cyprus 2N = 1000	Turkey 2N = 276
α⁰ Thalassemia	0.001	<0.005	0.007	0.01	>0.003
α⁺ Thalassemia (Deletions)	0.011 ± 0.007	0.05 ± 0.03	0.037 ± 0017	0.08 – 0.1	0.022
α⁺ Thalassemia (Point mutations)	< 0.001	< 0.001	≈ 0.015	≈ 0.05	≈ 0.01
α-globin gene Triplications	0.004	0.02	0.009	0.007	0.02
α⁺ (Relative frequencies)					
-α³·⁷	97%	70%	70%	61%	52%
-α⁴·²	2%	30%		22%	11%
α₂ IVS 1; 5 bp del		rare	3.75%	10%	15%
α₂ PA; 6 A→G			16%	7%	
α₂ PA; 4 A→G					18%
α₂ IN; T→C	<1%				
α₁ IN; A→G	1%		2%		
α₁ cd 59 G→A					4%

(continued)

Table 32.2 *continued*

α-Thalassemia determinants (gene frequency)	Spain 2N = 800	Portugal 2N = 200	Greece 2N = 454	Cyprus 2N = 1000	Turkey 2N = 276
α_1 cd 62 GTG del			rare		
α_2 TER; T→C(C.S.)			rare		
α_2 TER; T→A(lc)			3.75%		
α^0 (Relative frequencies)					
--Med I	≈ 100%	rare	73%	71%	35%
--Med II				4%	13%
-(α)20.5			27%	24%	52%
--Cal	rare				
--BR	rare				
--Span	rare				

α-Thalassemia determinants (gene frequency)	Israel (Middle East)	Israel (Yemen)	Israel (Arabs)	Egypt 2N = 124	Algeria
α^0 Thalassemia					
α^+ Thalassemia (Deletions)				0.08 ± 0.05	
α^+ Thalassemia (Point mutations)				0.006	
α-globin gene Triplications					
α^+ (Relative frequencies)					
$-\alpha^{3.7}$	50%	90%	20%	96%	75%
$-\alpha^{4.2}$				4%	
$-\alpha^{3.7}$ (HbG Philadelphia)					5%
$\alpha^{3.7II}$ ACCATC→-CATG					10%
α_2 IVS 1; 5 bp del	36%		60%		
α_2 PA; 6 A→G		10%			
α_2 cd 39–41 del/ins	15%		20%		
α cd 110; C→A (Petah Tikva)					10%
(α_2/α_1) T					
α^0 (Relative frequencies)					
--Med I	100%		75%		
--Yem		100%			
-(α)20.5			25%		66%
--?					33%

(Sardinia) Galanello et al., 1992, Masala, 1992 ; (Sicily) Fichera et al., 1997; (Calabria) Muglia et al., 1993, Di Rienzo et al., 1986 ; (Apulia) Massa et al., 1994 ; (Latium) Foglietta et al., 1995; (Spain) Villegas et al., 1992, Ayala et al., 1996, Villegas et al., 1997; (Portugal) Peres et al., 1995; (Greece) Kanavakis et al., 1986, Tzotzos et al., 1986, Traeger-Synodinos et al., 1993; (Cyprus) Baysal et al. 1995; Kyrri et al., 1997; (Turkey) Fei et al., 1989; Öner et al., 1997; (Israel) Shalmon et al., 1996, Rund et al., 1998, Tamary et al., 1998; (Egypt) Novelletto et al., 1989 – (Algeria) Henni et al., 1987.

Table 32.3. Arabian Peninsula

α-Thalassemia determinants (gene frequency)	Saudi Arabia 2N = 1688	Oman 2N = 254	Kuwait 2N = 120	U.A.E. 2N = 836
α⁰ Thalassemia				< 0.005
α⁺ Thalassemia (Deletions)	0.275 ± 0.02	0.67 ± 0.06	0.27 (27 S/S + 33 A/S people)	0.29 ± 0.03
α⁺ Thalassemia (Point mutations)			0.135	0.014
α-globin gene Triplications	0.005			
α⁺ (Relative frequencies)				
$-\alpha^{3.7}$	95%	95%	10%* 67%†	92%
$-\alpha^{4.2}$	5%	5%		2.3%
α_2 IVS 1; 5 bp del			3%* 25%†	2.3%
α_2 PA; 6 A→G			87%* 8%†	1%
α_2 PA; 4 A→G				<1%
α_2 TER; T→C (C.S.)				<1%
α⁰ (Relative frequencies)				
- -MED I				100%

(Saudi Arabia) El-Hazmi, 1994, 1999, Adekile, 1997; (Oman) White et al., 1993; (Kuwait) Adekile et al., 1994, Adekile and Haider, 1996; (U.A.E.) El-Kalla and Baysal, 1998.
* Alpha + alleles found in 15 patients of Hb H disease.
† alpha + alleles found in screening of S/S and A/S individuals.

cent are the $-\alpha^{4.2}$ type. Nondeletional α⁺ thalassemia mutations are less frequent, ranging from 0.135 in Kuwait to 0.014 in the United Arab Emirates. Nevertheless, the majority of patients with HbH disease are either homozygotes or compound heterozygotes for such determinants (Pressley et al., 1980; Adekile et al., 1994; El Kalla and Baysal, 1998) because of the prevalence of nondeletional defects of the α2-globin gene in which the production of α-globin mRNA is more severely reduced compared with the common α⁺ deletion haplotypes (Chapter 16). In Saudi Arabia, the frequency of the polyadenylation site mutation is unknown, but HbH disease is due either to the interaction of $-\alpha^{3.7}$ with $\alpha2^{PA;\ 6A\rightarrow G}$ or to homozygosity for the latter mutation. In Kuwait, one third of α⁺ thalassemia is nondeletional and is represented by $\alpha2^{IVS-1;\ 5\ bp\ del}$ (Hph 1) and the Saudi polyA mutation.

Table 32.3 shows the different proportions of α⁺ thalassemia alleles as estimated by the analysis of patients with HbH disease or by random screening. In the United Arab Emirates, the Mediterranean polyA site mutation ($\alpha2^{PA;\ 4A\rightarrow G}$) and Hb Constant Spring have been found in a few individuals with HbH disease. The α-globin gene haplotype associated with Hb Constant Spring in this region is uncharacterized. α⁰ Thalassemia determinants are absent or extremely rare in the Arabian peninsula. In the United Arab Emirates the - -MED I allele has been described in combination with the $-\alpha^{3.7}$ deletion (El Kalla and Baysal, 1998). To date, no cases of hydrops fetalis have been reported in patients from the Middle East.

Indian Subcontinent

The elevated levels of Hb Bart's observed in a variable proportion of newborns and sporadic reports of HbH disease have suggested, since the late 1950s, the presence of α thalassemia in India, Nepal, and Burma (reviewed by Weatherall and Clegg, 1981). Only after the application of recombinant DNA technology were the true frequencies of α thalassemia known and the prevalence of α thalassemia in tribal and nontribal populations from Nepal to Andhra Pradesh documented (Table 32.4). The data were obtained mainly by random screening and the α-globin genotypes characterized by DNA analysis. Both deletional and nondeletional α⁺ thalassemia occur in Indian populations. A deletion involving both α-globin genes (- -ᔆᴬ) has been reported in only one patient in northeast India (Drysdale and Higgs, 1988). Other α⁰ thalassemia determinants have not been found and are probably absent or very rare. Most of the tribal groups investigated live in rural areas or in the forest and are exposed (or were exposed until recently) to hyperendemic malaria. α⁺ Thalassemia reaches the highest frequencies in those populations, with values of 0.35 to 0.92 in Andhra Pradesh, 0.52 to 0.65 in Madhya Pradesh, and 0.83 in the Tharu people of the Terai region in Southern Nepal. The only exception is the Kachari population of Upper Assam, who show a gene frequency of 0.09. In nontribals, the frequency is much lower, ranging from 0.03 to 0.12. Both $-\alpha^{3.7}$ (types I and II) and $-\alpha^{4.2}$ contribute in variable proportions to the deletional α thalassemia found in tribal and nontribal populations. The $-\alpha^{3.5}$ haplotype is rare and to

Table 32.4. India

α-Thalassemia determinants (gene frequency)	Koya Dora 2N = 50	Konda Reddy 2N = 32	Konda Dora 2N = 22	Valmiki 2N = 50	Baghata 2N = 27	Konda Kammari 2N = 24	Kolam 2N = 13
Tribal population of Andhra Pradesh							
α^0 Thalassemia							
α^+ Thalassemia (Deletions)	0.680	0.350	0.500	0.460	0.700	0.630	0.920
α^+ Thalassemia (Point mutations)	0.120		0.050				
α-globin gene Triplications		0.060					
α^+ (Relative frequencies)							
$-\alpha^{3.7\,I}$	36%	100%	33%	57%	63%	46%	59%
$-\alpha^{3.7\,II}$	9%			26%		13%	16%
$-\alpha^{4.2}$	40%		58%	17%	37%	40%	25%
$-\alpha^{3.5}$							
α_1 IVSI-117 G→A							
α_2 TER; A→C (Hb Koya Dora)	15%		9%				

α-Thalassemia determinants (gene frequency)	Kachari (Assam) 2N = 102	Baiga (Madhya P.) 2N = 20	Gond (Madhya P.) 2N = 308	Tharu (Nepal) 2N = 36	Pan-Kond and non-tribals (Orissa)
Tribal populations of Assam, Madhya Pradesh, Nepal, and Orissa					
α^0 Thalassemia					
α^+ Thalassemia (Deletions)	0.09	0.65	0.52	0.72 (West) 0.83(Central)	0.28
α^+ Thalassemia (Point mutations)			0.08		
α-globin gene Triplications					0.016
α^+ (Relative frequencies)					
$-\alpha^{3.7\,I}$	89% (I + II)	46% (I + II)	49% (I + II)	93% (West) 100% (Central)	67% (I + II)
$-\alpha^{3.7\,II}$				7% (West)	
$-\alpha^{4.2}$	11%	54%	37%		30%
$-\alpha^{3.5}$					3%
α_1 IVSI-117 G→A			10%		
α_2 TER; A→C (Hb Koya Dora)			4%		

α-Thalassemia determinants (gene frequency)	Southern Nepal 2N = 34	Punjab 2N = 126	Madhya Pradesh 2N = 54	Andhra Pradesh 2N = 170
Nontribal populations of Nepal, Punjab, Madhya Pradesh, and Andhra Pradesh.				
α^0 Thalassemia				
α^+ Thalassemia (Deletions)	0.03 – 0.09	0.1	0.074	0.12 ± 0.05
α^+ Thalassemia (Point mutations)				
α-globin gene Triplications		0.02		
α^+ (Relative frequencies)				
$-\alpha^{3.7\,I}$	100%	100% ?	50% (I + II)	75%
$-\alpha^{3.7\,II}$				8%
$-\alpha^{4.2}$			50%	17%
$-\alpha^{3.5}$				
α_1 IVSI-117 G→A				
α_2 TER; A→C (Hb Koya Dora)				

Fodde et al., 1988, 1991.
(Assam) Hundrieser et al., 1987; (Madhya P.) Reddy et al., 1995, Gupta et al., 1991, Çürük et al., 1993; (Nepal) Modiano et al., 1991; (Orissa) Kulozik et al., 1988; (Nepal) Modiano et al., 1991; (Punjab) Garewal et al., 1994; (Madhya Pradesh) Gupta et al., 1991; (Andhra Pradesh) Fodde et al., 1991.

date has only been characterized in two related individuals from Orissa (Kulozik et al., 1988).

Nondeletional mutations are represented by α2^{TER}; $^{A→C}$ (Hb Koya Dora) (De Jong et al., 1975) and by the mRNA processing mutant, α1$^{IVS-1-117 G→A}$ (Çürük et al., 1993). The latter determinant has been found at an appreciable frequency only among the Gond people in Madhya Pradesh, whereas the former, originally reported among the Koya Doras in Andhra Pradesh, has also been found in other tribal groups. The extremely high frequencies of α$^+$ thalassemia correlate with the hyperendemicity of malaria, particularly in the tribal environment. Intense selection has driven the α-thalassemia allele almost to fixation in groups such as the Tharu and Koya Dora. The distribution and incidence of α-globin gene mutants, particularly among the tribal communities of Andhra Pradesh (Fodde et al., 1991), suggest, however, that factors other than malaria have played an important role in determining the frequency and clustering of α-thalassemia alleles. These factors may be identified in the consanguineous marriages and strict endogamy common in those populations, with random genetic drift and founder effects favored by isolation and the small size of the settlements.

A remarkable feature of the molecular heterogeneity of α thalassemia in the tribal people of Andhra Pradesh is the association of α thalassemia mutations with many haplotypes. The normal (αα) complement is associated with eleven haplotypes, whereas the deletion of a single gene (−α) is associated with twenty (Fodde et al., 1991). The presence of highly homologous sequences within the α-globin gene cluster has favored the generation, by unequal crossover and/or gene conversion, of several −α deletions. Attributing all the deletions to independent events, however, is difficult. More likely, the unique structure of the α-globin genes is responsible for both the occurrence of deletions and duplications, and for the reshuffling and redistribution of deletional mutations among most haplotypes. The frequency of the deletional haplotypes would, in turn, be increased by the selective pressure of malaria.

Southeast Asia

Southeast Asia is the only area of the world where the frequencies of α$^+$ and α^0 thalassemia are sufficiently high to cause a major public health problem. Because of the frequent presence of Hb Constant Spring, the clinical severity of HbH disease is usually more severe in Southeast Asia than in the Mediterranean area. The occurrence of Hb Bart's hydrops fetalis syndrome is quite high, causing an increase in perinatal mortality and frequent severe maternal complications (Chapter 18). Not surprising, therefore, is the fact that a great deal of early clinical and genetic research on α thalassemia was carried out in this area, particularly in Thailand. Table 32.5 shows a summary of α thalassemia allele frequencies, determined mostly by DNA analysis, in different regions of Thailand. As observed in other instances, the frequency of different alleles varies throughout the country. Both α^0 and α$^+$ thalassemia reach their highest frequencies in northern Thailand, whereas Hb Constant Spring is most frequent in the south and in the northeast, at the Laotian border. Most of the α$^+$ alleles are deletional, with a high prevalence of −α$^{3.7 I}$. DNA analysis confirmed that all the α^0 alleles were - -^{SEA}. Considering the frequencies reported in Table 32.5, the incidence of hydrops fetalis should range between 0.5 and 5 per 1,000 pregnancies and the prevalence of HbH disease in newborns, between 4 and 20 per 1,000 births. This means that in a population of 60 million with a birth rate of 20 per 1,000 there will be a minimum in southern Thailand of 570 hydropic pregnancies and 5,000 new patients with HbH disease each year.

Less information is available for the other Southeast Asian countries. In Indonesia, both α$^+$ and α^0 thalassemia are common, as shown by the finding of HbH disease and by the presence of Hb Constant Spring among the Batak people of Indonesia (Lie-Injo et al. quoted by Weatherall and Clegg, 1981). α^0 Thalassemia may be rare. In a random screening carried out by DNA analysis in Central Java (Tan et al., 1992) the frequency of α$^+$ thalassemia was low and limited to equal proportions of the common −α$^{3.7}$ and −α$^{4.2}$ deletions.

Recent population surveys by Weatherall and co-workers (communication of D. J. Weatherall at the 7th Congress on Thalassemia in Bangkok, 1999) suggested an extremely heterogeneous distribution of α$^+$ thalassemia among the islands of the Indonesian archipelago, with gene frequencies ranging from 0.01 to 0.14. Although precise frequency data are missing for the Philippines, α thalassemia is common, and its clinical consequences predominate over those of β thalassemia. Both HbH disease and hydrops fetalis have been documented (Dozy et al., 1977), and a large deletion of about 34 kb that includes all the α-like globin genes has been characterized (Fischel-Ghodsian et al., 1988). A screening carried out at the University of Hawaii (Hsia, 1992) on 1,655 Filipino immigrants revealed that about 30 percent were carriers of α$^+$ or α^0 thalassemia and 2 percent had HbH disease; three cases of hydrops fetalis were found. A recent population study in the Philippines (Ko et al. 1999 b) indicates a lower incidence of α thalassemia. The authors report gene frequencies of 0.012 for α^0 and of 0.004 for α$^+$ thalassemia. Most of the α$^+$ determinants are represented by the −α$^{3.7}$ deletion (98 percent compared with 2 percent −α$^{4.2}$), whereas the α^0 haplotypes consist of 60 percent - -^{FIL} and 40 percent - -^{SEA} deletions. Nondeletional mutations such as Hb Constant Spring and

Table 32.5. Southeast Asia

α-Thalassemia determinants (gene frequency)	Bangkok 2N = 812	Northern Th 2N = 430	Northeast Th 2N = 128	Southern Th 2N = 600	Singapore 2N = 792	Indonesia 2N = 206
Thailand, Singapore, and Indonesia						
α^0 Thalassemia	0.036 – 0.025	0.07 ± 0.02	0.03	0.022 ± 0.01	0.02 – 0.03 ?	< 0.01 ?
α^+ Thalassemia (Deletions)	0.08 ± 0.02	0.1 ± 0.03	0.164	0.065 ± 0.02	0.01 – 0.03 ?	0.03 ± 0.02
α^+ Thalassemia (Point mutations)		0.008	0.012	0.055	0.03 ± 0.01	
α-globin gene Triplications		0.007	0.008	0.005		0.01
α^+ (Relative frequencies)						
$-\alpha^{3.7}$	87%	89%	68%	68%	68%	50%
$-\alpha^{4.2}$	4%		7%		14%	50%
α_2 TER; T→C (CS)	9%	11%	25%	32%	8%	
α_2 cd 125 T→C (Quoug Sge)					3%	
α T-α					2%	
α^0 (Relative frequencies)						
- -SEA	100%	100%	100%	100%	98%	
- -THAI					1.6%	
- -FIL					0.3%	

α-Thalassemia determinants (gene frequency)	Laos 2N = 88	Vietnam 2N = 88	Kampuchea 2N = 116	Malaysia
Laos, Vietnam, Kampuchea, and Malaysia				
α^0 Thalassemia			0.009	0.045
α^+ Thalassemia (Deletions)	0.11	0.035	0.155	0.16
α^+ Thalassemia (Point mutations)				
α-globin gene Triplications				
α^+ (Relative frequencies)				
$-\alpha^{3.7}$	90%	100%	100%	28%
$-\alpha^{4.2}$	10%			7%
α_2 TER; T→C (CS)				58%
α_2 cd 125 T→C (Quoug Sze)				
α T-α				7%
α^0 (Relative frequencies)				
- -SEA				
- -THAI				
- -FIL				

(Thailand) Ausavarungnirun et al. 1998, O-Prasertsawat et al. 1990, Tanpaichitr et al. 1988, Thongiairoam et al. 1991, Lemmens-Zygulska et al. 1996, Hundrieser et al. 1990, Sriroongrueng et al. 1997; (Singapore) Tan et al. 1999; (Indonesia) Tan et al. 1992; (Laos and Vietnam) Dodé et al. 1988; (Kampuchea) Hundrieser et al. 1988; (Malaysia) George et al., 1992, 1999.

Hb Quong Sze, frequent in Southeast Asia, were not found. It is likely that in this survey the occurrence of α^+ thalassemia has been underestimated because the carriers were identified primarily by the analysis of hematologic parameters. In continental Southeast Asia, α thalassemia occurs frequently in Malaysia. According to the observations of George et al. (1992) on HbH disease patients, α^0 thalassemia is caused by the - -SEA determinant, whereas α^+ thalassemia is caused about equally by deletions and point mutations.

In the survey of Hsia (1992), 13 percent of 712 Laotian immigrants screened for the presence of hemoglobinopathies and thalassemia were carriers of α^0 or α^+ thalassemia, and 1 percent had HbH disease. Of 3,000 patients screened, Hb Constant Spring was found almost exclusively in Laotians (four of five cases) (PCR and slot blot hybridization were used for its detection). Another termination codon mutation, Hb Paksé (α_2 TER; TAA→TAT) has been found in the same ethnic group (Waye et al., 1994). Screenings carried out at the end of the 1980s on a very limited number of individuals (Dodé et al., 1988; Hundrieser et al., 1988) had revealed the occurrence of deletional α^+ thalassemia in Vietnam, Laos, and Kampuchea (see Table 32.5). Because of the sample size the frequency of α^0 thalassemia was probably underestimated. In Singapore, the population consists of 78 percent Chinese from the southern provinces, 14 percent Malays, and 7 percent southern Indians. The gene frequency of α thalassemia is about 3 to 4 percent, in keeping with the data from southern China (Tan et al., 1999). Analysis of DNA from a large group of unrelated individuals suspected of carrying α thalassemia has provided the results reported in Table 32.5. Most of the α^+ thalassemia mutations are deletional and caused by the $-\alpha^{3.7}$ haplotype, whereas point mutations are represented by Hb Constant Spring, Hb Quong Sze, and Hb Paksè. The haplotype $-^{-SEA}$ makes up most of the α^0 thalassemia mutations, with a few $-^{-Thai}$ and $-^{-Fil}$ haplotypes.

In summary, both α^0 and α^+ thalassemia occur at variable (mostly high) levels throughout Southeast Asia. Unfortunately, except for Thailand, few accurate data obtained by random screening and DNA analysis have been published.

China

In China, α thalassemia occurs mainly in the southern provinces, particularly Guangxi, where raised levels of Hb Bart's are found in the cord blood of 15 percent of newborns. Guangdong and Jangxi provinces follow with percentages of 4.1 and 2.6, respectively (Zeng and Huang, 1987). As shown in Table 32.6, in Guangxi the $-\alpha^{3.7}$ and $-\alpha^{4.2}$ deletions account for most deletional α^+ thalassemias, with $-\alpha^{2.7}$ accounting for the rest. Nondeletional α^+ mutations are represented by Hb Constant Spring and Hb Quong Sze. The large deletions, $-^{-SEA}$ and, infrequently, $-^{-THAI}$ account for the α^0 thalassemias (Zhao et al., 1992; Liang et al., 1994). In Hong Kong, where the population originates mostly from Southern China, the gene frequency of α^0 thalassemia is between 0.02 and 0.03, with (apparently) lower values for α^+ thalassemia (Lau et al., 1997). The $-\alpha^{3.7}$ deletion is most prevalent, but the Hb Constant Spring mutation was not detected by PCR or dot blot hybridization. The sole deletion causing α^0 thalassemia is $-^{-SEA}$. Data consistent with those of Lau had been reported earlier (Chan et al., 1986) following a random screening in Hong Kong of people originating from the Guangdong province of China.

In Taiwan, the resident population is almost entirely of Southern Chinese origin, and the prevalence of α thalassemia is similar to that found on the Chinese mainland (Peng et al., 1989). About 300,000 individuals represent the aboriginal population of the island. The main aboriginal groups have remained linguistically and geographically isolated, and their α thalassemia frequencies differ from those of Chinese immigrants, with higher values in the Ami people and lower ones in the other three main groups (Ko et al., 1993). The groups migrated to Taiwan from the mainland at different times and through different routes, and they settled in areas where malaria was either endemic or sporadic, depending on the altitude. All those differing circumstances may account for the nonuniform distribution of α thalassemia among Taiwanese.

Oceania

Over the last 15 years, the prevalence of α thalassemia in Pacific Islanders has been intensely studied by random, DNA-based screening of thousands of individuals. α^0 Thalassemia is virtually absent, even though rare cases of HbH disease caused by nondeletional mutations have been observed in Papua, New Guinea (Hill et al., 1987). α^+ Thalassemia is represented by two subtypes (I and III) of the $-\alpha^{3.7}$ allele and by $-\alpha^{4.2}$ deletions (Table 32.7). The frequency distribution of α^+ thalassemia follows a pattern consistent with the degree of malaria endemicity. The prevalence of α^+ thalassemia is low in the Papua New Guinea highlands and reaches its highest levels in coastal areas and the lowlands, where malaria is hyperendemic. Likewise, both malaria endemicity and α^+ thalassemia prevalence decrease southward across the Vanuatu archipelago, attaining a minimum value (6 percent) in New Caledonia, which has always been malaria free (Flint et al., 1986).

The three α^+ deletions occurring in the Pacific area are found on three ($-\alpha^{3.7}$ I) and six ($-\alpha^{4.2}$) different haplotypes, respectively; the $-\alpha^{3.7}$ III mutation is associated with a single haplotype and has been found only in Oceania. All the haplotypes associated with the α^+ deletions common in the area belong to the III-V group, whereas those associated with the same deletions in Southeast Asia belong to the I-II group (O'Shaughnessy et al., 1990). In addition, the $-^{-SEA}$ deletion does not occur in Oceania. On this basis, Flint et al. (1998) hypothesized that not only the type III $-\alpha^{3.7}$ deletion but also the other mutations have an autochthonous origin, and their frequency increased because of the selective pressure of malaria. The regional distribution of $-\alpha^{3.7}$, $-\alpha^{4.2}$, and the HbJ Tongariki haplotype further support the hypothesis. Malaria has never been endemic in Micronesia and Polynesia. Nevertheless α^+ thalassemia occurs in both areas but at much lower frequencies than in Melanesia, and with a nonuniform frequency distribution. This situation could be explained by gene flow from Melanesians to a migrant population on its way to colonize new regions. Founder effect and random drift might have considerably increased the frequency of α thalassemia alleles even in the absence of malaria. The gene frequency of α+ thalassemia is the same in aboriginals from central and northwestern Australia (see Table 32.7). The analysis of α-globin gene haplotypes indicates, however, a close relationship between central Australian aboriginals and

Table 32.6. China

α-Thalassemia determinants (gene frequency)	Southern China (Guangxi) 301 newborns	Hong Kong 2N = 3600	Taiwan (Chinese)	Taiwan (Ami) 2N = 1044	Taiwan (Bunun) 2N = 492	Taiwan (Atayal) 2N = 454	Taiwan (Paiwan) 2N = 428
α^0 Thalassemia	0.15 (frequency of raised Hb Bart's in newborns)	0.023	0.02	0.042 ± 0.012	0.002	0.002	0.009
α^+ Thalassemia (Deletions)		0.003	0.01	0.041	0.004		
α^+ Thalassemia (Point mutations)							
α-globin gene Triplications		0.001					
α^+ (Relative frequencies)							
$-\alpha^{3.7}$	23%	66%		98%	100%		
$-\alpha^{4.2}$	27%	33%		2%			
$-\alpha^{2.7}$	3%						
α_2 TER; T→C (Hb CS)	42%						
α_2 Cd 125; T→C (Hb Quoug Sge)	5%						
α^0 (Relative frequencies)							
--SEA	97%	100%	97%	21%	100%		57%
--THAI	3%			77%			43%
--FIL			3%	2%		100%	

(Southern China) Zeng and Huong, 1987, Liang et al., 1994; (Hong Kong) Chan et al. 1986, Lau et al., 1997; (Taiwan) Peng et al, 1989, Lin et al., 1991, Ko et al, 1991, 1993, Ko et al. 1999a.

Table 32.7. Oceania

α-Thalassemia determinants (gene frequency)	Australia (Central) 2N = 238	Australia (N.W.) 2N = 292	Papua N.G. (Highlands) 2N = 226	Papua N.G. (Lowlands) 2N = 753
α^0 Thalassemia				
α^+ Thalassemia (Deletions)	0.03 ± 0.02	0.034	0.053 (0 – 0.07)	0.38 (0.03 – 0.91)
α^+ Thalassemia (Point mutations)				
α-globin gene Triplications	0.005	0.007	0.004	0.03
α^+ (Relative frequencies)				
$-\alpha^{3.7\ I}$	100%	90%	19%	14%
$-\alpha^{3.7\ II}$				
$-\alpha^{3.7\ III}$		10%		3%
$-\alpha^{4.2}$			81%	83%

α-Thalassemia determinants (gene frequency)	Vanuatu 2N = 1079	Micronesia (overall) 2N = 844	Polynesia (West-Centr) 2N = 458	French Polynesia 2N = 2112	Tahiti 2N = 1732
α^0 Thalassemia					
α^+ Thalassemia (Deletions)	0.26 (0.09 – 0.68)	0.026	0.06	0.14 (0.05 – 0.19)	0.114 ± 0.015
α^+ Thalassemia (Point mutations)	0.05				
α-globin gene Triplications		0.006	0.002		0.002
α^+ (Relative frequencies)					
$-\alpha^{3.7\ I}$	9%	6%			1%
$-\alpha^{3.7\ II}$					
$-\alpha^{3.7\ III}$	68%	67%	96%	100%	97%
$-\alpha^{4.2}$	23%	27%	4%		2%

(Australia) Roberts-Thompson et al. 1996; Tsintsof et al. 1990; (Papua N.G.) Yenchitsomanus et al. 1986.
(Vanuatu) Hill et al. 1985; Ganczakowski et al. 1995; (Micronesia – Polynesia) O'Shaughnessy et al. 1990; Philippon et al. 1995

New Guinea highlanders. This suggests a common origin of the two populations (Roberts-Thomson et al., 1996). Central Australia is not a malarial area and the occurrence of α thalassemia is most probably due to gene flow from the northern coastal regions.

References

Abdalla, SH, Corrah, PT, and Higgs, DR. (1989). α-Thalassaemia in The Gambia. *Trans. Ro. Soc. Trop. Med. Hyg.* 83: 420.

Adekile, AD, Liu, JC, Sulzer, AJ et al. (1993). Frequency of the α-thalassemia-2 gene among Nigerian SS patients and its influence on malaria antibody titers. *Hemoglobin* 17: 73–79.

Adekile, AD, Gu, LH, Baysal, E et al. (1994). Molecular characterization of alpha-thalassemia determinants, beta-thalassemia alleles, and beta S haplotypes among Kuwaiti Arabs. *Acta Haematol.* 92: 176–181.

Adekile, AD and Haider, MZ. (1996). Morbidity, βs haplotype and α-globin gene patterns among sickle cell anemia patients in Kuwait. *Acta Haematol.* 96: 150–154.

Adekile, AD. (1997). Historical and anthropological correlates of βs haplotypes and α- and β-thalassemia alleles in the Arabian Peninsula. *Hemoglobin* 21: 281–296.

Ausavarungnirun, R, Winichagoon, P, Fucharoen, S et al. (1998). Detection of ζ-globin chains in the cord blood by ELISA (enzyme-linked immunoadsorbent assay): Rapid screening for alpha-thalassaemia 1 (South East Asian type). *Am. J. Hematol.* 57: 283–266.

Ayala, S, Colomer, D, Aymerich, M et al. (1996). Non-deletional alpha-thalassemia: First description of alpha[Hph] alpha and alpha[Nco] alpha mutations in a Spanish population. *Am. J. Hematol.* 52: 144–149.

Baysal, E, Kleanthous, M, Bozkurt, G et al. (1995). Alpha-thalassemia in the population of Cyprus. *Br. J. Haematol.* 89: 496–499.

Bento, MC, Gonçalves, P, Rebelo, U et al. (1997). A study of hemoglobinopathies in Sâo Tomé e Principe. Abstract 128, 6th *International. Conference on Thalassaemia*, April 1997, Malta.

Bernini, LF and Harteveld, CL. (1998). α-Thalassaemia. *Baillières Clin. Haematol.* 11: 53–90.

Bowden, DK, Vickers, MA, and Higgs, DR. (1992). A PCR based strategy to detect the common severe determinants of alpha thalassaemia. *Br. J. Haematol.* 81: 104–108.

Bowden, DK, Hill, AVS, Higgs, DR et al. (1985). Relative roles of genetic factors, dietary deficiencies and infection in anaemia in Vanuatu, South West Pacific. *Lancet* ii: 1025–1028.

Camaschella, C, Bertero, MT, Serra, A et al. (1987). A benign form of thalassaemia intermedia may be determined by the interaction of triplicated alpha locus and heterozygous beta-thalassaemia. *Br. J. Haematol.* 66: 103–107.

Chan, V, Chan, TK, Cheng, MY et al. (1986). Organization of the ζ-α genes in Chinese. *Br. J. Haematol.* 64: 97–105.

Chui, DH, Luo, HY, Clarke, BJ et al. (1988). Potential application of a new screening test for alpha-thalassaemia-1 carriers. *Hemoglobin* 12: 459–463.

Çürük, MA, Baysal, E, Gupta, RB et al. (1993). An IVS-1-117 G→A acceptor splice mutation in the α1-globin gene is a non-deletional α-thalassaemia-2 determinant in an Indian population. *Br. J. Haematol.* 85: 148–152.

De Jong, WWW, Meera Khan, P, and Bernini, LF. (1975). Hemoglobin Koya Dora: High frequency of a chain termination mutant. *Am. J. Hum. Genet.* 27: 81–90.

Di Rienzo, A, Novelletto, A, Aliquò, MC et al. (1986). Molecular basis for HbH disease in Italy: Geographical distribution of deletional and non-deletional α-thalassemia haplotypes. *Am. J. Hum. Genet.* 39: 631–639.

Dodé, C, Berth, A, Rochette, J et al. (1988). Analysis of crossover type in the α-3.7 haplotype among sickle anemia patients from various parts of Africa. *Hum. Genet.* 78: 193–195.

Dodé, C, Labie, D, and Rochette, J. (1988). Types of α + thalassaemia in Southeast Asia refugees. *Ann. Génét.* 31: 201–204.

Dodé, C, Rochette, J, and Krishnamoorthy, R. (1990). Locus assignment of human α-globin mutations by selective amplification and direct sequencing. *Br. J. Haematol.* 76: 275–281.

Dozy, AM, Kabisch, H, Baker, J et al. (1977). The molecular defects of alpha-thalassemia in the Filipino. *Hemoglobin* 1: 539–546.

Dozy, AM, Forman, EN, Abuelo, DN et al. (1979). Prenatal diagnosis of homozygous α-thalassemia. *J. Am. Med. Assoc.* 24: 1610–1612.

Drysdale, HC and Higgs, DR. (1988). α-Thalassaemia in an Asian Indian. *Br. J. Haematol.* 68: 264.

Efremov, GD. (1992). Hemoglobinopathies in Yugoslavia: An update. *Hemoglobin* 16: 531–544.

El Hazmi, MAF. (1994). Genetic red cell disorders in Saudi Arabia: A multifaceted problem. *Hemoglobin* 18: 257–268.

El Hazmi, MAF and Warsy, AS. (1996). Hemoglobinopathies in Arab Countries. In: Teebi, AS and Farag, TI, editors. *Genetic disorders among Arab populations. Oxford Monographs on Medical Genetics,* Vol 30. New York: Oxford University Press, pp 83–110.

El Hazmi, MAF. (1999). α-Thalassaemia deletion pattern in the Saudi population. Abstract T009, 7th International Conference on Thalassemia, May-June 1999, Bangkok, Thailand.

El Kalla, S and Baysal, E. (1998). Alpha-thalassemia in the United Arab Emirates. *Acta Haematol.* 100: 49–53.

Falusi, AG, Esan, GJF, Ayyub, H et al. (1987). Alpha-thalassaemia in Nigeria: Its interaction with sickle cell disease. *Euro. J. Haematol.* 38: 370–375.

Fei, YJ, Kutlar, F, Harris, HF et al. (1989). A search for anomalies in the ζ,α,β and γ globin gene arrangements in normal Black, Italian, Turkish and Spanish newborns. *Hemoglobin* 13: 45–65.

Fessas, P, Lie Injo, LE, Na-Nakorn, S et al. (1972). Identification of slow-moving hemoglobins in haemoglobin H disease from different racial groups. *Lancet* i: 1308.

Fichera, M, Spalletta, A, Fiorenza, F et al. (1997). Molecular basis of α-thalassemia in Sicily. *Hum. Genet.* 99: 381–386.

Fischel-Ghodsian, N, Vickers, MA, Seip, M et al. (1988). Characterization of two deletions that remove the entire human zeta-alpha globin gene complex (- -THAI and - -FIL). *Br. J. Haematol.* 70: 233–238.

Flint, J, Hill, VS, Bowden, DK et al. (1986). High frequencies of α-thalassemia are the result of natural selection by malaria. *Nature* 321: 744–750.

Flint, J, Harding, RM, Boyce, AJ et al. (1998). The population genetics of haemoglobinopathies. *Ballières Clin. Haematol.* 11: 1–51.

Fodde, R, Losekoot, M, van den Brook, MH et al. (1988). Prevalence and molecular heterogeneity of α + -thalassemia in two tribal populations from Andhra Pradesh, India. *Hum. Genet.* 80: 157–160.

Fodde, R, Harteveld, CL, Losekoot, M et al. (1991). Multiple recombination events are responsible for the heterogeneity of α + -thalassemia haplotypes among the forest tribes of Andhra Pradesh, India. *Ann. Hum. Genet.* 55: 43–50.

Foglietta, E, Grisanti, P, Lerone, M et al. (1995). Prime indagini sulla frequenza e l'eterogeneità delle α microcitemie nel Lazio. *Il Progresso Medico* 51: 45–45.

Folayan-Esan, GJ. (1972). Haemoglobin Bart's in newborn Nigerians. *Br. J. Haematol.* 22: 73.

Fortina, P, Dianzani, I, Serra, A et al. (1991). A newly characterized α-thalassaemia-1 deletion removes the entire α-like globin gene cluster in an Italian family. *Br. J. Haematol.* 78: 529–534.

Galanello, R, Ruggeri, R, Paglietti, E et al. (1983). A family with segregating triplicated alpha globin loci and beta thalassemia. *Blood* 62: 1035–1040.

Galanello, R, Maccioni, L, Ruggeri, R et al. (1984). Alpha thalassaemia in Sardinian newborns. *Br. J. Haematol.* 58: 361–368.

Galanello, R, Sanna, MA, Maccioni, L et al. (1990). Fetal hydrops in Sardinia: Implications for genetic counselling. *Clin. Genet.* 38: 327–331.

Galanello, R, Aru, B, Dessi, C et al. (1992). HbH disease in Sardinia: Molecular, hematological and clinical aspects. *Acta Haematol.* 88: 1–6.

Ganczakowski, M, Bowden, DK, Maitland, K et al. (1995). Thalassaemia in Vanuatu, South-West Pacific: Frequency and haematological phenotypes of young children. *Br. J. Haematol.* 89: 485–495.

Garewal, G, Fearon, CW, Warren, TC et al. (1994). The molecular basis of β-thalassemia in Punjabi and Maharastran Indians includes a multilocus aetiology involving triplicated α-globin loci. *Br. J. Haematol.* 86: 372–276.

George, E, Li, HJ, Fei, YJ et al. (1992). Types of thalassemia among patients attending a large university clinic in Kuala Lumpur, Malaysia. *Hemoglobin* 16: 51–66.

Gupta, RB, Tiwary, RS, Kutlar, F et al. (1991). Hemoglobinopathies among the Gond tribal groups of central India: Interaction of α-and β-thalassemia with β-chain variants. *Hemoglobin* 15: 441–458.

Harteveld, CL, Heister, JGAM, Giordano, PC et al. (1996). Rapid detection of point mutations and polymorphisms of the α-globin genes by DGGE and SSCA. *Hum. Mutat.* 7: 114–122.

Henni, T, Morlé, F, Lopez, B et al. (1987). α-Thalassemia haplotypes in the Algerian population. *Hum. Genet.* 75: 272–276.

Higgs, DR, Pressley, L, Old, JM et al. (1979). Negro α-thalassaemia is caused by deletion of a single α-globin gene. *Lancet* ii: 272–276.

Higgs, DR, Pressley, L, Clegg, JB et al. (1980a). Detection of α-thalassaemia in Negro infants. *Br. J. Haematol.* 46: 39–46.

Higgs, DR, Pressley, L, Clegg, JB et al. (1980b). α-Thalassemia in Black populations. *Johns Hopkins Med. J.* 146: 300–310.

Higgs, DR, Pressley, L, Serjeant, GR et al. (1981). The genetics and molecular basis of α-thalassaemia in association with Hb S in Jamaican Negroes. *Br. J. Haematol.* 47: 43–56.

Hill, AVS, Bowden, DK, Trent, RJ et al. (1985). Melanesians and Polynesians share a unique α-thalassemia mutation. *Am. J. Hum. Genet.* 37: 571–580.

Hill, AVS, Thein, SL, Mavo, B et al. (1987). Non-deletion haemoglobin disease in Papua New Guinea. *J. Med. Genet.* 24: 767–771.

Hill, AVS. (1992). Molecular epidemiology of the thalassaemias (including haemoglobin E). *Baillières Clin. Haematol.* 5: 209–238.

Hsia, YE. (1992). Hereditary anemias in Hawaii: An update. *Hawaii Med. J.* 51: 17–19.

Hundrieser, J, Deka, R, and Gogoi, BC. (1987). α-Thalassaemia in the Kachari population of Assam (India). *Hemoglobin* 11: 517–519.

Hundrieser, J, Sanguansermsri, T, Flatz, SD et al. (1988). Frequency of deletional types of α-thalassemia in Kampuchea. *Ann. Genaet.* 31: 205–210.

Hundrieser, J, Laig, M, Yongvanit, P et al. (1990). Study of alpha-thalassemia in Northeastern Thailand at the DNA level. *Hum. Hered.* 40: 85–88.

Kanavakis, E, Tzotzos, S, Liapaki, A et al. (1986). Frequency of α-thalassemia in Greece. *Am. J. Hematol.* 22: 225–232.

Kar, BC, Satapathy, RK, Kulozik, AE et al. (1986). Sickle cell disease in Orissa State, India. *Lancet* ii: 1198–1201.

Kattamis, AC, Camaschella, C, Sivera, P et al. (1996). Human α-thalassemia syndromes: Detection of molecular defects. *Am. J. Hematol.* 53: 81–91.

Ko, TM, Hsieh, FJ, Hsu, PM et al. (1991). Molecular characterization of severe α-thalassemias causing hydrops fetalis in Taiwan. *Am. J. Med. Genet.* 39: 317–320.

Ko, TM, Chen, TA, Hsieh, MI et al. (1993). Alpha-thalassemia in the four major aboriginal groups in Taiwan. *Hum. Genet.* 92: 79–80.

Ko, TM and Li, SF. (1999a). Molecular characterization of the - -FIL determinant of alpha-thalassemia (corrigendum). *Am. J. Hematol.* 60: 173.

Ko, TM, Hwa, HL, Liu, CW et al. (1999b). Prevalence study and molecular characterization of α-thalassemia in Filipinos. *Annals of Hematology* 78: 355–357.

Kulozik, AE, Kar, BC, Serjeant, GR et al. (1988). The molecular basis of α-thalassemia in India. Its interaction with the sickle cell gene. *Blood* 71: 467–472.

Kyrri, A, Kleanthous, M, Kyriacou, K et al. (1997). α-Thalassemia in Cyprus: Epidemiologic and molecular aspects. Abstract 155, 6th International Conference on Thalassaemia, April.

Lau, YL, Chan, CL, Chan, YYA et al. (1997). Prevalence and genotypes of α- and β-thalassemia carriers in Hong Kong: Implications for population screening. *N. Engl. J. Med.* 336: 1298–1301.

Lemmens-Zygulska, M, Eigel, A, Helbig, B et al. (1996). Prevalence of α-thalassemias in Northern Thailand. *Hum. Genet.* 98: 354–347.

Liang, R, Liang, S, Jiang, NH et al. (1994). α and β thalassaemia among Chinese children in Guangxi Province, PR China: Molecular and haematological characterization. *Br. J. Haematol.* 86: 351–354.

Lin, CK, Lee, SH, Wang, CC et al. (1991). Alpha-thalassemic traits are common in the Taiwanese population: Usefulness of a modified hemoglobin H preparation for prevalence studies. *J. Lab. Clin. Med.* 118: 599–603.

Liu, TC, Chiou, SS, Lin, SF et al. (1994). Molecular basis and hematological characterization of HbH disease in South East Asia. *Am. J. Hematol.* 45: 293–297.

Livingstone, FB. (1985). *Frequencies of haemoglobin variants.* Oxford: Oxford University Press.

Masala, B. (1992). Hemoglobinopathies in Sardinia. *Hemoglobin* 16: 331–351.

Massa, A, Pecci, G, Grubessi, R et al. (1994). -(α)20.5 is the most frequent large deletion in the Puglia region of Italy. *Hemoglobin* 18: 353–357.

Mears, JG, Lachman, HM, Labie, D et al. (1983). Alpha thalassemia is related to prolonged survival in sickle cell anemia. *Blood* 62: 286–291.

Modiano, G, Morpurgo, G, Terrenato, L et al. (1991). Protection against malaria morbidity: Near fixation of the α-thalassemia gene in a Nepalese population. *Am. J. Hum. Genet.* 48: 390–397.

Morlé, F, Lopez, B, Henni, T et al. (1985). α-Thalassemia associated with the deletion of two nucleotides at position −2 and −3 preceding the AUG codon. *EMBO J.* 4: 1245–1250.

Muglia, M, Annesi, G, Gabriele, AL et al. (1993). α-Thalassemia in a Southern Italian population (detection by a non-radioactive procedure). *Hemoglobin* 17: 285–287.

Muklwala, EC, Banda, J, Siziva, S et al. (1989). Alpha thalassaemia in Zambian newborn. *Clin. Lab. Haematol.* 11: 1–6.

Nhonoli, AM, Kujwalile JM, Mmari, PW et al. (1979). Haemoglobin Bart's in newborn Tanzanians. *Acta Haematol.* 61: 114.

Novelletto, A, Hafez, M, Di Rienzo, A et al. (1989). Frequency and molecular types of deletional α-thalassemia in Egypt. *Hum. Genet.* 81: 211–213.

Öner, C, Gürgey, A, Öner, R et al. (1997). The molecular basis of Hb H disease in Turkey. *Hemoglobin* 21: 41–51.

O-Prasertsawat, P, Suthutvoravut, S, and Chaturachinda, K. (1990). Hydrops fetalis due to Bart's hemoglobinopathy at Ramathibodi Hospital (1978–1987): A 10 year review. *J. Med. Assoc. Tha.* 73: 65–68.

O'Shaughnessy, DF, Hill, AVS, Bowden, DK et al. (1990). Globin genes in Micronesia: Origins and affinities of Pacific Island peoples. *Am. J. Hum. Genet.* 46: 144–155.

Pagnier, J, Dunda-Belkhodja, O, Zohoun, I et al. (1984). α-Thalassemia among sickle cell anemia patients in various African populations. *Hum. Genet.* 68: 318–319.

Peng, HW, Choo, KB, Ho, CH et al. (1989). Arrangement of α-globin gene cluster in Taiwan. *Acta Haematol.* 82: 64–68.

Peres, MJ, Romao, L, Carreiro, H et al. (1995). Molecular basis of alpha-thalassemia in Portugal. *Hemoglobin* 19: 343–352.

Philippon, G, Martinson, JJ, Rugless, MJ et al. (1995). α-Thalassemia and globin gene rearrangements in French Polynesia. *Eur. J. Haematol.* 55: 171–177.

Pirastu, M, Lee, KY, Dozy, AM et al. (1982). Alpha thalassemia in two Mediterranean populations. *Blood* 60: 509–512.

Pressley, L, Higgs, DR, Clegg, JB et al. (1980). A new genetic basis for hemoglobin H disease. *N. Engl. J. Med.* 303: 1383–1388.

Ramsay, M and Jenkins, T. (1984). α-Thalassaemia in Africa: The oldest malaria protective trait? *Lancet* 2: 410.

Ramsay, M and Jenkins, T. (1987). Globin gene-associated restriction-fragment-length polymorphisms in Southern African peoples. *Am. J. Hum. Genet.* 41: 1132–1144.

Reddy, PH, Petrou, M, Reddy, PA et al. (1995). Hereditary anaemias and iron deficiency in a tribal population (the Baiga) of central India. *Eur. J. Haematol.* 55: 103–109.

Roberts-Thomson, JM, Martinson, JJ, Norwich, JT et al. (1996). An ancient common origin of Aboriginal Australians and New Guinea Highlanders is supported by α-globin haplotype analysis. *Am. J. Hum. Genet.* 58: 1017–1024.

Rund, D, Oron-Karni, V, Filon, D et al. (1998). α-Globin mutations and rearrangements in Israel. *Ann. N. Y. Acad. Sci.* 850: 426–428.

Segbena, AY, Prehu, C, Wajcman, H et al. (1998). Hemoglobins in Togolese newborns: Hb S, Hb C, Hb Bart's and α-globin gene status. *Am. J. Hematol.* 59: 208–213.

Shalmon, L, Kirschmann, C, and Zaizov, R. (1996). Alpha-thalassemia genes in Israel: Deletional and non-deletional mutations in patients of various origins. *Hum. Hered.* 46: 15–19.

Sriroongrueng, W, Pornpatkul, M, Panich, V et al. (1997). Alpha-thalassemia incidence in Southern Thailand by restriction endonuclease analysis of globin from placental blood at Songklanagarind Hospital. *Southeast Asian J. Trop. Med. Public Health* 28: 93–96.

Tamary, H, Klinger, G, Shalmon, L et al. (1998). The diverse molecular basis and mild clinical picture of HbH disease in Israel. *Ann. N. Y. Acad. Sci.* 850: 432–435.

Tan, JAMA, Tay, JSH, Soemantry, A et al. (1992). Deletional types of alpha-thalassemia in Central Java. *Hum. Hered.* 42: 289–292.

Tan, GP, Chee, M, Huan, PT et al. (1999). A strategy for screening alpha-thalassemia in Singapore. Abstract T007, 7th International Conference on Thalassemia, May-June 1999 Bangkok, Thailand.

Tang, W, Luo, HY, Eng, B et al. (1993). Immunocytological test to detect adult carriers of (- -SEA/) deletional α-thalassaemia. *Lancet* 342: 1145–1147.

Tanpaichitr, VS, Pung-Amritt, P, Puchaiwatanon, O et al. (1988). Studies of Hemoglobin Bart's and deletion of α-globin genes from cord blood in Thailand. *Birth Defects* 23: 15–21.

Thonglairoam, V, Winichagoon, P, Fucharoen, S et al. (1991). Hemoglobin Constant Spring in Bangkok: Molecular screening by selective enzymatic amplification of the α2 globin gene. *Am. J. Haematol.* 38: 277–280.

Traeger-Synodinos, J, Kanavakis, E, Tzetis, M et al. (1993). Characterization of non-deletion thalassemia mutations in the Greek populations. *Am. J. Hematol.* 44: 162–167.

Tsintsof, AS, Hertzberg, MS, Prior, JF et al. (1990). α-Globin gene markers identify genetic differences between Australian Aborigines and Melanesians. *Am. J. Hum. Genet.* 46: 138–143.

Tzotzos, S, Kanavakis, E, Metaxotou-Mavromati, A et al. (1986). The molecular basis of HbH disease in Greece. *Br. J. Haematol.* 63: 263–271.

Villegas, A, Sanchez, J, and Sal del Rio, E. (1992). α-Globin genotypes in a Spanish population. *Hemoglobin* 16: 427–429.

Villegas, A, Sanchez, J, Gonzalez, FA et al. (1994). Alpha-thalassemia-1 (- -CAL mutation) in a Spanish family. *Am. J. Hematol.* 46: 367–368.

Villegas, A, Sanchez, J, Armada, B et al. (1997). Non-deletional α-thalassemia in a Spanish population. *Am. J. Hematol.* 54: 342–343.

Waye, JS, Eng, B, Patterson, M et al. (1994). Identification of a novel termination codon mutation (TAA- -> TAT, Term- -> Tyr) in the alpha 2 globin gene of a Laotian girl with hemoglobin H disease. *Blood* 83: 3418–3420.

Weatherall, DJ and Clegg, JB. (1981). *The thalassaemia syndromes,* 3rd ed. Oxford: Blackwell Publishing.

Weatherall, DJ. (1963). Abnormal hemoglobins in the neonatal period and their relationship to thalassaemia. *Br. J. Haematol.* 9: 265–277.

White, JM, Christie, BS, Nam, D et al. (1993). Frequency and clinical significance of erythrocyte genetic abnormalities in Omanis. *J. Med. Genet.* 30: 396–400.

Williams, TN, Maitland, K, Ganczakowski, M et al. (1996). Red blood cell phenotypes in the alpha + thalassaemias from early childhood to maturity. *Br. J. Haematol.* 95: 266–272.

Wongchanchailert, M, Laosombat, U, and Maipang, M. (1992). Hemoglobin H disease in children. *J. Med. Assoc. Thai.* 75: 611–618.

Yenchitsomanus, P, Summers, KM, Board, PG et al. (1986). Alpha-thalassemia in Papua New Guinea. *Hum. Genet.* 74: 432–437.

Zeng, YT and Huang, SZ. (1987). Disorders of haemoglobin in China. *J. Med. Genet.* 24: 578–583.

Zhao, JB, Zhao, L, Gu, YC et al. (1992). Types of α-globin gene deficiencies in Chinese newborn babies in the Guangxi region, P.R. China. *Hemoglobin* 16: 325–328.

33

Geographic Heterogeneity of Sickle Cell Disease

GRAHAM SERJEANT

DISTRIBUTION OF THE SICKLE CELL GENE

A close relationship with the distribution of falciparum malaria determines the primary distribution of the sickle cell gene (see Chapter 30). The prevalence of the sickle cell trait reaches frequencies of 20 percent to 25 percent throughout equatorial Africa, the eastern part of Saudi Arabia, and central India (see Chapter 29). As detailed in Chapter 26, the gene was secondarily carried to the American continent (North America, South America, and the Caribbean) during the slave trade between 1650 and 1830, around the Mediterranean and Middle East (Sicily, Greece, Turkey, Jordan, Iran, Israel) much earlier during the Phoenician civilization of approximately 1000 B.C., and northern Europe (United Kingdom, France, Germany) since the 1950s. Sickle cell disease now occurs against a variety of genetic and environmental backgrounds and the study of geographic differences in expression of the disease provides insights into the determinants of clinical severity. Genetic factors contributing to disease variability include β-globin gene haplotype, α thalassemia, and hereditary persistence of high fetal hemoglobin (HbF) levels (see Chapter 26), whereas environmental factors are less well documented but include infections, especially malaria; nutrition; climate; socioeconomic conditions; and medical care.

GENETIC FACTORS

β-Globin Gene Haplotype

Studies of the regions flanking the β-globin locus on chromosome 11 have revealed variations in DNA structure (polymorphisms or haplotypes) associated with HbS that are discussed in detail in Chapter 26. Major haplotypes are recognized in Africa, and named after the areas where they were first described: the Senegal haplotype, the Benin haplotype in central West Africa, and the Bantu or Central African Republic haplotype. A fourth haplotype is associated with the HbS mutation in eastern Saudi Arabia (El-Hazmi, 1990; Padmos et al., 1991) and central India (Kar et al., 1986; Kulozik et al., 1986; Labie et al., 1989) and is known as the Asian or Arab-India haplotype. The Benin haplotype is predominant in most sickle cell populations in North America and the Caribbean (Antonarakis et al., 1984), with 60 percent of Jamaican patients with sickle cell disease being homozygotes for Benin and 20 percent heterozygotes. The frequency of the Bantu haplotype exceeds that of the Benin haplotype in most of Brazil (Zago et al., 1992) reflecting the origin of that African population from areas now known as Zaire and Angola. The Benin haplotype accounts for the HbS genes in Sicily (Ragusa et al., 1988), Greece (Boussiou et al., 1991), Turkey (Aluoch et al., 1986), and southwest Saudi Arabia (El-Hazmi, 1990; Padmos, 1991).

Although the distribution of β-globin haplotypes is well documented, the degree to which these haplotypes modify hematologic and clinical expression of sickle cell disease is less clear. These studies are difficult to perform because any haplotype-related effects may be confounded by the selection of patients based on their symptoms and other biases of the populations studied. These difficulties are illustrated in the interpretation of HbF levels in the different β-globin haplotypes. In the Senegal haplotype, HbF levels are believed to be increased (Nagel et al., 1991) although it is unclear whether this effect is confined to homozygotes for the haplotype. In the Bantu haplotype, mean HbF levels are believed to be lower than in the Benin haplotype (Nagel et al., 1987). In the Benin haplotype, HbF levels are highly variable and the β-globin haplotype plays a relatively minor role (Chang et al., 1995). In the Asian haplotype, high HbF levels are common in sickle cell anemia and even sickle cell trait subjects in an Indian study (Kulozik et al., 1987) demonstrated increasing HbF level in homozygotes compared to heterozygotes for this haplotype. However, among sickle cell anemia patients homozygous for the Arab-India

Martin H. Steinberg, Bernard G. Forget, Douglas R. Higgs, and Ronald L. Nagel, editors. *Disorders of Hemoglobin: Genetics, Pathophysiology, and Clinical Management.* © 2001 Cambridge University Press. All rights reserved.

Table 33.1. Comparison of Some Hematologic Indices in Jamaican Patients with Sickle Cell Anemia with and without α Thalassemia

	Normal controls (αα/αα), n = 88, mean ± SD (range)	Heterozygous α⁺ thalassemia (α–/αα), n = 44, mean ± SD (range)	Homozygous α⁺ thalassemia (α–/α–), n = 44, mean ± SD (range)
Hb (g/dL)*	7.8 ± 1.1 (6.0–10.5)	8.1 ± 1.0 (5.8–10.8)	8.8 ± 1.3 (6.9–11.5)
HbA$_2$ (%)[†]	2.8 ± 0.4 (2.1–3.8)	3.1 ± 0.3 (2.4–3.9)	3.9 ± 0.4 (3.0–4.7)
HbF (%)[‡]	5.3 (0.6–18.0)	4.8 (0.9–15.0)	3.8 (0.8–18.4)
MCHC (g/dL)[†]	34.8 ± 1.7 (31–39)	34.3 ± 1.6 (30–39)	32.8 ± 1.3 (30–36)
RBC (× 10^{12}/L)[†]	2.6 ± 0.4 (1.8–3.7)	2.9 ± 0.5 (2.1–4.5)	3.9 ± 0.6 (2.8–5.0)
MCV (fl)[†]	90.1 ± 6.1 (69–101)	84.4 ± 7.8 (63–96)	71.2 ± 3.2 (63–78)
Reticulocytes (%)[†]	11.9 (5–25)	9.3 (4–17)	6.4 (3–12)

* Significant differences between α–/αα and α–/α– and between αα/αα and α–/α–.
[†] Significant differences between all groups.
[‡] Significant differences only between αα/αα and α–/α–.
Adapted from Higgs et al. (1982), with permission.

haplotype in eastern Saudi Arabia, although the mean HbF level was elevated at 13.3 percent, the range was 4.9 percent to 22.1 percent, suggesting that factors other than haplotype were important for setting the HbF level (Padmos et al., 1991). These observations, and other data discussed in Chapter 26, imply that the β-globin gene haplotype has a relatively minor effect on the HbF level and although the mechanism of any effect is unclear, data from the Asian haplotype patients are consistent with close linkage with a separate gene determining HbF. The influence of haplotype on HbF levels is therefore unclear at the present time and even greater uncertainty attends the possible effects of haplotype on clinical course.

α Thalassemia

Since the genes determining α thalassemia are on chromosome 16 and those determining sickle cell disease on chromosome 11, both abnormalities may be coinherited. In practice, severe α⁰ thalassemia (dele-

tion of both α-globin genes) occurs predominantly in Southeast Asia and rarely, if ever, coincides with HbS. The mild α⁺ thalassemia (deletion of a single α-globin gene), on the other hand, is common in populations with HbS, and in peoples of West African ancestry in the United States 35 percent were heterozygotes and 3 percent to 4 percent homozygotes for this abnormality (Dozy et al., 1979). In eastern and southwestern Saudi Arabia (El-Hazmi et al., 1990; Padmos et al., 1991) and in India (Labie et al., 1989; Kulozik et al., 1988) α⁺ thalassemia occurs in over 50 percent of populations with sickle cell disease, and in Saudi Arabia, nondeletional forms of α thalassemia may occur. Greece has the only documented population with sickle cell disease in which α thalassemia is rare (Christakis et al., 1990). In sickle cell anemia, α⁺ thalassemia modifies the hematologic and clinical expression (Embury et al., 1982; Higgs et al., 1982; Steinberg et al., 1984). As discussed in Chapters 24, 26, and 28 (Tables 33.1 and 33.2) α thalassemia lowers the mean corpuscular hemoglobin concentration (MCHC), inhibiting poly-

Table 33.2. Comparison of Some Clinical Features in Sickle Cell Anemia with and without α Thalassemia

	Normal controls (αα/αα)	Heterozygous α⁺ thalassemia (α–/αα)	Homozygous α⁺ thalassemia (α–/α–)
Painful episode frequency	+	+	++
Acute chest syndrome (% affected)*	34	30	16
Leg ulceration*	45	36	23
Splenomegaly*	14	24	45
Avascular necrosis of femoral head	+	?	++

* Percent affected were significantly different between αα/αα and α–/α– groups (data from Higgs et al., 1982).
Data derived from Embury et al. (1982), Higgs et al. (1982), Platt et al. (1991), Bailey et al. (1991), Steinberg et al. (1984), Ballas et al. (1989), Sebes (1989).

merization of HbS and sickling and might be expected to promote flow in capillaries and small vessels, but the viscosity effects of the increased total hemoglobin level may impair flow in larger vessels. It therefore presents a particularly interesting model that may allow differentiation of the effects of flow in the small and larger vessels. In homozygous α^+ thalassemia, the deleterious effects of the increase in total hemoglobin override the beneficial effects of inhibition of intravascular sickling, leading to an increase in bone pain episodes, whereas the protective effects of the reduced sickling allow persistence of splenomegaly and reduce the frequency of leg ulcers, and at least in some studies, acute chest syndrome and stroke.

Hereditary Persistence of High Fetal Hemoglobin Levels

Patients with sickle cell anemia maintain elevated levels of γ-globin chain synthesis into adult life, resulting in elevated HbF levels that vary markedly between patients. Since HbF molecules interfere with polymerization of HbS molecules and inhibit sickling, patients with high HbF levels are protected from many of the early life-threatening complications of the disease (Stevens et al., 1981; Bailey et al., 1992). Hematologically, the effects of high levels of HbF are complex but probably decrease hemolysis and generally result in higher total hemoglobin levels (Maude et al., 1987). Clinically, high HbF levels are associated with persistence of splenomegaly (Serjeant, 1970) and probably persistence of normal splenic function (Al-Awamy et al., 1984; Mallouh et al., 1984) protecting against acute splenic sequestration (Stevens et al., 1981) and reducing the susceptibility to overwhelming septicemia. Other effects of high HbF levels include more normal growth (Ashcroft et al., 1972; Lowry et al., 1977), less leg ulceration (Koshy et al., 1989), acute chest syndrome (Castro et al., 1994), and painful episodes (Platt et al., 1991), a milder clinical course (Jackson et al., 1961; Thomas et al., 1997), and probably greater survival (Gelpi, 1979; Platt et al., 1994).

The inheritance of genes determining high levels of HbF is not well understood (see Chapters 15 and 26). In most sickle cell subjects with high HbF levels, either one or both parents show a modest elevation of HbF within the normal range. However, since HbF levels decline with age and are higher in females than males, it has not been possible to define the regulatory gene(s) on the basis of a set HbF level. Based on current evidence it seems likely that HbF levels in sickle cell disease are determined by several factors, some environmental and some genetic. Since HbF protects against sickling, red cells with high HbF levels persist for longer in the circulation, tending to elevate

hemolysate HbF levels because of cell selection (Dover et al., 1978). Possible genetic factors that may contribute to the elevation of HbF levels are discussed in Chapters 15 and 26.

Total Hemoglobin Levels

In sickle cell anemia associated with the Benin haplotype, steady-state hemoglobin levels are most commonly 6 to 9 g/dL (range, 5 to 12 g/dL). Determinants of the steady-state hemoglobin level in sickle cell anemia include HbF, α thalassemia, β-globin gene haplotype, red cell survival, and oxygen dissociation curve (Serjeant et al., 1996), and although the first three factors have a clear genetic basis, it is likely that genetic factors contribute to other determinants of hemoglobin level (see Chapter 20). High hemoglobin levels may contribute to morbidity as a risk factor for bone pain episodes (Baum et al., 1987; Platt et al., 1991), avascular necrosis of the femoral head (Hawker et al., 1982), proliferative sickle retinopathy (Fox et al., 1990), and acute chest syndrome (Castro et al., 1994). High hemoglobin levels as a result of high HbF levels (Maude et al., 1987) do not carry these risks but the combination of high total hemoglobin and low HbF is potentially deleterious.

Conversely, a low total hemoglobin level may be beneficial because of the associated hyperdynamic circulation. Patients with such a condition are less prone to bone pain episodes but cardiovascular function may be compromised earlier with the declining hemoglobin levels consequent on renal impairment common with advancing age. Stroke in childhood may be more common because of increased cerebral blood flow (see Chapter 24).

ENVIRONMENTAL FACTORS

Infections

Malaria. Malaria is a major factor contributing to the morbidity and mortality of sickle cell disease, and its control reduces symptoms and improves survival. The sickle cell trait manifests a relative resistance to falciparum malaria (see Chapter 30), but in patients with sickle cell disease, malaria is a common precipitant of painful episodes (Konotey-Ahulu, 1971; Maharajan et al., 1983) and prophylaxis reduced their frequency to that observed among patients in the United States (Oyejide et al., 1982). By causing an additional severe hemolytic anemia, malaria is probably a major contributor to death (Maharajan et al., 1983).

Encapsulated Organisms. The early loss of splenic function renders patients more prone to invasive infection by encapsulated organisms, especially *Streptococcus pneumoniae, Haemophilus influenzae* type b, and *Salmonella* spp. The morbidity and mortality from pneumococcal septicemia has been reduced or prevented by prophylactic penicillin in early childhood and pneumococcal vaccine at later ages (John et al., 1984; Gaston et al., 1986), although these policies may require modification with the increasing frequency of penicillin-resistant pneumococci and the development of a conjugated pneumococcal vaccine that may be effective when given in the first 6 months of life (see Chapter 24). Bacteremia from the pneumococcus may be less prevalent under tropical conditions. Studies in equatorial Africa (Akinyanju et al., 1987; Akuse, 1996) and eastern Saudi Arabia (Mallouh and Salamah, 1985b) have noted the prominence of Salmonella spp, Staphylococcus, and Klebsiella, and the relative rarity of *Streptococcus pneumoniae* infection. The mechanisms contributing to this different pattern of bacteremia in tropical areas is unknown although it has been postulated that persistence of splenomegaly and possibly splenic function may be promoted in Nigeria by malaria-induced splenomegaly (Akuse, 1996) and in Saudi Arabia by the high HbF levels (Mallouh and Salamah, 1985b). The conjugated vaccine against *Hemophilus influenzae* type b is likely to reduce the incidence of septicemia from this cause. Salmonella septicemia and osteomyelitis are potentially life-threatening complications, the incidence of which reflects the frequency of Salmonella carriage in the general population and are consequently likely to be reduced by proper piped water supplies and sewage disposal (Adeyokunnu and Hendrickse, 1980; Maharajan et al., 1983). Animal vectors of Salmonella such as chickens may also represent a public health problem and could contribute to the increasing frequency of Salmonella infections (30 percent *Salmonella enteritidis*) observed in Jamaica. An analysis of 55 Salmonella isolations from blood, pus, or aspirates over a 22-year period in Jamaica noted that 28 were associated with osteomyelitis and 27 with septicemia without clinical evidence of bone involvement (Wright et al., 1997). The long established association of Salmonella with osteomyelitis led to the early use of specific anti-Salmonella therapy in this group, but 22 percent of those with septicemia died because they received only penicillin on the assumption of pneumococcal disease.

Viral and Other Infections. There is no evidence of an increased susceptibility to viral infections in sickle cell disease, but human parvovirus infection is important because of its capacity to temporarily destroy red cell precursors in the bone marrow. Although this aplasia lasts only 7 to 10 days and is unimportant in hematologically normal subjects, the markedly shortened red cell survival in sickle cell disease implies that the aplastic crisis is a potential cause of mortality (Serjeant et al., 1981). In Jamaica, human parvovirus infection occurred in 30 percent of children by the age of 15 years (Serjeant et al., 1993), and although there is some evidence that the epidemiology of human parvovirus infection differs in other communities (Rao et al., 1983), this is likely to be an important contributor to childhood mortality. Awareness, early diagnosis, proper monitoring of siblings, and transfusion reduce mortality, and a human parvovirus vaccine has been developed but is awaiting clinical trial. Other common childhood infections are likely to carry a higher morbidity when superimposed on sickle cell disease, and reluctance to give immunization in children during intercurrent infections and febrile episodes, which are more common in sickle cell disease, implies that greater vigilance is needed to ensure complete immunization. Regimens for control of many of these infections are available and whether they are effectively implemented depends on the development of health care services in the individual countries. The relative sophistication of health services in North America, the Caribbean, and Europe implies that patients should be protected from such infections and consequently have less morbidity and greater survival. Unfortunately this is not the case in many developing countries.

Nutrition

The metabolic demands of the greatly expanded bone marrow and the increased cardiovascular work consequent on anemia are likely to contribute to the 20 percent increase observed in the resting metabolic rate of adolescents with sickle cell disease (Singhal et al., 1993). This does not appear to be compensated for by an increase in dietary intake. An increase in growth following relief of the hemolytic burden of hypersplenism (Singhal et al., 1995; Badaloo et al., 1996) or by dietary supplementation overriding appetite control (Heyman et al., 1985) is consistent with suboptimal nutrition. The reduction in physical activity of sickle cell patients is also consistent with an energy deficiency and calorie economy (Singhal et al., 1997). Furthermore this deficiency may affect not only growth but also cognitive development (Knight et al., 1995). These observations imply that failure to meet the increased nutritional demands may increase the potential morbidity of the disease, and provide a mechanism whereby socioeconomic status of the patient may modify clinical outcome. Folic acid requirements are also increased and must be met by increased dietary availability or by supplementation in order to avoid the marked anemia resulting from megaloblastic erythropoiesis. This is particularly important in West Africa (Hendricks et al., 1972) where dietary availability of folic acid appears to be low and megaloblastic change common. In North America, the Caribbean, and Europe folate deficiency appears less common even in the absence of supplementation (Rabb et al., 1983) and may reflect a lesser demand in the absence of malaria.

Climate

Climate may also be important through its effect in precipitating painful episodes that contribute to the morbidity and occasionally mortality of the disease (Platt et al., 1994). Cold wet weather or the rainy season is an important precipitant for the painful episode in West Africa (Addae, 1971) and this relationship has also been shown in the Caribbean (Redwood et al., 1976) and North America (Resar and Oski, 1991). Theoretically, exposure of patients to more extreme conditions should be followed by more frequent pains although this relationship may be obscured by modification of the microclimate with warm clothing and central heating. On the other hand, a hot dry climate such as Saudi Arabia may predispose to dehydration as a risk factor for painful episodes.

Leg Ulceration

Chronic leg ulceration occurs in approximately 70 percent of postpubertal Jamaican patients with sickle cell disease (Serjeant, 1974) compared with 5 percent in the United States (Koshy et al., 1989), 10 percent to 15 percent in West Africa (Adedeji and Ukoli, 1987), less than 5 percent in Greece (Christakis et al., 1990), and less than 1 percent in India and Saudi Arabia (Padmos et al., 1991; Kar et al., 1986). Although some of these geographic differences may be attributable to genetic factors such as different haplotypes or HbF levels, the much higher prevalence among the predominantly Benin haplotype in Jamaica compared to that in the United States, West Africa, and Greece is strongly suggestive of an environmental effect. The pathologic basis of this effect is currently unclear but leg ulceration with its chronicity, impact on education, and subsequent employment potential is a major determinant of morbidity of sickle cell disease in Jamaica (Alleyne et al., 1977).

Socioeconomic Status

There can be little doubt that the socioeconomic status of the patient is a major determinant of the clinical course although only limited data are available. Services such as private transport and telephone allow earlier consultation and easier access to medical care, as well as better immunization, nutrition, and malarial prophylaxis. Smaller families allow greater attention to be paid to sickle cell offspring and better housing implies better public health measures with clean water and sewage disposal. High socioeconomic status has been claimed to improve survival and any effects are likely to be multifactorial (Konotey-Ahulu, 1973).

Medical Care

The provision of specialized medical services for patients in sickle cell clinics is likely to alter the morbidity and outcome of the disease. Such clinics act as centers for education about the disease for both patients and their families. Acute splenic sequestration provides an example of the importance of parental education. This complication is of unknown etiology but sudden enlargement of the spleen traps red cells, resulting in a sudden severe anemia and often death (Topley et al., 1981). Early diagnosis and prompt blood transfusion relieve the initial symptoms and, if complications recur, prophylactic splenectomy is advocated. Parental education at early diagnosis and clinic attendance has reduced mortality from this complication by 90 percent in Jamaica (Emond et al., 1985) and has also been effective in the United States.

Sophisticated facilities may, ironically, increase morbidity and possibly mortality if incorrectly used. Exploratory surgery is sometimes performed for acute cholestasis or abdominal painful episode when greater clinical experience would favor conservative management. There appears to be little evidence for the removal of asymptomatic gallstones yet cholecystectomy, especially laparoscopic, is commonly performed. Transfusion is sometimes overused for a multitude of clinical complications when alternative management is available. Transfusion programs may be used in the management of pregnancy without good evidence for their beneficial effect, and chronic transfusion programs, although justified in the prophylaxis of stroke, have been proposed for other complications with the resultant risks of alloimmunization, transfusion-borne infections, iron accumulation, and permanent implanted ports to obtain venous access (see Chapter 37).

AGE AND SECULAR CHANGES

Prognosis and survival in sickle cell disease are also influenced by the age of the patient at the onset of clinical symptoms. The greatest mortality in sickle cell disease occurs in the second 6 months of life and mortality declines for each individual subsequent year (Lee et al., 1995). This implies that the prognosis for a

10-year-old patient is better than that of a newborn who has yet to traverse the early high-risk period. Furthermore, the morbidity may also improve with advancing age, with the susceptibility to infection appearing to wane and painful episodes becoming less frequent and less severe in most patients after the age of 30 years. Interpretation of these age effects may be further confounded by secular changes since improving management of the disease improves survival, as illustrated in the Jamaican Cohort Study in which survival of the last 210 subjects was significantly greater than the first 105 subjects (Lee et al., 1995). In the Cooperative Study in the United States, among 3,764 patients aged from birth to 66 years at enrollment, it was estimated that the median age at death for sickle cell anemia males was 42 years and for sickle cell anemia females 48 years (Platt et al., 1994). In the Jamaican Cohort Study based on 315 sickle cell subjects detected by newborn screening, 83 percent of the first 207 children have currently survived beyond 20 years.

GEOGRAPHIC VARIATION OF SICKLE CELL DISEASE

The interaction of these various genetic and environmental influences determines the clinical pattern of sickle cell disease in its different locations. The disease falls into two broad genetic patterns: patients of West African origin (predominantly Benin haplotype) and those in eastern Saudi Arabia and India, carriers of the Arab-India haplotype.

Areas with the Benin Haplotype

Within areas affected by the Benin haplotype, there is some genetic variation in the prevalence of α^+ thalassemia and of high HbF levels, but much of the variability in disease severity and outcome results from environmental effects.

West Africa. The frequency of sickle cell trait varies from 15 percent to 25 percent and of α^+ thalassemia from 35 percent to 40 percent; malaria is common and general public health measures are poor outside major cities. The affected population is predominantly young with high early mortality, and survival to adulthood is uncommon. The early clinical picture is dominated by infections, especially with Salmonella spp, *Klebsiella,* and *Staphylococcus,* but *Streptococcus pneumonia* appears uncommon. Malaria is a major influence and effective prophylaxis improves both morbidity and mortality. The hemolytic rate of sickle cell disease will be accelerated by malaria, and the limited dietary availability of folic acid (Fleming et al., 1969) implies that megaloblastic change from folate deficiency is common, with one study reporting folate deficiency in 11 percent of newly referred patients (Watson-Williams, 1962). Otherwise the major causes of death are not well documented and autopsy data are limited. Complications of adolescence or adult life such as leg ulceration, priapism, or pregnancy appear less common than in Jamaica and end organ damage such as renal failure is rare, but these observations reflect a patient population not surviving long enough to develop these complications. There is a clinical impression that socioeconomic factors are very important in both morbidity and mortality from the disease (Trowell et al., 1957; Konotey-Ahulu, 1973; Konotey-Ahulu, 1974; Ohene-Frempong and Nkrumah, 1994).

Jamaica. The disease is almost entirely of West African origin; the sickle cell trait occurs in 10 percent of the population and α^+ thalassemia in 35 percent to 40 percent. Malaria has been eradicated and public health measures are generally well developed. The greatest mortality is in the second 6 months of the first year of life, falling for each succeeding year, although it may rise again in early adult life. Causes of early mortality are acute splenic sequestration, pneumococcal septicemia, aplastic crisis, acute chest syndrome, and stroke, but mortality from the first two causes has significantly decreased over the past 20 years (Lee et al., 1995). Leg ulceration occurs in 70 percent of sickle cell adults and is particularly characteristic of the disease in Jamaica. Stuttering priapism occurs in 40 percent of postpubertal males. The painful episode is an important problem especially in young adult males, although over 90 percent of affected patients are managed as outpatients (Serjeant et al., 1994; Ware et al., 1999). In the absence of malaria, splenomegaly is an indicator of mildness representing persistence of a capillary bed that has not been destroyed by intravascular sickling, and this persists in approximately 10 percent of sickle cell patients beyond the age of 15 years. At later ages, end organ damage, especially chronic renal failure (Morgan and Sergeant, 1981) from glomerular fibrosis, increasingly contributes to morbidity, the falling erythropoietin levels and consequent lower hemoglobin compromising cardiovascular function. The overall clinical course is very variable with many patients mildly affected, survival beyond 40 years being common, and estimates of average survival exceeding 50 years (Wierenga, personal communication).

North America. The disease reported from North America is almost entirely of West African origin; the sickle cell trait occurs in 8 percent of this population and α^+ thalassemia in 35 percent to 40 percent. Generally disease expression is similar to that in Jamaica although only 5 percent develop leg ulceration. Painful episodes dominate the clinical picture in young adults, but better epidemiologic data suggest that frequent admissions for painful episodes are due to a small subgroup of severely affected or poorly coping patients (Platt et al., 1991). With advancing age, organ damage results in both renal and chronic pulmonary failure (Powars et al., 1988). Median survival in a study conducted between 1978 and 1988 was calculated at 42 years for males and 48 years for females (Platt et al., 1994).

South America. Most of the disease occurs in Brazil where the affected population is of West of Central African origin as reflected in the approximately equal proportions of Benin and Bantu haplotypes (Zago et al., 1992). Manifestations of the disease appear to be similar to those in Jamaica although only limited clinical data are available and there is no information on survival.

Northern Europe. In the United Kingdom, sickle cell disease is of West African origin, partly via the Caribbean and partly direct. In France the disease is mostly imported directly from Africa, and in Germany it occurs mostly in patients of Turkish origin who carry the Benin haplotype. No studies are available on the natural history of sickle cell disease in Europe but observations in the United Kingdom and France suggest that the expression of the disease does not differ from that observed in Jamaica except for a lower prevalence of leg ulceration. Average survival of patients is currently unknown.

Greece. The sickle cell gene in Greece is linked to the Benin haplotype consistent with a West African origin, but carriers of the gene do not have African physical characteristics. It is most common in villages in northern Greece where up to 30 percent may have the sickle cell trait (Deliyannis and Tavalarakis, 1955). Despite this high frequency, sickle cell disease is not common because of the tendency of young people to move away from these villages, and the high prevalence of β thalassemia genes in southern Greece implies that sickle cell-β⁰ thalassemia is equally common. A study comparing Greek and Jamaican sickle cell disease found that Greek subjects had higher hemoglobin levels and red cell counts and lower MCHC and reticulocyte counts (Christakis et al., 1990). The higher hemoglobin and lower reticulocyte counts are consistent with less hemolysis, but Greek subjects have neither of the genetic factors recognized to ameliorate hemolysis in patients of African origin, α thalassemia or high levels of HbF. The low MCHC, which was not attributable to iron deficiency or α thalassemia, might be expected to retard sickling and its mechanism is of potential interest. Clinically, Greek sickle cell subjects showed persistence of splenomegaly, a more normal body build, and less leg ulceration and priapism.

Painful episodes were an important cause of morbidity but are probably limited to a severely affected subset of patients. Data are limited on the causes of death and no data are available on survival.

Areas with the Asian Haplotype

Saudi Arabia. The sickle cell gene occurs in two major areas, the Eastern Province where some communities such as Qatif and Hofuf have sickle cell trait frequencies of 25 percent, and the southwest where sickle cell trait frequencies are 5 percent. The Arab-India haplotype, representing an independent occurrence of the HbS gene, characterizes the sickle cell gene in the Eastern Province, and the Benin haplotype, imported from Africa, that in the southwest. Both areas have deletional α⁺ thalassemia in over 50 percent of the population and nondeletional forms also occur. High levels of HbF characterize the Arab-India haplotype. These features result in two different hematologic forms of sickle cell anemia disease: a hematologically milder form occurring in the Eastern Province and a hematologically more severe disease characterizing the southwest (El Mouzan et al., 1989; Padmos et al., 1991). Saudi Arabia therefore offers an opportunity to compare the effects of the two haplotypes within a similar environment.

Compared to southwestern patients, eastern patients have higher hemoglobin and HbF, and lower HbA₂, MCHC, mean cell volume (MCV), and reticulocyte counts. Clinically splenomegaly persisted for longer, and leg ulceration and priapism were rare. Yet painful episodes are seen in both groups of patients.

Sickle cell disease in the Orissa State of India is very similar to that in the Eastern Province of Saudi Arabia.

COMPARISON OF FOUR SICKLE CELL PATIENT GROUPS

The results of these differing genetic and environmental backgrounds are illustrated by comparisons of sickle cell disease in four different areas: Jamaica, Greece, Eastern Saudi Arabia, and Central India (Table 33.3). α⁺ Thalassemia is rare in Greece, common in Jamaica, and even more common in Saudi Arabia and India. β-Globin gene haplotypes are predominantly Benin in Jamaica, entirely Benin in Greece, and almost entirely Asian in the other two groups. The resulting hematologic differences (Table 33.4) are largely but not entirely attributable to these genetic differences and the clinical differences (Table 33.5) in large part reflect the hematologic differences. Some clinical features such as the high prevalence of leg ulceration in Jamaica or of Salmonella osteomyelitis in Saudi Arabia are presumed to result from environmental factors and others such as the high

Table 33.3. α Thalassemia and β-Globin Gene Haplotype in Homozygous Sickle Cell Disease in Four Geographic Areas

	Jamaica	Greece	Eastern Saudi Arabia	Orissa State, India
α Thalassemia (α-gene) frequency	0.185	0.037	0.375	0.317
Predominant β-globin haplotype	Benin	Benin	Arab-Indian	Arab-Indian

Data derived from Padmos et al. (1991), Kar et al. (1986), Christakis et al. (1990).

prevalence of avascular necrosis of the femoral head in Saudi Arabia may be exaggerated by symptomatic selection in the studied population.

Comparable and reliable incidence data for painful episodes in the four populations are not available, but painful episodes remain a major source of morbidity even in eastern Saudi Arabia and India despite the high HbF levels characterizing these groups. The high frequency of α^+ thalassemia would be expected to increase the risk (Bailey et al., 1991; Platt et al., 1991) and high HbF levels decrease the risk (Castro et al., 1994) of painful events.

The low prevalence of leg ulceration in Saudi Arabia and India is consistent with a protective effect of α^+ thalassemia or high HbF levels as supported by data from Jamaica and the United States (Higgs et al., 1982; Koshy et al., 1989). However, leg ulceration remains extremely common in Jamaica despite a high prevalence of α^+ thalassemia, and the assumption that poor socioeconomic conditions were responsible was not supported by data from India where such conditions are common but leg ulceration rare. One must conclude that some other factor, not yet recognized, in Jamaican conditions is responsible.

The infrequency of priapism in Saudi Arabia and India is consistent with their high HbF levels and observations that low HbF levels are a risk factor for this complication in Jamaica (Emond et al., 1980).

The data on avascular necrosis of the femoral head are difficult to interpret and subject to symptomatic selection in the study groups, although it seems unlikely that this could account entirely for the high prevalence observed in Saudi Arabia (Padmos et al., 1991). α^+ Thalassemia is a risk factor (Steinberg et al., 1984; Ballas et al., 1989) from studies in the United States but did not account for the high prevalence in Saudi Arabia (Padmos et al., 1995), which currently remains unexplained.

High levels of HbF and α^+ thalassemia are associated with persistence of splenomegaly (Serjeant 1970; Higgs et al., 1982) implying persistence of splenic function (Al-Awamy et al., 1984; Mallouh et al., 1984). Subjects in eastern Saudi Arabia and India should therefore be protected from pneumococcal septicemia and acute splenic sequestration (Stevens et al., 1981; Edmond et al., 1985) but may be at greater risk of hypersplenism (Kar et al., 1986; Mallouh and Salamah, 1985a).

The ultimate significance of these differences lies in their effect on mortality, and although data are limited, it wold be anticipated that sickle cell patients in eastern Saudi Arabia and India would be relatively protected from the serious early complications of acute splenic sequestration and pneumococcal septicemia. The greater red cell survival in α^+ thalassemia (De Ceulaer et al., 1983) and high HbF levels should decrease mortality

Table 33.4. Comparison of Some Hematologic Indices in Sickle Cell Anemia in Four Geographic Areas

	Jamaica	Greece	Eastern Saudi Arabia	Orissa State, India
HbA_2	3.0 (1.5–4.7)	2.8 (1.9–4.0)	2.2 (1.2–4.0)	1.9 (1.1–3.4)
Corrected HbA_2%*	3.2 (1.8–4.8)	3.0 (2.1–4.0)	2.5 (1.4–4.7)	2.3 (1.4–3.7)
HbF (%)	6.1 (0.4–33.2)	5.6 (0.7–13.6)	13.3 (4.9–22.1)	16.6 (4.6–31.5)
Hb (g/dL)	8.0 (4.1–13.5)	9.4 (5.7–11.9)	10.3 (6.5–12.9)	8.7 (3.9–13.5)
MCHC (g/dL)	33.9 (27–41)	32.8 (30–38)	32.9 (27–39)	31.5 (25–42)
MCV (fl)	87.3 (62–115)	92.8 (68–108)	82.4 (52–105)	83.6 (60–113)
Reticulocytes (%)	10.5 (1–31)	7.9 (2–16)	5.9 (2–14)	6.5 (1–29)

* Corrected HbA_2 refers to HbA_2 level expressed as a percentage of total adult hemoglobin; this measure therefore introduces a correction for varying HbF levels (depicted as mean [range]).

Data derived from Padmos et al. (1991), Kar et al. (1986), Christakis et al. (1990).

Table 33.5. Some Clinical Features of Sickle Cell Anemia in Four Geographic Areas

	Jamaica	Greece	Eastern Saudi Arabia	Orissa State, India
Painful episode	++	++	++	++
Osteonecrosis	8	12	27	?10
Leg ulceration	75	2	0	1
Priapism (% males)	40	8	6	0
Splenomegaly	5	19	53	69

Note: Figures represent percentage of patients affected.
Data derived from Padmos et al. (1991), Kar et al. (1986) Christakis et al. (1990).

from the aplastic crisis and stroke. Data on the incidence of stroke in eastern Saudi Arabia and India are not available but this complication might be predicted to be less common. Finally, the progressive end organ damage resulting in chronic pulmonary fibrosis (Powars et al., 1988) and renal impairment (Morgan and Serjeant, 1981), which are major determinants of mortality in sickle cell adults from Jamaica and the United States, do not appear to be common in eastern Saudi Arabia or India. These observations are consistent with the low mortality reported from eastern Saudi Arabia in both children (Perrine et al., 1981) and adults (Perrine et al., 1978) and the calculations for near normal survival (Gelpi, 1979) in that area.

References

Addae, SK. (1971). Mechanism for the high incidence of sickle-cell crisis in the tropical cool season. *Lancet* 2: 1256.

Adedeji, MO and Ukoli, FAM. (1987). Hematological factors associated with leg ulcer in sickle cell disease. *Trop. Geogr. Med.* 39: 354–356.

Adeyokunnu, AA and Hendrickse, RG. (1980). Salmonella osteomyelitis in childhood. A report of 63 cases seen in Nigerian children of whom 57 had sickle cell anemia. *Arch. Dis. Child.* 55: 175–184.

Akinyanju, O and Johnson, AO. (1987). Acute illness in Nigerian children with sickle cell anemia. *Ann. Trop. Pediatr.* 7: 181–186.

Akuse, RM. (1996). Variation in the pattern of bacterial infection in patients with sickle cell disease requiring admission. *J. Trop. Pediatr.* 42: 318–323.

Al-Awamy, B, Wilson, WA, and Pearson, HA. (1984). Splenic function in sickle cell disease in the Eastern Province of Saudi Arabia. *J. Pediatr.* 104: 714–717.

Alleyne, SI, Wint, E, and Serjeant, GR. (1977). Social effects of leg ulceration in sickle cell anemia. *South. Med. J.* 70: 213–214.

Aluoch, JR, Kilinc, Y, Aksoy, M et al. (1986). Sickle cell anemia among Eti-Turks: Haematological, clinical and genetic observations. *Br. J. Haematol.* 64: 45–55.

Antonarakis, SE, Boehm, CD, Serjeant, GR et al. (1984). Origin of the β^S-globin gene in blacks: The contribution of recurrent mutation or gene conversion or both. *Proc. Natl. Acad. Sci. U.S.A.* 81: 853–856.

Ashcroft, MT, Serjeant, GR, and Desai, P. (1972). Height, weights, and skeletal age of Jamaican adolescents with sickle cell anemia. *Arch. Dis. Child.* 47: 519–524.

Badaloo, AV, Singhal, A, Forrester, TE et al. (1996). The effect of splenectomy for hypersplenism on whole body protein turnover, resting metabolic rate and growth in sickle cell disease. *Eur. J. Clin. Nutr.* 50: 672–675.

Bailey, K, Morris, J, and Serjeant, GR. (1992). Fetal hemoglobin and early manifestation of homozygous sickle cell disease. *Arch. Dis. Child.* 67: 517–520.

Bailey, S, Higgs, DR, Morris, J, and Serjeant GR. (1991). Is the painful crisis of sickle cell disease due to sickling? *Lancet* 337: 735.

Ballas, SK, Talacki, CA, Rao, VM, and Steiner, RM. (1989). The prevalence of avascular necrosis in sickle cell anemia: Correlation with α-thalassemia. *Hemoglobin* 13: 649–655.

Baum, KF, Dunn, DT, Maude, GH, and Serjeant, GR. (1987). The painful crisis of sickle cell disease. A study of risk factors. *Arch. Intern. Med.* 147: 1231–1234.

Boussiou, M, Loukopoulos, D, Christakis, J, and Fessas, Ph. (1991). The origin of the sickle cell mutation in Greece: Evidence from β^S-globin gene cluster polymorphisms. *Hemoglobin* 15: 459–467.

Castro, O, Brambilla, DJ, Thorington, B et al. (1994). The acute chest syndrome in sickle cell disease: Incidence and risk factors. *Blood* 84: 643–649.

Chang, YC, Smith, KD, Moore, RD et al. (1995). An analysis of fetal hemoglobin variation in sickle cell disease: The relative contributions of the X-linked factor, β-globin haplotypes, α-globin gene number, gender and age. *Blood* 85: 1111–1117.

Christakis, J, Vavatsi, N, Hassapopoulou, H et al. (1990). Comparison of homozygous sickle cell disease in Northern Greece and Jamaica. *Lancet* 335: 637–640.

De Ceular, K, Higgs, DR, Weatherall, DJ et al. (1983). α-thalassemia reduces the hemolytic rate in homozygous sickle-cell disease. *N. Engl. J. Med.* 309: 189–190.

Deliyannis, G and Tavalarakis, N. (1955). Sickling phenomenon in Northern Greece. *Br. Med. J.* 2: 299–301.

Dover, GJ, Boyer, SH, Charache, S, and Heintzelman, K. (1978). Individual variation in the production and survival of F cells in sickle-cell disease. *N. Engl. J. Med.* 229: 1428–1435.

Dozy, AM, Kan, YW, Embury, SH et al. (1979). Alpha gene organization in blacks precludes the severe form of α-thalassaemia. *Nature* 280: 605–607.

Edmond, AM, Holman, R, Hayes, RJ, and Serjeant, G. (1980). Priapism and impotence in homozygous sickle cell disease. *Arch. Intern. Med.* 140: 1434–1437.

Emond, AM, Collis, R, Darvill, D et al. (1985). Acute splenic sequestration in homozygous sickle cell disease; natural history and management. *J. Pediatr.* 107: 201–206.

El-Hazmi, MAF. (1990). β-globin gene haplotypes in the Saudi sickle cell anemia patients. *Hum. Hered.* 40: 177–186.

El Mouzan, Ml, Al Awamy, BH, Al Torki, MT, and Niazi, GA. (1989). Variability of sickle cell disease in the Eastern Province of Saudi Arabia. *J. Pediatr.* 14: 973–976.

Embury, SH, Dozy, AM, Miller, J et al. (1982). Concurrent sickle-cell anemia and α-thalassemia. Effect on severity of anemia. *N. Engl. J. Med.* 306: 270–274.

Fleming, AF, Allan, NC, and Stenhouse, NS. (1969). Folate activity, vitamin B12 concentration and megaloblastic erythropoiesis in anemic pregnant Nigerians. *Am. J. Clin. Nutr.* 22: 755–766.

Fox, PD, Dunn, DT, Morris, JS, and Serjeant, GR. (1990). Risk factors for proliferative sickle retinopathy. *Br. J. Ophthalmol.* 74: 172–176.

Gaston, MH, Verter, JI, Woods, G et al. (1986). Prophylaxis with oral penicillin in children with sickle cell anemia. *N. Engl. J. Med.* 314: 1593–1599.

Gelpi, AP. (1979). Benign sickle cell disease in Saudi Arabia: Survival estimate and population dynamics. *Clin. Genet.* 15: 307–310.

Hawker, H, Neilson, H, Hayes, RJ, and Serjeant, GR. (1982). Hematological factors associated with avascular necrosis of the femoral head in homozygous sickle cell disease. *Br. J. Haematol.* 50: 29–34.

Hendricks, JPdeV, Harrison, KA, Watson-Williams, EJ, Luzzatto, L et al. (1972). Pregnancy in homozygous sickle-cell anemia. *J. Obstet. Gynecol. Br. Comm.* 79: 396–440.

Heyman, MB, Vichinsky, E, Katz, R et al. (1985). Growth retardation in sickle-cell disease treated by nutritional support. *Lancet* 1: 903–906.

Higgs, DR, Aldridge, BE, Lamb, J et al. (1982). The interaction of α-thalassemia and homozygous sickle-cell disease. *N. Engl. J. Med.* 306: 1441–1446.

Jackson, JF, Odom, JL, and Bell, WN. (1961). Amelioration of sickle cell disease by persistent fetal hemoglobin. *J. Am. Med. Assoc.* 177: 867–869.

John, AB, Ramlal, A, Jackson, H et al. (1894). Prevention of pneumococcal infection in children with homozygous sickle cell disease. *Br. Med. J.* 288: 1567–1570.

Kar, BC, Satapathy, RK, Kulozik, AE et al. (1986). Sickle cell disease in Orissa State, India. *Lancet* 2: 1198–1201.

Knight, S, Singhal, A, Thomas, P, and Serjeant, G. (1995). Factors associated with lowered intelligence in homozygous sickle cell disease. *Arch. Dis. Child.* 73: 316–320.

Konotey-Ahulu, FID. (1971). Treatment and prevention of sickle-cell crisis. *Lancet* 2: 1255.

Konotey-Ahulu, FID. (1973). Effect of environment on sickle cell disease in West Africa: Epidemiologic and clinical considerations. In Abramson, H, Bertks, JF, and Wethers, DL, editors. *Sickle cell disease, diagnosis, management, education, and research.* St Louis: CV Mosby. pp. 20–38.

Konotey-Ahulu, FID. (1974). The sickle cell diseases. *Arch. Intern. Med.* 133: 611–619.

Koshy, M, Entsuah, R, Koranda, A et al. (1989). Leg ulcers in patients with sickle cell disease. *Blood* 74: 1403–1408.

Kulozik, AE, Waiscoat, JS, Serjeant, GR et al. (1986). Geographical survey of β^S-globin gene haplotypes: Evidence for an independent Asian origin of the sickle-cell mutation. *Ann. J. Hum. Genet.* 39: 239–244.

Kulozik, AE, Kar, BC, Satapathy, RK et al. (1987). Fetal hemoglobin levels and β^S-globin haplotypes in an Indian population with sickle cell disease. *Blood* 69: 1724–1726.

Kulozik, AE, Kar, BC, Serjeant, BE et al. (1988). The molecular basis of α-thalassemia in India. Its interaction with the sickle cell gene. *Blood* 71: 467–472.

Labie, D, Srinivas, R, Dunda, O et al. (1989). Haplotypes in tribal Indians bearing the sickle gene: Evidence for the unicentric origin of the β^S mutation and the unicentric origin of the tribal populations of India. *Hum. Biol.* 61: 479–491.

Lee, A, Thomas, P, Cupidore, L et al. (1995). Improved survival in homozygous sickle cell disease: Lessons from a cohort study. *Br. Med. J.* 311: 160–162.

Lowry, MR, Desai, P, Ashcroft, MT et al. (1977). Heights and weights of Jamaican children with homozygous sickle cell disease. *Hum. Biol.* 49: 429–436.

Maharajan, R, Fleming, AF, and Euler, L. (1983). Pattern of infections among patients with sickle-cell anemia requiring hospital admissions. *Nig. J. Pediatr.* 10: 13–17.

Mallouh, AA and Salamah, MM. (1985a). Hypersplenism in homozygous sickle-cell disease in Saudi Arabia. *Ann. Trop. Pediatr.* 5: 143–146.

Mallouh, AA and Salamah, MM. (1985b). Pattern of bacterial infections in homozygous sickle-cell disease. A report from Saudi Arabia. *Am. J. Dis. Child.* 139: 820–822.

Mallouh, AA, Burke, GM, Salamah, M, and Ahmad, MS. (1984). Splenic function in Saudi children with sickle cell disease. *Ann. Trop. Pediatr.* 4: 87–91.

Maude, GH, Hayes, RJ, and Serjeant, GR. (1987). The hematology of steady state homozygous sickle cell disease: Interrelationships between hematological indices. *Br. J. Hematol.* 66: 549–558.

Morgan, AG and Serjeant, GR. (1981). Renal function in patients over 40 with homozygous sickle-cell disease *Br. Med. J.* 282: 1181–1183.

Nagel, RL, Rao, SK, Dunda-Belkohdja, O et al. (1987). The hematological characteristics of sickle cell anemia bearing the Bantu haplotype: The relationship between ^{G}γ and HbF level. *Blood* 69: 1026–1030.

Nagel, RL, Erlingsson, S, Fabry, ME et al. (1991). The Senegal DNA haplotype is associated with the amelioration of anemia in African-American sickle cell anemia patients. *Blood* 77: 1371–1375.

Ohene-Frempong, K and Nkrumah, FK. (1994). Sickle cell disease in Africa. In Embury, SH, Hebbe, RP, Mohandas, N, and Steinberg MH, editors. *Sickle cell disease: Basic princi-*

ples and clinical practice. New York: Raven Press. pp. 423–435.

Okuonghae, HO, Nwankwo, MU, and Offor, EC. (1993). Pattern of bacteraemia in febrile children with sickle cell anemia. Ann. Trop. Pediatr. 13: 55–64.

Oyejide, OC, Adeyokunnyu, AA, Kraus, JF, and Fanti, C. (1982). A comparative study of the morbidity associated with sickle cell anemia among patients in Ibadan (Nigeria) and Oakland (United States). Trop. Geogr. Med. 34: 341–345.

Padmos, A, Roberts, G, Lindahl, S et al. (1995). Avascular necrosis of the femoral head in Saudi Arabians with homozygous sickle cell disease—risk factors. Ann. Saudi Med. 15: 21–24.

Padmos, MA, Roberts, GT, Sackey, K et al. (1991). Two different forms of homozygous sickle cell disease occur in Saudi Arabia. Br. J. Hematol. 79: 93–98.

Perrine, RP, Pembrey, ME, John, P et al. (1978). Natural history of sickle anemia in Saudi Arabs. A study of 270 subjects. Ann. Intern. Med. 88: 1–6.

Perrine, RP, John, P, Pembrey, M, and Perrine, S. (1981). Sickle cell disease in Saudi Arabs in early childhood. Arch. Dis. Child. 56: 187–192.

Platt, OS, Thorington, BD, Brambrilla, DJ et al. (1991). Pain in sickle disease. Rates and risk factors. N. Engl. J. Med. 325: 11–16.

Platt, OS, Brambilla, DJ, Rosse, WF et al. (1994). Mortality in sickle cell disease. Life expectancy and risk factors for early death. N. Engl. J. Med. 330: 1639–1644.

Powars, DR, Weidman, JA, Odom-Maryon, T et al. (1988). Sickle cell chronic lung disease: Prior morbidity and the risk of pulmonary failure. Medicine 67: 66–76.

Rabb, LM, Grandison, Y, Mason, K et al. (1983). A trial of folate supplementation in children with homozygous sickle cell disease. Br. J. Hematol. 54: 589–594.

Ragusa, A, Lombardo, M, Sortino, G et al. (1988). β^S gene in Sicily is in linkage disequilibrium with the Benin haplotype: Implications for gene flow. Am. J. Hematol. 27: 139–141.

Rao, KRP, Patel, AR, Anderson et al. (1983). Infection with parvovirus-like virus and aplastic crisis in chronic hemolytic anemia. Ann. Intern. Med. 98: 930–932.

Redwood, AM, Williams, EM, Desai, P, and Serjeant, GR. (1976). Climate and painful crisis of sickle-cell disease in Jamaica. Br. Med. J. 1: 66–68.

Resar, LMS and Oski, FA. (1991). Cold water exposure and vaso-occlusive crisis in sickle cell anemia. J. Pediatr. 118: 407–409.

Sebes, JI. (1989). Diagnostic imaging of bone and joint abnormalities associated with sickle cell hemoglobinopathies. AJR 152: 1153–1159.

Serjeant, GR. (1970). Irreversibly sickled cells and splenomegaly in sickle-cell anemia. Br. J. Hematol. 19: 635–641.

Serjeant, GR. (1974). Leg ulceration in sickle cell anemia. Arch. Intern. Med. 133: 690–694.

Serjeant, GR. (1975). Fetal hemoglobin in homozygous sickle cell disease. Clin. Hematol. 4: 109–122.

Serjeant, GR and Ashcroft, MT. (1973). Delayed skeletal maturation in sickle cell anemia in Jamaica. Johns Hopkins Med. J. 132: 95–102.

Serjeant, GR, Topley, JM, Mason, K et al. (1981). Outbreak of aplastic crisis in sickle cell anemia associated with parvovirus-like agent. Lancet 2: 595–597.

Serjeant, GR, Serjeant, BE, Thomas, P et al. (1993). Human parvovirus infection in homozygous sickle cell disease. Lancet 341: 1237–1240.

Serjeant, GR, De Ceulaer, C, Lethbridge, R et al. (1994). The painful crisis of homozygous sickle cell disease—clinical features. Br. J. Hematol. 87: 586–591.

Serjeant, G, Serjeant, B, Stephens, A et al. (1996). Determinants of hemoglobin level in steady-state homozygous sickle cell disease. Br. J. Hematol. 92: 143–149.

Singhal, A, Davies, P, Sahota, A et al. (1993). Resting metabolic rate in homozygous sickle cell disease. Am. J. Clin. Nutr. 57: 32–34.

Singhal, A, Thomas, P, Kearney, T et al. (1995). Acceleration in linear growth after splenectomy for hypersplenism in homozygous sickle cell disease. Arch. Dis. Child. 72: 227–229.

Singhal, A, Wierenga, KJJ, Byford, S et al. (1997). Is there an energy deficiency in homozygous sickle cell disease? Am. J. Clin. Nutr. 66: 386–390.

Steinberg, MH, Rosenstock, W, Coleman, MB et al. (1984). Effects of thalassemia and microcytosis on the hematologic and vaso-occlusive severity of sickle cell anemia. Blood 63: 1353–1360.

Stevens, MCG, Hayes, RJ, Vaidya, S, and Serjeant, GR. (1981). Fetal hemoglobin and clinical severity of homozygous sickle cell disease in early childhood. J. Pediatr. 98: 37–41.

Thomas, PW, Higgs, DR, and Serjeant, GR. (1997). Benign clinical course of homozygous sickle cell disease—a search for predictors. J. Clin. Epidemiol. 50: 121–126.

Topley, JM, Rogers, DW, Stevens, MCG, and Serjeant, GR. (1981). Acute splenic sequestration and hypersplenism in the first five years in homozygous sickle cell disease. Arch. Intern. Med. 56: 765–769.

Trowell, HC, Raper, AB, and Welbourn, HF. (1957). The natural history of homozygous sickle-cell anemia in Central Africa. Q. J. Med. 26: 410–422.

Ware, ME, Hambleton, I, Ochaya, I, and Serjeant, GR. (1999). Day care management of sickle cell painful crises in Jamaica: A model applicable elsewhere? Br. J. Haematol. 104: 93–96.

Watson-Williams, EJ. (1962). Folic acid deficiency in sickle-cell anemia. E. Afr. Med. J. 39: 213–221.

Wright, J, Thomas, P, and Serjeant, GR. (1997). Septicemia caused by salmonella infection; an overlooked complication of sickle cell disease. J. Pediatr. 130: 394–399.

Zago, MA, Figueiredo, MS, and Ogo, SH. (1992). Bantu β^S cluster haplotype predominates among Brazilian Blacks. Am. J. Phys. Anthropol. 88: 295–298.

SECTION VI

DIAGNOSIS AND SPECIAL TREATMENT FOR SICKLE CELL DISEASE AND β THALASSEMIA

MARTIN H. STEINBERG
RONALD L. NAGEL

Several reliable laboratory methods can be used to confirm the diagnosis of sickle cell disease and β thalassemia and to define the genotypes that underlie the phenotype. These include traditional methods—based on the detection of sickle hemoglobin, HbF, and HbA$_2$—and newer DNA-based methods that define the disorder by its genetic abnormality. Often, protein-based and DNA-based diagnostic tests are complementary. Although often perceived as not needed for management of the individual patient, for purposes of genetic counseling or for establishing risk categories, a genotype-based diagnosis is mandatory. With background information from the patient's history, physical examination, blood counts, and erythrocyte indices, protein-based methods such as hemoglobin electrophoresis, isoelectric focusing (IEF), and high-performance liquid chromatography (HPLC) can suggest the genotype of sickle cell disease, and studies of informative members of the patient's family can establish this definitively, obviating the need for DNA-based testing.

As the mutations for β thalassemia are multitudinous, only DNA-based studies can pinpoint the genotype of this disease. An approach to the diagnosis of sickle cell disease and β thalassemia is shown in Figure 1. Protein-based studies have the ability of measuring simultaneously levels of HbA, HbS, HbF, and HbA$_2$. DNA-based tests cannot do this and cur-

rently are less available and more expensive than traditional methods of evaluation such as hemoglobin electrophoresis. DNA-based tests have the advantage that a diagnosis can be established from DNA in any available nucleated cell—even fetal cells in maternal blood can be used—making it possible to do prenatal diagnosis by the expedient method of maternal blood sampling. Trophoblast, amniocytes, or blood provide suitable tissue for examination and DNA diagnosis can be applied antenatally, neonatally, in children, and in adults. High concentrations of HbF and little HbA may confound antenatal and neonatal protein-based diagnostic methods. The incredibly rapid pace of technological advances in molecular biological methods makes it likely that the level of skill required for DNA-based diagnosis, the time involved, and the costs will all fall, making DNA tests more widely practical and available. It is well within our current expectations as the human genome sequencing project nears completion that all genetic diseases will be rapidly and inexpensively ascertainable before or at birth.

Three of the following chapters discuss laboratory methods used for the diagnosis of sickle cell disease and the β thalassemias. They cover methods used for the clinical laboratory evaluation of sickle cell disease and β thalassemia and include hemoglobin electrophoresis, HPLC, IEF, measurement of HbF concentration and F-cells. Differences in the application of these tests for antenatal, neonatal, and adult diagnosis are clarified. Some laboratory methods are used primarily in research on hemoglobinopathies and the thalassemias. We include some of these methods to provide a perspective of the current range of possible diagnostic studies.

Transgenic animal models of thalassemia and sickle cell anemia are becoming useful as new treatments are being evaluated and the complex pathophysiology of these diseases is being unraveled. These models, with their benefits and liabilities, are presented.

Elements of successful establishment and implementation of programs for antenatal diagnosis of the thalassemias and the hemoglobinopathies—beyond the methods of disease detection—are discussed in Chapter 36. Neonatal screening programs directed at disease detection, and population screening aimed at the finding of heterozygous carriers are also covered.

During the past decade—at least in industrialized countries—new, highly specialized treatment for sickle cell disease and the β thalassemias have evolved to reach clinical application. These include

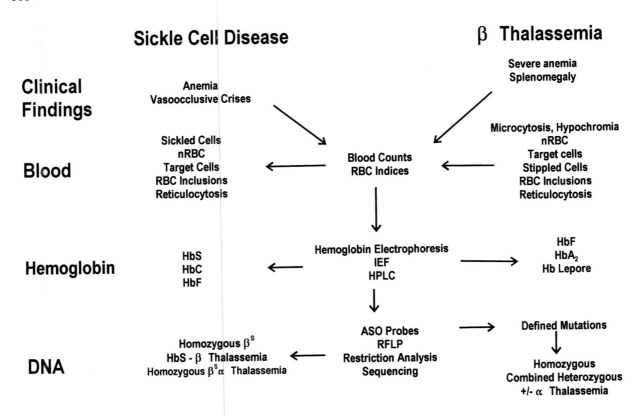

Section VI. Diagnosis of sickle cell disease and β thalasemmia.

the use of myelosuppressive agents, such as hydroxyurea, to perturb the bone marrow and increase HbF levels, bone marrow transplantation, and new approaches to blood transfusion and iron chelation. Included in four chapters on new treatments are details of the use of transfusions for specific indications in sickle cell anemia and for the treatment of the severe β thalassemias. In sickle cell anemia, preoperative, intrapartum, and prophylactic use of transfusions are topics of much recent study while hypertransfusion regimens still form the mainstay of management for β thalassemia.

Transfusions are not innocuous and are complicated by alloimmunization, the transmission of unsuspected viral diseases, and iron overload. Their use has to be parsimonious. The current state-of-the-art of iron chelation therapy is presented with protocols for the use of parenteral chelating agents and a discussion of the current status of oral chelating agents. The issues and the controversy involving the use of L1 as a chelator in thalassemia will also be addressed.

Stem cell transplantation has been used successfully in sickle cell anemia and β thalassemia. Chapters on transplantation should permit the

clinician to know when to refer patients with sickle cell anemia and β thalassemia for transplantation. They include criteria for patient selection, conditioning regimens, complications and their management, and the most recent results of transplantation. Transplantation is a dynamic field and its future includes the use of nonmyeloblastive conditioning regimens, cord blood stem cells, inducing stable mixed chimerism, and new possibilities for immunosuppresion. Bone marrow stem cell transplantation, if successful, provides the sole cure for sickle cell disease and β thalassemia. In sickle cell anemia, the mortality risk is between 5 percent and 15 percent. Children below age 16, with severe complications—stroke, acute chest syndrome, refractory pain—and an HLA-matched donor are presently the best candidates for bone marrow transplantation but few patients meet these requirements. Event-free survival is good but follow-up is still short and the full toxicity of transplantation and the attendant immunosuppressive treatment is unknown.

The propitious consequences of high HbF in sickle cell anemia stimulated studies on the potential of drug treatment to increase HbF in patients with sickle cell anemia and ameliorate their disease. Hydroxyurea has been successfully used for this purpose. A double-blind, placebo-controlled trial of hydroxyurea in adults with several crises yearly showed that hydroxyurea reduced by nearly half the incidence of pain episodes, acute chest syndrome, frequency of hospitalization, and blood transfusion. Hydroxyurea-treated patients had an increase in HbF from a baseline of 5 percent to about 9 percent after 2 years. HbF increased to a mean of 18 percent in the best responders and to 9 percent in the next highest response group but changed little in other patients. Surprisingly, the trial of hydroxyurea raised questions as to the mechanism by which this drug ameliorated the disease. A picture is emerging that HbF elevation is only a part of the story, and that other effects of this cytotoxic agent could be operative.

Studies of hydroxyurea in young children or adolescents—where therapeutic benefits should be greatest—are just beginning, yet to date these trials have reached remarkably similar conclusions. HbF increased from 5 percent before treatment to 16 to 19 percent after 6 months to 1 year of treatment. As in adults, hemolysis and neutrophil counts decreased. Short-term toxicity was minor. Early interruption of the vasoocclusive process in young patients may also prevent damage to the central nervous system, lungs, kidneys, and bones that end in disability or death.

We do not yet know the long-term negative effects of hydroxyurea—is it mutagenic, carcinogenic, or leukemogenic? To date, leukemia or cancer has not occurred in sickle cell anemia patients treated with hydroxyurea but follow-up is still short. In children, we do not know if this drug has adverse effects on growth and development. Even with a small risk, the benefits of this treatment in seriously ill patients may be dominant. We hope—but do not presently know—that hydroxyurea will prevent organ damage, restore function to already injured organs, and reduce mortality. Hydroxyurea appears as effective in HbS-β thalassemia as in sickle cell anemia. In HbSC disease hydroxyurea increased mean corpuscular volume and hemoglobin level and reduced reticulocyte counts, "stress" reticulocytes, and serum bilirubin. Hydroxyurea may affect HbSC disease cells independently of increasing HbF but further studies are needed.

As Dan Quayle aptly put it, making predictions is difficult, especially of the future. As we mentioned in our introduction to the pathophysiology of sickle syndromes, the future probably holds a better understanding of the modifier or epistatic genes that underlie the multiple pleiotropic effects found in these diseases and that are the major basis for interindividual variability of the phenotype. In terms of diagnosis, the counterpart of this future development is the emergence of diagnostic tests for polymorphic modifier genes that will allow, in addition to the genotype diagnosis of the hemoglobinopathy, the determination of the future level of severity and the type of pleiotropic effects more likely to occur in that particular patient. This knowledge will make prenatal diagnosis and the selection of patients for risky procedures more rational. In addition, it might allow us to predict drug response, and make this type of therapeutic indication safer for the patient.

Other areas that will most likely flourish in the near future are gene therapy and the experimental approaches to preventing complications of sickle cell disease and β thalassemia. Two chapters cover these topics. Discussed are the principles of gene therapy, approaches to sickle cell disease and β thalassemia using gene therapy-based methods, and the current problems of gene therapy, foremost among them being how to achieve stable and robust transgene expression.

There is more to sickle cell anemia than polymerization of HbS, and the final chapter in this section discusses membrane active agents, such as clotrimazole and Mg, that may rehydrate the "dry" sickle cell. Other experimental agents may favorably alter hemoglobin-oxygen affinity, interfere with the adhesivity of the sickle cell or the interaction of sickled cells with endothelial cells, or modulate the endothelial cell. These novel treatments offer many new possibilities for interrupting the pathophysiology of sickle cell anemia.

Those interested in hemoglobinopathies should welcome the new millennium as a harbinger of exciting developments.

34

Laboratory Diagnosis of Hemoglobin Disorders, and Animal Models for Their Study

MARY E. FABRY

INTRODUCTION

Normal adult blood contains predominantly HbA_0 ($\alpha_2\beta_2$) and small amounts of HbF ($\alpha_2\gamma_2$) and HbA_2 ($\alpha_2\delta_2$). After they are synthesized, the monomeric globin chains form $\alpha\beta$ dimers that do not dissociate under physiologic conditions (see Chapter 8). In the presence of oxygen, hemoglobin tetramers rapidly dissociate into very low concentrations of $\alpha\beta$ dimers that can then form new tetramers (Park, 1970; Shaeffer et al., 1984). This implies that when more than one α- or β-globin chain is present, the predominant form in the red cell will be the heterotetramer (for example, in red cells with HbS and HbC the dominant species will be $\alpha_2\beta^S\beta^C$) (Fig. 34.1). However, most separation techniques detect only the homotetramer because the migratory properties of the individual dimers are similar to those of the homotetramers (identical $\alpha\beta$ subunits); hence following dissociation of the heterotetramer into dimers, the two dimers will move apart toward the region where the respective homotetramers are found and recombine. This process will continue until all heterotetramers have dissociated. Heterotetramers can be detected by conventional separation techniques if oxygen is rigorously excluded, because exchange is greatly slowed in deoxyhemoglobin (Park, 1970).

Characterization of mutant hemoglobins and thalassemias described throughout this book takes place in a number of contexts: very large newborn screening laboratories that need to positively identify the most common mutants; general adult hematology laboratories; and smaller research settings that may deal with less common human mutant globins or even hemoglobins of transgenic mice. Approaches that are necessary in one setting may not be practical in other settings.

DETECTION AND QUANTITATION OF MUTANT HEMOGLOBINS

Laboratory Safety

Safety of personnel working in hematology laboratories is a major consideration. The primary risks are hepatitis and human immunodeficiency virus (HIV), and although most personnel are aware of and concerned about the dangers of HIV, the most probable and potentially serious risk is still hepatitis because of its highly transmissible nature. Any human sample, regardless of origin, should be regarded as a potential source of infection. The first line of defense is care in sample handling: avoiding aerosol formation; wearing gloves; and observing precautions to avoid transferring material from gloves to other surfaces that may be touched by exposed skin. Strict separation of sample handling areas and areas where food may be consumed is critical. Periodic lectures on the dangers of blood-borne pathogens and immunization against hepatitis B are required of all personnel involved in handling human samples. For more detailed discussion of laboratory safety, see the Occupational Safety and Health Agency (OSHA) site on the Internet at www.osha.gov.

Sample Preservation and Preparation

Any analytical technique is only as good as the starting material. Starting samples vary widely in the techniques described below and include recovery of hemoglobin from dried filter paper blots obtained from infants for screening. However, the usual sample arrives as anticoagulated whole blood that should be refrigerated and processed within 24 to 48 hours. In this time range hemoglobin is best stored as red cells in plasma because the red cell contains the enzyme methemoglobin reductase, which will convert any methemoglobin formed to deoxyhemoglobin. Plasma contains glucose and albumin, which stabilize the red cell and its membrane and ensure that enzyme activity will be maintained. Longer periods of storage are possible, but over time methemoglobin will be generated and there is a possibility of selective loss of less stable mutant hemoglobins.

Martin H. Steinberg, Bernard G. Forget, Douglas R. Higgs, and Ronald L. Nagel, editors. *Disorders of Hemoglobin: Genetics, Pathophysiology, and Clinical Management.* © 2001 Cambridge University Press. All rights reserved.

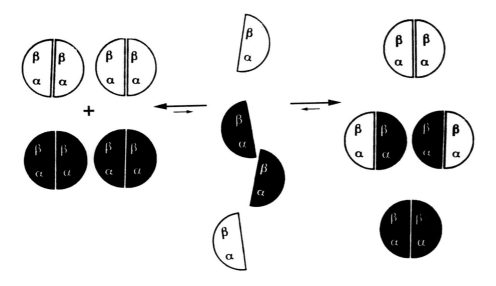

Figure 34.1. Hemoglobin is a tetramer made up of two $\alpha\beta$ dimers that do not dissociate under physiologic conditions. However, the tetramers rapidly dissociate and re-associate, generating very low concentrations of dimers under physiologic conditions. Mixing two hemoglobins, represented by black and white, rapidly leads to an equilibrium mixture in which the original homotetramers and the heterotetramer exist in a ratio of 1:2:1.

Hemoglobin for analysis is usually prepared by hypotonic lysis with shaking. The media for hypotonic lysis may include a detergent to facilitate rupture of the red cell membrane, and the membranes may be further disrupted by the addition of toluene or a similar organic solvent. Care must be taken that all cells undergo lysis. These precautions are particularly important for samples, such as those from sickle cell disease patients, where the red cells are heterogeneous in their properties and some cells—which may have a different hemoglobin composition (see Chapter 10)—may be particularly resistant to lysis. Long-term storage of hemoglobin samples requires first washing the cells in isotonic saline to remove plasma proteins, after which the cells are stored immersed in liquid nitrogen (the gas phase is not cold enough) or stored in a freezer at a temperature of $-135°C$ or less. Hemoglobin stored at higher temperatures gradually loses heme and becomes insoluble.

Electrophoresis

Proteins are composed of amino acids that bear side chains that may be capable of ionizing; the C-terminal COOH and the N-terminal NH$_2$ are also capable of ionization. The side chains of aliphatic amino acids, such as alanine, glycine, valine, and isoleucine, do not ionize. The pH at which a side chain is half-ionized is its pK, which may be altered by the structure of the protein. Proteins are amphoteric; that is, they bear both positively or negatively charged side chains. The net charge of a protein will depend on the pH of the solution and the pKs of its amino acids. Because proteins are charged molecules, they will migrate in an electric field and the relative speed and direction will depend on the sign and magnitude of the net charge.

At pH 8.6, all human hemoglobins will have a net negative charge and will migrate in an electric field toward the positive pole or anode. Separation of hemoglobins by electrophoresis is based on the relative charge of the $\alpha\beta$ dimer and hence mutations that do not alter the charge may be "silent" and not detectable by electrophoresis. However, interaction with the matrix (such as cellulose acetate or agar) may also affect the rate of migration. Most electrophoretic methods separate hemoglobin tetramers, but only tetramers composed of two identical $\alpha\beta$ dimers, or homotetramers, are seen at the end of the separation process.

Because different hemoglobins may migrate similarly under a given set of conditions, electrophoresis is usually performed at two different pHs and on two different supporting mediums. The usual choice is cellulose acetate electrophoresis at pH 8.4 and citrate agar electrophoresis at pH 6.0 (Dacie and Lewis, 1995). On citrate agar, in addition to the net charge, there is some selective interaction with the substrate, which further aids in resolution of hemoglobins with similar electrophoretic properties. This is based on the interaction of the central cavity of the hemoglobin with agaropectin in agar (Winter and Yodh, 1983). Some commercial kits for agar electrophoresis substitute maleic acid for citrate, which results in altered migration for some hemoglobins. Charts accompanying these kits should be used to assess which hemoglobins are present. In all cases, a set of reference hemoglobins, usually HbsA, A$_2$, F, S, and C should be included with each run. It is useful to mix these known standards with the test sample when the presence of mutants with electrophoretic properties similar to normal and common variants is suspected. Electrophoresis can also be carried out on separated globin chains if denaturing conditions are used (Ueda and Schneider, 1969; Schneider, 1974). In these cases urea is added to the electrophoresis buffer and the diluent in which the hemoglobin is dissolved. Another approach that sometimes allows separation of overlapping hemoglobins, one of which contains cysteine, is treatment of the sample with cystamine (Whitney, 1978). This simplifies analysis for samples with multiple α- and β-globin chains; however, at this point it is reasonable to turn to a higher resolution technique such as isoelectric focusing, high-performance liquid chromatography (HPLC), or mass spectroscopy.

Method. Most laboratories use commercially prepared kits that contain the hemolyzing agent, buffers, support media (cellulose acetate or agar), a means for applying multiple samples, and a stain. The sample is hemolyzed and applied to the cathodic or negative side. Sample left at the point of application usually indicates poorly hemolyzed sample or an unstable hemoglobin. Samples may be stained with protein or hemoglobin specific stains (based on peroxidase activity), or the color of the hemoglobin itself can be used for visualization.

Advantages and Limitations. Both equipment and reagents are relatively inexpensive and multiple samples can be placed on a single support or gel. These properties made electrophoresis one of the earliest methods of screening and it is still useful for quick screening of small numbers of human samples. However, the sample bands are relatively wide, and many abnormal hemoglobins overlap (for example, on cellulose acetate, HbS overlaps with HbD and HbG, and HbA$_2$ overlaps with HbsC, E, and O); however, citrate agar electrophoresis will separate HbC from HbE. Inquiry about the patient's ethnic background is also useful. For example, HbC originated in Africa, whereas HbE originated in Southeast Asia, facts that may point to one of these variants. Quantitation by densitometry is possible and widely used but is somewhat inaccurate at low percent (<5 percent) of abnormal hemoglobins; hence other techniques are used to detect low levels of HbF or HbA$_2$ (see below). Migration and resolution on citrate agar are strongly dependent on the concentration of the material applied. Finally, these methods are not suitable for automated application of samples or automated analysis of results. An example of hemoglobin electrophoresis in some sickle hemoglobinopathies is shown in Figure 24.3.

Isoelectric Focusing

Historically, isoelectric focusing (IEF) was developed as a preparative technique and was performed in fluid-filled columns with baffles to stabilize compartments with different pHs (Rilbe, 1995). Subsequently, gel-filled tubes and thin acrylic flatbed systems were used for high-resolution separations and thick flatbed systems were used for preparative separations. More recently, IEF has been adapted to capillary technology, which allows separation of very small samples and automation of sampling.

IEF is capable of much higher resolution than the electrophoretic techniques described above. If a molecule has two or more ionizable groups, at least one of which has a pK in the acidic range and another in the basic range, then there will be a pH at which the net charge is zero. Proteins and amino acids all have a pH at which the net charge is zero, which is called the isoelectric point or pI. At this pH there is no net movement in the presence of an externally applied electric field. In order to separate proteins based on their isoelectric points, a stable pH gradient needs to be created. This is achieved by applying a set of ampholites with pIs that cover the range of pIs of the proteins that are to be separated on a support matrix. During the initial period after the current is applied, both the ampholites and the proteins to be separated move as the pH gradient is formed. If a protein molecule finds itself on the acidic side of its isoelectric point it will migrate to the cathode, and if it finds itself on the basic side of its isoelectric point it will migrate toward the anode (hence the term isoelectric focusing). Sharp bands of individual proteins are thus formed. If focusing is continued, the pH gradient is eventually degraded and the protein bands begin to spread. A major factor that degrades the pH gradient is the effect of heat; therefore, efficient cooling is a crucial aspect of all IEF systems. With optimization, methods using free ampholites can resolve two proteins with a pI difference of about 0.01 pH unit (Righetti et al., 1983) (Fig. 34.2). Even higher resolution can be attained if the ampholites are covalently bound to the matrix and the pH gradient is preformed by casting the gel with a two-vessel gradient mixer, thus preforming a stable pH gradient before the protein is applied. This type of gel is capable of resolution of proteins with pIs differing by about 0.001 pH units and has been described by Righetti and co-workers, who have written comprehensive reviews on the subject (Righetti et al., 1996; Righetti and Bossi, 1997).

A recent development is adaptation of IEF to capillary electrophoresis instrumentation. This technology is currently undergoing rapid evolution and standard-

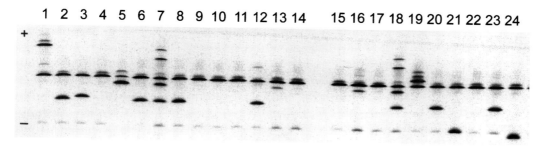

Figure 34.2. Separation of various mutant hemoglobins by isoelectric focusing. A precast agarose gel (Resolve Systems, Wallac Inc., Akron, OH) was used at 75 mA, 1,200 V, 14°C, for 90 minutes. Present on the gel are: lane 1, HbA-HbN Baltimore; lanes 2, 6, 8, 12, 20, 23, sickle cell trait; lane 3 HbA-HbD Punjab; lane 5 normal newborn; lanes 7, 18 controls (HbA₂, HbF, HbS, HbF, HbA, HbJ Baltimore, HbI Texas); lane 16 β-thalassemia trait; lane 19 HbA-Hb Hope; lane 21 HbE trait; lane 24 HbC trait. (Gel contributed by H. Wajcman, Director of Reseach INSERM, Hopital Henri Mondor, Paris, France.)

ized systems are not yet available; however, the combination of the high resolution attainable with IEF, the potential for automation, and the ability to utilize extremely small samples promises that this will be an important technique in the future. Capillary electrophoresis combined with mass spectrometry has been applied to analysis of proteins present in single cells (Hofstadler et al., 1995; Cao and Moini, 1999). A wide variety of detection systems have been used, including conventional UV/visible detection similar to that used by HPLC instruments (Mario et al., 1997), absorption imaging (Wu and Pawliszyn, 1995), and mass spectroscopy (Banks, 1997).

Advantages and Limitations. IEF uses somewhat more expensive materials than conventional electrophoresis, but resolution is much higher. Heating and distortion due to contamination of the sample or the gel with the anodic or cathodic buffer solutions are common sources of error. The most commonly used IEF technique is application of multiple samples to a commercially prepared thin layer gel, which precludes automated technology. However, the development of capillary IEF has opened the way for its use in automated systems; this technology is undergoing rapid development and may become as important in automated systems as HPLC. Tables of isoelectric points of abnormal hemoglobins are available (Basset et al., 1982).

HPLC

The techniques described so far depend primarily on the ionization (pKs) of the amino acid side chains of intact hemoglobin molecules and their migration in an electric field. In HPLC, ionic and hydrophobic interactions of the sample with the supporting matrix are the basis of separation. The sample is applied as a thin layer to the top of the column under conditions wherein it interacts strongly with the matrix. The proteins are then eluted with a developing solution (buffer) of gradually increasing strength, until all of the proteins are eluted. In cation and anion exchange chromatography, the properties of the developing solution that are varied are pH and ionic strength (salt concentration) and in reverse phase chromatography, the hydrophobicity (organic solvent) content is also varied. Hemoglobin may be separated as the intact tetramer or, under denaturing conditions, the individual globin chains can be separated. Human hemoglobins usually have a relatively small number of possible homotetramers and analysis of the intact tetramer generally yields readily interpretable results.

Dedicated clinical systems based on HPLC separation of tetrameric hemoglobin with very rapid automated sampling are available that allow preprogrammed detection of hemoglobin variants (Mario et al., 1997). Hemoglobin from transgenic mice—because of the possible formation of human-mouse chimeric αβ dimers and hence a wide variety of homotetramers—and less common human variants yield a more readily interpretable chromatogram when denaturing conditions are used and the isolated α and β chains are detected (Fig. 34.3). The usual HPLC setup consists of columns, reservoirs, highly accurate mixing pumps, and a UV/visible detector. In most systems the pumps and the detector are computer controlled and the area under each detectable peak is automatically calculated. Very small internal diameters increase column resolution and decrease the amount of sample required at the cost of increased time per sample (Huisman, 1987).

Advantages and Limitations. Under the appropriate conditions HPLC readily separates proteins that cannot be resolved by other means. However, resolution may depend on the characteristics of commercially supplied columns and may require adjustment of the developing buffer to cope with variation in the quality

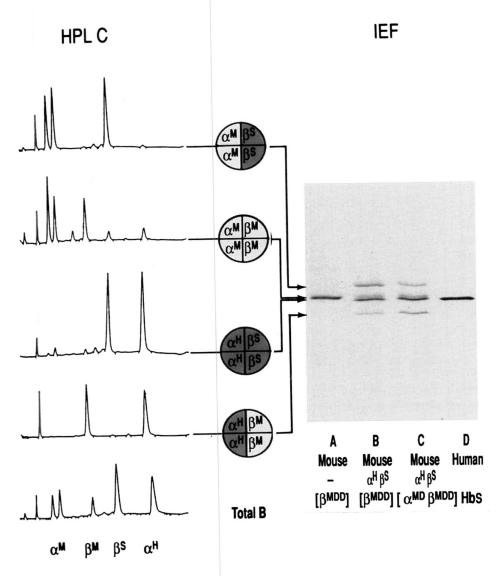

Figure 34.3. Isoelectric focusing (IEF) and HPLC of hemoglobins from several transgenic mice expressing human HbS and mouse globins (Fabry et al., 1992a). The bands representing homotetramers composed of dimers of mouse α and human β^S chains, mouse α and mouse β chains, human α and human β^S chains, and human α and mouse β chains were separated by isoelectric focusing, isolated from the gel, and separated by denaturing HPLC to allow identification of the tetramers present in the isoelectric focusing gel. (From Fabry et al., 1992, with permission.) For full color reproduction, see color plate 34.3.

of the available columns. The equipment used for HPLC is much more expensive, sophisticated, and difficult to maintain than that used for electrophoresis or IEF, but is still well within the reach of individual research laboratories. HPLC screening techniques have been developed in which individual samples can be run in approximately 3 minutes with very high reproducibility (Mario et al., 1997).

Mass Spectroscopy

Modern mass spectroscopy can start with a hemolysate and return the molecular weights of individual globin chains to within ± one atomic mass unit (amu). This level of accuracy allows detection of posttranslational modification and verification of mutant and recombinant hemoglobins and, in contrast to electrophoretic techniques, mass spectroscopy can separate similarly charged samples. Individual bands or peaks from IEF or HPLC can also serve as the starting sample. Sample requirements are very small—a few picomoles of protein. Hemoglobin is an ideal molecule for mass spectroscopy since it has a favorable size, an adequate number of protonation sites, distinct mass differences between mutants, and few posttranslational modifications (Shackleton and Witkowska, 1996).

Mass spectroscopy is based on the principle that charged particles moving through a magnetic field will undergo deflection proportional to the charge to mass ratio. Particles with the smallest charge to mass ratio are the least affected. The sample is first converted to gaseous ions and an accelerating voltage is applied. The particles are focused through a slit into a highly evacuated area, where they are subject to the magnetic field that causes them to separate. The defining advances that allowed mass spectroscopy of biological samples were those that allowed ionization of single, intact, underivatized proteins and biopolymers. The most important methods of ionization are electrospray ionization (ESI), which was discovered by Dole in 1968 (Dole et al., 1968) and re-introduced by Yamashita and Fenn in 1984 (Yamashita and Fenn, 1984), and matrix-assisted laser desorption (MALDI). ESI is most suitable for intact globin chain analysis and MALDI is the method of choice for peptide identification. ESI allows mass spectrometers to be interfaced with HPLC and capillary IEF focusing devices, which frequently allows immediate positive identification of the separated species and is also useful for identification of small peaks that may represent derivatives or degradation products.

More recently, mass spectroscopy has been used for complete sequencing of proteins based on identification of fragments. This approach is particularly useful for hemoglobins since sequence homology allows good working approximations to be formulated even for hemoglobins from rare or unusual species. Fragments can be produced classically by proteolytic digestion and then exposed to MALDI mass spectroscopy. The abnormal fragments can be identified, and in many cases, the mutation deduced. With a few exceptions, whole blood hemolysates can be subjected to digestion without further separation. Separation is necessary when the variant is present at a low level, a mass difference of 1 d is suspected, or high levels of HbF are present. In these cases the sample can be purified by IEF or HPLC prior to digestion (Witkowska et al., 1991). Alternatively, the protein can be fragmented in the spectrometer itself without resorting to wet chemistry and the fragments produced in the spectrometer can be used to identify the portion bearing the mutant amino acid (Ferranti et al., 1993; Light-Wahl et al., 1993; Bakhtiar et al., 1994).

An interesting application of mass spectroscopy to a hemoglobin variant was the detection of Hb Quebec-Chori, an electrophoretically silent substitution that migrates in IEF at the position of HbA, but, in combination with HbS, results in a severe form of sickle trait (Fig. 34.4) (see Chapter 29). Mass spectrometry combined with capillary electrophoresis has been applied to analysis of proteins present in single or small numbers of red cells (Hofstadler et al., 1995; Cao and Moini, 1999).

Advantages and Limitations. The most commonly used techniques for separating and, in many cases, identifying hemoglobin mutants, HPLC and IEF, rely on relative position on a gel or column that is nonspecific. Mass spectroscopy provides a means of positive identification that is particularly important for minor components and unusual mutants. A major limitation is access to instrumentation, which can usually be found in dedicated service divisions of major research institutions or at commercial enterprises. Mass spectroscopy is most useful when it is necessary to verify a proposed hemoglobin variant or decide between a small number of possible choices. However, given a molecular weight for an abnormal α or β chain and the list of known mutants, it is possible to deduce candidates. Although accuracy of a single mass unit is readily attainable, the effective resolution of most nonresearch grade mass spectrometers is of the order of 8 to 10 mass units. Therefore, mixtures with closely matched masses may require a combination of techniques for resolution.

HbF

HbF (see Chapter 10) is the dominant hemoglobin during the last two trimesters of gestation and immediately after birth. In adult blood the normal level of HbF is less than 2 percent; however, it is elevated in hemolytic anemia, some malignancies, and hereditary persistence of fetal hemoglobin (HPFH). It interferes with polymerization of HbS due to exclusion of both HbF and the heterotetramer $(\alpha_2\gamma\beta^S)$ from the polymer. An interesting feature of HbF is that it is unevenly distributed among red cells. Cells with high levels of HbF are called F-cells and, in sickle cell disease, are seldom found in the most dense (highest mean cell hemoglobin concentration [MCHC]), irreversibly sickled cell (ISC)-rich fractions. This implies that, when either HbF or F-cells are measured, care must be taken to avoid biasing the sample; careful mixing into the suspension of any cells that have settled at the bottom of the tube is sufficient. Several methods may be used for quantitation of HbF, including alkaline denaturation, electrophoresis, or IEF followed by densitometry, disposable minicolumns, and HPLC.

HbF is more resistant to denaturation by alkaline conditions than is HbA. In the alkaline denaturation method, potassium hydroxide is added to a known concentration of hemoglobin and, after a predetermined time interval, the reaction is stopped by adding a known volume of ammonium sulfate, which lowers the pH and precipitates the denatured hemoglobin that is removed by filtration. The concentration of hemoglobin remaining in solution is then determined.

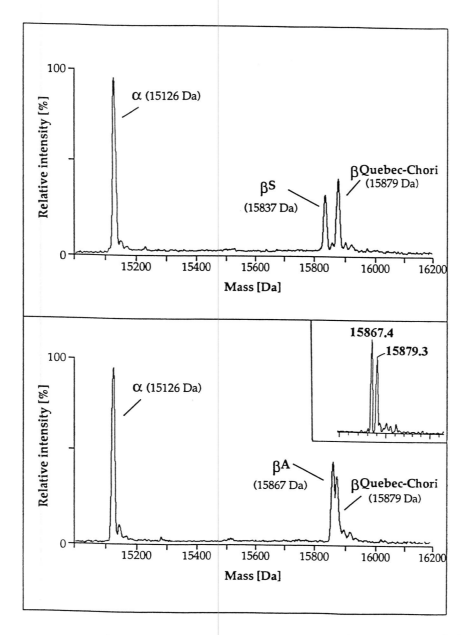

Figure 34.4. Transformed electrospray mass spectra of globins from a child (top panel) who presented with sickle cell–like symptoms and a sickle cell trait pattern on isoelectric focusing and from the child's mother (bottom panel) whose isoelectric focusing pattern indicated the presence of HbA only. The inset in the bottom panel shows the β-globin range of the spectrum that was deconvoluted to the zero charge state utilizing a high-resolution maximum entropy algorithm (Ferrige et al., 1992), which shows a difference of 12 mass units from HbA. The new hemoglobin was named Hb Quebec-Chori and was found to have a mutation at the β87 position (Thr→Ile) (see Chapter 28). In this case, although isoelectric focusing failed to resolve the mutant hemoglobin from HbA, HPLC clearly indicated the presence of a second hemoglobin. (Spectrum provided by E. Witkowska, Children's Hospital of Oakland Research Institute, Oakland, California.)

Two versions of the alkaline denaturation protocol exist: that of Betke et al (Betke et al., 1959), which is reliable for HbF less than 10 percent to 15 percent and thereafter systematically underestimates the percentage, and that of Jonxis and Visser (Jonxis and Visser, 1956), which is only accurate when HbF is greater than 10 percent. Commercially prepared kits are available for alkaline denaturation. HPLC also allows accurate quantitation of HbF and for large-scale screening there are dedicated screening systems that are capable of identifying and quantitating HbF (Papassotiriou et al., 1998; Prehu et al., 1998). Electrophoresis or IEF followed by densitometry are less reliable than HPLC. For detection of very low levels of HbF radioimmunoassay (RIA) (Garver et al.,

1976; Rutland et al., 1983) and enzyme-linked immunoassay (ELISA) (Moscoso et al., 1989; Epstein et al., 1996) are alternative techniques suitable for screening large numbers of samples.

Advantages and Limitations. The materials for alkaline denaturation are inexpensive, but the technique is labor intensive. The most commonly used method for alkaline denaturation systematically underestimates HbF in samples with high levels, such as cord blood, and an alternative method has been developed to deal with this limitation (Jonxis and Visser, 1956). HPLC is accurate for samples with levels of HbF down to about 0.5 percent and has no upper limit of detection, but requires access to the appropriate equipment. Some hemoglobin components that are present at low concentrations elute in the position of HbF under some HPLC conditions, but a recent work describes the use of potassium hydrogen phthalate buffer for hemolysis, which eliminates the reversibly glycated hemoglobins, outlines the need to consider acetylated HbF (which may be as high as 8 percent to 15 percent), and lists some possible variants that may overlap with HbF in the commercial HPLC systems (Prehu et al., 1998).

Since HbF is almost always unevenly distributed among erythrocytes—an exception is some types of hereditary persistence of HbF—immunologic techniques that allow the determination of F-cells are also useful and can provide a reasonable surrogate for whole blood HbF levels (Steinberg et al., 1997). However, see Thein and Craig (1998) for variation in the ratio of HbF/F-cell level in adults due to heterocellular HPFH.

HbA$_2$

Electrophoresis on polyacrylamide gels or cellulose acetate membranes widely separates HbA$_2$ from HbA and HbF, enabling accurate measurement of this minor hemoglobin component. Acid agar gel electrophoresis does not resolve HbA$_2$ from HbA. The low level of HbA$_2$ in erythrocytes, and its narrow range, cause methods of measurement that are facile from the standpoint of the clinical laboratory, such as densitometric tracings of electropherograms, to be inaccurate (Steinberg and Adams, 1991). For acceptable accuracy, the HbA$_2$ fraction must be eluted from electrophoresis gels and the eluate measured spectrophotometrically (Anonymous, 1978).

Refrigeration and freezing may reduce the HbA$_2$ percentage in stored hemolysates. The differential elution of HbA$_2$ in minicolumns is reliable, rapid, and inexpensive (Steinberg and Adams, 1991).

HbA$_2$ cannot be separated from hemoglobin variants with similar positive charges—such as HbC and HbE—by electrophoresis and many column-chromatographic methods. In the company of abnormal globins that contain only a single additional positive charge, such as the sickle β-globin chain, the HbA$_2$ level has been reported to be higher than normal (Craver et al., 1997). Good laboratory technique and the choice of appropriate separation methods can circumvent this overestimation of HbA$_2$ and permit the use of electrophoresis and some methods of chromatography to measure HbA$_2$ in the presence of HbS (Steinberg and Adams, 1991).

HPLC can separate HbA$_2$ from other hemoglobins and the δ-globin chain of HbA$_2$ from α-, β-, and γ-globin chains. Cation exchange columns afford excellent resolution of HbA$_2$ from HbS and HbC (Wilson, 1989) but the expense of the method and the time it takes detract from its usefulness. The quantification of non-α-globin chains with a Vydac C$_4$ column provides a useful surrogate for the measurement of intact hemoglobins and contributes an effective way of assessing HbA$_2$ in the presence of HbC or HbE (Shelton and Schroeder, 1984; Schroeder et al., 1986).

In the presence of HbS, the level of HbA$_2$ measured by cation-exchange HPLC may be falsely elevated, probably due to the co-elution of HbS adducts (Such et al., 1996). In the absence of HbS, HbA$_2$ concentrations determined by HPLC and microcolumn chromatography are similar.

HbA$_2$ may be measured immunologically (Garver et al., 1976, 1984). This technique has the virtue of specificity. The levels obtained correlate well with the more traditional methods of measurement.

Capillary IEF has been used to measure HbA$_2$ in normal subjects and in those with β-thalassemia trait, sickle cell trait, and sickle cell anemia (Craver et al., 1997; Jenkins et al., 1997). Accurate measurements are possible, although in one study HbA$_2$ levels in sickle cell trait and sickle cell anemia were slightly elevated (2.8 ± 1.0 and 2.9 ± 0.9 percent) compared to normals (2.4 ± 0.9 percent) but clearly separated from β-thalassemia trait (4.3 percent to 7.3 percent) (Craver et al., 1997).

Glycosylated forms of HbA$_2$, analogous to the minor components of HbA are present and can be quantified by HPLC and IEF (Tegos and Beutler, 1980). Like HbA$_{1c}$, these glycohemoglobins are elevated in poorly controlled diabetics (see Chapter 10).

HEMOGLOBIN PROPERTIES

p^{50} and Other Measurements of Oxygen Saturation

The partial pressure at which hemoglobin is half-saturated with oxygen, or p^{50}, is an important property of hemoglobin in solution and in the red cell. The p^{50} is extremely sensitive to the presence of 2,3-bisphosphoglycerate (2,3-BPG), inorganic phosphate or other phosphates, pH (Bohr effect), CO_2, anions, and, in the case of HbS, polymer formation. The p^{50} of dilute solutions of HbA and HbS are equal. In the red cell and in plasma, HbA has a p^{50} of 25 ± 2 mm Hg when equilibrated with gases containing 5 percent CO_2. The increase in p^{50} (or decrease in oxygen affinity) is primarily due to the effect of 2,3-BPG on the oxygen affinity of hemoglobin. However, if blood is inadvertently equilibrated with gases lacking CO_2 the pH increases as CO_2 is lost and the apparent p^{50} can reach values of greater than 50 mm Hg. The p^{50} of HbS in the red cell is higher, ranging from 25 to 45 mm Hg. Benesch et al. (1978) showed that the polymerization of HbS increases p^{50} in proportion to the amount of polymer formed because polymer has a lower p^{50}. In blood with HbA, the association curve (Hb $\rightarrow$ HbO$_2$) is identical to the dissociation curve (HbO$_2$ $\rightarrow$ Hb); there is no hysteresis. However, the p^{50} in blood samples with HbS depends on whether equilibrium with polymer has been reached, that is, whether polymer formation or polymer melting is complete before the next level of oxygenation is tested. Eaton and Hofrichter (1990) found that the delay time for polymer formation is dependent to the 30th power on the deoxyhemoglobin concentration. These properties are described in greater detail in Chapters 9 and 23. In the absence of equilibrium there is hysteresis and the p^{50} for the association and dissociation curves will differ. Changing the PO$_2$ at a slower rate will bring the two curves closer together.

The most common measurements of p^{50} are based on measurement of oxygen association curves. Two parameters are simultaneously measured: the partial pressure of oxygen (PO$_2$), which is continuously varied, and the percentage hemoglobin, which is saturated with oxygen. In these measurements, the hemoglobin is first fully deoxygenated and then oxygen is gradually reintroduced while the PO$_2$ is measured with an oxygen electrode. At the same time hemoglobin saturation with oxygen is measured optically. Most current systems employ a dual wavelength (or multiple wavelength) method to measure the percentage of oxyhemoglobin. A single p^{50} determination typically takes about 30 minutes. The Aminco Hemoscan, which is no longer manufactured, equilibrated hemoglobin or whole blood samples between layers of gas-permeable membranes; this had the advantage of allowing measurement of whole blood in the original plasma. The Hemox-Analyzer by TCS Medical Products uses 30 to 50 μL of blood or an equivalent concentration of hemoglobin suspended in

4 mL of solution with an antifoaming agent. Gases are bubbled through the stirred solution or red cell suspension and the percentage oxyhemoglobin is measured with a dual wavelength spectrophotometer at 560 nm, which is sensitive to the transition between deoxyhemoglobin and oxyhemoglobin, and at 570 nm, an isobestic point at which the absorption is sensitive to the hemoglobin concentration, but insensitive to the oxygenation state. Dual wavelength systems cannot discriminate between oxyHb and several other forms of hemoglobin such as CO, NO, metHb, or sulfHb, which may lead to systematic errors (see Chapter 46).

Blood gas analyzers measure the pH, PO$_2$, and PCO$_2$ for samples of whole blood and then calculate hemoglobin saturation with oxygen and a number of other parameters based on the normal p^{50}. This will systematically overestimate the percentage of oxyhemoglobin present in the blood of sickle cell disease patients and any other hemoglobinopathies that result in elevated p^{50}. Similarly, a low p^{50} such as is found for HbF will result in systematic underestimation of the percentage of oxyhemoglobin. The presence of met- and carbonmonoxy hemoglobin are not accounted for in these measurements.

Arterial hemoglobin saturation with oxygen can be measured in vivo by use of a pulse oximeter. The pulse oximeter estimates arterial hemoglobin saturation by measuring the light absorbance of pulsating vascular tissue at two wavelengths. The relationship between measured light absorbance and saturation was developed empirically and is built into the oximeter software. The presence of methemoglobin and carbonmonoxy hemoglobin (CO-Hb) will lead to systematic overestimation of oxygen saturation by pulse oximetry.

Instrumentation Laboratories makes a CO-Oximeter that uses multiple wavelengths to measure the hemoglobin concentration, percentage oxyhemoglobin, hemoglobin, percentage methemoglobin, and percentage carbonmonoxy hemoglobin that can be used in conjunction with blood gas analyzers to give a more accurate, but still incomplete, picture of hemoglobin saturation.

It is also necessary to measure 2,3-BPG content of the red cell in order to evaluate the significance of p^{50} measurements because altered p^{50} may be the result of a hemoglobin abnormality or altered 2,3-BPG content.

Limitations and Methods. If a hemoglobin with a p^{50} different from that of HbA is present (such as HbS or HbF), the hemoglobin saturation cannot be obtained from a blood gas analyzer, which uses the p^{50} of HbA to calculate hemoglobin saturation from the measured oxygen partial pressure. 2,3-BPG is usually assayed by use of a commercially available kit.

DETECTION AND ESTIMATION OF POLYMER FORMATION IN RED CELLS AND SOLUTIONS CONTAINING HbS

Solubility

The insolubility of deoxyhemoglobin S in high phosphate solutions is the basis of a fast, nonquantitative test that when combined with the results of cellulose acetate electrophoresis results in a positive identification of HbS. The reagents are commercially available in kit form or can be prepared as described by Dacie and Lewis (1995). Twenty μL whole blood is added to 2 mL high phosphate buffer (2.3 M) with saponin and sodium dithionite and allowed to stand at room temperature for 5 minutes. Homozygous HbA and HbS blood should always be included as positive controls. A clear sample indicates the absence of HbS and a turbid sample indicates the presence of HbS. The sample can then be centrifuged and observed again; if the solution under the precipitate is clear and colorless then the sample is from a patient who may be homozygous for HbS; precipitate and pale solution indicates the presence of a large percentage of another hemoglobin as is found in sickle cell trait, HbSC disease, or even HbS with a high percentage of HbF. Dithionite solutions are subject to oxidation, and failure of the HbS positive control to yield a clear solution indicates the need to prepare a new solution or to obtain a fresh stock of sodium dithionite. Solid sodium dithionite should be divided into small aliquots in screwcap vials and stored in a desiccator to avoid water uptake and subsequent oxidation.

Solubility tests should never be used in place of a DNA-based diagnosis of sickle cell disease, the ideal for patient counseling and management or even hemoglobin electrophoresis, IEF, or HPLC. Conducted correctly, they can identify the presence of a sickling hemoglobin (see Chapter 28) and this may be important clinically when all that needs to be known is if this type of hemoglobin is present (see Chapters 24 and 29).

C_{SAT}

The solubility of a substance is the concentration of that substance in equilibrium with a condensed phase that may be crystalline, polymer, or particulate. In the case of HbS, the solubility is important because it allows estimation of the percentage of the HbS content of the red cell that will be converted to polymer under fully deoxygenated conditions. The concentration of deoxyhemoglobin S in equilibrium with the polymer phase (C_{SAT}) is useful for characterizing sickle hemoglobins that contain a second mutation and for characterizing mixtures of HbS with other hemoglobins.

There are two major methods in use at the present time. One employs quasiphysiologic conditions and the other relies on high phosphate to precipitate sickle hemoglobins. Formation of protein crystals and polymers is extremely sensitive to the nature and concentration of the counter ions present. Either the crystal structure itself or the rate of nucleation can be affected. In the low phosphate method, the hemoglobin is concentrated versus 0.1 M potassium phosphate buffer (pH 7.35) at 25° C and then deoxygenated on ice, first by alternating vacuum and nitrogen, and then by adding enough sodium dithionite solution to give a final concentration equal to three times the heme concentration. The samples are transferred anaerobically to C_{SAT} tubes filled with paraffin oil, incubated at 25°C overnight in a nitrogen atmosphere, and centrifuged for 2 hours at 35,000 rpm at 25°C with purified HbS used as a control. The supernatants are removed anaerobically and concentrations and deoxy pHs are determined; solubility is expressed in g/dL of HbS in equilibrium with the polymer.

An alternative method is based on the turbidity of a microparticulate suspension that is formed when HbS is introduced into a solution at pH 7.0 and 27°C with a high (2.48 to 2.86 M) phosphate concentration that has been deoxygenated with dithionite (Adachi and Asakura, 1979b). Water is then added until the turbidity clears. Relative solubilities can be expressed in terms of the phosphate concentration 50 percent of the way to a completely clear solution. Alternatively, relative solubilities at a constant phosphate concentration can be given in g/dL after the suspension has been centrifuged; it should be emphasized, however, that because of decreased solubility, only the relative values are physiologically meaningful.

Recently another approach has been proposed that uses 50 mM phosphate in the presence of 70 kd dextran to decrease polymer solubility (Bookchin et al., 1999). The polymer fibers formed were electron microscopically indistinguishable from those formed in the absence of dextran. Since solubility is determined by the residues in the contact area between the tetramers, this method offers a great advantage over the high phosphate method, in which the insoluble phase does not have a fiber structure.

Advantages and Limitations. The low phosphate method requires relatively large sample size, access to an ultracentrifuge, and is technologically demanding; however, conditions closer to those found in the red cell govern polymer formation, and solubilities can be compared to those found in the red cell. The high phosphate method uses much smaller samples and is technologically less demanding; however, because of the sensitivity of microparticulate formation to the type and concentration of counter ions present, high phosphate may result in relative solubilities that do not reflect those found in the red cell. Indeed, it was noted in the original article describing the high phosphate method that the pH dependence of solubility is opposite to that found in the minimum gelling concentration method (Adachi and Asakura, 1979a).

CHARACTERIZING THE RED CELL

Complete Blood Count (CBC)

Manual Measurement. Although red cell indices are determined by automated methods in most laboratories, manual methods are still used for small numbers of samples and for some hemoglobinopathies. The ratio of hemoglobin to hematocrit (PCV) can be used to calculate an MCHC that may be more reliable than that determined by automated measurements. The most accurate way to measure hemoglobin concentration is by the cyanmethemoglobin method, which is insensitive to oxygenation and pH. Hemoglobin is oxidized to methemoglobin by ferricyanide and then interacts with cyanide to form cyanmethemoglobin. In this method a measured aliquot of red cells is lysed by shaking in a known volume of Drabkin's reagent, which is commercially available. When stored in a brown bottle at room temperature, the reagent is stable for several months. The resulting lysate is allowed to stand for 5 minutes to allow complete conversion of the hemoglobin to cyanmethemoglobin, and its absorbance at 540 nm is read in a spectrophotometer. A dedicated microhematocrit centrifuge that generates a force of 12,000 g and microhematocrit tubes with or without heparin are used. The sample is carefully mixed and drawn up into the tube and the dry end of the tube is capped with sealing material. Centrifugation for 3 to 5 minutes is sufficient for most samples and results in a transparent column of cells that has a trapped plasma volume of less than 1 percent in most cases. For samples from patients with high PCV and those with sickle cell anemia or hereditary spherocytosis, an additional 5 minutes of centrifugation may be required. If MCHC is to be calculated from hemoglobin and hematocrit, multiple measurements should be made.

Automated Measurements. Current automated CBC methods measure properties of single cells flowing through a detector (Bentley et al., 1993). Two general types of detection are currently used: Coulter-type detectors based on impedence and high-frequency conductivity and detectors based on optical properties of the cell. Most instruments measure several variables and present results as an average value; the averaging of samples with red cell heterogeneity, therefore, such

as those from sickle cell anemia or hereditary spherocytosis, may yield values that seem normal. All instruments count particles, estimate their size, and hemolyze the cells and measure hemoglobin. The results of the direct measurements (hemoglobin, red blood cell count, white blood cell count [WBC], and platelet count) are the most accurate values, but failure to hemolyze all cells may lead to error in hemoglobin concentration in hemoglobinopathies such as sickle cell disease and in hereditary spherocytosis. Since identification of erythrocytes and platelets is based on their size, fragmentation may lead to misclassification. Most systems measure hemoglobin by the cyanmethemoglobin method. Coulter detectors are based on the observation that the electrical conductivity of cells is lower than that of saline solutions and measurement of the impedance across a small orifice with cells flowing through allows cell size [mean corpuscular volume (MCV)] to be estimated. High-frequency impedance measurements are used in some instruments primarily for white cell differential counts. Factors that lead to deviations are cellular asymmetry and loss of an intact cell membrane, both of which may be features in samples with abnormal red cells.

Cell volume measurements using light scattering (Mie principle) are based on the observation that the intensity of light scattered at small angles in the forward direction is proportional to cell size. Two major factors lead to deviations: cell shape and variation in refractive index, which is related to hemoglobin concentration. Bayer has approached the first problem by sphering the cells at constant volume, and the second problem has been addressed directly by measuring at two wavelengths, which allows intracellular hemoglobin concentration and refractive index to be estimated. Incomplete sphering is a problem for some samples such as those from sickle cell disease patients. PCV, mean corpuscular hemoglobin (MCH), MCHC, and red cell distribution width (RDW), and also other functions that provide information on dense cells and the amount of hemolysis are calculated from measured variation in red cell size. For most instruments, the least reliable measurement is the MCHC, which is calculated from the whole blood hemoglobin concentration divided by the mean cell volume times the number of cells. Since the calculation requires three measurements in most instruments, the error from all of them enters into the calculation.

Advantages and Limitations. The major advantages of automated methods are speed, low manpower requirements, high precision, and low exposure of technologists to pathogens. Comparisons of available instruments have been made by several groups (Gulati et al., 1992; Bentley et al., 1993; Jones et al., 1995).

Automated systems have high reproducibility (repeating the same sample several times results in little error); however, the accuracy is sensitive to errors in calibration that systematically affect the results so that absolute values may vary between instruments. All systems generate flags to call attention to unusual values, which may be taken either as indications of pathology or a need to examine the sample more closely. In general all instruments performed all tests satisfactorily with the exception of estimation of MCHC, which was the least reliable. Analyzers employing the Mie principle, by measuring density of individual red cells, are able to generate histograms of variation in cell density (cell hemoglobin distribution) of individual red cells in a given blood sample (see below). This is useful for following changes in the distribution of dense red cells in sickle cell anemia.

Reticulocyte Count

Reticulocyte counts, along with PCV measurements, are useful for evaluating the efficacy of hematopoiesis and the extent of processes that lead to red cell destruction. Reticulocytes are immature red cells that still contain remnants of messenger RNA (mRNA); they continue to synthesize hemoglobin for 1 to 2 days in the marrow and for another day after being released into the circulation. The peripheral blood of normal adults has less than 2 percent reticulocytes, but the count varies with the method. If the individual is under hematopoietic stress, the peripheral blood may contain stress reticulocytes, cells prematurely released from the bone marrow when severe hypoxia is present, or even nucleated erythrocytes. All reticulocyte counts are based on the presence of RNA in the cell. In the manual method, the cells are stained with new methylene blue, which precipitates the RNA, rendering it visible as blue granules or filaments. The amount and distribution of the precipitate allow the degree of immaturity of the reticulocyte to be estimated, and stress reticulocytes have a characteristic appearance (see Chapter 20). After staining, the cells are spread on a microscope slide and reticulocytes are counted as a percentage of all red cells. A major source of error in counting hand-smeared slides is the necessity of choosing the best region of the slide for counting, since the percentage reticulocytes varies with location. This can be avoided by using an automated slide maker. The next major source of error is counting too few cells. Manual counts using acridine orange, which causes RNA to fluoresce, and fluorescence microscopy are also possible. Automated reticulocyte counts use fluorescent-stained cells that are read in a flow cytometer, which may be either dedicated to reticulocyte counting or part of a larger automated system.

Red cells are usually discriminated from white cells and platelets by size, and a maximum fluorescence gate is usually set that may exclude nucleated red cells. The relative age of reticulocytes can be estimated by the degree of fluorescence. One drawback of these methods is that staining with the most frequently used reagent, thiazole orange, requires about 30 minutes incubation and variation in the chosen time of incubation may affect the final reticulocyte count. Based on the intensity of the reaction between the dye Oxazine 750 and reticulocyte mRNA, reticulocytes can be classified as low-, medium-, or high-staining intensity reticulocytes. An increase in the number of high-staining intensity reticulocytes indicates the presence of "stress" reticulocytes. Reticulocytes can also be stained with a labeled antibody to the transferrin receptor (Frazier et al., 1982).

Advantages and Limitations. Automated determination of reticulocyte counts has a much higher reproducibility and precision than manual methods and is far less labor intensive; however, results are sensitive to factors such as the incubation time used and the method used to calibrate the system.

Measures of Cell Heterogeneity

1. **RDW and HDW.** Most automated counters produce an indication of red cell heterogeneity called the red cell distribution width (RDW), which is calculated from the measured variation in red cell size by a nonlinear formula that magnifies heterogeneity. A correlation between the RDW and percentage of cells in the densest part of density gradient separations has been shown (Lawrence et al., 1985). Bayer counters compute a hemoglobin distribution width (HDW) that is based on variation of the hemoglobin content of the red cells. Bayer counters can also measure reticulocyte volume (MCVr), reticulocyte hemoglobin concentration (CHCMr), total reticulocyte hemoglobin (retHb), ratio of total hemoglobin to retHb (Hb/retHb), absolute reticulocyte count, mature red cell hemoglobin (rbcHb), rbcHb/retHb ratio, and numbers of erythrocytes with MCHC more than 38%. From the absolute reticulocyte count and the CHr, the retHb is calculated which expresses in g/L, the hemoglobin content of all reticulocytes. (Brugnara et al., 1997) The ratio of rbcHb to retHb defines the ratio between the hemoglobin contained in mature red cells and in the reticulocytes. Under steady-state conditions, erythrocyte survival may be estimated indirectly from the ratio of hemoglobin contained in mature red cells and in reticulocytes. A reduction in retHb and a concomitant increase in rbcHb/retHb ratio, provide indirect evidence for prolonged red cell survival.

2. Detection of variation in MCHC, red cell density distribution.

MCHC has distinct characteristics in many hemoglobinopathies. Early and comprehensive studies on red cell MCHC were done by Ponder (1948), who was able to detect the small increase in red cell MCHC that occurs when normal human red cells are deoxygenated, which was later visually demonstrated on continuous density gradients (Fabry and Nagel, 1982b). Hemoglobin concentration in the red cell is directly proportional to cell density, but is not necessarily correlated with cell volume unless cells from the same source are compared at different osmolarities. For example, the red cells of patients with HbE are microcytic, but have a narrow range of densities identical to that of individuals with HbA (Nagel et al., 1981). Red cells from normal adults have an MCHC of 33 ± 1.5 g/dL by conventional measurements; however, more sensitive measurements show that there are consistent differences between males and females and between African Americans and Caucasians (Blumenfeld et al., 1988). Several hemoglobinopathies have altered MCHC with a narrow range of densities: For example, in $\delta\beta$-thalassemia trait the cells are uniformly less dense by about 2g/dL and in homozygous HbC disease, the cells are uniformly more dense by about 4 g/dL. In other diseases, such as sickle cell disease, hereditary spherocytosis, and some of the thalassemias, there is a broad, but characteristic, distribution of red cells that include both high- and low-density red cells.

MCHC is one of the red cell indices measured by instruments used for the CBC. It is the least reliable of all automated measurements, and is frequently considered uninformative. Therefore, several alternative methods have been devised to analyze and isolate red cells according to density. These can be broken into three broad classes: methods using microhematocrit tubes filled with materials of different densities, methods that rely on discontinuous or layered density of supporting media for separation, and techniques that rely on continuous density gradients. All methods take advantage of the fact that cells will move under the influence of centrifugal force until they find a region of density the same as that of the cell—continuous gradients—or stop when they encounter a region of higher density—at the boundaries in discontinuous gradients. The red cell is unique among cells in its extraordinarily high protein concentration, which leads to a higher density than that of other cell types. Therefore, a further requirement for red cell separations is a much higher density than that used for separation of other cell types.

Discontinuous gradients based on a number of substances have been used in density-based separation. The most successful of these methods are based on substances that are nontoxic to the cell, have a low osmolarity, neutral pH, and low viscosity. Phthalate esters, Percoll®, Hypaque®, Stractan® (Larex®), and others have all been used for red cell separations. Some of the earliest separations of red cells were based on discontinuous albumin gradients, which are expensive and highly viscous. Danon and co-workers (Marikovsky et al., 1976) devised a simple method of generating density profiles and isolating cells of defined density using mixtures of phthalate esters that cover the density range of red cells. A series of solutions with different densities are made by mixing n-butyl phthalate with dimethyl phthalate. The phthalate solution is drawn into a microhematocrit tube, then red cells are drawn into the tube, the tube is sealed and centrifuged, and the percentage cells that are less dense and more dense than the phthalate solution are calculated. When these values are plotted for a series of densities, a density profile is generated. A disadvantage of the phthalate ester method is that the separated cells are not viable for transport or other physiologic studies. Stractan® (arabinopolygalactan, now marketed as Larex®) is a high-molecular-weight product made from the bark of the larch tree. It is physiologically benign and has a low osmotic contribution, which allows the ionic content of solutions to be adjusted freely. Clark used discontinuous Stractan gradients (Clark et al., 1978). A disadvantage of discontinuous gradients is that they usually have four or fewer densities. This can either mask relatively large changes in density of cells at the upper boundary between density levels or exaggerate small changes in cells at the lower boundary.

Percoll® is a commercially available product that spontaneously generates a continuous density gradient when centrifuged. Percoll® is composed of silica particles coated with polyvinyl pyrolidone that have a range of sizes. The rate of sedimentation of these particles under the influence of centrifugal force is determined by their size. The density at any depth in the tube is determined by the number and size of the particles. For this reason the density profile of Percoll® gradients depends on the duration of centrifugation, viscosity (which is temperature dependent), and g force applied. The density range of Percoll® is suitable for separation of white cells and needs to be increased before it can be applied to red cells. Vettore combined Renografin® with Percoll® to produce a continuous density gradient capable of resolving red cells on the basis of density (Vettore et al., 1984). A disadvantage of Renografin® is its high osmolarity, which results in a final osmolarity of the mixture of more than 360 mOsm. Fabry et al. (Fabry and Nagel, 1982a) combined Stractan® with Percoll® to produce continuous density gradients with physiologic pH, osmolarity, and ionic composition. These gradients are sensitive to very small changes in red cell density and can be used both preparatively and analytically. Assignment of density is based on position relative to density marker beads and on measured MCHC of cells isolated from defined positions in the gradient. An example of the power of separation of Percoll®-Larex® gradients is given in Figure 34.5, in which the red cell density distributions of several common hemoglobinopathies are compared.

Advantages and Limitations. All separations based on red cell MCHC (density) are sensitive to the pH and osmolarity of the solutions because these variables will change the MCHC of the cells. The microhematocrit approach is technologically undemanding; however, it does not yield viable cells for further experimentation and the accuracy of the density distribution determined is dependent on the accuracy of formulating the individual solutions. Sedimentation through the interface may depend on red cell deformability (Corry and Meiselman, 1978), leading to systematic underestimation of the density of poorly deformable cells. Stractan® (Larex®) is tedious to prepare, but cells isolated from these gradients are suitable for transport measurements and other protocols requiring physiologically intact cells. For discontinu-

ous separations, reproducibility for separations based on a single set of solutions is high, but the accuracy of assigned densities is dependent on the accuracy of formulating and calibrating individual solutions. Separations on continuous gradients are usually based on position relative to density marker beads and normal red cells and accuracy depends on the original calibration of the marker beads for the Percoll®-Larex® mixture. Because the Percoll®-Larex® mixture has a composition that is different from the Percoll® mixtures contemplated by the manufacturer, the density marker beads need to be recalibrated for the mixture in use.

F-Cells

HbF is not uniformly distributed among red cells with the exception of gene deletion hereditary persistence of HPFH, and cells with detectable amounts of HbF are called F-cells (see Chapter 10) (Kleihauer, 1974). In some individuals the level of HbF and F-cells may increase under conditions of hematopoietic stress or following administration of cytotoxic drugs such as hydroxyurea. F-cells can be detected by two techniques. The original technique was developed by Kleihauer and Betke and relied on resistance of precipitated HbF to acid elution (Betke and Kleihauer, 1969). Cells are spread on a slide, fixed with alcohol, and then incubated with citric acid-phosphate buffer. HbF remains precipitated while all other hemoglobins are eluted from the cell. When stained with hematoxylin-eosin F-cells are stained; in gene deletion HPFH all erythrocytes are uniformly stained.

Development of monoclonal antibodies to HbF in several laboratories (Zago et al., 1979; Boyer et al., 1984) allowed a more quantitative detection of HbF. Cells are first lightly fixed and the membrane permeabilized with detergents and/or organic solvents. This procedure is sensitive to too little fixation or too vigorous permeabilization where hemoglobin is lost or the cells fragment. With too much fixation or too little permeabilization antibodies do not penetrate effectively. After fixation and permeabilization, the cells are stained with antibody and may be observed either by microscopy or in a fluorescence-activated cell sorter (FACS) (Fig. 34.6). The earliest measurements used immunodiffusion to create a ring of precipitated HbF-antibody around the positive cells (Boyer et al., 1984). Fluorescent labels may be attached directly to the antibodies and cells observed by fluorescence microscopy (Stamatoyannopoulos et al., 1983). More recently, monoclonal antibodies against several hemoglobins including HbF have become commercially available. These antibodies can be used for immunofluorescent labeling of F-cells in fixed smears on slides, including

Figure 34.5. Percoll®-Larex® continuous density gradient. Red cell density is directly proportional to the mean corpuscular hemoglobin concentration (MCHC). The least dense (lowest MCHC) cells are at the top of the gradient and the highest density cells are at the bottom. This technique provides a method for directly visualizing the distribution of red cell density in a sample of whole blood. The example shows a continuous density gradient with density marker beads and red cells from patients with normal hemoglobin (AA), HbC trait (AC), HbC disease (CC), sickle cell anemia (SS), HbS-O Arabia, and hereditary spherocytosis (HS). For full color reproduction, see color plate 34.5.

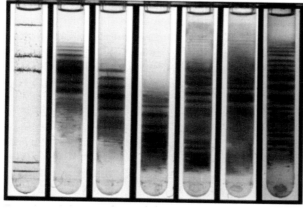

Beads   AA   AC   CC   SS   SOArab   HS

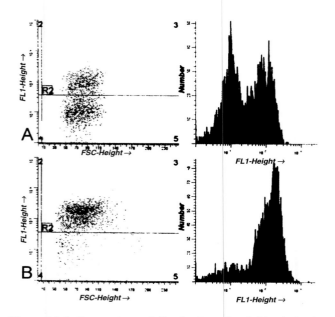

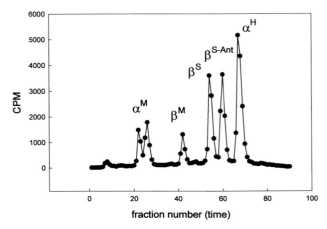

Figure 34.7. Chain synthesis as measured by incorporation of radioactive leucine followed by separation of globin chains by denaturing reverse-phase HPLC. In this case the sample studied was from a transgenic mouse expressing both human α, β^S, and $\beta^{S-Antilles}$ as well as mouse α and β globins.

Figure 34.6. Comparison of distribution of γ-globin chains in red cells by FACS analysis using FITC-labeled antibody specific for human γ-globin chains (supplied by Thomas Campbell of EG&G Wallac). In this case, the examples are two different types of transgenic mice expressing exclusively human hemoglobin and either a low level of γ globin (panel **A**) or a high level of γ globin (panel **B**). Left panels: fluorescence intensity versus cell size; right panels: number of cells versus fluorescence intensity. Note the presence of two populations of red cells that represent non-F-cells and F-cells (high fluorescence intensity).

archival samples, using a method described by Thein and Reittie (1998b)

Advantages and Limitations. Manual determination of F-cells requires little equipment, but is labor intensive and requires skill in making and reading smears. Use of FACS analysis greatly increases the precision of the measurement, but requires equipment and skill in preparing the cells to avoid lysis or understaining. Preparation of multiple samples can be time consuming despite the speed of the final counting.

Globin Chain Synthesis

Imbalance of synthesis of α- versus β-globin chains is the fundamental definition of thalassemia. Globin-chain synthesis occurs in erythrocyte precursors, including reticulocytes in the peripheral blood. It is usually assumed that the α- to β-globin ratio in blood was equivalent to that in bone marrow; however Cividalli et al. (1977) found a greater imbalance of non-α versus α-globin chain in bone marrow cells than in peripheral blood. This may be due to the greater proteolytic activity in nucleated erythrocytes. Globin-chain synthesis is measured by incubating reticulocytes

or bone marrow cells with ^3H leucine (Kan et al., 1972), washing the cells, lysing them, and separating their globin chains. The most convenient method currently used for chain separation is reverse-phase HPLC as that described by Galanello et al. (1998). Fractions containing globin chains are collected, mixed with scintillation fluid, and the radioactivity incorporated is counted using a liquid scintillation counter (Fig. 34.7). Various electrophoresis techniques based on denaturing gels have also been used to separate globin but the resolution obtainable by HPLC is superior and the sample size required is smaller by a factor of more than a hundred. The efficiency of labeling can be greatly improved if the percentage reticulocytes are enriched by a process such as layering whole blood on a discontinuous Stractan® gradient and collecting the lightest fraction that contains the most reticulocytes.

Advantages and Limitations. The combination of reticulocyte enrichment and HPLC allows chain synthesis on very small samples, 200 μL of packed cells for low reticulocyte samples and less for high reticulocyte samples, with minimal use of radioisotope. However, the investment in time, acquiring the technology, and equipment is significant.

Hemoglobin S Polymerization and Rate of Sickling

When the concentration of deoxy HbS exceeds the C_{SAT}, polymer is formed. However, polymer formation does not occur immediately because, prior to polymer formation, nucleation must occur, and because the nucleus consists of several hemoglobin molecules, there is a very high concentration dependence (see Chapter 23). The time between deoxygenation and the onset of polymer formation is called the delay time (Eaton and Hofrichter, 1987) which has one of the highest concentration dependencies in biology (to the 30th power; Eaton and Hofrichter, 1990) and may range from values of less than a microsecond at high hemoglobin concentrations to several minutes at low concentrations. The distortion of the red cell known as sickling is the result of intracellular polymer formation and may be used as an indirect endpoint for polymer formation. Three methods are currently used for measuring the rate of sickling and polymer formation: manual mixing, continuous flow (Harrington and Nagel, 1977), and the laser photolysis method developed by Eaton et al. (Murray et al., 1988). Only the laser photolysis method directly measures polymer formation and the time resolution of these methods varies from minutes, to seconds for the continuous flow method, to submilliseconds for the laser photolysis method. When delay times in the red cell exceed a few seconds, the process becomes stochastic, that is, the delay time is variable because at low concentrations of deoxyhemoglobin in the red cell the formation of a nucleus in a given red cell is determined by probability.

In the manual and stopped flow methods, oxygenated red cells are mixed with buffered sodium dithionite, which reacts with the oxygen and, at predetermined intervals, cells are removed, fixed with isotonic formalin; the number of cells which have sickled are counted, and the results plotted as a function of time. Since samples of blood from sickle cell disease patients may contain appreciable numbers of cells with unusual shapes, the number of deformed cells may be counted in a control sample and subtracted from the total of sickled cells. As with any method that relies on counting cells, the more cells counted, the more reliable the result. This method is capable of showing that cells from patients with HbSC disease deform less rapidly than sickle cell anemia cells and can detect retardation of polymer formation by antisickling agents (Harrington and Nagel, 1977).

Polymer formation in solution and in red cells can be directly measured by using laser photolysis of CO-Hb to produce deoxy-Hb followed by detection of polymer formation by light scattering (Coletta et al., 1982; Mozzarelli et al., 1987). The principle of this measurement is the observation that CO can be very rapidly flashed off the hemoglobin by exposure to a focused laser beam at 514.5 nm yielding deoxyhemoglobin, and polymerization of the deoxyhemoglobin can be monitored by light scattering (Coletta et al., 1982; Mozzarelli et al., 1987). This method allows direct measurement of polymer formation with very high time resolution. Currently, the data are collected on a cell-by-cell basis, so the time required to analyze a statistically significant number of cells is appreciable.

Advantages and Limitations. The manual mixing and continuous flow methods are not as technologically demanding as laser photolysis, but they are only able to differentiate between cells with relatively long delay times. They are useful for evaluating the effects of antisickling agents and the inhibitory effect of hemoglobins other than HbS on sickling. The laser photolysis approach is technologically demanding but can measure very short delay times in both cells and solutions of HbS.

TRANSGENIC MOUSE MODELS OF THALASSEMIA AND SICKLE CELL DISEASE

Transgenic mice are important in the study of the pathophysiology and treatment of hemoglobin disorders. While their small size is a disadvantage for some physiologic studies, it is an advantage for maintaining colonies and breeding. A large library of inbred strains, spontaneous and induced mutations, and engineered knockouts and insertions can be incorporated into transgenic animals. Mice that result from the embryonic stem cell (ES) technology that is used to generate gene knockout mice and most mice that are produced by injection of gene constructs into fertile eggs, are on mixed or even poorly characterized genetic backgrounds (cells or fertilized eggs are derived from more than one inbred strain) and must be bred onto another inbred strain to obtain sustainable lines and consistent physiology. The choice of genetic background or the presence of a mixed background may affect both hematology and other aspects of physiology. Different established inbred strains of mice, and male and female mice, may have quite different mean values for physiologic characteristics such as urine concentrating ability, other renal functions, body and organ weight, and average lifespan, further complicating the interpretation of some experiments. It should also be noted that mice have a higher plasma osmolarity than humans (330 versus 280 mOsm; Crispins, 1975) and that the 2,3-BPG content of mouse red cells is twice that of human red cells.

There are at least five common α-globin chains and three common β-globin chains among inbred strains (Whitney, 1982) and while the common C57 strain has only a single α- and β-globin chain, other strains may have two α-globin or two β-globin chains. When these are combined with proteins from human globin transgenes, a large number of homotetramers due to the presence of interspecies αβ dimers can result. One of the mouse β-globin variants, β^{minor}, also forms tetramers with unusually low p^{50}s (Roy et al., 1995),

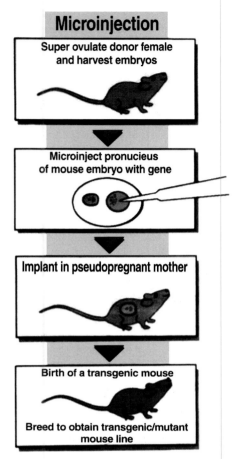

Microinjection

Super ovulate donor female and harvest embryos

Microinject pronucleus of mouse embryo with gene

Implant in pseudopregnant mother

Birth of a transgenic mouse

Breed to obtain transgenic/mutant mouse line

Figure 34.8. Creation of a transgenic mouse by injection of a construct into the pronucleus of a fertilized mouse egg. The injected eggs are then implanted into pseudopregnant females and the resulting pups are screened for the presence of the transgene. Pups positive for the transgene are bred to determine if the transgene is present in the germ line.

which may affect polymer formation and the pathophysiology of sickle mice.

The Technology of Transgenic and Knockout Mice

In the early 1980s several groups introduced cloned DNA into fertilized mouse embryos (Gordon et al., 1980; Costantini and Lacy, 1981) and succeeded in detecting gene expression. Rabbit β-globin genes were introduced into fertilized mouse embryos by Lacy et al. (1983), who observed hemoglobin expression but in tissues other than erythrocytes. Following the discovery of a locus control region (LCR) 5′ to the β-globin gene cluster by Tuan et al. (1985) (see Chapter 7), several groups of investigators (Chada et al., 1985; Townes et al., 1985; Kollias et al., 1986) linked the cloned LCR to various β-globin gene constructs and achieved erythroid expression in transgenic animals. The generalized scheme now used for producing trans-

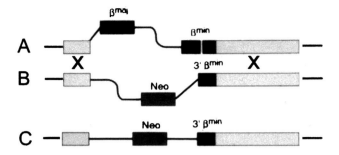

Figure 34.9. Targeted insertional deletion of the mouse β-globin genes. Line A is a simplified representation of the β-globin locus in the diffuse mouse, which makes two β globins: βmajor and βminor. Line B represents the replacement vector, which has an area of homology on the 5′ side, a Neo fragment capable of conferring resistance to G418, which also contains thymidine kinase genes driven by a promoter, and another area of homology corresponding to a portion of the βminor gene and extending beyond it. Line C shows the result of a crossover that contains the Neo fragment and an inactive remnant of the βminor gene.

genic mice from constructs injected into fertilized mouse embryos is illustrated in Figure 34.8 and was reviewed in Hogan et al., 1986.

Knockout or knockin technology, a means of deleting endogenous genes or introducing new genes into a genome by homologous recombination, is illustrated in Figure 34.9. Homologous sequences flanking the gene of interest are isolated and inserted into a targeting construct that contains selectable markers—in the illustration, neomycin resistance and herpes simplex virus thymidine kinase driven by a promoter. This targeting vector is transfected into a line of ES cells that are selected by exposure to neomycin and ganciclovir. Colonies are picked, expanded, and analyzed by Southern blot analysis for fragments of the predicted size. Cells with the mutated β-globin gene are then injected into blastocysts to generate chimeric animals that are screened for the mutation and bred to detect animals with the mutation in their germ line (Fig. 34.10). Full knockouts of both the mouse α- and β-globin genes using this general approach were complicated by the presence of two genes in each cluster requiring large deletions of DNA.

Thalassemic Mice

Mouse models of thalassemia due to either deletions or knockouts of the α- and β-globin genes are available. These contrast with human thalassemia that has multiple causes (see Chapters 12 and 17). A non-lethal deletion of the βmajor globin gene of a mouse with so-called diffuse hemoglobin (Hbbth-1), that can be bred to homozygosity, was detected by electrophoretic screening by Skow et al. (1983), who

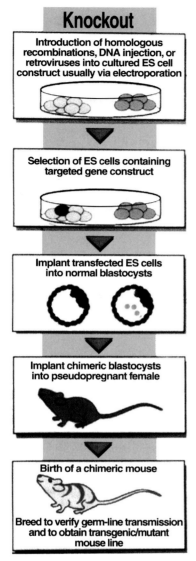

Knockout

Introduction of homologous recombinations, DNA injection, or retroviruses into cultured ES cell construct usually via electroporation

Selection of ES cells containing targeted gene construct

Implant transfected ES cells into normal blastocysts

Implant chimeric blastocysts into pseudopregnant female

Birth of a chimeric mouse

Breed to verify germ-line transmission and to obtain transgenic/mutant mouse line

Figure 34.10. Creation of a knockout mouse using ES cell technology. The targeting vector is introduced into ES cells, which are then selected by exposure to neomycin and ganciclovir. The selected cells are implanted into normal blastocysts that are then implanted into pseudopregnant females. The resulting pups are then screened and bred to verify transmission of the mutated genes into the germ line.

noticed the excess of mouse β^{minor} although whether the increased β^{minor} is a general response to anemia or a more specific response to the deletion that generated the thalassemia (see below) still needs to be determined. Mice homozygous for the β^{major} deletion have a high reticulocyte count (20 percent versus 2 percent for C57Bl), anemia (Hct 33 versus 48 for C57Bl), microcytosis (MCV 39 fl versus 45 fl), low MCH (12.7 pg Hb/cell versus 14.5 for C57Bl mice), and a low MCHC with a broad distribution of red cell densities that looks much like the density distribution

obtained for human patients with β thalassemia intermedia. Three α-globin chain mutations causing thalassemia have been described, all due to deletions (Whitney et al., 1981). However, the deletions are sufficiently large so that they are lethal when homozygous even in the presence of a rescuing human transgene. In the heterozygous state the α/β-chain ratio is about 0.75 and hence the induced thalassemia is relatively mild. If a single α-globin gene deletion is bred into mice homozygous for the β^{major} deletion, much of the red cell pathology is corrected; reticulocyte counts decrease from about 20 percent to 5 percent and red cell density is normalized, an observation akin to that observed when human α thalassemia and β thalassemia coexist.

Mouse models have been advocated as models for human thalassemia (Martinell et al., 1981; Skow et al., 1983; Rouyer Fessard et al., 1990). Parallels between human β thalassemia intermedia and the effect of the homozygous mouse β^{major} deletion (Hbb^{th-1}) have been pointed out (Rouyer Fessard et al., 1990). Normally, the mouse β^{major} gene contributes 80 percent of the β-globin chains, but in the presence of its deletion, synthesis of β^{minor} globin increases from 20 percent to 70–80 percent of the α-globin synthesis rate (Whitney and Popp, 1984). While increased β^{minor} synthesis should result in partial reversal of the phenotype, membrane content of α-globin, reduction of spectrin, and protein oxidation are comparable to that found in human thalassemia intermedia (Rouyer Fessard et al., 1990). Mice with deletional thalassemia have been used to study treatments with erythropoietin, clotrimazole, and hydroxyurea (de Franceschi et al., 1996b) (see Chapter 42).

A disruption of the β^{major}-chain was generated in 1993 (Shehee et al., 1993) by inserting a bacterial *(neo)* gene into the second exon of the mouse β^{major} gene and then using ES cell technology to generate knockout mice. This results in a more severe form of thalassemia than the previously described β^{major} deletion and is lethal in the homozygous state despite the continued production of β^{minor} globin. When this is bred into mice expressing the human β-globin gene, the percentage human β-globin chain is higher than that obtained with the β^{major} deletion (Fabry et al., 1995b). Shehee et al. proposed that the reduced severity of the deletion model when compared to the disruption model was due to the ability of the remaining β^{minor} gene to interact directly with the LCR without competition from the missing β^{major} gene, which would result in increased transcription and β^{minor} globin synthesis. In contrast to the deletion, with a disrupted gene, not only is the β^{major} promoter intact, but, in addition, the inserted *tk* promoter driving the *neo* gene is present, possibly resulting in further competition for the LCR and reduced transcription of the β^{minor} globin gene. A similar hypothesis has been proposed to account for the higher levels of HbA_2 and HbF when the β-globin gene promoter is deleted in some type of human β thalassemia (see Chapter 10).

In 1995, two groups (Ciavatta et al., 1995; Yang et al., 1995) succeeded in generating full β-globin gene knockout mice. A full knockout of the α-globin gene was generated in the same year (Paszty et al., 1995), making possible the generation of transgenic mice with exclusively human hemoglobins by breeding transgenic mice with α- and β-globin knockouts. The knockouts are lethal in the homozygous state unless rescued by a transgene. The hemizygous form of the α-globin gene knockout is equivalent to the common Asian form of α thalassemia in humans, - -/$\alpha\alpha$, or the Mediterranean/African form, $-\alpha/-\alpha$, and has a small but detectable effect in mice with reticulocytes increased to 7 percent, MCV decreased to 39 fl (45 fl for normal C57BI mice), and MCH decreased from 14.5 pg Hb/cell to 12.6 pg/cell. In homozygotes without a rescuing transgene the α knockout mouse has a condition similar to human hydrops fetalis (Paszty et al., 1995).

Sickle Transgenic Mice

The pathophysiology of sickle cell anemia is complex (see Chapters 20 to 22) and modulated by many genetic, epistatic, and environmental elements (Chapter 26). Because of the wide range of pathology and the variety of factors that modulate sickle cell disease—many of which may be different in mice—and because of differences in physiology between mice and humans, it is unlikely that a single animal model will adequately represent all aspects of the disease; nonetheless, animal models have already made significant contributions to our understanding of sickle cell disease.

Following the introduction of cloned human DNA into fertilized mouse embryos, incorporation of the LCR into human globin gene constructs was required before high levels of erythroid-specific expression were achieved. Higher expression of human β globin was achieved by introduction of the homozygous mouse β^{major} deletion (Costantini et al., 1986) and by engineering sufficient human β^A expression to ameliorate mouse deletional β-thalassemia. In 1988 Rubin and co-workers introduced human β^S into transgenic mice, but observed no pathology; these authors suggested trying a "super β^S" such as HbS-Antilles (see Chapter 28) to induce sickle pathology. Rhoda et al. (1988) demonstrated that the mouse α-globin chain is as effective as human γ-globin chain at inhibiting polymerization of HbS. This indicated the necessity of introducing the human α-globin gene for a successful mouse model of sickle cell

anemia, and, since the existing mouse α-globin deletions could not be bred to homozygosity, it also set a goal for a selective knockout of the mouse α-globin genes that was not realized until 1995.

The first models expressing moderately high levels of both human α- and β^S-globin chains were reported by Greaves et al. (1990) and Ryan et al. (1990). Subsequently, many different lines of mice with variable degrees of severity became available, allowing more detailed studies of pathology. These strains included mice expressing the "super β^S" HbS-Antilles, which failed to exhibit the expected level of pathology in part because of low human α-globin expression (Rubin et al., 1991); the SAD mouse expressing the β^S mutation and two additional "super" β^S mutations, HbS-Antilles and HbD-Punjab (Trudel et al., 1991); mice expressing both human α and β^S globins in the presence of homozygous mouse β-globin gene deletion and heterozygous α-globin gene deletion (Fabry et al., 1992a; Fabry et al., 1992); mice expressing human α- and β^S-globin genes in the presence of homozygous mouse β^{major} deletion (Reilly et al., 1994); mice expressing human α-, β^S-, and $\beta^{S-Antilles}$, which balanced the high human α-globin gene expression of the Costantini β^S line against the low human α-globin gene expression of the Rubin $\beta^{S-Antilles}$ line (Fabry et al., 1995a); and mice with high O_2 affinity mouse globins and HbS-Antilles (Popp et al., 1997). Full deoxygenation produced sickled cells and intracellular polymer formation in most of these models (Fig. 34.11).

The enhanced effect on polymer formation of mice expressing the "super" β^S globins are due to two

Figure 34.11. Electron microscopy of slowly deoxygenated red cells from a mouse expressing the Costantini $\alpha^H\beta^S$ transgene and homozygous for the β^{major} deletion. Left panel: scanning electron microscopy showing sickled cells. Right panel: transmission electron microscopy showing intracellular polymer (long dark fibers). Bars are 1 μm. (From Fabry et al., 1992a, with permission.)

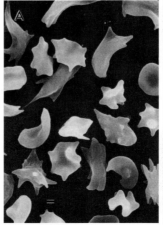
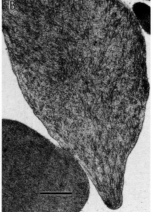

features: reduction in oxygen affinity, which shifts the conformation of the hemoglobin to the T-state and favors polymer formation; and reduced solubility, which suggests that new contact sites in the polymer have been created. HbS-Antilles has, in addition to the β^S mutation at β-6 (Glu $\rightarrow$ Val), a second mutation in the same chain at β-23 (Val $\rightarrow$ Ile). The second mutation results in a lower oxygen affinity and lower solubility under deoxygenated conditions than HbS (Monplaisir et al., 1986). In contrast to patients heterozygous for HbS who are well, patients who are heterozygous for HbS-Antilles have significant clinical disease. The HbD Punjab mutation at β-121 (Glu $\rightarrow$ Gln) results in a severe sickle syndrome in the compound heterozygote state with HbS due to the very low solubility of the deoxygenated hybrid tetramer $\alpha_2\beta^S\beta^D$ (Milner et al., 1970) (see Chapter 28).

A long-standing objection to all of the early transgenic mouse models of sickle cell anemia was that they exhibited either no anemia or very mild anemia. The SAD mice of Trudel et al. and the S+S-Antilles mice of Fabry et al. have a modest reduction of PCV that was most evident neonatally. In sickle cell anemia, increased blood viscosity, a function of PCV, increases the probability of slow flow, deoxygenation, and vasoocclusion (see Chapter 20). Therefore, the absence of anemia in these early mouse models probably contributed to increased pathology rather than the reverse.

The effect of γ-globin chains on transgenic mouse models is important both for understanding the mechanism of the protective effect of γ-globin chains and as a baseline for evaluating anti-sickling hemoglobins proposed for use in gene therapy. Trudel and co-workers (Blouin et al., 2000) have explored the effect of γ-globin chains on pathology in the SAD mouse by breeding four different levels of human γ-chains into the SAD mouse. SAD mice expressing 5.2, 10.6, 18.4, and 24.4 percent γ-globin as a percent of all β-like chains were studied. Some properties were found to be improved in proportion to the amount of γ chains expressed: such as, the density gradient profile and the percent of hyperdense cells (which are related) and the percent of microcytic cells. Interestingly, several other properties—lifespan, percent of viable pups, and glomerular profile area (which relates to kidney pathology)—exhibited improvement with just 5.2 percent γ-globin chains and little additional benefit was conferred with higher levels. Other factors such as spleen size and percent red pulp in the spleen were unresponsive to the presence of γ chains at any level. The varied responses of different forms of pathology to percent γ chains may indicate that the protective effect of γ globin has mechanisms that vary from tissue to tissue.

The most recent stage of creating mouse models of human sickle cell disease has been the creation of mice expressing exclusively human hemoglobins; the first two models were announced simultaneously in 1997 by Pàszty et al. and by Ryan et al. Both lines of mice incorporate the mouse α-globin gene knockout described by Pàszty et al. (1995) and the mouse β-globin gene knockout described by Ciavatta et al. (1995) and transgenes expressing human α-, β-, and γ-globin genes. Pàszty et al. described a single line of mice expressing HbS and, in adults, very low levels of human HbF. Ryan et al. described six different lines expressing HbS and varying levels of human HbF. Another line of mice expressing exclusively human hemoglobin has been described by Gaensler and co-workers (Chang et al., 1998) based on a single copy of a 240-kb yeast artificial chromosome which contains the β-gene cluster with the β^S mutation and a separate introduction of two copies of the human α2-globin gene driven by a 6.5-kb mini-LCR. The mouse β^{maj}-β^{min} knockout was obtained from Smithies and co-workers (Detloff et al., 1994) and a knockout of the mouse α-globin genes was generated by Gaensler and co-workers. These mice have the advantage that the normal structure of the β-globin locus is preserved. They are anemic (PCV 22), have an elevated reticulocyte count (20%), and have a low MCH (10.4 pg/cell) which may be comparable to that of the Berkeley mouse (Pàszty et al., 1997) since the MCH of control mice is given as 16.1 pg/cell. They have prenatal expression of γ-globin chains that decrease to 1 percent to 5 percent at birth. This line of mice may be an excellent model to study hemoglobin switching.

Although mice expressing exclusively human hemoglobins have many useful similarities to human sickle cell disease including anemia, reticulocytosis, loss of urine concentrating ability, and tissue damage, all strains examined to date have features of β thalassemia with very low MCH and low MCHC only partially explained by reticulocytosis. In contrast, most of the transgenic sickle mice that still express mouse globins have elevated MCHC, a feature attributed to the deoxygenation-induced potassium efflux (Romero et al, 1997). Very low MCH in these full knockout mice is coupled with low MCHC, neither of which is a feature of sickle cell disease. This combination will reduce both the rate and extent of HbS polymer formation and be protective against sickling-related pathology. It will also confound attempts to evaluate the effect of introducing antisickling globins into these mice because the presence of the antisickling β chains will correct the low MCH and raise the MCHC, which will be a strong pro-polymerization effect due to the great sensitivity of the delay time to intracellular Hb concentration. At the same time the antisickling globin will interfere with polymer formation. Evaluation of efficacy under these conditions will be difficult.

Mice expressing exclusively human hemoglobin are particularly desirable for testing anti-sickling hemoglobins proposed for use in gene therapy due to the absence of mouse α globins which may confound interpretation by interacting selectively with modified β-globin chains and by inhibiting polymer formation (Rhoda et al., 1988). However, most of the mice expressing exclusively human hemoglobin have both low MCH and low MCHC which may complicate evaluation of the efficacy of anti-sickling globins. An exception are mice based on the transgene generated by Costantini and co-workers (Fabry et al., 1992). By incorporation of three different human γ-globin gene expressing lines generated by Gilman (Gilman et al., 1995) and Forget and co-workers (Arcasoy et al., 1997), the Costantini line expressing the human α-globin gene and a β^S-globin gene (named the NYC1 line) has also been bred to a full knockout. In these mice, adults of the low γ-globin expressing line had >4 percent γ-globin as a percent of all β-like chains; an intermediate line had adult expression of 20 percent γ-globin (and an expression of only 7 percent at 15–30 days); and a high γ-globin expressing line had 37 percent γ-globin chains in mice that were over 60 days old (Fabry et al., 1999). The increase in γ chain expression in the mice expressing intermediate levels of γ globin is due to the presence of F-cells which are selectively spared and increase as a percent of all cells until the mice are <60 days of age. These mice have high reticulocyte counts and anemia. On the other hand, the MCHC of the 20 percent γ-globin chain mouse has an average value similar to that of C57 mice and that of the 37 percent γ-globin chain mice is elevated, similar to that observed for other mice expressing high levels of HbS (Fig. 34.12). Both of the γ-globin gene expressing lines generated by Gilman have much higher expression of γ-globin genes during the fetal and neonatal period (Gilman et al., 1995), as does the γ expressing line generated by Forget and co-workers (Arcasoy et al., 1997).

Because of their higher MCH and MCHC, these mice are generally more severe than Berkeley mice (Pàszty et al, 1997) expressing comparable levels of γ-globin chains. For example, as reported by Fabry and co-workers (Fabry et al, 1999), the reticulocyte count, PCV and urine concentrating defect for the Costantini mouse that express 20 percent γ-globin as adults were similar to original Berkeley mouse (reticulocyte count 30 percent ± 10 percent vs 37 percent ± 8 percent; PCV 33 ± 2 vs. 30 ± 4, respectively; and spontaneous loss of urine concentrating ability for both types of mice) even though the Berkeley mouse expresses essentially no detectable γ-globin chains after birth. The same transgene which resulted in 20 percent adult expression in

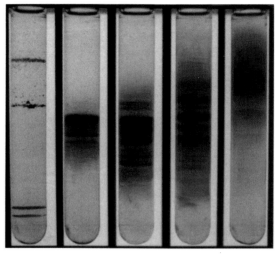

	Beads	C57Bl	Costantini Gilman G1 α^{H}β^{S}γ	Costantini Gilman G2 α^{H}β^{S}γ	Berkeley α^{H}β^S
Knockouts	–		α^{KK}β^{KK}	α^{KK}β^{KK}	α^{KK}β^{KK}
α^H	–		100	100	100
β^S	–		63	93	100
γ	–		27	7	<1
MCH	14.5		14.8	13.1	9.3

Figure 34.12. Percoll®-Larex® continuous density gradient of three types of transgenic mice expressing exclusively human hemoglobin. The lightest cells (at the top of the gradient) have low MCHC and are predominantly reticulocytes and the densest cells (at the bottom of the gradient) have high MCHC and are enriched in irreversibly sickled cells. The gradient has physiologic pH and osmolarity and is performed at 37°C. From left to right: density marker beads, C57Bl, Costantini mice with 27 percent γ-globin chains (expressing Gilman G1) at 15 to 30 days, Costantini mice with 7 percent γ globin (expressing Gilman G2) at 15 to 30 days, and the Berkeley mouse. Note the highest density (MCHC) cells in the Costantini G2 mouse and the lowest density (MCHC) cells in the Berkeley mouse. For full color reproduction, see color plate 34.12.

the NYC1 mouse, which has a spontaneous urine concentrating defect, was bred into the Berkeley mouse and resulted in adult γ-globin chain expression of 21 percent and normal urine concentrating ability. From these results and those of Trudel and co-workers (Blouin et al, 2000) discussed above, we can conclude that the level of γ-globin chains needed to correct various forms of pathology in transgenic mice will vary depending on the characteristics of each line and that no direct comparison to level of γ globin needed to ameliorate human disease can be made. However, evaluation of the level of γ gene expression needed to correct various pathological features is a necessary first step in establishing benchmarks for testing anti-sickling globins proposed for use in gene therapy.

All of the knockout sickle mice described are the products of hundreds of matings and once a successful line has been established it has been possible to propagate it. In contrast, a recently described line expressing exclusively HbC (Fabry et al., 1998) was fully knocked-out in a relatively small number of matings, which implies that mouse red cells tolerate the presence of exclusively human hemoglobins relatively well. One possible explanation for this contrast is that the many matings of the HbS mice are required to find an epistatic ameliorating feature that allows each line to survive. This speculation can only be validated by extensive analysis of the existing lines.

Red Cell Properties of Sickle Transgenic Mice. Human red cells live about 120 days whereas mouse red cells live about 40 days. Therefore, the baseline reticulocyte count in human blood is much lower than in mice. The oxygen affinity of murine hemoglobins is lower than that of human hemoglobins. Human red cells with HbA have a p^{50} of about 25 mm Hg, whereas C57Bl mouse red cells have a p^{50} of about 40 mm Hg. Mice do not have a high oxygen affinity HbF to cope with the low oxygen fetal environment. Instead, the red cells of fetal mice do not upregulate 2,3-BPG levels, which decreases oxygen affinity, until after birth and adult levels are not reached until about 3 weeks of age (Scott et al., 1976). Adult mouse red cells have much higher levels of 2,3-BPG (30μm/g of Hb) than human red cells (10 to 15 μm/g Hb), and mouse red cells that express exclusively human hemoglobin have even more elevated levels of 2,3-BPG (30 to 40 μm/g of Hb), which reduces the p^{50} from that found in humans. For example, the p^{50} of HbA in a fully knocked-out line expressing only human globins is 33 mm Hg due to the high level of 2,3-BPG. Polymer formation is enhanced by elevated levels of 2,3-BPG (Swerdlow et al., 1977) and the severity of pathology induced by HbS in mice may be due in part to elevation of BPG.

MCHC plays a crucial role in the pathophysiology of sickle cell disease since the rate of polymer formation is inversely proportional to the 30th power of the concentration of deoxy HbS (see Chapter 23) and the extent of polymer formation is directly proportional to the concentration of HbS. Two features of mouse erythrocytes would be expected to increase the pathology caused by introduced HbS: elevated MCHC due to the higher plasma osmolarity of mice (Crispins, 1975; Fabry et al., 1995a) and elevated red cell 2,3-BPG content.

Transgenic mice offer a unique opportunity to study the mechanisms of cation transport in sickle cell disease. One of the most exciting observations of the sickle transgenic mouse was the discovery that deoxy potassium efflux, first described by Tosteson (Tosteson et al., 1955) and unique to human sickle cells, is also found in the red cells of transgenic mice expressing high levels of HbS (Romero et al., 1997a). A calcium stimulated potassium channel appears to be similar in mouse and the human red cells (de Franceschi et al., 1994). This property has been used to advantage by Brugnara et al. to demonstrate the beneficial effects on red cell density of inhibition of the potassium channel by clotrimazole (de Franceschi et al., 1994) and putative inhibition of K:Cl cotransport by Mg^{++} supplementation (de Franceschi et al., 1996a) (see Chapters 22 and 42). The characteristics of K:Cl cotransport in the mouse red cell are more controversial. Romero et al. (1997a) have reported a number of differences between K:Cl cotransport in mouse and human red cells. These include lack of inhibition by NO_3^-, also described by Brugnara et al. (Armsby et al., 1995); lack of sensitivity to [(dihydroindenyl)oxy] alkanoic acid (DIOA); a long delay time for activation; lack of volume sensitive activation; and a large isotonic flux (Romero et al., 1997). These differences imply that the mouse red cell is not a perfect model for cation transport in sickle cell disease. However, following introduction of HbC and, in mice expressing exclusively human HbS and γ-globin chains, sensitivity to NO_3^- and DIOA are restored, strongly suggesting interaction of the K:Cl cotransporter or its modulators with both human and murine hemoglobin (Romero et al., 1999). Signs of oxidative damage have also been noted in erythrocytes of transgenic sickle mice (Reilly et al., 1994; de Franceschi et al., 1995) and may also contribute to mouse red cell pathology.

Pathophysiology of Sickle Transgenic Mice. Although mice are expected to have differences in pathology from the human, many similarities have been found and indeed, in some cases, the pathology found in mice has spurred the search for similar pathology in humans that was subsequently found.

Sickle cell anemia affects the kidney (see Chapter 24). Trudel et al. (1991; 1994) reported glomerular sclerosis and elevated blood urea nitrogen and proteinuria in the SAD mouse. Fabry et al reported that mice expressing human α and $β^S$ globin on a homozygous deletional background have an enhanced glomerular filtration rate (GFR) and a urine concentrating defect when exposed to hypoxia (Fabry et al., 1992a) (Fig. 34.13); the same investigators found that S+S-Antilles mice have a severe and spontaneous urine-concentrating defect (Fabry et al., 1995). S+S-Antilles mice are mice with both the Costantini $α^H β^S$ and the Rubin $α^H β^{S-Antilles}$ transgenes and a homozygous deletion of mouse $β^{major}$. Bank et al. (1996) found that mice expressing the Costantini $α^H β^S$ transgene on a

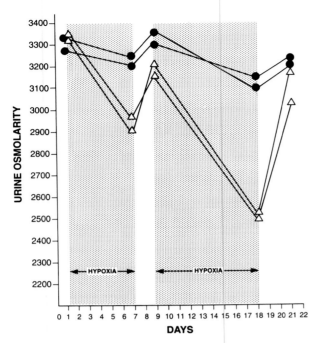

Figure 34.13. Urine-concentrating ability of mice expressing the Costantini $\alpha^H\beta^S$ transgene that are homozygous for the mouse β^{major} deletion (Fabry et al., 1992b). The mice were maintained under hypoxic conditions (8 percent O_2, 0.5 percent CO_2, balance N_2) during the periods indicated and urine-concentrating ability was measured after 24 hours of water deprivation. Transgenic animals are indicated by open triangles and control C57Bl mice, by filled circles. Note that significant but incomplete recovery occurred after 2 days at room air.

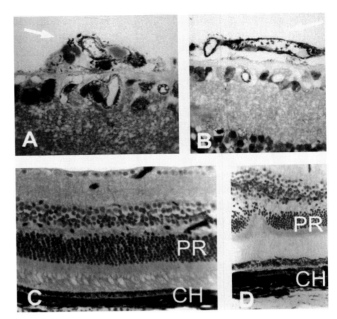

Figure 34.14. Examples of retinopathy in sickle transgenic mice expressing the Costantini $\alpha^H\beta^S$ transgene and homozygous for the β^{major} deletion. Panels A and B: pre-retinal neovascularization indicated by arrows. Panel C: a normal retina indicating choroid (CH) and photoreceptor (PR) layers. Panel D: a pathologic retina showing dilated obstructed CH with a disrupted PR layer above it. For full color reproduction, see color plate 34.14.

homozygous deletional background have elevated levels of nitric oxide synthase (NOS, both eNOS and iNOS) in the kidney, which become even higher when the mice are exposed to hypoxia. They speculated that this could explain the elevated GFR and could lead to other forms of renal damage as well as explain other symptoms of sickle cell disease.

Recent studies in isolated human renal tubular cells have shown that when L-arginine is depleted, the production of NO from NOS falls, and the production of O_2^- and peroxynitrite rises (Xia et al., 1996). A cytotoxic effect of peroxynitrite on tubular cells was evident by release of LDH, and nitrotyrosine staining was positive (Xia et al., 1996). These observations led Bank et al. to question whether the elevated expression of NOS (determined by Western blot analysis) in the kidneys of the β^S sickle cell mice was associated with increased NO production and/or peroxynitrite production. In order to determine this, immunohistochemistry studies of control and β^S mice were carried out, using an affinity purified polyclonal antibody directed against nitrotyrosine. Elevated nitrotyrosine was found co-localized with elevated iNOS in tubular epithelial cells of the kidney. These authors also observed moderate tubular cell apoptosis in transgenic sickle mice exposed to hypoxia in contrast to control mice that had minimal apoptosis after exposure to hypoxia (Bank et al., 1998). The potential role of NOS in the pathogenesis of sickle cell disease had not previously been appreciated, although it had been noted by Enwonwu (1989) that arginine, the precursor of nitric oxide (NO), is depleted in the plasma of sickle cell disease patients. Other possible symptoms of elevated NOS activity such as low systematic blood pressure have been found in both human sickle cell disease patients (Lipowsky et al., 1987; Rodgers et al., 1993; Pegelow et al., 1997) and in transgenic mice expressing HbS and HbS-Antilles (Kaul et al., 1998).

The retina of transgenic sickle mice is the first genetically induced animal model of pre-retinal neovascularization and has many of the features of the retina in sickle cell disease (see Chapters 20 and 27). Found in about 30 percent of transgenic mice over 1 year of age, the abnormalities include dropout of retinal vessels, structures reminiscent of black sunbursts that are due to invasion of pigmented epithelial cells from the choroid, and loss of photoreceptors in regions where the underlying choroid has been destroyed (Lutty et al., 1994, 1998) (Fig. 34.14). The role of destruction of the choroid in human sickle cell retinopathy had not previously been appreciated and

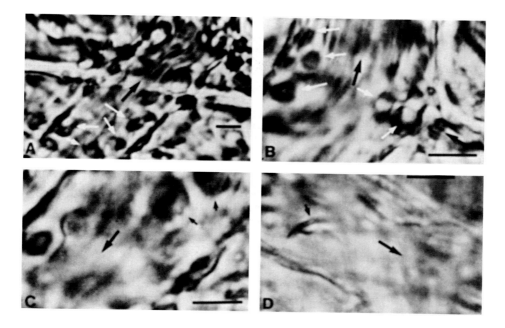

Figure 34.15. Videomicrograph showing in vivo adherence of red cells to the endothelium of postcapillary venules in the cremaster muscle preparation of an S + S-Antilles mouse. Adherent red cells during steady flow are indicated by small arrows and the direction of flow is indicated by a large arrow. Bar is 10 μm. In Panel C, leukocytes are indicated by small black arrows and can be distinguished from the mouse erythrocytes (~5 μm) by their larger size.

when Lutty et al. examined human eyes obtained at autopsy from sickle cell patients, he found evidence of choroidal damage (McLeod et al., 1997).

The microcirculation has been one of the most interesting areas of study in the sickle transgenic mouse. Adhesion of sickle cells to the endothelium and its potential role in sickle cell disease were first proposed by Hebbel (Hebbel et al., 1980), but were not observed in vivo until the cremaster muscle preparation of the S+S-Antilles mouse was examined (Fig. 34.15) (Kaul et al., 1995). Kaul et al. have demonstrated reduced red cell velocity and blood flow in the S+S-Antilles mouse when the mouse cremaster muscle was suffused with a solution equilibrated with room air. When the gas used to equilibrate the suffusate contained increased oxygen, red cell velocity increased, blood flow increased, and the vessel diameter was maintained (Kaul et al., 1995). This result was in contrast to normal (C57Bl) mice where a change to suffusion with oxygen-equilibrated solutions resulted in decreased flow and vasoconstriction. The simplest explanation of these observations is that in the transgenic mouse, with equilibration with room air, there is HbS polymer formation that increases viscosity and reduces flow; oxygenation reverses this condition.

This does not explain the failure to observe vasoconstriction under these conditions and has led to the speculation that vascular response is blunted in sickle transgenic mice, a condition long suspected in human subjects with sickle cell disease. This observation led to examination of other aspects of the vascular response in the S+S-Antilles mouse and it was found that these mice have constitutively low blood pressure, that vessel diameter does not respond to administration of acetylcholine, an endothelium-dependent vasodilator, or sodium nitroprusside (SNP), an NO-donor. However, L-NAME, a nonselective inhibitor of NOS, does cause a significant increase in blood pressure in both sickle and control mice (Kaul et al., 1998). It was concluded that increased NOS/NO activity results in hypotension and altered microvascular response to NO-mediated vasodilators in the S+S-Antilles mouse and that similar processes may also occur in sickle cell patients. Loss of vascular tone probably has both advantages and disadvantages for the sickle mouse and for human sickle cell patients. Vasodilation and/or lack of vasoconstriction will minimize chances for blockage by nondeformable cells, but at the cost of overexposure of tissues to oxygen with the consequent risk of oxidative damage.

In all sickle mouse models the liver is a major site of pathology. In humans, both chronic and acute pathology have been described (see Chapter 24), but the liver appears to be much less severely affected than in the mouse. In mice, the liver suffers from repeated infarcts that increase when mice are hypoxic (Osei et al., 1996) and occur with a greater frequency, as judged by both histology (Fabry et al., 1995a) and elevated levels of the serum enzyme alanine transaminase, in more severe mouse models such as the HbS-HbS-Antilles mouse (Fabry et al., 1992b, 1995). Liver pathology has also been described in full knockout mice (Pàszty et al., 1997; Ryan et al., 1997). Elevated levels of iNOS and eNOS have been found in livers of transgenic sickle mice and have been attributed to hypoxic damage and/or the effect of shear stress due to the effectively higher viscosity of sickle blood and possibly damage by adhesion of red cells (Osei et al., 1996). Extramedullary hematopoiesis has been detected in the liver of knockout transgenic sickle mice (Ryan et al., 1997).

Splenic enlargement, fibrosis, and expansion of the erythropoietic red pulp were noted even in mice with a relatively mild phenotype (Fabry et al., 1992a) and also in those with intermediate levels of severity (Trudel et al., 1991; Fabry et al., 1995a). More dramatic enlargement, from 7- to 20-fold with fibrosis and expanded red pulp, was detected in severe sickle transgenic mice with full knockouts (Pàszty et al., 1997; Ryan et al., 1997). A significant proportion of the total red cell mass is found in the spleen in these animals and may be partially responsible for the low PCV.

The lung in transgenic sickle mice with more severe pathology shows congestion, thickened septa (Fabry et al., 1995a), fibrosis, and thrombosis (Trudel et al., 1994). A similar pattern is found in transgenic sickle knockout mice (Pàszty et al., 1997). Study of the brain in transgenic sickle mice is relatively unexplored. Occasional red neurons and rare pycnotic neurons were observed in HbS, HbS-Antilles mice (Fabry et al., 1995). The red neurons may be indicative of hypoxic episodes secondary to vasoocclusion. They would not be regarded as significant in the absence of the more severe findings in two older animals that had neuronal dropout, pycnotic neurons and supporting cells, and pycnotic Purkinje cells in the cerebellum, findings compatible with intermittent ischemia.

Other Hemoglobinopathies. Other nonsickle, human globin transgenes have been introduced into the mouse. Among those reported are the β^A-globin gene (Chada et al., 1985; White et al., 1994); γ-globin gene (Gilman et al., 1995; Arcasoy et al., 1997); δ-globin gene (Nagel et al., 1995); and recently, the β^C-globin gene (Fabry et al., 1998). Some have been bred onto full knockout backgrounds. For example, a mouse expressing human α- and β^A-globin chains was generated by White et al., (1994) and bred onto a full knockout background by Pàszty et al. This mouse has features of β thalassemia with a low MCHC that can be corrected by introducing the γ-globin gene. More recently, a mouse expressing exclusively human HbC was described (Fabry et al., 1998). These mice have many features of human HbC disease (see Chapter 27) including dehydrated, high MCHC red cells, high K:Cl cotransport, circulating intracellular crystals of HbC that increase when the mice are splenectomized, and folded red cells.

An Overview of the Utility of Transgenic Mouse Models for Sickle Cell Disease

Despite the complex pathophysiology of sickle cell anemia and its modulation by multiple elements—that are likely to be different in mice—transgenic mice have already made significant contributions to our understanding of sickle cell disease. It is clear that much can be learned from imperfect models (for example, mice with some residual mouse globins) and that the characteristics of a perfect model will depend on which questions are asked. Yet, the quest for a more perfect mouse is reasonable since the rationale for animal models is the possibility of detecting the outcome of complex interactions that cannot be confidently predicted, or verified, from results obtained by in vitro experimentation.

In the effort to satisfy all demands for the "perfect" model, it is easy to lose sight of the compromises that have been made. Mice have some features that may make the physiologic consequences of sickle cell disease even more severe than they are in humans: High plasma osmolarity increases the MCHC of mouse red cells and favors polymer formation and high 2,3-BPG also favors polymer formation. Because of these known differences, and others that are yet to be discovered, it may not be possible to make a mouse with exclusively HbS, low levels of HbF in adults, and a normal MCHC without altering some other feature to ameliorate the disease.

It is worthwhile to bear in mind some of the hematologic features of transgenic mice that may confound analysis in terms of severity, the ameliorating effects of human γ-globin chains or other antisickling hemoglobins, and applicability of results to gene therapy in humans.

1. Although many transgenic lines have high expression of human HbF during the fetal period, the way that mice normally adapt to the hypoxia of the uterine environment is by delaying 2,3-BPG production until just after birth, and full 2,3-BPG expression is not reached until about 3 weeks of age. It is therefore necessary to be aware of two switches that occur in mice: the downregulation of the human γ-globin gene and the upregulation by the mouse gene governing 2,3 BPG production.

2. Many lines of transgenic mice express their human hemoglobins in a pancellular mode and this is also true for many lines that express γ-globin genes; however, F-cells do occur in some mouse lines that can both enhance the verisimilitude of the model and com-

plicate data analysis since the percentage γ-globin chains in whole blood may be a balance between the synthesis of γ chain and selective red cell destruction of non-F-cells.

3. The amount of hemoglobin in whole blood due to transgene expression may not be constant during the lifetime of the mouse. Gene expression, the site of erythropoiesis, hemoglobin assembly, and selective red cell destruction can all play a role in this outcome, and it is important to be aware of these complications and to measure transgene production as a function of mouse age by several methods such as HPLC and globin chain synthesis.

4. Effects of different mouse backgrounds: Inbred strains of mice do differ physiologically, for example, in renal function. In addition, some strains have a propensity to develop distinctive types of pathology. For example, nontransgenic C57Bl mice are noted for spontaneous occurrence of skin lesions and failure to retract the penis, which is usually ascribed to nerve damage.

5. Production of human hemoglobin in mouse red cells appears to require extremely high levels of mRNA (Alami et al., 1999). It is always necessary to measure actual globin chain synthesis before reaching conclusions about hemoglobin gene expression in transgenic mice.

Currently, the best way to demonstrate that the effect of γ-globin chains in a sickle cell mouse model is due to inhibition of HbS polymer formation is by producing a similar mouse that expresses β^A-globin chains at a comparable level. The β^A chains will dilute the concentration of HbS, but will not reduce polymer formation as effectively because heterotetramers containing γ chains, $\alpha_2\beta^S\gamma$, are excluded from the polymer while heterotetramers containing β^A chains, $\alpha_2\beta^S\beta^A$, are incorporated in the polymer, although with a lower efficiency (see Chapter 10). Similarly, antisickling hemoglobins intended for use in gene therapy need to be compared to γ-globin chains expressed at a similar level to validate their antisickling properties. However, a major obstacle to comparing the "same" mouse with β^A- or γ-globin chains is that every transgene is inserted in a different location in the chromosome and with a different copy number and potentially with a different level of expression at different ages in the mouse. This limitation can now be overcome with new technology based on site-specific recombination mediated by the CRE or FLP recombinase (Bouhassira et al., 1997; Seibler et al., 1998). It is now possible to first tag a locus with appropriate recombination sites and then use these enzymes to insert transgenes to be compared at a predetermined location, thereby eliminating position and variable copy number effects.

Hematologic severity may not correlate with physiologic severity. The full knockout HbC mouse has nearly the same level of hematologic severity as some of the full sickle knockout mice. That is, the PCV and reticulocyte counts are nearly the same. However, the physiologic impact of HbC is much milder and as a result these mice were bred to a full knockout with a very small number of matings, and both male and female mice with exclusively HbC are capable of breeding. This is in sharp contrast to the many matings required to produce full knockout mice with HbS, both with and without human γ-globin gene expression, and the general inability of female mice with high levels of β^S to reliably survive pregnancy and give birth to viable pups. In evaluating antisickling hemoglobins physiologic parameters should be evaluated along with strictly hematologic parameters.

The current generation of mice expressing exclusively human hemoglobin is technologically state-of-the-art, and yet these too have imperfections. Most of the full knockouts have low MCHC, a condition not associated with human sickle cell disease: even HbS-β^0 thalassemia has a "normal" MCHC. In these animals, low MCHC may be a necessary compensation to ameliorate the induced pathology and allow survival. Regulation of chain balance is imperfectly understood and in most transgenic lines chain balance is the result of chance, because whatever mechanisms are responsible for chain balance are probably circumvented in the creation of the transgenics. When chain balance is not achieved in mice expressing HbS and the mice suffer from thalassemia, the pathology observed will be a combination of polymer-related damage and oxidative damage, which may interact synergistically. Even in the absence of chain imbalance, low MCHC may confound the interpretation of results in experiments where breeding in an antisickling hemoglobin may alter red cell MCHC and hence affect polymer formation or other MCHC-related forms of pathology.

The final consideration is the need to examine more than one model before drawing conclusions. An example of this is the unexpectedly severe phenotype of the mouse expressing both HbS and HbS-Antilles and the unexpectedly strong antisickling effect of γ-globin chains in the presence of a "super" β^S such as HbS-Antilles. One way of coping with the limitations of individual mouse models is to look for features that are consistent over several different models.

REFERENCE RESOURCES

A number of useful Internet sites can be accessed to find characteristics of mutant hemoglobins and literature references as well as safety information about blood handling.

1. Globin database: http://globin.cse.psu.edu. Mutant hemoglobins and their properties.
2. Swiss protein database: www.expasy.ch. Protein sequences, molecular weights.
3. Protein Data Bank: www.rcsb.org/pdb. Protein sequences, crystallographic coordinates.
4. OSHA: www.osha.gov. Safety information about blood handling.

References

Adachi, K and Asakura, T. (1979a). Gelation of deoxyhemoglobin A in concentrated phosphate buffer. Exhibition of delay time prior to aggregation and crystallization of deoxyhemoglobin A. *J. Biol. Chem.* 254: 12273–12276.

Adachi, K and Asakura, T. (1979b). The solubility of sickle and non-sickle hemoglobins in concentrated phosphate buffer. *J. Biol. Chem.* 254: 4079–4084.

Alami, R, Gilman, JG, Feng, YQ et al. (1999). Anti-β^S ribozyme reduces β^S mRNA levels in transgenic mice: Potential application to the gene therapy of sickle cell anemia. *Blood Cells Mol. Dis.* 25: 110–119.

Anonymous. (1978). Recommendations for selected methods for quantitative estimation of HbA2 and for Hb A2 reference preparation. International committee for standardization in haematology. *Br. J. Haematol.* 38: 573–578.

Arcasoy, MO, Romana, M, Fabry, ME et al. (1997). High levels of human gamma-globin gene expression in adult mice carrying a transgene of deletion-type hereditary persistence of fetal hemoglobin. *Mol. Cell. Biol.* 17: 2076–2089.

Armsby, CC, Brugnara, C, and Alper, SL. (1995). Cation transport in mouse erythrocytes: Role of K(+)-Cl-cotransport in regulatory volume decrease. *Am. J. Physiol.* 268 (Pt 1): C894–902.

Bakhtiar, R, Wu, Q, Hofstadler, SA, and Smith, RD. (1994). Charge state specific facile gas-phase cleavage of Asp 75-Met 76 peptide bond in the alpha-chain of human apohemoglobin probed by electrospray ionization mass spectrometry. *Biol. Mass. Spectrom.* 23: 707–710.

Bank, N, Aynedjian, HS, Qiu, JH et al. (1996). Renal nitric oxide synthases in transgenic sickle cell mice. *Kidney Int.* 50: 184–189.

Bank, N, Kiroycheva, M, Ahmed, F et al. (1998). Peroxynitrite formation and apoptosis in transgenic sickle cell mouse kidneys. *Kidney Int.* 54: 1520–1528.

Banks, JF. (1997). Recent advances in capillary electrophoresis/electrospray/mass spectrometry. [Review] [104 refs]. *Electrophoresis* 18: 2255–2266.

Basset, P, Braconnier, F, and Rosa, J. (1982). An update on electrophoretic and chromatographic methods in the diagnosis of hemoglobinopathies. [Review] [174 refs]. *J. Chromatog.* 227: 267–304.

Benesch, RE, Edalji, R, Kwong, S, and Benesch, R. (1978). Oxygen affinity as an index of hemoglobin S polymerization: A new micromethod. *Anal. Biochem.* 89: 162–173.

Bentley, SA, Johnson, A, and Bishop, CA. (1993). A parallel evaluation of four automated hematology analyzers. *Am. J. Clin. Pathol.* 100: 626–632.

Betke, K and Kleihauer, E. (1969). The acid elution technique and the question of the influence of membrane qualities on its results. *Ann. Soc. Belge Med. Trop.* 49: 151–156.

Betke, K, Marti, HQ, and Schlicht, I. (1959). Estimation of small percentages of foetal haemoglobin. *Nature* 184: 877.

Blouin, MJ, Beauchemin, H, Wright, A et al. (2000). Genetic correction of sickle cell disease: insights using transgenic mouse models. *Nat. Med.* 6: 177–182.

Blumenfeld, N, Fabry, ME, Thysen, B, and Nagel, RL. (1988). Red cell density is sex and race dependent in the adult. *J. Lab. Clin. Med.* 112: 333–338.

Bookchin, RM, Balazs, T, Wang, Z et al. (1999). Polymer structure and solubility of deoxyhemoglobin S in the presence of high concentrations of volume-excluding 70-kDa dextran. *J. Biol. Chem.* 274: 6689–6697.

Bouhassira, EE, Westerman, K, and Leboulch, P. (1997). Transcriptional behavior of LCR enhancer elements integrated at the same chromosomal locus by recombinase-mediated cassette exchange. *Blood* 90: 3332–3344.

Boyer, SH, Dover, GJ, Serjeant, GR et al. (1984). Production of F cells in sickle cell anemia: Regulation by a genetic locus or loci separate from the beta-globin gene cluster. *Blood* 64: 1053–1058.

Brugnara, C, Zelmanovic, D, Sorette, M et al. (1997). Reticulocyte hemoglobin: An integrated parameter for evaluation of erythropoietic activity. *Am. J. Clin. Path.* 108: 133–142.

Cao, P and Moini, M. (1999). Separation and detection of the alpha- and beta-chains of hemoglobin of single intact red blood cells using capillary electrophoresis/electrospray ionization time-of-flight mass spectrometry. *J. Am. Soc. Mass Spectrom.* 10: 184–186.

Chada, K, Magram, J, and Costantini, F. (1985). Tissue- and stage-specific expression of a cloned adult beta globin gene in transgenic mice. *Prog. Clin. Biol. Res.* 191: 305–319.

Chang, JC, Lu, R, Lin, C et al. (1998). Transgenic knockout mice exclusively expressing human hemoglobin S after transfer of a 240-kb beta-globin yeast artificial chromosome: A mouse model of sickle cell anemia. *Proc. Natl. Acad. Sci. U.S.A.* 95 14886–14890.

Ciavatta, DJ, Ryan, TM, Farmer, SC, and Townes, TM. (1995). Mouse model of human beta zero thalassemia: Targeted deletion of the mouse beta maj- and beta min-globin genes in embryonic stem cells. *Proc. Natl. Acad. Sci. U.S.A.* 92: 9259–9263.

Cividalli, G, Kerem, H, and Rachmilewitz, EA. (1977). Homozygous beta-0 and beta-+ thalassemia in Kurdish Jews and Arabs. *Hemoglobin* 1: 333–347.

Clark, MR, Morrison, CE, and Shohet, SB. (1978). Monovalent cation transport in irreversibly sickled cells. *J. Clin. Invest.* 62: 329–337.

Coletta, M, Hofrichter, J, Ferrone, FA, and Eaton, WA. (1982). Kinetics of sickle haemoglobin polymerization in single red cells. *Nature* 300: 194–197.

Corry, WD and Meiselman, HJ. (1978). Modification of erythrocyte physiochemical properties by millimolar concentrations of glutaraldehyde. *Blood Cells* 4: 465–480.

Costantini, F and Lacy, E. (1981). Introduction of a rabbit beta-globin gene into the mouse germ line. *Nature* 294: 92–94.

Costantini, F, Chada, K, and Magram, J. (1986). Correction of murine beta-thalassemia by gene transfer into the germ line. *Science* 233: 1192–1194.

Craver, RD, Abermanis, JG, Warrier, RP et al. (1997). Hemoglobin A2 levels in healthy persons, sickle cell disease, sickle cell trait, and beta-thalassemia by capillary isoelectric focusing. *Am. J. Clin. Pathol.* 107: 88–91.

Crispins, CG. (1975). *Handbook on the Laboratory Mouse.* Springfield, IL: Charles C Thomas.

Dacie, JV and Lewis, SM. (1995). *Practical Hematology.* Edinburgh: Churchill Livingstone.

de Franceschi, L, Saadane, N, Trudel, M et al. (1994). Treatment with oral clotrimazole blocks Ca(2+)-activated K+ transport and reverses erythrocyte dehydration in transgenic SAD mice. A model for therapy of sickle cell disease. *J. Clin. Invest.* 93: 1670–1676.

de Franceschi, L, Beuzard, Y, and Brugnara, C. (1995). Sulfhydryl oxidation and activation of red cell K(+)-Cl-cotransport in the transgenic SAD mouse. *Am. J. Physiol.* 269 (Pt 1): C899–906.

de Franceschi, L, Beuzard, Y, Jouault, H, and Brugnara, C. (1996a). Modulation of erythrocyte potassium chloride cotransport, potassium content, and density by dietary magnesium intake in transgenic SAD mouse. *Blood* 88: 2738–2744.

de Franceschi, L, Rouyer-Fessard, P, Alper, SL et al. (1996b). Combination therapy of erythropoietin, hydroxyurea, and clotrimazole in a beta thalassemic mouse: A model for human therapy. *Blood* 87: 1188–1195.

Detloff, PJ, Lewis, J, John, SW et al. (1994). Deletion and replacement of the mouse adult beta-globin genes by a "plug and socket" repeated targeting strategy. *Mol. Cell. Biol.* 94: 6936–6943.

Dole, M, Mack, LL, Hines, RL et al. (1968). Molecular beams of macroions. *J. Chem. Phys.* 49: 2240–2249.

Eaton, WA and Hofrichter, J. (1987). Hemoglobin S gelation and sickle cell disease. *Blood* 70: 1245–1266.

Eaton, WA and Hofrichter, J. (1990). Sickle cell hemoglobin polymerization. *Adv. Protein. Chem.* 40: 63–279.

Enwonwu, CO. (1989). Increased metabolic demand for arginine in sickle cell anemia. *Med. Sci. Res.* 17: 997–998.

Epstein, N, Epstein, M, Boulet, A et al. (1996). Monoclonal antibody-based methods for quantitation of hemoglobins: Application to evaluating patients with sickle cell anemia treated with hydroxyurea. *Eur. J. Haematol.* 57: 17–24.

Fabry, ME, Costantini, F, Pachnis, A et al. (1992a). High expression of human β^S- and α-globins in transgenic mice: Erythrocyte abnormalities, organ damage, and the effect of hypoxia. *Proc Nat. Acad. Sci. U.S.A.* 89: 12155–12159.

Fabry, ME and Nagel, RL. (1982a). Heterogeneity of red cells in the sickler: A characteristic with practical clinical and pathophysiological implications. *Blood Cells* 8: 9–15.

Fabry, ME and Nagel, RL. (1982b). The effect of deoxygenation on red cell density: Significance for the pathophysiology of sickle cell anemia. *Blood* 60: 1370–1377.

Fabry, ME, Nagel, RL, Pachnis A et al. (1992). High expression of human β^S and α-globins in transgenic mice: Hemoglobin composition and hematological consequences. *Proc. Natl. Acad. Sci. U.S.A.* 89: 12150–12154.

Fabry, ME, Sengupta, A, Suzuka, SM et al. (1995a). A second generation transgenic mouse model expressing both hemoglobin S (HbS) and HbS-Antilles results in increased phenotypic severity. *Blood* 86: 2419–2428.

Fabry, ME, Suzuka, SM, Rubin, EM, Costantini, E et al. (1995b). Strategies for amelioration of sickle cell disease: Use of transgenic mice for validation of anti-sickling strategies. In Beuzard, Y, Lubin, B, and Rosa, J, editors. *Sickle cell disease and thalassemias: New trends in therapy.* London: John Libbey Eurotext Ltd, p. 253.

Fabry, ME, Romero, JR, Suzuka, SM et al. (1998). Hemoglobin C in transgenic mice with full mouse globin knockouts. *Blood* 92: 330a (abstract).

Fabry, ME, Suzuka, SM, Gilman, JG et al. (1999). Second generation knock-out mice are useful for validation of gene therapy strategies. *Blood* 94: 645a.

Ferranti, P, Carbone, V, Sannolo, N et al. (1993). Mass spectrometric analysis of rat hemoglobin by FAB-overlapping. Primary structure of the alpha-major and of four beta constitutive chains. *Int. J. Biochem.* 25: 1943–1950.

Ferrige, AG, Seddon, MJ, Green, BN et al. (1992). Disentangling electrospray spectra with maximum entropy. *Rapid Communications in Mass. Spectrometry.* 6: 707–711.

Frazier, JL, Caskey, JH, Yoffe, M, and Seligman, PA. (1982). Studies of the transferrin receptor on both human reticulocytes and nucleated human cells in culture: Comparison of factors regulating receptor density. *J. Clin. Invest.* 69: 853–865.

Galanello, R, Satta, S, Pirroni, MG et al. (1998). Globin chain synthesis by high performance liquid chromatography in the screening of thalassemia syndromes. *Hemoglobin* 22: 501–508.

Garver, FA, Jones, CS, Baker, MM et al. (1976). Specific radioimmunochemical identification and quantitation of hemoglobins A2 and F. *Am. J. Hematol.* 1: 459–469.

Garver, FA, Singh, H, Moscoso, H et al. (1984). Identification and quantification of hemoglobins A2 and Barts with an enzyme-labeled immunosorbent assay. *Clin. Chem.* 30: 1205–1208.

Gilman, JG, Fabry, ME, Suzuka, SM, and Nagel, RL. (1995). Human G-gamma:A-gamma globin ratios switch during prenatal development in a transgenic mouse with HS4-G-gamma (–158T)-A-gamma. *Blood* 86: 648a.

Gordon, RE, Hanley, PE, Shaw, D et al. (1980). Localization of metabolites in animals using 31P topical magnetic resonance. *Nature* 287: 736–738.

Greaves, DR, Fraser, P, Vidal, MA et al. (1990). A transgenic mouse model of sickle cell disorder. *Nature* 343: 183–185.

Gulati, GL, Hyun, BH, and Ashton, JK. (1992). Advances of the past decade in automated hematology. [Review] [55 refs]. *Am. J. Clin. Pathol.* 98(Suppl 6). S11–6.

Harrington, JP and Nagel, RL. (1977). The effects of alkylureas and nitrogen mustards on the kinetics of red cell sickling. *J. Lab. Clin. Med.* 90: 863–872.

Hebbel, RP, Boogaerts, MAB, Eaton, JW, and Steinberg, MH. (1980). Erythrocyte adherence in sickle cell disorders. *N. Engl. J. Med.* 302: 992.

Hofstadler, SA, Swanek, FD, Gale, DC et al. (1995). Capillary electrophoresis-electrospray ionization Fourier transform ion cyclotron resonance mass spectrometry for direct analysis of cellular proteins. *Anal. Chem.* 67: 1477–1480.

Hogan, BLM, Costantini, F, and Lacy, E. (1986). *Manipulating the Mouse Embryo: A Laboratory Manual.* Cold Spring Harbor: Cold Spring Harbor Laboratory.

Huisman, TH. (1987). Separation of hemoglobins and hemoglobin chains by high-performance liquid chromatography. [Review] [53]. *J. Chromatogr.* 418: 277–304.

Jenkins, MA, Hendy, J, and Smith, IL. (1997). Evaluation of hemoglobin A2 quantitation assay and hemoglobin variant screening by capillary electrophoresis. *J. Capillary Electrophoresis* 4: 137–143.

Jones, RG, Faust, AM, and Matthews, RA. (1995). Quality team approach in evaluating three automated hematology analyzers with five-part differential capability. *Am. J. Clin. Pathol.* 103: 159–166.

Jonxis, JHP and Visser, HKA. (1956). Determination of low percentages of fetal hemoglobin in blood of normal children. *Am. J. Dis. Child.* 92: 588.

Kan, YW, Dozy, AM, Alter, BP et al. (1972). Detection of the sickle gene in the human fetus. Potential for intrauterine diagnosis of sickle-cell anemia. *N. Engl. J. Med.* 287: 1–5.

Kaul, DK, Fabry, ME, Costantini, F et al. (1995). In vivo demonstration of red cell-endothelial interaction, sickling and altered microvascular response to oxygen in the sickle transgenic mouse. *J. Clin. Invest.* 96: 2845–2853.

Kaul, DK, Liu, XD, Fabry, ME, and Nagel, RL. (1998). Increased nitric oxide synthase expression in transgenic sickle mice is associated with relative hypotension and altered microvascular response. *Blood* 92: 330a (abstract).

Kleihauer, E. (1974). Determination of fetal hemoglobin: Elution technique. In Schmidt, RM, Huisman, TH, and Lehman, H, editors. *The detection of hemoglobinopathies.* Cleveland: CRC Press.

Kollias, G, Wrighton, N, Hurst, J, and Grosveld, F. (1986). Regulated expression of human A gamma-, beta-, and hybrid gamma beta-globin genes in transgenic mice: Manipulation of the developmental expression patterns. *Cell* 46: 89–94.

Lacy, E, Roberts, S, Evans, EP et al. (1983). A foreign beta-globin gene in transgenic mice: Integration at abnormal chromosomal positions and expression in inappropriate tissues. *Cell* 34: 343–358.

Lawrence, C, Fabry, ME, and Nagel, RL. (1985). Red cell distribution width parallels dense red cell disappearance during painful crises in sickle cell anemia. *J. Lab. Clin. Med.* 105: 706–710.

Light-Wahl, KJ, Loo, JA, Edmonds, CG et al. (1993). Collisionally activated dissociation and tandem mass spectrometry of intact hemoglobin beta-chain variant proteins with electrospray ionization. *Biol. Mass. Spectrom.* 22: 112–120.

Lipowsky, HH, Sheikh, NU, and Katz, DM. (1987). Intravital microscopy of capillary hemodynamics in sickle cell disease. *J. Clin. Invest.* 80: 117–127.

Lutty, GA, McLeod, DS, Pachnis, A et al. (1994). Retinal and choroidal neovascularization in a transgenic mouse model of sickle cell disease. *Am. J. Pathol.* 145: 490–497.

Lutty, GA, Merges, C, McLeod, DS et al. (1998). Nonperfusion of retina and choroid in transgenic mouse models of sickle cell disease. *Curr. Eye Res.* 17: 438–444.

Marikovsky, Y, Lotan, R, Lis, H et al. (1976). Agglutination and labeling density of soybean agglutinin on young and old human red blood cells. *Exp. Cell Res.* 99: 453–456.

Mario, N, Baudin, B, Aussel, C, and Giboudeau, J. (1997). Capillary isoelectric focusing and high-performance cation-exchange chromatography compared for qualitative and quantitative analysis of hemoglobin variants. *Clin. Chem.* 43: 2137–2142.

Martinell, J, Whitney, JB III, Popp, RA et al. (1981). Three mouse models of human thalassemia. *Proc. Natl. Acad. Sci. U. S. A.* 78: 5056–5060.

McLeod, DS, Merges, C, Fukushima, A et al. (1997). Histopathologic features of neovascularization in sickle cell retinopathy. *Am. J. Ophthalmol.* 124: 455–472.

Milner, PF, Miller, C, Grey, R et al. (1970). Hemoglobin O arab in four negro families and its interaction with hemoglobin S and hemoglobin C. *N. Engl. J. Med.* 283: 1417–1425.

Monplaisir, N, Merault, G, Poyart, C et al. (1986). Hemoglobin S Antilles: A variant with lower solubility than hemoglobin S and producing sickle cell disease in heterozygotes. *Proc. Natl. Acad. Sci. U.S.A.* 83: 9363–9367.

Moscoso, H, Shyamala, M, Kiefer, CR, and Garver, FA. (1989). Monoclonal antibody to the gamma chain of human fetal hemoglobin used to develop an enzyme immunoassay. *Clin. Chem.* 35: 2066–2069.

Mozzarelli, A, Hofrichter, J, and Eaton, WA. (1987). The problem of describing gelation in vivo. *Prog. Clin. Biol. Res.* 240: 237–244.

Murray, LP, Hofrichter, J, Henry, ER, and Eaton, WA. (1988). Time-resolved optical spectroscopy and structural dynamics following photodissociation of carbonmonoxyhemoglobin. *Biophys. Chem.* 29: 63–76.

Nagel, RL, Raventos Suarez, C, Fabry, ME et al. (1981). Impairment of the growth of Plasmodium falciparum in HbEE erythrocytes. *J. Clin. Invest.* 68: 303–305.

Nagel, RL, Sharma, A, Kumar, R, and Fabry, ME. (1995). Severe red cell abnormalities in transgenic mice expressing high levels of normal human delta chains. *Blood* 86: 990a (abstract).

Osei, SY, Ahima, RS, Fabry, ME et al. (1996). Immunohistochemical localization of hepatic nitric oxide synthase in normal and transgenic sickle cell mice: The effect of hypoxia. *Blood* 88: 3583–3588.

Papassotiriou, I, Ducrocq, R, Prehu, C et al. (1998). Gamma chain heterogeneity: Determination of Hb F composition by perfusion chromatography. *Hemoglobin* 22: 469–481.

Park, CM. (1970). The dimerization of deoxyhemoglobin and of oxyhemoglobin. Evidence for cleavage along the same plane. *J. Biol. Chem.* 245: 5390–5394.

Pàszty, C, Mohandas, N, Stevens, ME et al. (1995). Lethal alpha-thalassaemia created by gene targeting in mice and its genetic rescue. *Nat. Genet.* 11: 33–39.

Pàszty, C, Brion, CM, Manci, E et al. (1997). Transgenic knockout mice with exclusively human sickle hemoglobin and sickle cell disease. *Science* 278: 876–878.

Pegelow, CH, Colangelo, L, Steinberg, M et al. (1997). Natural history of blood pressure in sickle cell disease: Risks for stroke and death associated with relative hypertension in sickle cell anemia. *Am. J. Med.* 102: 171–177.

Ponder, E. (1948). *Hemolysis and Related Phenomena.* New York: Grune & Stratton.

Popp, RA, Popp, DM, Shinpock, SG et al. (1997). A transgenic mouse model of hemoglobin S Antilles disease. *Blood* 89: 4204–4212.

Prehu, C, Ducrocq, R, Godart, C et al. (1998). Determination of Hb F levels: The routine methods. *Hemoglobin* 22: 459–467.

Reilly, MP, Chomo, MJ, Obata, K, and Asakura, T. (1994). Red blood cell membrane and density changes under ambient and hypoxic conditions in transgenic mice producing human sickle hemoglobin. *Exp. Hematol.* 22: 501–509.

Rhoda, MD, Domenget, C, Vidaud, M et al. (1988). Mouse alpha chains inhibit polymerization of hemoglobin induced by human beta S or beta S Antilles chains. *Biochim. Biophys. Acta* 952: 208–212.

Righetti, PG and Bossi, A. (1997). Isoelectric focusing in immobilized pH gradients: Recent analytical and preparative developments [Review] *Anal. Biochem.* 247: 1–10.

Righetti, PG, Gianazza, E, and Bjellqvist, B. (1983). Modern aspects of isoelectric focusing: Two-dimensional maps and immobilized pH gradients [Review] *J. Biochem. Biophys. Methods* 8: 89–108.

Righetti, PG, Gelfi, C, and Chiari, M. (1996). Isoelectric focusing in immobilized pH gradients. *Methods Enzymol.* 270: 235–255.

Rilbe, H. (1995). Some reminiscences of the history of electrophoresis. *Electrophoresis* 16: 1354–1359.

Rodgers, GP, Walker, EC and Podgor, MJ. (1993). Is "relative" hypertension a risk factor for vasoocclusive complications in sickle cell disease? *Am. J. Med. Sci.* 305: 150–156.

Romero, J, Fabry, ME, Suzuka, SM et al. (1997a). Red blood cells of a transgenic mouse expressing high levels of human hemoglobin S exhibit deoxy-stimulated cation flux. *J. Membrene Biol.* 159: 187–196.

Romero, JR, Fabry, ME, Suzuka, SM et al. (1997b). K:Cl cotransport in red cells of transgenic mice expressing high levels of human hemoglobin S. *Am. J. Hematol.* 55: 112–114.

Romero, JR, Suzuka, SM, Romero-Gonzalez, GV et al. (1999). Full knockout mouse red cells expressing HbC or HbS and γ have high K:Cl cotransport in contrast to low expression in HbA mouse red cells. *Blood.* 94: 198a.

Rouyer Fessard, P, Leroy Viard, K, Domenget, C et al. (1990). Mouse beta thalassemia, a model for the membrane defects of erythrocytes in the human disease. *J. Biol. Chem.* 265: 20247–20251.

Roy, RP, Nacharaju, P, Nagel, RL, and Acharya, AS. (1995). Symmetric interspecies hybrids of mouse and human hemoglobin: Molecular basis of their abnormal oxygen affinity. *J. Protein Chem.* 14: 81–88.

Rubin, EM, Lu, RH, Cooper, S et al. (1988). Introduction and expression of the human β^S-globin gene in transgenic mice. *Am. J. Hum. Genet.* 42: 585–591.

Rubin, EM, Witkowska, HE, Spangler, E et al. (1991). Hypoxia-induced in vivo sickling of transgenic mouse red cells. *J. Clin. Invest.* 87: 639–647.

Rutland, PC, Pembrey, ME, and Davies, T. (1983). The estimation of fetal haemoglobin in healthy adults by radioimmunoassay. *Br. J. Haematol.* 53: 673–682.

Ryan, TM, Townes, TM, Reilly, MP et al. (1990). Human sickle hemoglobin in transgenic mice. *Science* 247: 566–568.

Ryan, TM, Ciavatta, DJ, and Townes, TM. (1997). Knockout-transgenic mouse model of sickle cell disease. *Science* 278: 873–876.

Schneider, RG. (1974). Differentiation of electrophoretically similar hemoglobins—such as S, D, G, and P; or A2, C, E, and O—by electrophoresis of the globin chains. *Clin. Chem.* 20: 1111–1115.

Schroeder, WA, Shelton, JB, Shelton, JR, and Huynh, V. (1986). The estimation of Hb A2 in the presence of Hb C or Hb E by reverse phase high performance liquid chromatography. *Hemoglobin* 10: 253–257.

Scott, AF, Bunn, HF, and Brush, AH. (1976). Functional aspects of hemoglobin evolution in the mammals. *J. Mol. Evol.* 8: 311–316.

Seibler, J, Schubeler, D, Fiering, S et al. (1998). DNA cassette exchange in ES cells mediated by Flp recombinase: An efficient strategy for repeated modification of tagged loci by marker-free constructs. *Biochemistry* 37: 6229–6234.

Shackleton, CH and Witkowska, HE. (1996). Characterizing abnormal hemoglobin by MS [Review]. *Anal. Chem.* 68: 29A–33A.

Shaeffer, JR, McDonald, MJ, Turci, SM et al. (1984). Dimer-monomer dissociation of human hemoglobin A. *J. Biol. Chem.* 259: 14544–14547.

Shehee, WR, Oliver, P, and Smithies, O. (1993). Lethal thalassemia after insertional disruption of the mouse major adult beta-globin gene. *Proc. Natl. Acad. Sci. U.S.A.* 90: 3177–3181.

Shelton, JB and Schroeder, WA. (1984). Separation of globin chains on a large pore C4 column. *J. Liq. Chromatogr.* 1: 1969–1977.

Skow, LC, Burkhart, BA, Johnson, FM et al. (1983). A mouse model for beta-thalassemia. *Cell* 34: 1043–1052.

Stamatoyannopoulos, G, Farquhar, M, Lindsley, D et al. (1983). Monoclonal antibodies specific for globin chains. *Blood* 61: 530–539.

Steinberg, MH and Adams, JG. (1991). Hemoglobin A2: Origin, evolution, and aftermath [Review]. *Blood* 78: 2165–2177.

Steinberg, MH, Lu, ZH, Barton, FB et al. (1997). Fetal hemoglobin in sickle cell anemia: Determinants of response to hydroxyurea. Multicenter Study of Hydroxyurea. *Blood* 89: 1078–1088.

Suh, DD, Krauss, JS, and Bures, K. (1996). Influence of hemoglobin S adducts on hemoglobin A2 quantification by HPLC. *Clin. Chem.* 42: 1113–1114.

Swerdlow, PH, Bryan, RA, Bertles, JF et al. (1977). Effect of 2, 3-diphosphoglycerate on the solubility of deoxy-sickle hemoglobin. *Hemoglobin* 1: 527–537.

Tegos, C and Beutler, E. (1980). Glycosylated hemoglobin A2 components. *Blood* 56: 571–572.

Thein, SL and Craig, JE. (1998). Genetics of Hb F/F cell variance in adults and heterocellular hereditary persistence of fetal hemoglobin [Review]. *Hemoglobin* 22: 401–414.

Thein, SI and Reittie, JE. (1998). F cells by immunofluorescent staining of erythrocyte smears. *Hemoglobin* 22: 415–417.

Tosteson, DC, Carlsen, E, and Dunham, ET. (1955). The effect of sickling on ion transport. I. The effect of sickling on potassium transport. *J. Gen. Physiol.* 39: 31–53.

Townes, TM, Lingrel, JB, Chen, HY et al. (1985). Erythroid-specific expression of human beta-globin genes in transgenic mice. *EMBO J.* 4: 1715–1723.

Trudel, M, Saadane, N, Garel, M-C et al. (1991). Towards a transgenic mouse model of sickle cell disease: Hemoglobin SAD. *EMBO J.* 10: 3157–3168.

Trudel, MC, De Paepe, ME, Chretien, N et al. (1994). Sickle cell disease of transgenic SAD mice. *Blood* 84: 3189–3197.

Tuan, D, Solomon, W, Li, Q, and London, IM. (1985). The "beta-like-globin" gene domain in human erythroid cells. *Proc. Natl. Acad. Sci. U.S.A.* 82: 6384–6388.

Ueda, S and Schneider, RG. (1969). Rapid differentiation of polypeptide chains of hemoglobin by cellulose acetate electrophoresis of hemolysates. *Blood* 34: 230–235.

Vettore, L, Zanella, A, Molaro, GL et al. (1984). A new test for the laboratory diagnosis of spherocytosis. *Acta Haematol.* 72: 258–263.

White, SP, Birch, P, and Kumar, R. (1994). Interactions at the alpha 1 beta 1 interface in hemoglobin: A single amino acid change affects dimer ratio in transgenic mice expressing human hemoglobin. *Hemoglobin* 18: 413–426.

Whitney, JB. (1978). Simplified typing of mouse hemoglobin (Hbb) phenotypes using cystamine. *Biochem. Genet.* 16: 667–672.

Whitney, JB III. (1982). Mouse hemoglobinopathies: Detection and characterization of thalassemias and globin-structure mutations. *Prog. Clin. Biol. Res.* 94: 133–142.

Whitney, JB III and Popp, RA. (1984). Animal model of human disease: Thalassemia: Alpha-thalassemia in laboratory mice. *Am. J. Pathol.* 116: 523–525.

Whitney, JB. 3rd, Martinell, J, Popp, RA et al. (1981). Deletions in the alpha-globin gene complex in alpha-thalassemic mice. *Proc. Natl. Acad. Sci. U.S.A.* 78: 7644–7647.

Wilson, JB. (1989). Separation of human hemoglobin variants by HPLC. In Gooding, K and Reymer, F, editors. *HPLC of biological macromolecules: Methods and application.* New York: Marcel Dekker, p. 1.

Winter, WP and Yodh, J. (1983). Interaction of human hemoglobin and its variants with agar. *Science* 221: 175–178.

Witkowska, HE, Lubin, BH, Beuzard, Y et al. (1991). Sickle cell disease in a patient with sickle cell trait and compound heterozygosity for hemoglobin S and hemoglobin Quebec-Chori. *N. Engl. J. Med.* 325: 1150–1154.

Wu, J and Pawliszyn, J. (1995). Application of capillary isoelectric focusing with absorption imaging detection to the quantitative determination of human hemoglobin variants. *Electrophoresis* 16: 670–673.

Xia, Y, Dawson, VL, Dawson, TM et al. (1996). Nitric oxide synthase generates superoxide and nitric oxide in arginine-depleted cells leading to peroxynitrite-mediated cellular injury. *Proc. Natl. Acad. Sci. U.S.A.* 93: 6770–6774.

Yamashita, M and Fenn, JB. (1984). Electrospray ion source. Another variation on the free-jet theme. *J. Phys. Chem.* 88: 4451–4459.

Yang, B, Kirby, S, Lewis, J et al. (1995). A mouse model for β^0-thalassemia. *Proc. Natl. Acad. Sci. U.S.A.* 92: 11608–11612.

Zago, MA, Wood, WG, Clegg, JB et al. (1979). Genetic control of F cells in human adults. *Blood* 53: 977–986.

35

DNA-Based Diagnosis of the Hemoglobin Disorders

J. M. OLD

INTRODUCTION

The hemoglobinopathies are a diverse group of autosomal recessive disorders characterized by either the synthesis of a structurally abnormal globin (the hemoglobin variants) or the reduced synthesis of one or more of the globin chains (the thalassemias). As a group they are the most common single gene disorder in the world and are found at high frequencies in many populations as a result of positive selection pressure due to falciparum malaria. Heterozygous individuals are easily identifiable by hematologic and molecular analysis, permitting the control of the serious hemoglobinopathies by a program of carrier screening, counseling, and prenatal diagnosis by fetal DNA analysis. The most important disorders for which prenatal diagnosis is considered are α^0 thalassemia, β thalassemia, sickle cell anemia, and the various compound heterozygous states that result in a clinically significant disease.

Although almost a thousand mutant alleles resulting in hemoglobin disorders have now been characterized at the molecular level, mutation analysis for the hemoglobin disorders is simplified because the molecular defects are regionally specific. Each local population has its own characteristic spectrum of a small number of hemoglobin variants and thalassemia mutations. These have been characterized for most at-risk ethnic groups and the allele frequencies are known. Therefore, knowledge of the ethnic origin of a patient under study usually enables the quick identification of the underlying molecular defects by the application of molecular biology techniques. The majority of the molecular defects can be diagnosed using a variety of techniques based on the amplification of DNA by the polymerase chain reaction (PCR). In most cases there are several methods available for the diagnosis of any one particular mutation and this chapter provides an overview of the methods currently being used. The methods described with primer sequences are the ones I have had most experience with in my laboratory.

SOURCES OF DNA

Blood

DNA is normally prepared from 5 to 10 mL of peripheral blood that is anticoagulated with heparin or, preferably, EDTA. The DNA can be isolated by the standard method of phenol-chloroform extraction and ethanol precipitation, or by using one of the several kits on the market based on salt extraction, protein precipitation, and so forth. Sufficient DNA is obtained for molecular analysis and subsequent storage in a DNA bank at $-20°C$. If this is not required, a much smaller quantity of blood may be used for PCR diagnosis of the globin gene disorders. Mutation analysis may be carried out by simply adding 1 μL of boiled whole blood to the PCR reaction mixture (Liu et al., 2000).

Amniotic Fluid

DNA can be prepared from amniotic fluid cells directly or after culturing. It takes 2 to 3 weeks to grow amniocytes to confluence in a 25-mL flask, but culturing has the advantage that a large amount of DNA is obtained (in our experience, the yield from such a flask has varied from 15 to 45 μg, enough DNA for all types of analyses). However, not all laboratories have the facilities for cell culture and diagnosis can be made using DNA from noncultivated cells in most cases. Approximately 5 μg of DNA is obtained from 15 mL of amniotic fluid and this is sufficient for any PCR-based method of analysis. However, for genotype analysis by Southern blotting it is only enough for one attempt and thus a small portion should be prudently set aside for culturing in case of failure. The method of DNA preparation for both cultured and noncultivated cells is essentially the same as that for chorionic villi (Old, 1986).

Martin H. Steinberg, Bernard G. Forget, Douglas R. Higgs, and Ronald L. Nagel, editors. *Disorders of Hemoglobin: Genetics, Pathophysiology, and Clinical Management.* © 2001 Cambridge University Press. All rights reserved.

Chorionic Villi

The two main approaches to chorionic villus sampling, ultrasound-guided transcervical aspiration and ultrasound-guided transabdominal sampling, both provide good quality samples of chorionic villi for fetal DNA diagnosis. Sufficient DNA is normally obtained for both PCR and Southern blot analysis of the globin genes. For our first 200 CVS DNA diagnoses the average yield of DNA was 46 µg and only in one instance was less than 5 µg obtained (Old, 1986).

The main technical problem with this source of fetal DNA is the risk of contamination with maternal DNA, which arises from the maternal decidua that is sometimes obtained along with the chorionic villi. However, by careful dissection and removal of the maternal decidua with the aid of a phase-contrast microscope, pure fetal DNA samples can be obtained, as shown by Rosatelli et al. (1992) who reported no misdiagnoses in a total of 457 first trimester diagnoses for β thalassemia in the Italian population. Maternal contamination can be ruled out in most cases by the presence of one maternal and one paternal allele following the amplification of highly polymorphic repeat markers (Decorte et al., 1990). The risk of misdiagnosis through maternal DNA contamination can be further reduced by the preparation of DNA from a single villus frond.

Fetal Cells in Maternal Blood

Fetal cells have long been known to be present in the maternal circulation and they provide an attractive noninvasive approach to prenatal diagnosis. However attempts to isolate the fetal cells using immunologic methods and cell sorters have had little success in providing a population of cells pure enough for fetal DNA analysis. Until recently analysis of fetal cells in maternal blood could only be applied for the prenatal diagnosis of β thalassemia in women whose partners carried a different mutation, as reported for the diagnosis of Hb Lepore (Camaschella et al., 1990). However, the development of the technique of isolation of single nucleated fetal erythrocytes by micromanipulation under microscopic observation (Sekizawa et al., 1996) has permitted the analysis of both fetal genes in single cells from maternal blood. This approach has now been tried successfully for prenatal diagnosis in two pregnancies at risk for sickle cell anemia and β thalassemia (Cheung et al., 1996).

Preimplantation Diagnosis

Preimplantation genetic diagnosis (PGD) for the globin gene disorders is now possible by either DNA analysis of single cells biopsied from cleaving embryos or by analysis of polar body DNA obtained from the two polar bodies extruded during the maturation of the oocyte. Both approaches use nested PCR and appear to be subject to the problem of allele dropout, which, like the problem of maternal contamination, is overcome by the simultaneous analysis of other maternal and paternal markers. The birth of five healthy children following PGD for β thalassemia by polar body analysis has recently been reported (Kuliev et al., 1999).

DNA DIAGNOSIS OF α THALASSEMIA

α-Thalassemia results from either deletion mutations affecting the α-globin gene cluster or point mutations within one of the two α-globin genes (see Chapter 17). The deletion breakpoints of seven of the most common deletions have been sequenced and these alleles can now be diagnosed by PCR using the technique sometimes known as gap PCR. The other deletion alleles are diagnosed by Southern blot analysis and this approach remains in use in many laboratories for the molecular diagnosis of α-thalassemia because of its ability to diagnose all alleles in one test and for confirmation of prenatal diagnosis for α^0-thalassemia by gap PCR.

Diagnosis of Deletion Mutations by PCR

The two most common α^+-thalassemia deletion genes, the $-\alpha^{3.7}$ and $-\alpha^{4.2}$ alleles, together with five α^0-thalassemia deletion genes, the $- -^{FIL}$, $- -^{THAI}$, $- -^{MED}$, $-(\alpha)^{20.5}$, and the $- -^{SEA}$ alleles, can be diagnosed by gap PCR (Bowden et al., 1992; Dode et al., 1992; Baysal and Huisman, 1994; Ko and Li, 1999; Liu et al., 1999) (Table 35.1). Gap PCR is the simplest of amplification techniques, using two primers complementary to the sense and antisense strand of the DNA regions that flank the deletion. Amplified product is only obtained from the α-thalassemia deletion allele as the primers are located too far apart on the normal DNA sequence for successful amplification. Therefore the normal allele (αα) is detected by amplifying across one of the breakpoints, using one primer complementary to the deleted sequence and one to the normal sequence. An example of the use of gap PCR for the diagnosis of the Mediterranean α^0-thalassemia mutation $- -^{MED}$ is illustrated in Figure 35.1.

Gap PCR provides a quick diagnostic test for α^0-thalassemia trait but requires careful application for prenatal diagnosis. Amplification of sequences in the α-globin gene cluster is technically more difficult than that of the β-globin gene cluster, requiring more stringent conditions for success due to the higher G+C nucleotide content. Experience in my laboratory and others (Ko et al., 1997) has shown some of the pub-

Table 35.1. Thalassemia Deletion Mutations that Have Been Diagnosed by Gap PCR

Disorder	Deletion mutation	Reference
α^0 thalassemia	$- -^{SEA}$	(Molchanova et al., 1994)
	$- -^{MED}$	(Molchanova et al., 1994)
	$-(\alpha)^{20.5}$	(Molchanova et al., 1994)
	$- -^{FIL}$	(Ko and Li, 1999)
	$- -^{THAI}$	(Liu et al., 1999)
α^+ thalassemia	$-\alpha^{3.7}$	(Baysal and Huisman, 1994)
	$-\alpha^{4.2}$	(Baysal and Huisman, 1994)
β^0 thalassemia	290 bp deletion	(Faa et al., 1992)
	532 bp deletion	(Waye et al., 1991)
	619 bp deletion	(Old et al., 1990)
	1,393 bp deletion	(Thein et al., 1989)
	1,605 bp deletion	(Dimovski et al., 1993)
	3.5 kb deletion	(Lynch et al., 1991)
	10.3 kb deletion	(Craig et al., 1992)
	45 kb deletion	(Waye et al., 1994)
Hb Lepore	Hb Lepore	(Craig et al., 1994)
$(\delta\beta)^0$ thalassemia	Spanish	(Craig et al., 1994)
	Sicilian	(Craig et al., 1994)
	Vietnamese	(Craig et al., 1994)
	Macedonian/Turkish	(Craig et al., 1994)
$^G\gamma(^A\gamma\delta\beta)^0$ thalassemia	Indian	(Craig et al., 1994)
	Chinese	(Craig et al., 1994)
HPFH	HPFH1	(Craig et al., 1994)
	HPFH2	(Craig et al., 1994)
	HPFH3	(Craig et al., 1994)

selective amplification of the α-globin genes (Molchanova et al., 1994). This technique allows the amplified product from each α-globin gene to be analyzed for the expected known mutation according to the ethnic origin of the patient or the gene to be sequenced to identify new ones. Several of the nondeletion α^+-thalassemia mutations create or destroy a restriction enzyme site and may be analyzed for by restriction enzyme digestion of the amplified product. For example, Hb Constant Spring mutation can be diagnosed by Mse I digestion (Ko et al., 1993). In theory any technique for the direct detection of point mutations such as allele-specific oligonucleotide hybridization or allele-specific priming may be used for the diagnosis of nondeletion α^+-thalassemia mutations. However, no simple strategy to diagnose all the known mutations has been developed. The only published approach to date is a complex strategy involving the combined application of the indirect detection methods of denaturing gradient gel electrophoresis (DGGE) and single-strand conformation analysis (SSCA), followed by direct DNA sequencing (Hartveld et al., 1996).

lished primer pairs to be unreliable, resulting occasionally in unpredictable reaction failure and causing the problem of allele dropout.

For more reliable diagnosis of the carrier state by gap PCR, amplification of the GC-rich α-globin locus may be improved by utilizing betaine and dimethyl sulfoxide in the PCR reaction. These agents enhance the reaction by disrupting the base pairing of the GC-rich region and lead to the destabilization of the secondary structure by making the GC and AT base pairs equally stable in the DNA duplex. The application of these agents with redesigned primers has led to the development of multiplex assay to detect heterozygosity and homozygosity of the seven deletion mutations (Chong et al., 2000; Liu et al., 2000).

Diagnosis of Point Mutations by PCR

The nondeletion α^+-thalassemia mutations can be identified by PCR techniques following the

Southern Blot Analysis

Southern blot analysis, using a combination of restriction enzyme digests and gene probes, can be used to diagnose all the common deletion mutations and the triple and quadruple α-gene alleles. The enzymes BamH I and Bgl II are used routinely to diagnose most α-thalassemia deletions (Fig. 35.2). A list of the characteristic abnormal restriction fragments used in my laboratory for diagnostic purposes is presented in Table 35.2. The single, double, triple, and quadruple α-globin gene alleles are identified by a BamH I digest hybridized to an α-globin gene probe and this digest also provides a diagnostic test for the Mediterranean α^0-thalassemia deletion gene $-(\alpha)^{20.5}$. BamH I digested DNA hybridized to a ζ-globin gene probe provides a diagnostic test for the $- -^{SEA}$ α^0-thalassemia allele and, similarly, a Bgl II digest hybridized to a ζ-globin gene probe provides a diagnostic test for the $- -^{MED}$ allele. Diagnosis of most of the α-thalassemia alleles requires the interpretation of

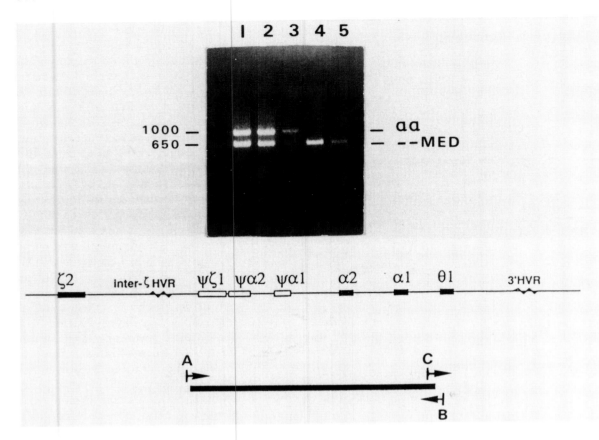

Figure 35.1. Prenatal diagnosis of the - -^MED α⁰-thalassemia allele using gap PCR. The amplification products after agarose gel electrophoresis and ethidium bromide staining are shown as follows: lane 1, maternal DNA; lane 2, paternal DNA; lane 3, normal DNA; lanes 4 and 5, different concentrations of chorionic villi DNA. The diagram below shows the location of the - -^MED deletion with respect to the α-globin gene cluster. Primers A and B span the deletion and amplify - -^MED allele to give a 650-bp product; primers B and C span one breakpoint and amplify the normal allele to give a 1,000-bp product.

the results obtained with two different enzyme digests and probe hybridizations, usually a *BamH* I/α-probe blot and a *Bgl* II/ζ-probe blot. This is because several alleles have similar sized abnormal *Bgl* II/ζ-probe fragments, and in addition, some alleles generate fragments with similar sizes to normal gene fragments. For example, both the –α³·⁷ and αααα alleles yield a 16-kb *Bgl* II/ζ fragment, the –α⁴·², - -^SA, and - -^BRIT alleles yield similar sized 7- to 8-kb *Bgl* II/ζ fragments, and the - -^SEA allele yields fragments that can be confused with a 10.5-kb normal fragment. A combination of *BamH* I and *Bgl* II digestions can be used for the diagnosis of all the common α-thalassemia deletion genes except for the - -^THAI and - -^FIL deletions. These two alleles are diagnosed using an *Sst* I digest hybridized to a DNA probe (named LO) located downstream of the ζ-globin gene (Fischel-Ghodsian et al., 1988).

DNA DIAGNOSIS OF β THALASSEMIA

Diagnostic Strategy

Although more than 175 different β thalassemias have been characterized (see Chapter 12), only approximately thirty mutations are found in at-risk groups at a frequency of 1 percent or greater (as listed in Table 35.3) and thus just a small number account for the majority of the mutations worldwide (Huisman, 1990). All of the mutations are regionally specific and the spectrum of mutations has now been determined for most at-risk populations. Each population has been found to have just a few of the common mutations together with a larger and more variable number of rare ones. This makes it easy to screen for β-thalassemia mutations in most cases if the ethnic origin of the patient is known.

The strategy for identifying β-thalassemia mutations in most diagnostic laboratories is to screen for the common ones first by using a PCR-based technique that allows the detection of multiple mutations simultaneously. This approach will identify the mutation in more than 90 percent of cases and then a further screening for the possible rare mutation will identify the defect in most of the remaining cases. Mutations remaining unknown after this second screening are characterized by direct DNA sequence

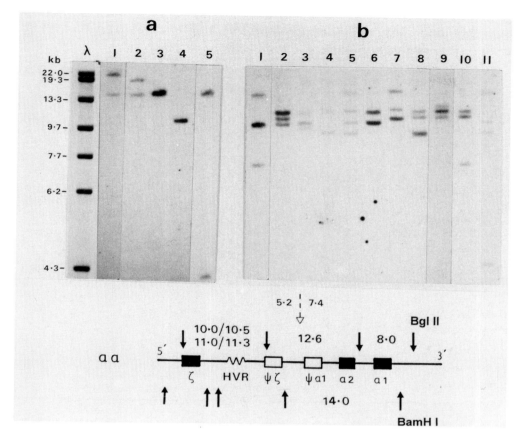

Figure 35.2. Southern blots showing the characterization of various α-thalassemia alleles: (a) shows *Bam*H I/α-probe hybridization; (b) shows *Bgl* II/ζ-probe hybridization. The first lane (λ) contains DNA marker fragments. The genotypes (and fragment sizes in kilobase pairs) illustrated for each lane are: (a) 1: ααααα/αα (22/14); 2: αααα/αα (18/14); 3: αα/αα (14); 4: −α³·⁷/−α³·⁷ (10.3); 5: −(α)²⁰·⁵/αα (14/4). (b) 1: −α³·⁷/−α⁴·² (16/11.0/8); 2: αα/αα (12.6/11.3/11.0); 3: −(α)²⁰·⁵/αα (12.6/11.0/10.8); 4: αα/αα (12.6/10.5); 5: −α³·⁷/αα (16/12.6/11.0/10.5); 6: αα/αα (12.6/11.0); 7: αα/αα (16/12.6/11.3); 8: − −ˢᴱᴬ/αα (12.6/11.3/10.5); 9: − −ᴹᴱᴰ/αα (13.9/12.6/11.3); 10: − −ᴮᴿᴵᵀ/αα (12.6/11.3/8); 11: −α³·⁷/−α³·⁷ (16/11.0/10.5/5.2). The diagram below the blots shows the positions of the *Bgl* II and *Bam*H I sites in normal DNA. The inter-ζ gene hypervariable region (HVR) gives rise to fragments of variable band sizes. There are four common *Bgl* II band sizes (10.0, 10.5, 11.0, and 11.3 kb) of which three are shown here. The ψζ gene also contains two small variable regions that give rise to occasional variation in the size of the 12.6-kb *Bgl* II fragment (lane 7). There is a polymorphic *Bgl* II site that, when present, reduces the 12.6-kb and −α³·⁷ 16-kb fragments to 5.2 kb (lane 11).

analysis. The β-globin gene can be amplified simultaneously in three sections of about 500 bp in length for direct DNA sequence analysis using an automatic DNA sequencer. Alternatively the site of the mutation may be localized first by the application of a nonspecific detection method such as denaturing gradient gel electrophoresis and then the mutation identified using just one sequencing reaction. Although a bewildering variety of PCR techniques have been described for the molecular diagnosis of point mutations, most diagnostic laboratories are using one or more of the techniques described below.

PCR: Allele-Specific Oligonucleotides

The hybridization of allele-specific oligonucleotide probes (ASOs) to amplified genomic DNA bound to a nylon membrane in the form of dots was the first PCR method to be developed. The method is based on the use of two oligonucleotide probes for each mutation, one complementary to the mutant DNA sequence and the other complementary to the normal β-gene sequence at the same position. The probes are usually 5′ end-labeled with either ³²P-labeled labeled deoxynucleoside triphosphates, biotin, or horseradish peroxidase. The genotype of the DNA sample is diagnosed by observing the presence or absence of a hybridization signal from the mutation specific and normal probes. The technique has been applied in many laboratories with great success, especially for populations with just one common mutation and a small number of rare ones, as in the example of Sardinia (Ristaldi et al., 1989). However, when screening for a large number of different mutations the method becomes limited by the

Table 35.2. The Diagnosis of α Thalassemia and Other Alleles by Southern Blotting

Allele	Restriction enzyme/gene probe				
	BamH I/α	Bgl II/α	BamH I/ζ	Bgl II/ζ	Sst I/LO
αα	14	12.6 7.4	10–11.3 5.9	12.6 or 5.2 10, 10.5, 11, or 11.3	5.0
ααα	18	12.6 7.4	10–11.3 5.9	12.6 or 16 10, 10.5, 11, or 11.3	5.0
αααα	22	12.6 7.4	10–11.3 5.9	12.6 or 20 10, 10.5, 11, or 11.3	5.0
$-\alpha^{3.7}$	10.3	16	10–11.3 5.9	16 10, 10.5, 11, or 11.3	5.0
$-\alpha^{4.2}$	9.8	8.0 7.4	10–11.3 5.9	10, 10.5, 11, or 11.3 8.0	5.0
$-(\alpha)^{20.5}$	4.0	10.8	5.9	10.8	5.0
- -MED	None	None	5.9	13.9	5.0
- -SEA	None	None	20 5.9	10.5	5.0
- -SA	None	None	5.9	7.0	5.0
- -BRIT	None	None	5.9	8.0	5.0
- -THAI	None	None	None	None	8.0
- -FIL	None	None	None	None	7.4

Note: Fragment sizes are given in kilobase pairs. Characteristic abnormal fragments are underlined.
LO: DNA probe located downstream of the ζ-globin gene (Fischel-Ghodsian et al., 1988.

need for separate hybridization and washing step for each detection of each mutation.

To overcome this problem of screening for multiple mutations, a method of reverse dot blotting has been developed in which the roles of the oligonucleotide probe and the amplified genomic DNA are reversed (Saiki et al., 1989). Unlabeled oligonucleotide probes complementary to the mutant and normal DNA sequences are fixed to a nylon membrane strip in the form of dots or slots. Amplified genomic DNA, labeled by either the use of end-labeled primers or the internal incorporation of biotinylated dUTP, is then hybridized to the filter. This procedure allows multiple mutations to be tested for in one hybridization reaction. It has been applied to the diagnosis of β-thalassemia mutations in Mediterranean individuals (Maggio et al., 1993), African Americans (Sutcharitchan et al., 1995), and Thais (Newton et al., 1989), using a two-step procedure with one nylon strip for the common mutations and another for the less common ones.

Reversed hybridization screening is the only technique for the diagnosis of β-thalassemia mutations to have been developed commercially with some success and currently there are two competing systems on the market. ViennaLab (Vienna, Austria) has a strip with oligonucleotide probes for eight common Mediterranean mutations fixed to it, together with probes to detect HbS and HbC mutations in amplified DNA. Bio-Rad (Hercules, CA) has developed a different system

with the oligonucleotides complementary to mutant and normal sequences immobilized on the wells of a microplate; this is a more complex system requiring a dedicated microplate incubator, washer, and reader to carry out the test. There are two kits on the market, one for eight common Mediterranean mutations and one for the eight most common Southeast Asian β-thalassemia mutations (including HbE).

PCR: Primer-Specific Amplification

A number of different diagnostic methods have been developed based on the principle of primer-specific amplification, which is that a perfectly matched PCR primer is much more efficient in annealing and directing primer extension than a mismatched one. The most widely used method is known as the amplification refractory mutation system (ARMS), in which a primer will only permit amplification to take place when it perfectly matches the target DNA sequence at the 3′ terminal nucleotide (Newton et al., 1989). The target DNA is amplified using a common primer and either of two allele-specific primers, one complementary to the mutation to be detected (the β-thalassemia primer) and the other complementary to normal DNA sequence at the same position. The method provides a quick screening assay that does not require any form of labeling as the amplified products are visualized simply by agarose gel electrophoresis and ethidium bromide staining.

Table 35.3. The Distribution of the Common β-Thalassemia Mutations Expressed as Percentage of Gene Frequencies of the Total Number of Thalassemia Chromosomes Studied

| Mutation | Mediterranean | | | India | | Chinese | | African |
	Italy	Greece	Turkey	Pakistan	India	China	Thailand	African American
−88(C→T)					0.8			21.4
−87(C→G)	0.4	1.8	1.2					
−30(T→A)			2.5					
−29(A→G)						1.9		60.3
−28(A→G)						11.6	4.9	
CAP+1(A→C)					1.7			
CD5(−CT)		1.2	0.8					
CD6(−A)	0.4	2.9	0.6					
CD8(−AA)		0.6	7.4					
CD8/9(+G)				28.9	12.0			
CD15(G→A)				3.5	0.8			0.8
CD16(−C)				1.3	1.7			
CD17(A→T)						10.5	24.7	
CD24(T→A)								7.9
CD30(G→A)				0.9				
CD30(G→C)				3.5	0.9			
CD39(C→T)	40.1	17.4	3.5					
CD41/42(−TCTT)				7.9	13.7	38.6	46.4	
CD71/72(+A)						12.4	2.3	
IVSI-1(G→A)	4.3	13.6	2.5					
IVSI-1(G→T)				8.2	6.6			
IVSI-5(G→C)				26.4	48.5	2.5	4.9	
IVSI-6(T→C)	16.3	7.4	17.4					
IVSI-110(G→A)	29.8	43.7	41.9					
IVSII-1(G→A)	1.1	2.1	9.7					
IVSII-654(C→T)						15.7	8.9	
IVSII-745(C→G)	3.5	7.1	2.7					
619 bp deletion				23.3	13.3			
Others	4.1	2.2	9.7	0.5	0.9	6.8	7.9	10.6

Abbreviations: CD, codon; IVS, intervening sequence; bp, base pairs.

ARMS primers were first developed for the screening and prenatal diagnosis of β-thalassemia mutations in the Asian Indian and Cypriot populations in the United Kingdom (Old et al., 1990). Subsequently ARMS primers have been designed to screen for the common mutations of all ethnic groups (Old, 1996). Figure 35.3 shows the results of screening a Cypriot individual with β-thalassemia trait for seven common mutations by ARMS-PCR. Details of the mutation-specific and normal sequence-specific primers used in my laboratory to diagnose the common β-thalassemia mutations are presented in Tables 35.4 and 35.5. ARMS-PCR is currently the main approach for mutation detection and prenatal diagnosis in the United Kingdom for β thalassemia, HbE thalassemia, and the sickling disorders. The technique has been established in other countries such as India because of its rapid and inexpensive properties, making the development of a prenatal diag-

nostic service in developing countries realistic for the first time (Saxena et al., 1998).

Other variations on the primer-specific amplification theme are multiplex ARMS, COP-PCR, and MS-PCR. More than one mutation may be screened for at the same time in a single PCR reaction by multiplexing the ARMS primers provided that they are coupled with the same common primer (Tan et al., 1994). Fluorescent labeling of the common primer allows the sizing of the amplification products on an automated DNA fragment analyzer (Zschocke and Graham, 1995). If the normal and mutant ARMS primers for a specific mutation are co-amplified in the same reaction they compete with each other to amplify the target sequence. This technique is called competitive oligonucleotide priming (COP) and requires the two ARMS primers to be labeled differently. Fluorescent labels permit a diagnosis to be made by means of color com-

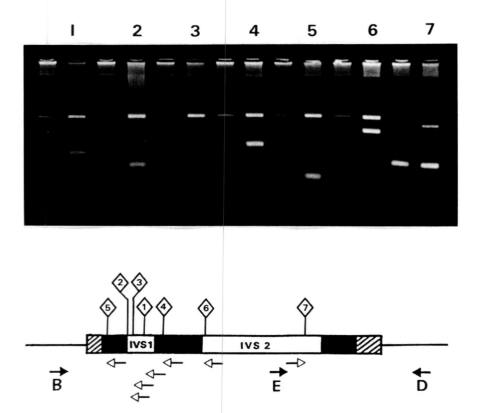

Figure 35.3. ARMS-PCR screening of a DNA sample for seven common Mediterranean mutations. The gel shows alternating tracks containing the amplification products from DNA of a patient with β-thalassemia trait and those from control DNAs for each of the seven mutations (labeled 1–7). The mutations screened for are: 1, IVSI-110 (G→A); 2, IVSI-1 (G→A); 3, IVSI-6 (T→C); 4, codon 39 (C→T); 5, codon 6 (–A); 6, IVSII-1 (G→A); 7, IVSII-745 (C→G); locations are shown in the diagram of the β-gene. In the first twelve lanes, the control primers D and E (Table 35.4) were used (producing an 861-bp fragment), and in the last two lanes, the $^{G}\gamma$-*Hin*d III RFLP control primers were used (producing a 323-bp fragment).

plementation assay (Chehab and Kan, 1989). A variation of this method is to use ARMS primers that differ in length instead of the label. The primers compete with each other to produce fragments that can be distinguished simply by agarose gel electrophoresis. Normal, heterozygous, and homozygous DNA are diagnosed by simple analysis of the presence/absence of the two products. This technique, called mutagenetically separated polymerase chain reaction (MS-PCR), has been applied to the prenatal diagnosis of β thalassemia in Taiwan (Chang et al., 1995).

PCR: Restriction Enzyme Analysis

More than forty β-thalassemia mutations are known to create or abolish a restriction endonuclease site (Table 35.6). The majority of these can be detected

quickly by restriction endonuclease analysis of amplified DNA. The presence or absence of the enzyme recognition site is determined from the pattern of digested fragments after agarose or polyacrylamide gel electrophoresis. As a screening method, this approach is limited by the small fraction of β-thalassemia mutations that affect a restriction enzyme site. In addition, in some cases there is another restriction enzyme site very close to the mutation site and hence the fragment sizes produced by normal and mutant DNA are difficult to resolve.

Mutations that do not naturally create or abolish restriction sites may be diagnosed by the technique of amplification-created restriction sites (ACRS). This method uses primers that are designed to insert new bases into the amplified product in order to create a restriction enzyme recognition site adjacent to the mutation sequence. This permits known mutations that normally do not alter a recognition site to be detected by restriction enzyme digestion of the PCR product. This technique has been applied to the detection of Mediterranean β-thalassemia mutations (Linderman et al., 1991).

Gap PCR

Small deletion mutations in the β-globin gene sequence (see Chapter 12) may be detected by PCR using two primers complementary to the sense and anti-

Table 35.4. Primer Sequences Used for the Detection of the Common β-Thalassemia Mutations by the Allele-Specific Priming Technique

Mutation	Oligonucleotide sequence	Second primer	Product size (bp)
−88(C→T)	TCACTTAGACCTCACCCTGTGGAGCCTCAT	A	684
−87(C→G)	CACTTAGACCTCACCCTGTGGAGCCACCCG	A	683
−30(T→A)	GCAGGGAGGGCAGGAGCCAGGGCTGGGGAA	A	626
−29(A→G)	CAGGGAGGGCAGGAGCCAGGGCTGGGTATG	A	625
−28(A→G)	AGGGAGGGCAGGAGCCAGGGCTGGGCTTAG	A	624
CAP+1(A→G)	ATAAGTCAGGGCAGAGCCATCTATTGGTTC	A	597
CD5(−CT)	TCAAACAGACACCATGGTGCACCTGAGTCG	A	528
CD6(−A)	CCCACAGGGCAGTAACGGCAGACTTCTGCC	B	207
CD8(−AA)	ACACCATGGTGCACCTGACTCCTGAGCAGG	A	520
CD8/9(+G)	CCTTGCCCCACAGGGCAGTAACGGCACACC	B	225
CD15(G→A)	TGAGGAGAAGTCTGCCGTTACTGCCCAGTA	A	500
CD16(−C)	TCACCACCAACTTCATCCACGTTCACGTTC	B	238
CD17(A→T)	CTCACCACCAACTTCAGCCACGTTCAGCTA	B	239
CD24(T→A)	CTTGATACCAACCTGCCCAGGGCCTCTCCT	B	262
CD30(G→A)	TAAACGTGTCTTGTAACCTTGATACCTACT	B	280
CD30(G→C)	TAAACCTGTCTTGTAACCTTGATACCTACG	B	280
CD39(C→T)	CAGATCCCCAAAGGACTCAAAGAACCTGTA	B	436
CD41/42(−TCTT)	GAGTGGACAGATCCCCAAAGGACTCAACCT	B	439
CD71−72(+A)	CATGGCAAGAAAGTGCTCGGTGCCTTTAAG	C	241
IVSI-1(G→A)	TTAAACCTGTCTTGTAACCTTGATACCGAT	B	281
IVSI-1(G→T)	TTAAACCTGTCTTGTAACCTTGATACCGAAA	B	281
IVSI-5(G→C)	CTCCTTAAACCTGTCTTGTAACCTTGTTAG	B	285
IVSI-6(T→C)	TCTCCTTAAACCTGTCTTGTAACCTTCATG	B	286
IVSI-110(G→A)	ACCAGCAGCCTAAGGGTGGGAAAATAGAGT	B	419
IVSII-1(G→A)	AAGAAAACATCAAGGGTCCCATAGACTGAT	B	634
IVSII-654(C→T)	GAATAACAGTGATAATTTCTGGGTTAACGT*	D	829
IVSII-745(C→G)	TCATATTGCTAATAGCAGCTACAATCGAGG*	D	738
βˢCD6(A→T)	CCCACAGGGCAGTAACGGCAGACTTCTGCA	B	207
βᶜCD6(G→A)	CCACAGGGCAGTAACGGCAGACTTCTCGTT	B	206
βᴱCD26(G→A)	TAACCTTGATACCAACCTGCCCAGGGCGTT	B	236

Note: The above primers are coupled as indicated with primers A, B, C or D:
A: CCCCTTCCTATGACATGAACTTAA
B: ACCTCACCCTGTGGAGCCAC
C: TTCGTCTGTTTCCCATTCTAAACT; or
D: GAGTCAAGGCTGAGAGATGCAGGA.

The control primers used for all of the above mutation-specific ARMS primers, except the two marked*, are primers D plus E: CAATG-TATCATGCCTCTTTGCACC. For IVSII-654(C→T) and IVSII-745(C→G), the ᴳγ-*Hind* III RFLP primers (see below) are used as control primers.

Hind III/ᴳγ:
Forward: AGTGCTGCAAGAAGAACAACTACC
Reverse: CTCTGCATCATGGGCAGTGAGCTC

sense strand in the DNA regions that flank the deletion (Faa et al., 1992). For large deletions, amplified product using flanking primers is obtained only from the deletion allele because the distance between the two primers is too great to amplify normal DNA. As is the case with the α-thalassemia deletions, the normal allele may be detected by amplifying sequences spanning one of the breakpoints, using a primer complementary to the deleted sequence and one complementary to flanking DNA (Waye et al., 1994). As well as deletion β thalassemia, the deletions in the β-globin gene cluster that

result in Hb Lepore and a number of δβ-thalassemia and hereditary persistence of fetal hemoglobin (HPFH) mutations (see Chapter 15) can be diagnosed by this method (Table 35.1) (Craig et al., 1994).

PCR Methods for Unknown Mutations

A number of techniques have been applied for the characterization of β-thalassemia mutations without prior knowledge of the molecular defect. The most widely used of these methods is denaturing gradient

Table 35.5. Primer Sequences Used for the Detection of the Corresponding Normal DNA Sequence in the Allele-Specific Priming Technique for Diagnosis of the Indicated Mutations

Mutation	Oligonucleotide sequence	Second primer	Product size (bp)
−88 (C→T)	TCACTTAGACCTCACCCTGTGGAGCCACTC	A	684
−87 (C→G)	CACTTAGACCTCACCCTGTGGAGCCACCCC	A	683
CD5 (−CT)	CAAACAGACACCATGGTGCACCTGACTCCT	A	528
CD6 (−A)	CACAGGGCAGTAACGGCAGACTTCTCCTCA	B	207
CD8 (−AA)	ACACCATGGTGCACCTGACTCCTGAGCAGA	A	520
CD8/9 (+G)	CCTTGCCCCACAGGGCAGTAACGGCACACT	B	225
CD15 (G→A)	TGAGGAGAAGTCTGCCGTTACTGCCCAGTA	A	500
CD30 (G→C)	TAAACCTGTCTTGTAACCTTGATACCTACC	B	280
CD39 (C→T)	TTAGGCTGCTGGTGGTCTACCCTTGGTCCC	A	299
CD41/42 (−TCTT)	GAGTGGACAGATCCCCAAAGGACTCAAAGA	B	439
IVSI-1 (G→A)	TTAAACCTGTCTTGTAACCTTGATACCCAC	B	281
IVSI-1 (G→T)	GATGAAGTTGGTGGTGAGGCCCTGGGTAGG	A	455
IVSI-5 (G→C)	CTCCTTAAACCTGTCTTGTAACCTTGTTAC	B	285
IVSI-6 (T→C)	AGTTGGTGGTGAGGCCCTGGGCAGGTTGGT	A	449
IVSI-110 (G→A)	ACCAGCAGCCTAAGGGTGGGAAAATACACC	B	419
IVSII-1 (G→A)	AAGAAAACATCAAGGGTCCCATAGACTGAC	B	634
IVSII-654 (C→T)	GAATAACAGTGATAATTTCTGGGTTAACGC	D	829
IVSII-745 (C→G)	TCATATTGCTAATAGCAGCTACAATCGAGC	D	738
βSCD6 (A→T)	AACAGACACCATGGTGCACCTGACTCGTGA	A	527
βECD26 (G→A)	TAACCTTGATACCAACCTGCCCAGGGCGTC	B	236

Note: See Table 35.4 for details of primers A–D and control primers.

gel electrophoresis (DGGE), which allows the separation of DNA fragments differing by a single base change according to their melting properties (Losekoot et al., 1991). The technique involves the electrophoresis of double-stranded DNA fragments through a linearly increasing denaturing gradient until the lowest melting temperature domain of the fragment denatures, creating a branched molecule that effectively becomes stationary in the gel matrix. DNA fragments differing by one base pair in the low melting temperature domain have different melting temperatures and can be separated in most (but not all) cases by this technique. The β-globin gene is amplified in segments using five to seven pairs of primers, one of each pair having a GC-rich sequence added to it to create a high melting domain. Heterozygous DNA creates four bands, two heteroduplexes of normal and mutant sequences and two homoduplexes, one of normal sequence and the other of mutant sequence. DGGE has been used for prenatal diagnosis of β thalassemia in India (Gorakshaker et al., 1997) and also for the analysis of point mutations resulting in δ thalassemia and nondeletion HPFH (Gottardi et al., 1992; Papadakis et al., 1997).

Another approach is by heteroduplex analysis using nondenaturing gel electrophoresis. Unique heteroduplex patterns can be generated for each mutation by

annealing an amplified target DNA fragment with an amplified heteroduplex generator molecule, a synthetic oligonucleotide of about 130 bases in length containing deliberate sequence changes or identifiers at known mutation positions (Savage et al., 1995). Other methods such as mismatch cleavage (CMC), single-stranded conformational polymorphism analysis (SSCP), and the protein truncation test are also good methods of detecting unknown mutations but they have not been applied specifically to the diagnosis of the hemoglobinopathies.

The above techniques simply pinpoint the presence of a mutation or DNA polymorphism in the amplified target sequence. Sequencing of the amplified product may then be carried out manually or automatically to identify the localized mutation. This can now be done very efficiently using an automated DNA sequencing machine utilizing fluorescence detection technology. The specialized equipment required for this technique is currently very expensive, but as the more efficient second-generation machines are developed, the cost will come down and direct DNA sequencing will probably become the primary method of mutation detection. Once a rare or novel mutation has been identified through DNA sequencing, the DNA sample can be used as a control to develop ASO or ARMS primers for the more rapid and less expensive screening of further cases.

Table 35.6. β-Thalassemia Mutations Detectable by Restriction Enzyme Digestion of Amplified Product

Position	Mutation	Ethnic group	Affected site*
−88	C→T	African/Asian Indian	+Fok I
−87	C→G	Mediterranean	−Avr II
−87	C→T	Italian	−Avr II
−87	C→A	African/Yugoslavian	−Avr II
−86	C→G	Lebanese	−Avr II
−86	C→A	Italian	−Avr II
−29	A→G	African/Chinese	+Nla III
+43 to +40	(−AAAC)	Chinese	+Dde I
Initiation CD	T→C	Yugoslavian	−Nco I
Initiation CD	T→G	Chinese	−Nco I
Initiation CD	A→G	Japanese	−Nco I
CD 5	(−CT)	Mediterranean	−Dde I
CD 6	(−A)	Mediterranean	−Dde I
CD 15	(−T)	Asian Indian	+Bgl I
CD 17	A→T	Chinese	+Mae I
CD 26	G→T	Thai	−Mnl I
CD 26	G→A	Southeast Asian (HbE)	−Mnl I
CD 27	G→T	Mediterranean (Hb Knossos)	−Sau96 I
CD 29	C→T	Lebanese	−BspM I
CD 30	G→C	Tunisian/African	−BspM I
CD 30	G→A	Bulgarian	−BspM I
IVSI-1	G→A	Mediterranean	−BspM I
IVSI-1	G→T	Asian Indian/Chinese	−BspM I
IVSI-2	T→G	Tunisian	−BspM I
IVSI-2	T→C	African	−BspM I
IVSI-2	T→A	Algerian	−BspM I
IVSI-5	G→A	Mediterranean	+EcoR V
IVSI-6	T→C	Mediterranean	+SfaN I
IVSI-116	T→G	Mediterranean	+Mae I
IVSI-130	G→C	Turkish	−Dde I
IVSI-130	G→A	Egyptian	−Dde I
CD 35	C→A	Thai	−Acc I
CD 37	G→A	Saudi Arabian	−Ava II
CD 38/39	(−C)	Czechoslovakian	−Ava II
CD 37/8/9	(−GACCCAG)	Turkish	−Ava II
CD 39	C→T	Mediterranean	+Mae I
CD 43	G→T	Chinese	−Hinf I
CD 47	(+A)	Surinamese	−Xho I
CD 61	A→T	African	−Hph I
CD 74/75	(−C)	Turkish	−Hae III
CD 121	G→T	Polish, French, Japanese	−EcoR I
IVSII-I	G→A	Mediterranean	−Hph I
IVSII-4,5	(−AG)	Portuguese	−Hph I
IVSII-745	C→G	Mediterranean	+Rsa I

* +, cretes; −, abolishes restriction site.

β-globin Gene Haplotype Analysis

At least eighteen RFLPs have been characterized within the β-globin gene cluster (Kazazian and Boehm, 1988), (see Chapter 12). Conveniently, most of these RFLP sites are nonrandomly associated with each other and they combine to produce just a handful of haplotypes (Antonarakis et al., 1982). In particular, they form a 5′ cluster from the ε-gene to the δ-gene and a 3′ cluster around the β-globin gene. In between is a 9-kb stretch of DNA containing a relative hot spot for meiotic recombination. The recombination between the two clusters has been calculated to be approximately 1 in 350 meioses (Chakravarti et al., 1984). Hybridization studies have shown that each β-thalassemia mutation is strongly associated with just one or two haplotypes (Orkin et al., 1982), probably because of their recent origin as compared to the haplotypes, and thus haplotype analysis has been used to study the origins of identical mutations found in different ethnic groups.

The β-globin gene cluster haplotype normally consists of 5 RFLPs located in the 5′ cluster (Hinc II/ε-gene; Hind III/Gγ-gene; Hind III/Aγ-gene; Hinc II/3′ψβ; and Hinc II/5′ψβ) and two RFLPs in the 3′ cluster (Ava II/β-gene; BamH I/β-gene) (Old et al., 1984). Although originally analyzed by Southern blotting, all the RFLPs except the BamH I polymorphism can be easily analyzed by PCR. The primer sequences together with the sizes of the fragments generated are listed in Table 35.7. The BamH I RFLP is located within a L1 repetitive element creating amplification problems and a Hinf I RFLP located just 3′ to the β-globin gene is used instead, because these two RFLPs have been found to exist in linkage disequilibrium (Semenza et al., 1989).

Three other RFLPs are included in Table 35.7. An Ava II RFLP in the ψβ-gene is extremely useful in haplotype analysis of Mediterranean β-thalassemia heterozygotes. The (−) allele for this RFLP is frequently found on chromosomes carrying the IVSI-110 mutation, whereas it is very rare on normal β-globin chromosomes (Wainscoat et al., 1984) and thus is a very useful informative marker for individuals heterozygous for this mutation. The Rsa I RFLP located just 5′ to the β-globin gene is useful for link-

Table 35.7. Primers Used for the Analysis of β-Globin Gene Cluster RFLPs

RFLP and Primers: 5′ primer 3′ primer	Product size (bp)	Coordinates on GenBank sequence U01317	Absence of site (bp)	Presence of site (bp)	Annealing temperature (°C)
Hinc II/ε 5′TCTCTGTTTGATGACAAATTC 5′AGTCATTGGTCAAGGCTGACC	760	 18652–18672 19391–19411	760	315 445	55
Xmn I/Gγ 5′AACTGTTGCTTTATAGGATTTT 5′AGGAGCTTATTGATAACCTCAGAC	657	 33862–33883 34495–34518	657	455 202	55
Hind III/Gγ 5′AGTGCTGCAAGAAGAACAACTACC 5′CTCTGCATCATGGGCAGTGAGCTC	326	 35677–35700 35981–36004	326	235 91	65
Hind III/Aγ 5′ATGCTGCTAATGCTTCATTAC 5′TCATGTGTGATCTCTCAGCAG	635	 40357–40377 40971–40991	635	327 308	65
Hinc II/5′ψβ 5′TCCTATCCATTACTGTTCCTTGAA 5′ATTGTCTTATTCTAGAGACGATTT	795	 46686–46709 47457–47480	795	691 104	55
Ava II/ψβ Sequence as for *Hind* 5′ψβ RFLP	795	 46686–46709 47457–47480	795	440 355	55
Hinc II/3′ψβ 5′GTACTCATACTTTAAGTCCTAACT 5′TAAGCAAGATTATTTCTGGTCTCT	913	 49559–49582 50448–50471	913	479 434	55
Rsa I/β 5′AGACATAATTTATTAGCATGCATG 5′CCCCTTCCTATGACATGAACTTAA	1200	 61504–61527 62680–62703	411 plus constant fragments of 694 and 95	330 81 plus 694 and 95	55
Ava II/β 5′GTGGTCTACCCTTGGACCCAGAGG 5′TTCGTCTGTTTCCCATTCTAAACT	328	 62416–62439 62720–62743	328	228 100	65
Hinf I/β 5′GGAGGTTAAAGTTTTGCTATGCTGTAT 5′GGGCCTATGATAGGGTAAT	474	 63974–64001 64429–64447	320 plus constant fragment of 154	213 107 and 154	55

age analysis because it appears to be unlinked to either the 5′ cluster or the 3′ cluster RFLPs and thus may be informative when the 5′ haplotype and the 3′ haplotype are not. Finally, the $^G\gamma$-*Xmn* I RFLP, created by the nondeletion HPFH C→T mutation at position −158, is included because of its use in the analysis of sickle cell gene haplotypes and in individuals with thalassemia intermedia.

DNA DIAGNOSIS OF δβ THALASSEMIA, HB LEPORE, AND HPFH

The δβ-thalassemia, Hb Lepore, and HPFH deletion mutations (see Chapter 15) were characterized origi-

nally by restriction enzyme mapping and Southern blotting. Consequently each deletion mutation may be diagnosed by the identification of characteristic abnormal DNA fragments that span the breakpoint of the deletion. Selection of the right restriction enzyme digest and gene probe depends on identifying the ethnic origin of the individual to be studied and characterization of the phenotype in the heterozygous state. A similar strategy is required when these mutations are diagnosed by gap PCR. Gap PCR can now be used for Hb Lepore (Camaschella et al., 1990) and eight δβ-thalassemia and HPFH deletion mutations (Craig et al., 1994) as described in Table 35.1.

DNA DIAGNOSIS OF ABNORMAL HEMOGLOBINS

More than 700 hemoglobin variants have been described to date (see Section VII), although only a few are clinically important and require routine diagnosis by DNA analysis methods. These variants are HbS, HbC, HbE, HbD Punjab, and HbO Arab. The mutations for these five abnormal hemoglobins can be diagnosed by a variety of techniques as described below. The majority of the other abnormal variants have never been sequenced at the DNA level and although the mutations can be presumed from the amino acid change in most cases, DNA sequencing is required to confirm the nucleotide change before other diagnostic methods can be developed for screening purposes. This can be performed in the same manner as that described for the identification of thalassemia point mutations in the β gene and both α genes, or by the sequencing of cDNA produced by the reverse transcription of globin mRNA (Smetanina et al., 1997).

HbS

HbS (β Glu$\rightarrow$Val) is caused by an A$\rightarrow$T substitution in the second nucleotide of the sixth codon of the β-globin gene (see Section IV). The mutation destroys the recognition site for three restriction enzymes, *MnI* I, *Dde* I, and *Mst* II. *Mst* II is now unavailable commercially and an isoschizomer such as *Cvn* I, *OxaN* I, or *Sau* I may be used instead. *Mst* II was the enzyme of choice for detection of the β^S allele by Southern blot analysis (Orkin et al., 1982) because it cuts infrequently around the β-globin gene producing large DNA fragments. However, this is not a problem when the analysis is done by PCR and the enzyme *Dde* I is very suitable (Old et al., 1989). *Dde* I is a frequent cutter and several constant sites can be included in the amplified β-gene fragment to act as a control for the complete digestion of the amplified product, as illustrated in Figure 35.4. The primer sequences currently used in my laboratory are listed in Table 35.8. The β^S mutation can also be detected by a variety of other PCR-based techniques such as ASO/dot blotting or the ARMS method. The latter technique is always used in my laboratory as a second diagnostic method for confirmation of a prenatal diagnosis result obtained by *Dde* I PCR. The primer sequences for this ARMS assay are included in Tables 35.4 and 35.5.

HbC

The HbC ($\beta6$ Glu$\rightarrow$Lys) mutation, a G$\rightarrow$A substitution at codon 6, also occurs inside the recognition sites for *MnI* I, *Dde* I, and *Mst* II. However, it does not abolish the site for *Dde* I or *Mst* II because the muta-

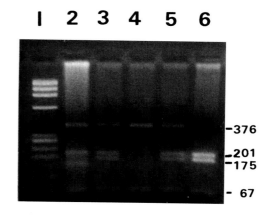

5' β-globin gene Dde I sites

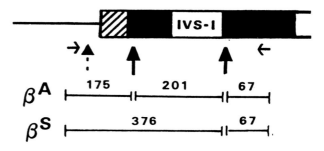

Figure 35.4. The diagnosis of the sickle cell gene mutation by *Dde* I digestion of amplified DNA. The gel shows *Dde* I-digested fragments of: AS individuals (lane 2, 3, and 5); AA individual (lanes 6); SS individual (track 4). Lane 1 contains φX174 – *Hae* III DNA markers. The primers used are listed in Table 35.8. The *Dde* I site 5' to the one at codon 6 (marked by the dotted arrow) is a rare polymorphic site caused by the sequence change G$\rightarrow$A at position −83 to the β-globin gene. When present, the fragment of 175 bp is cleaved to give 153-bp and 27-bp fragments as shown in lane 2.

tion occurs at a nonspecific nucleotide in the enzyme recognition sequences. Thus *Dde* I or *Mst* II cannot be used to detect the β^C mutation and another method such as ASO/dot blotting or the ARMS technique must be used. The primer sequences used for the ARMS method are included in Tables 35.4 and 35.5.

HbD Punjab and HbO Arab

The mutations giving rise to the abnormal variants HbD Punjab ($\beta121$ Glu$\rightarrow$Gln) and HbO Arab ($\beta121$ Glu$\rightarrow$Lys) both abolish an *EcoR* I site at codon 121 (Trent et al., 1984). Mutation detection is carried out very simply by amplification of a fragment containing the site and digesting with *EcoR* I. As there are no other *EcoR* I sites within several kilobases of the β-globin gene, care should be taken to always run appro-

Table 35.8. Oligonucleotide Primers for the Detection of β^S, β^E, β^D Punjab, and β^O Arab Mutations as RFLPs

Mutation and affected RE site	Primer sequence 5'–3'	Annealing temperature (°C)	Product size (bp)	Absence of site (bp)	Presence of site (bp)
β^{S}CD6 (A→T)	ACCTCACCCTGTGGAGCCAC	65	443	386	201
(Loss of Dde I site)	GAGTGGACAGATCCCCAAAGGACTCAAGGA	65		67	175
					67
β^{E}CD26 (G→A)	ACCTCACCCTGTGGAGCCAC	65	443	231	171
(Loss of Mnl I site)	GAGTGGACAGATCCCCAAAGGACTCAAGGA			89	89
				56	60
				35	35
				33	33
β^D Punjab					
CD121 (G→C)	CAATGTATCATGCCTCTTTGCACC	65	861	861	552
(Loss of EcoR I site)	GAGTCAAGGCTGAGAGATGCAGGA	65			309
β^O Arab					
CD121 (G→A)	CAATGTATCATGCCTCTTTGCACC	65	861	861	552
(Loss of EcoR I site)	GAGTCAAGGCTGAGAGATGCAGGA	65			309

priate control DNA samples. The primer sequences used for this approach are listed in Table 35.8.

HbE

The HbE mutation, a G→A mutation at codon 26, abolishes an *Mnl* I site and may be diagnosed by amplification of exon 1 and restriction enzyme analysis (Thein et al., 1987). The primer sequences used for this approach are listed in Table 35.8. The HbE mutation may also be diagnosed easily using ASO probes or ARMS primers. The primer sequences for the latter technique are listed in Tables 35.4 and 35.5.

GENERAL STRATEGY

The variety of techniques for the DNA-based diagnosis of the hemoglobinopathies creates a problem for laboratories wishing to start molecular analysis of the globin gene mutations: What is the best method to adopt? It is clear that ASO hybridization and the ARMS currently form the linchpins for the diagnosis of β-thalassemia. Both offer a rapid, inexpensive, and convenient method to test for multiple mutations simultaneously. Whether one chooses the dot-blot method or the reverse dot-blot approach will depend on a number of factors, including the range of mutations to be diagnosed, the ability to use radioactivity, or the need to go for the nonisotopic approach (and thus to consider the use of one of the kits on the market). The laboratory also needs to become proficient in a number of other techniques, such as gap PCR, and be able to sequence a β-globin gene for the rare cases in which no common mutations can be identified in individuals with clear-cut phenotypic evidence of β thalassemia. In addition, when these techniques are used for prenatal diagnosis a number of precautionary measures must be used, such as the analysis of fetal DNA samples for maternal DNA contamination when necessary and the confirmation of a diagnosis by a different approach. Therefore the answer to the question is that each laboratory must carry out preliminary studies utilizing a number of these approaches and work out for itself which are the best techniques suited to its needs and population.

References

Antonarakis, SE, Boehm, CD, Diardina, PJV, and Kazazian, HHJ. (1982). Non-random association of polymorphic restriction sites in the β-globin gene cluster. *Proc. Natl. Acad. Sci. U.S.A.* 79: 137–141.

Baysal, E and Huisman, THJ. (1994). Detection of common deletional α-thalassaemia-2 determinants by PCR. *Am. J. Hematol.* 46: 208.

Bowden, DK, Vickers, MA, and Higgs, DR. (1992). A PCR-based strategy to detect the common severe determinants of α-thalassaemia. *Br. J. Haematol.* 81: 104–108.

Camaschella, C, Alfarano, A, Gottardi, E et al. (1990). Prenatal diagnosis of fetal hemoglobin Lepore-Boston disease on maternal peripheral blood. *Blood* 75: 2102–2106.

Chakravarti, A, Buetow, KH, Antonarakis, SE, Waber, PG et al. (1984). Non-uniform recombination within the human β-globin gene cluster. *Am. J. Hum. Genet.* 71: 79.

Chang, JG, Lu, JM, Huang, JM et al. (1995). Rapid diagnosis of β-thalassaemia by mutagenically separated polymerase chain reaction (MS-PCR) and its application to prenatal diagnosis. *Br. J. Haematol.* 91: 602.

Chehab, FF and Kan, YW. (1989). Detection of specific DNA sequence by fluorescence amplification: A colour complementation assay. *Proc. Natl. Acad. Sci. U.S.A.* 86: 9178.

Cheung, M-C, Goldberg, JD, and Kan, YW. (1996). Prenatal diagnosis of sickle cell anemia and thalassemia by analysis of fetal cells in maternal blood. *Nat. Genet.* 14: 264–268.

Chong, SS, Boehm, CD, Higgs, DR, and Cutting, GR. (2000). Single-tube multiplex-PCR screen for common deletional determinants of α-thalassaemia. *Blood* 95: 360–362.

Craig, JE, Kelly, SJ, Barnetson, R, and Thein, SL. (1992). Molecular characterisation of a novel 10.3 kb deletion causing β-thalassaemia with unusually high Hb A_2. *Br. J. Haematol.* 82: 735–744.

Craig, JE, Barnetson, RA, Prior, J, Raven, JL et al. (1994). Rapid detection of deletions causing δβ thalassaemia and hereditary persistence of fetal hemoglobin by enzymatic amplification. *Blood* 83: 1673–1682.

Decorte, R, Cuppens, H, Marynen, P, and Cassiman, J-J. (1990). Rapid detection of hypervariable regions by the polymerase chain reaction technique. *DNA Cell. Biol.* 9: 461–469.

Dimovski, AJ, Efremove, DG, Jankovic, L et al. (1993). A $β^0$ thalassaemia due to a 1605 bp deletion of the 5′ β-globin gene region. *Br. J. Haematol.* 85: 143–147.

Dode, C, Krishnamoorthy, R, Lamb, J, and Rochette, J. (1992). Rapid analysis of $-α^{3.7}$ thalassaemia and $ααα^{anti}$ $^{3.7}$ triplication by enzymatic amplification analysis. *Br. J. Haematol.* 82: 105.

Faa, V, Rosatelli, MC, Sardu, R et al. (1992). A simple electrophoretic procedure for fetal diagnosis of β-thalassaemia due to short deletions. *Prenat. Diagn.* 12: 903–908.

Fischel-Ghodsian, N, Vickers, MA, Seip, M et al. (1988). Characterization of two deletions that remove the entire human ζ-α globin gene complex (- -Thai and - -Fil). *Br. J. Haematol.* 70: 233–238.

Gorakshaker, AC, Lulla, CP, Nadkarni, AH et al. (1997). Prenatal diagnosis of β-thalassaemia using denaturing gradient gel electrophoresis among Indians. *Hemoglobin* 21: 421–435.

Gottardi, E, Losekoot, M, Fodde, R et al. (1992). Rapid identification of denaturing gradient gel electrophoresis of mutations in the γ-globin gene promoters in non-deletion type HPFH. *Br. J. Haematol.* 80: 533–538.

Hartveld, KL, Heister, AJGAM, Giordano, PC et al. (1996). Rapid detection of point mutations and polymorphisms of the α-globin genes by DGGE and SSCA. *Hum. Mutat.* 7: 114–122.

Huisman, THJ. (1990). Frequencies of common β-thalassaemia alleles among different populations: Variability in clinical severity. *Br. J. Haematol.* 75: 454–457.

Kazazian, HH Jr and Boehm, CD. (1988). Molecular basis and prenatal diagnosis of β-thalassaemia. *Blood* 72: 1107.

Ko, T-M and Li, S-F. (1999). Molecular characterization of the - -FIL determinant of alpha-thalassaemia. *Am. J. Hematol.* 60: 173.

Ko, TM, Tseng, LH, Hsieh, FJ, and Lee, TY. (1993). Prenatal diagnosis of HbH disease due to compound heterozygosity for south-east Asian deletion and Hb Constant Spring by polymerase chain reaction. *Prenat. Diagn.* 13: 143.

Ko, T-M, Tseng, L-H, Hsu, P-M et al. (1997). Molecular characterization of β-thalassemia in Taiwan and the identification of two new mutations. *Hemoglobin* 21: 131–142.

Kuliev, A, Rechitsky, S, Verlinsky, O et al. (1999). Birth of healthy children after preimplantation diagnosis of thalassemias. *J. Assist. Reprod. Genet.* 16: 207–211.

Linderman, R, Hu, SP, Volpato, F, and Trent, RJ. (1991). Polymerase chain reaction (PCR) mutagenesis enabling rapid non-radioactive detection of common β-thalassaemia mutations in Mediterraneans. *Br. J. Haematol.* 78: 100.

Liu, YT, Old, JM, Fisher, CA et al. (2000). Rapid detection of α-thalassaemia deletions and α-globin gene triplication by multiplex PCRs. *Br. J. Haematol.* 108: 295–299.

Losekoot, M, Fodde, R, Harteveld, CL et al. (1991). Denaturing gradient gel electrophoresis and direct sequencing of PCR amplified genomic DNA: A rapid and reliable diagnostic approach to beta thalassaemia. *Br. J. Haematol.* 76: 269–274.

Lynch, JR, Brown, JM, Best, S et al. (1991). Characterisation of the breakpoint of a 3.5 kb deletion of the β-globin gene. *Genomics* 10: 509–511.

Maggio, A, Giambona, A, Cai, SP et al. (1993). Rapid and simultaneous typing of hemoglobin S, hemoglobin C and seven Mediterranean β-thalassaemia mutations by covalent reverse dot-blot analysis: Application to prenatal diagnosis in Sicily. *Blood* 81: 239–242.

Molchanova, TP, Pobedimskaya, DD, and Postnikov, YV. (1994). A simplified procedure for sequencing amplified DNA containing the α-2 or α-1 globin gene. *Hemoglobin* 18: 251.

Newton, CR, Graham, A, and Heptinstall, LE. (1989). Analysis of any point mutation in DNA. The amplification refractory mutation system (ARMS). *Nucleic Acids Res.* 17: 2503–2516.

Old, JM. (1986). Fetal DNA analysis. In Davies, KE, editor. *Genetic analysis of the human disease: A practical approach.* Oxford, England: IRL Press. p. 1.

Old, J. (1996). Haemoglobinopathies. *Prenat. Diagn.* 16: 1181–1186.

Old, JM, Petrou, M, Modell, B, and Weatherall, DJ. (1984). Feasibility of antenatal diagnosis of β-thalassaemia by DNA polymorphisms in Asian Indians and Cypriot populations. *Br. J. Haematol.* 57: 255–263.

Old, JM, Thein, SL, Weatherall, DJ et al. (1989). Prenatal diagnosis of the major haemoglobin disorders. *Mol. Biol. Med.* 6: 55–63.

Old, JM, Varawalla, NY, and Weatherall, DJ. (1990). The rapid detection and prenatal diagnosis of β thalassaemia in the Asian Indian and Cypriot populations in the UK. *Lancet* 336: 834–837.

Orkin, SH, Little, PFR, Kazazian, HH, Jr, and Boehm, CD. (1982). Improved detection of the sickle mutation by DNA analysis. *N. Engl. J. Med.* 307: 32–36.

Papadakis, M, Papapanagiotou, E, and Loutradi-Anagnostou, A. (1997). Scanning methods to identify the molecular heterogeneity of δ-globin gene especially in δ-thalassemias: Detection of three novel substitutions in the promoter region of the gene. *Hum. Mutat.* 9: 465–472.

Ristaldi, MS, Pirastu, M, Rosatelli, C, and Cao, A. (1989). Prenatal diagnosis of β-thalassaemia in Mediterranean populations by dot blot analysis with DNA amplification and allele specific oligonucleotide probes. *Prenat. Diagn.* 9: 629–638.

Rosatelli MC, Tuveri, T, Scalas MT et al. (1992). Molecular screening and fetal diagnosis of β-thalassaemia in the Italian population. *Hum. Genet.* 89: 585–589.

Saiki, RK, Walsh, PS, Levenson, CH, and Erlich, HA. (1989) Genetic analysis of amplified DNA with immobilized sequence-specific oligonucleotide probes. *Proc. Natl. Acad. Sci. U.S.A.* 86: 6230–6234.

Savage, DA, Wood, NAP, Bidwell, JL et al. (1995). Detection of β-thalassaemia mutations using DNA heteroduplex generator molecules. *Br. J. Haematol.* 90: 564.

Saxena, R, Jain, PK, Thomas, E, and Verma, IC. (1998). Prenatal diagnosis of β-thalassaemia: Experience in a developing country. *Prenat. Diagn.* 18: 1–7.

Sekizawa, A, Watanabe, A, Kimwa, T et al. (1996). Prenatal diagnosis of the fetal RhD blood type using a single fetal nucleated erythrocyte from maternal blood. *Obstet. Gynaecol.* 87: 501–505.

Semenza, GL, Dowling, CE, and Kazazian, HH Jr. (1989). Hinf I polymorphisms 3′ to the human β globin gene detected by the polymerase chain reaction (PCR). *Nucleic Acids Res.* 17: 2376.

Smetanina, NS, Molchanova, TP, and Huisman, THJ. (1997). Analysis of mRNA from red cells of patients with thalassemia and hemoglobin variants. *Hemoglobin* 21: 437–467.

Sutcharitchan, P, Saiki, R, Huisman, THJ et al. (1995). Reverse dot-blot detection of the African-American β-thalassaemia mutations. *Blood* 86: 1580.

Tan, JAMA, Tay, JSH, Lin, LI et al. (1994). The amplification refractory mutation system (ARMS): A rapid and direct prenatal diagnostic technique for β-thalassaemia in Singapore. *Prenat. Diagn.* 14: 1077.

Thein, SL, Lynch, JR, Old, JM, and Weatherall, DJ. (1987). Direct detection of haemoglobin E with Mnl I. *J. Med. Gene.* 24: 110–111.

Thein, SL, Hesketh, C, Brown, KM et al. (1989). Molecular characterisation of a high A₂ β thalassaemia by direct sequencing of single strand enriched amplified genomic DNA. *Blood* 73: 924–930.

Trent, RJ, Davis, B, Wilkinson, T, and Kronenberg, H. (1984). Identification of β variant hemoglobins by DNA restriction endonuclease mapping. *Hemoglobin* 8: 443–462.

Wainscoat, JS, Old, JM, Thein, SL, and Weatherall, DJ. (1984). A new DNA polymorphism for prenatal diagnosis of β-thalassaemia in Mediterranean populations. *Lancet* 2: 1299–1301.

Waye, JS, Cai, S-P, Eng, B et al. (1991). High haemoglobin A$_2$ β^0 thalassaemia due to a 532 bp deletion of the 5′ β-globin gene region. *Blood* 77: 1100–1103.

Waye, JS, Eng, B, Hunt, JA et al. (1994). Filipino β-thalassaemia due to a large deletion: Identification of the deletion endpoints and polymerase chain reaction (PCR)-based diagnosis. *Hum. Genet.* 94: 530–532.

Zschocke, J and Graham, CA. (1995). A fluorescent multiplex ARMS method for rapid mutation analysis. *Mol. Cell. Probes* 9: 447.

36

Prenatal Diagnosis and Screening for Thalassemia and Sickle Cell Disease

ANTONIO CAO
MARIA CRISTINA ROSATELLI
JAMES R. ECKMAN

INTRODUCTION

About 250 million people—4.5 percent of the world population—are carriers of a defective globin gene, and about 300,000 affected homozygotes, equally divided between sickle cell disorders and thalassemia syndromes, are born each year (WHO, 1996). Bone marrow transplantation from HLA-identical siblings is presently the sole definitive cure for some homozygotes with β thalassemia and sickle cell anemia, although, for the large majority of patients, only supportive management is actually available (see Chapters 39 and 40). Life expectancy varies according to the type of thalassemia or sickle cell disease but does not usually extend beyond the third to fifth decade. Prevention of these disorders is therefore estimable. Thalassemia and sickle cell disease have a high incidence in the Mediterranean basin, the Middle East, the Indian subcontinent, Asia, and Tropical Africa, where they have gained the status of major public health problems (see Chapters 30 to 33). Due to population flow and the slave trade, both thalassemia and sickle cell disease now also occur with a high frequency in Northern Europe, North and South America, and in the Caribbean region.

In the 1970s, prevention of thalassemia major and sickle cell anemia was attempted in Northern Italy and in a small Greek community by carrier screening and genetic counseling, respectively, supporting the principle that these diseases can be prevented by birth con-trol, mate selection, or adoption in lieu of childbearing (Stamatoyannopoulos, 1974). This approach, how-ever, produced no significant difference in the propor-tion of marriages between heterozygotes, the numbers of affected individuals expected by random mating, or the incidence of homozygotes. The effectiveness of screening and counseling, at least for β thalassemia, changed drastically in the mid-1970s with the advent of prenatal diagnosis, which provided a new option to couples at risk (Cao et al., 1997).

POPULATION SCREENING AND COUNSELING FOR THALASSEMIA AND HEMOGLOBINOPATHIES

Identification of couples at risk for hemoglobin disor-ders may be done retrospectively following the birth of an affected child, or prospectively, by analyzing spouses who are still childless. Prospective identifica-tion is obviously more advantageous since it allows families to be free from disease and society to avoid the health and economic burdens of affected patients. This approach can be accomplished by population screen-ing. To date, prospective identification and counseling of couples at risk for inherited hemoglobinopathies has been carried out only in geographic areas with popula-tions at risk for β thalassemia. Programs are ongoing in several areas in the Mediterranean basin, such as Cyprus, Greece, and various regions of continental Italy and Sardinia (Angastiniotis et al., 1995; Cao et al., 1996; Loukopoulos, 1996). Some prospective screening programs—in Sardinia, Cyprus, and Greece, for example—have operated for a long time and a large amount of data are available for analysis. Prospective screening to prevent α thalassemia hydrops fetalis is available in South Asia where this disorder is common.

SCREENING FOR β THALASSEMIA

Education and Involvement of the Population

Long-term screening programs have been character-ized by the extensive involvement of the population at large. These populations were educated by the mass media, posters, and information booklets as well as by lectures for community leaders and for the general pop-ulation. To transmit messages as efficiently and simply as possible—and also to avoid potential adverse effects on carriers and parents—the educational campaign was designed together with parents' or patients' associa-tions. Specific educational meetings on the disease and the screening program were held with physicians and particularly with pediatricians, obstetricians, family

Martin H. Steinberg, Bernard G. Forget, Douglas R. Higgs, and Ronald L. Nagel, editors. *Disorders of Hemoglobin: Genetics, Pathophysi-ology, and Clinical Management.* © 2001 Cambridge University Press. All rights reserved.

planning associations, nurses, and social workers. Details on where and how to be examined were published in special booklets that were left at key places, such as marriage registries and obstetrics, pediatric, general practice, and family planning clinics. The booklets contained the following messages:

1. The carrier state, which may be identified by appropriate methods, has no disadvantages.
2. The homozygous state produces a severe disease with survival requiring continuous transfusions in combination with iron chelation. Cure is possible by bone marrow transplantation only in the limited case of a homozygote having an HLA-identical donor.
3. Different options are available to avoid having affected children when both members of a couple have been identified as carriers. These options include fetal diagnosis, which is safe both for the mother and the fetus.

Additionally, a thalassemia meeting is organized in Cyprus every year, and a magazine and information pamphlets are published regularly. More recently, formal education on inherited anemias with particular emphasis on thalassemia has been introduced in the school curricula of the above Mediterranean countries. The Orthodox Church, particularly in Cyprus, contributed greatly to the overall success of the campaign by encouraging premarital carrier screening, while the Catholic Church in Italy did not participate in the preventive campaign.

Experience indicates that population screening campaigns should accommodate the cultural values and religious beliefs of the target populations. A critical evaluation of the channels used to inform the general public in Sardinia has been carried out twice: once at the beginning of the program, and again at an intermediate point in the program. At the beginning, the information on β thalassemia was made known to 44 percent of the population via the mass media, to 31 percent via a general practitioner, and to 23 percent via an obstetrician. This trend has changed, and the information is now passed through physicians—family doctors, obstetricians, genetic counselors—and reaches more than 70 percent of the target population.

Finally, an important prerequisite for a successful campaign is that adequate facilities must be organized to meet the demand for screening and prenatal diagnosis before the educational campaign begins.

Target Population

Although the target population is predominantly couples contemplating marriage, diagnostic testing is often requested—before or after conception—by couples starting a family. Now, as in the early days of screening, the anticipation and results of this testing can cause considerable emotional stress. The number of young unmarried people requesting screening in Cyprus and Italy, including Sardinia, is growing, suggesting that the population is becoming more aware of β thalassemia and of the methodology for its prevention. In Cyprus and Italy, adolescent schoolchildren have been screened recently, while screening of army personnel has proven unsuccessful, because the examinees usually forget their test results by the time they are ready to start a family. In the above populations, heterozygote screening has been carried out on a voluntary basis. According to ethical principles, informed consent and informative counseling should precede genetic screening. However, although formal informed consent was not requested in these programs, every effort was made to inform those screened on the meaning of the carrier state and the potential for adverse effects associated with its detection. Experience so far suggests that all mandatory population screening and counseling should be discouraged since their outcomes can have a negative impact.

Counseling

Nondirective counseling, based on a private interview with the individual or couple, is aimed at providing information to help couples make reproductive choices relating to birth control, mate selection, adoption as opposed to childbearing, fetal testing with selective abortion, or artificial insemination via an unaffected donor. The details of fetal testing, including sampling, the risk to the fetus, and the chances for failure and misdiagnosis have been particularly emphasized. An explanatory booklet is usually provided, where the predicted natural history of the disease based on the genotype at the α-, β-, and γ-globin gene loci (see below) is described in great detail.

In cases with an existing normal or heterozygous β-thalassemia child, HLA typing on the fetal DNA is proposed to the parents, and if the circumstances warrant it, carried out to determine whether or not a sibling may be HLA identical and thus a suitable bone marrow donor. This information helps parents make an informed decision about interrupting the pregnancy. Since first trimester diagnosis became available, prenatal diagnosis is often used. Lastly, part of the counseling service is to inform the counselee about the risk to relatives and to recommend that they be informed as well so that they too can choose to undergo testing. In Sardinia many relatives so informed have opted for testing. This type of inductive screening is very efficient in detecting heterozygous β thalassemia. In Sardinia, for example, by inductive screening—that is, screening only 11% of the population at childbearing age—a large percentage of couples at risk—approximately 90 percent of those predicted on the basis of the carrier rate—have been detected.

SCREENING FOR α THALASSEMIA

Hydrops fetalis, the most severe form of α thalassemia, is caused by the deletion of all four α-globin genes and is lethal in utero or shortly after birth (see Chapters 17 and 18). Retrospective screening for hydrops fetalis has been carried out because of the severe complications that occur frequently in pregnancies with hydropic fetuses (Weatherall and Clegg, 1981). Limited prospective screening of α thalassemia in high-risk populations, such as Southeast Asians, is now being carried out in Hong Kong, southern China, Thailand, and Taiwan (Lau et al., 1997). This represents a high-priority health measure aimed at reducing the health burden caused by α thalassemia. Due to its mild phenotype, prevention of HbH disease is not justified and should usually be discouraged.

SCREENING FOR SICKLE CELL ANEMIA AND SICKLE CELL TRAIT

Population-based screening programs for sickle cell trait were started in many regions of the United States in the early 1970s (see Chapter 29). These programs, misguided in retrospect, often led to restricted occupational choice, denials of health and life insurance for some found to carry the HbS gene, and the stigmatization of carriers. Sickle cell trait screening is now directed to targeted groups such as couples who are most likely to carry HbS genes and who are considering beginning a family. Screening in patients at risk for sickle cell trait can also be recommended before major thoracic and cardiovascular surgery and when hyphema is present (see Chapter 29). The U.S. Armed Forces have a variable approach to sickle cell trait screening that differs by service and even by military installation. Screening individuals assigned to flight duty may be prudent. Screening the general population for the presence of sickle cell trait is not useful. Recommendations for counseling individuals with sickle cell trait are discussed in Chapter 29.

Prenatal diagnosis of sickle cell anemia has been limited to couples living in the Western world and in Third World countries to those who have had a high level of education and who can afford access to sophisticated genetic services (Wang et al., 1994). Nevertheless, an ongoing prospective program for sickle cell anemia detection in the Republic of Cuba and Guadeloupe, based on mass education, screening, and

genetic counseling as for β thalassemia, has given encouraging results so far (WHO, 1989; Granda et al., 1991). Many genetic and environmental factors modify the clinical course of sickle cell anemia so that the behavior of this disease can be extremely variable. Most of these factors are poorly understood. In carrier screening, therefore, it is essential to investigate the known genetic modifying determinants in order to be able to predict the clinical phenotype as accurately as possible (see Chapter 26).

SCREENING FOR HbE

Simple HbE heterozygotes are unaffected clinically and HbE disease has a very mild phenotype. Screening efforts are therefore directed at detecting severely affected individuals with HbE-β^0 thalassemia. HbE concentrations are very low in cord blood. In HbE disease, HbE cord blood levels are between 3.9 percent and 14.95 percent, while in HbE heterozygotes levels of 2.1 percent and 10.3 percent (mean, 4.5 percent) are found. Individuals with homozygous HbE and HbE-β^0 thalassemia had similar amounts of HbE and HbF and DNA analysis is necessary to differentiate between these two syndromes. Prenatal diagnosis of HbE syndromes can be performed, as for β thalassemia, by villocentesis at the gestational ages of 10 to 11 weeks. Screening for HbE and the vast complexity of the HbE disorders are discussed in Chapter 43.

METHODS OF CARRIER DETECTION

Carrier detection should not miss even a single couple at risk, since this could discredit the entire preventive genetics program. Heterozygous β thalassemia, whether it be the β^0 or the β^+ type, is characterized by a high red blood cell count, microcytosis, hypochromia, increased HbA$_2$ levels, and unbalanced α/non-α-globin chain synthesis (see Chapter 12). However, several environmental or genetic factors may modify this hematologic phenotype and confound carrier identification (Table 36.1).

Although the high HbA$_2$ levels typical of heterozygous β thalassemia may decrease as a result of iron deficiency, in our experience they remain within the range usually present in β-thalassemia carriers unless severe anemia is present (Galanello et al., 1981). Iron studies may nevertheless exclude associated iron deficiency.

In many carrier detection procedures, a preliminary selection of individuals at risk for heterozygosity for thalassemia is based on the mean corpuscular volume (MCV) and mean corpuscular hemoglobin (MCH) values. However, since combined heterozygotes for β thalassemia and α thalassemia could have normal MCV and

Table 36.1. Heterozygous β Thalassemia: Phenotype Modification

Phenotype	Genotype
Normal RBC indices	α and β thalassemia interaction
Normal HbA$_2$ level	Co-inheritance of δ and β thalassemia
	Some mild β-thalassemia mutations
	γδβ thalassemia
	Iron deficiency
Normal RBC indices and HbA$_2$ level	Silent β-thalassemia mutations
	(Silent) α-globin gene triplication
	α, β, and δ thalassemia mutations
Severe heterozygous β thalassemia	Co-inheritance of heterozygous β thalassemia and triplicated α-globin gene
	Hyperunstable hemoglobin

Table 36.2. Silent β-Thalassemia Mutations

Transcriptional mutants
β$^+$, −101 C→T
β$^+$, −92 C→T
β$^+$, + 10 (−T)
β$^+$, + 33 (C→G)

Cap site
β$^+$, + 1 (A→C)

RNA processing mutants (consensus sequence)
β$^+$ IVS II −844 (C→G)

3′UTR (3′ untranslated region)
β$^+$ + 1480 (C→G)

RNA cleavage and polyadenylation
Poly A, AATAA<u>A</u>→AATAA<u>G</u>

MCH, this approach is not foolproof (Melis et al., 1983). It is therefore essential—at least where both α and β thalassemia are prevalent—that the initial tests for carrier detection should also include the quantitation of HbA$_2$. A high frequency of α and β thalassemia is common in many populations at risk in the Mediterranean area, the Middle East, and the Far East.

Although elevation of HbA$_2$ is the most important feature in identifying heterozygous thalassemia (Weatherall and Clegg, 1981), a number of heterozygotes for β thalassemia, including carriers of mild β-thalassemia mutations and combined heterozygotes for δ and β thalassemia, may have normal or borderline HbA$_2$ levels (Rosatelli et al., 1992a; Galanello et al., 1994).

Silent β thalassemia and the triplicated α-globin gene arrangement—both of which may lead to the production of intermediate forms of thalassemia by interacting with typical heterozygous β thalassemia—are important problems in carrier screening. Some of the mutations causing silent β thalassemia are listed in Table 36.2. The condition is characterized by normal MCV and MCH and normal HbA$_2$ and F levels, and can only be identified by the slight unbalance in the α/non-α-globin biosynthesis ratios (Gonzales-Redondo et al., 1989; Galanello et al., 1994). A similar silent phenotype results from the presence of a triplicated α-globin gene locus. The co-occurrence of α, δ, and β thalassemia genes is rare and may lead to a completely silent phenotype, resulting in pitfalls in carrier detection (Galanello et al., 1988). Figure 36.1 presents a flow chart for carrier identification (Cao and Rosatelli, 1993).

Sickle cell trait is easily identified (see Chapter 29). Its phenotype is modified by co-inherited α thalassemia, which leads to a variable reduction in HbS levels depending on the number of missing α-globin genes, but this does not lead to difficulty in carrier identification (Higgs et al., 1982) (see Chapter 29).

Initial tests include MCV and MCH and high-performance liquid chromatography (HPLC) (see Chapter 34). HPLC can detect the most common, clinically relevant hemoglobin variants, such as HbS, HbC, HbD-Punjab, HbO-Arab, and HbE, and can also detect Hb Knossos, which is a mild β-thalassemia allele not defined by the commonly used electrophoretic procedure for hemoglobin analysis. HPLC may also be used to quantitate HbA$_2$ and HbF (Galanello et al., 1995). Only silent β thalassemia and the triplicated α-globin gene arrangement are missed by this approach. When the levels of MCH and MCV are low and those of HbA$_2$ high, a diagnosis of heterozygous β thalassemia is made.

Iron deficiency, α thalassemia, γδβ thalassemia, β and δ thalassemia, or mild β thalassemia may lead to a phenotype characterized by microcytosis, hypochromia, normal/borderline HbA$_2$, and normal HbF. After iron deficiency is excluded by measuring erythrocyte zinc protoporphyrin and evaluation of transferrin saturation, the different thalassemia determinants leading to this phenotype are discriminated by globin-chain synthesis analysis and eventually by α-, δ-, and β-globin gene analysis.

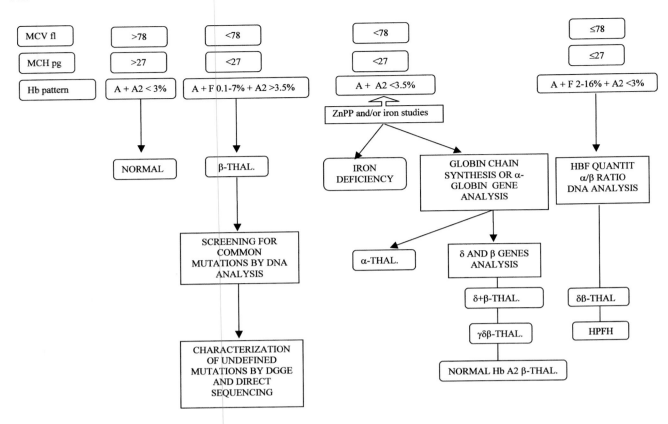

Figure 36.1. Flow chart for β-thalassemia carrier screening.

When normal MCV and borderline HbA₂ levels are found, a silent β-thalassemia mutation such as β⁺ –101 C→T (Gonzales-Redondo et al., 1989), β⁺ –92 C→T (Rosatelli et al., 1995), or β⁺ IVS2 nt 844 C→G (Rosatelli et al., 1994) should be suspected or a triplicated α-globin gene arrangement might be present. In these instances proceeding directly to α- and β-globin gene analysis should be considered since the α/β ratio may be normal in many of these cases. Only when carriers of these mutations mate with a typical high HbA₂ β-thalassemia heterozygote or with a carrier of an undetermined type of thalassemia is it recommended that the thalassemia mutation be defined.

In rare instances where normal or low MCH and MCV, normal or reduced HbA₂, and high HbF levels are observed, δβ thalassemia should be suspected and differentiated from hereditary persistence of fetal hemoglobin (HPFH). This distinction can be made by analyzing the red blood cell distribution of HbF, by globin-chain synthesis analysis, or by gene mapping the β-globin-gene-like cluster (see Chapter 15).

Screening by MCV and MCH or osmotic fragility is acceptable in populations with a relatively low incidence of both β and α thalassemia, because the number of false negatives resulting from combined heterozygosity for α and β thalassemia are likely to be very low.

MOLECULAR DIAGNOSIS

Specific mutations identified by carrier detection procedures are defined by one of the several polymerase chain reaction (PCR)-based procedures listed in Table 36.3 (see Chapter 35).

β Thalassemia

β Thalassemia is remarkably heterogeneous at the molecular level (Huisman and Carver, 1998) (see Chap-

---

Table 36.3. PCR-Based Procedures Used for the Detection of β Thalassemia

Known mutations
    Amplification refractory mutation system
    Reverse dot blot analyses
    Oligonucleotide ligation assay
    Restriction enzyme digestion
    Primer-specific restriction map modification
Unknown mutations
    Denaturing gradient gel electrophoresis
    Single-strand conformation polymorphism
    Protein truncation test
    Chemical cleavage method
    Enzyme cleavage method

ter 12), but a limited number of molecular defects are prevalent in each of the populations most at risk for severe thalassemia (Fig. 36.2). In practice this permits the most appropriate probes or primers to be selected according to the carrier's ethnic origin. Mutation detection is carried out on the PCR-amplified β-globin gene. The most commonly used screening procedures for known mutations are the reverse dot blot analysis (Saiki et al., 1989) with allele-specific oligonucleotide probes (Fig. 36.3), or primer-specific amplification (ARMS)(Newton et al., 1989). Other methodologies that could be used for mutation detection in carriers of thalassemia are the oligonucleotide ligation assay (Nickerson et al., 1990), restriction enzyme analysis (Pirastu et al., 1989), and the primer-specific restriction map modification (Gasparini et al., 1992). When a β-thalassemia mutation cannot be defined by one of the above procedures, characterization of the mutation is most commonly done by denaturing gradient gel electrophoresis (DGGE) (Myers et al., 1985; Cai and Kan, 1990; Rosatelli et al., 1992b), chemical mismatch cleavage analysis (Cotton et al., 1988), or single-strand conformation polymorphism (SSCP) analysis (Orita et al., 1989), followed by direct sequencing on amplified single-strand DNA (Gyllensten and Erlich, 1988; Sanger et al., 1977). After localization by DGGE, the mutation is defined by direct sequencing of the DNA contained in the fragment (Fig. 36.4). Direct β-globin gene sequencing may be carried out manually or automatically. If a mutation is not detected by DGGE analysis, small deletions are searched for by polyacrylamide gel electrophoresis of the PCR-amplified products prepared for ARMS or reverse dot blot analysis. Small deletions are suggested by very high HbA₂ levels (see Chapter 12). Larger deletions may be identified by RFLP analysis by Southern blot or PCR-based procedures. DNA-based diagnosis of hemoglobin disorders is discussed in Chapter 35.

Prediction of a Mild Phenotype

Although homozygosity or compound heterozygosity for β thalassemia usually results in the clinical phenotype of transfusion-dependent thalassemia major, a consistent proportion of these homozygotes have milder phenotypes that range in severity from the asymptomatic carrier state to thalassemia intermedia (Thein et al., 1988; Ho et al., 1998). Since the main pathophysiologic determinant of the severity of the thalassemia syndrome is the extent of α/non-α-globin-chain synthesis unbalance, any factor capable of reducing this unbalance may have an ameliorating effect. Homozygosity or compound heterozygosity for a silent or mild β thalassemia is the most important clinical mechanism resulting in thalassemia intermedia. By contrast, compound heterozygotes for a

mild or silent and a severe mutation may result in a large number of phenotypes, including severe and mild forms. Other mechanisms of thalassemia intermedia are co-inheritance with homozygous β thalassemia or α thalassemia or one of many determinants resulting in the continuous production of HbF in adult life (Chang et al., 1995; Craig et al., 1996) (see Chapters 12, 13, and 15). Despite the significant progress in this field, molecular mechanisms for a large number of cases of thalassemia intermedia have not yet been defined. Practically, since none of the above mechanisms result in a consistent effect, only co-inheritance of the mild or silent β-thalassemia alleles can be used to predict a mild phenotype.

δ Thalassemia

Compound heterozygotes for δ and β thalassemia may be confused with α thalassemia because of normal or borderline HbA₂ levels. The condition is defined by δ-globin gene analysis. Interacting δ thalassemia is first suspected when a borderline HbA₂ level is present or when family studies show segregating δ thalassemia— normal red cell indices and low HbA₂ concentrations— and β thalassemia. These compound heterozygotes for δ and β thalassemia should be definitively identified on the basis of globin-chain synthesis analysis and/or α-, δ-, and β-globin gene analysis. δ Thalassemia has been defined at the molecular level and most δ thalassemia determinants are in *trans* to β-thalassemia mutations; however, a few have also been detected in *cis* (Huisman and Carver, 1998). Each population at risk is likely to have a limited number of δ-thalassemia mutations and these are discussed in Chapter 10. In the Sardinian population, for instance, only two δ-thalassemia mutations have been detected so far, δ⁺27 (G→T) and a δ-thalassemia deletion, the so-called Corfù δβ thalassemia (Moi et al., 1988, 1992; Galanello et al., 1990). A limited number of allele-specific primers or probes can be used, therefore, to detect δ-thalassemia mutations in each population at risk (see below).

α Thalassemias

Deletion α thalassemias are detected by the use of two primers, flanking the deletion breakpoints, that permit amplification of a DNA segment only in the presence of the specific deletions. The DNA is then amplified by PCR (reviewed in Kattamis et al., 1996). As a control, the DNA from a normal chromosome is amplified simultaneously using one of the primers flanking the breakpoint together with a primer homologous to a DNA region deleted by the mutation. In addition, restriction enzyme analysis on selectively amplified α₁- and α₂-globin genes is used to detect nondeletion α thalassemias, and when this method is

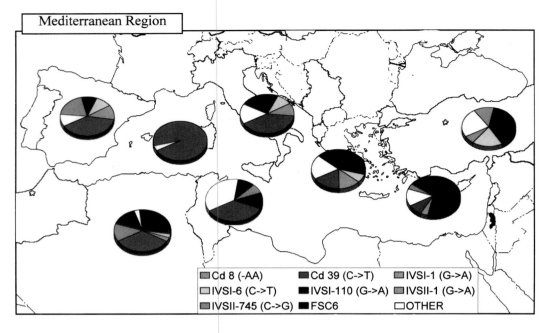

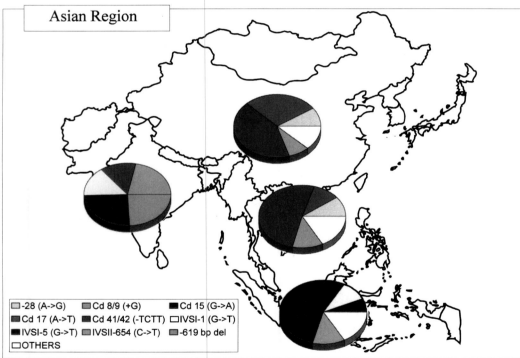

Figure 36.2. Population distribution of common β-thalassemia mutations. For full color reproduction, see color plate 36.2

not applicable, dot blot analysis with allele-specific oligonucleotide probes is used. α-Globin gene analysis is used both in defining the molecular defect in carriers of α thalassemia and in discriminating between heterozygous α thalassemia and compound heterozygos-

ity for δ and β thalassemia or γδβ thalassemia. Definition of the α-globin gene arrangement could also be useful in predicting the clinical phenotype of homozygous β thalassemia.

Sickle Cell Anemia

Sickle cell anemia is caused by homozygosity for the HbS mutation but compound heterozygous forms of

GENOMIC DNA

β-gene

PCR 5'— —3'

A B

A:5'-TAAGCCAGTGCCAGAAGAGCC-3'
B:5'-CACTGACCTCCCACATTCCC-3'

MUTATION DETECTION BY RDB HYBRIDIZATION

β39 βI–110 βI–1 βI–6 βII–1 βII–745 β6 β–87 β44 β76 βII–654 β8

WT
M

Figure 36.3. Screening for the most common β-thalassemia mutations by reverse dot blot analysis (RDB). Top: the whole β-globin gene is enzymatically amplified using primer A and B Bottom: A β-thalassemia carrier, heterozygote for IVSII-745 mutation. WT, wild type oligonucleotide hybridization; M, mutated oligonucleotide hybridization.

sickle cell disease are also common (see Chapter 28). Procedures similar to those used in β thalassemia are used in the molecular diagnosis of carriers of these hemoglobinopathies, especially dot blot analysis with allele-specific probes or primer specific amplification. Co-inherited modifying genes, the most noteworthy being α thalassemia and HPHF, may modulate the severity of sickle cell anemia (Steinberg, 1996) (see Chapter 26). The only determinant consistently associated with a milder phenotype is the presence of high levels of HbF. These modifying factors should be defined by appropriate procedures so that during genetic counseling couples at risk can be given the best possible prediction of the clinical phenotype.

PRENATAL DIAGNOSIS

The first prenatal diagnosis of both α and β thalassemia dates back to the 1970s and was carried out by globin-chain synthesis analysis of fetal blood obtained by fetoscopy or placental aspiration (Kan et al., 1975). Molecular definition of the thalassemias, the development of procedures for their detection by DNA analysis, and the introduction of chorionic villus sampling in the last decade have produced a dramatic improvement in the prenatal detection of these disorders. For a brief period after the first description of restriction fragment length polymorphisms (RFLP) thalassemia was diagnosed either indirectly by RFLP analysis (Kan et al.,

Figure 36.4. Molecular screening for rare or uncommon mutation of the β-globin gene. Left: denaturing gradient gel electrophoresis (DGGE) of a 3' fragment of the β-globin gene; WT/WT, normal subject; WT/Poly A = a β-thalassemia heterozygote for the polyadenylation signal mutation AATAAA→AATGAA. Right: Automated sequence analysis (Applied Biosystem 377 DNA sequencer) in the same subject.

WT/WT   WT/WT   WT/ poly A

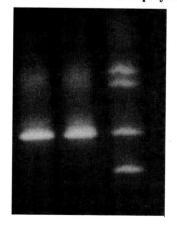

Poly (A) consensus sequence

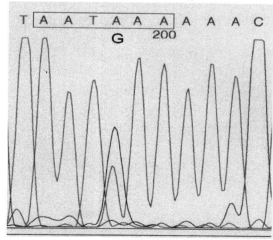

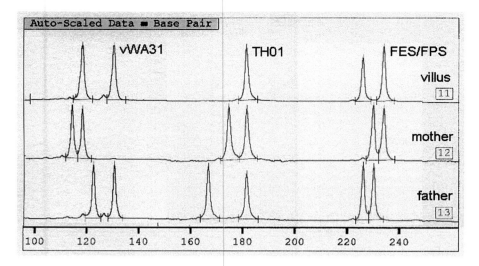

Figure 36.5. DNA polymorphism analysis in the prenatal diagnosis of a fetus at risk for β thalassemia. vWA31, short tandem repeat (TCTA) in the intron 40 of the human WF gene; THO1, short tandem repeat (AATG) in human chromosome (11p15.5); FES/FPS, short tandem repeat (ATTT) in the intron 5 of the human c-fes/fps protooncogene. For all the three markers examined fetal DNA shows the absence of double maternal contribution thus excluding maternal contamination.

fetal mortality associated with this method is acceptably low at about 1 percent. Chorionic villi may be obtained transcervically or transabdominally. We prefer the transabdominal route for several reasons: It has a lower infection rate and a lower incidence of amniotic fluid leakage, it is a simple procedure, and it is generally preferred by the patient.

1980) or directly by oligonucleotide hybridization on electrophoretically separated DNA fragments (Pirastu et al., 1983). Nowadays, thalassemias are detected directly by the analysis of amplified DNA from fetal trophoblasts or from amniotic fluid cells.

Sampling

Fetal DNA for analysis can be obtained from amniocytes or from chorionic villi. At present chorionic villus sampling is by far the most widely used procedure, mainly because it can be carried out within the first trimester of pregnancy, generally at the 10th to 12th week of gestation (Hogge et al., 1986; Cao et al., 1987; Brambati et al., 1988) and because the risk of

Fetal Analysis

Fetal DNA analysis is carried out as described above and in Chapter 35. To reduce the probability of a misdiagnosis, we analyze chorionic villus DNA using two different procedures: reverse dot blot hybridization and primer-specific amplification. Figure 36.5 is an example of a fetus at risk for combined heterozygosity for the $\beta^0 39$ and $\beta^+ IVSI-110$ mutations that was tested by both procedures, and Table 36.4 shows the overall results obtained in one genetic unit in Sardinia.

The sole instance of misdiagnosis was when prenatal diagnosis was carried out by oligonucleotide hybridization on electrophoretically separated nonamplified DNA fragments. Misdiagnosis may occur for several reasons. These include failure to amplify the target

Table 36.4. Results of Prenatal Diagnosis of β Thalassemia in Sardinia

Fetal DNA	Pregnancies monitored	Homozygous fetuses	Failures		Misdiagnoses	
			No.	%	No.	%
• PCR-based analysis	2,902	731	—	—	—	—
	1,194	325	7	0.6	1	0.08
• EDD with ASO probes fetal blood	1,131	286	10	0.9	2	0.2
Total	5,227	1,342	17	0.3	3	0.05

Abbreviations: EDD, enzymatically digested DNA; ASO, allele-specific oligonucleotide.

DNA fragment, false paternity, contamination with maternal cells, and sample exchange. Misdiagnosis because of failure of DNA amplification is obviously limited by the above duplicative approach. To avoid misdiagnosis from false paternity or contamination with maternal cells, we carry out DNA polymorphism analysis in parallel with mutation analysis (Fig. 36.5). Maternal cell contamination can be reduced by careful dissection under the inverted microscope of the maternal decidua from the fetal trophoblasts, by using a minimal amount (at least 3 μg) of chorionic villus DNA, and by a limited number of PCR cycles in order to reduce the chances of co-amplifying DNA from the maternal decidua.

With the advent of DNA amplification it became possible to analyze the genotype of a single cell. This paved the way for preimplantation or even preconception diagnosis (Monk and Holding, 1990). Preimplantation diagnosis may be carried out by biopsy of the blastula, obtained by washing the uterine cavity after in vivo fertilization, or by analysis of a single blastomere from an eight-cell embryo after in vitro fertilization (Handyside et al., 1992). Successful pregnancies have been reported following the transfer of human embryos in which a single gene defect has been excluded.

Preconception Diagnosis

Preconception diagnosis is based on the analysis of the first polar body of the unfertilized egg. With this method, unfertilized eggs that carry the defective gene and those without the defect can be identified. By fertilizing in vitro only the eggs without the defect and implanting them in the mother, a successful pregnancy with a normal fetus can be obtained. Of course, the genotype of the fetus should be checked further by chorionic villus biopsy.

In vitro embryo and preconception diagnosis are useful to couples for whom religious or ethical beliefs will not permit pregnancy termination, and for those who have already had several therapeutic abortions. At present, however, its use in the routine monitoring of pregnancies at risk is precluded by the technical demands of these procedures, the difficulty in organizing the service, and a high cost.

EFFECTIVENESS OF PREVENTION PROGRAMS

Thalassemia prevention programs have been successful because of a well-informed population and because the methodology for prevention had no consistent adverse effect on those found to be carriers. A marked decline in the incidence of thalassemia major has been documented in all populations at risk in the Mediterranean area where screening and counseling

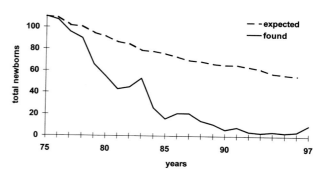

Figure 36.6. Fall of the birth rate of babies with homozygous β thalassemia in Sardinia.

has been introduced (Angastiniotis et al., 1995). Figure 36.6 presents an example of this trend in the Sardinian population, where the incidence of thalassemia major declined from 1:250 live births in the absence of a prevention program, to 1:4,000 with an effective prevention program, a reduction of 94 percent of the cases who would have been born on the basis of the prevalence of thalassemia heterozygotes. The residual Sardinian cases are attributable to the following: misinformation and/or absence of information (67 percent); false paternity (13 percent); choice to carry on the pregnancy without any prenatal test or choice to continue the pregnancy of an affected fetus (20 percent). Similar results have been obtained in other populations (Angastiniotis et al., 1995). These data suggest the necessity of educating health workers and the population at large in preventive genetics. The introduction of teaching on thalassemia in secondary schools may also be very instrumental in further reducing the incidence of this disorder.

FUTURE PROSPECTS

In carrier screening and prenatal diagnosis, it is realistic from a technical point of view to predict further simplification and full automation of the procedures used to detect the genes for thalassemia and other hemoglobinopathies. Primer-specific amplification and reverse oligonucleotide hybridization, for instance, may easily become fully automated. An oligonucleotide microchip assay has recently been proposed for the large-scale detection of mutations in genetic diseases including β thalassemia. Given the alternative features of a high throughput, automation, and modest cost, the DNA chip has the potential to become a valuable method in future applications of mutation detection in medicine. It is foreseeable that the cost of DNA analysis may be progressively reduced and that it may lead to using mutation detection as a screening method in the future, thus skipping steps based on hematologic analysis in carrier detection. Simplification of preimplantation embryo and preconception diagnosis may lead to a more extensive use of the procedure in the future, especially by those couples who are against pregnancy termination.

The most relevant advance would be fetal diagnosis by analysis of fetal cells in the maternal circulation. At present, several methods have been proposed for analysis, but none have given reliable results (Bianchi et al., 1990; Ganshirt-Ahlert et al., 1993). A procedure based on the density gradient separation of mononuclear cells from maternal blood, enriching fetal cells by magnetic-activated cell sorting with antitransferrin receptor antibody, identification of fetal cells by immunostaining with antifetal or antiembryonic hemoglobin antibodies, isolation of nucleated fetal red cells by microdissection under light microscopy, and nonradioactive PCR analysis, has detected point mutations responsible for β thalassemia or HbS (Cheung et al., 1996). Simplification and partial automation of this procedure may lead to the introduction of prenatal diagnosis by analysis of fetal cells in the maternal circulation in clinical practice.

Another important challenge for the future is the organization of genetic preventive programs, like those ongoing in the Mediterranean area, in other parts of the world with a high prevalence of β thalassemia, namely the Middle East, the Indian subcontinent, and the Far East. Yet, presently, the resources for population education and the state of technical development seem to preclude the materialization of such programs.

SCREENING FOR SICKLE CELL DISEASE

Population-based screening for sickle hemoglobin was initiated in the early 1970s in the United States. Only one mutation causes HbS, simplifying its detection compared to the thalassemias, yet the many compound heterozygous variants of sickle cell disease and the epistatic modifiers of these disorders add their own complexities to screening and counseling programs. The goals of these early programs initially focused on increasing awareness, providing accurate education about sickle cell disease, and detecting carriers so couples could make reproductive decisions based on accurate information about the risk of having an affected child (Whitten et al., 1981). These programs increased public awareness and knowledge about sickle cell anemia and trait but did less to directly impact on management of infants with disease.

The newborn screening for hemoglobinopathies that began in the 1930s and 1940s depended on the induction of sickling in red cell preparations (Diggs et al., 1933; Scott, 1948). These pioneer efforts identi-

fied infants with sickle hemoglobin but could not accurately differentiate carriers from individuals with disease (Scott et al., 1954). In the 1960s hemoglobin electrophoresis using cord blood samples was shown to be effective for identifying structural β-globin variants despite the preponderance of HbF at birth (Gilman et al., 1976; Pearson, 1989). Newborn screening programs using cellulose acetate and agar gel electrophoresis on cord blood samples were initiated in the early 1970s to determine the incidence of variants, document the early natural history of the disease, and provide early health care to affected infants (Pearson, 1973; Pearson et al., 1974; Sergeant et al., 1974, 1981; Gilman et al., 1976; Sexauer et al., 1976). Demonstration that hemoglobin identification could be accomplished using hemolysates prepared from the filter paper spots and collected for metabolic screening allowed testing for sickle cell conditions to be added to newborn screening programs that detected PKU and hypothyroidism (Garrick et al., 1973). New York State implemented the first statewide screening program from 1975 through 1978 (Grover et al., 1978; Grover 1989; Schedlbauer and Pass, 1989). The New York program and early screening programs in Jamaica, Colorado, Georgia, and Texas documented the feasibility of newborn screening, provided critical information about complications in the first years of life, and collected data suggesting early detection may reduce morbidity and mortality (Grover et al., 1978; John et al., 1984; Grover, 1989; Harris and Eckman, 1989; Schedlbauer and Pass, 1989; Therrell et al., 1989; Githens et al., 1990).

Screening newborns for sickle cell anemia was not thought to be effective in modifying outcome until Powars and others showed that early diagnosis and comprehensive care could reduce morbidity and mortality (Powars et al., 1981; Grover et al., 1983; John et al., 1984; Pearson, 1986). Publication of the results of the blinded, randomized, and controlled trial of penicillin prophylaxis in sickle cell anemia early documented the benefit of newborn diagnosis and prophylaxis with penicillin in preventing *Streptococcus pneumoniae* septicemia (Gaston et al., 1986). This landmark study provided a firm rationale for newborn screening (Gaston et al., 1986). In early 1987, an NIH Consensus Development Conference on Newborn Screening for Sickle Cell Disease and Other Hemoglobinopathies concluded that every newborn should be screened for sickle cell disease so that death during infancy could be prevented (Consensus Conference, 1987). The primary public health benefits are reduction in the high mortality during the first 5 years of life from treatable infection (Barret-Connor, 1971; Seeler, 1972; Diggs, 1973; Powars, 1975; Overturf et al., 1977; Pearson,

1977; Seeler and Jacobs, 1977; Lobel and Bove, 1982; O'Brien et al., 1976; Thomas et al., 1982; Zarkowsky et al., 1986; Lobel et al., 1989) and prevention of death from splenic sequestration (Emond et al., 1985). Rapid development of programs in the United States occurred because of direct federal funding for newborn screening (Sundall, 1987). By 1990 in the United States, 43 states, Puerto Rico, and the Virgin Islands had statewide programs (CORN, 1995). Thirty-nine states test all infants and six presently target "higher risk" populations (CORN, 1995). In 1992, over 2.9 million newborns were tested and about 2,800 were detected with clinically significant hemoglobin variants, documenting the rapid implementation of screening (CORN, 1995). Screening programs for hemoglobinopathies are being established in many countries in Europe, Africa, the Americas, and Asia.

PROGRAMMATIC ISSUES IN NEWBORN SCREENING FOR SICKLE CELL DISEASE

The goal of newborn hemoglobinopathy screening is to reduce morbidity and mortality in affected infants. There is proven benefit from early intervention in sickle cell anemia and HbS-β^0 thalassemia (Powars et al., 1981; Gaston et al., 1986; Lee et al., 1995; CDC, 1998; Eckman et al., 1997). Infants with HbSC disease have increased mortality (Rogers et al., 1978; Thomas et al., 1982; Gill et al., 1995) and incidence of bacterial infection (Zarkowsky et al., 1986; Lane et al., 1994) and will, therefore, also likely benefit from early intervention. Infants with many other hemoglobin variants and thalassemias that may be detected at birth may also benefit from early detection and entry into health care programs. The five programmatic elements required in newborn screening programs to maximize prevention of morbidity and mortality from hemoglobinopathies are outlined in Table 36.5.

NEONATAL SCREENING FOR SICKLE CELL ANEMIA

Mandating the availability of universal testing of infants born in the program area ensures that all infants with disease are identified. Universal testing also reduces potential discrimination or stigmatization (Consensus Conference, 1987). Integrating of sickle cell screening into established newborn screening programs for metabolic disorders, using hemolysates prepared from the filter paper spot as the analyte, increases efficiency and effectiveness (McCabe, 1982; Steinberg et al., 1991; AAP, 1992; Therrell et al., 1992). Targeted screening of infants considered to be at increased risk has been advocated to increase the

---

Table 36.5. Newborn Hemoglobin Screening Program—Elements Required to Minimize Morbidity and Mortality

Screening—Universal testing of neonates for hemoglobin variants

Follow-up—Rapid confirmation of positive screens and entry of infants with disease into health care

Diagnosis—Laboratory and clinical evaluation of neonates with positive screen results

Management—Comprehensive health care, education, and social support to provide and maintain therapy for all affected individuals

Evaluation—Ongoing assessment of screening and diagnostic methods, effectiveness of follow-up and management, and impact on the individual, family, and society

Modified from CORN (1999), with permission.

---

cost effectiveness of programs (Tsevat et al., 1991; Gessner et al., 1996; Panepinto et al., 2000); however, such approaches clearly increase the number of infants who are missed and puts them at risk for unnecessary death (Harris and Eckman, 1989).

LABORATORY APPROACHES TO SCREENING FOR HbS

Diagnosis of sickle syndromes in newborns is practical because a number of approaches for screening are sensitive and cost effective. There are few studies that directly compare the sensitivity, specificity, and cost/benefit of various methods of sample collection and techniques for hemoglobin analysis (Galacteros et al., 1980; Jacobs et al., 1986; Kinney et al., 1989; Papadea et al., 1994). False-negative tests result in the nonidentification of infants with disease and must be avoided. Retesting using a second sample collected from all infants with any abnormality on initial screening minimizes the occurrence of false negatives, but collecting samples on excessive numbers of carriers and infants with false-positive results causes unnecessary anxiety for parents, increases cost of follow-up, and reduces the credibility of the screening program (McCabe, 1982; AAP, 1992; Therrell et al., 1992). Therefore, a two-tiered approach in the screening laboratory is recommended where all initial abnormals are retested using a second sample obtained from the original filter paper or cord blood specimen (Therrell et al., 1992).

Newborn screening samples for hemoglobin analysis used in most statewide screening programs consist of hemolysates obtained from dried blood spots collected on filter paper by heel stick while a few programs use liquid blood collected from the umbilical cord at birth (CORN, 1998). Despite a few reports that suggest that filter paper samples do not provide an analyte that allows sufficient resolution of hemoglobin bands for accurate diagnosis (Kleman et al., 1989; Kutlar et al., 1990), a number of studies show filter paper samples are satisfactory for newborn screening (Jacobs et al., 1986; Kinney et al., 1989; Schedlbauer and Pass, 1989; Therrell et al., 1989; Papadea et al., 1994). Most programs use filter paper spots because hemoglobin testing can be integrated into metabolic newborn screening programs, simplifying sample collection, specimen processing, and data management.

There are a number of approaches to identification of sickle cell anemia and other hemoglobinopathies by the newborn screening laboratory that provide excellent results. A two-tiered approach to analysis is recommended where all abnormal samples are retested using a different analytic technique on a second hemolysate obtained from the original filter paper or cord blood sample (Therrell et al., 1992). Early programs utilized cellulose acetate electrophoresis at alkaline pH with initial confirmation by citrate agar electrophoresis at acid pH (Garrick et al., 1973; Pearson et al., 1974; Serjeant et al., 1974; Harris and Eckman, 1989; Schedlbauer and Pass, 1989; Therrell et al., 1989; Githens et al., 1990). Four programs in the United States still use cellulose acetate electrophoresis as the primary screening method (CORN, 1998). Isoelectric focusing (IEF) is presently used in most programs (Galacteros et al., 1980). HPLC is also being used as the primary screening technique using automated techniques and rapid run programs (Eastman et al., 1996). Report of a large experience using HPLC as the primary screening technique validates the accuracy and the utility of quantitative data in diagnosing infants who are compound heterozygotes for structural variants and thalassemia during primary screening (Lorey et al., 1994). Three states use HPLC as the primary screening method (CORN, 1998).

Protocols for the second tier testing to confirm the initial abnormal results show considerable variation between programs. Approaches for this initial screening laboratory confirmation include electrophoresis on citrate agar at acid pH, IEF, HPLC, immunologic-based techniques, and DNA/RNA determination of genotype (Steinberg et al., 1991; CORN, 1992). Use of HPLC as a confirmatory method is increasing because of superior separation of hemoglobin variants and because this technique provides quantitative data of use in diagnosing compound heterozygotes with structural variants and thalassemia (Wilson et al., 1983, 1996; Huisman, 1989; Steinberg et al., 1991).

A number of programs are using DNA- or RNA-based molecular genetic diagnostic techniques for con-firmation of the genotype on the initial screening sample (McCabe et al., 1987; Rubin et al., 1989; Jinks et al., 1989; Zhang and McCabe, 1992). Initial confirmation of the genotype has the potential to reduce the number of false positives and the time to definitive confirmation of the sickle phenotype (Steinberg et al., 1991; Zhang et al., 1994).

Accurate diagnosis of phenotype and genotype using the initial screening sample is desirable; however, all infants with suspected disease still must be confirmed using a separate sample collection because clerical and transcription errors are among the most common encountered causes of an erroneous diagnosis (Papadea et al., 1994). In some cases, physical examination, extended hematologic testing, family studies, and time may be required for diagnosis if the genotype is not determined directly by DNA analytic techniques (Sickle Cell Disease Guideline Panel, 1993).

FOLLOW-UP

Newborn screening programs should not be initiated without adequate provisions for follow-up services to establish a definitive diagnosis and provide for ongoing medical management of all infants detected with suspected disease. Such follow-up requires a well-organized newborn screening system and effective communication between components. Follow-up is initiated by prompt reporting of abnormal screening results by the screening laboratory to individuals responsible for retrieval, diagnosis, and management. Retrieval of infants with abnormal results requires the coordinated effort of many individuals in the health care system. Well-designed protocols are essential to provide such coordination. One individual, usually in public health, should be responsible for developing protocols, supervising implementation, and monitoring compliance. Effective communication between components is critical and best accomplished through a steering committee composed of individuals who represent all program components. Such committees develop protocols for improving the newborn screening system, solve problems, provide advocacy, and encourage respect among individuals in the program. Education of the public and health care providers is a critical component of follow-up. The need for screening and the goals and objectives, benefits, and limitations of the screening program should be communicated before a program is initiated (Therrell et al., 1992). Follow-up is facilitated if prospective parents are educated about the rationale for newborn screening well in advance of the birth (CORN, 1998). They should also be informed about the purpose of all repeat and diagnostic testing in an effective and sensitive manner so they understand the need for testing without becoming unnecessarily concerned. Health care providers need to be educated so they respond appropriately to notification that an infant in their care has an abnormal screening result.

Newborn screening for sickle cell syndromes provides unique challenges because a large number of other hemoglobin variants are identified that may cause clinical problems or may be of no clinical significance. In addition, approximately 50 heterozygous carriers of HbS and HbC are identified for every infant with sickle cell disease. Although there may be no immediate benefit to the infant, results that show a child is a carrier may provide information of use to the parents (CORN, 1998). Most agree that a mechanism should exist to provide results to the parents of all infants who are screened. If notified, parents of carriers of hemoglobin variants should have access to testing for themselves and other family members. Appropriate education and genetic counseling of the parents about their reproductive risks are based on their test results, not the results of the newborn screen (CORN, 1998). Parental and extended family testing requires a complete blood count with red cell indices in addition to hemoglobin electrophoresis IEF, or HPLC. Defining the parent's genotype may also require quantifying hemoglobin variants, HbA_2, and HbF or DNA-based testing. Each newborn screening program needs to develop protocols that address follow-up of carriers of sickle cell trait and those with other hemoglobin variants based on program goals, objectives, and resources (Table 36.6). Follow-up of hemoglobin variants depends on their clinical relevance in the population being screened. Although unsatisfactory samples for hemoglobin testing are less common than those for metabolic screening, procedures for prompt retesting of infants with unsatisfactory samples should have the same priority as follow-up of infants with suspected sickle cell disease.

DIAGNOSIS

Hemoglobinopathy confirmation testing should be performed on a second blood specimen obtained as soon as possible after the initial screen with a goal of initiating medical management of infants with sickle cell disease by 2 months of age. Diagnostic hemoglobin testing, complemented by clinical, hematologic, and family studies, should be coordinated by a physician knowledgeable in the diagnosis of hemoglobin disorders in infants. When DNA-based diagnosis or extended family testing is not available, confirmation may require repeated testing after the child reaches 6 months of age and occasionally definitive diagnosis may be delayed for several years. All children with phenotypes suggestive of sickle cell disease should be maintained on prophylactic peni-

---

Table 36.6. CORN Guidelines for Follow-Up of Carriers of Hemoglobin Variants Detected by Newborn Screening for Sickle Cell Disease

- Ideally, education about newborn sickle cell testing, which usually includes testing for sickle cell disease, should be provided to families during prenatal care, well in advance of the time of delivery.
- A mechanism should be in place in state newborn screening programs so that results of newborn screening for sickle cell disease can be made available to the parents of all infants who are tested.
- Parents of all infants who are detected to be carriers of hemoglobin variants should be offered appropriate education, counseling, and testing.
- Individuals who counsel should have appropriate training and credentialing in order to ensure the highest quality of services for families of carriers detected by newborn screening.
- Programs for follow-up of normals and carriers of hemoglobin variants should have a mechanism for monitoring and assessing the approaches to, response to, and costs of providing carrier education and counseling services.

From CORN (1998b), with permission.

---

cillin and treated as sickle cell anemia until definitive diagnostic testing is completed.

Initial screening results that suggest a clinically important hemoglobinopathy are usually confirmed using liquid blood samples and comprehensive laboratory testing that includes a variable combination of a complete blood count with red cell indices, a reticulocyte count, and hemoglobin electrophoresis, IEF, HPLC, or DNA-based diagnosis. Family studies and repeat testing up to age 2 years may be required to differentiate sickle cell anemia from HbS-β thalassemia or HbS HPFH. Confirmatory testing may be carried out by the initial screening laboratory or sent to a laboratory that specializes in hemoglobin identification.

Quantifying hemoglobin fractions is usually helpful and sometimes necessary for diagnosis (see Table 36.7). For example, quantifying of HbS and HbA distinguishes HbS-β+ thalassemia from sickle cell trait (Fairbanks, 1980). Levels of HbA_2 are useful in differentiating those who are homozygous for structural variants from those who are compound heterozygotes for a structural variant and β thalassemia (Fairbanks, 1980). The quantity and cellular distribution of HbF is useful in differentiating sickle cell anemia, HbS-β thalassemia, and HbS-HPFH syndromes in individuals over 2 years of age (Fairbanks, 1980). The proportion of HbS in sickle cell trait is often reduced in the presence of α thalassemia (see Chapters 28 and 29).

Table 36.7. Diagnosis of Infants with Newborn Screening Results Suggesting Sickle Cell Disease or Other Clinically Significant Hemoglobin Disorders

Screen result	Disease suggested	Confirmatory test results: Hb electrophoresis, HPLC, MCV
Hb FS	Sickle cell anemia	HbS, MCV normal or increased for age,* $A_2 < 3.5\%$, F < 20% at 2 years. DNA analysis = sickle cell anemia
Hb FS	HbS-β^0 thalassemia	HbS, MCV low for age,* $A_2 > 3.5\%$ at 2 years, DNA analysis = AS[†]
Hb FS	HbS-HPFH	HbS, $A_2 < 3.5\%$, F > 20% at 2 years. KB = pancellular, DNA analysis = S-, little or no hemolysis
Hb FSA	HbS-β^+ thalassemia	Hb SA, MCV low,* $A_2 > 3.5\%$, DNA analysis = AS[†]
Hb FSC	HbSC disease	HbSC, F < 20% at 6 mo. DNA analysis = SC
Hb FSD, FSO, FSE, FS-other	Hb SD, SO^Arab, SE, S-other	Special evaluation by hematology consultation with CBC, Hb ELP, IEF, HPLC, DNA-based studies[†]
Hb FC	HbC disease or C-β^0 thalassemia	Special evaluation by hematology consultation with CBC, Hb ELP, IEF, HPLC, DNA-based studies[†]
Hb FCA	HbC-β^+ thalassemia	Hb CA, MCV low,* DNA analysis = AC[†]
Hb FE	HbE disease or E-β^0 thalassemia	Special evaluation by hematology consultation with CBC, Hb ELP, IEF, HPLC, DNA-based studies[†]
Hb FA or FA-other + Bart's	α thalassemia	Special evaluation if Bart's > 10% or if family studies are indicated

Abbreviations: KB, Kleihauer Betke; ELP, electrophoresis.

* HbA_2 levels must be interpreted using the normal and abnormal values for each laboratory (see Chapter 10). Normal MCV (fl) at 1 mo > 85; 2 mo > 77; 3 to 6 mo > 74; 0.5 to 2 y > 70; 2 to 6 y > 75; 6 to 12 y > 77; 12 to 18 y > 78; > 18 y > 80 (Nathan and Oski, 1987).

† Thalassemia mutation may be diagnosed by allele-specific oligonucleotide probes based on ethnic origin.

HPLC allows automated, computer-assisted resolution and quantification of hemoglobin variants. Alternatively, HbA_2 can be quantified by microcolumns and HbF by alkali resistance or immunologically based assays. DNA-based diagnosis can reliably establish the genetic basis of most structural hemoglobin variants (Steinberg et al., 1991). The approach to definitive laboratory diagnosis is presented in Chapters 34 and 35.

Newborn screening identifies a large number of infants who are carriers for hemoglobin variants. The initial confirmation by the screening laboratory using HPLC, IEF, other electrophoretic techniques, immunologic assays, or DNA/RNA-based techniques using a second sample obtained from the initial filter paper specimen can usually accurately confirm the carrier status. Extent of further evaluation of unknown variants is determined by the presence of clinical or laboratory abnormalities in the infant and the resources and goals of the newborn screening program.

Because α thalassemias are very common in the African, Mediterranean, and Asian populations, Hb Bart's is a common abnormality detected by newborn screening in those areas (Papadea et al., 1994). Hb Bart's may be present in neonates with one, two, or three gene deletion α thalassemia (Fairbanks, 1980). The percentage of Hb Bart's in the cord blood sample may be a guide to the number of α-globin genes that have been lost but lacks precision (see Chapter 18). If the percentage of Hb Bart's is less than 5 percent to 10 percent, the infant most likely has lost one or two α-globin genes and will be a silent carrier or have α-thalassemia trait. Hb Bart's levels of about 10 percent usually indicate α-thalassemia trait with loss of two α-globin genes (Fairbanks, 1980; Ohene-Frempong et al., 1980; Lie-Injo et al., 1982). Hb Bart's levels of greater than 10 percent suggest HbH disease and should have further evaluation (Fairbanks, 1980). Filter paper samples are less sensitive than cord blood and not reliable for differentiating one and two gene deletion α thalassemias (Papadea et al., 1992).

Detecting Hb Bart's at birth may suggest α-thalassemia as the cause of microcytic anemia in the individual or his or her family. α-Thalassemia detected in Asian infants may indicate the presence of more serious forms of α thalassemia in the family. Extended family testing and genetic counseling may be indicated in these populations when the newborn screen shows Hb Bart's.

Detection of both HbF and HbE is common in Southeast Asian populations and may indicate homozygous HbE that is clinically benign or HbE-β^0 thalassemia that may cause severe clinical manifestations (Table 36.7; Lorey et al., 1994). DNA-based techniques allow reliable differentiation (Johnson et al., 1992). Detecting a very low percentage of HbE using HPLC suggests HbE-β thalassemia and may reduce the need for DNA-based diagnosis (Lorey et al., 1993).

Hemoglobin "F only" can be seen as a normal variation in prematurity, in homozygous β thalassemia, and in homozygous HPFH. Persistence of "F only" requires confirmatory testing to differentiate homozygous β thalassemia from HPFH (Table 36.7).

MANAGEMENT

Clinical management of sickle cell anemia in the newborn period is discussed in Chapter 24. Services for affected infants should include comprehensive health care by knowledgeable providers, education of parents, prophylaxis with twice daily oral penicillin, routine health maintenance, access to acute care, genetic counseling of parents, and psychosocial support for families (CORN, 1999). All infants with an HbFS pattern should be started on penicillin 125 mg orally twice a day by 2 months of age and those with confirmed sickle cell anemia and HbS-β⁰ thalassemia are continued on penicillin prophylaxis. Many programs also treat infants with hemoglobin HbSC disease and HbS-β⁺ with prophylactic penicillin (see Chapters 27 and 28). Whenever prophylactic penicillin is used in children at age 3 and above, the dose is increased to 250 mg twice a day and it is continued at least until the fifth birthday (Reid et al., 1995). Erythromycin is an alternative for children with penicillin allergy (Reid et al., 1995). Regular administration of long-acting penicillin by injection has also been shown to be effective (John et al., 1984). Management of acute and chronic complications requires that all infants diagnosed with a hemoglobin disease by newborn screening have unimpeded access to specialized care (CORN, 1999).

Detection of disease at birth allows early education of parents so they can participate in preventing complications and be prepared to cope with the challenges of raising a child with serious, life-long illness. The pathophysiology of the disease and complications, prognosis for the child, need for regular health care, and the genetic implications for their family should be the initial priorities for education. Education about prevention and early treatment of infection through regular administration of antibiotics, routine and special immunizations, and the response to febrile illness is a critical early priority. Parents should be taught to evaluate the spleen size in their child. Signs and symptoms that require urgent medical care to reduce complications and death from splenic sequestration, acute chest syndrome, stroke, and aplastic crisis must be taught (see Chapter 24). Parents need education about the social and psychological impact of the child's disease on their family. Education is reinforced during every health care encounter. Health maintenance requires regular preventive care and immediate access to knowledgeable care for acute illness.

Routine immunizations should be provided based on the recommendations of the World Health Organization, Centers for Disease Control, and American Academy of Pediatrics. Pneumococcal vaccine is recommended at age 2 years and again at age 5 years (Reid et al., 1995). Because of numerous reports of failure with the polysaccharide vaccine (Ammann et al., 1977; Cowan et al., 1978; Ahonkhai et al., 1979; Broome et al., 1980; Buchanan and Schiftman, 1980), the recently developed conjugated vaccines may replace or complement the 23-valent vaccine (Dagan et al., 1996; Vernacchio et al., 1998). Annual administration of influenza vaccine is also recommended and some advocate meningococcal vaccination (Reid et al., 1995).

Newborn screening will detect homozygotes and compound heterozygotes for a number of different hemoglobin variants and thalassemias. Although many may have significant disease, management is usually different than sickle syndromes. In addition, the ethnic background of the families will often differ from that of those with sickle cell disease. Newborn screening programs need to identify health care providers who are knowledgeable and culturally competent in managing infants with thalassemia major, HbE-β⁰ thalassemia, and HbH-Constant Spring disease.

Parents and other family members should have access to diagnostic testing and genetic counseling. Discussion of testing should be initiated with the mother and should include informed consent that provides information on the potential for determining nonpaternity to reduce the risk of disrupting familial integrity. Testing requires both an electronic hematology profile and hemoglobin electrophoresis, IEF, an HPLC to detect most carriers of hemoglobin variants and thalassemias. Sickle preparations and solubility testing are never indicated in screening for carriers to provide genetic counseling. Resources required to establish genotype before providing genetic counseling are similar to those required for disease diagnosis. If resources are ample, mothers of all carriers can also be contacted for individual counseling, education, and extended family testing (Consensus Conference, 1987). Because of limited resources, most programs provide written test results to the health care provider who submits the sample, and mechanisms are developed to notify parents of the test results and to provide information on resources available for counseling and education (CORN, 1998).

Psychosocial support systems are required for affected individuals and their families to maximize adjustment to the financial, social, and psychological impact of potential life-long illness. Parent/patient support groups and community-based sickle cell and thalassemia programs provide invaluable resources.

Professional resources for social support are also needed to address funding of health care, transportation, educational needs, and vocational training. Psychological support services are provided as needed to support individuals and families.

EVALUATION

Newborn screening programs should collect and analyze data to determine prevalence of disorders, ascertain coverage, document benefits, and monitor costs and problems in providing for diagnosis, education, counseling, and health care. Detailed recommendations for data collection have been published (CORN, 1999). Ongoing assessment of morbidity and mortality is helpful in documenting the impact of the program on the health of the affected individuals. Cost-benefit information is important for justifying funding and allocating resources to accomplish programmatic goals and objectives. Cost analysis should include estimates of expenses for sample collection, laboratory analysis, follow-up, and program administration (Therrell et al., 1992; Steinberg et al., 1991).

Quality assurance monitors should be established for every aspect of the newborn screening program (Steinberg et al., 1991; Therrell et al., 1992). Data on missed cases, time to retrieval of positives, percentage of patients lost to follow-up, compliance to treatment protocols, and outcome can be used to assess the effectiveness of the follow-up program. Quality assurance of screening laboratory procedures can be accomplished by following clinical laboratory regulatory guidelines, participating in proficiency testing programs, and determining screening accuracy by comparing initial screening results to those from final diagnostic testing (CORN, 1999). Electronic data exchange and management facilitate accomplishing and evaluating program goals and objectives (Therrell et al., 1992). Periodic review of testing and follow-up quality assurance results by advisory groups or steering committees provides inexpensive and effective evaluation (Steinberg et al., 1991; Therrell et al., 1992).

SUMMARY

Ideally, newborn hemoglobin screening programs should detect all infants with sickle cell anemia, HbS-β^0 thalassemia, and HbSC disease by testing all infants using screening procedures with high sensitivity and reasonable specificity. Infants detected who may have significant disease are retrieved for diagnostic confirmation and entry into ongoing health care programs. Management to minimize morbidity and mortality and optimize individual and family adjustment to the disease requires comprehensive health care by knowledgeable providers, education of parents, twice daily oral penicillin, routine health maintenance, access to acute care, genetic counseling, and psychosocial support for families. Parents should be educated about the disease and its major complications. Resources for nondirective genetic counseling and psychosocial support of the patient and their families should be available. Evaluation includes developing quality assurance guidelines, monitoring of all aspects of the program, and assessing outcome to maximize the utilization of resources and the public health benefit.

ACKNOWLEDGMENTS

We thank Rita Loi and Anton Gerada for editorial assistance. The research reported here was sponsored by the World Health Organization and was supported in part by grants from Assessorato Igiene e Sanità Regione Sardegna (Legge Regionale n. 11 30 Aprile 1990 anno 1998) (A. Cao).

References

Ahonkhai, VI, Landesman, SH, Fikrig, SM et al. (1979). Failure of pneumococcal vaccine in children with sickle-cell disease. N. Engl. J. Med. 301: 26–27.

American Academy of Pediatrics Committee on Genetics. (1992). Issues in newborn screening. Pediatrics 89: 345–349.

Ammann, AJ, Addiego, J, Wara, DW et al. (1977). Polyvalent pneumococcal-polysaccharide immunization of patients with sickle-cell anemia and patients with splenectomy. N. Engl. J. Med. 297: 897–900.

Angastiniotis, M, Modell, B, and Boulinzhenkov, V. (1995). Prevention and control of haemoglobinopathies. Bull. W. H. O. 73: 375–386.

Barret-Connor, E. (1971). Bacterial infection and sickle cell anemia: An analysis of 250 infections in 166 patients and a review of the literature. Medicine 50: 97–112.

Bianchi, DW, Flint, AF et al. (1990). Isolation of fetal DNA from nucleated erythrocytes in maternal blood. Proc. Natl. Acad. Sci. U.S.A. 87: 3279–3283.

Brambati, B, Lanzani, A, and Oldrini, A. (1988). Transabdominal chorionic villus sampling, clinical experience of 1159 cases. Prenat. Diagn. 8: 609–613.

Broome, CV, Facklam, RR, and Fraser, DW. (1980). Pneumococcal disease after pneumococcal vaccination. An alternative method to estimate the efficacy of pneumococcal vaccine. N. Engl. J. Med. 303: 549–552.

Buchanan, GR and Schiffman, G. (1980). Antibody responses to polyvalent pneumococcal vaccine in infants with sickle cell anemia. J. Pediatr. 96: 264–266.

Cai, SP and Kan, YW. (1990). Identification of the multiple β-thalassemia mutations by denaturing gradient gel electrophoresis. J. Clin. Invest. 85: 550–553.

Cao, A and Rosatelli, C. (1993). Screening and prenatal diagnosis of the haemoglobinopathies. In Higgs, DR and

Weatherall, DJ, editors. *Baillière's clinical haematology. The haemoglobinopathies.* Vol. 6. No. 1. London: Baillière Tindall, pp. 263–286.

Cao, A, Cossu, P, Monni, G, and Rosatelli, C. (1987). Chorionic villus sampling and acceptance rate of prenatal diagnosis. *Prenat. Diagn.* 7: 531–533.

Cao, A, Rosatelli, C, and Galanello, R. (1996). Control of β-thalassemia by carrier screening, genetic counselling and prenatal diagnosis: The Sardinian experience. *Ciba Found. Symp.* 197: 137–155.

Cao, A, Galanello, R, Saba, L, and Rosatelli, C. (1997). β-thalassemias: Molecular diagnosis, carrier screening and prevention. A review for clinicians. *JAMA* 278: 1273–1277.

Centers for Disease Control. (1998). Mortality among children with sickle cell disease identified by newborn screening during 1990–1994—California, Illinois, and New York. *MMWR Morb. Mortal. Wkly. Rep.* 47: 169–172.

Chang, YC, Smith, KD, Moore, RD et al. (1995). An analysis of fetal hemoglobin variation in sickle cell disease: The relative contributions of the X-linked factor, β-globin haplotypes, α-globin gene number, gender, and age. *Blood* 85: 1111–1117.

Cheung, M-C, Goldberg, JD, and Kan, YW. (1996). Prenatal diagnosis of sickle cell anemia and thalassemia by analysis of fetal cells in maternal blood. *Nat. Genet.* 14: 264–268.

Consensus Conference. (1987). Newborn screening for sickle cell disease and other hemoglobinopathies. *JAMA* 258: 1205–1209.

Cotton, RGH, Rodrigues, NR, and Campbell, RD. (1988). Reactivity of cytosine and thymine in single-base-pair mismatches with hydroxylamine and osmium tetroxide and its application to the study of mutations. *Proc. Natl. Acad. Sci. U.S.A.* 85: 4397–4401.

Council of Regional Networks for Genetic Services (CORN). (1995). *The Council of Regional Networks for Genetic Services (CORN) Newborn screening report: 1992.* Maternal and Child Health Program (Title V, Social Security Act) Maternal and Child Health Bureau, Health Resources and Services Administration, United States Department of Health and Human Services. Rockville, MD, pp. 79–100.

Council of Regional Networks for Genetic Services (CORN). (1998a). *The Council of Regional Networks for Genetic Services (CORN) Newborn screening report: 1995.* Maternal and Child Health Program (Title V, Social Security Act) Maternal and Child Health Bureau, Health Resources and Services Administration, United States Department of Health and Human Services. Rockville, MD, pp. 54–63.

Council of Regional Networks for Genetic Services (CORN). (1998b). *Guidelines for the follow-up of carriers detected of hemoglobin variants detected by newborn screening.* Maternal and Child Health Program (Title V, Social Security Act) Maternal and Child Health Bureau, Health Resources and Services Administration, United States Department of Health and Human Services. Rockville, MD.

Council of Regional Networks for Genetic Services (CORN). (1999). *Guidelines for the newborn screening system: Follow-up of children, diagnosis, management, and evaluation.* Maternal and Child Health Program (Title V, Social Security Act) Maternal and Child Health Bureau, Health Resources and Services Administration, United States Department of Health and Human Services. Rockville, MD.

Cowan, MJ, Ammann, AJ, Wara, DJ et al. (1978). Pneumococcal polysaccharide immunization in infants and children. *Pediatrics* 62: 721–727.

Craig, JE, Rochette, J et al. (1996). Dissecting the loci controlling fetal haemoglobin production on chromosome 11p and 6q by the regressive approach. *Nat. Genet.* 12: 58–64.

Dagan, R, Melamed, R, Muallem, M et al. (1996). Reduction of nasopharyngeal carriage of pneumococci during the second year of life by a heptavalent conjugate pneumococcal vaccine. *J. Infect. Dis.* 174: 1271–1278.

Diggs, LW. (1973). Anatomic lesions in sickle cell disease. In Abramson, H, Bertles, JF, Wethers, DL, editors. *Sickle cell disease: Diagnosis, management, education, and research.* St. Louis: C.V. Mosby, pp. 189–229.

Diggs, L, Ahman, CF, and Bibb, AB. (1933). The incidence of sickle cell trait. *Ann. Intern. Med.* 7: 769–777.

Eastman, JW, Wong, R, Liao, CL, and Morales, DR. (1996). Automated HPLC screening of newborns for sickle cell anemia and other hemoglobinopathies. *Clin. Chem.* 42: 704–710.

Eckman, JR, Dent, D, Bender, D et al. (1997). Follow-up of infants detected by newborn screening in Georgia, Louisiana, and Mississippi. In *Sickle Cell Disease in the 21st Century.* Abstracts of the 25th Annual Meeting of the NIH Sickle Cell Program, Washington, D.C., September 15–20, 180a.

Emond, AM, Collins, R, Darville, D et al. (1985). Acute splenic sequestration in homozygous sickle cell disease; natural history and management. *J. Pediatr.* 107: 201–206.

Fairbanks, VF. (1980). *Hemoglobinopathies and Thalassemias.* New York: Thieme-Stratton, pp. 18–27.

Galacteros, F, Kleman, K, Caburi-Martin, J et al. (1980). Cord blood screening for hemoglobin abnormalities by thin layer isoelectric focusing. *Blood* 56: 1068–1071.

Galanello, R, Ruggeri, R, Addis, M et al. (1981). Hemoglobin A_2 in iron deficiency β thalassemia heterozygotes. *Hemoglobin* 5: 613–618.

Galanello, R, Paglietti, E, Addis, M et al. (1988). Pitfalls in genetic counselling for β-thalassemia: An individual with 4 different thalassemia mutations. *Clin. Genet.* 33: 151–155.

Galanello, R, Melis, MA et al. (1990). Deletion δ-thalassemia; the 7.2 kb deletion of Corfù δβ-thalassemia in a non-β-thalassemic chromosome [letter]. *Blood* 75: 1447–1449.

Galanello, R, Barella, S, Ideo, A et al. (1994). Genotype of subjects with borderline HbA_2: Implication for β-thalassemia carrier screening. *Am. J. Hematol.* 46: 79–81.

Galanello, R, Barella, S, Gasperini, D et al. (1995). Evaluation of a new automatic HPLC analyzer for thalassemia and hemoglobin variants screening. *J. Autom. Chem.* 17: 73–76.

Ganshirt-Ahlert, D, Borjesson-Stoll, R, Burschyk, M et al. (1993). Detection of fetal trisomies 21 and 18 from maternal blood using triple gradient and magnetic cell sorting. *Am. J. Reprod. Immunol.* 30: 194–201.

Garrick, MD, Dembure, P, and Guthrie, R. (1973). Sickle-cell anemia and other hemoglobinopathies. Procedures and strategy for screening employing spots of blood on filter paper as specimens. *N. Engl. J. Med.* 288: 1265–1268.

Gasparini, P, Bonizzato, A, Dognini, M, and Pignatti, PF. (1992). Restriction site generating-polymerase chain reaction (RG-PCR) for the probeless detection of hidden genetic variation: Application to the study of some common cystic fibrosis mutations. *Mol. Cell. Probes* 6: 1–7.

Gaston, MH, Verter, JI, Woods, G et al. (1986). Prophylaxis with oral penicillin in children with sickle cell anemia. *N. Engl. J. Med.* 314: 1593–1599.

Gessner, BD, Teutsch, SM, and Shaffer, PA. (1996). A cost-effectiveness evaluation of newborn hemoglobinopathy screening from the prospective of state health care systems. *Early Hum. Dev.* 45: 257–275.

Gill, FM, Sleeper, LA, Weiner, SJ et al. (1995). Clinical events in the first decade in a cohort of infants with sickle cell disease. Cooperative Study of Sickle Cell Disease. *Blood* 86: 776–783.

Gilman, PA, McFarlane, JM, and Huisman, HJ. (1976). Natural history (NHx) of sickle cell anemia: Re-evaluation of a 15 year cord blood testing program. *Pediatr. Res.* 10: 452.

Githens, JH, Lane, PA, McCurdy, RS et al. (1990). Newborn screening for hemoglobinopathies in Colorado. *Am. J. Dis. Child.* 144: 446–470.

Gonzales-Redondo, JM, Stoming, TA, Kutlar, A et al. (1989). A C→T substitution at nt −101 in a conserved DNA sequence of the promoter region of the β-globin gene is associated with "silent" β-thalassemia. *Blood* 73: 1705–1711.

Granda, H, Gispert, S, Dorticos, A et al. (1991). Cuban Programme for prevention of sickle cell disease. *Lancet* 337: 152–153.

Grover, R. (1989). Program effects on decreasing morbidity and mortality. Newborn screening in New York City. *Pediatrics* 83(Suppl 5, pt 2): 819–822.

Grover, R, Wethers, D, Shahidi, S et al. (1978). Evaluation of the expanded newborn screening program in New York City. *Am. J. Dis. Child.* 61: 740–749.

Grover, R, Shahidi, S, Fisher, B et al. (1983). Current sickle cell screening program for newborns in New York City, 1979–1980. *Am. J. Pub. Health.* 73: 249–252.

Gyllensten, UB and Erlich, HA. (1988). Generation of single stranded DNA by the polymerase chain reaction and its application to direct sequencing of the HLA-DQα locus. *Proc. Natl. Acad. Sci. U.S.A.* 85: 7652–7656.

Handyside, AM, Lesko, JG, Tarin, JJ et al. (1992). Birth of a normal girl after in vitro fertilization and preimplantation diagnostic testing for cystic fibrosis. *N. Engl. J. Med.* 327: 905–909.

Harris, MS and Eckman, JR. (1989). Approaches to screening. Georgia's experience with newborn screening: 1981 to 1985. *Pediatrics* 83(Suppl 5, pt 2): 858–860.

Higgs, DR, Aldridge, BE, Lamb, J et al. (1982). The interaction of alpha-thalassemia and homozygous sickle-cell disease. *N. Engl. J. Med.* 306: 1441–1446.

Ho, PJ, Hall, GW, Luo, LY et al. (1998). β thalassaemia intermedia: Is it possible consistently to predict phenotype from genotype? *Br. J. Haematol.* 100: 70–78.

Hogge, WA, Schonberg, SA, and Golbus, MS. (1986). Chorionic villus sampling: Experience of the first 1000 cases. *Am. J. Obstet. Gynaecol.* 154: 1249–1252.

Huisman, THJ. (1989). Usefulness of cation exchange high performance liquid chromatography as a testing procedure. *Pediatrics* 83 (Suppl 5, pt 2): 849–851.

Huisman, THJ, and Carver MFH. (1998). The β- and δ-thalassemia repository. 9th ed. *Hemoglobin* 22: 169–195.

Jacobs, S, Peterson, L, Thompson, L et al. (1986). Newborn screening for hemoglobin abnormalities. A comparison of methods. *Am. J. Clin. Pathol.* 85: 713–715.

Jinks, DC, Minter, M, Tarver, DA et al. (1989). Molecular genetic diagnosis of sickle cell disease using dried blood specimens on blotters used for newborn screening. *Hum. Genet.* 81: 363–366.

John, AB, Ramlal, A, Jackson, H et al. (1984). Prevention of pneumococcal infection in children with homozygous sickle cell disease. *Br. Med. J.* 288: 1567–1570.

Johnson, JP, Vichinsky, E, Hurst, D et al. (1992). Differentiation of homozygous hemoglobin E from compound heterozygous hemoglobin E-β-O thalassemia by hemoglobin E mutation analysis. *J. Pediatr.* 120: 775–779.

Kan, YW, Golbus, MS, Klein, P, and Dozy, AM. (1975). Successful application of prenatal diagnosis in a pregnancy at risk for homozygous β-thalassemia. *N. Engl. J. Med.* 292: 1096–1099.

Kan, YW, Lee, KY, Furbetta, M et al. (1980). Polymorphism of DNA sequence in the β-globin gene region: Application to prenatal diagnosis of β-thalassemia in Sardinia. *N. Engl. J. Med.* 302: 185–188.

Kattamis, AC, Camaschella, C, Sivera, P et al. (1996). Human α-thalassemia syndromes: Detection of molecular defects. *Am. J. Hematol.* 53: 81–91.

Kinney, TR, Sawtschenko, M, Whorton, J et al. (1989). Techniques comparison and report of the North Carolina experience. *Pediatrics* 83(Suppl 5, pt 2): 843–848.

Kleman, KM, Vichinsky, E, and Lubin, BH. (1989). Experience with newborn screening using isoelectric focusing. *Pediatrics* 83(Suppl 5, pt 2): 852–854.

Kutlar, A, Ozcan, O, Brisco, JT et al. (1990). The detection of hemoglobin variants by isoelectrofocusing using EDTA-collected and filter paper-dried cord blood specimens. *Am. J. Clin. Pathol.* 94: 199–202.

Lane, PA, Rogers, ZR, Woods, GM et al. (1994). Fatal pneumococcal septicemia in hemoglobin SC disease. *J. Pediatr.* 124: 859–862.

Lau, YL, Chan, L, Chan, YYA et al. (1997). Prevalence and genotypes of α- and β-thalassemia carriers in Hong Kong—Implications for population screening. *N. Engl. J. Med.* 336: 1298–1301.

Lee, A, Thomas, P, Cupidore, L et al. (1995). Improved survival of homozygous sickle cell disease: Lessons from a cohort study. *Br. Med. J.* 311: 1600–1602.

Lie-Injo, LE, Solai, A, Herrera, AR et al. (1982). Hb Bart's level in cord blood and deletions of α-globin genes. *Blood* 59: 370–376.

Lobel, JS and Bove, KE. (1982). Clinicopathologic characteristics of septicemia in sickle cell disease. *Am. J. Dis. Child.* 136: 543–547.

Lobel, JS, Cameron, BF, Johnson, E et al. (1989). Value of screening umbilical cord blood for hemoglobinopathy. *Pediatrics* 83(Suppl 5, pt 2): 823–826.

Lorey, F, Cunningham, G, Vichinsky, E et al. (1993). Detection of HbE/beta-thalassemia versus homozygous EE using high performance liquid chromatography results from newborns. *Biochem. Med. Metab. Biol.* 49: 67–73.

Lorey, F, Cunningham, G, Shafer, F et al. (1994). Universal screening for hemoglobinopathies using high-performance liquid chromatography: Clinical results of 2.2 million screens. *Eur. J. Hum. Genet.* 2: 262–271.

Loukopoulos, D. (1996). Current status of thalassemia and the sickle cell syndromes in Greece. *Sem. Hematol.* 33: 76–86.

McCabe, ERB. (1982). Principles of newborn screening for metabolic disease. *Perinat. Neonatal.* 6: 63–73.

McCabe, ERB, Huang, SZ, Seltzer, WK, and Law, ML. (1987). DNA microextraction from dried blood spots on filter paper blotters: Potential applications to newborn screening. *Hum. Genet.* 75: 213–216.

Melis, MA, Pirastu, M, Galanello, R et al. (1983). Phenotypic effect of heterozygous α and β⁰ thalassemia interaction. *Blood* 62: 226–229.

Moi, P, Paglietti, E, Sanna, A, Brancati, C et al. (1988). Delineation of the molecular basis of δ- and normal HbA$_2$ β-thalassemia. *Blood* 72: 530–533.

Moi, P, Loudianos, G, Lavihna, J et al. (1992). δ-thalassemia due to a mutation in an erythroid specific binding protein sequence 3′ to the δ-globin gene. *Blood* 79: 512–516.

Monk, M and Holding, C. (1990). Amplification of a β-haemoglobin sequence in individual human oocytes and polar bodies. *Lancet* 325: 985–988.

Myers, RM, Fisher, SG, Lerman, LS and Maniatis, T. (1985). Nearly all single base substitution in DNA fragments joined to a GC-clamp can be detected by denaturing gradient gel electrophoresis. *Nucleic Acids Res.* 13: 3131–3135.

Nathan, DG and Oski, FA. (1987). *Hematology of Infancy and Childhood.* 3rd Ed. Philadelphia: W. B. Saunders, p. 1680.

Newton, CR, Graham, A, Heptinstall, LE et al. (1989). Analysis of any point mutation in DNA. The amplification refractory mutation system (ARMS). *Nucleic Acids Res.* 17: 2503–2516.

Nickerson, DA, Kaiser, R, Loggin, S et al. (1990). Automated DNA diagnostic using an ELISA-based oligonucleotide ligation assay. *Proc. Natl. Acad. Sci. U.S.A.* 87: 8923–8927.

O'Brien, RT, McIntosh, S, Aspnes, GT, and Pearson, HA. (1976). Prospective study of sickle cell anemia in infancy. *J. Pediatr.* 89: 205–210.

Ohene-Frempong, K, Rappaport, E, Atwater, J et al. (1980). Alpha-gene deletions in Black newborn infants with Hb Bart's. *Blood* 56: 931–933.

Orita, M, Iwahana, H, Kanazawa, H et al. (1989). Detection of polymorphisms of human DNA by gel electrophoresis as single-strand conformation polymorphism. *Proc. Natl. Acad. Sci. U.S.A.* 86: 2766–2770.

Overturf, GD, Powars, D, and Baraff, LJ. (1977). Bacterial meningitis and septicemia in sickle cell disease. *Am. J. Dis. Child.* 131: 784–787.

Panepinto, J, Magid, D, Rewers, MJ, and Lane, PA. (2000). Universal versus targeted screening of infants for sickle cell disease: A cost-effectiveness analysis. *J. Pediatr.* 136: 201–208.

Papadea, C, Eckman, JR, Kuehner, R, and Platt, AP. (1994). Comparison of liquid cord blood and filter paper spots for newborn hemoglobin screening: Laboratory and programmatic issues. *Pediatrics* 93: 427–432.

Pearson, HA. (1973). Sickle cell anemia: Clinical management during the early years of life. In Abramson, H, Bertles, JF, Wethers, DL, editors. *Sickle cell disease: Diagnosis, management, education, and research.* St. Louis: C.V. Mosby, pp. 224–251.

Pearson, HA. (1977). Sickle cell anemia and severe infections due to encapsulated bacteria. *J. Infect. Dis.* 136: S25–S30.

Pearson, HA. (1986). A neonatal program for sickle cell anemia. *Adv. Pediatr.* 3: 381–400.

Pearson, HA. (1989). Neonatal testing for sickle cell diseases—a historic perspective. Pediatrics 83(Suppl 5, part2): 815–818.

Pearson, HA, O'Brien, RT, McIntosk, S et al. (1974). Routine screening of umbilical cord blood for sickle cell disease. *JAMA* 227: 420–421.

Pirastu, M, Kan, YW, Cao, A et al. (1983). Prenatal diagnosis of β-thalassemia. Detection of a single nucleotide mutation in DNA. *N. Engl. J. Med.* 309: 284–287.

Pirastu, M, Ristaldi, MS, and Cao, A. (1989). Prenatal diagnosis of β-thalassemia based on restriction endonuclease analysis of amplified fetal DNA. *J. Med. Genet.* 26: 363–367.

Powars, DR. (1975). Natural history of sickle cell disease—the first ten years. *Semin. Hematol.* 12: 267–285.

Powars, D, Overturf, G, Weiss, J et al. (1981). Pneumococcal septicemia in children with sickle cell anemia. Changing trend of survival. *JAMA* 245: 1839–1842.

Reid, CD, Charache, S, Lubin, B et al. (1995). *Management and Therapy of Sickle Cell Disease. Third Ed.* NIH Publication 96–2117. Rockville, MD: National Institutes of Health. National Heart, Lung, and Blood Institute. Public Health Service, U.S. Department of Health and Human Services.

Rogers, DW, Clarke, JM, Cupidore, L et al. (1978). Early deaths in Jamaican children with sickle cell disease. *Br. Med. J.* 1: 1515–1516.

Rosatelli, C, Leoni, GB, Tuveri, T et al. (1992a). Heterozygous β-thalassemia: Relationship between the hematological phenotype and the type of β-thalassemia mutation. *Am. J. Hematol.* 39: 1–4.

Rosatelli, MC, Dozy, A, Faa, V et al. (1992b). Molecular characterization of β-thalassemia in the Sardinian population. *Am. J. Hum. Genet.* 50: 422–426.

Rosatelli, MC, Pischedda, A, Meloni, A et al. (1994). Homozygous β-thalassaemia resulting in the β-thalassaemia carrier state phenotype. *Br. J. Haematol.* 88: 562–565.

Rosatelli, MC, Faa, V, Meloni, A et al. (1995). A promoter mutation, C→T at position −92, leading to silent β-thalassaemia. *Br. J. Haematol.* 90: 483–485.

Rubin, EM, Andrews, KA, and Kan, YW. (1989). Newborn screening by DNA analysis of dried blood spots. *Hum. Genet.* 82: 134–136.

Saiki, RK, Walsh, PS, Levenson, CH, and Erlich, HA. (1989). Genetic analysis of amplified DNA with immobilized sequence-specific oligonucleotide probes. *Proc. Natl. Acad. Sci. U.S.A.* 86: 6230–6234.

Sanger, F, Micklen, S, Coulson, AR. (1977). DNA sequencing with chain terminating inhibitors. *Proc. Natl. Acad. Sci. U.S.A.* 74: 5463–5467.

Schedlbauer, LM and Pass, KA. (1989). Cellulose acetate/citrate agar electrophoresis of filter paper hemolysates from heel stick. *Pediatrics* 83(Suppl 5, pt 2): 839–842.

Scott, R. (1948). Screening for sickle cell in newborn infants. *Am. J. Dis. Child.* 75: 842–846.

Scott, RB, Freeman, LC, and Ferguson, AD. (1954). Studies in sickle cell anemia: Effect of age (maturation) on the incidence of the sickling phenomenon. *Pediatrics* 14: 209–214.

Seeler, RA. (1972). Deaths in children with sickle cell anemia. A clinical analysis of 19 fatal instances in Chicago. *Clin. Pediatr.* 11: 634–637.

Seeler, RA and Jacobs, NM. (1977). Pyogenic infections in children with sickle hemoglobinopathy. *J. Pediatr.* 90: 161–162.

Serjeant, BE, Forbes, M, Williams, LL, and Serjeant, GR. (1974). Screening cord bloods for detection of sickle cell disease in Jamaica. *Clin. Chem.* 20: 666–669.

Serjeant, GR, Grandison, Y, Lowrie, Y et al. (1981). The development of hematologic changes in homozygous sickle cell disease: A cohort study from birth to six years. *Br. J. Haematol.* 48: 533–543.

Sexauer, CL, Graham, HL, Starling, KA and Fernbach, DJ. (1976). A test for abnormal hemoglobins in umbilical cord blood. *Am. J. Dis. Child.* 130: 805–806.

Sickle Cell Disease Guideline Panel. (1993). *Sickle Cell Disease: Screening, Diagnosis, Management, and Counseling in Newborns and Infants. Clinical Practice Guideline No. 6.* AHCPR Pub. No. 93–0562. Rockville, MD: Agency for Health Care Policy and Research, Public Health Service, U.S. Department of Health and Human Services.

Stamatoyannopoulos, G. (1974). Problems of screening and counselling in the hemoglobinopathies. Proc. *4th International Conference. Birth Defects* Vienna, 268–276.

Steinberg, MH. (1996). Modulation of the phenotypic diversity of sickle cell anemia. *Hemoglobin* 20: 1–19.

Steinberg MH, Adams, JG, Baine, RM et al. (1991). Ad Hoc Newborn Screening Committee, National Sickle Cell Disease Advisory Committee. *Newborn Screening for Hemoglobinopathies: Program Development and Laboratory Methods.* Bethesda, MD: Sickle Cell Disease Branch, National Institutes of Health.

Sundall, DN. (1987). Availability of funds for maternal and child health projects. *Fed. Reg.* 52: 29072.

Thein, SL, Hesketh, C, Wallace, RB, Weatherall, DJ. (1988). The molecular basis of thalassaemia intermedia in Asian Indians: Application to prenatal diagnosis. *Br. J. Haematol.* 70: 225–231.

Therrell, BL, Simmank, JL, and Wilborn, M. (1989). Experiences with sickle hemoglobin testing in the Texas newborn screening program. *Pediatrics* 83(Suppl 5, pt 2): 864–867.

Therrell, BL, Panny, SR, Davidson, A et al. (1992). U.S. newborn screening system guidelines: Statement of the Council of Regional Networks for Genetic Services. *Screening* 1: 135–147.

Thomas, AN, Pattison, C, and Serjeant, GR. (1982). Causes of death in sickle-cell disease in Jamaica. *Br. Med. J.* 285: 633–635.

Tsevat J, Wong JB, Pauker SG, and Steinberg MH. (1991). Neonatal screening for sickle cell disease: A cost-effectiveness analysis. *J. Pediatr.* 118: 546–554.

Vernacchio, L, Neufeld, EJ, Mac Donald, K et al. (1998). Combined schedule of 7-valent pneumococcal conjugate vaccine followed by 23-valent pneumococcal vaccine in children and young adults with sickle cell disease. *J. Pediatr.* 133: 275–278.

Vichinsky, E, Hurst, D, Earles, A et al. (1988). Newborn screening for sickle cell disease: Effect on mortality. *Pediatrics* 81: 749–755.

Wang, X, Seaman, C, Paik, M et al. (1994). Experience with 500 prenatal diagnoses of sickle cell diseases: The effect of gestational age on affected pregnancy outcome. *Prenat. Diagn.* 14: 851–857.

Weatherall, SJ and Clegg, JB (editors). (1981). *The Thalassaemia Syndromes.* 3rd ed. Oxford: Blackwell Scientific Publications.

Whitten, CF, Thomas, JF, and Nishiura, EN. (1981). Sickle cell trait counseling-evaluation of counselors and counselees. *Am. J. Hum. Genet.* 33: 802.

WHO Working Group (1989). Feasibility Study on Hereditary Disease Community Control Programmes, Cagliari, Sardinia, April 8–9, 1989 (WHO/HDP/HA/WG/89.1).

WHO Scientific Group. (1996). Control of hereditary diseases. WHO Technical Report Series 865.

Wilson, JB, Headlee, ME, and Huisman, THJ. (1983). A new high performance liquid chromatographic procedure for the separation and quantitation of various hemoglobin variants in adults and newborn babies. *J. Lab. Clin. Med.* 102: 174–186.

Wilson, JB, Wrightstone, RN, and Huisman, THJ. (1986). A rapid cation-exchange high performance liquid chromatographic procedure for the separation and quantitation of hemoglobin variants in cord blood samples. *J. Lab. Clin. Med.* 108: 138–141.

Zarkowsky, HS, Gallagher, D, Gill, F et al. (1986). Bacteremia in sickle hemoglobinopathies. *J. Pediatr.* 109: 579–585.

Zhang, YH and McCabe, ERB. (1992). RNA analysis from newborn screening dried blood specimens. *Hum. Genet.* 89: 311–314.

Zhang, YH, McCabe, LL, Wilborn, M et al. (1994). Application of molecular genetics in public health: Improved follow-up in a neonatal hemoglobinopathy screening program. *Biochem. Med. Metab. Biol.* 52: 27–35.

37

Transfusion and Iron Chelation Therapy in Thalassemia and Sickle Cell Anemia

ALAN R. COHEN
JOHN B. PORTER

TRANSFUSION THERAPY

Thalassemia Major (Cooley's Anemia)

Seventy-five years ago, Dr. Thomas Cooley and his colleagues at the Children's Hospital of Michigan administered blood transfusions to children with a newly recognized clinical entity whose features included severe anemia, splenomegaly, and peculiar facies (Cooley et al., 1927). Five years later, Cooley's name had become indelibly associated with the disease, and transfusions were administered along with ferrous carbonate, ultraviolet rays, and extract of pituitary gland (Whipple and Bradford, 1932). Not surprisingly, given the state of crossmatching at the time, the response to transfusion was at best variable and at worst nonexistent. Another 30 years elapsed before improvements in blood banking and recognition of the benefits of a higher hemoglobin level came together to initiate the era of modern transfusion therapy for thalassemia major.

Transfusion Programs. In 1963, at the first Cooley's Anemia Symposium of the New York Academy of Sciences, Wolman (1964) presented the results of his evaluation of thirty-five children with thalassemia major, ages 12 years or less, whose pretransfusion hemoglobin levels fell into three categories: 4.0 to 5.9 g/dL, 6.0 to 7.9 g/dL, and 8.0 to 9.9 g/dL. Children in

the highest hemoglobin group had better linear growth, less enlargement of the liver and spleen, less thickening of the skull and overgrowth of the maxilla, fewer fractures, and less cardiomegaly than children in the two lowest hemoglobin groups. At the same meeting, Schorr and Radel (1964) described two patients who received regular red cell transfusions to maintain their hemoglobin level above 10 g/dL at all times. Nearly 4 decades later, this regimen—hypertransfusion—remains the standard of care for the treatment of thalassemia major. General guidelines for hypertransfusion therapy are presented in Tables 37.1 and 37.2 and discussed in detail later.

By the second Cooley's Anemia Symposium in 1968, several reports confirmed the benefits of hypertransfusion (Beard et al., 1969; Piomelli et al., 1969; Wolman and Ortolani, 1969). Notably, all investigators found that patients were leading normal, active lives. However, their satisfaction with the benefits of hypertransfusion therapy was tempered by a growing appreciation of the problem of transfusional iron overload and the need for iron chelation therapy.

The choice of a particular pretransfusion hemoglobin level continues to vary among thalassemia centers, but usually falls between 9.0 and 10.5 g/dL. The goal is to select a target hemoglobin level that achieves the important physiologic benefits while minimizing the rate of iron accumulation. In regard to the first issue, no significant difference in appearance, cardiac size, occurrence of splenomegaly or feeling of well-being has been identified with higher or lower hemoglobin levels in a hypertransfusion regimen. Because some of the complications of thalassemia may be related directly or indirectly to erythroid hyperplasia in the bone marrow, the level of bone marrow suppression achieved by different target hemoglobin levels may have clinical significance. Both ferrokinetic studies and measurements of serum transferrin receptor levels have shown an inverse relationship between mean pretransfusion hemoglobin level and marrow erythroid activity (Cavill et al., 1978; Propper et al., 1980; Cazzola et al., 1995). When anemia is severe—hemoglobin level 4 to 7 g/dL—the marrow erythroid activity increases to ten times normal. One important clinical consequence is impaired bone metabolism with osteomalacia (Pootrakul et al., 1981). However, when the selected mean pretransfusion hemoglobin level is 9 g/dL rather than 10.5 g/dL, erthyroid activity increases only threefold (Cazzola et al., 1995), and this level of erythroid expansion is associated with little or no impairment of bone metabolism (Pootrakul et al., 1981). Thus, no significant physiologic difference

Table 37.1. **General Guidelines for Transfusion Therapy for Thalassemia Major**

Variable	Range
Pretransfusion hemoglobin level	9–10.5 g/dL
Blood product	Leukodepleted red cells
Amount of blood	1 to 3 units
Interval between transfusions	2 to 4 weeks

between a target pretransfusion hemoglobin level of 9 and 10.5 g/dL is known at this time.

Hemoglobin Level and Blood Requirements. The relationship between target hemoglobin level, blood requirements, and rate of iron accumulation in patients with thalassemia major is controversial. In a study of 166 splenectomized and nonsplenectomized patients, transfusion requirements remained constant at mean transfusion hemoglobin levels of 10 to 14 g/dL (equivalent to pretransfusion hemoglobin levels of approximately 8 to 12 g/dL) (Gabutti et al., 1980). A subsequent expansion of this study to include 392 patients from three Italian centers confirmed the earlier findings and concluded that the maintenance of higher hemoglobin levels in transfusion programs for thalassemia major did not require a higher blood requirement (Gabutti et al., 1982). Additional supportive evidence came from a study of "supertransfusion" where maintenance of pretransfusion packed cell volumes (PCVs) of 27 and 35 percent required similar amounts of blood (Propper et al., 1980).

In contrast with these findings, several studies have found that the maintenance of higher hemoglobin levels requires more blood. For example, the transfusion requirements of fourteen French patients were directly proportional to the mean hemoglobin levels and nearly doubled between 9.6 and 13.4 g/dL (Brunengo and Girot, 1986). Among 3,468 patients in Greece and Italy, transfusion requirements in 1985 were propor-

tional to mean hemoglobin level in both splenectomized and nonsplenectomized patients (Rebulla and Modell, 1991). In only one large study has the annual transfusion requirement been measured repeatedly in the same patients under two different transfusion regimens (Cazzola et al., 1997). From 1982 to 1986, when the mean pretransfusion hemoglobin level of thirty-two Italian patients was 11.3 g/dL, the mean annual transfusion requirement was 137 mL/kg (Table 37.3). After modification of the transfusion regimen in 1987 to 1992, the mean transfusion hemoglobin level fell to 9.4 g/dL, and the mean blood requirement decreased to 104 mL/kg. Of particular note, the change in target hemoglobin level from 11.3 to 9.4 g/dL was associated with a reduction in excessive iron stores, suggesting that this improvement in overall iron status at the lower hemoglobin level may have been a combined effect of decreased transfusion iron loading, enhanced deferoxamine-induced iron excretion, and maintenance of an acceptable level of gastrointestinal iron absorption.

Beginning Transfusion Therapy. The decision to begin chronic transfusion therapy in an infant or young child with homozygous β thalassemia rests on a combination of laboratory and clinical data. The specific molecular defect may provide a general, albeit imperfect, prognostic clue, and the course of an affected sibling may strengthen this clue. The hemoglobin level alone, unless extremely low, is not a sufficient determinant of the need for transfusion. Clinical factors and other laboratory findings in addition to the hemoglobin level determine whether the interests of the patient are better served by a chronic hemolytic anemia or a chronic transfusion program. For example, the development of Cooley's facies, growth retardation, pathologic fractures, or persistent fatigue is a strong indication for transfusion, even when the hemoglobin level is 8 g/dL. On the other hand, for a patient with none of these problems despite a lower hemoglobin level, the marginal benefits of transfusions may be outweighed by the associated risks. Clinicians

Table 37.2. **Estimation of Blood Requirements According to Hematocrit of Donor Units**

Hematocrit of packed red cell units (%)	Amount of packed red cells to raise Hb by 1 g/dL (mL/kg)
60	3.7
65	3.5
70	3.2
75	3.0

Table 37.3. **Effect of Target Hemoglobin Level on Transfusion Requirements in Thalassemia**

Years	Mean pre-transfusion hemoglobin level (g/dL)	Mean transfusion requirements (mL/kg/yr)	Median serum ferritin (µg/L)
1981–1986	11.3 ± 0.5	137 ± 26	2,280
1987–1992	9.4 ± 0.4	104 ± 23	1,004

From Cazzola et al., 1997.

should regularly assess growth and, in conjunction with the family, the overall well-being of the child. In addition, the nucleated red cell count or other laboratory indicators of the degree of erythropoiesis should be monitored because the consequences of excessive bone marrow expansion may be as important as those of anemia in prompting regular transfusions. Later initiation of transfusion therapy may delay the need for iron chelation therapy until an age at which side effects are less common. However, earlier initiation of transfusion therapy may prevent irreversible facial changes and may lower the risk of alloimmunization (see later). When the indications for transfusion therapy are equivocal but a decision is made to proceed, the treatment should be reevaluated if the patient later undergoes splenectomy. In some patients, removal of the spleen may make the difference between dependency and nondependency on regular administration of red cells.

Choice of Blood Product. Patients with thalassemia should receive leukoreduced red blood cells to decrease or eliminate febrile reactions. The reduction of white cells to less than 5×10^6 per unit of red cells may carry the additional benefit of delaying sensitization to human leukocyte antigens (HLA) in patients who may later be candidates for bone marrow transplantation. Filtration of the blood product, before storage or at the time of administration, is the method most commonly used for removal of white cells. Prestorage leukoreduction is usually more efficient than bedside filtration (Sprogoe-Jakobsen et al., 1995). Prestorage leokoreduction may also decrease cytokine accumulation in the blood product during storage, further diminishing the chance of a febrile reaction. One study has suggested that prestorage leukoreduction has the additional advantage of reducing the proliferation of *Yersinia enterocolitica* in blood products inoculated with the organism (Buchholz et al., 1992). Because infection with *Y. enterocolitica* may be a particularly serious event in patients with iron overload receiving chelation therapy, decreasing the likelihood of its transmission from asymptomatic donors may reduce the risk of one of the more serious infectious complications of thalassemia. Whether leukoreduction removes prions from potentially infected units is still being investigated.

Additive solutions containing saline, glucose, adenine, and phosphate or mannitol have reduced the detrimental effects of storage on red cells. Even after 42 days of storage, red cell recovery 24 hours after transfusion is 75 percent or greater (Hogman, 1998). Little information is available, however, regarding the survival of these red cells after the first 24 hours. Earlier studies showed that the survival of red cells

stored in acid-citrate-dextrose for 28 days was less than red cells stored for 14 days (Mollison et al., 1997). Although this difference is not important for a patient receiving a single transfusion perioperatively, it may have a marked effect on the overall blood requirements of a patient with thalassemia major receiving long-term transfusion therapy. Until more is known about the effect of storage time on red cell survival after transfusion with current blood products, it seems prudent to use red cells less than 7 to 14 days old for patients with thalassemia major.

Frequency and Amount of Transfusion. When using donor units with a PCV of 75 percent, transfusion of 10 to 15 mL of red cells per kilogram body weight at 3- or 4-week intervals usually maintains a minimum hemoglobin level of 9.0 to 10.5 g/dL. The new additive solutions described here have reduced the PCV of packed red cells from 75 to 80 percent to 60 to 65 percent, and therefore larger volumes of the blood product are necessary to achieve the same target hemoglobin level. This may pose problems for small children or for older patients with heart disease, and in these instances hemoconcentration of the donor units may be necessary. Whereas intervals between transfusions of 3 to 4 weeks accommodate the school or work schedule of most patients with thalassemia major, shorter intervals would more closely mimic the physiologic situation by reducing fluctuations in hemoglobin level. Moreover, mathematical modeling suggests that maintenance of a pretransfusion hemoglobin level of 9 g/dL with transfusions every 2 weeks rather than every 4 weeks would reduce overall blood requirements by 20 percent (Piomelli, 1995). However, in a large group of Italian patients who had undergone splenectomy, a shorter interval of 2 weeks between transfusions had no measurable effect on transfusion requirements compared with an interval of 3 or 4 weeks (Rebulla and Modell, 1991).

Other conditions may increase the frequency of transfusion or the amount of blood needed to maintain the target hemoglobin level. For example, transfusion requirements rise during pregnancy in women with β thalassemia major (Kumar et al., 1997; Skordis et al., 1998). Patients undergoing treatment for hepatitis C infection with ribavirin need additional blood owing to drug-induced hemolysis. In eleven patients with thalassemia major who received ribavirin in combination with interferon α, transfusion requirements increased by 25 to 94 percent (median 41 percent) compared with the pretreatment period (Telfer et al., 1997).

Young Red Cells. During the last 20 years, several groups have evaluated the effect of young red cell (neocyte) transfusions on overall blood requirements

Table 37.4. Comparison of Simple Transfusion and Red Cell Exchange Transfusion in Thalassemia

	Mean pretransfusion hemoglobin level (g/dL)	Mean posttransfusion hemoglobin level (g/dL)	Mean transfusion interval (days)	Transfusion requirement (mL/kg/day)
Simple transfusion	9.7	14.2	35.7	0.41
Red cell exchange transfusion	9.6	14.5	50.8	0.29

From Berdoukas et al., 1986.

and therefore on the rate of iron loading. The theoretical benefit of this modified blood product lies in the assumption that although all red cells contribute the same amount of iron on senescence, younger red cells from the donor will circulate longer in the recipient before the iron is inevitably released. Thus, enhancement of the blood product for younger donor red cells should reduce the transfusion requirements and the rate of iron loading. Studies in animals have confirmed that age-dependent separation of red cells by density gradient centrifugation has a marked effect on red cell survival (Piomelli et al., 1978). Both simple centrifugation of single donor units and neocyte enhancement during continuous centrifugation apheresis of the donor have yielded red cells with younger estimated mean ages and, in labeled erythrocyte survival studies, longer half-lives than conventional units (Propper et al., 1980; Corash et al., 1981; Graziano et al., 1982; Klein, 1982; Bracey et al., 1983). Several factors have impeded the clinical application of young red cell transfusions. In particular, preparation of neocytes by continuous flow centrifugation is costly, and trials using neocytes prepared from single donor units have been disappointing. In three studies, the reduction in the rate of iron loading was only 13 to 20 percent, and both the preparation costs and donor exposures were significantly higher in transfusion regimens involving neocytes compared with conventional red cell units (Cohen et al., 1984b; Marcus et al., 1985; Collins et al., 1994; Spanos et al., 1996).

Partial Exchange Transfusion. Partial exchange transfusion, whether performed manually or by erythrocytapheresis, decreases the net blood requirement by combining the administration of donor red cells with the removal of red cells from the patient. The rationale for the use of partial exchange transfusion to prevent complications of sickle cell disease is straightforward (see later). Donor HbA-containing cells directly replace endogenous HbS-containing cells, and because the goal of lowering the HbS level is largely independent of the total hemoglobin level, little or no net gain of red cells occurs. The goal of transfusion therapy for thalassemia major differs from that for

sickle cell disease. The critical outcome is maintaining a particular hemoglobin level. Although the rationale for the use of partial exchange transfusion for this purpose is less obvious, studies from Australia support this approach in thalassemia major (Berdoukas et al., 1986). Seventeen patients with thalassemia, as well as one with sickle cell anemia and one with Diamond-Blackfan anemia, underwent regular partial exchange transfusion for 6 to 7 months. The investigators used continuous flow centrifugation, and they enriched the returned blood for younger red cells. Compared with simple transfusion, the net rate of iron loading fell by 29 percent (Table 37.4). The mean interval between transfusions increased from 36 to 51 days. Serum ferritin levels decreased by 20 percent during partial exchange transfusion therapy, in contrast with an increase of 12 percent during a comparable period of conventional transfusion therapy. The authors noted the disadvantages of a 40 to 60 percent increase in exposure to donor units and a 1.5- to 2.0-fold increase in transfusion-associated costs. Subsequently, the investigators reported the successful extension of this program without neocyte enrichment (Berdoukas and Moore, 1990).

Pilot studies of partial exchange transfusion in Philadelphia confirmed these earlier findings. In three patients with thalassemia major, automated partial exchange transfusion at 3-week intervals for 1 to 2 years decreased net red cell requirements and thus transfusional iron loading by a mean of 44 percent compared with simple transfusion (Cohen et al., 1998). Donor blood exposure increased 2.5- to 3.0-fold. Age-dependent separation of pretransfusion blood samples by density gradient analysis showed a significant increase in younger red cells during partial exchange transfusion compared with simple transfusion. This finding suggests that the benefit of partial exchange transfusion in thalassemia may be derived primarily from the replacement of previously administered donor red cells with new donor red cells that have a younger mean age. By reducing the rate of new iron accumulation, this means of transfusion may enhance the overall management of transfusional iron overload in thalassemia major.

Other Thalassemia Disorders. By definition, patients with thalassemia intermedia do not need regular blood transfusions, at least until adolescence or adulthood. However, they may need occasional transfusions during illnesses, with pregnancy, or at the time of surgery. Patients with HbH disease (Chapter 18), in particular, often have a significant decrease in their hemoglobin level during febrile illnesses, and the exacerbation of the anemia, in combination with the poor oxygen delivery by HbH, may warrant red cell transfusion. With advancing age, patients with thalassemia intermedia sometimes become transfusion-dependent as a result of a further decline in the hemoglobin level, a reduced tolerance of the anemia, or complications such as bone pain, recurrent fractures, or extramedullary hematopoiesis.

Fetuses without functional α-globin genes (homozygous α^0 thalassemia, α thalassemia hydrops fetalis) are severely anemic and usually succumb before birth (Liang et al., 1985) (Chapter 18). Administration of red cell transfusions in utero has, on rare occasions, sustained fetal life (Chui and Waye, 1998). Early delivery with immediate transfusion has rescued other fetuses. However, the frequent occurrence of congenital anomalies and delayed development in surviving infants require careful consideration of the ethics of transfusion therapy in this disease. Furthermore, the rescue of the fetus with homozygous α^0 thalassemia is only the beginning of a lifetime of transfusion dependency or a prelude to the need for bone marrow transplantation.

Sickle Cell Disease

Transfusion therapy in sickle cell disease has two important goals. First, transfusions restore the hemoglobin level in patients with an acute exacerbation of the underlying anemia such as occurs during a splenic sequestration crisis. Second, transfusions reduce the proportion of HbS-containing erythrocytes, thereby decreasing the likelihood of vasoocclusive complications, such as stroke. As described later, the appropriate choice of one of these two goals will guide other features of therapy such as the choice of blood product, method of transfusion, and selection of tests for monitoring the transfusion program. In some situations, such as severe acute chest syndrome, the two goals of transfusion therapy overlap; in other situations, such as preparation for surgery under general anesthesia, the benefits of transfusion therapy cannot be attributed with certainty to one goal or the other.

Choice of Blood Product. The same considerations used in selecting a blood product in thalassemia also apply to sickle cell disease. Leukoreduction is important for preventing febrile reactions and reducing the risk of sensitization to HLA antigens. The latter effect may be particularly important in light of the increasing application of bone marrow transplantation to the treatment of this hemoglobinopathy. Selection of blood with a shorter storage time is as important for patients with sickle cell disease who undergo long-term transfusion as it is for patients with thalassemia. Ironically, the administration of large amounts of very fresh blood, particularly in an exchange transfusion, may pose a theoretical risk to the patient with sickle cell disease by producing a sudden leftward shift of the oxygen dissociation curve and resulting in decreased tissue oxygenation (White et al., 1976b). However, adverse clinical consequences of exchange transfusion with fresh red cells remain unproven. Moreover, the improved blood viscosity resulting from the increase in HbA cells after exchange transfusion probably maintains or even improves oxygen delivery despite the decrease in the p^{50} (Schmalzer et al., 1987).

Extended red cell antigen typing before the first transfusion is particularly important in sickle cell disease because as discussed later, alloantibodies are common. The use of the original antigen profile to accurately determine the specificity of new antibodies and to eliminate the possibility of an autoantibody will help prevent hemolytic reactions after subsequent transfusions. Several investigators have advocated the use of blood matched for multiple red cell antigens for patients with sickle cell disease (Ambruso et al., 1987; Vichinsky et al., 1990). This approach may be particularly useful when the racial composition of the donor and recipient pool differ as they do in the United States, and certain blood group antigens are common in donors but rare in recipients. In a prospective study, the initiation of complete matching of donor blood for the Rh, Kell, Kidd, and Duffy systems and less stringent matching for other minor groups resulted in a tenfold reduction in the rate of new alloantibody formation per unit (Ambruso et al., 1987). Because of the high cost associated with extended antigen matching, other investigators have proposed using this approach only after patients have developed one or two alloantibodies (Luban, 1989; Orlina et al., 1991). A less expensive and less labor-intensive strategy involves the use of racially matched blood (Orlina et al., 1991; Sosler et al., 1993). Units donated by African Americans have an eightfold greater likelihood of antigen identity than units from predominantly Caucasian donor pools (Sosler et al., 1993). Programs to increase blood donations by African Americans would strengthen either strategy (Beattie and Shafer, 1986).

Patients with sickle cell disease on chronic transfusion programs should not receive blood from donors with sickle cell trait. As discussed later, the target of such transfusion programs is a reduction in the percentage of endogenous HbS-containing cells to a particular level, and this is measured in the laboratory by the relative amounts of HbA (from the donor) and HbS (from the recipient). The administration of sickle cell trait rather than normal cells will obscure the laboratory assessment of the proportion of the patient's cells that remain in the circulation.

Administration of Blood. When administering red cells to relieve anemia, the physician must first determine whether there is accompanying hypovolemia. If the patient's blood volume is reduced, as in an acute splenic sequestration crisis, sufficient red cells to raise the hemoglobin concentration to the desired level can be given without undue concern about circulatory overload. In contrast, in a more slowly developing anemia such as an aplastic crisis, the patient's blood volume is maintained, and the volume of administered red cells must be carefully considered so as not to trade improvement in oxygen-carrying capacity for congestive heart failure. One simple approach to this situation is to use the hemoglobin level to determine the volume of the transfusion product. For example, if the hemoglobin level is 3 g/dL, the volume of packed red cells 3 mL/kg of body weight (Chapter 24). In most clinical situations, even a small rise in the hemoglobin level is sufficient to address the immediate problem. However, as noted previously, the use of newer additive solutions has reduced the PCV of donor red cell units, leaving an even more delicate balance between raising the hemoglobin concentration and preventing volume overload. A rapidly acting diuretic may be helpful in this situation.

For chronic transfusion programs, the administration of one or two units of red cells every 3 or 4 weeks will reduce the HbS level to the commonly chosen target of 30 to 50 percent. Compared with simple transfusion, manual or automated partial exchange transfusion decreases the net amount of blood needed to lower HbS levels by combining the administration of donor red cells with the removal of the patient's red cells (Cohen et al., 1992; Kim et al., 1994; Adams et al., 1996; Hilliard et al., 1998). This technique has proven to be a valuable tool in the management of iron overload in patients with sickle cell disease on long-term transfusion programs for the prevention of stroke or other complications. New iron accumulation is stopped or profoundly reduced. A single partial exchange transfusion is also a useful tool for the rapid reduction of HbS levels in the patient with sickle cell disease who has an acute complication or who needs surgery (see later). Partial exchange transfusion can decrease the HbS level below 30 percent in less than 2 hours without the problems of volume overload or hyperviscosity that would accompany repeated simple

transfusions for this purpose (Klein et al., 1980; Janes et al., 1997).

Monitoring Transfusion Therapy. Hemoglobin levels reflect the success of transfusion to relieve anemia and to improve oxygen-carrying capacity. Clinical improvement often follows even small increases in the hemoglobin level. Administration of an excessive amount of red cells may cause serious problems owing to hyperviscosity (Jan et al., 1982; Schmalzer et al., 1987); and when transfusion is used to relieve anemia, the target hemoglobin level should generally not exceed the patient's baseline value and usually should be considerably less.

The percentage of the total hemoglobin accounted for by HbS reflects the success of transfusions to reduce the likelihood of vasoocclusion. The specific target level of HbS varies with the clinical situation but is most commonly 30 to 50 percent. Measurement of the percentage of HbS is usually performed by high-pressure liquid chromatography (HPLC) or by hemoglobin electrophoresis with scanning of the bands by densitometry (Chapter 34). The hemoglobin level and reticulocyte count are imprecise measures of the level of suppression of endogenous erythropoiesis and should not be used in place of the HbS level (Zinkham et al., 1994). The serum transferrin receptor concentration reflects erythropoietic activity (Tancabelic et al., 1999), but as a surrogate marker of the patient's production of HbS-containing erythrocytes, it holds no advantage over direct measurement of blood HbS levels.

Even when the goal of transfusion in sickle cell disease is to reduce the HbS level rather than to correct the anemia, the hemoglobin level should be monitored to prevent problems of hyperviscosity. Simple transfusions to reduce the HbS level to less than 30 percent may have the unintended consequence of raising the hemoglobin above 11 to 12 g/dL. Early detection of this possibility allows modification of the simple transfusion program or substitution of partial exchange transfusion.

Clinical Application of Transfusion Therapy in Sickle Cell Disease. In the discussions of specific complications of sickle cell disease (Chapters 24, 25, and 27 through 29), the reader can find a review of available therapies, including red cell transfusions. The following section focuses on the data for and against transfusion therapy for these complications. Particular attention is devoted to randomized, prospective studies of transfusion therapy, but few such studies are available. The specific clinical indications for transfusion therapy are divided into those that require treatment of anemia, those that require a reduction in cells capable of sickling, and those for which the rationale for transfusion therapy is uncertain.

Relief of Anemia

Aplastic Crisis. Exacerbation of anemia during a period of erythroid hypoplasia may require red cell transfusion if accompanied by hemodynamic compromise or deteriorating clinical status (e.g., extreme weakness, syncope) in the absence of laboratory evidence of imminent bone marrow recovery. A mild decline in hemoglobin level alone is not an indication for transfusion, and even hemoglobin levels of 4 to 5 g/dL during an aplastic crisis may be well tolerated. When the need for a transfusion is uncertain, evidence of imminent bone marrow recovery, such as nucleated red cells in the peripheral blood or the reappearance of reticulocytes, may favor waiting. If red cells are necessary, the slow administration of one or two transfusions of small volume, raising the hemoglobin by 2 to 3 g/dL over 4 to 8 hours, is usually sufficient to improve the clinical condition of the patient until spontaneous recovery occurs.

Acute Splenic Sequestration Crisis. Sudden, massive enlargement of the spleen with pooling of large amounts of blood within the organ may cause profound anemia and hypovolemia. Transfusion therapy carries two benefits: restoration of intravascular volume and improvement in oxygen-carrying capacity. Acute splenic sequestration crisis is one of the few complications of sickle cell disease in which rapid administration of red cells is not only safe but may also be lifesaving. Occasionally, transfusion with O negative or Rh and ABO specific, noncrossmatched blood may be necessary to prevent death from shock and severe anemia. Hypovolemia makes consideration of the volume of the transfused red cells relatively unimportant. However, small amounts of blood are usually sufficient to reverse the process of sequestration, releasing trapped blood back into the circulation and further improving the intravascular volume and the hemoglobin level (Chapter 24).

Reduction of Sickling

Prevention of Stroke. Regular red cell transfusions to maintain the HbS level below 30 percent reduce the risk of recurrent thrombotic stroke from 50 to 90 percent to less than 15 percent (Powars et al., 1978; Russell et al., 1984; Balkaran et al., 1992; Pegelow et al., 1995). In the United States, this finding has led to the initiation of transfusion therapy after a first stroke in children with sickle cell disease. In a French study of ten children who did not receive transfusions after their initial stroke, the absence of recurrence prompted the recommendation by these investigators that a chronic transfusion program

begin only after a second stroke (de Montalambert et al., 1993). Unfortunately, no studies have successfully identified clinical, laboratory, or radiologic characteristics that distinguish patients at risk for a recurrent stroke.

Transfusion therapy for prevention of recurrent stroke usually begins at the time of the first episode. Partial exchange transfusion is commonly used to quickly reduce the HbS level to 30 percent. The alternative of frequently repeated simple transfusions at the time of the acute event may raise the total hemoglobin level above 11 to 12 g/dL, risking further central nervous system damage from hyperviscosity. Therapy continues with a long-term transfusion program generally designed to maintain the HbS level below 30 percent by simple transfusions of one or two units of red cells every 3 or 4 weeks, or by partial exchange transfusion at similar intervals.

Although the value of transfusion in preventing recurrent stroke is clear, the optimal duration of therapy is uncertain. Most recurrences in patients who have not had transfusions are in the first 3 years after the initial event (Powars et al., 1978), suggesting that lowering the HbS level is particularly important during this period. This view is supported by the recurrence of stroke in seven of ten patients who stopped transfusion therapy after 1 or 2 years (Wilimas et al., 1980) and in four of ten patients who stopped after 1 to 4 years (de Montalembert et al., 1993). The benefits of longer transfusion therapy are debatable. In one study, stopping transfusions even after 5 to 12 years resulted in a 50 percent recurrence rate within 1 year (Wang et al., 1991), but in another study, stopping transfusions after a mean duration of 6 years resulted in no recurrences during the next 3 to 18 years (Rana et al., 1997). At present, most pediatric sickle cell centers continue transfusion therapy indefinitely for the prevention of recurrent stroke. This therapy, however, frequently ends when patients transfer to adult centers. The determination of the optimal duration of transfusion therapy for prevention of recurrent stroke awaits a prospective, randomized trial that avoids the pitfall of selection bias and that accounts for the potential impact of transfusions administered for other purposes.

Because the major reason for discontinuing transfusions is the concern about iron overload, an alternative to stopping therapy is to modify the transfusion program to reduce the rate of iron accumulation. In a study of fifteen patients with no recurrence of stroke and no progressive neurologic deterioration during at least 4 years of conventional transfusion therapy, a subsequent increase in the pretransfusion HbS level from 30 to 50 percent reduced blood requirements and thus the rate of iron loading by 24 percent without raising the risk of recurrent stroke (Cohen et al., 1992). A second study supported the safety and benefits of this modified simple

Table 37.5. Comparison of Annual Net Red Cell Loading and Annual Donor Red Cell Usage with Simple Transfusion and Erythrocytapheresis to Prevent Recurrent Stroke in Sickle Cell Disease

Transfusion protocol	Annual net red cell load	Annual donor red cell usage
Simple transfusion (target HbS < 30%)	133.0 ± 29.3 mL RBC/kg/yr	176.9 ± 39.3 mL PRBC/kg/yr
Simple transfusion (target HbS < 50%)	99.4 ± 37.7 mL RBC/kg/yr	132.8 ± 49.5 mL PRBC/kg/yr
Erythrocytapheresis (target HbS < 50%)	17.8 ± 12.9 mL RBC/kg/yr	214.6 ± 45.0 mL PRBC/kg/yr

RBC, red blood cell; PRBC, packed red blood cell

transfusion program (Miller et al., 1992), and even greater reductions in net blood requirements have been achieved with manual or automated exchange transfusions (Table 37.5) (Cohen et al., 1992; Adams et al., 1996; Hilliard et al., 1998). Novel transfusion programs that prevent recurrent stroke and reduce the risk of iron overload may increase the clinician's level of comfort with long-term therapy.

The potential application of transfusion therapy to the prevention of an initial rather than a recurrent stroke has awaited an acceptably sensitive and specific method for identifying patients at risk. The demonstration of the diagnostic value of transcranial Doppler ultrasonography for this purpose (Adams et al., 1992, 1997) led to a prospective, randomized trial in which transfusion therapy significantly reduced the risk of first stroke in patients with abnormal cerebral blood flow (Table 37.6) (Adams et al., 1998) (Chapter 24). Applying these results to clinical practice may sharply increase—at least in the short run—the number of children receiving regular blood transfusions for stroke prevention. However, the unwillingness of families and physicians to enter patients in the transfusion arm of the study and the dropout rate from this arm because of alloimmunization, poor compliance, rapidly rising ferritin levels, and other reasons illustrate the problems that continue to confront transfusion therapy for stroke (Cohen, 1998).

Pregnancy. When pregnant women with sickling disorders develop complications such as toxemia, septicemia, severe acute chest syndrome, exacerbation of anemia, stroke, acute renal failure, or the need for emergency surgery, red cell transfusions are commonly administered to raise the hemoglobin level or decrease the HbS percentage (Koshy and Burd, 1991; Koshy et al., 1995) (Chapter 24). Greater controversy surrounds the use of prophylactic transfusion therapy during pregnancy (Morrison and Wiser, 1976a, 1976b; Charache et al., 1980; Morrison et al., 1980; Miller et al., 1981; Cunningham et al., 1983; Tuck et al., 1987; Koshy et al., 1988; Morrison et al., 1991; Howard et al., 1995). Assessment of the effectiveness of this approach is hindered by differing transfusion protocols and by retrospective analyses. Even if one limits the additional confounding effect of general improvements in obstetrical care by considering only those studies reported in the last 20 years, conclusions differ widely. For example, in a retrospective review of 101 women with sickling disorders treated between 1981 and 1990 at a single institution, the investigators concluded that the early (mean 19 weeks) introduction of partial exchange transfusions to maintain the HbS below 50 percent resulted in fewer crises, a lower incidence of pneumonia, a reduction in preterm deliveries, a lower perinatal death rate, and fewer low birth weight infants (Morrison et al., 1991). In contrast, two retrospective British studies covering similar periods found no beneficial effect of prophylactic transfusions on either maternal or fetal outcome (Tuck et al., 1987; Howard et al., 1995). One study involved partial exchange transfusions from the first or second trimester but no consistent target hemoglobin level or HbS percentage (Howard et al., 1995); the other used simple transfusion to reduce the HbS level below 25 percent and raise the hemoglobin to 11 g/dL (Tuck et al., 1987).

The most informative data regarding the role of prophylactic transfusions during pregnancy in women with

Table 37.6. Effect of Transfusion Therapy on Prevention of First Stroke in Children with Sickle Cell Disease and Abnormal Transcranial Doppler Ultrasonograph

	Patient-months	Cerebral infarctions	Intracerebral hematoma
Transfusion (n = 63)	1,321	1	0
No Transfusion (n = 67)	1,229	10	1

From Adams et al., 1998.

sickle cell disease come from a multicenter, prospective, randomized, controlled study (Koshy et al., 1988). Thirty-six women received prophylactic simple or partial exchange transfusions beginning before 28 weeks to maintain the hemoglobin level between 10 and 11 g/dL and to reduce the HbS level to less than 35 percent. An equal number of women received transfusions only for medical or obstetrical emergencies. Although women receiving prophylactic transfusions had fewer painful crises and a lower cumulative incidence of sickle cell disease-related complications, the two treatment groups did not differ in obstetric complications or perinatal outcome. The investigators noted that pregnant patients with sickle cell disease and their fetuses were at high risk, with or without prophylactic transfusions; the perinatal death rate was 10 percent. Perhaps this is what has led clinicians to continue the use of prophylactic transfusions during pregnancy in many centers, causing Serjeant to conclude that "even when evidence is available, it seems that the appeal of transfusion is so strong that ... data [such as those of Koshy] are disregarded" (Serjeant, 1997).

Acute Chest Syndrome. Many patients with acute chest syndrome receive one or two simple transfusions to raise the hemoglobin level and augment oxygen-carrying capacity (Poncz et al., 1985; Emre et al., 1993). Exchange transfusion is now being used with increasing frequency in patients with progressive acute chest syndrome in an attempt to reduce the morbidity and mortality of this often devastating complication of sickle cell disease. Case reports and uncontrolled series describe rapid clinical and radiologic improvement and higher PaO_2 levels after exchange transfusion (Lanzkowsky et al., 1978; Kleinman et al., 1981; Davies et al., 1984; Mallouh and Asha, 1988; Emre et al., 1995). In the largest series to date, thirty-five patients with acute chest syndrome and clinical deterioration underwent exchange transfusion (Wayne et al., 1993). Thirty-two of the thirty-five patients, including five of seven on assisted ventilation, had rapid and dramatic improvement in oxygenation and other clinical parameters, leading the investigators to recommend exchange transfusion for patients with diffuse pulmonary involvement. In 671 episodes of acute chest syndrome, phenotypically matched transfusions improved oxygenation, with a 1 percent rate of alloimmunization (Vichinsky et al., 200).

The role of transfusion therapy for acute chest syndrome may extend to the prevention of recurrences in patients with severe or repeated episodes. This long-term application is predicated on the finding that recurrent acute chest syndrome may be immediately life-threatening or may contribute to chronic pulmonary failure, pulmonary hypertension, and cor pulmonale (Collins and Orringer, 1982; Powars et al., 1988). Regular red cell transfusions reduced the rate of acute chest syndrome (Styles and Vichinsky, 1994); their effect on late pulmonary outcomes is unknown.

Prevention of Sequestration Crises. Chronic transfusion therapy may reduce the risk of recurrent acute splenic sequestration crisis and delay but not necessarily prevent the need for splenectomy. Only two of ten children had a recurrence of splenic sequestration crisis while receiving regular transfusions to maintain the HbS below 30 percent for 6 to 12 months (Kinney et al., 1990). However, recurrences were frequent when the transfusion program was interrupted or completed. Chronic splenic enlargement and hypersplenism also improve during long-term transfusion therapy but recur after treatment is stopped (Rao and Gooden, 1985). These findings suggest that transfusion therapy may be particularly beneficial in the management of recurrent acute splenic sequestration crisis or chronic hypersplenism in very young children by delaying the need for splenectomy until a later age when the risk of post-splenectomy sepsis has diminished.

Painful Episodes. Five percent of patients with sickle cell disease have three to ten episodes of intense pain each year and account for 33 percent of all painful episodes requiring hospital visits (Platt et al., 1991) (Chapter 25). No study to date has directly addressed the value of transfusion therapy in reducing the physical and social consequences of such a severe course. However, the experience gained from transfusion therapy for prevention of recurrent stroke demonstrates that reduction of the HbS level to 30 percent reduces the rate of painful crises by tenfold (Styles and Vichinsky, 1994).

The value of transfusion therapy in the management of acute painful episode is less certain. Partial exchange transfusion to reduce the HbS below 50 percent improved the clinical condition and reduced the length of hospitalization in eight patients (Brody et al., 1970). However, no subsequent study has confirmed or disproved these old but intriguing findings. Acute painful crisis may occasionally progress to catastrophic multiorgan failure associated with a falling hemoglobin level. In seventeen such episodes, transfusion therapy quickly and dramatically improved the encephalopathy, urine output, oxygenation, and general clinical condition (Hassell et al., 1994). Improvement after exchange transfusion was particularly rapid, suggesting that the benefit derived from transfusion therapy was due to a reduction in sickle cells rather than, or in addition to, a restoration of oxygen-carrying capacity.

Priapism. Small, uncontrolled studies of simple and exchange transfusion in the treatment of priapism have yielded inconsistent results (Seeler, 1973; Kinney et al., 1975; Baron and Leiter, 1978; Rifkind et al., 1979; Noe et al., 1981; Walker et al., 1983; Karayalcin et al., 1984; Tarry et al., 1987; Hamre et al., 1991; Miller et al., 1995). Overall, approximately one third of patients who were treated with transfusions went on to have a shunt procedure. No difference between the results with simple and exchange transfusion is readily discernible, aside from descriptions of individual patients who had immediate detumescence or relief of pain during erythrocytapheresis. Neurologic events, including seizures and strokes, have occurred in a small but worrisome number of patients within 1 to 14 days of simple or exchange transfusion for priapism (ASPEN syndrome) (Royal and Seeler, 1978; Rackoff et al., 1992; Siegel et al., 1993; Miller et al., 1995). Whether the risk of such events is greater after transfusion therapy for priapism than for other complications of sickle cell disease is uncertain, and no pathophysiologic explanation is apparent. However, the limited benefit of transfusion therapy for priapism and the possible risk of neurologic sequelae should be carefully considered in managing this acute problem. Long-term transfusion therapy may help prevent recurrent episodes of priapism (Miller et al., 1995).

Relief of Anemia or Reduction of Sickling

Perioperative Management. The use of transfusions to prevent complications of general anesthesia and surgery is particularly controversial (Chapter 24). To reduce the high risk of perioperative complications, some investigators have favored routine or selective administration of red cells to correct the anemia, whereas others have favored administration of red cells to decrease the HbS level. Uncontrolled studies of these

approaches have yielded perioperative complication rates of 0 to 20 percent and a very low death rate (Holzmann et al., 1969; Morrison et al., 1978; Lanzkowsky et al., 1978; Homi et al., 1979; Janik and Seeler, 1980; Fullerton et al., 1981; Coker and Milner, 1982; Bischoff et al., 1988; Ware et al., 1988; Derkay et al., 1991; Griffin and Buchanan, 1983; Bhattacharyya et al., 1993; Halvorson et al., 1997). Other investigators have argued that the key to an equally successful outcome, at least in minor surgical procedures, is careful attention to hydration and oxygenation rather than administration of red cells (Oduro and Searle, 1972; Griffin and Buchanan, 1993; Serjeant, 1997). Partial resolution of the role of perioperative transfusion therapy comes from a large, multiinstitutional, randomized study of two approaches (Vichinsky et al., 1995). Patients in Group 1 received simple or exchange transfusions to reduce the HbS level below 30 percent and to raise the total hemoglobin level to 10 g/dL, and patients in Group 2 received simple transfusions to raise the total hemoglobin level to 10 g/dL irrespective of the HbS level. Clinical characteristics, type of surgical procedure, and supportive management were similar in the two groups. The type of transfusion therapy did not affect the rate of minor or major perioperative complications other than those related to transfusion itself (Table 37.7). Acute chest syndrome occurred in 11 percent of patients in Group 1 and 10 percent of patients in Group 2. Both deaths occurred in Group 1. The reduction in HbS level in Group 1 required twice as much donor blood as the increase in hemoglobin level in Group 2. As a result, patients in Group 1 had a significantly higher rate of alloimmunization.

Although this study randomly assigned patients only to one of two transfusion arms, the investigators concurrently followed a group of patients who, for dif-

Table 37.7. Effect of Goal of Perioperative Transfusions on Outcome

Complications	Group 1 (HbS < 30%, Hb = 10 g/dL)	Group 2 (Hb = 10 g/dL)
Serious or life-threatening postoperative complications	21%	22%
Acute chest syndrome	10%	10%
Fever or infection	7%	5%
Painful crisis	4%	7%
Neurologic event	1%	< 1%
Death	1%	0%
Transfusion-related complications	14%	7%
New antibody	10%	5%
Hemolysis	6%	1%

From Vichinsky et al., 1995.

ferent reasons, did not receive transfusions. In a sub-analysis of patients undergoing cholecystectomy, the most common surgical procedure, the rate of sickling-related complications was higher in patients who did not receive a transfusion than in those receiving either of the two transfusion regimens (Haberkern et al., 1997). Acute chest syndrome occurred in 19 percent of the thirty-seven patients who did not receive transfusions, and two patients died. In other series of patients who did not routinely receive transfusions preoperatively, retrospective analyses have shown complication rates of 13 to 26 percent (Homi et al., 1979; Griffin and Buchanan, 1993; Koshy et al., 1995). Adverse events were generally more common in patients undergoing major surgery (e.g., cholecystectomy, splenectomy) or emergency surgery.

Based on current data, preoperative transfusion to raise the hemoglobin level to 10 g/dL generally appears to be as effective as a transfusion program to reduce the HbS below 30 percent and to cause less alloimmunization. However, with either approach, acute chest syndrome remains a substantial risk, especially in patients with a history of lung disease who are undergoing a high-risk operation. Their management is discussed in Chapter 24. Transfusions before minor, elective procedures such as placement of tympanostomy tubes may convey no advantage in patients without chronic lung disease or other significant complications. In one special instance, retinal reattachment, transfusions to reduce the HbS level below 30 percent may be particularly important to prevent postoperative ischemia of the anterior segment (Brazier et al., 1986). Currently available data do not address some issues such as the management of the patient with sickle cell anemia and a baseline hemoglobin of 10 g/dL or the value and goal of preoperative transfusions in HbSC (Chapter 27), and transfusion strategies in these and other instances will vary among sickle cell centers.

Other Proposed Indications. Case reports and uncontrolled series have suggested a possible therapeutic role for red cell transfusions in the management of other complications of sickle cell anemia such as leg ulcers, avascular necrosis, and persistent hematuria. In some of these descriptions, the benefit of transfusion has appeared to be dramatic, but specific recommendations must await more extensive clinical trials.

Other Views and Other Approaches. Not everyone accepts a major role for transfusion therapy in sickle cell disease. In Jamaica, none of the 4,000 patients with sickle cell anemia receives prophylactic transfusions preoperatively, during pregnancy, or to prevent recurrent complications (Serjeant, 1997). The director of this center argues that, with the exception of pre-

vention of recurrent stroke, alternative methods for managing these clinical situations are equally effective. Furthermore, in many parts of the world, blood fully tested for viral contamination is not readily available.

New approaches to the management of sickle cell disease may redefine the role of transfusion therapy. For example, hydroxyurea therapy (Chapter 38) is now an alternative to transfusions for the treatment of recurrent painful episodes. Bone marrow transplantation is being offered with increasing frequency as an alternative to transfusion therapy for patients with stroke or other severe or recurrent complications (Chapter 40). These advances, as well as progress in the general management of pregnancy, general anesthesia, and other medical and surgical conditions, will require regular reevaluation of the effectiveness and safety of transfusions.

Other Hemoglobinopathies

Patients with unstable hemoglobins may need occasional red cell transfusion during exacerbations of anemia (Chapter 44). If the unstable hemoglobin has an increased oxygen affinity, the decision to transfuse reaches a higher level of complexity (Larson et al., 1997). In this situation, the chronic hemolysis resulting from the unstable hemoglobin blocks the usual compensatory polycythemia in response to the hemoglobin's abnormally increased oxygen affinity. The resultant "normal" hemoglobin level may have only half the normal oxygen delivery capacity. Simple transfusions to achieve normal oxygen delivery at the time of surgery or acute illnesses may raise the hemoglobin to unacceptably high levels. Alternatively, exchange transfusion carries the dual benefits of improving oxygen delivery while maintaining a normal total hemoglobin level, and replacing the unstable hemoglobin variant with HbA.

Complications of Transfusion Therapy

Most adverse consequences of transfusion therapy for thalassemia, sickle cell anemia, and other hemoglobinopathies are independent of the underlying blood disorder, although they may occur with differing frequency in each of these diseases. The following sections focus on complications that are particularly problematic for patients with hemoglobinopathies receiving long-term transfusion therapy. A detailed discussion of other complications such as febrile or allergic reactions and acute hemolytic transfusion reactions can be found in textbooks of transfusion medicine. Iron overload, the leading and most complex clinical problem of long-term transfusion therapy, is discussed in the second major section of this chapter.

Alloimmunization. Alloantibodies have been detected in 3 to 23 percent of patients with thalassemia (Coles et al., 1981; Sirchia et al., 1985; Spanos et al., 1990; Rebulla and Modell, 1991). Variations between centers are probably due to different degrees of discordance of red cell antigen frequencies between donors and recipients, different approaches to antigen matching, and different definitions of clinically significant antibodies. Development of more than two alloantibodies is uncommon (Sirchia et al., 1985; Rebulla and Modell, 1991). Antibodies are most commonly directed against antigens of the Rh and Kell systems, (Sirchia et al., 1985; Spanos et al., 1990), and extension of antigen matching beyond these systems may not be helpful (Michail-Merianou et al., 1987).

The age at which transfusion therapy is initiated in thalassemia major has a consistent effect on the rate of alloimmunization. In two studies from Greece, alloimmunization occurred more than twice as often in children beginning transfusion therapy after age 3 years (Spanos et al., 1990), and four times as often in children beginning transfusion therapy after age 1 year (Michail-Merianou et al., 1987). In a study of 110 alloimmunized patients in Greece and Italy, alloantibodies developed in fewer than 3 percent of children who began transfusion therapy in the first year of life, but in more than 15 percent of children who received their first transfusion after age 4 years (Rebulla and Modell, 1991). Because alloimmunization by itself is rarely a significant clinical problem in thalassemia, these findings of the influence of age may not have a substantial impact on the decision to initiate or delay transfusion therapy. However, in some children receiving regular transfusions, alloantibodies are accompanied by red cell autoantibodies (see later), presenting additional and often serious clinical problems. This unusual but severe complication is worthy of consideration in deciding at what age to initiate transfusion therapy in the child with a marginal hemoglobin level or clinical status.

Red cell alloimmunization occurs in 8 to 38 percent of patients with sickle cell disease who have received transfusions (Orlina et al., 1978; Coles et al., 1981; Sarnaik et al., 1986; Davies et al., 1986; Ambruso et al., 1987; Cox et al., 1988; Patten et al., 1989; Rosse et al., 1990; Vichinsky et al., 1990). In the large Cooperative Study of Sickle Cell Disease (Chapter 24), the overall rate of alloimmunization in 1,814 patients transfused before and/or after study entry was 18.6 percent (Rosse et al., 1990). In a subanalysis of 604 patients who had no alloantibodies at study entry and who subsequently received transfusions, the investigators found a significantly higher incidence of alloimmunization in patients with sickle cell anemia compared with patients with

other sickling disorders. The relationship between age and risk of alloimmunization, described earlier for thalassemia, also exists in sickle cell disease. Patients with sickle cell disease who received their first transfusion at 10 years of age or older had a higher rate of alloimmunization (20.7 percent) than those who received then first transfusion at less than age 10 years (9.6 percent). Alloimmunization rose continuously with an increasing number of transfusions; however, patients who underwent their first transfusion at a young age consistently required more transfusions to become alloimmunized than those whose first transfusions occurred when they were older.

Red cell antigens causing alloimmunization in patients with sickle cell disease most commonly belong to the Rh, Kell, Duffy, and Kidd systems. Antibodies to E, C, K, Jk[b], and Fy[a] account for approximately 80 percent of clinically significant alloantibodies, reflecting the differences in red cell phenotype between blood donors who are predominantly Caucasian and patients with sickle cell disease who are predominantly African American (Rosse et al., 1990; Vichinsky et al., 1990). For example, in northern California, the red cells of 68 percent of blood donors are positive for C antigen, whereas 72 percent of patients with sickle cell disease from the same area are C-negative and therefore susceptible to immunization by this antigen (Vichinsky et al., 1990). Reflecting the importance of racial differences between blood donors and recipients is the low rate of alloimmunization (5.4 percent among Caucasian patients with sickle cell disease in Italy who have received transfusions) (Russo-Mancuso et al., 1998).

Alloimmunization has consequences that range from a modest amount of extra work and expense in the blood bank to severe hemolysis. Delayed hemolytic transfusion reactions pose a particularly important problem for patients with sickle cell disease (Cox et al., 1988; Orlina et al., 1991; Syed et al., 1996; Petz et al., 1997). This complication arises when an alloantibody is not present in sufficient quantity to be detected by direct or indirect antiglobulin testing or when the antibody is directed against a low-frequency antigen that is not present on the screening cells used for the indirect antiglobulin test (Larson et al., 1996). On reexposure to the offending antigen, an anamnestic response occurs, and hemolysis begins in 3 to 10 days. Fever and back pain may accompany the delayed hemolysis, mimicking a vasoocclusive episode (Diamond et al., 1980). The timing of this event in relationship to a recent transfusion, an unexpected fall in the hemoglobin level, and a less than expected reduction in the percentage of HbS should prompt a search for a new alloantibody. In two prospective studies, delayed hemolytic transfusion reactions occurred in 38 and 44 percent of newly alloimmunized patients with sickle cell disease. (Vichinsky et al., 1990, 1995).

Red cell alloantibodies in patients with thalassemia or sickle cell disease may be accompanied by autoantibodies (Chapin and Zarkowsky, 1981; King et al., 1997; Castellino et al., 1999). The mechanism underlying the formation of autoantibodies is unclear, but possible causes include antigenic changes in the erythrocyte membrane or more generalized immune dysregulation. Erythrocyte autoantibodies occur in 7.6 percent of multiply transfused children with sickle cell disease but cause hemolysis in only 2 percent (Castellino et al., 1999). The autoimmune hemolysis is readily recognizable by the precipitous decrease in hemoglobin level to less than pretransfusion levels and the development of a new antibody with broad reactivity. Treatment with steroids and intravenous immune globulin is sometimes effective; further transfusions, even using apparently compatible blood, should be carefully considered in light of the risk of life-threatening hemolysis.

Platelet alloimmunization is also common in sickle cell disease, affecting 85 percent of patients who have received more than fifty transfusions (Friedman et al., 1996). The risk of developing platelet alloantibodies is related to the number of red cell transfusions but not to the presence or absence of red cell alloantibodies. As bone marrow transplantation becomes more important in sickle cell disease and thalassemia, it is particularly important to prevent refractoriness to the platelet transfusions that are often required for supportive care during transplantation. Current methods of leukoreduction have greatly reduced the risk of platelet alloimmunization, and patients with hemoglobinopathies should, if possible, receive only leukoreduced red cells.

Transfusion-Transmitted Infections. Because patients with thalassemia major and those with sickle cell anemia who undergo transfusions regularly usually receive 12 to 50 units of red cells each year, they are at higher risk than most blood recipients for transfusion-transmitted infections such as hepatitis and human immunodeficiency virus (HIV). Rates of seropositivity for hepatitis C vary from 12 percent of patients with thalassemia who receive their transfusions in the United Kingdom to 91 percent of patients who receive their transfusions in Italy (Wonke et al., 1990; Rebulla et al., 1992). Antibodies to hepatitis C are present in 23 to 30 percent of patients with sickle cell anemia who have received more than 10 units of red cells (DeVault et al., 1994; Hasan et al., 1996). Hepatitis C may have particularly grave clinical consequences in regularly transfused patients with hemoglobinopathies because iron overload aggravates the liver damage and

diminishes the response to antiviral therapy (Clemente et al., 1994; Di Marco et al., 1997). Hepatitis G virus is also prevalent in patients with thalassemia major but appears to be an infrequent cause of liver disease (Prati et al., 1998). The newly discovered TT virus is extremely common among patients with thalassemia, suggesting transmission by transfusion (Prati et al., 1999). New cases of transfusion-transmitted hepatitis B are rare in the United States as a result of vaccination programs. However, many patients in other countries have not been vaccinated and remain at risk for this major cause of chronic liver disease (de Montalembert et al., 1992).

The risk of transfusion-transmitted HIV infection in patients with thalassemia and sickle cell anemia has varied with time and geographic location. In 1984, when donor testing was still unavailable, 12 percent of patients with thalassemia at one center in New York were seropositive for HIV (Robert-Guroff et al., 1987). In contrast, in a 1987 study of 3,633 patients with thalassemia in Europe, only 1.56 percent were seropositive for HIV (Lefrere and Girot, 1987). After the introduction of routine donor screening programs and serologic testing for HIV, new seroconversions have become extremely rare in many countries (Lefrere and Girot, 1989; Mozzi et al., 1992). However, in those countries with the unfortunate combination of high HIV prevalence and inadequate blood safety programs, the rate of HIV infection is still as high as 22 percent in repeatedly transfused children with sickle cell disease (Ouattara et al., 1998). One Indian center that continues to rely on unscreened blood from paid donors who have high seropositivity rates foresees transfusion-associated HIV infection as a persistent, major hazard for patients with thalassemia (Kumar et al., 1996).

Iron overload, as assessed by serum ferritin level, may contribute to the progression of HIV infection in patients with thalassemia (Salhi et al., 1998). The iron chelator desferrioxamine, on the other hand, may have a dose-dependent inhibitory effect on disease progression (Costagliola et al., 1994). Both of these observations require confirmatory studies.

Red cell transfusions infrequently transmit bacterial infections (Menitove, 1996). However, *Y. enterocolitica*, the organism responsible for seven of the eight fatal red cell-transmitted bacterial infections reported to the Food and Drug Administration between 1986 and 1991, deserves special attention. This contaminant represents a particular problem for patients who have undergone long-term transfusions because iron overload and the iron chelator desferrioxamine enhance its pathogenicity. *Y. enterocolitica* enters the blood supply when blood donation coincides with asymptomatic bacteremia, making efforts at preven-

Table 37.8. Effect of Splenectomy on Transfusion Requirements

Spleen status	Transfusion requirements
Nonsplenectomized	230 ± 56 mL PRBC/kg/yr (range 131–382)
Splenectomized	129 ± 21 mL PRBC/kg/yr (range 80–155)

From Cohen et al., 1980.
PRBC = packed red blood cell.

tion difficult. Evaluating febrile transfusion reactions or persistent unexplained fevers in patients with hemoglobinopathies undergoing transfusions long-term should include careful consideration of systemic or localized *Yersinia* infection.

Hypersplenism and Increased Transfusion Requirements. A sustained increase in transfusion requirements is a strong indication for splenectomy in patients with thalassemia major (Table 37.8) (Modell, 1977; Cohen et al., 1980). When the annual blood requirement exceeds 200 mL of packed red cells (PCV 75 percent) per kilogram of body weight, a minimum reduction of at least 20 percent usually follows removal of the spleen. The role of splenectomy in reducing transfusion requirements may be less important in patients who are well chelated and should be weighed against potential complications such as postsplenectomy sepsis and thrombosis. Moreover, other causes of increased blood requirements, such as alloimmunization or different preparation of donor units, should be sought before removing the spleen for this purpose.

Regular red cell transfusions may have the unintended consequence of reversing partial splenic atrophy in children and adults with sickle cell disease. As the newly restored spleen enlarges, transfusion requirements sometimes increase substantially (Cohen et al., 1991; Campbell et al., 1997). In such cases, removal of the spleen reduces the need for donor blood (and therefore the accumulation of iron) by 39 to 51 percent. Careful monitoring of spleen size and annual transfusion requirements assists in identifying patients with hypersplenism who may benefit from surgical intervention.

Hypertension and Encephalopathy. Hypertension, accompanied or followed shortly after by headache, changes in mental status, and seizures, is an unusual but potentially devastating complication of transfusion therapy in thalassemia, especially when the hemoglobin is raised from very low levels to normal or high levels (Wasi et al., 1978; Yetgin and Hicsonmez, 1979). A similar constellation of findings may occur after transfusion in sickle cell anemia (Royal and Seeler, 1978; Warth, 1984). The cause is unknown. Autopsy findings in six cases showed brain edema and congestion, gross or microscopic hemorrhage, and microdissecting aneurysms (Sonakul and Fucharoen, 1992). No underlying vascular disease distinguished these patients from those without encephalopathy. Complaints of headache or weakness after transfusion should prompt careful evaluation for neurologic abnormalities including cerebral hemorrhage; hypertension, if present, should be treated aggressively.

IRON OVERLOAD AND CHELATION THERAPY

Pathophysiology of Iron Overload

Rates of Iron Loading. A healthy human has an average iron content of 40 to 50 mg per kg body weight, the majority of which is present in hemoglobin (30 mg/kg). About 4 mg/kg is present in myoglobin in muscle tissue and 2 mg/kg is present in cells as iron-containing enzymes. The remaining body iron is present in the storage form of ferritin or hemosiderin, predominantly in liver, spleen, and bone marrow. Storage iron is usually between 0 and 2,000 mg (mean, 769 mg for men and 323 mg for women)(Jacobs, 1974), depending on the balance between available dietary iron and the iron requirements of the individual (Bothwell et al., 1979). A healthy individual absorbs about 10 percent of the iron in the diet, or 1 to 2 mg/day. This intake is matched by insensible losses through exfoliation of skin, urinary tract, and gut mucosal cells, together with gastrointestinal and menstrual loss of red blood cells. Humans have a limited capacity to modulate iron absorption and have no physiologic mechanism for excreting excess iron.

Total body iron may accumulate as a consequence of increased gastrointestinal absorption or from repeated red cell transfusions. In thalassemia major, iron loading predominantly derives from blood transfusion but excess iron absorption may also contribute. A unit of red cells, processed from 420 mL of donor blood, contains approximately 200 mg of iron. Patients with thalassemia major who have undergone splenectomy receive the red cells derived from approximately 300 mL of whole blood per kg per annum (Modell, 1977) to maintain a mean hemoglobin level of 12 g/dL. This volume of transfused blood is equivalent to 0.4 mg/kg of transfused iron daily or 28 mg of iron in an adult weighing 70 kg. The transfusion requirements in patients who have not had a splenectomy may be higher (Modell, 1977). Added to the transfusional iron is gastrointestinal iron absorption, accounting for a further 1 to 4 mg/day (Pippard and

Weatherall, 1984). Thus, iron will accumulate at a rate of 0.4 to 0.5 mg/kg/day or 28 to 35 mg/day in an adult patient with thalassemia major who weighs 70 kg and has undergone splenectomy.

In thalassemia intermedia, blood transfusion is intermittent or not required, and the increased iron loading is mainly a consequence of excess iron absorption. The degree of excess iron absorption depends on several factors such as the degree of ineffective erythropoiesis, the extent of erythroid expansion, and the severity of the anemia, all of which are highly variable in thalassemia intermedia syndromes. In one study, patients with thalassemia intermedia absorbed 26 to 73 percent of food iron (Pippard et al., 1979). In another study, patients with this form of thalassemia absorbed 60 percent (range 17 to 90 percent) of a 5 mg dose of ferrous sulfate, whereas healthy control subjects absorbed 10 percent (range 5 to 15 percent) (Modell 1979; Pippard et al., 1979). In yet another study, absorption varied from 20 to 75 percent in HbE-β thalassemia and correlated with plasma iron turnover, transferrin saturation, and liver iron concentration (Pootrakul et al., 1988). Iron absorption in thalassemia intermedia can thus be up to five to ten times normal, or 0.1 mg/kg/day (Gordeuk et al., 1987).

In sickle cell disorders, there is little evidence of iron overload in the absence of blood transfusion (O'Brien, 1978). Indeed, a variable proportion of untransfused patients may be iron deficient (Vichinsky et al., 1981; Rao et al., 1984; Davies et al., 1984a). Repeated simple blood transfusions will inevitably lead to iron overload, but exchange transfusions will not result in iron loading if performed in such a way that transfusional iron input is matched by that removed during manual exchanges (Porter and Huehns, 1987) or by automated red cell exchanges (Cohen et al., 1992).

Distribution of Excess Iron. The tissue distribution and clinical manifestations of excess iron are influenced by the mode and rate of iron loading and by the absolute levels of tissue iron within the body. Increased iron absorption leading to a predominantly parenchymal distribution of iron loading is a feature of genetic hemochromatosis but is also found in many conditions associated with ineffective erythropoiesis (Cavill 1975; Pippard and Weatherall 1984; Pootrakul et al., 1988).

Postmortem examination of patients with thalassemia major (Modell and Matthews, 1976) showed striking variability in iron concentrations in different tissues. Iron was found at high concentrations in liver, heart, and endocrine glands, with very little present in striated muscle and none in the brain and nervous tissue. In the absence of chelation therapy, siderosis in liver macrophages and hepatocytes correlated with the number of units of blood transfused, age, and liver iron concentration (Risdon et al., 1975). With more advanced iron overload or in patients who have undergone splenectomy, hepatocyte iron predominated.

In transfusional iron overload, cardiac iron is preferentially distributed to the ventricular myocardium compared with atrial myocardium or conducting tissue (Buja and Roberts, 1971). Ventricular myocardial iron distribution is uneven, being maximal in the subepicardium, intermediate in the subendocardial region and papillary muscles, and least in the middle third of the ventricular myocardium. Focal areas of fibrosis may also be seen in papillary muscles or ventricles. This uneven distribution of iron makes endocardial biopsy an unreliable tool for assessing cardiac iron concentration and iron-mediated cardiac damage (Fitchettt et al., 1980; Barosi et al., 1989). The reasons for the uneven distribution of body iron are not fully understood but likely reflect variable tissue distribution of both transferrin and nontransferrin iron uptake mechanisms. In heart cells in vitro there is evidence for both transferrin-mediated (Fava et al., 1981) and nontransferrin-mediated uptake of iron (Link et al., 1985; Parkes et al., 1993), consistent with the finding that cardiac iron correlates with both serum iron and transferrin saturation in thalassemia (Barosi et al., 1989). Nontransferrin iron appearing in plasma could be a key prerequisite to iron loading of tissues that lack significant numbers of transferrin receptors but possess uptake mechanisms for nontransferrin iron.

Clinical Consequences of Excess Iron. In thalassemia major, if chelation treatment is withheld, death from iron-induced cardiac failure is common starting in the second decade of life (Table 37.9) (Wolfe et al., 1985; Zurlo et al., 1989; Brittenham et al., 1994). In contrast, in conditions such as genetic hemochromatosis where iron loading is slower, cirrhosis is a common presenting feature, usually in the fourth and fifth decades of life, and commonly leads to death from liver failure or hepatocellular cancer. Cirrhosis is also a common feature in thalassemia major, being present in 50 percent of patients at postmortem and is particularly likely if chronic infective hepatitis (e.g., hepatitis C) is also present. However, historically, cirrhosis is a relatively uncommon cause of death in thalassemia major (Zurlo et al., 1989).

Liver fibrosis may develop early in the course of thalassemia major, even in the absence of infective hepatitis. For example, fibrosis has been observed as early as age 3 years after starting transfusion (Angelucci et al., 1994). Fibrosis correlates with age, the number of units of blood transfused, and liver iron concentration (Risdon et al., 1975).

Table 37.9. Causes of Death in Thalassemia

Age (years)	0–4	5–9	10–14	15–19	>20	Total
Heart disease	0	6	39	35	16	96
Infection	2	6	9	3	0	20
Liver disease	0	0	2	7	1	10
Malignancy	2	2	1	1	2	8
Endocrine disease	0	0	2	1	1	4
Accident	0	0	2	2	0	4
Thromboembolism	0	1	1	0	0	2
Anemia	2	0	0	0	0	2
Other	0	1	1	0	1	3
Unknown	0	1	3	3	1	8
Total	6	16	61	53	23	159

From Zurlo et al., 1989.

Hypogonadism is common, occurring in 62 percent of patients over age 12 years (Piga et al., 1997) and leading to disturbances of growth and sexual maturation. Hypogonadism is typically secondary to anterior pituitary dysfunction (hypogonadotrophic hypogonadism); hence in many women with thalassemia and secondary amenorrhea (Chatterjee et al., 1993), induction of ovulation and successful pregnancy are often achievable (Chatterjee et al., 1995).

Other complications such as diabetes, hypothyroidism (Landau et al., 1993), and hypoparathyroidism (McIntosh, 1976) are seen in a variable proportion of patients, and their frequency is falling with improved chelation therapy. Indeed, in optimally treated patients who receive more than 260 infusions of desferrioxamine yearly, these complications are absent at a 15-years follow-up (Gabutti and Piga, 1996). Low levels of adrenal androgen secretion with normal glucocorticoid reserve have also been reported (Sklar et al., 1987). Other features of iron overload include skin pigmentation, arthropathy, ascorbic acid deficiency, and osteoporosis (Gordeuk et al., 1987).

Infections are the second most frequent cause of death in thalassemia and are particularly common in younger age groups (Zurlo et al., 1989). Postsplenectomy sepsis resulting from encapsulated organisms is an important contributor (Pinna et al., 1988). However iron overload also appears to play a central role in increasing susceptibility to infection. There are several case reports of infection with *Y. enterocolitica, Vibrio vulnificus, Listeria monocytogenes, Escherichia coli,* and *Candida klebsiella* and species (Barry and Reeve, 1977; Hwang et al., 1994). This increased infective risk partly results from the saturation of transferrin with iron, depriving the body of an important mechanism to withhold this nutrient from bacteria. There is also evidence for defective neutrophil and macrophage function (Skoutelis et al., 1984; Ballart et

al., 1986; Kutukculer et al., 1996), presumably secondary to excess iron. Some bacteria such as *Yersinia* are able to utilize iron from iron complexes of chelators (Robins-Browne and Prpic, 1985). This is particularly likely if the chelator is a naturally occurring siderophore such as desferrioxamine.

Illustrating the relevance of the rate of iron loading to the clinical manifestations of iron overload is the contrasting complications of excessive iron in thalassemia major and thalassemia intermedia. Thalassemia intermedia is a heterogeneous collection of disorders with varying rates of hemolysis and iron absorption and different requirements for intermittent transfusions (Pootrakul et al., 1988). Because of the slower buildup of iron in thalassemia intermedia, damaging levels of iron loading typically develop later in life than in thalassemia major and may not affect pituitary function until the third or fourth decade or beyond. Therefore, in thalassemia intermedia, growth and sexual development are typically unaffected by iron overload per se and, when present, are more likely to be the consequences of ineffective erythropoiesis and anemia.

In sickle cell diseases, where there is typically no requirement for regular blood transfusions to correct anemia, iron overload develops only in individuals who receive repeated blood transfusions to prevent selected disease complications. In the minority of patients who receive sufficient repeated transfusions to cause significant iron overload, clinical consequences begin later than in thalassemia major and thus effects on growth and sexual development are uncommon. Indeed much documented evidence for iron overload in sickle cell disease is confined to case studies. There is, however, evidence of transfusion-induced iron loading in the liver (Brittenham et al., 1993), with cirrhosis (Comer et al., 1991), siderosis in the heart (Buja and Roberts, 1971), hypothyroidism (Phillips et al., 1992), and increased pancreatic deposition of iron (Siegelman et al., 1994). Portal fibrosis has been noted in one third of patients after 1 to 4 years of regular transfusion without chelation and in a similar proportion of patients receiving long-term transfusion and chelation therapy. Fibrosis occurs at widely varying hepatic iron concentrations of 9 to 38 mg/g dry weight in the absence of hepatitis C infection (Olivieri et al., 1999). Once regular transfusion therapy has begun, there is no theoretical reason why any given degree of iron loading should result in a significantly different risk of organ damage than in thalassemia major. It should be remembered that the use of the serum ferritin to estimate iron loading may be particularly problematic in sickle cell disease. The ferritin level is disproportionately increased in relation to iron loading for several weeks after a painful sickle cell episode (Brownell et al., 1986; Porter and Huehns, 1987) and generally correlates poorly with hepatic iron concentration (Olivieri et al., 1999; Hartmatz et al., 1999).

Mechanisms of Toxicity of Iron Overload. In the absence of iron overload, iron is unavailable to participate in the generation of harmful free radicals because of its binding to physiologic ligands such as transferrin. However, when iron overload develops, these protective mechanisms become saturated, and plasma nontransferrin bound iron (Hershko et al., 1978b) and increased quantities of labile low molecular weight intracellular iron (Breuer et al., 1995) may participate in the generation of harmful free radicals.

A free radical is defined as any species capable of independent existence that contains one or more unpaired electrons. The products formed sequentially during the reduction of molecular oxygen (O_2) to water are superoxide (O_2^-), hydrogen peroxide (H_2O_2), and the hydroxyl radical ($OH^\bullet$), the reduction of the latter resulting in the formation of water. Hydroxyl radical has a great affinity for electrons and will oxidize all substances within its immediate vicinity (diffusion radius of 2.3 nm) (Marx and van Asbeck, 1996). H_2O_2 by itself is relatively stable and nontoxic. However, it is an important precursor of hydroxyl radicals requiring the availability of catalytic trace elements such as iron, copper, or cobalt. Iron is particularly important because it is present at sufficient concentrations in tissues and because of the favorable redox potential of the Fe^{+2}/Fe^{+3} couple (between +0.35 and −0.5V). Oxidation of Fe^{+2} to Fe^{+3}, with the concomitant generation of the hydroxyl radical from water, is referred to as the Fenton reaction:

$$H_2O_2 + Fe^{+2} \rightarrow OH- + OH^\bullet + Fe^{+3} \text{ (Fenton reaction)}$$

Within cells are physiologic scavengers of toxic oxygen products such as superoxide dismutase, which dismutates O_2^- to H_2O_2, and catalase, which scavenges H_2O_2. Tissue damage depends on the relative rates of formation and scavenging of toxic free radicals. The hydroxyl radical $OH^\bullet$ can damage biomolecules including proteins, DNA, and membrane lipids by peroxidation. Particularly important is the initiation of peroxidation of lipid (Lp) by hydrogen abstraction (Gutteridge and Halliwell, 1989):

$$LpH + OH^\bullet \rightarrow Lp^\bullet + H_2O$$

Because iron is concentrated in hepatocyte lysosomes in both primary and secondary iron overload, these organelles are particularly susceptible to lipid peroxidation (Kornbrust and Mavis 1980; Bacon et al., 1983). Lysosomal fragility results and is directly proportional to the degree of iron overload (Le Sage, 1986; Myers et al., 1991) (Fig. 37.1). Lipid peroxidation and damage to organelles and lysosomal fragility may lead to cell death but may also encourage fibrogenesis. Iron-induced aldehyde lipid peroxidation products such as malondialdehyde (MDA) (Houglum et al., 1990) and 4-hydroxynonenal (HNE) (Parola et al., 1993) promote collagen gene expression and fibrogenesis in cultured fibroblasts and perisinusoidal stellate (ito) cells. Fibrogenesis is also associated with autocrine production of TGFβ-1 in stellate cells (Bissell et al., 1995), and increased levels of TGFβ-1 and procollagen al(I) mRNA have been observed in a model of iron and alcohol induced fibrogensis (Tsakamota et al., 1995). Increased TGFβ-1 expression and MDA protein adducts have also been reported in hepatocytes and sinusoidal cells of patients with genetic hemochromatosis (Houglum et al., 1997), suggesting that iron overload increases both lipid peroxidation and TGFβ-1 expression, which together may promote hepatic injury and fibrogenesis. In other tissues, similar mechanisms are likely to be involved, although the concentration and distribution of intracellular iron differ between tissues.

Objectives of Chelation Therapy

Chelation therapy for iron overload has two major objectives; (1) to induce sufficient iron excretion to achieve safe tissue iron levels and (2) to detoxify the excess iron until the first objective is achieved.

Achievement of Safe Tissue Iron Concentrations by Promoting Negative Iron Balance. Iron loading in transfusion-dependent anemia ranges from 0.4 to 0.5 mg/kg/day. Thus, a target iron excretion of approximately 0.4 mg/kg/day in patients who have undergone splenectomy and approximately 0.5 mg/kg/day in patients with intact spleens is usually required to

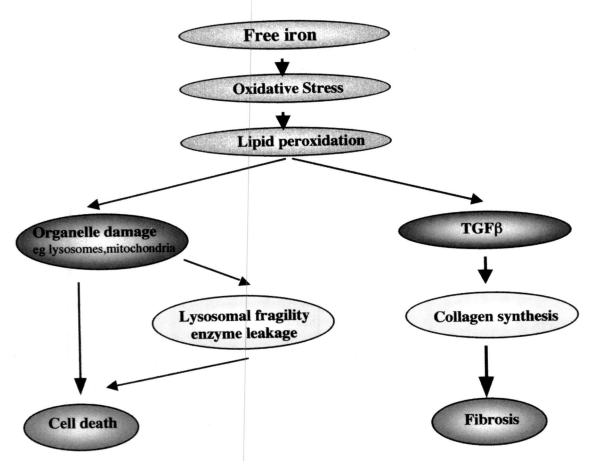

Figure 37.1. Mechanisms of liver damage in iron overload.

maintain iron balance in transfusion-dependent anemia. Both urinary and fecal iron excretion in response
to chelation therapy contribute, in principle, to iron
balance. After administration of desferrioxamine, the
relative proportions of iron excretion by these two
routes vary considerably, both between patients and
also at different times of the transfusion cycle (Pippard
et al., 1982a). Theoretically, the efficiency of iron
chelation may decrease as iron overload is reduced,
but ideally negative iron balance should be achieved at
all excess tissue iron concentrations that are likely to
be harmful. If desferrioxamine were 100 percent efficient, a dose of 6 mg/kg/dy would be sufficient to
achieve iron balance. However, the usual dose of the
drug is 40 to 60 mg/kg/dy, reflecting only 10 percent
efficiency (Porter et al., 1998). Orally active hydroxypyridinone, deferiprone (L1, CP20), is even less efficient (3.8 percent) (Al-Refaie et al., 1995b).

Desirable target ranges of tissue iron with chelation
therapy have been based partly on observations in heterozygotes with genetic hemochromatosis. Normal
concentrations of liver iron are less than 1.6 mg/g dry
weight (wt). In heterozygotes for hereditary hemochro-

matosis, mildly increased liver iron concentrations (3
to 7 mg/g dry wt) are associated with normal life
expectancy without cardiac or liver complications. In
thalassemia major, a liver iron concentration above 15
mg/g dry wt (about 80 μmol/g wet wt) is an approximate threshold for development of cardiac disease and
early death (Brittenham et al., 1994). Because of the
inefficiency of iron chelation and the increased risk of
chelator-induced toxicity as iron levels decline, a realistic goal with chelation therapy is to achieve liver iron
concentrations in the range of 3 to 7 mg/g dry wt,
which although higher than normal, are not known to
be harmful. Indeed, liver iron concentrations within or
below this range can be achieved with standard doses
of desferrioxamine (Aldouri et al., 1987; Olivieri,
1996). In principle, a similar target range should be
sought with any new chelator regimen, although the
precise relationship between liver iron concentration
and clinical complications of transfusional iron overload remains uncertain.

Detoxification of Harmful Iron Species. Although it
may take months or years to remove all the excess iron
from iron-loaded subjects, a well-designed chelator
should ideally decrease the damage caused by the iron
until all the excess iron has been removed. To do this,

potentially harmful iron pools (see later) must be removed rapidly by chelation and rendered harmless. For iron to be made unavailable to participate in the generation of free radicals, it must be fully coordinated at each of its six ligand-binding sites. If any of these remain partially coordinated, iron may participate in the Fenton reaction, resulting in lipid peroxidation with organelle and cell damage from hydroxyl radicals. The design of a chelator is crucial to preventing these events. In general, hexadentate ligands, which have six coordination sites and hence bind iron in a 1:1 ratio, scavenge iron at low chelator concentrations more efficiently and are more stable in their iron complexed forms than bidentate or tridentate chelators (Fig. 37.2). These chelator classes have two or three iron coordinating sites per ligand, respectively, and therefore require three or two chelating molecules, respectively, to coordinate iron (III) completely. EDTA, which coordinates only one free electron, does not diminish the reactivity of iron salts in the Fenton reaction and indeed may catalyze such reactions (Gutteridge and Halliwell, 1989). By contrast the hexadentate desferrioxamine and physiologic ligands, such as lactoferrin and transferrin, which surround the iron more completely, are powerful inhibitors of lipid peroxidation in several experimental systems (Gutteridge et al., 1979). The iron-chelate complexes of bidentate hydroxypyridinones, being less stable than the hexadentate desferrioxamine, can generate free radicals and damage cell membranes with increased lipid peroxidation and loss of cell viability, particularly if the chelators have high lipid solubility (Dobbin et al., 1993).

Iron Pools Available for Chelation. Studies involving the labeling of iron pools both in experimental animals

(Hershko et al., 1978a, 1978b) and in patients (Hershko and Rachmilewitz, 1979) showed that only a small proportion of total body iron is available for chelation at any moment in time. This has a fundamental bearing on the strategies adopted for chelation therapy because it follows that escalation of chelation doses will have a finite impact on increasing iron excretion. This can be understood by considering both extracellular and intracellular iron turnover.

Extracellular Iron

Body iron turnover—20 to 30 mg/day in healthy individuals—is predominantly through the plasma compartment from the breakdown of effete red cells in macrophages of the spleen, liver, and bone marrow. Iron is released onto transferrin for subsequent delivery to erythroid precursors in the bone marrow (Finch et al., 1970). This may increase up to sevenfold when hemolysis and ineffective erythropoiesis are pronounced, such as in thalassemia intermedia (Pootrakul et al., 1988). Considerable evidence both from animal studies (Hershko et al., 1978) and in humans (Hershko and Rachmilewitz, 1979) shows that iron derived from the breakdown of hemoglobin in macrophages is chelated directly by desferrioxamine and other compounds such as DTPA (Hershko, 1975) before binding to transferrin (Fig. 37.3). Whether this interception occurs extracellularly or within the macrophages is not certain, but in vitro studies suggest the former is more likely with desferrioxamine (Saito et al., 1986); however, this will presumably vary depending on rates of access of the chelator to intracellular iron pools in macrophages. Studies using selective ^{59}Fe cell labeling techniques in iron overloaded rats (Hershko et al., 1973, 1978; Hershko 1978) and ferrokinetic data in humans (Hershko and Rachmilewitz, 1979) suggest that most urinary iron excretion with desferrioxamine is derived from catabolized red cells (Fig. 37.3).

Figure 37.2. Denticity of iron chelation.

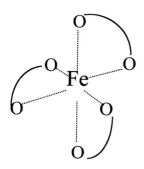

BIDENTATE

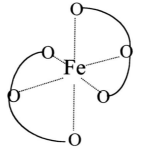

TRIDENTATE

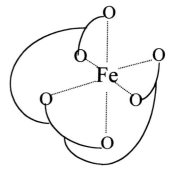

HEXADENTATE

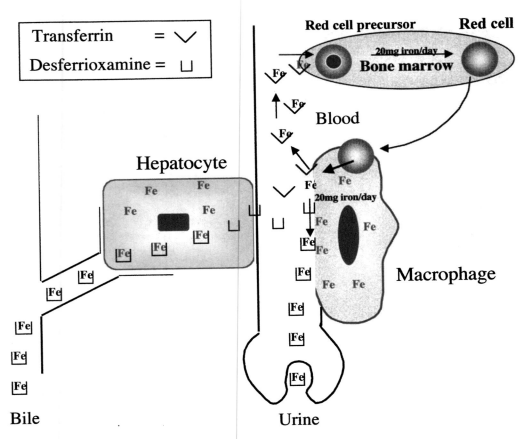

Figure 37.3. Scheme of desferrioxamine mechanism of action.

Plasma iron is tightly bound to transferrin and is virtually unavailable for chelation by desferrioxamine (Hershko et al., 1973). Hydroxypyridinones can remove iron from transferrin, but the concentrations required to do so at an effectual rate make this an unlikely mode of action in vivo. For example, at 100 μmol/L concentrations of deferiprone, approximately one fourth of the iron is removed from 90 percent saturated transferrin and only 12 percent from 30 percent saturated transferrin after 24 hours (Stefanini et al., 1991). Furthermore, because at any moment only approximately 4 mg of iron is bound to transferrin, this is unlikely to be a major source of chelatable iron (Fig. 37.3). It must also be remembered that at clinically relevant concentrations of transferrin and chelator, iron can also be donated to transferrin by bidentate hydroxypyridin-4-ones but not by desferrioxamine (Stefanini et al., 1991). This is because the iron complexes of bidentate chelators are inherently less stable than those of hexadentate ligands such as desferrioxamine (see later). Thus, following orally administered chelators such as deferiprone or CP94, as plasma concentrations are only transiently above 100 μmol/L (Kontoghiorghes et al., 1990; Porter et al.,

1994) (Table 37.10), donation of iron to transferrin may be as likely as iron removal, particularly when transferrin is not saturated in the steady state.

Another important potentially chelatable extracellular iron pool is plasma non-transferrin-bound iron (Hershko et al., 1978b), which is found at concentrations of up to 10 μmol/L when transferrin becomes saturated in iron overload. The exact chemical nature of non-transferrin-bound iron is uncertain. In experimental models, non-transferrin-bound iron is rapidly taken up by hepatocytes (Brissot et al., 1985) and myocytes (Link et al., 1989). In the absence of potentially detoxifying intracellular enzymes such as superoxide dismutase, catalase, and glutathione reductase, non-transferrin-bound iron may promote the formation of free hydroxyl radicals and may accelerate the peroxidation of membrane lipids as has been shown in vitro (Gutteridge et al., 1985). In cultured heart cells, non-transferrin-bound iron is taken up at 200 times the rate of transferrin iron and causes lipid peroxidation, organelle dysfunction, and abnormal rhythmicity (Link et al., 1989, 1993). The contribution of chelation of non-transferrin-bound iron to iron balance has not been determined, but removal of non-transferrin bound by chelation therapy is potentially important for the detoxification of iron. It is not known whether non-transferrin-bound iron is directly chelated by des-

Table 37.10. Pharmacology of Deferiprone and Desferrioxamine.

	Deferiprone	Desferrioxamine
Denticity	Bidentate	Hexadentate
Molecular weight	175	657
pM* for Iron 3+	20 (Hider et al., 1996)	27.6 (Raymond* et al., 1981)
Route of absorption	Oral	Parenteral (SC, IV, or IM)
Peak plasma concentration at clinical doses	90–450 µmol/L (Kontoghiorghes et al., 1990) 73–317 µmol/L after 50 mg/kg (Al-Refaie, 1995b)	7 µmol/L (Lee et al., 1993)
Elimination	Rapid $t^1/_2$ = 1.52h (Al-Refaie, 1995b)	Rapid Initial $t^1/_2$ = 0.3h (Lee et al., 1993) Terminal $t^1/_2$ = 3h (Lee et al., 1993)
Excretion of free ligand	Urine	Urine + feces (30–50% fecal) (Pippard et al., 1982)
Excretion of iron complex	Urine (Olivieri et al., 1990)	Urine + feces (Pippard et al., 1982a)
Metabolism	Glucuronidation in liver	Oxidative deamination in liver (Singh et al., 1990)
Major metabolite in plasma	Inactive glucuronide (Al-Refaie, 1995b)	Metabolite B (iron binding)
Major species in urine	Inactive glucuronide (40% unmetabolized)	Metabolite B (iron binding) (Singh et al., 1990)
Efficiency of chelation (% of dose that chelates iron)	3.8% (Al-Refaie, 1995b)	~10% (Porter et al., 1998)
Ascorbic acid	Increases urinary iron (Pippard et al., 1982a)	No consistent effect

SC, subcutaneous; IV, intravenous, IM, intramous culor.
* Where pM is -log of the uncoordinated metal (iron) concentration calculated under the conditions: pH 7.4, 10 µmol/L ligand, 1 µmol/L iron(III).

ferrioxamine or hydroxypyridinones in the plasma compartment, although its removal in vitro at clinically achievable concentrations of desferrioxamine is slow (Srichairatanakool et al., 1997). In thalassemia major and intermedia, non-transferrin-bound iron is highly labile and is detectable within minutes of stopping intravenous desferrioxamine infusions (Porter et al., 1996), suggesting that chelation regimens that achieve continuous presence of chelator in the plasma compartment may be preferable to regimens where the chelator is intermittently available.

Intracellular Iron

Iron chelators can be considered as interacting with three potential intracellular iron pools. These are the labile "transit" iron pool or LIP (pool 1), which is generally of low molecular weight, finite, and rapidly chelatable; the storage iron pool of hemosiderin and ferritin (pool 2), which is relatively slowly chelatable but larger at any moment in time than pool 1; and, thirdly, functional iron pools (pool 3), which are iron-containing molecules essential for normal cellular function (e.g., hemoglobin, myoglobin, and enzymes such as

lipoxygenase and ribonucleotide reductase). Pool 1 is in dynamic exchange with the other two iron pools. The goal of chelation therapy is to chelate pool 1 without affecting the important functions of iron in pool 3. In principle, some of pool 2 may be depleted directly, but this is relatively slow because chelators cannot remove iron from ferritin cores at a clinically useful rate.

Transit iron can theoretically be chelated at any point during its uptake into cells by receptor-mediated endocytosis of transferrin, liberation from transferrin in the acidic endosome, egress from the endosome possibly using the Nramp2 transporter system (Fleming et al., 1998), (divalent metal transporter 1) and ultimate entry into a cytosolic labile iron pool. Labile chelatable intracellular iron has been shown in a variety of cells including reticulocytes, marrow cells, intestinal epithelial cells, blood leukocytes, alveolar macrophages, and hepatocytes, although evidence has been largely indirect and the nature of the pool is uncertain (Jacobs, 1977; Weaver and Pollack, 1989; Pollack, 1992). It is clear however that iron entering the cell, either from transferrin or by other mechanisms, becomes transiently chelatable before it is incorporated into ferritin (Pippard et al., 1982b). Early studies in Chang cells showed approximately 20 percent of cellular iron was present as a non-heme, non-ferritin soluble form after 24 hours of incubation (Bailey-Wood et al., 1975) and was rapidly chelatable with EDTA, desferrioxamine, or transferrin (White et al., 1976a). Mulligan et al. (1986) quantitated this pool from tissue homogenate iron extracted by desferrioxamine and found that it correlated with an ultrafilterable fraction bound to low molecular weight ligand(s). More recent work using a fluorescent probe (calcein) in K562 cells suggests that the labile intracellular iron pool is present at 0.4 mmol/L with an estimated transit time of 24 hours (Breuer et al., 1995). Similar values have been obtained with rat hepatocytes labeled with $^{59}FeCl_3$ and analyzed for desferrioxamine-chelatable ^{59}Fe (Rothman et al., 1992). The same properties of chelators that favor mobilization of intracellular iron (Porter 1988), such as lipid solubility, also favor chelation of the labile intracellular pool (Zanninell et al., 1997). However, finite labile intracellular iron is always available for chelation, and by increasing chelator concentrations above those required to coordinate this, pool 3 may be compromised without significant further enhancement of total intracellular iron removal.

Iron in pool 2 can be mobilized from ferritin by desferrioxamine in vitro, but the rate is less than 0.5 percent/hr, even when desferrioxamine is present in 15 molar excess (Crichton et al., 1980). Furthermore, acidic pH values, such as those present in the lysosome, do not appear to enhance this rate (Brady et al., 1988). Bidentate hydroxypyridinones can gain access to the ferritin core directly by virtue of their smaller size (Brady et al., 1988; Dobbin et al., 1993). However, at neutral pH values, iron mobilization from rat ferritin is still only 1 percent/hr even in the presence of fifteenfold chelator excess (Brady et al., 1988). Thus, in vivo access by chelators to ferritin iron will occur at useful rates only when this protein is being degraded by proteolysis with the subsequent release of iron to the labile intracellular transit pool. It has been estimated that ferritin is turned over intracellularly with a half-life of about 72 hours (Drysdale and Munro, 1966) and that proteolysis is predominantly lysosomal rather than cytosolic (Cooper et al., 1988).

The physicochemical properties of chelators have a major influence on their rate of access to iron in pool 3. By virtue of its hexadentate structure, relatively high molecular weight (Table 37.10), and its hydrophilicity compared with the clinically studied hydroxypyridinones, desferrioxamine accesses intracellular iron and iron within organelles more slowly than hydroxypyridinones (Porter et al., 1988; Hoyes and Porter, 1993). Interactions with key enzymes in pool 3, such as lipoxygenase (Abeysinghe et al., 1996) and ribonucleotide

reductase (Cooper et al., 1996), are significantly slower for desferrioxamine than for hydroxypyridinones. Because of the pivotal role of ribonucleotide reductase in DNA synthesis and cell proliferation, its rapid inhibition by hydroxypyridinones is a putative mechanism for the leukopenia and marrow hypoplasia associated with this class of chelators (Hoyes et al., 1992, 1993; Cooper et al., 1996). Hydroxypyridinones designed to interact at a reduced rate with enzymes of pool 3 have reduced antiproliferative effects and effects on apoptosis while maintaining their ability to mobilize intracellular iron (Kayyali et al., 1997).

Constraints of Chelator Design

Hexadentate chelators tend to have greater ability to scavenge iron at low concentrations, lesser potential to redistribute iron, and slower access to iron in pool 3 than bidentate and tridentate ligands. Unfortunately, it is difficult to design hexadentate molecules with molecular weights less than 400, thus severely limiting their absorption from the gastrointestinal tract; and hexadentate chelators have yet to be identified with sufficient oral bioavailability for clinical use (Hider et al., 1994).

Many bidentate and tridentate chelators have sufficiently low molecular weights for acceptable oral bioavailability. To minimize the inherent disadvantages of their lower denticity, novel chelators with greater stability of the iron-chelate complex are being sought. Clinically useful iron chelators should possess a sufficiently high iron binding (stability) constant (Porter et al., 1988) and have specificity of iron binding over other metals (e.g., zinc and copper). A more clinically relevant expression of iron binding than the stability constant is the pM, defined as -log of the uncoordinated metal (iron) concentration calculated at pH 7.4, 10μmol/L ligand concentration and 1 μmol/L iron (III) (Table 37.10). This measure takes into account the tendency of bidentate chelators to dissociate at low concentrations and is a more useful indicator of the ability of a chelator to scavenge iron at low chelator concentrations. Chelators with high pM values therefore are desirable.

The distribution of chelators to different tissues and subcellular compartments will inevitably affect their potential toxicity. Ideally a compound should have low penetration of the central nervous system, where adverse effects have been observed with desferrioxamine (see later), and should have a high extraction of iron from liver cells where iron is present in high concentrations (Hider et al., 1994, 1996). The rate at which chelators gain access to intracellular iron pools is determined by their lipid solubility, charge, shape, and molecular weight (Porter et al., 1988, 1990; Zanninelli et al., 1997). Once within cells, the structure of iron chelators also determines the rate of interaction with key iron-containing enzymes in pool 3.

Finally, the metabolism of chelators has a key bearing on their efficacy and toxicity in both laboratory animals (Porter et al., 1993) and humans (Porter et al., 1994). Both deferiprone and CP94, another hydroxypyridinone that has been evaluated clinically, are rapidly inactivated by glucuronidation of the iron-binding site, thereby limiting their efficacy (Table 37.10). By designing prodrugs of hydroxypyridinones, rapid liver extraction of the prodrug followed by metabolism to a hydrophilic active drug could maximize removal of hepatic iron while minimizing potential toxicity owing to penetration of the central nervous system and bone marrow (Hider et al., 1994).

PARENTERAL CHELATION THERAPY WITH DESFERRIOXAMINE

Pharmacology of Desferrioxamine

Desferrioxamine is a hexadentate siderophore isolated from *Streptomyces pilosus*. Its hexadentate structure results in a relatively high molecular weight (657) that limits its absorption from the gut, and parenteral routes of administration are the only realistic methods of delivery. However, its hexadentate coordination helps desferrioxamine to scavenge Fe^{3+}, particularly at low concentrations of iron, as evidenced by the high pM (Table 37.10). A hexadentate structure and high pM also contribute to stabilization of the iron complex, and iron redistribution or partial iron complexation is insignificant.

Elimination is fast, with an initial half-life of 0.3 hours and a terminal half-life of 3 hours (Lee et al., 1993). With an intravenous infusion of 50 mg/kg/day, mean steady state concentrations of 7.4 μmol/L are achieved (Lee et al., 1993) (Table 37.10). The major iron-binding metabolite (metabolite B) occurs by oxidative deamination (Singh et al., 1990), and levels of metabolite B are generally lower than those of desferrioxamine (Lee et al., 1993). Desferrioxamine and its major metabolites are cleared by the liver and the kidney in their iron-free forms. However, once iron is bound to form ferrioxamine in the plasma, clearance is almost exclusively renal, as ferrioxamine is not cleared by the liver; therefore, in renal disease, levels of ferrioxamine may accumulate. However, ferrioxamine is highly stable and does not redistribute iron significantly within the body.

Fecal iron excretion as ferrioxamine is thus almost entirely due to intrahepatic iron chelation, whereas urinary iron is mainly derived from plasma iron turnover (Hershko et al., 1973) (Fig. 37.3). Uptake of desferrioxamine into hepatocytes results in chelation of cytosolic and possible lysosomal iron to form ferrioxamine that is then excreted in the bile (Hershko et al., 1978). At conventional doses, about a third of the iron is excreted through this route into the feces, and this amount increases with higher desferrioxamine doses (Pippard et al., 1982a; Pippard 1989), reflecting a greater proportion of intrahepatic chelation.

Other metals are bound by desferrioxamine with a much lower affinity; only the chelation of aluminum has clinical significance. Desferrioxamine has been successfully used to treat aluminum overload in renal dialysis patients at doses of 5 to 10 mg/kg once a week (Andriani et al., 1996).

Historical Perspective of Clinical Desferrioxamine Use

Desferrioxamine was first given as single intramuscular injections in 1962 and was shown to increase urinary iron excretion in a dose-dependent manner, proportional to iron stores (Sephton-Smith, 1962). It was then shown that by giving daily intramuscular injections to children (mean age, 6 years) at 500 mg 6 days a week over 7 years, liver iron could be kept at approximately 3 percent dry weight and liver fibrosis could be stabilized (Barry et al., 1974). Later, Propper and associates (1976) showed that 24-hour intravenous infusions resulted in more urinary iron than the same dose given as an intramuscular bolus. Twenty-four-hour subcutaneous desferrioxamine infusions resulted in urinary iron excretion nearly equivalent to that achieved with intravenous infusions (Hussain et al., 1976; Propper et al., 1977). Pippard and co-workers (1978a, 1978b) established that urinary iron excretion was not appreciably decreased in most patients by giving the same dose over 12 hours rather than 24 hours, and this was generally sufficient to achieve iron balance. Metabolic iron balance studies revealed that between 30 and 50 percent of total iron excretion with desferrioxamine was in the feces and that the proportion in the feces increased with increasing desferrioxamine doses and after suppression of erythropoiesis by blood transfusion (Pippard et al., 1982a). Nightly 8- to 12-hour subcutaneous infusions of desferrioxamine gradually became standard practice for transfusion-dependent thalassemia. Ascorbate (2 to 3 mg/kg/day) given on the same day as desferrioxamine increased urinary iron excretion (Pippard et al., 1982a), but higher doses were possibly associated with cardiac toxicity (Nienhuis, 1981).

In the 1980s, progressively larger doses of desferrioxamine were tried, often by the intravenous route, in an attempt to reverse massive iron overload or to reverse cardiac failure (Marcus et al., 1984; Cohen et al., 1987; Freeman et al., 1989). Although some of these objectives were achieved, significant toxicity, most noticeably retinal and auditory, began to be reported (Davies et al., 1983; Olivieri et al., 1986) followed by effects on bone and growth in children (De Virgillis et al., 1988; Piga et al., 1988). From these and other studies, as well as from clinical observations, a "standard" dosing regimen for desferrioxamine has emerged, aimed at balancing the beneficial effects of chelation with unwanted effects of excessive dosing. Still, some aspects of "standard therapy" recommendations, such as when to begin chelation and the dose recommended to maximize growth potential, have been arrived at by empirical retrospective analysis rather than by prospective randomized trials.

Evidence of Efficacy of Desferrioxamine

Evidence for the efficacy of desferrioxamine is summarized in Table 37.11. Iron balance, based on urine iron alone, is obtained at a dose of approximately 30 mg/kg/day when given as a 12-hour infusion (Pippard et al., 1978a). Fecal excretion contributes a further 30 to 50 percent to total desferrioxamine-induced iron output (Pippard et al., 1982a). Urine iron excreted has been shown to correlate with transferrin saturation (Modell and Beck 1974), the number of transfusions (Modell and Beck, 1974) and

the dose of desferrioxamine (Sephton-Smith 1962; Pippard et al., 1978a; Modell and Beck, 1974). It is clear that subcutaneous infusions of 40 mg/kg and above maintain liver iron at safe levels (Cohen et al., 1981, 1984a; Aldouri et al., 1987; Olivieri, 1996; Olivieri et al., 1998). Intensification of therapy by combining subcutaneous and intravenous therapy can normalize liver iron levels (Cohen et al., 1987).

Evidence of prevention of iron-mediated organ damage is also persuasive. Intramuscular desferrioxamine at relatively modest doses stabilizes hepatic fibrosis (Modell et al., 1982), and there was no progression of hepatic fibrosis over an 8-year period in patients receiving subcutaneous infusions of desferrioxamine (Aldouri et al., 1987). It is also clear that desferrioxamine can prevent (Zurlo et al., 1989; Olivieri et al., 1994; Brittenham et al., 1994) and can also reverse cardiac toxicity from iron overload (Marcus et al., 1984; Freeman et al., 1989; Rahko et al., 1986; Aldouri et al., 1990). Introduction of subcutaneous infusions of desferrioxamine before age 10 years significantly reduces gonadal dysfunction from iron overload, with improvement in pubertal status and growth (Bronspeigel-Weintrob et al., 1990). Concomitant improvement in fertility has also been seen, although secondary amenorrhea is still common

---

Table 37.11. Clinical Efficacy of Desferrioxamine

Variable	Effect
Urine iron excretion at 50 mg/kg	18.2 mg (Olivieri et al., *1990*)
Effect on iron balance in thalassemia major	Balance at 30 mg/kg as 12 hour subcutaneous infusion but efficacy under-estimated (urine only) Pippard et al., 1978a,b)
Iron excretion correlates with	Number of transfusions (Modell and Beck, 1974) DFO dose (Sephton-Smith, 1962) Tf saturation (Modell and Beck, 1974)
Cardiac toxicity	Prevents (Zurlo et al., *1989*; Brittenham et al., 1994) Reverses (Freeman et al., *1989*; Marcus et al., 1984)
Liver iron	Maintained at safe levels at 40 mg/kg/sc. (Olivieri, 1996) Combined SC and IV DFO normalizes (Cohen et al., 1984a)
Liver fibrosis	Decreases risk IM (Barry et al., 1974) No progression over 8 y SC (Aldouri et al., 1987)
Survival	Prolongs (Modell et al., *1982*; Zurlo et al., 1989; Brittenham, et al. 1994) Cardiac event-free survival related to % time ferritin <2500 Related to liver iron and frequency of use (Brittenham, 1994) Prolongation related to compliance (Gabutti and Piga, 1996)
Hypogonadotrophic hypogonadism	Decreasing frequency but still common (Chatterjee, 1993)
Diabetes, hypothyroidism, hypoparathyroidism	Absent at 15-year follow-up if started on standard protocol and >260 infusions/year (Gabutti and Piga, 1996)

SC, subcutaneous; IV, intravenous; IM, intramuscular.

(Chatterjee et al., 1993). The onset of glucose intolerance is delayed, glucose intolerance may be improved, and hypothyroidism may also be reversed by the timely use of desferrioxamine. (Fosburg and Nathan, 1990; Flynn et al., 1982).

By the 1980s, the impact of desferrioxamine on overall survival began to emerge (Modell et al., 1982). However, only recently has the full impact on survival been clearly documented (Zurlo et al., 1989; Brittenham et al., 1994; Olivieri et al., 1994; Gabutti and Piga, 1996). Life table analysis shows that patients who adhere well with treatment can have 100 percent survival at age 25 years, whereas survival for patients who comply poorly is only 32 percent (Brittenham et al., 1994). More recent studies show that for patients who administer subcutaneous infusions of desferrioxamine more than 250 times yearly, survival is 95 percent at age 30 years. If the frequency of infusion falls below 250 times a year (equivalent to about five times a week), survival at age 30 years is only 12 percent (Gabutti and Piga, 1996).

The immediate challenge in desferrioxamine treatment is to improve the compliance of patients who find it difficult to administer the chelator regularly. New delivery systems, discussed later, the use of anesthetic creams, improved formulations, and better support to patients and relatives may help increase compliance.

Tolerability of Desferrioxamine

Toxicity from desferrioxamine in thalassemia major is unlikely at doses up to 40 mg/kg/day. When body iron levels decline, as measured by lowering of serum ferritin or liver iron, the risk of desferrioxamine toxicity increases (Porter et al., 1989c; Olivieri and Brittenham, 1997). It is important to monitor these patients particularly carefully and to consider lowering the dose as iron levels fall. Clinical monitoring for the tolerability of desferrioxamine is summarized in Table 37.12.

Injection Site Reactions. Local mild reactions often caused by desferrioxamine being reconstituted above the recommended concentration of 10 percent may occur with skin reddening and soreness at the site of subcutaneous infusions. Increasing the volume of water used to dilute the desferrioxamine can substantially decrease reactions. The frequency of such side effects has been further decreased recently by the introduction of new manufacturing techniques for desferrioxamine. On occasions when local reactions remain a problem, the addition of a small dose of hydrocortisone (5 to 10 mg) to the desferrioxamine solution may be effective.

Effects on Growth and Bone. Desferrioxamine usually improves growth in thalassemia major by decreasing iron overload; however, if too much is given, growth may be retarded. Young age (< 3 years at commencement of treatment), higher doses of desferrioxamine (De Virgillis et al., 1988), and lower levels of iron overload are risk factors. It is advisable to monitor height velocity and sitting and standing height twice a year and adjust dosing as necessary. A quick resumption in growth follows reduction in desferrioxamine dosing without the need to stop treatment (Piga et al., 1988). Rickets-like bony abnormalities have been described in association with decreased growth (De Virgillis et al., 1988), and radiographic abnormalities of the distal ulnar, radial, and tibial metaphases appear to be associated features. Vertebral growth retardation or milder changes involving vertebral demineralization and flatness of vertebral bodies have also been noted in well-chelated patients (Gabutti and Piga, 1996). It may be advisable to undertake regular surveillance for the toxic effects of desferrioxamine on bone (De Sanctis et al., 1996) with annual radiologic assessment of the thoracolumbar-sacral spine, forearm, and knees and to reduce the dose of drug if significant changes are noted.

Table 37.12. Monitoring for Desferrioxamine Tolerability

Effect	Monitoring	Frequency
Local skin reactions	History and examination	Clinic visits
Ototoxicity	Audiometry therapeutic ratio	Yearly unless symptomatic; 3 monthly with ferritin results
Retinal toxicity	Clinical history	Clinic visits
	Funduscopy	Yearly
	Electroretinography	Yearly
Growth	Height (sitting and standing)	6 monthly
	Dose/therapeutic Index	3 monthly
Bone	X-ray study of knees, wrists, spine	Every 1 to 2 years unless abnormal
Yersinia infection	Stool/blood culture, serology	Clinical suspicion

Retinal and Auditory Toxicity. Retinal and optic nerve disturbances, sometimes associated with pigmentary retinal changes, were originally described in patients receiving very high doses of desferrioxamine (125 mg/kg/day) (Davies et al., 1983) but are rare at currently recommended doses. Other abnormalities that have been linked to excessive use of desferrioxamine include blurred vision, loss of central vision, night blindness, and optic neuropathy (Olivieri et al., 1986). The risk may be higher in patients with diabetes or other factors affecting the blood-retinal barrier (Arden et al., 1984), so these groups should be monitored more carefully using electroretinography. Desferrioxamine therapy should be withdrawn until symptoms partially or fully resolve when treatment can usually be resumed at a reduced dose with close monitoring by electroretinography.

High frequency sensorineural hearing loss was initially described in approximately 25 percent of well-chelated patients on high desferrioxamine regimens but may be reversible if diagnosed early (Olivieri et al., 1986; Porter et al., 1989c). The risk is greatest in patients with low degrees of iron overload receiving high doses of desferrioxamine. By keeping the therapeutic index (mean daily desferrioxamine dose in mg/kg divided by serum ferritin level in $\mu g/L$) (Porter et al., 1989c) below 0.025 and by monitoring regularly by audiometry, the risks can be minimized. It is advisable to perform audiometry before starting treatment and about once a year during treatment.

Infections. There is an increased risk of *Yersinia* infection in iron overload, and this risk increases further with desferrioxamine treatment, as *Yersinia* does not make a natural siderophore and uses iron from ferrioxamine to facilitate its growth (Robins-Browne and Prpic, 1983; Gallant et al., 1986). Patients who present with diarrhea, abdominal pain, or fever should stop desferrioxamine until *Yersinia* infection can be reasonably excluded by appropriate stool samples, blood cultures, and serologic testing. If *Yersinia* infection is proven or seriously suspected, desferrioxamine should be withheld until the infection has been eliminated by antibiotic treatment. Prolonged treatment with antibiotics such as cotrimoxazole or ciprofloxacin is occasionally necessary to prevent recurrence, but it is rarely necessary to withhold desferrioxamine after the initial infection has been treated. Very rarely other infections such as *Pneumocystis carinii* (Kouides et al., 1988) and mucormycosis (Boelaert et al., 1987) have been associated with desferrioxamine use. In any patient with undiagnosed fever, it is wise to consider stopping the desferrioxamine until the cause is identified.

Miscellaneous Effects. Generalized reactions such as fever, muscle aches, and arthralgia occur rarely.

True systemic allergic reactions are uncommon but can include anaphylaxis. Some patients can be successfully desensitized using published procedures to prevent further allergic reactions (Miller, et al., 1981; Bosquet et al., 1983).

Renal impairment, characterized by a reduction in the glomerular filtration rate, has been reported in occasional patients given high doses of desferrioxamine (Koren et al., 1990, 1991). A fatal respiratory syndrome similar to acute respiratory distress syndrome (ARDS) has been described in patients with acute iron poisoning given high dose (15 mg/kg/hr) desferrioxamine infusions for longer than 24 hours; lower doses and shorter infusions are recommended for acute iron poisoning (Tenenbein et al., 1992). Pulmonary injury with fibrosis has also been reported in patients with chronic iron overload receiving high doses of desferrioxamine (10 to 22 mg/kg/hr) (Freedman et al., 1990).

In non-iron-overloaded patients, the use of desferrioxamine potentiated the action of prochlorperazine, a phenothiazine derivative, leading to reversible coma in two patients receiving this combination (Blake et al., 1985). Lens opacities observed rarely in patients receiving high doses of desferrioxamine improved when the chelator was withdrawn (Davies et al., 1983). Thrombocytopenia has been observed with desferrioxamine in two patients on renal dialysis (Walker et al., 1985). It is important to avoid a sudden bolus infusion of desferrioxamine in patients receiving intravenous treatment through an indwelling catheter or during blood transfusions, as this may lead to nausea, vomiting, hypotension with acute collapse (Modell, 1979), or even transient aphasia (Dickerhoff, 1987).

Indications for Initiating Desferrioxamine Therapy

Iron chelation is indicated when body iron has increased to levels where it is potentially harmful and where erythropoietic reserve does not allow the removal of excess iron by venesection. Numerically, the most important group of patients to benefit from iron chelation therapy are those with transfusion-dependent anemia, of which thalassemia major is the largest group. Chelation therapy also has a role in other transfusion-dependent anemias such as pure red cell aplasia, aplastic anemia, and myelofibrosis. A variety of chronic anemias associated with iron loading, where regular transfusion is not necessary but erythropoietic reserve may be marginal (e.g., pyruvate kinase deficiency, sideroblastic anemias, thalassemia intermedia) may also benefit from chelation therapy if venesection is not feasible. Patients with sickle cell disease who receive long-term transfusion therapy to prevent its complications will eventually require iron chelation therapy unless exchange transfusions are used in preference to simple transfusions.

The exact timing and dosing of a desferrioxamine regimen depend on the rate and degree of iron loading for each individual. These variables are better defined for transfusion-dependent β thalassemia major than for other disorders (Table 37.13). However, although it is now clear that the introduction of desferrioxamine at excessive doses or at too early an age increases the risks of desferrioxamine toxicity such as growth retardation and bony lesions, the optimal dosing and timing have not been the subjects of prospective, randomized trials; therefore recommendations are to some extent are empirically based.

Uncertainties remain about the optimal age for starting therapy in thalassemia major. Delay in treatment until after age 3 years has been recommended because of observations that poor growth and metaphyseal dysplasia may occur when treatment is started earlier (De Sanctis et al., 1996; Rodda et al., 1995; Piga et al., 1988; De Virgillis et al., 1988; Olivieri et al., 1992b). Conversely, delay in starting treatment increases the risk of iron-mediated toxicity; as noted previously, hepatic fibrosis associated with liver iron loading has been reported in children as young as 3 years old (Angelucci

et al., 1994; Berkovitch et al., 1993). It is possible that very low doses given from an earlier age could prevent buildup of liver iron without concomitant desferrioxamine toxicity, but data that address this issue directly are not available. Furthermore, failure to start treatment sufficiently early increases the risk of growth retardation owing to the well-established effects of iron overload on growth and sexual development. Under current practice, desferrioxamine in β thalassemia major should begin at age 3 years or when the ferritin reaches 1,000 μg/L, whichever is sooner, and should not exceed 30 mg/kg until response to this regimen can be assessed. Others (Olivieri and Brittenham, 1997) have argued that because of the variability of serum ferritin as a measure of iron overload and because of the apparent safety of liver biopsies when performed under ultrasound guidance, even in children 5 years old or younger (Angelucci et al., 1994), direct measurement of iron burden by assessment of hepatic iron concentration should be considered 1 year after starting regular transfusion (Table 37.13). Whether or not liver biopsy is used to support clinical decision making at this stage, regular assessment of desferrioxamine-related effectiveness and toxicity is important (Table 37.12).

Indications for starting desferrioxamine are less well defined for sickle cell disease and thalassemia intermedia than for β thalassemia major. Hitherto, liver biopsy

Table 37.13. Use of Ferritin or Liver Iron for DFO Dose Adjustment in Thalassemia Major

Variable	Finding	Action
Ferritin (μg/L)	<1000 or age <3	Wait before starting DFO *or* quantitate liver iron
	>1000 and age >3 and not taking DFO	Start at 25–30 mg/kg SC 5 times a week 8–12h infusion

	>1500 consistently and on DFO	Increase dose and/or frequency but;
		  – Keep therapeutic index < 0.025
		  – Do not exceed 35 mg/kg if < 5 years
		  – Do not exceed 40 mg/kg until fully grown
		  – Do not exceed 50 mg/kg in adults

	> 2500 consistently and not responding to above	Consider 24-hr continuous DFO;
		  – IV with portacath
		  – or SC via light-weight infusor
		  – dose to keep therapeutic index <0.025
		  – monitor ferritin monthly

Liver Iron (mg/g dry wt)	<3.2	No treatment, reassess in 6 months
	3.2–7	Give SC 8–12hr DFO 5 times a week at standard doses for age as above
	7–15	Increase DFO dose and/or frequency but do not exceed dose for age as above; keep therapeutic index (<0.025)
	>15	Consider 24-hr continuous treatment with DFO IV with portacath or SC via light weight infusor monitor as above for ferritin

SC, subcutaneous; IV, intravenous.

Treatment is 8–12 hr SC infusion unless otherwise stated. Ferritin values given assume that inflammation and infection have been reasonably excluded. Doses given are the mean daily dose (i.e., dose × weekly frequency divided by 7).

has not been used extensively or routinely in these conditions, and there has been a reliance on the serum ferritin as a guide for initiation of desferrioxamine therapy. Ferritin is a particularly unreliable guide to levels of iron loading in sickle cell disorders, leading to disproportionally high values unless care is taken avoid samples taken within 3 months of a vasoocclusive episode (Brownell et al., 1986; Porter and Huehns, 1987). In two recent reports of the relationship between serum ferritin and liver iron in patients with sickle cell disease who have undergone transfusions long term, the correlations (r = 0.49 and 0.48) were lower than in other groups of patients previously reported (Hartmatz et al., 1999; Olivieri et al., 1999). Because of the variability of serum ferritin levels in sickle cell disease, this measurement and the related therapeutic index (ratio of dose to serum ferritin) should be used with caution to determine the need for chelation therapy and to adjust the dose of desferrioxamine, respectively (Styles and Vichinsky, 1995).

Serum ferritin is disproportionately low in relation to biochemically measured liver iron concentration in thalassemia intermedia compared with thalassemia major (Galanello et al., 1999; Saxon et al., 1999). This discordance detracts from the value of the ferritin level in contributing to the decision to begin chelation therapy in thalassemia intermedia. Because initiation of desferrioxamine in thalassemia intermedia and sickle cell disease is usually required later in life than in thalassemia major, consideration of adverse effects of the chelator on growth are generally less critical. However, other toxic effects must be carefully considered. Therapy could be commenced when transferrin becomes saturated and non-transferrin-bound iron is present, although no studies address this issue directly. Therefore, in both thalassemia intermedia and sickle cell disease, it may be advisable to quantitate liver iron before making a decision to initiate therapy, and to repeat liver iron quantitation at regular intervals while treatment continues. Regular monitoring for desferrioxamine-related toxicities (Table 37.14) is particularly important in these conditions.

Dosing and Clinical Monitoring of Desferrioxamine Therapy

Optimizing Dose Regimen

For transfusion-dependent thalassemia, 8- to 12-hour subcutaneous infusions (maximum 10 percent solution in water) at 30 to 50 mg/kg, a minimum of 5 nights a week, is currently recommended standard practice. This level maintains iron loading at levels below those regarded as toxic (Olivieri, 1996). Downward dose adjustment is advisable with young age and low levels of iron loading (Table 37.13). In patients younger than 5 years old, doses in excess of 35 mg/kg/day may be inadvisable. Serum ferritin can be used as an approximate indicator of falling iron levels, and doses of desferrioxamine should be reduced accordingly so as to keep the therapeutic index less than 0.025 (mean daily dose in mg/kg, divided by the serum ferritin in μg/L) (Porter and Huehns, 1989). If liver iron quantitation is

Table 37.14. Monitoring for Complications of Iron Overload in Thalassemia

Effect	Monitoring	Frequency
Cardiac complications	ECG, 24-hr tape	Yearly More frequently if complications
	MUGA or ECHO	Yearly More frequently if complications
Growth	Height and weight sitting and standing height	Each clinic visit until growth ceases 6 monthly
Bone	Bone densitometry scan for osteoporosis	Yearly after 8 years
	Bone age (x-ray study of knees, wrists)	At start of chelation treatment and every 1-2 yr until growth complete
	Spine x-ray study	Every 3 years
Sexual development	Tanner staging	Yearly from 10 years
	FSH, LH, estradiol, testosterone	Yearly
Diabetes	Urine for glucose	Each visit
	GTT	Yearly
Hypothyroidism	T$_4$, TSH	6 monthly
Hypoparathyroidism	Ca, PO$_4$ PTH and vitamin D if low calcium level	3 monthly

ECG, electrocardiogram; MUGA, multiple gated acquisition; ECHO, echocardiogram; FSH, follicle-stimulating hormone; LH, leutinizing hormone; GTT, glucose tolerance test; TSH, thyroid-stimulating hormone; PTH, parathyroid hormone.

available, a scheme for dose adjustment has been suggested (Olivieri and Brittenham, 1997) (Table 37.13). It must also be borne in mind that liver iron determinations are unlikely to be available more frequently than yearly even in centers performing these measurements routinely and that ferritin measurements will still be useful in dose adjustment. In patients with consistently high levels of iron overload or in those who develop cardiac or other serious complications of iron overload, 24-hour continuous chelation therapy should be considered, either using subcutaneous infusion if the patient will tolerate such a regimen or an implanted intravenous device.

Subcutaneous infusions of standard doses of desferrioxamine two to three times weekly will generally achieve negative iron balance in thalassemia intermedia. Lower doses (e.g., 10 to 20 mg/kg) given continuously would, in principle, give better protection against non-transferrin-bound iron (Porter, 1996).

Few data are available about dose optimization in sickle cell disease. Iron balance with desferrioxamine and the proportions of fecal and urinary iron excretion appear similar to those seen in thalassemia (Collins et al., 1994). Although the general principles used in thalassemia are broadly applicable, for reasons discussed earlier the use of serum ferritin as a guide to dose adjustment may be particularly problematic. Liver iron concentrations above 7 mg/g dry wt are a clear indication for starting treatment. Maximal doses should not exceed those given in thalassemia syndromes, and careful monitoring for desferrioxamine-induced toxicity is advisable.

Delivery of Subcutaneous Desferrioxamine. The mode of delivery of desferrioxamine is critical for compliance and hence the success of therapy. Desferrioxamine solutions of more than 10 percent may increase the risk of irritation to the skin. If the patient continues to experience irritation, pain, or bruising at the sites of infusion despite dilution of desferrioxamine to a 10 percent or less solution, 5 to 10 mg of hydrocortisone added to the infused solution may be helpful. The needle used for infusion may contribute to local reactions in some individuals, and it is sometimes worth trying different types (e.g., butterfly or vertical).

Several delivery systems are now available for intravenous or subcutaneous treatment. Historically, the most widely used have been the battery-operated syringe driver systems, delivering between 10 and 30 mL, depending on the manufacturer. These are best suited to subcutaneous infusions for 8 to 12 hours daily, but some can also be used for intravenous infusions. Recently, lighter or smaller systems have been developed that may be better suited to continuous

infusion. Some battery-operated pumps can take larger volumes of desferrioxamine solution (50 to 100 mL), allowing continuous intravenous treatment for up to 1 week. An alternative is to use disposable pumps that expel fluid under the pressure produced by filling an expandable balloon (Araujo et al., 1996). These devices are light and silent, making them attractive to patients who need continuous infusions, but they are expensive. Recently introduced mechanical delivery devices and gas-operated systems are also lighter and more compact than conventional syringe driver models.

Subcutaneous bolus injections are a recently evaluated alternative approach to chelation therapy with desferrioxamine if pumps are not available or if they are impractical. Studies suggest that iron excretion with twice daily subcutaneous injections of desferrioxamine may be comparable to that observed with the same total dose given as an 8-hour subcutaneous infusion (Jensen et al., 1996; Borgna-Pignatti and Cohen, 1997). At present, however, no data on fecal iron excretion or effects on liver iron are available, and additional studies are indicated to assess the long-term effects of such an approach on iron balance and iron-mediated tissue damage.

Intravenous Desferrioxamine for High-Risk Patients. Some patients may have been poorly chelated because of delay in starting treatment or because of poor compliance after desferrioxamine was commenced. Measures should be introduced to reverse the iron loading and its effects and to establish a regimen with which the patients can better comply. If serum ferritin or liver iron values are persistently high, despite such measures to improve compliance with subcutaneous treatment, or if patients develop serious complications of iron overload, then continuous intravenous therapy should be considered. Higher doses, still keeping the therapeutic index <0.025 (Porter et al., 1989), may be appropriate in such patients. Doses in excess of 50 to 60 mg/kg/day have been used successfully but increase the risk of pulmonary (Freedman et al., 1990) and retinal toxicity (Davies et al., 1983).

Continuous intravenous therapy is best given through a subcutaneously placed port that can stay in for many months and allow outpatient therapy. The risk of thrombosis and infection of the line necessitates careful management in a specialized unit (Cohen et al., 1987; Davis and Porter, 2000). In patients who develop cardiac complications, continuous 24-hour intravenous therapy 7 days a week is preferable (Cohen et al., 1987) to minimize the duration of cardiac exposure to non-transferrin-bound iron (Davis and Porter, 2000). Continuous intravenous treatment can reverse established cardiac failure (Marcus et al.,

1984; Freeman et al., 1989) and cardiac dysrhythmias (Davis and Porter, 2000), although the response may be unpredictable in advanced cardiac failure.

New Approaches for Desferrioxamine Use. Because of the potential advantages of continuous treatment during which plasma concentrations are kept at a constant level, and because of the variable compliance with standard subcutaneous therapy, a new approach using a slow release subcutaneous depot formulation of desferrioxamine was developed. In this formulation, a salt of desferrioxamine that has greater lipid solubility than the standard mesylate salt is suspended in mygliol, an oil that has been previously used in other depot preparations. This formulation results in a slow release of desferrioxamine from the oily subcutaneous depot over several days. The desferrioxamine released into plasma has the same structure as in standard subcutaneous infusions. After single bolus subcutaneous injections of this formulation to patients with thalassemia major, plasma levels and urinary iron excretion are sustained over several days (Porter et al., 1997). A depot dose of approximately 7.5 mg/kg promoted equivalent urinary iron excretion to an 8-hour subcutaneous infusion of 40 mg/kg (Porter et al., 1997). The proportion of the drug excreted in the iron bound form (chelation efficiency) is significantly greater than with standard desferrioxamine therapy, and there is a parallel reduction in the proportion of desferrioxamine metabolites (Porter et al., 1998). Results of repeat dose administration failed to show a significant increase in urinary iron excretion, and repeat administration was found by many patients to be uncomfortable. For these reasons, the development of this formulation was discontinued.

Monitoring Desferrioxamine Therapy

Monitoring desferrioxamine therapy requires assessment of the degree of iron overload with appropriate dose adjustments (Table 37.13), evaluation of the clinical consequences of iron overload (Table 37.14), and regular monitoring of the effects of excessive chelation treatment (Table 37.12). Efficacy of desferrioxamine in removing excessive iron is most reliably monitored by liver iron quantitation, although serum ferritin is of value prognostically and in making dose adjustments. Measurement of desferrioxamine-induced urinary iron may be helpful in "fine-tuning" dose schedules in individual cases.

Use and Limitations of Serum Ferritin. The serum ferritin level is influenced by body iron stores, recent compliance with chelation therapy, and tissue damage and inflammation; therefore the ferritin level must be used with caution to assess iron loading and to adjust desferrioxamine dosing.

Serum ferritin levels correlate with iron loading. In normal subjects (Walters et al., 1973) and in genetic hemochromatosis (Beamish et al., 1974), a good correlation (r = 0.75) exists between the amount of iron mobilized by quantitative phlebotomy and the serum ferritin level. In children with thalassemia and transfusional iron overload, early studies showed a correlation between liver iron concentration, measured by liver biopsy, and serum ferritin level, as well as a close correlation (r = 0.88) between serum ferritin level and the number of units of transfused blood in children who had not received iron chelation therapy (Letsky et al., 1974). In subsequent studies of adults and children with thalassemia major receiving desferrioxamine, investigators have found similar relationships between serum ferritin level and liver iron concentration (Aldouri et al., 1987; Olivieri et al., 1995). In HbE-β thalassemia and HbH disease, the log value of the serum ferritin level correlated strongly with the liver iron concentration measured by a superconducting quantum interface device (SQUID) (r = 0.82) (Pootrakul et al., 1988). Prieto and co-workers found a weak correlation (r = 0.11) between serum ferritin level and liver iron concentration in a diverse group of patients with liver disease, but they found a much closer correlation after dividing the ferritin level by the aspartate aminotransferase (AST) level to correct for liver inflammation (Prieto et al., 1975). Recent literature, although confirming the relationship between serum ferritin and liver iron concentration, has emphasized that the ferritin level, in patients undergoing transfusions long term, many of whom have hepatitis, fails to give a clinically reliable prediction of the liver iron concentration (Olivieri et al., 1995; Olivieri and Brittenham, 1997).

Despite these limitations and because measurement of serum ferritin can be repeated frequently, it remains a useful test, and repeated measurements have prognostic value in identifying patients at risk of iron-induced heart disease (Olivieri et al., 1994). The target ferritin level should be approximately 1,000 to 2,000 µg/L, as the risk of complications from iron overload increases when values exceed 2,500 µg/L on more than one third of annual measurements (Olivieri et al., 1994). Serial ferritin measurements are more reliable than single values and ideally should be obtained every 3 months. It is important to discuss the results with patients so they are encouraged and rewarded by decreasing and warned by increasing ferritin values. If the ferritin alone is used to monitor treatment, care should be taken to lower the dose as the ferritin falls below 1,000 µg/L, keeping the therapeutic index below 0.025 (Porter et al., 1989c) and regularly monitoring for ototoxicity, retinal toxicity, and effects on growth.

Liver Biopsy for Iron Quantitation. A more reliable but less convenient way to monitor efficacy is by serial liver biopsies and measurement of hepatic iron concentration. Some authors have expressed doubts about the reproducibility of iron measurement by liver biopsy, owing to uneven distribution of liver iron, particularly with advanced liver disease (Villeneuve et al., 1996). Iron concentrations may be higher peripherally than centrally (Ambu et al., 1995). The size of the biopsy sample also affects the accuracy of the measurement. If the measurement is performed by established methods (Barry and Sherlock, 1971) on samples of adequate size and with no advanced fibrotic or cirrhotic changes, the coefficient of variation on duplicate specimens is acceptable at 6.6 percent (Barry et al., 1974). Comparison of multiple biopsy samples from patients with cirrhosis showed that samples weighing more than 4 mg dry wt gave a significantly lower coefficient of variation (20 percent) than smaller samples (Villeneuve et al., 1996).

A scheme of dose adjustment for desferrioxamine has been suggested using yearly measurement of hepatic iron concentration (Olivieri and Brittenham, 1997). In this scheme, the trigger hepatic iron concentration for starting or ceasing desferrioxamine is 3.2 mg/g dry wt, and the target concentration is between 3.2 and 7 mg/g dry wt. The maximum dose given for this range of hepatic iron concentration is 25 mg/kg five nights a week if under age 5 years, increasing to 40 mg/kg five nights a week above this age. Patients with hepatic iron concentration between 7 and 15 mg/g dry wt may be at increased risk of organ damage from iron overload. The frequency of administration of desferrioxamine for these patients should be adjusted accordingly without increasing doses above those recommended for the patient's age range. If the liver iron exceeds 15 mg/g dry wt, the patient is said to be at high risk for serious iron-related complications, and daily or continuous treatment should be strongly considered.

The case for using hepatic iron concentration to monitor treatment with desferrioxamine is based on the strong link between liver iron and prognosis in patients with thalassemia major, a link obtained using SQUID measurement of hepatic iron concentration (Brittenham et al., 1994). Biochemical measurement of hepatic iron concentration in liver biopsies may be less helpful prognostically because of uneven distribution of tissue iron, especially in the presence of cirrhosis (Villeneuve et al., 1996). Moreover, in many clinics worldwide, the regular measurement of hepatic iron concentration by biopsy is organizationally difficult, and many patients who have been monitored successfully for many years using the serum ferritin level are reluctant to undergo yearly liver biopsies. On the other hand, liver biopsy yields additional information about inflammation and fibrosis that may be particularly important in monitoring the activity of hepatitis C or in evaluating experimental chelation regimens. In recent years, there has been a trend in clinical practice toward increased use of liver biopsy, both to quantitate liver iron and to assess liver inflammation and damage. Because of the increased use of hepatic iron concentration to monitor treatment, there is a need to harmonize both the techniques used to measure hepatic iron concentration and the units in which it is expressed. For example, some laboratories weigh the wet samples but use a conversion factor from wet to dry weight and express results in the latter units. A variety of conversion factors from wet to dry weight have been used by different centers. Implementing an internationally accepted standard and methodology would help interpret outcome studies of chelation treatment.

Noninvasive Measurement of Liver Iron. The most sensitive, accurate, and reproducible noninvasive measurement of liver iron is the SQUID, which relies on the principle that the paramagnetic field produced by the liver is proportional to storage iron concentration. Only three such devices are in use worldwide (United States, Germany, and Italy), and they have been calibrated using different approaches. These devices are also expensive to purchase and maintain. In hemochromatosis, iron measurements by SQUID show an excellent correlation (r = 0.98) with liver iron measured by biopsy (Brittenham et al., 1982). Less impressive correlation has been obtained in thalassemia (Nielsen et al., 1995), but biochemical measurements of liver iron were performed by a variety of methods in several different centers.

Other techniques for noninvasive measurement of liver iron concentration, such as magnetic resonance imaging (MRI) (Bonetti et al., 1996) and computed tomography scanning, have been evaluated, but have been insufficiently reproducible or sensitive in the required range of liver iron concentration to be clinically useful (Mazza et al., 1995).

Desferrioxamine-Induced Urinary Iron Excretion. A relationship between 24-hour urinary iron excretion after administration of intramuscular desferrioxamine and iron stores was recognized soon after the drug was introduced (Balcerzac et al., 1968). Later, it was suggested that 24-hour urinary iron excretion could be used to titrate an individual's therapy with desferrioxamine by "tailoring the dose" for that patient, because the dose at which the urinary iron excretion plateaus varies considerably among patients (Pippard et al., 1978a, 1978b). Several limitations to this approach exist. First, many families have difficulty obtaining reliable sequential 24-hour urine collections outside the hospital. Considerable day-to-day variability in urinary iron excretion with desferrioxamine is present, even under controlled conditions of collection, and this may be compounded by variable daily ascorbate intake (Pippard et al., 1978a). Any impact of this approach on desferrioxamine-mediated toxicity has not been formally assessed. Finally, the proportion of urinary iron excretion relative to fecal iron excretion is not constant. Urinary iron excretion decreases after blood transfusion and suppression of erythropoiesis and is proportionately smaller at higher doses of desferrioxamine (Pippard et al., 1982). Despite these caveats, measurement of urinary iron has an important role in the assessment of new chelation therapies and a supplementary role in modifying the desferrioxamine regimen in selected patients.

Tissue Iron in Other Organs. Accurate measurement of cardiac iron by biopsy is difficult because of its uneven distribution (Buja and Roberts, 1971; Fitchett et al., 1980; Barosi et al., 1989). Using MRI to quantitate heart iron is technically feasible (Olivieri et al., 1992c) and measurement by gated T_2 relaxation time correlates with liver T_2 relaxation time and serum ferritin (Mavrogeni et al., 1998), but presently there are insufficient data and experience to recommend MRI for routine monitoring of cardiac iron. MRI of the pituitary gland shows a correlation between anterior pituitary size and biochemical markers of anterior pituitary function (Chatterjee et al., 1998), but its value in routine practice has yet to be defined.

Monitoring the Clinical Complications of Iron Overload. Regular monitoring of patients for adverse clinical effects of iron overload on the heart, liver, endocrine organs, and growth and development is an essential part of the management of chelation therapy (Table 37.14).

Monitoring for Desferrioxamine-Mediated Toxicity. After 30 years of experience, the short- and long-term toxic effects of desferrioxamine are now well known (Porter and Huehns, 1989) and have been detailed previously. Although the risk factors for some toxicities are understood—high desferrioxamine dose and low iron loading for retinal, audiologic, and growth effects—there is considerable clinical variability, and it is wise to regularly monitor patients for these complications. Although toxicity from dissociation of the iron-chelate complex is unlikely to occur because of the stability of ferrioxamine at neutral pH values, ferrioxamine promotes some infections such as *Yersinia*. These infections are more likely when the iron complex cannot be eliminated efficiently as in renal failure. The frequency and intensity of monitoring clearly depend on available resources, but a suggested scheme for monitoring for desferrioxamine-related tolerability is shown in Table 37.12.

ORAL CHELATION THERAPY

The only orally active iron chelator that has undergone prolonged clinical trials is deferiprone (L1 or CP20), a member of the hydroxypyridinone family of bidentate iron chelators.

Pharmacology of Deferiprone

Deferiprone (L1) molecules are small, neutrally charged, and more lipophilic than desferrioxamine. With a molecular weight approximately one third that of desferrioxamine (Table 37.10), oral absorption is rapid, with the drug appearing in plasma within 5 to 10 minutes of ingestion. High concentrations are achieved at commonly prescribed doses, reaching levels in excess of 300 μmol/L after oral ingestion of a 50 mg/kg dose (Kontoghiorghes et al., 1990b; Al-Refaie et al., 1995b). These levels are short-lived, with an elimination half-life of 1.52 hours (Al-Refaie et al., 1995) (Table 37.10). L1 is metabolized to the inactive glucuronide that is the predominant form recovered in the urine (Kontoghiorghes et al., 1990; Lange et al., 1993). In contrast to desferrioxamine, deferiprone-induced iron excretion is almost exclusively urinary (Kontoghiorghes et al., 1988; Olivieri et al., 1990; Collins et al., 1994).

The bidentate nature of chelation with deferiprone with a low pM compared with desferrioxamine increases the potential to redistribute iron within the body (Pippard et al., 1989). The bidentate chelator may also form incomplete 1:1 and 1:2 iron-chelate complexes at low chelator concentrations that have the potential to participate in the generation of hydroxyl radicals, increasing the risk of lipid peroxidation (Dobbin et al., 1993) and DNA damage in the presence of high concentrations of intracellular iron (Cragg et al., 1996).

Historical Perspective of Deferiprone (L1) Usage

Hydroxypyridinones were first described by Hider and colleagues in 1982 (Hider et al., 1982). Preclinical toxicologic evaluation was limited and did not conform to conventional practices before the commencement of clinical studies. This was partly because initial clinical trials were carried out by clinical investigators without the backing of a major pharmaceutical company. Early trials, discussed later, showed promising effects on urinary iron excretion in myelodysplasia and in patients with transfusional iron overload (Kontoghiorghes et al., 1987a,b).

Subsequent animal toxicology showed a dose and time-dependent suppression of the bone marrow in several animal species, both in iron overloaded and nonoverloaded states (Porter et al., 1989b; Porter et al., 1991). Thymic atrophy and teratogenic effects at doses close to the effective clinical therapeutic range were later identified (Berdoukas et al., 1993). Several cases of agranulocytosis were also reported in humans (Hoffbrand et al., 1989; Al-Refaie et al., 1992, 1993). Other effects in animal models, such as redistribution of iron from the liver to the heart and liver fibrosis, were later reported with the closely related hydroxypyridinone, CP94, in an iron overloaded gerbil model (Carthew et al., 1993, 1994). Ciba-Geigy declined to develop the drug in 1993 because of their findings of animal toxicology (Berdoukas et al., 1993). Apotex then undertook the development of this drug, and trials were begun between 1993 and 1995 to establish the efficacy of deferiprone and the frequency of complications. The original efficacy study was discontinued in 1996 after disagreements between the company and the clinical investigators (Olivieri and Brittenham, 1997). Results of the first year of the toxicity trial have been reported, other clinical trials are in progress in Europe, and it is anticipated that a limited license will be granted Europe by the end of 1999 (Cohen et al., 1998a, 2000).

Evidence of Efficacy of Deferiprone

Evidence of efficacy with deferiprone has been based on the effects of the drug on iron excretion, serum ferritin, and liver iron concentration. Insufficient data exist to make clear conclusions about the long-term effects on morbidity and mortality.

Effects on Iron Excretion. Early observations showed sufficiently increased urinary iron excretion to promote negative iron balance at doses between 75 and 100 mg/kg/day in previously poorly chelated individuals (Kontoghiorghes et al., 1987). A dose of 75 mg/kg/day but not 50 mg/kg/day promoted negative iron balance in the urine (Olivieri et al., 1990). Urinary iron excretion correlated with the serum ferritin and with desferrioxamine-induced urinary iron excretion (Olivieri et al., 1990) (Table 37.15). Iron balance studies (Collins et al., 1994; Olivieri et al., 1990) showed that, in contrast to desferrioxamine, fecal iron excretion induced with deferiprone was insignificant (Table 37.15). A similar pattern of low fecal iron excretion with deferiprone was also observed in iron balance studies of patients with sickle cell disease who experienced iron overload (Collins et al., 1994). Total iron excretion at doses of 75 mg/kg/day is about 60 percent of that seen with desferrioxamine at 50 mg/kg/day given as a 12-hour subcutaneous infusion, but sufficient to induce negative iron balance (Collins et al., 1994). Urinary iron excretion did not change significantly in a group of patients receiving 75 mg/kg/day with a mean follow-up of 39 months (Hoffbrand et al., 1998). Dose equivalence for desferrioxamine and deferiprone has not been determined in iron balance studies.

Effects on Serum Ferritin. Serum ferritin values fell in the most heavily iron overloaded subjects with initial levels above 5000 µg/L (Al-Refaie et al., 1992). In India, where there are relatively large numbers of patients who otherwise have little access to chelation treatment, the serum ferritin fell from initially very high levels to an average of more than 3,500 µg/L over 20 months (Agarwal et al., 1992). In a Canadian study of twenty-one patients, the serum ferritin declined from 3,975 to 2,546 µg/L ($P < .005$) after a mean follow-up period of 3 years at a dose of 75 mg/kg/day (Olivieri et al., 1995). The changes were most marked in patients starting with high ferritin values. In patients with ferritin values below 2,500 µg/L before treatment, there was no significant further change. In a study from London, there was no overall change in serum ferritin level in twenty-six patients treated for 3 years at 75 mg/kg (initial value 2,937 µg/L, final value 2,323 µg/L). In fifty-two patients from Turin with a median pretreatment ferritin value of 1,826 µg/L, there was no significant change in the serum ferritin level after 2 years of therapy with deferiprone at a dose of 75 mg/kg/day (Longo et al., 1998). Thus, it appears that ferritin levels will decline if pretreatment values are high, but at values below approximately 2,500 µg/L, serum ferritin levels remain unchanged, a finding confirmed in a large multicenter study (Cohen et al., 2000).

Effect on Liver Iron. The response of liver iron concentration to deferiprone was first reported in twenty-one patients with a 3-year follow-up period (Olivieri et al., 1995). In ten previously suboptimally chelated patients, mean hepatic iron concentrations declined from 125 µmol/g wet wt (23 mg/g dry wt) to 60 µmol/g wet wt (11 mg/g dry wt) ($P < .005$), with values above 80 µmol/g wet wt (15 mg/g dry wt) in only two patients. In the eleven patients in whom desferrioxamine had been effectively taken before the use of deferiprone, hepatic iron concentrations remained below 80 µmol/g wet wt (15 mg/g dry wt). In a more recent follow-up study of the same patients, now treated for a mean of 4.6 years, hepatic iron was greater than 80 µmol/g wet wt (15 mg/g dry wt) in seven of eighteen patients (39 percent) (Olivieri et al., 1998).

These latter findings are in broad agreement with other work (Hoffbrand et al., 1998) where hepatic

Table 37.15. Clinical Efficacy of Deferiprone

Variable	Effect

Urine iron excretion
  at 50 mg/kg
  at 75 mg/kg
	Mean 12 mg/day (Olivieri et al., 1990)
	Mean 27 mg/day (Olivieri et al., 1990)
	No change in urine iron over 2–4 year follow-up (Hoffbrand et al., 1998)
	Excretion correlates with serum ferritin (Olivieri et al., 1990) and DFO induced
	  iron excretion (Olivieri et al., 1990)
	Falls with decreased iron loading (Olivieri, 1996)

Iron balance at 75 mg/kg in thalassemia major	Variable in metabolic balance study; 9–25 mg/day (Olivieri et al., 1990) Positive in 69% of patients (n = 52) over 2y by SQUID (Longo et al., 1998)
Iron balance in SS at 75 mg/kg	Negative (0.53 ± 0.17 mg/kg/day, 23% in feces) (Collins et al., 1994) significantly less than DFO (0.88 mg/kg/day, 59% in feces) at 50 mg/kg
Serum ferritin (at 75 mg/kg)	Rapid fall in minimally chelated patients (Agarwal et al., 1992) Fall in poorly chelated patients (Al-Refaie et al., 1992) Fall in poorly chelated patients over 3 years (Olivieri et al., 1995) Rise in well-treated patients over 2–3 years (Longo, 1998 Longo, 1999)
Liver iron (at 75 mg/kg)	Initial fall in poorly chelated patients over 3 years (Olivieri et al., 1995) Stabilizes at "high risk" levels in 39% (>15 mg/g dry wt) at 4.6 years (Olivieri, 1998) Above 15 mg/g dry wt in 58% at 2–4 year follow-up (Hoffbrand et al., 1998) Increase in well-chelated patients: by 41% at 2 years (Longo, 1998) by 56% at 3 years (Longo, 1999)
Liver fibrosis (at 75 mg/kg)	Progression in 5/12 patients at 3.2 years (Olivieri, 1996) No progression in 16/16 patients at 2.3 years (Piga et al., 1998) Mild fibrosis in 1/12 HCV mRNA–ve and severe in 5/5 HC+ve at 2–4 years (Hoffbrand et al., 1998)
Cardiomyopathy	Unknown, not recommended if cardiac dysfunction
Effect on survival	Unknown

SS, sickle cell anemia; HCV, hepatitis C virus.

iron was greater than 15 mg/g dry wt in ten of seventeen patients (58 percent) in a 2- to 4-year follow-up period and below 7 mg/g dry wt in only two patients. Urine iron excretion did not change significantly over this period. In a 7- to 8-year follow-up period of seven patients treated in Switzerland, there was an "unexplained resurgence" of serum ferritin after 4 to 5 years, which was associated with a concomitant increase in liver iron in three of these patients (Tondury et al., 1998). In another study of fifty-two previously well-chelated patients from Italy, treated for 2 years at 75 mg/kg/day, the hepatic iron concentration increased in 69 percent of patients by a mean of 43 percent (Longo et al., 1998). In a follow-up report, mean values had increased by 56 percent from 5.1 to 8.0 mg/g dry wt after 3 years.

It is not necessary to invoke a loss of drug activity to explain these findings. When the data from various studies are considered together, they are consistent with a declining efficiency of chelation as the hepatic iron concentration falls from high values in previously poorly chelated patients. In patients who had low hepatic iron concentrations before commencing deferiprone, levels of hepatic iron appear to rise slowly until a new equilibrium is achieved at values significantly greater than starting concentrations. The final hepatic iron concentration may be undesirably high in about half the patients but will take several years to reach equilibrium, particularly if starting levels are low. Considerable variation in responses among patients is also present, possibly owing to differences in the rates of chelator inactivation by glucuronidation. Liver iron measurement should be carefully considered as an integral part of the monitoring of the effectiveness of therapy with deferiprone. At higher doses of deferiprone, for example 100 mg/kg/day, equilibrium levels may be more acceptable in a higher proportion of patients (Wonke et al., 1998). However, the toxicity profile has not been established at such doses.

In conditions where the rate of iron loading is slower than in thalassaemia major, it would be anticipated that deferiprone could achieve acceptable levels of liver iron at doses of 75 mg/kg or less. Indeed in a case report of a patient with thalassaemia intermedia, liver iron was reduced from 14.6 to 1.9 mg/g dry wt after 9 months of deferiprone therapy. This reduction of liver iron to normal levels was accompanied by normalization of the serum ferritin and a possible qualitative reduction in cardiac iron measured by T_1-weighted spin echo MRI (Olivieri et al., 1992c).

Effects on Other Long-Term Complications of Iron Overload. Although more than 30 years of follow-up data are available for desferrioxamine-treated patients using untreated patients as historical control subjects, there are no data on the relative effects of deferiprone and desferrioxamine on survival and on morbidity from iron overload. There are also insufficient data to indicate whether deferiprone has an effect on cardiac toxicity from iron overload. In a recent large study, five of fifty-one patients treated with deferiprone died after a mean time of 18 months, four with congestive heart failure (Hoffbrand et al., 1998). By contrast, ample data suggest that desferrioxamine, if used regularly, can prevent or reverse cardiac toxicity, indicating that this chelator should be recommended for heavily iron overloaded patients with a high risk of cardiac complications.

Neutropenia and Agranulocytosis. Agranulocytosis was initially reported in 3 to 4 percent of patients treated with deferiprone, and mild neutropenia occurred in an additional 4 percent (Al-Refaie et al., 1992, 1995). In humans, unlike in laboratory animals (Porter et al., 1989b), this effect appears unpredictable. Neutropenia may last from 4 to 124 days (Hoffbrand et al., 1989; Hoffbrand, 1994; Cohen et al., 1998a, 2000). Hematopoietic growth factors have been used in some cases of severe or protracted neutropenia, but their value is uncertain. Reintroduction of deferiprone leads to a rapid fall in the neutrophil count in some patients; therefore its use is contraindicated in patients with agranulocytosis and should be retried only in patients with milder forms of neutropenia and carefully monitored. It may be wise to avoid deferiprone in patients in whom stem cell or progenitor function is compromised, such as those with Diamond-Blackfan anemia. In one case report, agranulocytosis was associated with a vasculitic syndrome and disturbances of immune function (Castriota-Scanderbeg and Sacco, 1997).

The results of a 1-year multicenter safety trial of 187 patients showed that if the blood count is monitored weekly and the drug is stopped at the first signs of neutropenia, the risk of agranulocytosis (absolute neutrophil count $<500/\mu L$) is as low as 0.6 percent (Cohen et al., 1998a). In this study, the one patient who developed agranulocytosis did so after 15 weeks of treatment and the condition resolved during treatment with G-CSF. Neutropenia, as defined by a neutrophil count of 500 to $1,500/\mu L$, occurred in nine subjects (4.8 percent). The lower incidence of agranulocytosis compared with some earlier studies suggests that this may be decreased by monitoring the white count weekly and stopping therapy in a timely manner. At present, it is not possible to predict whether the neutropenia is part of an independent fluctuation in the neutrophil count, more likely in unsplenectomized patients, or is the first sign of deferiprone-induced agranulocytosis.

Arthropathy. Painful swelling of the joints, particularly the knees, occurs in 6 to 39 percent of patients treated with deferiprone and usually, but not always, resolves after stopping therapy (Al-Refaie et al., 1992; Agarwal et al., 1992; Cohen et al., 1998a). Arthritis was most common in the Indian study, where many patients were heavily iron overloaded (Agarwal et al., 1992), raising the possible explanation of redistribution of iron to the joints.

Other Unwanted Effects. Other unwanted effects in pooled data on eighty-four patients from several centers were nausea (8 percent), mild zinc deficiency (14 percent), and fluctuation in liver function tests (44 percent) (Al-Refaie et al., 1995). As a result of unwanted effects, treatment has been discontinued in 13 to 30 percent of patients in various studies (Al-Refaie et al., 1992, 1995; Hoffbrand et al., 1998; Cohen et al., 1998a). A number of other events have been reported to have occurred during therapy with deferiprone such as a fatal systemic lupus erythematosus (Mehta et al., 1991), increased antinuclear antibodies and rheumatoid factors (Mehta et al., 1993), and a fatal varicella infection; but any relationship of these events to deferiprone is uncertain (Berdoukas et al., 1993). No significant changes in antinuclear or rheumatoid factors have been confirmed by other studies (Cohen et al., 2000), and anti-DNA and anti-histone antibodies have been persistently negative (Olivieri et al., 1995). Progression of audiometric disturbances has been described in five of nine patients who were switched from desferrioxamine to deferiprone (Chiodo et al., 1997). In the same study, however, seven patients without audiometric disturbance who were switched to deferiprone developed no new abnormalities.

Recent concern has been expressed about possible increasing liver fibrosis in deferiprone-treated patients (Olivieri et al., 1998). In a retrospective analysis, progression of fibrosis was compared between twelve patients treated with deferiprone and a contemporary group of age-matched control subjects receiving regular desferrioxamine. Fibrosis progressed in five patients on deferiprone and in none of twelve patients on desferrioxamine, with an estimated median time to progression of fibrosis of 3.2 years in deferiprone-treated patients. Four of the five patients with increasing fibrosis were seropositive for hepatitis C. The frequency of antibody to hepatitis C was the same (6/14) in the deferiprone-treated group and the desferrioxamine-treated group (5/12).

In another study (Hoffbrand et al., 1998), liver biopsies taken at 2 to 4 years of follow-up in patients who were hepatitis C RNA negative showed no fibrosis in eleven of twelve and mild fibrosis in one of twelve patients. In all five patients who were hepatitis C RNA positive, cirrhosis was present. Results of the control group who were hepatitis C RNA positive and received desferrioxamine were not reported. In another study, hepatic fibrosis was found in seven of eleven patients on long-term deferiprone, and the fibrosis was greater in the hepatitis C positive group than in the hepatitis C negative group (Tondury et al., 1998). No desferrioxamine-treated control subjects were reported in this study. Preliminary data from a retrospective study of sixteen patients from Turin with paired liver biopsies show no progression of fibrosis over a median time of 2.3 years of observation (Piga et al., 1998). At present, therefore, there is lack of consensus about whether deferiprone adds to the known fibrotic risks from hepatitis C and iron overload. These questions can be answered conclusively only with a prospective trial with carefully chosen control subjects.

FUTURE PERSPECTIVES WITH CHELATION THERAPY

Neither desferrioxamine nor deferiprone offers an ideal long-term solution to the treatment of iron overload. In its currently available formulation, treatment with desferrioxamine is a demanding regimen that challenges good compliance, and patients die from insufficient treatment. Those who comply with chelation treatment, however, have an excellent chance of surviving to the fifth decade.

Insufficient data about any long-term effects of deferiprone on morbidity and mortality from iron overload are available to recommend this treatment as an alternative to desferrioxamine. On the basis of available information, deferiprone should be considered only in circumstances where desferrioxamine cannot be given, either for reasons of availability or because of serious intractable tolerability problems.

There remains a need for an orally available alternative to desferrioxamine with a higher therapeutic safety margin than that of deferiprone. Several candidates are in various stages of development.

Other Hydroxypyridinones

The one hydroxypyridinone other than deferiprone that has been evaluated clinically is 1,2 diethyl-3-hydroxypyridin-4-one, CP94. This bidentate hydroxypyridinone is highly active in animal models, particularly in the rat (Porter et al., 1993). In humans, however, the drug was not sufficiently effective to induce negative iron balance owing to rapid inactivation by glucuronidation (Porter et al., 1994). New generations of hydroxypyridinones with improved pM values and improved biodistribution properties are in preclinical development. Novartis has identified one such compound, but this is currently not their first choice for clinical development. Hider and colleagues (1994) have identified a number of hydroxypyridinones with less inactivation by glucuronidation than deferiprone or with improved pM values. Other derivatives have been identified with slower interaction with iron-containing intracellular enzymes and slower induction of apoptosis in proliferating cells (Kayyali et al., 1998). These compounds are in preclinical evaluation.

HBED and Derivatives

HBED (N, N′-bis(2-hydroxybenzyl)ethylenediamine-N,N′-diacetic acid) is one of a group of hexadentate chelators containing both aminocarboxylate and phenolic functions, first sythesized by Martell and co-workers (Frost et al., 1958; L'Eplattenier et al., 1967) in an attempt to provide more selectivity of iron chelation than is offered with simpler aminocarboxylates such as diethylentriamine pentaacetate (DTPA). The stability constant for iron(III) is 10^{40}, although there are still appreciable affinities for copper (10^{21}), zinc (10^{18}), and calcium (10^{9}) as a consequence of its two carboxylate functions.

Early rodent studies showed that HBED was associated with relatively low toxicity ($LD_{50} = 800$ mg/kg), but still lacked significant oral activity (Hershko et al., 1984; Pitt et al., 1986). A subchronic toxicity study of the HBED monosodium salt has been reported in rodents, and iron excretion has been evaluated in primates (Bergeron et al., 1999). In the latter model, the subcutaneous injection of HBED in buffer or its monosodium salt, 75 to 324 μmol/kg, produced a net iron excretion that was nearly three times that observed after similar doses of subcutaneous desferrioxamine.

In human studies HBED has poor oral absorption, leading to insufficient iron excretion for negative iron balance (5.4 to 8.1 mg/day) at doses up to 80 mg/kg/day in three divided doses (Grady and Hershko, 1990a,b; Grady et al., 1994). Two patients have received 120 mg/kg, resulting in twice as much iron excretion as at 80 mg/kg, but negative iron balance was still not achieved (Grady and Giardina, 1997).

The dimethyl ester of HBED is well absorbed and effective via the oral route in animal models (Hershko et al., 1984; Pitt et al., 1986). For this reason, Grady and colleagues investigated the efficacy of ester and other prodrug derivatives to improve oral bioavailability. (Grady and Giardina, 1997). Novartis has investigated dimethyl and other derivatives of HBED preclinically. Some of these have good oral bioavailability in rat and primate (marmoset) models.

PIH and Derivatives

PIH, a tridentate chelator formed by the addition of isoniazid to equimolar quantities of pyridoxal, was originally investigated following the observation that it mobilized ^{59}Fe from reticulocytes (Ponka et al., 1979a, 1981). A large series of pyridoxal hydrazones has been synthesized and evaluated preclinically (Ponka et al., 1979b; Hoy et al., 1979; Blaha et al., 1998). These compounds are uncharged at neutral pH and by varying the aromatic acyl function, it is possible to vary their partition coefficient. Unlike other iron chelators, these compounds bind both iron(III) and iron(II) (Sarel et al., 1986), which theoretically could lead the iron complex to redox cycle, thereby generating free radicals. Although PIH has a relatively low stability constant for iron (logK = 8.67) (Avramovici-Grisaru and Sarel, 1983), it removes iron from transferrin at a rate similar to desferrioxamine at equal binding equivalents (Ponka et al., 1979b). A further theoretical disadvantage of this series of compounds is their possession of a "Schiff-base link", which increases their susceptibility to hydrolysis and therefore to breakdown in the gastrointestinal tract.

Oral administration of PIH to rats, at a dose of 100 mg/kg/24 hr, failed to show any reduction in hepatic iron stores after 10 weeks of administration (Williams et al., 1982). Detailed toxicity testing suggests that PIH is without significant toxicity macroscopically, biochemically, or histologically in rats and hamsters (Brittenham, 1990). A limited clinical trial with PIH showed no significant toxicity at a dose of 30 mg/kg/day for 6 days, although iron excretion was not impressive and total iron excretion at this dose was insufficient to produce negative iron balance in regularly transfused patients (Brittenham, 1990).

More recently, more than 40 analogs of PIH have been synthesized and evaluated in rodent models. These chelators significantly enhance biliary excretion of iron following their intraperitoneal and/or oral administration to rats (Blaha et al., 1998). The most effective is PFBH, which increased iron concentration in the bile about 150-fold, compared with basal biliary iron concentration, within 1 hour after a single intraperitoneal dose of 0.2 mmol/kg. This compared with a 20- to 30-fold increase with desferrioxamine under the same conditions.

Other Chelators

Novartis has begun phase I clinical trials of a tridentate orally active chelator (ICL670A), an N-substituted bis-hydroxyphenyltriazole, which is a novel class of chelator (Schnebli, 1997). The compound was twice as effective as desferrioxamine and five times as effective as deferiprone in the rat, and ten times more effective than deferiprone in the marmoset. Toxicity has been assessed in both marmosets and rats with a "no adverse effect level" of 130 mg/kg/day in females and 65 mg/kg/day in males. Potential target organs for toxicity are the kidney, gastrointestinal tract, and heart; but most of the effects were interpreted as secondary to extreme iron deprivation. Results of phase I clinical studies are awaited as work progresses to make a safe and effective oral iron chelator available to patients.

References

Abeysinghe, RD, Roberts, PJ, Cooper, CE et al. (1996). The environment of the lipoxygenase iron binding site explored with novel hydroxypyridinone iron chelators. *J. Biol. Chem.* 271: 7965–7972.

Adams, DM, Schultz, WH, Ware, RE, and Kinney, TR. (1996). Erythrocytapheresis can reduce iron overload and reduce the need for chelation therapy in chronically transfused pediatric patients. *J. Pediatr. Hematol. Oncol.* 18: 46–50.

Adams, R, McKie, V, Nichols, F et al. (1992). The use of transcranial ultrasonography to predict stroke in sickle cell disease. *N. Engl. J. Med.* 326: 605–610.

Adams, RJ, McKie, VC, Carl, EM et al. (1997). Long-term stroke risk in children with sickle cell disease screened with transcranial doppler. *Ann. Neurol.* 42: 699–704.

Adams, RJ, McKie, VC, Hsu, L et al. (1998). Prevention of a first stroke by transfusions in children with sickle cell anemia and abnormal results on transcranial Doppler ultrasonography. *N. Engl. J. Med.* 339: 5–11.

Agarwal, MB, Gupte, SS, Viswanathan, C et al. (1992). Long term assessment of efficacy and safety of L1, an oral iron chelator in transfusion dependent thalassaemia. *Br. J. Haematol.* 82: 460–466.

Al-Refaie, FN, Hershko, C, Hoffbrand, AV et al. (1995a). Results of long-term deferiprone (L1) therapy: A report by the International Study Group on Oral Iron Chelators. *Br. J. Haematol.* 91: 224–229.

Al-Refaie, FN, Sheppard, LN, Nortey, P et al. (1995b). Pharmacokinetics of the oral iron chelator (L1) in patients with iron overload. *Br. J. Haematol.* 89: 403–408.

Al-Refaie, FN, Veys, PA, Wilkes, S et al. (1993). Agranulocytosis in a patient with thalassaemia major during treatment with the oral iron chelator, 1,2-dimethyl-3-hydroxypyrid-4-one. *Acta Haematol.* 89: 86–90.

Al-Refaie, FN, Wonke, B, Hoffbrand, AV et al. (1992). Efficacy and possible adverse effects of the oral iron chelator 1,2-dimethyl-3-hydroxypyridin-4-one (L1) in thalassemia major. *Blood* 80: 593–599.

Aldouri, MA, Hoffbrand, AV, Flynn, DM et al. (1990). High incidence of cardiomyopathy in beta-thalassemia patients receiving transfusion and iron chelation: Reversal by intensified chelation. *Acta Haematol.* 84: 113–117.

Aldouri, MA, Wonke, B, Hoffbrand, AV et al. (1987). Iron state and hepatic disease in patients with thalassaemia major, treated with long term subcutaneous desferrioxamine. *J. Clin. Pathol.* 40: 1353–1359.

Ambruso, DR, Githens, JH, Alcorn, R et al. (1987). Experience with donors matched for minor blood group antigens in patients with sickle cell anemia who are receiving chronic transfusion therapy. *Transfusion,* 27: 94–98.

Ambu, R, Crisponi, G, Sciot, R et al. (1995). Uneven hepatic iron and phosphorus distribution in beta-thalassemia. *J. Hepatol.* 23: 544–549.

Andriani, M, Nordio, M, and Saporiti, E. (1996). Estimation of statistical moments for desferrioxamine and its iron and aluminum chelates: Contribution to optimisation of therapy in uremic patients. *Nephron* 72: 218–224.

Angelucci, E, Baronciani, D, Lucarelli, G et al. (1994). Needle liver biopsy in thalassaemia: Analyses of diagnostic accuracy and safety in 1184 consecutive biopsies. *Br. J. Haematol.* 89: 757.

Araujo, A, Kosaryan, M, MacDowell, A et al. (1996). A novel delivery system for continuous desferrioxamine infusion in transfusional iron overload. *Br. J. Haematol.* 93: 835–837.

Arden, GB, Wonke, B, Kennedy, C, and Huehns, ER. (1984). Ocular changes in patients undergoing long term desferrioxamine treatment. *Br. J. Ophthalmol.* 68: 873–877.

Avramovici-Grisaru, S and Sarel, S. (1983). Syntheses of iron bis (pyridoxal isonicotinoyl hydrazones) and the in vivo iron-removal properties of some pyridoxal derivatives. *J. Med. Chem.* 26: 298–302.

Bacon, BR, Tacvill, AS, Brittenham, GM et al. (1983). Hepatic lipid peroxidation in vivo in rats with chronic iron overload. *J. Clin. Invest.* 71: 429–439.

Bailey-Wood, R, White, G, and Jacobs, A. (1975). The use of Chang cells in vitro for the investigation of cellular iron metabolism. *Br. J. Exp. Pathol.* 56: 358–362.

Balcerzac, S, Westerman, M, Heihn, E, and Taylor, FH. (1968). Effect of desferrioxamine and DTPA in iron overload. *Br. Med. J.* 2: 1573–1576.

Balkaran, B, Char, G, Morris, JS et al. (1992). Stroke in a cohort of patients with sickle cell disease. *J. Pediatr.* 120: 360–366.

Ballart, IJ, Estevez, ME, Sen, L et al. (1986). Progressive dysfunction of monocytes associated with iron overload and age in patients with thalassemia major. *Blood* 67: 105–109.

Baron, M and Leiter, E. (1978). The management of priapism in sickle cell anemia. *J. Urol.* 119: 610–611.

Barosi, G, Arbustini, E, Gavazzi, A et al. (1989). Myocardial iron grading by endomyocardial biopsy. A clinico-pathologic study on iron overloaded patients. *Eur. J. Haematol.* 42: 382–388.

Barry, DMJ and Reeve, AN. (1977). Increased incidence of gram-negative neonatal sepsis with intramuscular iron administration. *Pediatrics* 60: 908–912.

Barry, M, Flynn, DM, Letsky, EA, and Risdon, RA. (1974). Long term chelation therapy in thalassaemia: effect on liver iron concentration, liver histology and clinical progress. *Br. Med. J.* 2: 16–20.

Barry, M and Sherlock, S. (1971). Measurement of liver-iron concentration in needle biopsy specimens. *Lancet* 1: 100–103.

Beamish, MR, Walter, R, and Miller, F. (1974). Transferrin iron, chelatable iron and ferritin in idiopathic haemochromatosis. *Br. J. Haematol.* 27: 219–228.

Beard, MEJ, Necheles, TF, and Allen, DM. (1969). Clinical experience with intensive transfusion therapy in Cooley's anemia. *Ann. NY Acad. Sci.* 165: 415–422.

Beattie, KM and Shafer, AW. (1986). Broadening the base of a rare donor program by targeting minority populations. *Transfusion* 26: 401–404.

Berdoukas, V, Bentley, P, Frost, H, and Schnebli, HP. (1993). Toxicity of oral chelator L1 (Letter). *Lancet* 341: 1088.

Berdoukas, VA, Kwan, YL, and Sansotta, ML. (1986). A study on the value of red cell exchange transfusion in transfusion dependent anaemias. *Clin. Lab. Haematol.* 8: 209–220.

Berdoukas, VA and Moore, RC. (1990). Automated red cell exchange transfusions in transfusion dependent anemias. *Proceedings of the 5th Annual Meeting of the Cooleycare Group,* Athens, Greece.

Bergeron, RJ, Wiegand, J, and Brittenham, GM. (1999). HBED: The continuing development of a potential alternative to desferrioxamine for iron-chelating therapy. *Blood* 93: 370–375.

Berkovitch, M, Collins, AF, Papadouris, D et al. (1993). Need for early, low-dose chelation therapy in young children with transfused homozygous beta thalassemia. *Blood* 82: 359a.

Bhattacharyya, N, Wayne, AS, Kevy, SV, and Shamberger, RC. (1993). Perioperative management for cholecystectomy in sickle cell disease. *J. Pediatr. Surg.* 28: 72–75.

Bischoff, RJ, Williamson, A, Dalali, MJ et al. (1988). Assessment of the use of transfusion therapy perioperatively in patients with sickle cell hemoglobinopathies. *Ann. Surg.* 207: 434–438.

Bissell, DM, Wang, SS, Jarnagin, WR, and Roll, FJ. (1995). Cell specific expression of transforming growth factor-β in the rat liver. *J. Clin. Invest.* 96: 447–455.

Blaha, K, Cikrt, M, Nerudova, J, and Ponka, HF. (1998). Biliary iron excretion in rats following treatment with analogs of pyridoxal isonicotinoyl hydrazone. *Blood* 91: 4368–4372.

Blake, DR, Winyard, P, Lunec, J et al. (1985). Cerebral and ocular toxicity induced by desferrioxamine Q. *J. Med.* 56: 345–355.

Boelaert, JR, Verauwe, PL, and Vandepitte, JM. (1987). Mucormycosis infections in dialysis patients. *Ann. Intern. Med.* 107: 782–783.

Bonetti, MG, Castriota-Scanderbeg, A, Criconia, GM et al. (1996). Hepatic iron overload in thalassemic patients: proposal and validation of an MRI method of assessment. *Pediatr. Radiol.* 26: 650–656.

Borgna-Pignatti, C and Cohen, A. (1997). Evaluation of a new method of administration of the iron chelating agent deferoxamine. *J. Pediatr.* 130: 86–88.

Bosquet, J, Navarro, M, Robert, G et al. (1983). Rapid desensitisation for desferrioxamine anaphylactoid reaction. *Lancet* 2: 859–860.

Bothwell, T, Charlton, RW, Cook, JD, and Finch, CA. (1979). *Iron metabolism in man.* Oxford: Blackwell.

Bracey, AW, Klein, HG, Chambers, S, and Corash, L. (1983). Ex vivo selective isolation of young red blood cells using the IBM-2991 cell washer. *Blood* 61: 1068–1071.

Brady, MC, Lilley, KS, Treffry, A et al. (1988). Release of iron from ferritin molecules and the iron cores by 3-hydroxypyridinone chelators in vitro. *J. Inorg. Biochem.* 32: 1–14.

Brazier, DJ, Gregor, ZJ, Blach, RK et al. (1986). Retinal detachment in patients with proliferative sickle cell retinopathy. *Trans. Ophthalmol. Soc. U.K.* 105: 100–105.

Breuer, W, Epsztejn, S, and Cabantchik ZI. (1995). Iron acquired from transferrin by K562 cells is delivered into a cytoplasmic pool of chelatable iron (II). *J. Biol. Chem.* 270: 24209–24215.

Brissot, P, Wright, TL, Ma, WL, and Weisiger, RA. (1985). Efficient clearance of non-transferrin-bound iron by rat liver. *J. Clin. Invest.* 76: 1463–1470.

Brittenham, G. (1990). Pyridoxal isonicotinoyl hydrazone: An effective iron-chelator after oral administration. *Semin. Hematol.* 27: 112–116.

Brittenham, GM, Cohen, AR, McLaren, CE et al. (1993). Hepatic iron stores and plasma ferritin concentration in patients with sickle cell anemia and thalassemia major. *Am. J. Hematol.* 42: 81–85.

Brittenham, GM, Farrell, DE, Harris, JW et al. (1982). Magnetic-susceptibility measurement of human iron stores. *N. Engl. J. Med.* 307: 1671–1675.

Brittenham, GM, Griffith, PM, Nienhuis, AW et al. (1994). Efficacy of desferioxamine in preventing complications of iron overload in patients with thalassemia major. *N. Engl. J. Med.* 331: 567–573.

Brody, JI, Goldsmith, MH, Park, SK, and Soltys, HD. (1970). Symptomatic crises of sickle cell anemia treated by limited exchange transfusion. *Ann. Intern. Med.* 72: 327–330.

Bronspeigel-Weintrob, N, Olivieri, NF, Tyler, BJ et al. (1990). Effect of age at the start of iron chelation therapy on gonadal function in β-thalassemia major. *N. Engl. J. Med.* 323: 713–719.

Brownell, A, Lowson, S, and Brozovic, M. (1986). Serum ferritin concentration in sickle cell crisis. *J. Clin. Pathol.* 39: 253–255.

Brunengo, MA and Girot, R. (1986). Apports transfusionnels et taux d'hemoglobine moyen annuel dans la thalassemie majeure. *Nouvelle Revue Francaise d'Hematologie* 28: 309–313.

Buchholz, DH, AuBuchon, JP, Snyder, EL et al. (1992). Removal of *Yersinia enterocolitica* from AS-1 red cells. *Transfusion* 32: 667–672.

Buja, LM and Roberts, WC. (1971). Iron in the heart. *Am. J. Med.* 51: 209–221.

Campbell, PJ, Olatunji, PO, Ryan, KE, and Davies, SC. (1997). Splenic regrowth in sickle cell anaemia following hypertransfusion. *Br. J. Haematol.* 96: 77–79.

Carthew, P, Dorman, BM, Edwards, RE et al. (1993). A unique rodent model for both cardiotoxic and heptatotoxic effects of prolonged iron overload. *Lab. Invest.* 69: 217–222.

Carthew, P, Smith, AG, Hide, RC et al. (1994). Potentiation of iron accumulation in cardiac myocytes during the treatment of iron overload in gerbils with the hydroxypyridinone iron chelator CP94. *Biometals* 7: 267–270.

Castellino, SM, Combs, MR, Zimmerman, SA et al. (1999). Erythrocyte autoantibodies in paediatric patients with sickle cell disease receiving transfusion therapy: Frequency, characteristics and significance. *Br. J. Haematol.* 104: 189–194.

Castriota-Scanderbeg, A and Sacco, M. (1997). Agranulocytosis, arthritis and systemic vasculitis in a patient receiving the oral iron chelator L1 (deferiprone). *Br. J. Haematol.* 96: 254–255.

Cavill, I. (1975). Internal regulation of iron absorption. *Nature* 256: 328–329.

Cavill, I, Ricketts, C, Jacobs, A, and Letsky, E. (1978). Erythropoiesis and the effect of transfusion in homozygous β-thalassemia. *N. Engl. J. Med.* 298: 776–778.

Cazzola, M, Borgna-Pignatti, C, Locatelli, F et al. (1997). A moderate transfusion regimen may reduce iron loading in β-thalassemia major without producing excessive expansion of erythropoiesis. *Transfusion* 37: 135–140.

Cazzola, M, De Stefano, P, Ponchio, L et al. (1995). Relationship between transfusion regimen and suppression of erythropoiesis in β-thalassaemia major. *Br. J. Haematol.* 89: 473–478.

Chapin, H and Zarkowsky, HS. (1981). Combined sickle cell disease and autoimmune hemolytic anemia. *Arch. Intern. Med.* 141: 1091–1093.

Charache, S, Scott, J, Niebyl, J, and Bonds, D. (1980). Management of sickle cell disease in pregnant patients. *Obstetr. Gynecol.* 55: 407–410.

Chatterjee, R, Katz, M, Cox, TF, and Porter, JB. (1993). Prospective study of the hypothalamic-pituitary axis in thalassaemic patients who develop secondary amenorrhoea. *Clin. Endocrinol.* 39: 287.

Chatterjee, R, Katz, M, Oatridge, A et al. (1998). Selective loss of anterior pituitary volume with severe pituitary-gonadal insufficiency in poorly compliant male thalassemic patients with pubertal arrest. *Ann. NY. Acad. Sci.* 850: 479–482.

Chatterjee, R, Wonke, B, Porter, JB, and Katz, M. (1995). Correction of primary and secondary amenorrhoea and induction of ovulation by pulsatile infusion of gonadotrophin releasing hormone (GnRH) in patients with beta thalassaemia major. In Beuzard, Y, Lubin, B, and Rosa, J, editors. *Sickle cell disease and thalassaemia: New trends in therapy.* Colloq. Inserm., 234: 451–455.

Chiodo, AA, Alberti, PW, Sher, GD et al. (1997). Desferrioxamine ototoxicity in an adult transfusion dependent population. *J. Otolaryngol.* 26: 116–122.

Chui, DHK and Waye, JS. (1998). Hydrops fetalis caused by α-thalassaemia: An emerging health care problem. *Blood* 91: 2213–2222.

Clemente, MG, Congia, M, Lai, ME et al. (1994). Effect of iron overload on the response to recombinant interferon-alfa treatment in transfusion-dependent patients with thalassemia major and chronic hepatitis C. *J. Pediatr.* 125: 123–128.

Cohen, A, Galanello, R, Piga, A et al. (1998a). A multi-center safety trial of the oral iron chelator deferiprone. *Ann. NY. Acad. Sci.* 850: 223–226.

Cohen, A, Markenson, AL, and Schwartz, E. (1980). Transfusion requirements and splenectomy in thalassemia major. *J. Pediatr.* 97: 100–102.

Cohen, A, Martin, M, and Schwartz, E. (1981). Response to long term desferrioxamine therapy in thalassemia. *J. Pediatr.* 99: 689–694.

Cohen, A, Martin, M, and Schwartz, E. (1984a). Depletion of excessive iron stores with desferrioxamine. *Br. J. Haematol.* 58: 369–373.

Cohen, AR. (1998). Sickle cell disease: New treatments, new questions. *N. Engl. J. Med.* 339: 42–44.

Cohen, AR, Buchanan, GR, Martin, M, and Ohene-Frempong, K. (1991). Increased blood requirements during long-term transfusion therapy for sickle cell disease. *J. Pediatr.* 118: 405–407.

Cohen, AR, Friedman, DF, Larson, PJ et al. (1998b). Erythrocytapheresis to reduce iron loading in thalassemia. *Blood* 92 (Suppl 1): 532a–533a.

Cohen, AR, Galanello, R, Piga, A et al. (2000). Safety profile of the oral iron chelator deferiprone: a multi-centre study. *Br. J..Haematol.* 108: 305–312.

Cohen, AR, Martin, MB, Silber, JH et al. (1992). A modified transfusion program for prevention of stroke in sickle cell disease. *Blood* 79: 1657–1661.

Cohen, AR, Mizanin, J, and Schwartz, E. (1987). Rapid removal of excessive iron with daily high dose intravenous chelation therapy. *J. Pediatr.* 115: 151–155.

Cohen, AR, Schmidt, JM, Martin, MB et al. (1984b). Clinical trial of young red cell transfusions. *J. Pediatr.* 104: 865–868.

Coker, NJ and Milner, PF. (1982). Elective surgery in patients with sickle cell anemia. *Arch. Otolaryngol.* 108: 574–576.

Coles, SM, Klein, HG, and Holland, PV. (1981). Alloimmunization in two multitransfused patient populations. *Transfusion* 21: 462–466.

Collins, AF, Fassos, FF, Stobie, S et al. (1994). Iron-balance and dose-response studies of the oral iron chelator 1,2-dimethyl-3-hydroxypyrid-4-one (L1) in iron-loaded patients with sickle cell disease. *Blood* 83: 2329–2333.

Collins, AF, Goncalves-Dias, C, Haddad, S et al. (1994). Comparison of a transfusion preparation of newly formed red cells and standard washed red cell transfusions in patients with homozygous β-thalassemia. *Transfusion* 34: 517–520.

Collins, FS and Orringer, EP. (1982). Pulmonary hypertension and cor pulmonale in the sickle hemoglobinopathies. *Am. J. Med.* 73: 814–821.

Comer, GM, Ozick, LA, Sachdev, RK et al. (1991). Transfusion-related chronic liver disease in sickle cell anemia. *Am. J. Gastroenterol.* 86: 1232–1234.

Cooley, TB, Witwer, ER, and Lee, P. (1927). Anemia in children with splenomegaly and peculiar changes in the bones. *Am. J. Dis. Child.* 34: 347–363.

Cooper, C, Lynagh, G, Hider, RC et al. (1996). Inhibition of ribonucleotide reductase by intracellular iron chelation as monitored by electron paramagnetic resonance. *J. Biol. Chem.* 271: 20291–20299.

Cooper, PJ, Iancu, TC, Ward, RJ et al. (1988). Quantitative analysis of immunogold labelling for ferritin in liver from control and iron-overloaded rats. *Histochem. J.* 20: 499–509.

Corash, L, Klein, H, Deisseroth, A et al. (1981). Selective isolation of young erythrocytes for transfusion support of thalassemia major patients. *Blood* 57: 599–606.

Costagliola, DG, de Montalembert, M, Lefrere, JJ et al. (1994). Dose of desferrioxamine and evolution of HIV-1 infection in thalassaemic patients. *Br. J. Haematol.* 87: 849–852.

Cox, JV, Steane, E, Cunningham, G, and Frenkel, EP. (1988). Risk of alloimmunization and delayed hemolytic transfusion reactions in patients with sickle cell disease. *Arch. Intern. Med.* 148: 2485–2489.

Cragg, L, Hebbel, RP, Solovey, A et al. (1996). The iron chelator L1 potentiates iron-mediated oxidative DNA damage. *Blood* 88 (Supplement 1): 646a (abstract).

Crichton, RR, Roman, F, and Roland, F. (1980). Iron mobilisation from ferritin by chelating agents. *J. Inorg. Biochem.* 13: 305–316.

Cunningham, FG, Pritchard, JA, and Mason, R. (1983). Pregnancy and sickle cell hemoglobinopathies; Results with and without prophylactic transfusions. *Obstet. Gynaecol.* 62: 419–424.

Davies, S, Hentroth, JS, and Brozovic, M. (1984a). Effect of blood transfusion on iron status in sickle cell anaemia. *Clin. Lab. Haematol.* 6: 17–22.

Davies, SC, Luce, PJ, Win, AA et al. (1984b). Acute chest syndrome in sickle-cell disease. *Lancet* 1: 36–38.

Davies, SC, Marcus, RE, Hungerford, JL et al. (1983). Ocular toxicity of high-dose intravenous desferrioxamine. *Lancet* 2: 181–184.

Davies, SC, McWilliam, AC, and Hewitt, PE. (1986). Red cell alloimmunization in sickle cell disease. *Br. J. Haematol.* 63: 241–245.

Davies, B and Porter, JB. (2000). Long-term outcome of continuous 24-hour deteroxamine infusion via indwelling intraveneous catheters in high risk β-thalassemia. *Blood* 25: 1229–1236.

de Montalembert, M, Beauvais, P, Bachir, D et al. (1993). Cerebrovascular accidents in sickle cell disease. Risk factors and blood transfusion influence. *Eur. J. Pediatr.* 152: 201–204.

de Montalembert, M, Costagliola, DG, Lefrere, JJ et al. (1992). Prevalence of markers for human immunodeficiency virus types 1 and 2, human T-lymphotropic virus type 1, cytomegalovirus, and hepatitis B and C virus in multiply transfused thalassemia patients. The French Study Group on Thalassaemia. *Transfusion* 32: 509–512.

De Sanctis, V, Pinamonti, A, Di Palma, A et al. (1996). Growth and development in thalassaemia major patients with severe bone lesions due to desferrioxamine. *Eur. J. Paediatr.* 155: 368–372.

De Virgillis, S, Congia, M, Frau, F et al. (1988). Desferrioxamine-induced growth retardation in patients with thalassemia major. *J. Pediatr.* 113: 661–669.

Derkay, CS, Bray, G, Milmoe, GJ, and Grundfast, KM. (1991). Adenotonsillectomy in children with sickle cell disease. *South. Med. J.* 84: 205–208.

DeVault, KR, Friedman, LS, and Westerberg, S. (1994). Hepatitis C in sickle cell anemia. *J. Clin. Gastroenterol.* 18: 206–209.

Di Marco, V, Lo Iacono, O, Almasio, P et al. (1997). Long-term efficacy of α-interferon in β-thalassemics with chronic hepatitis C. *Blood* 90: 2207–2212.

Diamond, WJ, Brown, FL, Bitterman, P et al. (1980). Delayed hemolytic reaction presenting as sickle cell crisis. *Ann. Intern. Med.* 93: 231–233.

Dickerhoff, R. (1987). Acute aphasia and loss of vision with desferrioxamine overdose. *J. Pediatr. Hematol. Oncol.* 9: 287–288.

Dobbin, PS, Hider, RC, Hall, AD et al. (1993). Synthesis, physicochemical properties and biological evaluation of N-substituted-2-alkyl-3-hydroxy-4(1H)-pyridinones. *J. Med. Chem.* 36: 2448–2458.

Drysdale, JW and Munro, JE. (1966). Regulation of synthesis and turnover of ferritin in rat liver. *J. Biol. Chem.* 241: 3630–3637.

Emre, U, Miller, ST, Gutierez, M et al. (1995). Effect of transfusion in acute chest syndrome of sickle cell disease. *J. Pediatr.* 127: 901–904.

Emre, U, Miller, ST, Rao, SP, and Rao, M. (1993). Alveolar-arterial oxygen gradient in acute chest syndrome of sickle cell disease. *J. Pediatr.* 123: 272–275.

Fava, RA, Comeau, RD, and Woodworth, RC. (1981). Specific membrane receptors for diferric-transferrin in cultured rat skeletal myocytes and chick-embryo cardiac myocytes. *Bioscience Reports* 1: 377–385.

Finch, CA, Deubelbeiss, K, Cook, JD et al. (1970). Ferrokinetics in man. *J. Clin. Invest.* 49: 17–53.

Fitchett, DH, Coltart, DJ, Littler, WA et al. (1980). Cardiac involvement in secondary haemochromatosis: A catheter biopsy study and analysis of myocardium. *Cardiovasc. Res.* 14: 719–724.

Fleming, MD, Romano, MA, Su, MA et al. (1998). Nramp2 is mutated in the anemic Belgrade (b) rat: Evidence of a role for Nramp2 in endosomal iron transport. *Proc. Natl. Acad. Sci. U.S.A.* 95: 1148–1153.

Flynn, DM, Hoffbrand, AV, and Politis, D. (1982). Subcutaneous desferrioxamine in thalassaemia major. The effects of three years treatment on liver iron, serum ferritin and comments on echocardiography. *Birth Defects* 18: 347–353.

Fosburg, M and Nathan, DG. (1990). Treatment of Cooleys anemia. *Blood* 76: 435–444.

Freedman, MH, Grisaru, D, Olivieri, NF et al. (1990). Pulmonary syndrome in patients with thalassemia receiving intravenous desferrioxamine infusions. *Am. J. Dis. Child.* 144: 565–569.

Freeman, AP, Giles, RW, Berdoukas, VA et al. (1989). Sustained normalisation of cardiac function by chelation therapy in thalassaemia major. *Clin. Lab. Haematol.* 11: 299–307.

Friedman, DF, Lukas, MB, Jawad, A et al. (1996). Alloimmunization to platelets in heavily transfused patients with sickle cell disease. *Blood* 88: 3216–3222.

Frost, AE, Freedman, HH, Westerback, SJ, and Martell, AE. (1958). Chelating tendencies of N,N′-ethylenbis [2-(o-hydroxyphenyl)]-glycene. *J. Am. Chem. Soc.* 80: 530–536.

Fullerton, MW, Philippart, AI, and Lusher, JM. (1981). Preoperative exchange transfusion in sickle cell disease. *J. Pediatr. Surg.* 16: 297–300.

Gabutti, V and Piga, A. (1996). Results of long term chelation therapy. *Acta Haematol.* 95: 26–36.

Gabutti, V, Piga, A, Fortina, P et al. (1980). Correlation between transfusion requirement, blood volume and haemoglobin level in homozygous β-thalassaemia. *Acta Haematol.* 64: 103–108.

Gabutti, V, Piga, A, Nicola, P et al. (1982). Haemoglobin levels and blood requirement in thalassaemia. *Arch. Dis. Child.* 57: 156–157.

Galanello, R, De Virgillis, S, Giagu, N et al. (1999). Evaluation of iron overload in thalassemia intermedia. *Proceedings of the 9th International Conference on Iron Chelation*, Hamburg, Germany.

Gallant, R, Freedman, MH, Vellend, H, and Francome, WH. (1986). *Yersinia* sepsis in patients with iron overload treated with desferrioxamine (letter). *N. Engl. J. Med.* 314: 1643.

Gordeuk, VR, Bacon, BR, and Brittenham, GM. (1987). Iron overload: Causes and consequences. *Ann. Rev. Nutr.* 7: 485–508.

Grady, R and Giardina, P. (1997). Oral iron chelation: Further progress with HBED. *Blood* 90 (Supplement 1): 14b.

Grady, RW and Hershko, C. (1990a). An evaluation of the potential of HBED as an orally effective iron-chelating drug. *Semin. Hematol.* 27: 105–111.

Grady, RW, Hershko, C. (1990b). HBED: A potential oral iron chelator. *Ann. NY. Acad. Sci.* 612: 361–368.

Grady, RW, Salbe, AD, Hilgartner, MW, and Giardina, PJ. (1994). Results from a phase 1 clinical trial of HBED. *Adv. Exp. Med. Biol.* 356: 351–359.

Graziano, JH, Piomelli, S, Hilgartner, M et al. (1981). Chelation therapy in beta-thalassemia major. III. The role of splenectomy in achieving iron balance. *J. Pediatr.* 99: 695–699.

Graziano, JH, Piomelli, S, Seaman, C et al. (1982). A simple technique for preparation of young red cells for transfusion from ordinary blood units. *Blood* 59: 865–868.

Griffin, TC and Buchanan, GR. (1993). Elective surgery in children with sickle cell disease without preoperative blood transfusion. *J. Pediatr. Surg.* 28: 681–685.

Gutteridge, JMC and Halliwell, B. (1989). Iron toxicity and oxygen radicals. *Baillieres Clin. Haematol.* 2: 195–256.

Gutteridge, JMC, Richmond, R, and Halliwell, B. (1979). Inhibition of iron catalysed formation of hydroxyl radicals from superoxide and of lipid peroxidation by desferrioxamine. *Biochem. J.* 184: 469–472.

Gutteridge, JMC, Rowley, DA, Griffiths, E, and Halliwell, B. (1985). Low molecular weight iron complexes and oxygen radical reactions in idiopathic haemochromatosis. *Clin. Sci.* 68: 463–467.

Haberkern, CM, Neumayr, LD, Orringer, EP et al. (1997). Cholecystectomy in sickle cell anemia patients: Perioperative outcome of 364 cases from the National Preoperative Transfusion Study. *Blood* 89: 1533–1542.

Halvorson, DJ, Mckie, V, McKie, K et al. (1997). Sickle cell disease and tonsillectomy: Preoperative management and postoperative complications. *Arch. Otolarngol. Head Neck Surg.* 123: 689–692.

Hamre, MR, Harmaon, EP, and Kirkpatrick, DV. (1991). Priapism as a complication of sickle cell disease. *J. Urol.* 145: 1–5.

Hartmatz, P, Quirolo, K, Singer, T et al. (1999). Development of hemochromatosis in patients with sickle cell disease (SCD) receiving chronic RBC transfusion therapy. *Proceedings of 9th International Conference on Oral Iron Chelation*, Hamburg, Germany.

Hasan, MF, Marsh, F, Posner, G et al. (1996). Chronic hepatitis C in patients with sickle cell disease. *Am. J. Gastroenterol.* 91: 1204–1206.

Hassell, KL, Eckman, JR, and Lane, PA. (1994). Acute multi-organ failure syndrome: A potentially catastrophic complication of severe sickle cell pain episodes. *Am. J. Med.* 96: 155–162.

Hershko, C. (1975). A study of the chelating agent diethyl-enetriaminepentacetic acid using selective radioiron probes of reticuloendothelial and parenchymal iron stores. *J. Lab. Clin. Med.* 85: 913–921.

Hershko, C. (1978). Determinants of fecal and urinary iron excretion in rats. *Blood* 51: 415–423.

Hershko, C, Cook, JD, and Finch, CA. (1973). Storage iron kinetics III. Study of desferrioxamine action by selective radioiron labels of RE and parenchymal cells. *J. Lab. Clin. Med.* 81: 876–886.

Hershko, C, Grady, R, and Link, G. (1984). Phenolic ethyl-enediamine derivatives: A study of orally effective iron chelators. *J. Lab. Clin. Med.* 103: 337–346.

Hershko, C, Grady, RW, and Cerami, A. (1978a). Mechanism of desferrioxamine-induced iron excretion in the hypertransfused rat: Definition of two alternative pathways of iron mobilisation. *J. Lab. Clin. Med.* 92: 144–151.

Hershko, C, Graham, G, Bates, GW, and Rachmilewitz, EA. (1978b). Non-specific serum iron in thalassaemia: An abnormal serum fraction of potential toxicity. *Br. J. Haematol.* 40: 255–263.

Hershko, C and Rachmilewitz, EA. (1979). Mechanism of desferrioxamine induced iron excretion in thalassaemia. *Br. J. Haematol.* 42: 125–132.

Hider, RC, Choudhury, R, Rai, BL et al. (1996). Design of orally active iron chelators. *Acta Haematol.* 95: 6–12.

Hider, RC, Kontoghiorghes, G, and Silver, J. (1982). Pharmaceutical compositions. UK Patent GB 2118176A.,

Hider, RC, Porter, JB, and Singh, S. (1994). The design of therapeutically useful iron chelators. In RJ Bergeron and G. Brittenham, eds, *The development of iron chelators for clinical use*. Boca Raton, FL: CRC Press.

Hilliard, LM, Williams, BF, Lounsbury, AE, and Howard, TH. (1998). Erythrocytapheresis limits iron accumulation in chronically transfused sickle cell patients. *Am. J. Hematol.* 59: 28–35.

Hoffbrand, AV. (1994). Prospects for oral iron chelation. *J. Lab. Clin. Med.* 21: 86–92.

Hoffbrand, AV, Al-Refaie, F, Davis, B et al. (1998). Long-term deferiprone in 51 transfusion-dependent iron over-loaded patients. *Blood* 91: 295–300.

Hoffbrand, AV, Bartlett, AN, Veys, PA et al. (1989). Agranulocytosis and thrombocytopenia in patients with Blackfan-Diamond anaemia during oral chelator trial (letter). *Lancet* 2: 457.

Hogman, CF. (1998). Preparation and preservation of red cells. *Vox Sang.* 74 (Suppl 2): 177–187.

Holzmann, L, Finn, H, Lichtman, HC, and Harmel, MH. (1969). Anesthesia in patients with sickle cell disease: A review of 112 cases. *Anesth. Anal.* Z48: 566–572.

Homi, J, Reynolds, J, and Skinner, A et al. (1979). General anesthesia in sickle cell disease. *Br. Med. J.* 1: 1599–1601.

Houglum, K, Filip, M, Witztum, JL, and Chojkier, M. (1990). Malondialdehyde and 4-hydroxynonenal protein adducts in plasma and liver of rats with iron overload. *J. Clin. Invest.* 86: 1991–1998.

Houglum, K, Ramm, GA, Crawford, DH et al. (1997). Excess iron induces hepatic oxidative stress and trans-forming growth factor beta 1 in genetic hemochromatosis. *Hepatology* 26: 605–610.

Howard, RJ, Tuck, SM, and Pearson, TC. (1995). Pregnancy in sickle cell disease in the UK: Results of a multicentre survey of the effect of prophylactic blood transfusion on maternal and fetal outcome. *Br. J. Obstetr. Gynaecol.* 102: 947–951.

Hoy, T, Humphrys, J, Jacobs, A et al. (1979). Effective iron chelation following oral administration of an isoniazid-pyridoxal hydrazone. *Br. J. Haematol.* 43: 443–449.

Hoyes, KP, Abeysinghe, RD, Jones, HM et al. (1993). In vivo and in vitro effects of 3-hydroxypyridin-4-one chelators on murine haemopoeisis. *Exp. Hematol.* 21: 86–92.

Hoyes, KP, Hider, RC, and Porter, JB. (1992). Cell cycle syn-chronisation and growth inhibition by 3-hydroxypyridi-none iron chelators in leukaemia cell lines. *Cancer Res.* 52: 4591–4599.

Hoyes, KP and Porter, JB. (1993). Subcellular distribution of desferrioxamine and hydroxypyridin-4-one chelators in K562 cells affects chelation of intracellular iron pools. *Br. J. Haematol.* 85: 393–400.

Hussain, MAM, Flynn, DM, Green, N et al. (1976). Subcutaneous infusion and intramuscular injection of des-ferrioxamine in patients with transfusional iron overload. *Lancet* 2: 1278–1280.

Hwang, CF, Lee, CY, Lee, PI et al. (1994). Pyogenic liver abscess in beta-thalassemia major- -report of two cases. *Chung Hua Min Kuo Hsiao Erh Ko I Hsueh Hui Tsa Chih* 35: 466–467.

Jacobs, A. (1974). The pathology of iron overload. In A. Jacobs and M. Worwood, editors, *Iron in biochemistry and medicine*. London: Academic Press.

Jacobs, A. (1977). Low molecular weight intracellular iron transport compounds. *Blood* 50: 433–439.

Jan, K, Usami, S, and Smith, JA. (1982). Effects of transfu-sion on rheological properties of blood in sickle cell ane-mia. *Transfusion* 22: 17–20.

Janes, SL, Pocock, M, Bishop, E, and Bevan, DH. (1997). Automated red cell exchange in sickle cell disease. *Br. J. Haematol.* 97: 256–258.

Janik, J and Seeler, RA. (1980). Perioperative management of children with sickle hemoglobinopathy. *J. Pediatr. Surg.* 15: 117–120.

Jensen, PD, Heickendorff, L, Pedersen, B et al. (1996). The effect of iron chelation on haemopoiesis in MDS patients with transfusional iron overload. *Br. J. Haematol.* 94: 288–299.

Karayalcin, G, Shende, A, Festa, R, and Lanzkowsky, P. (1984). Partial exchange transfusion for treatment of priapism in children with sickle cell disease. *Pediatr. Res.* 18: 242a.

Kayyali, RS, Porter, JB, and Hider, RC. (1997). Design of 3-hydroxypyridin-4-one chelators with minimal inhibitory properties towards iron-containing metalloenzymes. *J. Pharmaceut. Pharmacol.* 49: 97a.

Kayyali, RS, Porter, JB, and Hider, RC. (1998). The design of low toxicity 3-hydroxypyridin-4-one iron chelators. *J. Pharm. Pharmacol.* 50: 261a.

Kim, HC, Dugan, NP, Silber, JH et al. (1994). Erythrocytapheresis therapy to reduce iron overload in chronically transfused patients with sickle cell disease. *Blood* 83: 1136–1142.

King, KE, Shirey, RS, Lankiewicz, MW et al. (1997). Delayed hemolytic transfusion reactions in sickle cell disease: simultaneous destruction of recipients' red cells. *Transfusion* 37: 376–381.

Kinney, TR, Harris, MB, and Russell, MO. (1975). Priapism in association with sickle hemoglobinopathies in children. *J. Pediatr.* 86: 241–242.

Kinney, TR, Ware, RE, Schultz, WH, and Filston, HC. (1990). Long-term management of splenic sequestration in children with sickle cell disease. *J. Pediatr.* 117: 194–199.

Klein, HG. (1982). Transfusions with young erythrocytes (neocytes) in sickle cell anemia. *Am. J. Pediatr. Hematol. Oncol.* 4: 162–165.

Klein, HG, Garner, RJ, Miller, DM et al. (1980). Automated partial exchange transfusion in sickle cell anemia. *Transfusion* 20: 578–584.

Kleinman, S, Thompson-Breton, R, Breen, D et al. (1981). Exchange red blood cell pheresis in a pediatric patient with severe complications of sickle cell anemia. *Transfusion* 21: 443–446.

Kontoghiorghes, GJ, Aldouri, MA, Hoffbrand, AV et al. (1987a). Effective chelation of iron in β thalassaemia with the oral chelator 1,2,dimethyl-3-hydroxypyridin-4-one. *Br. Med. J.* 295: 1509–1512.

Kontoghiorghes, GJ, Aldouri, MA, Sheppard, L, and Hoffbrand, AV. (1987b). 1,2-dimethyl-3-hydroxypyrid-4-one, an orally active chelator for treatment of iron overload. *Lancet* 1: 1294–1295.

Kontoghiorghes, GJ, Goddard, JG, Bartlett, AN, and Sheppard, L. (1990). Pharmacokinetic studies in humans with the oral iron chelator 1,2-dimethyl-3-hydroxypyrid-4-one. *Clin. Pharmacol.* 48: 255–261.

Kontoghiorghes, GJ, Sheppard, L, and Barr, J. (1988). Iron balance studies with the oral chelator 1,2,dimethyl-3-hydroxypyridin-4-one. *Br. J. Haematol.* 69: 129a.

Koren, G, Bentur, Y, Strong, D et al. (1990). Acute changes in renal function associated with desferrioxamine therapy. *Am. J. Dis. Child.* 143: 1077–1080.

Koren, G, Kochavi Atiya, Y, Bentur, Y, and Olivieri, NF. (1991). The effects of subcutaneous deferoxamine administration on renal function in thalassemia major. *Int. J. Hematol.* 54: 371–375.

Kornbrust, DJ and Mavis, RD. (1980). Microsomal lipid peroxidation. 1. Characterisation of the role of iron and NADPH. *Mol. Pharmacol.* 17: 400–407.

Koshy, M and Burd, L. (1991). Management of pregnancy in sickle cell syndromes. *Hematol. Oncol. Clin. North Am.* 5: 585–596.

Koshy, M, Burd, L, Wallace, D et al. (1988). Prophylactic red-cell transfusions in pregnant patients with sickle cell disease. A randomized cooperative study. *N. Engl. J. Med.* 319: 1447–1452.

Koshy, M, Weiner, SJ, Miller, ST et al. (1995). Surgery and anesthesia in sickle cell disease. Cooperative study of sickle cell diseases. *Blood* 86: 3676–3684.

Kouides, PA, Slapak, CA, Rosenwasser, LJ, and Miller, KB. (1988). *Pneumocystis carinii* pneumonia as a complication of desferrioxamine therapy. *Br. J. Haematol.* 70: 382–384.

Kumar, RM, Rizk, DEE, and Khuranna, A. (1997). β-Thalassemia major and successful pregnancy. *J. Reprod. Med.* 42: 294–298.

Kumar, RM, Rizk, DEE, and Khuranna, AK. (1996). Unscreened transfusion related human immunodeficiency virus type-1 infection amongst Indian thalassemic children (letter). *Am. J. Hematol.* 53: 51–52.

Kutukculer, N, Kutlu, O, Nisli, G et al. (1996). Assessment of neutrophil chemotaxis and random migration in children with thalassemia major. *Pediatr. Hematol. Oncol.* 13: 239–245.

L'Eplattenier, F, Murase, I, and Martell, AE. (1967). New multidentate ligands. VI. Chelating tendencies of N,N'-do(2-hydroxybenzyl) ethylenediamine-N-N'diacetic acid. *J. Am. Chem. Soc.* 89: 837–843.

Landau, H, Matoth, I, Landau-Cordova, Z et al. (1993). Cross-sectional and longditudinal study of the pituitary-thyroid axis in patients with thalassaemia major. *Clin. Endocrinol.* 38: 55–61.

Lange, R, Lameijer, W, Roozendaal, KL, and Kersten, M. (1993). Pharmaceutical analysis and pharmacokinetics of the oral iron chelator 1,2-dimethyl-3-hydroxypyridi-4-one (DMHP). *Proceedings of 4th International Conference on Oral Chelation,* Limasol, Cyprus,

Lanzkowsky, P, Shende, A, Karayalcin, G et al. (1978). Partial exchange transfusion in sickle cell anemia. Use in children with serious complications. *Am. J. Dis. Child.* 32: 1206–1208.

Larson, PJ, Freidman, DF, Reilly, MP et al. (1997). The presurgical management with erythrocytapheresis of a patient with a high-oxygen-affinity, unstable Hb variant (Hb Bryn Mawr). *Transfusion* 37: 703–707.

Larson, PJ, Lukas, MB, Freidman, DF, and Manno, CS. (1996). Delayed hemolytic transfusion reaction due to anti-Go(a), an antibody against the low-prevalence gonzales antigen. *Am. J. Hematol.* 53: 248–250.

Le Sage, GD, Kost, LJ, Barham, SS, and LaRusso, NF. (1986). Biliary excretion of iron from hepatocyte lysosomes in the rat: A major excretory pathway in experimental iron overload. *J. Clin. Invest.* 77: 90–97.

Lee, P, Mohammed, N, Abeysinghe, RD et al. (1993). Intravenous infusion pharmacokinetics of desferrioxamine in thalassaemia patients. *Drug Metab. Dispos.* 21: 640–644.

Lefrere, JJ, Girot, R. (1987). HIV infection in polytransfused thalassemic patients. *Lancet*, 2, 686 (letter).

Lefrere, JJ and Girot, R. (1989). Risk of HIV infection in polytransfused thalassemic patients (letter). *Lancet* 2: 813.

Letsky, EA, Miller, F, Worwood, M, and Flynn, DM. (1974). Serum ferritin in children with thalassaemia regularly transfused. *J. Clin. Pathol.* 27: 1213–1216.

Liang, ST, Wong, VCW, So, WWK et al. (1985). Homozygous α-thalassaemia: Clinical presentation, diagnosis and management. A review of 46 cases. *Br. J. Obstetr. Gynaecol.* 92: 680–684.

Link, G, Pinson, A, and Hershko, C. (1985). Heart cells in culture: A model of myocardial iron overload and chelation. *J. Lab. Clin. Med.* 106: 147–153.

Link, G, Pinson, A, and Hershko, C. (1993). Iron loading of cultured cardiac myocytes modifies sarcolemmal structure and increases lysosomal fragility. *J. Lab. Clin. Med.* 121: 127–134.

Link, G, Pinson, A, Kahane, I, and Hershko, C. (1989). Iron loading modifies the fatty acid composition of cultured rat myocardial cells and liposomal vesicles: Effect of ascorbate and alpha-tocopherol on myocardial lipid peroxidation. *J. Lab. Clin. Med.* 114: 243–249.

Longo, F, Fischer, R, Engelbert, R et al. (1998). Iron balance in thalassemia patients treated with deferiprone. *Blood* 92: 235a.

Longo, F, Fischer, R, Engelbert, R et al. (1998). Iron balance in thalassemia patients treated with deferiprone. *Blood* 92. Supplement 1.235a abstract 1333.

Longo, F, Vol, V, Gaglioti, R et al. (1999). Factors Influencing the efficacy of deferiprone treatment. Proceedings of the 9th International conference on oral iron chelation. *Hamburg*, p. 24.

Luban, NLC. (1989). Variability in rates of alloimmunization in different groups of children with sickle cell disease: Effect of ethnic background. *Am. J. Pediatr. Hematol. Oncol.* 11: 314–319.

Mallouh, AA and Asha, A. (1988). Beneficial effect of blood transfusion in children with sickle cell chest syndrome. *Am. J. Dis. Child.* 142: 178–182.

Marcus, RE, Davies, SC, Bantock, HM et al. (1984). Desferrioxamine to improve cardiac function in iron overloaded patients with thalassaemia major. *Lancet* 1: 392–393.

Marcus, RE, Wonke, B, Bantock, HM et al. (1985). A prospective trial of young red cells in 48 patients with transfusion-dependent thalassaemia. *Br. J. Haematol.* 60: 153–159.

Marx, JJM and van Asbeck, BS. (1996). Use of chelators in preventing hydroxyl radical damage: Adult respiratory distress syndrome as an experimental model for the treatment of oxygen-radical-mediated tissue damage. *Acta Haematol.* 95: 49–62.

Mavrogeni, SI, Maris, T, Gouliamos, A et al. (1998). Myocardial iron deposition in beta-thalassemia studied by magnetic resonance imaging. *Int. J. Cardiol. Imag.* 14: 117–122.

Mazza, P, Giua, R, De Marco, S et al. (1995). Iron overload in thalassemia: comparative analysis of magnetic resonance imaging, serum ferritin and iron content of the liver. *Haematologica* 80: 398–404.

McIntosh, N. (1976). Endocrinopathy in thalassaemia major. *Arch. Dis. Child.* 51: 195–201.

Mehta, J, Chablani, A, Reporter, R et al. (1993). Autoantibodies in thalassaemia major: Relationship with oral iron chelator L1. *J. Assoc. Physicians India* 41: 339–341.

Mehta, J, Singhal, S, Revanker, R et al. (1991). Fatal systemic lupus erythematosus in patient taking oral iron chelator L1 (letter). *Lancet* 337: 298.

Menitove, JE. (1996). Transfusion-transmitted infections: Update. *Semin. Hematol.* 33: 290–301.

Michail-Merianou, V, Pamphili-Panousopoulou, L, Piperi-Lowes, L et al. (1987). Alloimmunization to red cell antigens in thalassemia: Comparative study of usual versus better-match transfusion programmes. *Vox Sang.* 52: 95–98.

Miller, KB, Rosenwasser, LJ, Bessette, JM et al. (1981). Rapid desensitization for desferrioxamine anaphylactic reaction (letter). *Lancet* 1: 1059.

Miller, ST, Jensen, D, and Rao, SP. (1992). Less intensive long-term transfusion therapy for sickle cell anemia and cerebrovascular accident. *J. Pediatr.* 120: 54–57.

Miller, ST, Rao, SP, Dunn, EK, and Glassberg, KI. (1995). Priapism in children with sickle cell disease. *J. Urol.* 154: 844–847.

Modell, B. (1977). Total management of thalassaemia major. *Arch. Dis. Child.* 52: 485–500.

Modell, B. (1979). Advances in the use of iron-chelating agents for the treatment of iron overload. *Prog. Haematol.* 11: 267–312.

Modell, B, Letsky, EA, Flynn, DM et al. (1982). Survival and desferrioxamine in thalassaemia major. *Br. Med. J.* 284: 1081–1084.

Modell, B and Matthews, R. (1976). Thalassemia in Britain and Australia. *Birth Defects Original Article Series* 12: 13–29.

Modell, CB and Beck, J. (1974). Long term desferrioxamine therapy in thalassaemia. *Ann. NY Acad. Sci.* 232: 201–210.

Mollison, PL, Engelfriet, CP, and Contreras, M. (1997). *Blood transfusion in clinical medicine* (10th ed.). Oxford: Blackwell Science.

Morrison, JC, Morrison, FS, and Floyd, RC. (1991). Use of continuous flow erythrocytapheresis in pregnant patients with sickle cell disease. *J. Clin. Apheresis* 6: 224–229.

Morrison, JC, Schneider, JM, and Whybrew, WD. (1980). Prophylactic transfusions in pregnant patients with sickle hemoglobinopathies: Benefit versus risk. *Obstetr. Gynecol.* 56: 274–280.

Morrison, JC, Whybrew, WD, and Bucovaz, ET. (1978). Use of partial exchange transfusion perioperatively in patients with sickle hemoglobinopathies. *Am. J. Obstetr. Gynecol.* 132: 59–63.

Morrison, JC and Wiser, WL. (1976a). The use of prophylactic partial exchange transfusion in pregnancies associated with sickle cell hemoglobinopathies. *Obstetr. Gynecol.* 48: 516–520.

Morrison, JC and Wiser, WL. (1976b). The effect of maternal partial exchange transfusion on the infants of patients with sickle cell anemia. *J. Pediatr.* 89: 286–289.

Mozzi, F, Rebulla, P, Lillo, F et al. (1992). HIV and HTLV infections in 1305 transfusion-dependent thalassemis in Italy. *AIDS* 6: 505–508.

Mulligan, MM, Althus, B, and Linder, MC. (1986). Non-ferritin, non-heme iron pools in rat tissues. *Int. J. Biochem.* 18: 791–798.

Myers, BM, Prendergast, FG, Holman, R et al. (1991). Alterations in the structure, physicochemical properties, and pH of hepatocyte lysosomes in experimental iron overload. *J. Clin. Invest.* 88: 1207–1215.

Nielsen, P, Fischer, R, Engelhardt, R et al. (1995). Liver iron stores in patients with secondary haemosiderosis under iron chelation therapy with deferoxamine or deferiprone. *Br. J. Haematol.* 91: 827–833.

Nienhuis, AW. (1981). Vitamin C and iron. *N. Engl. J. Med.* 304: 170–171.

Noe, HN, Wilimas, J, and Jerkins, GR. (1981). Surgical management of priapism in children with sickle cell anemia. *J. Urol.* 126: 770–771.

O'Brien, RT. (1978). Iron burden in sickle cell anemia. *J. Pediatr.* 92: 579–588.

O'Brien, RT, Pearson, HA, and Spencer, RP. (1972). Transfusion-induced decrease in spleen size in thalassemia major: Documentation by radioisotopic scan. *J. Pediatr.* 81: 105–107.

Oduro, A and Searle, JF. (1972). Anaesthesia in sickle cell states: A plea for simplicity. *Br. Med. J.* 4: 596–598.

Olivieri, NF. (1996). Randomised trial of deferiprone and DFO in thalassemia major. *Blood* 88 (supplement 1): 651a.

Olivieri, NF, Berriman, AM, Tyler, BJ et al. (1992a). Reduction in tissue iron stores with a new regimen of continuous ambulatory intravenous deferoxamine. *Am. J. Hematol.* 41: 61–63.

Olivieri, NF and Brittenham, GM. (1997). Iron-chelating therapy and the treatment of thalassemia. *Blood* 89: 739–761.

Olivieri, NF, Brittenham, GM, Matsui, D et al. (1995). Iron-chelation therapy with oral deferiprone in patients with thalassemia major. *N. Engl. J. Med.* 332: 918–922.

Olivieri, NF, Brittenham, GM, McLaren, CE et al. (1998). Long-term safety and effectiveness of iron-chelation therapy with deferiprone for thalassemia major. *N. Engl. J. Med.* 339: 417–423.

Olivieri, NF, Buncic, JR, Chew, E et al. (1986). Visual and auditory neurotoxicity in patients receiving subcutaneous desferrioxamine infusions. *N. Engl. J. Med.* 314: 869–873.

Olivieri, NF, Koren, G, Harris, J et al. (1992b). Growth failure and bony changes induced by deferoxamine. *Am. J. Pediatr. Hematol. Oncol.* 14: 48–56.

Olivieri, NF, Koren, G, Herman, C et al. (1990). Comparison of oral iron chelator L1 and desferrioxamine in iron loaded patients. *Lancet* 336: 1275–1279.

Olivieri, NF, Koren, G, Matsui, D et al. (1992c). Reduction of tissue iron stores and normalization of serum ferritin during treatment with the oral iron chelator L1 in thalassemia intermedia. *Blood* 79: 2741–2748.

Olivieri, NF, Nathan, DG, MacMillan, JH et al. (1994). Survival in medically treated patients with homozygous beta-thalassemia. *N. Engl. J. Med.* 331: 574–578.

Olivieri, NF, Saxon, BR, Nisbet-Brown, E et al. (1999). Quantitative assessment of tissue iron in patients with sickle cell disease. *Proceedings of 9th International Conference on Oral Iron Chelation*, Hamburg, Germany.

Orlina, AR, Sosler, SD, and Koshy, M. (1991). Problems of chronic transfusion in sickle cell disease. *J. Clin. Apheresis*, 6: 234–240.

Orlina, AR, Unger, PJ, and Koshy, M. (1978). Post-transfusion alloimmunization in patients with sickle cell disease. *Am. J. Hematol.* 5: 101–106.

Ouattara, SA, Gody, M, Rioche, M et al. (1998). Blood transufsions and HIV infections in Ivory Coast. *J. Trop. Med. Hyg.* 91: 212–215.

Parkes, JG, Hussain, RA, Olivieri, NF, and Templeton, DM. (1993). Effects of iron loading on uptake, speciation, and chelation of iron in cultured myocardial cells. *J. Lab. Clin. Med.* 122: 36–47.

Parola, M, Pinzani, A, Casini, E et al. (1993). Stimulation of lipid peroxidation or 4-hydroxynonenal treatment increased procollagen (I) gene expression in human fat storing cells. *J. Biol. Chem.* 264: 16957–16962.

Patten, E, Patel, SN, Soto, B, and Gayle, RA. (1989). Prevalence of certain clinically significant alloantibodies in sickle cell disease patients. *Ann. NY. Acad. Sci.* 565: 443–445.

Pegelow, CH, Adams, RJ, McKie, V et al. (1995). Risk of recurrent stroke in patients with sickle cell disease treated with erythrocyte transfusions. *J. Pediatr.* 126: 896–899.

Petz, LD, Calhoun, L, Shulman, IA et al. (1997). The sickle cell hemolytic transfusion reaction syndrome. *Transfusion,* 37: 382–392.

Phillips, G, Becker, B, Keller, VA, and Hartman, J. (1992). Hypothyroidism in adults with sickle cell anemia. *Am. J. Med.* 92: 567–570.

Piga, A, Facello, O, Gaglioti, G et al. (1998). No progression of liver fibrosis in thalassaemia major during deferiprone or desferrioxamine iron chelation. *Blood* 92 (supplement 2): 21b.

Piga, A, Longo, F, Consolati, A et al. (1997). Mortality and morbidity in thalassemia with conventional treatment. *Bone Marrow Transplant.* 19 (Supplement 2): 11–15.

Piga, A, Luzzatto, L, Capalbo, P et al. (1988). High dose desferrioxamine as a cause of growth failure in thalassaemic patients. *Eur. J. Haematol.* 40: 380–381.

Pinna, AD, Argiolu, F, Marongiu, L, and Pinna, DC. (1988). Indications and results for splenectomy for beta thalassemia in two hundred and twenty-one pediatric patients. *Surg. Gynecol. Obstetr.* 167: 109–113.

Piomelli, S. (1995). The management of patients with Cooley's anemia: Transfusions and splenectomy. *Semin. Hematol.* 32: 262–268.

Piomelli, S, Danoff, SJ, Becker, MH et al. (1969). Prevention of bone malformations and cardiomegaly in Cooley's anemia by early hypertransfusion regimens. *Ann. NY. Acad. Sci.* 165: 427–436.

Piomelli, S, Seaman, C, Reibman, J et al. (1978). Separation of younger red cells with improved survival *in vivo*: An approach to chronic transfusion therapy. *Proc. Natl. Acad. Sci.* 75: 3474–3478.

Pippard, MJ. (1989). Desferrioxamine-induced iron excretion in humans. *Baillieres Clin. Haematol.* 2.2: 323–343.

Pippard, MJ, Callender, ST, Warner, GT, and Weatherall, DJ. (1979). Iron absorption and loading in β-thalassaemia intermedia. *Lancet* 2: 819–821.

Pippard, MJ, Callender, ST, and Weatherall, DJ. (1978a). Intensive iron-chelation with desferrioxamine in iron-loading anaemias. *Clin. Sci. Mol. Med.* 54: 99–106.

Pippard, MJ, Johnson, DK, Callender, ST, and Finch, CA. (1982a). Ferrioxamine excretion in iron loaded man. *Blood* 60: 288–294.

Pippard, MJ, Johnson, DK, and Finch, CA. (1982b). Hepatocyte iron kinetics in the rat explored with an iron chelator. *Br. J. Haematol.* 52: 211–224.

Pippard, MJ, Letsky, EA, Callender, ST, and Weatherall, DJ. (1978b). Prevention of iron loading in transfusion dependent thalasaemia. *Lancet* 1: 1179–1181.

Pippard, MJ, Pattanapanyssat, K, Tiperkae, J, and Hider, RC. (1989). Metabolism of the iron chelates of desferrioxamine and hydroxypyridinones in the rat. *Proceedings of the European Iron Club,* Budapest, Hungary.

Pippard, MJ and Weatherall, DW, (1984). Iron absorption in iron-loading anaemias. *Haematologica* 17: 407–414.

Pitt, CG, Bao, Y, Thompson, J et al. (1986). Esters and lactones of phenolic amino carboxylic acids: Prodrugs for iron chelation. *J. Med. Chem.* 29: 1231–1237.

Platt, OS, Thorington, BD, Brambilla, DJ et al. (1991). Pain in sickle cell disease. *N. Engl. J. Med.* 325: 11–16.

Pollack, S. (1994). Intracellular iron. *Adv. Exp. Med. Biol.* 356: 165–171.

Poncz, M, Kane, E, and Gill, FM. (1985). Acute chest syndrome in sickle cell disease: Etiology and clinical correlates. *J. Pediatr.* 107: 861–866.

Ponka, P, Borova, J, Neuwirt, J, and Fuchs, O. (1979a). Mobilisation of iron from reticulocytes. Identification of pyridoxal isonicotinoyl hydrazone as a new iron chelating agent. *FEBS Lett.* 97: 317–321.

Ponka, P, Borova, J, Neuwirt, J et al. (1979b). A study of intracellular iron metabolism using pyridoxal isonicotyl hydrazone and other synthetic chelating agents. *Biochim. Biophys. Acta.* 586: 278–297.

Pootrakul, P, Hungsprenges, S, Fucharoen, S et al. (1981). Relation between erythropoiesis and bone metabolism in thalassemia. *N. Engl. J. Med.* 304: 1470–1473.

Pootrakul, P, Kitcharoen, K, Yansukon, P et al. (1988). The effect of erythroid hyperplasia on iron balance. *Blood* 71: 1124–1129.

Porter, JB. (1996). Evaluation of chelators for clinical use. *Acta Haematol.* 95: 13–25.

Porter, JB, Abeysinghe, RD, Hoyes, KP et al. (1993). Contrasting interspecies efficacy and toxicology of 1,2-diethyl-3-hydroxypyridin-4-one, CP94, relates to differing metabolism of the iron chelating site. *Br. J. Haematol.* 85: 159–168.

Porter, JB, Abeysinghe, RD, Marshall, L et al. (1996). Kinetics of removal and reappearance of non-transferrin-bound plasma iron with desferrioxamine therapy. *Blood* 88: 705–714.

Porter, JB, Alberti, D, Hassan, I et al. (1997). Subcutaneous depot desferrioxamine (CGH 749B): Relationship of pharmacokinetics to efficacy and drug metabolism. *Blood* 90: 265a.

Porter, JB and Faherty, AM. (1996). 12 years experience of intravenous desferrioxamine using indwelling intravenous devices in thalassaemia. *Br. J. Haematol.* 93 (supplement 1): 86a.

Porter, JB, Gyparaki, M, Burke, LC et al. (1988). Iron mobilization from hepatocyte monolayer cultures by chelators: The importance of membrane permeability and the iron binding constant. *Blood* 72: 1497–1503.

Porter, JB, Hider, RC, and Huehns, ER. (1989a). The development of iron chelating drugs. *Baillieres Clin. Haematol.* 2: 257–292.

Porter, JB, Hoyes, KP, Abeysinghe, R et al. (1989b). Animal toxicology of iron chelator L1 (letter). *Lancet* 2: 156.

Porter, JB, Hoyes, KP, Abeysinghe, RD et al. (1991). Comparison of the subacute toxicity and efficacy of 3-hydroxypyridin-4-one iron chelators in overloaded and non-overloaded mice. *Blood* 79: 2727–2734.

Porter, JB and Huehns, ER. (1987). Transfusion and exchange transfusion in sickle cell anaemia, with particular reference to iron metabolism. *Acta Haematol.* 78: 198–205.

Porter, JB and Huehns, ER. (1989). The toxic effects of desferrioxamine. *Baillieres Clin. Haematol.* 2: 459–474.

Porter, JB, Jaswon, MS, Huehns, ER et al. (1989c). Desferrioxamine ototoxicity: evaluation of risk factors in thalassaemic patients and guidelines for safe dosage. *Br. J. Haematol.* 73: 403–409.

Porter, JB, Morgan, J, Hoyes, KP et al. (1990). Relative oral efficacy and acute toxicity of hydroxypyridin-4-one iron chelators in mice. *Blood* 76: 2389–2396.

Porter, JB, Singh, S, Hoyes, KP. (1994). Lessons from preclinical and clinical studies with hydroxypyridinone chelators. *Adv. Exp. Med. Biol.* 356: 361–370.

Porter, JB, Weir, DT, Davis, B et al. (1998). Iron balance and chelation efficiency following single dose depot desferrioxamine. *Blood* 92 (supplement 1): 325a.

Powars, D, Weidman, JA, Odom-Maryon, T et al. (1988). Sickle cell chronic lung disease: Prior morbidity and the risk of pulmonary failure. *Medicine* 67: 66–76.

Powars, D, Wilson, B, Imbus, C et al. (1978). The natural history of stroke in sickle cell disease. *Am. J. Med.* 65: 461–471.

Prati, D, Lin, Y, De Mattei, C et al. (1999). A prospective study on TT virus infection in transfusion-dependent patients with β-thalassemia. *Blood* 93: 1502–1505.

Prati, D, Zanella, A, Bosoni, P et al. (1998). The incidence and natural course of transfusion-associated GB virus C/hepatitis G virus infection in a cohort of thalassemic patients. The Cooleycare Cooperative Group. *Blood* 91: 774–777.

Prieto, J, Barry, M, and Sherlock, S. (1975). Serum ferritin in patients with iron overload and with acute and chronic liver disease. *Gastroenterology* 68: 525–533.

Propper, RD, Button, LN, and Nathan, DG. (1980). New approaches to the transfusion management of thalassemia. *Blood* 55: 55–60.

Propper, RL, Cooper, B, Rufo, RR et al. (1977). Continuous subcutaneous administration of desferrioxamine in patients with iron overload. *N. Engl. J. Med.* 297: 418–423.

Rackoff, WR, Ohene-Frempong, K, and Month, S. (1992). Neurological events after partial exchange transfusion for priapism in sickle cell disease. *J. Pediatr.* 120: 882–885.

Rahko, PS, Salerni, R, and Uretsky, BF. (1986). Successful reversal by chelation therapy of congestive cardiomyopathy due to iron overload. *J. Am. Coll. Cardiol.* 8: 436–440.

Rana, S, Houston, PE, Surana, N et al. (1997). Discontinuation of long-term transfusion therapy in patients with sickle cell disease and stroke. *J. Pediatr.* 131: 757–760.

Rao, KRP, Ashok, RP, McGinnis, P, and Patel, MK. (1984). Iron stores in adults with sickle cell anemia. *J. Lab. Clin. Med.* 103: 792–797.

Rao, S and Gooden, S. (1985). Splenic sequestration in sickle cell disease: Role of transfusion therapy. *Am. J. Pediatr. Hematol. Oncol.* 7: 298–301.

Rebulla, P and Modell, B. (1991). Transfusion requirements and effects in patients with thalassaemia major. *Lancet* 337: 277–280.

Rebulla, P, Mozzi, F, Contino, G et al. (1992). Antibody to hepatitis C virus in 1,305 Italian multiply transfused thalassaemics: A comparison of first and second generation tests. *Transfus. Med.* 2: 69–70.

Rifkind, S, Waisman, J, Thompson, R, and Goldfinger, D. (1979). RBC exchange pheresis for priapism in sickle cell disease. *JAMA* 242: 2317–2318.

Risdon, RA, Barry, M, and Flynn, DM. (1975). Transfusional iron overload: The relationship between tissue iron concentration and hepatic fibrosis in thalassaemia. *J. Pathol.* 116: 83–95.

Robert-Guroff, M, Giardina, PJ, Robey, WG et al. (1987). HTLV-III neutralizing antibody development in transfusion-dependent seropositive patients with beta-thalassemia. *J. Immunol.* 138: 3731–3736.

Robins-Browne, RM and Prpic, JK. (1983). Desferrioxamine and systemic yersiniosis (letter). *Lancet* 2: 1372.

Robins-Browne, RM and Prpic, JK. (1985). Effects of iron and desferrioxamine on infections with *Yersinia enterocolitica. Infect. Immun.* 47: 774–779.

Rodda, CP, Reid, ED, Johnson, S et al. (1995). Short stature in homozygous beta-thalassaemia is due to disproportionate truncal shortening. *Clin. Endocrinol.* 42: 587–592.

Rosse, WF, Gallagher, D, and Kinney, TR. (1990). Transfusion and alloimmunization in sickle cell disease. *Blood* 76: 1431–1437.

Rothman, RJ, Serroni, A, and Farber, JL. (1992). Cellular pool of transient ferric iron, chelatable by deferoxamine and distinct from ferritin, that is involved in oxidative cell injury. *Mol. Pharmacol.* 42: 19–28.

Royal, JE and Seeler, RA. (1978). Hypertension, convulsions, and cerebral haemorrhage in sickle-cell anaemia patients after blood transfusions (letter). *Lancet* 2: 1207.

Russell, MO, Goldberg, HI, Hodson, A et al. (1984). Effects of transfusion therapy on arteriographic abnormalities and on recurrence of stroke in sickle cell disease. *Blood* 63: 162–169.

Russo-Mancuso, G, Sciotto, A, Munda, SE et al. (1998). Alloimmunization and autoimmunity in caucasian patients with sickle cell disease. *Int. J. Pediatr. Hematol. Oncol.* 5: 443–447.

Saito, K, Nishisato, T, Grasso, JA, and Aisen, P. (1986). Interaction of transferrin with iron loaded rat peritoneal macrophages. *Br. J. Haematol.* 62: 275–286.

Salhi, Y, Costagliola, D, Rebulla, P et al. (1998). Serum ferritin, desferrioxamine, and evolution of HIV-1 infection in thalassemic patients. *J. Acqu. Immune Defic. Syndr. Hum. Retrovirol.* 18: 473–478.

Sarel, S, Avramovici-Grisaru, S, and Cohen, S. (1986). The formation and double decomposition of pyridoxyl isonicotinyl hydrazone dimethiodide mediated by iron (II) salts. *J. Chem. Soc. Commun.* 24: 952–967.

Sarnaik, S, Schornack, J, and Lusher, JM. (1986). The incidence of development of irregular red cell antibodies in patients with sickle cell anemia. *Transfusion* 26: 249–252.

Saxon, BR, Nisbet-Brown, E, Klein, NC et al. (1999). Evaluation of body iron burden in thalassaemia intermedia. *Proceedings of 9th International Conference on Iron Chelation,* Hamburg, Germany.

Schmalzer, EA, Lee, JO, Brown, AK et al. (1987). Viscosity of mixtures of sickle and normal red cells at varying hematocrit levels. Implications for transfusion. *Transfusion* 27: 228–233.

Schnebli, H. (1997). Novel, potent and well tolerated iron chelators from Novartis. *8th International Conference on Oral Chelation in the Treatment of Thalassaemia and Other Diseases,* Corfu, Greece.

Schorr, JB and Radel, E. (1964). Transfusion therapy and its complications in patients with Cooley's anemia. *Ann. NY. Acad. Sci.* 119: 703–708.

Seeler, RA. (1973). Intensive transfusion therapy for priapism in boys with sickle cell anemia. *J. Urol.* 110: 360–361.

Sephton-Smith, R. (1962). Iron excretion in thalassaemia major after administration of chelating agents. *Br. Med. J.* 2: 1577–1580.

Serjeant, GR. (1997). Chronic transfusion programmes in sickle cell disease: Problem or panacea? *Br. J. Haematol.* 97: 253–255.

Siegel, JF, Rich, MA, and Brock, WA. (1993). Association of sickle cell disease, priapism, exchange transfusion and neurological events: ASPEN syndrome. *J. Urol.* 150: 1480–1482.

Siegelman, ES, Outwater, E, Hanau, CA et al. (1994). Abdominal iron distribution in sickle cell disease: MR findings in transfusion and nontransfusion dependent patients. *J. Comput. Assist. Tomog.* 18: 63–67.

Singh, S, Hider, RC, and Porter, JB. (1990). Separation and identification of desferrioxamine and its iron chelating metabolites by high-performance liquid chromatography and fast atom bombardment mass spectrometry. *Anal. Biochem.* 187: 1–8.

Sirchia, G, Zanella, A, Parravicini, A et al. (1985). Red cell alloantibodies in thalassemia major. Results of an Italian cooperative study. *Transfusion* 25: 110–112.

Sklar, CA, Lew, LQ, Yoon, DJ, and David, R. (1987). Adrenal function in thalassemia major following long-term treatment with multiple transusions and chelation therapy. Evidence for dissociation of cortisol and adrenal androgen secretion. *Am. J. Dis. Child.* 141: 327–330.

Skordis, N, Christou, S, Koliou, M et al. (1998). Fertility in female patients with thalassemia. *J. Pediatr. Endocrinol. Metab.* 11 (Suppl 3): 935–943.

Skoutelis, AT, Lianou, E, Papavassiliou, T et al. (1984). Defective phagocytic and bactericidal function of polymorphonuclear leucocytes in patients with beta-thalassaemia major. *J. Infect.* 8: 118–122.

Sonakul, D and Fucharoen, S. (1992). Brain pathology in 6 fatal cases of post-transfusion hypertension, convulsion and cerebral hemorrhage syndrome. *Southeast Asian J. Trop. Med. Public Health* 23 (supplement 2): 116–119.

Sosler, SD, Jilly, BJ, Saporito, C, and Koshy, M. (1993). A simple, practical model for reducing alloimmunization in patients with sickle cell disease. *Am. J. Hematol.* 43: 103–106.

Spanos, T, Karageorga, M, Ladis, V et al. (1990). Red cell alloantibodies in patients with thalassemia. *Vox Sang.* 58: 50–55.

Spanos, T, Ladis, V, Palamidou, F et al. (1996). The impact of neocyte transfusion in the management of thalassaemia. *Vox Sang.* 70: 217–233.

Sprogoe-Jakobsen, U, Saetre, AM, and Georgsen, J. (1995). Preparation of white cell-reduced red cells by filtration: Comparison of a beside filter and two blood bank filter systems. *Transfusion* 35: 421–426.

Srichairatanakool, S, Kemp, P, and Porter, JB. (1997). Evidence for "shuttle" effect of NTBI onto desferrioxamine in thalassaemic plasma in the presence of NTA. *International Symposium: Iron in Biology and Medicine,* St. Malo, France.

Stefanini, S, Chiancone, E, Cavallo, S et al. (1991). The interaction of hydroxypyridinones with human serum transferrin and ovotransferrin. *J. Inorg. Biochem.* 44: 27–37.

Styles, L and Vichinsky, E. (1995). The effect of low dose desferrioxamine on ototoxicity in hemoglobinopathy patients. *Colloque INSERM* 234: 377–378.

Styles, LA and Vichinsky, E. (1994). Effects of a long-term transfusion regimen on sickle cell-related illnesses. *J. Pediatr.* 125: 909–911.

Syed, SK, Sears, DA, Werch, JB et al. (1996). Delayed hemolytic transfusion reaction in sickle cell disease. *Am. J. Med. Sci.* 312: 175–181.

Tancabelic, J, Sheth, S, Paik, M, and Piomelli, S. (1999). Serum transferrin receptor as a marker of erythropoiesis suppression in patients on chronic transfusion. *Am. J. Hematol.* 60: 121–125.

Tarry, WF, Duckett, JW, and Snyder, HM. (1987). Urological complications of sickle cell disease in a pediatric population. *J. Urol.* 138: 592–594.

Telfer, PT, Garson, JA, Whitby, K et al. (1997). Combination therapy with interferon alpha and ribavirin for chronic hepatitis C virus infection in thalassemic patients. *Br. J. Haematol.* 98: 850–855.

Tenenbein, M, Kowalski, S, Sienko, A et al. (1992). Pulmonary toxic effects of continuous desferrioxamine administration in acute iron poisoning. *Lancet* 339: 699–701.

Tondury, P, Zimmermann, A, Nielsen, P, and Hirt, A. (1998). Liver iron and fibrosis during long-term treatment with deferiprone in Swiss thalassaemic patients. *Br. J. Haematol.* 101: 413–415.

Tsakamota, H, Horne, W, Kamimura, S et al. (1995). Experimantal liver cirrhosis induced by alcohol and iron. *J. Clin. Invest.* 96: 620–630.

Tuck, SM, James, CE, and Brewster, EM. (1987). Prophylactic blood transfusion in maternal sickle cell syndromes. *Br. J. Obstetr. Gynaecol.* 94: 121–125.

Vichinsky, E, Kleman, K, Embury, S, and Lubin, B. (1981). The diagnosis of iron deficiency anemia in sickle cell disease. *Blood* 58: 963–968.

Vichinsky, EP, Earles, A, Johnson, RA et al. (1990). Alloimmunization in sickle cell anemia and transfusion of racially unmatched blood. *N. Engl. J. Med.* 322: 1617–1621.

Vichinsky, EP, Haberkern, CM, Neumayr, L et al. (1995). A comparison of conservative and aggressive transfusion regimens in the perioperative management of sickle cell disease. *N. Engl. J. Med.* 333: 206–213.

Vichinsky, EP, Styles, LA, Colangelo, LH et al. (1997). Acute chest syndrome in sickle cell disease: Clinical presentation and course. Cooperative study of sickle cell disease. *Blood* 89: 1787–1792.

Vichinsky, EP, Neumayr, LD, Earles AN et al. (2000). Causes and outcomes of the acute chest syndrome in sickle cell disease. *N. Engl. J. Med.* 343: 1855–1865.

Villeneuve, JP, Bilodeau, M, Lepage, R et al. (1996). Variability in hepatic iron concentration measurement from needle-biopsy specimens. *J. Hepatol.* 25: 172–177.

Walker, EM, Mitchum, EN, and Rous, SN. (1983). Automated erythrocytapheresis for relief of priapism in sickle cell hemoglobinopathies. *J. Urol.* 130: 912–916.

Walker, JA, Sherman, RA, and Eisinger, RP. (1985). Thrombocytopenia associated with intravenous desferrioxamine. *Am. J. Kidney Dis.* 6: 254–256.

Walters, GO, Miller, R, and Worwood, M. (1973). Serum ferritin concentration and iron stores in normal subjects. *J. Clin. Pathol.* 26: 770–772.

Wang, W, Kovnar, EH, Tonkin, IL et al. (1991). High risk of recurrent stroke after discontinuance of five to twelve years of transfusion therapy in patients with sickle cell disease. *J. Pediatr.* 118: 377–382.

Ware, R, Filston, HC, Schultz, WH, and Kinney, TR. (1988). Elective cholecystectomy in children with sickle hemoglobinopathies. *Ann. Surg.* 208: 17–22.

Warth, JA. (1984). Hypertension and a seizure following transfusion in an adult with sickle cell anemia. *Arch. Intern. Med.* 144: 607–608.

Wasi, P, Pootrakul, P, Piankijagum, A et al. (1978). A syndrome of hypertension, convulsion, and cerebral haemorrhage in thalassaemic patients after muliple blood transfusions. *Lancet* 2: 602–604.

Wayne, AS, Kevy, SV, and Nathan, DG. (1993). Transfusion management of sickle cell disease. *Blood* 81: 1109–1123.

Weaver, J and Pollack, S. (1989). Low-Mr iron isolated from guinea pig reticulocytes as AMP-Fe and ATP-Fe complexes. *Biochem. J.* 261: 787–792.

Whipple, GH and Bradford, WL. (1932). Racial or familial anemia of children. *Am. J. Dis. Child.* 44: 336–365.

White, GP, Bailey-Wood, R, and Jacobs, A. (1976a). The effect of chelating agents on cellular iron metabolism. *Clin. Sci. Mol. Med.* 50: 145–152.

White, JM, White, YS, Buskard, N, and Gillies, IDS. (1976b). Increasing whole blood oxygen affinity during rapid exchange transfusion: A potential hazard. *Transfusion,* 16: 232–236.

Wilimas, J, Goff, JR, Anderson, HRJ et al. (1980). Efficacy of transfusion therapy for one to two years in patients with sickle cell disease and cerebrovascular accidents. *J. Pediatr.* 96: 205–208.

Williams, A, Hoy, T, Pugh, A, and Jacobs, A. (1982). Pyridoxal complexes as potential chelating agents for oral therapy in transfusional iron overoad. *J. Pharm. Pharmacol.* 34: 730–732.

Wolfe, L, Olivieri, N, Sallan, D et al. (1985). Prevention of cardiac disease by subcutaneous desferrioxamine in patients with thalassaemia major. *N. Engl. J. Med.* 312: 1600–1601.

Wolman, IJ. (1964). Transfusion therapy in Cooley's anemia: Growth and health as related to long-range hemoglobin levels. A progress report. *Ann. NY Acad. Sci.* 119: 736–747.

Wolman, IJ and Ortolani, M. (1969). Some clinical features of Cooley's anemia patients as related to transfusion schedules. *Ann. NY Acad. Sci.* 165: 407–414.

Wonke, B, Hoffbrand, AV, Brown, D, and Dusheiko, G. (1990). Antibody to hepatitis C virus in multiply transfused patients with thalassaemia major. *J. Clin. Pathol.* 43: 638–640.

Wonke, B, Wright, C, and Hoffbrand, AV. (1998). Combined therapy with deferiprone and desferrioxamine. *Br. J. Haematol.* 103: 361–364.

Yetgin, S and Hicsonmez, G. (1979). Hypertension, convulsions and purpuric skin lesions after blood-transfusions (letter). *Lancet* 1: 610.

Zanninelli, G, Glickstein, H, Breur, W et al. (1997). Chelation and mobilization of cellular iron by different classes of chelators. *Mol. Pharmacol.* 51: 842–852.

Zinkham, WH, Siedler, AJ, and Kickler, TS. (1994). Variable degrees of suppression of hemoglobin S synthesis in subjects with hemoglobin SS disease on a long-term transfusion regimen. *J. Pediatr.* 124: 215–219.

Zurlo, MG, Stefano, P, Borgna-Pignatti, C et al. (1989). Survival and causes of death in thalassaemia major. *Lancet* 2: 27–30.

38

Pharmacologic Treatment of Sickle Cell Disease and Thalassemia: The Augmentation of Fetal Hemoglobin

GRIFFIN P. RODGERS
MARTIN H. STEINBERG

Research rarely traverses a straight path from a germinal hypothesis to a final result. The evolution of pharmacologic therapy whose goal is to increase the concentration of fetal hemoglobin (HbF) in erythrocytes of patients with sickle cell anemia and β thalassemia illustrates this observation. This story started more than 50 years ago when it was recognized that there was a "paucity" of sickle cell anemia symptoms during infancy and that the red cells of infants with sickle cell trait failed to sickle to the same extent as did their mother's cells when the mother also had the trait (Watson et al., 1948). Watson hypothesized that these observations were due to elevated HbF levels in infant blood (Watson et al., 1948). Soon afterwards, Edington noted that combined heterozygotes for sickle cell trait and hereditary persistence of HbF were clinically normal despite the high HbS concentrations in their red cells (Edington and Lehmann 1955) (Chapters 15 and 28). This work triggered studies that showed that HbF interfered with HbS polymerization (Chapter 23). It was recognized that enough HbF, widely distributed among sickle erythrocytes or the red cells of severe β thalassemia, would "cure" these diseases (Chapters 10, 13, and 24). A search for agents to reverse the switch from γ- to β-globin chain synthesis was launched. Clinical use of a nucleoside analog, 5-azacytidine, was postulated to work by a direct effect on γ-globin gene expression. Although it

increased HbF concentration, it was toxic and difficult to use. Other cytotoxic drugs that might promote HbF production indirectly by perturbing the maturation kinetics of erythroid precursors were tried. When used in sickle cell anemia, these drugs—hydroxyurea is the prototype—increased HbF levels in some patients, and in preliminary studies there were indications of clinical benefits. Controlled clinical trials confirmed that hydroxyurea improved some symptoms of sickle cell anemia. In β thalassemia patients treated with these agents, the total hemoglobin concentration rose in some individuals. Finally, careful appraisal of the effects of hydroxyurea raised the possibility that the benefits of treatment could be due to factors other than increased HbF.

Reactivating HbF synthesis in cells where it is dormant is a problem in the regulation of expression in a gene cluster under tight developmental control (Chapters 4, 5, and 15). DNA modification has long been proposed as one mechanism of gene regulation (Holliday and Pugh, 1975). Among the DNA alterations postulated to have an important influence on gene expression is cytosine methylation and demethylation at CpG (cytosine-guanine dinucleotide) sites (Felsenfeld and McGhee, 1982, 1990; Bhattacharya et al., 1999; Singhal and Ginder, 1999). Cytosine methylation may repress transcription (Singhal and Ginder, 1999). It was observed that inducers of globin synthesis in erythroid cell lines caused hypomethylation of some CpG dinucleotides; that hypomethylated DNA surrounded the expressed chicken β-globin gene, but that these same sites were methylated when this gene was not expressed; that the human γ-globin gene is hypomethylated in fetal tissues; and that promoter methylation silences transcription of embryonic globin genes (Christman et al., 1977; McGhee and Ginder, 1979; van der Ploeg and Flavell, 1980; Singal et al., 1997). Methylation may affect gene expression because of chromatin remodeling (Davey et al., 1997). However, hypomethylation does not accompany all expressed genes in all life forms and is mainly a feature of organisms with large genomes; whether gene hypomethylation is a cause or an effect of gene expression is not totally clear (Felsenfeld and McGhee, 1982; Enver et al., 1988; Garrick et al., 1996). Gene methylation is mediated by DNA methyltransferase. Methyltransferases are most efficient when DNA is hemimethylated so that the methylation pattern of a gene is heritable and replicated on the daughter strand when the parental strand is methylated; however, genes are also capable of de novo methylation. Hypomethylation can be induced by the use of cyti-

Martin H. Steinberg, Bernard G. Forget, Douglas R. Higgs, and Ronald L. Nagel, editors. *Disorders of Hemoglobin: Genetics, Pathophysiology, and Clinical Management.* © 2001 Cambridge University Press. All rights reserved.

dine analogs (e.g., 5-azacytidine) that are incorporated into DNA. Less than 5 percent incorporation results in more than 95 percent hypomethylation. Nitrogen in the 5 position of the pyridine ring resists methylation and inactivates DNA methyltransferase. Other cytidine analogs with similar modifications can also induce hypomethylation but analogs without substitution at position 5 do not cause hypomethylation. Inducing hypomethylation activates transcription of many tissue-specific genes, such as myotubule formation from mouse embryo cells, and, under certain conditions, reactivates inactive X-chromosome genes (Jones and Taylor, 1980; Mohandas et al., 1998). Hypomethylation is a general feature of the "housekeeping" genes that are usually expressed in all cells (Stein et al., 1983).

DeSimone and co-workers (1982) phlebotomized baboons and measured changes in HbF concentration and the frequency of F cells with and without administration of 5-azacytidine. Their results (Fig. 38.1), showed that phlebotomy alone caused a rapid increase in F cells, with a maximum HbF concentration of 2 to 10 percent of total hemoglobin. When 5-azacytidine was administered, HbF concentration increased to 67 to 81 percent in "high" HbF responders and to about 30 percent in "low" responders. Increased HbF was due to an elevation in HbF per F cell. Packed cell volume (PCV) fell to 18 to 24, whereas reticulocyte counts and mean corpuscular volume (MCV) increased substantially. High doses of hydroxyurea (25 to 50 mg/kg/day) did not increase HbF concentration and reduced the response to 5-azacytidine.

These exciting results were rapidly applied to clinical trials of 5-azacytidine in patients with sickle cell anemia and β thalassemia (Fig. 38.2). In sickle cell anemia, HbF levels increased; in β thalassemia, hemoglobin concentration increased (Ley et al., 1982, 1983a, 1983b; Charache et al., 1983). Hypomethylation of CpG dinucleotides in the γ-globin gene promoters was not present before treatment. After treatment there were areas of hypomethylation in total genomic DNA, and one site—107 bp 5′ to both $^G\gamma$- and $^A\gamma$-globin genes—became less methylated (Charache et al., 1983). The era of therapeutic modulation of gene expression for hemoglobinopathies thus began (Benz, 1982). However, 5-azacytidine is toxic, probably carcinogenic, and has a narrow window of therapeutic efficacy. That 5-azacytidine might stimulate HbF production via cytotoxicity rather than a regulatory effect prompted a search for easier to manage "switching" agents. Among the drugs studied, which included cytosine arabinoside, vinblastine, methotrexate, and hydroxyurea, the latter generated interest even though in the first baboon studies it did not increase HbF when given alone and depressed the HbF response when given in conjunction with 5-azacytidine (Torrealba-de Ron et al., 1984; Veith et al., 1985a, 1985b).

Figure 38.1. Effects of 5-azacytidine on HbF levels and F cells in baboons. A reciprocal relationship exists between the fall in HbA and the increase in HbF and F cells after beginning administration of 5-azacytidine. (From DeSimone et al. 1982, with permission.)

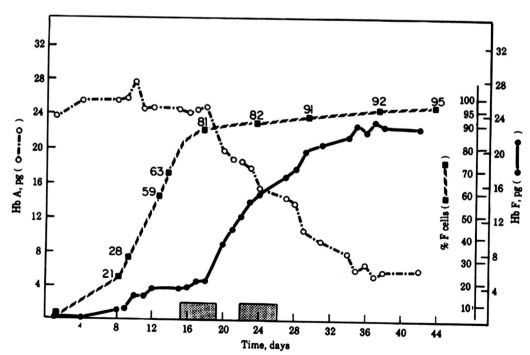

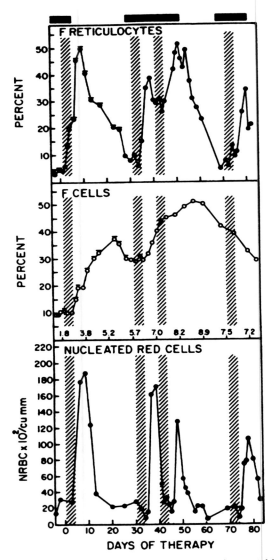

Figure 38.2. Effects of 5-azacytidine on HbF in sickle cell anemia. Solid bars represent treatment with 5-azacytidine. HbF concentrations in the hemolysates are shown beneath the percent F cells. (From Charache et al., 1983, with permission.)

Anemic monkeys treated with hydroxyurea increased their HbF levels (Letvin et al., 1984). When given to two patients with sickle cell anemia at doses of 50 to 100 mg/kg/day in three divided doses for 5 days, hydroxyurea increased F reticulocytes and HbF concentrations with little myelotoxicity. Methylation at several sites 5′ to the γ-globin genes was decreased (Fig. 38.3) (Platt et al., 1984). Hydroxyurea, unlike 5-azacytidine, is not incorporated into DNA, does not inhibit DNA methyltransferase, and does not have a primary effect on DNA methylation. This strongly suggested that HbF was increased by mechanisms other than primary γ-globin gene hypomethylation (Chapter 7) and that γ-globin gene hypomethylation

could be a secondary effect of increased γ-globin gene expression. With the findings that easier to use drugs could increase HbF concentrations and the perception that 5-azacytidine was associated with an increased risk of carcinogenesis, its use has been restricted to individuals with end-stage β thalassemia and alloantibodies that preclude transfusion.

An analog of 5-azacytidine, 5-aza-2′-deoxycytidine, may have fewer adverse effects than the original drug and may resurrect studies of this potentially useful "switching" agent. In preliminary trials, nine patients who failed to respond to hydroxyurea with an increase in HbF synthesis were given 0.15 mg/kg/day 5-aza-2′-deoxycytidine 5 days a week for 2 weeks. All patients responded with a mean increase of HbF of nearly 7 percent by 4 weeks after treatment initiation. Mild and reversible neutropenia was the sole adverse effect (Koshy et al., 1998). These results are encouraging and suggest that a 5-azacytidine analog may stimulate HbF production when hydroxyurea cannot, but they are only preliminary.

HYDROXYUREA IN SICKLE CELL ANEMIA

Hydroxyurea, a ribonucleotide reductase inhibitor, impedes DNA synthesis by preventing formation of deoxyribonucleotides from their ribonucleoside precursors. Hydroxyurea has long been used to treat neoplastic disorders, most often chronic granulocytic leukemia, polycythemia vera, and head and neck cancer. It has nearly complete oral bioavailability with little interindividual variability, making it a simple drug to use (Young and Hodas, 1968; Rodriguez et al., 1998). After it was established that hydroxyurea could safely (at least in the short term) increase HbF in sickle cell anemia patients (Dover et al., 1986; Charache et al., 1987, 1992) and with ample evidence for the favorable effects of high HbF levels in this disease (Chapters 20, 23–25, and 28), studies were initiated to see if this drug could increase HbF in larger numbers of patients with sickle cell anemia and ameliorate their disease. Hydroxyurea did both (DeSimone et al., 1982; Ley et al., 1983a; Platt et al., 1984; Rodgers et al., 1990; El-Hazmi et al., 1992; Charache et al., 1995a).

Our most reliable information on the effectiveness of hydroxyurea in sickle cell anemia comes from a double-blind, placebo-controlled multicenter trial of hydroxyurea in 299 adults with sickle cell anemia who had experienced at least three acute painful episodes in the year preceding the trial. Hydroxyurea reduced by nearly half the frequency of hospitalization and the incidence of pain episodes, acute chest syndrome, and blood transfusion (Charache et al., 1995a). Red cell survival and iron clearance increased, whereas reticulocyte count and plasma iron turnover fell (Ballas et

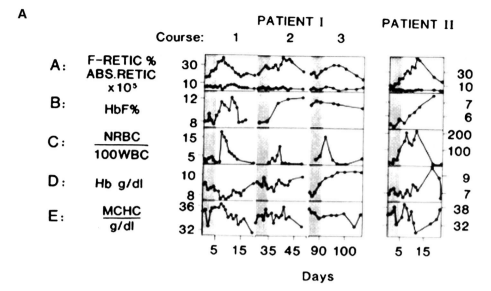

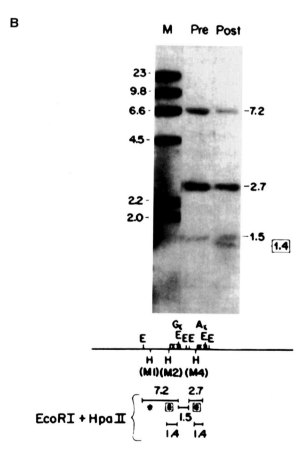

Figur 38.3. Effects of hydroxyurea on HbF in sickle cell anemia. (A) Reticulocyte counts, percent HbF, nucleated red cells, hemoglobin concentration, and MCHC in two patients with sickle cell anemia treated with hydroxyurea. (B) Posttreatment with hydroxyurea, a 1.4kb band that hybridizes with a γ-globin gene-specific probe appears. This represents cleavage by Hpa II at hypomethylated sites 5′ to the γ-globin genes. M denotes size markers and lanes 2 and 3 are pretreatment and posttreatment. (From Platt et al., 1984 with permission.)

al., 1999). Some patients had improved physical capacity with increased anaerobic muscular performance and aerobic cardiovascular fitness (Hackney et al., 1997). Several estimates of quality of life, including general perceptions of health and social function and recall of pain, improved in hydroxyurea-treated patients compared with control subjects at 2 years of observation after the controlled phase of this trial was stopped, although the improvement was modest (Terrin et al., 1999). Hydroxyurea appeared to be cost-effective and clinically beneficial (Moore et al., 2000). Cost estimates were obtained for all outpatient, emergency department, and hospitalizations associated with painful episodes and acute chest syndrome and for managing hydroxyurea therapy. Annual mean costs for painful episodes were $12,000 for hydroxyurea-treated patients and $17,000 for placebo-treated patients. When emergency department visits, costs of analgesics, and blood transfusion were included, the costs were $16,800 for hydroxyurea and $22,000 for placebo patients.

Hydroxyurea-treated patients had an increase in HbF from a baseline of 5 percent to about 9 percent after 2 years of treatment (Charache et al., 1995a). HbF increased to a mean of 18 percent in the top quartile of HbF responders and to 9 percent in the next quartile but changed little in the lower two quartiles of HbF response (Steinberg et al., 1997a). These results may not be typical of all patients with sickle cell anemia because the patients selected for this study were adults with a mean age of about 30 years who had severe disease and who were treated to the brink of myelotoxicity with escalating doses of the drug (Charache et al., 1995b). In other studies, especially in children (see later), hydroxyurea was associated with higher levels of HbF, and perhaps more patients responded favorably to treatment with an increase in HbF concentration.

Predicting who will respond to this treatment would be desirable. In the multicenter trial, the best HbF-responding patients had the highest initial neutrophil and reticulocyte counts and the largest treatment-associated decrements in these counts (Table 38.1). Patients with the greatest reduction in granulocyte, monocyte, and reticulocyte counts also had the largest reduction in acute pain episodes (Charache et al., 1996) (Fig. 38.4). In poor HbF responders, HbF levels and blood counts changed little from the baseline values (Steinberg et al., 1997a). Individuals with the best HbF response were less likely to have a Bantu haplotype chromosome (Chapter 26) (Charache et al., 1996).

Variations in F cells, MCV, neutrophil counts, and reticulocyte counts over time in the four quartiles of HbF response are shown in Figure 38.5. Most patients responded initially to hydroxyurea with increased

Table 38.1. HbF Level and F Cells According to Neutrophil and Reticulocyte Counts After 2 Years of Treatment with Hydroxyurea

Quartile of HbF response

	1st	2nd	3rd	4th
2-year HbF change (%)	−1.5	0.6	3.7	11.7
2-year F-cell change (%)	−1.1	8.1	17.7	36.2
Neutrophil decrement ($10^3/\mu$L)	−0.3	−1.0	−2.2	−4.1
Reticulocyte decrement ($10^3/\mu$L)	−37	−37	−95	−233

numbers of F cells, but there was a divergence between patients who were long-term responders and those who did not sustain their F-cell response. Among patients with little change in final HbF level, neutrophil and reticulocyte counts returned to baseline early during the course of treatment and percent F cells decreased. Patients in quartiles 1 and 2 had early changes in F cells. Perhaps, because of marrow "scarring," some patients are unable to tolerate continual myelosuppressive doses of hydroxyurea. Blood cell counts decline with aging in sickle cell anemia, an observation that may reflect cumulative vasoocclusive damage to the bone marrow (Hayes et al., 1985; West et al., 1992). F-cell production (FCP) locus phenotype (Chapters 10 and 26) was a determinant of baseline HbF levels, but did not predict the HbF response to hydroxyurea. Earlier studies suggested that individuals with low baseline HbF and F-reticulocyte levels were less likely to have an increase in HbF (Charache et al., 1987), an observation not confirmed when more patients were studied.

Myelosuppression—perhaps a prerequisite for hydroxyurea enhancement of HbF synthesis—is determined by an interplay between the myelotoxic effects of the drug and the proliferative capacity of the bone marrow. Patients with the highest baseline granulocyte and reticulocyte counts, who also had the largest decreases in these counts during treatment, had the greatest increases in HbF. In earlier studies, the initial leukocyte count and change in leukocytes with treatment were also determinants of the final HbF level after treatment with hydroxyurea (Charache et al., 1992). In these other studies as in the multicenter trial, some patients did not respond to treatment or had a minor increase in HbF. However, the dosing regimens, final dosages achieved, and length of treatment in all of these studies differed (Rodgers et al., 1990; Charache et al., 1992).

These results suggested that in adults, the ability to respond to hydroxyurea is dependent on bone marrow

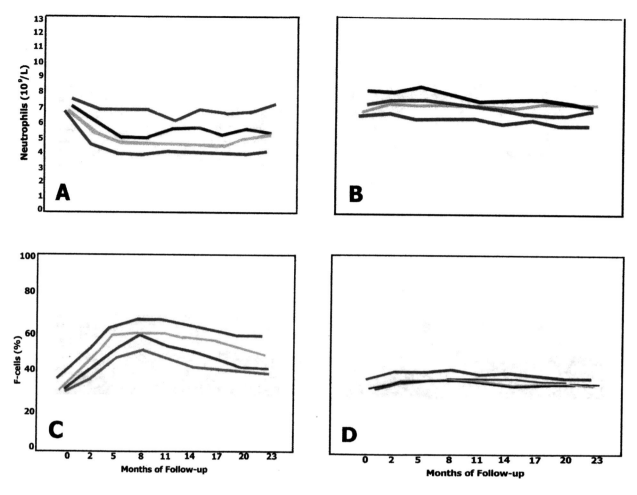

Figure 38.4. Changes in neutrophil counts (**A and B**) and F cells (**C and D**) during treatment of sickle cell anemia with hydroxyurea or placebo. Red lines indicate 0 to < 2 pain episodes/year; yellow lines, 2 to < 5 episodes/year; blue lines, 5 to < 10 episodes/year; and green lines, ≥ 10 episodes/year. (Panels A and C) Hydroxyurea-treated patients. (Panels B and D) Placebo-treated patients. For color reproduction, see color plate 38.4. (Adapted from Charache et al., 1996.)

"reserve" or the capacity of the marrow to withstand moderate doses of hydroxyurea with acceptable myelotoxicity. Baseline reticulocyte and neutrophil counts may reflect marrow "reserve." Sustained HbF increases during hydroxyurea treatment can occur in individuals with bone marrow "reserve" sufficient to cope with the myelotoxicity of this agent as a population of erythroblasts with the capacity to make substantial amounts of HbF repopulate the marrow. Responding patients showed evidence of cyclic hematopoiesis reminiscent of individuals with myeloproliferative disease, whereas nonresponding patients had little evidence of cyclical variations in blood counts (Fig. 38.6).

The chemokine receptor Duffy (Fy) antigen is present in about one third of African Americans. In children

with sickle cell anemia, Fy-positive patients had baseline HbF levels nearly twice as high as Fy-negative individuals (10.1 ± 9.1 vs. 5.3 ± 3.8 percent). Fy-positive patients had higher HbF levels after treatment with hydroxyurea than Fy-negative patients and tolerated higher doses of the drug without toxicity (Raphael et al., 1997). These studies should be repeated, and if the observations are confirmed, the mechanism needs to be clarified.

Studies of hydroxyurea in young children or adolescents, where therapeutic benefits should be greatest, lag behind adult studies. Fewer than 300 children with clinically severe sickle cell disease treated with hydroxyurea have been reported, some only in abstract form (deMontalembert et al., 1994; Ferster et al., 1996; Jayabose et al., 1996; Scott et al., 1996; Olivieri and Vichinsky, 1998; Koren et al., 1999). Most were teenagers treated in unblinded pilot studies; but twenty-five patients, ages 2 to 22 years (median 9 years), were treated in a single-blinded crossover study with drug or placebo (Ferster et al., 1996). These trials had remarkably similar outcomes. HbF increased from 5 percent before treatment to 16 percent after 6 months to 1 year of treatment. As in adults, hemolysis and neutrophil

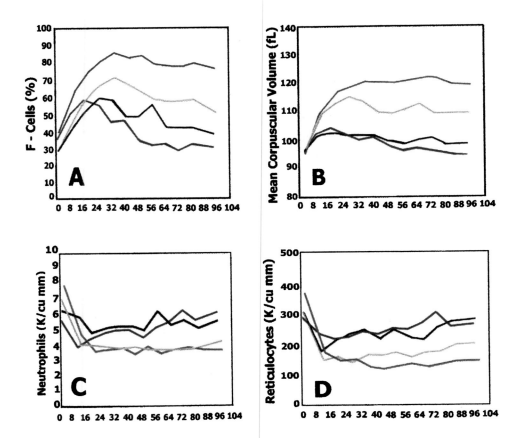

Figure 38.5. Variation in F cells, MCV, neutrophil counts, and reticulocyte counts during 2 years of treatment with hydroxyurea. Patients are grouped by the quartile of the final HbF response after two years of treatment (Red-top quartile of HbF response; yellow, third quartile; purple, second quartile; green, lowest [first] quartile). For color reproduction, see color plate 38.5. (Adapted from Steinberg et al., 1997a.)

counts decreased. Short-term toxicity in these and other trials (deMontalembert et al., 1999) was minor. A trial of hydroxyurea in eighty-four children ages 5 to 15 years of age (mean age ~10 years) has been completed (Kinney, 1999), and the results are similar to those seen in adults. Entry criteria were similar to those for the multicenter adult study, and hydroxyurea was titrated to maximally tolerated doses of 15 to 30 mg/kg/day. Sixty-eight patients reached the maximally tolerated dose, and fifty-two completed 1 year of treatment. About 20 percent of enrolled patients withdrew from the study, predominantly because of lack of compliance, not because of drug toxicity. At baseline, mean HbF was 6.8 percent and at the maximally tolerated dose, it increased to 19.8 percent. Other hematologic changes included increases in MCV from 86 to 99.5 fl, hemoglobin concentration from 7.8 to 8.8 g/dL, and a decline in leukocyte count from 13.6 to 9.3 × 10⁹/L. These changes, apparent after 6 months of treatment, were sustained at 24 months.

Limited pharmacokinetic studies of children with a median age of 12.8 years showed somewhat higher clearance, distribution volume, and area under the curve (AUC) than reported for adults (Parasuraman et al., 1998). There is no reason to think that the hematologic effects of hydroxyurea in children with sickle cell anemia will not, at least in the short term, result in clinical benefits similar to those seen in adults. Early interruption of the vasoocclusive process may also prevent or delay damage to the central nervous system, lungs, kidneys, and bones that end in disability or death, but this has not yet been shown.

Eight children, ages 2 to 5 years, who had frequent painful episodes and acute chest syndrome received a maximally tolerated daily dose of 27 mg/kg and were treated for 143 ± 85 weeks. HbF in these patients increased from 7 to 19 percent and total hemoglobin from 8.5 to 10.7 g/dL. In this uncontrolled study, the number of hospitalizations declined from 4.2 ± 2.3 yearly to 1.9 ± 0.9 and hospital days from 23 ± 13 to 10 ± 7. There were no growth or developmental delays. One individual had a stroke despite an increase in HbF (Aessopos et al., 1999).

Twenty-nine infants, ages 6 to 27 months (median 14 months), were treated with a set daily dose of 20 mg/kg of a hydroxyurea solution made up to 100 mg/mL. After a 12 month follow-up period, the predicted

A.

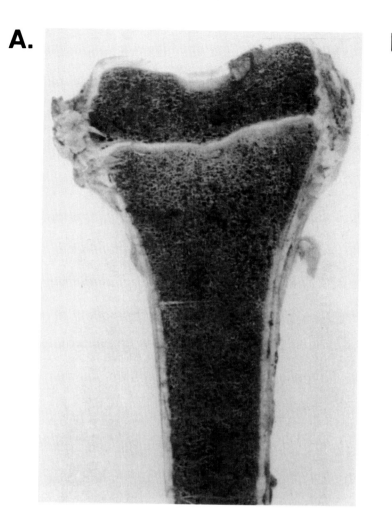

B.

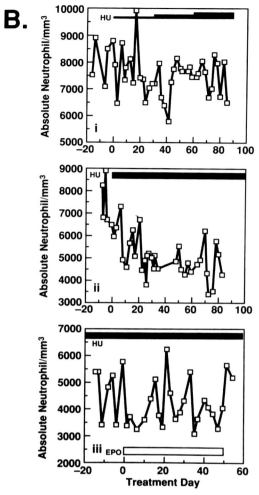

Figure 38.6. Cyclic erythropoiesis in sickle cell anemia patients responding to hydroxyurea with increased HbF level. (A) Hypercellular marrow from postmortem examination of a patient with sickle cell anemia illustrating the typical expanded marrow cellularity reminiscent of a myeloproliferative disease. (Courtesy of Professor A. V. Hoffbrand.) (B) In another patient, absolute neutrophil count before and during increasing doses of hydroxyurea and with the addition of erythropoietin to this treatment.

changes for sickle cell anemia infants in hemoglobin concentration, MCV, HbF, and leukocyte count were compared with observed changes. Hemoglobin increased from 8.5 to 9.1 g/dL (predicted, decline of 4 percent), MCV increased from 82 to 91 fl (predicted, increase of 2 percent), HbF increased from 21.3 to 23.2 percent (predicted, decline of 32 percent), and leukocytes decreased from 12.6 to 10.6/10⁹/L (predicted, increase of 3 percent (Wang et al., 1999). Nine patients were dropped from the study for poor compliance or parental refusal to continue, and one child died from splenic sequestration syndrome. One patient had a transient ischemic attack, seven patients had episodes of acute chest syndrome, two had splenic sequestration, and two had episodes of sepsis. Growth was normal. Despite impressive levels of HbF, acute complications of sickle cell anemia were still seen in these very young patients, but the total number of patients studied was small, the observation period was short, and there were no concurrent placebo control subjects.

Several reports recommend hydroxyurea as an alternative to transfusion to prevent new or recurrent stroke, especially when the blood transfusion is not feasible for reasons of patient preference or compliance, alloimmunization or autoimmunization, iron overload with ineffective chelation, drug allergy, or lack of venous access (Ware et al., 1995, 1999a; Adams et al., 1999). In one report of sixteen children, treatment with hydroxyurea raised HbF to 20 percent and phlebotomy reduced serum ferritin from 2,630 to 636 ng/mL (Ware et al., 1999a). Three patients had a new neurologic event early in the course of treatment before HbF response was maximized. In another report, one patient, age ~20 years, had begun tranfusions at age 6 years after a stroke but discontinued them recently against medical advice (Vichinsky and Lubin, 1994). Before stopping transfusions and starting hydroxyurea, a cerebral arteriogram showed total occlusion of both anterior cerebral arteries and moya-moya. After a year of treatment and with an HbF value of 21 percent, he had a fatal intracerebral hemorrhage. Whether intracerebral hemorrhage in adults can be prevented by transfusion is unknown (Chapters 24 and 37). There have been other instances of stroke, some mentioned previously, in patients with sickle cell anemia treated with hydroxyurea who had HbF levels that most would deem "therapeutic." There is little information on the distribution of HbF among erythrocytes in these instances (or in most cases of hydroxyurea treatment of sickle cell anemia) or the concentration of HbF/F-cell, but one study reported 78.5 percent F cells. If these cells all contained HbF concentrations sufficient to prevent cellular damage, the effects of this level of HbF should be equivalent to a transfusion in which 80 percent of cells are incapable of sickling and only ~20 percent of cells were HbS-cells. It is not clear if or why high HbF levels in hydroxyurea-treated patients with sickle cell anemia do not absolutely protect from stroke. HF levels of 20 percent do not protect absolutely from other disease events, and perhaps stroke is no exception, but just a more dramatic example of the shortcomings of a treatment that does not deal with all the pathology of the disease. Alternatively, the pathogenesis of cerebral vasculopathy differs from that of vasoocclusive pain episodes and other complications and is not responsive to the beneficial effects of increasing HbF concentration.

Side Effects

Aside from the expected and manageable myelotoxicity, side effects of hydroxyurea treatment have been few. Renal and hepatotoxicity are minimal or absent. Pigmentation of the nails (Adams-Graves et al., 1996), generalized or in the form of longitudinal bands, has been observed and may disappear despite continued treatment. Some localized increase in skin pigmentation has also been observed. Leg and oral ulcers have been reported in patients with myeloproliferative diseases treated with hydroxyurea (Norhaya et al., 1997; Best et al., 1998; Ravandi-Kashani et al., 1998; Kido et al., 1998). Ankle ulcers were seen when these patients received hydroxyurea for an average of 6 years. They healed when the drug was stopped but recurred when it was restarted. In sickle cell anemia, hydroxyurea was thought by some to help heal persistent leg ulcers. In the multicenter trial, hydroxyurea had no effect on healing or occurrence of leg ulcers, but, compared to the observations in myeloproliferative diseases, the follow-up interval was short.

Hydroxyurea is a teratogen in rats, cats, and rhesus monkeys and should not be used if pregnancy is planned (Ware et al., 1999b). Pregnancy has been reported in at least fourteen women receiving hydroxyurea, most with myeloproliferative disorders, but four with sickle cell anemia (Charache et al., 1995a, 1995b; Steinberg et al., 1998b; Diav-Citrin et al., 1999). There were no adverse outcomes in this small series. Contraception should be practiced by both women and men receiving hydroxyurea and the uncertain outcome of unplanned pregnancy discussed frankly. If a patient who is taking hydroxyurea becomes pregnant, there is little information on which to base a decision for continuation or termination.

Long-Term Prospects

Hydroxyurea needs to be taken indefinitely, and we do not yet know its long-term effects. Is it mutagenic or carcinogenic? To date, increases in chromosome breakage, recombination events, or mutations in the p53, n-ras, k-ras, or hprt genes, have not been found in hydroxyurea-treated sickle cell anemia patients compared to control subjects (Mougiou et al., 1997; Ware et al., 1998). A study was done of hprt gene mutations and "illegitimate" recombination events between the β and γ gene loci of the T-cell receptor in adults with sickle cell anemia exposed to hydroxyurea for 24 months, children with sickle cell anemia exposed for 7 or 30 months, and adults with myeloproliferative disorders exposed for 11 years. No differences in DNA mutations were found between these groups and unexposed matched control subjects or normal adults, suggesting that the leukemogenic potential of the drug is low (Ware et al., 1999b). Hydroxyurea appears to reduce extrachromosomally amplified genes, including c-myc, from tumor cells, thereby reducing their tumorigenicity (Eckardt et al., 1994).

About 5 to 10 percent of patients with polycythemia vera, a neoplastic myeloproliferative disease, treated with hydroxyurea develop acute leukemia (Weinfeld et al., 1994; Nand et al., 1996; Najean and Rain, 1997). In essential thrombocythemia, 3.4 percent of 201 patients given hydroxyurea as the sole treatment progressed to acute leukemia (Sterkers et al., 1998). Nine percent of fifty-six patients with essential thrombocythemia randomized to treatment with hydroxyurea developed leukemia after a median follow-up time of 73 months and 5.2 percent of 58 cases had a leukemic transformation, (Liozon et al., 1997; Barbul et al., 1998). Among the cases with leukemic transformation, two had nonrandom complex cytogenetic abnormalities, suggesting therapy-associated changes. It seems inescapable that there is a potential for leukemogenicity when hydroxyurea is used in myeloproliferative disorders. How and if the myeloproliferative disorders equate to a disease without cancer-promoting mutations but with lifelong expanded erythropoiesis remains to be seen. Acute leukemia has developed in patients with sickle cell anemia treated with hydroxyurea (Rauch et al., 1999). We also know of additional unreported cases. Whether these cases represent therapy-induced leukemogenesis is unknown.

Before its use in sickle cell anemia, hydroxyurea was occasionally given for "benign" diseases. It was given to sixty-four children with cyanotic congenital heart disease for a mean treatment duration of more than 5 years without any reports of malignancies (Triadou et al., 1994).

At the conclusion of the randomized treatment phase of the multicenter trial described previously, 2 hydroxyurea-assigned and 6 placebo-assigned patients had died. This difference was not statistically significant. After the randomized treatment phase of the study ended, the observation phase began. (Steinberg et al., 1997b; Steinberg et al., 1999a) Patients were free to continue, start, or stop hydroxyurea and were asked to participate in a long-term follow-up with particular attention focused on the development of neoplasia and cerebrovascular disease and to birth defects in offspring. Determining whether a treatment reduces mortality in any setting other than a randomized, placebo-controlled trial is difficult. Patients in this multicenter trial form the largest reported series of sickle cell anemia patients treated with hydroxyurea and have been followed for nearly 8 years. Because patient follow-up is less than 100 percent, certain assumptions must be made in the data analysis. Patients who were taking hydroxyurea for 2 months or more at the start of the follow-up phase were considered "on-hydroxyurea" while patients with less than 2 months of drug use were deemed "off-hydroxyurea." At the time of death, patients who were taking the drug or who were taking hydroxyurea when last seen alive or up to 1 year before death were considered "on-hydroxyurea."

Thirty-one of the 147 patients originally assigned to take a placebo had died (21.1 percent) compared with 22 of the 152 hydroxyurea-assigned patients (14.5 percent) ($P = 0.13$). Death due to pulmonary disease and crisis was twice as high in the original placebo group as in the hydroxyurea group. Cancer, leukemia, and birth defects have not occurred. When the assumption is made that the 40 patients whose hydroxyurea use was unknown are not taking this drug, the relative risk of death while off hydroxyurea compared with being on hydroxyurea was 1.5 ($P = 0.13$). When 40 patients whose hydroxyurea use is unknown are excluded from the analysis, the

relative risk of death off hydroxyurea (0.031 deaths/patient year) compared with being on hydroxyurea (0.026) was 1.8 ($P = 0.04$). Cumulative mortality since the conclusion of the randomized study, assuming that unless known to be dead, patients were alive, showed that the patients "on-hydroxyurea" had reduced mortality compared with individuals "off-hydroxyurea" ($P = 0.056$). Currently, it is unlikely that any other studies of adults with sickle cell anemia treated with hydroxyurea can answer the question of this drug's effect on mortality more conclusively than this one can. Mortality was unaffected by age or sex. To date, β-globin gene haplotype, α-globin genotype, F-cell production locus phenotype, HbF level, and crisis rate were unrelated to mortality but this may be a consequence of the small numbers of deaths and the selected nature of the patient population. These data suggest, but cannot unequivocally prove, that in moderately-to-severely affected adults with sickle cell anemia, treatment with hydroxyurea may be associated with a reduction of mortality. These data must be interpreted with the caveats that the effect of hydroxyurea on mortality was not specified as an a priori hypothesis of the multicenter study, comparisons of "off-hydroxyurea" vs. "on-hydroxyurea" are not randomized, and that the ability to take or not to take hydroxyurea (predictor) is dependent on being alive (outcome). Continued observation, especially with complete follow-up is critical.

Some hematological effects of hydroxyurea are sustained. In 132 patients on hydroxyurea compared with 32 patients off hydroxyurea mean hemoglobin concentration was 8.7 ± 1.8 vs. 8.2 ± 1.2 g/dL ($P = 0.08$); MCV 100.8 ± 12.8 vs. 94.9 ± 9.4 fl ($P = 0.004$); reticulocytes 189 ± 122.3 vs. $259 \pm 116.2 \times 10^3/\mu$L ($P = 0.008$); bilirubin 3.3 ± 4.8 vs. 4.8 ± 5.1 mg/dL ($P = 0.16$).

These observations—ones that will be continued—must be viewed in the perspective of the likelihood of finding adverse effects of hydroxyurea in the multicenter study sample. Between ages 20 and 40 years, the incidence of acute leukemia in African-American men and women is three to five cases/100,000 patients/year (0.003 to 0.005/1,000 patient-years). The incidence of cancer is between 50 and 250 cases/10,0000 patients/year (0.05 to 2.5 cases/1,000 patient-years). The multicenter study will have about 2,000 patient-years of follow-up data for all patients and 1,000 patient-years of follow-up data for patients initially randomized to receive hydroxyurea. Assuming that the baseline rate of leukemia and cancer in adults with sickle cell anemia does not vary greatly from that observed in the general population, we will be able to detect only hundred-fold increases in the incidence of leukemia or cancer in the follow-up studies.

In contrast, for example, intracerebral hemorrhage in adults with sickle cell anemia occurs at a rate of about 1/400 patient-years (0.5/1000 patient-years). By the same calculations discussed previously, it should be possible to detect a doubling in the incidence of intracerebral hemorrhage (or other more common complications) in patients initially randomized to receive hydroxyurea. A large registry of all patients treated with hydroxyurea should be established so that any adverse effects of this treatment can more rapidly be uncovered.

We do not know if hydroxyurea has adverse effects on growth and development (none have yet been reported [Scott et al., 1996]), or if continued exposure starting at a very young age will be especially hazardous. Very high doses of hydroxyurea, 2.5- to 50-fold higher than doses used to treat sickle cell anemia, retarded the proliferation of brain cells and development in mice 3 to 5 days postnatally, but it is not possible to extrapolate these observations to humans (Horiuchi, 1998). If hydroxyurea poses a carcinogenic risk, it is most likely a small one and will take many patient-years of observation to uncover. Even with a small risk, the benefits of this treatment in seriously ill patients may be dominant.

We hope, but do not presently know, that hydroxyurea will prevent organ damage and reduce mortality. After 1 year of treatment, splenic function in children who averaged 12 years of age did not change (Olivieri and Vichinksy, 1998). Of ten patients with sickle cell anemia who received hydroxyurea for 21 months and had an increase in HbF from 8 to 17 percent, only one patient recovered splenic function as determined by "pit" counts, Howell-Jolly bodies, and ^{99m}TC labeled heat-damaged erythrocyte scans. Splenic regeneration was reported in two adults with sickle cell anemia who had HbF levels of about 30 percent after hydroxyurea treatment (Claster and Vichinsky, 1996; Muraca et al., 1998). Recovery or improvement of splenic function is not likely in most older children or adults. Transplantation and hypertransfusion may also reestablish splenic function (Ferster et al., 1993; Campbell et al., 1997). Splenic tissue has a propensity to regenerate so that its regrowth may not be a good indicator of potential rejuvenation of other organs.

Mechanisms of Clinical Benefit

Hydroxyurea may work by multiple mechanisms as shown in Figure 38.7. We do not understand how this agent benefits patients with sickle cell anemia, but there are many hypotheses. Initially, hydroxyurea was believed to act solely by increasing HbF levels. Indeed, in most open-label trials improvement in clinical symptoms mirrored or slightly preceded the increase in HbF levels. Further studies suggested that the reduction in neutrophils, monocytes, and reticulocytes may also be important (Charache et al., 1996). Neutrophils from patients having a painful episode had increased adherence to cultured endothelial cells and expressed higher levels of CD64, an epitope than may promote vascular adherence (Fadlon et al., 1998). By reducing blood neutrophils, hydroxyurea may lessen the chance of vasoocclusive events. Diminishing the numbers of "stress" reticulocytes may be therapeutically beneficial, as these cells may also initiate vasoocclusive complications (Hebbel et al., 1980; Sugihara et al., 1992; Brittain et al., 1993; Joneckis et al., 1993; Swerlick et al., 1993; Wick et al., 1993; Gee et al., 1995). A decrease in the number of normal reticulocytes and "stress" reticulocytes occurred in patients with sickle cell anemia and HbSC disease treated with hydroxyurea. In those with sickle cell anemia, this reduction was correlated with the reduction in pain crises.

During treatment, many changes take place simultaneously in the sickle erythrocyte (Bridges et al., 1996). Indisputably, the increase in HbF is a primary effect of treatment. It is difficult to say if the other myriad effects are primary or secondary to increased HbF. As expected, with increasing HbF there is a reduced rate and extent of polymerization. Sickle cell-endothelial cell adherence decreases before a measured increase in HbF occurs, suggesting a direct effect on red cell membrane or endothelial cell adhesive properties. Hydroxyurea may have a direct effect on endothelial cells, changing their morphology and cation content and, at least in vitro, rendering them a less attractive site for sickle cell adherence (Adragna et al., 1994). Dense cell numbers decline as K^+ content increases (Bridges et al., 1996). Two reticulocyte adhesion receptors, $\alpha_4\beta_1$ intergrin, or the very late activation antigen-4, and CD36 also decline early in the course of hydroxyurea treatment before measurable increases in HbF (Styles et al., 1997). Improved cellular hydration and deformability are likely to be secondary to increased HbF and may play a role in the reduction of vasoocclusive episodes and also the reduced hemolysis accompanying treatment (Ballas et al., 1991).

Several reports suggest a novel method of action based on the generation of nitric oxide (NO) by peroxidation of hydroxyurea (Sato et al., 1997; Jiang et al., 1997; Xu et al., 1998). NO, or endothelial-derived relaxing factor, is a potent vasodilator. When given to rats, hydroxyurea urea leads to S-nitrosohemoglobin formation. Nitrosyl hemoglobin complex could also be detected as early as 30 minutes after administration of hydroxyurea to patients with sickle cell anemia and persisted up to 4 hours (Glover et al., 1999). NO may increase the O_2 affinity of HbS by reducing its polymerization potential but these results are unconfirmed (Head et al., 1997; Gladwin et al., 1999). In vitro

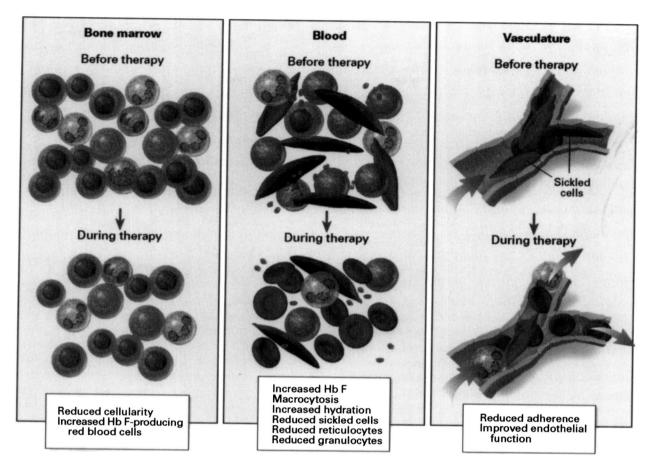

Figure 38.7 Mechanisms of action of hydroxyurea. Hydroxyurea acts on the bone marrow and, by its cytotoxic effects, selects a population of erythroblasts that can synthesize increased amounts of HbF. It has no known direct effects on gene expression. Bone marrow cellularity may also be diminished. Higher concentrations of HbF reduce the level of HbS polymer and the numbers of deformed, dense, and damaged erythrocytes. Cells with a high HbF content survive longer, attenuating hemolysis and leading to a reduction in reticulocytes. Circulating granulocytes, monocytes, and platelets are diminished. Fewer dense, poorly adhesive erythrocytes are less apt to adhere to and perturb the endothelium, reducing the likelihood of vasoocclusion. (From Steinberg, 1999 with permission.) For full color reproduction, see color plate 38.7.

studies have shown that HbS is also able to form sickle nitrosylhemoglobin and that the NO group of this modified molecule derives from the NHOH moiety of hydroxyurea (Xu, et al., 1998). Normally, S-nitrosohemoglobin is formed in the lung, whereas in tissues, NO is transferred to the vessel wall promoting vasodilation (Hofstra et al., 1996). Perhaps hydroxyurea, by increasing the O_2 affinity of HbS or by promoting vasodilation, reduces polymerization and the propensity for microvascular occlusion.

Preliminary studies have shown that hydroxyurea can induce methemoglobin formation and perhaps reduce deoxyHbS concentrations (Kim-Shapiro et al., 1997). An early attempt to treat sickle cell anemia by inducing methemoglobinemia using sodium nitrite was unsuccessful (Beutler and Mikus, 1961).

Other work has raised the possibility that hydroxyurea increases erythropoietin production up to 30-fold over baseline levels 2 to 10 days after beginning treatment. It was hypothesized that this enhances the proliferation of erythroid precursors with the capacity to synthesize HbF (Papassotiriou et al., 1998).

HYDROXYUREA IN OTHER SICKLE HEMOGLOBINOPATHIES

In HbS-β thalassemia, hydroxyurea appears to work as well as in sickle cell anemia (Voskaridou et al., 1995; Loukopoulos, 1996). In one reported trial in Greeks with HbS-$β^0$ thalassemia and $β^+$ thalassemia, HbF responses were higher than in African Americans with sickle cell anemia, increasing to 23 percent from 3.6 percent. Few patients were treated and the studies were uncontrolled, but pain episodes were said to stop. African Americans with HbS-$β^+$ thalassemia usually have 20 to 30 percent HbA and less severe disease. Most of these patients will not develop symptoms that warrant hydroxyurea treatment under the current guidelines for treatment.

Pilot studies of HbSC disease indicated that hydroxyurea (10 to 20 mg/kg/day) was associated with sustained erythrocyte volume increases, a decline in absolute reticulocyte counts, "stress" reticulocytes and dense red cells, and a small increase in PCV. Two additional measurements provided further indirect evidence that hydroxyurea may reduce hemolysis in HbSC disease; there was a significant decline in serum bilirubin and a reduction in the total hemoglobin content of all reticulocytes accompanied by increases in the ratio of the total hemoglobin content of all erythrocytes to reticulocyte hemoglobin content. This ratio is an indirect measure of red cell survival (Steinberg et al., 1997c).

There was no statistically significant mean increase in percent HbF and absolute HbF levels, but some individual patients did sustain and increase HbF levels. Perhaps a larger patient sample, treatment of younger patients, a longer period of treatment, or the use of higher doses of hydroxyurea may be needed before a consistent increase in HbF is observed in HbSC disease. Baseline HbF levels are lower in HbSC disease than in sickle cell anemia, and efforts to modify the phenotype of HbSC disease by increasing HbF levels may be unrewarding.

Five children with HbSC disease whose average age was 13.5 years and an additional six adults were treated with hydroxyurea, median dose of 1,000 mg/day, for 5 to 25 months. Hemoglobin concentration increased by about 1 g/dL, MCV increased from 80 to 94 to 103 fl, and HbF in children increased from 1.9 to 9.9 percent (Ware et al., 1999c).

The mechanism by which hydroxyurea alters the HbSC cell is unknown; however, based on our understanding of the pathophysiology of HbSC disease, reduced numbers of dense cells should favorably modulate the course of this disorder. Reduced cell density should diminish the polymerization tendency of HbS within HbSC cells in vivo as it does in vitro. Diminishing the number of high-intensity staining or "stress" reticulocytes may also be therapeutically beneficial, as these cells display adhesive ligands that facilitate erythrocyte-endothelial interactions and promote vasoocclusive complications (Hebbel et al., 1980; Sugihara et al., 1992; Brittain et al., 1993; Joneckis et al., 1993; Swerlick et al., 1993; Wick et al., 1993; Gee and Platt, 1995).

Because hydroxyurea was associated with advantageous cellular changes in HbSC disease additional studies in children were started to see if this treatment affected their ability to concentrate urine. Stabilization of the renal concentrating defect or its improvement in individuals who had not sustained irreversible renal medullary damage would be some indication that the cellular benefits of hydroxyurea were translated into an effect on vasoocclusive disease. Eight children (three male, five female) with HbSC disease, ages 10 to 17 years (mean 11 years), were given hydroxyurea 15 mg/kg as a single daily dose. Before determining the maximal urine concentrating ability, nonsteroidal anti-inflammatory drugs, and aspirin were discontinued for at least 1 week. Maximum urine concentrating ability was measured after an overnight fast and 0.08 μg/kg of subcutaneous desmopressin acetate (dDAVP) (Iyer, 2000). The next 30-minute voided urine sample was discarded, and urine voided at 2 and 4 hours after dDAVP administration was collected for osmolality measurement. Patients were treated for a mean of 14 months (12 to 15 months). Before beginning treatment and before receiving dDAVP, no patient had an overnight urine concentration greater than 545 mOsm (mean 445 mOsm; normal 800 to 1,000 mOsm). Seven of eight patients increased their urine concentration after receiving dDAVP, although none increased urine concentration to normal. In no patient did hydroxyurea appear to increase the maximal urine concentration ability beyond that of the baseline value. Two girls, 10 and 17 years old, increased their concentration of HbF during treatment. The first increased HbF from 6.3 to ~15 percent after 2 to 3 months of treatment; the second patient increased HbF from 1 to about 6 percent after 5 to 6 months of treatment.

These patients, whose average age was 11 years when treatment began, had pretreatment maximum urine concentrations, about half the expected normal value, and treatment with hydroxyurea did not increase the ability to concentrate urine. There were no increases in urine-concentrating ability in individual patients, even those who had increases in HbF concentration or who showed reduction in mean cell hemoglobin concentration (MCHC) and increases in MCV. Hemolysis appeared to be reduced in all patients, as estimated by the fall in reticulocyte count; yet there were no changes in PCV, and the Hb/rHb ratio changed little. These data suggest that at the time of study entry, the ability to concentrate urine was compromised, perhaps irreversibly, owing to structural damage to the countercurrent concentrating mechanism. Alternatively, treatment may have been given for too short a time interval or any effects of this drug on the sickle cell may have been too small to return the renal medullary circulation to normal. Perhaps higher doses of drug given for a longer time would have proven effective.

In one patient with HbSD$_{Los Angeles (Punjab)}$ who had a long history of frequent admissions for painful episodes and used about 140 tablets of codeine and acetaminophen monthly, 500 mg of hydroxyurea daily abolished pain and analgesic use (Udden et al., 1999).

Table 38.2. Use of Hydroxyurea in Sickle Cell Anemia

Indication for treatment

Adults, adolescents, and after consultation with parents and expert pediatricians, children with frequent pain episodes, history of acute chest syndrome, other severe vasoocclusive complications. Severe symptomatic anemia.

Baseline evaluation

Blood counts, red cell indices, HbF, serum chemistries, pregnancy test, willingness to adhere to all recommendations for treatment, absence of chronic transfusion program.

Initiation of treatment

Hydroxyurea 10 to 15 mg/kg/day or 500 mg qAM for 6–8 weeks, CBC q2weeks, HbF q6-8weeks.

Continuation of treatment

If counts are acceptable, escalate dose to 1,500 mg qAM in increments of 500 mg every 6 to 8 weeks.

Failure of HbF (or MCV) to increase

Consider biological inability to respond to treatment or poor compliance with treatment. Increase dose very cautiously to 2,000 to 2,500 mg daily (maximum dose 30 mg/kg). Absent transfusion support or intercurrent illness suppressing erythropoiesis, a trial period of 6 to 8 months is probably adequate.

Treatment endpoints

Less pain, increase in HbF (or MCV), increased hemoglobin level if severely anemic; acceptable toxicity.

Special caution should be exercised in patients with compromised renal or hepatic function and when patients are habituated to narcotics. Contraception should be practiced by both men and women because hydroxyurea is a teratogen, and its effects in pregnancy are unknown. After a stable and nontoxic dose of hydroxyurea is reached, blood counts should be completed at 4- to 8-week intervals. Granulocytes should be $\geq 2{,}000/mm^3$, platelets $\geq 80{,}000/mm^3$. A decline in hemoglobin level (in most patients who respond, the hemoglobin level increases slightly) and absolute reticulocyte count to $< 80{,}000/mm^3$ should be carefully evaluated. A hemoglobin < 5.5 g/dL before treatment is not a contraindication to treatment.
CBC, complete blood count; MCV, mean cell volume.

HbF increased form 3.6 to 11 percent. One pediatric patient with HbSO$_{Arab}$ who was treated for 8 months showed an increase in HbF from 6.6 to 11.8 percent (Rogers et al., 1997).

On the basis of these reports, it is impossible to know the rate of response to and effectiveness of hydroxyurea in varied compound heterozygous sickle hemoglobinopathies. It is unlikely that controlled trials will be done in less common types of sickle cell disease, other than HbSC disease. As suggested by the preliminary studies in HbSC disease, hydroxyurea may have alternative mechanisms of action in conditions where the pathophysiology is determined primarily by cell density. Treatment might best be reserved for patients whose illness is of sufficient severity to warrant a trial of this potentially hazardous drug.

Treatment Recommendations

Indications for hydroxyurea treatment are likely to change as more information on safety and benefits accrue and the results of trials in children are completed. Presently, hydroxyurea should be reserved for patients whose complications are sufficiently severe to warrant the burdens of treatment and who can comply with the treatment regimen. Adults and teenagers are the most suitable patients for treatment. Children with severe disease complications should be enrolled in clinical trials where possible and if they are eligible. Outside the context of controlled trials, consultation with expert pediatricians and a detailed explanation to parents of the unknown attributes of this treatment and its alternatives should precede therapy. Patients suitable for treatment and a method of therapy are outlined in Table 38.2.

There is no urgency to arrive rapidly at a final dose, especially because some patients have myelotoxicity at quite low doses. Therapy can be started with 10 to 15 mg/kg given in a single daily dose or be started on 500 mg/day. Rare adult patients cannot tolerate a 500 mg daily dose. After 6 to 8 weeks, if blood counts are stable, the dose may be increased to 1,000 mg/day. Most patients who respond to hydroxyurea maintain tolerable blood counts at doses between 1,000 and 2,000 mg/day (20 to 30 mg/kg). Because of the availability of 200, 300, and 400 mg hydroxyurea capsules (Droxia®), it is now possible to more precisely titrate the dose of hydroxyurea. In principle, this should allow the same dose to be given each day. Many different dosing schemes have been recommended, but the sole controlled study gave the drug daily and pushed the dose just short of toxicity (Charache et al., 1995b). Whether this is needed for a satisfactory therapeutic effect is not known. The therapeutic endpoint should strike a balance between nontoxic doses of hydroxyurea and increases of HbF. Because MCV rises when hydroxyurea is used and usually parallels the increase in HbF, this inexpensive measurement is a useful surrogate for HbF level and can be serially followed, although HbF should be measured at baseline and at 6- to 8-week intervals during the first 6 months of treatment. Blood transfusions suppress erythropoiesis, and active erythropoiesis is necessary for hydroxyurea to increase HbF. It is probably not efficacious to use this drug in patients on frequent or regular transfusion programs, although a preliminary report indicated that some children undergoing long-term transfusions may have a modest HbF increase when given hydroxyurea (Nadvi et al., 1998). Nine children with a mean age of 12.5 years on chronic transfusions for more than 3 years were given 30 mg/kg/day of hydroxyurea for 6 months. Four patients had an HbF increase ≥ 5 percent. In another study to test a modified transfusion-hydroxurea regimen for secondary stroke prevention, where erythrocytapheresis was used monthly to keep HbS levels at or below 50 percent with a hemoglobin concentration of 10 g/dL, hydroxyurea was given daily at a dose of 15 to 25 mg/kg (Hannah et al., 1999). HbF was between 7.3 and 13 percent, and in four of six patients who had been on hydroxyurea for more than 15 months, HbF was more than 10 percent. HbF levels before beginning drug treatment were not reported, so it is unclear whether any increment in HbF was associated with treatment.

Until a stable dose is achieved, blood counts should be monitored biweekly. Even when the final dose is reached, counts should be checked at 4- to 8-week intervals to forestall complications from the occasionally capricious decline in leukocyte or platelet counts. Some adult patients will not respond to treatment with an increase in HbF or MCV, even when they faithfully take their prescribed medication (Rodgers et al., 1990; El-Hazmi et al., 1995b, Steinberg et al., 1997a). The percentage of such patients may range from 10 to 25 percent of treated patients and is dependent on the dosing regimen, condition of the bone marrow, genetic determinants, and drug metabolism (Steinberg et al., 1997a). Patients should be explicitly counseled that (1) not everyone will respond, (2) responses differ among patients, (3) many months may be needed to find the best dose of drug, (4) medication must be taken exactly as directed with frequent blood tests, and (5) the long-term toxicities and effects of treatment are

unknown. When HbF and MCV do not increase, either the optimal dose has not been reached, the patient is biologically unable to respond to treatment, or compliance is poor. Rapid plasma clearance hinders monitoring compliance by blood sampling (Rodriguez et al., 1998). If a patient has not received blood transfusions or had an intercurrent illness that suppresses erythropoiesis, it is likely that a 6- to 8-month trial is sufficient to assess whether hydroxyurea will be an effective treatment.

HYDROXYUREA IN β THALASSEMIA

Very high doses of hydroxyurea were given to mice with β thalassemia caused by homozygous deletion of the β major-globin genes, increased PCV, and β minor-globin chain synthesis (Sauvage et al., 1993). Mice have no fetal hemoglobin, and β minor-globin gene expression has some features that resemble that of the human γ-globin genes. Compared with the many propitious studies of hydroxyurea in sickle cell anemia, a therapeutic role for this agent in the severe β thalassemias is questionable. In β thalassemia the goal of treatment is to reduce globin chain synthesis imbalance by enhancing non-α-globin chain synthesis and not to reduce polymerization potential by increasing HbF. To date, HbF increases have been unimpressive, although there is evidence that β-globin gene expression can be increased. In some types of β thalassemia intermedia, hydroxyurea has had hematologic benefit.

Two patients with β thalassemia intermedia, both heterozygous for the common Asian IVS-2-654 C→T mutation, responded to hydroxyurea with increases in hemoglobin levels and improvement in the β/α biosynthesis ratio (Zeng et al., 1995). HbF levels decreased. These patients received very low doses of hydroxyurea, and the authors speculated that this may have been responsible for the preferential increase in β-chain synthesis. Three other patients with β thalassemia intermedia given hydroxyurea had small and transient increases in HbF and PCV (Hajjar and Pearson, 1994). A 41-year-old man with a thalassemia intermedia phenotype, homozygous for the position 848 C→A mutation, had a 65 percent increase in absolute HbF level and 1.5 g/dL increase in hemoglobin concentration on a dose of 9 to 11 mg/kg/day of hydroxyurea (Saxon et al., 1998). Paraspinal extramedullary hematopoietic masses resolved with treatment. Five of six patients with β thalassemia intermedia given 10 to 15 mg/kg of hydroxyurea daily had an increase in hemoglobin concentration from 1.3 to 3.5 g/dL (Alberto, 1998). Thirteen patients with HbE-β⁰ thalassemia were treated with 10 to 20 mg/kg/day of hydroxyurea for 20 weeks (Fucharoen et al., 1996). HbF increased from 42 to 56 percent as

HbE fell from 59 to 49 percent. A small but significant increase in hemoglobin level from 6.6 to 7.3 g/dL was accompanied by indications of reduced hemolysis. In case reports, one patient with homozygous β^0 thalassemia and one with Hb Lepore/β^0 thalassemia were treated with hydroxyurea and had good clinical results (Arruda et al., 1997; Rigano et al., 1997). Extramedullary hematopoiesis was reduced and the hemoglobin level increased from 5.8 to 9.7 g/dL and HbF from 4.9 to 9.1/dL in the Hb Lepore/β^0 thalassemia patient, whereas the β thalassemia homozygote became transfusion independent.

Few reports of clinical efficacy in the most severe, transfusion-dependent types of β thalassemia suggest that hydroxyurea is not a generally useful treatment for these disorders. In some types of β thalassemia intermedia, there appears to be a modest effect on total hemoglobin concentration and HbF. There may be a reduction in hemolysis and regression of extramedullary hematopoiesis. Although the future for hydroxyurea, as presently used, as a sole treatment of β thalassemia major does not look promising, based on preliminary observations expanded trials of its use in thalassemia intermedia syndromes for more extended periods seem warranted.

HYDROXYUREA IN OTHER HEMOGLOBINOPATHIES

Because of thrombocytosis and extramedullary hematopoiesis, two patients with unstable hemoglobin hemolytic anemia were treated with hydroxyurea (Rose and Bauters, 1996). In both individuals, HbF increased to about 30 percent, and in one the amount of unstable hemoglobin fell from 12 to 3 percent. Hemoglobin levels remained stable or increased. Most cases of hemolytic anemia secondary to unstable hemoglobins do not require treatment to increase their PCV (Chapter 44). Whether other patients with the disorder will respond in the same way is unknown.

SHORT-CHAIN FATTY ACIDS

Sodium butyrate, a 4-carbon fatty acid analog, can induce reversible gene expression in cultured cells when present in millimolar concentrations (Kruh, 1982). Accompanying gene expression is an inhibition of histone deacetylase, histone hyperacetylation, and changes in chromatin structure. Other histone deacetylase inhibitors can also induce gene expression (McCaffrey et al., 1997). Sodium butyrate activated the embryonic ρ-globin gene in adult chicken cells treated with 5-azacytidine. 5-Azacytidine alone had little effect on gene expression even though hypomethylation occurred (Ginder et al., 1984). Both agents were required for Dnase hypersensitivity to appear 5′ to the

ρ-globin gene and for ρ-globin gene mRNA to be detected. Butyrate cannot reactivate inactive γ-globin genes in transgenic mice. 5-Azacytidine can reactivate γ-globin gene expression in this model and is synergistic with butyrate, suggesting that γ gene activation by butyrate may require an active chromatin structure (Pace et al., 1994). Butyrates appear to directly modulate globin gene expression by binding to transcriptionally active elements in the 5′ flanking region of the gene (Glauber et al., 1991). These so-called butyrate response elements have been mapped in mice with $^A\gamma$-globin transgenes and truncation mutations of the $^A\gamma$-globin gene promoter, to sequences −382 to −730 and −730 to −1350 of the γ gene promoter (Pace et al., 1996). However, the physiologic relevance of experiments using small constructs in limited numbers of transgenic lines is unclear. Unlike hydroxyurea and other myelosuppressive agents, butyrate does not appear to be cytotoxic and therefore is unlikely to affect HbF level by cell selection. Increased γ-globin mRNA and γ-globin chains were noted in nucleated red cell precursors isolated from seven patients with β thalassemia and a patient with sickle cell anemia before and during their treatment with butyrate (Ikuta et al., 1998). New in vivo footprints were present in four areas of the γ-globin gene promoter, designated BRE-G1-4, in the seven butyrate-responsive patients. These promoter sites, on the basis of other studies, were deemed to have functional importance and BRE-G3 (between −170 and −150 5′ to the transcription start site) and G4 (−209 to −203) were in areas where nondeletion hereditary persistence of fetal hemoglobin (HPFH) mutations had been found (Chapter 15). Two possible erythroid-specific and one ubiquitous transcription factor, αCP2, bound to BRE-G1 only in butyrate-responsive patients, suggesting that the response to butyrate involves alterations in DNA-transcription factor interactions in the γ-globin gene promoter.

Perrine and her co-workers noted that infants of diabetic mothers had a delayed switch from γ- to β-globin gene expression (Perrine et al., 1985; Bard and Prosmanne, 1985). It was postulated that this delay resulted from increased serum levels of α amino-n-butyric acid. In erythroid cell cultures and in ovine fetuses, α amino-n-butyric acid delayed the γ- to β-globin gene switch (Perrine et al., 1987, 1988). Sodium butyrate increased HbF in baboons and enhanced γ-globin gene expression in erythroid cells of patients with sickle cell anemia and β thalassemia (Constantoulakis et al., 1989; Perrine et al., 1989). Clinical trials of butyrate in sickle cell anemia and β thalassemia soon followed these encouraging studies.

Initial butyrate trials in β thalassemia and sickle cell anemia were inconsistent and disappointing. Few patients were treated and some had increased hemoglobin level, F cells, and HbF. However, it was unclear what proportion of patients had these effects, whether they were sustained, and if any clinical benefit resulted (Blau et al., 1993; Perrine et al., 1993; Dover et al., 1994; Sher et al., 1995). The first trials using arginine butyrate in β thalassemia involved continuous infusion of drug over 2 to 3 weeks, hardly a practical regimen for clinical use (Perrine et al., 1993). F cells, and γ-globin synthesis, and, in some cases, PCV increased. Butyrate can arrest growth at the G1 phase of the cell cycle, suggesting that its continued administration might induce myelosuppression and abrogate the initial HbF response associated with its use (Toscani et al., 1988). In baboons, continued administration of butyrate or acetate, a metabolite of butyrate, was responsible for the loss of an initial increase in HbF (Stamatoyannopoulos et al., 1994). Because of the antiproliferative effects of this agent, a regimen of intermittent exposure to butyrate was tested in sickle cell anemia.

When pulse treatments with arginine butyrate were given once or twice monthly, results were more encouraging (Sutton et al., 1998; Atweh et al., 1999). Eleven of fifteen patients with sickle cell anemia responded to a regimen of pulse intravenous butyrate treatment with a mean increase in HbF from 7 percent to 21 percent, and in some individuals this level was maintained for 1 to 2 years (Atweh et al., 1999). Responding patients had a baseline HbF above 2 percent, but all nonresponders had initial HbF levels less than 2 percent. These preliminary studies also suggested that there was no cross-resistance between butyrate and hydroxyurea and that pretreatment with hydroxyurea may, by selecting a population of erythroid precursors with active γ-globin genes, make them responsive to the actions of butyrate.

Kinetics of the HbF response to arginine butyrate showed that by 24 hours there was a threefold to sixfold increase in γ-globin chain synthesis, with even larger increments in γ-globin mRNA, suggesting a posttranscriptional mode of action (Weinberg et al., 1998). These were pilot studies involving few patients, but this regimen deserves further study.

Pulse butyrate given 4 nights twice a month increased the hemoglobin concentration from 1.3 to 4.0 g/dL (mean 2.9 g/dL) in four patients with β thalassemia intermedia and three with β thalassemia major (Bergsage et al., 1998). Four patients became transfusion independent and in some of them, the response to treatment has been sustained for over nearly 4 years. No response to oral sodium phenylbutyrate was seen in five infants and one 4-year-old child with β thalassemia (Sharma et al., 1998). Further trials are not planned for the oral analog, isobutyramide,

which has been reported to increase γ-globin synthesis in vitro and in vivo (Brown et al., 1994).

Presently, the use of butyrate or its analogs in sickle cell anemia or β thalassemia remains experimental and cannot be recommended for treatment outside of clinical trials.

Antiproliferative effects of buytrate and other short-chain fatty acids have prompted a search for similar agents that do not inhibit the metabolic transporters needed for cellular proliferation, are not rapidly metabolized, and can be used orally. In vitro studies of 0.2 mmol/L thiophenoxyacetic acid, phenoxyacetic acid, 2,2-dimethybutyric acid, and derivatives of cinnamic acid—compounds that inhibited the metabolic transporter System A pump less than did butyrate—increased γ-globin production 12 to 38 percent in erythroid progenitor cell cultures (Torkelson et al., 1996). Other short-chain fatty acids and their analogs also affect γ-globin gene expression in vitro and in vivo. (Stamatoyannopoulos et al., 1994; Perrine et al., 1994; Liakopoulou et al., 1995; Little et al., 1995; Hudgins et al., 1996; Torkelson et al., 1996; Selby et al., 1997). Acetate, a 2-carbon product of butyrate catabolism, stimulates γ-globin gene expression in erythroid progenitor colonies, transgenic mice bearing an ^{A}γ-globin gene construct, and in baboons. Fatty acids of 3, 5, 6, 7, 8, and 9 carbon length all have an effect on γ-globin gene expression, suggesting their possible development as therapeutic agents. HbF levels were elevated in patients receiving the anticonvulsant valproic acid. HbF levels were increased to 3 to 10 percent in four patients with clinical disorders of propionate metabolism with hemolytic anemia. Young women with starvation ketosis had higher HbF levels than control subjects, and this was associated with increased blood levels of β-hydroxybutyrate (Peters et al., 1998). Short-chain fatty acid derivatives of proprionic acid and butyric acid had half-lives of more than 7 hours after oral dosing with millimolar plasma concentration and increased F reticulocytes, γ-globin chain synthesis, and PCV in baboons, suggesting that they might be therapeutically useful (Boosalis et al., 1997, 1999). Clinical studies of other short-chain fatty acids lag far behind those of butyric acid analogs.

COMBINATION OF HbF-INDUCERS

Rapid regeneration of the erythroid progenitor pool during "stress erythropoiesis" has been associated with transient increases of HbF. On the basis of these observations, erythropoietin was given in conjunction with hydroxyurea in nonhuman primates and exerted an additive (or synergistic) augmentation in HbF levels (al-Khatti et al., 1988a, 1988b; McDonagh et al., 1992). Subsequently, a further increase in HbF levels

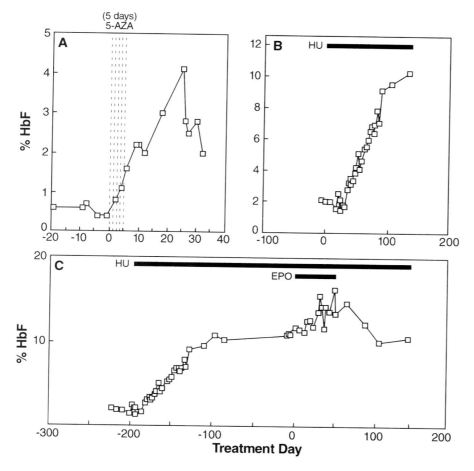

Figure 38.8. Kinetics of the HbF response to 5-azacytidine, hydroxyurea, and hydroxyurea plus erythropoietin in a single patient.

has been shown in hydroxyurea-treated patients with sickle cell disease when it is coadministered with erythropoietin (Rodgers et al., 1993; Voskaridou et al., 1995; El-Hazmi et al., 1995a). Recent availability of erythropoietin in a concentrated dosage of 40,000 unit/mL makes it feasible to restudy the effects of combined therapy with hydroxyurea and erythropoietin. An example of the synergistic effects seen when erythropoietin is added to hydroxyurea in shown in Figure 38.8. Also shown are the kinetics of the HbF response of a single patient with three different pharmacologic approaches.

In β thalassemia, erythropoietin levels are inappropriately low for the level of anemia. Erythropoietin alone and in combination with hydroxyurea—supplemental iron and folic acid were also given—was given to patients with β thalassemia intermedia to increase their hemoglobin concentration (Rachmilewitz and Acker, 1998; Rachmilewitz et al., 1995). In one trial of ten patients, six of whom had undergone splenectomy

increased their hemoglobin levels from about 7 to 9 g/dL in a dose-dependent fashion while receiving between 500 and 950 units/kg three times a week, an increase that was sustained for 11 months (Rachmilewitz et al., 1995). HbF levels did not change, but in some patients, the number of F cells increased. Two responding patients no longer required blood transfusions. Insufficient data are available to predict who will respond to this treatment by becoming transfusion-independent.

Preliminary trials of erythropoietin plus hydroxyurea (20 mg/kg/day of hydroxyurea 4 days a week followed by 500 units/kg/day erythropoietin on the remaining 3 days) showed a slight additive effect of these agents in two of seven patients (Rachmilewitz and Aker, 1998). Increasing the dose of erythropoietin and hydroxyurea appeared to give a better response rate, but the data were too scant to be conclusive. Some patients had increases in HbF; however, these results were in short-term studies, and do not suggest a major role for this type of combination treatment in the management of β thalassemia.

Although other cytokines, including GM-CSF and IL-3, may elevate HbF in the primate model, neither appears to work synergistically with hydroxyurea; moreover their potential to greatly increase the neutrophil count precludes their use in the context of the severe β-globin gene disorders (McDonagh et al., 1992).

Combination therapy with hydroxyurea and butyrate in two patients with hemoglobin Lepore has resulted in significant long-term increases in both the fetal hemoglobin and total hemoglobin concentrations (Olivieri et al., 1997). The magnitude of these responses, together with a similar response in a compound heterozygote for hemoglobin Lepore and β thalassemia, poses the obvious question of the role of the molecular defect in Hb Lepore and response to hydroxyurea (Rigano et al., 1997). Further studies using erthyroid cell culture or transgenic mice may clarify this issue. Three patients with sickle cell anemia treated with hydroxyurea had butyrate added to their drug regimen. In all three patients, HbF concentrations increased when butyrate was started including a patient who was resistant to treatment with butyrate alone (Atweh, GF, personal communication, 1999). In two of three patients who were unresponsive to butyrate, addition of hydroxyurea led to an increase in HbF (Atweh, GF, personal communication, 1999).

SUMMARY

Hydroxyurea is the first drug shown to prevent at least some complications of sickle cell disease in a majority of patients. The drug is still early in development. In the next decade, its value in younger patients, who stand to benefit most, should be defined and its long-term toxicity and effects on survival better delineated. This agent appears to have only marginal utility in the severe β thalassemias. Few would argue that hydroxyurea will be the final word in sickle cell disease treatment because its ability to increase HbF beyond 20 to 30 percent of total hemoglobin seems doubtful. Studies are needed to find new applications of current treatments and to devise new treatments to disrupt multiple facets of the pathophysiology of the sickle cell disease and β thalassemia, or to increase HbF to levels at which it constitutes a majority of the hemoglobin present.

References

Adams-Graves, P, Heltsley, C, and Deitcher, S. (1996). Hydroxyurea in sickle cell disease. *N. Engl. J. Med.* 334: 333–334.

Adams, RJ, Carl, EJ, McKie, VC et al. (1999). A pilot trial of hydroxyurea to prevent strokes in children with sickle cell anemia. *23rd Annual Meeting of the National Sickle Cell Disease Program*, San Francisco.

Adragna, NC, Fonseca, P, and Lauf, PK. (1994). Hydroxyurea affects cell morphology cation transport and red blood cell adhesion in cultured vascular endothelial cells. *Blood* 83: 553–560.

Aessopos, A, Karabatsos, F, Farmakis, D et al. (1999). Pregnancy in patients with well-treated β-thalassemia: Outcome for mothers and newborn infants. *Am. J. Obstet. Gynecol.* 180: 360–365.

al-Khatti, A, Papayannopoulou, T, Knitter, G et al. (1988a). Cooperative enhancement of F-cell formation in baboons treated with erythropoietin and hydroxyurea. *Blood* 72: 817–819.

al-Khatti, A, Umemura, T, Clow, J et al. (1988b). Erythropoietin stimulates F-reticulocyte formation in sickle cell anemia. *Trans. Assoc. Am. Physicians* 101: 54–61.

Alberto, FL, Arruda, VR, Lima, CSP et al. (1998). Long-term hydroxyurea therapy in thalassemia intermedia and thalassemia major patients. *Blood* 92: 36b.

Arruda, VR, Lima, CSP, Saad, STO, and Costa, FF. (1997). Successful use of hydroxyurea in β-thalassemia major. *N. Engl. J. Med.* 336: 964–964.

Atweh, GF, Sutton, M, Nassif, I et al. (1999). Sustained induction of fetal hemoglobin by pulse butyrate therapy in sickle cell disease. *Blood* 93: 1790–1797.

Ballas, SK, Dover, GJ, and Charache, S. (1991). Effect of hydroxyurea on the rheological properties of sickle erythrocytes in vivo. *Am. J. Hematol.* 32: 104–111.

Ballas, SK, Marcolina, MJ, Dover, GJ, and Barton, FB. (1999). Erythropoietic activity in patients with sickle cell anaemia before and after treatment with hydroxyurea. *Br. J. Haematol.* 105: 491–496.

Barbul, T, Finazzi, G, Ruggeri, M, and Rideghiero, F. (1998). Secondary leukemia following hydroxyurea in patients with essential thrombocythemia: Long-term results of a randomized clinical trial. *Blood* 92: 489a.

Bard, H and Prosmanne, J. (1985). Relative rates of fetal hemoglobin and adult hemoglobin synthesis in cord blood of infants of insulin-dependent diabetic mothers. *Pediatrics* 75: 1143–1147.

Benz, EJ Jr. (1982). Clinical management of gene expression. *N. Engl. J. Med.* 307: 1515–1516.

Bergsage, J, Li, Q, Boosalis, V et al. Pulse butyrate therapy in beta thalassemia. *Blood* 92: 529a.

Best, PJ, Daoud, MS, Pittelkow, MR, and Petitt RM. (1998). Hydroxyurea-induced leg ulceration in 14 patients. *Ann. Intern. Med.* 128: 29–32.

Beutler, E and Mikus, BJ. (1961). Effect of methemoglobin formation in sickle cell disease. *J. Clin. Invest.* 40: 1856–1871.

Bhattacharya, SK, Ramchandani, S, Cervoni, N, and Szyf, M. (1999). A mammalian protein with specific demethylase activity for mCpG DNA. *Nature* 397: 579–583.

Blau, CA, Constantoulakis, P, Shaw, CM, and Stamatoyannopoulos, G. (1993). Fetal hemoglobin induction with butyric acid: Efficacy and toxicity. *Blood* 81: 529–537.

Boosalis, M, Bandyopadhay, R, Pace, B et al. (1999). Fatty acid derivatives stimulating erythropoiesis & HbF. *23rd Annual Meeting of the National Sickle Cell Disease Program*, San Francisco.

Boosalis, M, Ikuta, T, Pace, B et al. (1997). Abrogation of IL-3 requirements and stimulation of hematopoietic cell proliferation in vitro and in vivo by carboxylic acids. *Blood Cells Mol. Dis.* 23: 434–442.

Bridges, KR, Barabino, GD, Brugnara, C et al. (1996). A multiparameter analysis of sickle erythrocytes in patients undergoing hydroxyurea therapy. *Blood* 88: 4701–4710.

Brittain, HA, Eckman, JR, Swerlick, RA et al. (1993). Thrombospondin from activated platelets promotes sickle erythrocyte adherence to human microvascular endothelium under physiologic flow: A potential role for platelet activation in sickle cell vaso-occlusion. *Blood* 81: 2137–2143.

Brown, AK, Sleeper, LA, Pegelow, CH et al. (1994). The influence of infant and maternal sickle cell disease on birth outcome and neonatal course. *Am. J. Dis. Child.* 148: 1156–1162.

Campbell, PJ, Olatunji, PO, Ryan, KE, and Davies, SC. (1997). Splenic regrowth in sickle cell anaemia following hypertransfusion. *Br. J. Haematol.* 96: 77–79.

Charache, S, Dover, G, Smith, K et al. (1983). Treatment of sickle cell anemia with 5-azacytidine results in increased fetal hemoglobin production and is associated with nonrandom hypomethylation of DNA around the γ–δ–β globin gene complex. *Proc. Natl. Acad. Sci. U.S.A.* 80: 4842–4846.

Charache, S, Dover, GJ, Moyer, MA, and Moore, JW. (1987). Hydroxyurea-induced augmentation of fetal hemoglobin production in patients with sickle cell anemia. *Blood* 69: 109–116.

Charache, S, Dover, GJ, Moore, RD et al. (1992). Hydroxyurea: Effects on hemoglobin F production in patients with sickle cell anemia. *Blood* 79: 2555–2565.

Charache, S, Terrin, ML, Moore, RD et al. (1995a). Effect of hydroxyurea on the frequency of painful crises in sickle cell anemia. *N. Engl. J. Med.* 332: 1317–1322.

Charache, S, Terrin, ML, Moore, RD et al. (1995b). Design of the multicenter study of hydroxyurea in sickle cell anemia. *Controlled Clin. Trials* 16: 432–446.

Charache, S, Barton, FB, Moore, RD et al. (1996). Hydroxyurea and sickle cell anemia: Clinical utility of a myelosuppressive "switching" agent. *Medicine (Baltimore)* 75: 300–326.

Christman, JK, Price, P, Pedrinan, L, and Acs, G. (1977). Correlation between hypomethylation of DNA and expression of globin genes in Friend erythroleukemia cells. *Eur. J. Biochem.* 81: 53–61.

Claster, S and Vichinsky, E. (1996). First report of reversal of organ dysfunction in sickle cell anemia by the use of hydroxyurea: Splenic regeneration. *Blood* 88: 1951–1953.

Constantoulakis, P, Knitter, G, and Stamatoyannopoulos, G. (1989). On the induction of fetal hemoglobin by butyrates: In vivo and in vitro studies with sodium butyrate and comparison of combination treatments with 5-AzaC and AraC. *Blood* 74: 1963–1971.

Davey, C, Pennings, S, and Allan, J. (1997). CpG methylation remodels chromatin structure in vitro. *J. Mol. Biol.* 267: 276–288.

deMontalembert, M, Belloy, M, Bernaudin, F et al. (1994). Clinical and hematological response of sickle cell children to treatment with hydroxyurea. *Blood* 84(Suppl 1): 219a.

deMontalembert, M, Begue, P, Bernaudin, F et al. (1999). Preliminary report of a toxicity study of hydroxyurea in sickle cell disease. French Study Group on Sickle Cell Disease. *Arch Dis Child* 81: 437–439.

DeSimone, J, Heller, P, Hall, L, and Zwiers, D. (1982). 5-Azacytidine stimulates fetal hemoglobin synthesis in anemia baboons. *Proc. Natl. Acad. Sci. U.S.A.* 79: 4428–4431.

Diav-Citrin, O, Hunnisett, L, Sher, GD, and Koren, G. (1999). Hydroxyurea use during pregnancy: A case report in sickle cell disease and review of the literature. *Am. J. Hematol.* 60: 148–150.

Dover, GJ, Humphries, RK, Moore, JG et al. (1986). Hydroxyurea induction of hemoglobin F production in sickle cell disease: Relationship between cytotoxicity and F cell production. *Blood* 67: 735–738.

Dover, GJ, Brusilow, S, and Charache, S. (1994). Induction of fetal hemoglobin production in subjects with sickle cell anemia by oral sodium phenylbutyrate. *Blood* 84: 339–343.

Eckardt, SG, Dai, A, Davidson, KK et al. (1994). Induction of differentiation in HL-60 cells by the reduction of extrachromosomally-amplified c-*myc*. *Proc. Natl. Acad. Sci. U.S.A.* 91: 6674.

Edington, GM and Lehmann, H. (1955). Expression of the sickle-cell gene in Africa. *Br. Med. J.* 1: 1308–1311.

El-Hazmi, MAF, Warsy, AS, Al-Momen, A, and Harakati, M. (1992). Hydroxyurea for the treatment of sickle cell disease. *Acta Haematol.* 88: 170–174.

El-Hazmi, MAF, Al-Momen, A, Warsy, AS et al. (1995a). The pharmacological manipulation of fetal haemoglobin: Trials using hydroxyurea and recombinant human erythropoietin. *Acta Haematol.* 93: 57–61.

El-Hazmi, MAF, Al-Momen, A, Kandaswamy, S et al. (1995b). On the use of hydroxyurea erythropoietin combination therapy for sickle cell disease. *Acta Haematol.* 94: 128–134.

Enver, T, Zhang, J-W, Papayannopoulou, T, and Stamatoyannopoulos, G. (1988). DNA methylation: A secondary event in globin gene switching? *Genes Dev.* 2: 698–706.

Fadlon, E, Vordermeier, S, Pearson, TC et al. (1998). Blood polymorphonuclear leukocytes from the majority of sickle cell patients in the crisis phase of the disease show enhanced adhesion to vascular endothelium and increased expression of CD64. *Blood* 91: 266–274.

Felsenfeld, G and McGhee, J. (1982). Methylation and gene control. *Nature* 296: 602–603.

Ferster, A, Bujan, W, Corazza, F et al. (1993). Bone marrow transplantation corrects the splenic reticuloendothelial dysfunction in sickle cell anemia. *Blood* 81: 1102–1105.

Ferster, A, Vermylen, C, Cornu, G et al. (1996). Hydroxyurea for treatment of severe sickle cell anemia: A pediatric clinical trial. *Blood* 88: 1960–1964.

Fucharoen, S, Siritanaratkul, N, Winichagoon, P et al. (1996). Hydroxyurea increases hemoglobin F levels and improves the effectiveness of erythropoiesis in β-thalassemia hemoglobin E disease. *Blood* 87: 887–892.

Garrick, D, Sutherland, H, Robertson, G, and Whitelaw, E. (1996). Variegated expression of a globin transgene correlates with chromatin accessibility but not methylation status. *Nucleic Acids Res.* 24: 4902–4909.

Gee, BE and Platt, OS. (1995). Sickle reticulocytes adhere to VCAM-1. *Blood* 85: 268–274.

Ginder, GD, Whitters, MJ, and Pohlman, JK. (1984). Activation of a chicken embryonic globin gene in adult erythroid cells by 5-azacytidine and sodium butyrate. *Proc. Natl. Acad. Sci. U.S.A.* 81: 3954–3958.

Gladwin, MT, Schechter, AN, Shelhamer, JH et al. (1999). Inhaled nitric oxide augments nitric oxide transport on sickle cell hemoglobin without affecting oxygen affinity. *J. Clin. Invest.* 104: 937–945.

Glauber, JG, Wandersee, NJ, Little, JA, and Ginder, GD. (1991). 5′-Flanking sequences mediate butyrate stimulation of embryonic globin gene expression in adult erythroid cells. *Mol. Cell. Biol.* 11: 4690–4697.

Glover, RE, Ivy, ED, Orringer, EP et al. (1999). Detection of nitrosyl hemoglobin in venous blood in the treatment of sickle cell anemia with hydroxyurea. *Mol. Pharmacol.* 55: 1006–10010.

Hackney, AC, Hezier, W, Gulledge, TP et al. (1997). Effects of hydroxyurea administration on the body weight, body composition and exercise performance of patients with sickle-cell anaemia. *Clin. Sci.* 92: 481–486.

Hajjar, FM and Pearson, HA. (1994). Pharmacologic treatment of thalassemia intermedia with hydroxyurea. *J. Pediatr.* 125: 490–492.

Hannah, A, McKie, V, McKie, KM et al. (1999). Combination of hydroxyurea and a modified transfusion regimen in secondary stroke prevention on sickle cell disease. *23rd Annual Meeting of the National Sickle Cell Disease Program.*

Hayes, RJ, Beckford, M, Grandison, Y et al. (1985). The haematology of steady state homozygous sickle cell disease: Frequency distribution variation with age and sex, longitudinal observations. *Br. J. Haematol.* 59: 369–382.

Head, CA, Brugnara, C, Martinez-Ruiz, R et al. (1997). Low concentrations of nitric oxide increase oxygen affinity of sickle erythrocytes in vitro and in vivo. *J. Clin. Invest.* 100: 1193–1198.

Hebbel, RP, Boogaerts, MA, Eaton, JW, and Steinberg, MH. (1980). Erythrocyte adherence to endothelium in sickle-cell anemia. A possible determinant of disease severity. *N. Engl. J. Med.* 302: 992–995.

Hofstra, TC, Kalra, VK, Meiselman, HJ, and Coates, TD. (1996). Sickle erythrocytes adhere to polymorphonuclear neutrophils and activate the neutrophil respiratory burst. *Blood* 87: 4440–4447.

Holliday, R and Pugh, JE. (1975). DNA modification mechanisms and gene activity during development. *Science* 187: 226–232.

Holliday, R, Monk M, and Pugh, JE. (1990). DNA methylation and gene regulation. *Philos. Trans. R. Soc. Lond. B. Biol. Sci.* 326: 177–338.

Horiuchi, K, Golden, JA, Das, SK et al. (1998). Adverse effects of hydroxyurea on growth and development of young mice. *Blood* 92: 160a.

Hudgins, WR, Fibach, E, Safaya, S et al. (1996). Transcriptional upregulation of gamma-globin by phenylbutyrate and analogous aromatic fatty acids. *Biochem. Pharmacol.* 52: 1227–1233.

Ikuta, T, Kan, YW, Swerdlow, PS et al. (1998). Alterations in protein-DNA interactions in the gamma-globin gene promoter in response to butyrate therapy. *Blood* 92: 2924–2933.

Iyer, R, Baliga, R, Nagel, RL et al. (2000). Maximum urine concentrating ability in children with Hb SC disease: Effects of hydroxyurea. *Am. J. Hematol.* 64: 47–42.

Jayabose, S, Tugal, O, Sandoval, C et al. (1996). Clinical and hematologic effects of hydroxyurea in children with sickle cell anemia. *J. Pediatr.* 129: 559–565.

Jiang, J, Jordan, SJ, Barr, DP et al. (1997). In vivo production of nitric oxide in rats after administration of hydroxyurea. *Mol. Pharmacol.* 52: 1081–1086.

Joneckis, CC, Ackley, RL, Orringer, EP et al. (1993). Integrin $\alpha_4\beta_1$ and glycoprotein IV (CD36) are expressed on circulating reticulocytes in sickle cell anemia. *Blood* 82: 3548–3555.

Jones, PA and Taylor SM. (1980). Cellular differentiation cytidine analogs and DNA methylation. *Cell* 20: 85–93.

Kido, M, Tago, O, Fujiwara, H et al. (1998). Leg ulcer associated with hydroxyurea treatment in a patient with chronic myelogenous leukaemia: Successful treatment with prostaglandin E_1 and pentoxifylline. *Br. J. Dermatol.* 139: 1124–1126.

Kim-Shapiro, DB, King, SB, Bonifant, CL, and Ballas, SK. (1997). Hydroxyurea reacts with sickle cell hemoglobin to form methemoglobin and other minor species. *Blood* 90: 28b.

Kinney, TR, Helms, RW, O'Branski, EE et al. (1999). Safety of hydroxyurea in children with sickle cell anemia: results of the HUG-KIDS study, a phase I/II trial. Pediatric Hydroxyurea Group. *Blood* 94: 1550–1554.

Koren, A, Segal-Kupershmit, D, Zalman, L et al. (1999). Effect of hydroxyurea in sickle cell anemia: A clinical trial in children and teenagers with severe sickle cell anemia and sickle cell beta thalassemia. *Pediatr. Hematol. Oncol.* 16: 221–232.

Koshy, M, DeSimone, J, Molokie, R et al. (1998). Augmentation of fetal hemoglobin (HbF) by low dose short-duration 5′-aza-deoxycytidine (decitabine) administration in sickle cell anemia patients who had no HbF elevation following hydroxyurea therapy. *Blood* 92(Supplement 1): 30b.

Kruh, J. (1982). Effects of sodium butyrate a new pharmacological agent on cells in culture. *Mol. Cell. Biochem.* 42: 65–82.

Letvin, NL, Linch, DC, Beardsley, P et al. (1984). Augmentation of fetal hemoglobin in anemic monkeys by hydroxyurea. *N. Engl. J. Med.* 310: 869–874.

Ley, TJ, DeSimone, J, Anagnou, NP et al. (1982). 5-Azacytidine selectively increases gamma-globin synthesis in a patient with beta+ thalassemia. *N. Engl. J. Med.* 307: 1469–1475.

Ley, TJ, DeSimone, J, Noguchi, CT et al. (1983a). 5-Azacytidine increases gamma-globin synthesis and reduces the proportion of dense cells in patients with sickle cell anemia. *Blood* 62: 370–380.

Ley, TJ, Anagnou, NP, Noguchi, CT et al. (1983b). DNA methylation and globin gene expression in patients treated with 5-azacytidine. *Prog. Clin. Biol. Res.* 134: 457–474.

Liakopoulou, E, Blau, CA, Li, QL et al. (1995). Stimulation of fetal hemoglobin production by short chain fatty acids. *Blood* 86: 3227–3235.

Liozon, E, Brigaudeau, C, Trimoreau, F et al. (1997). Is treatment with hydroxyurea leukemogenic in patients with essential thrombocythemia? An analysis of three new cases of leukaemic transformation and review of the literature. *Hematol. Cell Ther.* 39: 11–18.

Little, JA, Dempsey, NJ, Tuchman, M, and Ginder, GD. (1995). Metabolic persistence of fetal hemoglobin. *Blood* 85: 1712–1718.

Loukopoulos, D. (1996). Current status of thalassemia and the sickle cell syndromes in Greece. *Semin. Hematol.* 33: 76–86.

McCaffrey, PG, Newsome, DA, Fibach, E et al. (1997). Induction of gamma-globin by histone deacetylase inhibitors. *Blood* 90: 2075–2083.

McDonagh, KT, Dover, GJ, Donahue, RE et al. (1992). Hydroxyurea-induced HbF production in anemic primates: Augmentation by erythropoietin, hematopoietic growth factors, and sodium butyrate. *Exp. Hematol.* 20: 1156–1164.

McGhee, JD and Ginder, GD. (1979). Specific DNA methylation sites in the vicinity of the chicken β-globin genes. *Nature* 280: 419–420.

Mohandas, T, Sparkes, RS, and Shapiro, LJ. (1998). Reactivation of an inactive human X chromosome: Evidence for X inactivation by DNA methylation. *Science* 211: 393–396.

Moore, RD, Charache, S, Terrin, ML et al. (2000). Cost-effectiveness of hydroxyurea in sickle cell anemia. *Am. J. Hematol.* 64: 26–31.

Mougiou, A, Kouka, M, Mavromani, E et al. (1997). Cytogenetic and molecular (p53 and ras) studies in sickle cell patients receiving hydroxyurea over long time periods do not indicate and increased risk for leukemia. *Blood* 90: 29b.

Muraca, MF, Schinkel, H, Brown, E, and Olivieri, NF. (1998). Splenic function in patients with sickle cell disease treated with hydroxyurea. *Blood* 92: 32b.

Nadvi, SZ, Panchoosingh, H, Thomas, R, and Sarnaik, S. (1998). Use of hydroxyurea in patients with sickle cell anemia on chronic transfusion. *Blood* 92: 32b.

Najean, Y and Rain, J-D. (1997). Treatment of polycythemia vera: Use of ^{32}P alone or in combination with maintenance therapy using hydroxyurea in 461 patients greater than 65 years of age. *Blood* 89: 2319–2327.

Nand, S, Stock, W, Godwin, J, and Fisher, SG. (1996). Leukemogenic risk of hydroxyurea therapy in polycythemia vera, essential thrombocythemia, and myeloid metaplasia with myelofibrosis. *Am. J. Hematol.* 52: 42–46.

Norhaya, MR, Cheong, SK, Ainoon O, and Hamidah, NH. (1997). Painful oral ulcers with hydroxyurea therapy. *Singapore Med J* 38: 283–284.

Olivieri, NF, Rees, DC, Ginder, GD et al. (1997). Treatment of thalassaemia major with phenylbutyrate and hydroxyurea. *Lancet* 350: 491–492.

Olivieri, NF and Vichinksy, EP. (1998). Hydroxyurea in children with sickle cell disease: Impact on splenic function and compliance with therapy. *J. Pediatr. Hematol. Oncol.* 20: 26–31.

Pace, B, Li, Q, Peterson, K, and Stamatoyannopoulos, G. (1994). α-Amino butyric acid cannot reactivate the silenced gamma gene of the β locus *YAC* transgenic mouse. *Blood* 84: 4344–4353.

Pace, BS, Li, QL, and Stamatoyannopoulos, G. (1996). In vivo search for butyrate responsive sequences using transgenic mice carrying $^{A}\gamma$ gene promoter mutants. *Blood* 88: 1079–1083.

Papassotiriou, I, Stamoulakatou, A, Voskaridou, E et al. (1998). Hydroxyurea induced erythropoietin secretion in sickle cell syndromes may contribute in their HbF increase. *Blood* 92: 160a.

Parasuraman, S, Rodman, JH, Ware, RE et al. (1998). Pharmacokinetics (PK) of hydroxyurea (HU) in children with sickle cell anemia (SCA). *Blood* 92: 32b.

Perrine, SP, Greene, MF, and Faller, DV. (1985). Delay in the fetal globin switch in infants of diabetic mothers. *N. Engl. J. Med.* 312: 334–338.

Perrine, SP, Miller, BA, Greene, MF et al. (1987). Butyric acid analogues augment γ globin gene expression in neonatal erythroid progenitors. *Biochem. Biophys. Res. Commun.* 148: 694–700.

Perrine, SP, Rudolph, A, Faller, DV et al. (1988). Butyrate infusions in the ovine fetus delay the biologic clock for globin gene switching. *Proc. Natl. Acad. Sci. U.S.A.* 85: 8540–8542.

Perrine, SP, Miller, BA, Faller, DV et al. (1989). Sodium butyrate enhances fetal globin gene expression in erythroid progenitors of patients with Hb SS and beta thalassemia. *Blood* 74: 454–459.

Perrine, SP, Ginder, GD, Faller, DV et al. (1993). A short-term trial of butyrate to stimulate fetal-globin- gene expression in the β-globin disorders. *N. Engl. J. Med.* 328: 81–86.

Perrine, SP, Dover, GH, Daftari, P et al. (1994). Isobutyramide, an orally bioavailable butyrate analogue, stimulates fetal globin gene expression in vitro and in vivo. *Br. J. Haematol.* 88: 555–561.

Peters, A, Rohloff, D, Kohlmann, T et al. (1998). Fetal hemoglobin in starvation ketosis of young women. *Blood* 91: 691–694.

Platt, OS, Orkin, SH, Dover, G et al. (1984). Hydroxyurea enhances fetal hemoglobin production in sickle cell anemia. *J. Clin. Invest.* 74: 652–656.

Rachmilewitz, EA and Aker, M. (1998). The role of recombinant human erythropoietin in the treatment of thalassemia. *Ann. NY Acad. Sci.* 850: 129–138.

Rachmilewitz, EA, Aker, M, Perry, D, and Dover, G. (1995). Sustained increase in haemoglobin and RBC following long-term administration of recombinant human erythropoietin to patients with homozygous beta-thalassaemia. *Br. J. Haematol.* 90: 341–345.

Raphael, R, Ohene-Frempong, K, and Horiuchi, K. (1997). Influence of Duffy blood type on hydroxyurea (HU) therapy in pediatric sickle cell disease (SCD) patients. *Blood* 90: 444a.

Rauch, A., Borromeo, M., and Ghafoor, A et al. (1999). Leukemogenesis of hydroxyurea in the treatment of sickle cell anemia. *Blood* 94: 415a.

Ravandi-Kashani, F, Cortes, J, Cohen, P et al. (1998). Cutaneous ulcers associated with hydroxyurea (HU) therapy in myeloproliferative disorders. *Blood* 92: 248b.

Rigano, P, Manfre, L, La Galla, R et al. (1997). Clinical and hematological response to hydroxyurea in a patient with Hb Lepore/β-thalassemia. *Hemoglobin* 21: 219–226.

Rodgers, GP, Dover, GJ, Noguchi, CT et al. (1990). Hematologic responses of patients with sickle cell disease to treatment with hydroxyurea. *N. Engl. J. Med.* 322: 1037–1045.

Rodgers, GP, Dover, GJ, Uyesaka, N et al. (1993). Augmentation by erythropoietin of the fetal-hemoglobin response to hydroxyurea in sickle cell disease. *N. Engl. J. Med.* 328: 73–80.

Rodriguez, GI, Kuhn, JG, Weiss, GR et al. (1998). A bioavailability and pharmacokinetic study of oral and intravenous hydroxyurea. *Blood* 91: 1533–1541.

Rogers, ZR. (1997). Hydroxyurea therapy for diverse pediatric populations with sickle cell disease. *Semin. Hematol.* 34: 42–47.

Rose, C and Bauters, F. (1996). Hydroxyurea therapy in highly unstable hemoglobin carriers. *Blood* 88: 2807–2808.

Sato, K, Akaike, T, Sawa, T et al. (1997). Nitric oxide generation from hydroxyurea via copper-catalyzed peroxidation and implications for pharmacological actions of hydroxyurea. *Jpn. J. Cancer Res.* 88: 1199–1204.

Sauvage, C, Rouyer-Fessard, P, and Beuzard, Y. (1993). Improvement of mouse β thalassaemia by hydroxyurea. *Br. J. Haematol.* 84: 492–496.

Saxon, BR, Rees, D, and Olivieri, NF. (1998). Regression of extramedullary haemopoiesis and augmentation of fetal haemoglobin concentration during hydroxyurea therapy in β thalassaemia. *Br. J. Haematol.* 101: 416–419.

Scott, JP, Hillery, CA, Brown, ER et al. (1996). Hydroxyurea therapy in children severely affected with sickle cell disease. *J. Pediatr.* 128: 820–828.

Selby, R, Nisbet-Brown, E, Basran, RK et al. (1997). Valproic acid and augmentation of fetal hemoglobin in individuals with and without sickle cell disease. *Blood* 90: 891–893.

Sharma, S, Nisbet-Brown, E, Rees, DR, and Olivieri, NF. (1998). Sodium phenylbutyrate therapy in infants and children with thalassemia. *Blood* 92: 530a.

Sher, GD, Ginder, GD, Little, J et al. (1995). Extended therapy with intravenous arginine butyrate in patients with β-hemoglobinopathies. *N. Engl. J. Med.* 332: 1606–1610.

Singal, R, Ferris, R, Little, JA et al. (1997). Methylation of the minimal promoter of an embryonic globin gene silences transcription in primary erythroid cells. *Proc. Natl. Acad. Sci. U.S.A.* 94: 13724–13729.

Singhal, R and Ginder, GD. (1999) DNA methylation. *Blood* 93: 4059–4070.

Stamatoyannopoulos, G, Blau, CA, Nakamoto, B et al. (1994). Fetal hemoglobin induction by acetate, a product of butyrate catabolism. *Blood* 84: 3198–3204.

Stein, R, Sciaky-Gallili, N, Razin, A, and Cedar, H. (1983). Pattern of methylation of two genes coding for housekeeping functions. *Proc. Natl. Acad. Sci. U.S.A.* 80: 2422–2426.

Steinberg, MH, Lu, Z-H, Barton, FB et al. (1997a). Fetal hemoglobin in sickle cell anemia: Determinants of response to hydroxyurea. *Blood* 89: 1078–1088.

Steinberg, MH, Ballas, S, Barton, F, and Terrin, M. (1997b). Mortality at 4–5 years: Results from the the multicenter study of hydroxyurea in sickle cell anemia (MSH). *Blood* 90: 444a.

Steinberg, MH, Barton, F, Castro, O et al. (2000). Risks and benefits of hydroxyurea (HU) in adult sickle cell anemia. Effects at 6 to 7 years. *Blood* 94: 644a.

Steinberg, MH. (1999) Management of sickle cell disease. *N. Engl. J. Med.* 340: 1021–1030.

Steinberg, MH, Barton, F, Castro, O et al. (1999). Risks and benefits of hydroxyurea (Hydroxyurea) in adult sickle cell anemia. Effects at 6- to 7-years. *Blood* 94: 644a.

Sterkers, Y, Preudhomme, C, Laï, JL et al. (1998). Acute myeloid leukemia and myelodysplastic syndromes following essential thrombocythemia treated with hydroxyurea: High proportion of cases with 17p deletion. *Blood* 91: 616–622.

Styles, LA, Lubin, B, Vichinsky, E et al. (1997). Decrease of very late activation antigen-4 and CD36 on reticulocytes in sickle cell patients treated with hydroxyurea. *Blood* 89: 2554–2559.

Sugihara, K, Sugihara, T, Mohandas, N, and Hebbel, RP. (1992). Thrombospondin mediates adherence of $CD36^+$ sickle reticulocytes to endothelial cells. *Blood* 80: 2634–2642.

Sutton, M, Nassif, I, Stamatoyannopoulos, G et al. (1998). Absence of cross-resistance to the Hb F stimulating activities of butyrate & hydroxyurea. *Blood* 92: 694a.

Swerlick, RA, Eckman, JR, Kumar, A et al. (1993). $\alpha_4\beta_1$-Integrin expression on sickle reticulocytes: Vascular cell adhesion molecule-1-dependent binding to endothelium. *Blood* 82: 1891–1899.

Terrin, ML, Barton, FB, Bonds, D et al. (1999). Effect of hydroxyurea on quality of life: 2-year results from the multicenter study of hydroxyurea in sickle cell anemia. *23rd Annual Meeting of the National Sickle Cell Disease Program*, San Francisco.

Torkelson, S, White, B, Faller, DV et al. (1996). Erythroid progenitor proliferation is stimulated by phenoxyacetic and phenylalkyl acids. *Blood Cells Mol. Dis.* 22: 150–158.

Torrealba-de Ron, AT, Papayannopoulou, T, Knapp, MS et al. (1984). Perturbations in the erythroid marrow progenitor cell pools may play a role in the augmentation of HbF by 5-azacytidine. *Blood* 63: 201–210.

Triadou, P, Maier-Redelsperger, M, Krishnamoorthy, R et al. (1994). Fetal hemoglobin variations following hydroxyurea treatment in patients with cyanotic congenital heart disease. *Nouv. Rev. Fr. Hematol.* 36: 367–372.

Udden, MM, Lo, MN, and Sears, DA. (1999). Successful hydroxyurea treatment of a patient with SD hemoglobinopathy. *Am. J. Hematol.* 60: 84–85.

van der Ploeg, LH and Flavell, RA. (1980). DNA methylation in the human gamma delta beta-globin locus in erythroid and nonerythroid tissues. *Cell* 19: 947–958.

Veith, R, Papayannopoulou, T, Kurachi, S, and Stamatoyannopoulos, G. (1985a). Treatment of baboon with vinblastine: Insights into the mechanisms of pharmacologic stimulation of Hb F in the adult. *Blood,* 66: 456–459.

Veith, R, Galanello, R, Papayannopoulou, T, and Stamatoyan-nopoulos, G. (1985b). Stimulation of F-cell production in patients with sickle-cell anemia treated with cytarabine or hydroxyurea. *N. Engl. J. Med.* 313: 1571–1575.

Vichinsky, EP and Lubin, BH. (1994). A cautionary note regarding hydroxyurea in sickle cell disease. *Blood* 83: 1124–1128.

Voskaridou, E, Kalotychou, V, and Loukopoulos, D. (1995). Clinical and laboratory effects of long-term administration of hydroxyurea to patients with sickle-cell/β-thalassaemia. *Br. J. Haematol.* 89: 479–484.

Wang, W, Wynn, L, Rogers, Z et al. (1999). Effects of hydroxyurea in very young children with sickle cell disease: A pilot trial. *23rd Annual Meeting of the National Sickle Cell Disease Program*, San Francisco.

Ware, RE, Hanft, VN, Pickens, CV et al. (1998). Acquired DNA mutations and the leukemogenic potential of hydroxyurea therapy. *Blood* 92: 424a.

Ware, RE, Zimmerman, SA, and Schultz, WH. (1999a). Hydroxyurea as an alternative to blood transfusions for the prevention of recurrent stroke in children with sickle cell disease. *Blood* 94: 3022–3026.

Ware, RE, Hanft, VN, Pickens, CV et al. (1999b). Acquired DNA mutations associated with in vitro and in vivo exposure to hydroxyurea. *23rd Annual Meeting of the National Sickle Cell Disease Program*, San Francisco.

Ware, RE, Sommerich, M, Zimmerman, SA et al. (1999c). Hydroxyurea therapy for pediatric patients with Hemoglobin SC disease: Laboratory and clinical effects. *23rd Annual Meeting of the National Sickle Cell Disease Program*, San Francisco.

Ware, RE, Steinberg, MH, and Kinney, TR. (1995). Hydroxyurea: An alternative to transfusion therapy for stroke in sickle cell anemia. *Am. J. Hematol.* 50: 140–143.

Watson, J, Stahman, AW, and Bilello FP. (1948). Significance of paucity of sickle cells in newborn negro infants. *Am. J. Med. Sci.* 215: 419–423.

Weinberg, RS, Sutton, M, Galperin, Y et al. (1998). Kinetics of fetal hemoglobin (HbF) induction by arginine butyrate in sickle cell disease (SCD). *Blood* 92: 12a.

Weinfeld, A, Swolin, B, and Westin, J. (1994). Acute leukaemia after hydroxyurea therapy in polycythemia vera and allied disorders: Prospective study of efficacy and leukaemogenicity with therapeutic implications. *Eur. J. Haematol.* 52: 134–139.

West, MS, Wethers, D, Smith, J et al. (1992). Laboratory profile of sickle cell disease: A cross-sectional analysis. *J. Clin. Epidemiol.* 45: 893–909.

Wick, TM, Moake, JL, Udden, MM, and McIntire, LV. (1993). Unusually large von Willebrand factor multimers preferentially promote young sickle and nonsickle erythrocyte adhesion to endothelial cells. *Am. J. Hematol.* 42: 284–292.

Xu, YP, Mull, CD, Bonifant, CL et al. (1998). Nitrosylation of sickle cell hemoglobin by hydroxyurea. *J. Organic. Chem.* 63: 6452–6453.

Young, CW and Hodas, S. (1968). Hydroxyurea: Inhibitory effect on DNA metabolism. *Science* 146: 1172–1174.

Zeng, YT, Huang, S-Z, Ren, Z-R et al. (1995). Hydroxyurea therapy in β-thalassaemia intermedia: Improvement in haematological parameters due to enhanced β-globin synthesis. *Br. J. Haematol.* 90: 557–563.

39

Bone Marrow Transplantation in β Thalassemia

EMANUELE ANGELUCCI
GUIDO LUCARELLI

INTRODUCTION

Homozygous β thalassemia is a worldwide distributed inherited disease characterized by absent or defective β-globin chain synthesis. The defect in β-globin chain synthesis causes imbalance in chain production and accumulation of free α-globin chain in red blood cells or red blood cell precursors, leading to intramedullary destruction (Schrier et al., 1997), apoptosis (Yuan et al., 1993), ineffective erythropoiesis, and hemolytic anemia. According to the World Health Organization, approximately 180 million people are carriers for one of the forms of genetic disorders of hemoglobin synthesis (Anonymous, 1981) and over 300,000 infants with major syndromes are born every year (Angastiniotis and Modell, 1998). Because of migration, β thalassemia has spread from its original geographic distribution in the Mediterranean, Africa, and Asia and is now endemic throughout Europe, America, and Australia.

The development of regular transfusion regimens and of chelation treatment with deferoxamine (Giardini, 1997; Olivieri and Brittenham, 1997) (see Chapter 37) has led to the transformation of this disease in developed countries from a fatal disease in infancy to a chronic disease associated with prolonged survival (Brittenham et al., 1994; Olivieri et al., 1994; Lucarelli et al., 1995; Giardini, 1997). Medical treatment is expensive and requires a complex multidisciplinary approach. Therefore, thalassemia remains a fatal dis-

ease early in life in underdeveloped countries where most patients are born.

BONE MARROW TRANSPLANTATION FOR THALASSEMIA

In simple terms, the purpose of treating β thalassemia by allogeneic bone marrow transplantation (BMT) is to cure it, that is, to replace ineffective erythropoiesis with effective erythropoiesis capable of producing sufficient number of circulating red cells containing an adequate amount of hemoglobin. However, this simple statement implies several major problems: biological, clinical, and ethical (Giardini, 1995).

The Initial Experience

In December 1981, a 14-month-old child with β thalassemia who had been transfused with a total of 250 mL of packed red blood cells received a bone marrow transplant from his HLA identical sister in Seattle (Thomas et al., 1982). The transplant was successful and the child is now over 18 years old, in excellent health without any hematologic manifestations of thalassemia. Two weeks later, a 14-year-old patient with advanced thalassemia who had received more than 150 red blood cell transfusions was transplanted in Pesaro but had recurrence of thalassemia after rejection of the graft (Lucarelli et al., 1984).

The Pesaro Experience

In the early 1980s, the initial Pesaro studies were concentrated on patients with advanced β thalassemia and short life expectancy (Zurlo et al., 1989; Ehlers et al., 1991). Of the first six patients over age 16 years transplanted after conditioning using high doses of cyclophosphamide and total body irradiation, four died of causes related to graft-versus-host disease within the first 100 days, one died of infection on day 235, and one had recurrence of thalassemia on day 48 and died of thalassemia-related cardiac disease more than 6 years later (Lucarelli et al., 1984).

In view of this experience, studies then concentrated on patients under age 17 years. Results in young patients were encouraging (Lucarelli et al., 1984, 1985, 1987) and in 1990 the Pesaro group reported experience through August 1988 in treating 222 consecutive patients under age 16 years (Lucarelli et al., 1990). All of these patients received HLA-identical marrow, in ten cases from parents, and in the other cases from siblings. All patients were prepared for transplantation after conditioning with regimens containing busulfan (14 mg/kg) followed by cyclophosphamide (200 mg/kg). In this series, the probability of survival and thalassemia-free survival plateaus after 1 year at 82 percent and 75 percent, respectively (Lucarelli et al., 1990). Analysis of the influence of pretransplant characteristics on the outcome of transplantation was conducted in 116 patients who were all treated with exactly the same regimen. It was demonstrated that hepatomegaly and portal fibrosis were associated with a significantly reduced probability of survival. In a multivariate analysis, history of poor compliance with iron chelation therapy could not be distinguished from hepatomegaly as a predictor of survival and thalassemia-free survival. The influence of pretransplant characteristics on the outcome of transplantation was reexamined in late 1989 (Lucarelli et al., 1991) by which time 161 patients under the age of 17 had been treated with the same regimen. The quality of chelation therapy was characterized as regular when deferoxamine therapy was initiated not later than 18 months after the first transfusion and administered subcutaneously for 8 to 10 hours continuously for at least 5 days each week. Chelation therapy was defined as irregular for any deviation from this requirement. The degree of hepatomegaly (greater than or not greater than 2 cm), the presence or absence of portal fibrosis in the pretransplant liver biopsy (Angelucci et al., 1995), and the quality of chelation (regular or irregular) given through the years before transplant were identified as variables permitting the categorization of patients aged less than 17 years into three risk classes. Class 1 patients had none of these adverse risk factors, Class 3 patients had all three, and Class 2 patients had one or two adverse risk factors (Table 39.1).

Table 39.1. Pesaro Risk Classification for Bone Marrow Transplantation in Thalassemia

	Hepatomegaly	Irregular chelation	Liver fibrosis
Class 1	No	No	No
Class 2	One or two of the 3 risk factors		
Class 3	Yes	Yes	Yes

Note: Hepatomegaly was defined as enlargement of the liver of more than 2 cm below the costal margin. Chelation was characterized as regular when deferoxamine therapy was initiated not later than 18 months after the first transfusion and administered subcutaneously for 8 to 10 hours continuously for at least 5 days each week. Chelation was defined as irregular for any deviation from this requirement.

Updated Results

From December 17, 1981 through February 28, 1997, 785 consecutive patients with homozygous β thalassemia received marrow transplants from HLA-identical related donors (761 siblings, 24 parents). Patients' mean age was 10 ± 6 years (range 1 to 35 years). Analysis was performed on June 30, 1998, with survival updated at the time of last contact. Overall Kaplan-Meier survival and thalassemia-free survival are, respectively, 78 percent and 71 percent at 16 years after transplant. Results are shown in Figure 39.1. Of these 785 consecutive patients, 165 (21 percent) died; Table 39.2 lists all of the causes of death.

Figure 39.1. The Kaplan-Meier probabilities of survival and thalassemia-free survival for all of the 785 patients with thalassemia, ages 1 through 35 years (mean ± SD = 10.4 ± 6), who received HLA-identical transplants from December 17, 1981 through February 28, 1997. Analysis was performed on June 30, 1998. Survival was updated on the day of last contact.

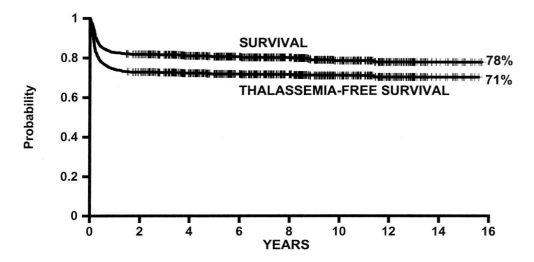

Table 39.2. Causes of Death (165 Deaths Among 785 Consecutive Transplants)

Transplant-related deaths	
Acute grade III–IV GVHD and related complications	53
Marrow aplasia and related complications	15
Infectious diseases	40
Respiratory diseases (3 adult respiratory distress syndrome, 2 idiopathic interstitial pneumonia)	5
Liver disease (3 venoocclusive disease, 7 liver failure)	10
Cardiac diseases (7 cardiac tamponade, 1 heart failure)	8
Bleeding (4 central nervous system, 1 gastrointestinal)	5
B-lymphoproliferative disease	2
Chronic GVHD and related complications	15
Unknown	1
Thalassemia-related deaths (occurring >1 year after BMT in absence of chronic GVHD)	
Heart failure (in autologous reconstitution)	4
Overwhelming postsplenectomy infection (4 and 6 years after transplant with functioning graft without chronic GVHD)	2
Other causes of deaths	
Car accident	4
Mushroom poisoning	1

Note: Deaths occurring in uncontrolled GVHD have been considered caused by GVHD as the major cause.

Table 39.3. Preparative Regimen, GVHD Prophylaxis, and Infectious Disease Prophylaxis in Use for Class 1 and 2 Patients

Preparative regimen
  Busulfan PO 14 mg/kg over 4 days
  Cyclophosphamide IV 200 mg/kg over 4 days
Graft-versus-host prophylaxis
  Cyclosporin A 5 mg/kg IV from day −5/−2 to day +5
  Cyclosporin A 3 mg/kg IV from day +6 to day +21
  Cyclosporin A 12.5 mg/kg PO from day +21 to day +60 then gradual tapering up to +1 year
  Methylprednisolone 0.5 mg/kg IV from day −1
Antiinfectious prophylaxis
  Third-generation cephalosporin IV from day −1
  Amikacin 15 mg/kg/day IV from day −1
  Amphotericin B 0.3 mg/kg/day IV from day +8
  Acyclovir 15 mg/kg/day IV from day −7
  Polyspecific human immunoglobulin 500 mg/kg IV on day −1
  Polyspecific human immunoglobulin 250 mg/kg IV on day +8 and +22

(busulfan 14 mg/kg, cyclophosphamide 200 mg/kg, and cyclosporin A alone for graft-versus-host disease prophylaxis; the detailed protocol is reported in Table 39.3). Survival, thalassemia-free survival, transplant-related mortality, and rejection rate were 94 percent, 87 percent, 6 percent, and 7 percent, respectively (Fig. 39.2)

Class 2. Class 2 patients are characterized by the presence of one or two of the three risk factors. Two

Class 1. Class 1 patients are characterized by the absence of hepatomegaly and portal fibrosis and by a history of regular chelation therapy. Up to February 28, 1997, 116 patients (mean age 5 ± 3 years, range 1 to 16 years) who met the criteria for Class 1 were transplanted in Pesaro using the conditioning regimen actually in use

Figure 39.2. The Kaplan-Meier probabilities of survival, thalassemia-free survival, rejection, and nonrejection mortality for the 116 Class 1 thalassemia patients transplanted using the same conditioning regimen (mean age 5 ± 3 years, range 1 to 16 years).

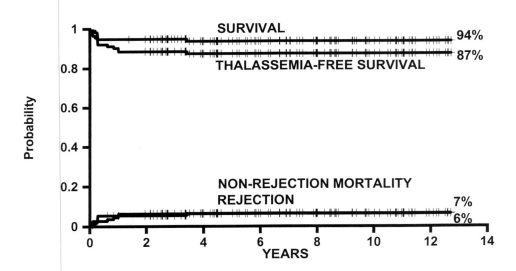

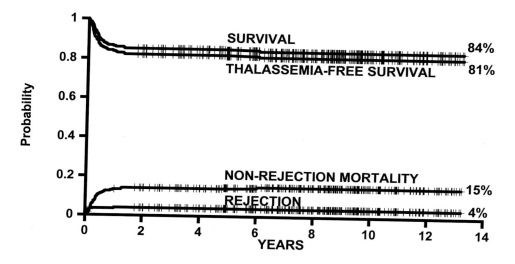

Figure 39.3. The Kaplan-Meier probabilities of survival, tha-lassemia-free survival, rejection and nonrejection mortality for the 276 Class 2 patients transplanted using the same condition-ing regimen (mean age 9 ± 4 years, range 2 to 16 years).

hundred seventy-six consecutive Class 2 patients, mean age 9 ± 4 years (range 2 to 16 years) were transplanted using the above specified regimen. Survival, thalassemia-free survival, transplant-related mortality, and rejection rate were 84 percent, 81 percent, 15 percent, and 4 per-cent, respectively (Fig. 39.3).

Class 3. At the time of the initial classification in 1989 (Lucarelli et al., 1990), 24 Class 3 patients had been prepared for transplant with the standard busulfan (14 mg/kg) and cyclophosphamide (200 mg/kg) regi-men. Their 3-year survival and thalassemia-free survival were 61 percent and 53 percent, respectively. This group of patients was characterized by a high transplant-related mortality (Lucarelli et al., 1990, 1996), which affected 39 percent of the patients. Therefore, at that time, admission of Class 3 patients to transplant was closed. Because of the high transplant-related mortality new protocols were explored, including a reduced dose of cyclophosphamide or use of other agents for immunosuppressive therapy. A large experience (Lucarelli et al., 1996) showed that survival, tha-lassemia-free survival, transplant-related mortality, and rejection rates were 74 percent, 49 percent, 24 percent, and 35 percent, respectively. From March 1989 to Feb-ruary 1998, 122 Class 3 patients (mean age 11 ± 3 years, range 3 to 16 years) were transplanted with busulfan (14 mg/kg), a reduced dose of cyclophosphamide (120 to 160 mg/kg), and various regimens for graft-versus-host disease prophylaxis. In this cohort, survival, tha-lassemia-free survival, transplant-related mortality, and rejection rate were 80 percent, 56 percent, 18 percent, and 33 percent, respectively (Fig.39.4).

Adult Patients. In the 1990 report (Lucarelli et al., 1990), children were defined as those patients up to 15 years of age. After that report, the definition of child-hood was changed to up to 16 years of age. Therefore, in all subsequent reports (and in this chapter), children are those patients up to 16 years of age and adults are those patients ages 17 years or more. As described above, the early experience with transplantation for patients older than 16 years was poor. Most adult patients presenting for transplantation have disease characteristics that place them in Class 3, and because of the improved results in treating young Class 3 patients using protocols with lower doses of cyclophosphamide, transplantation studies were resumed for patients ages 17 years or older.

Since February 1997, 108 patients ages 17 to 35 years (mean age 21 ± 4 years) have been transplanted from an HLA-identical sibling donor. Twenty of these patients were classified as Class 2 and 88 as Class 3. Adult Class 2 patients received standard conditioning regimen for Class 2 (busulfan 14 mg/kg and cyclophosphamide 200 mg/kg) while adult Class 3 patients received busulfan 14 mg/kg and cyclophos-phamide 120 mg/kg or 160 mg/kg. Survival, tha-lassemia-free survival, transplant-related mortality, and rejection rate were 67 percent, 63 percent, 35 per-cent, and 4 percent, respectively (Fig. 39.5). Because of the different numbers of patients in the two classes and the use of different conditioning regimens, no analyses could be performed on the effect of the classes on transplant outcome. In adult patients, the presence of active chronic hepatitis at the time of liver biopsy was a poor prognostic factor for transplant outcome (Lucarelli et al., 1999).

Experience of Other Transplant Centers

Marrow transplant programs for thalassemia have now been established in several parts of the world

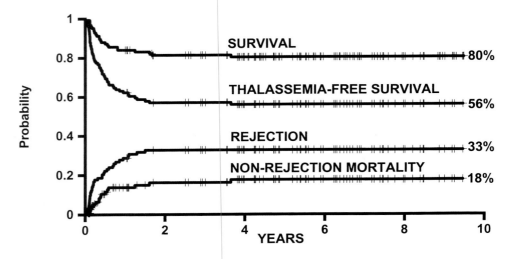

Figure 39.4. The Kaplan-Meier probabilities of survival, thalassemia-free survival, rejection and nonrejection mortality for the 122 Class 3 patients transplanted after March 1989 using a conditioning regimen with a reduced dose of cyclophosphamide (<200 mg/kg) (mean age 11 ± 3 years, range 3 to 16 years).

where the disease is prevalent. Overall, around 80 percent of patients survive long term and of these, nearly 90 percent are cured (Roberts, 1997). Table 39.4 lists results obtained in several centers worldwide, demonstrating that the Pesaro results have been widely reproduced (Olivieri et al., 1995).

Figure 39.5. The Kaplan-Meier probabilities of survival, thalassemia-free survival, rejection, and nonrejection mortality for the 108 patients older than 16 years of age (mean 21 ± 4 years, range 17 to 35 years). Twenty of these patients were in Class 2 and were transplanted using the regimen for Class 2 patients (cyclophosphamide 200 mg/kg); 88 were in Class 3 and were transplanted with regimens containing a decreased dose of cyclophosphamide (<200 mg/kg).

HLA-Nonidentical Related Donor Transplant

Approximately 60 percent to 70 percent of children with β thalassemia do not have HLA-identical family members (Delfini et al., 1986) and therefore are not candidates for marrow transplantation. Expanding the number of available donors would have a major impact on the management of this disease. The use of HLA-nonidentical family member donors in the treatment of β thalassemia has not been comprehensively studied in recent years because the results in leukemia were not good enough to justify a large trial. Reported results are anecdotal and therefore it is difficult to extrapolate useful information.

In Pesaro, as of December 1998, twenty-nine thalassemia patients had transplantation from an alternative family member donor. Six donors were phenotypically identical relatives and two were mismatched relatives (four cousins, two aunts, one uncle and one grandmother); thirteen were mismatched siblings and eight were mismatched parents. The

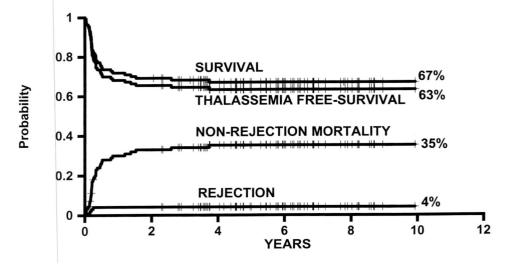

Table 39.4. Reported Transplants for Thalassemia

Center	Patients	Survival (%)	Thalassemia-free survival (%)
Pescara (Di Bartolomeo et al., 1997)	102	91	87
Cagliari (Pediatric Dept.) (Argiolu et al., 1997)	37	88	88
Cagliari (Internal Medicine Dept.)*	40	85	75
Pavia†	14	95	95
U.S. (Clift and Johnson, 1997)	68	87	69
U.K. (Roberts et al., 1997)	50	90	76
Tehran (Ghavamzadeh et al., 1997)	70	83	71
Vellore (Dennison et al., 1997)	50	76	68
Malaysia (Lin et al., 1997)	28	86	75
Hong Kong (Li et al., 1997)	25	86	83
Bangkok (Issaragrisil et al., 1997)	21	76	53
New York (Boulad et al., 1998)	13	92	85
Stanford (Lee et al., 1998)	11	100	91

* G. La Nasa, personal communication.
† F. Locatelli, personal communication.

number of mismatched HLA antigens was one in fifteen cases, two in five cases, and three in three cases. Results have not been very rewarding, with only six successes, ten transplant-related deaths, and thirteen patients with recurrence of thalassemia (Gaziev et al., 2000b).

Between 1969 and 1996, sixty cases were reported by twenty-two different teams to the International Bone Marrow Transplant Registry (IBMTR) but only eleven (17 percent) were transplanted since 1993. Forty-seven of the sixty patients survived and sixteen of the survivors had recurrence of thalassemia. Overall survival was 65 percent and disease-free survival was 50 percent. Incomplete information was available on the degree of HLA mismatching, but in this cohort of sixty patients, twenty-four were transplanted from an HLA phenotypically matched parental donor (this category of transplant is reported together with that of HLA-identical siblings in the reported Pesaro experience), eleven had related donors with one antigen mismatch, and four had donors with two antigen mismatches (Sullivan et al., 1998). Although most of these patients have not benefited from improved supportive care techniques (Goodrich et al., 1993) and DNA typing technologies (Choo et al., 1993; Petersdorf et al., 1994; Santamaria et al., 1994), it is clear that mismatched related donor transplant is not an attractive option at present in the early management of patients who can obtain and tolerate optimal medical therapy. For those patients who cannot avail themselves of optimal medical treatment, the decision to undergo HLA-nonidentical related donor transplant should be made on the basis of the risk/benefit ratio for the individual patient and the degree of HLA disparity (Anasetti et al., 1989).

THE THALASSEMIA PATIENT UNDERGOING BONE MARROW TRANSPLANTATION

Patient Selection and Classes of Risk

All patients undergoing chronic transfusion to survive are potential candidates for BMT. Patients with advanced liver [Child-Pugh grade B-C (Pugh et al., 1973)] and cardiac disease are not eligible for BMT. Thalassemia intermedia patients can be considered for marrow transplantation in selected situations (Baronciani et al., 1996).

The development of a regimen of regular transfusions (Cazzola et al., 1995; Giardini, 1997) combined with regular iron chelation therapy has transformed the prognosis for thalassemia children in industrialized countries from a disease fatal in infancy to a chronic disease permitting prolonged survival (Zurlo et al., 1989; Olivieri et al., 1994; Borgna-Pignatti et al., 1998) (see Chapter 37). The critical factor for survival of thalassemic patients undergoing transfusion and chelation therapy is control of the iron overload. If good compliance is obtained with chelation therapy, iron overload can be controlled but not abolished (Olivieri and Brittenham, 1997). In the majority of centers treating thalassemia, adequate chelation with deferoxamine was initiated between 1976 and 1977 and the first patients treated with the regimen since infancy are now in their mid-twenties. Several groups have recently published their own unicentric results assessing Kaplan-Meier survival with medical therapy: 85 percent at age 17 years in New York (Giardina et al., 1997), 66 percent at age 25 years in Torino (Piga et al., 1997), 75 percent at age 25 years in Catania (Di Gregorio et al., 1997), and 72 percent at age 26 years in Cagliari (Lai et al., 1997). Three North American groups reported a 55 percent cardiac disease-free survival after 15 years of chelation therapy in a cohort of ninety-seven patients (mean age at the end of the study, 23 years) (Olivieri et al., 1994). A recent large multicenter analysis updated in February 1997 and including 820 Italian patients born after 1970 and treated in seven Italian hospitals showed a Kaplan-Meier probability of survival of 85 percent at age 24 years without any evidence of a plateau (Borgna-Pignatti et al., 1998). In the same cohort, the probability of complication-free survival was dramatically lower (about 64 percent at 24 years) and the complications that were analyzed did not include hypothyroidism, treated hypogonadism, hepatitis virus infections, and liver fibrosis. All of these reports refer to groups of patients heterogeneous for age as well as duration of and compliance to chelation therapy. Comparison of these statistics with transplant results is impossible because (1) any classification assessing treatment outcome should be performed on the basis of pretreatment characteristics and intention to treat and cannot be based on treatment response, and (2) there are no survivors with medical therapy who are disease free. In this situation, the decision to submit a thalassemic child to a curative but potentially fatal procedure may be difficult. Classification of patients in pretransplant classes of risk permits an assessment of an individual patient's probability of cure by marrow transplantation independently of the patient's response to treatment and therefore adequate information can be obtained from survival curves.

The clinical significance of the Pesaro classification has been sometimes misinterpreted. This classification has been developed for transplant purposes and reflects advancement of thalassemia. Even if it is mainly based on liver status, it does not reflect a liver-related cause of death. Liver status has to be considered a "window" on the patient's global health situation. In fact, it was not possible to identify any complication that was particularly related to the different classes or to the status of liver disease but the probability of survival from a certain complication was markedly different between the classes. Overall incidence of grade III–IV acute graft-versus-host disease was 13.5 percent without a significantly different incidence between the classes in multivariate analyses; on the contrary, an impressive difference in mortality from grade III–IV acute graft-versus-host disease was recorded between the classes (27 percent in Class 1, 48 percent in Class 2, and 84 percent in Class 3) (Gaziev et al., 1997a).

A major criticism of the Pesaro classification is that two of the variables are qualitative (quality of chelation and hepatomegaly) and subject to variability between observers and this would lead to a different classification of the same patient by different observers (Olivieri et al., 1995). This is an important criticism and obviously quantitatively defined risk factors based on a defined unit of measure would increase the accuracy and reproducibility of the classification. Unfortunately, all of the attempts to introduce such criteria failed. Variables such as serum ferritin or hepatic iron concentration did not achieve significance in the statistical analyses as predictors of transplant outcome (Lucarelli et al., 1990, 1999). This reflects the complexity in assessing the global clinical condition of a thalassemic patient. Any quantitative laboratory value reflecting iron overload (i.e., serum ferritin or hepatic iron concentration) reflects the situation at a certain moment in life and does not necessarily reflect the impact of years of exposure to a toxic agent such as iron. This means that it is possible to find a patient with good control of body iron obtained in adulthood but with advanced stage of liver damage up to cirrhosis due to prior years of severe iron overload. In addition, the presence of a criterion such as regularity of chelation and how this criterion has been defined (any deviation during the time from regular treatment) makes it impossible to return to Class 1 once a patient has been classified as Class 2 or Class 3. The inclusion of a patient in Class 2 and particularly in Class 3 represents failure of conventional therapy and this reflects the clinically progressive nature of the disease whose optimal treatment is based on a delicate balance between the degree of anemia, body iron content, and iron chelation treatment. Prospective analyses of the probability to progress from one risk class to another with medical treatment would be very useful to decide on the best treatment for thalassemia patients, but unfortunately this kind of information is not available.

In the cohort of 785 patients reported in this chapter, 140 were Class 1 but only 13 of these were age 11 years or older, 360 were Class 2, and 275 were Class 3 (ten patients could not be classified due to the lack of an evaluable liver biopsy). These results are shown in Figure 39.6. Because patients represented very different conditions, this figure cannot be interpreted as a demonstration of the clinically progressive nature of β thalassemia. The figure reports the condition of thalassemia patients at the time they were admitted for bone marrow transplant, over the 15 years of the program.

Patient Evaluation Before Transplantation

The main purpose of the pretransplant evaluation is assessment of the patient's risk class. Nevertheless, all of the possible consequences of chronic transfusional therapy must be evaluated prior to BMT. This is very useful in assessing the patient's individual transplant

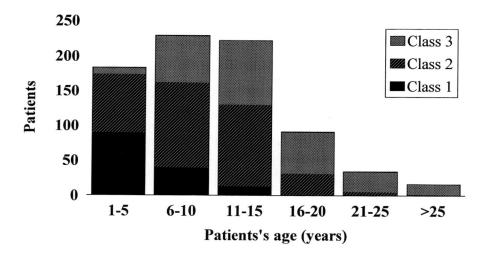

Figure 39.6. Class distribution of 785 thalassemic patients who underwent allogeneic BMT in Pesaro from December 17, 1981 through February 28, 1997 (in 10 cases, class could not be assessed).

prognosis and to guide long-term posttransplant treatment. The liver is the main site of iron deposition. Liver biopsy permits an accurate evaluation of liver fibrosis, liver iron, and chronic hepatitis (Angelucci et al., 1995). The risk of nonfatal bleeding complication of this procedure in thalassemia is 0.6 percent without ultrasound guidance (Angelucci et al., 1995) and less than 0.1 percent with ultrasound guidance (personal observation). None of the noninvasive diagnostic techniques available today, such as ultrasound, magnetic resonance imaging (Angelucci et al., 1997a), or magnetic susceptibility (Brittenham et al., 1982) provide adequate and complete information on hepatic status. Therefore, all patients should be submitted to liver biopsy before considering BMT. In our institution, thalassemia patients ages 3 years or less are not submitted to routine liver biopsy before transplantation and risk class is assessed on the basis of only two criteria.

Although seropositivity for hepatitis B and C virus are not contraindications for transplantation, serologic tests for these blood-borne viral infections must be done. Many thalassemic patients have splenomegaly. Hypersplenism can complicate the posttransplant course by increasing duration of cytopenias and the need for platelet and red blood cell transfusions. A pretransplant splenectomy should be considered for patients with severe splenomegaly (spleen extending to or below the traverse umbilical line). Cardiac evaluation should include a 12-lead ECG, 24-hour Holter monitor, and resting echocardiogram. More accurate diagnostic tests, such as low-dose dobutamine echostress, can identify alterations of cardiac contractility in some asymptomatic patients (Mariotti et al., 1996) but these early alterations do not have a statistically significant influence on transplant outcome. Complete endocrine evaluation including thyroid function tests, growth hormone releasing hormone stimulation test for hypothalamic anterior-pituitary function, and pancreatic β-cell function should be performed in patients older than age 10 years. For male patients with normal semen analyses, sperm bank storage is recommended. From the hematologic point of view, patient and donor globin-chain synthesis studies or DNA analysis should be studied to determine whether the patient has β⁰, β⁺, or HbS-β thalassemia and if the donor is normal or has β thalassemia minor. A sibling with thalassemia minor can be a bone marrow donor, but the diagnosis should be known in order to monitor the posttransplant course.

Preparative Regimens

Conditioning regimens for marrow transplantation of patients with diseases other than aplastic anemia must achieve two objectives: (1) eradication of the diseased marrow and (2) establishment of a tolerant environment that will permit donor stem cells to survive. Although total body irradiation can achieve these results there are many reasons to avoid the use of this marrow ablative modality. These include the growth-retarding effect of radiation in young children (Giorgiani et al., 1995) and the increased risk of secondary malignancies reported in patients treated for leukemia (Witherspoon et al., 1989), lymphoma, and aplastic anemia (Socie et al., 1992; Witherspoon et al., 1992; Curtis et al., 1997). There is extensive experience with the use of busulfan and its derivatives in ablating marrow in patients undergoing BMT for the treatment of nonmalignant diseases such as Wiskott-Aldrich syndrome (Parkman et al., 1978; Kapoor et al., 1981) and various inborn errors of metabolism (Hobbs et al., 1986).

Busulfan is an alkylating agent with exquisite specificity for the most primitive precursors of the myeloid-erythroid axis. It has been used in low doses for many years in the treatment of chronic myeloid leukemia. Studies in animals demonstrated that marrow-lethal doses of busulfan have minor toxic effects on the lymphoid system and cause only minor immunosuppression (Floersheim and Elson, 1961). Pharmacokinetic parameters of busulfan have been assessed in β-thalassemia patients: mean absorption half-time is 26 ± 17 minutes, mean area under the curve is 700 ± 390 M/min, average steady-state level is 478 ± 266 ng/mL, and mean elimination half-time is 1.9 ± 0.9 hours. No relationship between the pharmacokinetic parameters of busulfan and toxicity or transplant outcome has been found (Pawlowska et al., 1997). Studies on dogs transplanted from DLA-identical littermates demonstrated a 50 percent engraftment rate after busulfan alone and a 95 percent engraftment rate when antithymocyte serum was included in the preparative regimen (Storb et al., 1977). Busulfan is able to eradicate an expanded erythron but if used alone is not likely to be sufficiently immunosuppressive to permit sustained allogeneic engraftment.

Cyclophosphamide is an agent that is well established as providing adequate immunosuppression to permit allogeneic engraftment of patients with aplastic anemia (Thomas et al., 1972; Storb and Champlin, 1991). Cyclophosphamide has been a component of a large number of preparative regimens for marrow transplantation in patients with various hematologic malignancies. The dose-limiting toxicity of cyclophosphamide is to the heart and not to the marrow. High doses of cyclophosphamide (200 mg/kg over 4 consecutive days) as sole antitumor agent in patients receiving allogeneic transplant for leukemia were sufficiently immunosuppressive to permit sustained allogeneic engraftment (Santos et al., 1971). However, hematopoiesis in mice, monkeys, and humans recovers promptly after the highest doses of cyclophosphamide because it does not eliminate hematopoietic stem cells.

The combination of oral busulfan (16 mg/kg) and cyclophosphamide (200 mg/kg) as a preparative regimen for marrow transplant in adult acute myeloid leukemia was developed by Santos and associates (Santos et al., 1983). Early results were encouraging and in the attempt to reduce toxicity-related mortality, Tutschka and colleagues (1987) reduced the total dose of cyclophosphamide to 120 mg/kg over 2 days. Although there are no clinical studies on this specific issue, it is widely believed that cyclophosphamide alone at the reported dose of 120 mg/kg does not provide sufficient immunosuppression to allow permanent stem cell engraftment in a host with normal immune competence. The success of marrow trans-

plantation with the Tutschka regimen suggests that busulfan can increase the immunosuppressive properties of cyclophosphamide.

Experience in the use of "chemotherapy-only" transplant regimens for the treatment of malignancy (Santos et al., 1971; Tutschka et al., 1980, 1989, 1991; Santos et al., 1983; Appelbaum et al., 1984) has been pivotal in developing regimens appropriate for the treatment of β thalassemia. The combination of busulfan and cyclophosphamide (the so-called BU-CY regimen) is able to eradicate the expanded thalassemic erythron and permit sustained allogeneic engraftment.

Graft-Versus-Host Disease—Infectious Diseases Prophylaxis and Specific Complications

In regards to BMT, thalassemia patients are characterized by two features that make clinical management different from that of leukemia patients: chronic blood transfusions and the absence of previous chemotherapy and immunosuppression. In thalassemia, no graft-versus-leukemia effect is required for success and no evidence of graft-versus-thalassemia has been observed. This should be kept in mind in modeling immunosuppressive prophylaxis and treatment.

Cyclosporin A is used as graft-versus-host disease prophylaxis in our institution. Use of cyclosporin is continued for 1 year after transplantation; low-dose methylprednisolone (0.5 mg/kg) is added in the early posttransplant phase. The detailed schedule of cyclosporin use is shown in Table 39.3. Class 3 patients receive a modified "short methotrexate" regimen (cyclophosphamide 7.5 mg/kg intravenously on day +1 and then methotrexate at 10 mg/m² on days 3 and 6 after transplantation). We no longer use antilymphocyte globulin. Despite the risk of blood-borne infections from prior transfusions, thalassemia patients do not have increased risk of infectious diseases if compared to other patients undergoing marrow transplant. No specific infection was associated with iron overload or its severity (unpublished observation). A low incidence of cytomegalovirus infections and associated mortality has been encountered in very young patients (Baronciani et al., 1990). During the course of transplantation, patients receive standard intravenous antibiotic prophylaxis, including third-generation cephalosporin, aminoglycoside, and low-dose amphotericin B (0.3 mg/kg). Prophylactic acyclovir and preemptive ganciclovir are also given (Goodrich et al., 1993).

Detailed guidelines for clinical management of thalassemia patients undergoing marrow transplantation have been published elsewhere (Angelucci and Lucarelli, 1996). Liver and cardiac complications are briefly discussed here. Despite prior liver damage due to iron overload and viral hepatitis (Erer et al., 1994), venoocclusive disease of the liver has not been a major problem. On the other hand, transplant can acutely aggravate the course of iron-induced liver failure. Particularly in adult patients (Lucarelli et al., 1999), the differential diagnosis of hyperbilirubinemia must include liver failure. Even if cardiac failure is rarely seen during the course of transplantation—in our experience cardiac failure was the major cause of death in only one patient, see Table 39.2—impaired cardiac function secondary to iron overload can lead to fluid accumulation. Specific recommendations include keeping patients in a negative water balance, low-dose continuous infusion of dopamine, and digitalization. A particular complication encountered in transplanting thalassemia patients is cardiac tamponade. This event affects 2 percent of thalassemia patients undergoing marrow transplant (Angelucci et al., 1992). It is characterized by sudden and unheralded cardiac decompensation caused by rapid fluid accumulation (Angelucci et al., 1994) in the pericardial space without concurrent myocardial disease. The fluid is a sterile, colorless transudate. This is an early complication and has been observed immediately after cyclophosphamide infusion and up until day +62 after transplant. Treatment consists of emergency periocardiocentesis and the event is fatal unless drainage of the pericardial space is immediately carried out.

Recurrence of Thalassemia

In a variable percentage of cases, the patient can reject the graft after marrow transplantation. Rejection can be followed by persistent aplasia or by return of β thalassemia. The first situation is relatively rare and can be reversed only with a second transplant. The second situation is more frequent and its incidence varies with the conditioning regimen and the general condition of the patients. With the standard conditioning regimen (busulfan 14 mg/kg and cyclophosphamide 200 mg/kg) return to β thalassemia occurred in 7 percent of Class 1 patients, in 4 percent of Class 2, and in 13 percent of Class 3 patients (Lucarelli et al., 1990, 1996). As discussed above, the dose of cyclophosphamide was decreased to 120 to 160 mg/kg in children of Class 3. In such patients, the incidence of recurrence of thalassemia increased significantly from 13 percent to 35 percent (Lucarelli et al., 1996). In contrast to these results in younger Class 3 patients receiving regimens with lower cyclophosphamide dosages, the cumulative incidence of recurrence of thalassemia in adult patients was only 4 percent. The reason for this difference is unknown but it is noteworthy that adult patients had a history of more red

cell transfusions than did the Class 3 patients who were less than age 17 years. It seems that the likelihood of rejection is inversely related to the transfusion burden (Lucarelli et al., 1996). The latest recurrence of thalassemia occurred on day + 548 after transplantation. Recurrence never occurred in patients 2 years or later after transplant.

By analogy to the behavior of malignant tissue, it might be supposed that a largely expanded hematopoietic tissue mass would be difficult to eradicate and likely to recur after transplantation. However, leukemic relapse is characterized by the reappearance of leukemia in the presence of a persistent immune system of donor origin. In contrast, the return of thalassemia usually occurs in the context of a return of host-type immune reconstitution. This event has aspects of both rejection and relapse.

Second Transplant

If β thalassemia recurs a second transplant can be proposed to patients starting at least 2 years after the first transplant. In this situation, marrow transplantation is associated with a higher rejection and mortality rate. Through November 1998, twenty-one second transplants were performed in Pesaro: five patients died of transplant-related complications, nine had recurrence of thalassemia, and seven are alive and well, cured without chronic graft-versus-host disease (Gaziev et al., 2000).

Mixed Chimeric State

Contrary to what was commonly believed, complete donor hematopoiesis is not essential for sustained engraftment. The presence of hematopoietic cells of donor as well of recipient origin is not a rare event after marrow transplant for thalassemia. This situation is defined as mixed chimerism.

The first observations of the presence of mixed chimerism were made during studies of posttransplant engraftment (Olivieri et al., 1990) and warranted the establishment of a prospective study of the phenomenon. The cells of 295 patients evaluable for engraftment for a minimum period of 2 years after transplant were examined at predetermined times (2, 6, 12, and 24 months after transplant) by molecular genetic techniques, such as determination of restriction fragment length polymorphisms and variable number of tandem repeats (RFLP-VNTR) (Nesci et al., 1992), or by fluorescence in situ hybridization (FISH) for Y chromosome, if applicable. Mixed chimerism was observed in 95 of 295 (32 percent) thalassemic patients within the first 2 months after the transplant. By the second year after the transplant, 42 of the 95 mixed chimeric patients evolved to complete engraftment (residual host cells were no longer detectable), 33 showed a progressive loss of donor-engrafted cells and had recurrence of thalassemia, while 20 patients had persistence of mixed chimerism. During the same period of observation, none of the 200 patients who had complete engraftment at the second month of follow-up subsequently developed graft failure or recurrence of thalassemia, while 6 of these patients developed a status of persistent mixed chimerism (Andreani et al., 2000). After the second year of follow-up, these 26 patients were submitted to yearly assessment of mixed chimerism for a period of time between 2 and 11 years. Although the percentage of donor-engrafted cells was variable (30 percent to 90 percent) and in some instances was particularly low (30 percent), all patients survived in a state of persistent mixed chimerism with a stable hemoglobin level between 8.3 and 16.7 g/dL, a $\beta/\beta + \gamma$ chain synthetic ratio of between 0.7 and 1, in excellent clinical condition, and transfusion free.

On the basis of these results, we characterized a condition of transient chimerism (in the first 24 months after transplant) and a condition of persistent chimerism (after the 24th month of follow-up). Transient mixed chimerism was more frequent following the conditioning regimen using 120 mg/kg of cyclophosphamide (Manna et al., 1993; Nesci et al., 1998) than following the regimen using 200 mg/kg. When the situation of transient chimerism was quantitatively analyzed by dilution experiments of DNA or by the number of cells carrying the Y chromosome (in sex-mismatched transplants) it was clear that the number of residual host cells in the early phase was an important factor determining transplant outcome. The rate of autologous reconstitution was 95 percent for chimeric patients with residual host cells greater then 25 percent and 20 percent for those with a level of residual host cells less than 25 percent (Andreani et al., 2000). When the 26 persistently chimeric patients were analyzed in more detail, they demonstrated that mixed chimerism was present in bone marrow at the same level as that in the peripheral blood, with the exception of one case in whom there were 25 percent donor cells in the bone marrow, but approximately 70 percent donor cells in the peripheral blood (Andreani et al., 1996). In some of these patients with mixed chimerism, it was possible to demonstrate the presence of a large number of recipient myeloid and erythroid progenitor cells [by PCR-VNTR analyses of the DNA extracted from single plucked erythroid burst-forming units (BFU-e) and granulocyte-macrophage colony-forming units (CFU-GM) colonies] demonstrating that a relatively low number of donor erythroid progenitors (down to 30 percent of the total BFU-e) carrying "normal" hemoglobin genes is nevertheless able to produce large numbers of red cells with a

sufficient amount of hemoglobin to avoid the need for transfusion (Fig. 39.7). Selective survival of the nonthalassemic red cells is without doubt an important factor in this phenomenon.

Cost

The issue of cost may influence the choice between medical treatment and transplantation. The estimated cost of bone marrow transplant for a hemoglobinopathy patient (in 1990 dollars) was $173,250 in 1991 (Kirkpatrick et al., 1991). Additional costs can be anticipated for the first 5 years after transplantation (Welch and Larson, 1989), but they are less than those calculated for leukemia (unpublished observation). The cost of transfusion and chelation therapy was estimated to be about $32,000/year in 1991 for a 30 kg patient (Kirkpatrick et al., 1991). This cost would be expected to increase as the patient grew and required more transfusions and more chelation (Olivieri et al., 1994) and does not include the cost of treating various complications.

β-THALASSEMIA PATIENTS AFTER BONE MARROW TRANSPLANTATION (EX-THALASSEMIC)

Transplantation in β thalassemia provided what is probably a permanent cure for the marrow defect in nearly all patients, but prolonged follow-up is necessary to determine the long-term outcome. However, thalassemia patients who have acquired normal bone marrow as a result of transplantation cannot be accurately described as cured. They have homozygosity for the mutant gene in every cell of the body except for their hematopoietic cells and are carriers of all the clinical complications acquired during prior years of transfusion and chelation therapy. The treatment of

Figure 39.7. Evaluation of donor/recipient origin by PCR amplification for the D1S80 minisatellite locus of single BFU-e-derived colonies obtained from a patient with persistent mixed chimerism after BMT for thalassemia. For full color reproduction, see color plate 39.7.

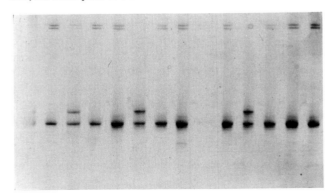

patients with thalassemia is not always complete once successful marrow transplants have been achieved. Health and a normal life expectancy can only be achieved after the cure of the organ damage acquired during years with thalassemia and its treatment (mainly iron overload and hepatitis C virus infection). Transplanted β-thalassemia patients have been defined as "ex-thalassemic" to indicate a patient cured from the genetic disease but still affected by all of the thalassemia-related complications.

The care of the patients after transplantation should be divided into transplant-related complications and thalassemia-related complications.

Transplant-Related Complications

Transplant-related complications include chronic graft-versus-host disease and secondary malignancy.

Chronic Graft-Versus-Host Disease. The most severe long-term marrow transplant complication is chronic graft-versus-host disease (GVHD), which is associated with significant morbidity and mortality (Shulman et al., 1980; Sullivan et al., 1981). A recent retrospective study was performed in Pesaro on 734 consecutive thalassemic patients, 614 of whom were evaluable for chronic GVHD (Gaziev et al., 1997a). Overall incidence of chronic GVHD was 27.3 percent (168 of 614 evaluable patients). In 70 percent of the cases, chronic GVHD developed as a continuation of acute GVHD, while in 30 percent it presented as de novo chronic GVHD. In 49 percent of the cases, chronic GVHD developed within the first 6 months after transplantation, in 39 percent between 6 months and 1 year, and in 12 percent after the discontinuation of cyclosporin 1 year after transplantation. The probability of mild, moderate, and severe chronic GVHD were 20 percent, 8 percent, and 2 percent, respectively. In 67 percent of the affected patients, chronic GVHD was limited and in 33 percent it was extensive. No difference in incidence was observed between the three classes of risk.

All of the patients with mild chronic GVHD recovered from the complication. Of the 53 with the moderate to severe form of GVHD 15 died with chronic GVHD, 28 completely recovered by the time therapy was discontinued, and 10 were still under immunosuppressive treatment at the end of the study. In summary, of the 168 patients who developed chronic GVHD, 85.1 percent recovered from the complication, 8.9 percent died, and 6 percent were still under treatment at the end of the study.

Secondary Malignancies. At the time of this writing four cases of early malignancies (within the 1st year after transplant) have been recorded: three cases of B-

cell lymphoproliferative disease and one case of cardiac myxoma. Two of the patients with B-cell lymphoproliferative disease died of progressive disease and one is alive and well more than 10 years after radiotherapy (Gaziev et al., 1997b); the patient with cardiac myxoma survived and is alive and well more than 5 years after surgical removal of the tumor (Baronciani et al., 1998).

Two cases of late malignancies (solid tumors) were recorded: one patient who developed Kaposi sarcoma while on treatment for mild chronic GVHD [the sarcoma spontaneously reversed after discontinuation of immunosuppressive treatment (Erer et al., 1997b)] and one case of lip spinocellular cancer in a patient with chronic mucosal GVHD (Gaziev et al., 1997b). Overall, the incidence of secondary long-term solid tumors in the ex-thalassemic is less than 7/100,000/year. The incidence of secondary malignancies does not appear to be, so far, more than the incidence reported in patients undergoing medical treatment (Miniero et al., 1985; Stricker et al., 1986; Das Gupta et al., 1988; Borgna-Pignatti et al., 1998) and therefore it should not be a reason to deny transplantation. These data are in accordance with the data reported by the International Bone Marrow Transplant Registry (Curtis et al., 1997) in patients receiving BMT for nonmalignant diseases in whom secondary malignancies were not significantly increased when compared to the expected incidence in the normal population. A prospective study is ongoing in Pesaro on this issue and it would be very useful if a similar prospective study were carried out in medically treated patients.

Thalassemia-Related Complications

Thalassemia-related complications are those acquired during years of thalassemia and its treatment.

Iron Overload. Once BMT has replaced ineffective with effective erythropoiesis, the patient is cured of thalassemia. However, there is no reason to expect that marrow transplant could eliminate excess iron acquired during years of thalassemia. Spontaneous decrement of iron stores is limited after BMT (Lucarelli et al., 1993; Muretto et al., 1994). Heavily iron overloaded patients with acquired tissue damage maintain high level of iron throughout the years following transplantation.

Iron overload causes significant morbidity and mortality as seen in hereditary hemochromatosis (Niederau et al., 1985) and progression of liver disease to the stage of cirrhosis has been documented in some Class 3 patients years after transplantation (Angelucci et al., 1993a). Interestingly, no patients presented with deterioration of cardiac status during follow-up despite several of them having hepatic iron concentration above the

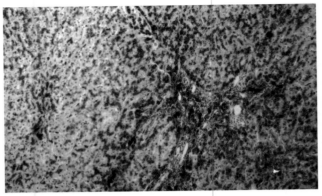

Figure 39.8. Pretransplant liver biopsy of a thalassemia patient. The biopsy was prepared by Perls's technique. Hepatic iron concentration was 23 mg/g dry weight. For full color reproduction, see color plate 39.8.

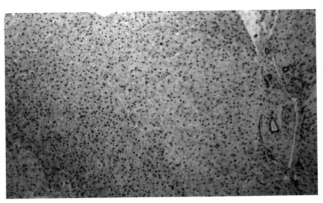

Figure 39.9. Liver biopsy (Perls's technique) of the same patient as in Figure 39.8, 8 years after BMT. Hepatic iron concentration was 1.41 mg/g dry weight, normal value <1.6 mg/g (Weinfeld, 1964). The patient had been treated by a course of sequential phlebotomies starting during the third year after transplant. For full color reproduction, see color plate 39.9.

threshold level predictive of cardiac disease (15 mg/g dry weight) (Lucarelli et al., 1993); a limited role of hemosiderin-iron in the generation of free radicals has been postulated as the reason for this finding (Lucarelli et al., 1993).

In the ex-thalassemic, because of the presence of normal erythropoiesis, phlebotomy appeared to be the appropriate mechanism to remove excess iron (Angelucci et al., 1997b). Phlebotomy is safe, inexpensive, and highly efficient and therefore is the treatment of choice in this situation even in those patients who received a transplant from a donor with thalassemia minor. With this approach, excess iron can be completely mobilized from the body without any relevant side effect (Figs. 39.8 and 39.9). Following completion of the program, significant improvement in liver function was observed particularly in patients infected with hepatitis C virus (Angelucci et al., 1997b). Patients with early cardiac involvement (left ventricular diastolic dysfunction and impaired left ventricular contractility) demonstrated regression of subclinical cardiac disease after iron depletion (Mariotti et al., 1998).

In those ex-thalassemic patients with high iron levels who cannot be treated with phlebotomies because of their young age or difficult access to peripheral veins, daily subcutaneous administration of deferoxamine has proved to be useful in reducing iron stores (Giardini et al., 1995).

A strategy for iron treatment after marrow transplantation has been developed: liver biopsy is performed 18 months after BMT and the hepatic iron concentration is determined. No significant progression of liver disease has been observed comparing the 18th month biopsy to the pretransplant biopsy (unpublished observation) and therefore early treatment has not been considered necessary. Eighteen months after BMT, patients are no longer taking

cyclosporin or other transplant-related medications and the iron problem can be addressed.

The therapeutic strategy is based on the value of hepatic iron concentration and on the basis of the experience acquired in subjects homozygous and heterozygous for hereditary hemochromatosis. Subjects heterozygous for hereditary hemochromatosis develop a low level of iron loading, hepatic iron concentration of about 3.2 to 7 mg/g dry weight without significant organ damage, and have a normal life expectancy (Cartwright et al., 1979; Bulay et al., 1996). This range has been defined as the "optimal" level of iron overload in thalassemia patients receiving transfusions and chelation therapy (Olivieri and Brittenham, 1997). Patients with higher levels of iron burden are at risk of complications such us diabetes mellitus and liver fibrosis (Loreal et al., 1992; Niederau et al., 1996). A hepatic iron concentration exceeding 22 mg/g has been associated with liver cirrhosis (Basset et al., 1986) but more recently, liver fibrosis and cirrhosis have been documented in patients with lower levels of hepatic iron concentration: hepatic iron concentration was 21 ± 8 mg/g dry weight in patients with cirrhosis, 18 ± 9 mg/g dry weight in patients with fibrosis, and 13 ± 6 mg/g dry weight in the prefibrotic stage (Loreal et al., 1992). Patients with hereditary hemochromatosis could be a good clinical model to predict iron-related complications and guide therapy in the ex-thalassemic, but this model should be interpreted as a conservative model because several factors influencing iron damage (age, rate of iron accumulation, duration of exposure, presence of cofactors for liver disease) are different in the two diseases. Also, partition of iron burden is different: At the same level of hepatic iron concentration, the total body iron burden

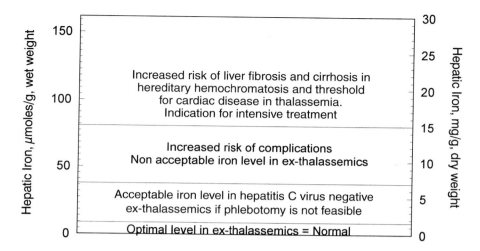

Figure 39.10. Guidelines for iron treatment in the "ex-thalassemic." Optimal liver iron concentration is that of normal individuals: <1.6 mg/g dry weight (Weinfeld, 1964). A hepatic iron concentration of up to 7 mg/g dry weight is acceptable in those patients who are anti–hepatitis C-virus negative. Higher values of hepatic iron concentration are not acceptable and should be treated. Patients with a hepatic iron concentration exceeding 15 mg/g dry weight should be intensively treated. (Modified from Olivieri and Brittenham, 1997, with permission.)

is almost twice as high in thalassemia as in hereditary hemochromatosis (Angelucci et al., 1998a).

The optimal iron level in the ex-thalassemic is the "normal level," that is, a hepatic iron concentration of less than 1.6 mg/g dry weight (Weinfeld, 1964) and this should be the theoretical goal for any patient. All patients with active hepatitis C virus infection should be treated to a normal liver iron content (see below). A hepatic iron concentration between 1.6 and 7 mg/g dry weight can be acceptable in a hepatitis C virus negative patient if phlebotomy is not feasible. We do not recommend deferoxamine in this situation but schedule a repeat liver biopsy after 5 to 6 years of follow-up. All patients with liver iron content within the range of that associated with increased complications (i.e., 7 and 15 mg/g dry weight) should be treated until they fall under this level. Patients with a hepatic iron concentration exceeding 15 mg/g dry weight should be intensively treated. Figure 39.10 has been modified from the original figure of Olivieri and Brittenham (1997) and adapted to the case of the ex-thalassemic.

Chronic Hepatitis and Liver Fibrosis. Hepatitis C virus infection is common in thalassemic patients, particularly in those transfused before second-generation enzyme-linked immonosorbent assay (ELISA) tests became available. Approximately 25 percent of thalassemic patients in the United Kingdom have antibodies to hepatitis C virus (Wonke et al., 1990) and in some parts of Italy the prevalence is greater than 70 percent and proportional to the amount of blood transfusions received (Angelucci, 1994). Hepatitis C virus infection gives rise to chronic hepatitis (Kiyosawa et al., 1990), cirrhosis (Koretz et al., 1993), and finally to hepatocarcinoma (Tong et al., 1995), even if the precise risk of developing one of these complications is controversial (Seeff et al., 1992; Alter, 1995). In thalassemia, liver damage due to hepatitis C virus infection is exacerbated by iron overload and liver disease is a recognized cause of mortality (Zurlo et al., 1989) and morbidity (Angelucci et al., 1993b). After BMT, 10 percent to 15 percent of patients became hepatitis C virus seronegative (Erer et al., 1997a); however, the problem of hepatitis C virus infection usually remains. Transplanted thalassemics have a long (probably normal) life expectancy and mild chronic liver disease has to be considered in this prospective. Viral liver disease is probably the only factor potentially limiting survival in ex-thalassemics, thus avoidance of progression of liver damage to cirrhosis in long-term follow-up (over 20 to 30 years) is fundamental.

Reduction or normalization of the iron pool results in marked improvement in serum levels of liver enzymes and in liver histopathology in the majority of the ex-thalassemics (Angelucci et al., 1997b; Lucarelli et al., 1998). In about half the hepatitis C virus seropositive patients, transaminase normalized and the histologic activity index significantly improved after iron depletion (Angelucci et al., 1998b), resulting in the dilemma of whether to recommend interferon therapy (Desmet et al., 1994). Also, in patients presenting with active hepatitis after iron removal, interferon treatment has proved to be a rational approach several years after transplant, with a success rate not different from that obtained in the normal population (Giardini et al., 1997).

The absence of thalassemia and of iron overload makes it easier to treat other complications such us viral hepatitis, somewhat contradicting the assessment that the cure of thalassemia by transplantation does not modify the other complications already acquired at the time of transplant (Olivieri et al., 1995).

Endocrine Dysfunction. Hypogonadism is the most common endocrine disorder in medically treated patients with thalassemia major, involving approximately half the patients (De Sanctis et al., 1995b, 1997b). In a study involving sixty-eight transplanted thalassemics, 32 percent reached an advanced or complete puberty spontaneously (34 percent of the females and 63 percent of the males) (De Sanctis et al., 1997a) despite clinical and hormonal evidence of gonadal impairment in most of them (De Sanctis et al., 1993). In this cohort, age, iron overload, and endocrine dysfunction were not uniform before transplantation. Iron overload and conditioning regimen were the major factors influencing endocrine function. Recently, a young woman transplanted at age 10 years became pregnant naturally and delivered a normal (thalassemia minor) child (Borgna-Pignatti et al., 1996). Preliminary observations of young children transplanted in the early phase of thalassemia indicate a good prognosis for growth and gonadal function.

Another well-recognized complication in thalassemia major is impaired glucose tolerance and diabetes mellitus (De Sanctis et al., 1988), which is due to a combination of insulin deficiency (caused by pancreatic β-cell exhaustion or damage related to iron overload) and insulin resistance. In a prospective study, it has been demonstrated that transplantation using busulfan, cyclophosphamide, and cyclosporin does not affect pancreatic β-cell function (Galimberti et al., 1995). Of ninety-three patients studied, only three patients with an impaired oral glucose tolerance test and liver cirrhosis before transplant demonstrated worsening of glucose intolerance, while more than half of the patients with an impaired oral glucose tolerance test before transplant showed improvement of pancreatic β-cell function after marrow transplant.

From preliminary unpublished observations, even thyroid function seems not to be affected by transplantation after conditioning regimens without radiation.

FUTURE APPROACHES

In Utero Transplantation in β Thalassemia and α Thalassemia

In utero hamatopoietic stem cell transplantation differs from postnatal BMT because engraftment depends on competitive population of receptive sites in the recipient bone marrow. There is ample evidence from experimental (Fleischman and Mintz, 1979; Flake et al., 1986; Harrison et al., 1989) and natural models (Owen, 1945) that donor cells can effectively compete with recipient cells in the fetal microenvironment to permanently engraft hematopoietic stem cells. Effective prenatal treatment depends on the ability of normal cells to engraft and compete in the thalassemic microenviroment. Advantages of this approach compared to postnatal transplantation should be (1) immunologic tolerance, (2) absence of myeloablation and related mortality and morbidity, and (3) absence of thalassemia-related organ or tissue damage.

Engraftment is favored in diseases where there is a selective advantage for donor cells (e.g., congenital immunodeficiency disorders) but where there is normal recipient microenviroment. Clinical success is thus far limited to immunodeficiency disorders (Linch et al., 1986; Cowan and Golbus, 1994; Touraine, 1996; Wengler et al., 1996; Flake and Zanjani, 1997). All of the reported attempts to date in thalassemia have failed. There have been eight attempts to treat thalassemia by in utero transplantation: five fetuses with β thalassemia and three with α thalassemia. Of the five fetuses with β thalassemia two died due to procedure-related complications and two were transplanted at 18 and 19 weeks of gestational age and failed on immunologic grounds. One fetus transplanted at 12 weeks gestation with fetal liver derived cells was initially reported as engrafted on the basis of a Y chromosome by polymerase chain reaction (PCR) and 0.9 percent HbA at birth. HbA increased to 30 percent at age 1 year but no additional follow-up engraftment data have been published (Flake and Zanjani, 1997). In terms of competition for marrow engraftment, α thalassemia has a theoretical biological disadvantage due to the early fetal anemia (α-globin-dependent hemoglobin production begins at 8 weeks gestation), early development of fetal hydrops (12 to 14 weeks), and hypercellular fetal hematopoietic microenviroment, which may not be optimal in terms of available receptive sites or donor cell competition. Of the three α-thalassemic fetuses, one was transplanted at 18 weeks of gestation with T-cell-depleted maternal marrow. There was no evidence of engraftment at 24 weeks by percutaneous umbilical blood sampling and the pregnancy was terminated (Cowan and Golbus, 1994). Analysis at autopsy revealed marked extramedullary hematopoiesis with donor cells identified in extramedullary sites, confirming results obtained in sheep where donor cells do not appear in the peripheral circulation until later in gestation. A second case was transplanted at 15 weeks gestation by a single injection of cryopreserved fetal liver-derived cells (Westgren et al., 1996) without detectable engraftment. The third case of α thalassemia was transplanted by a series of three samples of CD34-enriched paternal marrow cells at 13, 18, and 23 weeks gestation (Hayward et al., 1996). The fetus required repeated intrauterine transfusions to survive to term and had only a trace positive PCR signal for α-globin genes in cord blood and bone marrow cells and evidence of donor-specific tolerance by mixed lymphocyte reaction. The child remained healthy but transfusion dependent at age 1 year. Clinical observations of correction of anemia by relatively low degrees of mixed chimerism after postnatal transplant (Andreani et al., 2000) and the apparent selective advantage of donor erythropoiesis are the basis for the development of in utero transplantation. At the moment, there is no convincing evidence for the efficacy of in utero transplantation in the treatment of the hemoglobinopathies, but it does not appear to have been adequately tested, particularly regarding the choice of appropriate gestational age for transplantation, source of stem cells, number of transplants, and so on.

Transplant From Matched Unrelated Donors

The most serious limitation for the general applicability or use of allogeneic BMT in thalassemia is the availability of a related HLA-identical donor. There is a 25 percent chance that any given sibling could be HLA identical to a potential patient and a calculated probability of 33 percent for a thalassemic patient to have an HLA-identical sibling within the family (Delfini et al., 1986). In our experience, 8.5 percent of thalassemic patients were found to be phenotypically HLA identical to one parent (Delfini et al., 1986). Unrelated donor transplant has great potential in thalassemia because of the possibility for many patients to remain healthy for a long time under medical treatment until an "optimal" marrow donor is identified. It is possible that due to the geographic distribution of thalassemia in selected areas (i.e., Sardinia), the probability of finding an unrelated identical donor would be higher than in the general population if in those areas large and representative marrow donor registries were established. In Sardinia, due to the high incidence of patients with similar extended HLA haplotypes, the probability of finding a matched unrelated marrow donor identical for two extended haplotypes was estimated to be around 8.5 to 9 percent with a regional donor registry of 15,000 volunteer donors (Contu et al., 1992).

In recent years, improvements in HLA typing technology, increased control of graft-versus-host disease and infectious diseases, and expanded pools of unrelated volunteer donors (Anasetti et al., 1995; Anasetti, 1997) have led to a significant improvement in the outcome of unrelated marrow transplant in patients affected by malignancies and by inborn errors (Miano et al., 1998). In chronic myeloid leukemia, unrelated transplant results are now not much different from those achieved using a related HLA-identical donor (Hansen et al., 1998).

On the basis of this finding a program of matched unrelated donor transplantation for thalassemia involving two Italian transplant centers was established in 1996. To proceed to transplant patients should not have cirrhosis or cardiac disease, and a high degree of histocompatibility between patient and potential donor should be present. The clinical trial requires extended haplotype identity, which means identity from locus HLA-A to locus HLA-Dq on the same chromosome. Due to the phenomenon of linkage disequilibrium it is reasonable to believe that such unrelated subjects could be reasonably well matched (Contu et al., 1994; La Nasa et al., 1997).

At the time of this writing, twenty patients have been transplanted in this program: three had recurrence of thalassemia, four died, and thirteen had successful transplants with a median follow-up of more than 2 years. Incidence of grade II–III acute graft-versus-host disease was 35 percent and incidence of limited chronic GVHD was 35 percent (none developed extensive chronic GVHD). Median Karnofky score is 100 percent (G. La Nasa, personal communication).

Chimerism

The experience of mixed chimerism demonstrates that "partial engraftment" can be sufficient to sustain prolonged and probably permanent erythroid function capable of rendering the patient transfusion-free. Even though we were not able to identify any treatment-related variable (preparative regimen, GVHD prophylaxis, etc.) correlated with the development of persistent mixed chimerism, this observation opens new therapeutic possibilities such as the use of minimally ablative preparative regimens to obtain partial engraftment but avoiding or significantly diminishing transplant-related morbidity and mortality, particularly in adult patients with advanced disease. The potential use of minimally myeloablative therapy in this condition has been supported by studies using animal models (Stewart et al., 1998).

Gene Therapy

Gene therapy is comprehensively discussed in Chapter 41 but we believe that if replacement of the affected gene will become a clinically effective treatment option, this should be considered as an evolution of the bone marrow transplant experience against which the results of any other therapeutic option should be compared. The experience of persistent mixed chimerism after transplantation suggests that, if gene therapy becomes a clinically practical option, it may not be necessary to completely eradicate the thalassemic marrow in order to permit clinical control of the disease.

References

Alter, HJ. (1995). To C or not to C: These are the questions. *Blood* 85: 1681–1695.

Anasetti, C. (1997). Marrow transplantation from unrelated volunteer donors. *Bone Marrow Transplant.* 19: 183–185.

Anasetti, C, Amos, D, Beatty, PG et al. (1989). Effect of HLA compatibility on engraftment of bone marrow transplants in patients with leukemia or lymphoma. *N. Engl. J. Med.* 320: 197–204.

Anasetti, C, Etzioni, R, Petersdorf, EW et al. (1995). Marrow transplantation from unrelated volunteer donors. *Ann. Rev. Med.* 46: 169–179.

Andreani, M, Manna, M, Lucarelli, G et al. (1996). Persistence of mixed chimerism in patients transplanted for the treatment of thalassemia. *Blood* 87: 3494–3499.

Andreani, M, Nesci, S, Lucarelli, G et al. (2000). Long-term survival of ex-thalassemic patients with persistent mixed chimerism after bone marrow transplantation. *Bone Marrow Transplant.* 25: 401–404.

Angastiniotis, M and Modell, B. (1998). Global epidemiology of hemoglobin disorders. *Ann. N. Y. Acad. Sci.* 850: 251–269.

Angelucci, E. (1994). Antibodies to hepatitis C virus in thalassemia. *Haematologica* 79: 353–355.

Angelucci, E and Lucarelli, G. (1996). The clinical management of thalassemia patients undergoing bone marrow transplantation. In Burt, RK, Deeg, HJ, Lothian, ST, and Santos, G, editors. *Bone marrow transplantation.* Austin: R.G. Landes. p. 286.

Angelucci, E, Mariotti, E, Lucarelli, G et al. (1992). Sudden cardiac tamponade after chemotherapy for marrow transplantation in thalassemia. *Lancet* 339: 287–289.

Angelucci, E, Baronciani, D, Lucarelli, G et al. (1993a). Bone marrow transplantation in class 3 thalassemia patients. *Bone Marrow Transplant.* 12 (Suppl 1): 63–64.

Angelucci, E, Baronciani, D, Lucarelli, G et al. (1993b). Liver iron overload and liver fibrosis in thalassemia. *Bone Marrow Transplant.* 12: 29–31.

Angelucci, E, Mariotti, E, Lucarelli, G et al. (1994). Cardiac tamponade in thalassemia. *Bone Marrow Transplant.* 13: 827–829.

Angelucci, E, Baronciani, D, Lucarelli, G et al. (1995). Needle liver biopsy in thalassaemia: Analyses of diagnostic accuracy and safety in 1184 consecutive biopsies. *Br. J. Haematol.* 89: 757–761.

Angelucci, E, Giovagnoni, A, Valeri, G et al. (1997a). Limitation of magnetic resonance imaging in measurements of hepatic iron. *Blood* 90: 4736–4742.

Angelucci, E, Muretto, P, Lucarelli, G et al. (1997b). Phlebotomy to reduce iron overload in patients cured of tha-

lassemia by bone marrow transplantation. *Blood* 90: 994–998.

Angelucci, E, Fargion, S, Ripalti, M et al. (1998a). Total body iron stores are greater in thalassemia major than in genetic hemochromatosis at equivalent hepatic iron concentrations. *Blood* 92: 3134a.

Angelucci, E, Muretto, P, Lucarelli, G et al. (1998b). Treatment of iron overload in the "ex-thalassemic": Report from the phlebotomy program. *Ann. N. Y. Acad. Sci.* 850: 288–293.

Anonymous. (1981). Community control of hereditary anemias. *Bull. W. H. Or.* 61: 63.

Appelbaum, FR, Storb, R, Ramberg, RE et al. (1984). Allogeneic marrow transplantation in the treatment of preleukemia. *Ann. Intern. Med.* 100: 689–693.

Argiolu, F, Sanna, MA, Cossu, F et al. (1997). Bone marrow transplant in thalassemia. The experience of Cagliari. *Bone Marrow Transplant.* 19: 65–67.

Baronciani, D, Angelucci, E, Lucarelli, G et al. (1990). Cytomegalovirus infections in thalassemic patients after bone marrow transplantation. *Bone Marrow Transplant.* 167–172.

Baronciani, D, Angelucci, E, Agostinelli, F et al. (1996). Bone marrow transplantation in a thalassemia patient with congenital heart disease. *Bone Marrow Transplant.* 17: 119–120.

Baronciani, D, Angelucci, E, Martinelli, F et al. (1998). An unusual marrow transplant complication: Cardiac myxoma. *Bone Marrow Transplant.* 21: 825–827.

Basset, M, Halliday, WJ, and Powell, LW. (1986). Value of hepatic iron measurements in early hemochromatosis and determination of the critical iron level associated with fibrosis. *Hepatology* 6: 24–29.

Borgna-Pignatti, C, Marradi, P, Rugolotto, S, and Marcolongo, A. (1996). Successful pregnancy after bone marrow transplantation for thalassemia. *Bone Marrow Transplant.* 18: 235–236.

Borgna-Pignatti, C, Rugolotto, S, DeStefano, P et al. (1998). Survival and disease complications in thalassemia major. *Ann. N. Y. Acad. Sci.* 850: 227–231.

Boulad, F, Giardina, PJ, Gillio, A et al. (1998). Bone marrow transplantation for homozygous beta-thalassemia. The Memorial Sloan-Kettering Cancer Center Experience. *Ann. N. Y. Acad. Sci.* 850: 498–502.

Brittenham, GM, Farrel, DE, Harris, JW et al. (1982). Magnetic-susceptibility measurement of human iron stores. *N. Engl. J. Med.* 307: 1671–1675.

Brittenham, GM, Griffith, PM, Nienhuis, AW et al. (1994). Efficacy of deferoxamine in preventing complications of iron overload in patients with thalassemia mayor. *N. Engl. J. Med.* 331: 567–573.

Bulay, ZJ, Griffen, LM, Jorde, LB et al. (1996). Clinical and biochemical abnormalities in people heterozygous for hemochromatosis. *N. Engl. J. Med.* 335: 1799–1805.

Cartwright, GE, Edwards, CQ, Kravitz, K et al. (1979). Hereditary hemochromatosis: Phenotypic expression of the disease. *N. Engl. J. Med.* 301: 175–179.

Cazzola, M, Locatelli, F, and DeStefano, P. (1995). Deferoxamine in thalassemia major. *N. Engl. J. Med.* 332: 271.

Choo, SY, Starling, GC, Anasetti, C, and Hansen, JA. (1993). Selection of an unrelated donor for marrow transplantation facilitated by the molecular characterization of a novel HLA-A allele. *Hum. Immunol.* 36: 20–26.

Clift, RA and Johnson, FL. (1997). Marrow transplants for thalassemia. The USA experience. *Bone Marrow Transplant.* 19: 57–59.

Contu, L, Arras, M, Mulargia, M et al. (1992). Study of HLA segregation in 479 thalassemic families. *Tissue Antigens* 2: 58–67.

Contu, L, La Nasa, G, Arras, M et al. (1994). Successful unrelated bone marrow transplantation in beta-thalassemia. *Bone Marrow Transplant.* 13: 329–331.

Cowan, M and Golbus, M. (1994). In utero hematopoietic stem cell transplants for inherited disease. *Am. J. Pediatr. Hematol. Oncol.* 16: 35–42.

Curtis, RE, Rowlings, PA, Deeg, HJ et al. (1997). Solid cancers after bone marrow transplantation. *N. Engl. J. Med.* 336: 897–904.

Das Gupta, A, Nair, L, and Barbhaya, SA. (1988). Association of hematologic malignancies with hemoglobinopathies. *Am. J. Hematol.* 28: 130.

De Sanctis, V, Zurlo, MG, Senesi, E et al. (1988). Insulin-dependent diabetes in thalassemia. *Arch. Dis. Child.* 63: 58–62.

De Sanctis, V, Galimberti, M, Lucarelli, G et al. (1993). Pubertal development in thalassemic patients after allogeneic bone marrow transplantation. *Eur. J. Pediatr.* 152: 1–5.

De Sanctis, V, Pintor, C, Gamberini, MR et al. (1995). Multicentre study on prevalence of endocrine complications in thalassemia major. *Clin. Endocrinol.* 42: 581–586.

De Sanctis, V, Galimberti, M, Lucarelli, G et al. (1997a). Growth and development in ex-thalassemic patients. *Bone Marrow Transplant.* 19: 126–127.

De Sanctis, V, Urso, L, Govoni, R et al. (1997b). Growth, pubertal development and fertility in severe beta-thalassemia: The Ferrara's experience. *Bone Marrow Transplant.* 19: 30–31.

Delfini, C, Donati, M, Marchionni, D et al. (1986). HLA compatibility for patients with thalassemia: Implications for bone marrow transplantation. *Int. J. Cell Cloning* 4: 274–278.

Dennison, D, Srivastava, A, and Chandy, M. (1997). Bone marrow transplantation for thalassaemia in India. *Bone Marrow Transplant.* 19: 70.

Desmet, VJ, Gerber, M, Hoofnagle, JH et al. (1994). Classification of chronic hepatitis. Diagnosis, grading and staging. *Hepatology* 19: 1513–1520.

Di Bartolomeo, P, Di Girolamo, G, Olioso, P et al. (1997). The Pescara experience of allogenic bone marrow transplantation in thalassemia. *Bone Marrow Transplant.* 19: 48–53.

Di Gregorio, F, Pizzarelli, G, Romeo, MA, and Russo, G. (1997). Mortality and morbidity in thalassemia major: The experience of Catania. *Bone Marrow Transplant.* 19: 14–15.

Ehlers, KH, Giardina, PJ, Lesser, ML et al. (1991). Prolonged survival in patients with beta-thalassemia major treated with deferoxamine. *J. Pediatr.* 118: 540–545.

Erer, B, Angelucci, E, Lucarelli, G et al. (1994). Hepatitis C virus infection in thalassemia patients undergoing allogeneic bone marrow transplantation. *Bone Marrow Transplant.* 14: 369–372.

Erer, B, Angelucci, E, Lucarelli, G et al. (1997a). HCV infection in thalassemia before and after BMT. *Bone Marrow Transplant.* 19: 155–157.

Erer, B, Angelucci, E, Muretto, P et al. (1997b). Kaposi's sarcoma after allogeneic bone marrow transplantation. *Bone Marrow Transplant.* 19: 629–631.

Flake, AW, Harrison, MR, Adzick, NS, and Zanjani, ED. (1986). Transplantation of fetal hematopoietic stem cells in utero. *Science* 233: 776–778.

Flake, AW and Zanjani, ED. (1997). In utero hematopoietic stem cell transplantation. A status report. *J. Am. Med. Assoc.* 278: 932–937.

Fleischman, R and Mintz, B. (1979). Prevention of genetic anemias in mice by microinjection of normal hematopoietic cells into the fetal placenta. *Proc. Natl. Acad. Sci. U.S.A.* 76: 5736–5740.

Floersheim, GL and Elson, LA. (1961). Restoration of hematopoiesis following a lethal dose of dimethyl myleran by isologic bone marrow transplantation in mice. Experiments on modification of intolerance to homologous bone marrow by 6-mercaptopurine, amino-chlorambucil and cortisone. *Acta Haematol.* 26: 233–245.

Galimberti, M, De Sanctis, V, Lucarelli, G et al. (1995). Pancreatic beta-cell function before and after bone marrow transplantation for thalassemia. In Andò, S. and Brancati, C., editors, Endocrine Disorders in Thalassemia. Physiopathological and Therapeutic Aspects. Berlin: Springer-Verlag, p. 69–72.

Gaziev, D, Polchi, P, Galimberti, M et al. (1997a). Graft-versus-host disease after bone marrow transplantation for thalassemia. An analysis of incidence and risk factors. *Transplantation* 63: 854–860.

Gaziev, D, Lucarelli, G, Galimberti, M et al. (1997b). Malignancies after bone marrow transplantation for thalassemia. *Bone Marrow Transplant.* 19: 142–144.

Gaziev, D, Polchi, P, Lucarelli, G et al. (2000a). Second marrow transplants for graft failure in patients with thalassemia. *Bone Marrow Transplant.* 24: 1299–1306.

Gaziev, D, Galimberti, M, Lucarelli, G et al. (2000b). Bone marrow transplantation from alternative donors for thalassemia: HLA-phenotypically identical relative and HLA-nonidentical sibling or parent transplants. *Bone Marrow Transplant.* 25: 815–822.

Ghavamzadeh, A, Bahar, B, Djahani, M et al. (1997). Bone marrow transplantation of thalassemia, the experience in Tehran (Iran). *Bone Marrow Transplant.* 19: 71–73.

Giardina, PJ, Ehlers, KH, Grady, RW et al. (1997). Progress in the management of thalassemia: Over a decade and a half of experience with subcutaneous desferrioxamine. *Bone Marrow Transplant.* 19: 9–10.

Giardini, C. (1995). Ethical issue of bone marrow transplantation for thalassemia. *Bone Marrow Transplant.* 15: 657–658.

Giardini, C. (1997). Treatment of β-thalassemia. *Curr. Opin. Hematol.* 4: 79–87.

Giardini, C, Galimberti, M, Lucarelli, G et al. (1995). Desferioxamine therapy accelerates clearance of iron deposits after bone marrow transplantation. *Br. J. Haematol.* 89: 868–873.

Giardini, C, Galimberti, M, Lucarelli, G, et al. (1997). Alfa-interferon treatment of chronic hepatitis C after bone marrow transplantation for homozygous beta-thalassemia. *Bone Marrow Transplant.* 20: 767–772.

Giorgiani, G, Bozzola, M, Locatelli, F et al. (1995). Role of busulfan and total body irradiation on growth of prepubertal children recieving bone marrow transplantation and result of treatment with recombinant human growth hormone. *Blood* 86: 825–831.

Goodrich, JM, Bowden, RA, Fisher, L et al. (1993). Ganciclovir prophylaxis to prevent cytomegalovirus disease after allogeneic marrow transplant. *Ann. Intern. Med* 118: 173–178.

Hansen, JA, Gooley, TA, Martin, PJ et al. (1998). Bone marrow transplantation from unrelated donors for patients with chronic myeloid leukemia. *N. Engl. J. Med.* 338: 962–968.

Harrison, MR, Slotnick, RN, Crombleholme, TM et al. (1989). In-utero transplantation of fetal liver haemopoietic stem cells in monkeys. *Lancet* 2: 1425–1427.

Hayward, A, Hobbins, R, Quinones, R et al. (1996). Microchimerism and tolerance following intrauterine transplantation and transfusion for α-thalassemia-1. Presented at the 'In utero stem cell transplantation and gene therapy conference'. Reno, NV

Hobbs, JR, Hugh-Jones, K, Shaw, PJ et al. (1986). Engraftment rates related to busulphan and cyclophosphamide dosages for displacement bone marrow transplants in fifty children. *Bone Marrow Transplant.* 1: 201–208.

Issaragrisil, S, Suvatte, V, Visuthisakchai, S et al. (1997). Bone marrow and cord blood stem cell transplantation for thalassemia in Thailand. *Bone Marrow Transplant.* 19: 54–56.

Kapoor, N, Kirkpatrick, D, Oleske, J et al. (1981). Reconstitution of normal megakaryocytopoiesis and immunologic functions in Wiskott-Aldrich syndrome by marrow transplantation following myeloablation and immunosuppression with busulfan and cyclophosphamide. *Blood* 57: 692–696.

Kirkpatrick, DV, Barrios, NJ, and Humbert, JH. (1991). Bone marrow transplantation for sickle cell anemia. *Semin. Hematol.* 28: 240–243.

Kiyosawa, K, Sodeyama, T, Tanaka, E et al. (1990). Interrelationship of blood transfusion, non-A, non-B hepatitis and hepatocellular carcinoma: Analysis by detection of antibody to hepatitis C virus. *Hepatology* 12: 671–675.

Koretz, RL, Abbey, H, Coleman, E, and Gitnick, G. (1993). Non-A, non-B post-transfusion hepatitis: Looking back in the second decade. *Ann. Intern. Med.* 119: 110–115.

Lai, ME, Belluzzo, N, Muraca, M et al. (1997). The prognosis for adults with thalassemia major treated with medical therapy: An interim report: Cagliari 1995. *Bone Marrow Transplant.* 19: 18–19.

La Nasa, G, Vacca, A, Pizzati, A et al. (1997). Role of HLA extended haplotypes in unrelated bone marrow transplantation. *Bone Marrow Transplant.* 19: 186–189.

Lee, YS, Kristovich, KM, Ducore, JM et al. (1998). Bone marrow transplantation in thalassemia. A role for radiation? *Ann. N. Y. Acad. Sci.* 850: 503–505.

Li, CK, Yuen, PMP, Shing, MK et al. (1997). Stem cell transplant for thalassaemia patients in Hong Kong. *Bone Marrow Transplant.* 19: 62–64.

Lin, HP, Chan, LL, Lam, SK et al. (1997). Bone marrow transplantation for thalassemia. The experience from Malaysia. *Bone Marrow Transplant.* 19: 74–77.

Linch, D, Rodeck, C, and Nicolaides, K. (1986). Attempted bone marrow transplantation in a 17 week fetus. *Lancet* 1: 1382.

Loreal, O, Deugnier, Y, Moirand, R et al. (1992). Liver fibrosis in genetic hemochromatosis. Respective roles of iron and non-iron related factors in 127 homozygous patients. *J. Hepatol.* 16: 122–127.

Lucarelli, G, Polchi, P, Izzi, T et al. (1984). Allogeneic marrow transplantation for thalassemia. *Exp. Hematol.* 12: 676–681.

Lucarelli, G, Polchi, P, Galimberti, M et al. (1985). Marrow transplantation for thalassemia following busulphan and cyclophosphamide. *Lancet* 1: 1355–1357.

Lucarelli, G, Galimberti, M, Polchi, P et al. (1987). Marrow transplantation in patients with advanced thalassemia. *N. Engl. J. Med.* 316: 1050–1055.

Lucarelli, G, Galimberti, M, Polchi, P et al. (1990). Bone marrow transplantation in patients with thalassemia. *N. Engl. J. Med.* 322: 417–421.

Lucarelli, G, Galimberti, M, Polchi, P et al. (1991). Bone marrow transplantation in Thalassemia. *Hematol. Oncol. Clin. North. Am.* 5: 549–556.

Lucarelli, G, Angelucci, E, Giardini, C et al. (1993). Fate of iron stores in thalassemia after bone marrow transplantation. *Lancet* 342: 1388–1391.

Lucarelli, G, Clift, R, and Angelucci, E. (1995). Deferoxamine in thalassemia major. *N. Engl. J. Med.* 332: 271.

Lucarelli, G, Clift, RA, Galimberti, M et al. (1996). Marrow transplantation for patients with thalassemia. Results in class 3 patients. *Blood* 87: 2082–2088.

Lucarelli, G, Galimberti, M, Giardini, C et al. (1998). Bone marrow transplantation in thalassemia: The experience of Pesaro. *Ann. N. Y. Acad. Sci.* 850: 270–275.

Lucarelli, G, Clift, RA, Galimberti, M et al. (1999). Bone marrow transplantation in adult thalassemic patients. *Blood* 93: 1164–1167.

Manna, M, Nesci, S, Andreani, M et al. (1993). Influence of the conditioning regimens on the incidence of mixed chimerism in thalassemic transplanted patients. *Bone Marrow Transplant.* 12 (Suppl 1): 70–73.

Mariotti, E, Agostini, A, Angelucci, E et al. (1996). Reduced left ventricular contractile reserve identified by low dose dobutamine echocardiography as an early marker of cardiac involvement in asymptomatic patients with thalassemia major. *Echocardiography* 13: 463–472.

Mariotti, E, Angelucci, E, Agostini, A et al. (1998). Evaluation of cardiac status in iron-loaded thalassemia patients following bone marrow transplantation: Improvement in cardiac function during reduction in iron burden. *Br. J. Haematol.* 103: 916–921.

Miano, M, Porta, E, Locatelli, F et al. (1998). Unrelated donor marrow transplantation for inborn errors. *Bone Marrow Transplant.* 21: S37–S40.

Miniero, R, Pastore, G, Saracco, P, and Terracini, B. (1985). Homozygous beta thalassemia and cancer. *Haematologica* 70: 78–79.

Muretto, P, Del Fiasco, S, Angelucci, E, and Lucarelli, G. (1994). Bone marrow transplantation in thalassemia: Modification of hepatic iron overload and related pathologies after long-term engrafting. *Liver* 14: 14–24.

Nesci, S, Manna, M, Andreani, M et al. (1992). Mixed chimerism in thalassemic patients after bone marrow transplantation. *Bone Marrow Transplant.* 10: 143–146.

Nesci, S, Manna, M, Lucarelli, G et al. (1998). Mixed chimerism after bone marrow transplantation in thalasemia. *Ann. N. Y. Acad. Sci.* 850: 495–497.

Niederau, C, Fisher, R, Sonnenberg, A et al. (1985). Survival and causes of death in cirrhotic and in noncirrhotic patients with primary hemochromatosis. *N. Engl. J. Med.* 313: 1256–1262.

Niederau, C, Fisher, R, Purschel, A et al. (1996). Long term survival in patients with hereditary hemochromatosis. *Gastroenterology* 110: 1107–1119.

Olivieri, NF and Brittenham, GM. (1997). Iron-chelation therapy and the treatment of thalassemia. *Blood* 89: 739–761.

Olivieri, NF, Freedman, MH, Saunders, EF et al. (1990). Graft rejection without clinical relapse in patients with homozygous beta-thalassemia following bone marrow transplantation. *Blood* 76 (10 Suppl 1): 559a(Abstract).

Olivieri, NF, Nathan, DG, MacMillan, JH et al. (1994). Survival in medically treated patients with homozygous β-thalassemia. *N. Engl. J. Med.* 331: 574–578.

Olivieri, NF, Nathan, DG, and Cohen, AR. (1995). Deferoxamine in thalassemia major. *N. Engl. J. Med.* 332: 272.

Owen, RD. (1945). Immunogenetic consequences of vascular anastomoses between bovine cattle twins. *Science* 102: 400–401.

Parkman, R, Rappeport, J, Geha, R et al. (1978). Complete correction of the Wiskott-Aldrich syndrome by allogeneic bone-marrow transplantation. *N. Engl. J. Med.* 298: 921–927.

Pawlowska, AB, Blazar, BR, Angelucci, E et al. (1997). Relationship of plasma pharmacokinetics of high-dose oral busulfan to the outcome of allogeneic bone marrow transplantation in children with thalassemia. *Bone Marrow Transplant.* 20: 915–920.

Petersdorf, EW, Stanley, JF, Martin, PJ, and Hansen, JA. (1994). Molecular diversity of the HLA-C locus in unrelated marrow transplantation. *Tissue Antigens* 44: 93–99.

Piga, A, Longo, F, Consolati, A et al. (1997). Mortality and morbidity in thalassemia with conventional treatment. *Bone Marrow Transplant.* 19: 11–13.

Pugh, RNH, Murray-Lyon, IM, Dawson, JL et al. (1973). Transsection of the oesophagus for bleeding of oesophageal varices. *Br. J. Surg.* 60: 646–649.

Roberts, IAG. (1997). Current status of allogeneic transplantation for haemoglobinopathies. *Br. J. Haematol.* 98: 1–7.

Roberts, IAG, Darbyshire, PJ, and Will, AM. (1997). BMT for children with B-thalassemia major in the UK. *Bone Marrow Transplant.* 19: 60–61.

Santamaria, P, Reinsmoen, NL, Lindstrom, AL et al. (1994). Frequent HLA class I and DP sequence mismatches in serologically (HLA-A, HLA-B, HLA-DR) and molecularly (HLA-DRB1, HLA-DQAI, HLA-DQBI) HLA-identical unrelated marrow transplant pairs. *Blood* 83: 280–287.

Santos, GW, Sensenbrenner, LL, Burke, PJ et al. (1971). Marrow transplantation in man following cyclophosphamide. *Transplant. Proc.* 3: 400–404.

Santos, GW, Tutschka, PJ, Brookmeyer, R et al. (1983). Marrow transplantation for acute nonlymphocytic leukemia after treatment with busulfan and cyclophosphamide. *N. Engl. J. Med.* 309: 1347–1353.

Schrier, S, Ma, L, Angelucci, E, and Lucarelli, G. (1997). Advances in understanding of the abnormal cell biology in the thalassemias. *Bone Marrow Transplant.* 19: 1–3.

Seeff, LB, Buskett-Bales, Z, Wright, EC et al. (1992). Long-term mortality after transfusion-associated non-A, non-B hepatitis. *N. Engl. J. Med.* 327: 1906–1911.

Shulman, HM, Sullivan, KM, Weiden, PL et al. (1980). Chronic graft-versus-host syndrome in man. A long-term clinicopathologic study of 20 Seattle patients. *Am. J. Med.* 69: 204–217.

Socie, G, Henry-Amar, M, Cosset, JM et al. (1992). Increased incidence of solid malignant tumors after bone marrow transplantation for severe aplastic anemia (Letter). *Blood* 79: 290.

Stewart, FM, Zhong, S, Wuu, J et al. (1998). Lymphohematopoietic engraftment in minimally myeloablated hosts. *Blood* 91: 3681–3687.

Storb, R and Champlin, RE. (1991). Bone marrow transplantation for severe aplastic anemia. *Bone Marrow Transplant.* 8: 69–72.

Storb, R, Weiden, PL, Graham, TC et al. (1977). Hemopoietic grafts between DLA-identical canine littermates following dimethyl myleran. Evidence for resistance to grafts not associated with DLA and abrogated by antithymocyte serum. *Transplantation* 24: 349–357.

Stricker, RB, Linker, CA, Crowley, TJ, and Embury, SH. (1986). Hematologic malignancy in sickle cell disease: Report of four cases and review of the literature. *Am. J. Hematol.* 21: 223–230.

Sullivan, KM, Shulman, HM, Storb, R et al. (1981). Chronic graft-versus-host disease in 52 patients: Adverse natural course and successful treatment with combination immunosuppression. *Blood* 57: 267–276.

Sullivan, KM, Anasetti, C, Horowitz, M et al. (1998). Unrelated and HLA-nonidentical related donor marrow transplantation for thalassemia and leukemia. *Ann. N. Y. Acad. Sci.* 850: 312–351.

Thomas, ED, Buckner, CD, Storb, R et al. (1972). Aplastic anaemia treated by marrow transplantation. *Lancet* 1: 284–289.

Thomas, ED, Buckner, CD, Sanders, JE et al. (1982). Marrow transplantation for thalassaemia. *Lancet* 2: 227–229.

Tong, MJ, El-Farra, NS, Reikes, AR, and Co, RL. (1995). Clinical outcomes after transfusion-associated hepatitis C. *N. Engl. J. Med.* 332: 1463–1466.

Touraine, JL. (1996). Treatment of human fetuses and induction of immunological tolerance in humans by in utero transplantation of stem cells into fetal recipients. *Acta Haematol.* 96: 115–119.

Tutschka, PJ, Elfenbein, GJ, Sensenbrenner, LL et al. (1980). Preparative regimens for marrow transplantation in acute leukemia and aplastic anemia. Baltimore experience. *Am. J. Pediatr. Hematol. Oncol.* 2: 363–370.

Tutschka, PJ, Copelan, EA, and Klein, JP. (1987). Bone marrow transplantation for leukemia following a new busulfan and cyclophosphamide regimen. *Blood* 70: 1382–1388.

Tutschka, PJ, Copelan, EA, and Kapoor, N. (1989). Replacing total body irradiation with busulfan as conditioning of patients with leukemia for allogeneic marrow transplantation. *Transplant. Proc.* 21: 2952–2954.

Tutschka, PJ, Copelan, EA, Kapoor, N et al. (1991). Allogeneic bone marrow transplantation for leukemia using chemotherapy as conditioning: 6-year results of a single institution trial. *Transplant. Proc.* 23: 1709–1710.

Weinfeld, A. (1964). Storage iron in man. *Acta Med. Scand.* 427: 1–155.

Welch, HG and Larson, EB. (1989). Cost effectiveness of bone marrow transplantation in acute nonlymphocytic leukemia. *N. Engl. J. Med.* 321: 807–812.

Wengler, GA, Lanfranchi, A, Frusca, T et al. (1996). In-utero transplantation of parental CD34 haemopoietic progenitor cells in a patient with X-linked severe combined immunodeficiency (SCIDX1). *Lancet* 348: 1484–1487.

Westgren, M, Ringden, O, Eik-Nes, S et al. (1996). Lack of evidence of permanent engraftment after in utero fetal stem cell transplantation in congenital hemoglobinopathies. *Transplantation* 61: 1176–1179.

Witherspoon, RP, Fisher, LD, Schoch, G et al. (1989). Secondary cancers after bone marrow transplantation for leukemia or aplastic anemia. *N. Engl. J. Med.* 321: 784–789.

Witherspoon, RP, Storb, R, Pepe, M et al. (1992). Cumulative incidence of secondary solid malignant tumors in aplastic anemia patients given marrow grafts after conditioning with chemotherapy alone (Letter). *Blood* 79: 289–292.

Wonke, B, Hoffbrand, AV, Brown, D, and Dusheiko, G. (1990). Antibodies to hepatitis C virus in multiply transfused patients with thalassemia major. *J. Clin. Pathol.* 43: 638–640.

Yuan, J, Angelucci, E, Lucarelli, G et al. (1993). Accelerated programmed cell death (apoptosis) in erythroid precursors of patients with severe beta-thalassemia (Cooley's anemia) (see comment). *Blood* 82: 374–377.

Zurlo, MG, De Stefano, P, Borgna-Pignatti, C et al. (1989). Survival and causes of death in thalassemia major. *Lancet* 2: 27–30.

40

Bone Marrow Transplantation in Sickle Cell Anemia

CHRISTIANE VERMYLEN

INTRODUCTION

Bone marrow transplantation (BMT) for hemoglobinopathies was first proposed for thalassemia major (Thomas et al., 1982) and is now the therapy of choice for young patients affected by the disorder when a suitable donor is available (Lucarelli, 1997) (see Chapter 39). BMT for sickle cell anemia was first performed in a young girl who also had acute myeloid leukemia (Johnson et al., 1984). Minimal complications followed the procedure, and hemoglobin electrophoresis indicated conversion to the donor phenotype (sickle cell trait).

In developed countries, and with optimal care, many sickle cell anemia patients can be well for many years, but the disease—which is affected by genetic and environmental factors, socioeconomic status, and the level of medical support—follows an unpredictable course (Serjeant, 1995). The Cooperative Study of Sickle Cell Disease, a prospective study of 3,764 U.S. patients, showed that sickle cell anemia in Black Americans decreased life expectancy by 25 to 30 years (Platt et al., 1994). Morbidity is also a source of concern, with a devastating stroke sometimes the first symptom of the disease and cognitive impairment, a problem the magnitude of which is just beginning to be appreciated (see Chapter 24). Episodes of pain, accompanied by progressive organ damage and fail-

ure, may occur throughout the patient's life (Vichinsky and Styles, 1996; Wong et al., 1996) (see Chapters 23 to 25). Sickle cell anemia may also bring about social and psychological problems, leading, as do other chronic illnesses, to dependence, lack of self-confidence, difficulties in competing for jobs, and poor social skills (Kinney and Ware, 1996).

Hydroxyurea dramatically improves the clinical course of the disease for some adults and children by enhancing the level of HbF and producing other effects (Charache et al., 1995; Ferster et al., 1996) (see Chapter 38). All patients do not respond similarly. The drug must be taken continually and monitored carefully. Its long-term complications are unknown, and its use in developing countries is difficult.

CRITERIA FOR PATIENT SELECTION

Disease and Patient-Related Criteria

Because it carries its own mortality risk, BMT for nonmalignant diseases was initially used only for life-threatening disorders such as aplastic anemia and severe combined immunodeficiency disease. When better supportive care became available and clinical outcomes improved, the treatment was applied to genetic diseases with less immediate mortality, such as thalassemia major. The decision to perform hematopoietic stem cell transplantation in patients with sickle cell anemia, however, was surrounded by controversy. The lack of reliable prognostic factors made it difficult to know when transplantation was warranted and to balance the immediate risk against the potential long-term gain. In 1990, a consensus conference established selection criteria for transplantation in children with sickle cell anemia (Sullivan and Reid, 1991). It seemed reasonable to limit marrow transplantation to those patients who had clinical evidence of severe and potentially mortal complications but who were not so severely affected as to reduce significantly the chance of the procedure to succeed (Nagel, 1991). In the words of E.D. Thomas (1991), "In sickle cell anemia, we really do not want patients with renal failure, severe neurological impairment, or pulmonary failure. If we are going to do this [bone marrow transplantation], we ought to do it correctly. We ought to take young patients in whom the risk of graft-versus-host disease is minimal. Patients who have end-stage complications of vasculopathy are going to cloud the issue."

A multicenter collaborative study of allogeneic marrow transplantation for sickle cell anemia was initiated in 1991 with the following selection criteria (Walters et al., 1996a):

1. Children should have sickle cell anemia or HbSC disease or HbS-β^0 thalassemia.
2. They should be less than 16 years old and have an HLA-identical related donor.
3. At least one of the following signs or symptoms must be present:
   a. Stroke or a central nervous system (CNS) event lasting longer than 24 hours
   b. Acute chest syndrome
   c. Recurrent severe pain episodes
   d. Impaired neuropsychological function and abnormal cerebral magnetic resonance imaging (MRI) scan (but not severe residual functional neurologic impairment)
   e. Stage I or II sickle lung disease
   f. Sickle nephropathy (glomerular filtration rate less than 30 percent of the predicted normal value)
   g. Bilateral proliferative retinopathy and major visual impairment
   h. Osteonecrosis of multiple joints
   i. Red-cell alloimmunization during long-term transfusion therapy

In the United States and in Europe, the majority of patients with sickle cell disease have one or more of those complications. Eight patients who met the criteria—two in Belgium and six in the United States—were given transplants. They were well aware of the risks of the procedure but were unwilling to accept the morbidity of their disease.

Other Selection Criteria

The primary barrier to stem cell transplantation is the lack of an HLA-identical donor. Among the 4,848 sickle cell anemia patients under 16 years of age who were followed in twenty-two collaborating centers, 315 (6.5 percent) met protocol entry criteria for transplantation. Of those, 128 (41 percent) had HLA typing performed, and 44 (14 percent of those meeting the entry criteria) had an HLA-identical sibling. The reasons for not proceeding with HLA typing in the remaining 187 patients included lack of a candidate sibling donor (76 patients; 24 percent of those meeting criteria), lack of financial or psychosocial support (33; 10.5 percent), parental refusal (30; 9.5 percent), physician refusal (13; 4 percent), history of medical noncompliance (2; <1 percent), and other reasons (33; 10.5 percent) (Walters et al., 1996b).

Kodish and colleagues (1991), in a study based in the United States, reviewed parental decision-making in relation to BMT for sickle cell anemia independently of the presence of a potential donor. Sixty-seven parents were asked to state the highest mortality risk at which they would consent to the curative procedure. Sixteen (24 percent) were unwilling to accept BMT even with a 100 percent probability of cure and 0 percent short-term mortality. Fifteen (22 percent) would consent if mortality did not exceed 5 percent. Twenty-five (37 percent) were willing to accept a 15 percent or greater risk of short-term mortality. Eight (12 percent) were willing to accept a 50 percent or greater risk of short-term mortality in exchange for a cure for sickle cell anemia. The decisions reflected socioeconomic factors rather than the severity of the child's disease. Parents were more willing to consider BMT if they had a high school education, were in full-time employment, or had more than one child with sickle cell anemia.

Adequate availability of preventive and supportive medical treatment also influences parental decisions. In Belgium, for example, many families with children with sickle cell anemia are in residence only temporarily, usually for professional reasons or to study. They have a high level of education, and their medical care is covered by Belgian social security. All of these families were willing to accept the risk of transplantation, even when the child was very young and still asymptomatic. Their awareness of the high mortality rate for sickle cell disease in their country and the risk of infections related to blood transfusions did not leave much room for doubt. In those families, the risk of transplantation weighed against the risks of having the disease in Africa, making them very much in favor of transplantation.

CONDITIONING REGIMENS AND PROPHYLACTIC THERAPY

Conditioning Regimens

In sickle cell anemia, the conditioning regimen used for hematopoietic stem cell transplantation is based on the experience of transplantation for thalassemia. Both of these hemolytic disorders have bone marrow that is highly proliferative and hypercellular. Preparative therapy must therefore provide both myeloablation and effective immunosuppression. Yet, it is desirable to reduce the long-term side effects of chemotherapy by reducing its cytotoxicity as much as possible. In sickle cell anemia, stable mixed chimerism may be sufficient to eradicate the symptoms.

Presently, the conditioning regimen consists of busulfan (3.5 to 4.0 mg/kg in 4 divided daily oral doses for 4 days; total dosage, 14 to 16 mg/kg); cyclophosphamide (50 mg/kg once daily intravenously for 4 days; total dosage, 200 mg/kg); horse antithymocyte globulin (ATG) (30 mg/kg once daily intravenously for 3 days, total dose 90 mg/kg). If possible, busulfan blood concentration should be monitored to maintain an average steady state of 400 to 600 ng/mL.

Graft-Versus-Host Prophylaxis

Graft-versus-host disease (GVHD) prevention should include a combination of cyclosporine and a short course of methotrexate (10 mg/m^2 on days 1, 3, and 6).

Prophylaxis of Neurologic Complications

There is a propensity for CNS events after transplantation for sickle cell disease (Walters et al., 1995). To forestall such complications, the following measures were adopted: intensified anticonvulsant prophylaxis with phenytoin, strict control of hypertension, control of magnesium levels, maintenance of hemoglobin concentrations between 9 and 11 g/dL, and platelet counts greater than 50×10^9/L.

Prophylaxis of Infections

Oral gut decontamination is necessary during the neutropenic period. Early detection of cytomegalovirus (CMV) by blood antigen screening or by polymerase chain reaction (PCR)-based techniques allows preemptive therapy, reducing the risk of CMV disease and CMV-associated morbidity and mortality (Einsele et al., 1995). Oral acyclovir and prophylactic intravenous immunoglobulin are given during the first year after transplantation. Emphasis should be placed on the risk of *S. pneumoniae* infection after transplantation, and the use of prophylactic penicillin needs to be considered until the recovery of spleen function can be demonstrated. The emergence of penicillin-resistant strains of the pneumococcus, however, now complicates this decision.

CURRENT RESULTS

The Belgian Experience

Fifty-four patients underwent transplantation with HLA-identical hematopoietic stem cells (bone marrow, fifty-two; cord blood, two) in Belgium between April 1986 and January 1997. Fifty (bone marrow, forty-eight; cord blood, two; twenty-seven female, twenty-three male) of the patients were followed for over 1 year. For forty-nine patients, the donors were HLA-genoidentical siblings and for one, the donor was the HLA-phenoidentical father. The countries of origin were Democratic Republic Congo (formerly Zaire): forty-three, Cameroon: three, Nigeria: two, Burundi:

one, and Central Republic of Africa: one. At the time of transplantation their ages ranged from 0.9 to 23 years (median: 7.5 years), and the follow-up ranged from 0.3 to 11 years (median: 5 years). Kaplan-Meier estimates of overall survival, event-free survival, and disease-free survival for all fifty patients were 93 percent, 82 percent, and 85 percent, respectively. All vasoocclusive manifestations of the disease and disease-associated hemolytic anemia disappeared in the successfully treated patients.

The fifty patients can be divided for analysis into two groups. Group 1—thirty-six patients (eighteen female, eighteen male, age range 1.7 to 23 years) with a median age of 8.6 years—received transplants because of the severity of their disease. They fulfilled the inclusion criteria for severity retrospectively. Two female patients did not fulfill the criteria of age less than 16 years; they were 17- and 23-year-old students, well aware of the inherent risks of the procedure but unable to accept the morbidity of the disease. Frequent painful episodes were present in all Group 1 patients, seizures or strokes were present in six, acute chest syndrome in twenty, and osteonecrosis in three. The overall survival, event-free survival, and disease-free survival rates were 88 percent, 76 percent, and 80 percent, respectively.

Group 2 (nine female and five male patients, ages 0.9 to 15 years with a median of 2.0 years) comprised the asymptomatic patients who were transplanted at a young age because their family was returning to Africa. The patients had minimal symptoms. While they had painful episodes, there was no acute chest syndrome, seizures, stroke, priapism, or chronic organ damage, and no more than three blood transfusions were received prior to transplantation. Early in the course of the disease, the overall survival, event-free survival, and disease-free survival rates were 100 percent, 93 percent, and 93 percent, respectively.

The conditioning regimens consisted of busulfan 16 mg/kg and cyclophosphamide 200 mg/kg (Bu16/Cy200) in twenty-two patients; Bu16/Cy200/total lymphoid irradiation (TLI) in six patients; Bu16/Cy200/ATG in fourteen patients; Bu14/Cy200 in six patients; and Bu 500 mg/m^2/Cy200 in two patients. Total lymphoid irradiation (TLI) was given as 750 cGy in one fraction over 6 hours with 18 MV x-rays produced by linear acceleration, the lungs being shielded. TLI was given to heavily transfused patients to reduce the risk of rejection. In later transplantations, TLI was replaced by ATG (Fresenius) given prior to the surgery at 15 to 90 mg/kg divided into three doses. One patient underwent a second BMT and was conditioned by a previously described regimen containing cyclophosphamide, ATG, and thoracoabdominal irradiation (Storb et al., 1987).

Following the observation of a high incidence of neurologic events posttransplantation, thirteen patients received a prophylactic anticonvulsant (phenytoin or carbamazepine). They also received blood transfusions to maintain the platelet count above $50 \times 10^9/L$ and hemoglobin concentrations between 9.0 and 11.0 g/dL. Blood pressure, cyclosporin A, and magnesium levels were strictly controlled (Walters et al., 1995).

To prevent GVHD, twenty-five patients were given cyclosporin A alone for a period of 6 to 18 months and twenty-five received cyclosporine A together with a short course of methotrexate. Acute GVHD was treated with corticosteroids. Chronic GVHD required the use of azathioprine in four patients and thalidomide in four patients. Prophylaxis of infections included gut decontamination and infusions of immunoglobulin during the first year posttransplantation. It was suggested that penicillin be continued until recovery of spleen function.

Chimerism was evaluated by cytogenetic techniques when donor and recipient were of the opposite sex, by residual HbS levels when the donor was homozygous for HbA, and by studies of variable numbers of tandem repeats in DNA if donor and recipient were of the same sex.

The functional status of the patients following transplantation was measured by the Lansky instead of the Karnofsky scale because it provides a better description of children's activities. Lansky scores of 100 to 80 indicate the ability to carry on normal activities without special care, 70 to 50 indicate mild to moderate restriction, and 40 to 10 moderate to severe restriction. For the Kaplan-Meier plots of overall survival, event-free survival, and disease-free survival, events included death, absence of engraftment, rejection, and recurrence of the disease. Disease-free survival was defined by the absence of clinical and biological signs and symptoms of sickle cell anemia. The Fisher exact test was used to compare event percentages, and the Wilcoxon rank-sum test was used to assess the significance of the age difference between Group 1 and Group 2.

Engraftment and Survival

Forty-eight patients were alive 16 months to 12 years after transplantation (median follow-up, 6 years). One patient died 3 months after BMT of acute GVHD complicated by CMV and *Aspergillus* infections, and one died suddenly 6 years after transplantation; this patient had been asymptomatic since transplantation with a normal hemoglobin level and complete chimerism (100 percent donor cells). Three patients never presented any sign of engraftment (Table 40.1). They were 6, 7, and 14 years old at the time of transplantation; two were on a chronic transfusion program for acute chest syndrome

Table 40.1. Results of Transplantation in Sickle Cell Anemia According to the Patient's Status at the Time of the Procedure

	Group 1*	Group 2†	P value
Number of patients	36	14	
Sex: F/M	18/18	9/5	
Age (yr): median (range)	8.6 (1.7–23)	2.0 (0.9–15)	.0016
Number of RBC transfusions	>3	≤3	
Survival	34	14	
Deaths	2	0	
Absence of engraftment	3	0	
Relapse	1	1	
Mixed chimerism (>30% recipient cells)	3	0	
Total	9 (25%)	1 (7%)	.001
Acute GVHD grade I–II	14	5	
Acute GVHD grade III–IV	1	0	
Chronic GVHD limited	5	2	
Chronic GVHD extensive	3	0	

Abbreviations: RBC, red blood cell; GVHD, graft-versus-host disease.

* Group 1: Patients severely affected by sickle cell anemia at the time of transplantation.

† Group 2: Patients transplanted at an early stage of the disease. blank

or stroke; the third patient had suffered vasoocclusive crises and had been transfused more than three times. The number of nucleated cells infused in these three patients was 2 (one patient), and 4×10^8 cells/kg (two patients). Their conditioning regimens consisted of Bu14/Cy200 in one patient and Bu16/Cy200/ATG in two patients. The patients remained free of symptoms for several years after an autologous recovery; this was attributed to a persistent high level of HbF (Ferster et al., 1995).

Rejection occurred in two patients. The first, a Group 1 patient, rejected the graft between day 30 and 60 although initial engraftment had been confirmed by cytogenetic studies. The donor was the father, and a second, successful, BMT was performed on day 60 (Storb et al., 1987). The second, a 4-year-old boy from Group 2, rejected the graft after 18 months; he had been conditioned with Bu14/Cy200. Mixed chimerism was present in six patients. In three from Group 1, the percentage of recipient cells was 35 percent, 30 percent, and 50 per-

Table 40.2. Cord Blood Transplantations in Sickle Cell Anemia

	Belgium		France
Recipient	UPN 38	UPN 43	
Sex	F	F	F
Age (y)	5.5	3.1	11.5
Weight (kg)	23.5	16.1	33
Cord blood			
Origin	HLA-id sister	HLA-id sister	HLA-id sibling
Volume (mL)	141	100	
Nucleated cells ($\times 10^7$/kg)	4.6	4.7	6.0
CD$_{34}$ ($\times 10^5$/kg)	0.9	0.9	1.3
CFU-GM ($\times 10^4$/kg)	3.3	3.6	0.5
Engraftment			
ANC ($>0.5 \times 10^9$/L)	Day 32	Day 31	no
Platelets ($>50 \times 10^9$/L)	Day 48	Day 54	no
Chimerism	100% donor	100% donor	100% recipient
GVHD			
Acute	0	0	1
Chronic	0	Skin (lichenoid)	0

Abbreviations: UPN, unique patient number; GVHD, graft-versus-host disease; ANC, absolute neutrophil count; CFU-GM, colony forming unit-granulocytes monocytes.

cent, respectively, 6, 13, and 60 months after transplantation. In three from Group 2, chimerism was stable at less than 10 percent recipient cells.

Engraftment in the two patients who received cord blood transplantation was slow. They were 5 and 3 years old and received growth factors (Filgrastim, Amgen Roche, Belgium) from day 23 and 17, respectively. Clinical data, number of cells infused, and time for recovery are summarized in Table 40.2. Acute GVHD was not present but the 5-year-old developed de novo chronic GVHD 18 months after transplantation, when cyclosporin A was stopped. A lichenoid type of chronic GVHD affecting only the skin was confirmed by biopsy. Psoralen plus ultraviolet A (PUVA) treatment was ineffective. HbF level in the two patients decreased slowly during the first months, in accordance with the intrinsic properties of stem cells of cord blood origin (Brichard et al., 1996).

TRANSPLANT-RELATED MORBIDITY

Graft-Versus-Host Disease

Grade I acute GVHD was diagnosed in ten patients from Group 2, grade II in nine from Group 2, and grade III in one from Group 1. Chronic GVHD was diagnosed in ten patients and was extensive in the three who were from Group 1. Two patients with chronic GVHD developed mild dyspnea related to bronchiolitis obliterans, confirmed by computed tomography (CT) scan and pulmonary function tests.

Neurologic Complications

Eighteen patients had seizures after transplantation; five (38 percent) were receiving prophylactic anticonvulsant therapy and thirteen (35 percent) were not. Four of the eighteen had presented with a history of seizures or strokes before transplantation. Of the thirty-two patients who did not have neurologic complications, two had a history of seizures before transplantation. There was no recurrence of strokes among the four patients who had had them before transplantation.

LONG-TERM BENEFITS AND SIDE EFFECTS

Forty-five patients had stable engraftment; disease-associated manifestations and hemolytic anemia disappeared in all of them, and they all had a Lansky score of 100. Two patients with chronic GVHD and bronchiolitis obliterans had a score of 90, and one with chronic GVHD and acute myeloid leukemia had a score of 60. Fourteen patients (28 percent) returned to their country of origin in Africa 12 months to 5 years (median: 21 months) after transplantation.

Growth was normal after transplantation except in two patients who had received intensive immune suppression, including corticosteroids, for chronic GVHD. Thyroid function was normal in twenty-seven of the twenty-eight evaluated patients. One patient had normal thyroid hormone levels with an elevated thyroid-stimulating hormone (TSH) level and received a conditioning regimen that included Bu16/Cy200, with-

Table 40.3. Gonadal Function in Adolescent Girls After Bone Marrow Transplantation (BMT) for Sickle Cell Anemia

	Age at BMT (y)	Preparative regimen	Age at evaluation (y)	Amenorrhea	LH (mU/mL); N: 1–13	FSH (mU/mL); N:1–24	Estradiol, (pg/mL); N: >35
UPN 4	9	BuCyTLI	18	Primary	37.2	105	<10
UPN 12	23	BuCy	ND	Secondary	ND	ND	ND
UPN 14	12	BuCyTLI	19	Primary	23.5	97.7	<10
UPN 15	10	BuCy	15	Spont men	49	51	15
			17*		5.9	5.1	121
UPN 21	13	BuCyATG	18	Primary	75	94	<10
UPN 22	17	BuCyTLI	22	Secondary	88	160	<10
UPN 28	15	BuCyATG	17	Primary	21	110	<10
UPN 40	12	BuCyATG	15	Primary	24	33	<10

Abbreviations: Bu, busulfan; Cy, cyclophosphamide; TLI, total lymphoid irradiation; ATG, antithymocyte globulin; UPN, unique patient number; Spont men, spontaneous menarche; LH, luteinizing hormone; FSH, follicle-stimulating hormone.
* UPN 15: measurements done at the age of 17 giving normal values.

out TLI. He developed chronic GVHD with bronchiolitis obliterans. The two young women (ages 17 and 23) who received transplants developed secondary amenorrhea. The levels of luteinizing hormone (LH), follicle-stimulating hormone (FSH), and estradiol in one individual (UPN 22) are shown in Table 40.3. If we consider that menarche occurs around the age of 15 in sickle cell patients, six others were evaluable; five had primary amenorrhea and delayed sexual maturation, and they required hormone replacement therapy. One had a spontaneous menarche at the age of 15. Her levels of LH and FSH were elevated at that time, but she had normal levels of LH, FSH, and estradiol at age 17 (Table 40.3). The six adolescent boys evaluated had normal sexual development, but four had decreased testosterone levels, four had elevated FSH levels, and one had an elevated LH level (Table 40.4). Fertility was not tested. Osteonecrosis of hips and shoulders was present in three patients who were 15, 17, and 23 years old at the time of transplantation. Three years after transplantation there was no radiologic improvement.

Spleen

The possibility of recovering splenic function became apparent when the first transplanted sickle cell anemia patient, 1 year posttransplantation, developed immune thrombocytopenia and isotopic studies showed splenic sequestration of platelets. In further studies, normal spleen isotope uptake was found in three patients transplanted for sickle cell anemia (Ferster et al., 1993). Spleen function was then prospectively studied in ten patients, ages 2.4 to 17 years (median: 13 years) at the time of transplantation, by using ^{Tc}99m-labeled erythrocytes and ^{51}Cr heat-damaged red blood cells. In seven patients, an increase of the splenic red cell pool was seen between 3 months and 3 years. Two of the seven also had increased phagocytosis of heat-damaged red blood cells. Three, however, showed no improvement in splenic function. One patient, who was transplanted at the age of 2.4 years and had residual splenic function at that time, had a decrease in his splenic function after transplantation. He developed severe chronic GVHD, received intensive immune suppression, and developed myelodysplasia and acute myeloid leukemia. Three years after transplantation, isotopic studies revealed an absence of splenic tissue. Another patient who was transplanted at the age of 5 years developed a localized chronic GVHD and had no detectable splenic function 2 years after transplantation.

Secondary Malignancy

One patient with extensive chronic GVHD required steroids, cyclosporin A, and azathioprine for 4 months and thalidomide for 30 months. He developed myelodysplasia 35 months after BMT and 18 months later, acute myeloid leukemia of donor cell origin.

THE TOTAL EUROPEAN EXPERIENCE

One hundred sixteen patients with sickle cell anemia have been transplanted in Belgium, France (Bernaudin et al., 1997; G. Souillet, personal communication), the United Kingdom (I. Roberts, personal communication), Italy (Giardini et al., 1997, and personal communication), Germany (R. Dickerhoff, personal communication), and Switzerland (P. Tuchschmid, personal communication). Of those, 95 (82%) are alive and well. In one case, a favorable outcome of osteonecrosis was

Table 40.4. Gonadal Function in Adolescent Boys After Bone Marrow Transplantation (BMT) for Sickle Cell Anemia

	Age at BMT (y)	Preparative regimen	Age at evaluation (y)	LH (mU/mL); N:1–10	FSH (mU/ml) N:1–8	Testosterone (nM/L); N:13–35
UPN 6	7	BuCy	16	4.6	4.4	10.7
UPN 23	13	BuCyTLI	17	2.4	11.6	6.6
UPN 24	11	BuCyTLI	16	2.8	10.9	9.1
UPN 29	14	BuCyATG	18	11	13	ND
UPN 32	15	BuCyATG	17	5.4	10.9	16
UPN 39	15	BuCyATG	17	2.3	7.9	14.2

Abbreviations: Bu, busulfan; Cy, cyclophosphamide; TLI, total lymphoid irradiation; ATG, antithymocyte globulin; UPN, unique patient number, ND, not determined.

observed with rapid humeral head reconstruction (Bernaudin et al., 1997).

Ten patients died, nine of GVHD and infectious complications and one of an unknown cause (see above). Ten patients did not engraft or rejected the transplant. Of those, four underwent a second transplantation, two of which were successful. One 11-year-old boy (33 kg) had received a cord blood transplantation in France when he was 13 months old that did not engraft (Table 40.5), and a second, bone marrow, transplantation from the same donor was done. That, too, failed. The boy finally had an autologous recovery (Bernaudin et al., 1997). Current Kaplan-Meier estimates of overall, event-free, and disease-free survival for the first 101 patients transplanted in Europe are 90 percent, 79 percent, and 81 percent, respectively.

THE UNITED STATES EXPERIENCE

By the mid-1990s, thirty-eight patients had been enrolled in the collaborative study of allogeneic marrow transplantation for sickle cell anemia (Walters et al., 1996a, 1997). Another twenty-four patients were transplanted but not as part of the study (F.L. Johnson, personal communication). Four of the sixty-two patients died, three of intraventricular hemorrhage and one of GVHD. Nine patients rejected the graft, and two of them had a successful second transplant (Table 40.6). Fifty-one (82 percent) of the transplanted patients are alive, well, and free of sickle cell disease. Kaplan-Meier estimates of survival, event-free survival, and rejection or recurrence for the patients included in the collaborative study are, respectively, 93 percent, 79 percent, and 14 percent. A higher incidence of cerebral hemorrhage in the United States as compared to Belgium may reflect differences in the patients selected for transplantation. Among Belgian patients, 12 percent had experienced strokes or seizures before transplantation, whereas in the United States study 50 percent of the patients had strokes prior to transplantation. The proportion of patients receiving chronic transfusions was thus also much higher in the United States study. Any differences observed in the Kaplan-Meier estimates of disease-free

Table 40.5. Hematopoietic Stem Cell Transplantation in Sickle Cell Anemia: European Data

	Number of patients	Deaths	No engraftment, relapse, and autologous recovery	Second transplantation	Alive, free of disease
Belgium	54	2	5	1	48
France (Bernaudin, 1997)	33	3	4	2	27
United Kingdom*	15	2	0	0	13
Italy (Giardini, 1997)	9	3	0	0	6
Germany†	3	0	1	1	2
Switzerland‡	2	0	0	0	2
Total	116	10	10	4	98

Unpublished data obtained by personal communication with *Irene Roberts (UK), †Roswitha Dickerhoff (Germany), and ‡Peter Tuchschmid (Switzerland).

Table 40.6. Hematopoietic Stem Cell Transplantation in Sickle Cell Anemia

	Number of patients	Deaths	No engraftment, relapse, and autologous recovery	Second transplantation	Alive, free of disease
Collaborative study	38	2	4	0	32
Johnson's study	24	2	5	2	19
Total	62	4	9	2	51

* Results from the Collaborative Group study of marrow transplantation for sickle cell anemia (Walters et al., 1997) and from another group of patients transplanted in the U.S. (personal communication with F.L. Johnson, Portland, Oregon).

survival between the Belgian and United States may be explained by the transplantation of patients with more severe disease in the United States study. A recent summary of 50 patients in the U.S. collaborative study showed 94 percent overall survival and 84 percent event-free survival. Twenty-two patients with stable engraftment and a mean follow-up of 57.9 months had no further episodes of pain, stroke, or acute chest syndrome. Patients with a prior history of stroke had stable or improved cerebral magnetic resonance imaging results and seven of eight patients transplanted for recurrent acute chest syndrome had stable pulmonary function (Walters et al., 2000).

Multicenter studies in the United States have been extended to the efficacy of transplantation in young adults. A female adult with sickle cell anemia and chronic renal failure was transplanted in Chicago. Because she required hemodialysis a kidney transplantation was proposed with a sibling as the donor. The sibling was HLA-identical and a BMT was successfully performed before the kidney transplantation (K. van Besien, personal communication) No series of transplantations in adults with sickle cell anemia have been reported.

COMPLICATIONS OF TRANSPLANTATION AND THEIR MANAGEMENT

The major complications encountered after hematopoietic stem cell transplantation for sickle cell anemia are the absence of engraftment, graft rejection, acute and chronic GVHD, cerebral hemorrhage, and gonadal dysfunction.

Absence of Engraftment and Graft Rejection

Absence of engraftment and graft rejection occurred mostly in patients who had not received ATG before transplantation. ATG appears to be an important factor in the conditioning regimen, especially for older children who have been transfused often. A sufficient number of hematopoietic progeni-

tor cells is also important for good engraftment. Methotrexate, which reduces the risk of GVHD, may have an adverse effect on engraftment and perhaps should be reserved for young patients, who are less at risk of developing GVHD. Stable mixed chimerism may be sufficient to reduce the level of HbS to where vasoocclusive disease and hemolysis do not provoke symptoms. When complete autologous recovery occurs, patients often remain symptom-free for a period of time due to the reactivation of HbF synthesis by the regenerating bone marrow (Ferster et al., 1995) (see Chapter 7). When bone marrow aplasia without autologous recovery occurs, an autologous BMT can be done provided that autologous bone marrow has been cryopreserved before chemotherapy, in anticipation of a rescue. Second BMTs are possible, but the risks of the procedure are increased. In Europe and the United States, six second transplants have been performed and four were successful.

Acute and Chronic Graft-Versus-Host Disease

Acute and chronic GVHD were the main causes of death and morbidity in transplanted sickle cell patients, despite the fact that all transplants—with the exception of one phenoidentical transplantation—were done with HLA-genoidentical sibling donors. Prophylaxis combining cyclosporine and methotrexate is recommended. Early detection of CMV and preemptive treatment is another way of reducing the risk of GVHD. When acute GVHD occurs, corticosteroids should be added to cyclosporine. ATG or monoclonal antibodies have been proposed in cases of grade III or IV acute GVHD unresponsive to the first line therapy, but that increases the risk of infectious complications. Extensive chronic GVHD is difficult to mange. Cyclosporine remains the gold standard with steroids given either daily or on alternate days by high-dose pulse therapy or topically. Second-line therapies include thalidomide, azathioprine, and perhaps in the future, mycophenolate mofetil (Storb et al., 1997). Another promising tool may be the use of extracorporeal photopheresis (Dall'Amico et al., 1997). In both acute and chronic GVHD, supportive care, including the prevention, early detection, and treatment of infections, adequate nutrition, prevention of osteoporosis, and good dental hygiene, is very important.

Cerebral Hemorrhage

The risk of developing a cerebral hemorrhage is elevated in sickle cell anemia because of the vasculopathy of the disease and the subclinical endothelial lesions in the cerebral vessels. High blood pressure and a low platelet count are additional posttransplantation risk factors. Prophylactic measures dramatically reduce those risks (Walters et al., 1995).

Gonadal Dysfunction

The alkylating agents included in the conditioning regimen, cyclophosphamide and busulfan, have been associated with ovarian failure and testicular dysfunction. In the Belgian series, gonadal dysfunction appeared in all females transplanted between the ages of 9 and 23 years, although it was transient in one. While boys experienced normal sexual maturation, most of them had abnormal LH, FSH, or testosterone levels and biochemical evidence of Leydig cell damage. Busulfan is known to induce gonadal insufficiency and the possibility of that outcome should be discussed with patients and their families (De Sanctis et al., 1991). It remains to be determined if patients transplanted early in life will develop gonadal failure later. A successful pregnancy was reported in a patient who had undergone BMT for thalassemia and had received the same conditioning regimen employed for sickle cell anemia (Borgna-Pignatti et al., 1996).

FUTURE DIRECTIONS

Transplantation of Very Young Patients

Lacking good prognostic markers that can predict the course of sickle cell anemia, it is difficult to know when to propose a hematopoietic stem cell transplantation for young patients who are still asymptomatic or nearly so. That is unfortunate because the risks of transplantation are less in young patients who have not yet suffered organ damage or received many blood transfusions. As mentioned previously, young patients had very encouraging results (Vermylen et al., 1998). Because of the potentially adverse late effects of the conditioning regimens, efforts should be made to find a less toxic therapy that can establish a level of stable mixed chimerism sufficient to reduce the level of HbS and complications of disease.

Transplantation of Adult Patients

Severely affected adults with sickle cell anemia often provoke a discussion of the possibility of transplantation. These individuals commonly have repetitive painful episodes and chronic organ damage, and because of their poor quality of life they are willing to face the risks of transplantation. The risks, unfortunately, are high in such cases. The incidence of GVHD increases with age, and the morbidity of the complication can be as bad as sickle cell anemia itself. Damage caused by many years of unrelenting vasoocclusive disease may make the affected organs targets for transplantation complications such as CNS hemorrhage, pulmonary fibrosis, hepatic venoocclusive disease, renal failure, cardiac disease, and infection. For patients well aware of all those problems and ready to accept them, transplantation is technically feasible, and a protocol has been developed for transplantation of patients between the ages of 16 and 21 years with a conditioning regimen of busulfan, cyclophosphamide, and ATG. Eligible patients must have a history of recurrent acute chest syndrome or early sickle cell lung disease, sickle nephropathy with proteinuria and a glomerular filtration rate between 30 percent and 50 percent of predicted, recurrent painful episodes, or be on chronic transfusion therapy with alloimmunization. Advanced liver, lung, renal, or cerebrovascular disease are among the exclusion criteria.

The Use of Volunteer Unrelated Donors

A minority of patients affected by sickle cell anemia are likely to have a healthy HLA-identical sibling suitable as a transplantation donor. Volunteer unrelated donors are used in malignant conditions with a poor prognosis. In sickle cell anemia, however, there is an imbalance between the immediate risk from the procedure and the long-term benefit. Therefore, transplantation using volunteer unrelated donors is not routinely recommended. In exceptional cases (i.e., when there is a severe clinical course and a poor prognosis) it might be considered. Such patients and adults considered for transplantation—in fact, all patients seeking transplantation for sickle cell disease—should be included in research protocols. In the future, better techniques for HLA typing may improve the search for a perfect match and make it easier to use unrelated donors. Including more members of at-risk minority populations in potential bone marrow donor pools would also improve the chances of finding a suitable donor.

Cord Blood

Cord blood transplantation can be considered if an HLA-genoidentical sibling without sickle cell anemia is born. Engraftment of cord blood is slower than engraftment of bone marrow or peripheral blood stem cells, and the risk of infections is increased. Cord blood transplantation has the advantage that the donor need not undergo general anesthesia for the collection of cells. To date, three cord blood transplantations have been performed, and two were successful (Bernaudin et al., 1997).

Restrictions associated with unrelated volunteer bone marrow donors also apply to unrelated cord blood transplantation, although some believe that the risk of GVHD is decreased when cord blood is used. This remains to be proven in large studies. Furthermore, the number of cord blood stem cells is limited so that cord blood transplantation should be reserved for young children with a low body weight.

Mixed Chimerism

Observations made after transplantation for thalassemia major or sickle cell anemia suggest that mixed chimerism can be considered persistent if it lasts for more than 2 years. The ratio of donor to recipient cells usually plateaus 3 years after transplantation. In thalassemia major, a 30 percent donor cell population is sufficient to maintain a stable level of hemoglobin and preclude the need for blood transfusions. In sickle cell anemia, one patient with only 10 percent donor cells in the bone marrow and an HbS fraction of 13 percent in the blood was symptom free (Walters et al., 1997).

New Conditioning Regimens

Because mixed chimerism may effectively abolish symptoms, it has been suggested that a less toxic regimen than the classical busulfan-cyclophosphamide combination be explored. A nonmyeloablative conditioning regimen including fludarabine, ATG, and low-dose busulfan (8 mg/kg) has been proposed as an alternative; it is well tolerated and produces no severe toxicity (Slavin et al., 1998). To prevent rejection, transient mixed chimerism can be reversed with graded increments of donor lymphocyte infusions.

CONCLUSION

When BMT for sickle cell disease is successful, it is curative, but it has a short-term mortality of about 10 percent. In the absence of predictors of prognosis, and knowing that with modern supportive care most patients will live into their fifth decade, proposing marrow transplantation is difficult. Transplantation, when undertaken, should be done in the context of an established clinical trial.

References

Bernaudin, F, Souillet, G, Vannier, JP, et al. for the Société Française de Greffe de Moelle. (1997). Report of the French experience concerning 26 children transplanted for severe sickle cell disease. *Bone Marrow Transplant.* 19 (Suppl 2): 112–115.

Borgna-Pignatti, C, Marradi, P, Rugolotto, S, and Marcolongo, A. (1996). Succesful pregnancy after bone marrow transplantation for thalassemia. *Bone Marrow Transplant.* 18: 235–236.

Brichard, B, Vermylen, C, Ninane, J, and Cornu, G. (1996). Persistence of fetal hemoglobin production after succesful transplantation of cord blood stem cells in a patient with sickle cell anemia. *J. Pediatr.* 128: 241–243.

Charache, S, Terrin, ML, Moore, RD et al. and the Investigators of the Multicenter Study of Hydroxyurea in Sickle Cell Anemia. (1995). Effect of hydroxyurea on the frequency of painful crises in sickle cell anemia. *N. Engl. J. Med.* 332: 1317–1322.

Dall'Amico, R, Rossetti, F, Zulian, F et al. (1997). Photopheresis in paediatric patients with drug-resistant chronic graft-versus-host disease. *Br. J. Haematol.* 97: 848–854.

De Sanctis, V, Galimberti, M, Lucarelli, G et al. (1991). Gonadal function after allogenic bone marrow transplantation for thalassemia. *Arch. Dis. Child.* 66: 517–520.

Einsele, H, Ehninger, G, Hebart, H et al. (1995). Polymerase chain reaction monitoring reduces the incidence of cytomegalovirus disease and the duration and side effects of antiviral therapy after bone marrow transplantation. *Blood* 86: 2815–2820.

Ferster, A, Bujan, W, Corazza, F et al. (1993). Bone marrow transplantation corrects the splenic reticuloendothelial dysfunction in sickle cell anemia. *Blood* 81: 1102–1105.

Ferster, A, Corazza, F, Vertonge, F et al. (1995). Transplanted sickle-cell disease patients with autologous bone marrow recovery after graft failure develop increased levels of fetal haemoglobin which corrects disease severity. *Br. J. Haematol.* 90: 804–808.

Ferster, A, Vermylen, C, Cornu, G et al. (1996). Hydroxyurea for treatment of severe sickle cell anemia: A pediatric clinical trial. *Blood* 88: 1960–1964.

Giardini, C, Galimberti, M, Lucarelli, G et al. (1997). Bone marrow transplantation in sickle cell disorders in Pesaro. *Bone Marrow Transplant.* 19 (Suppl 2): 106–109.

Johnson, FL, Look, AT, Gockerman, J et al. (1984). Bone marrow transplantation in a patient with sickle cell anemia. *N. Engl. J. Med.* 311: 780–783.

Kinney, T and Ware, R. (1996). The adolescent with sickle cell anemia. *Hematol. Oncol. Clin. North Am.* 10: 1255–1264.

Kodish, E, Lantos, J, Stocking, C et al. (1991). Bone marrow transplantation for sickle cell disease. A study of parents' decisions. *N. Engl. J. Med.* 325: 1349–1353.

Lucarelli, G. (1997). Bone marrow transplantation for thalassemia. *J. Inter. Med.* 242 (Suppl 740), 49–52.

Nagel, R. (1991). The dilemma of marrow transplantation in sickle cell anemia. *Semin. Hematol.* 28: 233–234.

Platt, OS, Brambilla, DJ, Rosse, WF et al. (1994). Mortality in sickle cell disease: Life expectancy and risk factors for early death. *N. Engl. J. Med.* 330: 1639–1644.

Serjeant, GR. (1995). Natural history and determinants of clinical severity of sickle cell disease. *Curr. Opin. Hematol.* 2: 103–108.

Slavin, S., Nagler, A, Naparstek, E et al. (1998). Non-myeloablative stem cell transplantation and cell therapy as an alternative to conventional bone marrow transplantation with lethal cytoreduction for the treatment of malignant and nonmalignant hematologic diseases. *Blood* 91: 756–763.

Storb, R, Weiden, PL, Sullivan, KM et al. (1987). Second marrow transplants in patients with aplastic anemia rejecting the first graft: Use of a conditioning regimen including cyclophosphamide and antithymocyte globulin. *Blood* 70: 116–121.

Storb, R, Yu, C, Wagner, JL et al. (1997). Stable mixed hematopoietic chimerism in DLA-identical littermate dogs given sublethal total body irradiation before and pharmacological immunosuppression after marrow transplantation. *Blood* 89: 3048–3054.

Sullivan, KM and Reid, CD. (1991). Introduction to a symposium on sickle cell anemia: Current results of comprehensive care and the evolving role of bone marrow transplantation. *Semin. Hematol.* 28: 177–179.

Thomas, ED. (1991). The pros and cons of bone marrow transplantation for sickle cell anemia. *Semin. Hematol.* 28: 260–262.

Thomas, ED, Buckner, CD, Sanders, JE et al. (1982). Marrow transplantation for thalassaemia. *Lancet* 2: 227–229.

Vermylen, C and Cornu, G. (1997). Hematopoietic stem cell transplantation for sickle cell anemia. *Curr. Opin. Hematol.* 4: 377–380.

Vermylen, C, Fernandez Robles, E, Ninane, J, and Cornu, G. (1988). Bone marrow transplantation in five children with sickle cell anaemia. *Lancet* 1: 1427–1428.

Vermylen, C, Cornu, G, Ferster, A et al. (1998). Haematopoietic stem cell transplantation for sickle cell anaemia: The first 50 patients transplanted in Belgium. *Bone Marrow Transplant,* 22: 1–6.

Vichinsky, E and Styles, L. (1996). Sickle cell disease: Pulmonary complications. *Hematol. Oncol. Clin. North Am.* 10: 1275–1287.

Walters, MC, Sullivan, KM, Bernaudin, F et al. (1995). Neurologic complications after allogeneic marrow transplantation for sickle cell anemia. *Blood* 85: 879–884.

Walters, MC, Patience, M, Leisenring, W et al. (1996a). Bone marrow transplantation for sickle cell anemia. *N. Engl. J. Med.* 335: 369–376.

Walters, MC, Patience, M, Leisenring, W et al. (1996b). Barriers to bone marrow transplantation for sickle cell anemia. *Biol. Blood Marrow Transplant.* 2: 100–104.

Walters, MC, Patience, M, Leisenring, W et al. (1997). Collaborative multicenter investigation of marrow transplantation for sickle cell disease: Current results and future directions. *Biol. Blood Marrow Transplant.* 3: 310–315.

Walters, MC, Storb, R, Patience, M et al. (2000). Impact of bone marrow transplantation for symptomatic sickle cell disease: An interim report. *Blood* 95: 1918–1924.

Wong, W, Elliot-Mills, D, and Powars, D. (1996). Renal failure in sickle cell anemia. *Hematol. Oncol. Clin. North Am.* 10: 1321–1331.

41

Prospects for Gene Therapy of Sickle Cell Disease and Thalassemia

BRIAN P. SORRENTINO
ARTHUR W. NIENHUIS

Inserting genes into repopulating hematopoietic stem cells and achieving lineage-specific expression after long-term reconstitution with genetically modified stem cells would create many therapeutic opportunities (Sorrentino and Nienhuis, 1999). Hemoglobin disorders were among the first diseases for which gene therapy was imagined. Indeed, sickle cell disease was the first molecularly defined disease (Pauling et al., 1949). Thalassemias, disorders of deficient synthesis of α- or β-globin chains, conceptually, would be directly correctable by gene replacement therapy (Weatherall, 1994). Exchange of genetic information between microorganisms had been well established as had the ability of naked DNA to transform the phenotypic properties of bacteria. Thus, at least in concept, gene therapy for the hemoglobin disorders seemed an ultimately achievable goal.

Until the basic molecular biology of gene expression in human cells was understood, the prospects for gene therapy remained distant. Progress toward this goal was rapid during the 1970s. Biologically active mRNA was isolated from human reticulocytes of normal individuals and those with hemoglobin disorders (Nienhuis and Anderson, 1971; Benz and Forget, 1971). Discovery of reverse transcriptase allowed these mRNAs to be converted into complementary (c) DNA and molecularly cloned using rapidly developing recombinant DNA techniques (Maniatis et al., 1976).

The genomic globin genes were among the first to be molecularly cloned from total cell DNA (Lawn et al., 1980). Within 10 years from the initial isolation of biologically active globin mRNA, the entire β-globin locus had been mapped and each of the individual genes cloned and sequenced (Efstratiadis et al., 1980).

Although naked plasmid DNA could be introduced into mammalian cells by physical techniques, the inefficiency of such processes required inclusion of a dominant selectable marker within the recombinant DNA molecule to simplify the recovery of successfully transduced cells (Pellicer et al., 1978). Such methodology was far too inefficient to apply to gene transfer into the rare hematopoietic stem cell population that represented no more than one in 10^5 bone marrow cells. Furthermore, stem cells are quiescent; therefore, the recovery of genetically modified cells by drug selection in vitro was simply not practical.

Viruses have succeeded evolutionarily in nature because of their ability to transfer and express their genetic information in eukaryotic cells. Experimentalists interested in gene transfer turned to viral systems to develop strategies potentially useful for therapeutic gene transfer. Murine retroviruses had been thoroughly characterized by studying their role in oncogenesis. Such viruses were known to carry genetic information in the form of transduced cellular genes, which in mutated form were oncogenic. Proviral genomes of murine tumor viruses, once available in recombinant DNA form, were genetically modified to serve as vehicles for the transfer of genetic markers into tissue culture cells (Tabin et al., 1982; Watanabe and Temin, 1983; Mann et al., 1983). Soon this technology was used to insert new genes into a physiologically relevant cell population, namely pluripotent murine hematopoietic cells capable of forming spleen colonies in irradiated animals (Williams et al., 1984). Shortly afterwards, similar vectors were used to insert genes into cells capable of establishing long-term hematopoiesis in murine recipients (Dick et al., 1985; Eglitis et al., 1985; Keller et al., 1985; Lemischka et al., 1986).

The stage seemed set for the rapid launch of gene therapy for treatment of hemoglobin disorders. Unfortunately, early hopes were dashed when studies in large animals (Bodine et al., 1993c; van Beusechem et al., 1992) and ultimately in humans (Dunbar et al., 1995; Hanania et al., 1996) proved that retroviral vectors suitable for gene transfer into murine stem cells were inefficient for transducing their primate counterparts. Furthermore, significant levels of globin expression could be achieved only through the use of the native genomic globin genes linked to distant regulatory elements from the locus control region (LCR) (Grosveld et al., 1987). Although such constructs worked well in transgenic animals, the combination of a native globin gene with required regulatory elements proved highly unstable when inserted into retroviral vectors (Sadelain et al., 1995; Sadelain, 1997). A decade of often frustrating effort made all too evident the many barriers to stem cell targeted gene transfer of globin genes for therapeutic purposes.

Recent progress again provides encouragement that gene therapy may ultimately be developed for hemoglobin disorders. Several viral vector systems are being characterized that have potential for gene insertion into primitive hematopoietic cells. The biological properties of repopulating stem cells are becoming much better understood so that their manipulation for achieving gene transfer may become more feasible. Globin gene configurations that survive vector-mediated gene transfer have been identified for several vector systems. Finally, growing knowledge of hemoglobin switching mechanisms (Chapter 7) and the identification of trans-acting factors that modulate expression of individual globin genes provide an alternative approach—the utilization of gene transfer to achieve reactivation of the fetal globin genes during postnatal life in patients with sickle cell anemia or thalassemia.

VIRAL VECTORS

Murine Retroviral Vectors

Retroviruses have a unique capacity to convert their single-stranded RNA genome into a double-stranded DNA molecule, which is then integrated through the action of host cell and viral proteins, particularly integrase, into a cellular chromosome. Increasing knowledge of the organization of the genome of murine oncoretroviruses suggested strategies for deriving vector particles free of replication-competent retroviruses that were potentially useful for gene therapy applications. In the description that follows, many technical terms are used. Please refer to the glossary of terminology at the end of this chapter for more details. Only the long terminal repeats (LTRs) and sequences at the 5' end of the viral genome are required for efficient packaging of RNA molecules into vector particles (Fig. 41.1A). Most of the coding sequences for the viral proteins, GAG, POL, and envelope (ENV) can be eliminated from the vector genome. Conversely, expression cassettes for the viral proteins have been constructed that allow their expression in packaging cells as RNA molecules that lack both the LTRs and packaging sequences (Mann et al., 1983; Cone and Mulligan, 1984). Separating the GAG and POL genes from the

ENV gene on two separate transcriptional units (so-called split packaging lines) substantially reduces the possibility for regeneration of replication-competent retrovirus (Fig. 41.1B) (Markowitz et al., 1988a, 1988b). Second- and third-generation vector genomes contain a larger packaging signal that extends into the GAG coding region, thereby improving vector production (Bender et al., 1987). Despite this extended overlap with the transcriptional unit encoding GAG, the risk of emergence of replication-competent retrovirus by homologous recombination has been controlled by introduction of mutations into the GAG sequences of the vector genome (Miller and Rosman, 1989) and by using split-function packaging lines. Most packaging lines and producer clones have been based on murine 3T3 fibroblast cell lines, but more recently packaging lines based on human cells have been generated using this general strategy (Ory et al., 1996; Davis et al., 1997). The vector particles produced by such cell lines are more resistant to destruction by human complement and thus may ultimately prove more useful for various gene therapy applications.

Figure 41.2 outlines the interaction of a retroviral vector particle with a target cell. Particle uptake is initiated by the binding of the viral envelope protein with cell surface molecules that act as receptors. Different classes of virus use different proteins for receptors. For example, ecotropic viruses that infect murine and other rodent cells rely on a cationic amino acid transporter to initiate cellular entry (Kim et al., 1991; Wang et al., 1991), whereas amphotropic viruses, whose broader host range includes human cells, use a sodium-dependent phosphate transporter (Kavanaugh et al., 1994; Miller et al., 1994a). Movement of the viral genome with associated matrix proteins and enzymatic activities into the nucleus requires dissolution of the nuclear membrane during mitosis (Miller et al., 1990). Thus, retroviral vectors that are based on the Moloney virus and other murine oncoretroviruses require cell division for genome integration. Furthermore, the preintegration nucleoprotein complex of oncoretroviruses is highly unstable (Lewis and Emerman, 1994); therefore successful transduction requires genome integration within hours of exposure of target cells to the retroviral vector particles.

After integration, expression of the genes encoded by the proviral genome requires continued activity of promoter and enhancer sequences within the LTR. Unfortunately, silencing is all too common and may be mediated both by methylation (Challita and Kohn, 1994) of proviral sequences and at the level of chromatin structure (Chen et al., 1997b). Murine leukemia virus LTRs seem particularly prone to silencing in embryonic stem cells and in primitive hematopoietic cells. Newer vectors have been designed to resist such

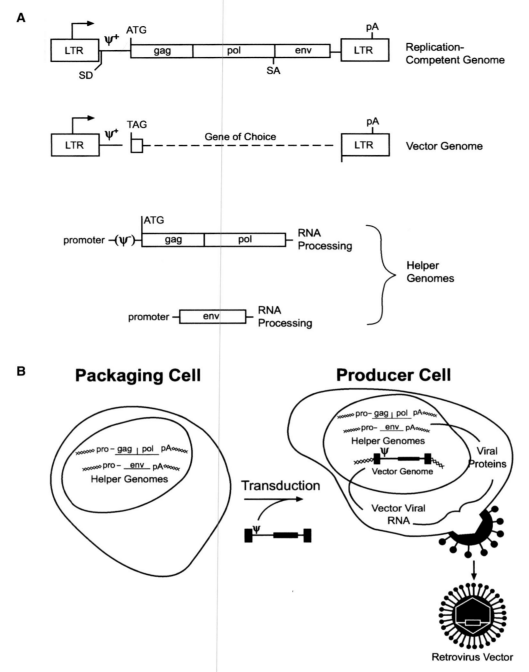

Figure 41.1. Packaging of murine retroviral vectors. (**A**) Retroviral vector and packaging genomes. Shown at the top is the structure of the wild-type replication competent genome from a murine retrovirus. The 5′ long terminal repeat (LTR) directs transcriptional initiation (arrow) and the 3′ LTR contains the polyadenlyation (pA) sequence. The ψ packaging sequence is required for incorporation of the genome into viral particles. The relative locations of the viral GAG, POL, and ENV genes are shown, with the translational start site for GAG indicated by the ATG initiation codon. Also shown are splice donor (SD) and acceptor (SA) sites, which result in a spliced subgenomic transcript. Vector genomes are made by deleting the viral genes and inserting an exogenous gene in their place. The ψ packaging sequence and the upstream portion of GAG are retained to enable efficient encapsidation of the vector genome. The initiation codon has been mutated to reduce the probability of generating replication-competent retrovirus as a result of recombination between the vector and packaging genomes. Helper genomes are generated by expressing the GAG, POL, and ENV genes from two separate plasmids under control of exogenous promoters and RNA processing elements. The ψ packaging sequence has been deleted in these helper genomes so that their transcripts are not encapsidated. (**B**) Packaging and producer cells. Packaging cells are made by stably inserting the helper genomes into mammalian cells. The vector genome is then stably inserted, typically by transduction with the vector genome, to derive vector-producing cells. In these cells, transcomplementation of the genomic vector RNA by viral proteins results in infectious, but replication-incompetent vector particles that are released into the medium. (Adapted from Sorrentino, BP and Nienhuis, AW. [1999]. In Friedmann, T, editor. *The development of gene therapy.* New York: Cold Spring Harbor Laboratory Press.)

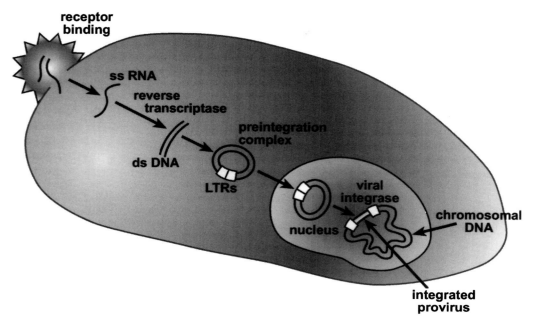

Figure 41.2. The retroviral life cycle. Binding of the virus to the cell is mediated by specific interactions with the viral envelope and cellular receptors. The diploid RNA genome is released into the cytoplasm, where a double stranded complementary DNA is formed through the action of viral reverse transcriptase. A circular double-stranded DNA intermediate is incorporated as part of the preintegration complex, which gains access to the nuclear contents either during mitosis or by direct nuclear transmigration in the case of lentiviruses. The proviral genome is subsequently integrated into the chromosomal DNA, a reaction mediated by the viral integrase protein. After integration, the provirus will be stably passed to subsequent daughter cells after host cell division.

silencing. These are based on the murine myeloproliferative sarcoma virus (MPSV) whose LTR is active in hematopoietic cells (Franz et al., 1986; Weiher et al., 1987). Further resistance to silencing is achieved by mutations in the enhancer region of the LTR (Hiberg et al., 1987); by alteration in the 5′ untranslated region encompassing the tRNA binding site, which functions in reverse transcription (Weiher et al., 1987; Grez et al., 1990); and in one case, by insertion of bacterial demethylating sequences in the promoter region (Challita et al., 1995). Such vectors have proved resistant to silencing in serial transplant experiments in murine recipients (Pawliuk et al., 1997). Retention of 5′ and 3′ splice sites that generate a subgenomic mRNA analogous to that which encodes the envelope protein in wild-type viruses also enhances vector mediated gene expression (Krall et al., 1996; Kaptein et al., 1997).

Expression of more than one gene product from a proviral genome is often desirable. Several designs have been tested for creating multigene vectors. One that has been tested extensively is the insertion of a second promoter downstream from the first open reading frame followed by the second open reading frame. Unfortunately, promoter interference often results in poor expression from the internal promoter (Emerman and Temin, 1984).

Another technique that has been much more successful involves the inclusion of an internal ribosomal entry site (IRES) between the two open reading frames, creating a vector genome that encodes a polycistronic transcript (Morgan et al., 1992). Using this design, several genes have been expressed in tandem with the coding sequences for green fluorescent protein, a readily assayable and selectable marker (Persons et al., 1997, 1998a).

Another approach is to place a complete transcriptional unit in reverse orientation within the 3′ LTR of the proviral genome (Hantzopoulos et al., 1989). After replication of such a genome and insertion into a target cell, the transcriptional unit within the 3′ LTR is duplicated, becoming part of the integrated 5′ LTR. Such double copy vectors often result in a much higher level of expression than can be achieved with an internal promoter configuration, particularly when a deletion mutation is introduced in the 3′ LTR to create a "self-inactivating vector" that lacks LTR promoter activity in target cells (Hantzopoulos et al., 1989).

As discussed in detail later, low levels of globin mRNA are generated by vectors that contain globin cDNA sequences. Vectors that incorporate an intact genomic globin gene in reverse transcriptional orientation with associated regulatory elements (Plavec et al., 1993; Leboulch et al., 1994; Sadelain et al., 1995; Ren et al., 1996) have been tested extensively in an effort to achieve therapeutically useful levels of globin in target hematopoietic cells.

Lentiviral Vectors

Human immunodeficiency virus (HIV) and other lentiviruses infect quiescent lymphocytes and monocytes (Lewis et al., 1992). In contrast to oncoretroviruses, lentiviruses can penetrate the nuclear membrane (Lewis and Emerman, 1994). Multiple nuclear localization signals within the matrix, vpr, and integrase proteins engage the nuclear import machinery, allowing the nucleoprotein preintegration complex to traverse nuclear pores (Bukrinsky et al., 1993; Heinzinger et al., 1994). The preintegration complex of lentiviral vectors is relatively stable. For example, a partial reverse transcriptase product formed in quiescent T lymphocytes can be rescued by cell activation for at least 7 to 8 days postinfection. In contrast, the nucleoprotein complex of oncoretroviruses disappears within 24 hours of infection of nondividing cells (Lewis and Emerman, 1994).

HIV-based vector development uses a general strategy similar to that used successfully with murine retroviral vectors. The vector genome includes *cis* active sequences necessary for generation of the RNA form of the viral genome and the sequences required for efficient packaging. Needed for these purposes are the LTRs, the 5′ end of the genome, which includes the 5′ splice donor site, a portion of the GAG gene required for efficient packaging, and ENV sequences that include the rev responsive element needed for nuclear to cytoplasmic transport of the unspliced RNA species (Parolin et al., 1996; Akkina et al., 1996; Naldini et al., 1996b). The packaging genome contains the sequences for GAG and POL under the control of a heterologous promoter (e.g., the cytomegalovirus [CMV] promoter and heterologous RNA processing signals). Because native HIV viral particles have a limited host range that is dependent on cell surface expression of CD4, a segment of the ENV gene is deleted from the helper vector. Pseudotyping of vector particles with the ENV protein of amphotropic oncoretrovirus or vesicular stomatitis virus creates vector particles with a broader host range. To date, most vector preparations have been derived by co-transfection of the two helper plasmids, one encoding the HIV proteins and the other an ENV protein, along with a vector plasmid into human kidney (293T) cells (Akkina et al., 1996).

Several of the HIV proteins are toxic, limiting the ability to derive packaging lines in which the helper components are stably integrated. This limitation has been overcome by placing both the GAG-POL and envelope genomes under the control of tetracycline

modulatable promoters (Kafri et al., 1999). Recent results suggest that it is possible to eliminate coding sequences for the accessory proteins, vif, vpr, vpu, and nef, and still generate vector particles capable of transducing quiescent cells (Zufferey et al., 1997; Kim et al., 1998). Elimination of these genes increases the safety of HIV-based lentiviral particles because each has a role in the pathogenicity of HIV. Furthermore, elimination of these protein products, which may be toxic to cells, should facilitate the derivation and use of stable packaging cell lines.

Safety will be a paramount concern if HIV-based vectors gain clinical application. As noted, elimination of the accessory and ENV genes greatly reduces the potential pathogenecity of any replication competent retroviruses (RCR) that may arise during packaging. As constructed, the vector and packaging genomes have limited homology, greatly reducing the probability of generation of RCR by homologous recombination.

Lentiviral vectors have been found to efficiently transduce quiescent cell populations in vivo, including myocytes and hepatocytes (Kafri et al., 1997), neurons (Naldini et al., 1996a, 1996b; Blomer et al., 1997), and retinal cells (Miyoshi et al., 1997). Lentiviral vectors can transduce quiescent human primitive hematopoietic cells that are capable of establishing human hematopoiesis in immunodeficient mice (Miyoshi et al., 1999).

One significant advantage of HIV vectors is their dependence on the expression of the *trans*-acting proteins, tet and rev, in packaging cells that are absent from the target cell population. Thus, the HIV LTR is naturally "self-inactivating." Self-inactivation may prove advantageous for deriving vector particles that include tissue-specific transcriptional regulatory elements because of the reduced possibility of promoter or transcript interference.

Foamy Virus Vectors

Human foamy virus (HFV), a retrovirus that is a member of the Spumavirus family, is also being explored for potential gene therapy applications. Although HFV was isolated from a nasopharyngeal carcinoma, seropositivity in humans is rare, and the virus is thought to be nonpathogenic (Ali et al., 1996). Recently, a vector production system has been derived that generates replication-defective particles free of RCR (Russell and Miller, 1996). The broad host range of HFV includes human clonogenic hematopoietic progenitors (Hirata et al., 1996). Expression of the HFV LTR requires a virally encoded transactivator, Bel-1, which can be provided in *trans* in packaging cells ensuring an inactive vector LTR in the target population (Bieniasz et al., 1997). Although HFV may be less dependent on cell division than oncoretroviruses, a direct comparison suggests that HIV is more efficient than oncoretroviruses at transducing $G_{1/S}$ or G_2-arrested cells (Bieniasz et al., 1995).

Adeno-Associated Virus Vectors

Adeno-associated virus (AAV) is a replication-defective parvovirus that depends on a helper virus, either adenovirus or herpes virus, for virus production during lytic infection. No disease has been associated with this virus, although 80 percent of humans have detectable antibodies. Recombinant AAV (rAAV) vector particles have been created and can transduce both quiescent and dividing cells. Direct injection of rAAV vector particles into muscle, liver, and brain results in transduction of fully differentiated, quiescent myocytes (Kessler et al., 1996; Fisher et al., 1997), hepatocytes (Synder et al., 1997; Koeberl et al., 1997; Nakai et al., 1998), or neurons (McCown et al., 1996), respectively. rAAV Vector particles have been used to transfer an intact genomic globin gene with associated regulatory elements into cultured human erythroleukemia cells (Walsh et al., 1992; Miller et al., 1993; Einerhand et al., 1995; Hargrove et al., 1997).

The AAV virus contains a single stranded DNA genome of 4,680 nucleotides including 145 bp inverted terminal repeats (ITRs) and encodes non-structural (Rep) proteins, p78, p68, p52, and p40, and the capsid proteins, VP1, VP2, and VP3. Each vector particle includes one of the two DNA strands; virus preparations are mixtures of both types of particles. Integration and persistence of a latent genome often occur after infection of susceptible cells by wild-type AAV in the absence of a helper virus. Many, but not all, wild-type AAV genome integration events occur within a preferred site (AAVS1) on human chromosome 19 (Kotin et al., 1992). The higher molecular weight Rep protein species, p78 and p68, mediate site-specific integration by virtue of sequence-specific interaction with sequences within the AAV ITRs and the host-cell AAV integration site. Only the ITRs are required for AAV genome replication and encapsidation (Samulski et al., 1983). Packaging of a rAAV genome is most efficient if its length is close to that of wild-type; shorter genomes are packaged less efficiently, and the upper limit of rAAV genome size is approximately 5,000 nucleotides (reviewed in Sorrentino and Nienhuis, 1999).

Production of rAAV vector particles remains problematic, although progress has recently been achieved. The initial strategy for deriving vector particles involved infection of HeLa or 293T cells with adenovirus at relatively low multiplicity of infection (MOI) followed by co-transduction with a helper plasmid encoding Rep and capsid functions and a vector plasmid that included the rAAV genome. After 48 hours, cells are lysed, releasing concentrated rAAV and adenoviral particles. Elimination of adenoviral particles can be accomplished by cesium chloride buoyant density gradient centrifugation or column chromatography followed by inactivation of any residual particles by heating the preparation at 55°C for 1 hour (Samulski et al., 1989). Such conventional rAAV vector preparations have particle titers of 10^9–10^{10}/mL. Both Rep and capsid proteins are highly toxic to dividing cells so that derivation of packaging lines has not been readily accomplished. Packaging lines have been created by integration of the wild-type AAV genome without ITRs, as well as the vector genome (Inoue and Russell, 1998). Adenovirus is required for helper functions including activation of latent helper genome. The presence of adenovirus and propensity for wild-type AAV generation by nonhomologous recombination have limited the titer and quality of the derived vector preparations. Progress in generating rAAV vector particles has been achieved by construction of a plasmid encoding the adenoviral genes required for AAV production (E1a, E1b, orf6 of the E4 region and VLA genes). Co-transfection of producer cells with this plasmid, the vector plasmid, and a plasmid encoding the AAV proteins (Fig. 41.3) results in the generation of rAAV vector particles devoid of adenovirus (Ferrari et al., 1997; Xiao et al., 1998). Because producer cells make only rAAV rather than rAAV and adenoviral particles, the yield of rAAV is improved by 10- to 100-fold. Rep and cap genes have been placed in opposite transcriptional orientations in a single plasmid (Allen et al., 1997) or individually expressed from separate plasmids (Nathwani et al., 1999a) to allow vector preparations that are free of wild-type AAV. These rAAV vector preparations are useful for experimental purposes, but scaling up of this process for derivation of materials for clinical protocols represents a formidable challenge.

rAAV Vectors have a broad host cell range. Recent work has shown that particle binding to target cells is mediated by a nearly ubiquitously expressed heparin sulfate proteoglycan (Summerford and Samulski, 1998). Particle entry appears to require a second molecule acting as a co-receptor; both fibroblast growth factor receptor 1 (Qing et al., 1999) and $\alpha v \beta 5$ integrin (Summerford et al., 1999) have been shown to perform this function. Although AAV particles are thought to enter cells by receptor-mediated endocytosis, little is know about this process or the subsequent steps of uncoding and translocation of the vector genome to the nucleus. Expression of a rAAV-encoded gene requires conversion of the single-stranded to a double-stranded genome. Second strand synthesis is

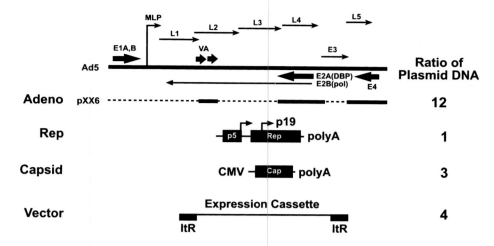

Figure 41.3. Production of AAV particles. System for production of rAAV particles without contamination by wild-type AAV or helper adenovirus. 293T cells, which express the adenoviral E1a and E1b proteins, are co-transfected with four plasmids encoding the following components in the indicated ratios: (1) adenoviral E2 and E4 proteins and VA RNAs, (2) AAV rep proteins, (3) AAV capsid proteins, and (4) the vector genome flanked by AAV inverted terminal repeats (ITRs). After 48 to 72 hours, the cells are lysed, releasing 10^3–10^4 vector particles per cell, which after purification and concentration, yield vector preparations having titers of up to 10^{12} particles per milliliter.

promoted by adenoviral proteins E1a, E2, and orf6 of the E4 region (Ferrari et al., 1996; Fisher et al., 1996). Promotion of second strand synthesis is also achieved by cytotoxic agents (e.g., hydroxyurea, γ irradiation, cold shock, or exposure of cells to DNA damaging agents) (Alexander et al., 1994, 1996; Russell et al., 1995). A cellular phosphoprotein binds to AAV ITRs; in its phosphorylated form, it inhibits second strand synthesis (Qing et al., 1998). These data in aggregate suggest that second strand synthesis is an important step in determining whether rAAV successfully transduce a target cell population.

Once second strand synthesis is complete, expression of the rAAV genome commences, and the target cell has been successfully transduced. In rapidly dividing cells, the episomal form of the rAAV genome persists for varying periods and is ultimately diluted out, and expression is lost as cells continue to proliferate. Only a minority of cells undergo genome integration and remain permanently transduced (Bertran et al., 1996; Malik et al., 1997). Increasing the MOI of rAAV expands the proportion of cells with an integrated genome (Hargrove et al., 1997). At high MOIs, genome integration occurs in a majority of cells. Inclusion of a matrix association region within the vector genome appears to enhance the innate propensity of rAAV to integrate in a head-to-tail tandem array (Hargrove et al., 1997).

rAAV vectors efficiently transduce quiescent neurons, muscle cells, retinal cells, and hepatocytes in vivo. Direct injection of vector particles results in transduction of a substantial portion of the cells at and around the injection point (Kessler et al., 1996; Fisher et al., 1997). In quiescent myocytes, the rAAV genome remains single stranded for up to 30 days before forming a head-to-tail, high-molecular-weight tandem array, which may or may not be integrated into the target cell chromosome (Fisher et al., 1997). The nature of the persistent rAAV genome in brain and retinal cells remains to be established; rAAV-mediated gene expression in these tissues persist for many months without evidence of cellular toxicity or an immune response (Snyder et al., 1999; Herzog et al., 1999).

Integration of the wild-type AAV genome is mediated by the high-molecular-weight Rep proteins, p78 and p68. Their ability to enhance integration of a rAAV genome has been evaluated using a tetracycline-modulated promoter system to achieve conditional expression of these Rep proteins. Target cells were co-transduced with two vectors, one containing a globin gene and the other containing the Rep gene under the control of the tetracycline-modulated promoter. Transient expression of the Rep protein for 72 hours after exposure to vector particles failed to increase the frequency of rAAV genome integration (Bertran et al., 1998). Disruption of the integration target site, AAVS1, on chromosome 19 was frequently observed; and in a minority of instances, the rAAV genome bearing a globin gene was integrated into the preferred site on chromosome 19. These data suggest that Rep-mediated, site-specific integration of a rAAV genome can be achieved; but under the conditions tested, this process was both inefficient and associated with Rep-mediated effects on the genome independent of vector integration.

Most work with rAAV vectors has involved viral components having AAV2 serotype specificity. Recently, the genome of several other AAV serotypes has been molecularly cloned, and the host range of vector particles constructed with these components has been evaluated (Chiorini et al., 1997; Rutledge et al., 1998). Variability with respect to transducibility of different cell lines with these alternative serotype rAAV suggests that different receptors may be involved. To date, no striking advantage over AAV2 vectors has been discovered.

Adenoviral Vectors

Because of their lack of genome integration, adenoviral vectors seem to have little application for transduction of highly proliferative hematopoietic cells. However, such vectors have been explored as a means to transiently express a gene product that facilitates transduction of primitive hematopoietic cells with an integrating vector particle.

Thirty-five kilobases in length, the adenoviral genome encodes multiple proteins expressed successively during early, intermediate, and late stages of infection. To date, most vectors have been constructed by eliminating sequences in the viral E1 and E3 region (Yang et al., 1994a; Grubb et al., 1994). E3 encoded proteins are not required for viral replication, whereas E1 products are provided in *trans* in 293T cells, which express the E1 genes. Vector preparations having particle titers of 10^{11}–10^{12} that are essentially free of wild-type adenovirus can be routinely derived.

Adenoviral vectors transduce quiescent, differentiated muscle cells (Wickham et al., 1996; Feero et al., 1997; Chen et al., 1997a), hepatocytes (Morsy et al., 1993; Engelhardt et al., 1994; Kay et al., 1994), neurons (Davidson et al., 1993), and retinal cells (Li et al., 1994; Sakamoto et al., 1998) efficiently in vivo. Because the first-generation vectors retain several of the adenoviral genes expressed at low levels in vivo, a potent immune response is often generated that destroys transduced cells (Yang et al., 1994b, 1995; Yang and Wilson, 1995). Much effort has focused on eliminating additional adenoviral genes from second- and third-generation vectors (Engelhardt et al., 1994; Yang et al., 1994b Gao et al., 1996; Morsy et al., 1998). This effort has been complicated by the ability of adenoviral vectors to invoke an immune response directed to the transgene product itself (Yang et al., 1996), a response that apparently is based on the efficient transduction of antigen presenting dendritic cells in vivo (Jooss et al., 1998).

Entry of adenoviral vector particles into target cells is mediated via a cellular receptor (CAR) (Bergelson et al., 1997), with subsequent vector internalization requiring interaction with specific integrins (Wickham et al., 1993). Targeting of adenoviral particles using bispecific antibodies that bind both the Ad-vector and alternative cell surface proteins has been used to facilitate transduction of cells that do not express the CAR receptor or the required specific integrins (Wickham et al., 1996; Douglas et al., 1996). An alternative approach to adenoviral targeting is to genetically modify the knob region of the adenoviral fiber thought to interact with the CAR receptor (Wickham et al., 1997; Dmitriev et al., 1998; Krasnykh et al., 1998). Substitution of this region of the adenovirus 5 fiber protein with the corresponding sequences from a virus having adenovirus 3 serotype specificity allows the generation of vector particles having much higher transducibility for a spectrum of cell lines. For example, vector particles having the Ad3 serotype specificity transduce human hematopoietic cells much more efficiently than conventional Ad5 vector particles (Nathwani et al., 1999b).

SV40 Vectors

This DNA virus was one of the first proposed for gene transfer. Early vectors contained a small expression cassette within the early, T-antigen region and retained the sequences encoding SV40 capsid proteins. Although such vectors transduced target cells efficiently, the genome failed to integrate; therefore these vectors were not useful for permanent genetic modification of target cell populations. Recent modifications allow generation of vector particles containing largely foreign DNA. Only a small segment of the SV40 genome is required for encapsidation, allowing expression cassettes of up to 5 kilobases to be pseudotyped with SV40 proteins (Oppenheim et al., 1986). Infectious particles are generated by transfecting COS cells with circularized vector DNA and wild-type SV40 DNA. Vector preparations generated by this strategy contain substantial amounts of wild-type SV40. Development of an in vitro packaging system that relies on vector assembly using recombinant capsid proteins produced in insect cells may allow the generation of vector preparations free of wild-type virus (Sandalon et al., 1997). Pseudotyped SV40 particles encoding the human MDR1 gene transduce primary human bone marrow cells very efficiently (Rund et al., 1998). The future utility of this system, if any, for transduction of human hematopoietic cells may rely on the generation of hybrid viral particles in which a genome with a capacity for integration (e.g., a rAAV genome) is encapsidated within SV40 proteins, which facilitate delivery of that genome into the target population.

Herpes Virus Vectors

A disabled infectious herpes virus vector has been adapted for transduction of human hematopoietic cells. This disabled infectious single-cycle (DISC) vector has been modified to eliminate a gene (gH) that is essential for viral replication (Forrester et al., 1992); this gene can be replaced with a marker or therapeutic gene in the DISC-HSV genome. DISC-HSV is produced in a helper cell line that is engineered to express gH protein. Both human primary hematopoietic cells and leukemic blasts were readily transduced with a DISC-HSV vector encoding β-galactosidase (Dilloo et al., 1997). Peak expression occurred at 2 days and declined over 2 weeks during the expansion of primary hematopoietic cells in culture. Whether this vector system is preferable to adenovirus for the transient expression of proteins (e.g., a retroviral receptor) is not known.

GENE TRANSFER INTO STEM CELLS

Murine Stem Cells

During the decade since stem cell-targeted gene transfer into the murine system was first demonstrated, refinements of the basic methodology have significantly improved the efficiency of genetic modification of repopulating stem cells with oncoretroviral vectors. Strategies have been developed to derive high-titer vector producer clones (Persons et al., 1998b). 5-Fluorouracil (5-FU) is routinely administered to donor animals 48 hours before marrow harvest to achieve stem cell activation as the maturing, rapidly cycling progenitor and precursor population is eliminated (Bodine et al., 1991). Using complex cytokine mixtures and extended 4- to 5-day cultures designed to induce stem cell division significantly improves the transduction efficiency of repopulating cells (Bodine et al., 1989; Luskey et al., 1992). Co-culture of vector-producing cells with the target bone marrow cell population substantially increases gene transfer efficiency (Bodine et al., 1991). As detailed previously, modifications in vector design have overcome many of the problems of sustaining gene expression in the murine model. Work in mice is now focused on issues of functional gene expression, often designed to correct specific genetic deficiencies in unique, gene knock-out mouse strains.

Proof of principle experiments in animal models have now been performed for a number of genetic diseases. Deficiencies in one of the various protein components of the phagocyte oxidase complex results in the human disorder chronic granulomatous disease (Dinauer et al., 1987). Effete phagocytes in affected patients lack the ability to kill aggressive microbial pathogens resulting in chronic suppurative infections. Mouse models of these disorders have been created by eliminating the function of the murine homologs of the human proteins through gene knock-out (Jackson et al., 1995; Pollock et al., 1995). Retroviral-mediated gene transfer corrects the genetic defect and allows restoration of adequate phagocyte function to combat experimental infections (Bjorgvinsdottir et al., 1997; Mardiney et al., 1997).

Mice whose genome has homozygous disruptions of the Jak3 allele have severe combined immune deficiency (SCID) characterized by very low numbers of T and B lymphocytes and severe defects in both cellular and humoral immunity (Nosaka et al., 1995; Thomis et al., 1995). Homozygous Jak3 deficiency in humans also causes SCID (Macchi et al., 1995). In the murine model, introduction of the Jak3 gene into repopulating stem cells from Jak3-deficient mice restores immune function after transplantation of these genetically modified cells into Jak3-deficient recipients (Bunting et al., 1998b). Substantial increases in T and B lymphocytes compared with homozygous null animals have been documented. More important, modified animals are resistant to pulmonary influenza virus challenge and are capable of mounting humoral immune responses to protein antigens (Bunting et al., 1999). Jak3-corrected lymphocytes were amplified in vivo, suggesting that gene correction of a relatively small number of hematopoietic stem cells may be sufficient to reconstitute physiologically significant levels of immunity in humans.

Despite the existence of several animal models for the hemoglobin disorders, sickle cell anemia and severe β thalassemia (Ciavatta et al., 1995; Ryan et al., 1997) (Chapter 34), gene therapy for these diseases remains to be tested. Failure to take on this challenge reflects the difficulties in creating vectors capable of transferring and expressing a native globin gene in primary hematopoietic cells.

Large Animal Models

Large animal models were developed to test the emerging principles for stem cell targeted gene transfer. Rhesus and cynomologous macaques, baboons, dogs, and sheep have been used to evaluate gene transfer into repopulating cells. Relatively sophisticated regimens of supportive care ensures survival of these animals during reconstitution with autologous cells after otherwise lethal irradiation. In the initial studies, gene transfer efficiency into repopulating cells, as reflected by the frequency of genetically modified cells in peripheral blood or bone marrow, was far lower than that achieved in the murine model. Only 1 to 2 percent of blood cells contained the proviral genome (van Beusechem et al., 1992; Bodine et al., 1993). An exception to the generally poor transduction of stem cells in large animals is the report that 20 percent of hematopoietic cells contain the vector genome in dogs that had received bone marrow exposed to fresh vector-containing medium weekly for 3 weeks under "long-term culture" conditions designed to trigger stem cell self-renewal (Bienzle et al., 1994). This important observation has not been reproduced in other species (Tisdale et al., 1997). As described in later sections, these large animal models have proved useful for devising strategies to overcome the barriers of stem cell-targeted gene transfer.

Human Stem Cells: Marking Studies and Early Clinical Trials

After being inserted into the target cell genome, the provirus becomes a stable element useful for in vivo tracking of genetically modified cells. Virus-marked cells have been used to determine whether tumor cells within autologous bone marrow contribute to relapse after high-dose chemotherapy and bone marrow rescue. Marking studies were initially performed to evaluate the potential of tumor cells to contribute to relapse in children who were receiving autologous bone marrow transplantation as part of their therapy for neuroblastoma or acute myeloid leukemia (Brenner et al., 1993a,b; Rill et al., 1994). Marking trials have also been performed in adults with myeloid leukemia (Deisseroth et al., 1994), breast cancer, or multiple myeloma (Dunbar et al., 1995). Future marking studies are likely to be useful for evaluating the effectiveness of various purging methodologies.

Marking studies provided the first opportunity to evaluate gene transfer into human repopulating cells. Genetically modified cells were detected in blood and bone marrow after transplantation, and these cells persisted for long periods after engraftment. Transduction was highest in pediatric cancer patients whose marrow had been harvested after two cycles of intensive chemotherapy. Up to 10 to 15 percent of the clonogenic progenitors in bone marrow were found to contain the proviral genome (Brenner et al., 1993a), and marking has persisted and has been stable more than 5 years after transplantation. In adults, the gene transfer efficiency—reflected by the proportion of genetically modified cells in peripheral blood or bone marrow—has been less than 1 percent (Dunbar et al., 1995; Hesdorffer et al., 1998).

Adenosine deaminase (ADA) deficiency provided the first test of the therapeutic efficacy of retrovirus-mediated gene transfer. This disorder can be cured by allogeneic bone marrow transplantation and emerged as the primary candidate for the initial gene therapy trials in the late 1980s. Three trials have been reported to date. The first used ex vivo-expanded peripheral blood lymphocytes as targets for retrovirus-mediated gene transfer (Blaese et al., 1995); the second trial used both transduced lymphocytes and bone marrow stem cells (Bordignon et al., 1995); in the third trial, three infants received autologous, cord blood cells transduced with a retroviral vector encoding the ADA gene (Kohn et al., 1995). None of the patients received any form of myeloablation. Gene-modified cells persisted in all patients for up to 4 years, although their frequency has remained low.

Early marking studies and therapeutic trials have established the potential for genetic modification of human repopulating hematopoietic cells. The low frequency of genetically modified cells present in reconstituted recipients attests to the generally inadequate means for gene transfer.

STRATEGIES TO OVERCOME THE BARRIERS TO HUMAN STEM CELL TARGETED GENE TRANSFER

During the last several years, significant progress has been made in understanding the biological characteristics of human hematopoietic stem cells and in using this knowledge to improve gene transfer efficiency. Murine repopulating cells are transduced at higher efficiency than are large animal cells and cells in the human clinical trials performed to date. Comparisons of the murine system and those of large animal models and humans have identified key barriers to retroviral transduction (Fig. 41.4) that may be amenable to experimental manipulation.

Why Are Mouse Stem Cells Transduced More Efficiently Than Human Stem Cells?

One factor that determines transduction efficiency is the level of expression of the receptor used for vector entry into stem cells. Ecotropic vectors used in the murine studies rely on a cationic amino acid transporter for cell entry (Kim et al., 1991). The human homolog of this protein does not support vector uptake. Rather, amphotropic vectors used in large animal models and human studies rely on a phosphate transporter (Kavanaugh et al., 1994; Miller et al., 1994) expressed at much lower levels in primitive hematopoietic cells. These differences in the level of receptor expression correlate with the efficiency of gene transfer into murine repopulating cells (Orlic et al., 1996b).

Gene transfer by oncoretroviruses requires cell division (Miller et al., 1990); mouse stem cells cycle more frequently than those of humans (Fleming et al., 1993; Shah et al., 1996). Initiation of cell cycle progression in the primitive murine hematopoietic cell population is routinely achieved by administration of a myeloablative dose of 5-FU to mice 48 hours before marrow harvest (Randall and Weissman, 1997). Differences in the pharmacokinetics of 5-FU and stem cell dynamics have prevented the ready adaption of this strategy in

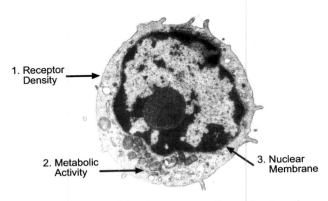

1. Receptor Density

2. Metabolic Activity

3. Nuclear Membrane

Figure 41.4. Biological barriers to stem cell transduction. Shown is an electron micrograph of a CD34+, CD38− human hematopoietic cell. The first barrier to stem cell transduction occurs at the level of the cell membrane and is due to limiting degrees of expression of retroviral receptor molecules. The second potential barrier occurs in the cytoplasm, where limiting amounts of nucleotide precursors associated with the G_0 state of the cell cycle may limit formation of the proviral cDNA. The third barrier occurs at the level of nuclear entry for the preintegration complex. Because mitosis is required for transduction with murine retroviral vectors, nuclear access is limited in most repopulating cells owing to cell cycle quiescence. (Photomicrograph provided by G. Murti.)

other animal models or humans. Co-culture of the target marrow cells with vector producer cells has achieved the highest level of gene transfer in the murine system (Bodine et al., 1991). However, after such co-culture, only the nonadherent subset of repopulating cells—about 25 percent of the total and most likely to be cycling—are recovered. In the syngeneic mouse model, more donors can be used to ensure that adequate cells are available for engraftment, whereas in larger animals and humans, the number of cells available for ex vivo manipulation and reconstitution is limited by the number of autologous cells that can be harvested from the recipient.

In summary, transduction of human stem cells is limited by the level of expression of the receptor utilized by standard amphotropic vectors and by the quiescent status of stem cells. Human stem cells are available in limited numbers, and minimal amplification of such stem cells has been achieved ex vivo without loss of repopulating potential (Bhatia et al., 1997). Much effort has been invested in overcoming these barriers to stem cell transduction with conventional oncoretroviral vectors. In the future, use of lentiviral vectors, which can transduce quiescent cells, may afford greater promise for efficient transduction.

Receptor Expression

Expression levels of the cell surface protein, which acts as a retroviral receptor, influences the frequency

of vector transduction of target cells. A variety of approaches have been explored to overcome the low levels of expression of the amphotropic receptor on human stem cells. Expression of the receptor is upregulated during culture of hematopoietic cells in the presence of cytokines (Crooks and Kohn, 1993) and may be enhanced by culture in phosphate-free medium. The amphotropic receptor is a phosphate transporter whose expression is increased in an environment of low phosphate (Kavanaugh et al., 1994). Cryopreservation and subsequent thawing of cord blood cells induce a large increase in receptor expression on CD34+ cells (Orlic et al., 1998). Cytokine mobilization of primitive hematopoietic cells in vivo releases a population that expresses higher levels of the amphotropic receptor (Orlic et al., 1998). Recent studies in nonhuman primates suggest that up to 10 percent of such repopulating cells can be transduced with an amphotropic vector (Tisdale et al., 1998).

Another strategy for overcoming the receptor barrier is to use a nonintegrating DNA viral vector, either an adenoviral or an adeno-associated viral vector, to express the ecotropic receptor gene followed by transduction of the population with an integrating, ecotropic retroviral vector. This sequential transduction strategy has been used successfully to introduce a retroviral vector genome encoding the green fluorescent protein into CD34+ (Qing et al., 1997) and CD34+, CD38− cells (Nathwani et al., 1999a) and clonogenic progenitors within the CD34+ population at efficiencies exceeding 50 percent (Nathwani et al., 1999a), although it has yet to be tested in the context of evaluating gene transfer into repopulating cells.

Retroviral vector particles may be formed with alternative ENV proteins; this mechanism, known as pseudotyping, creates vector particles with a modified host range reflecting, at least in part, that of the ENV protein. MLV pseudotyped with the Gibbon ape leukemia virus ENV protein (GALV) transduces hematopoietic cells more efficiently than conventional amphotropic vector particles (Bauer et al., 1995; Kiem et al., 1997). The GALV envelope binds to a phosphate transporter closely related to the amphotropic receptor, but which has a distinct expression pattern (Kavanaugh et al., 1994).

Another ENV protein that has been used for pseudotyping MLV vector particles is the G-protein from vesicular stomatitis virus (VSV-G) (Emi et al., 1991). This protein mediates viral binding through a membrane phospholipid thought to be present on all cells, as reflected by the extremely broad host range of wild-type VSV. VSV-G pseudotyped particles are more stable than conventional MLV particles and can be concentrated by ultracentrifugation (Burns et al., 1993). Although VSV-G pseudotyped MLV vectors transduce human CD34+ cells (Yang et al., 1995b), the transduction efficiency of repopulating cells has yet to be established. VSV-G envelope protein can also pseudotype HIV vectors expanding their host range (Akkina et al., 1996). In the future, it will be important to evaluate alternative envelope proteins for pseudotyping HIV vector particles to maximize their inherent biological advantages—relative stability of the preintegration nuclear matrix complex and the ability to traverse nuclear membranes.

Several other retroviral ENV proteins that appear to mediate cell entry via different receptors than those used by the amphotropic and GALV pseudotyped vector particles have been reported. To date, none have been extensively characterized for host range of appropriately pseudotyped vector particles. In the future, this may prove to be a productive avenue of investigation because the host range of MLV varies considerably, and the ENV proteins in current use were not selected from viruses having hematopoietic specificity.

Quiescent Stem Cells

Human primitive hematopoietic cells are largely in the G_0/G_1 phase of the cell cycle (Shah et al., 1996; Hao et al., 1996). Although such cells can be induced to cell cycle progression when cultured in vitro with complex cytokine mixtures, proliferation is generally associated with loss of repopulating activity (Tisdale et al., 1998). Only recently have conditions been identified that result in a twofold to fourfold increase in repopulating activity of human primitive hematopoietic cells as assayed in an immunodeficient mouse model (Bhatia et al., 1997). Uncertain at this time is whether this increase in repopulating activity reflects proliferation of cells or an increase in their marrow homing ability.

In principle, lentiviral vectors hold the greatest potential for transducing quiescent stem cells. Stability of the preintegration nucleoprotein complex and the ability of this complex to traverse the nuclear membrane are potentially powerful biological advantages for lentiviral vectors compared with those constructed with components of murine oncoretroviruses. Recent results have established that up to 70 percent of quiescent CD34+, CD38- cells can be transduced with an HIV-based lentiviral vector expressing a fluorescent marker (Uchida et al., 1998). A similar proportion of the colonies derived from clonogenic progenitors present in the cultured and transduced population expressed the marker. HIV vectors have been compared to a conventional oncoretroviral vectors for their ability to transduce cells capable of establishing human hematopoiesis in immunodeficient mice. Despite transduction under conditions in which there

was little potential for inducing cell cycle progression, up to 20 percent of the repopulating cells were successfully transduced with the lentiviral vector, whereas the oncoretroviral vector failed to transduce repopulating cells (Miyoshi et al., 1999). These results appear to verify the predicted biological advantages of the lentiviral vector system with respect to transduction of quiescent hematopoietic cells.

An alternative approach that has been pursued by many investigators is an attempt to identify conditions by which repopulating cells can be successfully transduced with conventional oncoretroviral vectors. One approach for increasing the transducibility of stem cells involves treatment of the donor with hematopoietic cytokines before collecting bone marrow or peripheral blood stem cells for transduction. Administration of stem cell factor (SCF) and granulocyte-colony stimulating factor (G-CSF) to mice results in a substantial amplification of stem cells in the bone marrow and peripheral blood (Bodine et al., 1994, 1996). Cytokine-activated stem cells were more efficiently transduced than conventional "post-5 FU" bone marrow stem cells, perhaps, in part, due to induction of cell cycling as a result of cytokine administration. Expression of the amphotropic retroviral receptor is also increased in stem cells recovered after cytokine stimulation (Orlic et al., 1998). Rhesus monkey stem cells mobilized with SCF and G-CSF and transduced with an amphotropic retroviral vector generated 5 percent genetically modified peripheral blood cells after transplantation (Tisdale et al., 1998).

Repopulating cells must be prestimulated with cytokines ex vivo for 48 to 72 hours before exposure to vector particles (Veena et al., 1998). Immediate exposure of hematopoietic cells to vector particles before induction of cell cycle progression by cytokines may result in vector particle uptake causing downmodulation of the retroviral receptor and rendering the target cells refractory to subsequent vector uptake when cell cycle progression has occurred (D. A. Williams, personal communication, June 1998). Oncoretroviruses have a highly unstable preintegration nucleoprotein complex, which decays in the cytoplasm before disruption of the nuclear membrane if taken up immediately by cells that may not undergo division for 48 to 96 hours after cytokine exposure. Relatively efficient transduction of umbilical cord blood cells capable of establishing hematopoiesis in immunodeficient mice has been achieved by prestimulating such cells for 3 days in serum-free cultures supplemented with hematopoietic cytokines before exposure to amphotropic vector particles (Schilz et al., 1998; Conneally et al., 1998).

Another approach for promoting cell cycle progression in culture is to modulate components of the cell cycle machinery. Downregulation of a cyclin-dependent kinase inhibitor, p27 (kip-1), has been achieved by adding specific antisense cyclin oligonucleotides to the culture medium (Dao et al., 1998b). Adding a neutralizing antibody directed against transforming growth factor β resulted in downregulation of p15 (INK4B), another cyclin-dependent kinase inhibitor that is a potent blocker of G_1 cell cycle progression. Manipulations like this have been shown to significantly enhance transduction of primitive hematopoietic cells capable of establishing human hematopoiesis in immunodeficient mice.

It is still uncertain whether in vitro manipulation of stem cells to enhance transduction with oncoretroviral vectors can overcome the inherent biological advantages of lentiviral vectors. Indeed many manipulations that enhance transduction with conventional MLV vectors may also increase transduction with lentiviral vectors.

rAAV Vectors have also been evaluated for their ability to transduce quiescent stem cells. Primary human CD34$^+$ cells have shown variable susceptibility to transduction with rAAV vectors (Ponnazhagan et al., 1997a), which may be due to different cell surface levels of heparan sulfate proteoglycan, a primary docking molecule for rAAV (Summerford and Samulski, 1998). Transducibility of target cells is also limited by the rate of conversion of the single-stranded rAAV genome into its double-stranded form (Fisher et al., 1996). Permanent genetic modification of a target cell requires integration of the double stranded rAAV genome, an inefficient process in most cells. Only at very high MOI have hematopoietic cell lines been permanently genetically modified with rAAV vectors (Hargrove et al., 1997). In murine (Ponnazhagan et al., 1997b) and large animal models (Schimmenti et al., 1998), studies show a low transduction efficiency of repopulating cells. Based on current knowledge, this vector system does not appear to hold promise for transduction of quiescent human hematopoietic stem cells.

Microenvironmental Influences

Hematopoietic stem cells exist within a complex bone marrow microenvironment that includes mesenchymal-derived stromal cells, extracellular matrix molecules, and a capillary network. Stromal cells produce a complex array of soluble and membrane-bound cytokines that influence the proliferative status and differentiation behavior of primitive hematopoietic cell populations. Efforts have been made to reproduce this microenvironment in vitro using long-term culture conditions in which a stromal layer is established to support hematopoiesis. Efficient transduction of long-term culture-initiating cells (LTC-IC) has been reported (Wells et al., 1995). Experience in animal

models is mixed. In dogs, a high transduction efficiency was reported (Bienzle et al., 1994), but efforts to reproduce these observations in Rhesus monkeys were unsuccessful (Tisdale et al., 1998). Clinical trials have suggested some enhancement of transduction when hematopoietic cells are co-cultured on autologous stroma (Hanania et al., 1996), although cytokines are also required to achieve a measurable level of stem cell marking (Emmons et al., 1997).

An experimental alternative to cumbersome stromal cell cultures is the use of extracellular matrix molecules. Fibronectin is an important mediator of gene transfer. Lately, a carboxyterminal 30/35 kD fragment with the capacity to co-localize retroviral vector particles and hematopoietic cells to distinct but closely approximate binding motifs has been identified (Moritz et al., 1994; Hanenberg et al., 1996). Fibronectin also supports proliferation of hematopoietic cells while maintaining stem cell regenerative capacity by signaling through integrin molecules on the stem cell surface (Dao et al., 1998d; Yokota et al., 1998). A commercially available human fibronectin fragment, CH296, contains both the stem cell binding motif and the binding site for vector particles (Hanenberg et al., 1997). Many protocols now incorporate coating of the culture plates with this fibronectin fragment to enhance transduction frequency, as documented in a baboon transplant model (Kiem et al., 1998).

STEM CELL SELECTION

Another strategy to overcome the limited transduction efficiency of hematopoietic stem cells is to use a selection strategy to recover successfully transduced cells. This can be accomplished in vitro using vectors expressing a protein detectable by fluorescent-activated cell sorting (FACS). Both CD24, a surface protein, and the cytoplasmic green fluorescent protein (GFP) have been used for this purpose in murine systems. Pretransplant transplant sorting of the expressing cell population and their subsequent transplantation into irradiated recipients result in reconstitution with more than 90 percent genetically modified cells (Pawliuk et al., 1994, 1997; Persons et al., 1997; 1998a). Using a drug selection marker for ex vivo selection is impractical because of the limiting proliferative potential of repopulating cells under currently used culture conditions. Even the FACS approach cannot be applied in large animal models or humans because of the limited availability of autologous cells and their low transduction efficiencies. A purified, successfully transduced population would be too small to reproducibly reconstitute the autologous host.

A more promising strategy for human application is the in vivo selection of genetically modified cells

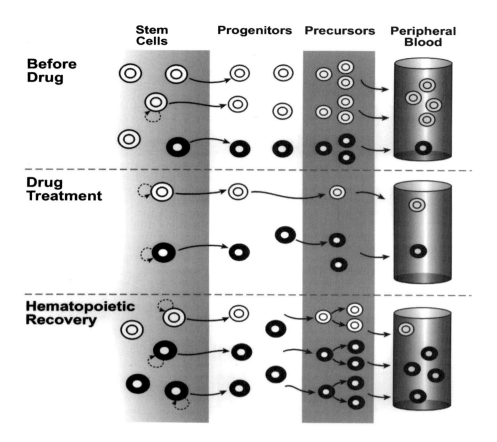

Figure 41.5. In vivo selection of stem cells transduced with a drug resistance gene vector. Schematic depiction of how stem cell selection with cytotoxic drugs can result in increased proportions of modified cells in the peripheral blood. Cells that contain a vector expressing a drug resistance gene are indicated with dark fill, whereas unmodified cells are open. Various stages of hematopoietic maturation are indicated and progression through these compartments is shown as solid arrows. Stem cell self-renewal divisions are shown as broken arrows. Before drug administration, a minority of cells contains the transferred drug resistance gene. When the animal is treated with the appropriate cytotoxic drug, stem cells expressing the resistance vector have a significant survival advantage and therefore are enriched by drug treatment. In the recovery phase, cell expansion results in an increased number and proportion of cells containing the drug resistance vector. If selection has occurred at the stem-cell level, increased numbers of genetically modified cells will be seen in all hematopoietic compartments, and will be stable over time. (Adapted from BP Sorrentino, 1996.)

expressing a gene-confering resistance to drugs with hematopoietic toxicity (Fig. 41.5). P-glycoprotein, which confers multidrug resistance (MDR-1), can confer selectable drug resistance in the murine system (Sorrentino et al., 1992). Attempts to extend these findings to larger animal models or in human clinical trials have been unsuccessful (Boesen et al., 1995; Hanania et al., 1996; Hesdorffer et al., 1998, in part

because of the low transduction efficiency and the proclivity of the MDR-1 gene to undergo rearrangement owing to splicing during the retroviral vector life cycle (Sorrentino et al., 1995). Recent results have shown that enforced, high level expression of MDR-1 in primitive hematopoietic cells substantially increases their self-renewal potential ex vivo, causing a myeloproliferative syndrome in transplanted mice (Bunting et al., 1998a). These findings would seem to preclude future use of the MDR-1 gene for in vivo amplification of genetically modified stem cells in humans.

Another system, based on the dihydrofolate reductase (DHFR) gene, appears to hold greater promise. The DHFR gene has several advantages; its cDNA is small and stable in retroviral vectors, and many drug-resistant variants have been characterized. An important limitation of this system, the resistance of primitive hematopoietic cells to antifolate toxicity (Blau et al., 1996), has been overcome by coincident administration of a nucleoside transport inhibitor that blocks nucleotide salvage pathways (Allay et al., 1997a). Co-administration of trimetrexate, a DHFR-specific antifolate, and nitro-benzyl mecaptopurine-riboside 5′monophosphate (NBMPR-P) is highly myelosuppressive in murine models, whereas the hematopoietic system is fully protected in mice reconstituted with genetically modified cells expressing a variant DHFR (L22Y) (Allay, J. A. and Sorrentino, B. P., unpublished data). Genetically modified hematopoietic cells can be amplified from fewer than 10 percent to greater than 80 percent by three cycles of trimetrexate/NBMPR-P administration (Allay et al., 1998). Serial transplant studies have shown that this amplification occurs at the stem cell level. Reproduction of these findings in a large animal model would support future development for clinical trials.

A third drug system that has been studied for stem cell selection uses alkyltransferase genes to confer protection against nitrosoureas such as BCNU or CCNU. Hematopoietic cells express low levels of alkyltransferases (Gerson et al., 1996) and can be made highly drug resistant by retroviral-mediated transfer of an alkyltransferase gene (Allay et al., 1995; Moritz et al., 1995; Harris et al., 1995). Nitrosoureas are highly toxic to hematopoietic stem cells as evidenced by prolonged and cumulative myelosuppression when used in cancer therapy. Amplification of transduced myeloid progenitors has been observed in mice first transplanted with methylguanine methyltransferase (MGMT)-transduced cells and subsequently treated with BCNU (Allay et al., 1997b). Variants of MGMT that are resistant to O^6-benzylguanine, a pharmacologic potentiator of nitrosourea toxicity, protect hematopoietic cells from a combination of BCNU and O^6BG and have also been used for selection (Davis et al., 1997).

An alternative strategy for achieving positive selection involves the construction of chimeric receptor molecules. Cytokine receptors achieve activation through ligand-induced dimerization. Dimerization can also be induced between chimeric molecules lacking the external ligand binding domain but including an internal binding domain for the drug, FK506. A dimeric form of this drug, designated FK1012, induces dimerization of such chimeric receptor molecules, resulting in generation of a mitogenic signal (Blau et al., 1997). Murine bone marrow cells expressing a chimeric receptor gene exhibit more than a 10^6-fold amplification during extended culture in FK1012 (Jin et al., 1998). The hormone-binding domain of the estrogen receptor has also been used to generate a variant G-CSF receptor that allows estrogen-induced growth of myeloid cells in vitro (Ito et al., 1997). Positive selection systems are currently being evaluated for their ability to induce amplification of pluripotent stem cells in mice.

In summary, various selection systems are undergoing development to provide a strategy for overcoming the limitation imposed by the low transduction efficiency of repopulating cells. Presently, the DHFR system appears to hold the most promise, but its future development is contingent on reproducing the success

achieved in the murine system in larger animal models. Alternative drug selection systems and the positive selection systems based on chimeric receptors are experimental strategies also worth pursuing.

GLOBIN GENE VECTORS

Effective gene therapy for hemoglobin disorders is likely to require expression vectors capable of supporting or stimulating a high level of globin synthesis. Maturing erythroblasts dedicate their protein synthetic material nearly exclusively to the production of hemoglobin. In postnatal humans, each erythroblast contains approximately 30,000 molecules of α- and β-globin mRNA. Some erythroblasts contain a small amount of γ-globin mRNA generated during the early stages of erythropoiesis. High levels of α- and β-globin mRNA are achieved by a high rate of transcription, efficient processing of the primary transcript, and great stability of mature globin mRNA (Volloch and Housman, 1981) (Chapter 8). Normal red cells have balanced α and non α globin synthesis, allowing virtually all globin chains to be assembled into hemoglobin tetramers ($\alpha_2\beta_2$, $\alpha_2\gamma\beta$ or $\alpha_2\gamma_2$) (Bunn, 1987).

Correction of the defect in β (or α) globin biosynthesis in the severe thalassemias will require production of an amount of globin equivalent to at least half, and preferably equal to, the output of a normal globin gene. The desired outcome of therapeutic intervention will be the conversion of a transfusion-dependent severe thalassemia to an asymptomatic thalassemia heterozygote. HbS-hereditary persistence of fetal hemoglobin (HPFH) (Chapters 15 and 28), where 20 percent fetal hemoglobin (HbF) is uniformly distributed among red cells, is asymptomatic (Bunn, 1997). Reproduction of this phenotype by insertion and expression of a provirally encoded globin gene will require expression equivalent to at least 20 percent the level of β^S globin production or 40 percent of the output of a single β^S gene. Because γ-globin chains compete favorably with β^S globin chains for available α chains (Bunn, 1987) (Chapter 8), vector-mediated addition of γ-globin should result in the displacement of an equivalent of β^S globin from the process of hemoglobin assembly. With a better understanding of the regulatory molecules that modulate expression of globin genes in maturing red cells of postnatal humans, expression cassettes may be designed that affect the activity of such molecules resulting in enhancement of γ-globin synthesis and a corresponding decrease in expression of the endogenous β-globin gene.

Much has been learned about the mechanisms of globin gene regulation that is relevant to vector design, but our understanding of this complex process is far from complete. Transcription factors are discussed in Chapter 4 and hemoglobin switching in Chapter 7.

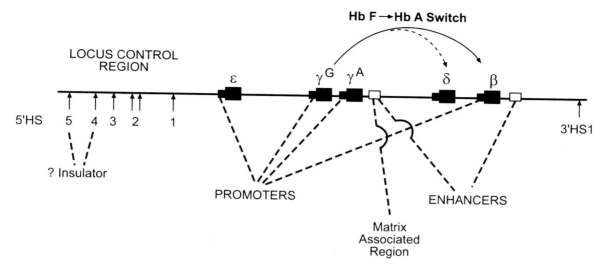

Figure 41.6. Organization of the human β-globin gene locus. Proximal regulatory elements include the promoters of the individual genes, as well as intragenic (not shown) and downstream, extragenic enhancers. The enhancer downstream from the γ-globin gene has been shown to bind to the nuclear matrix. Nuclease hypersensitive sites (HS) in chromatin are located upstream (5′ HS1 through 5′ HS5) and downstream (3′ HS1) from the gene cluster. The segment of DNA containing 5′ HS1, 5′ HS2, 5′ HS3, and 5′ HS4 constitutes the locus control region. The chicken homolog of 5′ HS5 has been shown to function as an insulator (Chung, et al., 1997), but human 5′ HS5 did not exhibit insulator activity in similar assays. No function has been ascribed to 3′ HS1. Certain regulatory elements are not shown (e.g. The ε-gene silencer, which overlaps with the promoter (Li et al., 1997), and sequences between the γ and β genes, which may have a role in hemoglobin switching (O'Neill et al., 1999).

Both the α- and β-globin loci include DNA regulatory elements within, or proximal to, each gene and additional regulatory elements that are located at some distance (Fig. 41.6). Gene proximal elements include the promoter sequences and intragenic and downstream enhancers (Grosveld et al., 1998; Li et al., 1998). Besides sequences directly involved in RNA splicing, the 3′ portion of the second intron contains sequences required for efficient 3′ end formation and polyadenylation (Antoniou et al., 1998) and the 3′ untranslated region contains sequences that confer stability on mature mRNA (Russell and Liebhaber, 1996; Holcik and Liebhaber, 1997).

In 1987, the locus control region (LCR) for the human β-globin gene cluster was defined (Grosveld et al., 1987) (see Chapters 5–7). First identified as a series of nuclease hypersensitive sites (HS) (Tuan et al., 1985; Forrester et al., 1987), functional studies suggested that the LCR confers position-independent, copy-number dependent expression of a β-globin gene in transgenic mice. Animals with the LCR linked to the β-globin gene

exhibited human β-globin gene expression at levels nearly equivalent to that of an endogenous mouse β-globin gene (Grosveld et al., 1987). The LCR has the properties of a powerful enhancer for which the individual globin gene promoters compete throughout development (Fraser and Grosveld, 1998; Reik et al., 1998). Regulatory elements outside the LCR are able to establish the open chromatic domain of the murine β-globin gene cluster (Epner et al., 1998). Insulators (Chung et al., 1997) and matrix attachment regions within the locus (Cunningham et al., 1994; Martin et al., 1996) are additional elements involved in formation of the open chromatin domain and in protecting the locus from the influence of regulatory elements outside of that domain (Fraser and Grosveld, 1998). Globin gene expression persists during terminal phases of erythroid maturation when most other genes are turned off. Little is known about the specific aspects of globin gene regulation that are responsible for persistent expression; therefore it is impossible to design expression cassettes that take into account this facet of globin gene expression and hemoglobin accumulation.

Retroviral Vectors

Design of retroviral vectors capable of highly efficient transfer of a globin gene into primitive hematopoietic cells and high level expression in differentiating erythroblasts is problematic. Initial attempts using globin cDNAs were unsuccessful because the level of expression was far too low for potential therapeutic benefit (Miller et al., 1988). An alternative strategy was incorporation of a genomic globin gene in the reverse transcription orientation to preserve intronic structure during generation of the viral genomic RNA (Table 41.1). Vector genomes having this configuration could be transmitted unrearranged

Table 41.1. Retroviral Vectors Tested for Globin Gene Transfer and Expression

1.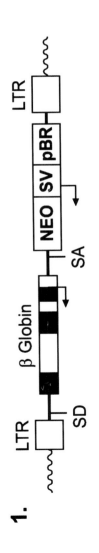

Cone et al., 1987; Weber-Benarous, et al., 1988; Dzierzak, Papayannopoulou and Mulligan, 1988.
Inducible expression of the human β-globin gene was demonstrated in murine and human erythroleukemia cells although the overall level of expression was very low. Transmission of the unrearranged vector genome into murine repopulating stem cells was demonstrated, resulting in tissue specific expression of the human β-globin gene in the erythroid lineage, albeit at very low levels.

2.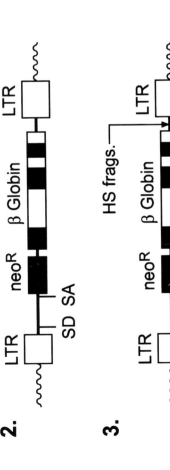

Karlsson et al., 1988; Bender, Gelinas and Miller, 1989.
Transmission of the unrearranged proviral genome into primitive murine repopulating cells was demonstrated. Expression persisted for up to four months at levels of 1% or less of a murine β-globin gene.

3.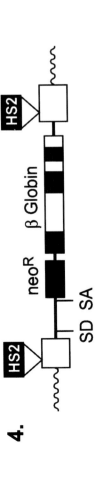

Novak et al., 1990.
Vectors containing HS1, HS2, HS3, HS4 or HS3 and HS4 were studied in murine erythroleukemia cells. Expression in individual clones was highly variable ranging from 35% to 132% of an endogenous murine β-globin gene compared to an average of 5.7% for the vector lacking LCR elements. Noteworthy is the fact that the producer clones were generally of low titer and frequently transmitted a rearranged proviral genome.

4.

Chang Liu and Kan, 1992.
HS2 sequences were inserted into the 3' LTR resulting in a "double copy" configuration following integration. Only a short, 36 base pair, fragment containing the tandem NF-E2 binding sites was stable in this configuration; longer HS2 fragments resulted in rearrangement during transfer of the vector genome. Producer clones were generally of low titer (10^3 to 10^5 neo^R units). Three murine erythroleukemia cell clones containing an unrearranged vector genome with the 36bp element expressed the human β-globin gene at 12% of the level a mouse α-gene compared to an average value of 6% for three clones containing a proviral genome without the HS2 element.

5.

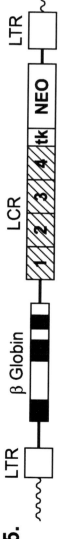

Plavec et al., 1993.

The LCR elements included in this vector genome ranged from 521 to 946 base pairs in size. Producer clones having titers in the range of 10^4 to 10^5 were isolated. Addition of the LCR elements increased expression of the β-globin gene approximately tenfold in murine erythroleukemia cells. Transmission of the proviral genome into repopulating cells was demonstrated in the majority of murine transplant recipients with expression in approximately 50%. From 0.4% to 12% of circulating erythrocytes contained human β-globin. Based on RNA levels, it was estimated that the human gene was expressed at approximately 10% to 39% of the level of a mouse β-globin gene.

6.

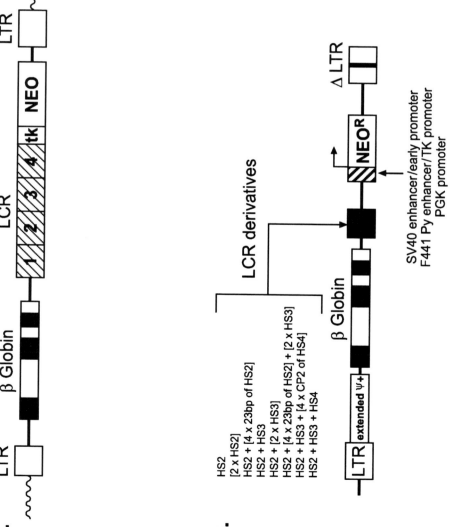

Leboulch et al., 1994; Raftopoulos et al., 1997.

Extensive, site-directed mutagenesis was performed to eliminate RNA processing signals from the DNA fragments included in this series of vector constructs. An approximate tenfold increase in titer was achieved as was an increased frequency of transmission of the unrearranged proviral genome. Transmission of selected vector genomes into repopulating murine stem cells was documented. In mouse erythroleukemia cells, the expression of the human β-globin gene was as high as 80% of a murine β-globin gene. In a second study, two mice having expression levels of 5% and 20% of that of the endogenous murine β-globin gene at six and eight months post-transplantation were described. Hematopoietic cells in several other transplant recipients contained a rearranged proviral genome.

(continued)

Table 41.1 (*continued*)

Takekoshi et al., 1995.
A hybrid δ/β gene was constructed to capitalize on the ability of δ-globin to inhibit polymerization of sickle hemoglobin. Expression in pools of mouse erythroleukemia cell clones was as high as 85% of a murine β-globin gene.

Sadelain et al., 1995; Rivella and Sadelain, 1998.
Empirical evaluation of multiple constructs containing a truncated β-globin gene and elements from the LCR identified the configuration shown on the left which allowed transmission of unrearranged proviral sequences with titers of greater than 10^6. Mouse erythroleukemia cells expressed the encoded human β-globin gene at levels between 4% and 46% of the level of a human β-globin gene within the normal locus on chromosome 11 in a erythroleukemia somatic cell hybrid. Although the human β-globin was initially expressed in mice repopulated with transduced hematopoietic cells, the level of expression diminished over time despite the persistence of maturing hematopoietic cells that contained the proviral genome.

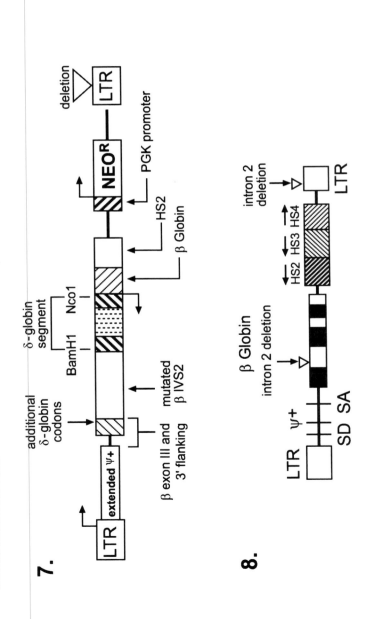

7.

8.

9.

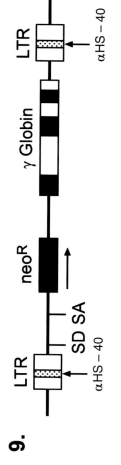

Ren et al., 1996.

This vector contains the human γ-globin gene in reverse transcription orientation between the LTRs, as shown, and a 255 base pair core element from the HS–40 site of the α-globin locus within the LTR in a "double copy" configuration. The γ-globin gene was expressed at levels comparable to that of a mouse β-globin gene in murine erythroleukemia cells. Subsequent work has shown that the γ-globin gene in this vector is expressed poorly in primary hematopoietic cells.

10.

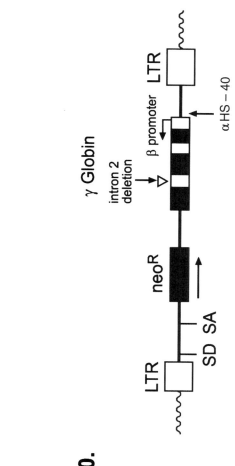

Li et al., 1999; Emery et al., 1999

In this vector, a segment of the large intron of the γ-globin gene has been deleted and the β-globin gene promoter has been substituted for the γ-promoter. The HS–40 core sequence from the α-globin locus has been tested in the configuration shown as well as within the LTR. High titer producer clones have been developed and the vector genome is transmitted into mouse erythroleukemia cells and murine erythroid progenitors where the hybrid globin gene is expressed at about 25% of the level of a mouse β-globin gene.

into murine repopulating cells, and the human globin gene was expressed specifically in the erythroid lineage. However, the level of expression was 1 percent or less of that of a murine β-globin gene.

Substantial effort was invested in defining the smallest fragments containing each of the HS sites that retained LCR activity (Philipsen et al., 1990; Talbot et al., 1990; Caterina et al., 1991; Pruzina et al., 1991; Liu et al., 1992; Philipsen et al., 1993). Core HS elements less than 1 kilobase in size were active in enhancing globin gene expression in transgenic mice. Unfortunately, incorporation of HS fragments into retroviral vectors proved highly problematic. Producer clones were generally of low titer and frequently transmitted a rearranged proviral genome. With effort, one could obtain erythroleukemia cell clones containing an intact proviral genome (Novak et al., 1990; Chang et al., 1992; Plavec et al., 1993). An increase in the expression of the encoded globin gene was observed from proviral genomes containing HS elements compared to control genomes, which did not (Table 41.1). Despite these apparent successes, such vectors have not been used in subsequent studies. None have been studied in the available murine models of human hemoglobin disorders (Ciavatta et al., 1995; Ryan et al., 1997; Nagel, 1998).

Two major efforts were undertaken to overcome the barriers associated with the development of useful globin retroviral vectors (Leboulch et al., 1994; Sadelain et al., 1995). Leboulch and colleagues (1994) used extensive site-directed mutagenesis to eliminate RNA processing signals from the β-globin gene and LCR fragments included in the vectors. Ultimately, a stable configuration was identified, and these vectors have now been studied in the murine transplant model. Expression of up to 20 percent of that of a mouse β-globin gene has been obtained (Raftopoulos et al., 1997). Sadelain et al., (1995) introduced a deletion of the second intron that eliminated RNA processing signals and empirically tested multiple orientations of several LCR fragments to identify an overall organization of the proviral genome that allowed transmission of unrearranged proviral sequences. Producer clones with titers more than 10^6 were obtained, but unfortunately the level of human β-globin gene expression diminished over time in the murine transplant model, suggesting silencing of the introduced gene (Rivella and Sadelain, 1998). Silencing of retroviral genomes may be caused by methylation of regulatory sequences. Histone deacetylation may also be involved in closing down the chromatin structure (Chen et al., 1997b). Studies in transgenic mice have shown that a retroviral LTR may result in silencing of a linked globin gene, which, without the LTR, is expressed at high levels in erythroid cells (McCune and Townes, 1994). Results in trans-

genic mice suggest that spacing and relative position and also the included sequences may be relevant to the influence of LTR elements on transgene expression (Ellis et al., 1997).

More recently, additional laboratories have begun to evaluate the ability to transfer a γ-globin gene with a retroviral vector (Ren, et al., 1996; Li, et al., 1999; Emery et al., 1999). Production of γ-globin chains in the red cells of patients with sickle cell disease is likely to be more effective therapeutically than production of normal β-globin because mixed tetramers (Hbα$_2$β^{S}γ) containing γ-globin do not participate in polymer formation (Chapters 10 and 23). Other genes for antisickling globins have been assembled (McCune et al., 1994; Takekoshi et al., 1995), although it is not clear that they have any advantage over γ-globin chains with respect to antisickling properties. Studies with γ-globin gene vectors have suggested that deletion of a large portion of the second intron improves vector stability and that the β-globin gene promoter is more active than that of the native γ-globin gene. HS–40 from the α-globin locus (Chapter 17) has been used as an "enhancer" either between the LTRs upstream from the β-globin gene promoter or within the LTRs in the double-copy configuration (Table 41.1). High titer producer clones transmit the proviral genome unrearranged into mouse erythroleukemia cells where the hybrid gene is expressed at levels up to 20 to 25 percent the level of a mouse β-globin gene. To date, no long-term studies in mice have been reported with respect to the transmission, stability, and expression of the encoded hybrid globin gene with this vector configuration.

The influence of insulator elements on globin gene expression within a retroviral genome has yet to be reported. Scaffold attachment regions (SARs) may enhance vector-encoded sequence expression in T lymphocytes and macrophages (Agarwal et al., 1998; Auten et al., 1999), but similar studies have not been reported for globin gene vectors. Of potential interest in this regard is the 3′ regulatory element downstream from the ^{A}γ-globin gene, which can function as a SAR (Cunningham et al., 1994).

As discussed, lentiviral vectors derived from HIV transduce quiescent cells more efficiently than conventional oncoretroviral vectors, the preintegration nucleoprotein complex of lentiviral vectors is stable over several days after transduction, and this complex can traverse this nuclear membrane without cell division. Based on the reports of successful transfer and expression of a γ-globin gene cassette derived from a genomic globin gene with oncoretroviral vectors (Table 41.1), we have tested similar designs in an HIV-based lentiviral vector system. The globin gene cassette was placed in a reverse transcriptional orientation upstream from the GFP coding sequences driven by the β-actin promoter. Vector particles were generated with a triple transection system consisting of a plasmid encoding the HIV components without envelope, a second plasmid encoding the vesicular stomatitis virus G envelope protein, and a third plasmid containing the vector genome. A vector encoding the full genomic $^A\gamma$-globin gene had very low titers, whereas a second vector with most of the second intron removed yielded vector preparations having higher titers. This vector genome could be transmitted unrearranged into erythroleukemia cells, although the level of expression of the encoded globin gene, which in this case was driven by the β-spectrin promoter, was relatively low. From these results, we tentatively conclude that the same issues that have arisen in the design and testing of oncoretroviral vectors containing globin genes will be relevant to the design of HIV-based vectors for globin gene transfer.

Recombinant Adeno-Associated Viral Vectors

Recombinant adeno-associated viral (rAAV) vectors were initially tested for globin gene transfer using a vector configuration that included a dominant selectable marker such as the phosphotransferase, which confers neomycin resistance (Neo) (Walsh et al., 1992; Miller et al., 1993; Einerhand et al., 1995; Zhou et al., 1996). Neo clones of transduced erythroleukemia cells could be recovered and many, but not all, contained an unrearranged proviral genome with an intact globin gene. When an element from HS2 was included, expression of the transferred globin gene in human erythroleukemia cells approximated that of an endogenous globin gene. Transduction of human primary erythroid progenitors with a vector lacking the Neo marker but containing additional elements from the LCR resulted in expression of the encoded γ-globin gene and measurable synthesis of HbF (Miller et al., 1994).

Discovery that rAAV may transduce cells relatively efficiently and express their encoded genes from an episomal form of the vector genome without subsequent genome integration (Bertran et al., 1996; Malik et al., 1997) raised concerns regarding the potential usefulness of rAAV for stem cell targeted gene transfer. A vector, rHS432$^A\gamma$*, was evaluated using human erythroleukemia cells as a model (Hargrove et al., 1997). Transduced cells were plated in semisolid medium, and 2 weeks later individual colonies were isolated and the cells analyzed, after expansion, for genome expression and integration. Two weeks after transduction, all colonies contained the $^A\gamma$*mRNA but only five of sixteen studied had an integrated, unrearranged rAAV genome. A second vector from which HS4 had been removed and a regulatory element (3′RE) downstream from the $^A\gamma$-globin gene added, rHS432$^A\gamma$*3′RE, was

also studied. At an MOI of 10^9, this vector integrated at high efficiency as an intact, tandem head-to-tail concatamer, with a median copy number of 6 and variable expression per copy ranging from approximately onefold to threefold that of an endogenous γ-globin gene. Others have reported transduction of primitive hematopoietic cells at lower MOIs (Lubovy et al., 1996; Chatterjee et al., 1999). These apparently contradictory results are unresolved.

Primary hematopoietic progenitor transduction with highly purified rAAV preparations free of wild-type AAV, and helper adenovirus has recently been reevaluated (Nathwani et al., 1999a). The rAAV studied encoded GFP and a drug-resistant variant of human DHFR. At an MOI of 10^7, 60 to 70 percent of CD34$^+$ cells expressed the GFP marker 48 hours after transduction, but only rare colonies formed during 2 weeks of culture in semisolid medium in the presence of trimetrexate. These result indicate that the rAAV genome was taken up and converted into an expressed, double-stranded episomal form, but that failure of integration accounted for the inability to achieve a drug-resistant phenotype during proliferation of the transduced progenitors. Earlier studies, where primary progenitors had been transduced at lower MOIs, were performed with crude preparations of vector particles that were highly contaminated with denatured adenoviral particles. These adenoviral particles may have facilitated uptake of the rAAV vector particles. As the methodology for making highly purified rAAV is improved (Conway et al., 1997; Xiao et al., 1998), it will be worthwhile to test the ability to transduce primary progenitors at MOIs of 10^9, levels, which resulted in vector genome integration in erythroleukemia cells.

Whether rAAV has potential value for gene transfer into hematopoietic stem cells appears highly problematic. Very high MOI, not achievable with current methods of virus production, may be required. The best results have been obtained with a vector that contains a MAR, although the multicopy head-to-tail tandem arrays integrated in erythroleukemia cells (Hargrove et al., 1997), if reproduced in primary hematopoietic cells, may not be optimal because of the resulting variable levels of globin gene expression in maturing erythroblasts. Presently, retroviral vectors appear to be more promising because of the predictable integration of one or at most two or three vector genomes of defined configuration.

STRATEGIES TO GENETICALLY ENHANCE HbF SYNTHESIS

An alternative approach to the development of effective gene therapy for hemoglobin disorders is to devise strategies to reactivate the γ-globin genes. HbF has nearly normal function and inhibits HbS polymerization (Chapter 10). In all HPFH, increased γ-globin synthesis is accompanied by a proportionate reduction in β-globin synthesis. This reciprocal change in the level of expression of the two genes presumably reflects competition between their proximal regulatory elements for the LCR, which in turn reflects the balance of transcriptional factor activity (Fraser and Grosveld, 1998). Therefore, genetic reactivation of HbF by modulation of specific transacting factor activity seems likely to result in an increase in γ and a turn down of β^S synthesis, preserving the overall balance between α and a non-α-globin chain production.

Another feature of hemoglobin synthesis, asynchronous production of γ- and β-globin chains during erythroid maturation in adult bone marrow, has provoked interest in targeting the γ-globin gene for genetic manipulation (Chui et al., 1980; Farquhar et al., 1981). This gene is incompletely silenced following the neonatal switch; normal adults have F cells containing 4 to 8 picograms of HbF (Wood et al., 1975; Boyer et al., 1975) (Chapter 10). Accumulation of γ globin occurs predominantly in the proerythroblast and basophilic erythroblast stages of erythropoiesis. As maturation progresses, there is a substantial increase in β-globin synthesis, leading to predominant accumulation of HbA (or HbS in sickle cell disease). Although there is heterogeneous distribution of HbF among mature erythrocytes, the capacity for γ-globin gene expression may be more uniformly distributed but effectively silenced in most earlier erythroblasts. The recapitulation of the γ to β switch during normal erythropoiesis and competition between the two genes for regulatory elements of the LCR suggests that a perturbation in transcriptional factor activity, tolerated by maturing erythroblasts, may be sufficient to substantially enhance γ-globin chain synthesis.

Switching Mechanism (Chapter 7)

Globin genes exhibit tissue-specific expression, and individual genes are selectively expressed during development. Low level, tissue-specific expression of individual globin genes in transgenic mice is mediated by their promoters and proximal enhancer sequences, but the LCR is required for high level expression (Fraser and Grosveld, 1998; Hardison et al., 1997) (Chapter 34). The LCR interacts with promoters of individual globin genes through formation of multicomponent complexes that include proteins that bind to the promoter or the HS with DNA sequence specificity. Competition for the LCR is determined in part by gene order and by the relative amounts of transcriptional factors and co-factors. Direct evidence that there is

alternative, competitive interaction of the LCR with the γ- and β-globin genes in human erythroid cells has been obtained by fluorescent in situ hybridization (Wijgerde et al., 1995).

Trans-Acting Factors (Chapter 4)

Only a few proteins have been directly implicated in controlling globin gene switching. These include GATA-1 and YY1 that interact with the ε-globin gene silencer in extinguishing ε-globin gene expression after the embryonic phase of erythropoiesis (Li et al., 1998). Enforced overexpression of GATA-1 in transgenic animals reduces expression of the ε-globin gene in yolk sac-derived erythroblasts (Li et al., 1997). Substantial evidence implicates erythroid Krüppel-like factor (EKLF), which interacts with the promoter CACCC box in achieving high levels of β-globin gene expression in adult red cells (Wijgerde et al., 1996; Bieker et al., 1998). Mice nullizygous for the EKLF gene have a severe deficiency of β-globin chain synthesis (Perkins et al., 1995; Nuez et al., 1995), but γ-globin gene expression is prolonged in EKLF (-/-) animals with the human β-globin locus present as a transgenic element. Conversely, overexpression of EKLF as a transgene results in accelerated γ to β switch in mice also harboring a β-locus transgene (Tewari et al., 1998). EKLF appears to activate the β promoter through interactions with CREB-binding protein (CBP), a co-activator with abilities to remodel chromatin through a histone acetylase domain and to directly interact with basal transcription machinery (J. Cunningham, unpublished observations). Further evidence suggests that a tripartite complex forms between EKLF, CBP, and TAF 130 (TATA-binding protein associated factor) in activating the β-globin gene promoter. Preliminary studies suggest that a transdominant mutant of EKLF (amino acids 250 to 362), when expressed by retroviral-mediated gene transfer in mice, which contain the human β-globin gene locus, increases γ-globin gene expression. A fetal stage-specific EKLF-like factor, FKLF, has been identified and molecularly cloned (Asano et al., 1999). FKLF interacts specifically with the γ-globin gene CACCC box. Its enforced overexpression in erythroleukemia cells results in augmented γ- and ε-globin gene production.

Sequences immediately upstream from the TATA box in the proximal γ-globin gene promoter are conserved in species in which there is fetal-specific expression of a γ-homologous gene (Chapter 5) and are thought to function as a stage selector element (SSE) (Jane et al., 1992). These sequences bind a heteromeric protein complex (SSP) that includes CP2, the chicken homolog of which has been implicated in the developmental control of globin gene expression (Jane et al.,

1995). SSP is thought to function by enhancing the attraction of the LCR to the transcription initiation complex assembled on the γ-globin gene promoter. Recent work has resulted in the identification of a protein termed NF-E4, which is the heterodimeric partner of CP2 in forming the SSP complex (Zhou et al., 1999). NF-E4 is a rare protein expressed in the fetal kidney and in the placenta only during the fetal stage of erythropoiesis. Current work is focused on evaluating the consequences of enforced overexpression of NF-E4 on the relative synthesis of γ- and β-globin in transgenic mice and maturing erythroblasts.

Another strategy for identifying novel γ-globin gene regulatory proteins involves screening with unique pharmacologic compounds defined in a high throughput drug screen for agents capable of inducing transcription specifically from the γ-globin gene promoter. A total of 54,656 compounds were screened using a stable human erythroleukemia cell line containing an HS2-γ-promoter/luciferase reporter gene (Holmes et al., 1999). This strategy was based on the hypothesis that many such compounds act directly through a transcriptional mechanism to induce γ-specific *trans*-acting factors that may be identified by representational difference analysis (RDA) of cDNAs derived from induced versus uninduced K562 cells. Using this strategy with one of the most active compounds (OSI-2040), marked enhancement of expression of a helix-loop-helix protein, Id2, was identified (Holmes et al., 1999). Retroviral-mediated enforced expression of Id2 in K562 cells resulted in a tenfold augmentation of γ-globin synthesis. A similar augmentation of γ-globin production has been shown in maturing erythroblasts derived from transduced human clonogenic progenitors.

SUMMARY

Gene therapy for the hemoglobin disorders will require substantial additional effort. Promising strategies to overcome the barriers to stem cell gene transfer must be integrated with efforts to design vectors that increase production of therapeutic levels of globin, either by transfer of a globin gene or by activation of the endogenous γ-globin genes. Significant efforts to achieve these goals over the last 15 years have been rewarded with gradual progress on which future advances will depend.

GLOSSARY OF GENE THERAPY TERMINOLOGY

Amphotropic. Amphotropic retroviruses are defined by the amphotropic envelope on the surface of the virion. Amphotropic retroviruses have a wide host range that includes both rodent and human cells. The host specificity is determined by the interaction of the amphotropic envelop protein with a specific phosphate transporter on the cell surface. Amphotropic retroviral vectors have been used in human and in monkey gene transfer experiments.

Cap Proteins. This refers to the capsid protein of the adeno-associated virus (AAV). The Cap protein is expressed on the coat of the AAV vector particles and mediates a specific interaction with cellular receptors on the target cell.

CH-296. This refers to a specific recombinant fragment of fibronectin. The CH-296 fragment contains the sequences for hematopoietic stem cell binding and immobilization of retroviral particles. Transduction in the presence of the CH-296 fragment greatly facilitates gene transfer into hematopoietic stem cells.

E1, E2, E3, E4. These refer to nonstructural genes in wild-type adenovirus that are required for the normal viral life cycle and infectivity. These early region genes can be deleted from third generation adenoviral vectors, however the E1 function must be provided in trans for vector particle formation.

Ecotropic. Ecotropic retrovirus is defined by the envelope protein present on the viral particle surface. Ecotropic retroviruses only infect rodent cells. This specificity is determined by the interaction of the ecotropic envelope protein with a specific amino acid transport molecule on the host cell surface that functions as a viral receptor. Ecotropic viruses are typically utilized for gene therapy experiments using mice.

env. This refers to the structural coat protein of the retroviral particle. The structure and sequence of the envelope protein will determine the host cell specificity of the retroviral vector. The specific envelope protein used in a retroviral vector can have an important effect in determining the transducibility of the target cell. The envelope protein interacts with specific cellular receptors on the target cell surface.

gag. The retroviral *gag* gene encodes a polyprotein that functions in both virion assembly and infection. The *gag* protein is made up of matrix, capsid and nucleocapsid proteins. In some viruses, the *gag* region may also contain additional small peptides. Processing of the poly *gag* protein into individual proteins is necessary for viral infectivity.

Gibbon Ape Leukemia Virus (GALV). GALV refers to an envelope protein derived from the Gibbon Ape leukemia virus. This envelope protein has a similar tropism to that derived from amphotropic retroviral vectors, with the exception that GALV pseudotyped vectors do not transduce murine cells. The

GALV envelope protein interacts with an alternate phosphate transporter distinct from that utilized by the amphotropic retroviruses. GALV pseudotyped vectors had been used to transduce primate hematopoietic cells.

Inverted Terminal Repeats (ITRs). This refers to a 145 base pair region that flanks the adeno-associated virus DNA genome. The ITRs are necessary for vector particle generation and integration into the target cell chromosome.

Lentivirus. This class of retroviruses has a more complex genome than oncoretroviruses. Lentiviral vectors have been derived from the human immunodeficiency (HIV) retrovirus. Lentiviruses typically express a number of accessory proteins necessary for the viral life cycle in addition to the gag, pol and env proteins. A potential advantage of lentiviral vectors is their ability to stably integrate into the chromosomes of non-dividing host cells.

Long Terminal Repeats (LTRs). Long terminal repeats comprise two sequences regions that flank both the 5′ and 3′ regions of the proviral DNA of a retrovirus. The LTR regions contain the promoter sequences necessary for transcription, a sequence for polyadenylation of the mRNA transcript, enhancer sequences that augment transcription, and sequences necessary for the integration into the host cell genome.

Moloney Virus. This refers to a specific type of murine leukemia virus that has been commonly used in retroviral-mediated gene transfer. Related mouse retroviruses that have been used in gene transfer experiments include the Harvey murine sarcoma virus, the myeloproliferative sarcoma virus, and the murine stem cell virus. These viruses have the same general structure of the Moloney virus but differ in specific sequences within the long terminal repeats, in primer binding sites, and in other non-coding sequences present within the viral vector backbone.

Oncoretrovirus. This refers to a class of retroviruses typified by the murine leukemia viruses. Oncoretroviruses have a relatively simple structure, and are one of the most commonly used types of retroviral vectors. One limitation with oncoretroviral vectors is that they require host cell mitosis for integration of a vector genome.

Packaging Cells. These refer to cells that have been genetically engineered to produce the viral proteins necessary for viral particle formation. These proteins are expressed from constructs encoding mRNAs that cannot be packaged. As a result, packaging cells do not produce infectious viral particles or vectors. As an example, retroviral packaging cells contain constructs that encode for gag, pol and env proteins.

pol. The *pol* gene encodes the retroviral reverse transcriptase enzyme necessary for formation of the DNA provirus using the genomic viral RNA as a template.

Producer Cells. Producer cells are packaging cells that have had a viral vector genome introduced. These cells will release vector particles into the supernatant that can be used for gene transfer into target cells.

Provirus. This refers to the double stranded DNA genome of a retrovirus. The provirus is formed after reverse transcription of the single stranded RNA genome. The double stranded DNA provirus then integrates into the host cell chromosome.

Pseudotyping. This refers to a process by which a retroviral vector is generated that expresses an alternate envelope protein on the viral particle surface. This is accomplished by introducing a heterologous envelope gene into the packaging cell that can function in packaging, particle formation, and infectivity in the target cell.

Rep Protein. This is a nonstructural protein component of the adeno-associated virus. A number of Rep proteins are expressed by wild-type AAV and their function has been associated with integration of the AAV genome into specific sites in the host cell chromosome.

Replication Competent Retrovirus (RCR). Replication competent retrovirus refers to viral particles that contain the viral proteins necessary for viral replication. Cells infected with replication competent retrovirus will produce infectious particles. In contrast, when a retroviral vector is inserted into a host cell, that host cell will no longer be able to produce retroviral particles. RCR can sometimes arise due to unintended homologous recombination between vector genome sequences and sequences present in packaging cells.

Self-Inactivating (SIN) Vector. These refer to vectors that contain deletions in the LTR promoter regions. SIN vectors lack LTR promoter activity after integration in target cells and have been used when other transcriptional cassettes are included in the vector.

Titer. This refers to the concentration of viral particles present in the supernatant of virus producing cells. The titer associated with individual producer cell clones is critically important for gene transfer efficiency. There are a number of different assays for measuring viral titers, and efficient stem cell transduction usually requires titers greater than 1×10^6 infectious particles per milliliter.

VSV-G. This refers to the vesicular stomatitis virus G protein. The G protein from VSV has been used for pseudotyping both retroviral and lentiviral vectors. The advantage of VSV-G is that it utilizes a ubiquitous phospholipid for cellular entry.

References

Agarwal, M, Austin, TW, Morel, F et al. (1998). Scaffold attachment region-mediated enhancement of retroviral vector expression in primary T cells. *J. Virol.* 72: 3720–3728.

Akkina, RK, Walton, RM, Chen, ML et al. (1996). High-efficiency gene transfer into CD34+ cells with a human immunodeficiency virus type 1-based retroviral vector pseudotyped with vesicular stomatitis virus envelope glycoprotein G. *J. Virol.* 70: 2581–2585.

Alexander, IE, Russell, DW, and Miller, AD. (1994). DNA-damaging agents greatly increase the transduction of nondividing cells by adeno-associated virus vectors. *J. Virol.* 68: 8282–8287.

Alexander, IE, Russell, DW, Spence, AM, and Miller, AD. (1996). Effects of gamma irradiation on the transduction of dividing and nondividing cells in brain and muscle of rats by adeno-associated virus vectors. *Hum. Gene Ther.* 7: 841–850.

Ali, M, Taylor, GP, Pitman, RJ et al. (1996). No evidence of antibody to human foamy virus in widespread human populations. *AIDS Res. Hum. Retroviruses* 12: 1473–1483.

Allay, JA, Davis, BM, and Gerson, SL. (1997b). Human alkyltransferase-transduced murine myeloid progenitors are enriched in vivo by BCNU treatment of transplanted mice. *Exp. Hematol.* 25: 1069–1076.

Allay, JA, Dumenco, LL, Koc, ON et al. (1995). Retroviral transduction and expression of the human alkyltransferase cDNA provides nitrosourea resistance to hematopoietic cells. *Blood* 85: 3342–3351.

Allay, JA, Persons, DA, Galipeau, J et al. (1998). In vivo selection of retrovirally transduced hematopoietic stem cells. *Nat. Med.* 4: 1136–1143.

Allay, JA, Spencer, HT, Wilkinson, SL et al. (1997a). Sensitization of hematopoietic stem and progenitor cells to trimetrexate using nucleoside transport inhibitors. *Blood* 90: 3546–3554.

Allen, JM, Debelak, DJ, Reynolds, TC, and Miller, AD. (1997). Identification and elimination of replication-competent adeno-associated virus (AAV) that can arise by nonhomologous recombination during AAV vector production. *J. Virol.* 71: 6816–6822.

Antoniou, M, Geraghty, F, Hurst, J, and Grosveld, F. (1998). Efficient 3′-end formation of human beta-globin mRNA in vivo requires sequences within the last intron but occurs independently of the splicing reaction. *Nucleic Acids Res.* 26: 721–729.

Asano, H, Li, XS, and Stamatoyannopoulos, G. (1999). FKLF, a novel kruppel-like factor that activates human embryonic and fetal-like globin genes. *Mol. Cell Biol.* 19: 3571–3579.

Auten, J, Agarwal, M, Chen, J et al. (1999). Effect of scaffold attachment region on transgene expression in retrovirus vector-transduced primary T cells and macrophages. *Hum. Gene Ther.* 10: 1389–1399.

Bauer, TRJ, Miller, AD, and Hickstein, DD. (1995). Improved transfer of the leukocyte integrin CD18 subunit into hematopoietic cell lines by using retroviral vectors having a gibbon ape leukemia virus envelope. *Blood* 86: 2379–2387.

Bender, MA, Gelinas, RE, and Miller, AD. (1989). A majority of mice show long-term expression of a human beta-globin gene after retrovirus transfer into hematopoietic stem cells. *Mol. Cell. Biol.* 9: 1426–1434.

Bender, MA, Palmer, TD, Gelinas, RE, and Miller, AD. (1987). Evidence that the packaging signal of Moloney murine leukemia virus extends into the gag region. *J. Virol.* 61: 1639–1646.

Benz, EJ Jr, and Forget, BG. (1971). Defect in messenger RNA for human hemoglobin synthesis in beta thalassemia. *J. Clin. Invest.* 50: 2755–2760.

Bergelson, JM, Cunningham, JA, Droguett, G et al. (1997). Isolation of a common receptor for Coxsackie B viruses and adenoviruses 2 and 5. *Science* 275: 1320–1323.

Bertran, J, Miller, JL, Yang, Y et al. (1996). Recombinant adeno-associated virus-mediated high-efficiency, transient expression of the murine cationic amino acid transporter (ecotropic retroviral receptor) permits stable transduction of human HeLa cells by ecotropic retroviral vectors. *J. Virol.* 70: 6759–6766.

Bertran, J, Yang, Y, Hargrove, P et al. (1998). Targeted integration of a recombinant globin gene adeno-associated viral vector into human chromosome 19. *Ann. N.Y. Acad. Sci.* 850: 163–177.

Bhatia, M, Bonnet, D, Kapp, U et al. (1997). Quantitative analysis reveals expansion of human hematopoietic repopulating cells after short-term ex vivo culture. *J. Exp. Med.* 186: 619–624.

Bieker, JJ, Ouyang, L, and Chen, X. (1998). Transcriptional factors for specific globin genes. *Ann. N.Y. Acad. Sci.* 850: 64–69.

Bieniasz, PD, Erlwein, O, Aguzzi, A et al. (1997). Gene transfer using replication-defective human foamy virus vectors. *Virology* 235: 65–72.

Bieniasz, PD, Weiss, RA, and McClure, MO. (1995). Cell cycle dependence of foamy retrovirus infection. *J. Virol.* 69: 7295–7299.

Bienzle, D, Abrams-Ogg, AC, Kruth, SA et al. (1994). Gene transfer into hematopoietic stem cells: long-term maintenance of in vitro activated progenitors without marrow ablation. *Proc. Natl. Acad. Sci. U.S.A.* 91: 350–354.

Bjorgvinsdottir, H, Ding, C, Pech, N et al. (1997). Retroviral-mediated gene transfer of gp91phox into bone marrow cells rescues defect in host defense against Aspergillus fumigatus in murine X-linked chronic granulomatous disease. *Blood* 89: 41–48.

Blaese, RM, Culver, KW, Miller, AD et al. (1995). T lymphocyte-directed gene therapy for ADA- SCID: Initial trial results after 4 years. *Science* 270: 475–480.

Blau, CA, Neff, T, and Papayannopoulou, T. (1996). The hematological effects of folate analogs: implications for using the dihydrofolate reductase gene for in vivo selection. *Hum. Gene Ther.* 7: 2069–2078.

Blau, CA, Peterson, KR, Drachman, JG, and Spencer, DM. (1997). A proliferation switch for genetically modified cells. *Proc. Natl. Acad. Sci. U.S.A.* 94: 3076–3081.

Blomer, U, Naldini, L, Kafri, T et al. (1997). Highly efficient and sustained gene transfer in adult neurons with a lentivirus vector. *J. Virol.* 71: 6641–6649.

Bodine, DM, Karlsson, S, and Nienhuis, AW. (1989). Combination of interleukins 3 and 6 preserves stem cell function in culture and enhances retrovirus-mediated gene transfer into hematopoietic stem cells. *Proc. Natl. Acad. Sci. U.S.A.* 86: 8897–8901.

Bodine, DM, McDonagh, KT, Seidel, NE, and Nienhuis, AW. (1991). Survival and retrovirus infection of murine hematopoietic stem cells in vitro: effects of 5-FU and method of infection. *Exp. Hematol.* 19: 206–212.

Bodine, DM, Moritz, T, Donahue, RE et al. (1993). Long-term in vivo expression of a murine adenosine deaminase gene in rhesus monkey hematopoietic cells of multiple lineages after retroviral mediated gene transfer into CD34+ bone marrow cells. *Blood* 82: 1975–1980.

Bodine, DM, Seidel, NE, Gale, MS et al. (1994). Efficient retrovirus transduction of mouse pluripotent hematopoietic stem cells mobilized into the peripheral blood by treatment with granulocyte colony-stimulating factor and stem cell factor. *Blood* 84: 1482–1491.

Bodine, DM, Seidel, NE, and Orlic, D. (1996). Bone marrow collected 14 days after in vivo administration of granulocyte colony-stimulating factor and stem cell factor to mice has 10-fold more repopulating ability than untreated bone marrow. *Blood* 88: 89–97.

Boesen, JJB, Brouwer, KB, Breems, DA et al. (1995). Transfer of the human multidrug resistance-1 (MDR-1) gene in primitive hemopoietic precursor cells in a rhesus monkey gene therapy model. *Blood* 86: A1170(Abstract).

Bordignon, C, Notarangelo, LD, Nobili, N, Ferrari, G, Casorati, G, Panina, P, Mazzolari, E, Maggioni, D, Rossi, C, and Servida, P. (1995). Gene therapy in peripheral blood lymphocytes and bone marrow for ADA-immunodeficient patients. *Science* 270: 470–475.

Boyer, SH, Belding, TK, Margolet, L, and Noyes, AN. (1975). Fetal hemoglobin restriction to a few erythrocytes (F cells) in normal human adults. *Science* 188: 361–363.

Brenner, MK, Rill, DR, Holladay, MS et al. (1993a). Gene marking to determine whether autologous marrow infusion restores long-term haemopoiesis in cancer patients. *Lancet* 342: 1134–1137.

Brenner, MK, Rill, DR, Moen, RC et al. (1993b). Gene-marking to trace origin of relapse after autologous bone-marrow transplantation. *Lancet* 341: 85–86.

Bukrinsky, MI, Haggerty, S, Dempsey, MP et al. (1993). A nuclear localization signal within HIV-1 matrix protein that governs infection of non-dividing cells [see comments]. *Nature* 365: 666–669.

Bunn, HF. (1987). Subunit assembly of hemoglobin: An important determinant of hematologic phenotype. *Blood* 69: 1–6.

Bunn, HF. (1997). Pathogenesis and treatment of sickle cell disease. *N. Engl. J.Med.* 337: 762–769.

Bunting, KD, Flynn, KJ, Riberdy, JM et al. (1999). Virus-specific immunity after gene therapy in a murine model of severe combined imunodeficiency. *Proc. Natl. Acad. Sci. U.S.A.* 96: 232–237.

Bunting, KD, Galipeau, J, Topham, D et al. (1998a). Transduction of murine bone marrow cells with an MDR1 vector enables ex vivo stem cell expansion, but these expanded grafts cause a myeloproliferative syndrome in transplanted mice. *Blood* 92: 2269–2279.

Bunting, KD, Sangster, MY, Ihle, JN, and Sorrentino, BP. (1998b). Restoration of lymphocyte function in Janus kinase 3-deficient mice by retroviral-mediated gene transfer [see comments]. *Nat. Med.* 4: 58–64.

Burns, JC, Friedmann, T, Driever, W et al. (1993). Vesicular stomatitis virus G glycoprotein pseudotyped retroviral vectors: Concentration to very high titer and efficient gene transfer into mammalian and nonmammalian cells [see comments]. *Proc. Natl. Acad. Sci. U.S.A.* 90: 8033–8037.

Caterina, JJ, Ryan, TM, Pawlik, KM et al. (1991). Human beta-globin locus control region: Analysis of the 5′ DNase I hypersensitive site HS 2 in transgenic mice. *Proc. Natl. Acad. Sci. U.S.A.* 88: 1626–1630.

Challita, PM and Kohn, DB. (1994). Lack of expression from a retroviral vector after transduction of murine hematopoietic stem cells is associated with methylation in vivo. *Proc. Natl. Acad. Sci. U.S.A.* 91: 2567–2571.

Challita, PM, Skelton, D, el-Khoueiry, A et al. (1995). Multiple modifications in cis elements of the long terminal repeat of retroviral vectors lead to increased expression and decreased DNA methylation in embryonic carcinoma cells. *J. Virol.* 69: 748–755.

Chang, JC, Liu, D, and Kan, YW. (1992). A 36-base-pair core sequence of locus control region enhances retrovirally transferred human beta-globin gene expression. *Proc. Natl. Acad. Sci. U.S.A.* 89: 3107–3110.

Chatterjee, S, Li, W, Wong, CA et al. (1999). Transduction of primitive human marrow and cord blood-derived hematopoietic progenitor cells with adeno-associated virus vectors. *Blood* 93: 1882–1894.

Chen, HH, Mack, LM, Kelly, R et al. (1997a). Persistence in muscle of an adenoviral vector that lacks all viral genes. *Proc. Natl. Acad. Sci. U.S.A.* 94: 1645–1650.

Chen, WY, Bailey, EC, McCune, SL et al. (1997b). Reactivation of silenced, virally transduced genes by inhibitors of histone deacetylase. *Proc. Natl. Acad. Sci. U.S.A.* 94: 5798–5803.

Chiorini, JA, Yang, L, Liu, Y et al. (1997). Cloning of adeno-associated virus type 4 (AAV4) and generation of recombinant AAV4 particles. *J. Virol.* 71: 6823–6833.

Chui, DH, Wong, SC, Enkin, MW et al. (1980). Proportion of fetal hemoglobin synthesis decreases during erythroid cell maturation. *Proc. Natl. Acad. Sci. U.S.A.* 77: 2757–2761.

Chung, JH, Bell, AC, and Felsenfeld, G. (1997). Characterization of the chicken beta-globin insulator. *Proc. Natl. Acad. Sci. U.S.A.* 94: 575–580.

Ciavatta, DJ, Ryan, TM, Farmer, SC, and Townes, TM. (1995). Mouse model of human β^0 thalassemia: targeted deletion of the mouse β^{maj}- and β^{min}-globin genes in embryonic stem cells. *Proc. Natl. Acad. Sci. U.S.A.* 92: 9259–9263.

Cone, RD and Mulligan, RC. (1984). High-efficiency gene transfer into mammalian cells: generation of helper-free recombinant retrovirus with broad mammalian host range. *Proc. Natl. Acad. Sci. U.S.A.* 81: 6349–6353.

Cone, RD, Weber-Benarous, A, Baorto, D, and Mulligan, RC. (1987). Regulated expression of a complete human beta-globin gene encoded by a transmissible retrovirus vector. *Mol. Cell. Biol.* 7: 887–897.

Conneally, E, Eaves, CJ, and Humphries, RK. (1998). Efficient retroviral-mediated gene transfer to human cord blood stem cells with in vivo repopulating potential. *Blood* 91: 3487–3493.

Conway, JE, Zolotukhin, S, Muzyczka, N et al. (1997). Recombinant adeno-associated virus type 2 replication and packaging is entirely supported by a herpes simplex virus type 1 amplicon expressing Rep and Cap. *J. Virol.* 71: 8780–8789.

Crooks, GM and Kohn, DB. (1993). Growth factors increase amphotropic retrovirus binding to human CD34+ bone marrow progenitor cells. *Blood* 82: 3290–3297.

Cunningham, JM, Purucker, ME, Jane, SM et al. (1994). The regulatory element 3′ to the A gamma-globin gene binds to the nuclear matrix and interacts with special A-T-rich binding protein 1 (SATB1), an SAR/MAR-associating region DNA binding protein. *Blood* 84: 1298–1308.

Dao, MA, Hashino, K, Kato, I, and Nolta, JA. (1998a). Adhesion to fibronectin maintains regenerative capacity during ex vivo culture and transduction of human hematopoietic stem and progenitor cells. *Blood* 92: 4612–4621.

Dao, MA, Taylor, N, and Nolta, JA. (1998b). Reduction in levels of the cyclin-dependent kinase inhibitor p27(kip-1) coupled with transforming growth factor beta neutralization induces cell-cycle entry and increases retroviral transduction of primitive human hematopoietic cells. *Proc. Natl. Acad. Sci. U.S.A.* 95: 13006–13011.

Davidson, BL, Allen, ED, Kozarsky, KF et al. (1993). A model system for in vivo gene transfer into the central nervous system using an adenoviral vector [see comments]. *Nat. Genet.* 3: 219–223.

Davis, BM, Reese, JS, Koc, ON et al. (1997). Selection for G156A O^6-methylguanine DNA methyltransferase gene-transduced hematopoietic progenitors and protection from lethality in mice treated with O^6-benzylguanine and 1,3-Bis(2-chloroethyl)-1-nitrosourea. *Cancer Res.* 57: 5093–5099.

Davis, JL, Witt, RM, Gross, PR et al. (1997). Retroviral particles produced from a stable human-derived packaging cell line transduce target cells with very high efficiencies. *Hum. Gene Ther.* 8: 1459–1467.

Deisseroth, AB, Zu, Z, Claxton, D et al. (1994). Genetic marking shows that Ph+ cells present in autologous transplants of chronic myelogenous leukemia (CML) contribute to relapse after autologous bone marrow in CML. *Blood* 83: 3068–3076.

Dick, JE, Magli, MC, Huszar, D et al. (1985). Introduction of a selectable gene into primitive stem cells capable of long-term reconstitution of the hemopoietic system of W/Wv mice. *Cell* 42: 71–79.

Dilloo, D, Rill, D, Entwistle, C et al. (1997). A novel herpes vector for the high-efficiency transduction of normal and malignant human hematopoietic cells. *Blood* 89: 119–127.

Dinauer, MC, Orkin, SH, Brown, R et al. (1987). The glycoprotein encoded by the X-linked chronic granulomatous disease locus is a component of the neutrophil cytochrome b complex. *Nature* 327: 717–720.

Dmitriev, I, Krasnykh, V, Miller, CR et al. (1998). An adenovirus vector with genetically modified fibers demonstrates expanded tropism via utilization of a coxsackievirus and adenovirus receptor-independent cell entry mechanism [In Process Citation]. *J. Virol.* 72: 9706–9713.

Douglas, JT, Rogers, BE, Rosenfeld, ME et al. (1996). Targeted gene delivery by tropism-modified adenoviral vectors. *Nat. Biotechnol.* 14: 1574–1578.

Dunbar, CE, Cottler-Fox, M, O'Shaughnessy, JA et al. (1995). Retrovirally marked CD34-enriched peripheral blood and bone marrow cells contribute to long-term engraftment after autologous transplantation. *Blood* 85: 3048–3057.

Dzierzak, EA, Papayannopoulou, T, and Mulligan, RC. (1988). Lineage-specific expression of a human beta-globin gene in murine bone marrow transplant recipients reconstituted with retrovirus-transduced stem cells. *Nature* 331: 35–41.

Efstratiadis, A, Posakony, JW, Maniatis, T et al. (1980). The structure and evolution of the human beta-globin gene family. *Cell* 21: 653–668.

Eglitis, MA, Kantoff, P, Gilboa, E, and Anderson, WF. (1985). Gene expression in mice after high efficiency retroviral-mediated gene transfer. *Science* 230: 1395–1398.

Einerhand, MP, Antoniou, M, Zolotukhin, S et al. (1995). Regulated high-level human beta-globin gene expression in erythroid cells following recombinant adeno-associated virus-mediated gene transfer. *Gene Ther.* 2: 336–343.

Ellis, J, Pasceri, P, Tan-Un, KC et al. (1997). Evaluation of beta-globin gene therapy constructs in single copy transgenic mice. *Nucleic Acids Res.* 25: 1296–1302.

Emerman, M and Temin, HM. (1984). Genes with promoters in retrovirus vectors can be independently suppressed by an epigenetic mechanism. *Cell* 39: 459–467.

Emery, DW, Morrish, F, Li, Q, and Stamatoyannopoulos, G. (1999). Analysis of γ-globin expression cassettes in retrovirus vectors. *Hum. Gene Ther.* 10: 877–888.

Emi, N, Friedmann, T, and Yee, JK. (1991). Pseudotype formation of murine leukemia virus with the G protein of vesicular stomatitis virus. *J. Virol.* 65: 1202–1207.

Emmons, RV, Doren, S, Zujewski, J et al. (1997). Retroviral gene transduction of adult peripheral blood or marrow-derived CD34+ cells for six hours without growth factors or on autologous stroma does not improve marking efficiency assessed in vivo. *Blood* 89: 4040–4046.

Engelhardt, JF, Ye, X, Doranz, B, and Wilson, JM. (1994). Ablation of E2A in recombinant adenoviruses improves transgene persistence and decreases inflammatory response in mouse liver. *Proc. Natl. Acad. Sci. U.S.A.* 91: 6196–6200.

Epner, E, Reik, A, Cimbora, D et al. (1998). The beta-globin LCR is not necessary for an open chromatin structure or developmentally regulated transcription of the native mouse beta-globin locus. *Mol. Cell* 2: 447–455.

Farquhar, MN, Turner, PA, Papayannopoulou, T et al. (1981). The asynchrony of gamma- and beta-chain synthesis during human erythroid cell maturation. III. gamma- and beta-mRNA in immature and mature erythroid clones. *Dev. Biol.* 85: 403–408.

Feero, WG, Rosenblatt, JD, Huard, J et al. (1997). Viral gene delivery to skeletal muscle: Insights on maturation-dependent loss of fiber infectivity for adenovirus and herpes simplex type 1 viral vectors. *Hum. Gene Ther.* 8: 371–380.

Ferrari, FK, Samulski, T, Shenk, T, and Samulski, RJ. (1996). Second-strand synthesis is a rate-limiting step for efficient transduction by recombinant adeno-associated virus vectors. *J. Virol.* 70: 3227–3234.

Ferrari, FK, Xiao, X, McCarty, D, and Samulski, RJ. (1997). New developments in the generation of Ad-free, high-titer rAAV gene therapy vectors. *Nat. Med.* 3: 1295–1297.

Fisher, KJ, Gao, GP, Weitzman, MD et al. (1996). Transduction with recombinant adeno-associated virus for gene therapy is limited by leading-strand synthesis. *J. Virol.* 70: 520–532.

Fisher, KJ, Jooss, K, Alston, J et al. (1997). Recombinant adeno-associated virus for muscle directed gene therapy. *Nat. Med.* 3: 306–312.

Fleming, WH, Alpern, EJ, Uchida, N et al. (1993). Functional heterogeneity is associated with the cell cycle status of murine hematopoietic stem cells. *J. Cell Biol.* 122: 897–902.

Forrester, A, Farrel, H, Wilkinson, G et al. (1992). Construction and properties of a mutant of herpes simplex virus type 1 with glycoprotein H coding sequences deleted. *J. Virol.* 66: 341–348.

Forrester, WC, Takagawa, S, Papayannopoulou, T et al. (1987). Evidence for a locus activation region: The formation of developmentally stable hypersensitive sites in globin-expressing hybrids. *Nucleic Acids Res.* 15: 10159–10177.

Franz, T, Hilberg, F, Seliger, B et al. (1986). Retroviral mutants efficiently expressed in embryonal carcinoma cells. *Proc. Natl. Acad. Sci. U.S.A.* 83: 3292–3296.

Fraser, P and Grosveld, F. (1998). Locus control regions, chromatin activation and transcription. *Curr. Opin. Cell Biol.* 10: 361–365.

Gao, GP, Yang, Y, and Wilson, JM. (1996). Biology of adenovirus vectors with E1 and E4 deletions for liver-directed gene therapy. *J. Virol.* 70: 8934–8943.

Gerson, SL, Phillips, W, Kastan, M et al. (1996). Human CD34+ hematopoietic progenitors have low, cytokine-unresponsive O6-alkylguanine-DNA alkyltransferase and are sensitive to 06-benzylguanine plus BCNU. *Blood* 88: 1649–1655.

Grez, M, Akgun, E, Hilberg, F, and Ostertag, W. (1990). Embryonic stem cell virus, a recombinant murine retrovirus with expression in embryonic stem cells. *Proc. Natl. Acad. Sci. U.S.A.* 87: 9202–9206.

Grosveld, F, De Boer, E, Dillon, N et al. (1998). The dynamics of globin gene expression and gene therapy vectors. *Semin. Hematol.* 35: 105–111.

Grosveld, F, van Assendelft, GB, Greaves, DR, and Kollias, G. (1987). Position-independent, high-level expression of the human beta- globin gene in transgenic mice. *Cell* 51: 975–985.

Grubb, BR, Pickles, RJ, Ye, H et al. (1994). Inefficient gene transfer by adenovirus vector to cystic fibrosis airway epithelia of mice and humans. *Nature* 37: 802–806.

Hanania, EG, Giles, RE, Kavanagh, J et al. (1996). Results of MDR-1 vector modification trial indicate that granulocyte/macrophage colony-forming unit cells do not contribute to posttransplant hematopoietic recovery following intensive systemic therapy [published erratum appears in *Proc. Natl. Acad. Sci. U.S.A.* 1997 May 13;94(10): 5495]. *Proc. Natl. Acad. Sci. U.S.A.* 93: 15346–15351.

Hanenberg, H, Hashino, K, Konishi, H et al. (1997). Optimization of fibronectin-assisted retroviral gene transfer into human CD34+ hematopoietic cells. *Hum. Gene Ther.* 8: 2193–2206.

Hanenberg, H, Xiao, XL, Dilloo, D et al. (1996). Colocalization of retrovirus and target cells on specific fibronectin fragments increases genetic transduction of mammalian cells. *Nat. Med.* 2: 876–882.

Hantzopoulos, PA, Sullenger, BA, Ungers, G, and Gilboa, E. (1989). Improved gene expression upon transfer of the adenosine deaminase minigene outside the transcriptional unit of a retroviral vector. *Proc. Natl. Acad. Sci. U.S.A.* 86: 3519–3523.

Hao, QL, Thiemann, FT, Petersen, D et al. (1996). Extended long-term culture reveals a highly quiescent and primitive human hematopoietic progenitor population. *Blood* 88: 3306–3313.

Hardison, R, Slightom, JL, Gumucio, DL et al. (1997). Locus control regions of mammalian beta-globin gene clusters: combining phylogenetic analyses and experimental results to gain functional insights. *Gene* 205: 73–94.

Hargrove, PW, Vanin, EF, Kurtzman, GJ, and Nienhuis, AW. (1997). High-level globin gene expression mediated by a recombinant adeno-associated virus genome that contains the 3′ γ globin gene regulatory element and integrates as tandem copies in erythroid cells. *Blood* 89: 2167–2175.

Harris, LC, Marathi, UK, Edwards, CC et al. (1995). Retroviral transfer of a bacterial alkyltransferase gene into murine bone marrow protects against chloroethylnitrosourea cytotoxicity. *Clin. Cancer Res.* 1: 1359–1368.

Heinzinger, NK, Bukinsky, MI, Haggerty, SA et al. (1994). The Vpr protein of human immunodeficiency virus type 1 influences nuclear localization of viral nucleic acids in nondividing host cells. *Proc. Natl. Acad. Sci. U.S.A.* 91: 7311–7315.

Herzog, RW, Yang, EY, Couto, LB et al. (1999). Long-term correction of canine hemophilia B by gene transfer of blood coagulation factor IX mediated by adeno-associated viral vector. *Nat. Med.* 5: 56–63.

Hesdorffer, C, Ayello, J, Ward, M et al. (1998). Phase I trial of retroviral-mediated transfer of the human MDR1 gene as marrow chemoprotection in patients undergoing high-dose chemotherapy and autologous stem-cell transplantation. *J. Clin. Oncol.* 16: 165–172.

Hilberg, F, Stocking, C, Ostertag, W, and Grez, M. (1987). Functional analysis of a retroviral host-range mutant: Altered long terminal repeat sequences allow expression in embryonal carcinoma cells. *Proc. Natl. Acad. Sci. U.S.A.* 84: 5232–5236.

Hirata, RK, Miller, AD, Andrews, RG, and Russell, DW. (1996). Transduction of hematopoietic cells by foamy virus vectors. *Blood* 88: 3654–3661.

Holcik, M and Liebhaber, SA. (1997). Four highly stable eukaryotic mRNAs assemble 3′ untranslated region RNA-protein complexes sharing cis and trans components. *Proc. Natl. Acad. Sci. U.S.A.* 94: 2410–2414.

Holmes, ML, Haley, JD, Cerruti, L et al. (1999). Identification of Id2 as a globin regulatory protein by representational difference analysis of K562 cells induced to express-globin with a fungal compound. *Mol. Cell Biol.* 19: 4182–4190.

Inoue, N and Russell, DW. (1998). Packaging cells based on inducible gene amplification for the production of adeno-associated virus vectors. *J. Virol.* 72: 7024–7031.

Ito, K, Ueda, Y, Kokubun, M et al. (1997). Development of a novel selective amplifier gene for controllable expansion of transduced hematopoietic cells. *Blood* 90: 3884–3892.

Jackson, SH, Gallin, JI, and Holland, SM. (1995). The p47phox mouse knock-out model of chronic granulomatous disease. *J. Exp. Med.* 182: 751–758.

Jane, SM, Ney, PA, Vanin, EF et al. (1992). Identification of a stage selector element in the human gamma-globin gene promoter that fosters preferential interaction with the 5′ HS2 enhancer when in competition with the beta-promoter. *EMBO J.* 11: 2961–2969.

Jane, SM, Nienhuis, AW, and Cunningham, JM. (1995). Hemoglobin switching in man and chicken is mediated by a heteromeric complex between the ubiquitous transcription factor CP2 and a developmentally specific protein [published erratum appears in *EMBO J.* 1995 Feb 15;14(4): 854]. *EMBO J.* 14: 97–105.

Jin, L, Siritanaratkul, N, Emery, DW et al. (1998). Targeted expansion of genetically modified bone marrow cells. *Proc. Natl. Acad. Sci. U.S.A.* 95: 8093–8097.

Jooss, K, Yang, Y, Fisher, KJ, and Wilson, JM. (1998). Transduction of dendritic cells by DNA viral vectors directs the immune response to transgene products in muscle fibers. *J. Virol.* 72: 4212–4223.

Kafri, T, Blomer, U, Peterson, DA et al. (1997). Sustained expression of genes delivered directly into liver and muscle by lentiviral vectors. *Nat. Genet.* 17: 314–317.

Kafri, T, van Praag, H, Ouyang, L et al. (1999). A packaging cell line for lentivirus vectors. *J. Virol.* 73: 576–584.

Kaptein, LC, van Beusechem, VW, Riviere, I et al. (1997). Long-term in vivo expression of the MFG-ADA retroviral vector in rhesus monkeys transplanted with transduced bone marrow cells. *Hum. Gene Ther.* 8: 1605–1610.

Karlsson, S, Bodine, DM, Perry, L et al. (1988). Expression of the human beta-globin gene following retroviral-mediated transfer into multipotential hematopoietic progenitors of mice. *Proc. Natl. Acad. Sci. U.S.A.* 85: 6060–6066.

Kavanaugh, MP, Miller, DG, Zhang, W et al. (1994). Cell-surface receptors for gibbon ape leukemia virus and amphotropic murine retrovirus are inducible sodium-dependent phosphate symporters. *Proc. Natl. Acad. Sci. U.S.A.* 91: 7071–7075.

Kay, MA, Landen, CN, Rothenberg, SR et al. (1994). In vivo hepatic gene therapy: Complete albeit transient correction of factor IX deficiency in hemophilia B dogs. *Proc. Natl. Acad. Sci. U.S.A.* 91: 2353–2357.

Keller, G, Paige, C, Gilboa, E, and Wagner, EF. (1985). Expression of a foreign gene in myeloid and lymphoid cells derived from multipotent haematopoietic precursors. *Nature* 318: 149–154.

Kessler, PD, Podsakoff, GM, Chen, X et al. (1996). Gene delivery to skeletal muscle results in sustained expression and systemic delivery of a therapeutic protein. *Proc. Natl. Acad. Sci. U.S.A.* 93: 14082–14087.

Kiem, HP, Andrews, RG, Morris, JA et al. (1998). Improved gene transfer into baboon marrow repopulating cells using recombinant human fibronectin fragment CH-296 in combination with interleukin-6, stem cell factor, FLT-3 ligand, and megakaryocyte growth and development factor. *Blood* 92: 1878–1886.

Kiem, HP, Heyward, S, Winkler, A et al. (1997). Gene transfer into marrow repopulating cells: Comparison between amphotropic and gibbon ape leukemia virus pseudotyped retroviral vectors in a competitive repopulation assay in baboons. *Blood* 90: 4638–4645.

Kim, JW, Closs, EI, Albritton, LM, and Cunningham, JM. (1991). Transport of cationic amino acids by the mouse ecotropic retrovirus receptor [see comments]. *Nature* 352: 725–728.

Kim, VN, Mitrophanous, K, Kingsman, SM, and Kingsman, AJ. (1998). Minimal requirement for a lentivirus vector based on human immunodeficiency virus type 1. *J. Virol.* 72: 811–816.

Koeberl, DD, Alexander, IE, Halbert, CL et al. (1997). Persistent expression of human clotting factor IX from mouse liver after intravenous injection of adeno-associated virus vectors. *Proc. Natl. Acad. Sci. U.S.A.* 94: 1426–1431.

Kohn, DB, Weinberg, KI, Nolta, JA et al. (1995). Engraftment of gene-modified umbilical cord blood cells in neonates with adenosine deaminase deficiency. *Nat. Med.* 1: 1017–1023.

Kotin, RM, Linden, RM, and Berns, KI. (1992). Characterization of a preferred site on human chromosome 19q for integration of adeno-associated virus DNA by non-homologous recombination. *EMBO J.* 11: 5071–5078.

Krall, WJ, Skelton, DC, Yu, XJ et al. (1996). Increased levels of spliced RNA account for augmented expression from the MFG retroviral vector in hematopoietic cells. *Gene Ther.* 3: 37–48.

Krasnykh, V, Dmitriev, I, Mikheeva, G et al. (1998). Characterization of an adenovirus vector containing a heterologous peptide epitope in the HI loop of the fiber knob. *J. Virol.* 72: 1844–1852.

Lawn, RM, Efstratiadis, A, O'Connell, C, and Maniatis, T. (1980). The nucleotide sequence of the human beta-globin gene. *Cell* 21: 647–651.

Leboulch, P, Huang, GM, Humphries, RK et al. (1994). Mutagenesis of retroviral vectors transducing human beta-globin gene and beta-globin locus control region derivatives results in stable transmission of an active transcriptional structure. *EMBO J.* 13: 3065–3076.

Lemischka, IR, Raulet, DH, and Mulligan, RC. (1986). Developmental potential and dynamic behavior of hematopoietic stem cells. *Cell* 45: 917–927.

Lewis, P, Hensel, M, and Emerman, M. (1992). Human immunodeficiency virus infection of cells arrested in the cell cycle [published erratum appears in *EMBO J.* 1992 Nov;11(11): 4249]. *EMBO J.* 11: 3053–3058.

Lewis, PF and Emerman, M. (1994). Passage through mitosis is required for oncoretroviruses but not for the human immunodeficiency virus. *J. Virol.* 68: 510–516.

Li, Q, Clegg, C, Peterson, K et al. (1997). Binary transgenic mouse model for studying the trans control of globin gene switching: Evidence that GATA-1 is an in vivo repressor of human epsilon gene expression. *Proc. Natl. Acad. Sci. U.S.A.* 94: 2444–2448.

Li, Q, Emery, DW, Fernandez, M et al. (1999). Development of viral vectors for gene therapy of beta-chain hemoglobinopathies: optimization of a gamma-globin gene expression cassette. *Blood* 93: 2208–2216.

Li, Q, Peterson, KR, and Stamatoyannopoulos, G. (1998). Developmental control of epsilon- and gamma-globin genes. *Ann. N.Y. Acad. Sci.* 850: 10–7, 10–17.

Li, T, Adamian, M, Roof, DJ et al. (1994). In vivo transfer of a reporter gene to the retina mediated by an adenoviral vector. *Invest. Ophthalmol. Vis. Sci.* 35: 2543–2549.

Liu, D, Chang, JC, Moi, P et al. (1992). Dissection of the enhancer activity of beta-globin 5′ DNase l-hypersensitive site 2 in transgenic mice. *Proc. Natl. Acad. Sci. U.S.A.* 89: 3899–3903.

Lubovy, M, McCune, S, Dong, JY et al. (1996). Stable transduction of recombinant adeno-associated virus into hematopoietic stem cells from normal and sickle cell patients. *Biol. Blood Marrow Transplant.* 2: 24–30.

Luskey, BD, Rosenblatt, M, Zsebo, K, and Williams, DA. (1992). Stem cell factor, interleukin-3, and interleukin-6 promote retroviral-mediated gene transfer into murine hematopoietic stem cells. *Blood* 80: 396–402.

Macchi, P, Villa, A, Gillani, S et al. (1995). Mutations of Jak-3 gene in patients with autosomal severe combined immune deficiency (SCID). *Nature* 377: 65–68.

Malik, P, McQuiston, SA, Yu, XJ et al. (1997). Recombinant adeno-associated virus mediates a high level of gene transfer but less efficient integration in the K562 human hematopoietic cell line. *J. Virol.* 71: 1776–1783.

Maniatis, T, Kee, SG, Efstratiadis, A, and Kafatos, FC. (1976). Amplification and characterization of a beta-globin gene synthesized in vitro. *Cell* 8: 163–182.

Mann, R, Mulligan, RC, and Baltimore, D. (1983). Construction of a retrovirus packaging mutant and its use to produce helper-free defective retrovirus. *Cell* 33: 153–159.

Mardiney, M, Jackson, SH, Spratt, SK et al. (1997). Enhanced host defense after gene transfer in the murine p47 phox-deficient model of chronic granulomatous disease. *Blood* 89: 2268–2275.

Markowitz, D, Goff, S, and Bank, A. (1988a). A safe packaging line for gene transfer: Separating viral genes on two different plasmids. *J. Virol.* 62: 1120–1124.

Markowitz, D, Goff, S, and Bank, A. (1988b). Construction and use of a safe and efficient amphotropic packaging cell line. *Virology* 167: 400–406.

Martin, DI, Fiering, S, and Groudine, M. (1996). Regulation of beta-globin gene expression: Straightening out the locus. *Curr. Opin. Genet. Dev.* 6: 488–495.

McCown, TJ, Xiao, X, Li, J et al. (1996). Differential and persistent expression patterns of CNS gene transfer by an adeno-associated virus (AAV) vector. *Brain Res.* 713: 99–107.

McCune, SL, Reilly, MP, Chomo, MJ et al. (1994). Recombinant human hemoglobins designed for gene therapy of sickle cell disease. *Proc. Natl. Acad. Sci. U.S.A.* 91: 9852–9856.

McCune, SL and Townes, TM. (1994). Retroviral vector sequences inhibit human beta-globin gene expression in transgenic mice. *Nucleic. Acids. Res.* 22: 4477–4481.

Miller, AD, Bender, MA, Harris, EA et al. (1988). Design of retrovirus vectors for transfer and expression of the human beta-globin gene [published erratum appears in *J. Virol.* 1989 Mar;63(3): 1493]. *J. Virol.* 62: 4337–4345.

Miller, AD and Rosman, GJ. (1989). Improved retroviral vectors for gene transfer and expression. *Biotechniques* 7: 980–986, 989.

Miller, DG, Adam, MA, and Miller, AD. (1990). Gene transfer by retrovirus vectors occurs only in cells that are actively replicating at the time of infection [published erratum appears in *Mol. Cell. Biol.* 1992 Jan;12(1): 433]. *Mol. Cell Biol.* 10: 4239–4242.

Miller, DG, Edwards, RH, and Miller, AD. (1994a). Cloning of the cellular receptor for amphotropic murine retroviruses reveals homology to that for gibbon ape leukemia virus. *Proc. Natl. Acad. Sci. U.S.A.* 91: 78–82.

Miller, JL, Donahue, RE, Sellers, SE et al. (1994b). Recombinant adeno-associated virus (rAAV)-mediated expression of a human gamma-globin gene in human progenitor-derived erythroid cells [published erratum appears in *Proc. Natl. Acad. Sci. U.S.A.* 1995 Jan 17;92(2): 646]. *Proc. Natl. Acad. Sci. U.S.A.* 91: 10183–10187.

Miller, JL, Walsh, CE, Ney, PA et al. (1993). Single-copy transduction and expression of human gamma-globin in K562 erythroleukemia cells using recombinant adeno-associated virus vectors: The effect of mutations in NF-E2 and GATA-1 binding motifs within the hypersensitivity site 2 enhancer [published erratum appears in *Blood* 1995 Feb 1;85(3): 862]. *Blood* 82: 1900–1906.

Miyoshi, H, Smith, KA, Mosier, DE et al. (1999). Efficient transduction of human CD34+ cells that mediate long-term engraftment of NOD/SCID mice by HIV vectors. *Science* 283: 682–686.

Miyoshi, H, Takahashi, M, Gage, FH, and Verma, IM. (1997). Stable and efficient gene transfer into the retina using an HIV-based lentiviral vector. *Proc. Natl. Acad. Sci. U.S.A.* 94: 10319–10323.

Morgan, RA, Couture, L, Elroy-Stein, O et al. (1992). Retroviral vectors containing putative internal ribosome entry sites: Development of a polycistronic gene transfer system and applications to human gene therapy. *Nucleic Acids Res.* 20: 1293–1299.

Moritz, T, Mackay, W, Glassner, BJ et al. (1995). Retrovirus-mediated expression of a DNA repair protein in bone marrow protects hematopoietic cells from nitrosourea-induced toxicity in vitro and in vivo. *Cancer Res.* 55: 2608–2614.

Moritz, T, Patel, VP, and Williams, DA. (1994). Bone marrow extracellular matrix molecules improve gene transfer into human hematopoietic cells via retroviral vectors. *J. Clin. Invest.* 93: 1451–1457.

Morsy, MA, Alford, EL, Bett, A et al. (1993). Efficient adenoviral-mediated ornithine transcarbamylase expression in deficient mouse and human hepatocytes. *J. Clin. Invest.* 92: 1580–1586.

Morsy, MA, Gu, M, Motzel, S et al. (1998). An adenoviral vector deleted for all viral coding sequences results in enhanced safety and extended expression of a leptin transgene. *Proc. Natl. Acad. Sci. U.S.A.* 95: 7866–7871.

Nagel, RL. (1998). A knockout of a transgenic mouse—animal models of sickle cell anemia. *N. Engl. J. Med.* 339: 194–195.

Nakai, H, Herzog, RW, Hagstrom, JN et al. (1998). Adeno-associated viral vector-mediated gene transfer of human blood coagulation factor IX into mouse liver. *Blood* 91: 4600–4607.

Naldini, L, Blomer, U, Gage, FH et al. (1996a). Efficient transfer, integration, and sustained long-term expression of the transgene in adult rat brains injected with a lentiviral vector. *Proc. Natl. Acad. Sci. U.S.A.* 93: 11382–11388.

Naldini, L, Blomer, U, Gally, P et al. (1996b). In vivo gene delivery and stable transduction of nondividing cells by a lentiviral vector [see comments]. *Science* 272: 263–267.

Nathwani, AC, Hanawa, H, Vandergriff, J et al. (2000). Efficient gene transfer into human cord blood CD34+ cells and the CD34+CD38− subset using highly purified recombinant adeno-associated viral vector preparations that are free of helper virus and wild-type AAV. *Gene Ther.* 7: 183–195.

Nathwani, AC, Persons, DA, Stevenson, SC et al. (1999). Adenoviral-mediated expression of the murine ecotropic receptor facilitates transduction of human hematopoietic cells with an ecotropic retroviral vector. *Gene Ther.* 6: 1456–1468.

Nienhuis, AW and Anderson, WF. (1971). Isolation and translation of hemoglobin messenger RNA from thalassemia, sickle cell anemia, and normal human reticulocytes. *J. Clin. Invest.* 50: 2458–2460.

Nosaka, T, van Deursen, JM, Tripp, RA et al. (1995). Defective lymphoid development in mice lacking Jak3 [published erratum appears in *Science* 1996 Jan 5: 271(5245): 17]. *Science* 270: 800–802.

Novak, U, Harris, EA, Forrester, W et al. (1990). High-level beta-globin expression after retroviral transfer of locus activation region-containing human beta-globin gene derivatives into murine erythroleukemia cells. *Proc. Natl. Acad. Sci. U.S.A.* 87: 3386–3390.

Nuez, B, Michalovich, D, Bygrave, A et al. (1995). Defective haematopoiesis in fetal liver resulting from inactivation of the EKLF gene. *Nature* 375: 316–318.

O'Neill, D, Yang, J, Erdjument-Bromage, H et al. (1999). Tissue-specific and developmental stage-specific DNA binding by a mammalian SWI/SNF complex associated with human fetal-to-adult globin gene switching. *Proc. Natl. Acad. Sci. U.S.A.* 96: 349–54.

Oppenheim, A, Peleg, A, Fibach, E, and Rachmilewitz, EA. (1986). Efficient introduction of plasmid DNA into human hemopoietic cells by encapsidation in simian virus 40 pseudovirions. *Proc. Natl. Acad. Sci. U.S.A.* 83: 6925–6929.

Orlic, D, Girard, LJ, Anderson, SM et al. (1998). Identification of human and mouse hematopoietic stem cell populations expressing high levels of mRNA encoding retrovirus receptors. *Blood* 91: 3247–3254.

Orlic, D, Girard, LJ, Jordan, CT et al. (1996). The level of mRNA encoding the amphotropic retrovirus receptor in mouse and human hematopoietic stem cells is low and correlates with the efficiency of retrovirus transduction. *Proc. Natl. Acad. Sci. U.S.A.* 93: 11097–11102.

Ory, DS, Neugeboren, BA, and Mulligan, RC. (1996). A stable human-derived packaging cell line for production of high titer retrovirus/vesicular stomatitis virus G pseudotypes. *Proc. Natl. Acad. Sci. U.S.A.* 93: 11400–11406.

Parolin, C, Taddeo, B, Palu, G, and Sodroski, J. (1996). Use of cis- and trans-acting viral regulatory sequences to improve expression of human immunodeficiency virus vectors in human lymphocytes. *Virology* 222: 415–422.

Pauling, L, Itano, H, Singer, SJ, and Wells, IC. (1949). Sickle cell anemia: A molecular disease. *Science* 110: 543.

Pawliuk, R, Eaves, CJ, and Humphries, RK. (1997). Sustained high-level reconstitution of the hematopoietic system by pre-selected hematopoietic cells expressing a transduced cell-surface antigen. *Hum. Gene Ther.* 8: 1595–1604.

Pawliuk, R, Kay, R, Lansdorp, P, and Humphries, RK. (1994). Selection of retrovirally transduced hematopoietic cells using CD24 as a marker of gene transfer. *Blood* 84: 2868–2877.

Pellicer, A, Wigler, M, Axel, R, and Silverstein, S. (1978). The transfer and stable integration of the HSV thymidine kinase gene into mouse cells. *Cell* 14: 133–141.

Perkins, AC, Sharpe, AH, and Orkin, SH. (1995). Lethal beta-thalassaemia in mice lacking the erythroid CACCC-transcription factor EKLF. *Nature* 375: 318–322.

Persons, DA, Allay, JA, Allay, ER et al. (1997). Retroviral-mediated transfer of the green fluorescent protein gene into murine hematopoietic cells facilitates scoring and selection of transduced progenitors in vitro and identification of genetically modified cells in vivo. *Blood* 90: 1777–1786.

Persons, DA, Allay, JA, Riberdy, JM et al. (1998a). Utilization of the green flourescent protein gene as a marker to identify and track genetically-modified hematopoietic cells. *Nat. Med.* 4: 1201–1205.

Persons, DA, Mehaffey, MG, Kaleko, M et al. (1998b). An improved method for generating retroviral producer clones for vectors lacking a selectable marker gene. *Blood Cells Mol. Dis.* 24: 167–182.

Philipsen, S, Pruzina, S, and Grosveld, F. (1993). The minimal requirements for activity in transgenic mice of hypersensitive site 3 of the beta globin locus control region. *EMBO J.* 12: 1077–1085.

Philipsen, S, Talbot, D, Fraser, P, and Grosveld F. (1990). The beta-globin dominant control region: Hypersensitive site 2. *EMBO J.* 9: 2159–2167.

Plavec, I, Papayannopoulou, T, Maury, C, and Meyer, F. (1993). A human beta-globin gene fused to the human beta-globin locus control region is expressed at high levels in erythroid cells of mice engrafted with retrovirus-transduced hematopoietic stem cells. *Blood* 81: 1384–1392.

Pollock, JD, Williams, DA, Gifford, MA et al. (1995). Mouse model of X-linked chronic granulomatous disease, an inherited defect in phagocyte superoxide production. *Nat. Genet.* 9: 202–209.

Ponnazhagan, S, Mukherjee, P, Wang, XS et al. (1997a). Adeno-associated virus type 2-mediated transduction in primary human bone marrow-derived CD34+ hematopoietic progenitor cells: Donor variation and correlation of transgene expression with cellular differentiation. *J. Virol.* 71: 8262–8267.

Ponnazhagan, S, Yoder, MC, and Srivastava, A. (1997b). Adeno-associated virus type 2-mediated transduction of murine hematopoietic cells with long-term repopulating ability and sustained expression of a human globin gene in vivo. *J. Virol.* 71: 3098–3104.

Pruzina, S, Hanscombe, O, Whyatt, D et al. (1991). Hypersensitive site 4 of the human beta globin locus control region. *Nucleic. Acids. Res.* 19: 1413–1419.

Qing, K, Bachelot, T, Mukherjee, P et al. (1997). Adeno-associated virus type 2-mediated transfer of ecotropic retrovirus receptor cDNA allows ecotropic retroviral transduction of established and primary human cells. *J. Virol.* 71: 5663–5667.

Qing, K, Khuntirat, B, Mah, C et al. (1998). Adeno-associated virus type 2-mediated gene transfer: correlation of tyrosine phosphorylation of the cellular single-stranded D sequence-binding protein with transgene expression in human cells in vitro and murine tissues in vivo. *J. Virol.* 72: 1593–1599.

Qing, K, Mah, C, Hansen, J et al. (1999). Human fibroblast growth factor receptor 1 is a co-receptor for infection by adeno-associated virus 2. *Nat. Med.* 5: 71–77.

Raftopoulos, H, Ward, M, Leboulch, P, and Bank, A. (1997). Long-term transfer and expression of the human beta-globin gene in a mouse transplant model. *Blood* 90: 3414–3422.

Randall, TD and Weissman, IL. (1997). Phenotypic and functional changes induced at the clonal level in hematopoietic stem cells after 5-fluorouracil treatment. *Blood* 89: 3596–3606.

Reik, A, Telling, A, Zitnik, G et al. (1998). The locus control region is necessary for gene expression in the human beta-globin locus but not the maintenance of an open chromatin structure in erythroid cells. *Mol. Cell Biol.* 18: 5992–6000.

Ren, S, Wong, BY, Li, J et al. (1996). Production of genetically stable high-titer retroviral vectors that carry a human gamma-globin gene under the control of the alpha-globin locus control region. *Blood* 87: 2518–2524.

Rill, DR, Santana, VM, Roberts, WM et al. (1994). Direct demonstration that autologous bone marrow transplantation for solid tumors can return a multiplicity of tumorigenic cells. *Blood* 84: 380–383.

Rivella, S and Sadelain, M. (1998). Genetic treatment of severe hemoglobinopathies: the combat against transgene variegation and transgene silencing. *Semin. Hematol.* 35: 112–125.

Rund, D, Dagan, M, Dalyot-Herman, N et al. (1998). Efficient transduction of human hematopoietic cells with the human multidrug resistance gene 1 via SV40 pseudovirions [see comments]. *Hum. Gene Ther.* 9: 649–657.

Russell, DW, Alexander, IE, and Miller, AD. (1995). DNA synthesis and topoisomerase inhibitors increase transduc-

tion by adeno-associated virus vectors. *Proc. Natl. Acad. Sci. U.S.A.* 92: 5719–5723.

Russell, DW and Miller, AD. (1996). Foamy virus vectors. *J. Virol.* 70: 217–222.

Russell, JE and Liebhaber, SA. (1996). The stability of human beta-globin mRNA is dependent on structural determinants positioned within its 3′ untranslated region. *Blood* 87: 5314–5323.

Rutledge, EA, Halbert, CL, and Russell, DW. (1998). Infectious clones and vectors derived from adeno-associated virus (AAV) serotypes other than AAV type 2. *J. Virol.* 72: 309–319.

Ryan, TM, Ciavatta, DJ, and Townes, TM. (1997). Knockout-transgenic mouse model of sickle cell disease [see comments]. *Science* 278: 873–876.

Sadelain, M. (1997). Genetic treatment of the haemoglobinopathies: Recombinations and new combinations. *Br. J. Haematol.* 98: 247–253.

Sadelain, M, Wang, CH, Antoniou, M et al. (1995). Generation of a high-titer retroviral vector capable of expressing high levels of the human beta-globin gene. *Proc. Natl. Acad. Sci. U.S.A.* 92: 6728–6732.

Sakamoto, T, Ueno, H, Goto, Y et al. (1998). Retinal functional change caused by adenoviral vector-mediated transfection of LacZ gene. *Hum. Genet. Ther.* 9: 789–799.

Samulski, RJ, Chang, LS, and Shenk, T. (1989). Helper-free stocks of recombinant adeno-associated viruses: normal integration does not require viral gene expression. *J. Virol.* 63: 3822–3828.

Samulski, RJ, Srivastava, A, Berns, KI, and Muzyczka, N. (1983). Rescue of adeno-associated virus from recombinant plasmids: Gene correction within the terminal repeats of AAV. *Cell* 33: 135–143.

Sandalon, Z, Dalyot-Herman, N, Oppenheim, AB, and Oppenheim, A. (1997). In vitro assembly of SV40 virions and pseudovirions: vector development for gene therapy. *Hum. Gene Ther.* 8: 843–849.

Schilz, AJ, Brouns, G, Knobeta, H et al. (1998). High efficiency gene transfer to human hematopoietic SCID-repopulating cells under serum-free conditions [In Process Citation]. *Blood* 92: 3163–3171.

Schimmenti, S, Boesen, J, Claassen, EA et al. (1998). Long-term genetic modification of Rhesus monkey hematopoietic cells following transplantation of adenoassociated virus vector-transduced CD34+ cells. *Hum. Gene Ther.* 9: 2727–2734.

Shah, AJ, Smogorzewska, EM, Hannum, C, and Crooks, GM. (1996). Flt3 ligand induces proliferation of quiescent human bone marrow CD34+CD38– cells and maintains progenitor cells in vitro. *Blood* 87: 3563–3570.

Snyder, RO, Miao, C, Meuse, L et al. (1999). Correction of hemophilia B in canine and murine models using recombinant adeno-associated viral vectors. *Nat. Med.* 5: 64–70.

Snyder, RO, Miao, CH, Patijn, GA et al. (1997). Persistent and therapeutic concentrations of human factor IX in mice after hepatic gene transfer of recombinant AAV vectors. *Nat. Genet.* 16: 270–276.

Sorrentino, BP. (1996). Drug resistance gene therapy. In MK Brenner and RC Moen, editors, *Gene Therapy in Cancer.* New York: Marcel Dekker.

Sorrentino, BP, Brandt, SJ, Bodine, D et al. (1992). Selection of drug-resistant bone marrow cells in vivo after retroviral transfer of human MDR1. *Science* 257: 99–103.

Sorrentino, BP, McDonagh, KT, Woods, D, and Orlic, D. (1995). Expression of retroviral vectors containing the human multidrug resistance 1 cDNA in hematopoietic cells of transplanted mice. *Blood* 86: 491–501.

Sorrentino, BP and Nienhuis, AW. (1999). The hematopoietic system as a target for gene therapy. In Friedmann, T, editor. *The development of gene therapy.* New York: Cold Spring Harbor Laboratory Press.

Summerford, C, Bartlett, JS, and Samulski, RJ. (1999). αVβ5 integrin: A co-receptor for adeno-associated virus type 2 infection. *Nat. Med.* 5: 78–82.

Summerford, C and Samulski, RJ. (1998). Membrane-associated heparan sulfate proteoglycan is a receptor for adeno-associated virus type 2 virions. *J. Virol.* 72: 1438–1445.

Tabin, CJ, Hoffmann, JW, Goff, SP, and Weinberg, RA. (1982). Adaptation of a retrovirus as a eucaryotic vector transmitting the herpes simplex virus thymidine kinase gene. *Mol. Cell Biol.* 2: 426–436.

Takekoshi, KJ, Oh, YH, Westerman, KW et al. (1995). Retroviral transfer of a human beta-globin/delta-globin hybrid gene linked to beta locus control region hypersensitive site 2 aimed at the gene therapy of sickle cell disease. *Proc. Natl. Acad. Sci. U.S.A.* 92: 3014–3018.

Talbot, D, Philipsen, S, Fraser, P, and Grosveld, F. (1990). Detailed analysis of the site 3 region of the human beta-globin dominant control region. *EMBO J.* 9: 2169–2177.

Tewari, R, Gillemans, N, Wijgerde, M et al. (1998). Erythroid Kruppel-like factor (EKLF) is active in primitive and definitive erythroid cells and is required for the function of 5'HS3 of the beta-globin locus control region. *EMBO J.* 17: 2334–2341.

Thomis, DC, Gurniak, CB, Tivol, E et al. (1995). Defects in B lymphocyte maturation and T lymphocyte activation in mice lacking Jak3. *Science* 270: 794–797.

Tisdale, JF, Hanazono, Y, Sellers, SE et al. (1998). Ex vivo expansion of genetically marked rhesus peripheral blood progenitor cells results in diminished long-term repopulating ability. *Blood* 92: 1131–1141.

Tisdale, JF, Moscow, J, Huang, H et al. (1997). Longterm culture retroviral transduction does not improve gene transfer efficiency into rhesus CD34+ PB cells. *Blood* 90 (Suppl. 1): 237a. (Abstract).

Tuan, D, Solomon, W, Li, Q, and London, IM. (1985). The "beta-like-globin" gene domain in human erythroid cells. *Proc. Natl. Acad. Sci. U.S.A.* 82: 6384–6388.

Uchida, N, Sutton, RE, Friera, AM et al. (1998). HIV, but not murine leukemia virus, vectors mediate high efficiency gene transfer into freshly isolated G0/G1 human hematopoietic stem cells. *Proc. Natl. Acad. Sci. U.S.A.* 95: 11939–11944.

van Beusechem, VW, Kukler, A, Heidt, PJ, and Valerio, D. (1992). Long-term expression of human adenosine deaminase in rhesus monkeys transplanted with retrovirus-infected bone-marrow cells. *Proc. Natl. Acad. Sci. U.S.A.* 89: 7640–7644.

Veena, P, Traycoff, CM, Williams, DA et al. (1998). Delayed targeting of cytokine-nonresponsive human bone marrow CD34(+) cells with retrovirus-mediated gene transfer enhances transduction efficiency and long-term expression of transduced genes. *Blood* 91: 3693–3701.

Volloch, V and Housman, D. (1981). Stability of globin mRNA in terminally differentiating murine erythroleukemia cells. *Cell* 23: 509–514.

Walsh, CE, Liu, JM, Xiao, X et al. (1992). Regulated high level expression of a human gamma-globin gene introduced into erythroid cells by an adeno-associated virus vector. *Proc. Natl. Acad. Sci. U.S.A.* 89: 7257–7261.

Wang, H, Kavanaugh, MP, North, RA, and Kabat, D. (1991). Cell-surface receptor for ecotropic murine retroviruses is a basic amino-acid transporter [see comments]. *Nature* 352: 729–731.

Watanabe, S and Temin, HM. (1983). Construction of a helper cell line for avian reticuloendotheliosis virus cloning vectors. *Mol. Cell. Biol.* 3: 2241–2249.

Weatherall, DJ. (1994). The thalassemias. In G. Stamatoyannopoulos G, Nienhuis, AW, Majerus, P, and Varmus, HE, editors. *Molecular basis of blood diseases.* Philadelphia: WB Saunders.

Weber-Benarous, A, Cone, RD, London, IM, and Mulligan RC. (1988). Retroviral-mediated transfer and expression of human beta-globin genes in cultured murine and human erythroid cells. *J. Biol. Chem.* 263: 6142–6145.

Weiher, H, Barklis, E, Ostertag, W, and Jaenisch, R. (1987). Two distinct sequence elements mediate retroviral gene expression in embryonal carcinoma cells. *J. Virol.* 61: 2742–2746.

Wells, S, Malik, P, Pensiero, M et al. (1995). The presence of an autologous marrow stromal cell layer increases glucocerebrosidase gene transduction of long-term culture initiating cells (LTCICs) from the bone marrow of a patient with Gaucher disease. *Gene Ther.* 2: 512–520.

Wickham, TJ, Mathias, P, Cheresh, DA, and Nemerow, GR. (1993). Integrins alpha v beta 3 and alpha v beta 5 promote adenovirus internalization but not virus attachment. *Cell* 73: 309–319.

Wickham, TJ, Segal, DM, Roelvink, PW et al. (1996). Targeted adenovirus gene transfer to endothelial and smooth muscle cells by using bispecific antibodies. *J. Virol.* 70: 6831–6838.

Wickham, TJ, Tzeng, E, Shears, LL et al. (1997). Increased in vitro and in vivo gene transfer by adenovirus vectors containing chimeric fiber proteins. *J. Virol.* 71: 8221–8229.

Wijgerde, M, Gribnau, J, Trimborn, T et al. (1996). The role of EKLF in human beta-globin gene competition. *Genes Dev.* 10: 2894–2902.

Wijgerde, M, Grosveld, F, and Fraser, P. (1995). Transcription complex stability and chromatin dynamics in vivo. *Nature* 377: 209–213.

Williams, DA, Lemischka, IR, Nathan, DG, and Mulligan, RC. (1984). Introduction of new genetic material into pluripotent haematopoietic stem cells of the mouse. *Nature* 310: 476–480.

Wood, WG, Stamatoyannopoulos, G, Lim, G, and Nute, PE. (1975). F-cells in the adult: normal values and levels in individuals with hereditary and acquired elevations of Hb F. *Blood* 46: 671–682.

Xiao, X, Li, J, and Samulski, RJ. (1998). Production of high-titer recombinant adeno-associated virus vectors in the absence of helper adenovirus. *J. Virol.* 72: 2224–2232.

Yang, Y, Jooss, KU, Su, Q et al. (1996). Immune responses to viral antigens versus transgene product in the elimination of recombinant adenovirus-infected hepatocytes in vivo. *Gene Ther.* 3: 137–144.

Yang, Y, Li, Q, Ertl, HC, and Wilson, JM. (1995a). Cellular and humoral immune responses to viral antigens create barriers to lung-directed gene therapy with recombinant adenoviruses. *J. Virol.* 69: 2004–2015.

Yang, Y, Nunes, FA, Berencsi, K et al. (1994a). Cellular immunity to viral antigens limits E1-deleted adenoviruses for gene therapy. *Proc. Natl. Acad. Sci. U.S.A.* 91: 4407–4411.

Yang, Y, Nunes, FA, Berencsi, K et al. (1994b). Inactivation of E2a in recombinant adenoviruses improves the prospect for gene therapy in cystic fibrosis. *Nat. Genet.* 7: 362–369.

Yang, Y, Vanin, EF, Whitt, MA et al. (1995b). Inducible, high-level production of infectious murine leukemia retroviral vector particles pseudotyped with vesicular stomatitis virus G envelope protein. *Hum. Gene Ther.* 6: 1203–1213.

Yang, Y and Wilson, JM. (1995). Clearance of adenovirus-infected hepatocytes by MHC class I-restricted CD4+ CTLs in vivo. *J. Immunol.* 155: 2564–2570.

Yokota, T, Oritani, K, Mitsui, H et al. (1998). Growth-supporting activities of fibronectin on hematopoietic stem/progenitor cells in vitro and in vivo: Structural requirement for fibronectin activities of CS1 and cell-binding domains. *Blood* 91: 3263–3272.

Zhou, SZ, Li, Q, Stamatoyannopoulos, G, and Srivastava, A. (1996). Adeno-associated virus 2-mediated transduction and erythroid cell-specific expression of a human beta-globin gene. *Gene Ther.* 3: 223–229.

Zhou, WL, Clouston, DR, Wang, X et al. (1999). Isolation and characterization of human NF-E4, the tissue restricted component of the stage selector protein complex. *Blood* 94 (Suppl 1): 614a (abstract).

Zufferey, R, Nagy, D, Mandel, RJ et al. (1997). Multiply attenuated lentiviral vector achieves efficient gene delivery in vivo. *Nat. Biotechnol.* 15: 871–875.

42

Experimental Therapies for Sickle Cell Anemia and β Thalassemia

YVES BEUZARD
LUCIA DE FRANCESCHI

INTRODUCTION

At first glance, for the following reasons, sickle cell disease and β thalassemia are ideal genetic disorders for which to design specific therapies at the cellular, protein, or gene levels. First, normal and abnormal differentiated cells, bone marrow precursors, progenitors, and hematopoietic stem cells are easily obtained for ex vivo studies. Second, the mechanisms and the pathophysiology of these diseases are well understood. Specific mutations of the β-hemoglobin gene, a relatively small gene, have been characterized; the abnormal structure of HbS detailed at atomic resolution is available; the secondary cellular defects and, beyond the erythrocyte itself, the interactions of the defective erythrocytes with other blood or vascular components are known in part. Third, mouse models are relevant for in vivo evaluation of new therapies. Lastly, a cooperative scientific and medical community has devoted substantial efforts during the last decades to define therapeutic targets and rationales as well as to design new experimental therapies.

The major goal of therapeutic approaches for sickle cell disease is to decrease the intracellular concentration of HbS, which polymerizes in the deoxy conformation and is responsible for vasoocclusion, sickle cell painful episodes, and many life- or organ-threatening complications (Bunn, 1997). The goal of therapies for β thalassemia major is to provide normal erythrocytes

as a substitute or to improve the survival and efficacy of production of diseased red cells by replacing the missing β-globin chain or by preventing secondary defects.

As described in other chapters of this book, cellular therapies—transfusions and hematopoietic stem cell transplantation—have important drawbacks and limitations. New agents activating fetal hemoglobin expression can ameliorate the disease of many sickle cell anemia patients but are not without risk and up to now have minor benefits in β thalassemia. Finally, hemoglobin gene therapy is far from being available in the near future (Table 42.1). Consequently, other therapies, which can alleviate the cellular and vascular defects of hemoglobinopathies, are under active research (Vichinsky et al., 1998). They can be classified according to their target and effects, as shown in Table 42.1. Many new experimental therapies are common for sickle cell disease and β-thalassemia syndromes, such as those given to prevent oxidation, membrane damage, apoptosis, hemolysis, adherence, cell-cell interactions and activation, procoagulant activity, and thrombosis or to promote hemoglobin chain proteolysis, iron or heme chelation within erythroid cells, and so forth.

HEMOGLOBIN MODIFIERS

Sickle Cell Disease

Initial attempts at developing specific therapies for sickle cell disease were aimed at decreasing HbS polymerization (Dean and Schechter, 1978). Hyperbaric oxygen was given to patients even before the discovery of the HbS molecule (Reinhardt et al., 1944). Nitrite generating methemoglobin (Beutler and Mikus, 1961) and carbon monoxide (Sirs, 1963) were tested in an attempt to decrease the proportion of HbS molecules in the deoxy conformation in which they polymerize. The incidence of sickle cell painful episodes, used as a criterion for efficacy, was not decreased in these clinical trials. Following the observation that urea inhibited HbS gelation and sickling of erythrocytes (Murayama, 1966) clinical trials with urea were undertaken. Their results were disappointing (Cooperative Urea Trials Group, 1974). However cyanate, derived from urea in solution, inhibited sickling and HbS polymerization (Cerami and Manning, 1971) and was tested as a potential treatment for sickle cell disease (Gillette et al., 1974). The initial attempt was encouraging, decreasing hemolysis and anemia. Carbamoylation of the N terminal amino

Table 42.1. Experimental Therapies of Hemoglobin Disorders

Hematopoietic stem cells
    Transplantation: cord blood
    Globin gene therapy:
        Addition, replacement, repair
        Knock out, inactivation
    Other gene therapies
        hematopoietins, transduction factors
Erythropoiesis
    Transacting factors
    γ genes: derepression (hydroxyurea, organic acid,
        erythropoietin)
    mRNA repair, trans-splicing, degradation
Hemoglobin
    Proteolysis, stabilization of hemoglobin chain
    Hemoglobin S modifiers
Cellular "stress"
    Erythrocyte dehydration inhibitors
    Iron chelators
    Hemin chelators
    Antioxidants
    Antiapoptotic agents
Therapies acting beyond erythrocytes
    Anticoagulants and antithrombotic agents
    Adherence inhibitors
    Vascular acting agents (NO)
    Erythrophagocytosis acting agents
    Erythrocyte replacement/blood substitute
    Nutrition supplement (arginine)
Organ-specific therapies

Table 42.2. Hemoglobin Modifiers As Antisickling Agents

Agents	Drawbacks
Noncovalent reagents	
Nonspecific reagents	
Urea, organic solvent	High concentration required
Aromatic alcohols or acids	Small and nonspecific effects
Stereospecific inhibitors	
Aromatic acid derivatives	Small effects
Peptides	High concentration required
Organic compounds	
Covalent reagents	
Targeting terminal residues (cyanate, pyridoxal, tucaresol)	Toxicity Immunostimulant
Targeting side chains (glyceraldehyde, nitrogen mustard)	Toxicity
Targeting 2,3 BPG binding site (Diaspirin)	Toxicity
Nitric oxide	Under evaluation

group of both α- and β-globin chains increased the oxygen affinity and the solubility of HbS directly. However, no significant reduction of painful episodes was observed, while side effects, such as cataracts and peripheral neuropathy, were detected. Thus, further clinical trials with oral potassium cyanate were stopped. To avoid systemic side effects, extracorporeal treatment of patient's blood with cyanate was tested (Diederich et al., 1976; Balcerzak et al., 1982). It did not decrease the frequency or the severity of painful episodes. The positive consequences of these negative attempts were the potential targeting of the α amino groups for covalent adducts and the discovery of gly-cosylated hemoglobin at the βNH$_2$ terminus as a con-sequence of elevated blood glucose concentrations in diabetes mellitus (Koenig et al., 1976).

The design of antisickling agents targeting the hemoglobin molecule was improved by the precise knowledge at the atomic level of hemoglobin tertiary structure and allosteric conformations (Perutz et al., 1951, Chapter 9). The intermolecular contacts were unveiled by x-ray crystallography (Wishner et al.,

1975). Twisted polymer composed of seven pairs of antiparallel strands was found in sickle cells by high-resolution microscopy (Dykes et al., 1978). The inter-molecular contacts have been confirmed by the changes in HbS solubility induced by various hemo-globin mutations located in the putative contact sites (Nagel et al., 1980; Benesch et al., 1982).

Table 42.2 summarizes the major potential antisick-ling agents that have been investigated. Various types of chemically reactive compounds were able to inhibit intermolecular contact or increase the oxygen affinity of HbS. Nitrogen mustards and other alkylating agents (Fung et al., 1975), pyridoxal and other aldehydes forming Schiff base adducts (Benesch et al., 1977; Zaugg et al., 1977; Acharya and Manning, 1980; Abraham et al., 1982), esterifying agents (Seetharam et al., 1983), sulfhydryl reagents targeting cysteine β93 (Garel et al., 1982), and bifunctional agents (Chao et al., 1976), that form intra- or intermolecular cross-links were found to be efficient antisickling com-pounds. Bis(3,5-dibromosalicyl)fumarate cross-linked β 82 lysine residues in the central cavity, preventing the binding of 2,3 biphosphoglycerate, (2,3 BPG) which stabilizes the deoxy conformation of HbS (Chatterjee et al., 1982). The poor specificity and the toxicity of many antisickling agents precluded clinical trials.

However, the cyclic aldehyde compounds were most promising. The initial reagent 12C79 (BW12C)

was very efficient in increasing the oxygen affinity of sickle erythrocytes in vitro (Keidan et al., 1989) or when infused in normal adults in a phase I study (Philip et al., 1993). It was specifically bound to the N terminus of α-globin chains (Wireko and Abraham, 1991) and prevented death induced by hypoxia in a transgenic model of sickle cell disease, the SAD mouse (Trudel et al., 1994). The orally active derivative 589C80 (tucaresol) was found to increase the oxygen affinity and to reduce hemolysis in six patients with sickle cell anemia (Arya et al., 1996). The oxygen affinity of HbS was increased between 10 percent and 20 percent in all patients, depending on the dose. Rises in hemoglobin concentration (mean 2.2 g/dL), a decrease in irreversibly sickled cells by one-half, and decreased hemolysis as shown by falls in lactate dehydrogenase (16 percent to 52 percent) were obtained within a few days and lasted for 1 to 2 weeks. However, three patients developed fever and tender lymphadenopathy, between days 7 and 11 from the start of the drug. Schiff base formation on specific amines of the T-cell surface provided a costimulatory signal that activated Na$^+$ and K$^+$ transport, enhancing T-cell receptor dependent interleukin (IL)-2 production (Rhodes et al., 1995; Rhodes, 1996; Chen et al., 1997). Tucaresol is in clinical trials as an immunopotentiator in chronic hepatitis B virus infection, human immuno deficiency virus (HIV) infection, and malignant melanoma (Chen and Rhodes, 1996) but not in sickle cell disease.

It may be possible to develop other cyclic aldehyde compounds that could have lower T-cell potentiation and maintain very efficient hemoglobin binding and a left shift of the red cell oxygen dissociation curve (Abraham et al., 1991, 1995). However, it should be noted that agents that increase the oxygen affinity of HbS may also increase the red cell mass and blood viscosity, a potentially adverse effect. They could be useful for very short-term therapy of severe sickle cell painful episodes in hospitalized patients. The specific inhibition of intermolecular contacts within the HbS molecule by agents that do not affect the oxygen affinity of HbS remains a major goal.

Fifty years after the discovery of the abnormal protein, despite the many experimental advantages available for studying sickle cell disease, none of the hundreds of antisickling agents that inhibit HbS polymerization in vitro are in clinical use. Unfortunately, the hemoglobin molecules are at a very high concentration within erythrocytes—5 mmol/L—representing one-third of the red cell mass. The abnormal red cells have a rapid turnover requiring large amounts of a potential therapeutic drug to be bound to the hemoglobin molecules. In addition, the agent should not affect the physiologic functions of hemoglobin. It must be specific for hemoglobin and nontoxic at an efficient dose.

Today, the tremendous progress of molecular drug design and the recently refined structure of HbS polymer at 2.05 angstrom resolution (Harrington et al., 1997) should be used with appropriate screening to search for hemoglobin modifiers with specific antisickling properties. Nitric oxide and NO-releasing compounds may be of special interest (see later in this chapter).

β Thalassemia

Hemoglobin modifiers targeting α-globin chains could be useful therapies in β thalassemia major, the severity of which is related to the excess of unpaired α-globin chains. These unstable α chains oxidize, precipitate, and form Heinz bodies in erythroid cells. Reduction in α-chain instability, heme oxidation, and release, could transform Cooley's anemia into a thalassemia intermedia syndrome, as shown by the clinical benefit of increasing the expression of γ-globin chains of HbF or by coinheritance of α-thalassemia determinants, both of which decrease the relative excess of α-globin chains. In HbH disease, despite a similar degree of hemoglobin chain imbalance, the self-association of β-globin chains into nonfunctional β$_4$ tetramers, or HbH, induces a less severe anemia that is mostly hemolytic, in contrast to the ineffective erythropoiesis prevalent in β thalassemia major.

INHIBITORS OF ERYTHROCYTE DEHYDRATION

In sickle cells, the amount and rate of formation of polymers are dependent on several variables: intracellular HbS concentration; PO$_2$; the amount of other hemoglobins such as HbF and HbA$_2$, which could antagonize HbS polymerization, temperature; pH; and the concentration of 2,3 BPG, which stabilizes the deoxy conformation in which HbS polymerizes (Poillon et al., 1998).

Pathophysiologic aspects of sickle cell anemia have been discussed in Chapters 20–22. Intracellular concentration of HbS is a major factor for polymerization as the delay time of polymer formation is dependent on the 15th to 30th power of hemoglobin concentration (Eaton and Hofrichter, 1987). In most physiologic conditions hemoglobin polymers are not present in erythrocytes of sickle cell trait carriers who are asymptomatic, because the HbS concentration is 13 to 14 g/dL of cells, below the threshold value for polymerization.

In sickle cell anemia patients, a vicious cycle between polymerization of HbS and cellular dehydration most probably plays a major role in the expression

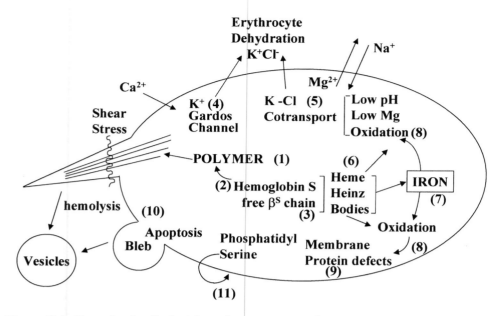

Figure 42.1. Sites of red cell physiology that are targets of experimental therapies. Sickle hemoglobin polymer and free β^S-globin chains, primary defects in sickle cell anemia are shown in red, secondary defects are shown in green, and tertiary defects in black. For full color reproduction, see color plate 42.1.

of the disease. A substantial number of abnormally dense erythrocytes results from polymerization-induced membrane damage, leading to cell dehydration (Glader and Nathan, 1978; Joiner, 1993). Because the polymerization process is highly dependent on HbS concentration, these dense erythrocytes are likely to rapidly accumulate HbS polymers at decreased PO_2, become distorted and rigid, and contribute to vasoocclusive and hemolytic defects.

Important contributors to sickle cell dehydration are potassium-chloride-cotransport (K-Cl efflux) and the calcium-activated K^+ channel, the so-called Gardos channel (Lew et al., 1991). Deoxygenation-induced HbS polymer formation leads to increased membrane permeability to cations, including Ca^{++} and Mg^{++}. The transient increase in cellular ionized calcium is sufficient to trigger activity of the K^+ channel (Gardos) resulting in water loss. In sickle cell disease, K-Cl cotransport is activated by low pH (Brugnara et al., 1986), low magnesium content of erythrocytes oxidative damage, positively charged hemoglobin (HbS, HbC), and cell swelling (Fig. 42.1).

Water retention using antidiuretic therapy (desmopressin) and a low-sodium diet was an initial attempt to decrease cellular HbS concentration by hypotonic swelling (Rosa et al., 1980). The practical difficulty was in maintaining a significant hyponatremia and a second trial (Charache and Walker, 1981) failed to confirm the initial beneficial results. This nonselective

approach to erythrocyte hydration was associated with neurotoxicity. Cetiedil, a membrane active agent that has a low affinity for the Gardos channel and that increases Na^+ permeability, was shown to have some beneficial effects in reducing sickle cell crises (Berkowitz and Orringer, 1981; Benjamin et al., 1986). However, no further clinical study of this agent has been carried out. Calcium channel blockers (verapamil, diltiazem, bepridil, nifedipine, nitrendipine) inhibit sickling and erythrocyte dehydration in vitro (Benjamin, 1989) but had little effects in vivo. Other membrane modifiers that have an erythrocyte swelling effect such as monensin, tellurite, nystatin, and chlorpromazine have been studied only in vitro.

Clotrimazole and Ca++ Activated K+ Channel (Gardos Channel)

Considerable progress has been made recently in the development of therapies that inhibit potassium and water loss from sickle erythrocytes and reduce the formation of abnormally dense and dehydrated sickle cells.

A recent development in the study of the Gardos channel has been the description of the inhibitory effect of clotrimazole (CLT) (Sawyer et al., 1975) and other imidazole antimycotics (Alvarez et al., 1992; Brugnara et al., 1995). Clotrimazole is the most potent inhibitor of the erythrocyte Gardos channel, whereas econazole and miconazole are the most potent inhibitors of plasma membrane Ca^{++} channels, (Alvarez et al., 1992). CLT specifically inhibits the Gardos channel of sickle cell erythrocytes as measured by the inhibition of Ca^{++}-activated Rb^+ influx (IC_{50} = 51 ± 15 nM). It displaces charybdotoxin, which is known to bind close to the opening of the channel, indicating that CLT acts as a pore blocker (Brugnara et al., 1993b). In vitro pharmacologic studies suggest that neither type I nor type II imidazole receptors are present on red cells, so that the action of CLT can be recognized as a specific inhibitory effect on the Gardos channel (Brugnara et al., 1995). In vitro studies with human sickle cells indicate that CLT can specifically prevent red cell dehydration and K+ loss through Gardos channel inhibition (Brugnara et al., 1993a).

The efficacy of CLT as a specific inhibitor of the Gardos channel has been evaluated in vivo in a mouse model for sickle cell disease: the SAD mouse (De Franceschi et al., 1994). The SAD mouse is characterized by the presence of the triply mutated HbSAD, which combines the β6 Val mutation of HbS with two additional mutations known to promote HbS polymerization, HbS-Antilles (β6 val, β23 Ile) and HbD-Punjab (β121 Gln). The SAD mice show clinical and biological features similar to those observed in HbSC disease. The effect of oral administration of CLT was studied in SAD mice during a 4 week period. Oral administration of CLT (160 mg/kg/d) induced a significant inhibition of the Ca++ activated-Rb+ transport measured in whole blood, and restored the red cell volume after 48 hours of administration. These effects persisted during the 28 days of treatment (De Franceschi et al., 1994). The inhibition of the Gardos channel was associated with increased erythrocyte K+ content, decreased mean corpuscular hemoglobin concentration (MCHC), and decreased red cell density. All of these changes were reversible within 2 days after CLT was withdrawn at day 7 or 28 of treatment. No toxicity and side effects were observed.

Studies with normal volunteers taking CLT orally have identified a dosage range (10 to 20 mg/kg of body weight/d) that leads to marked inhibition of the erythrocyte Gardos channel (Brugnara et al., 1994). This dosage is substantially lower than that used in the treatment of systemic mycosis (100 to 160 mg/kg/d) (Sawyer et al., 1975; Seo et al., 1977). CLT metabolites lacking the imidazole ring are detectable in plasma. These metabolites have no antimycotic effects but they maintain a substantial inhibitory activity on the Gardos channel.

A short-term study was carried out in sickle cell anemia patients, who were treated with CLT at a dosage of 10 to 30 mg/kg/d. The CLT treatment induced an inhibition of the Gardos channel, a decrease in red cell dehydration, and an increase in red cell K+ content (Brugnara et al., 1996). The effects of CLT on red cells were more evident in patients with a significant number of dense cells at baseline. Adverse side effects were limited to mild/moderate dysuria in all subjects, likely due to urinary excretion of CLT metabolites, and a reversible increase in plasma ala-

nine transaminase and aspartic transaminase levels in two subjects treated with CLT at the dosage of 30 mg/kg/d.

Clearly, further investigation of this potentially useful, nontoxic compound or its derivatives in preventing red cell dehydration is warranted. Current studies are addressing the issue of long-term treatment with CLT and combination therapy with hydroxyurea (see Chapter 38).

Magnesium and K-Cl Transport

K-Cl cotransport promotes loss of K+ and Cl- with subsequent erythrocyte dehydration and is activated when young erythrocytes are exposed to any of a number of different conditions: pH values lower than 7.40, swelling in hypotonic media, low intracellular magnesium content, and positively charged hemoglobin variants such as HbS or HbC (Canessa et al., 1986; Brugnara, 1995). Pharmacologic inhibitors of this pathway, which could be used to prevent cell dehydration in vivo, do not exist. [(Dihydroindenyl)oxy]alkanoic acid (DIOA) can inhibit the K-Cl cotransport system but it is not active at a low enough concentration to be used in vivo (Vitoux et al., 1989).]

However, K-Cl cotransport is exquisitely sensitive to cell magnesium concentration, and a slight increase in cell Mg induces marked inhibition of K-Cl cotransport (Brugnara and Tosteson, 1987). The Mg content of erythrocytes is an important modulator of red blood cell volume, volume regulatory mechanisms, and membrane functions (Rayssignier et al., 1991; Brugnara, 1995) (Fig. 42.2A). Cellular Mg content has a direct effect on erythrocyte volume and water content (Brugnara and Tosteson, 1987). When cell Mg++ is increased, Cl- moves into the cell to compensate for the positively charged ions, with an obligatory osmotic water influx and consequent cell swelling. There have been reports of abnormally low cell Mg content in sickle erythrocytes, especially in the dense fractions containing irreversibly sickled cells (ISC) (Olukoga et al., 1990; Ortiz et al., 1990).

The effects of oral Mg supplementation have been studied in the SAD mouse (De Franceschi et al., 1996). In this mouse strain, oral Mg supplementation (1,000 ± 20 mg/kg of body weight/d) restored red cell Mg and K contents, and reduced K-Cl cotransport activity, MCHC, and cell density. On the other hand a Mg-deficient diet led to worsening anemia, reticulocytosis, and dehydration of SAD mouse red cells, associated with increased K-Cl cotransport activity. Oral magnesium supplementation prevented additional erythrocyte dehydration and K loss caused by hypoxemia. The best protective effect against red cell dehydration and K loss was obtained by the use of magnesium sup-

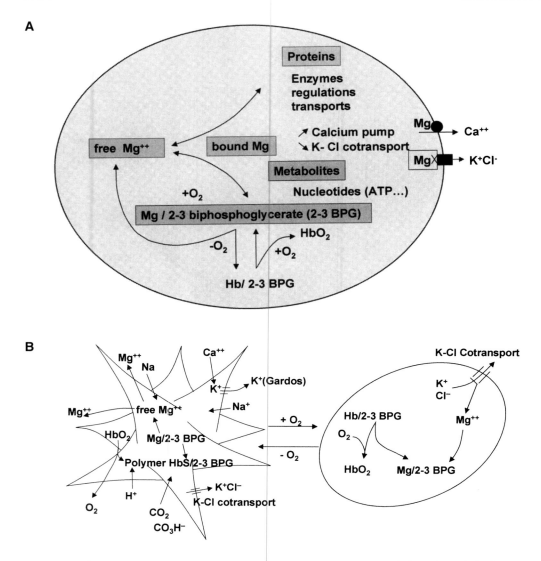

Figure 42.2. Magnesium and the erythrocyte. (A) Effects of Mg in the normal red cell. (B) Effects of Mg in the sickle erythrocyte.

plementation with clotrimazole (De Franceschi et al., 2000).

Studies in diabetic patients have shown that dietary Mg supplementation with Mg pidolate can increase red cell Mg content (Borella et al., 1993; Paolisso et al., 1994). Based on the SAD mouse experiments, the effects of oral Mg supplementation were evaluated on red cell dehydration in sickle cell anemia patients (De Franceschi et al., 1997a, 1997b, 2000) Mg pidolate at a dose of 0.6 mEq/kg/d was used as oral Mg supplementation in ten sickle cell anemia patients. Four weeks of treatment induced an increase in red cell Mg and K content, and a decrease in the activity of K-Cl cotransport. Ektacytometric analysis showed changes indicative of improved hydration of red cell in agreement with a reduction of red cell dehydration demonstrated by the phthalate ester density distribution curve. There were no laboratory or clinical signs of hypermagnesemia; mild, transient diarrhea was the only reported side effect. A pilot study, using Mg pidolate for 6 months, confirmed the beneficial effects on red cell dehydration of oral Mg pidolate supplementation and has demonstrated a 58 percent reduction in the number of painful days (De Franceschi et al., 2000).

Magnesium supplementation ameliorated the anemia in a mouse model of β thalassemia (de Franceschi et al., 1997c) and decreased red cell dehydration in human β thalassemia intermedia (de Franceschi et al., 1998).

These results represent a promising therapeutic approach for preventing red cell dehydration in sickle cell disease. Ongoing studies (randomized, placebo controlled) are currently evaluating the effects of long-term magnesium supplementation in sickle cell anemia patients.

Nitric Oxide (NO)

NO is a highly diffusible intercellular messenger in various tissues, having short range of action related to a very short life span. Its vasodilatory property is used for the treatment of heart ischemia. NO is released from NO donors, the first of which was nitroglycerin. Septic shock is associated with excess NO production (Lamas et al., 1998). NO affects blood cells. It inhibits leukocyte adherence to endothelium and platelet activation, and aggregation. It also interacts with hemoglobin. This last interaction will be discussed here because it has several implications in physiology, pathology, and therapy of hemoglobin disorders.

NO is generated from L-arginine by the endothelial NO synthases. NO activates soluble guanylate cyclase, to produce cyclic guanosine monophosphate (cGMP), a second messenger, involved in many cellular functions. NO diffuses out of the originating cells and into nearby target cells, where it binds the heme group of cytosolic guanylate cyclase and activates this enzyme by breaking the iron/proximal histidine bond, a similar mechanism as found in the binding of NO to the heme of hemoglobin The first known role of hemoglobin with regard to NO was to trap this free radical, preventing its diffusion after local release by endothelial cells. $Hb^{++}O_2$ reacts immediately with NO to form nitrate (NO_3^-), which is eliminated in the urine (Henry et al., 1996).

$$Hb^{++}O_2 + NO^\bullet = Hb^{+++} + NO_3^-$$

Oxidized hemoglobin (methemoglobin Hb^{+++}) is subsequently reduced by the hemoglobin reductase system to Hb^{++}, which is able to bind new oxygen molecules (see Chapter 46).

The second property of hemoglobin, when deoxygenated, is to immediately form a stable complex with NO, nitrosyl hemoglobin (Hb heme-NO), binding initially to the α-globin chain. The affinity of hemoglobin for NO is 1 million fold greater than that for oxygen. Until recently, study of this property has been restricted to the field of physical biochemistry.

A third type of reaction of hemoglobin with NO is to form nitrosothiols, which result from the binding of NO to the two thiol groups present at the surface of the hemoglobin molecule (i.e., the cysteine β93 residues). This reaction occurs when hemoglobin is in the oxy conformation, forming S nitrosyl hemoglobin (Hb-S-NO) (Jia et al., 1996).

Small nitrosothiol molecules are becoming of increasing interest and could be involved in the transfer of NO. The thiol groups of hemoglobin can exchange NO with small nitrosothiols derived from free cysteine and glutathione (Stamler et al., 1997).

Accordingly, the thiol groups of hemoglobin could bind and transfer NO or exchange NO with small shuttle molecules favoring better blood perfusion of hypoxic tissues. Besides its native NO form or nitrosyl (heme-NO, nitrosothiol) nitrogen monoxide gives rise to functional or toxic derivatives such as nitrite (NO_2^-) and peroxonitrite ($ONOO^-$), which can cross the red cell membrane and form NO and $OH^\bullet$, the most toxic radical of oxygen (Mallozi et al., 1997).

Low concentrations of NO may increase the oxygen affinity of sickle erythrocytes although this effect is controversial (Head et al., 1997; Gladwin et al., 1999). In one study (see Chapter 24) the left shift of the oxygen dissociation curve was obtained within 45 minutes after exposure of deoxygenated sickle cells to NO and was dose dependent in the range 20 to 80 ppm of NO. Breathing of NO, 80 ppm for 45 minutes, induced a restoration of the normal oxygen dissociation curve of sickle cells, in eight of nine patients homozygous for the sickle cell mutation. In contrast, NO did not affect the oxygen affinity of normal erythrocytes in vitro or in vivo. The formation of methemoglobin was negligible.

NO, a potent vasodilator, is an important regulator of vascular tone. The combination of hemoglobin polymerization, abnormal adherence of sickle erythrocytes to endothelial cells, and disturbed vasomotor tone regulation culminate in vasoocclusion. In rats, human sickle cells induced stroke and subsequent death only in animals in whom NO production was suppressed by NO synthase inhibitors (French et al., 1997). NO metabolites can be decreased during sickle cell vasoocclusive episodes associated with severe pain (Lopez et al., 1996, 1998) or with acute chest syndrome (Morris et al., 1998) and in association with reduced blood levels of arginine, the physiologic precursor of NO. The increase in NO derivatives in the blood of patients with sickle cell disease was described in an earlier study (Rees et al., 1995).

In patients with various types of anemia, NO derivatives increased by 54 percent in plasma, with low doses of oral arginine (0.1 mg/kg/d). However, this supplement did not modify the level of NO derivatives in plasma of sickle cell anemia patients (Morris et al., 1998). Interestingly, hydroxyurea, which can increase HbF expression and reduce the clinical severity of sickle cell disease (Charache et al., 1995) is also an NO donor (Jiang et al., 1998).

Thus, NO may have several beneficial effects: (1) at the erythrocyte level, by decreasing polymer formation, (2) by decreasing cell adherence and aggregation of platelets, and (3) as a vasomodulator in hypoxic areas. Further studies are required to determine the usefulness of NO breathing, arginine, and NO donors in the treatment of sickle cell painful episodes and acute ischemia of various organs.

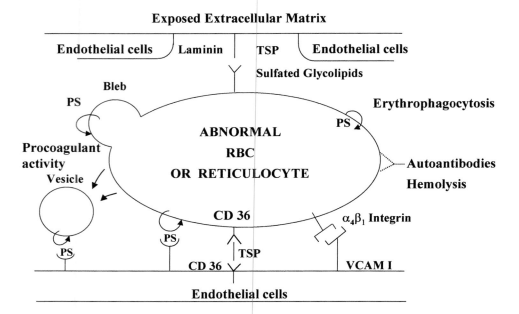

Figure 42.3. Potential targets for agents that interfere with adherence of erythrocytes to endothelial cells. PS, phosphatidyl serine; TSP, thrombospondin.

Antiadherence Therapy

Cellular interactions between erythrocytes, endothelial cells, leukocytes, and platelets are increased in sickle cell disease and in β thalassemia. The abnormal cell-cell interactions could be targets for new therapies (Fig. 42.3).

RheothRx (Poloxamer 188) is a nonionic surfactant block copolymer with hemorheologic properties that improve microvascular blood flow by lowering viscosity and frictional forces. RheothRx has been shown to block hydrophobic adhesive interactions (cell-cell, cell-protein, and protein-protein) in blood, resulting in the reduction of erythrocyte aggregation, adherence of erythrocytes to vascular endothelium, and an improvement in microvascular flow (Armstrong et al., 1995; Smith et al., 1987). In a randomized, double blind, placebo-controlled, pilot phase II study, RheothRx was well tolerated when fifty patients received 48 hour infusions of either RheothRx or placebo for moderate or severe pain lasting at least 4 hours, but less than 18 hours after presentation to the hospital (Adams-Graves et al., 1997). A 48 hour infusion at doses of 30 mg/kg/h of RheothRx significantly reduced total analgesic use and pain intensity and showed trends to shorter duration of painful episodes and total days of hospitalization. This first formulation of Poloxamer 188 was associated with reversible nephrotoxicity in patients with heart failure. This toxicity was shown to be due to impurities in the formulation and a new highly purified product, Flocor™, is now undergoing therapeutic trials (Adams-Graves, et al., submitted).

Iloprost and pentoxifylline may have similar antiadherence properties as Poloxamer 188, inhibiting the adherence of sickle erythrocytes to endothelial cells the mechanisms of action of which are not clarified.

Various types of compounds may impair intercellular adherence such as anionic polysaccharides, polyethylene glycol covalently bound to erythrocytes (Armstrong et al., 1997) or other erythrocyte "coating" molecules (Scott et al., 1997; Barabino et al., 1999).

An interesting potential therapeutic approach is the inhibition of the binding of naturally occurring adherence molecules to erythrocytes, endothelial cells, or platelets. Three types of adherence molecules should be considered: (1) the integrin α4β1 receptor of fibronectin and the vascular cell adhesion molecule 1 (VCAM1); (2) the receptor CD36, which binds thrombospondin and collagen and is present on the surface of endothelial cells, platelets, and a reticulocyte-rich subpopulation of normal and sickle erythrocytes; and (3) sulfated glycolipids, which bind thrombospondin, Von Willebrand factor multimers, and laminin (Hillery et al., 1996; Udani et al., 1998). Anti-integrin agents developed for the treatment of myocardial ischemia (Lefkovits et al., 1995) now provide the rationale for approaches to inhibit the pathologic adherence properties of erythrocytes, endothelial cells, and platelets in sickle cell disease. Adherence of sickle red cells to endothelial cells can be inhibited by antibodies to glycoproteins GPIIb/IIIa and GPIb. Antibodies to the integrins $\alpha_V \beta_3$ and $\alpha_{II} \beta_3$ (GP IIb IIIa) block platelet activating factor-induced sickle cell adhesion in the ex vivo vasculature of the rat (Kaul et al., 2000). Most probably, other mechanisms may be involved in abnormal cell-cell interactions in sickle cell disease and β thalassemia. Anti-$\alpha_4\beta_1$ and anti-VCAM therapies are under evaluation but not yet approved for human use. The use of RGD peptide has been shown to inhibit the adherence of sickle cells to endothelium, in vitro (Kumar et al., 1996). It could also be possible to inhibit the function or the release of receptors or factors that increase the adherence of erythrocytes by intercellular bridges, including platelet activation and secretion of products such as thrombospondin and Von Willebrand factor. Hydroxyurea therapy has been shown to inhibit sickle cell adherence (Bridges et al., 1996) and to reduce the expression of CD36 and $\alpha_4\beta_1$ molecules on red blood cells (Styles et al., 1997). By decreasing the leukocyte count and the number of erythrocytes with phagocytic membrane markers, hydroxyurea probably plays an important role in the improvement of the vascular pathology of sickle cell disease. A glycolytic pathway intermediate, fructose-1, 6-diphosphate (Cordox™) may have therapeutic effects in ischemic tissues by increasing the levels of ATP and creatine phosphate (Marangos et al., 1998). In a pilot randomized trial of forty-six patients with sickle cell disease and acute pain, patients receiving a single 30-minute infusion of 50 mg/kg had a significant reduction in pain intensity compared to placebo-treated patients in the first 4 hours postinfusion (Karwatowska-Prokopczuk et al., submitted). A more definitive efficacy trial of this agent is ongoing.

Anticoagulants and Antiplatelet Therapies

For the purpose of preventing sickle cell painful events, early trials of anticoagulant therapy were disappointing because high doses were used and bleeding episodes were frequent. However small doses of heparin prevented many episodes of pain or reduced hospital days (Chaplin et al., 1980). Low doses of warfarin were used to reduce thrombin generation without side effects (Wolters et al., 1995). A prospective trial of low-molecular-weight heparin is ongoing for sickle cell disease. Other new anticoagulants with specific activity against Factor Xa and thrombin are promising. Prevention of stroke and neurovascular complications of sickle cell disease are major targets for potential anticoagulant therapies as well as the acute chest syndrome, other acute complications, and organ dysfunction or damage, which may be improved by prevention of thrombosis and blood clotting within small or large vessels.

Placebo-controlled trials of low-dose aspirin as prophylaxis for sickle cell painful episode were not associated with any significant benefit in decreasing the frequency of pain episodes (Greenberg et al., 1983; Zago et al., 1984). However the in vivo effects of aspirin on platelet function were not evaluated and documentation of the effect of different doses is very important. High doses of aspirin inhibit prostacyclin production and may worsen sickle cell disease by reducing vasodilatation (Vichinsky et al., 1998). The aspirin-dipyridamole association showed a modest benefit (Chaplin et al., 1980). New agents that block GPIIb/IIIa and GPIb interactions with fibrinogen and Von Willebrand factor are of special interest.

PROTEOLYSIS

β Thalassemia

Pathophysiologic features of β thalassemia are discussed in Chapter 11. The cellular content of unpaired α-globin chains, resulting from the deficiency in β-globin chain expression, is a critical factor in the anemia and pathophysiology of β thalassemia. The number of free α-globin chains results from the balance between the relative excess of the α-globin chain synthesis and the rate of proteolysis of soluble α chains and of precipitated and aggregated α chains present in Heinz bodies or associated with the membrane (Table 42.3). In β-thalassemia heterozygotes the 50 percent relative excess of α-globin chains is proteolyzed. A larger excess of free α chains, as occurs with the additional inheritance of an α-globin gene triplication, is often associated with a β thalassemia intermedia syndrome characterized by transfusion-independent anemia (Gasperini et al., 1998).

A mild β thalassemia intermedia syndrome can replace severe Cooley's anemia in homozygotes for β^0 thalassemia who have coinherited either an α-thalassemia determinant, which reduces the α-globin chain excess, or an increase in γ-globin gene expression, which partially compensates for the β-globin chain deficiency. In both cases, the relative excess of α-globin chains should be reduced (Ratip et al., 1997).

Proteolysis of soluble α-globin chains is a major determinant of the severity of β thalassemia. A comparison between mouse and splenectomized human β-thalassemia patients showed that in both cases a similar degree of anemia was associated with a similar amount of insoluble α-globin chains in red cell ghosts. However, the fate of α chains was very different in the two species. In β-thalassemic mice, Hbb th₁/th₁, mouse α chains are in small excess, highly unstable and not proteolyzed (Rouyer-Fessard et al., 1990). In contrast, in the reticulocytes of β-thalassemic mice expressing human α-globin chains, the human α chains were more stable and much more proteolyzed than the mouse α chains (P. Rouyer-Fessard and Y. Beuzard,

Table 42.3. β-Thalassemic Erythrocytes: Therapeutic Targets

Gene, transcription, translation
↓ Increase in γ-globin expression
▼ Decrease in α-globin expression
α Hemoglobin chains
↓ Increase in proteolysis
▼ Blockade of iron redox cycle
Heme derivatives (free)
▼ Chelation of heme or hemin
Iron (free)
↓ Chelation
▼ Blockade of redox cycle
Oxidation
↓ Radical scavenger
▼ Oxidative chain blockers
Apoptosis/hemolysis/erythrophagocytosis
  Antiapoptotic agents
  Membrane protecting agents

unpublished results). Exposure to several antioxidants resulted in increased proteolysis of human α-globin chains in reticulocytes, indicating that oxidation can decrease the proteolytic process in β-thalassemic erythroid cells.

The proteolysis of α-globin chains has been mostly studied in reticulocytes or in erythrocyte lysates from β-thalassemia patients. One major system for the proteolysis of soluble α chain in reticulocytes is the ATP and ubiquitin-dependent 26S proteasome (Shaeffer and Kania, 1995). The proteolytic capabilities of hemolysates from β-thalassemic blood could be increased by the addition of Ub aldehyde, a synthetic inhibitor of isopeptidases, which hydrolyzes the bond between ubiquitin and the α-hemoglobin or α-globin chain targets, which are substrates for proteolysis when bound to ubiquitin (Shaeffer and Cohen, 1997). This result could be the basis for a therapeutic approach for β thalassemia in order to increase α-chain proteolysis. Proteolysis of α-globin chains in β-thalassemia reticulocytes is very sensitive to oxidation and thiol reagents. N-ethyl maleimide, which binds to the thiol group of cysteine residues, inhibits by 80 percent the proteolysis of soluble α-globin chains (Shaeffer, 1988).

Oxidized proteins, found in abnormal amounts in β-thalassemic cells, form aggregates, due to increased surface hydrophobicity and to cross-linking reactions. In most cells, oxidized proteins are proteolyzed in an ATP and ubiquitin-independent pathway, by the 20S "core" proteasome, which recognizes bulky or hydrophobic residues exposed at the surface of oxidized proteins (Grune and Davies, 1997). By removing potentially toxic proteins and peptides, the proteasome plays a key role in the overall antioxidant defense of erythrocytes as shown after oxidative marking or "hydrophobic" modification of hemoglobin in red blood cells exposed to H_2O_2 or hydroxyl radicals (Giulivi and Davies, 1993; Pacifici et al., 1993). However, protein oxidation induced by hemoglobin chains, heme derivatives, and iron decreases the rate of α-globin chain proteolysis and generates a vicious cycle. Breaking the oxidation/reduction cycle of proteolysis is an important therapeutic goal.

Sickle Cell Disease

By decreasing the HbS content of erythrocytes, the thalassemia determinants associated with the β^s mutations, either HbS-β thalassemia or sickle cell anemia-α thalassemia, would be expected to lessen the clinical severity of sickle cell disease. In fact, this is not necessarily the case (see Chapters 26 and 28). An excess of hemoglobin chains, either α-globin chains in HbS-β thalassemia or β^s-globin chains in sickle cell anemia-α thalassemia, is observed in these compound genotypes. This excess of hemoglobin chains induces defects that probably counteract the beneficial overall reduction in HbS content. Accordingly, for example in Jamaica, the favorable predictors for clinical expression are the absence of an α-thalassemia determinant and high HbF expression (Serjeant, 1997). Uncombined α- or β-globin chains are unstable and generate increased amounts of membrane-bound hemoglobin chains, heme, and iron, which catalyze cellular oxidative reactions and membrane defects. In these cases, increased proteolysis of the unpaired hemoglobin chains in the soluble or insoluble state should improve the physiologic state of the erythrocyte and reduce the clinical severity of the disease. However, this important therapeutic goal has not yet been addressed.

ANTIOXIDANTS

Intracellular Iron Chelators

β Thalassemia and sickle cell disease are characterized by abnormal erythrocyte oxidative reactions catalyzed by "free" iron associated with membrane, heme derivatives, and precipitated hemoglobin or hemoglobin chains (Hebbel, 1991; Repka and Hebbel, 1991; Sugihara et al., 1992; Repka et al., 1993; Scott et al., 1993; Loegering et al., 1996; Shalev and Hebbel, 1996a, 1996b; Browne et al., 1998) (see Chapter 20). To test the hypothesis that excess iron deposits are important to the pathophysiology of β thalassemia, the iron chelator deferiprone (L1) was administered to β-thalassemic mice for 4 weeks (Browne et al., 1997).

With L1 therapy, improvement of many thalassemic features were observed including decreased membrane free iron and protein oxidation, decreased immunoglobulin bound to erythrocytes, increased K content, erythrocyte hydration, and mean cell volume (MCV). The clearance of erythrocytes, biotinylated in vivo, showed an increased red blood cell survival in L1-treated β-thalassemic mice. This result provides an in vivo confirmation that free iron deposits in erythroid cells contribute to the pathophysiology of β thalassemia and that an iron chelator can remove free pathologic iron deposits from erythrocyte membranes and improve the physiologic state of the cell. In contrast to deferoxamine, deferiprone has been shown to chelate pathologic iron deposits from membranes of intact thalassemic or sickle erythrocytes both in vitro and in vivo (Shalev et al., 1995). However, to be efficient, the iron chelator L1 has to be in relative excess to iron, at least in a 3 to 1 ratio, to inhibit the generation of free radicals. At low concentration, L1 increases oxygen radical generation and potentiates oxidative DNA damage in iron-loaded liver cells (Cragg et al., 1998). An ideal iron chelator should be hexadented (like deferoxamine) for iron binding but it should be able to remove intracellular and membrane associated iron.

Heme Chelators

Heme derivatives released by abnormal and denatured hemoglobin or hemoglobin chains are pro-oxidants. Thus, agents that inhibit their redox activity may diminish erythrocyte injury. Chloroquine and dichloroquine compounds inhibit iron release from hemin or hemoglobin chains induced in the presence of glutathione or H_2O_2. The dichloroquine heme complex inhibits heme dependent peroxidation of membrane lipids and might be beneficial in the treatment of hemoglobinopathies (Scott et al., 1997b). Antioxidants and ferriheme binding agents have synergistic effects in inhibiting membrane peroxidation (Dailly et al., 1998).

Antioxidants

Chain-breaking antioxidants have been disappointing in the treatment of hemoglobin disorders, for example, tocopherol (vitamin E) for β thalassemia (Rachmilewitz et al., 1979) (see also Chapter 11) and vaniline for sickle cell disease (Aruoma 1992; Tresoriere et al., 1998).

The thiol compound N-acetyl cysteine acts as an antioxidant in sickle and normal erythrocytes under oxidative stress (Udupi and Rice-Evans, 1992). It was shown recently to inhibit, at the low concentration of 0.25 mmol/L, the formation of dense and irreversibly sickled cells in vitro and the formation of oxidized membrane proteins (Gibson et al., 1998). N-acetyl cysteine is converted to cysteine, a precursor of reduced glutathione, which is diminished by 20 percent in sickle erythrocytes, especially in dense sickle cells (Lachant and Tanaka, 1986). N-acetyl cysteine may also improve the plasma redox potential as found in senescence and in cancer patients (Hack et al., 1998). Another thiol compound, aminothiol (amifostine), a cytoprotective agent that decreases the toxicity of anticancer therapy, has been found to improve the blood counts in patients with myelodysplastic syndrome, including sideroblastic refractory anemia. This agent reduces by half the need for transfusions in one third of transfusion-dependent patients with myelodysplasia (List et al., 1997). Aminothiol has not yet been studied in patients with hemoglobinopathies.

Repletion of the redox potential of nicotinamide adenine dinucleotide (ratio of NADH to NAD^+ + NADH) was obtained in erythrocytes of seven sickle cell disease patients treated with oral L-glutamine (30 g/d). The NADH level increased from 47.05 ± 6.3 nmol/mL RBC to 72.1 ± 15.1 nmol/mL RBC ($P < .01$). These changes may decrease the oxidative susceptibility of sickle erythrocytes and result in clinical benefit (Nihara et al., 1998). The mechanisms leading to these changes are not fully understood.

Allopurinol, which inhibits uric acid formation, has been shown to decrease the peroxidation damage of sickle erythrocytes measured by the malondialdehyde level in blood (Sertac et al., 1997).

Sickle cell disease patients may have reduced antioxidant capacity in addition to increased oxidant stress in erythrocytes. One-half of sickle cell disease patients exhibit leukocyte vitamin C deficiency, which is due to increased vitamin C utilization and not to inadequate dietary intake of vitamin C (Chiu et al., 1990). Ascorbic acid protects sickle cells against oxidant stress, having a stimulatory effect on the rate of glucose oxidation by the pentose monophosphate shunt (Lachant and Tanaka, 1986), suggesting that clinical trials should be undertaken to examine the efficacy of ascorbic acid as a potential therapy for sickle cell disease.

Entrapment of α-globin chains in human erythrocytes is a pertinent in vitro model of β-thalassemic red blood cells (Scott et al., 1990, 1993). The amount of free heme and iron released in this model of β thalassemia can be as much as 20 times that which can be attributed to entrapped α chains alone. This excess of free heme and iron arises from hemoglobin and can be induced by intracellular glutathione and low amounts of H_2O_2 spontaneously generated in thalassemic erythrocytes. This self-amplifying oxidant chain depletes cellular reducing potential (glutathione in the reduced form) and increases red cell oxidation and destruction (Scott and Eaton, 1995).

β-thalassemia patients are subjected to peroxidative tissue injury by iron and heme derivatives released in and from erythroid cells and by secondary iron overload. Peroxidation products are increased about twofold in serum compared with normal control subjects. Serum levels of vitamin E, ascorbate, vitamin A, β carotene, and lycopene are decreased in these patients. Vitamin E levels were inversely related to ferritin levels, while vitamin E, vitamin A, and lycopene levels were inversely related to transaminase levels (Livrea et al., 1997). Plant flavonoids and polyphenols are antioxidants of potential interest, especially tea polyphenols (Grinberg et al., 1994, 1995, 1997). A therapeutic trial with tea, which may also decrease iron absorption, is ongoing in patients with β thalassemia intermedia (see also Chapter 11).

A new class of antioxidants, indolinic and quinolinic nitroxide, protect erythrocytes from hemolytic events and oxidative stress (Gabbianelli et al., 1997). Similarly, demethylisoeugenol protects normal and β-thalassemic erythrocytes against oxidative damage and its active reduced form is regenerated in the presence of reduced glutathione (Ko et al., 1997). The new antioxidant N-allylsecoboldine protects β thalassemic erythrocytes from peroxyl, hydroxyl radicals, and H_2O_2, decreasing hemolysis and lipid peroxidation, in vitro (Teng et al., 1996).

BLOOD SUBSTITUTES

In search of alternative sources of blood for transfusion, various blood substitutes are under development. Cross-linked hemoglobin solutions with the appropriate oxygen affinity and cooperativity are prepared from human blood, bovine hemoglobin (Gonzales et al., 1997), or from recombinant hemoglobin (Ming Swi Chang, 1997). Polymerized bovine hemoglobin infusions were well tolerated by eighteen adults with sickle cell disease, in a phase I/II study (Gonzales et al., 1997).

Regardless of the source of hemoglobin, its infusion must overcome several problems such as the induction of vasoconstriction, rapid oxidation, and loss of function of hemoglobin in plasma, as well as the short half-life of intravascular hemoglobin (Ming Swi Chang, 1997; Doherty et al., 1998). The polyhemoglobin-superoxide dismutase-catalase complex is a blood substitute with antioxidant properties (D'Agnillo and Chang, 1998)

A new source of hemoglobin and even of red blood cells can theoretically be obtained by culturing CD34+ hematopoietic progenitors or stem cells from umbilical cord blood. After culture in vitro, a 1 million-fold expansion in cell number can be obtained, with the production of 10 pg of hemoglobin per reticulocyte, close to the in vivo expression level. In the near future, long-term cultures of stem cells with full differentiation along the erythroid lineage may increase the yield of hemoglobin production 1,000-fold more and lead to the synthesis of up to 30 mg of hemoglobin or 10^9 erythrocytes per stem cell (Glaser, 1998; Malik et al., 1998).

CONCLUSION

In early clinical trials of specific therapies for sickle cell disease, the improvement of pain was the major criterion of efficacy even with molecules that were not pain relievers. In most cases, the results were disappointing. Today, continuous progress is being made in the understanding of the pathophysiology of disease and of the complex intravascular interplay of sickle erythrocytes, reticulocytes, endothelial cells, platelets, leukocytes, proteins, and regulatory factors, in particular inflammatory cytokines, thus allowing us to ask more specific questions in order to evaluate experimental therapies at different levels of complexity.

It is important to acknowledge the role of animal models which speed up answers to specific questions and confirm proof of principle in vivo, before performing clinical trials (see Chapter 34). Mouse models of hemoglobin disorders are very useful in many aspects of sickle cell disease and thalassemia, in particular to evaluate the role of various genetic or environmental factors. Now it is possible to change a single genetic or environmental factor in congenic mice, including nutrition, to modulate the expression of the disease and to define or confirm therapeutic targets.

Finally, with direct molecular approaches at the protein or the gene level and cellular replacement by transplantation, an array of therapies, compensating for the deleterious consequences of the primary defect, within the abnormal erythroid cells and beyond, should be beneficial for improving the survival and function of diseased erythrocytes, and the quality of life and probably the life expectancy of many patients with severe hemoglobin disorders.

References

Abraham, DJ, Mehanna, AS, Wireko, FC et al. (1991). Vanillin, a potential agent for the treatment of sickle cell anemia. *Blood* 77: 1334–1341.

Abraham, DJ, Safo, MK, Boyiri, T et al. (1995). How allosteric effectors can bind to the same protein residue and produce opposite shifts in the allosteric equilibrium. *Biochemistry* 34: 15006–15020.

Abraham, EC, Stallings, M, Abraham, A, and Garbutt GJ. (1982). Modification of sickle hemoglobin by acetaldehyde and its effect on oxygenation, gelation and sickling. *Biochem. Biophys. Acta* 705: 76–81.

Acharya, SA and Manning, JM. (1980). Reactivity of the amino groups of carbonmonoxy HbS to glyceraldehyde. *J. Biol. Chem.* 255: 1406–1412.

Adams-Graves, P, Cedar, A, Koshy, M et al. (1997). Rheoth Rx (Poloxamer 188) injection for the acute painful episode of sickle cell disease: A pilot study. *Blood* 90: 2041–2046.

Adams-Graves, P, Koshy, M, Steinberg, MH et al. (Submitted). Phase I study of FLOCOR™ (purified poloxamer 188) in patients with sickle cell disease in acute vaso-occlusive crisis.

Alvarez, J, Montero, M, and Garcia-Sancho, J. (1992). High affinity inhibition of Ca²⁺ dependent K channels by cytochrome P-450 inhibitors. *J. Biol. Chem.* 267: 11789–11793.

Armstrong, JK, Meiselman, HJ, and Fischer, TC. (1995). Inhibition of red blood cell-induced platelet aggregation in whole blood by a nonionic surfactant, poloxamer 188 (RheothRX injection). *Thromb. Res.* 79: 437–450.

Armstrong, JK, Meiselman, HJ, and Fisher, TC. (1997). Covalent binding of poly(ethylene glycol) (PEG) to the surface of red blood cells inhibits aggregation and reduces low shear blood viscosity. *Am. J. Hematol.* 56: 26–28.

Aruoma, OI. (1992). Dietary management of sickle cell anaemia with vanillin. *Free Rad. Res. Comm.* 17: 349–350.

Arya, R, Rolan, PE, Wootton, R et al. (1996). Tucaresol increases oxygen affinity and reduces haemolysis in subjects with sickle cell anemia. *Br. J. Haematol.* 93: 817–821.

Balcerzak, SP, Grever, MR, Sing, DE et al. (1982). Preliminary studies of continuous extracorporeal carbamylation in the treatment of sickle cell anemia. *J. Lab. Clin. Med.* 100: 345–355.

Barbarino, GA, Liu, XD, Ewenstein, BM, and Kauk, DK. Anionic polysaccharides inhibit adhesion of sickle cell erythrocytes to the vascuar endothelium and result in improved hemodynamic behavior. *Blood* 93: 1422–1429.

Benesch, R, Benesch, RE, Edalji, R, and Suzuki, T. (1977). 5′ deoxypridoxal as a potential anti-sickling agent. *Proc. Natl. Acad. Sci. U.S.A.* 74: 1721–1723.

Benesch, R, Kwong, S, and Benesch, R. (1982). The effects of alpha chain mutations *cis* and *trans* to the β6 mutation on the polymerization of sickle cell haemoglobin. *Nature* 299: 231–234.

Benjamin, LJ. (1989). Membrane modifiers in sickle cell disease. *Ann N. Y. Acad. Sci.* 565: 247–261.

Benjamin, LJ, Berkowitz, R, Orringer, EP et al. (1986). A collaborative, double-blind randomized study of cetidiel citrate in sickle cell crisis. *Blood* 67: 1442–1447.

Berkowitz, LR and Orringer, P. (1981). Effect of cetidiel, an in vitro anti-sickling agent, on erythrocyte membrane cation permeability. *J. Clin. Invest.* 68: 1215–1220.

Beutler, E and Mikus, BJ. (1961). The effect of methemoglobin formation in sickle cell disease. *J. Clin. Invest.* 40: 1856–1871.

Borella, P, Ambrosini, G, Concari, M, and Bargellini, M. (1993). Is magnesium content in erythrocytes suitable for evaluating cation retention after oral physiological supplementation in marginally magnesium-deficient subjects? *Magnes. Res.* 6: 149–153.

Browne, PV, Shalev, O, Kuypers, FA et al. (1997). Removal of erythrocyte membrane iron in vivo ameliorates the pathobiology of murine thalassemia. *J. Clin. Invest.* 100: 1459–1464.

Browne, P, Shalev, O, and Hebbel, RP. (1998). The molecular pathobiology of cell membrane iron: The sickle cell as a model. *Free Radic. Biol. Med.* 24: 1040–1048.

Brugnara, C. (1995). Erythrocyte dehydration in pathophysiology and treatment of sickle cell disease. *Curr. Opin. Hematol.* 2: 132–138.

Brugnara, C and Tosteson, DC. (1987). Inhibition of K transport by divalent cations in sickle erythrocytes. *Blood* 70: 1810–1815.

Brugnara, C, Bunn, HF, and Tosteson, DC. (1986). Regulation of erythrocyte cation and water content in sickle cell anemia. *Science* 232: 388–390.

Brugnara, C, De Franceschi, L, and Alper, SL. (1993a). Inhibition of Ca²⁺-dependent K⁺ transport and cell dehydration in sickle erythrocytes by clotrimazole and other imidazole derivatives. *J. Clin. Invest.* 92: 520–526.

Brugnara, C, De Franceschi, L, and Alper, SL. (1993b). Ca²⁺ activated-K transport of human and rabbit erythrocytes: Comparison of binding and transport inhibition by scorpion toxins. *J. Biol. Chem.* 268: 8760–8768.

Brugnara, C, Arsmby, CC, Sakamoto, M et al. (1994). In vivo blockade of Ca²⁺ activated K transport in normal human erythrocytes by oral administration of clotrimazole [abstract]. *J. Gen. Physiol.* 104: 15a.

Brugnara, C, De Franceschi, L, Armsby, CC et al. (1995). A new therapeutic approach for sickle cell disease. Blockade of the red cell Ca²⁺ activated K channel by clotrimazole. *Ann. N. Y. Acad. Sci.* 763: 262–271.

Brugnara, C, Gee, B, Armsby, CC et al. (1996). Therapy with oral clotrimazole induces inhibition of the Gardos channel and reduction of erythrocyte dehydration in patients with sickle cell disease. *J. Clin. Invest.* 97: 1227–1234.

Bunn, HF. (1997). Pathogenesis and treatment of sickle cell disease. *N. Engl. J. Med.* 337: 762–769.

Canessa, M, Spalvins, A, and Nagel, RL. (1986). Volume dependent and NEM-stimulated K-Cl cotransport is elevated in SS, SC and CC human red cells. *FEBS Lett.* 200: 197–202.

Cerami, A and Manning, JA. (1971). Potassium cyanate as an inhibitor of sickling of erythrocytes *in vitro*. *Proc. Natl. Acad. Sci. U.S.A.* 68: 1180–1183.

Chao, TL, Berenfeld, MR, and Gabuzda, TG. (1976). Inhibition of sickling by methyacetimidate. *FEBS Lett.* 62: 57–59.

Chaplin, H Jr, Alkjaersig, N, Fletcher, AP et al. (1980). Aspirin-dipyridamole prophylaxis of sickle cell disease pain crises. *Thromb. Haemost.* 43: 218–221.

Charache, S and Walker, WG. (1981). Failure of desmopressin to lower serum sodium or prevent crisis in patients with sickle cell anemia. *Blood* 58: 892–896.

Charache, S, Terrin, ML, Moore, RD et al. (1995). Effect of hydroxyurea on the frequency of painful crises in sickle cell anemia. Investigators of the Multicenter Study of Hydroxyurea in Sickle Cell Anemia. *N. Engl. J. Med.* 332: 1317–1322.

Chatterjee, R, Walder, RY, Arnone, A, and Walder, JA. (1982). Mechanism of the increase of solubility of deoxyHbS due to cross-linking the β chains between lysine-82β1 and lysine-82β2. *Biochemistry* 21: 5901–5909.

Chen, H and Rhodes, J. (1996). Schiff base forming drugs: Mechanisms of immune potentiation and therapeutic potential. *J. Mol. Med.* 74: 497–504.

Chen, H, Hall, S, Heffernan, B et al. (1997). Convergence of Schiff base costimulatory signaling and TCR signaling at the level of mitogen-activated protein kinase ERK2. *J. Immunol.* 159: 2274–2281.

Chiu, D, Vichinsky, E, Ho, SL et al. (1990). Vitamin C deficiency in patients with sickle cell anemia. *Am. J. Pediatr. Hematol. Oncol.* 12: 262–267.

Cooperative Urea Trials Group. (1974). Treatment of sickle cell crisis with urea in invert sugar—a controlled trial. *J. Am. Med. Assoc.* 228: 1125–1128.

Cragg, L, Hebbel, RP, Miller, W et al. (1998). The iron chelator L1 potentiates oxidative DNA damage in iron-loaded liver cells. *Blood* 92: 632–638.

D'Agnillo, F and Chang, TMS. (1998). Polyhemoglobin-superoxide dismutase-catalase as a blood substitute with antioxidant properties. *Nat. Biotech.* 16: 667–671.

Dailly, E, Urien, S, and Tillement, JP. (1998). Chain-breaking antioxidants and ferriheme-bound drugs are synergistic inhibitors of erythrocyte membrane peroxidation. *Free Radical Res.* 28: 205–214.

De Franceschi, L, Saadane, N, Trudel, M et al. (1994). Treatment with oral clotrimazole blocks Ca^{2+} activated K$^+$ transport and reverses erythrocytes dehydration in transgenic SAD mice: A model for therapy of sickle cell disease. *J. Clin. Invest.* 93: 1670–1676.

De Franceschi, L, Beuzard, Y, Jouault, H, and Brugnara, C. (1996). Modulation of erythrocyte potassium chloride cotransport, potassium content, and density by dietary magnesium intake in transgenic SAD mouse. *Blood* 88: 2738–2744.

De Franceschi, L, Bachir, D, Galactéros, F et al. (1997a). Oral magnesium supplements reduce erythrocyte dehydration in patients with sickle cell disease. *J. Clin. Invest.* 100: 1847–1852.

De Franceschi, L, Bachir, D, Galacteros, F et al. (1997b). Dietary magnesium supplementation reduces pain crisis in patients with sickle cell disease. *Blood* 90 (Suppl 1): 1159a.

De Franceschi, L, Brugnara, C, Jouault, H, and Beuzard, Y. (1997c). Dietary magnesium supplementation ameliorates anemia in a mouse model of β-thalassemia. *Blood* 90: 1283–1290.

De Franceschi, L, Cappellini, MD, Graziadei, G et al. (1998). The effect of dietary magnesium supplementation on the cellular abnormalities of erythrocytes in patients with beta thalassemia intermedia. *Haematologica* 83: 118–125.

De Franceschi, L, Bachir, D, Galacteros, F et al. (2000). Oral magnesium pidolate: Effects of long-term administration in patients with sickle cell disease. *Br. J. Haematol.* 108: 284–289.

Dean, J and Schechter, AN. (1978). Sickle cell anemia: Molecular and cellular bases of therapeutic approaches. *N. Engl. J. Med.* 299: 752–763; 804–811; 863–870.

Diederich, D, Trueworthy, RC, Gill, P et al. (1976). Hematologic and clinical responses in patients with sickle cell anemia after chronic extra-corporeal red cell carbamylation. *J. Clin. Invest.* 58: 642–653.

Doherty, DH, Doyle, MP, Curry, SR et al. (1998). Rate of reaction with nitric oxide determines the hypertensive effect of cell-free hemoglobin. *Nat. Biotech.* 16: 672–676.

Dykes, G, Crepeau, RH, and Edelstein, SJ. (1978). Three-dimensional reconstruction of the fibers of sickle-cell haemoglobin. *Nature* 272: 506–510.

Eaton, WA and Hofrichter, J. (1987). Hemogobin gelation and sickle cell disease. *Blood* 70: 1245–1266.

French, JA II, Dermot, K, Scott, JP, Hoffmann, RG et al. (1997). Mechanisms of stroke in sickle cell disease: Sickle erythrocytes decrease cerebral bood flow in rats after nitric oxide synthase inhibition. *Blood* 89: 4591–4599.

Fung, LWH, Ho, C, Roth, EF Jr, and Nagel, RL. (1975). The alkylation of HbS by nitrogen mustard. *J. Biol. Chem.* 250: 4786–4789.

Gabbianelli, R, Falcioni, G, Santroni, AM et al. (1997). Effect of aromatic nitroxides on hemolysis of human erythrocytes entrapped with isolated hemoglobin chains. *Free Radical Biol. Med.* 23: 278–284.

Garel, MC, Beuzard, Y, Thillet, J et al. (1982). Binding of 21 thiol reagents to human hemoglobin in solution and intact cells. *Eur. J. Biochem.* 123: 513–519.

Gasperini, D, Perseu, L, Melis, MA et al. (1998). Heterozygous beta-thalassemia with thalassemia intermedia phenotype. *Am. J. Hematol.* 57: 43–47.

Gibson, XA, Shartava, A, McIntyre, J et al. (1998). The efficacy of reducing agents or antioxidants in blocking the formation of dense cells and irreversibly sickled cells in vitro. *Blood* 91: 4373–4378.

Gillette, PN, Peterson, CM, Lu, YS, and Cerami, A. (1974). Sodium cyanate as a potential treatment of sickle cell disease. *N. Engl. J. Med.* 290: 654–660.

Giulivi, C and Davies, KJ. (1993). Dityrosine and tyrosine oxidation products are endogenous markers for the selective proteolysis of oxidatively modified red blood cell hemoglobin by (the 19S) proteasome. *J. Biol. Chem.* 268: 8752–8759.

Glader, BE and Nathan, NG. (1978). Cation permeability alteration during sickling: Relationship to cation composition and cellular dehydration of irreversibly sickled cell. *Blood* 51: 983–989.

Gladwin, MT, Schechter, AN, Shelhamer, JH et al. (1999). Inhaled nitric oxide augments nitric oxide transport on sickle cell hemoglobin without affecting oxygen affinity. *J. Clin. Invest.* 104: 937–945.

Glaser, V. (1998). Fake blood market gets hemoglobin transfusion from reticulocytes. *Nat. Biotechnol.* 16: 709.

Gonzales, P, Hackney, AC, Jones, S, Strayhorn, D et al. (1997). A phase I/II study of polymerized bovine hemoglobin in adult patients with sickle cell disease not in crisis at the time of study. *J. Invest. Med.* 45: 258–264.

Grinberg, LN, Rachmilewitz, EA, and Newmark, H. (1994). Protective effects of rutin against hemoglobin oxidation. *Biochem. Pharmacol.* 48: 643–649.

Grinberg, LN, Rachmilewitz, EA, Kitrossky, N, and Chevion, M. (1995). Hydroxyl radical generation in beta-thalassemic red blood cells. *Free Radic. Bio. Med.* 18: 611–615.

Grinberg, LN, Newmark, H, Kitrossky, N et al. (1997). Protective effects of tea polyphenols against oxidative damage to red blood cells. *Biochem. Pharmacol.* 54: 973–978.

Grune, T and Davies, KJ. (1997). Breakdown of oxidized proteins as a part of secondary antioxidant defenses in mammalian cells. *Biofactors* 6: 165–172.

Hack, V, Breitkreutz, R, Kinscherf, R et al. (1998). The redox state as a correlate of senescence and wasting and as a target for therapeutic intervention. *Blood* 92: 59–67.

Harrington, DJ, Adachi, K, and Royer, WE. (1997). The high resolution crystal structure of deoxyHbSJ. *Mol. Biol.* 272: 398–407.

Head, CA, Brugnara, C, Martinez-Ruiz, R, Kacmarek, RM et al. (1997). Low concentrations of nitric oxide increase oxygen affinity of sickle erythrocytes *in vitro* and *in vivo*. *J. Clin. Invest.* 100: 1193–1198.

Hebbel, RP. (1991). Beyond hemoglobin polymerization: The red blood cell membrane and sickle disease pathophysiology. *Blood* 77: 214–237.

Henry, Y, Guissani, A, and Ducastel, B. (1996). Nitric oxide research from chemistry to biology: EPR spectroscopy of nitrosylated compounds. Effects of nitric oxide on red blood cells. Springer Verlag, pp. 110–125.

Hillery, CA, Du, MC, Montgomery, RR, and Scott, JP. (1996). Increased adhesion of erythrocytes to components of the extracellular matrix: Isolation and characterization of a red blood cell lipid that binds thrombospondin and laminin. *Blood* 87: 4879–4886.

Jia, L, Bonaventura, C, Bonaventura, J, and Stamler, JS. (1996). S-nitrosohaemoglobin: A dynamic activity of blood involved in vascular control. *Nature* 380: 221–226.

Jiang, JJ, Jordan, SJ, Barr, DP, Gunther, MR et al. (1998). In vivo production of nitric oxide in rats after administration of hydroxyurea. *Eur. J. Haematol.* 60: 1–6.

Joiner, CH. (1993). Cation transport and volume regulation in sickle red blood cells. *Am. J. Physiol.* 264: 251–270.

Karwatowska-Prokopczuk, E, Dziewanowska, ZE, Fox, AW et al. (Submitted). A pilot study of Cordox™ (fructose 1, 6-diphosphate) for the treatment of acute painful episode of sickle cell anemia.

Kaul, DK, Tsai, HM, Liu, XD et al. (2000). Monoclonal antibodies to alphaVbeta3 (7E3 and LM609) inhibit sickle red blood cell-endothelium interactions induced by platelet-activating factor. *Blood* 95: 368–374.

Keidan, AJ, Sowter, MC, Johnson, CS et al. (1989). Pharmacological modification of oxygen affinity improves deformability of deoxygenated sickle erythrocytes: A possible therapeutic approach to sickle cell disease. *Clin. Sci.* 76: 357–362.

Ko, FN, Hsiao, G, and Kuo, YH. (1997). Protection of oxidative hemolysis by demethyldiisoeugenol in normal and beta-thalassemic red blood cells. *Free Radical Biol. Med.* 22: 215–222.

Koenig, RJ, Petersons, CM, Jones, RL et al. (1976). Correlation of glucose regulation and hemoglobin A_{1c} in diabetes mellitus. *N. Engl. J. Med.* 295: 417–420.

Kumar, A, Eckman, JR, and Wick, TM. (1996). Inhibition of plasma-mediated adherence of sickle erythrocytes to microvascular endothelium by conformationally constrained RGD-containing peptides. *Am. J. Hematol.* 53: 92–98.

Lachant, NA and Tanaka, KR. (1986). Antioxidants in sickle cell disease: The *in vitro* effects of ascorbic acid. *Am. J. Med. Sci.* 292: 3.

Lamas, S, Pérez-Sala, D, and Moncada, S. (1998). Nitric oxide: From discovery to the clinic. *TiPS* 19: 436–438.

Lefkovits, J, Plow, EF, and Topol, EJ. (1995). Platelet glycoprotein IIb/IIIa receptors in cardiovascular medicine. *N. Engl. J. Med.* 332: 1553–1559.

Lew, VL, Freeman, CJ, Ortiz, OE, and Bookchin, RM. (1991). A mathematical model of the volume, pH, and ion content regulation in reticulocytes: Application to the pathophysiology of sickle cell dehydration. *J. Clin. Invest.* 87: 100–112.

List, AF, Brasfield, F, Heaton, R et al. (1997). Stimulation of hematopoiesis by amifostine in patients with myelodysplastic syndrome. *Blood* 90: 3364–3369.

Livrea, MA, Tesoriere, L, Pintaudi, AM et al. (1996). Oxidative stress and antioxidant status in beta-thalassemia major: Iron overload and depletion of lipid soluble antioxidants. *Blood.* 88: 3608–3614.

Loegering, DJ, Raley, MJ, Reho, TA, and Eaton, JW. (1996). Macrophage dysfunction following the phagocytosis of IgG-coated erythrocytes: Production of lipid peroxidation products. *J. Leuk. Biol.* 59: 357–362.

Lopez, BL, Barnett, J, Ballas, SK et al. (1996). Nitric oxide metabolite levels in acute vaso-occlusive sickle-cell crisis. *Acad. Emerg. Med.* 3: 1098–1103.

Lopez, BL, Moon, LD, Ballas, SK, and Ma, KL. (1998). Sequential nitric oxide measurements during the emergency department treatment of acute vaso-occlusive sickle cell crisis. *Blood* 92(Suppl 1): 330a.

Malik, P, Fisher, TC, Barsky, LW et al. (1998). An *in vitro* model of human red blood cell production from hematopoietic progenitor cells. *Blood* 91: 2664–2671.

Mallozzi, C, Di Stasi, AM, and Minetti, M. (1997). Peroxynitrite modulates tyrosine-dependent signal transduction pathway of human erythrocyte band 3. *FASEB J.* 11: 1281–1290.

Marangos, PJ, Fox, AW, Riedel, BJ et al. (1998). Potential therapeutic applications of fructose-1, 6-diphosphate. *Exp. Opin. Invest. Drugs* 7: 6–15.

Ming Swi Chang, T. (1997). What are modified hemoglobin blood substitutes? In *Blood substitutes, principles, methods, products and clinical trials*. Karger Landes Systems, chapter 3.

Morris, C, Kuypers, F, Larkin, S et al. (1998). Patterns of L-arginine and nitric oxide production in SCD children hospitalized with vaso-occlusive crisis and acute chest syndrome. *Blood* 92 (Suppl 1): 160a.

Murayama, M. (1966). Molecular mechanism of red cell "sickling." *Science* 153: 145–149.

Nagel, RL, Johnson, J, Bookchin, RM et al. (1980). β-chain contact sites in the haemoglobin S polymer. *Nature* 283: 832–834.

Nihara, Y, Zerez, CR, Akiyama, DS, and Tanaka, KR. (1998). Oral L-glutamine therapy for sickle cell anemia: I. Subjective clinical improvement and favorable change in red cell NAD redox potential. *Am. J. Hematol.* 58: 117–121.

Olukoga, AO, Adewaye, HO, Erasmus, RT, and Adedayn, MA. (1990). Erythrocyte and plasma magnesium in sickle cell anemia. *J. East Afr. Med.* 67: 348–350.

Ortiz, OE, Lew, VL, and Bookchin, RM. (1990). Deoxygenation permeabilizes sickle cel anemia red cells to magnesium and reverse its gradient in the dense cells. *J. Physiol. (London)* 427: 211–216.

Pacifici, RE, Kono, Y, and Davies, KJ. (1993). Hydrophobicity as the signal for selective degradation of hydroxyl radical-modified hemoglobin by the multicatalytic proteinase complex, proteasome. *J. Biol. Chem.* 268: 15405–15411.

Paolisso, G, Scheen, A, Cazzolino, D et al. (1994). Changes in glucose turnover parameters and improvement of glucose oxidation after 4 weeks magnesium administration in elderly noninsulin-dependent (type II) diabetic patients. *J. Endocrinol. Meta.* 78: 1510–1514.

Perutz, MF, Liquori, AM, and Eirich, F. (1951). X-ray and solubility studies of the hemoglobin of sickle-cell anemia patients. *Nature* 167: 929–931.

Philip, PA, Thompson, CH, Carmichael, J et al. (1993). A phase I study of the left-shifting agent BW12C79 plus mitomycin C and the effect on the skeletal muscle metabolism using 31P magnetic resonance spectroscopy. *Cancer Res.* 53: 5649–5653.

Poillon, WN, Kim, BC, and Castro, O. (1998). Intracellular HbS polymerization and the clinical severity of sickle cell anemia. *Blood* 91: 1777–1783.

Rachmilewitz, EA, Shifter, A, and Kahane, I. (1979). Vitamin E deficiency in beta-thalassemia major: Changes in hematological and biochemical parameters after a therapeutic trial with alpha-tocopherol. *Am. J. Clin. Nutr.* 32: 1850–1858.

Ratip, S, Petrou, M, Old, JM et al. (1997). Relationship between the severity of beta-thalassemia syndromes and the number of alleviating mutations. *Eur. J. Haematol.* 58: 14–21.

Rayssignier Y, Gueux E, and Motta, R. (1991). Magnesium deficiency effects on fluidity and function of plasma and sub cellular memebranes. In Lasserre, B and Durlach, J, editors. *Magnesium, a relevant ion.* London: Libbey. pp. 311–316.

Rees, DC, Cervi, P, Grimwade, D et al. (1995). The metabolites of nitric oxide in sickle-cell disease. *Br. J. Haematol.* 91: 834–837.

Reinhardt, EH, Moore, VV, Dubach, R, and Wade, LJ. (1944). Depressant effect of high concentrations of inspired oxygen on erythrogenesis observations on patients with sickle cell anemia with a description of the observed toxic manifestations of oxygen. *J. Clin. Invest.* 23: 682–698.

Repka, T and Hebbel, RP. (1991). Hydroxyl radical formation by sickle erythrocyte membranes: Role of pathologic iron deposits and cytoplasmic reducing agents. *Blood* 78: 2753–2758.

Repka, T, Shalev, O, Reddy, R et al. (1993). Nonrandom association of free iron with membranes of sickle and beta-thalassemic erythrocytes. *Blood* 82: 3204–3210.

Rhodes, J, Chen, H, Hall, SR et al. (1995). Therapeutic potentiation of the immune system by costimulatory Schiff-base-forming drugs. *Nature* 377: 71–75.

Rhodes, J. (1996). Covalent chemical events in immune induction: Fundamental and therapeutic aspects. *Immunol. Today* 17: 436–441.

Rosa, RM, Bierer, BE, Thomas, R et al. (1980a). A study of induced hyponatremia in the prevention and treatment of sickle cell crisis. *N. Eng. J. Med.* 303: 1138–1143.

Rouyer-Fessard, P, Leroy-Viard, K, Domenget, C et al. (1990). Mouse beta thalassemia, a model for the membrane defects of erythrocytes in the human disease. *J. Biol. Chem.* 265: 20247–20251.

Sawyer, PR, Brogden, RN, Pinder, RM et al. (1975). Clotrimazole: A review of its antifungal activity and therapeutic afficacy. *Drugs* 9: 424–427.

Scott, MD and Eaton, JW. (1995). Thalassemic erythrocytes: Cellular suicide arising from iron and glutathione-dependent oxidation reactions? *Br. J. Haematol.* 91: 811–819.

Scott, MD, Rouyer-Fessard, P, Lubin, BH, and Beuzard, Y. (1990). Entrapment of purified alpha-hemoglobin chains in normal erythrocytes. A model for beta thalassemia. *J. Biol. Chem.* 265: 17953–17959.

Scott, MD, Van den Berg, JJ, Repka, R et al. (1993). Effect of excess alpha-hemoglobin chains on cellular and membrane oxidation in model beta-thalassemic erythrocytes. *J. Clin. Invest.* 91: 1706–1712.

Scott, MD, Murad, KL, Koumpouras, F et al. (1997a). Chemical camouflage of antigenic determinants: Stealth erythrocytes. *Proc. Natl. Acad. Sci. U.S.A.* 94: 7566–7571.

Scott, MD, Yang, L, Ulrich, P, and Shupe, T. (1997b). Pharmacologic interception of heme—a potential therapeutic strategy for the treatment of beta thalassemia. *Redox Report* 3: 159.

Seetharam, R, Manning, JM, and Acharya, AS. (1983). Specific modification of the carboxyl groups of HbS. *J. Biol. Chem.* 258: 14810–14815.

Seo M, Iida, H, and Miura, Y. (1977). Basic experiments with clotrimazole administered orally. *Curr. Med. Res. Opin.* 5: 169–178.

Sergeant, GR. (1997). Understanding the morbidity of sickle cell disease. *Br. J. Haematol.* 99: 976–977.

Sertac, A, Bingol, F, Aydin, S, and Uslu, A. (1997). Peroxidative damage in sickle-cell erythrocyte ghosts: Protective effect of allopurinol. *Gen. Pharmacol.* 28: 427–428.

Shaeffer, JR and Cohen, RE. (1997). Ubiquitin aldehyde increases adenosine triphosphate-dependent proteolysis of hemoglobin α-subunits in β-thalassemic hemolysates. *Blood* 90: 1300–1308.

Shaeffer, JR. (1988). ATP-dependent proteolysis of hemoglobin alpha chains in beta-thalassemic hemolysates is ubiquitin-dependent. *J. Biol. Chem.* 263: 13663–13669.

Shaeffer, JR and Kania, MA. (1995). Degradation of monoubiquitinated alpha-globin by 26S proteasomes. *Biochemistry* 34: 4015–4021.

Shalev, O and Hebbel, RP. (1996a). Catalysis of soluble hemoglobin oxidation by free iron on sickle red cell membranes. *Blood* 87: 3948–3952.

Shalev, O and Hebbel, RP. (1996b). Extremely high avidity association of Fe(III) with the sickle red cell membrane. *Blood* 88: 349–352.

Shalev, O, Repka, T, Goldfarb, A et al. (1995). Deferiprone (L1) chelates pathologic iron deposits from membranes of intact thalassemic and sickle red blood cells both *in vitro* and *in vivo*. *Blood* 86: 2008–2013.

Sirs, JA. (1963). The use of carbon monoxide on red cell life span in sickle cell disease. *Lancet* 1: 1971.

Smith CM, Hebbel, RP, Tukey, DP et al. (1987). Pluronic F-68 reduces the endothelial adherence and improves the rheology of liganded sickle erythrocytes. *Blood* 69: 1631–1636.

Stamler, JS, Jia, L, Jerry, PE et al. (1997). Blood flow regulation by S-nitrosohemoglobin in the physiological oxygen gradient. *Nature* 276: 2034–2036.

Styles, LA, Lubin, B, Vichinsky, E et al. (1997). Decrease of very late activation antigen-4 and CD36 on reticulocytes in sickle cell patients treated with hydroxyurea. *Blood* 89: 2554–2559.

Sugihara, T, Repka, T, and Hebbel, RP. (1992). Detection, characterization, and bioavailability of membrane-associated iron in the intact sickle red cell. *J. Clin. Invest.* 90: 2327–2332.

Sugihara, T, Rao, G, and Hebbel, RP. (1993). Diphenylamine: An usual antioxidant. *Free Radical Biol. Med.* 14: 381–387.

Teng, CM, Hsiao, G, Ko, FN et al. (1996). N-allylsecobol-dine as a novel antioxidant against peroxidative damage. *Eur. J. Pharmacol* 303: 129–139.

Tresoriere, L, Darpa, D, Maggio, A et al. (1998). Oxidation resistance of LDL is correlated with vitamin E status in beta-thalassemia intermedia. *Atherosclerosis* 137: 429–435.

Trudel, M, De Paepe, M, Chretien, N et al. (1994). Sickle cell disease of transgenic SAD mice. *Blood* 84: 3189–3197.

Udani, M, Zen, Q, Cottman, M, Leonard, N et al. (1998). Basal cell adhesion molecule/lutheran protein. The receptor critical for sickle cell adhesion to laminin. *J. Clin. Invest.* 101: 2550–2558.

Udupi, V and Rice-Evans, C. (1992). Thiol compounds as protective agents in erythrocytes under oxidative stress. *Free Radical Res. Commun.* 16: 315–323.

Vichinsky, E, Brugnara, C, and Styles, L. (1998). Future therapy for sickle cell disease. *Blood* 92 (Suppl 1, part 2): 112–135.

Vitoux, D, Olivieri, O, Garay, RP et al. (1989). Inhibition of K+ efflux and dehydration of sickle cells by [(dihydroindenyl) oxy] alkanoic acid]: An inhibitor of the K$^+$ CL$^-$ cotransport system. *Proc. Natl. Acad. Sci. USA.* 86: 4273–4276.

Wireko, FC and Abraham, DJ. (1991). X-ray diffraction study of the binding of the antisickling agent 12C79 to human hemoglobin *Proc. Natl. Acad. Sci. U.S.A.* 88: 2209–2211.

Wishner, BC, Ward, KB, Lattam, EE, and Love, WE. (1975). Crystal structure of sickle-cell deoxyhemoglobin at 5Å resolution. *J. Mol. Biol.* 98: 179–194.

Wolters, HJ, ten Cate, H, Thomas, LL et al. (1995). Low-intensity oral anticoagulation in sickle-cell disease reverses the prethrombotic state: Promises for treatment? *Br. J. Haematol.* 90: 715–717.

Zago, MA, Costa, FF, Ismael, SJ. (1984). Treatment of sickle cell diseases with aspirin. *Acta Haematol.* 72: 61–64.

Zaugg, RH, Walder, JA, and Klotz, IM. (1977). Schiff-base adducts of hemoglobin. Modifications that inhibit erythrocyte sickling. *J. Biol. Chem.* 252: 8542–8548.

SECTION VII

OTHER INHERITED DISORDERS OF HEMOGLOBIN

RONALD L. NAGEL

In the next three chapters, we discuss one very common hemoglobinopathy—perhaps the world's most common—and many rare hemoglobinopathies, some that are clinically important and others that are interesting biologically. Rare conditions like these have taught us much about the structure-stability-function relationships of hemoglobin. Studying hemoglobin mutants has provided the most comprehensive list of mutations of any system in human biology, providing a road map for understanding problems of other genetic loci. Globin gene mutations—these include nearly every class of mutation so far described—provided an early catalogue of the types of mutations that can cause genetic disease.

Hemoglobin E (HbE), the most common abnormal hemoglobin in Southeast Asians, is especially prevalent at the border of Thailand, Laos, and Cambodia, where its gene frequency may reach 0.5. Thirty million Southeast Asians are estimated to be heterozygous for HbE and one million are homozygotes. Like sickle cell disease and the thalassemias, HbE carriers have been "selected" by endemic malaria. Many syndromes are observed when HbE is combined with different genotypes of α and β thalassemia and with other abnormal hemoglobins. Asymptomatic and symptomatic forms of HbE-associated conditions exist. HbE heterozygotes and homozygotes are clinically normal with minor changes in blood counts. HbE forms 25 percent to 30 percent of the hemolysate in HbE hetyerozygotes and with compound heterozygosity for HbE and α thalassemia-2. In compound heterozygotes for α thalassemia-1 and HbE, the amount of HbE ranges between 19 percent and 21 percent whereas 13 percent to 15 percent HbE is observed in individuals who are compound heterozygotes for HbH disease and HbE. Microcytosis and target cells are the most prominent hematologic markers of homozygosity for HbE.

HbE-β thalassemia usually has the phenotype of thalassemia intermedia or thalassemia major. HbE-β^0 thalassemia is characterized by 40 percent to 60 percent HbE, with the remainder HbF. In HbE-β^+ thalassemia, a variable amount of HbA is detected in addition to HbE and HbF. Abnormal splicing of the β^E transcript results in reduced amounts of β^E-mRNA and β^E-globin chains, causing a mild β^+ thalassemia determinant accounting for the differences between homozygous HbE disease and HbE-β thalassemia. Despite apparently identical genotypes, compound heterozygotes for β thalassemia and HbE have remarkably variable phenotypes. Why such diversity exists is not always clear but the interactions of various genotypes of α thalassemia, different β-thalassemia mutations, and the ability to produce HbF are all important. Like patients with Cooley's anemia, patients with HbE-β thalassemia may have marked bone marrow expansion, osteoporosis, iron overload, heart failure, hepatomegaly, and be susceptible to infection. At death, thromboembolism seems common. Treatment of HbE-β thalassemia should not differ from that of β thalassemia major, but, unfortunately, regular transfusion and iron chelation is not possible for most patients with HbE-β thalassemia in developing countries.

Abnormal hemoglobins with high or low oxygen affinity, variants that have their heme iron oxidized to the ferric form causing methemoglobinemia (HbM), or hemoglobin variants that are unstable, are abnormalities seen rarely by the general physician and encountered uncommonly in the practice of hematology. High oxygen affinity hemoglobin variants cause erythrocytosis. Low oxygen affinity variants may be accompanied by cyanosis and anemia, and HbM variants present with cyanosis. Patients with unstable hemoglobins may have hemolytic anemia that can worsen during infection and when certain drugs are used, and can be accompanied by characteristically dark urine or pigmenturia due to the presence of dipyrroles. Since these uncommon variants are unusual causes of erythrocytosis, cyanosis, and hemolytic anemia their presence is often unsuspected. When they are present, their identification can prevent hazardous diagnostic tests, spare

Martin H. Steinberg, Bernard G. Forget, Douglas R. Higgs, and Ronald L. Nagel, editors. *Disorders of Hemoglobin: Genetics, Pathophysiology, and Clinical Management.* © 2001 Cambridge University Press. All rights reserved.

the institution of potentially dangerous treatments, permit reassurance of the patient, and provide counseling to the family.

A 1998 syllabus of Human Hemoglobin Variants listed 750 unique hemoglobin variants including 217 involving the α-globin gene, 362 involving the β-globin gene, 70 γ-globin gene variants, 32 δ-globin gene variants, and 69 variants caused by either two mutations in one globin gene, hybrid chains, elongated chains, or truncated chains. Mutations of hemoglobin can be classified in two categories: mutations with frequencies above 1 percent of an affected population, such as HbS, HbE, HbC, and the thalassemias; and hemoglobin mutations that are rare.

Comparatively few globin residues are critical for maintaining the structural integrity and functional performance of hemoglobin. Most hemoglobin gene mutations are, therefore, not associated with hematologic or clinical abnormalities and escape detection, especially when they are electrophoretically or chromatographically silent. Some mutations, while not medically important, illustrate interesting biological and anthropologic principles. Selected rare variants, discussed in Chapter 45, have little or no clinical phenotype and are interesting solely for the biological principles they illustrate. In the last 10 years, more than 100 recombinant hemoglobins have been generated and these have also proven useful for understanding the structure-function relationships of hemoglobin and the polymerization of HbS. Recombinant hemoglobins have also stimulated the field of hemoglobin-based blood substitutes by providing new and state-of-the art compounds of potential clinical interest.

Among the posttranslational modifications that can alter hemoglobin structure are deamidation of selected asparaginyl residues to aspartate that result in two species of globin caused by a single mutation, oxidation of leucine to hydroxyleucine, and acetylation of a retained N-terminal methionyl when normal cleavage of this residue malfunctions. Mutations may lead to elongated or shortened globins and more than one mutation in a single globin gene.

HbG Philadelphia is the most common α-globin gene variant in people of African descent, and is clinically benign. It is usually found with α thalassemia and can be present with different α-globin gene haplotypes; in heterozygotes its level in the hemolysate can vary from 20 percent to 50 percent. When present with HbS or HbC new hemoglobin species appear due to hybrid tetramer formation.

Hemoglobinopathy detection is often a part of the evaluation of anemia, microcytosis, or erythrocytosis; it should be determined if an abnormal variant is present, how abundant is the variant, and if the variant is relevant to the clinical picture that prompted the studies initially. Measurement of the hemoglobin-oxygen dissociation curve is vital when a hemoglobin variant is suspected of causing erythrocytosis.

Mutations of the β-globin gene usually change only one hemoglobin component and stable variants usually have a concentration of 40 percent to 50 percent. As a corollary, HbA levels are reduced by nearly half. In contrast, α-globin gene variants should produce abnormal "HbA," "HbA$_2$," and "HbF" fractions because each of these hemoglobins contains α-globin chains. As a first approximation, mutation of one α-globin gene might then be expected to create variants forming 20 percent to 25 percent of the total HbA, and similar fractions of the total HbA$_2$ and HbF. The actual amounts of different hemoglobin types that accumulate in vivo depend on the output from individual globin genes, the stability of the globin and hemoglobin products, and on the posttranslational assembly of αβ dimers that is dependent on the charge of the globin subunits. α-Globin chain abnormalities are expressed at birth and can produce signs of disease neonatally while β-globin chain mutations are clinically apparent after the first few months of life, although they can be detected before this with proper diagnostic techniques.

43

Hemoglobin E Disorders

SUTHAT FUCHAROEN

INTRODUCTION

Hemoglobin E (HbE) is the most common abnormal hemoglobin in Southeast Asians, especially among the Khmer, Laotians, Mon/Khmer speaking people, the Zhuang in Guangxi, People's Republic of China, and in India and Sri Lanka. However, the occurrence of HbE is most concentrated at the border of Thailand, Laos and Cambodia, an area dubbed the HbE triangle (Na-Nakorn et al., 1956; Flatz, 1965, 1967; Wasi, 1986). The gene frequency of HbE is between 0.05 and 0.10, reaching 0.5 percent in certain parts of Cambodia and the northeast of Thailand. It is estimated that 30 million Southeast Asians are heterozygous for HbE and 1 million are homozygous. The maintenance of so high a gene frequency indicates that the HbE variant somehow improves fitness. Correlation of HbE frequency with the incidence of malaria has been noted, suggesting the presence of a balanced polymorphism (Luzzatto, 1979). Studies of malaria and HbE are detailed in Chapter 30.

CLASSIFICATION OF HbE DISORDERS

In 1954, HbE became the fourth abnormal hemoglobin identified by electrophoresis (Itano et al., 1954), and a substitution of lysine for glutamic acid at position 26 of the β-globin chain was found in 1961 (Hunt and Ingram, 1961). Many different syndromes are observed when HbE is variously combined with different α and β thalassemias and with other abnormal hemoglobins. (Fig. 43.1) They can be classified into asymptomatic and symptomatic forms (Table 43.1).

Asymptomatic Forms

HbE Heterozygotes. HbE heterozygotes are clinically normal with minimal changes in blood counts and erythrocyte indices. Red cell morphology is similar to that in thalassemia minor with normocytic or slightly microcytic red cells [mean corpuscular volume (MCV) 84 ± 5 fl]. A few target cells may be present in the blood smear. Osmotic fragility curves may be within normal limits or moderately shifted to the right, indicating slightly decreased osmotic fragility. Hemoglobin electrophoresis reveals both HbA and HbE. Quantifying the amount of HbE is crucial for the diagnosis of various HbE syndromes that occur from the interaction of HbE with other genetic hemoglobin abnormalities and nongenetic factors (Table 43.2). HbE constitutes 25 percent to 30 percent of the hemolysate in HbE trait and with compound heterozygosity for HbE and α thalassemia-2 ($-\alpha/\alpha\alpha$). HbE-α thalassemia-2 cannot be differentiated from simple HbE trait by hematologic screening. The amount of HbE is reduced by coexistent α thalassemia. Lower levels of HbE suggest concomitant inheritance of the α thalassemia-1 (- -/αα) gene (Wasi et al., 1969; Fucharoen et al., 1988a). In compound heterozygotes for α thalassemia-1 and HbE, the amount of HbE ranges between 19 percent and 21 percent. A marked decrease of HbE to 13 percent to 15 percent is observed in individuals who are compound heterozygotes for HbH disease and HbE and have the HbAE Bart's disease syndrome (Wasi et al., 1967; Fucharoen et al., 1988c, 1998b; Thonglairuam et al., 1989). Interactions between HbE and various α-thalassemia genes are illustrated in Figure 43.2. HbE levels of 39 percent or above suggest the interaction of HbE with β thalassemia (Minnich et al., 1954; Chernoff et al., 1956; Fucharoen et al., 1988b; Rees et al., 1998). HbE heterozygotes who have iron deficiency anemia will have lowered amounts of HbE and further reduced MCV and mean corpuscular hemoglobin (MCH), depending on the degree of anemia (Wasi et al., 1968).

Homozygous HbE. Homozygotes for HbE usually have normal hemoglobin levels but some may be mildly anemic; clinical symptoms are rare. Most

Martin H. Steinberg, Bernard G. Forget, Douglas R. Higgs, and Ronald L. Nagel, editors. *Disorders of Hemoglobin: Genetics, Pathophysiology, and Clinical Management.* © 2001 Cambridge University Press. All rights reserved.

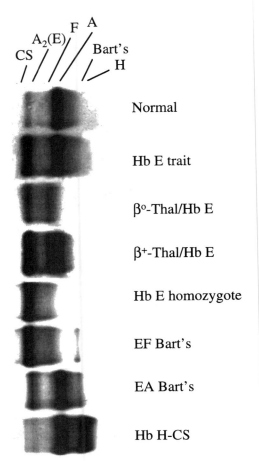

Figure 43.1. Hemoglobin types of various HbE syndromes performed by electrophoresis in an alkaline pH buffer.

mal RNA splicing caused by the HbE mutation (Orkin et al., 1982; Traeger et al., 1982) (see Chapter 12).

Symptomatic Forms

HbE-β Thalassemia. Generally, HbE-β thalassemia disease is a thalassemia syndrome of intermediate severity although the clinical spectrum can be very heterogeneous (Fucharoen et al., 1988b; Rees et al., 1998). Two types of HbE-β thalassemia disease have been described that depend on the presence or absence of HbA. In HbE-$β^0$ thalassemia, $β^A$-globin chains are not present. This genotype results in HbE-$β^0$ thalasemia disease characterized by HbE and HbF without detectable HbA (Fig. 43.1). HbE constitutes between 40 percent and 60 percent of the hemolysate with the remainder HbF (Table 43.2). Clinically, HbE-$β^0$ thalassemia and homozygous HbE are remarkably different; the latter is asymptomatic and the level of HbF much lower. In exceptionally rare cases the amount of HbE in HbE-$β^0$ thalassemia and homozygous HbE may overlap, requiring familial studies and further investigation to define the genotype. In HbE-$β^+$ thalassemia, some HbA is detected in addition to HbE and HbF. However, different $β^+$-thalassemia genes result in a variable severity of disease because of different levels of HbA (Fucharoen and Winichagoon, 1997).

HbAE Bart's Disease. This thalassemia syndrome, characterized by the presence of HbA, HbE, and Hb Bart's, results from the interaction of HbH disease with heterozygous HbE (Wasi et al., 1967; Fucharoen et al., 1988c, 1998b; Thonglairuam et al., 1989). Two common subtypes of HbAE Bart's disease have been observed: α thalassemia-1/α thalassemia 2-$β^A$ and α-thalassemia-1/Hb Constant Spring – $β^A/β^E$. The latter disorder was found to have a more severe clinical syndrome than the former type of HbAE Bart's disease. Usually, the HbE level ranged from 13 percent to 15 percent (Table 43.2). The presence of α thalassemia-1 and α thalassemia-2 genes leads to less availability of α-globin chain for HbE production. Small amounts of Hb Bart's are always present in this genotype. Intraerythrocytic inclusion bodies (HbH inclusions) can be demonstrated in 5 percent to 6 percent of the erythrocytes, indicating the presence of small amounts of HbH ($β_4$); this amount is insufficient to be resolved by electrophoresis.

HbEF Bart's Disease. HbEF Bart's disease is characterized by HbE, HbF, and Bart's Hb (Wasi et al., 1967). HbE constitutes 80 percent and HbF 10 percent of the hemolysate with the remainder Hb Bart's.

patients are not jaundiced and the liver and spleen are usually not enlarged. Reticulocyte counts are consistently normal, and nucleated red cells are not seen in the blood. Bone marrow examinations show a normal cellular pattern or minimal erythrocytic hyperplasia. Bone changes are not present. Osmotic fragility studies show a marked increase in the resistance of erythrocytes to hypotonic saline, indicating decreased osmotic fragility. Besides a slightly reduced hemoglobin level and microcytic, poorly hemoglobinized red cells (Table 43.2), the most unique finding is the red cell morphology with 20 percent to 80 percent target red cells (Fig. 43.3). Hemoglobin analysis reveals about 85 percent to 95 percent HbE with the remainder HbF (Na-Nakorn and Minnich, 1957). There is defective $β^E$-globin chain synthesis in all HbE homozygotes with an average α/non-α biosynthesis ratio of 2, equivalent to the ratio found in $β^+$-thalassemia heterozygotes (Pootrakul et al., 1976; Traeger et al., 1980; Wasi et al., 1982a). Defective $β^E$ chain synthesis is due to decreased $β^E$ mRNA production, a result of abnor-

Table 43.1. Summary of the Common HbE Syndromes in Thailand

Phenotype	Genotype	Anemia	Distinguishing features
Asymptomatic			
HbE heterozygote	β^N/β^E	No	Hbs E (25–30%)+A
HbE-α thalassemia-2 heterozygote	β^N/β^E- $-\alpha^N/\alpha^{thal\ 2}$	No	Hbs E (25–30%)+A
HbE-α thalassemia-1 heterozygote	β^N/β^E- $-\alpha^N/\alpha^{thal\ 1}$	No	Hbs E (19–21%)+A
HbE homozygote	β^E/β^E	No	Only HbE
HbE homozygote-α thalassemia heterozygote	β^E/β^E- $-\alpha^N/\alpha^{thal}$	No	Only HbE
HbE/HbC	β^E/β^C	No	HbE (32%)+HbC(56%)
Symptomatic			
HbE homozygote-Hb CS homozygote	β^E/β^E- -Hb CS/Hb CS	Mild	Hbs E ($\alpha_2\beta_2^E$)+$\alpha_2^{CS}\beta_2^E$
HbE-β^0 thalassemia	β^0/β^E	Moderate to severe	Hbs E+F
HbE-β^+ thalassemia	β^+/β^E	Mild	Hbs E+F+A
EA Bart's			
HbH disease with HbE heterozygote	α Thal 1/α thal 2- -β^N/β^E	Moderate	Hbs E+A+Bart's
HbH-CS disease with HbE heterozygote	α Thal 1/Hb CS- -β^N/β^E	Moderate	Hbs CS+E+A+Bart's
EF Bart's			
HbH disease with HbE homozygote	α Thal 1/α thal 2- -β^E/β^E	Moderate to severe	Hbs E+F+Bart's
HbH-CS disease with HbE homozygote	α Thal 1/Hb CS- -β^E/β^E	Moderate to severe	Hbs CS+E+F+Bart's
HbH disease with HbE-β thalassemia disease	α Thal 1/α thal 2- -β^0/β^E	Moderate to severe	Hbs E+F+Bart's
HbH-CS disease with HbE-β thalassemia disease	α Thal 1/Hb CS- -β^0/β^E	Moderate to severe	Hbs CS+E+F+Bart's

The superscript N indicates a normal β- and α-globin chain.

The presence of Hb Bart's indicates that there is excess γ-globin chain. However, no inclusion bodies or HbH were present, probably because the abnormal β^E-globin chains do not form tetramers. Four genotypes of HbEF Bart's disease can be found. These result from the interaction between HbH disease and either α thalassemia-1/α thalassemia-2 or α thalassemia-1/Hb Constant Spring genotypes, with either homozygous HbE or HbE-β thalassemia (Fucharoen et al., 1988e). Hb Constant Spring and small amounts of HbA may be observed in patients with the α thalassemia-1/Hb Constant Spring and HbE-β^+ thalassemia genotype. To differentiate among these genotypes, family studies and further investigation by DNA analysis are required.

Homozygous HbE – Homozygous Hb Constant Spring Syndrome. It is difficult to identify the existence of the α-thalassemia gene in homozygous HbE without DNA analysis. Individuals have been encountered who were homozygous for HbE and homozygous for Hb Constant Spring. They had thalassemia intermedia with a mild degree of anemia, jaundice, and splenomegaly. Their MCV ranged from 75 to 80 fl and MCH was between 23 and 25 pg (Table 43.2). Compared with homozygous HbE alone there were minimal red cell changes. This

may be due to the interaction of α thalassemia with the β-thalassemia-like reduced globin synthesis typical of HbE (see Chapters 11 and 13).

GENOTYPE-PHENOTYPE INTERACTIONS

Despite seemingly identical genotypes, compound heterozygotes for β thalassemia and HbE have remarkably variable phenotypes. Notable are variations in anemia, growth, development, hepatosplenomegaly, and transfusion requirements (Fig. 43.4). Disease severity has been assessed based on age at presentation, hemoglobin level in the steady state, age of first transfusion, frequency of transfusion, presence of hepatosplenomegaly, bone changes, and growth retardation. Using these criteria, the phenotypic severity of HbE-β thalassemia patients was classified into three groups: (1) mild; hemoglobin level $\geq$ 7.5 g/dL could be maintained without transfusion if the transfusion frequency was less than once every 2 years or less than every 6 months if transfusion was started after age 10; (2) severe; transfusion requirements began at age 4 or older with a frequency of transfusion between 6 weeks and 4 months, or between 3 and 4 months if transfusion commenced before age 4 years; (3) moderate; transfusion requirement began

Table 43.2. Hematologic Data in Various HbE Syndromes

	Hb (g/dL)	MCV (fl)	MCH (pg)	MCHC (g/dL)	RDW (%)	Osmotic fragility	DCIP	Alkaline denaturation test (%)	Hb typing
Normal	M 15.9 ± 0.9 F 12.5 ± 2.0	87 ± 6	31 ± 1.1	33 ± 0.9	13.1 ± 0.8	N	–	0.5 ± 0.2	A$_2$ (2.5 ± 0.2)+A
HbE trait	12.8 ± 1.5	84 ± 5	30 ± 2.4	33 ± 1.8	14.1 ± 0.6	N or D	+	0.9 ± 0.7	E (29.4 ± 2.3 %)+A
HbE-α thalassemia-2	13.1 ± 1.4	88 ± 4	ND	ND	ND	N or D	+		E (28.5 ± 1.5%)+A
HbE-α thalassemia-1	12.5 ± 1.4	77 ± 5	23 ± 1.1	32 ± 1.6	ND	D	+	0.9 ± 0.4	E (20.7 ± 1.2%)+A
Homozygous HbE	11.4 ± 1.8	70 ± 4	22 ± 1.9	33 ± 1.7	15.6	D	+	1.8 ± 1.4	EE (E87.7 ± 5.9%)
HbE-β^0 thalassemia	7.8 ± 2.6	67 ± 6	19 ± 3.6	28 ± 4.8	26.5 ± 5.6	D	+	42 ± 11.5	E (58 ± 11.5%)+F
EA Bart's disease HbE-α thalassemia 1/α thalassemia 2	9.1 ± 1.1	60 ± 3	17 ± 2	31 ± 4	ND	D	+	2.0 ± 0.7	E (13.0 ± 2.1%)+A +Bart's (2.2 ± 1.8%)
HbE-α thalassemia 1/Hb CS	8.0 ± 0.9	67 ± 4	19 ± 2	29 ± 2	ND	D	+	2.3 ± 1.4	CS (1.1 ± 0.4%)+E (13.9 ± 1.8%)+A+Bart's (3.9 ± 1.5%)
EF Bart's disease	8.0 ± 1.3	63 ± 6	18 ± 2	29 ± 2	ND	D	+	5.8 ± 3.7	E (80%)+F+Bart's (5%) or CS (1.9 ± 0.9%)+E (86.4 ± 8%)+F+Bart's (3.7 ± 1.9%)

Abbreviations: ND, not determined; N, normal; D, decreased; CS, Constant Spring; DCIP, dichlorophenolindophenol.

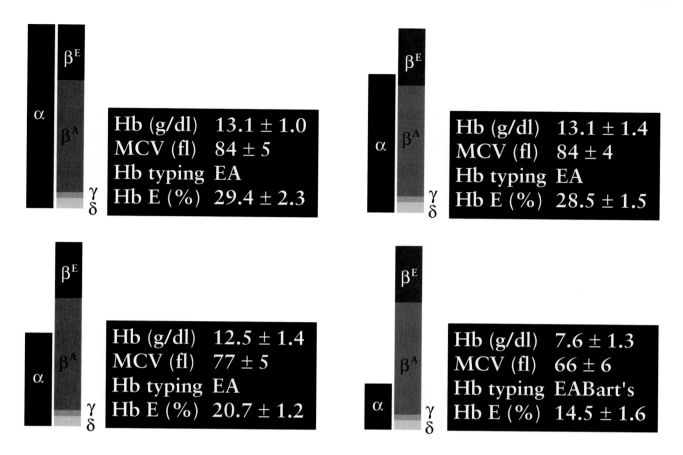

Figure 43.2. Hb E heterozygote versus α-thalassemia. Interaction of different α-thalassemia genes and HbE heterozygote leads to changes in the hematologic parameters.

between 1 and 2 years of age (Ho et al., 1998). A spectrum of severity with hemoglobin levels from 2.5 to 13.5 g/dL, in the steady state, was found in 803 patients with HbE-β⁰ thalassemia (Fucharoen et al., 1988b). Since β⁰ thalassemia is associated with an absence of β-globin chain synthesis, the causes of phenotype heterogeneity in these patients is likely to be a result of factors other than reduced β-globin chain synthesis.

Systematic studies of Thai patients may help us understand factors that determine the severity of anemia in HbE-β⁰ thalassemia. Analysis of concordance and discordance of hemoglobin levels in 216 sibling pairs from 98 families showed a remarkable skew toward the lower values with a mode at 0 to 0.5 g/dL (Fucharoen et al., 1984). Concordance of hemoglobin levels between sibling pairs greatly exceeded discordance, indicating that severity of anemia in these patients is determined by polygenic factors, rather than a single gene effect. Among the factors that influence the severity of anemia are the following.

β-Thalassemia Mutations

Although β⁰ thalassemia is caused by many mutations, all result in absence of β-globin chain production by the abnormal gene (see Chapter 12). β⁰ Thalassemia is usually more severe than β⁺ thalassemia, where a wide range of β-globin chain production is observed. Some β⁺-thalassemia mutations may produce only very small amounts of β-globin chains and have a phenotype similar to that of β⁰ thalassemia (e.g., C→T in IVS-II-654) (see Chapter 12). Alternatively, interaction between HbE and mild β⁺ thalassemia, such as A→G at position −28 or A→G in codon 19 of the β-globin gene, usually results in a mild thalassemic phenotype. Table 43.3 shows the hematologic data and hemoglobin analysis, in the steady state, in mild HbE-β⁺ thalassemia compared to homozygous HbE and severe types of HbE-β⁺ thalassemia (Fucharoen and Winichagoon, 1997). In mild HbE-β⁺ thalassemia, HbE formed about 60 percent of total hemoglobin and HbF levels were about 3 to 10 percent, which is the same effect produced by the mutation in codon 19 (Hb Malay, β19(B1) Asn→Ser). HbF is minimally increased in the absence of severe hemolytic stress. In a few cases, the hemoglobin phenotype was "HbE + HbA" with 60 percent HbE. In contrast, in the two types of

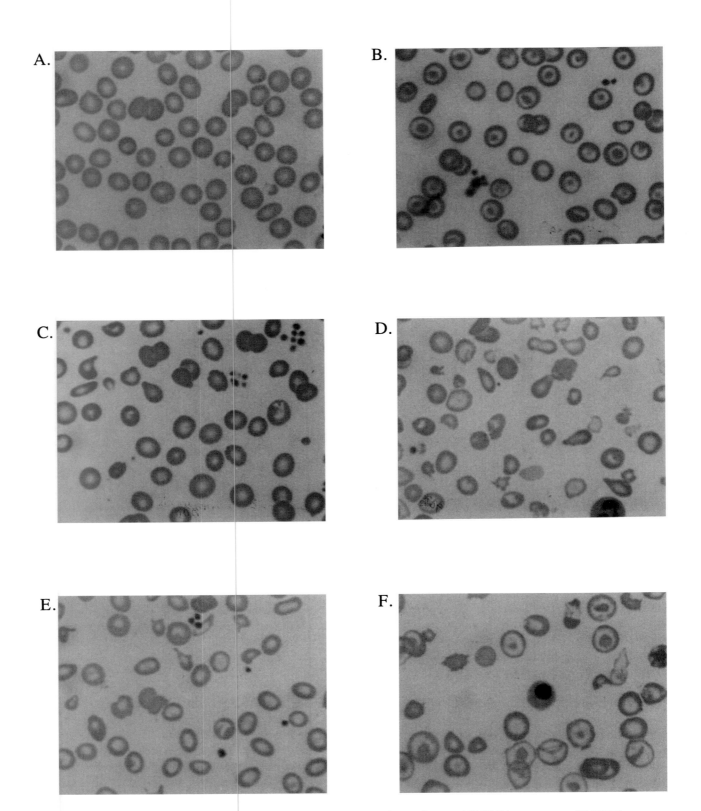

Figure 43.3. Morphology of red cells with Wright's staining in various HbE syndromes. **(A)** HbE heterozygote; **(B)** HbE homozygote; **(C)** HbE-α thalassemia-1; **(D)** Hb E-β thalassemia; **(E)** AE Bart's disease; **(F)** EF Bart's disease. For color reproduction, see color plate 43.3.

and HbE had moderate to severe disease. These observations suggest that additional factors may be involved in determining disease severity.

Co-inheritance of α Thalassemia

Concomitant inheritance of α thalassemia and Hb Constant Spring may be responsible for mildness of anemia in β thalassemia (Winichagoon et al., 1985, 1987). HbE-β⁰ thalassemia patients who have co-inherited α thalassemia-2 have hemoglobin levels of 7.4 g/dL or above whereas those without detectable α thalassemia have hemoglobin levels higher or lower than 7.4 g/dL. Co-inheritance of α thalassemia-1 with HbE-β⁰ thalassemia may lead to so mild a condition that the individuals do not have a clinical abnormality that requires medical attention (Winichagoon et al., 1985). However, this effect was more evident in the HbE-β⁰ thalassemia or β⁺ thalassemia/β⁰ thalassemia and minimal in β⁰ thalassemia/β⁰ thalassemia compound heterozygotes (Ho et al., 1998).

Association with Increased HbF

Co-inheritance of determinants that increase HbF expression can ameliorate the severity of β thalassemia. Inheritance of a β-thalassemia chromosome with the Xmnl cleavage site at position –158 5′ to the $^{G}\gamma$-globin gene is associated with increased HbF and milder anemia (Winichagoon et al., 1993). Two copies of this allele were necessary to produce a significant clinical effect. Hemoglobin levels of patients with an Xmnl +/+ genotype were greater than 8.5 g/dL whereas those of patients with the Xmnl –/– genotype were less than 7 g/dL. Increased expression of the $^{G}\gamma$-globin gene was also detected in the Xmnl +/+ patients. This increase of γ-globin gene activity would help to reduce the overall globin chain imbalance and thus ameliorate the anemia. However, a similar effect was not seen in individuals heterozygous for the Xmnl site

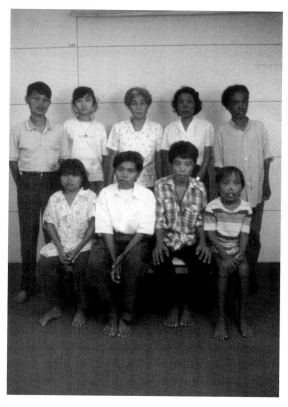

Figure 43.4. A group of β-thalassemia patients with variation of anemia and clinical phenotypes.

severe HbE-β⁺ thalassemia shown in Table 43.3 with mutations at IVS-II-654 and IVS-I-5, the mutations lead to severe hemolytic stress with HbF increased to a similar degree as in HbE-β⁰ thalassemia. Therefore, these severe HbE-β⁺ thalassemias act as HbE-β⁰ thalassemia. Compound heterozygotes for β⁺- and β⁰-thalassemia genes also show variable severity similar to HbE-β⁰ thalassemia (see Chapter 12). We can conclude that (1) patients with mild β⁺ thalassemia and HbE had mild disease; and (2) patients with severe β⁺- or β⁰-thalassemia alleles

Table 43.3. Hemoglobin Levels and Hemoglobin Analysis in Two Types of Mild HbE-β⁺ Thalassemia, Severe HbE-β⁺ Thalassemia, and Homozygous HbE

	Homozygous HbE	Mild HbE-β⁺ thalassemia		Severe HbE-β⁺ thalassemia	
		–28/HbE	Codon 19/HbE	IVS-II-654/HbE	IVS-I-5/HbE
Number	39	16	7	13	5
Hb type	EE	EFA	EF+Malay	EF	EF
Hb (g/dL)	11.4 ± 1.2	9.5 ± 1.5	9.2 ± 2.8	6.6 ± 0.9	7.9 ± 1.0
HbE (%)	95.2 ± 2.1	57.1 ± 5.9	58.2 ± 3.4	57.5 ± 11.6	52.2 ± 8.0
HbF (%)	4.8 ± 2.1	10.1 ± 5.6	3.4 ± 1.1	39.2 ± 13.7	47.7 ± 8.0

Table 43.4. Genetic Determinants for the Severity Difference in 80 Patients with HbE-β Thalassemia Disease

Phenotype	No.	Type of mutation		α-Genotype				Xmn I $^{G}\gamma$-gene			
		Hb E-β$^+$ thal	Hb E-β^0 thal	αα/αα	--αα	-α/αα	α^{CS}α/αα	+/+	+/-	-/-	ND
Mild	27	4	23	15	0	8	4	1	22	2	2
Moderate	42	0	42	40	0	0	2	1	32	6	3
Severe	11	0	11	11	0	0	0	0	8	3	0

polymorphism. Patients with a single copy of the Xmnl positive allele appeared to have a variable clinical course and a wide range of hemoglobin levels and HbF production.

Table 43.4 shows the effect of the type of β-thalassemia mutation, α thalassemia, and the Xmnl restriction site in determining severity in 80 Thai HbE-β thalassemia patients. The presence of a mild β-thalassemia mutation, α thalassemia, and homozygosity for the Xmnl restriction site was associated with a mild phenotype in seventeen of twenty-seven cases (63 percent) of patients. Although two cases were Xmnl negative, one had β$^+$ thalassemia/HbE and the other had the Hb Constant Spring gene. The above findings indicated that the three factors can account for the mildness of the disease in 21 percent of total cases. In severe cases, none had co-inherited α thalassemia or an Hb Constant Spring gene and three of eleven cases (27 percent) were also Xmnl negative. However, six of forty-two patients with moderate severity also lacked an Xmnl restriction site.

Amount of Alternative Spliced β^E-Globin mRNA

An underproduction of β-globin chains from the β^E-globin gene strongly suggests that alternative RNA splicing is of physiologic significance. We have determined the percentage of the alternative spliced β^E globin mRNA by the reverse transcriptase polymerase chain reaction (RT-PCR) technique in fourteen patients with the same β-thalassemia mutation (Winichagoon et al., 1995). Variation in clinical phenotype and degree of anemia were present. Preliminary results showed abnormally spliced β^E globin mRNA in patients with severe symptoms and low hemoglobin levels between 2.9 percent and 6.1 percent, whereas those with higher hemoglobin levels had values from 1.6 percent to 2.6 percent. The majority of patients with the Xmnl negative genotype had more severe anemia and a higher percentage of abnormally spliced β^E globin mRNA. This indicated that the amount of alternatively spliced β^E globin mRNA was a more predominant factor in determining severity of anemia than the pattern of Xmnl polymorphism or the level of HbF. If true, β-globin mutations resulting in abnormal pre-mRNA processing should result in variable degrees of gene expression and greater severity of anemia. Further investigation is needed to clarify this point.

In conclusion, the genotypic factors that can be used to predict a mild phenotype in HbE β thalassemia are mild β$^+$-thalassemia mutations, the co-inheritance of α thalassemia, and the homozygosity for Xmnl restriction site 5' to the $^{G}\gamma$ globin gene. However, the Xmnl-$^{G}\gamma$ site may not consistently predict the phenotype of HbE-β thalassemia.

Pyrimidine 5' Nucleotidase Deficiency

In one Bangladeshi family, an individual homozygous for both HbE and pyrimidine 5' nucleotidase deficiency was found. The patient had a severe hemolytic anemia in contrast with HbE homozygotes. Globin-chain synthesis experiments showed that the mechanism underlying the interaction between these two genotypes was a marked decrease in the stability of HbE in pyrimidine 5' nucleotidase-deficient red blood cells. In these cells, free α-globin chains but not β^E-globin chains accumulated on the membrane. It was hypothesized that the marked instability of HbE in the enzyme-deficient cells resulted from oxidant damage to mildly unstable HbE (Rees et al., 1996).

LABORATORY DIAGNOSIS

Diagnosis with Adult Blood

The diagnosis of HbE is based on the electrophoretic or chromatographic separation of hemoglobins from peripheral blood. In alkaline buffer (pH 8.6), HbE migrates like HbA$_2$ on cellulose-acetate membranes but can be distinguished from HbA$_2$ by its higher concentration—more than 10 percent of the total hemoglobin. HbE also migrates like HbA$_2$ on HPLC columns (Fucharoen et al., 1998a). Variable concentrations of HbE may reflect the genotypes of HbE disorders. In general, as mentioned above, HbE is 25 percent to 30 percent of the hemolysate from heterozygotes and lower amounts of HbE are found with co-inheritance of α thalassemia (Table 43.2) or with coexistence of iron deficiency anemia. Lower proportions of HbE in heterozygotes indicate a concomitant inheritance of the more pronounced defects of α-globin chain synthesis as in HbAE Bart's disease (Wasi et al., 1967; Fucharoen et al., 1988c, 1998b; Thonglairuam et al., 1989). In contrast, the amount of HbE is higher in HbE-β thalassemia and HbE levels of 85 percent to 95 percent of total hemoglobin are found with homozygous HbE. Compound heterozygotes with HbE and HbC also appear to have very high HbE levels because HbC ($\alpha_2\beta^{6Glu\rightarrow Lys}_2$) coelectrophoreses with HbE ($\alpha_2\beta^{6Glu\rightarrow Lys}_2$) in the standard alkaline buffer. These two variants can be distinguished by agar-gel electrophoresis at acid pH, or by reverse phase HPLC, and by the presence of about 45 percent HbC in the heterozygous state (Siriboon et al., 1993).

The blue dye dichlorophenolindophenol (DCIP) can be used as a screening test for HbE, which has a weakened $\alpha_1\beta_1$ contact and precipitates upon incubation with the dye at 37°C (Frischer and Bowman, 1975). Homozygous HbE produces heavy sediments at the bottom of the tube whereas heterozygous HbE, HbH disease, and HbE-β thalassemia produce a cloudy or evenly distributed particulate appearance.

PATHOPHYSIOLOGY

Individuals homozygous for HbE are usually clinically normal but compound heterozygotes with HbE-β thalassemia may have thalassemia major (Fucharoen et al., 1988b). The abnormal β^E gene results in reduced amounts of β^E-mRNA and β^E-globin chains, leading to a mild β^+-thalassemia phenotype (Traeger et al., 1982; Wasi et al., 1982a). This occurs because the G→A mutation in codon 26 (Glu→Lys) of the β^E-globin gene activates a cryptic splice site at codon 25, leading to alternative mRNA splicing with reduced β^E-globin chain production (Orkin et al., 1982) (see Chapter 12). A reduction in β^E-chain synthesis results in α/β synthesis ratios from 1.2 to 2.1 in HbE heterozygotes. Besides the reduction of β^E-globin chains, the tertiary conformation of the HbE molecule is also affected. This is because the inhibitory effect of the β-26 substitution on the α1β1 contact may lead to the exposure of certain sulfhydryl groups and precipitation under conditions of oxidative stress (Frischer and Bowman, 1975). Finally, the low percentage of HbE may also be partly attributed to the defective assembly of $\alpha_2\ \beta^E_2$ tetramers (Huisman, 1997) (see Chapter 8). The pathophysiology of thalassemia is reviewed in Chapters 11 and 17.

CLINICAL MANIFESTATIONS

HbE-β thalassemia is an important cause of childhood chronic disease in Southeast Asia. In contrast to thalassemia patients in developed countries, and for economic reasons, most Southeast Asian patients are not transfused or are suboptimally transfused, and iron chelation is uncommon. Patients show remarkable variability in the clinical expression of HbE-β thalassemia ranging from a mild form of thalassemia intermedia to transfusion-dependent conditions clinically indistinguishable from homozygous β^0 thalassemia (Fig. 43.4). About half of the patients have the thalassemia intermedia and half have the thalassemia major phenotype. In 803 HbE-β thalassemia patients, hemoglobin levels ranged from 3 to 13 g/dL and averaged 7.7 g/dL in the steady state (Fucharoen et al., 1988b). This remarkable variability in severity reflects the heterogeneity of β-thalassemia mutations present with HbE and other modulating factors. Similar disease heterogeneity has also been observed among the HbE-β thalassemia patients living in the United Kingdom and elsewhere (Rees et al., 1998).

Severe HbE-β thalassemia causes congenital hemolytic anemia. At birth, infants are asymptomatic because HbF levels are high. As HbF production wanes and is replaced by inefficient HbE production at 6 to 12 months of age, anemia with abdominal enlargement develops. Almost without exception, signs of impaired health were noted during the first decade of life. Clinical data in 378 patients with HbE-β thalassemia are shown in Table 43.5. The initial complaints varied from patient to patient, and several symptoms usually appeared simultaneously. Most common was the development of a mass in the left upper quadrant and pallor. Youngest patients had the smallest spleens but no correlation existed between the actual degree of organ enlargement and the state of the disease (Chernoff et al., 1956). With time and without transfusions, anemia, jaundice, hepatosplenomegaly, retardation of physical development, and thalassemic or Mongoloid facies are present. Absence of secondary sexual development was found in some patients and chronic leg ulcers were sometimes observed. These clinical manifestation are secondary to decreased oxygen delivery to tissues, ineffective erythropoiesis, and iron overload and resemble those of untreated β thalassemia major (see Chapter 13).

Erythropoiesis

Erythropoiesis is massively increased—to 10 to 15 times normal—because anemia stimulates erythropoietin production. Extensive erythropoiesis can be found in the liver, spleen, and bone, and in extramedullary

Table 43.5. Clinical Data in 378 Patients with HbE-β Thalassemia Disease

	Number	%
Age at onset (yr)		
0–9	299	79.10
10–19	49	12.96
20–29	23	6.09
30–39	7	1.85
Growth development		
Normal	94	24.87
Retardation	284	75.13
Mongoloid facies		
Absent	65	17.20
Slight	159	42.06
Obvious	154	40.74
Hepatomegaly		
Absent	41	10.85
<5 cm	247	65.34
5–8 cm	66	17.46
>8 cm	24	6.35
Splenomegaly		
Absent	9	2.38
<5 cm	132	34.92
5–8 cm	62	16.40
>8 cm	75	19.84
First menstruation (yr)		
10–14	15	8.72
15–19	86	50.00
20–24	10	5.81
None	54	31.40
No record	7	4.07
Splenectomy (yr)	134	35.45
0–9	52	38.81
10–19	63	47.01
20–29	12	8.96
>30	7	5.22
Blood transfusion	231	61.11
<5 units	115	49.78
5–9 units	47	20.35
10–14 units	22	9.52
15–19 units	11	4.76
>20 units	12	5.19
Unknown	24	10.39

Iron Overload

Iron overload occurs without exception (Pootrakul et al., 1981b). Excessive iron accumulates because of blood transfusions and enhanced gastrointestinal absorption (Vatanavicharn et al., 1983). The skin is darkened and iron deposition occurs in the bone marrow, liver, spleen, heart, pancreas, and elsewhere (Sonakul et al., 1988b; Thakerngpol et al., 1988; Tran et al., 1990). Arrhythmias are not as frequently encountered as in Cooley's anemia and while liver fibrosis from iron overload is common, ascites and other signs of cirrhosis are very rare. Diabetes mellitus secondary to iron deposition in the pancreas frequently develops in untreated adult patients if they live long enough (Vannasaeng et al., 1981). We have observed a terminal wasting stage in some patients who lived into their third and fourth decades. These patients developed more skin pigmentation, poor appetite, weight loss, and increasing anemia, and eventually died. This is believed to result from organ failure caused by uncontrolled tissue oxidation from chronic, severe iron overload. As iron overload is a constant complication of thalassemia and iron is a strong oxidant, reduced levels of antioxidants such as vitamins C and E are common in thalassemia patients (Vatanavicharn et al., 1985).

Heart Disease

Half of the patients with HbE-β thalassemia die of heart failure. This is associated with failure of other organs, delayed growth and sexual maturation, hepatomegaly, and endocrinopathies. Organ failure results from iron deposition in the heart and other tissues (Sonakul et al., 1984, 1988b; Thakerngpol et al., 1988; Tran et al., 1990). Myocardial iron deposition was mostly slight, occurring primarily as small granules in perinuclear areas, with later accumulation throughout the fibers, predominantly subepicardial, occasionally subendocardial. The small amount of iron deposited in the heart was in marked contrast to enormous iron deposition in the liver and pancreas. Other causes of death are anemia, constrictive pericarditis, and pulmonary artery occlusion. Cardiomegaly was proportional to the severity of anemia and systolic murmurs were frequently present (Yipinsoi et al., 1968; Sudhas Na Ayuthya et al., 1988; Jootar and Fucharoen, 1990).

Chronic pericarditis following upper respiratory tract infection is frequently encountered, more so in splenectomized patients. Because of chest pains, a pericardial rub may be detected or the rub is accidentally detected during physical examination. A pericardial rub lasts a few days to a few weeks. Intractable pericardial effusion may follow, causing cardiac tamponade and failure, and requires aspiration. In a very few cases

sites. Erythropoietic masses in the spinal canal have caused spinal cord compression and paraplegia, and when they occur intracranially convulsions may result (Fucharoen et al., 1981b, 1985; Issaragrisil et al., 1981). These symptoms can be reversed by radiation. Massive erythropoiesis leads to fragility and distortion of the bones and decreases bone density because of osteoporosis and osteomalacia as observed in irregularly transfused thalassemia major patients (Pootrakul et al., 1981a). Bone marrow expansion also increases blood volume, leading to high output cardiac failure.

chronic constrictive pericarditis develops, requiring surgical intervention. Histologic examination of the pericardium shows nonspecific pericarditis (Sonakul et al., 1984). Viral infection has been suspected as the cause of this pericarditis but has not been proven.

Infections

Prospective studies showed increased susceptibility to viral, bacterial, and fungal infection that may be causes of death in severe HbE-β thalassemia (Aswapokee et al., 1988b; Fucharoen et al., 1988d). In splenectomized patients, septicemia can be very acute and overwhelming, leading to death in a short period. Gram-negative and gram-positive bacteria are frequent causes of septicemia (Aswapokee et al., 1988a). Fungal infection with *Pythium* can lead to arterial occlusion and gangrene of the legs (Sathapatayavongs et al., 1989; Wanachiwanawin et al., 1993). Investigators have not yet pinpointed the mechanisms that cause increased susceptibility to infections but iron overload and severe anemia may be involved.

Gallstones

Stones are found in about 50 percent of patients (Chandcharoensin-Wilde et al., 1988). For the detection of biliary calculi, ultrasonography is more sensitive than oral cholecystography and plain abdominal films. Cholecystitis and ascending cholangitis may occur with abdominal pain, fever, and increasing jaundice (Vathanopas et al., 1988). Antibiotics alone are usually not effective and cholecystectomy is necessary.

Hypertension, Convulsions, and Cerebral Hemorrhage After Multiple Blood Transfusions

Some thalassemia patients developed hypertension, convulsions, and cerebral hemorrhage after transfusion of two or more units of blood and many of these patients died (Wasi et al., 1978). This complication may develop as late as 2 weeks after multiple transfusion, suggesting that blood volume overload is not the cause of hypertension. Monitoring blood pressure during and after blood transfusions with prompt antihypertensive intervention has reduced deaths from this complication.

Hypoxemia

A great majority of splenectomized HbE-β^0 thalassemia patients develop hypoxemia with low arterial PO_2 (Wasi et al., 1982b). Platelet counts in splenec-tomized thalassemia patients were double that of non-splenectomized patients; young and larger platelets were also observed in the absence of the spleen. Platelet microaggregates have been detected in the circulation of these splenectomized patients (Winichagoon et al., 1981). One hypothesis for the pathogenesis of hypoxemia in HbE-β^0 thalassemia is that platelets—increased in number, younger and more active after splenectomy—aggregate in the circulation, and in the pulmonary vasculature. Some substances released during platelet aggregation may cause constriction of the terminal bronchioles leading to decreased oxygenation and hypoxemia. A canine model showed that induction of platelet aggregation in the circulation reproduced the hypoxemia observed in splenectomized thalassemia patients.

Administration of aspirin to inhibit platelet aggregation reduced the degree of hypoxemia in the majority of cases (Fucharoen et al., 1981a), suggesting that these agents should be routinely given to splenectomized patients with HbE-β thalassemia.

Thromboembolism

Autopsy findings in a large number of patients with HbE-β thalassemia revealed striking pulmonary artery occlusion. Serial sections of the lungs revealed in some patients as many as 24 lesions/cm^2, the distribution of which indicated embolism (Sonakul et al., 1980, 1988a). Thromboembolism in HbE-β thalassemia seems to involve platelets, a reactive thalassemic red cell surface, coagulation factors, and abnormal endothelium but this problem is still under study.

Autoimmune Hemolytic Anemia

Some patients develop autoimmune hemolytic anemia with worsening anemia and a positive Coombs' test (Kruatrachue et al., 1980). The condition is responsive to corticosteroids. Studies of HbE thalassemia patients with this anemia showed that their red cell surface is an active site of complex immune reactions that are likely to be associated with many pathophysiologic phenomena (Malasit et al., 1997).

TREATMENT RECOMMENDATIONS

Principles of treatment are similar to those for patients with severe β thalassemia, with transfusions and chelation of iron (see Chapters 13 and 37). Standard management of severely anemic patients should consist of regular blood transfusions, if possible, to maintain hemoglobin levels of 10 to 12 g/dL. However, in those who have the phenotype of thalassemia intermedia, the need for transfusion should be carefully evaluated.

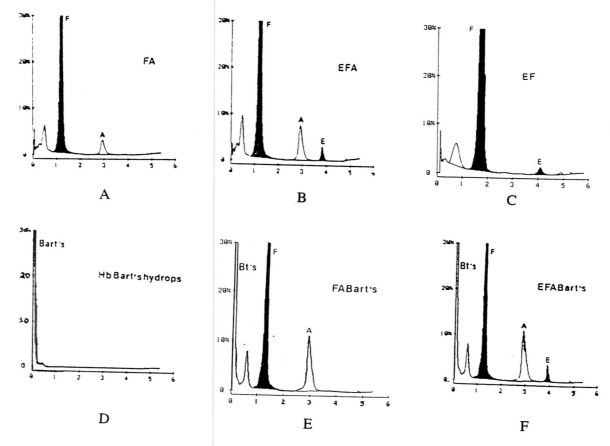

Figure 43.5. Chromatograms of newborns with HbE syndromes detected by automated HPLC. (**A**) Healthy newborn; (**B**) newborn with HbE trait; (**C**) newborn with HbE-β thalassemia; (**D**) newborn with Hb Bart's hydrops fetalis; (**E**) newborn with HbH disease; (**F**) newborn with HbAE Bart's disease.

Splenectomy is recommended for patients who have splenomegaly with hypersplenism.

Hydroxyurea may increase HbF levels in HbE-β thalassemia (Fucharoen et al., 1996) (see Chapter 38). Long-term benefit of hydroxyurea therapy needs further investigation. Erythropoietin may alleviate anemia and assist healing of leg ulcers. Bone marrow transplantation and cord blood transplantation have also been employed (Issaragrisil, 1994; Issaragrisil et al., 1995).

NEONATAL AND PRENATAL DIAGNOSIS

The amount of HbA_2 in normal newborns is lower than in adults and usually is not visualized by hemoglobin electrophoresis. Pootrakul et al. observed a "slow" hemoglobin component at the position of HbA_2 that proved to be HbE (Pootrakul et al., 1988). The mean HbE level, quantitated by cellulose-acetate electrophoresis, was 3.7 percent. An automatic HPLC system (Variant™, Bio-Rad) was used to study various HbE disorders in cord blood (Fig. 43.5). HbE concentrations in homozygous HbE ranged between 3.9 percent and 14.9 percent. In HbE heterozygotes, HbE was between 2.1 percent and 10.3 percent with a mean of 4.5 percent (Table 43.6) (Fucharoen et al., 1998). These data suggest that newborns with homozygous HbE have a tendency to have higher concentration of HbE than those with heterozygous HbE, but some overlap occurs. Furthermore, both homozygous HbE and $HbE-\beta^0$ thalassemia patients had similar chromatograms composed of HbE and HbF with similar amounts of HbE. DNA analysis is necessary to differentiate between these two syndromes.

Diagnosis of HbE syndromes can also be performed prenatally by cordocentesis at the gestational ages of 16 to 24 weeks (Fucharoen et al., 1998a). The chromatograms obtained from cordocentesis using the automatic HPLC system were similar to those of the cord blood specimens. In the HbE heterozygote, 0.8 percent to 1.5 percent of HbE was detected in addition to HbA. HbA was not present in fetuses homozygous for HbE or with $HbE-\beta^0$ thalassemia (Table 43.7). These two conditions were distinguished only by DNA analysis.

Table 43.6. Hematologic Data and Hemoglobin Analysis in Cord Blood Samples

| Phenotype | No. | Hb (g/dL) | MCV (fl) | MCH (pg) | MCHC (g/dL) | Hb type | % Hemoglobin (HPLC) | | | | Genotype |
							A$_2$ (E)	F	A	Bart's	
Normal	326	15.4 ± 1.7	105 ± 6.2	35 ± 2.2	33 ± 1.0	FA	0.6 ± 0.4	74.1 ± 6.4	17.8 ± 6.3	0.7 ± 0.4	$\alpha\alpha/\alpha\alpha$-$\beta^A/\beta^A$
EA Bart's disease	1	13..0	72	22	30	EFA Bart's	3.6	80.6	12.2	27.9	$-/-\alpha$-β^A/β^E
EF Bart's disease	1	11.2	70	21	30	EF Bart's	30.1	64.4	0.9	17.5	$-/-\alpha$-β^E/β^E
HbE-β thalassemia disease	1	13.1	99	33	34	EF	2.0	93.0	0.1	1.0	$\alpha\alpha/\alpha\alpha$-$\beta^{thal}/\beta^E$
HbE homozygote	9	14.5 ± 2.1	103 ± 6.7	34 ± 2.5	33 ± 1.2	EF	8.0 ± 3.6	81.4 ± 4.5	0.6 ± 0.6	0	$\alpha\alpha/\alpha\alpha$-$\beta^E/\beta^E$
HbE trait	114	15.4 ± 1.6	104 ± 7.5	35 ± 6.6	33 ± 1.0	EFA	4.5 ± 1.5	76.7 ± 4.8	10.1 ± 3.5	0.7 ± 0.4	$\alpha\alpha/\alpha\alpha$-$\beta^A/\beta^E$
EE-α thalassemia-2	1	13.8	96	31	33	EF Bart's	11.6	76.1	0.4	1.9	$-\alpha/\alpha\alpha$-β^E/β^E
EE-α thalassemia-1	1	13.5	82	27	33	EF Bart's	7.6	81.3	0.3	8.8	$-/\alpha\alpha$-β^E/β^E
HbE-α thalassemia-1	5	14.0 ± 1.3	89 ± 4.8	28 ± 1.5	32 ± 0.5	EFA Bart's	5.1 ± 1.1	72.8 ± 4.4	15.6 ± 3.6	8.6 ± 1.7	$-/\alpha\alpha$-β^A/β^E
HbE-α thalassemia-2/Hb CS	1	15.0	106	32	30	EFA Bart's	3.0	66.0	22.1	9.3	$-\alpha^{CS}\alpha$-β^A/β^E
HbE-α thalassemia-2/α thalassemia-2	3	13.2	78	25	32	EFA Bart's	5.6	72.0	15.9	3.7	$-\alpha/-\alpha$-β^A/β^E
		14.3	91	28	31	EFA Bart's	4.2	79.3	12.3	5.3	$-\alpha/-\alpha$-β^A/β^E
		14.9	98	31	31	EFA Bart's	2.2	88.2	4.9	2.8	$-\alpha/-\alpha$-β^A/β^E

Abbreviation: CS, Constant Spring.

Table 43.7. The Amounts of Hbs A₂ (E), F, and A From a Normal Fetus and Fetuses with Thalassemias and HbE

Phenotype	No.	Hb Type	Hb analysis (%)			
			A₂/E	F	A	Bart's
Normal	1	FA	0	94.0	5.8	–
β-thalassemia trait	6	FA	0	94.8–96.3	4.0–5.2	–
HbE-β thalassemia	7	EF	1.0–1.7	89.4–98.6	0	–
Homozygous HbE	2	EF	3.0, 2.1	96.8, 97.3	0	–
HbE trait	4	EFA	0.8–1.4	94.0–97.2	2.0–2.8	–
Hb Bart's hydrops fetalis	10	Portland and Bart's	0	0	0	85–90

CONCLUSIONS

Hemoglobin E and thalassemias are a major public health problem in Southeast Asia. Progress in biomedical research during recent years has clarified the molecular defects in the majority of cases. However, as in sickle cell anemia and β thalassemia, there is still considerable pathophysiology unexplained by the abnormal molecular findings. The clinical manifestations of thalassemia syndromes such as HbE-β thalassemia are very heterogeneous. Better understanding of factor(s) that modify severity will enable us to improve the quality of life for patients. Prevention programs by a good screening strategy with proper counseling and prenatal diagnosis will help to control the birth of patients with severe disease (see Chapter 36). However, not all couples at high risk for conceiving HbE-β thalassemia children need prenatal diagnosis. Expensive and risky treatments such as hypertransfusion, regular chelation, and bone marrow transplantation should be carefully evaluated for individual patients. If important therapeutic decisions are to be made using "predictors" of mild disease the prognostic factors upon which a decision is based must be very carefully validated. At present this is not usually possible.

Conventional treatment by regular transfusion and iron chelation is not possible for most patients in developing countries. A cure is still limited to the small number of patients who have undergone bone marrow stem cell transplantation. Disease modification may be possible with a better understanding and management of some of the complex pathophysiologic changes that occur in the HbE disorders. An understanding of the heterogeneity in severity, so complex in these disorders and often not understood, is also important for medical and paramedical personnel so they can provide proper counseling to patients and their families.

ACKNOWLEDGMENTS

This work was supported by the Prajadhipok Rambhai Barni Foundation and the National Science and Technology Development Agency. Pictures of red cell morphology in Figure 43.3 are kindly provided by Professor Among Piankijagum at Hematology Unit, Siriraj Hospital, Mahidol University.

References

Aswapokee, N, Aswapokee, P, Fucharoen, S, and Wasi, P. (1988a). A study of infective episodes in patients with β-thalassemia/Hb E disease in Thailand. *Birth Defects* 23(5A): 513–520.

Aswapokee, P, Aswapokee, N, Fucharoen, S et al. (1988b). Severe infection in thalassemia: A prospective study. *Birth Defects* 23(5A): 521–526.

Chandcharoensin-Wilde, C, Chairoongruang, S, Jitnuson, P et al. (1988). Gallstones in thalassemia. *Birth Defects* 23(5B): 263–267.

Chernoff, AI, Minnich, V, Na-Nakorn, S et al. (1956). Studies on hemoglobin E. I. The clinical, hematologic, and genetic characteristics of the hemoglobin E syndromes. *J. Lab. Clin. Med.* 47: 455–489.

Flatz, G. (1965). Hemoglobin E in Southeast Asia. In *Felicitation volumes of Southeast-Asian Studies,* Vol. 1. Bangkok: Siam Society. pp. 96–106.

Flatz, G. (1967). Hemoglobin E: Distribution and population dynamics. *Humangenetik* 3: 189–234.

Frischer, H and Bowman, J. (1975). Hemoglobin E, an oxidatively unstable mutation. *J. Lab. Clin. Med.* 85: 531–539.

Fucharoen, S and Winichagoon, P. (1997). Hemoglobinopathies in Southeast Asia: Molecular biology and clinical medicine. *Hemoglobin* 21: 299–319.

Fucharoen, S, Youngchaiyud, P, and Wasi, P. (1981a). Hypoxemia and the effect of aspirin in thalassemia. *Southeast Asian J. Trop. Med. Public Health* 12: 90–93.

Fucharoen, S, Tunthanavatana, C, Sonakul, D, and Wasi, P. (1981b). Intracranial extramedullary hematopoiesis in β⁰-thalassemia/hemoglobin E disease. *Am. J. Hematol.* 10: 75–78.

Fucharoen, S, Winichagoon, P, Pootrakul, P, and Wasi, P. (1984). Determination for different severity of anemia in thalassemia: Concordance and discordance among sib pairs. *Am. J. Med. Genet.* 19: 39–44.

Fucharoen, S, Suthipongchai, S, Poungvarin, N et al. (1985). Intracranial extramedullary hematopoiesis inducing epilepsy in a patient with β-thalassemia/hemoglobin E. *Arch. Intern. Med.* 145: 739–742.

Fucharoen, S, Winichagoon, P, and Thonglairoam, V. (1988a). β-Thalassemia associated with α-thalassemia in Thailand. *Hemoglobin* 12: 581–592.

Fucharoen, S, Winichagoon, P, Pootrakul, P et al. (1988b). Variable severity of Southeast Asian β-thalassemia/Hb E disease. *Birth Defects* 23(5A): 241–248.

Fucharoen, S, Winichagoon, P, Prayoonwiwat, W et al. (1988c). Clinical and hematologic manifestations of AE Bart's disease. *Birth Defects* 23(5A): 327–332.

Fucharoen, S, Piankijagum, A, and Wasi, P. (1988d). Deaths in β-thalassemia/Hb E patients secondary to infections. *Birth Defects* 23(5A): 495–500.

Fucharoen, S, Winichagoon, P, Thonglairuam, V, and Wasi, P. (1988e). EF Bart's disease: Interaction of the abnormal α- and β-globin genes. *Eur. J. Haematol.* 40: 75–78.

Fucharoen, S, Siritanaratkul, N, Winichagoon, P et al. (1996). Hydroxyurea increases Hb F levels and improves the effectiveness of erythropoiesis in β-thalassemia/Hb E disease. *Blood* 87: 887–892.

Fucharoen, S, Winichagoon, P, Wisedpanichkij, R et al. (1998a). Prenatal and postnatal diagnoses of thalassemias and hemoglobinopathies by HPLC. *Clin. Chem.* 44: 740–748.

Fucharoen, S, Winichagoon, P, Siritanaratkul, N et al. (1998b). Alpha and beta thalassemia in Thailand. *Ann. N. Y. Acad. Sci.* 850: 412–414.

Ho, PJ, Hall, GW, Luo, LY et al. (1998). Beta-thalassaemia intermedia: Is it possible consistently to predict phenotype from genotype? *Br. J. Haematol.* 100: 70–78.

Huisman, THJ. (1997). Hb E and α-thalassemia; variability in the assembly of β^E chain containing tetramers. *Hemoglobin* 21: 227–236.

Hunt, JA and Ingram, VM. (1961). Abnormal human haemoglobins. VI. The chemical difference between Hb A and E. *Biochim. Biophys. Acta* 49: 520–546.

Issaragrisil, S. (1994). Bone marrow transplantation in Thailand. *Bone Marrow Transplan.* 13: 721–723.

Issaragrisil, S, Piankijagum, A, and Wasi, P. (1981). Spinal cord compression in thalassemia. Report of 12 cases and recommendations for treatment. *Arch. Intern. Med.* 141: 1033–1036.

Issaragrisil, S, Visuthisakchai, S, Suvatte, V et al. (1995). Brief report: Transplantation of cord-blood stem cells into a patient with severe thalassemia. *N. Engl. J. Med.* 332: 367–368.

Itano, HA, Bergren, WR, and Sturgeon, P. (1954). Identification of a fourth abnormal human hemoglobin. *J. Am. Chem. Soc.* 76: 2278.

Jootar, P and Fucharoen, S. (1990). Cardiac involvement in beta-thalassemia/hemoglobin E disease: Clinical and hemodynamic findings. *Southeast Asian J. Trop. Med. Public Health* 21: 269–273.

Kruatrachue, M, Sirisinha, S, Pacharee, P et al. (1980). An association between thalassaemia and autoimmune haemolytic anaemia (AIHA). *Scand. J. Haematol.* 25: 259–263.

Luzzatto, L. (1979). Genetics of red cells and susceptibility to malaria. *Blood* 54: 961–966.

Malasit, P, Mahasorn, W, Mongkolsapaya, J et al. (1997). Presence of immunoglobulins, C3 and cytolytic C5b-9 complement components on the surface of erythrocytes from patients with β-thalassaemia/haemoglobin E disease. *Br. J. Haematol.* 96: 507–513.

Minnich, V, Na-Nakorn, S, Thongchareonsuk, S, and Kochaseni, S. (1954). Mediterranean anemia: A study of thirty-two cases in Thailand. *Blood* 9: 1–23.

Na-Nakorn, S and Minnich, V. (1957). Studies on hemoglobin E. III. Homozygous hemoglobin E and variants of thalassemia and hemoglobin E. A family study. *Blood* XII: 529–538.

Na-Nakorn, S, Minnich, V, and Chernoff, A.I. (1956). Studies on hemoglobin E. II. The incidence of hemoglobin E in Thailand. *J. Lab. Clin. Med.* 47: 490–498.

Orkin, SH, Kazazian, HH Jr, Antonarakis, SE et al. (1982). Abnormal RNA processing due to the exon mutation of the β^E-globin gene. *Nature* 300: 768–769.

Pootrakul, P, Hungsprenges, S, Fucharoen, S et al. (1981a). Relation between erythropoiesis and bone metabolism in thalassemia. *N. Engl. J. Med.* 304: 1470–1473.

Pootrakul, P, Vongsmasa, V, La-ongpanich, P, and Wasi, P. (1981b). Serum ferritin levels in thalassaemias and the effect of splenectomy. *Acta Haematol.* 66: 244–250.

Pootrakul, S, Assawamunkong, S, and Na-Nakorn, S. (1976). β^+-Thalassemia trait: Hematologic and hemoglobin synthesis studies. *Hemoglobin* 1: 75–83.

Pootrakul, S, Muang-sup, V, Fucharoen, S, and Wasi, P. (1988). Cord blood study on β-thalassemia and hemoglobin E. *Am. J. Med. Genet.* 29: 49–57.

Rees, DC, Duley, J, Simmonds, HA et al. (1996). Interaction of hemoglobin E and pyrimidine 5′ nucleotidase deficiency. *Blood* 88: 2761–2767.

Rees, DC, Styles, L, Vichinsky, EP et al. (1998). The hemoglobin E syndromes. *Ann. N. Y. Acad. Sci.* 850: 334–343.

Sathapatayavongs, B, Leelachaikul, P, Prachaktam, R et al. (1989). Human pythiosis associated with thalassemia hemoglobinopathy syndrome. *J. Infect. Dis.* 159: 274–280.

Siriboon, W, Srisomsap, C, Winichagoon, P et al. (1993). Identification of Hb C [β6 (A3) Glu→Lys] in a Thai male. *Hemoglobin* 17: 419–425.

Sonakul, D, Pacharee, P, Laohapand, T et al. (1980). Pulmonary artery obstruction in thalassemia. *Southeast Asian J. Trop. Med. Public Health* 11: 516–523.

Sonakul, D, Pacharee, P, Wasi, P, and Fucharoen, S. (1984). Cardiac pathology in 47 patients with beta thalassemia/hemoglobin E. *Southeast Asian J. Trop. Med. Public Health* 15: 554–563.

Sonakul, D, Suwanagool, P, Sirivaidyapong, P, and Fucharoen, S. (1988a). Distribution of pulmonary thromboembolic lesions in thalassemic patients. *Birth Defects* 23(5A): 375–384.

Sonakul, D, Pacharee, P, and Thakerngpol, K. (1988b). Pathologic findings in 76 autopsy cases of thalassemia. *Birth Defects* 23(5B): 157–176.

Sudhas Na Ayuthya, P, Pongpanich, B, Damrongwatna, T et al. (1988). Cardiac study in thalassemic children. *Birth Defects* 23(5B); 351–354.

Thakerngpol, K, Sonakul, D, Fucharoen, S et al. (1988). Histochemical study of liver tissue from thalassemic patients. *Birth Defects* 23(5B): 193–198.

Thonglairuam, V, Winichagoon, P, Fucharoen, S, and Wasi, P. (1989). The molecular basis of AE-Bart's disease. *Hemoglobin* 13: 117–124.

Traeger, J, Wood, WG, Clegg, JB et al. (1980). Defective synthesis of Hb E is due to reduced levels of β^E-mRNA. *Nature* 288: 497–499.

Traeger, J, Winichagoon, P, and Wood, W.G. (1982). Instability of β^E-messenger RNA during erythroid cell maturation in hemoglobin E homozygotes. *J. Clin. Invest.* 69: 1050–1053.

Tran, KC, Webb, J, Macey, DJ, and Pootrakul, P. (1990). β-Thalassemia/hemoglobin E tissue ferritins. II. A comparison of heart and pancreas ferritins with those of liver and spleen. *Biol. Metals* 3: 227–231.

Vannasaeng, S, Ploybutr, S, Visutkul, P et al. (1981). Endocrine function in thalassemia. *Clin. Endocrinol.* 14: 165–173.

Vatanavicharn, S, Anuwatanakulchai, M, Tuntawiroon, M et al. (1983). Iron absorption in patients with β-thalassaemia/haemoglobin E disease and the effect of splenectomy. *Acta Haematol.* 69: 414–416.

Vatanavicharn, S, Yenchitsomanus, P, and Siddhikol, C. (1985). Vitamin E in β-thalassaemia and α-thalassaemia (Hb H) diseases. *Acta Haematol.* 73: 183.

Vathanopas, V, Fucharoen, S, Chandcharoensin-Wilde, C et al. (1988). Cholecystectomy in thalassemia. *Birth Defects* 23(5B): 269–273.

Wanachiwanawin, W, Thianprasit, M, Fucharoen, S et al. (1993). Fatal arteritis due to pythium insidiosum infection in patients with thalassemia. *Trans. R. Soc. Trop. Med. Hyg.* 87: 296–298.

Wasi, P. (1986). Geographic distribution of hemoglobin variants in Southeast Asia. In Winter, WP, editors. *Hemoglobin variants in human populations,* Vol. 2. Florida: CRC Press. pp. 111–127.

Wasi, P, Sookanek, M, Pootrakul, S et al. (1967). Haemoglobin E and α-thalassaemia. *Br. Med. J.* 4: 29–32.

Wasi, P, Disthasongchan, P, and Na-Nakorn, S. (1968). The effect of iron deficiency on the levels of hemoglobin A_2 and E. *J. Lab. Clin. Med.* 71: 85–91.

Wasi, P, Na-Nakorn, S, Pootrakul, S et al. (1969). Alpha- and beta-thalassemia in Thailand. *Ann. N. Y. Acad. Sci.* 165: 60–82.

Wasi, P, Na-Nakorn, S, Pootrakul, P et al. (1978). A syndrome of hypertension, convulsion and cerebral hemorrhage in thalassemic patients after multiple blood-transfusions. *Lancet* 2: 602–604.

Wasi, P, Winichagoon, P, Baramee, T, and Fucharoen, S. (1982a). Globin chain synthesis in heterozygous and homozygous hemoglobin E. *Hemoglobin* 6: 75–78.

Wasi, P, Fucharoen, S, Youngchaiyud, P, and Sonakul, D. (1982b). Hypoxemia in thalassemia. *Birth Defects* 18: 213–217.

Winichagoon, P, Fucharoen, S, and Wasi, P. (1981). Increased circulating platelet aggregates in thalassemia. *Southeast Asian J. Trop. Med. Public Health* 12: 556–560.

Winichagoon, P, Fucharoen, S, Weatherall, DJ, and Wasi, P. (1985). Concomitant inheritance of α-thalassemia in β^0-thalassemia/Hb E disease. *Am. J. Hematol.* 20: 217–222.

Winichagoon, P, Fucharoen, S, Thonglairoam, V, and Wasi, P. (1987). Different severity of homozygous β-thalassemia among siblings. *Hum. Genet.* 76: 296–297.

Winichagoon, P, Thonglairoam, V, Fucharoen, S et al. (1993). Severity differences in β-thalassaemia/haemoglobin E syndromes: Implication of genetic factors. *Br. J. Haematol.* 83: 633–639.

Winichagoon, P, Fucharoen, S, Wilairat, P et al. (1995). Role of alternatively spliced β^E-globin mRNA on clinical severity of β-thalassemia/hemoglobin E disease. *Southeast Asian J. Trop. Med. Public Health* 26(Suppl 1): 241–245.

Yipinsoi, T, Haraphongse, M, Wasi, P, and Na-Nakorn, S. (1968). Cardiological examinations in hemoglobin E and thalassemia diseases. *J. Med. Assoc. Thailand* 51: 131–141.

44

Disorders of Hemoglobin Function and Stability

RONALD L. NAGEL

Mutations of the coding sequence of globin genes may alter the function or stability of the hemoglobin molecule, and understanding these hemoglobin mutants is medically useful for physicians who must diagnose and treat patients with hemoglobinopathies. Hemoglobin mutants provide the most comprehensive list of human mutations for any protein, creating a road map for understanding problems of other genetic loci. Studies of these mutant hemoglobins have provided unsuspected insight into the structure-function relationships of normal hemoglobins.

This chapter does not provide a complete listing of functionally abnormal or unstable hemoglobins. In 1998, the Globin Gene Server (http://globin.cse.psu.edu) listed close to 800 different hemoglobin mutations; twenty-six were associated with increased oxygen affinity and the potential for causing erythrocytosis; forty-one were unstable and associated with hemolytic anemia. New variants with these properties are continually being described. Instead, this discussion is limited to examples that are illustrative of interesting aspects of either the protein chemistry, physiology, clinical presentation, or diagnosis of unstable hemoglobins or hemoglobin variants with altered oxygen affinity. Chapters 14 and 17 discuss β- and α-globin gene coding region mutations, which, unlike the variants covered in this chapter, have little or no abnormal protein and consequently

have a thalassemic phenotype. They are part of the dominant thalassemia syndrome. Chapter 45 describes mutant hemoglobins of biological interest that are not often accompanied by a clinical phenotype.

The term *ligand* is used here to denote small molecules capable of binding heme—usually O_2, CO, and NO—generally at its iron center. The R→T transition refers to the switching of two hemoglobin conformers, one with high affinity (R) and the other with low affinity (T) for a ligand (Ferni et al., 1989). This fully defines the two state working model hemoglobin discussed in detail in Chapter 9, which provides important background information for this and Chapter 10.

HIGH OXYGEN AFFINITY HEMOGLOBINS: ERYTHROCYTOSIS

Mutations causing changes in the primary structure of the α- or β-globin chains (also the γ- and δ-globin chains, although mutations of these globins are not often recognized clinically) can change hemoglobin-ligand affinity. Single point substitutions, double point substitutions, deletions, insertions, reading frameshift mutations, and fusion genes can all result in hemoglobins with increased oxygen affinity. Most, but not all, of these high affinity hemoglobins, as noted later, can be understood with our present knowledge of the structure-function relationships in hemoglobin.

Underlying all known molecular mechanisms accounting for the generation of high ligand affinity hemoglobin mutants is the furtherance of the R state, or high affinity conformer of the molecule (Chapter 9). This can occur by stabilizing the R state or destabilizing the T state. The molecular basis of this conformational change can be one of the following:

1. An alteration in critical areas of the molecule that are directly involved in the R→T transition. These areas are the switch region, the flexible joint, or the C-termini located in the α1β2 interface between the two dissociable dimers.
2. A more drastic conformational change, also favoring the R state, can arise from a mutation of the α1β1 interface, which is not normally dissociable and does not participate in the R→T conformational change.
3. A mutation reducing the affinity of the hemoglobin for 2,3 BPG.
4. R→T transition can also be biased toward the R state by constraining the molecule through limited polymerization, unlike that of HbS.

Martin H. Steinberg, Bernard G. Forget, Douglas R. Higgs, and Ronald L. Nagel, editors. *Disorders of Hemoglobin: Genetics, Pathophysiology, and Clinical Management.* © 2001 Cambridge University Press. All rights reserved.

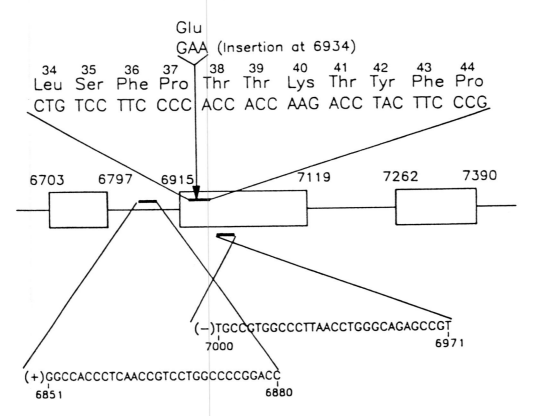

Figure 44.1A. Schematic representation of the DNA sequencing of the PCR-generated fragments from Hb Catonsville, showing the insertion of the glutamyl residues (GAA) between Pro-37 and Thr-38. All other codons are in phase and are normal. The locations of the synthesis primers are also shown as black bars. (Figure continues next page.)

5. Elongation of chains by termination codon or frame-shift mutations can disrupt the overall conformation of hemoglobin, favoring the R state.

Examples of each of these mechanisms follow. Mutations for high affinity hemoglobin variants have been described only in the heterozygous form. It is likely that these mutations are lethal in the homozygote state, particularly if they affect the α-globin chains.

Alterations of Critical Molecular Regions Directly Involved in the Conformational Transition between the R and T State, Resulting in the Stabilization of the R State or Destabilization of the T State

α-Chain Abnormalities. Hb Catonsville (Glu inserted between α37 (C2) and Thr (C3)) (Moo-Penn et al., 1989) is an insertional mutation in which the codon GAA, an alternate codon for Glu, is inserted into the beginning of the C helix. The mechanism of this insertion is not well understood, but a nonallelic gene conversion is a good possibility. This event disturbs the

critical α1β2 interface that is pivotal for the conformational changes involved in the R→T transition causing high oxygen affinity, reduced cooperativity, reduced Bohr effect, and instability.

The insertion in Hb Catonsville occurs in the anomalous 3_{10} helical region at the beginning of the C helix (Kavanaugh et al., 1993) (Fig. 44.1A). Each globin subunit of hemoglobin is composed of eight predominantly α-helical structures (labeled A to H) separated by non-helical, or elbow regions (Chapter 9). All α helices are right handed, and the amide (-CO-NH-) backbone forms a helical structure with 3.6 residues per turn, stabilized by hydrogen bonds between a -C=O with the NH four residues further down the chain (Fig. 44.1B). The helices vary in length between four amino acids (the minimum number of members required to construct an α-helix) and as many as twenty-eight amino acids. Nevertheless, the initial or terminal portions of the α helices are anomalous because they fit either a 3_{10} helix (four residues per turn) or a π helix (five residues per turn). Usually, insertions or deletions can be theoretically accommodated in protein helices by two alternative mechanisms: (1) the register shift mechanism, where the helical geometry is preserved at the expense of requiring all residues preceding the insertion to rotate by 100 degrees in a plain α-helix and by 120 degrees in a 3_{10} helix and (z) bulge (called also indentation), where the helical geometry but not the helix register is disturbed.

High resolution x-ray diffraction analysis of deoxy-hemoglobin Catonsville (Moo-Penn et al., 1989)

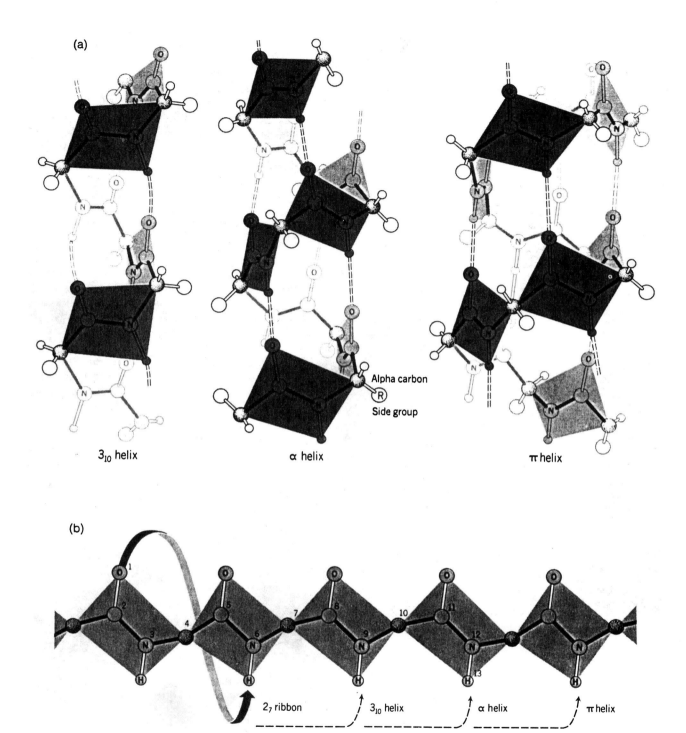

Figure 44.1B. Coiling of polypeptide chains into helices. (a) The 3_{10} α, and π helices differ in their patterns of hydrogen bonding, shown in (b). Hydrogen bonds in the α helix are particularly unstrained, making the α helix especially stable. The α carbons are stippled, with small attached spheres for hydrogens and larger spheres for side chains. (b) Hydrogen-bonding pattern forms one turn of the helix to the next, for four related helices. Only the α helix is found extensively in proteins; the others are found only occasionally for very short stretches, usually winding down or unwinding the last turn of an α helix.

In figure (a), labels: 3_{10} helix, α helix, π helix; Alpha carbon, Side group, R.

In figure (b), labels: 2_7 ribbon, 3_{10} helix, α helix, π helix.

shows that the inserted residue is accommodated as a bulge, validating this mechanism. Data also show that the insertion converted the first turn of the C helix from a 3_{10} helix to a α-helix-type geometry, leading to the speculation that a common "handling" of insertions and deletions in mutated proteins might be interconversion between 3_{10}, α and π helices.

Hb Chesapeake (α92 (FG4) Arg→Leu) (Clegg et al., 1963; Charache et al., 1966; Nagel et al., 1967) was the first high affinity mutant described in a classic paper by Charache et al. (1966). Upon alkaline hemoglobin electrophoresis, Hb Chesapeake was a fast-moving electrophoretic variant, representing about 20 percent of the total hemoglobin. Oxygen affinity studies revealed a whole blood p^{50} of 19 mm Hg; (normal, 26 mm Hg) with a normal Bohr effect and normal 2,3-BPG binding (Benesch and Benesch, 1967; Arnone et al., 1972). Hb Chesapeake produced moderate erythrocytosis. The α92 Leu mutation is a substitution of an invariant residue—a residue conserved among most α-globin chains analyzed, regardless of species—that stabilizes the R state at the α1β2 area of contact, making T conformer contacts less favored (Fig. 44.2).

HbJ Capetown (α92 (FG4) Arg→Gln) is a mutation at the same site as Hb Chesapeake and has similar characteristics, although there is less stabilization of the R state. Initially, this abnormal hemoglobin was reported to have a very low Hill coefficient (n) value (Lines and McIntosh, 1967). This result was based on studies of whole hemolysate that contained two hemoglobins with very different oxygen affinities, HbA and HbJ Capetown, but very similar n values (Nagel et al., 1971a). When combined, HbA and HbJ Capetown generated a flattened oxygen equilibrium curve since Hb Capetown will begin loading oxygen first because of its high ligand affinity. As a result, a reliable n value for each individual hemoglobin cannot be calculated.

Hb Montefiore (α126 (H9) Asp→Tyr) produces mild erythrocytosis. This hemoglobin variant migrated close to HbF on electrophoresis at pH 8.6 and accounts for 20.3 percent of the hemolysate, explaining the mild phenotype. Oxygen binding of Hb Montefiore erythrocytes revealed a 40 percent decrease in the p^{50} at pH 7.4 and an n value of 1.6 (normal: 2.6). Depletion of red cell 2,3 BPG did not alter these results. When studied at pH 7.2, Hb Montefiore showed an eightfold reduction in p^{50} and further reduction in the Hill coefficient. Heterotropic effectors, such as 2,3 BPG and inositol hexaphosphate, reacted normally, and, interestingly, they increased cooperativity of oxygen binding. Cl⁻ ion effect and the Bohr effect were moderately reduced. A benzafibrate derivative, (L345), known to bind α126, increased the p^{50} of normal hemoglobin ninefold but barely affected

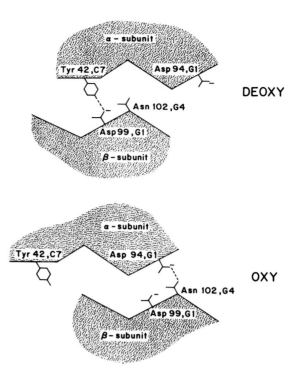

Figure 44.2. Diagram showing the $α_1β_2$ area of contact in the oxy and deoxy conformation is stabilized by the H bond between Tyr 42α and Asp 99β. When oxygenation occurs, this bond is broken and a new one is formed between Asp94α and Asn 102β. In hemoglobins Beth Israel, Kansas, and Titusville, substitutions of one of these residues apparently interfere with this H bond that normally stabilizes the oxy (R) conformation; hence the T state (low affinity) is favored.

the p^{50} of Hb Montefiore. These functional studies, along with intrinsic fluorescence and Resonance Raman spectroscopy, suggested that the very low n value and the high oxygen affinity for Hb Montefiore were a result of both a destabilized T state and a deoxy T state that intrinsically bound ligand with higher affinity than deoxy HbA. While Hb Montefiore still bound ligand cooperatively, the difference in ligand binding properties of the two quaternary states was drastically reduced. The intrinsic affinity for ligand by additional structural changes around the heme group suggested that more than one mechanism was involved. An increased n value from 1.2 to 1.4 produced by 2,3 BPG was the consequence of this heterotropic effector partially restabilizing the T state.

Hb Nunobiki (α141 (HC3) Arg→Cys) (Shimasaki, 1985) is one of four mutations of this invariant residue, all of which exhibit high affinity for oxygen, significantly decreased heterotropic interactions, and moderate to mild erythrocytosis. At pH 8.6, Hb Nunobiki is an electrophoretically fast-moving hemoglobin, accounting for 13 percent of the hemolysate.

A cysteine residue at α141 has a pleotropic effect. During storage, Hb Nunobiki develops more rapid electrophoretic mobility, presumably through the oxidation of the cysteine residue to a negatively charged sulfoxide (-SO⁻) or sulfitic acid (-SOO⁻). Paradoxically, it is more resistant to autoxidation. This protection from oxidants is caused by its high oxygen affinity; the addition of a new cysteine residue for the consumption of oxidants might explain this paradox.

The low percentage of Hb Nunobiki is the consequence of being a mutant of the α_1 gene, which is known to be expressed one-third to two-thirds less than the α_2 gene. (Kazanetz et al., 1996). Finally, as with other α N-terminal mutations, this variant is accompanied by only mild erythrocytosis despite drastically abnormal ligand binding, perhaps a result of its low concentration. High ligand affinity is due to the breaking of the C terminal to C terminal salt bridge indispensable for the stabilization of the T state, favoring the R state.

Other mutations at the same site have different phenotypes. **Hb Suresnes** (α141 Arg→His) (Saenz et al., 1977; Poyart et al., 1976) was present at a level of 22 to 25 percent. The hemoglobin concentration was normal, but oxygen affinity was increased with decreased cooperativity and Bohr effect. **Hb Legnano** (α141 Arg→Leu) (Mavilio et al., 1978) was expressed at 32 to 35 percent and associated with erythrocytosis and increased oxygen affinity, decreased cooperativity, and Bohr effect; it was also slightly unstable. **Hb Camaguey** (α141 Arg→Gly) (Martinez et al., 1978) was expressed at a low level (18 to 20 percent), and erythrocytosis was not present; functional studies were not reported. **Hb Cubujuqui** (α141 Arg→Ser) was present at levels of 25 to 29 percent. Although its oxygen affinity was increased and the Bohr effect and cooperativity decreased, erythrocytosis was absent. **Hb Singapore** (α141 Arg→Pro) (306) forms 25 percent of the hemolysate. Erythrocytosis was absent, but functional studies were not reported. This group of mutations represents an interesting cluster of variants that illustrate the effects of different mutations at the same amino acid residue on hemoglobin function.

Beta Chain Abnormalities. Hb Poissy (β56 (D7) Gly→Arg; β86 (F2) Ala→Pro) (Lacombe et al., 1985) contains two mutations in the same β-globin gene. One mutation, at β56, had been previously described as Hb Hamadan, a variant with no functional abnormalities. A second case of "Hb Hamadan" was found, but the patient had erythrocytosis. When the structure of this variant was reexamined (Lacombe et al., 1985), a second, silent mutation, β86 Ala→Pro, in the same β chain was found. Hb Poissy had a threefold increase in oxygen affinity, a low n, and a diminished Bohr effect. The auto-oxidation rate was biphasic, suggesting an inequivalency in the propensity for methemoglobin formation (conversion of heme iron from ferrous to ferric) of the α and the β hemes. Nuclear magnetic res-

onance (NMR) studies suggested that the insertion of the prolyl residue into the α helix displaced the F helix toward the heme group, destabilizing this helix toward the critical FG corner and interfering with the α1β2 contact area. This displacement favored the R state and modified the environment of the heme groups.

Hb Howick (β37 (C3) Trp→Gly)(Owen et al., 1993) is one of three mutations at codon β37. Hb Howick and Hb Hirose (Trp→Ser) have increased oxygen affinity, whereas Hb Rothchild (Trp→Gly) has low oxygen affinity (see later). Hb Howick accounts for 29 percent of the hemolysate and migrates electrophoretically with HbD at alkaline pH and with HbF on citrate agar electrophoresis. The red cell p⁵⁰ of the heterozygote carrier was 20 mm Hg, and the Bohr effect was reduced. Oxygen affinity was very high at low pH. β37 sits in the α1β2 area of contact, and the absence of Trp is expected to alter the bonds between the two dimers critical in the R→T transition, destabilizing the T conformer. Purified Hb Howick is nearly totally dimerized in the R state (associated equilibrium constant = 35 mmol/L), whereas the T form is highly tetrameric (associated equilibrium constant of 3 μmol/L (Brittain, 1994). These vastly different values are due to the large increase in the dissociation rate of oxyHb Howick. Simulation of the protein concentration dependence of O_2 binding fits well with experimental data and are also consistent with the free-energy change associated with the change of the Gly residue from a hydrophilic to a hydrophobic environment during dimerization.

The pivotal role of β37 has stimulated studies of recombinant hemoglobins at this site (Chapter 45). Kavanaugh et al (Moo-Penn et al., 1989) have studied the high resolution crystal structure of four recombinant mutants: β37 Trp→Tyr, β37 Trp→Ala, β37 Trp→Glu, and β37 Trp→Gly (Hb Howick). None of these mutations altered tertiary structure at the mutation site. However, they altered the α1β2 interface, caused distal tertiary structural change involving α94 Asp-α95 Pro, produced distal tertiary changes involving β99 Asp and β102 Asn, increased the mobility of the α-globin subunit C-terminal dipeptide, and shortened the Fe-Nϵ 2 His in both chains in the β37 Tyr and β37 Glu mutants. Overall, the magnitude of the structural changes increased in the order: β37 Trp→Tyr>β37 Trp→Ala>β37 Trp→Glu and β37 Trp→Gly (Hb Howick) and paralleled the disruption of function detected in these recombinant mutants.

Six known mutations of the β99 (Gl) site exist: **Hb Kempsey** (β99 Asp→Asn; GAT→AAT) (Reed et al., 1968), **Hb Yakima** (Asp→His) (Jones et al., 1967), **Hb Radcliffe** (Asp→Ala) (Weatherall et al., 1977), **Hb Ypsilanti** (Asp→Tyr) (Rucknagel et al., 1967), **Hb Hotel-Dieu** (Asp→Gly) (Blouquit et al., 1981), and **Hb Chemilly** (Asp→Val) (Rochette et al., 1984).

These six mutations are all present at about 40 to 50 percent of the hemolysate, can be separated electrophoretically, exhibit moderately high oxygen affinity, show a 25 to 60 percent decrease in the Bohr effect, and are characterized clinically by erythrocytosis. All have disturbances in the α1β2 area of contact.

In Yakima, x-ray crystallography of the deoxy form shows that the intersubunit deoxy bonds between β99 (G1) and α C7 and α G4 are broken, a situation that favors the R conformation. Crystallography of COHb Ypsilanti at 3.0 Å resolution revealed a novel feature, a different and stable quaternary structure along the α1β2 interface. The two stable dimers in the liganded form of this hemoglobin rotated beyond the limits observed in the R/T difference. As a consequence of this rotation, many of the salt bridges stabilizing the R structure are lost, but the H bonding between β94 Asp and β102 is retained and new bonds are formed by the mutated β99 Tyr with α97 Asn and α38 Thr. This new quaternary conformation, termed Y, to differentiate it from the R and T conformers, could be a transient conformation attained during normal R→T transition, which, in the presence of the Asp→Tyr mutation, becomes stabilized. Two carriers of Hb Yakima had different levels or erythrocytosis because of iron deficiency in one affected member of the pedigree.

Other properties of this group of mutants include moderately decreased response to 2,3-BPG of Hbs Kempsey (Ricco et al., 1992) and Radcliffe and slightly decreased response to 2,3-BPG in Hb Hotel Dieu. Hb Ypsilanti and Radcliffe form stable hybrids in the hemolysates in which the abnormal β chains coexist with normal β chains.

Hb Alberta (β101 (G3) Glu→Gly) (Wong et al., 1978) affects the dimer interaction across the α1β2 interface of both R and T states of the molecule. Purified, striped Hb Alberta has a p^{50} of 0.75 versus 2.3 mm Hg for HbA under the same conditions, slightly reduced cooperativity, and normal Bohr effect. Inositol hexaphosphate decreased the oxygen affinity to 8 mm Hg, normalized cooperativity, and increased the Bohr effect. Spectroscopic kinetic techniques applied to conditions in which the R and T state of the molecule could be observed separately revealed that the liganded Alberta tetramer was less dissociated into dimers than the HbA tetramer.

Hb Puttelange (β140 (H18) Ala→Val) (Wajcman et al., 1995) was found as an apparent de novo mutation in a French family where affected members had erythrocytosis. Upon isoelectric focusing, Hb Puttelange migrated slightly cathodically to HbA. Although high oxygen affinity was present, more interesting was that β-globin gene DNA analysis strongly suggested that the mutation was not de novo, but rather an example of paternal germ line mosaicism, leading to a recurrent risk of transmission.

Hb Osler (originally described as 145 (HC2) Tyr→Asp) (Charache et al., 1975; Kattamis et al., 1997) is expressed at 30 percent level. It has increased oxygen affinity with a decreased Bohr effect and cooperativity. Erythrocytosis was present with a packed cell volume (PCV) between 62 and 69 percent. The true structure of Hb Osler, an example of hemoglobin deamidation, is discussed in Chapter 45.

Four mutations have been described at β146 (HC3): **Hb Hiroshima** (His→Asp) (Imai, 1968; Nagel et al., 1971b), **Hb York** (His→Pro) (Suzuki et al., 1966), **Hb Cowtown** (His→Leu) (Udem et al., 1970), and **Hb Cochin-Port Royal** (His→Arg) (Wajcman et al., 1975; Russu and Ho, 1986). The first three are accompanied by erythrocytosis, and the highest PCV (51 to 54 percent) was associated with Hb Cowtown. All of these variants are present at levels of 40 to 45 percent and are detectable by electrophoresis. Hb Hiroshima, Hb York, and Hb Cowtown have moderately increased oxygen affinity and reduced Bohr effect. Hb Cowtown has normal cooperativity, but cooperativity is reduced in the other two mutants. In addition, Hb Cowtown has a decreased 2,3 BPG effect. Hb Cochin-Port Royal has normal oxygen affinity but a very reduced Bohr effect. All of these mutants disrupt a salt bridge that stabilizes the T state and the absence of the β146 His reduces the Bohr protons by half. Reduced 2,3 BPG binding might be secondary to the reduction of positive charges in the central cavity and/or to the destabilization of the T state.

Alteration of the α1β1 Area of Contact with Major Disruption of the Overall Conformation of Hemoglobin, Favoring the R State

Hb San Diego (β109 (G11) Val→Met) (Nute et al., 1974) is an electrophoretically silent mutation with moderately high oxygen affinity, a normal Bohr effect, and clinically apparent erythrocytosis. It may be the result of a C→T transition of a CpG dinucleotide (Chapter 45) (Coleman et al., 1993). The molecular mechanism of high oxygen affinity probably involves a stearic hindrance, induced by the larger bulk of the methionine residue, compared with valine, in the α1β1 contact, particularly in the deoxy (T) configuration, there by biasing the molecule toward the R state.

Hb Crete (β129 (H7) Ala→Pro) (Maniatis et al., 1979) presented with a curious syndrome of erythrocytosis, hemolysis, splenomegaly, abnormal red cell morphology, and marked erythroid hyperplasia. This index case was a combined heterozygote for Hb Crete and δβ thalassemia, with 67 percent Hb Crete and 30 percent HbF. The unique red cells had a p^{50} of 11.3, whereas isolated Hb Crete had a p^{50} of 2.2 mm Hg at pH 7.3 compared with 5.4 for HbA, moderately decreased cooperativity, and a normal Bohr effect. Hb Crete was also mildly unstable. Proline is not accommodated in the α helix and disturbs H helix while also having a longer range effect on nearby residues in the α1β1 interface, perturbing this area of subunit contact.

This case is instructive for several reasons. Splenomegaly is not usually associated with erythrocytosis caused by high oxygen affinity hemoglobins; however, in this instance it was caused by δβ thalassemia. The high affinity of Hb Crete may have complex origins. Another family member who was heterozygous for Hb Crete alone had only 38 percent of this variant and a PCV of 50 percent. In the proband, the magnitude of the erythrocytosis is greater because the level of Hb Crete is much higher and HbF also has high oxygen affinity.

Mutations That Decrease the Affinity of Hemoglobin for 2,3-BPG

Three mutations of β82 Lys (EF6) have been described: **Hb Rahere** (Lys→Thr) (Lorkin et al., 1975), **Hb Helsinki** (Lys→Met) (Ikkala et al., 1976), and **Hb Providence** (Lys→Asn→Asp) (Lorkin et al., 1975; Bonaventura et al., 1976). All have moderately high oxygen affinity and moderate erythrocytosis. The asparaginyl residue of Hb Providence is deamidated in vivo (Chapter 45). These mutants have drastically reduced 2,3-BPG binding owing to the elimination of one of the normal binding sites for this allosteric effector. β82 Lys is an invariant residue, suggesting the importance that evolution places on the binding of polyphosphates.

Hb Old Dominion (β143 (H21) His→Tyr) (Elder et al., 1998), found among Scotts/Irish individuals, has a mild increase in oxygen affinity hemoglobin and no clinical consequences. This hemoglobin elutes before HbA by reverse phase high performance liquid chromatography (HPLC) and forms 50 percent of the hemolysate. A CAC→TAC at codon β143 disrupts the 2,3 BPG binding site in the central cavity of hemoglobin. Hb Old Dominion co-elutes with HbA$_{1C}$ on ion exchange chromatography and therefore may lead to the erroneous diagnosis of diabetes or mismanagement of a diabetic patient with this variant.

Reducing Heme-Heme Interaction by Restraining the Quaternary Conformation Through Polymerization

Hb Porto Alegre (β9 (A6) Ser→Cys) (Bonaventura and Riggs, 1967; Tondo et al., 1974) is an interesting mutant with higher than normal oxygen affinity and a tendency to aggregate. Erythrocytosis is not present in carriers. Polymerization of Hb Porto Alegre is based on the formation of disulfide bonds in oxygenated samples and is fundamentally different from HbS

polymerization. Polymerization of this mutant diminishes heme-heme interaction and increases the oxygen affinity.

A "silent" variant undetectable by isoelectric focusing, **Hb Olympia** (β20 (B2) Val→Met [GTG→ATG]) (Stamatoyannopoulos et al., 1973; Edelstein et al., 1986) produces erythrocytosis owing to a moderately increased oxygen affinity with a normal Bohr effect and cooperativity. Difficulties in isolation impaired the study of this mutation, which is particularly intriguing because the mutation affects an exterior residue that is not involved in any of the areas of contact associated with quaternary conformational changes. A combined heterozygote for β thalassemia and Hb Olympia had nearly 100 percent Hb Olympia. In this patient, Edelstein and collaborators confirmed the high oxygen affinity, low n value, and normal heterotropic interactions with 2,3 BPG and Cl$^-$. Analysis of the oxygen equilibrium curve showed a pH dependency of the n value, suggesting that the tetramer self-aggregates in the T state at high pH, a property confirmed by centrifugation studies in the liganded and unliganded state. This property, observed in fish hemoglobins, is called the Root effect. The actual size of the aggregates is unknown (Edelstein et al., 1986).

Elongation of the Globin Chain Disrupting the Quaternary Structure

Hb Tak β147 (+CA) is an abnormal hemoglobin with elongation of the β-globin chain by eleven amino acid residues probably resulting from unequal crossing-over and a resulting frameshift that eliminated a stop codon. Consequently the mRNA is read until the next new stop codon, which happens to occur thirty-three nucleotides downstream (Flatz et al., 1971; Imai and Lehmann; 1975; Lehmann et al., 1975; Hoyer et al., 1998). Hb Tak constitutes 40 percent of the hemolysate, has a very high oxygen affinity with no cooperativity (n=0), and has no allosteric interaction with pH or 2,3 BPG. This is not surprising, as the C-terminal of the β chain is actively involved in the conformational changes of the hemoglobin molecule by stabilizing the T state. Because these stabilizing interactions are disrupted, Hb Tak, is totally frozen in the R state. It is also slightly unstable. Despite these severe functional abnormalities, the heterozygous patient did not have erythrocytosis. The extreme biphasic nature of the hemoglobin-oxygen affinity curve observed in mixtures of Hb Tak and HbA suggested that hybrid ($\alpha_2\beta^A\beta^T$) formation is absent. The top portion of the oxygen equilibrium curve is normal and begins to be abnormal only below 40 percent saturation. Because physiologic oxygen exchange occurs most commonly above that level of saturation, the tissues might not be hypoxic, thereby removing the stimulus for increased erythropoiesis.

Hb Saverne (Delano et al., 1984; Delanoe-Garin et al., 1988) is an elongated β chain of 156 amino acid residues, probably caused by a frameshift mutation involving a deletion of the second base of the triplet coding for His 143. This abnormal hemoglobin amounts to 30 percent of the hemolysate; is electrophoretically slightly faster than HbA; and has high oxygen affinity, no cooperativity, and a low Bohr effect. As in Hb Tak, the disruption of the C-termini resulting from the excess residues destabilizes the T conformer, favoring the R state. A compensated hemolytic anemia is present, which could be the consequence of the conflicting effects of high oxygen affinity and instability.

Another extended globin with high oxygen affinity is **Hb Thionville** (α1 Val→Glu). The mechanism for this and similar N-terminal elongations is discussed in Chapter 45. Hb Thionville has intrinsically high affinity owing to changes in the α1β2 contact surface, but since this variant forms only 21 percent of the total hemoglobin, it has little functional or clinical importance. Hb Thionville is interesting for other reasons. Allosteric interactions in which α chains participate—the Bohr effect and Cl⁻ binding—are reduced and can be separated from β chain allosteric interaction such as 2,3 BPG binding, that is normal. Also illustrated is the interference of an acetylated N-terminus, with the R→T transition showing the importance of an unblocked N-terminus for the conformational changes of hemoglobin. Several β-globin chain variants also have N-terminal extensions, but oxygen equilibrium studies have not been reported (Chapter 45).

High Affinity Hemoglobins That Lack An Explanation for Their Functional Behavior

Hb Heathrow (β103 (G5) Phe→Leu) (White et al., 1973) is an electrophoretically silent mutant with moderately high oxygen affinity and erythrocytosis. The mutation affects an invariant residue that guards the entrance to the heme pocket; the molecular mechanism accounting for high oxygen affinity is unknown. A smaller side chain at the bottom of the heme pocket might alter ligand access or the electronic environment of the prosthetic group.

DIAGNOSIS OF HIGH OXYGEN AFFINITY HEMOGLOBINS

Charache (Charache et al., 1966) described an 81-year-old patient who presented with erythrocytosis, an abnormal hemoglobin on hemoglobin electrophoresis, and erythrocytes with increased oxygen affinity. This abnormal hemoglobin, called Hb Chesapeake, proved to be a substitution of leucine for arginine at residue 92 of the α-globin chain. Its discovery opened a new chapter in the study of hemoglobinopathies by showing that a hemoglobin variant could generate yet another clinical syndrome and contribute to the elucidation of the molecular mechanisms underlying the function of normal hemoglobin. Because the propositus of the Hb Chesapeake pedigree presented with mild angina, it is legitimate to ask if this a characteristic of the carriers of high affinity hemoglobin. Studies of other members of the same pedigree and a large number of carriers of other high affinity hemoglobins have convinced most observers that the presence of these variants is largely without clinical consequence, except when inappropriate iatrogenic interventions are undertaken or a mistaken diagnosis of polycythemia vera or another cause of erythrocytosis is made.

High affinity hemoglobin patients do *not* have increased white cell and platelet counts. Sometimes there is a family history of "thick blood," suggesting the existence of a genetic disease. High oxygen affinity hemoglobins have often been detected as "new mutations," that is, in the absence of the abnormal hemoglobin among parents or siblings.

A differential diagnosis of increased red cell mass—the bench mark of erythrocytosis—without elevation of white cells and platelets and no splenomegaly includes the following:

A. Primary increase of erythropoietin (inappropriately high erythropoietin levels)
   1. Erythropoietin producing neoplasms
   2. Erythropoietin producing renal lesions
B. Mutations of the erythropoietin receptor
C. Secondary increases in erythropoietin (appropriately high erythropoietin levels)
   1. Hypoxemia secondary to
      a. Chronic pulmonary disease
      b. Right ro left cardiac shunts
      c. Sleep apnea
      d. Massive obesity (Pickwickian syndrome)
      e. High altitude
   2. Hypoxemia secondary to red cell defects
      a. High oxygen affinity hemoglobins
      b. Absence or decrease in 2,3 BPG mutase
      c. Some cases of congenital methemoglobinemia
      d. Chronic carbon monoxide poisoning (smoking and work-related exposures)
      e. Methemoglobinemia
      f. Chronic CO poisoning (including heavy smoking)
D. Idiopathic familial erythrocytosis (not known if appropriate or inappropriate erythropoietin levels)

Diagnosis of these entities requires different methodologic approaches. For example, a primary increase of erythropoietin can be suspected in the appropriate clinical environment, but can be certified only by measuring blood erythropoietin levels. Hypoxia of pulmonary or cardiovascular origin can be excluded on the basis of blood gases because these patients characteristically have low PO_2 and low O_2 saturations. Patients with red cells that have an altered capacity to transport oxygen have normal PO_2.

Individuals with erythrocytosis caused by high oxygen affinity hemoglobin variants have erythrocytes with high oxygen affinity, high oxygen affinity of the hemolysate, and near normal 2,3 BPG concentrations. With 2,3 BPG mutase deficiency, erythrocytes have high oxygen affinity red cells, the oxygen affinity of the hemolysate is normal, and levels of 2,3 BPG are very low (Rosa et al., 1978). In both instances, the absorption spectrum of the hemolysate is normal.

Congenital methemoglobinemia has an abnormal peak at 620 nm, and the level of CO hemoglobin can be assayed by a three-wave length calculation, as the spectra of COHb and O_2Hb differ significantly. Several gas measuring apparatuses are available in hospitals (e.g., the CO oximeter) and, except with some M hemoglobins, can give an accurate reading of methemoglobinemia and carboxyhemoglobinemia in whole blood (for further details see Chapter 46).

Defects of the erythropoietin receptor (EpoR) include truncation of the intracytoplasmic C-terminal domain, which negatively regulates the erythropoietin/EpoR signal transduction pathway (Prchal and Sokol, 1996). These patients have decreased or normal serum erythropoietin levels and increased sensitivity of burst-forming units (BFU-e) and colony-forming units (CFU-e)(erythroid precursors) to erythropoietin in vitro. Future research will determine if the yet unrecognized defects in idiopathic familial erythrocytosis could be the product of alterations of the oxygen-sensing system tied to erythropoietin (the hypoxic inducible factor or Hinf1) or other constituents of the EpoR signaling pathway (JAK-2, HCP, STAT 5).

Some forms of familial erythrocytosis have normal oxygen affinity of red cells and hemolysate and are inherited recessively. It should therefore be expected among siblings, but not among parents or descendants (Adamson, 1975). Recent reports have described high frequency of this ailment among the Chuvash of Russia, where it is not linked to the EpoR gene (Seryeva, 1997).

Laboratory Studies

With some caveats, determination of the red cell oxygen equilibrium curve is the benchmark for the diagnosis of erythrocytosis owing to high oxygen affinity hemoglobins. An accurate p^{50} value cannot be "calculated" from PO_2 data. Measuring directly the saturation of hemoglobin and PO_2 is necessary obtain an accurate p^{50}. The Hemoscan types of apparatus are perfectly adequate for this purpose, but the state of the art equipment is the Imai cell as an attachment to a recording spectrophotometer. Also, an oxygen equilibrium of the dialyzed hemolysate is indispensable to exclude cytosol effects on ligand binding (e.g., genetic reduction of 2,3 BPG). If this is not possible, a repeat of the red cell oxygen equilibrium in 2,3 BPG depleted red cells is useful.

Once a low p^{50} is documented, a search for abnormal hemoglobins can begin using method discussed in Chapter 34. Cellulose acetate hemoglobin electrophoresis at alkaline pH has a low sensitivity for detecting high affinity mutants, because many have a migration indistinguishable from HbA. Citrate agar electrophoresis and isoelectric focusing can improve detection, but some high affinity hemoglobins with neutral substitutions cannot be detected by these methods. High-performance liquid chromatography (HPLC) is sometimes useful for detecting electrophoretically silent variants (Chapter 34). A normal electrophoresis or HPLC does *not* exclude the diagnosis of a high affinity hemoglobin, and more sensitive protein-based testing may be needed.

When all protein-based studies fail to detect an abnormal hemoglobin and the clinical and oxygen equilibrium studies strongly suggest the existence of such a variant, determining the DNA sequence of the globin genes will detect any mutations present.

Pathophysiologic and Clinical Aspects of High Affinity Hemoglobins

Patients with high affinity hemoglobins accompanied by erythrocytosis have a benign clinical course and no apparent complications apart from a ruddy complexion. Splenomegaly is absent except when a confounding disorder is present. Hemoglobin concentration and PCV are increased only moderately. Some patients with Hb Malmo have been reported to be symptomatic and benefit from phlebotomy and the transfusion of normal blood, but this is an exception. Many cases of high oxygen affinity hemoglobins are diagnosed in the course of a routine hematologic examination or when the family of a proband is examined. Some have suspected that carriers of these variants may have enhanced athletic performance under some circumstances, and this has lead to the unfortunate and sometimes fatal use of erythropoietin or transfusion to enhance performance in competitive athletics.

By early diagnosis of high affinity hemoglobins, unnecessary invasive diagnostic procedures and inappropriate and often dangerous therapeutic interventions can be avoided. Some patients have undergone expensive and unnecessary cardiac catheterization. Others have received several courses of ^{32}P treatment based on a mistaken diagnosis of polycythemia vera. Generally, any patient suspected of having polycythemia vera and about to undergo a serious therapeutic intervention should undergo whole blood oxygen equilibrium measurement.

Several questions about the clinical effects of high oxygen affinity hemoglobins remain. Do they interfere with the delivery of oxygen to the tissues? Patients heterozygous for physiologically significant high oxygen affinity hemoglobins are from birth onwards probably reasonably compensated for this abnormality. Any reduction of tissue O_2 delivery (Fig. 44.3) is primarily compensated for by increases in red cell mass induced by erythropoietin, probable increases in tissue blood flow, and perhaps changes in perfusion patterns in selected regions of the body that appear to negate any adverse effect of increased blood viscosity.

Erythropoietin mediates increases in red cell mass in response to hypoxic stimuli (Adamson and Finch, 1968; Adamson et al., 1972; Adamson and Finch, 1975). Patients with different high oxygen affinity hemoglobins and erythrocytosis had normal erythropoietin levels in their urine, but showed dramatic increases in erythropoietin when phlebotomized to a normal red cell mass. This effect was not observed in patients with familial erythrocytosis, which is in some cases, the result of a defect in the erythropoietin receptor.

Patients with high oxygen affinity hemoglobins have normal oxygen consumption, normal arterial PO_2, a reduced mixed venous PO_2 in some cases, and decreased resting cardiac output (Charache et al., 1978). Phlebotomy or measured exercise induced increases in cardiac output and lowered mixed venous PO_2. A patient with Hb Malmö had increased myocardial blood flow, and patients with Hb Yakima had increased cerebral flow, indicating increased perfusion efficiency.

Is there an added risk involved in pregnancy for women with high oxygen affinity hemoglobins? Increased morbidity or mortality in mothers or their offspring has not been observed, suggesting that either the affinity of the mother's hemoglobin is irrelevant with respect to oxygen delivery to the fetus or other compensatory mechanisms in addition to the differences in oxygen affinity between HbF and HbA must be operative in pregnancies in where the woman has a hemoglobin whose oxygen affinity is greater than that of HbF (Charache et al., 1985).

Why does the magnitude of erythrocytosis vary among carriers of high oxygen affinity hemoglobins with similar p^{50}? Carriers of Hb Osler had the same p^{50} as patients with **Hb McKees Rocks** ($\beta145$ Tyr→termination codon), but had a hemoglobin level

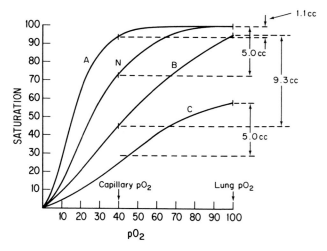

Figure 44.3. Extraction of O_2 from hemoglobin binding curves with different p^{50}. Curve N: normal, resulting in a O_2 extraction at the tissue level of 5.0 mL of O_2. Curve A = high affecting Hb: *Reduction* in oxygen extraction to 1.1 mL; Curve B = moderate shift to the right (low affinity) of O_2 binding curve: *Increase* of oxygen extraction to 9.3; Curve C = intense shift to the right (very low affinity) of O_2 binding curve: return to a *normal* extraction 5.0 mL.

more than 4 g/dL higher. When oxygen transport was assessed in these two patient groups, only a small decrease in mixed venous PO_2 was observed (Butler et al., 1982). Perhaps this was a consequence of better O_2 extraction by carriers of Hb McKee Rocks who did not require any higher red cell mass. Alternatively these patients may have differed in their ability to increase their red cell mass. While acquired abnormalities such as iron deficiency could account for these differences, a genetic basis of this phenomenon would require a polymorphic gene linked to the β-like globin gene cluster. Such an epistatic genetic effect might be present because adaptation to hypoxia of high altitude also differs among ethnic groups (Butler et al., 1982). Sherpas of Nepal have a lower PCV, an absence of chronic mountain sickness, and a normal oxygen equilibrium curve. Quechuas and Aymaras, populations adapted to the Andes, exhibited a higher PCV, chronic mountain sickness, and right-shifted oxygen equilibrium curves. These findings suggest that adaptation to hypoxia, regardless of the cause, may be complex.

Treatment Recommendations

Is phlebotomy indicated in the erythrocytosis of high oxygen affinity hemoglobins? Patients with high oxygen affinity hemoglobins have reasonable compensation for their abnormality with correction of the delivery of oxygen to the tissues despite increases in blood viscosity. Therefore, it appears that no intervention is needed. Exercise studies before and after phlebotomy in patients with Hb Osler did not show a need for phlebotomy (Butler et al., 1982). Although rare individuals appear to have benefitted from phlebotomy, other unknown factors might be interfering with their normal compensation for high hemoglobin oxygen affinity, and increased blood viscosity might have become a burden. Prudence dictates that before embarking on a regimen of chronic phlebotomy, one should be conservative and review the hematologic and physiologic findings at 6-month intervals during the first few years after diagnosis. In older patients, special attention should be directed to blood flow to the heart and central nervous system.

Low ambient PO_2, as occurs in unpressurized airplanes and ascent to altitude, does not represent a risk because high affinity hemoglobins are avid for oxygen. Hypothetically, carriers would be less prone to "the bends" during deep sea diving because of slower oxygen release during ascension.

LOW OXYGEN AFFINITY HEMOGLOBIN MUTANTS: CYANOSIS

Patients with low ligand affinity hemoglobin variants can have a slate gray color of their skin and mucous membranes. Cyanosis is present from birth in some carriers of α-globin chain abnormalities. In carriers of β-globin chain mutants, cyanosis may appear from the middle to the end of the first year of life because β-globin gene expression begins later in development than α-globin gene expression, peaking at about 6 months of age (Chapters 10 and 15). Patients with low oxygen affinity hemoglobins do not always have cyanosis. Cyanosis secondary to abnormal hemoglobins must be distinguished from cyanosis of other causes.

Clinical Features of Low Affinity Hemoglobins

Fewer low oxygen affinity hemoglobins have been described than have high oxygen affinity variants. Only sixteen of these variants, about 2 percent of all hemoglobin variants, have been characterized. They can be classified as follows.

Alterations of Critical Molecular Regions Directly Involved in the Conformational Transition Between the R and T State, Resulting in the Stabilization of the T State or Destabilization of the R State. Hb Bruxelles (β42 Phe (CD1) Phe→0) (Hargrove et al., 1997) is a deletion of the most conserved amino acid residue of hemoglobin. Phenylalanine residues at β41 and β42 are conserved in all normal mammalian non-α-globin chains and are indispensable for the structural integrity and oxygen-

binding functions of the molecule (Fig. 44.4). Sequence analysis was insufficient to differentiate between phenylalanine β41 and β42 as the site of the deletion Hb Bruxelles deletion. DNA analysis showed that the missing codon was the TTT of β42.

The index case of Hb Bruxelles was a patient who from 4 years of age had severe hemolytic anemia and cyanosis, requiring blood transfusion on one occasion. Later in life, her hemoglobin concentration stabilized at about 10 g/dL. Reasons for this "switch" of phenotype are unknown. Other mutations of β41 and β42, which are predominately unstable hemoglobins, are discussed later.

The striking feature of the oxygen equilibrium curve of Hb Bruxelles (Griffin et al., 1996) (Fig. 44.5) is that unlike the normal curve, which is roughly symmetric with maximum cooperativity at half saturation, Hb Bruxelles has almost nonexistent cooperativity and a shift of the allosteric equilibrium almost entirely to the T or deoxy state. Confirming the latter, even at low photolysis levels, CO rebinding kinetics showed the T conformation; hence the switch between R and T occurs after the third heme is liganded, not after second

Figure 44.4. Structure of the heme pocket of the β chain in deoxy normal HbA using Quanta 4.0 (Molecular Simulation, Inc) taken from the crystallographic coordinate file 3 hhb of the Protein Data Bank. Arrow indicates location of β42 Phe residue (deleted in Hb Bruxelles).

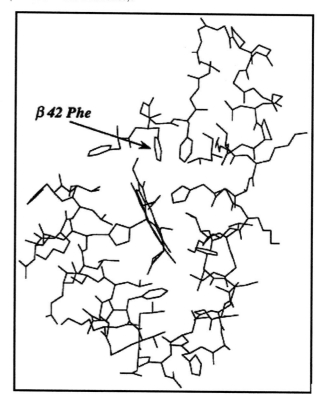

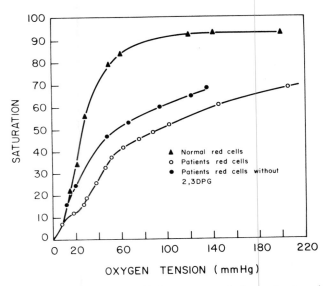

Figure 44.5. Oxygen equilibrium curves of the patient's red cells, red cells deprived of 2,3 BPG, and a normal control sample (temperature 37°C, pH 7.40).

heme ligation as in normal hemoglobin. Hb Bruxelles provides a fine example of the separation of ligand affinity and allosteric effects. The shift to T state is so large (allosteric effect) that the oxygen equilibrium/CO kinetics show essentially T-state properties. Because cooperativity is minimal in the absence of effectors, the shift in p^{50} observed with 2,3 BPG is a ligand affinity effect. In HbA, the contributions of allosteric effects and ligand affinity contribute equally to the 2,3 BPG shift in oxygen affinity. In Hb Bruxelles, the p^{50} shift caused by allosteric effectors is due entirely to ligand affinity changes because the molecule is already nearly totally in the T state.

Hb Titusville (α94 (G1) Asp→Asn) (Schneider et al., 1975) is the sole described α-globin chain mutation with low oxygen affinity. Separable from HbA by electrophoresis, this α-globin chain variant formed 35 percent of the total hemoglobin. Cyanosis was not present, probably because of the relative anemia (hemoglobin concentration 12.5 g/dL) secondary to more efficient oxygen delivery to the tissues. Hb Titusville had a p^{50} of 16 mm Hg compared with the normal control level of 5 mm Hg, and a Bohr effect reduced by more than 60 percent. The molecular defect involved the α1β2 area of contact, and the substitution favored the T state. There was a tendency of this variant to dimerize.

Three low oxygen affinity variants have been described at β102 (G4): **Hb Kansas** (Asn→Thr) (Reismann et al., 1961; Bonaventura and Riggs, 1968), **Hb Beth Israel** (Asn→Ser) (Nagel et al., 1976), and **Hb St Mande** (Asn→Tyr) (Arous et al., 1981).

These three abnormal hemoglobins all have low oxygen affinity and produce clinically apparent cyanosis.

Hb Kansas, the first low affinity hemoglobin described and the best studied, has a whole blood p^{50} of about 70 mm Hg compared with the normal values of p^{50} of 26 mmHg, decreased cooperativity, and a normal Bohr effect. The β102 Asn residue is invariant among β-globin chains and participates in the only hydrogen bond between Asn102 and Asp94 across the α1β2 interface in oxyHb. This bond is broken when the molecule assumes the T state (Fig. 44.2). Examination of deoxyHb Kansas by difference Fourier x-ray diffraction analysis at 5.5 Å resolution has shown that the new Thr residue is incapable of forming this bond (Greer, 1971a). Thus, the low oxygen affinity results from destabilization of the R conformer. In addition, other structural changes occur at the α1β2 interface, which accounts for the increased tendency of Hb Kansas to dissociate into $\alpha\beta$ dimers. It is the mirror image, pathogenetically, of Hb Chesapeake.

It is interesting to note that replacement of the same β102 Asn residue by Lys in **Hb Richmond** is not accompanied by abnormal oxygen binding properties (Efremov, 1961). Crystallography has shown that the introduced Lys residue is capable of bridging the α1β2 region and forming a salt bridge with the Asp 94, providing further evidence for the defect in Hb Kansas (Greer, 1971a). Nevertheless, because there are some abnormalities in the α1β2 region on the different Fourier maps, it has been suggested that reexamination of the oxygen equilibrium curve of Hb Richmond might be appropriate.

Hb Beth Israel was found in a patient with cyanosis of the fingers, lips, and nail beds. The patient had been severely disciplined for constantly having "dirty hands," and neither he nor his parents noticed his abnormal skin color. Cyanosis was detected by an observant surgeon about to repair a hernia. This hemoglobin is difficult to separate by electrophoresis. Whole blood p^{50} was 88 mm Hg, and arterial blood was only 63 percent saturated despite a normal PO_2 of 97 mm Hg (Fig. 44.2). Hemolysate also had a low oxygen affinity and a normal Bohr effect. Erythrocyte 2,3 BPG was mildly elevated. The molecular mechanism of reduced oxygen affinity is the same as for Hb Kansas, although the defect might be more disruptive locally as the serine side chain is shorter than that of threonine.

Hb Saint Mande makes up 38 percent of the hemolysate and migrates electrophoretically like HbF. It was found in an individual who exhibited labial cyanosis and a hemoglobin of 9.6 g/dL. The p^{50} was 52 mm Hg. Oxygen saturation of arterial blood was 81 percent. NMR spectroscopy showed that the quaternary structure of the liganded conformer was different from the R state but also different from the T state (Andersen, 1975). This special ligand quaternary structure also differed from Hb Kansas, which had an NMR spectrum similar to the T-state quaternary structure in the liganded molecule. Of interest was that the tertiary conformation around the heme of both chains was altered, suggesting that the β chain mutation propagated a conformation modification to the other subunit (long range interaction) involving β141 Leu.

Because there are several mutations of the β102 site, their phenotypes can be compared. The intensity of the cyanosis and extent of the decrease in oxygen affinity are inversely proportional to the length of the substituted side chain: maximal for serine, less for threonine, and least for tyrosine.

Hb Rothschild (β37 (C3) Trp→Arg) (Gacon et al., 1977) is a remarkable example of a hemoglobin with altered oxygen affinity (Sharma et al., 1980). It has alternatively low and high oxygen affinity, depending on the conditions of study. This mutant exhibits generally low affinity. Nevertheless, the situation is far more complicated (Sharma et al., 1980) because the molecule is extensively dissociated into dimers in the liganded state, which explains the low affinity, fully liganded dimers, have lower oxygen affinity than partially unsaturated dimers. The T state of Hb Rothschild has a higher affinity for ligands than the T state of HbA, accounting for the low/high affinity description of this mutant. The molecular basis of this unique set of properties is probably due the β37 Arg, which interacts with β92 (FG4) Arg. This clash of positive charges destabilizes the subunit contacts at the level of the α1β2 interface with extensive dissociation into αβ dimers. There is also less constraint of the T state, which explains the higher affinity of the deoxy form, and monoliganded tetramers probably have increased dissociation, again conspiring against a true T-state behavior. Considerable alteration in the intradimer stability alters the refolding capacity (Craik et al., 1980). These findings predict small, but potentially significant, long-range interactions in the areas of the molecule distal to the substitution. Polarized absorption microspectroscopy of crystals of T-state Hb Rothschild was used to show it that Cl⁻ decreases the oxygen affinity, most likely binding to the new arginyl residue, an effect not seen in crystals of HbA (DeFuria and Miller, 1972; Rivetti et al., 1993).

Hb Aalborg (β74 (E18) Gly→Arg) (Williamson et al., 1990) accounting for 21 percent of the hemolysate, has decreased oxygen affinity, increased affinity for 2,3 BPG, and is moderately unstable. Clinically, it is associated with mild anemia. Electrophoretically it has a mobility between that of HbF and HbS. Further understanding of this mutant has been provided by

crystallographic analysis (Fermi et al., 1992) and a comparison with **Hb Shepard's Bush** (β74 (E18) Gly→Asp), an unstable high oxygen affinity mutant. Hb Shepard's Bush has an opposite charge substitution and exhibits increased ligand affinity, diminished affinity for phosphate, and instability. Fermi et al. (1992), superimposed the B, G, and H helix of HbA known not to be affected by ligand binding on those of Hb Aalborg. This maneuver revealed a shift of the F helix of deoxyHb Aaborg toward the EF corner, a movement opposite the normal change with ligand binding. On transition to the R state, this is linked to an increased tilt of the proximal histidine away from the heme axis, accounting for the bias toward the T state and the low oxygen affinity. The opposite effects of 2,3 BPG binding between Hb Aalborg and Shepard's Bush are the consequence of the opposite charges of the introduced residues.

Steric Hindrance Causing Decreased Affinity for Ligands. **Hb Connecticut** (β21 (B3) (Asp→Gly)) (Moo-Penn et al., 1981) is an electrophoretically separable mutation amounting to 39 percent of the hemolysate. Whole blood p⁵⁰ was elevated at 28.5 mm Hg, but the Bohr effect and 2,3 BPG interactions were normal. Neither cyanosis nor anemia was present. This mutation is of special interest because it involves a residue not critical for the ligand-dependent conformational changes. Moo-Penn et al. (1981) have suggested, on the basis of preliminary x-ray data, that the molecular abnormality probably involves the disruption of the salt bridges between β21 Asp and the β61 β65 lysine residues. This event might allow the E helix to come closer to the heme plate, inducing stearic hindrance to the binding of ligands.

Hb Bologna (β61 (E5) Lys→Met (Marinucci et al., 1981) is separable electrophoretically and forms 48 percent of the hemolysate. The propositus was neither anemic nor cyanotic. This mutation has also been found in conjuction with β⁰ thalassemia, where it accounts for 90 percent of the hemolysate. Remarkably, affected patients had no apparent cyanosis, despite a whole blood p⁵⁰ of 37.6 mm Hg in the compound heterozygotes and 31 mm Hg in the simple heterozygotes.

β61 Lys is an external residue, close to the distal heme-linked E7 histidine, and forms a salt bridge with asparagine at position 21 of the same β-globin chain. It also contacts β25 of the B helix and β55 and β56 in the D helix. The disruption of any or all of these contacts is likely to alter the oxygen binding properties of the β heme. Interestingly, compensatory erythroid expansion, observed commonly in thalassemia, is not evident in the compound heterozygote for β⁰ thalassemia and Hb Bologna, showing the effect of increased tissue oxygen delivery because of the right-shifted oxygen equilibrium curve.

In **Hb Chico** (β66 (E10) Lys→Thr)(Bonaventura et al., 1991), low oxygen affinity is not limited to the tetramer but is also present in the isolated β Chico globin chain. This supports the notion that the mutation induces decreased affinity for ligands by changes in the heme environment unrelated to the R→T transition. The most economical explanation is the rupture of the salt bridge that β66 Lys forms with one of the propionate side chains of the β heme. Crystallographic studies show the hydrogen bonding of the introduced β66 Thr to the distal histidine β63 (E7). Nevertheless, site-directed mutagenesis studies have shown that although distal histidines are important in ligand binding in R state α-chains, they are not significant in β chains (Olson et al., 1988). Hence, the low affinity of Hb Chico must be secondary to direct steric hindrance.

Alteration of the $\alpha1\beta1$ Area of Contact with Major Disruption of the Overall Conformation of Hemoglobin that Favors the T State

Two mutant hemoglobins have been described at β108 (G10): **Hb Yoshizuka** (Asn→Asp) (Imamura et al., 1969) and **Hb Presbyterian** (Asn→Lys) (Moo-Penn et al., 1978). **Hb Yoshizuka**, which constitutes 51 percent of the hemolysate, has significantly lower oxygen affinity and a 30 percent decreased Bohr effect. Carriers usually have mild anemia but lack cyanosis. β108 Asn lies in the central cavity and is hydrogen bonded to β103 His, a residue located in the $\alpha1\beta1$ contact. In addition, this residue is linked extensively through hydrogen bonding via water molecules to other residues both in the α- and β-globin chains. The introduction of the carbonyl group of the asparaginyl residue severely disrupts this contact and changes the electrostatic properties of the central cavity, resulting in the destabilization of the oxy conformation. In Hb Presbyterian, the mutated residue has the opposite charge of Hb Yoshizuka (Lys instead of Asp). Hb Presbyterian forms 40 percent of the hemolysate, is electrophoretically fast moving, has low oxygen affinity, a 30 percent increased Bohr effect, and normal interactions with 2,3 BPG. Carriers are mildly anemic. This hemoglobin does not dissociate normally in the R state, suggesting that the molecule is biased toward the T state (Moo-Penn et al., 1978).

These two hemoglobins illustrate that any charge, positive or negative, disrupts drastically the $\alpha1\beta1$ area of contact, but, some aspects of the pathophysiology of the mutant hemoglobins can be quite different. Understanding the basis for the Bohr effect differences will require high resolution crystallography.

Both Hb Yoshizuka and Hb Presbyterian have been expressed in transgenic pigs and purified to homogeneity (O'Donnell et al., 1994). Their study showed

that Hb Presbyterian has a dramatic Cl$^-$ effect, exhibiting a p^{50} almost identical to HbA at low Cl$^-$ concentrations but increased to more than 40 mm Hg at 0.5 M Cl$^-$. This effect was completely abolished when Hb Presbyterian was stabilized at the central cavity by interdimeric cross-linking. Molecular modeling suggested that Cl$^-$ can bridge the ϵ-amino group of β108 Lys with either the guanidino group of β104 Arg or the ϵ-amino of β99 Lys, resulting in the stabilization of the T structure. In contrast, Hb Yoshizuka is insensitive to Cl$^-$, showing the great effect of the nature of the introduced side chain.

Mutations of **Hb Vancouver** (β73 (E17) Asp→Tyr) (Jones et al., 1976), **Hb Korle Bu** (β73 Asp→Asn) (Konotey-Ahulu et al., 1968), and **Hb Mobile** (β73 Asp→Val) (Schneider et al., 1975) are similar. All amount to close to 40 percent of the hemolysate without apparent cyanosis. Hb Vancouver has a whole blood p^{50} of 29.5 mm Hg; this variant and Hb Mobile have a 20 percent increased Bohr effect. In isolated mutant hemoglobins, the order of p^{50}'s is: Hb Vancouver>Hb Mobile>Hb Korle Bu>HbA (Wajcman and Jones, 1977). A molecular mechanism for these differential effects is not obvious. Residue β73 is on the surface and is known for its capacity to interfere with the polymerization of HbS (Bookchin and Nagel, 1973; Wishner et al., 1975). The bulkier side chain could perhaps interfere with the entrance of ligands into the heme pocket and alter the oxygen affinity by stearic hindrance (Jones et al., 1976). Others have argued that since the size of asparaginyl and the aspartyl residues is almost identical, this cannot explain the observed differences in p^{50} (Wajcman and Jones, 1977). The increase in p^{50} is proportional to the hydrophobicity of the newly introduced residue, making it likely that the effect is the result of the formation of a hydrophobic bond of increasing strength that perturbs the normal conformation (Wajcman and Jones, 1977). A good candidate for the receptor for this interaction is β84 Thr located in the EF segment, that is, in the junction segment between helics E and F.

Pathophysiologic Considerations

Low affinity hemoglobins deliver more O_2 to the tissues. Figure 44.3 illustrates O_2 extraction from a hemoglobin with an oxygen dissociation curve situated to the right of normal. When hemoglobin has a right-shifted or low affinity curve, the difference between oxygen binding in the lungs at a PO_2 levels of 100 mm Hg and unloading in the tissues at 40 mm Hg can be twice as great as the differences in a hemoglobin with a normal oxygen equilibrium curve. Oxygen extraction does not increase monotonically with increases in p^{50}. After reaching a maximum level it decreases to a normal extraction at a p^{50} of about 80 mm Hg. Patients with moderately right-shifted red cell oxygen equilibrium curves could be anemic (p^{50} between 35 and 55), but anemia should not be expected in patients with severely right-shifted curves (p^{50} approximately 80). The clinical picture observed with Hb Kansas, Beth Israel, Titusville, and Seattle is in accord with this analysis. Clinically apparent cyanosis is observed only in carriers of low oxygen affinity variants with greatly right-shifted curves, beyond 50 mm Hg, and where the variant accounts for a substantial portion of the hemolysate.

The effect of a right-shifted oxygen equilibrium curve on the level of 2,3 BPG is of interest. In erythrocytes, about 20 percent of the conversion of 1,3-diphosphoglycerate to 3-phosphoglycerate is indirect through the formation of 2,3 BPG. Erythrocyte 2,3 BPG is known to rise in many conditions associated with hypoxia.

Desaturation increases intraerythrocytic pH as a result of the Bohr effect, where deoxyhemoglobin binds more protons than oxyhemoglobin. This slight intraerythrocytic alkalosis, in turn, stimulates two enzymes involved in 2,3 BPG synthesis: phosphofructokinase, which controls the overall glycolytic rate, and diphosphoglycerate mutase, which directly controls the rate of 2,3 BPG synthesis. High pH also inhibits 2,3 BPG phosphatase, simultaneously increasing the synthesis of 2,3 BPG and decreasing its destruction. Release of endproduct inhibition, as low oxygen affinity hemoglobins with an increased proportion of deoxyhemoglobin binds more 2,3 BPG, decreases free 2,3 BPG and inhibits diphosphoglycerate mutase, also may increase 2,3 BPG (Nagel et al., 1976).

Diagnosis of Low Affinity Hemoglobin Variants

Detection of a low oxygen affinity hemoglobin is part of the differential diagnosis of patients with cyanosis, particularly when cardiopulmonary causes can be excluded. Before undertaking expensive or risky invasive diagnostic procedures in cases of cyanosis, it is advisable to obtain a hemoglobin electrophoresis and a whole blood p^{50}. A search for low affinity hemoglobins as an explanation for anemia in the absence of cyanosis is less compelling, as the yield is very low. If other investigations prove fruitless, however, unexplained normocytic anemia deserves exploration at least by measuring the whole blood p^{50}.

A simple beside test to distinguish cyanosis caused by low oxygen affinity hemoglobins, and cardiopulmonary cyanosis from that of methemoglobinemia, M hemoglobins, and sulfhemoglobinemia is to expose blood from the patient to pure oxygen. When cyanosis is due to low oxygen affinity hemoglobins or cardiopulmonary disease, blood will turn from purplegreenish to the bright red color of fully oxygenated

blood. In contrast, blood of patients with methemoglobinemia, sulfhemoglobinemia, and M hemoglobins will retain its abnormal color despite exposure to pure O_2.

Treatment Recommendations

No treatment is needed because the condition is totally benign in the heterozygous case, and no homozygous patients have been described with low oxygen affinity hemoglobins. The importance of early diagnosis is *to avoid* unnecessary evaluation, some of which involves serious risks, and unnecessary concern for the patient and family.

M HEMOGLOBINS: PSEUDOCYANOSIS

Pathophysiologic Features of the M Hemoglobins

In the first report of methemoglobinemia caused by an M hemoglobin, published 1 year before Pauling's discovery of HbS, Horlein and Weber (1948) described a family with congenital cyanosis resulting from abnormal red cells. They determined that the defect was autosomal dominant, caused by red cells with an abnormal pigment, that was similar but not identical to methemoglobin, and showed that the genetic defect resided in the globin, not heme.

Additional M hemoglobins were characterized by Gerald and Efron (1961). Simultaneously, Shibata et al. (1960 and 1981) in Japan solved the problem of the hereditary nigremia (*kuroko* or "black child"), which had been observed by clinicians in the Shiden village of the Iwate prefecture for more than 160 years. They found a brownish colored hemoglobin in the hemolysate of a patient, later characterized as **HbM Iwate** ($\alpha_1$87 or $\alpha_2$87 (F8) His→Tyr).

In the M hemoglobins, the mutant globin chain creates an abnormal microenvironment for the heme iron, displacing the equilibrium toward the oxidized or ferric state. A combination of Fe^{+3} and its abnormal coordination with the substituted amino acid generates an abnormal visible spectrum that resembles, but is clearly different from, methemoglobin in which the heme iron is oxidized but an associated amino acid substitution is absent. The strength of attachment of ferric heme to globins differs among M hemoglobins. Table 44.1 shows HbM mutations.

In four of the five known M hemoglobins, affecting either the α- or β-globin chain, the distal or proximal histidine interacting with the heme iron is replaced by tyrosine. In the fifth HbM, HbM Milwaukee, β67 Val is replaced by a glutamic acid residue whose longer side chain can reach and perturb the heme iron. Some properties of M hemoglobins are shown in Table 44.2. M hemoglobin mutations have also been described in

Table 44.1. Hemoglobin M Variants

HbM Hyde Park	β92 (F8) his→tyr
HbM Saskatoon	β63 (E7) his→tyr
HbM Iwate	α87 (F8) his→tyr
HbM Boston	α58 (E7) his→tyr
HbM Milwaukee	β67 (E11) val→glu
Fetal HbM Osaka	γ63 (E7) his→tyr

the ^{G}γ-globin chain as HbF-M Osaka (^{G}γ63 His→Tyr) and HbF-M Fort Ripley (^{G}γ92 His Tyr) and have been associated with neonatal "cyanosis" that disappears with maturation.

Several shared molecular abnormalities are associated with the M hemoglobins. They can be classified as either weak heme attachment or binding of the iron to the remaining histidine and to the newly introduced tyrosine.

Weak Heme Attachment. X-ray crystallographic studies (Greer, 1971b) of deoxy HbM Hyde Park (β92 (F8) His→Tyr) showed a loss of 20 to 30 percent of the heme. A minor hemoglobin component of about 5 percent migrated between HbA$_2$ and HbA/Hyde Park (Shibata and Iuchi, 1977). α-Globin chains of the abnormal component were normal, but only one of the two β^{HP} chains contained heme.

Binding of the Iron To the Remaining Histidine and To the Newly Introduced Tyrosine. An intriguing question has been the nature of the interaction of the newly introduced tyrosine with the heme iron. The status of the proximal histidine (F8) in the β^M chains (Hb Hyde Park) and the α^M-chains (Hb Iwate) provides an interesting contrast. It was first suggested that the β heme of Hb Hyde Park moves toward the E helix, allowing the

iron to be bound by the distal histidine, accommodating the bulkier side chain of the new tyrosine, and generating a phenolic bond to the sixth coordinating position of the iron, thereby stabilizing it in the ferric form (Gerald and Efron, 1961). Crystallographic studies contradicted this interpretation (Greer, 1971b), showing that heme was not displaced toward the E helix and suggesting that the tyrosine residue must be accommodated by movements of the F helix, which appeared largely destabilized. Independent confirmation was provided by electron nuclear double resonance spectroscopy (Feher et al., 1973) where examination of the ^{14}N interactions in HbM Hyde Park did not show any of the high frequency peaks assigned to the proximal histidines, indicating that the distal histidines did not take over the role of the proximal histidine. It is likely that the β92 tyrosine of HbM Hyde Park binds the heme iron through a phenolic anion.

In the example of HbM Iwate, crystallographic studies (Greer, 1971b) did find displacement of the E helix of the α chains toward the heme plate by approximately 2Å, which is the distortion expected if the distal histidine (E7) of the α-globin chain had moved to bind the fifth coordinating position in the α-heme iron. No direct data exist with regard to the position of the tyrosine α87 (F8), but presumably it interacts with the heme iron (Gerald and Efron, 1961). NMR studies (Peisach and Gersonde, 1977; LaMar et al., 1980) indicated that when the abnormal heme is reduced and bound to a ligand, the iron can bind the distal histidine.

Interactions of the tyrosine-substituted distal histidines (E7) in the β^M-chain of HbM Saskatoon and the α^M-chain in HbM Boston are also known. Data for HbM Boston are more precise (Fig. 44.6). Pulsinelli et al. (1973) demonstrated by x-ray crystallography that the new residue, α58 (E7) Tyr, fills the fifth coordination position of the heme iron despite the presence of a normal proximal histidine. This bond moves the plane

Table 44.2. Some Properties of HbM

Variant	Percent	Hb (g/dl)	Reticulocytes (%)	T$_{1/2}$ of reduction of Fe^{+3} by dithionate	p50	Bohr effect	Conversion of abnormal units to cyanmetHb with KCN
HbM Hyde Park	—	10–13	4–6	55	Normal	Present	Slow
HbM Iwate	19	17	—	—	Decreased	Decreased	Very slow
HbM Boston	—	—	—	260	Decreased	Decreased	Slow
HbM Milwaukee	50	14–15	1–2	23	Decreased	Present	Fast
HbM Saskatoon	35	13–16	0.8–3.2	15	Normal	Present	Fast
HbA	97	15	1	Very rapid			Very fast

Hill's constant (n) is between 1.1 and 1.3 for all variants (normal 2.7).

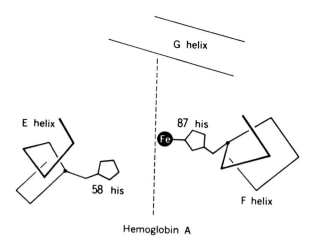

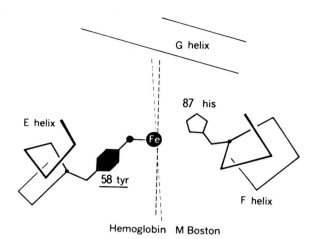

Figure 44.6. Alteration of the heme and surroundings in hemoglobin M Boston in which His α58(E7) is replaced by Tyr. Normal molecule at the left, mutant at right. Tyrosine becomes the fifth heme ligand in the mutant, the heme moves toward it, and the former heme ligand, His α87(F8), moves away from the heme. With the coupling between heme and F helix broken, the subunits remain in the T configuration, so the oxygen affinity of all subunits is decreased.

of the heme sufficiently to make the interaction between the proximal histidine and the heme iron impossible, an interpretation confirmed by NMR spectroscopy (LaMar et al., 1980).

HbM Milwaukee is the sole example of an M hemoglobin caused not by mutation of the proximal or distal histidine residues, but by the nearby β67 (E11) Val. When this residue is replaced by a residue with an appropriate side chain, as is the case with a glutaminyl residue, it perturbs the heme iron and generates an M hemoglobin. Other mutations of that site, such as Hb Bristol (Asp) or Hb Sidney (Ala), are unstable or have low affinity but do not lead to heme iron oxidation. X-ray crystallography showed that the carboxylic group of the new glutamine residue occupies the sixth coordination position of the iron, and that the proximal histidine maintains its role as the tenant of the fifth coordinating position (Perutz et al., 1972). This stabilizes the abnormal ferric state of HbM Milwaukee.

Oxygen-Binding Properties and the R→T Transition of M Hemoglobins

HbM Milwaukee-1, Hyde Park (Milwaukee-2), and Boston all adopt deoxy or deoxy-like conformation upon the deoxygenation of the two normal chains even though the abnormal chains cannot offload oxygen. This event as well as crystallographic, electron paramagnetic resonance, and NMR spectroscopy

(Raftery and Huestis, 1973); 2,3 BPG binding studies (Raftery and Huestis, 1973); and an examination of the copolymerization of deoxy HbC Harlem (Raftery and Huestis, 1973) affirm that after two heme groups become deoxygenated, the entire molecule adopts the deoxy T conformation.

A normal Bohr effect and p^{50} strongly suggest that in HbM Milwaukee-1, Hb M Saskatoon, and HbM Hyde Park, the molecule adopts the R state when the two normal chains are oxygenated. NMR studies of HbM Milwaukee-1 (Lindstrom et al., 1972; Hayashi et al., 1969) support the notion that the conformational changes take place when the normal heme groups are oxygenated. In contrast, HbM Iwate is in the crystallographic T configuration (Greer, 1971b) when its normal heme groups are in the ferric state, explaining its decreased oxygen affinity. The molecule does not shift to the R state when the normal heme groups are liganded and remains in the low affinity T state. A similar situation probably exists in HbM Boston (LaMar et al., 1980), as the habit of the deoxy crystal remains intact after oxygenation, suggesting that no conformational change has occurred that would require a different crystal structure.

HbM Saskatoon and HbM Boston have different properties despite the common substitution of the distal histidine, because the former variant does not change its conformation when oxygenated but the latter variant does (Susuki et al., 1966). Why properties of the β-globin chains differ from that of the α-globin chains when their distal histidine is substituted is unresolved (Hayashi, et al., 1968).

Iron Oxidation and Spectral Characteristics

In all M hemoglobins, the affected heme groups are stabilized in the ferric state and have an abnormal microenvironment. They exhibit an abnormal visible absorption spectrum that can be easily distinguished from methemoglobin (Fig. 44.7A). This characteristic separates these variants from some unstable hemoglobin mutants that have a tendency to form methemoglobin, such as Hb St. Louis (Thillet et al., 1976), Hb Bicetre (Wajcman et al., 1976), HbI Toulouse (Rose et al., 1969), and Hb Seattle (Kurachi et al., 1973).

Heme iron in the abnormal subunits of the M hemoglobin exhibit an abnormally low redox potential. They are oxidized more rapidly by molecular oxygen (Bunn and Forget, 1986) and are resistant to a variable degree to reduction by dithionite. Differences exist in the rate of reduction of the five M hemoglobins with various reductases, including the enzyme active in the normal erythrocyte, NADH-cytochrome b_5 reductase (Nagai et al., 1980). HbM Iwate, HbM Hyde Park, and HbM Boston are not reduced at all; but HbM Milwaukee is reduced slowly and HbM Saskatoon is reduced normally by this reductase. These last two variants might be less oxidized in vivo than expected. Full ferric conversion might occur only in vitro, owing to the high auto-oxidation rate of these abnormal hemoglobins. Nevertheless, older red cells may have fully oxidized abnormal chains consistent with the presence of clinically apparent cyanosis. Column chromatography that separates the HbM from HbA shows differences in the oxidation state of iron of the two hemoglobins, as does the separation of globin chains after paramercurobenzoate treatment and starch gel separation (see later).

Clinical Aspects and Diagnosis

Clinically, the skin and mucous membranes of HbM carriers have an appearance similar to, but not identical with, cyanosis, which is called *pseudocyanosis*. Skin and mucosal surfaces are brownish/slate colored, more like methemoglobinemia, but not as slate blue-purple as true cyanosis. This distinction is subtle and might not be apparent without simultaneously comparing the two conditions. Skin reflects hemoglobin molecules with an abnormal ferric heme and abnormal spectrum, whereas cyanosis is caused by the presence of more than 5 g/dL of deoxyhemoglobin. Pseudocyanosis is present from birth in α-globin chain abnormalities and from the middle of the first year of life in the β-chain mutants. A mixture of the abnormal pigment and true cyanosis, resulting from hemoglobin desaturation of the normal chains, is observed in the low oxygen affinity HbM Boston and HbM Hb Iwate.

Pseudocyanosis is not associated with dyspnea or clubbing, and carriers have a normal life expectancy. A mild hemolytic anemia and reticulocytosis have been observed in HbM Hyde Park and can be explained by the instability of the hemoglobin induced by partial heme loss.

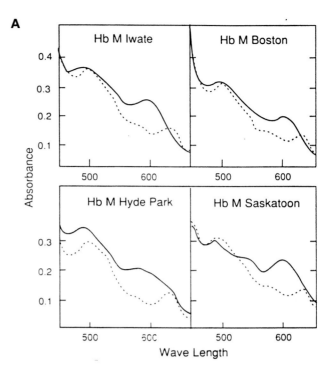

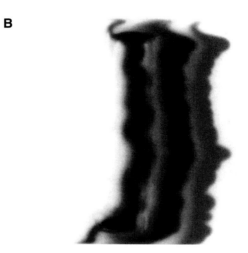

Figure 44.7. (A) Spectra between 450 and 650 μm of the oxidized form of four M hemoglobins are compared in each case with the normal methemoglobin spectra. In these spectra, the normal chains are met, and the abnormal chains have their own particular spectral properties. (After Shibata et al., 1967.) (B) Separation of chains from tetramers of Hb M Boston (α58(E7)His→Tyr), using the P-chloride mercuric benzoate (PCMB) method, and starch block electrophoresis at pH 8.6. Notice that the band to the right has a bright red color and hence the hemes are normal; that is, β chains. The band to the left is dark brown, that is, α^{Boston} chain. The band in the middle is a combination of both colors because it is the undissociated tetramer. For full color reproduction, see color plate 44.7B.

HbM should be considered in all patients with abnormal homogenous coloration of the skin and mucosa, particularly if pulmonary and cardiac function is normal. The diagnosis can be suspected by observing an abnormal brown coloration of the blood in a tube. To distinguish this coloration from methemoglobin, the addition of KCN to the hemolysate is useful. KCN will turn blood containing methemoglobin red but has little if any effect on HbM-containing hemolysates (see Table 44.2 for the differences among M hemoglobins). Lack of color conversion with KCN is diagnostic for HbM.

A spectrophotometric recording of the visible spectrum of the hemolysate is critical for the diagnosis. Figure 44.7A illustrates the differences in the spectrum observed between the M hemoglobins and their differences from the spectrum of methemoglobin A. M hemoglobins do not have an absorbance peak at 630 to 635 nm, which is typical of methemoglobin A. In the presence of HbM, accurate measurement of oxygen saturation and CO hemoglobin is difficult with most instruments. Absorption maxima at different wavelengths of all hemoglobin M variants have been reported (Shimasaki, 1985).

Electrophoresis has limited value for detection of M hemoglobins as the oxy forms are not separable from normal hemoglobin on cellulose acetate at alkaline pH. Agar electrophoresis and isoelectric focusing can distinguish some M hemoglobins. Ion exchange chromatography on Biorex 70 columns, equilibrated and developed with 0.196 M $NaPO_4$, pH 6.42, can separate the brown M hemoglobin from the normal hemoglobin. Hemoglobin chains can be prepared by blocking the cysteine thiols with p-chloromercuricbenzoate and separating the chains electrophoretically or chromatographically. This procedure can determined which chain is abnormally colored (Fig. 44.7B).

Perhaps the greatest hazard for carriers of a HbM is misdiagnosis and the risk of expensive and hazardous medical studies. We are aware of one instance in which a 1-week-old infant was misdiagnosed as having a pseudotruncus arteriosus and underwent cardiovascular surgery. Only when the father was identified many years later as a carrier of HbM Boston and the family study was completed was the child also recognized as a carrier of this abnormal hemoglobin.

Distinction of Red Cell-Induced Cyanosis From Low Oxygen Affinity Hemoglobins and Pseudocyanosis from M Hemoglobins From Other Conditions

Although cyanosis is most often due to cardiac or pulmonary disease, the differential diagnosis includes two classes of abnormal hemoglobins with a normal visible spectrum but a markedly right-shifted p^{50} resulting in significant arterial desaturation (Reismann et al., 1961; Moo-Penn et al., 1977). In cases of sulfhemoglobin, methemoglobin (Chapter 46), and hemoglobin M, the altered visible spectrum of the abnormal pigments is responsible for the brownish/slate skin color (Chapter 46). The spectral properties of sulfhemoglobin differ from those of methemoglobin so that it is not surprising that patients can be markedly cyanotic with 12 percent (1.6 g/dL) sulfhemoglobin (Park and Nagel, 1984; Park et al., 1986), whereas cyanosis requires 5 g/dL of deoxyhemoglobin.

Dyspnea is not associated with the mutant hemoglobins with right-shifted oxygen dissociation curves (Reismann et al., 1961; Moo-Penn et al., 1977) or with M hemoglobins (Bunn, 1986; Beutler, 1983) but can be present with even relatively mild degrees of methemoglobinemia (Finch, 1948). Little data are available for sulfhemoglobinemia (Finch, 1948) (Chapter 46).

Because the altered hemes in HbM, sulfhemoglobin, and methemoglobin do not transport oxygen, affected individuals with all three conditions may have normal hemoglobin concentrations but are functionally anemic simply because of insufficient operational heme groups. This effect is clinically significant only in extreme cases of methemoglobinemia and sulfhemoglobinemia or when the overall hemoglobin level is low (Pinkas et al., 1963; Rose, 1980). In HbM, the proportion of normal to abnormal heme is genetically determined and fixed so that decreased oxygen delivery is problematical only when superimposed on an underlying anemia.

Clinical effects of nonfunctional heme groups are not limited to an inability to transport oxygen. Small amounts of nonfunctional heme can have clinical significance if their presence in partially modified tetramers produces a physiologically dysfunctional shift in the oxygenation curve of neighboring unmodified subunits. This is the molecular basis of the left-shifted oxygenation curve, the impaired oxygen delivery to the tissues, and the resulting respiratory distress seen in relatively mild degrees of methemoglobinemia. This phenomenon, called the Darling-Roughton effect (Lorkin et al., 1975; Bonaventura et al., 1976), occurs as oxidized subunits in partially oxidized tetramers are held in an R-like (or liganded) conformation, increasing the oxygen affinity of the remaining subunits. Although mixed venous blood is unusually saturated, the abnormal spectrum of the methemoglobin dominates this effect causing cyanosis. An analogous left shift in oxygenation curve, although to a more pronounced degree, is present with carbon monoxide poisoning; here also, impaired oxygen delivery exacerbates dyspnea.

In the hemoglobins M, abnormal nonfunctional hemes in the affected tetramers result in a marked flattening of the oxygen affinity curve. The curve is also right shifted, particularly in the most physiologically relevant PO_2 range (Darling and Roughton, 1942; Bunn and Forget, 1986). This leads to normal or even enhanced ability to deliver oxygen to the periphery, which is consistent with the absence of respiratory insufficiency in these syndromes.

Treatment Recommendations

Treatment is neither possible nor necessary. A correct diagnosis is most important because it will forestall therapeutic and diagnostic misadventures.

UNSTABLE HEMOGLOBIN VARIANTS: THE CONGENITAL HEINZ BODY HEMOLYTIC ANEMIA SYNDROME

Some hemoglobin mutants have substitutions that alter their solubility. Intraerythrocytic precipitates derived from these unstable abnormal hemoglobins are detectable by supravital staining as dark globular aggregates called Heinz bodies. These inclusions reduce the life span of the erythrocyte and generate a hemolysis of varied severity called the Heinz body hemolytic anemia syndrome. Heinz body hemolytic anemia is not exclusive to unstable hemoglobins but can also be generated by congenital erythrocyte enzyme deficiencies. In mid-1998, according to Globin Gene Server, 225 of more than 800 mutations of hemoglobin, or more than 25 percent, were designated as "unstable." Some of these unstable variants, classified according to the level of reticulocytosis and other properties, are listed in Table 44.3.

Cathie (1952) first described a case with a congenital hemolytic anemia. At age 10 months, this child presented with jaundice, splenomegaly, and pigmenturia. Because this syndrome did not respond to splenectomy, the authors concluded that it was not hereditary spherocytosis. Schmid et al. (1959) described a similar case. Eighteen years later, an unstable hemoglobin, Hb Bristol, was identified. In the intervening years, other unstable hemoglobins were described and a simple diagnostic test, the heat stability test, was devised. **Hb Köln** (β98 (FG5) Val→Met) was first described in Europeans (Pribilla et al., 1965; Carrell et al., 1966) and has become the prototype and most commonly reported unstable hemoglobin (Miller et al., 1971; Egan and Fairbanks, 1973; Ohba et al., 1973; Allen et al., 1984). Variable anemia, reticulocytosis, splenomegaly, and 10 to 25 percent Hb Köln are the major clinical features.

Structural Abnormalities Causing Unstable Hemoglobins

Substitutions in the primary sequence of globin can lead to alterations in the tertiary or quaternary structure of hemoglobin and result in a globin polypeptide chain, or a hemoglobin tetramer that is unstable and precipitates intracellularly. Different structural alterations can cause hemoglobin instability.

Mutations That Weaken or Modify the Heme-Globin Interactions. Binding of heme to the globin is important, not only for the oxygen binding properties of the molecule but also for its stability and solubility. Figure 44.8 depicts several of the mutations involving residues with defined interactions with the heme groups that result in an unstable hemoglobin. These include (1) substitutions that introduce into the heme pocket a charged side chain where a nonpolar side chain existed previously (e.g., Hb Boras, Hb Bristol, Hb Olmsted, and Hb Himeji), (2) deletions involving residues that directly interact with the heme (e.g., Hb Gun Hill), and (3) mutations of the nontyrosine substitutions of the (F8) proximal histidine such as Hbs Saint Etienne (also known as Istanbul), J-Altgeld Gardens, Mozhaizk, Newcastle, Iwata, Redondo (also known as Hb Isehara), or of the (E7) distal histidine such as Hb Zürich and Hb Bicetre.

In **Hb Zürich** (β63 (E7) His→Arg), the substitution of an arginine for the distal histidine in the β-globin chains enlarges the space available for ligand binding around the iron, fundamentally changing some of its ligand properties (Robinson, 1974; Asakura et al., 1975; Roth et al., 1976; Tucker et al., 1978; Virshup et al., 1983). Although the extra space in the heme pocket has little consequences for the oxygen molecule that binds iron at an angle, a significant difference for CO becomes apparent. The biatomic CO binds perpendicular to the heme, and owing to stearic constraints present in the normal heme pocket, its binding constant to iron is reduced with respect to oxygen. This reduction of the binding constant is a normal adaptation to the endogenous generation of CO (one CO molecule evolves from each heme catabolized) and protects hemoglobin from being bound to CO in excess. The toxicity of CO stems from the significant reduction in the dissociation constant compared with oxygen, making COHb a particularly stable ligand species.

Carriers of Hb Zürich exhibit an increased affinity for CO owing to the increase in binding constant. This molecular pathology is, in effect, a protective mechanism that does not allow the abnormal β-globin chain heme group to be oxidized to the ferric form increasing its instability. Smokers with Hb Zürich have high levels of COHb, but nonsmoking carriers also have

Table 44.3. Unstable Hemoglobin Variants

	Mutation	Name	Molecular mechanism*	Reticulocytes and additional abnormalities
α-CHAIN SITE				
α6 (A3)	Asp → O	Boyle Heights		HA
α24 (B5)	Tyr → His	Luxembourg	4	Low
α26 (B7)	Ala → Glu	Shenyang		
α27 (B8)	Glu → Lys	Shuangfeng		Medium
α31 (B12)	Arg → Ser	Prato		
α43 (CE1)	Phe → Val	Torino	1	Medium, LA
	Phe → Leu	Hirosaki		
α47 (CE5)	Asp → Gly	Kokura, Umi, Beilinson	2	Medium, HA
	Asp → His	Hasharon, Sealy, L-Ferrara		Low
	Asp → Asn	Arya		Low
	Asp → Ala	Cordele		Low
α50 (CE8)	His → Arg	Aichi		
α53 (E2)	Ala → Asp	J-Rovigo		Low
α59 (E8)	Gly → Val	Tettori		Medium
α62 (E11)	Val → Met	Evans	1	High
α63 (E12)	Ala → Asp	Pontoise		
α80 (F1)	Leu → Arg	Ann Arbor	2	Medium
α86 (F7)	Leu → Arg	Moabit	1	Medium, LA
α87 (F8)	His → Arg	Iwata		Low, met
α91 (FG3)	Leu → Pro	Port Philip	2	Low
α103 (G10)	His → Arg	Contaldo		Medium
α109 (G16)	Leu → Arg	Suan-Dok	2	Thal
α110 (G17)	Ala → Asp	Petah Tikva		Low
α112 (G19)	His → Asp	Hopkins II	2	Low, HA
α130 (H13)	Ala → Pro	Sun Prairie	2	High, hypo
α131 (H14)	Ser → Pro	Questembert		
α136 (H19)	Leu → Pro	Bibba	2	Medium
	Leu → Arg	Toyama		
β-CHAIN MUTATIONS				
β6 or 7 (A3)	Glu → O	Leiden	3b	Low
β7 (A4)	Glu → Gly	G-San Jose		
β11 (A8)	Val → Asp	Windsor	1	Low, HA
β14 (A11)	Leu → Arg	Sogn		
	Leu → Pro	Saki	2	Low
β15 (A12)	Trp → Arg	Belfast	2	Low, LA
	Trp → Gly	Radwick	3	Low
β22 (B4)	Glu → Lys	E-Saskatoon	3	
β23 (B5)	Val → Gly	Miyashiro		Low, HA
β24 (B6)	Gly → Arg	Riverdale-Bronx	3	Medium, HA
	Gly → Val	Savannah	3	High, HA
	Gly → Asp	Moscva	3	
β26 (B8)	Glu → Lys	E		Thal
	Glu → Val	Mondor		
β27 (B9)	Ala → Asp	Volga, Drenthe	3a	H
β28 (B10)	Leu → Gin	St Louis	1	HA
	Leu → Arg	Chesterfield		Thal
	Leu → Pro	Genova, Hyogo	2	HA
β29 (B11)	Gly → Asp	Lufkin		Medium
β30 (B12)	Arg → Ser	Tacoma	2	Low
β31 (B13)	Leu → Pro	Yokohama	2	Medium
β32 (B14)	Leu → Pro	Perth, Lincoln	2	High
	Leu → Arg	Kobe	3a	High
	Leu → Val	Castilla Muscat		

(continued)

Table 44.3 *(continued)*

	Mutation	Name	Molecular mechanism*	Reticulocytes and additional abnormalities
β33 (B15) or β34 (B 16)	Val → O	Korea		
β35 (C1)	Tyr → Phe	Philly	4	Low, HA
β36 (C2)	Pro → Thr	Linkoping		
β38 (C4)	Thr → Pro	Hazebrouck	2	Medium
β39 (C5)	Gln → Glu	Vassa		Low
β41 (C7)/β42 (CD1)	Phe → O	Bruxelles		
β42 (CD1)	Phe → Ser	Hammersmith		High, LA
	Phe → Leu	Chiba		Medium, LA
	Phe → Val	Louisville, Bucaresti Sendagi, Warsaw		LA
β43 (CD2)	(Phe-Glu-Ser) → O or (Glu-Ser-Phe) → O	Niteroi		LA
β45 (CD4)	Phe → Ser	Cheverly		Low, LA
β48 (CD7)	Leu → Arg	Okaloosa	3a	Low, LA
β49 (CD8)	Phe → Val	Las Palmas		Low
β54 (D5)	Sen → Pro	Jacksonville	3a, 4	High, HA
β55 (D6)	Met → Lys	Matera		
β56 (D7)	Gly-Asn-Pro-Lys) → O	Tochigi		
β57 (E1)	Asn → Lys	G-Ferrara	2	
β60 (E4)	Val → Ala	Collingwood		
	Val → Glu	Cagliari		High, thal
β62 (E6)	Ala → Pro	Duarte	2	Medium, HA
β63 (E7)	His → Pro	Bicetre	2	Medium, met
	His → Arg	Zurich		
β64 (E8)	Gly → Asp	J-Calabria, J Bari		Low, HA
β66 (E10)	Lys → Glu	I.Tolouse	1	Low, met
β67 (E11)	Val → Asp	Bristol	1	High, LA
	Val → Ala	Sydney	1	Medium
β68 (E12)	Leu → Pro	Mizuho	2	
β70 (E14)	Ala → Asp	Seattle	1	Low
β71 (E15)	Phe → Ser	Christchurch	3c	Medium
β74 (E18)	Gly → Val	Bushwick		Low
	Gly → Arg	Aalborg	3a	Low
	Gly → Asp	Shepherds Bush	3	Medium, HA
β74–β75	(Gly-Leu) → O	St Antoine	3b	Medium
β75 (E19)	Leu → Pro	Atlanta	2	
	Leu → Arg	Pasadena		HA
β81 (EF5)	Leu → Arg	Baylor	3a	Low, HA
β83 (EF7)	Gly → Cys	Ta-Li		Polym
β85 (F1)	Phe → Ser	Buenos Aires, Bryn Mawr	1	Medium, HA
β87 (F3)	Thr → O	Tours	2	Medium
β88 (F4)	Leu → Arg	Boros	1	
	Leu → Pro	Santa Ana	2	High
β91 (F7)	Leu → Pro	Sabrine	2	High
	Leu → Arg	Carribean	1	Low, LA
β91–β95 (F7-FG1)	(Leu-His-Cys-Asp-Lys) → O	Gun Hill	3b	Medium
β92 (F8)	His → Gln	St Etienne, Istanbul	1	Low, HA
	His → Asp	J-Altgeld Gardens		Low
	His → Pro	Newcastle	2	Medium, HA
	His → Arg	Mozhaisk		Medium
	His → Asn → Asp	Redondo, Isehara	1	

(continued)

Table 44.3 (continued)

	Mutation	Name	Molecular mechanism*	Reticulocytes and additional abnormalities
β97 (FG4)	His → Pro	Nagoya		
β98 (FG5)	Val → Met	Koln, San Francisco, Ube 1	1, 4	Medium, HA
	Val → Gly	Nottingham	1, 3c	High, HA
	Val → Ala	Djelfa	1, 3c	
β101 (G3)	Glu → Gln	Rush		Low
β106 (G8)	Leu → Pro	Southampton, Casper	2	High, HA
	Leu → Gln	Tubingen	1, 3a	High, HA
	Leu → Arg	Terre Haute		Thal
β107 (G9)	Gly → Arg	Burke		Medium, LA
β111 (G13)	Val → Phe	Peterborough	3, 4	Low, LA
	Val → Ala	Stanmore		LA
β112 (G14)	Cys → Arg	Indianapolis	3a, 4	High
β113 (G15)	Val → Glu	New York, Kaohsiung		LA
β115 (G17)	Ala → Pro	Madrid	2	High
β117 (G19)	His → Pro	Saitama	2	High
β119 (GH2)	Gly → Asp	Fannin-Lubbock		
	Gly → Val	Bougardirey-Mali		
β124 (H2)	Pro → Arg	Khartoum	4	
β126 (H4)	Val → Glu	Hofu		
	Val → Gly	Dhonburi, Neapolis	2	M, thal
β127 (H5)	Gln → Lys	Brest	4	High
β128 (H6)	Ala → Asp	J-Guantanamo	4	Low
β129 (H7)	Ala → Pro	Crete		
	Ala → Val	LaDesirade		LA
β130 (H8)	Tyr → Asp	Wien	3a	High
β131 (H9)	Gln → Lys	Shelby	2	
	Gln → Pro	Shanghai		
	Gln → Arg	Samebourg		
β134 (H12)	Val → Glu	North Shore	3	Low, Thal
β135 (H13)	Ala → Pro	Altdort	2	Medium
	Ala → Glu	Beckman		
β136 (H14)	Gly → Asp	Hope		LA
β138 (H16)	Ala → Pro	Brockton	2	Medium
β139 (H17)	Asn → Asp	Geelong		
β140 (H18)	Ala → Asp	Himeji		LA
β141 (H19)	Leu → Arg	Olmsted	3	Low
	Leu → O	Coventry	3b	Medium
β142 (H20)	Ala → Pro	Toyoake	2	Low

δ CHAIN

	Mutation	Name		
δ98 (FG5)	Val → Met	A₂ Wrens		
δ121 (GH4)	Glu → Val	A₂ Manzanares		

Gγ CHAIN

	Mutation	Name		
γ130 (H8)	Trp → Gly	F-Poole		

AγT CHAIN

	Mutation	Name		
AγT25 (B7)	Gly → Arg	F-Xin Jiang		

(continued)

Table 44.3 *(continued)*

Mutation	Name	Molecular mechanism*	Reticulocytes and additional abnormalities
EXTENSION (FRAMESHIFT)			
144 (β) Lys-Ser-Ile-Thr-150 Lys-Leu-Ala-Phe-Leu-Leu-Ser-Asn-155 Phe-Tyr-COOH	Cranston	3	Medium

Low, <5% reticulocytes; medium, 5%–15% reticulocytes; high, 15% reticulocytes
HA, high affinity:
LA, low affinity; polym, tendency to polymerize; thal, thalassemia: met, tendency to methemoglobin formation; hypo, hypochromia.
* 1, heme environment; 2, secondary structure; 3, tertiary structure; 3a, change residue in interior; 3b. deletion; 3c, steric hindrance; 4, $\alpha_1 \beta_1$ contact.

Figure 44.8. Diagram of the heme pocket, showing the replacement site of several of the unstable hemoglobins. Valine E4 is at the corner of the pocket, and its side chain does not make contact with the heme but does affect the placement of adjacent amino acid side chains. (After Williamson et al., 1990.)

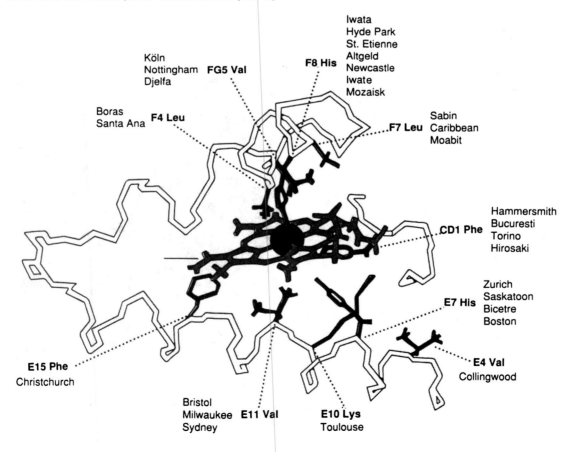

abnormal COHb levels. Owing to the partially protective effect of COHb Zürich, Heinz bodies are found less often among smokers than nonsmokers with this abnormal hemoglobin.

Hb Zürich carriers have a special susceptibility to hemolytic crisis induced by sulfanilamide. The increased aperture of the heme pocket also explains this phenomenon. Sulfanilamide becomes capable of binding to the heme and producing methemoglobin directly, a reaction also inhibited by CO.

Substitutions involving the proximal (F8) β histidine are of interest. Tyrosine substitutions lead to M hemoglobins, but other residues have other consequences. **Hb Redondo** (β92 His→Asn→Asp) (Wajcman et al., 1994) has a phenotype that includes compensated hemolytic anemia and macrocytosis. Two abnormal hemoglobin bands were present with alkaline electrophoresis, a major band migrating in the position of HbA$_2$ forming 10 percent of the total hemoglobin and a minor component measuring about 6 percent that migrated close to HbS. Addition of heme to the hemolysate showed that both bands lacked β-heme groups and were semi-hemoglobins. A phenotypic consequence of this phenomenon was an artifactual low MCH and total hemoglobin concentration when determined spectrophotometrically. The slower electrophoretic band increased during storage, suggested posttranslation modification that was due to deamidation of the asparaginyl residue (Chapter 45).

Contiguous phenylalanine residues at β41 and β42 are conserved in all mammalian globins. Hb Bruxelles, where β42 is deleted, has high oxygen affinity (see previously). **Hb Bucaresti** (β42 (CDI) Phe→Leu) (Bratu et al., 1971) was discovered in a family with two affected members and was characterized by anemia, reticulocytosis, Heinz bodies, splenomegaly, and a heat unstable hemolysate. **Hb Hammersmith** (β42 (CD1) Phe→Ser) (Wajcman et al., 1973) was discovered in a similar patient. **Hb Warsaw/Sendagi** (β42 (CD1) Phe→Val) (Honig et al., 1990; Ogata et al., 1986) was found in an individual with moderate hemolytic anemia and thermoinstability of the hemolysate. This variant was purified by reverse-phase HPLC and had low oxygen affinity and normal response to 2,3 BPG. Five to 6 percent of the hemolysate consisted of partially heme-depleted tetramers. A heme-intact fraction of Hb Warsaw had a high oxygen affinity, decreased cooperativity, and 2,3 BPG interaction and a very low Bohr effect. A heme-depleted fraction was consisted mainly of dimers. **Hb Mequon** (β41 (C7) Phe→Tyr) (Burket et al., 1976) presented with episodic hemolytic anemia. Heinz bodies and instability of the hemolysate. **Hb Denver** (β41 (C7) Phe→Ser) (Stabler et al., 1994) was present in an

individual with chronic cyanosis, moderate reticulocytosis, and mild anemia. Although this hemoglobin did not separate from HbA by standard electrophoretic means, it was separated by isoelectric focusing and HPLC. A hemolysate was heat unstable and the isolated variant had low oxygen affinity.

These mutants illustrate the importance of conserved amino acid residues for the function of the molecule. Short-term globin biosynthesis studies of Hb Warsaw (Honig et al., 1990) revealed that a major portion of radiolabeled L-leucine was recovered from the dimeric heme-depleted fraction, strongly suggesting that subunit association preceded the incorporation of heme into the β subunit. Structural studies of deoxyhemoglobin containing half normal and half variant β-globin chains revealed that the mutation leaves a cavity next to the heme large enough to accommodate a water molecule, which could account for the instability of Hb Warsaw and other mutants of the same site. Heme and the pyrrol nearest to the CD1 Val in Hb Warsaw tilts into the cavity. This tilt results in an increase of the tilt of the proximal histidine relative to the heme plane, which in turn could stretch the Fe-Nε toward this histidine, accounting for the lower oxygen affinity.

A fascinating posttranslation modification, leucine hydroxylation, has been postulated from the study of the unstable variants **Hb Coventry** (originally described as β141 (H19) Leu→0) and **Hb Atlanta** (β75 (E19) Leu→Pro) and is discussed in detail in Chapter 45. Hb Atlanta (Brennan et al., 1983) is an internal mutation that produces a mild hemolytic anemia with Heinz bodies and reticulocytosis. Not separable by standard electrophoresis but well resolved by isoelectric focusing, it is expressed at a level of 33 percent. This hemoglobin is unstable, but further functional studies are not available. The mutation is a CTG→CCG change at codon 75. The molecular mechanism of the instability presumably is disruption of the H α-helix. Splenectomy improved the anemia.

Mutations That Interfere with the Secondary Structure of the Subunits. Hemoglobin is more than 75 percent α helix, and any disruption of this secondary structure reduces subunit solubility. Unstable hemoglobin mutants can result from the introduction of proline in the helical structure or the substitution of glycine by a mutation in invariant positions in the interhelical bends. Twenty-seven of 272 unstable hemoglobins with single or double substitutions involve the introduction of a proline residue.

Hb Brockton (β138(H16) Ala→Pro) (Russu and Ho, 1986) is associated with mild anemia. It cannot be separated from HbA with standard electrophoretic procedures. Crystallographic examination showed that the tertiary structure was disrupted in the vicinity of the mutated residue. Molecular instability was probably the result of the breakage of a buried H bond, normally tying β138 Ala with β134 Val, a task that the proline side chain cannot accomplish.

In **Hb Singapore** (α141 (HC3) Arg→Pro), the introduction of a prolyl residue is not accompanied by instability. Here, the substituted residue is the last amino acid of the α chains, Arg 141, so there is no disruption of α-helix. Generally, prolyl residues can be accommodated at the terminal residues of an α helix.

Mutations That Interfere with the Tertiary Structure of The Subunit. Because hemoglobin is a tight globular protein, α-helical regions must be folded into a solid sphere, a design introducing enormous architectural constraints. Amino acid substitutions can occur with no change in solubility as long as (1) no charged residues (hydrophilic) are allowed to point inward, (2) no bulky side chains are allowed to substitute for less bulky residues inside the molecule, and (3) critical nonpolar residues are not lost from the surface of the subunit. A special case is what has been termed the *loss of nonpolar plug*. This term is a reference to hydrophobic residues that are located on the surface and prevent water from invading the interior of the molecule, which is a common cause of hemoglobin instability. About half of these cases result from the substitution of arginine for leucine.

HbJ Biska results from an eight-residue deletion between either α50–57 and α52-59, the longest described amino acid deletion of the hemoglobin molecule (Prchal and Sokol, 1996; Wacjman et al., 1998). Although the deletion includes the distal histidine and neighboring residues, the hemoglobin is only mildly unstable in vitro, hemolysis is absent, and the concentration of this variant is approximately that expected for a variant of the α_1-globin gene. X-ray crystallography, not yet reported, should provide information regarding alternative secondary/tertiary/quaternary structures that retain the basic properties of the molecule.

Mutations That Affect Subunit Interactions: Interference with the Quaternary Structure. This class of mutations involves the introduction of charged residues in the interior, or the loss of intersubunit contact hydrogen bonds or salt bridges in the α1β1 contact area. This area of contact is critical for stability, as it does not dissociate as does the α1β2 contact. Globin subunit dimerization is a first-order reaction (concentration independent), but tetramerization is a second-order reaction (concentration dependent). Dimer concentration in the concentrated hemoglobin milieu of the red cell is quite small. Nevertheless, dissociation is possible and constantly occurring.

Breakdown of α1β1 dimers into monomers, which normally occurs to a vanishingly small extent, is a threat to molecular integrity as it generates methemoglobin and consequent instability. Dissociation of chains along the α1β1 contact generates α- and β-globin chains that uncoil, loosening their heme-globin interaction and favoring methemoglobin formation. Several unstable hemoglobin mutations involve residues located in the α1β1 area of contact: **Hb Philly** (Reider et al., 1969), **Hb Peterborough** (King et al., 1972), **Hb Stanmore** (Como et al., 1991), **Hb Linkoping** (Wada et al., 1987), **Hb J Guantanamo** (Martinez et al., 1977), and **Hb Khartoum** (Clegg et al., 1969).

Hyperunstable Hemoglobins

Hyperunstable hemoglobins are either barely detectable or undetectable in the hemolysate. These hemoglobins, discussed in Chapters 14 and 17, are presumably synthesized normally but are rapidly destroyed, creating the phenotype of dominant inherited thalassemia.

Clinical Characteristics of the Congenital Heinz Body Hemolytic Anemias

Unstable hemoglobins are uncommon mutational events, generally limited to a single pedigree (Ohba, 1990). There are two exceptions. Hb Köln has been detected in several different pedigrees and geographic locations. α-Globin chain mutants, such as **Hb Hasharon** (α(CE5) Asp→His), are found predominantly among Ashkenazi Jews and cause hemolysis in newborns (Ohba et al., 1987). In some adult carriers, Hb Hasharon produces mild anemia, but no hemolysis is observed in other carriers with the same pedigree (Levine et al, 1995). Epistatic effects of other nonlinked genes may be responsible for these differences.

Unstable γ-chain variants, such as **Hb Poole** ($^G\gamma$130 Trp→Gly)(24), have been associated with hemolysis in infants, but they disappear as β-globin chain synthesis increases.

Hemolytic anemia, the chief feature of unstable hemoglobins, varies considerably in its intensity depending on the nature of the mutation. Hemolytic crises, an abrupt increase in hemolysis beyond the steady state, sometimes occur and are often associated with bacterial or viral infections, or with exposure to chemical oxidants (Nagel and Ranney, 1973). The mechanism of the infection-mediated hemolysis is not clear, but pyrexia and transient acidosis may contribute, as both are capable of increasing hemoglobin denaturation. Drugs such as sulfonamides have been directly implicated in a hemolytic crisis associated with Hb Zürich, Hb Hasharon (Tatsis et al., 1972), Hb Shepards Bush, and Hb Peterbourough. These crises are generally self-limited and stopping all possible offending drugs is wise. As in all patients with chronic hemolysis, B19 parvovirus can induce an aplastic crisis with severe anemia.

Patients with unstable hemoglobins may have characteristically dark urines or pigmenturia. This color change is not due to bilirubinuria but rather to the presence of dipyrrole methenes of the mesobilifucsin group (Reider et al., 1972). The origin of these fluorescent compounds is not clear. Their structure, two pyrrole rings still bound to each other by a methenyl bridge, suggests the malfunctioning of methenyl oxygenase, the enzyme involved in the breaking of -CH= bridges. Fluorescent dypyrroles are also present in Heinz bodies (Eisinger et al., 1985).

The absence of pigmenturia does not exclude the diagnosis of unstable hemoglobin, because not all unstable mutants exhibit pigmenturia, and severity of the hemolysis is unrelated to pigmenturia. For example, carriers of Hb Köln and Hb Zürich can have pigmenturia (Kolski and Miller, 1976); hemolysis may be severe with Hb Köln and is usually very mild in Hb Zürich.

Pathophysiology of the Heinz Body Hemolytic Syndrome Produce by Unstable Hemoglobins

Thermostability of Hemoglobins. When heat-unstable hemoglobins were related to the presence of a Heinz body hemolytic anemia by Grimes and Meisler (1962), a conceptual framework for understanding this syndrome was generated. Homeothermic mammals and birds have relatively thermostable hemoglobins. If a hemolysate is incubated for 1 or 2 hours at 50°C, little protein precipitate occurs. This property is observed, to a lesser degree, even in reptilian hemoglobins. In amphibians and fish, the thermostability of hemoglobin decreases substantially.

As a first approximation, these differences may be related to the mean environmental temperature. Poikilotherm hemoglobin exposed to low mean temperatures must have evolved to homeotherm hemoglobin exposed to higher mean temperatures by accumulating mutations that provide thermostable proteins (Borgese et al., 1982; Tondo et al., 1980).

Perutz and Raidt (1975) suggested that the thermostability of some proteins, including hemoglobin, can be attributed to electrostatic interactions and salt bridge formation, whereas Bigelow (1967) contended that hydrophobic interactions are most critical. Others believe that both electrostatic and hydrophobic interactions are contributory (Kauzmann, 1959). Most supporting evidence comes from the structural analysis of homologous proteins obtained from thermophilic and mesophilic bacteria (Argos et al., 1979), or by comparing amino acid sequence in hemoglobins of organisms of different temperature preference (Perutz and Raidt, 1975). Fish hemoglobins can be classified into four categories of stability: stable at all pHs (skate hemoglobins), stable at acid but unstable at alkaline pH (mustelus cains or dogfish hemoglobins), unstable at acid but stable at alkaline pH (toadfish hemoglobins), and unstable at all pHs (most fish hemoglobins) (Borgese et al., 1982). The effect of salt, which interferes with electrostatic interactions, and alkylureas, chemicals that interfere with hydrophobic interactions, is revealing. Electrostatic interactions are not consistently related to thermostability, but all hemoglobins show increased thermoinstability in the presence of alkylureas. In this model system, hydrophobic interactions are at the heart of the thermostability properties of hemoglobins.

Other contributions to the thermostability come from the strength of the heme-globin bonds. Bunn and Jandl (1968) showed that heme exchange between hemoglobin and albumin and between different hemoglobin molecules decreases considerably when methemoglobin heme is ligated with cyanide. Presumably, cyanmethemoglobin has a stronger heme-globin attachment than methemoglobin and is more similar in this regard to liganded hemoglobin.

Heme Dissociation from Hemoglobin. Heme loss is reduced in hemoglobin encapsulated in a red cell compared with hemoglobin solutions stored at 37°C for 120 days, the approximate life span of the red cell. Heme loss is inhibited, but not prevented, by maintaining heme in the reduced ferrous state. This involves the action of methemoglobin reductases and antioxygen radical enzymes. In the very high intercellular concentration of hemoglobin, these enzymes reduce the extent of dimerization and prevent the dispersion and precipitation of free heme (Brennan et al., 1993). When hemoglobin is lost from cell in the circulation, it becomes almost completely dimerized because of its great dilution, and it is bound specifically by haptoglobin until the availability of this serum protein is exhausted, at which time hemoglobin dimers are filtered through the glomerulus into the urine, producing hematuria.

Dimers autoxidize and lose heme more readily than ferrous dimers or tetramers. In pioneering work on the exchange of hemes between HbA and HbF and between HbA and albumin, β-globin chains lost heme fivefold to tenfold more readily than γ and α chains (Bunn and Jandl, 1968). Using a genetically engineered heme-free apomyoglobin to measure time course of heme dissociation, where the distal histidine was replaced by tyrosine producing a green holoprotein signature when heme was bound, β heme dissociation in native hemoglobin increased tenfold when going from high to low concentration, whereas dissociation was three times less in α subunits and concentration independent. In monomeric α and β chains, dissociation increased considerably compared with β subunit in tetramers and also exhibited a chain-dependent difference.

Aggregation of monomers into tetramers decreased heme loss twentyfold, but dimerization did not change, suggesting that hemoglobin has evolved to lose heme rapidly after cell lysis, swiftly eliminating this toxic compound (Fig. 44.9).

Auto-oxidation of Hemoglobin. Generation of methemoglobin increases the thermoinstability of hemoglobin, indicating that the pathways and events accompanying the conversion of Fe^{+2} to Fe^{+3} in hemoglobin are important for understanding unstable hemoglobins (Miura et al., 1987).

When hemoglobin solutions are left at room temperature, they turn a brownish hue owing to methemoglo-

bin formation, a reaction that happens even faster a 37°C. Chemically, this auto-oxidation is probably a result of superoxide anion (O_2^-) generation. This is an infrequent event because oxyhemoglobin usually gives up dimolecular oxygen (O_2) and converts itself partially into deoxyhemoglobin. Superoxide anion generation results from the transfer of a d electron from the heme iron to the unoccupied pi2* orbital that converts iron into the low spin ferric state. This reaction is catalyzed

Figure 44.9. Denaturation and clearance of hemoglobin in vivo (as per Hargrove et al., 1998; scheme modified from a figure in Bunn and Forget, 1986). Because the dissociation of hemoglobin to dimers is a first-order reaction, few dimers are found in red cell because of the very high concentration of hemoglobin (34 g/dL). Potent reduction systems keep the heme-iron hemoglobin in the ferrous state. When hemoglobin leaves the red cell during intravascular hemolysis, there is a drastic reduction in hemoglobin concentration and hence the dramatic increase in the dimer compartment. Dimers are more likely to auto-oxidize and to lose heme. Holohemoglobin and apohemoglobin dimers are removed by haptoglobin (Nagel and Gibson, 1971), and free heme is rapidly take up by serum albumin (metalbumin), with low affinity (Morgan et al., 1976), and apohemopexin, with affinity, as shown by Muller-Eberhard (1988).

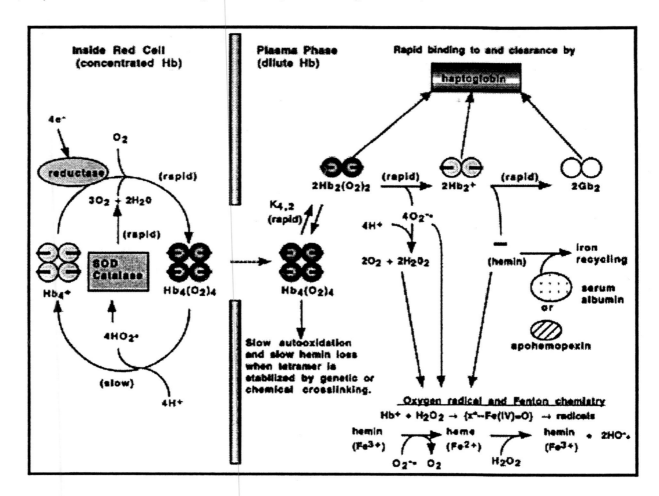

Reversible Hemichromes

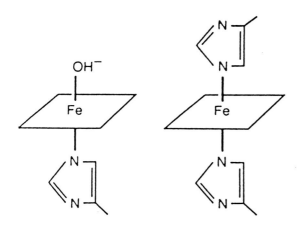

Irreversible Hemichromes

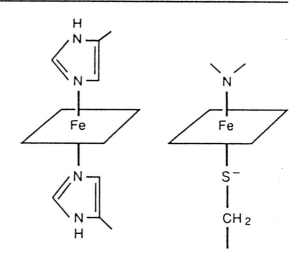

Figure 44.10. Diagrammatic structure of different hemichromes from Peisach et al. (1975). The figures depict the proximal histidine below the plane of the heme and the distal histidine above the plane.

by H⁺, Cl⁻, superoxide anion itself, and probably by the T state of hemoglobin, all of which favor autoxidation (Fig. 44.9). Totally deoxygenated hemoglobin, although in the T state, has no oxygen to contribute to the reaction and is more stable and less likely to undergo auto-oxidation (Brooks, 1935).

EDTA decreases auto-oxidation of hemolysates, indicating that divalent cations could play a catalytic role in this process. Copper, a known hemoprotein binder (Gurd et al., 1967), binds specifically to β93 cysteine oxidizing β heme (Bemski et al., 1969; Nagel et al., 1970; Rifkind, 1974; Winterbourne and Carrell; 1977). In contrast, the α chains are a preferred site for auto-oxidation (Mansouri and Winterhalter, 1973). Isoelectric focusing is an excellent tool to separate and quantify the different products of autoxidation. Auto-oxidation of hemoglobin is favored by increased temperature, 2,3 BPG, trace metals, and low pH.

Denaturation of Hemoglobin and Hemichrome Formation. Heinz bodies are the product of hemoglobin denaturation. First suggested to be heme-depleted globin chains (Jacob and Winterhalter, 1970a, b), these inclusions were subsequently identified as hemichromes. Hemichromes are derivatives of the low spin forms of ferric hemoglobin that have the sixth coordination position occupied by a ligand provided by the globin. This ligand can be a hydroxyl group (–OH) or protonated histidyl in reversible hemichromes, or an unprotonated histidyl in irreversible hemichromes (Rachmilewitz et al., 1971; Rachmilewitz and Harari, 1972; Rachmilewitz and White, 1973; Rachmilewitz, 1974; Peisach et al., 1975). Another type of irreversible hemichrome can be generated by having the fifth coordination posi-

tion occupied by a cysteine and the sixth by an aliphatic amine (Fig. 44.10). All of these compounds can be resolved by electron spin resonance spectroscopy, but not absorption spectroscopy, as their visible spectra are quite similar. Hemichromes are generated when the heme is dissociated from the heme pocket and rebinds elsewhere in the globin after the α or the β chains have suffered some form of uncoiling or denaturation. Irreversible hemichromes seem to be an indispensable stage in the formation of Heinz bodies. Winterbourne and Carrell (1974) have found both α- and β-globin chains in Heinz bodies and have worked out a scheme for the process involved in the generation of Heinz bodies (Winterbourne et al., 1976) (Fig. 44.11). As a rule, weakening of the heme-globin bond will accelerate hemoglobin denaturation.

Anemia in the Unstable Hemoglobin Heinz Bodies Hemolytic Syndrome. Heinz body-containing erythrocytes have a reduced life span. Evidence indicates that Heinz bodies at least partially adhere to the cytosolic face of the erythrocyte membrane by hydrophobic interactions and not through covalent bonds, as first suggested (Rifkind, 1965; Schnitzer et al., 1971; Winterbourne and Carrell, 1972; Chan and Desforges, 1974).

Band 3 (AE-1, or the anion exchanger) is one of the most abundant erythrocyte transmembrane proteins. Piercing the membrane, it has a highly glycosylated portion on the red cell surface, a hydrophobic portion

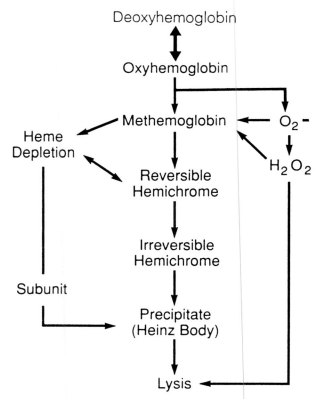

Figure 44.11. Description of the intraerythrocytic denaturation of unstable hemoglobins as proposed by Winterbourne and Carrell (1974).

spanning the lipid bilayer, and an N-terminal cytosolic domain that has two conformationally independent portions separated by a protease sensitive hinge region. This domain, highly negatively charged, has a high content of proline and other amino acid residues not accommodated in an α helix. Hemoglobin and hemichromes bind the most N-terminal portion of the cytosolic domain of Band 3 (Low, 1989; Low et al., 1984; Walder et al., 1984).

Band 3 sequences can thread into the positively charged central cavity of hemoglobin, which is why it preferentially and reversibly binds deoxyhemoglobin. Hemoglobins with the greatest positive charge have the highest affinity for Band 3. HbA_2 (Chapter 10) and HbC attach tenaciously to the membrane, and HbS has an affinity intermediate between HbA and HbC (Reiss et al., 1982)(Chapter 27).

Unstable hemoglobins generate considerable hemichrome that may bind Band 3. Erythrocytes containing unstable hemoglobins have decreased deformability (Miller et al., 1971), a characteristic that condemns them to be preferentially trapped in the spleen. It is possible that the inclusions of Heinz body-containing red cells are initially pitted in the spleen.

Pitting refers to the mechanism by which a portion of the membrane with the Heinz body inclusion is excised from the cell during their passage through the sinusoidal slits of the spleen. In the process, membrane loss progressively converts discoid erythrocytes into spherocytes. Rigid spherocytes are eventually removed from the circulation.

Other sources of potential membrane damage are a result of peroxidation and protein cross-linking of membrane proteins. These are probably secondary to the presence of free heme, iron that acts as a Fenton reagent, decompartalization of iron, and the generation of free radicals secondary to methemoglobin formation and hemoglobin denaturation (Chou and Fitch, 1981; Flynn et al., 1983). Other evidence of membrane alteration is the presence of abnormal K^+ efflux in some cells (Jacob et al., 1968; Miller et al., 1971).

A further determinant of the anemia is the oxygen equilibrium curve. Although 2,3 BPG levels are generally normal (DeFuria and Miller, 1972), some of the unstable variants have a high or low oxygen affinity. High ligand affinity, unstable hemoglobins would tend to have milder anemia and the low ligand affinity unstable hemoglobins would be characterized by more severe anemia (Monod et al., 1967).

The phenotype of unstable hemoglobin hemolytic anemia is affected by their synthesis and catabolism. Hyperunstable variants (Chapters 14 and 17) are synthesized normally but catabolized immediately and are associated with a thalassemic phenotype. Less dramatic phenotypes are represented by unstable hemoglobins with lower than normal synthesis: **Hb Boras, Hb Abraham Lincoln**, and **Hb Riverdale-Bronx**.

In **Hb Gun Hill** (β91 (F7)-β95 (FG1) Leu-His-Cys-Asp-Lys deleted)(Bradley et al., 1967; Rieder, 1971), unstable α-chain monomers can exchange with stable α-globin chains from the surplus α-globin chain pool. Unstable hemoglobins, where recently synthesized isolated chains are incapable of dimer assembly, would paradoxically tend to have more abnormal hemoglobin present, more Heinz bodies, and more severe hemolysis.

Some unstable hemoglobins are linked to α or β thalassemia genes. The α-chain mutants Hb Suan-Dok and Hb Petah Tikva coexist in *cis* with α-thalassemia, and the β-chain mutant Hb Leiden coexists in *cis* with a β thalassemia mutation.

Diagnosis

Any single test for unstable hemoglobins may be negative so that multiple tests are often needed. A differential diagnosis of an adult with unstable hemoglobinopathy includes other causes of the congenital

---

Table 44.4. Diagnosis of Unstable Hemoglobins

• Heinz bodies spontaneously present in blood (less frequent) or induced by incubation of a sterile blood sample for 24 hours followed by staining with a supravital dye
• Hemoglobin electrophoresis: Only a positive result is useful and negative results do not exclude an unstable variant. Sometimes a smeared band is present
• Positive heat stability test

Heinz body hemolytic syndrome, such as erythrocyte enzymopathies, and acquired forms of Heinz body hemolytic anemias, such as acquired methemoglobinemia caused by chemicals and drugs. In rare cases, several of these entities may interact (Bradley and Ranney, 1973). In young adults and children, Wilson's disease and erythropoietic porphyria must be considered. Often, Heinz bodies cannot be found suggesting the possibility of autoimmune hemolytic anemia. Diagnosis of these disorders is summarized in Table 44.4.

Blood Smear and Heinz Body Preparation. Abnormalities of the blood smear are not specific for unstable hemoglobins. Anisocytosis, sometimes hypochromia, often prominent basophilic stippling, Howell-Jolly bodies, nucleated red blood cells, and microspherocytes may be found.

Heinz body detection requires the incubation of erythrocytes with a supravital stain such as new methylene blue or crystal violet. Heinz bodies appear as single or multiple pale purple inclusions of 2 μm in diameter or less and frequently appear membrane attached. Heinz bodies may be found in fresh blood, but in most cases, incubation for 24 hours in the absence of glucose is required for their formation. A normal control sample should always be run simultaneously. After splenectomy, Heinz bodies become easier to detect.

Electrophoresis. Between 25 and 30 percent of unstable hemoglobins are not detectable by electrophoresis or other methods of hemoglobin separation. Hemoglobin electrophoresis can sometimes show an abnormal hemoglobin component, but many times the unstable hemoglobin appears as a diffuse band. This alteration is probably secondary to the partial denaturation of hemoglobin molecules during electrophoresis or during preelectrophoresis processing of the hemolysate. Occasionally, only precipitated material at the origin is observed.

Heat Stability Test. The heat denaturation test, where a hemolysate is incubated for 1 or 2 hours at 50°C, is a simple and reliable procedure described more than 25 years ago (Grimes and Meisler, 1962; Grimes et al., 1964). Under these conditions, normal hemolysates are stable, and a visible precipitate signals the presence of an unstable hemoglobin. Some abnormal hemoglobins, such as Hb Hasharon, precipitate at temperatures higher than 50°C, but control samples are indispensable as normal hemoglobin begins to precipitate at about 55°C.

Other similar laboratory procedures for determining hemoglobin instability are available. An isopropanol test (Carrell and Kay, 1972) is used by many laboratories, but gives false-positive results when the sample contains more than 5 percent HbF. A zinc acetate precipitation is free of interference from HbF but is rarely used (Ohba et al., 1981). Mechanical agitation can also precipitate some unstable hemoglobins (Asakura et al., 1975; Roth et al., 1976).

Treatment Recommendations

Congenital Heinz body hemolytic anemias resulting from unstable hemoglobins are generally mild disorders and do not require therapy, except for supportive and preventive measures. Administration of folic acid to ensure that an overworked marrow does not become deficient in this nutrient, prevention and prompt treatment of infections, treatment of fever with aspirin, and avoidance of oxidant drugs, including acetaminophen, are generally useful steps in management.

In cases with more severe hemolysis the question of splenectomy arises. The spleen undoubtedly plays an important pathophysiologic role in the destruction of Heinz body-containing red cells. This must be balanced with the role of the spleen as a defense against pneumococcal infections early in life and the need for antipneumococcal vaccines and prophylactic penicillin in cases in which splenectomy was performed in childhood. According to Koler et al. (1973), on balance, splenectomy is beneficial for the most severe cases of unstable hemoglobinopathies, and partial correction of the anemia has been achieved in some instances.

However, splenectomy does not always reduce hemolysis or anemia.

Hydroxyurea has been used to stimulate HbF production in two cases of unstable hemoglobin disease (Chapter 38).

CONCLUSION

Hemoglobin variants with high or low oxygen affinity, which form methemoglobin or are unstable, are rare abnormalities infrequently seen by the general physician and uncommonly encountered in the practice of hematology. Because they are unusual causes of erythrocytosis, cyanosis, and hemolytic anemia, their presence is often unsuspected. When they are present, their identification can prevent hazardous diagnostic tests, spare the institution of potentially dangerous treatments, and permit reassurance of the patient and counseling to the family.

References

Adamson, JW. (1975). Familial polycythemia. *Semin. Hematol.* 12: 383.

Adamson, JW and Finch, CA. (1968). Erythropoietin and the polycythemias. *Ann. NY Acad. Sci.* 149: 560.

Adamson, JW, Hayashi A, Stamatoyannopoulos, G et al (1972). Erythrocyte function and marrow regulation in hemoglobin Bethesda (β 145 Histidine). *J Clin Invest* 51: 2883

Adamson, JW and Finch, CA. (1975). Hemoglobin function, oxygen affinity and erythropoietin. *Ann. Rev. Physiol.* 37: 351.

Allen, DW, Burgoyne, CF, Groat, JD et al. (1984). Comparison of hemoglobin Koln erythrocyte membranes with malondialdehyde-reacted normal erythrocyte membranes. *Blood* 64: 1263.

Allen, DW, Wyman, J, and Smith, CA. (1953). The oxygen equilibrium of foetal and adult human hemoglobin. *J. Biol. Chem.* 203: 81–85.

Andersen, L. (1975). Structures of deoxy and carbonmonoxy hemoglobin Kaissas in the deoxy quaternary conformation *J. Mol Biol.* 94: 33–49.

Argos, P, Rossman, MG, Grau, UM et al. (1979). Thermal stability and protein structure. *Biochemistry* 18: 5698–5703.

Arnone, A. (1972). X-ray diffraction study of binding of 2,3-diphosphoglycerate to human deoxyhaemoglobin. *Nature* 237: 146–153.

Arous, N, Braconnier, F, Thillet, J et al. (1981). Hemoglobin Saint Mande β102 (G4) Asn → Tyr: A new low oxygen affinity variant. *FEBS Lett.* 126: 114–120.

Asakura, T, Adachi, K, Shapiro, M et al. (1975). Mechanical precipitation of hemoglobin Koln. *Biochim. Biophys. Acta* 412: 197–203.

Baldwin, JM. (1980). The structure of human carbonmonoxyhaemoglobin at 2.7 A resolution. *J. Mol. Biol.* 136: 103–112.

Baldwin, J and Chothia, C. (1979). Haemoglobin: the structural changes related to ligand binding and its allosteric mechanism. *J. Mol. Biol.* 129: 175–183.

Bemski, G, Arends, T, and Blanc, G. (1969). Electron spin resonance of Cu (II) in copper hemoglobin complexes. *Biochem. Biophys. Res. Commun.* 35: 599–606.

Benesch, R and Benesch, RE. (1967). The effect of organic phosphates from the human erythrocyte on the allosteric properties of hemoglobin. *Biochem. Biophys. Res. Commun.* 26: 162–167.

Bigelow, C. (1967). On the average hydrophobicity of proteins and the relation between it and protein structure. *J. Theor. Biol.* 16: 187–194.

Blouquit, Y, Braconnier, F, Galacteros, F et al. (1981). Hemoglobin Hotel-Dieu β 99 Asp → Gly (G1). A new abnormal hemoglobin with high oxygen affinity. *Hemoglobin* 5: 19–25.

Bonaventura, J and Riggs, A. (1967). Polymerization of hemoglobins of mouse and man. Structural basis. *Science* 158: 800–809.

Bonaventura, J, Bonaventura, C, Amiconi, G et al. (1975). Allosteric interactions in non-α chains isolated from normal human hemoblobin fetal hemoglobin, and hemoglobin Abruzzo [β 143 (H21) His→Arg]. *J. Biol. Chem.* 250: 6278–6285.

Bonaventura, J, Bonaventura, C, Sullivan, B et al. (1976). Hemoglobin Providence. Functional consequences of two alterations of the 2,3-diphosphoglycerate binding site at position β82. *J. Biol. Chem.* 251: 7563–7571.

Bonaventura, C, Cashon, R, Bonaventura, J et al. (1991). Involvement of the distal histidine in the low affinity exhibited by Hb Chico (Lysβ66→Thr) and its isolated β chains. *J. Biol. Chem.* 266: 23033–23040.

Bonaventura, J and Riggs, A. (1968). Hemoglobn Kansas, a human hemoglobin with a neutral amino acid substitution and an abnormal oxygen equilibrium. *J. Biol. Chem.* 243: 980–986.

Bookchin, RM and Nagel, RL. (1973). Molecular interactions of sickling hemoglobin. In Abramson, H, Bertles, JF, and Wethers, DC, editors. *Sickle cell disease*, St. Louis: Mosby.

Borgese, TA, Harrington, J, Borgese, JM, and Nagel, RL. (1982). Thermostability of fish hemoglobins. *Comp. Biochem. Physiol.* 72B: 7.

Bouhassira, EE, Lachman, H, Labie, D, and Nagel, RL. (1989). A gene conversion located 5′ to ^Aγ gene is in linkage disequilibrium with the Bantu haplotype in sickle cell anemia. *J. Clin. Invest.* 83: 2070–2073.

Bradley, TB, Wohl, RC, and Rieder, RF. (1967). Hemoglobin Gun Hill: Deletion of five amino acid residues and impaired heme-globin binding. *Science* 157: 1581–1588.

Bratu, V, Lorkin, PA, Lehman, H, and Predescu, C. (1971). Haemoglobin Bucaresti β42 (CD1) Phe→Leu, a cause of unstable haemoglobin haemolytic anemia. *Biochem. Biophys. Acta* 251: 1–6.

Brennan, SO, Williamson, D, Symmans, WA, and Carrell, RW. (1983). Two unstable hemoglobins in one individual: Hb Atlanta (β 75 Leu leads to Pro) and

Hb Coventry (β141 Leu deleted) *Hemoglobin* 7: 303–712.

Brennan, SO, Shaw, JG, George, PM, and Huisman, THJ. (1993). Post-translational modification of beta 141 Leu associated with the β75(E19) Leu→Pro mutation in Hb Atlanta. *Hemoglobin* 17: 1–7.

Brittain, T. (1994). Role of dimerization in the control of the functioning of the human haemoglobin mutant haemoglobin Howick (β 37 Trp→Gly). *Biochem. J.* 300: 553–556.

Brooks, J. (1935). The oxidation of haemoglobin to methaemoglobin by oxygen. II. The relation between the rate of oxidation and the partial pressure of oxygen. *Proc. R. Soc. London B Ser.* 118: 560.

Bunn, HF and Drysdale, JW. (1971). The separation of partially oxidized hemoglobins *Biochem. Biophys. Acta* 229: 51–59.

Bunn, HF and Forget, BG. (1986). *Hemoglobin: Molecular, genetic and clinical aspects.* Philadelphia: WB Saunders.

Bunn, FH and Jandl, JH. (1968). Exchange of heme among hemoglobins and between hemoglobin and albumin. *J. Biol. Chem.* 243: 465–472.

Burket, LB, Sharma, VS, Pisciotta, AV et al. (1976). Hemoglobin Mequon beta 41 (C7) phenylalanine leads to tyrosine. *Blood* 48: 645–651.

Burscaux, E, Poyart, C, Guesnon, P, and Teisseire, B. (1979). Comparative effects of CO_2 on the affinity for O_2 of fetal and adult hemoglobins. *Pfluegers Arch.* 378: 197–1002.

Butler, WM, Spratling, L, Kark, JA et al. (1982). Hemoglobin Osler: Report of a new family with exercise studies before and after phlebotomy. *Am. J. Hematol.* 13: 293–304.

Card, R and Brain, M. (1973). The "anemia" of childhood. *N. Engl. J. Med* 288: 338–389.

Caldwell, PRB and Nagel, RL. (1973). The binding of 2,3 diphosphoglycerate as a conformational probe of human hemoglobins. *M. Mol. Biol.* 74: 605–702.

Carrell, RW, Lehmann, H, and Hutchison, HE. (1966). Haemoglobin Köln (β-98 Valine->Methionine): An unstable protein causing inclusion-body anaemia. *Nature* 210: 915–916.

Carrell, RW and, Kay R. (1972). A simple method for the detection of unstable hemoglobins. *Br. J. Haematol.* 23: 615.

Cathie, AB. (1952). Apparent idiopathic Heinz body anemia. *Treat Ormond Sta. J.* 3: 43–49.

Chan, E and Desforges, J. (1974). Role of disulfide bonds in Heinz body attachment to membranes. *Blood* 44: 921–928.

Chanutin, A and Curnish, RR. (1967). Effect of organic and inorganic phosphates on the oxygen equilibrium of human erychrocytes. *Arch. Biochem. Biohys.* 121: 96–103.

Charache, S, Achuff, S, Winslow, R et al. (1978). Variability of the homeostatic response to altered p$_{50}$. *Blood* 52: 1156–1162.

Charache, S, Brimhall, B, and Jones, RT. (1975). Polycythemia produced by hemoglobin Osler (beta-145

(HC2) Tyr yields Asp). *Johns Hopkins Med. J.* 136: 132–136.

Charache, S, Catalano, P, Burns, S et al. (1985). Pregnancy in carriers of high-affinity hemoglobins. *Blood* 65: 713–719.

Charache, S, Weatherall, DJ, and Clegg, JB. (1966). Polycythemia associated with a hemoglobinopathy. *J. Clin. Invest.* 45: 813–819.

Chothia, C, Janin, J, and Wodak, S. (1976). Hemoglobin: The structural changes related to ligand binding and its allosteric mechanism. *Proc. Natl. Acad. Sci. U.S.A.* 73: 3793–38402.

Chou, AC and Fitch, CD. (1981). Mechanism of hemolysis induced by ferriprotoporphyrin IX. *J. Clin. Invest.* 68: 672–678.

Clegg, JB, Naughton, MA, and Weatherall, DJ. (1966). Abnormal human haemoglobins. Separation and characterization of the α and β chains by chromatography, and the determination of two new variants, Hb Chesapeake and Hb J (Bangkok). *J. Mol. Biol* 19: 91–96.

Clegg, JB, Weatherall, DJ, Wong HB, and Mustafa, D. (1969). Two new haemoglobin variants involving proline substitutions. *Nature* 22: 379–384.

Codringron, JF, Kutlar, F, Harris, HF et al. (1989). Hb A$_2$-Wrens or α$_2$898 (FG5) Val→Met, an unstable δ chain variant identified by sequence analysis of amplified DNA. *Biochem. Biophys. Acta* 1009: 87–89.

Coleman, MB, Adams, LG III, Walker, AM et al. (1993). Hb San Diego [beta 109(G11) Val→Met] in an Iranian: further evidence for a mutational hot spot at position 109 of the beta-globin gene. *Hemoglobin* 17: 543–554

Como, PF, Wylie, BR, Trent, RJ et al. (1991). A new unstable and low oxygen affinity hemoglobin variant: Hb Stanmore [β111(G13)Val→Ala]. *Hemoglobin* 15: 53–65.

Craik, CS, Valette, I, Beychok, A, and Waks, M. (1980). Refolding defects in hemoglobin Rothschild. *J. Biol. Chem.* 255: 6219–6224.

Darling, RC and Roughton, FJW. (1942). The effect of methemoglobin on the equilibrium between oxygen and hemoglobin. *Am. J. Physiol.* 137: 56–62.

DeFuria, FG and Miller, DR. (1972). Oxygen affinity in hemoglobin Koln disease. *Blood* 39: 398–404.

Delano, J, North, ML, Arous, N et al. (1984). Hb Saverne: a new variant having an elongated β chain. *Blood* 64(Suppl): 56a.

Delanoe-Garin, J, Blouquit, Y, Arous, N et al. (1988). Hemoglobin Saverne. A new variant with elonged β chains: Structural and functional properties. *Hemoglobin* 12: 337–352.

Dover, GJ, Boyer, SH, and Bell, WR (1978). Microscopic method for assaying F cell production: Illustrative changes during infancy and in aplastic anemia. *Blood* 52: 664–671.

Dover, GJ, Boyer, SH, and Pembrey, ME. (1981). F cell production in sickle cell anemia: Regulation by genes linked to β-hemoglobin locus. *Science* 211: 1441–1449.

Dover, GJ, Boyer, SH, Charache, S, and Heintzelman, K, (1978b). Individual variation in the production and survival of F-cells in sickle cell disease. *N. Engl. J. Med.* 299: 1428–1434.

Dumoulin, A, Manning, LR, Jenkins, WT et al. (1997). Exchange of subunit interfaces between recombinant adult and fetal hemoglobins. Evidence for a functional inter-relationship among regions of the tetramer. *J. Biol. Chem.* 272: 31326–31334.

Edelstein, SJ, Poyart, C, Blouquit, Y, and Kister, J. (1986). Self-association of haemoglobin Olympia ($\alpha_2\beta_2$ 20 (B2) Val → Met). A human haemoglobin bearing a substitution at the surface of the molecule. *J. Mol. Biol.* 187: 277–283.

Efremov, GD, Huisman, THJ, Smith, LL et al. (1961). Hemoglobin Richmond, a human hemoglobin which forms asymmetric hybrids with other hemoglobins. *J. Biol. Chem.* 244: 6105–6122.

Egan, EL and Fairbanks, VF. (1973). Postsplenectomy erythrocytosis in hemoglobin Köln disease. *N. Engl. J. Med.* 288, 929–931.

Eisinger, J, Flores, J, Tyson, JA, and Shohet, SB. (1985). Fluorescent cytoplasm and Heinz bodies of Koln erythrocytes. Evidence for intracellular heme catabolism. *Blood* 65: 886–894.

Elder, GE, Lappin, TR, Horne, AB et al. (1998). *Mayo Clin. Proc.* 73: 321–328.

Elder, GE, Lappin, TR, Horne, AB et al. (1998). Hemoglobin Old Dominion/Burton-upon-Trent, beta 143 (H21) His→Tyr, codon 143 CAC→TAC- -a variant with altered oxygen affinity that compromises measurement of glycated hemoglobin in diabetes mellitus: structure, function, and DNA sequence. *Mayo Clin Proc* 73: 321–328.

Feher, G, Isaacson, RA, and Scholes, CP. (1973). Electron nuclear double resonance (ENDOR) studies on normal and abnormal hemoglobins. *Ann NY Acad. Sci.* 222: 86–93.

Fermi, G, Perutz, MF, Williamson, D et al. (1992). Structure-function relationships in the low affinity mutant haemoglobin Aaborg (Gly74(E18)β→ Arg) *J. Mol. Biol.* 226: 883–888.

Fermi, G, Perutz, MF, Shaanan, B et al. (1989). The crystal structure of human deoxyhemoglobin at 1.7 A resolution. *J. Mol. Biol.* 175: 159–165.

Finch, CA. (1948). Methemoglobinemia and sulfhemoglobinemia. *N. Engl. J. Med.* 239: 470–476.

Fischer, S, Nagel, RL, Bookchin, RM et al. (1975). The binding of hemoglobin to membranes of normal and sickle erythrocytes. *Biochem. Biophys. Acta* 375: 422–430.

Flatz, G, Kinderlerer, JL, Kilmartin, JV et al. (1971). Haemoglobin Tak: a variant with additional residues at the end of the β-chains. *Lancet* 10: 732–739.

Flynn, TP, Allen, DW, Johnson, GJ, and White, JG. (1983). Oxidant damage of the lipids and proteins of the erythrocyte membranes in unstable hemoglobin disease. Evidence for the role of lipid peroxidation. *J. Clin. Invest.* 71: 1215–1222.

Frier, JA and Perutz, M. (1977). Structure of human foetal deoxyhaemoglobin. *J. Mol. Biol.* 112: 97–102

Gacon, G, Belkhodja, O, Wajcman, H et al. (1977). Structural and functional studies of Hb Rothschild beta (C3) Trp replaced by Arg. A new variant of the alpha1 beta2 contact. *FEBS Lett* 15: 82: 243–246.

Garcia, CR, Navarro, JL, Lam, H et al. (1983). Hb A$_2$-Manzanares or $\alpha_2\delta_2$ 121 (GH4) Glu→Val, an unstable δ chain variant observed in a Spanish family. *Hemoglobin* 7: 435–442.

Gerald, DS and Efron, ML. (1961). Chemical studies of several varieties of Hb M. *Proc. Natl. Acad. Sci. U.S.A.* 47: 1758–1762.

Glader, BE, Hemoglobin FM-Fort Ripley. Another lesson from the neonate. (1989). *Pediatrics* 83: 792–793.

Goosens, M, Lee, KY, Liebhaber, SA, and Kan, YW. (1982). Globin structural mutant α125 Leu→Pro is a novel cause of α-thalassmeia. *Nature* 296: 864–865.

Greenberg, HB. (1964). Syncope and shock due to methemoglobinemia. *Arch. Environ. Health* 9: 762–766.

Greer, J. (1971a). Three dimensional structure of abnormal haemoglobins Kansas and Richmond. *J. Mol. Biol.* 59: 99–107.

Greer, J. (1971b). Three dimension studies of abnormal human hemoglobins M Hyde Park and M Iwate. *J. Mol. Biol.* 59: 107–206.

Griffon, N, Badens, C, Lena-Russo, D et al. (1996). Hb Bruxelles, deletion of Phe42, shows a low oxygen affinity and low cooperativity of ligand biding. *J. Biol. Chem.* 271: 25916–25920.

Grimes, AJ, Meisler, A, and Dacie, JV. (1964). Congenital Heinz-body anaemia: further evidence on the cause of Heinz-body production in red cells. *Br. J. Haematol.* 10: 281–294.

Gros, G and Bauer, C. (1978). High pK value of the N-terminal amino group of the γ chains cause low CO$_2$ binding of human fetal hemoglobin. *Biochem. Biophys. Res. Commin.* 80: 56–59.

Guang, W, Ma, M, and Qian, D. (in press). Hb F-Xin-Jin or $^G\gamma^I$119(GH2)Gly→Arg. A new unstable fetal hemoglobin variant. *Hemoglobin.*

Grimes, AJ and Meisler, A. (1962). Possible cause of Heinz bodies in congenital Heinz body anaemia. *Nature* 194: 190.

Gurd, FRN, Falk, KE, Malmstrom, BG, and Vanngard, T. (1967). The conformational transition of sperm whale ferrimyoglobin in the presence of several equivalents of cupric ion. *J. Biol. Chem.* 242: 5731–7739.

Hargrove, MS, Whitaker, T, Olson, JS et al. (1997). Quaternary structure regulates hemin dissociation from human hemoglobin. *J. Biol. Chem.* 272: 17385–17389.

Hayashi, A Fujita, T, Fujimura, M, and Titani, K. (1979). A new fetal hemoglobin, HbF M Osaka (α_2 γ_2 63 His→Leu). A mutant with high oxygen affinity and erythrocytosis. *Am. J. Clin. Pathol.* 72: 1028–1032.

Hayashi, A, Suzuki, T, Shimizu, A, and Yamamura, Y. (1968). Properties of hemoglobin M. Unequivalent nature of the α and β subunits in the hemoglobin molecule. *Biochim. Biophys. Acta* 168: 262.

Hayashi, A, Suzuki, T, Imai, K et al. (1969). Properties of hemoglobin M Milwaukee I variant and its unique characteristics. *Biochem. Biophys. Acta* 194: 6.

Ho, C and Russu, IM. (1978). Biochemical and clinical aspects of hemoglobin abnormalities. In Caughey, WS, editor. New York: Academic Press.

Honig, GR, Vida, LN, Rosenblum, BB et al. (1990). Hemoglobin Warsaw (Phe beta42 (CD1)→Val), an unstable variant with decreased oxygen affinity. Characterization of its synthesis, functional properties, and structure. *J. Biol. Chem.* 265: 126–132.

Hoyer, JD, Wick, MJ, and Thibodeau, SN, et al. (1998). Hb Tak confirmed by DNA analysis: not expressed as thalassemia in a Hb Tak/Hb E compound heterozygote. *Hemoglobin* 22: 45–52.

Horlein, H and Weber, G. (1948). Uber chronisch famil-iare methamoglobinanue and eine neue modifikation des Methamoglobins. *Dtsch. Med. Wochenschr.* 73: 476.

Huchns, ER, Hecht, F, Keil, JV, and Motulsky, AG. (1964). Developmental hemoglobin anomalies in a chromoso-mal triplication: D_1 trisomy syndrome. *Proc. Natl. Acad. Sci. U.S.A.* 51: 89.

Ikkala, E, Koskela, J, Pikkarainen, P et al. (1976). Hb Helsinki: A variant with a high oxygen affinity and a substitution at a 2,3-DPG binding site (β 82 [EF6] Lys → Met). *Acta Haematol* 56: 257.

Imai, K. (1968). Oxygen-equilibrium characteristics of abnormal Hemoglobin Hiroshima ($\alpha_2\beta_2$ 143 Asp). *Arch. Biochem. Biophys.* 127: 543.

Imai, K and Lehmann, H. (1975). The oxygen affinity of Haemoglobin Tak, a variant with elongated β chain. *Biochim. Biophys. Acta* 412: 288–293.

Imamura, T, Fujita, S, Ohta, Y et al. (1969). Hemoglobin Yoshizuka (G10 (108) β Asparagine → Aspartic acid): A new variant with a reduced oxygen affinity from a Japanese family. *J. Clin. Invest.* 48: 2341–2349.

Jacob, HS, Brain, MK, and Dacie, JV. (1968). Altered sulfhydryl reactivity of hemoglobins and red blood cell membranes in congenital Heinz body hemolytic anemia. *J. Clin. Invest.* 47: 2664–2671.

Jacob, HS and Winterhalter, KH. (1970a). Unstable hemo-globins: the role of heme loss in Heinz body formation. *Proc. Natl. Acad. Sci. U.S.A.* 65: 697–702.

Jacob, HS and Winterhalter, KH. (1970b). The role of hemo-globin heme loss in Heinz body formation: Studies with a partially heme-deficient hemoglobin and with genetically unstable hemoglobin. *J. Clin. Invest.* 49: 2008–2013.

Jandl, JH, Simmons, RL, and Castle, WB. (1961). Red cell fil-tration and the pathogenesis of certain hemolytic anemias. *Blood* 18: 133–139.

Jones RT, Osgood, EE, Brimhall, B et al. (1967). Hemoglobin Yakima. I. Clinical and biochemical stud-ies. *J. Clin. Invest.* 46: 1840–1846.

Jones, RT, Brimhall, B, Pootrakul, S, and Gray, G. (1976). Hemoglobin Vancouver [$\alpha_2\beta_2$ 73 (E17) Asp → Tyr]: Its structure and function. *J. Mol. Evol.* 9: 37–43.

Jope, EM. (1945). The ultra-violet spectral absorption of haemoglobin inside and outside the red blood cell. In Roughton, FJW and Kendrew, JC, editors. *Haemoglobin.* London: Butterworth.

Kattamis, AC, Kelly, KM, Ohene-Frempong, K et al. (1997). Hb Osler (β145(HC23)Tyr→Asp) results

from translational modification. *Hemoglobin* 21: 109–120.

Kauzmann, W. (1959). Some factors in the interpretation of protein denaturation. *Adv. Protein Chem.* 14: 1–5.

Kavanaugh, JS, Moo-Penn, WF, and Arnone, A. (1993). Accomodation of insertions in helices: The mutation in hemoglobin Catonsville (Pro37) (C2)alpha-Glu-Thr38 (C3) alpha generates a 3_{10} →alpha bulge. *Biochemistry* 32: 2509–2513.

Kazanetz, EG, Leonova, JY, Huisman, THJ et al. (1996). Hb Nunobiki or α2 141 (HC3)Arg→Cysβ2 in a Belgian female results from a CGT→TGT mutation in the α2-globin gene. *Hemoglobin* 20: 443–445.

Kendrew, JC, Dickerson, RE, Strandberg, BE et al. (1960). Structure of myoglobin. A three-dimensional Fourier synthesis at 2 A resolution. *Nature* 185: 422–432.

Kilmartin, JV, Fogg, JH, and Perutz, ME (1980). Role of C-terminal histidine in the alkaline Bohr effect of human hemoglobin. *Biochemistry* 19: 3189–3194.

King, MAR, Wiltshire, BG, Lehmann, H, and Moriomoto, H. (1972). An unstable haemoglobin with reduced oxy-gen affinity: Haemoglobin Peterborough, β 111 (G13) Valine → Phenylalanine, its interaction with normal haemoglobin and with Haemoglobin Lepore. *Br. J. Haematol.* 22: 125–131.

Kleinhauer, E, Braun, H, and Berke, K. (1957). Demonstration von fetalem Haemoglobin in den Erythrozyten eines Blutausstrichs. *klin. Wochensshr.* 35: 637–642.

Kohne, E, Krause, M, Leopold, D et al. (1977). Koelliker (alpha2 minus 141 (HC3) Arg gamma2: A modification of fetal hemoglobin. *Hemoglobin* 1: 257–266.

Komiyama, N, Shih, DT, Looker, D et al. (1991). Was the loss in alpha globin a functional neutral mutant? *Nature* 352: 349–351.

Koler, RD, Jones, RT, Bigley, RH et al. (1973). Hemoglobin Casper: β 106 (G8) Leu → Pro, a contem-porary mutation. *Am. J. Med.* 55: 549–555.

Kolski, GB and Miller, DR. (1976). Heme synthesis in hereditary hemolytic anemias: Decreased δ-amino-lev-ulinic acid synthetase in hemoglobin Koln disease. *Pediatr. Res.* 10: 702–709.

Konotey-Ahulu, FID, Gallo, E, Lehmann, H, and Ringelhann, B. (1968). Haemoglobin Korle-Bu (β73 Aspartic acid → Asparagine) showing one of the two amino acid substitutions of Haemoglobin C. Harlem. *J. Med. Genet.* 5: 107–115.

Koshland, DE, Jr, Nemethy, G, and Filmer, D. (1966). Comparison of experimental binding data and theoreti-cal model in proteins containing subunits. *Biochemistry* 5: 365–374.

Kurachi, S, Hermodson, M, Hornung, S, and Stamatoyan-nopoulos, G. (1973). Struture of Haemoglobin Seattle. *Nature (London) New Biol* 243: 275–304.

Lacombe, C, Craescu, CT, Blouquit, Y et al. (1985). Structural and functional studies of hemoglobin Poissy alpha 2 beta 2(56). *Eur. J. Biochem.* 153: 655–662.

LaMar, GR, Nagai, K, Jue, T et al. (1980). Assignment of proximal histidyl imidazole exchangeable proton NMR resonances to individual subunits in HbA, Boston, Iwate and Milwaukee. *Biochem. Biophys. Res. Commun.* 96: 1177–1184.

Lee-Potter, JP, Deacon-Smith, RA, Simpkiss, MJ et al. (1975a). A new cause of haemolytic anemia in the new-born. A description of an unstable fetal haemoglobin: F Poole α2^{G}γ2 130 Tryptophan→Glycine. *J. Clin. Pathol.* 28: 317–323.

Lee-Potter, JP, Deacon-Smith, RA, Simpkiss, MJ et al. (1975b). A new cause of haemolytic anemia in the new-born. Adescription of an unstable fetal haemoglobin: F Poole α2^{G}γ2 130 Tryptophan→Glycine. *J. Clin. Pathol.* 28: 317–323.

Lehmann, H, Casey, R, Lang, A et al. (1975). Haemoglobin Tak: A β-chain elongation. *Br. J. Haematol.* 31: 119–125.

Levine, RL, Lincoln, DR, Buchholz, WM et al. (1975). Hemoglobin Hasharon in a premature infant with hemolytic anemia. *Pediatr. Res.* 9: 7.

Lindstrom, TR, Ho, C, and Pisciotta, AV. (1972). Nuclear magnetic resonance studies of haemoglobin M Milwaukee. *Nature* 237: 263–270.

Lines, JG and McIntosh, R. (1967). Oxygen binding by Haemoglobin J Cape Town (α2 92 Arg → Gln). *Nature* 215: 297–300.

Lorkin, PA, Stephens, AD, Beard, MEJ et al. (1975). Haemoglobin Rahere (β82 Lys → Thr): A new high affinity haemoglobin associated with decreased 2,3-diphosphoglycerate binding and relative polycythaemia. *Br. Med. J.* 4: 200–202.

Low, P. (1989). Interaction of native and denatured hemoglobins with Band 3: Consequences for erythrocyte structure and function. In Agre, P and Parker, JC, editors. *Red blood cell membranes.* New York: Marcel Dekker, Inc.

Low, PS, Westfall, MA, Allen, DP, and Appell, KC. (1984). Characterization of the reversible conformational equilibrium of the cytoplasmic domain of erythrocyte membrane band 3. *J. Biol. Chem.* 259: 13070–13075.

Maniatis, A, Bousios, T, Nagel, RL et al. (1979). Hemoglobin Crete (β129 Ala → Pro): A new high affinity variant interacting with β^0 and (δβ)^0 thalassemia. *Blood* 54: 54–61.

Mansouri, A and Winterhalter, KH. (1973). Nonequivalence of chains in hemoglobin oxidation. *Biochemistry* 12: 4946–4952.

Marinucci, M, Giuliani, A, Maffi, D et al. (1981). Hemoglobin Bologna (α$_2$β$_2$ 61 (E5) Lys → Met), an abnormal human hemoglobin with low oxygen affinity. *Biochim. Biophys. Acta.* 668: 209–215.

Martinez, G, Lima, F, and Colombo, B. (1977). Haemoglobin J Guantanamo (α$_2$β$_2$ 128 (H6) Ala → Asp). A new fast unstable haemoglobin found in a Cuban family. *Biochim. Biophys. Acta* 491: 1–10.

Martinez, G, Lima, F, Residenti, C, and Colombo, B. (1978). Hb J Camaguey alpha 2 141(HC3) Arg replaced by Gly beta 2: A new abnormal human hemoglobin. *Hemoglobin* 2: 47–53.

Mavilio, F, Marinucci, M, Tentori, L et al. (1978). Hemoglobin Legnano (alpha2 141 (HC3) Arg replaced by Leu beta2): A new abnormal human hemoglobin with high oxygen affinity. *Hemoglobin* 2: 249–259.

Miller, DR, Weed, RI, Stamatoyannopoulos, G, and Yoshida, A. (1971). Hemoglobin Köln disease occurring as a fresh mutation: erythrocyte metabolism and survival. *Blood* 38: 71–80.

Miura, S, Ikeda-Saito, T, Yonetani, T, and Ho, C. (1987). Oxygen equilibrium studies of cross-linked asymmetrical cyanomet valency hybrid hemoglobins: models for partially oxygenated species. *Biochemistry* 26: 2149–2155.

Miyoshi, K, Kaneto, Y, Kawai, H. et al. (1988). X-linked dominant control of F-cells in normal adult life: Characterization of the Swiss type as hereditary persistence of fetal hemoglobin regulated dominantly by gene(s) on X chromosome. *Blood* 72: 1854–1860.

Monod, J, Wyman, J, and Changeaux, JP. (1967). On the nature of allosteric transition: A plausible model. *J. Mol. Biol.* 12: 88–97.

Moo-Penn, WF, Bechtel, KC, Schmidt, RM et al. (1977). Hemoglobin Raleigh (β1 Valine → acetylamine). *Biochemistry* 16: 4872–4881.

Moo-Penn, WF, McPhedran, P, Bobrow, S et al. (1981). Hemoglobin Connecticut (β21 (β3) Asp → Gly): A hemoglobin variant with low oxygen affinity. *Am. J. Hematol.* 11: 137–145.

Moo-Penn, WF, Swan, DC, Hine, TK et al. (1978). Hb Catonsville (glutamic acid inserted between Pro-37(C2)alpha and Thr-38(C3)alpha). Non allelic gene conversion? *J. Biol. Chem.* 264: 21454–21457.

Moo-Penn, WF, Wolff, JA, Simon, G et al. (1989). Hemoglobin Presbyterian (1978): β108 (G10) Asparagine → Lysine. A hemoglobin variant with low oxygen affinity. *FEBS Lett.* 92: 53–61.

Nagai, M, Yubisui, T, and Yoneyama, Y. (1980). Enzymatic reduction of hemoglobin M Milwaukee I and M Saskatoon by NADH-cytochrome b$_5$ reductase and NADPH flavin reductase purified from human erythrocytes. *J. Biol. Chem.* 255: 4599–4609.

Nagel, RL, Bemski, G, and Pincus, P. (1970). Some aspects of the binding of Cu (II) to human hemoglobin and its subunits. *Arch. Biochem. Biophys.* 137: 428–437.

Nagel, RL and Bookchin, RM. (1974). Human hemoglobin mutants with abnormal oxygen binding. *Semin. Hematol.* 11: 385–394.

Nagel, RL, Gibson, QH, and Charache, S. (1967). Relation between structure and function in Hemoglobin Chesapeake. *Biochemistry* 6: 2395.

Nagel, RL, Ranney, HM, and Kucinskis, LL. (1966). Tyrosine ionization in human CO and deoxyhemoglobin. *Biochemistry* 5: 1934.

Nagel, RL and Ranney, HM. (1973). Drug-induced oxidative denaturation of hemoglobin. *Semin. Hematol.* 10: 269.

Nagel, RL and Gibson, QH (1971). The binding of hemoglobin to haptoglobin and its relation to subunit dissociation of hemoglobin. *J. Biol. Chem.* 246: 69–73.

Nagel, RL, Gibson, QH, and Jenkins, T. (1971a). Ligand binding in the Hb J Capetown. *J. Mol. Biol.* 58: 643.

Nagel, RL, Gibson, QH, and Hamilton, HB. (1971b). Ligand kinetics in Hemoglobin Hiroshima. *J. Clin. Invest.* 50: 1772.

Nagel, RL, Lynfield, J, Johnson, J et al. (1976). Hemoglobin Beth Israel: A mutant causing clinically apparent cyanosis. *N. Engl. J. Med.* 295: 125–130.

Nute, PE, Stamatoyannopoulos, G, Hermodson, MA et al. (1974). Hemoglobinopathic erythrocytosis due to a new electrophoretically silent variant, Hemoglobin San Diego (β 109 (G11) Val → Met). *J. Clin. Invest.* 53: 320.

O'Donnell, JK, Birch, P, Parsons, CT et al. (1994). Influence of the chemical nature of the side chain at beta 108 of hemoglobin A on the modulation of the oxygen affinity by chloride ions. Low oxygen affinity variants of human hemoglobins in transgenic pigs: hemoglobins Presbyterian and Yoshizuka. *J. Biol. Chem.* 269: 27692–27699.

Ogata, K, Ito, T, Okazaki, T et al. (1986). Hemoglobin Sendagi (beta 42 Phe→Val: A new unstable hemoglobin variant having an amino acid substitution at CD1 of the beta-chain. *Hemoglobin* 10: 469–481.

Ohba, Y. (1990). Unstable hemoglobins. *Hemoglobin* 14: 353–388.

Ohba, Y, Hattori, Y, Yoshinaka, H et al. (1981). Urea polyacrylamide gel electrophoresis of PCMB precipitate as a sensitive test for the detection of the unstable hemoglobin subunit. *Clin. Chim. Acta* 119: 179–185.

Ohba, Y, Miyaji, T, Matsuoka, M et al. (1975). S: Hemoglobin Hirosaki [α43 (CE1) Phe→Leu] a new unstable variant. *Biochem. Biophys. Acta* 405: 155–160.

Ohba, Y, Yamamoto, K, Kawata, R, and Miyaji, T. (1987). Hyperunstable Hemoglobin Toyama $\alpha_2 136$ (H19) leu→Arg β_2: Detection and identification by in vitro biosynthesis with radioactive aminoacids. *Hemoglobin* 11: 539–556.

Olson, JS, Mathews Rohlfs, RJ, Springer, BA et al. The role of the distal histidine in myoglobin and haemoglobin. *Nature* 336: 265–266.

Owen, MC, Ocelford, PA, Wells, RM, Howick, HB, (1993). (beta 37(C3) Trp→Gly): A new high oxygen affinity variant of the alpha 1 beta 2 contact. *Hemoglobin* 17: 513–521.

Park, CM and Nagel, RL. (1984). Sulfhemoglobin. Clinical and molecular aspects. *N. Engl. J. Med.* 310: 1579–1584.

Park, CM, Nagel, RL, Blumberg, WE et al. (1986). Sulfhemoglobin. Properties of partially sulfurated tetramers. *J. Biol. Chem.* 261: 8805–10.

Peisach, J and Gersonde K. (1977). Binding of CO to mutant α chains of HbM Iwate: Evidence for distal imidazole ligation. *Biochemistry* 16: 2539–2547.

Peisach, J, Blumberg, WE, and Rachmilewitz, EA. (1975). The demonstration of ferrihemochrome intermediates in Heinz body formation following the reduction of oxyhemoglobin A by acetylphenylhydrazine. *Biochem. Biophys. Acta* 393: 404–405.

Pembrey, ME, Weatherall, DJ, and Clegg, JB. (1973). Maternal synthesis of haemoglobin F in pregnancy. *Lancet* 16: 1351–1359.

Perrella, M, Bresciani, D, and Rossi-Bernardi, L. (1975a). The binding of CO_2 to human hemoglobin. *J. Biol. Chem.* 250: 5413–5421.

Perrella, M, Kilmartin, JV, Fogg, J et al. (1975b). Identification of the high and low affinity CO_2 binding sites of human haemoglobin. *Nature* 256: 759–767.

Perutz, MF. (1978). Electrostatic effects in proteins. *Science* 201: 1187–1195.

Perutz, MF. (1970). Stereochemistry of the cooperative effects in haemoglobin. *Nature (London) New Biol.* 288: 726–734.

Perutz, MF and Raidt, H. (1975). Sterochemical bases of heat stability in bacterial ferredoxins and in hemoglobin A_2. *Nature (London)* 255: 256–265.

Perutz, MF, Rossman, MG, Cullis, AF et al. (1960). Structure of haemoglobin. A three-dimensional Fourier synthesis at 5.5 A resolution, obtained by X-ray analysis. *Nature* 185: 416–423.

Perutz, MF, Sanders, JKM, Chenery, DH et al. (1978). Interactions between the quaternary structure of the globin and the open state of the heme in ferric mixed spin derivatives of hemoglobin. *Biochemistry* 17: 3640–3649.

Perutz, MF, Pulsinelli, PD and Ranney, HM. (1972). Structure and subunit interaction of haemoglobin M Milwauke. *Nature (London) New Biol.* 237: 259–267.

Pinkas, J, Pjaldetti, M, Joshua, H et al. (1963). Sulfhemoglobinemia and acute hemolytic anemia with Heinz bodies following contact with a fungicide-zinc ethylanol bisthiocarbamate-in a subject with glucose-6-phosphate dehydrogenase deficiency and hypocatalasemia. *Blood* 21: 484–496.

Poyart, C, Burseaux, E, Guesnon, P, and Teissiere, B. (1978). Chloride binding and Bohr effect of human fetal erythrocytes and HbFH solutions. *Pfluegers Arch.* 37: 169–173.

Poyart, C, Krishnamoorthy, R, Burseaux, E et al. (1976). Structural and functional studies of haemoglobin Suresnes or alpha2 141 (HC3) Arg replaced by His beta2, a new high oxygen affinity mutant. *FEBS Lett.* 69: 103–109.

Prchal, JT and Sokol, L. (1996). "Benign erytrocytosis" and other familial and congenital polycythemias. *Eur. J. Haematol.* 57: 263–268.

Pribilla, W, Klesse, P, and Betkle, K. (1965). Hämoglobin-Köln-krankheit: Familiäre hypochrome hämolytische anämie mit hämoglobinanomalie. *Klin. Wochenschr.* 43: 1049–1053.

Priest, JR, Watterson, J, Jones, RT et al. (1989). Mutant fetal hemoglobin causing cyanosis in a newborn. *Pediatries* 83: 734–736.

Pulsinelli, PD, Perutz, MF, and Nagel, RL. (1973). Structure of hemoglobin M Boston, a variant with a five-coordinated ferric heme. *Proc. Natl. Acad. Sci. U.S.A.* 70: 3870–3879.

Purcell, Y and Brozovic, B. (1974). Red cell 2,3 diphosphoglycerate concentration in man decreases with age. *Nature* 251: 511–513.

Rachmilewitz, EA. (1974). Denaturation of the normal and abnormal hemoglobin molecule. *Semin. Hematol.* 11: 441–452.

Rachmilewitz, EA, Peisach, J, and Blumberg, WE. (1971). Studies on the stability of oxyhemoglobin A and its constituent chains and their derivatives. *J. Biol. Chem.* 246: 3356–3364.

Rachmilewitz, EA and Harari, E. (1972). Intermediate hemichrome formation after oxidation of three unstable hemoglobins (Freiburg, Riverdale-Bronx and Koln). *Haematol. Bluttransfus.* 10: 241–249.

Ranney, HM, Nagel, RL, Heller, P, and Udem, L. (1968). Oxygen equilibrium of hemoglobin M_{Hyde} Park. *Biochim Biophys Acta* 160: 112–119.

Raftery, MA and Huestis, WH. (1973). Molecular conformation and cooperativity in hemoglobin. *Ann. NY Acad. Sci.* 222: 40–48.

Reed, CS, Hampson, R, Gordon, S et al. (1968). Erythroytosis secondary to increased oxygen affinity of a mutant hemoglobin, Hemoglobin Kempsey. *Blood* 31: 623–632.

Rieder, RF, Oski, FA, and Clegg, JB. (1969). Hemoglobin Philly (β35 Tyrosine → Phenylalanine): Studies in the molecular pathology of hemoglobin. *J. Clin. Invest.* 48: 1627–1632.

Rieder, RF. (1971). Synthesis of hemoglobin Gun Hill: Increased synthesis of the heme-free β^{GH} globin chain and subunit exchange with a free alpha chain pool. *J. Clin. Invest.* 50: 388–394.

Reismann, KR, Ruth, WE, and Nomura, T. (1961). A human hemoglobin with lowered oxygen affinity and impaired heme-heme interactions. *J. Clin. Invest.* 40: 182–195.

Reiss, GH, Ranney, HM, and Shaklai, N. (1982). Association of Hb C with erythrocyte ghosts. *J. Clin. Invest.* 70: 946–952.

Ricco, G, Scaroina, F, Amprimo, MC et al. (1992). Molecular characterization and functional studies on Hb Kemsey, β99(G-1) Asp→Asn, a high affinity variant. *Hematologica* 77: 215–220.

Rifkind, J. (1974). Copper and the autoxidation of hemoglobin. *Biochemistry* 13: 2475–2484.

Rifkind, RA. (1965). Heinz body anemia: an ultrastructural study. II. Red cell sequestration and destruction. *Blood* 26: 433–441.

Rivetti, C, Mozzarelli, A, Rossi, C et al. (1993). Effect of chloride on oxygen binding to crystals of hemoglobin Rothchild (β37 Trp→Arg) in the T quaternary structure. *Biochemistry* 32: 6411–6418.

Robinson, AB. (1974). Evolution and the distribution of glutamyl and asparaginyl residues in proteins. *Proc. Natl. Acad. Sci.* 71: 885–888.

Rochette, J, Poyart, C, Varet, B et al. (1984). A new hemoglobin variant altering the $\alpha_2\beta_2$ contact: Hb Chemilly $\alpha_2\beta_2$ 99 (G1) Asp → Val. *FEBS Lett.* 166: 8–14.

Rosa, J, Labie, D, Wajcman, H et al. (1969). Haemoglobin I Toulouse: β66 (E10) Lys → Glu: A new abnormal haemoglobin with a mutation localized on the E10 porphyrin surrounding zones. *Nature* 223: 190–199.

Rosa, R, Prehu, OM, Beuzard, Y, and Rosa, J. (1978). The first case of a complete deficiency of diphosphoglycerate mutase in human erythrocytes. *J. Clin. Invest.* 62: 907–914.

Rose, ZB. (1980). The enzymology of 2,3-bisphosphoglycerate. *Adv. Enzymol.* 51: 211–219.

Roth, EF Jr, Elbaum, D, Bookchin, RM, and Nagel, RL (1976). The conformational requirements for the mechanical precipitation of hemoglobin S and other mutants. *Blood* 48: 265–273.

Rucknagel, DL, Glynn, KP, and Smith, JR. (1967). Hemoglobin Ypsilanti characterized by increased oxygen affinity, abnormal polymerization and erythremia. *Clin. Res.* 15: 270–278.

Russu, IM and Ho, C. (1986). Assessment of role of beta 146-histidyl and other histidyl residues in the Bohr effect of human normal adult hemoglobin. *Biochemistry* 25: 1706–1816.

Russu, Ho, NT, and Ho, C. (1980). Role of the β 146 histidyl residue in the alkaline Bohr effect of hemoglobin. *Biochemistry* 19: 1043–1052.

Saenz, GF, Elizondo, J, Alvarado, MA et al. (1977). Chemical characterization of a new haemoglobin variant haemoglobin J Cubujuqui (alpha2141 (HC3)Arg replaced by Ser beta2). *Biochem. Biophys. Acta* 494: 48–56.

Salkie, ML, Gordon, PA, Rigal, WM et al. (1982). HbA2-Canada or $\alpha_2\delta_2$ 99 (G1) Asp → Asn, a newly discovered delta chain variant with increased oxygen affinity occurring in cis to β-thalassemia. *Hemoglobin* 6: 223–231.

Shaklai, N, Sharma, VS, and Ranney, HM. (1981). Interaction of sickle cell hemoglobin with erythrocyte membrane. *Proc. Natl. Acad. Sci. U.S.A.* 78: 65–68.

Schmid, R, Brecher, G, and Clemens, T. (1959). Familial hemolytic anemia with erythrocyte inclusion bodies and a defect in pigment metabolism. *Blood* 14: 991–1002.

Schneider, RG, Atkins, RJ, Hosty, TS et al. (1975). Haemoglobin Titusville: α94 Asp → Asn, a new haemoglobin with a lowered affinity for oxygen. *Biochem. Biophys. Acta* 400: 365–372.

Schneider, RG, Hosty, TS, Tomlin, G et al. (1975). Hb Mobile ($\alpha_2\beta_2$ 73 (E17) Asp → Val): A new variant. *Biochem. Genet.* 13: 411–419.

Schnitzer, B, Rucknagel, DL, Spencer, HH, and Aikawa M. (1971). Erythrocytes: pits and vacuoles as seen with transmission and scanning electron microscopy. *Science* 173: 251–254.

Schroeder, WA, Cua, JT, Matsuda, G, and Fenninger, WD. (1962). Hemoglobin F_1, and acetyl-containing hemoglobin. *Biochem. Biophys. Acta* 63: 532–536.

Shroeder, WA, Shelton, JR, Shelton, JB et al. (1963). The amino acid sequence of the γ-chain of human fetal hemoglobin. *Biochemistry* 2: 992–1002.

Shroeder, WA, Huisman, THJ, Efremov, GD et al. (1979). Further studies on the frequency and significance of the $^T\gamma$ chain of human fetal hemoglobin. *J. Clin. Invest.* 63: 268–274.

Sharma, NS, Newton, GL, Ranney, HM et al. (1980). Hemoglobin Rothschild (β37(C3) Trp → Arg): A high/low affinity haemoglobin variant. *J. Mol. Biol.* 144: 267–274.

Sherwood, JB and Goldwasser, E. (1979). Radio-immunoassay for erthropoietin. *Blood* 54: 885–894.

Shibata, S. (1981). Hemoglobinopathies in Japan. *Hemoglobin* 5: 509–606.

Shibata, S, Mijaji, T, and Iuchi, I. (1967). Methemoglobin M's of the Japanese. *Bull. Yamaguchi Med. Sch.* 14: 141–149.

Shibata, N and Iuchi, I. (1977). Characterization of a red minor component of abnormal hemoglobin found in HbM of Hyde Park disease. *Hemoglobin* 1: 829.

Shibata, S, Tanuira, A, and Iuchi, I. (1960). Hemoglobin M₁ demonstration of a new abnormal hemoglobin in hereditary nigremia. *Acta Haematol. Jpn.* 23: 96–104.

Shimasaki, S. (1985). A new hemoglobin variant, Hemoglobin Nunobiki [α 141 (HC3) Arg → Cys]. Notable influence of the carboxy-terminal cysteine upon various physico-chemical characteristics of hemoglobin. *J. Clin. Invest.* 75: 695–705.

Slightom, JL, Blechl, AE, and Smithies, O. (1980). Human fetal ᴳγ- and ᴬγ-globin genes: Complete nucleotide sequences suggest that DNA can be exchanged between these duplicated genes. *Cell* 21: 627–638.

Stabler, SP, Jones, RT, Head, C et al. (1994). Hemoglobin Denver [alpha 2 beta 2 (41) (C7) Phe→ Ser: A low O₂ affinity variant associated with chronic cyanosis and anemia. *Mayo Clin. Proc.* 69: 237–243.

Stamatoyannopoulos, G, Nute, PE, Adamson, JW et al. (1973). Hemoglobin Olympia (β20 Valine → Methionine): An electrophoretically silent variant associated with high oxygen affinity and erythrocytosis. *J. Clin. Invest.* 52: 342–351.

Suzuki, T, Hayashi, A, Shimizu, A, and Yamamura, Y. (1966). The oxygen equilibrium of hemoglobin M Saskatoon. *Biochim. Biophys. Acta* 127: 280–289.

Suzuki, T, Hayashi, A, Yamamura, Y et al. (1965). Functional abnormality of hemoglobin M_Oskaka. *Biochem. Biophys. Res. Commun.* 19: 691–699.

Seryeva, A, Gordeuk, VR, Tokarev, YN et al. (1997). Congenital polycythemia in Chuvashia. *Blood* 89: 2148–2154.

Tatsis, B, Dosik, H, Rieder, R et al. (1972). Hemoglobin Hasharon: Severe hemolytic anemia and hypersplenism associated with a mildly unstable hemoglobin. *Birth Defects Orig. Artic. Ser.* 8: 25–32.

Tetradeau, C, Lavalette, D, Momenteau, M, and Lhoste, JM. (1983). Energy barriers in the CO and O₂ bindings to heme model compounds. *Proc. Natl. Acad. Sci. U.S.A.* 84: 2267–2277.

Thillet, J, Cohen-Solal, M, Seligmann, M, and Rosa, J. (1976). Functional and physiochemical studies of Hemoglobin St. Louis β 28 (B10) Leu → Gln. *J. Clin. Invest.* 58: 1098–1104.

Tondo, C, Bonaventura, J, Bonaventura, C et al. (1974). Functional properties of Hemoglobin Porto Alegre (α₂Aβ₂9 Ser → Cys) and the reactivity of its extra cysteinyl residue. *Biochim. Biophys. Acta* 342: 15–22.

Tondo, CV, Mendez, HM, and Reischl, E. (1980). Thermostability of hemoglobins in homeothermic and non-homeothermic vertebrates. *Comp. Biochem. Physiol.* 66B: 151–159.

Tucker, PW, Phillips, SEV, Perutz, MF et al. (1978). Structure of hemoglobins Zürich [His E7(63)β-Arg] and Sydney [ValE11(67) β-Ala] and role of the distal residues in ligand binding. *Proc. Natl. Acad. Sci. U.S.A.* 75: 1076–1084.

Tyuma, I and Shamizu, N. (1969). Different response to organic phosphates of human fetal and adult hemoglobins. *Arch. Biochem. Biophys.* 129: 404–407.

Udem, L, Ranney, HM, Bunn, HF, and Pisciotta, A. (1970). Some observations on the Properties of hemoglobin M_Milwaukee. *J. Mol. Biol.* 48: 489–495.

Virshup, DM, Zinkham, WH, Sirota, RL, and Caughey, WS. (1983). Unique sensitivity of Hb Zürich to oxidative injury by phenazopyridine: Reversal of the effects by elevating carboxyhemoglobin in vivo and in vitro. *Am. J. Hematol.* 14: 315–324.

Wajcman, H and Jones, RT. (1977). Propietes fonctionelles des hemoglobins humaines mutees in position 73. *INSERM* 70: 269–275.

Wajcman, H, Krishnamoorthy, R, Gacon, G et al. (1976). A new hemoglobin variant involving the distal histidine: Hb Bicetre (β63 (E7) His → Pro). *J. Mol. Med.* 1: 187–196.

Wajcman, H, Dahmane, M, Prehu, C et al. (1998). Haemoglobin J-Briska: A new mildly unstable α1 gene variant with a deletion of eight residues (α50–57 or α5–5 or α52–59) including the distal histidine. *Br. J. Haematol.* 100: 401–406.

Wajcman, H, Girondon, E, Prome, D et al. (1995). Germline mosaicism for an alanine to valine substitution at residue beta 140 in hemoglobin Puttelange, a new variant with high oxygen affinity. *Hum. Genet.* 96: 711–716.

Wajcman, H, Kilmartin, JV, Najman, A, and Labie, D. (1975). Hemoglobin Cochin-Port-Royal: Consequences of the replacement of the beta chain C-terminal by an arginine. *Biochim. Biophys. Acta* 400: 354–363.

Wajcman, H, Leroux, A, and Labie, D. (1973). Functional properties of hemoglobin Hammersmith. *Biochemie* 55: 119–125.

Wacjman, H, Vasseur, C, Blouquit, Y et al. (1994): F. Hemoglobin Redondo [β92(F8)His→Asn]: An unstable hemoglobin variant associated with heme loss which occurs in two forms. *Am. J. Hematol.* 38: 194–200.

Wada, Y, Ikkala, E, Imai, K et al. (1987). Structure and function of a new hemoglobin variant, Hb Meilahti α2β236(C2)Pro→Thr), characterized by mass spectrometry. *Acta Haematol.* 78: 109–113.

Walder, JA, Chatterjee, R, Steck, T et al. (1984). The interaction of hemoglobin with the cytoplasmic domain of band 3 of the human erythrocyte membrane. *J. Biol. Chem.* 259: 10238–10246.

Weatherall, DJ, Clegg, JB, Callender, ST et al. (1977). Haemoglobin Radcliffe (α₂β₂99 (Gl) Ala): A high oxygen-affinity variant causing familial polycythaemia. *Br. J. Haematol.* 35: 177–185.

White, JM, Brain, MC, Lorkin, PA et al. (1970). Mild "unstable haemoglobin haemolytic anaemia" caused by haemoglobin Shepherds Bush (B74(E18) gly- -asp). *Nature* 225: 939–941.

White, JM, Szur, L, Gillies, IDS et al. (1973). Familial poly-cythaemia caused by a new haemoglobin variant. Hb Heathrow: β103 (G5) Phenylalanine → Leucine. *Br. Med. J.* 3: 665–672.

Williamson, D, Nutkins, J, Rosthoj, S et al. (1990). Characterization of Hb Aalborg, a new unstable hemoglo-bin variant, by fast atom bombardment mass spectrometry *Hemoglobin* 14: 137–145.

Winterbourne, CC and Carrell, RW. (1972). Characterization of Heinz bodies in unstable haemoglobin haemolytic anaemia. *Nature* 240: 150–154.

Winterbourne, CC and Carrell, RW. (1974). Studies of hemo-globin denaturation and Heinz body formation in the unsta-ble hemoglobins. *J. Clin. Invest.* 54: 678–686.

Winterbourne, CC and Carrell, RW. (1977). Oxidation of human hemoglobin by copper. *Biochem. J.* 165: 141–150.

Winterbourne, CC, McGrath, BM, and Carrell, RW. (1976). Reactions involving superoxide and normal and unstable haemoglobins. *Biochem. J.* 155: 503–509.

Wishner, BC, Ward, KB, Lattman, EE, and Love, WE. (1975). Crystal structure of sickle-cell deoxy hemoglo-bin at 5 Å resolution. *J. Mol. Biol.* 98: 179–185.

Wood, WG, Stamatoyannopoulos, G, Lim, G, and Nute, PE. (1975). F-cells in the adult: Normal values and levels in individuals with hereditary and acquired elevations of Hb F. *Blood* 46: 671–776.

45

Native and Recombinant Mutant Hemoglobins of Biological Interest

MARTIN H. STEINBERG
RONALD L. NAGEL

INTRODUCTION

Mutations of hemoglobin can be classified in two categories: mutations with frequencies above 1 percent of an affected population, such as HbS, HbE, HbC, and the thalassemias; and hemoglobin mutations that are relatively or extraordinarily rare. Malaria is responsible for the high prevalence of HbS, HbE, HbC, and thalassemia—also numerous other erythrocyte membrane and enzyme variants outside the subject matter of this book—in certain of the world's populations (see Chapter 30). Carriers of rare hemoglobin mutations may be clinically affected (see Chapter 44) but the diseases associated with these variants are not public health problems. Other rare variants, discussed in this chapter, are important solely for the biological principles they illustrate.

The 1998 *Syllabus of Human Hemoglobin Variants* listed 750 unique hemoglobin variants (Huisman et al., 1998). These included 217 involving the α-globin gene, 362 involving the β-globin gene, 70 γ-globin gene variants, 32 δ-globin gene variants, and 69 variants caused by either two mutations in one globin gene, hybrid chains, elongated chains, or truncated chains. This variant list is accessible on the World Wide Web at http://globin.cse.psu.edu. Not always included in this compilation, but also found on the Web and in a companion volume on thalassemia mutations, are variants caused by mutations within the coding portion of a globin gene and associated with the phenotype of thalassemia (Huisman et al., 1997). These interesting thalassemic hemoglobinopathies are discussed in Chapters 14 and 17.

Globin gene mutations, which include nearly every class of mutation so far described—except for trinucleotide repeats and other nucleotide expansions associated with neuromuscular disorders, uniparental disomy, and genetic imprinting—provided an early catalogue of the types of mutations that can cause genetic disease. Many of these mutations—affecting gene expression and producing thalassemia, altering hemoglobin solubility and producing sickle cell disease, affecting hemoglobin stability and causing premature red cell destruction, interfering with normal oxygen binding kinetics and producing erythrocytosis, and permitting heme iron oxidation, causing cyanosis—have been described in earlier chapters.

Comparatively few globin residues are critical for maintaining the structural integrity and functional performance of the molecule (see Chapter 9). Most hemoglobin gene mutations are, therefore, not associated with hematologic or clinical abnormalities and escape detection, especially when they are electrophoretically or chromatographically silent. Some mutations, while not medically important, illustrate interesting biological and anthropologic principles. This chapter will discuss some of these more interesting variant hemoglobins.

Large-scale population screening programs have defined the worldwide prevalence of medically important hemoglobinopathies and thalassemias. Most of the hemoglobin variants known today were discovered as a by-product of this extensive effort. Unlike some thalassemia mutations and HbS, HbE, and HbC, almost none of these variant hemoglobins are present at polymorphic frequencies (over 1 percent gene frequency) since they are genetically neutral and their carriage does not provide a selective advantage. Sometimes, in population isolates, there is a founder effect leading to a higher than expected prevalence of a particular mutation. In 1986, Winter edited a two-volume compendium of the geographic distribution of hemoglobin variants in the Americas, Europe, Africa, the former USSR, the Middle East, India, Southeast Asia, China, Japan, the Antipodes, and Oceania (Winter, 1986). These valuable volumes discuss the racial and ethnic makeup of each region surveyed and the distribution of hemoglobinopathies and thalassemia found in large population surveys. While this information in some respects is dated, it is unlikely that new globin mutations that reach polymorphic frequencies will be found.

In unexamined population isolates, some new variants present at high frequency may yet be uncovered and sporadic examples of new and already described variants will continue to be unearthed. The world's distribution of HbS, HbC, and HbE reflects one or a few origins of these mutations that were initially localized and attained polymorphic frequency because of selection. As a result of war, population migrations, and slave trading, these mutants then spread throughout the world. Our world is no longer pristine in the sense that populations remain confined to their native locales. Common hemoglobinopathies in many geographic areas, especially industrialized countries and regions with a history of slave importation, reflect the spread of ancient mutations and not mutations indigenous to that area.

MUTATION MECHANISM AND DISTRIBUTION

Over 90 percent of hemoglobinopathies are due to single base pair substitutions, or point mutations. How do single base pair mutations arise? DNA replication is not foolproof and has an inherent rate of error that is dependent on the fidelity of DNA polymerases and the efficiency of error correction mechanisms. Mutation is also sequence dependent. Bases may be misincorporated during replication. Repair enzymes may have a codon bias for mismatch repair so that certain misincorporations are more efficiently repaired than others. These sequence-dependent differences may account for the observation that some globin gene codons are associated with up to seven different mutations while others have one or no described mutations. That is, there may be "hot spots" for mutations and sites especially resistant to mutation.

Depurination occurs when the purine-deoxyribose bond is disrupted. Depurination can arise spontaneously and the rate of G cleavage is greater than that of A. Consistent with depurination as a cause of mutation, deoxyadenosine is the base most often misincorporated by DNA polymerases and G→A transitions are the most commonly observed human point mutations. About 10 percent of α- and β-globin gene structural mutants are due to G→A transitions.

Perhaps the best understood cause of point mutation is the methylation-mediated deamination of 5-methylcytosine to thymine. Thirty-eight percent of 880 base changes associated with genetic disease involved CpG dinucleotides (Cooper and Krawczak, 1993). G→A transitions result from the C→T transition on the antisense or mRNA coding strand leading to G→A miscorrection on the sense or noncoding strand. In eukaryotes, 5-methylcytosine usually occurs in a CpG dinucleotide. CpG dinucleotides are rare in vertebrates (about 20 percent of the expected fre-

quency) and usually methylated except in hypomethylated CpG islands often associated with active transcription. With a few exceptions, mutations are randomly distributed throughout the α- and β-globin gene without an evident "hot spot." Perutz has found that both methylated CpG in the β-globin genes and the unmethylated CpG in the α-globin genes appear to act as "hot spots" (Perutz, 1990). Hb San Diego may be the result of a C→T transition of a CpG dinucleotide. Increased susceptibility of CpG dinucleotides to mutation may account for the diverse populations in which Hb San Diego has been described (Coleman et al., 1993).

Up to four synonymous codons for each amino acid residue are permitted by the degeneracy of the genetic code. For twelve of the twenty-three amino acids present in hemoglobin—isoleucine is used only once in the γ-globin chain—codon usage is clearly biased (Bunn and Forget, 1986). Selective codon use is apparent in twelve instances for the α-globin gene, in seven instances for the β-globin gene, and in four instances for the γ-globin gene.

As of 1998, mutations at 105 of the 141 codons determining the α-globin chain amino acid sequence have been described, with a total of 217 different variants. In the β-globin gene, 362 mutations have been described for 138 of the 146 sequence-determining codons. Some codons have undergone as many as seven different mutations. Residues with multiple substitutions are usually, but not always, those forming important contacts between α- and β-globin chains or between globin and the heme groups. Substitutions at these residues produce a hematologic and clinical phenotype and are more likely to reach clinical attention. For example, seven mutations have been described at β99, all associated with high O$_2$ affinity variants and erythrocytosis. Four of the six variants of α141 where information is available, have increased O$_2$ affinity. Six mutations at β92 are all associated with unstable hemoglobins and hemolytic anemia. In contrast, the five mutations described at the β22 codon are all stable and functionally normal. It is not known if these sites are particularly prone to mutational events or if we are witnessing examples of bias of ascertainment where these mutations are identified because of their obvious phenotype.

More than 2,500 single base substitutions are possible in the α- and in the β-globin gene coding regions. Only 20 percent of these possible mutations have been described. Despite the advent of powerful new technologies for mutation discovery, the pace of description of new hemoglobin variants may have slowed because population surveys are less often done than in the past, clinically silent variants are still likely to escape notice, and many of the variants that cause a change in the charge of the molecule, simplifying their detection by isoelectric focusing or electrophoresis, have been already delineated. Neutral substitutions, where the charge of the molecule is unchanged, and without a clinical phenotype, will not be detected by protein-based screening.

Among all hemoglobin mutants, β-globin gene variants are most frequently described while α-, γ-, and δ-globin gene variants, respectively, are reported 65 percent, 20 percent, and 10 percent as often. This distribution has several explanations: (1) This preponderance of β-globin gene variants might reflect the fact that because of their higher concentration, there is greater likelihood that β-globin gene variants associated with a phenotype will be clinically apparent; (2) α-globin gene variants are encoded on one of four α-globin genes (or one of three when the variant is linked to α thalassemia) so their levels in the hemolysate are less than those of β-globin gene mutants. A high oxygen affinity variant present at 50 percent concentration, as are most β-globin gene mutants, is more likely to cause clinically apparent erythrocytosis than a similar α-globin gene variant present at 20 percent concentration. When insensitive tests are used, even with a clinical phenotype, some α-globin variants may go unnoticed because of their low levels in the blood; (3) It is possible that α-chain mutations are more likely to be lethal, because α-chains are essential for functional hemoglobin formation both in the embryo and fetus, increasing the chance of altering developmental or physiologic functions. α-Globin chains must also bind three types of non-α-globin chains, β, γ, and δ-globin chains, to form tetramers, increasing their chance of being functionally incompetent if mutated.

Very low concentrations of HbA$_2$ and HbF in adults often preclude the detection of an abnormal variant. Mutations of these genes are discussed in Chapter 10. γ-Globin gene mutations can affect either the $^\mathrm{g}$γ-globin gene or the $^\mathrm{A}$γ-globin gene. Only rarely do γ-globin chain abnormalities have a clinical phenotype in neonates and this usually is due to methemoglobinemia and cyanosis. γ-Globin variants can also be unstable, have increased or decreased oxygen affinity, be acetylated, and have "thalassemic" features. Due to gene duplication, four γ-globin genes are normally present and since there is differential expression of the linked $^\mathrm{G}$γ- and $^\mathrm{A}$γ-globin genes with the switch from fetal to adult expression, different levels of γ-globin gene variants are found. In babies, most variants of the $^\mathrm{G}$γ-globin gene are present at 23 percent of total hemoglobin while $^\mathrm{A}$γ-globin gene variants comprise about 10 percent of the hemolysate. Sometimes, different γ-globin gene arrangements including triplications, quadruplications, and chromosomes with a $^\mathrm{G}$γ-$^\mathrm{G}$γ or $^\mathrm{A}$γ-$^\mathrm{A}$γ arrangement, can alter the level of mutant γ- globins.

Structural variants of the embryonic ε and ζ globins have not been described at the DNA or protein level, although undoubtedly they occur.

CLASSIFICATION OF MUTATIONS

Post-translational Modifications

Changes induced by posttranslational modification of globin are broadly illustrative of the secondary modifications possible in all proteins and give rise to an interesting group of abnormal hemoglobins.

Deamidation. Under certain conditions, mutant asparaginyl residues can be deamidated to aspartate and result in two species of globin caused by a single mutation (Wright, 1991). Aspartic acid to asparagine mutants may be deamidated causing reduced quantities of the asparagine-containing globin (Jue et al., 1979). Usually, deamidation occurs when a histidine residue is adjacent to the asparagine substitution or when changes in the tertiary structure of a variant globin can bring a histidine into the proximity of a normally present asparagine. Other factors favoring asparagine deamidation are glycine, serine, or alanine residues with nonbulky side chains on either side of the asparagine or brought near the asparagine because of tertiary structure, a basic or acidic residue on one side and a serine or cysteine on the other side of asparagine, and peptide chain flexibility (Wright, 1991). Not all aspartic acid to asparagine mutants are subjected to posttranslational deamidation. Two abnormal hemoglobins may be present when variants susceptible to deamidation are analyzed: A native form containing the encoded asparagine and a deamidated form containing aspartic acid. When a variant of this type is present in a compound heterozygote with another variant hemoglobin, a confusing electrophoretogram or HPLC profile with three hemoglobin bands representing two globins resulting from the asparagine substitution and another from the other β-globin gene variant can be present. Hemoglobin abnormalities resulting from deamidation are shown in Table 45.1.

Hb Providence (β82 Lys→Asn). Deamidation of an asparaginyl residue was first noted in Hb Providence (Charache et al., 1977). Deamidation occurred slowly and was documented by globin biosynthesis studies that showed that only β$^\mathrm{A}$ and β$^\mathrm{asn}$ chains were synthesized.

Hb Osler (β145 Tyr→Asn [Asp]). First described as arising from a substitution of an aspartic acid residue for tyrosine, this high oxygen affinity variant is more complex (Charache et al., 1975; Hutt et al., 1996). Three major hemoglobin bands, migrating like Hb "J",

Table 45.1. Hemoglobin Variants with Deamidated Asparaginyl Residues

Variant	DNA mutation	Phenotype	Reference
La Roche-sur-Yon (β81 Leu→His)	CTC→CAC (?)	Unstable, decreased p^{50}, mild hemolysis. β81 Leu→His facilitates β80 Asn deamidation	Wajcman et al., 1992a
Providence (β82 Lys→Asn)	AAG→AAC/T (?)	Increased O_2 affinity but normal PCV	Charache et al., 1977
Redondo (β92 His→Asn)	CAC→AAC (?)	Heme loss, unstable, hemolysis, migrates like HbS and HbA_2	Wajcman et al., 1991
Osler (β145 Tyr→Asn)	TAT→AAT	Increased O_2 affinity, migrates like HbJ and HbA	Charache et al., 1975; Hutt et al., 1996
J Sardegna (α50 His→Asn)	CAC→AAC	Functionally normal. Present in 0.09% of Sardinians	Paleari et al., 1999
J Singapore ($\alpha_2$79 Ala→Gly)	GCG→GGG (?)	Normal, ~22%. The mutation may allow deamidation of α78 asn	Blackwell et al., 1972
Wayne (α139 –A)	–A in either α_1–α_2 globin gene with 5 codon elongation (?)	Normal hematology, either ~14% or ~6% present	Seid-Akhaven et al., 1976

Note: The DNA mutation has been confirmed only for Hb Osler and HbJ Sardegna. Migration refers to electrophoresis at alkaline pH.

Hb "A", and HbS and three different β-globin chains were present. When the granddaughter of the original case and the index case were restudied, DNA sequencing showed an HbS mutation and at codon 145, a TAT→AAT, corresponding to an asparagine substitution. In reality, the Hb "J" band is the deamidated Hb Osler (β145 Tyr→Asp) and the Hb "A" band is unmodified Hb Osler (β145 Tyr→Asn) (Fig. 45.1). Since Hb Osler (Asp) migrates with HbA, the amount of both forms of this variant in the heterozygote is near 60 percent rather than the reported 30 percent.

Hb La Roche-sur-Yon and J-Singapore. In the examples of **Hb LaRoche-sur-Yon** (β81 Leu→His) the normal asparagine at position 80 is deamidated and in **J-Singapore** (α79 Ala→Gly), α78 is deamidated. The EF segment of globin may provide a "hot spot" for deamidation since half the variants with this property are in this vicinity.

Hb Wayne. Hb Wayne, a frame shift variant, where the deletion of an A in codon α139 causes the α-globin chain to be extended by five residues until a new termination codon is encountered, has an asparagine at α139 (Fig. 45.2). Its deamidation leads to two Hb Wayne peptides, one of which contains aspartic acid

(Seid-Akhaven et al., 1976). Two families have been reported with Hb Wayne. In the first, Hb Wayne chains constituted 6 percent of the total hemoglobin and in the second family, Hb Wayne made up 14 percent of all hemoglobin. α-Globin gene haplotype was not known in the index case but was normal in the second family (Huisman et al., 1984). It is possible that the different concentrations of Hb Wayne were due to the mutations occurring on the α_2-globin gene in family 2 and the α_1-globin gene in family 1.

Figure 45.1. Electrophoretic separation of Hb Osler showing the "native" Hb Osler (Asn) and the deamidated Hb Osler (Asp). This sample was from a mixed heterozygote with HbS accounting for the absence of true HbA and the presence of HbS. (From Hutt et al., 1996, with permission.)

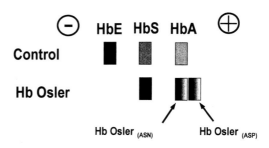

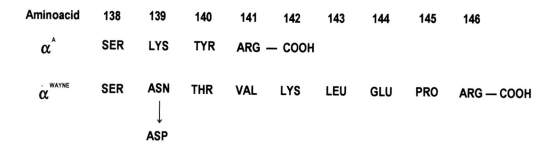

Aminoacid	138	139	140	141	142	143	144	145	146
α^A	SER	LYS	TYR	ARG — COOH					
α^{WAYNE}	SER	ASN ↓ ASP	THR	VAL	LYS	LEU	GLU	PRO	ARG — COOH

Figure 45.2. Structure of Hb Wayne. Because of the reading frameshift, an asparagine residue replaces the usual lysine at position 139 and the α-globin chain is extended by five amino acid residues until an in-phase termination codon is encountered. The α139 asparagine can be deamidated to aspartic acid.

HbJ Sardegna. HbJ Sardegna (α$_2$50 His→Asn) is found in nearly 0.1 percent of all Sardinians, and in the northern part of the island, in over twice this number (Paleari et al., 1999). Bands representing the native and deamidated form of this variant can be resolved by isoelectric focusing but not by HPLC. Functionally normal, this hemoglobin is often present with α thalassemia and β thalassemia. The former increases and the latter decreases its concentration.

Oxidation

Hb Coventry (β141 Leu→Hydroxyleu). A young girl with hemolytic anemia was found to have two unstable hemoglobins: Hb Sidney (β67 Val→Asp), a previously known unstable variant, and a new variant, Hb Coventry, suspected to be due to the deletion of β141 leucine. Hb Coventry formed less than 10 percent of the hemolysate. As the patient also had HbA, three β-globin genes were postulated, one being a βδ gene where a β141 deletion occurred during crossing over (Casey et al., 1978). Another patient with unstable hemoglobin hemolytic anemia was also found with three putative β-globin chains: Hb Atlanta (β75 Leu→Pro), Hb Coventry, and β^A (Brennan et al., 1983). These observations, and a third instance of Hb Coventry in a similar clinical setting, suggested that this variant was widespread and only became apparent when present with another unstable hemoglobin. Hb Coventry was hypothesized to result from a posttranslational change, laboratory artifact, or somatic mutation. Its broad distribution argued against the presence of a βδ anti-Lepore gene. Using new methods of HPLC these same investigators later proposed that the two mutations were in a single β-globin chain, Hb Atlanta-Coventry (β75 Leu→Pro; β141 Leu→Del), that was the product of a βδ anti-Lepore gene, the leucine 141 being deleted in the crossover event (Moo-Penn et al.,

1975). Two genetic events must have occurred to explain these findings: a de novo β75 Leu→Pro mutation and a sister chromatid exchange in a somatic cell.

Doggedly pursuing the basis for their findings, researchers applied newly available DNA techniques were applied to study the structure of the β-globin gene cluster and the nucleotide sequence of the β-globin genes (George et al., 1992). Only two normal β-globin genes were present! An expected β75 Leu→Pro mutation was found but the codon for β141 was intact in genomic DNA and in mRNA. Finally, by mass spectroscopy, the peptide containing β141 leucine was found to contain a novel amino acid of 129 daltons instead of the 113 daltons of leucine. This was postulated to be hydroxyleucine (Brennan et al., 1992). Hydroxyleucine cannot be detected by amino acid analysis so its presence remains conjectural. It was proposed that perturbation of the heme pocket by the β75 Leu→Pro mutation in the E helix, perhaps via the generation of activated oxygen species, led to oxidation of some β141 leucine residues. Peptides of similar abnormal mass were found in cases of Hb Christchurch (β71 Phe→Ser) and Hb Manukau (β67 Val→Gly)—other unstable hemoglobins of the E helix—and also in the original case of Hb Atlanta. This notion provides a parsimonious explanation for the existence of the Hb Coventry anomaly in the same globin chain as Hb Atlanta and other unstable variants (Brennan et al., 1993).

Acetylation

Hb Raleigh (β1 Val→Ala). Hb Raleigh is acetylated and migrates with HbA$_1$C (Moo-Penn et al., 1977). Proteins with an N-terminal alanine are often acetylated. Acetylation of a retained N-terminal methionyl occurs when normal cleavage of this residue malfunctions (see below). Acetylated hemoglobins can be mistaken for Hb A$_1$C.

Elongated Globins

By different mechanisms, hemoglobin chains may be extended beyond the expected 141 amino acid residues for the α-globin chain and 146 amino acid residues for the β-globin chain. Mechanistically, small insertions may

Table 45.2. Hemoglobin Variants with Elongated Globin Chains

Variant	Mutation	Mechanism	Phenotype
N-terminal extension			
South Florida (Boissel et al., 1985)	β1 Val→Met	Initiator met retained, chain extended by 1 residue	Acetylated at the NH_2 terminus and appears as HbA_1C
Doha (Kamel et al., 1985)	β1 Val→Glu	Initiator met retained, chain extended by 1 residue	21% in heterozygote, acetylated
Long Island (Prchal et al., 1986)	β2 His→Pro	Initiator met retained, chain extended by 1 residue	No clinical phenotype but appears as HbA_1C
Thionville (Vasseur et al., 1992)	α1 Val→Glu	Initiator met retained, chain extended by 1 residue	50% in heterozygote, acetylated
Insertions			
Catonsville (Kavanaugh et al., 1993)	Insertion between α37 and α38	Glu inserted	Increased O_2 affinity, unstable
Zaïre (Wajcman et al., 1992b)	Insertion between α116 and 117	5 residues inserted	Normal
Grady (Huisman et al., 1974)	Insertion between α118 and 119	3 residues inserted	Normal
Koriyama (Kawata et al., 1988)	Insertion between β95 and 96	5 residues inserted by possible out of frame base pairing. In Hb Gun Hill the same 15 bp segment is deleted	Severe instability and anemia. Resembles a thalassemic hemoglobinopathy
C-terminal extensions			
α-globin gene termination mutants	See Chapter 17	Termination codon mutations	α Thalassemia
Tak (Flatz et al., 1971; Hoyer et al., 1998)	β147 (+ AC)	2 bp insertion and frameshift	~Normal
Wayne (Seid-Akhaven et al., 1976)	α139 (−A)	1 bp deletion and frameshift	See Table 45.1

occur by a mechanism similar to that invoked for small deletions—slipped mispairing at the replication fork of DNA at the site of direct repeats or inverted repeats. Nonsense to missense mutations at the termination codon, reading frame shifts, failure to cleave the initiator methionine residue from the amino terminus of globin, amino acid insertions, and combined deletions and insertions have been reported. Many of the resulting variants are not associated with hematologic abnormalities and some are accompanied by hemolytic anemia that can be severe. Distortion of tertiary structure because of chain elongation not unexpectedly can provoke different degrees of globin instability. Examples of elongated chains associated with the phenotype of α thalassemia and unstable hemoglobins are discussed in Chapters 17 and 44. Table 45.2 highlights some other variants with extended globin chains.

Several mutations of the NH_2 terminal valine of both the α- and β-globin chain and a His→Pro mutation at β2 result in a globin elongated by one residue because of the failure to cleave the initiator methionyl residue (Table 45.3). Translation usually begins at an initiator methionine residue that is later enzymatically cleaved from the growing polypeptide chain. Subsequently, the N-terminal amino acid residue is acetylated. Removal of this initiator methionyl residue is normally a posttranslational modification except in secreted proteins, where it forms part of a signal sequence that is cleaved after protein translocation. Valine is a common NH_2 terminal residue in proteins where the initiator methionine is removed. There is no abnormal hematologic phenotype associated with these variants but the NH_2-terminal methionine is acetylated and appears as HbA_1C by some methods of hemoglobin separation. It has interfered with the assessment of diabetes in carriers of these variants.

Shortened Globins. Almost without exception, the deletion of one or more amino acid residues results in an unstable globin. When one or two residues are missing, the clinical phenotype is usually mild with slight anemia. One variant, **Hb Higashitochigi** (β24 or 25 Gly→O)(Fugisawa et al., 1993) leads to methemoglobinemia and **Hb Bruxelles** (β41 or 42 Phe→O) is

Table 45.3. α-Globin Gene Mutations Encoded on Both α-Globin Genes

Variant	α_2	Genotype	Percent	α_1	Genotype	Percent
J Paris (12 Ala→Asp)	GCC→GAC	$\alpha^x\alpha/\alpha\alpha$	24	GCC→GAC	$\alpha\alpha^x/\alpha\alpha$	20.7
Hekinan (27 Glu→Asp)	GAG→GAC	$\alpha^x\alpha/-\alpha$	27.9	GAG→GAT	$\alpha\alpha^x/\alpha\alpha$	13.9
G Philadelphia (68 Asn→Lys)*	AAC→AAA	$\alpha^x\alpha/\alpha\alpha$	25.1	AAC→AAG	$\alpha\alpha/-\alpha^{x*}$	33.4
J Broussais (90 Lys→Asn)	AAG→AAT	$\alpha^x\alpha/\alpha\alpha$	25	AAG→AAC	$\alpha\alpha^x/\alpha\alpha\alpha$	18
				AAG→AAC	$\alpha\alpha^x/\alpha\alpha$	20.6
Manitoba (102 Ser→Arg)	AGC→CGC	$\alpha^x\alpha/\alpha\alpha$	18.7	AGC→AGA	$\alpha\alpha^x/\alpha\alpha^x$	23.9
J Meerut (120 Ala→Glu)	GCG→GAG	$\alpha^x\alpha/\alpha\alpha$	23	GCG→GAG	$\alpha\alpha^x/\alpha\alpha$	18.4

* This variant is usually present on the $-\alpha^{3.7}$ rightward deletion chromosome.
From Molchanova et al. (1994a), with permission.

accompanied by severe Heinz body hemolytic anemia (Blouquit et al., 1989). When more than one or two amino acids are deleted the phenotype is apt to be more severe. These variants are discussed with the unstable hemoglobins in Chapter 44.

β-Globin Gene Variants with Point Mutations

Only two β-globin genes are normally present and gene deletion is a rare cause of β thalassemia. Therefore, the concentration of stable β-globin gene variants is quite constant at 40 percent to 50 percent. An exception, **Hb Dhofar** (β58 Pro→Arg), is linked in *cis* to a β+-thalassemia mutation and makes up only 15 percent of total hemoglobin (Williamson et al., 1995).

Hemoglobin G Coushatta (β22 Glu→Ala). This β-globin chain variant has no clinical or hematologic manifestations and has been found in geographically separated racial and ethnic groups (Schneider et al., 1964). Common in China and United States Coushatta Indians, it has also been described in Japan, Korea, and Turkey. It is the most common variant hemoglobin described along the Chinese Silk Road, a venerable trade route between the Orient and Europe. Its presence in Asia, the Old World, and in Amerindians, raised the question of whether this variant had a unicentric origin and spread to the New World over the ancient Bering land bridge or originated multicentrically in Asia and in Amerindians. To answer this query, the haplotype of the β-globin gene cluster was examined in Coushatta Indians from Louisiana and native Chinese who were carriers of HbG Coushatta. It was hypothesized that identical haplotypes associated with the HbG Coushatta mutation in both Coushatta Indians and Chinese would favor a single origin of this mutation in Asia, which then spread to North America by migration. Chinese families and Coushatta Indians had different haplotypes associated with the identical HbG Coushatta mutation defined by the presence of a Hind III restriction site in the $^A\gamma$-globin gene and an Ava II restriction site in the β-globin gene in Chinese and their absence in the Coushatta. In addition, DNA sequencing showed that Chinese individuals had a CAC at codon β 2 (β-globin gene framework 1 or 2) linked to the HbG gene while Coushatta Indians had a CAT (framework 3) indicating different β-globin gene frameworks. Both the HbG Coushatta mutation (GAA→GCA) and the codon 2 CAC→CAT polymorphism are normal δ-globin gene sequences suggesting the possibility of gene conversion. HbG Coushatta had at least two independent origins. These could be due to two separate mutations at codon β22, a mutation at this codon and a β→δ gene conversion, or two β→δ gene conversion events (Li et al., 1999). Recently, this variant has been reported in the Thai population on yet another β-globin gene haplotype, one that is predominant in Thais, suggesting yet another possible origin for this ostensibly genetically "neutral" variant (Itchayanan et al., 1999).

Hb Vicksburg (β75 Leu→deleted). In 1981, 8 percent of an abnormal hemoglobin was found in a young boy with the phenotype of β thalassemia intermedia (Adams et al., 1981). HbF was 90 percent, HbA$_2$, 3.4 percent, and HbA was absent. Both parents had β-thalassemia trait but in neither could Hb Vicksburg be detected. Hb Vicksburg was stable and β Vicksburg globin was not subject to posttranslational degradation. A marked deficit of β- compared with α-globin mRNA was found. It was hypothesized that the patient was a compound heterozygote for β^0 thalassemia and a gene containing a β^+-thalassemia mutation in *cis* to the Hb Vicksburg deletion. Recently, the -88 C→T β^+-thalassemia mutation was found in *cis* to the sickle mutation (Baklouti et al., 1989).

With the arrival of new technology that allowed direct confirmation of this hypothesis, this patient was reexamined 6, 8, and 10 years after the initial studies (Adams et al., 1991). At 6 years a small amount of HbA was also detected with Hb Vicksburg. At 8 and 10 years, Hb Vicksburg was not detectable and only HbA, HbF, and HbA$_2$ were found. Examination of the patients' DNA when both HbA and Hb Vicksburg were detectable in the hemolysate, showed that he was a compound heterozygote for the -88 C→T β^+ thalassemia and IVS II position 849 A→G mutation that causes β^0 thalassemia. On three separate occasions over a span of 5 years and employing several different means of detection, including allele-specific amplification, genomic sequencing, and restriction analysis of genomic DNA from blood leukocytes and erythroid colonies, the predicted Hb Vicksburg deletion was not present (Adams et al., 1991).

A simple explanation for these observations was not forthcoming but the following hypotheses were advanced. It was proposed that Hb Vicksburg arose as a stem cell mutation on the β^+-thalassemia chromosome. When first studied, only Hb Vicksburg was present, then both HbA and Hb Vicksburg were found, and finally, only HbA was seen. This suggested that over time there were at least two clones of erythroid progenitors contributing to erythropoiesis (Adams et al., 1991). Stem cells are known to cycle, and, conceivably, the clone containing the Hb Vicksburg mutation either was inactive or exhausted when the last studies were done (Abkowitz et al., 1990).

Unfortunately, erythroid colonies could not be studied when Hb Vicksburg was present in the blood. A leucine deleted in Hb Vicksburg calls to mind the origin of Hb Coventry (see above). Mass spectroscopy of Hb Vicksburg peptides was not done. There was no additional E helix mutation that could serve as the catalyst for leucine oxidation. It is still possible that some technical artifact was responsible for the failure to find a $\beta75$ leucine residue when Hb Vicksburg was present.

Studies of the stable variant, **Hb Costa Rica** ($\beta77$ His→Arg), provided some support for the notion of a somatic mutation causing traces of abnormal hemoglobin (Romero et al., 1996; Smetanina et al., 1996). Six to 8 percent Hb Costa Rica was found in a young woman but not any of her relatives. A mutation corresponding to the CAC→CGC transversion expected to code for this variant could not be detected in her genomic DNA. Yet, small amounts of Hb Costa Rica mRNA were present in reticulocytes. Globin gene structure was normal. A somatic mutation causing genetic mosaicism was hypothesized. In follow-up studies where erythroid burst-forming units (BFU-e) were grown from the blood of this patient, only 12 percent to 15 percent of these erythroid colonies contained both HbA and Hb Costa Rica mRNA while the remainder had mRNA only for HbA.

α-Globin Gene Variants with Point Mutations

Duplicated α-globin genes with identical coding regions make it possible for a mutation to occur in either the 5′ α$_2$-globin gene or the 3′ α$_1$-globin gene and for the identical mutation to be present in both α-globin genes. Where information is available, mutations are equally divided between both α-globin genes (Molchanova et al., 1994a). Depending on whether they are encoded on the α$_2$- or α$_1$-globin gene, there is a small difference in the levels of stable α-globin gene mutants. α$_2$-Globin mutants usually form about 24 percent and α$_1$-globin mutants about 20 percent of the hemolysate (Molchanova et al., 1994a). This level is influenced by the transcription rate of each α-globin gene, translational efficiency of the mRNA from each gene, the assembly of αβ dimers, the presence of deleted or triplicated α-globin loci, and the presence of nondeletion types of α thalassemia (see Chapter 17). Some identical amino acid substitutions encoded on both the α$_1$- and α$_2$-globin genes, often by different mutations, are shown in Table 45.3.

HbG Philadelphia (α68 Asn→Lys). HbG Philadelphia is the most common α-globin gene variant in Blacks and is found in about 1 in 5,000 African Americans. No clinical phenotype is associated with this variant, but, because it is usually found with α thalassemia and can be present on many different α-globin gene arrangements, its level in the hemolysate varies widely. Levels of this variant have a bimodal or trimodal distribution (Baine et al., 1976; Milner and Huisman, 1976). Interactions of HbG Philadelphia with sickle cell anemia are discussed in Chapter 28. Most often, in the Black population, HbG Philadelphia is present on the $-\alpha^{3.7}$ chromosome as an AAC→AAG transversion. It is also found in Italians on the α$_2$-globin gene in a normal α-globin gene locus ($\alpha^G\alpha/\alpha\alpha$) where the mutation is AAC→AAA (Brudzinski et al., 1984; Molchanova et al., 1994b). Different proportions of HbG Philadelphia found with different α-globin gene haplotypes are shown in Table 45.4. Besides the α-globin genotypes shown, it is likely that HbG Philadelphia will be found in *trans* to chromosomes with both α-globin genes deleted and associated with triplicated and quadruplicated α-globin loci. In the latter case, the percentage of HbG should be lower than usual.

Table 45.4. Levels of HbG Philadelphia in Different α-Globin Genotypes

α-Globin genotype	Percent HbG Philadelphia
$\alpha^x\alpha/\alpha\alpha$	25
$-\alpha^G/\alpha\alpha$	33
$-\alpha/\alpha^G\alpha$	33
$-\alpha/-\alpha^G$	50
$-\alpha^G/-\alpha^G$	100
$-\alpha^T/-\alpha^G$*	100
$--/-\alpha^G$†	HbG + HbH

* α^T denotes a dysfunctional α-globin gene that is not expressed because of a frameshift and new in-phase termination codon (Safaya and Rieder, 1988).
† In HbG/HbH disease, both HbH and HbG are present.
Data from Molchanova et al., 1994a, 1994b; Safaya and Rieder, 1988.

Other α-globin gene variants present at levels near 50 percent are probably also present on an α-thalassemia-2 chromosome. Hb J-Tongariki (α115 Ala→Asp) is commonly found in Melanesians and always present on a $-\alpha^{3.7}$ chromosome. Heterozygotes have about 50 percent and homozygotes nearly 100 percent of this variant (Abramson et al., 1970; Old et al., 1978; Bowden et al., 1982). This mutation was likely to have occurred on a $-\alpha^{3.7}$-thalassemia chromosome that is prevalent in Vanuatuans (Bowden et al., 1982).

HbI (α16 Lys→Glu). HbI may polymerize in vitro (Atwater et al., 1960; Beale and Lehmann, 1965). This was described in a pregnant woman who was well clinically but had mild anemia. Seventy percent of the hemoglobin was HbI and she was suspected also to have thalassemia, despite macrocytic red cells. A test for sickling using sodium metabisulfite was positive. These "sickled" cells closely, but not identically, resembled HbS-containing cells while the kinetics of cell deformation seemed much retarded compared with HbS-containing cells. Deoxygenation and acidification of HbI did not lead to gel formation and blood viscosity did not change when HbI was made to "sickle." This report contains many unknowns, including the structure of the abnormal globin and whether there is some sort of hemoglobin polymer in the cell. Some features of HbI resemble those of Hb Setif (see below).

HbI has been reported encoded on both linked α-globin genes of a single individual and considered an example of concerted evolution—the parallel development of related closely linked genes (Liebhaber et al., 1984). In a hematologically normal Black woman, 65 percent of the hemolysate was HbI. Her α-globin gene haplotype revealed a normal α-globin gene locus and an α-globin gene locus with the common $-\alpha^{3.7}$ dele-

tion. Genetic studies showed she transmitted to a daughter, who had only HbA, the $\alpha^{-3.7}$ deletion, suggesting that HbI was encoded on the normal α-globin gene locus. When mRNAs from the linked α_1- and α_2-globin gene were selectively isolated and translated in vitro, both were shown to encode a glutaminyl residue at position 16; α_1 mRNA also encoded normal α globin, the product of the chromosome with the $-\alpha^{3.7}$ deletion. These observations suggested a gene conversion event between the highly homologous α-globin genes. Two of the three α-globin genes present in the proband produced HbI accounting for the very high concentration of the variant.

Hb Setif (α22 Asp→Tyr). Only hemoglobin variants with the β6 Glu→Val mutation of sickle hemoglobin polymerize when deoxygenated and cause vasoocclusive disease. Hb Setif—a variant found in North Africa and the Middle East—forms pseudosickled cells in vitro, not in vivo, when it is oxygenated because of the aggregation of Hb Setif. Aggregation can be induced in cells with as little as 15 percent Hb Setif, the concentration of this variant in heterozygotes (Wajcman et al., 1972; Drupt et al., 1976; Raik et al., 1983; Charache et al., 1987; Noguchi et al., 1991). Pseudosickled Hb Setif cells can be distinguished from sickled HbS cells by many physical characteristics although they have several features in common. The C_{sat} of a 40/60 percent hemolysate of Hb Setif/HbA at 290 mOsm was 24 g/dL at 24°C. During incubation in NaCl buffer at 450 mOsm, polymer in pseudosickled cells required more than 30 minutes to begin formation, and, after 24 hours, nearly all cells contained aggregated Hb Setif (Noguchi et al., 1991). HbS polymer forms in fractions of a second to seconds. Deoxygenation inhibits pseudosickling of Hb Setif cells but is required for HbS polymerization. Pseudosickled Hb Setif cells have been described as twisted cigars with a monotonous morphology in contrast to the eclectic conformation of sickle cells (Fig. 45.3). In common with HbS erythrocytes, cell deformability decreased with increasing Hb Setif concentrations and increasing osmolality of the suspending buffer, while the amount of Hb Setif polymer increased under these conditions.

These observations provide insights into hemoglobin solubility and polymerization. However, pseudosickling of Hb Setif is strictly an in vitro phenomenon. Whether Hb Setif was present at levels of less than 20 percent—attributable to mild instability—or at concentrations near 40 percent—because of a coexistent α-thalassemia deletion—there was no evidence of hemolysis and vasoocclusive disease was not observed. Urine-concentrating ability in carriers of Hb Setif seemed unimpaired, whereas this is abnormal in sickle cell trait and

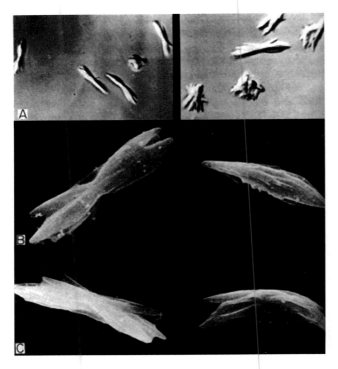

Figure 45.3. Pseudosickling of Hb Setif erythrocytes by (A) light microscopy and Nomarsky optics and (B and C) scanning electron microscopy. (From Charache et al., 1987, with permission.)

sickle cell anemia (Charache et al., 1987). Curiously, "pseudosickling" has been observed only with HbI and Hb Setif, two α-globin gene variants. It is not known how strenuous a search has been made for this phenomenon in other hemoglobin variants.

Five stable α-globin variants formed by mutations of codon α6 (Asp)—HbSarawa (Ala), Hb Dunn (Asn), Hb Ferndown (Val), Hb Woodville (Tyr), and HbSwan River (Gly)—are all present in lower than expected amounts that average about 10 percent. Four stable to mildly unstable variants with α27 (Glu) mutations— Hb Fort Worth (Gly), HbSpanish Town (Val), HbShuanfeng (Lys), and Hb Hekinan (Asp)—are present at concentrations of 4 percent to 14 percent (Huisman et al., 1998). In no case has it been established whether the mutant is on the α_2- or the α_1-globin gene or whether the α-globin gene loci are duplicated. Other than Hb Dunn, whose asparaginyl residue may be deamidated, it is not clear why variants with uncommonly low blood levels are clustered at these sites.

Two Point Mutations in One Globin Chain

Some hemoglobin variants have two amino acid substitutions in a single globin chain. Those involving the sickle and another mutation have been described in Chapter 28. In the sole α-globin chain variant originally described with two mutations, Hb J-Singapore (α78 Asn→Asp; α79 Ala→Gly), α78 asparagine is likely to be deamidated, but DNA studies have not been reported. β-Globin gene variants with two amino acid substitutions are shown in Table 45.5.

There are two origins for these double substitution variants: recombination between homologous chromosomes each containing a different mutation and a new mutation in a gene already containing one mutation. When both mutations are common in a population, such as the HbC mutation and HbN Baltimore mutation that together characterize Hb Arlington Park (Adams and Heller, 1977), or the HbE mutation and HbD Los Angeles mutation of HbT Cambodia, then the doubly substituted variant most likely arose by recombination (Baklouti et al., 1989; Anonymous, 1993). In the family with Hb Duino, the father of the proband had only Hb Camperdown (β104 Arg→Ser) while the proband, with both this mutation and the β92 His→Pro of Hb Newcastle, was likely to have acquired the second abnormal hemoglobin by de novo mutation (Wajcman et al., 1992b).

Hb Fannin-Lubbock was first reported to be a β119 Gly→Asp mutation (Huisman et al., 1996). DNA and amino acid analysis of hematologically normal propositi from five separate Spanish families with a fast migrating variant showed that this variant actually contained both β119 Gly→Asp (GGC→GAC) and a previously undescribed β111 Val→Leu (GTC→CTC) mutation (Qin et al., 1994). The original families have not been restudied but their heritage and the observation that the β111 Val→Leu was more likely to be responsible for the mild hemoglobin instability, suggests that this mutation may also have been present. Hb Masuda (β114 Leu→Met; β119 Gly→Asp), also slightly unstable, is reported to have one of the Hb Fannin-Lubbock mutations and the mutation of Hb Zengcheng (Ohba et al., 1998). DNA analysis was not done so that the presence of the β111 Val→Leu (GTC→CTC) cannot be excluded. However, these studies were in a Japanese family, making any relationship to Hispanic carriers of Hb Fannin-Lubbock unlikely.

Hb Medicine Lake (β98 Val→Met; β32 Leu→Gln) has the phenotype of severe β thalassemia since the β-globin chain, containing both the Hb Köln and the β32 mutation, is likely to be highly unstable and rapidly catabolized (Coleman et al., 1995) (Chapter 14). Lacking a detectable protein, it was not possible to explore directly the properties of the abnormal hemoglobin containing the β32 CTG→CAG mutation, but some predictions were made. Since the

Table 45.5. β-Globin Gene Variants with Two Amino Acid Substitutions*

Variant	Substitutions	Hemoglobins involved	Hematology
Arlington Park	β6 Glu→Lys	HbC	Normal
	β95 Lys→Glu	HbN Baltimore	
T-Cambodia	β26 Glu→Lys	HbE	?
	β121 Glu→Gln	HbD Los Angeles	
Grenoble	β51 Pro→Ser	–	?
	β52 Glu→Lys	Hb Osu Christiansborg	
Poissy	β56 Gly→Arg	Hamadan	Erythrocytosis
	β86 Ala→Pro	–	Hemolysis
Villeparisis	β77 His→Tyr	Fukuyama	Normal
	β80 Asn→Ser	–	
Duino	β92 His→Pro	Newcastle	Hemolysis
	β104 Arg→Ser	Camperdown	
Medicine Lake	β98 Val→Met	Köln	Severe β thalassemia
	β32 Leu→Gln	–	
Fannin-Lubbock	β111 Val→Leu	–	Normal
	β119 Gly→Asp	–	
Masuda	β114 Leu→Met	Zengcheng	Normal
	β119 Gly→Asp	–	
Cleveland	β121 Glu→Gln	D-Los Angeles	Normal
	β93 Cys→Arg	Okazaki	

* Variants with the sickle cell mutation and another amino acid substitution are discussed in Chapter 28 and listed in Table 28.5.

Leu→Gln mutation does not alter the charge of the β subunit, the electrophoretic mobility of Hb Medicine Lake may not differ from Hb Köln. A hydrophilic glutamine residue contains an uncharged polar side chain that could distort the B helix. Also, perturbation of the adjacent β31 leucine that contacts the heme group could result in instability (Honig et al., 1973; Garel et al., 1975). A definitive assessment of the inheritance of Hb Medicine Lake was not possible, but the most plausible cause of this abnormal hemoglobin was a new mutation in the germ cell of the father or in the proband.

Nonthalassemic Fusion Globins

Anti-Lepore βδ-fusion globins and **Hb Kenya**, a γβ-fusion globin, are not usually associated with hematologic abnormalities because a normal β-globin gene is present on the chromosome with the hybrid gene. These variants are shown in Table 45.6. **Hb Parchman** (δ1-12; β13-22; δβ22-50; β87-146) was first described as a double crossover but could, perhaps more plausibly, be due to gene conversion (δ22 Ala→Glu, 50 Ser→Thr) (Adams et al., 1982).

EVALUATION OF HEMOGLOBINOPATHIES

Hemoglobinopathy detection is often a part of the evaluation of anemia, microcytosis, or erythrocytosis.

The major clinical questions to be resolved are (1) Is an abnormal variant present? (2) What is (are) the abnormal variant(s)? (3) How abundant is (are) the variant(s)? (4) Is (are) the variant hemoglobin(s) relevant to the clinical picture that prompted the studies initially? Laboratory tests used for evaluating hemoglobinopathies are discussed in Chapter 34.

In summary, mutations of the β-globin gene usually change only one electrophoretic hemoglobin band,

Table 45.6. βδ and γβ Fusion Globins

Variant	Crossover	Features
Miyada	β through 12 δ from 12	17% in heterozygotes; normal hematology
P-Congo	β through 22 δ from 116	Normal hematology
P-Nilotic*	β through 22 δ from 50	Normal hematology
P-India	β through 87 δ from 116	23% in heterozygotes
Kenya	Aγ through 81 β from 86	6% in heterozygotes; 5% HbF (100%Gγ) Normal hematology

* Hb Lincoln Park is identical to HbP Nilotic but is associated with reticulocytosis. It contains a deletion of δ137 valine and was hypothesized to result from multiple crossing over events (Honig et al., 1978).

and stable variants usually have a concentration of 40 percent to 50 percent. As a corollary, HbA levels are reduced by nearly half. In contrast, α-globin variants should produce altered HbA, HbA$_2$, and HbF bands because each of these hemoglobins contains α globin. As a first approximation, mutation of one α-globin gene might then be expected to create variants forming 20 percent to 25 percent of the total HbA, and similar fractions of the total HbA$_2$ and HbF. γ-Globin variants will alter a single major hemoglobin band during fetal and neonatal life but, after the first year of life, will alter only the faint HbF band and are rarely detected. Mutants of the δ-globin gene will alter only the HbA$_2$ band and are never clinically significant. The actual amounts of different hemoglobin types that accumulate in vivo depend on the output from individual globin genes, the stability of the globin and hemoglobin products, and the posttranslational assembly of $\alpha\beta$ dimers that is dependent on the charge of the globin subunits (Chapter 8).

RECOMBINANT HEMOGLOBINS

Methods

Bacterial Expression Systems. First efforts to produce recombinant hemoglobins in *Escherichia coli* involved fusing globin cDNA to the coding region of a bacteriophage repressor protein that could then be digested to recover an intact globin chain (Olins and Lee, 1993). Expression levels were 10 percent to 20 percent. The insolubility of the fused globin was a useful feature that permitted its isolation. After recovery, the globin needed to be reconstituted in vitro with heme. Also, unintended deamination, acetylation, or incorporation of unusual amino acids such as norleucine or norvaline, were observed with this technique (Apostol et al., 1997). Misfolding of the tertiary structure of globin also occurred so that, for example, a small fraction of the recombinant hemoglobin had heme inserted with an abnormal tilt (Shen et al., 1997). Fortunately, this abnormal heme insertion could be easily corrected by deoxygenating the fraction with dithionate in the presence of CO, forming a ligand that can be subsequently removed by photolysis.

Second-generation efforts involved the coexpression of individual globins at a 2 percent to 10 percent level, but faced two problems: lack of N-terminal processing where the N-terminal methionine was not cleaved as usual; and unequal production of α- and β-globin chains. The first difficulty was surmounted by two alternative strategies (Hoffman et al., 1990). In one, valine was substituted for the initiator methionine, a change that resulted in a globin of correct sequence. Alternatively, methionyl aminopeptidase

was coexpressed in *E. coli*, with cleavage of the extra methionine. This approach, however, produced a mixture of processed and nonprocessed globin chains that needed further purification.

Yeast Expression Systems. An alternative to the *E. coli* approach was the use of yeast as an expression system for the cogeneration of α- and β-globin chains. N-terminal processing was present since yeasts have the required enzymes for this function, but the expression level was only 1 percent to 3 percent. Some evidence of misfolding was detected in a fraction of the human hemoglobins generated. Both types of unicellular expression experiments produced interesting recombinant mutants (see below).

Transgenic Mice and Pigs. Transgenic mice have been generated by microinjecting mouse oocytes with constructs containing the human β-globin gene cluster locus control region (LCR), a promoter, and either wild type or mutated globin genes. Constructs can be coinjected or a single construct can contain both α- and β-globin genes. Different lines of animals with the same globin gene-containing construct generate different levels of expression, probably because of different sites of transgene integration. Increased expression of the transgene can be achieved by crossing into the founder line and deletions or knockouts of the murine globins. Levels of transgene expression between 30 percent and 100 percent have been achieved in mice.

While transgenic mice can be useful for studying mutant hemoglobins and the pathogenesis of hemoglobinopathies (Chapter 34) or to test pharmacologic interventions or gene therapy strategies, they are ill-suited as a source of recombinant hemoglobins with potential utilization as blood substitutes. For this latter purpose, a transgenic pig model has been generated. Among the advantages of transgenic pigs are that large quantities of blood can be harvested containing high levels of human hemoglobin indistinguishable from the native form (Manjula et al., 1996). Pigs can grow to phenomenal sizes if fed sufficiently and a very large herd can be obtained from the founder in a few years due to high fecundity and short duration of pregnancy. Hemoglobin purification is much easier than with microbial expression systems (Kumar, 1995). An interesting aspect of the pig transgenic hemolysate is the absence of $\alpha_2{}^P\beta_2{}^H$ hybrids (Rao et al., 1996). This is not a result of the inability of pig α chain and human β chain to form dimers, because these dimers do form in vitro.

Interestingly, the $\alpha^P\beta^H$ dimer disappears in the presence of α^H at pH 6.0 and with MgCl at pH 7.0, conditions that dissociate $\alpha\beta$ dimer; only HbA is generated. This experiment suggests a lower thermodynamic sta-

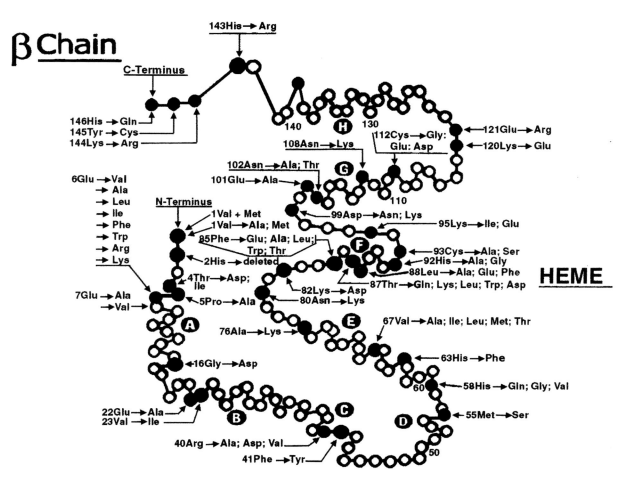

Figure 45.4. Recombinant mutations according to number of mutations introduced and type of globin chains modified. (From Huisman and Carver, 1998, with permission.)

bility of the $\alpha^P\beta^H$ dimer, since α^H chains are very successful in replacing α^P in the dimer. The other interspecies tetramer, $\alpha_2^H\beta_2^P$, is more stable than the human HbA tetramer.

In vivo, this effect will be seen in the formation of the dimer from isolated chains, and if there are enough α^H chains, they combine preferentially with β^P globin, compared to α^P chains, to form interspecies tetramers, because the interspecific tetramer is more stable than normal HbA.

Uses For and Types of Recombinant Hemoglobins

In the past 10 years, over 100 recombinant hemoglobins have been generated. Huisman and Carver (1998) have classified them according to the number of mutations introduced and the type of globin chain modified (Fig. 45.4). Recombinant hemoglobin molecules can be used to examine amino acid residues that assist or retard the polymerization of HbS (see Chapter 23). They have helped verify previous data on polymerization obtained using native mutants and have extended these types of studies to amino acid residues in globin not naturally substituted. Structure-function relationships of hemoglobin may also be further understood using recombinant hemoglobins, which have been useful in testing the two-state model, some allosteric interactions such as Cl⁻ binding to hemoglobin, and the structural basis of some of the other functions of hemoglobin

rMb(–D); rMb(–D→Ala⁵¹⁻⁵⁵) or rMb(–D)→Ala⁵¹⁻⁵⁴, Met⁵⁵) (Whitaker et al, 1995). These recombinants represent the deletion of the D helix (D-) in myoglobin and its substitution by 5 Ala or 4 Ala and 1 Met. Myoglobin and β-globin chains have a D helix while α-globin chains do not. The D helix is not involved in ligand binding. Its deletion or substitution did not affect the heme pocket. Instead, the crystal structure demonstrated a diffuse electron density between C and E helices in Mb(–D), indicating highly mobile or heterogeneous conformation in this region when the D helix was absent. This observation, plus the fiftyfold increase of heme lost from

Mb(–D), demonstrated that the D helix stabilizes the heme attachment to myoglobin and, by extension, β-hemoglobin chains (Whitaker et al., 1995). Heme loss was also high in Mb(–D)→Ala$^{51-55}$ but not in Mb(–D)→Ala$^{51-54}$, Met^{55}. In accordance with the previous interpretation was the observation that the crystal structure of Mb(–D)→Ala$^{51-54}$, Met^{55} had a well-defined and stable D helix. Deletion of the D helix in human β-globin chains also caused a marked increase in heme loss, which was not stabilized when an α-globin chain is engineered to contain a D helix. This suggested that the D helix of β-globin chains stabilizes both its own heme and α-chain heme.

rHbβ67(E11) Val→Thr (Perchik et al., 1996). Residues E7 and E11 are directly involved with the structural features of the distal heme pocket and engaged directly in ligand binding. Replacement of αHis E7 by recombinant hemoglobins that alter the size or polarity of the side chain have dramatic effects on ligand binding. The same is not true for recombinant substituted βHis E7. Functional studies of E11 substitutions with increasingly bulkier side chains (Val>Ile>Phe) showed decreased ligand binding pari-passu in α chains but not in β chains, except that ile sterically blocks access to the heme. Perchik and colleagues studied the rHbβ67 (E11) Val→Thr crystal structure and other properties to test by modeling the prediction that β67 Thr will form a hydrogen bond with a carbonyl of β63 His (E7) and possibly to a δN of the same residue (Perchik et al., 1996). The crystal structure showed very little tertiary alteration in the vicinity of the mutation, confirming these predictions, but this isosteric substitution does not accept an extra water molecule in the heme pocket, as found in **Hb Chico** (β66 Lys→Thr). A twofold increase in oxygen affinity and rate of oxidation must come from the increase in polarity introduced in the heme pocket by the bond between β67 Thr and β63 His.

rHb α96 Val→Trp. rHb α96 Val→Trp affects the α$_1$β$_2$ interface (Kim et al, 1995). This nonisosteric substitution produces a hemoglobin with low oxygen affinity but high cooperativity, which does not dissociate abnormally into dimers. The CO (R) form of this recombinant can be turned into the T state by the addition of inositol hexaphosphate and low temperature without changing the ligand state. No spectroscopic evidence was found for tertiary changes around the heme group or at the α$_1$β$_2$ interface. Dynamic modeling suggested that this is the consequence of a new H bond between α96 Trp and β99 Asp in the α$_1$β$_2$ interface. Fourier maps demonstrated that the α96 trp is in a different conformation than that predicted by modeling, underscoring the limitations of this technique. The indol N is engaged in a

novel water-mediated H bond across the α$_1$β$_2$ T interface with β101 Glu, providing stabilization of the T state as the structural basis for its low oxygen affinity (Puius et al., 1998).

Recombinant hemoglobins have the potential to be used as hemoglobin-based blood substitutes. Hemoglobin-based blood substitutes are a reasonable approach to fulfill the need for a shelf-storable oxygen carrying solution for use in surgery, trauma, and other emergencies. They have the advantages of ready availability, long shelf life, absence of the need for typing and cross matching, sterility, lack of immunosuppressive effects, and lower viscosity compared to blood (Cohn, 1997). Hemoglobin-based blood substitutes have developed rapidly and after passing myriad safety studies are in the process of efficacy evaluation. Most of the compounds presently being studied are cross-linked forms of human or bovine hemoglobin. Recombinant hemoglobins must be designed to overcome the very high oxygen affinity of free hemoglobin that hampers oxygen delivery. They should not readily dissociate into dimers, their molecular size should allow retention in the vascular compartment, and the tendency of free hemoglobin to turn into methemoglobin should be reduced.

An example of this type of molecular engineering, besides the α96 Trp recombinant mutant discussed above, is **rHb β108 Asn→Lys (rHb 1.1)** (Olson et al., 1997). In this low oxygen affinity hemoglobin, dimer formation inhibition was accomplished by introducing a glycine residue between two normal α-globin chains to produce one covalently continuous di-α chain. At a 2.0 Å resolution, crystal structure of this recombinant showed that the deoxy form of the molecule adopted the classic T state. At 2.6 Å resolution, the liganded state adopted a new quaternary state, the B form. Most strikingly, an H bond between β108 Lys and β35 Tyr was blocked in the T→B transition. The B state structure appears to be the consequence of the glycine bridge between the two α-globin chains. In another example using myoglobin, the distal portions of the heme pocket were modified to generate low oxygen affinity and decreased methemoglobin formation. Oxygen affinity was adjusted by mutating residues Leu (B10), His (E7), and Val (E11) with large polar residues that inhibit NO-induced changes and autooxidation.

Recombinant hemoglobins may be used to develop efficient synthesis of pharmaco-peptides. Chemical synthesis of peptides is hindered by high cost, difficulty in achieving purity, and lack of efficiency. Alternatively, fusion proteins involving α-globin chains fused with the pharmaco-active peptide has been accomplished. (Sharma et al., 1994). In one construct, an α-globin gene was fused with a recombination protein cleavage site and the 16 mer α-endorphin or the 26 mer magainin as an extension under the control of the β-globin gene LCR. Transgenic mouse red cells expressed this fused protein at more than 25 percent of total hemoglobin without apparent side effects.

CONCLUSION

In conclusion, recombinant hemoglobins have opened the door for extended testing of hypotheses of how normal hemoglobin works (structural-functional interactions), but have also stimulated the field of hemoglobin-based blood substitutes, by providing new and state-of-the art compounds of potential clinical interest. We should expect a rapid expansion of both of these avenues of research in the next decade.

References

Abkowitz, JL, Linenberger, ML, Newton, MA et al. (1990) Evidence for the maintenance of hematopoiesis in a large animal by sequential activation of stem-cells. *Proc. Natl. Acad. Sci. U.S.A.* 87: 9066.

Abramson, RK, Rucknagel, DL, Shreffler, DC, and Saave, JJ. (1970). Homozygous Hb J Tongariki: Evidence for only one alpha chain structural locus in Melanesians. *Science* 169: 194–196.

Adams, JG III and Heller, P. (1977). Hemoglobin Arlington Park: A new hemoglobin variant with two amino acid substitutions in the β chain. *Hemoglobin* 1: 419–426.

Adams, JG, Steinberg, MH, Newman, MV et al. (1981). β-Thalassemia present in *cis* to a new β-chain structural variant, Hb Vicksburg [β 75 (E19)Leu→0]. *Proc. Natl. Acad. Sci. U.S.A.* 78: 469–473.

Adams, JG, Morrison, WT, and Steinberg, MH. (1982). Hemoglobin Parchman: Double crossover within a single human gene. *Science* 218: 291–293.

Adams, JG, Hardy, CL, and Steinberg, MH. (1991). Disappearance of the protein of a somatic mutation: A possible example of stem cell inactivation. *Am. J. Physiol. Cell Physiol.* 261: C448–C454.

Anonymous. (1993). IHIC variants list. *Hemoglobin* 17: 89–177.

Apostol, I, Levine, J, Lippincott, J et al. (1997). Incorporation of norvaline to leucine positions in recombinant human hemoglobin expressed in *Escherichia coli. J. Biol. Chem.* 272: 28980–28988.

Atwater, J, Schwartz, E, Erslev, AJ et al. (1960). Sickling of erythrocytes in a patient with thalassemia-hemoglobin-1 disease. *N. Engl. J. Med.* 263: 1215.

Baine, RM, Rucknagel, DL, Dublin, PA, and Adams, JG III. (1976). Trimodality in the proportion of hemoglobin G Philadelphia in heterozygotes: Evidence for heterogeneity in the number of human alpha chain loci. *Proc. Natl. Acad. Sci. U.S.A.* 73: 3633–3636.

Baklouti, F, Ouzana, R, Gonnet, C et al. (1989). β⁺ Thalassemia in *cis* of a sickle gene: Occurrence of a promoter mutation on a beta S chromosome. *Blood* 74: 1817–1822.

Beale, D and Lehmann, H. (1965). Abnormal haemoglobins and the genetic code. *Nature* 207: 259–261.

Blackwell, RQ, Boon, WH, Liu, C, and Weng, MI. (1972). Hemoglobin J Singapore: Alpha 78 asn-Asp; alpha 70 ala-gly. *Biochim. Biophys. Acta* 278: 482–490.

Blouquit, Y, Bardakdjian, J, Lena-Russo, D et al. (1989). Hb Bruxelles: α₂ᴬ β₂ 41 Or 42(C7 or CD1) phe deleted. *Hemoglobin* 13: 465–474.

Boissel, J-P, Kasper, TJ, Shah, SC et al. (1985). Amino-terminal processing of proteins: HbSouth Florida a variant with retention of initiator methionine and Nᵃ-acetylation. *Proc. Natl. Acad. Sci. U.S.A.* 82: 8448–8452.

Bowden, DK, Pressley, L, Higgs, DR et al. (1982). Alpha-globin gene deletions associated with Hb J Tongariki. *Br. J. Haematol.* 51: 243–249.

Brennan, SO, Williamson, D, Symans, WA, and Carrell, RW. (1983). Two unstable hemoglobins in one individual: Hb Atlanta (β75 Leu→Pro) and Hb Coventry (β141 Leu deleted). *Hemoglobin* 7: 303–312.

Brennan, SO, Shaw, J, Allen, J, and George, PM. (1992). β 141 Leu is not deleted in the unstable haemoglobin Atlanta-Coventry but is replaced by a novel amino acid of mass 129 daltons. *Br. J. Haematol.* 81: 99–103.

Brennan, SO, Shaw, JG, George, PM, and Huisman, THJ. (1993). Posttranslational modification of β141 Leu associated with the β9 Leu→Pro mutation in Hb Atlanta. *Hemoglobin* 17: 1–7.

Brudzinski, CJ, Sisco, KL, Ferrucc, SJ, and Rucknagel, DL. (1984). The occurrence of the αᴳ Philadelphia-globin allele on a double-locus chromosome. *Am. J. Hum. Genet.* 36: 101–109.

Bunn, HF and Forget, BG. (1986). *Hemoglobin: Molecular, Genetic and Clinical Aspects*. Philadelphia: W.B. Saunders.

Casey, R, Kynoch, AM, Lang, A et al. (1978). Double heterozygosity for two unstable hemoglobins: HbSydney (β 67[E11] Val→Ala) and HbCoventry (β 141 [H9] Leu deleted). *Br. J. Haematol.* 38: 195–209.

Charache, S, Brimhall, B, and Jones, RT. (1975). Polycythemia produced by hemoglobin Osler (β 145 (HC2) tyr→Asp). *Johns Hopkins Med. J.* 136: 132–136.

Charache, S, Fox, J, McCurdy, PR et al. (1977). Postsynthetic deamidation of hemoglobin Providence (Beta 82 lys replaced by asn, Asp) and its effect on oxygen transport. *J. Clin. Invest.* 59: 652–658.

Charache, S, Raik, E, Holtzclaw, D et al. (1987). Pseudosickling of hemoglobin Setif. *Blood* 70: 237–242.

Cohn, SM. (1997). The current status of haemoglobin-based blood. *Ann. Med.* 29: 371–376.

Coleman, MB, Adams, JG III, Walker, AM et al. (1993). HbSan Diego [β 109(G11)Val→Met] in an Iranian: Further evidence for a mutational hot spot at position 109 of the β-globin gene. *Hemoglobin* 17: 543–545.

Coleman MB, Lu, Z-H, Smith, CM II et al. (1995) Two missense mutations in the β-globin gene can cause severe β thalassemia. Hemoglobin Medicine Lake (β32[B14]leucine→glutamine; 98 [FG5] valine→methionine). *J. Clin. Invest.* 95: 503–509.

Cooper, DN and Krawczak, M. (1993). *Human Gene Mutation*. Oxford: BIOS Scientific Publishers.

Drupt, F, Poillot, M-H, Leclerc, M et al. (1976). Hemoglobine instable (mutant alpha) se singularisant par la formation de pseudo-drapanocytes in vitro. *Nouv. Presse Med.* 5: 1066.

Flatz, G, Kinderlerer, J, Kilmartin, JV, and Lehmann, H. (1971). Haemoglobin Tak: A variant with additional residues at the end of the β-chains. *Lancet* 1: 732–733.

Fugisawa, K, Yamashiro, Y, Hattori, Y et al. (1993). Hb Higashitochigi (Hb HT) [β 24(B6) or β 25 (B7) glycine deleted]: A new unstable hemoglobin expressing cyanosis. *Hemoglobin* 17: 463–466.

Garel, MC, Blouquitt, Y, Rosa, J, and Romero Garcia, C. (1975). Hemoglobin Castilla β 32 (B14) Leu→Arg; a new unstable variant producing severe hemolytic disease. *FEBS Lett.* 58: 145–148.

George, PM, Myles, T, Williamson, D et al. (1992). A family with haemolytic anaemia and three β-globins: The deletion in haemoglobin Atlanta-Coventry (β 75 Leu→Pro, 141 Leu deleted) is not present at the nucleotide level. *Br. J. Haematol.* 81: 93–98.

Hoffman, SJ, Looker, DL, Roehrich, JM et al. (1990). Expression of fully functional tetrameric human hemoglobin in Escherichia Coli. *Proc. Natl. Acad. Sci. U.S.A.* 87: 8521–8525.

Honig, GR, Green, D, Shamsuddin, M et al. (1973). Hemoglobin Abraham Lincoln β 32 (B14) Leucine→Proline. An unstable variant producing severe hemolytic disease. *J. Clin. Invest.* 52: 1746–1755.

Honig, GR, Shamsuddin, M, Mason, RG, and Vida, LN. (1978). Hemoglobin Lincoln Park: A βδ (anti-Lepore) variant with an amino acid deletion in the δ chain derived segment. *Proc. Natl. Acad. Sci. U.S.A.* 75: 1475–1479.

Hoyer, JD, Wick, MJ, Thibodeau, SN et al. (1998). Hb Tak confirmed by DNA analysis: Not expressed as thalassemia in a Hb Tak/Hb E compound heterozygote. *Hemoglobin* 22: 45–52.

Huisman, THJ and Carver, MF. (1998). Recombinant hemoglobin variants [editorial]. *Hemoglobin* 22: 99–112.

Huisman, THJ, Wilson, JB, Gravely, M, and Hubbard, M. (1974). Hemoglobin Grady: The first example of a variant with elongated chains due to an insertion of residues. *Proc. Natl. Acad. Sci. U.S.A.* 71: 3270–3273.

Huisman, THJ, Headlee, MG, Wilson, JB et al. (1984). HbWayne the frameshift variant with extended α chains observed in a caucasian family from Alabama. *Hemoglobin* 8: 1–15.

Huisman, THJ, Carver, MFH, and Baysal, E. (1997). *A Syllabus of Thalassemia Mutations (1997).* Augusta: The Sickle Cell Anemia Foundation. pp. 1–309.

Huisman, THJ, Carver, MFH, and Efremov, GD. (1998). *A Syllabus of Human Hemoglobin Variants (Second Edition).* Augusta: Sickle Cell Anemia Foundation. p. 396.

Hutt, PJ, Donaldson, MH, Khatri, J et al. (1996). Hemoglobin S hemoglobin Osler: A case with 3 β globin chains. DNA sequence (AAT) proves that Hb Osler is β 145 Tyr→Asn. *Am. J. Hematol.* 52: 305–309.

Itchayanan, D, Svasti, J, Srisomsap, C et al. (1999). Hb G-Coushatta [β22(B4)Glu→Ala] in Thailand. *Hemoglobin* 23: 69–72.

Jue, DJ, Johnson, MH, Patchen, LC, and Moo-Penn, W. (1979). Hemoglobin Dunn: α6 (A4) apartic acid→asparagine. *Hemoglobin* 3: 137–143.

Kamel, K, el-Najjar, A, Chen, SS et al. (1985). Hb Doha or alpha 2 beta 2[X-N-Met-1 (NA1)Val→Glu] a new beta-chain abnormal hemoglobin observed in a Qatari female. *Biochim. Biophys. Acta* 831: 257–260.

Kavanaugh, JS, Moo-Penn, WF, and Arnone, A. (1993). Accommodation of insertions in helices: The mutation in hemoglobin Catonsville (Pro 37α-Glu-Thr 38α) generates a $3_{10} \rightarrow \alpha$ bulge. *Biochemistry* 32: 2509–2513.

Kawata, R, Ohba, Y, Yamamoto, K et al. (1988). Hyperunstable hemoglobin Korriyama anti-Hb Gun Hill insertion of five residues in the β chain. *Hemoglobin* 12: 311–321.

Kim, H-W, Shen, TJ, Sun, DP et al. (1995). A novel low oxygen affinity recombinant hemoglobin (alpha 96 val→trp): Switching quaternary structure without changing the ligation state. *J. Mol. Biol.* 248: 867–882.

Kumar, R. (1995). Recombinant hemoglobins as blood substitutes: A biotechnology prospective. Mini-review. *Proc. Soc. Exp. Biol. Med.* 208: 150–158.

Li, C, Wilson, D, Plonczynski, M et al. (1999). Genetic studies suggest a multicentric origin for hemoglobin G-Coushatta [β22(B4)Glu→Ala]. *Hemoglobin* 23: 57–67.

Liebhaber, SA, Rappaport, EF, Cash, FE et al. (1984). Hemoglobin I mutation encoded at both alpha-globin loci on the same chromosome: Concerted evolution in the human genome. *Science* 226: 1449–1451.

Manjula, BN, Kumar, R, Sun, DP et al. (1996). Correct assembly of human normal adult hemoglobin when expressed in transgenic swine: Chemical, conformational and functional equivalence with the human-derived protein. *Protein Sci.* 5: 956–965.

Milner, PF and Huisman, THJ. (1976). Studies on the proportion and synthesis of haemoglobin G Philadelphia in red cells of heterozygotes a homozygote and a heterozygote for both haemoglobin G and α thalassaemia. *Br. J. Haematol.* 34: 207–220.

Molchanova, TP, Pobedimskaya, DD, and Huisman, THJ. (1994a). The differences in quantities of α2- and α1-globin gene variants in heterozygotes. *Br. J. Haematol.* 88: 300–306.

Molchanova, TP, Pobedimskaya, DD, Ye, Z, and Huisman, THJ. (1994b). Two different mutations in codon 68 are observed in Hb G- Philadelphia heterozygotes. *Am. J. Hematol.* 45: 345–346.

Moo-Penn, W, Bechtel, K, Jue, D et al. (1975). The presence of hemoglobin S and C Harlem in an individual in the United States. *Blood* 46: 363–367.

Moo-Penn, W, Bechtel, K, Schmidt, RM et al. (1977). Hemoglobin Raleigh (β 1 valine→acetylalanine). structural and functional characterization. *Biochemistry* 16: 4872–4879.

Noguchi, CT, Mohandas, N, Blanchette-Mackie, J et al. (1991). Hemoglobin aggregation and pseudosickling in vitro of hemoglobin Setif-containing erythrocytes. *Am. J. Hematol.* 36: 131–139.

Ohba, Y, Ami, M, Imai, K, Komatsu, K et al. (1998). Hb Masuda [β 114 (G16) Leu→Met, 119 (GH2) gly→Asp]: A hemoglobin with two substitutions in the β globin chain. *Hemoglobin* 13: 753–759.

Old, JM, Clegg, JB, Weatherall, DJ, and Booth, PB. (1978). Haemoglobin J Tongariki is associated with α thalassaemia. *Nature* 273: 319–320.

Olins, PO and Lee, SC. (1993). Recent advances in heterologous gene expression in *Escherichia col. Curr. Opin. Biotechnol.* 4: 520–525.

Olson, JS, Eich, RF, Smith, LP et al. (1997). Protein engineering strategies for designing more stable hemoglobin-based blood substitutes. *Artific. Cell Blood Substitute Immob. Biotechnol.* 2: 227–241.

Paleari, R, Paglietti, E, Mosca, A et al. (1999). Post-translational deamidation of proteins: The case of hemoglobin J Sardegna [α50(CD8)His→Asn→Asp]. *Clin. Chem.* 45: 21–28.

Perchik, I, Ji, X, Fidelis, K et al. (1996). Crystallographic, molecular modeling, and biophysical characterization of the Valine β67 (E11)→ Threonine variant of hemoglobin. *Biochemistry* 35: 1935–1945.

Perutz, MF. (1990). Frequency of abnormal human haemoglobins caused by C→T transitions in CpG dinucleotides. *Biophys. Chem.* 37: 25–29.

Prchal, JT, Cashman, DP, and Kan, YW. (1986). Hemoglobin Long Island is caused by a single mutation (adenine to cytosine) resulting in a failure to cleave amino-terminal methionine. *Proc. Natl. Acad. Sci. U.S.A.* 83: 24–27.

Puius, YA, Zou, M, Ho, NT et al. (1998). Novel water-mediated hydrogen bonds as the structural basis of the low oxygen affinity of the blood substitute candidate rHb (alpha 96 Val→Trp). *Biochemistry* 37: 9258–9265.

Qin, WB, Pobedimskaya, DD, Molchanova, TP et al. (1994). Hb Fannin-Lubbock in five Spanish families is characterized by two mutations: β 111 GTC→CTC (Val→Leu) and β 119 GGC→GAC (Gly→Asp). *Hemoglobin* 18: 297–306.

Raik, E, Powell, E, Fleming, P, and Gordon, S. (1983). Hemoglobin Setif and in vitro pseudosickling noted in a family with co-existent alpha and beta thalassemia. *Pathology* 15: 453–456.

Rao, NJ, Manjula, BN, Kumar, R, and Acharya AS. (1996). Chimeric hemoglobins-hybrids of human and swine hemoglobin: Assembly and stability of interspecies hybrids. *Protein Sci.* 5: 956–965.

Romero, WER, Castillo, M, Chaves, MA et al. (1996). HbCosta Rica or α$_2$ β$_2$77(EF1)His→Arg: The first example of a somatic cell mutation in a globin gene. *Hum. Genet.* 97: 829–833.

Safaya, S and Rieder, RF. (1988). Dysfunctional α-globin gene in hemoglobin H disease in blacks: A dinucleotide deletion produces a frameshift and a termination codon. *J. Biol. Chem.* 263: 4328–4332.

Schneider, RG, Haggard, ME, McNutt, CW et al. (1964). Hemoglobin G$_{Coushatta}$: A new variant in an American Indian family. *Science* 143: 197.

Seid-Akhaven, M, Winter, WP, Abramson, R, and Rucknagel, DL. (1976). Hemoglobin Wayne: A frameshift mutation detected in human hemoglobin alpha chains. *Proc. Natl. Acad. Sci. U.S.A.* 73: 882–886.

Sharma, A, Khoury-Christianson, AM, White, S et al. (1994). High efficiency synthesis of human α-endorphin and magainin in the erythrocytes of transgenic mice: A production system for therapeutic peptides. *Proc. Natl. Acad. Sci. U.S.A.* 91: 9337–9341.

Shen, TJ, Ho, NT, Zou, M et al. (1997). *Protein Eng.* 10: 1085–1097.

Smetanina, NS, Gu, LH, Romero, WER et al. (1996). The relative levels of different types of β-mRNA and β-globin in BFU-E derived colonies from patients with β chain variants; further evidence for somatic mosaicism in the HbCosta Rica carrier [β 77(EF1)His→Arg]. *Hemoglobin* 20: 199–212.

Vasseur, C, Blouquit, Y, Kister, J et al. (1992). Hemoglobin Thionville. An α-chain variant with a substitution of a glutamate for valine at NA-1 and having an acetylated methionine NH$_2$ terminus. *J. Biol. Chem.* 267: 12682–12691.

Wajcman, H, Belkhodja, O, and Labie, D. (1972). HbSetif: αG1(94)Asp→Tyr. A new alpha chain hemoglobin variant with substitution of the residue involved in a hydrogen bond between unlike subunits. *FEBS Lett* 27: 298.

Wajcman, H, Vasseur, C, Blouquit, Y et al. (1991). Hemoglobin Redondo [β 92(F8) His→Asn]: An unstable hemoglobin variant associated with heme loss which occurs in two forms. *Am. J. Hematol.* 38: 194–200.

Wajcman, H, Kister, J, Vasseur, C et al. (1992a). Structure of the EF corner favors deamidation of asparaginyl residues in hemoglobin: The example of Hb La Roche-sur- Yon [β 81 (EF5) Leu → His]. *Biochim. Biophys. Acta Mol. Basis Dis.* 1138: 127–132.

Wajcman, H, Blouquit, Y, Vasseur, C et al. (1992b). Two new human hemoglobin variants caused by unusual mutational events: Hb Zaïre contains a five residue repetition within the α-chain and Hb Duino has two residues substituted in the β-chain. *Hum. Genet.* 89: 676–680.

Whitaker, TL, Berry, MB, Ho, EL et al. (1995). The D helix in myoglobin and in the subunit of hemoglobin is required for the retention of heme. *Biochemistry* 34: 8221–8226.

Williamson, D, Brown, KP, Langdown, JV, and Baglin, TP. (1995). Haemoglobin Dhofar is linked to the codon 29 C → T (IVS- 1 nt- 3) splice mutation which causes β$^+$ thalassaemia. *Br. J. Haematol.* 90: 229–231.

Winter, WP. (1986). *Hemoglobin Variants in Human Populations.* Boca Raton, FL: CRC Press.

Wright, HT. (1991). Sequence and structure determinants of nonenzymatic deamidation of asparagine and glutamine residues in proteins. *Protein Eng.* 4: 283–294.

ACQUIRED DISORDERS OF HEMOGLOBIN

RONALD L. NAGEL

Hemoglobins modified by carbon monoxide (CO) or oxidized to methemoglobin are the basis of a group of acquired and genetic diseases, the "dyshemoglobinemias." While rare, they can have serious clinical implications, and because effective treatments are available their timely identification is clinically important.

Most—not all—hemoglobin disorders that are clinically encountered result from globin gene mutations. In the following chapter we discuss abnormal hemoglobins that are not a consequence of disordered globin structure or synthesis. Hemoglobin can bind CO besides binding oxygen. CO, while having a lower binding constant for hemoglobin than oxygen, has a much lower dissociation rate, resulting in a high equilibrium constant, precluding normal oxygen binding. High levels of COHb, a result of CO-heme binding,

may cause life-threatening toxicity. COHb can cause accidental death and is a common method of suicide. The most common cause of high COHb levels is tobacco smoking. One example of an acquired hemoglobin disorder interacting with a genetic trait is seen in the carriers of the unstable Hb Zurich, who may have inordinately high levels of COHb Zurich, particularly if they are smokers. Ironically, this feature decreases the level of hemolysis.

Heme iron can be oxidized from its usual ferrous form to ferric heme that forms methemoglobin. Methemoglobin, like COHb, is also not capable of transporting oxygen. Methemoglobin can be produced by exogenous agents and methemoglobinemia can be found in people with mutant forms of the enzyme that mediates its reduction.

We also consider pathophysiologic, genetic, and clinical aspects of carboxyhemoglobinemia, methemoglobinemia, and sulfhemoglobinemia. NOHb (NO binding at the heme level) and nitrosohemoglobin (NO binding side chains of amino acid residues—for example, S-nitrosation of β 93 Cys), the result of nitric oxide-hemoglobin interaction, a subject of physiologic interest and perhaps clinical importance, is also discussed.

As we come to better understand the nature of genetic diversity, the distinction between environmental and genetic causes of dyshemoglobinemia is often blurred because many acquired dyshemoglobins are in effect the consequence of an environmental challenge in a genetically predisposed individual. Well-known examples of this interaction are the effects of primaquine and fava beans in G-6-PD-deficient individuals. One problem in understanding the clinical consequences of noxious environmental agents is that most of them are dangerous only to the susceptible subset of the population having the permissive genetic background. Without knowing who is at risk, the dangers of certain environmental toxins are not easily identifiable.

46

CO-, NO-, Met-, And Sulf-Hemoglobinemias: The Dyshemoglobins

RONALD L. NAGEL
ERNST R. JAFFÉ

Hemoglobin can bind gases in the environment and in blood plasma other than oxygen, including carbon monoxide (CO) and nitric oxide (NO). Carboxyhemoglobin (COHb) precludes normal oxygen transport and is toxic. Nitrosohemoglobin has critical physiologic functions. Normal hemoglobin can be oxidized to methemoglobin by exogenous agents, and methemoglobinemia can be found in people with mutant forms of the enzyme, which mediates its reduction. Hemoglobins that are modified by CO or oxidation are the basis of a group of acquired and genetic diseases that are rare but can have serious clinical implications. We call these disorders the dyshemoglobinemias.

CARBON MONOXIDE POISONING: CARBOXY (CO)-HEMOGLOBINEMIA

Background

CO, a toxic gas, is unusually dangerous because it is odorless, colorless and tasteless, increasing the probability of serious and life-threatening accidents when high concentrations are present in the environment (Vreman et al., 1995). CO has a low solubility in water and is relatively inert because of its high bond enthalpy, the highest of any molecule. Still, it combines with high affinity to the heme of hemoglobin—and with lesser affinities to

myoglobin and cytochromes—at the iron core, a site that it shares with oxygen (Antonini and Brunori, 1971). Binding of CO to hemoglobin is the root of its toxicity. An excellent summary of CO chemistry is provided by Bunn and Forget (1986).

At equilibrium in physiologic conditions, its affinity for hemoglobin is about 240 times greater than that of oxygen. This very high equilibrium constant is the result of reaction kinetics. Contrary to popular belief, CO reacts more slowly than oxygen with the heme of hemoglobin. At 20°C and pH 7.0, the "on" rate for CO is 20 mol/L^{-1} sec^{-1} versus 470 mol/L^{-1} sec^{-1} for O$_2$. It was long suspected that the steric constraints present in the heme pocket make it more difficult for CO to reach the heme group. Indeed, x-ray crystallography and neutron crystal structure showed that the Fe-C-O geometry was not "linear" as supposed, but "bent," an uncomfortable position for CO (Cheng and Schoenborn, 1991). Once CO is bound to heme, its "off" rate is only 0.015 sec^{-1} versus 35 sec^{-1} for O$_2$ (Antonini and Brunori, 1971). This extraordinarily slow process produces a very high affinity constant of CO for heme and a life-threatening danger for organisms exposed to high levels of CO. A precise and alternative picture of the steric mechanisms involved in the inhibition of CO binding to heme proteins has recently been proposed (Kachalova et al., 1999). These authors compared unliganded myoglobin and CO myoglobin at a resolution of 1.15 Å, and found perfect linearity of the Fe-C-O complex, not a "bent" configuration. This geometry was possible because a concerted motion of heme, iron, and helices E and F relieved the steric constraints (Fig. 46.1).

Once two molecules of CO are bound to hemoglobin, the molecule switches to the relaxed (R) state, further endangering those exposed to CO, and the two globin chains that remain capable of binding oxygen will be in their high affinity conformation. This high ligand affinity will make more difficult the delivery of oxygen to the tissues by the remaining oxygen binding sites. As a consequence of this phenomenon, called the Darling-Roughton effect (Darling and Roughton, 1942), the oxygen equilibrium curve of blood will be shifted to the left pari passu with increasing CO levels.

In the absence of environmental CO, the blood of adults contains about 1 to 2 percent COHb. This represents about 80 percent of the total body CO, the rest is probably sequestered in myoglobin and cytochromes. This CO is endogenously produced (Sjostrand, 1949). Its predominant origin is the degradation of heme by the rate-limiting heme oxygenase/cytochrome P-450 complex, which produces CO and biliverdin. CO levels in expired air have

Martin H. Steinberg, Bernard G. Forget, Douglas R. Higgs, and Ronald L. Nagel, editors. *Disorders of Hemoglobin: Genetics, Pathophysiology, and Clinical Management.* © 2001 Cambridge University Press. All rights reserved.

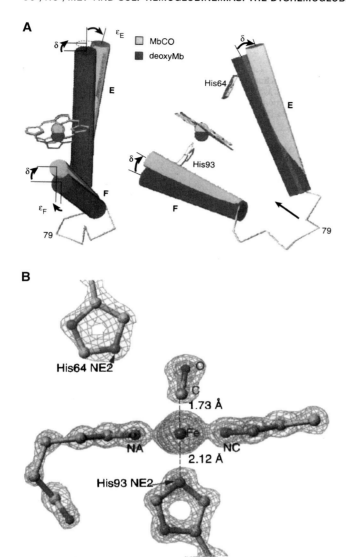

Figure 46.1. CO binding to myoglobin. (A) Binding of CO at the heme group. (B) CO binding to heme is possible because the E helix (and His 64) moves away, making space for the CO molecule without the need for bending.

hematomas, and infection tend to increase CO production up to threefold. Age and development also have an effect. Fetuses and newborns have double the normal adult levels of COHb, and levels can be much higher with hemolytic disease of the newborn.

Not all endogenous CO is the product of normal metabolism. Drugs such as diphenylhydantoin and phenobarbital, by inducing the cytochrome P-450 complex, increase CO production, as does any drug that causes low level hemolysis.

Endogenous CO production might have important physiologic consequences (EPA, 1991). Like its analog, NO, a vasoactive agent that participates in signal transduction, CO can bind to the heme of soluble guanylate cyclase and to the iron/sulfur centers of macrophage enzymes. Guanylate cyclase regulates cyclic guanosine-3′, 5′-monophosphate (cGMP), a second messenger involved in many cellular functions, which in turn regulates kinases, transport proteins, and phosphodiesterases. Any physiologic significance of CO in these reactions remains to be determined.

Exogenous sources of CO include atmospheric CO, which is a product of incomplete combustion and oxidation of hydrocarbons, and natural sources (Marks et al., 1991). COHb can be increased at high altitude when ambient CO is increased by improperly ventilated wood burning stoves. High altitude erythrocytosis and hypoxemia and our imperfect adaptation to high altitude decrease oxygen intake and prolong CO excretion, increasing COHb levels (McGrath, 1992).

Carbon Monoxide: Chronic Intoxication

In adults, symptoms of CO-hemoglobinemia might include irritability, nausea, lethargy, headaches, and sometimes a flulike condition. Higher COHb levels produce somnolence, palpitations, cardiomegaly, and hypertension and may contribute to atherosclerosis.

Chronic CO poisoning can produce erythrocytosis whose magnitude varies with the level of COHb. By increasing red cell production, chronic CO poisoning can mask the mild anemia of thalassemia trait or other acquired or genetic chronic hemolytic disorders.

Elimination of CO from the body is achieved by two mechanisms. Pulmonary excretion is by far the principal means of CO elimination. As the "off" rate of CO from hemoglobin is exceedingly slow, at 1 atmosphere, the half-life of COHb is 5 hours and 20 minutes; breathing 100 percent O_2 in a hyperbaric chamber can reduce it to 23 minutes. CO is catabolized by cytochrome oxidase, but this comprises a very small component of the CO elimination process.

Range of CO Levels. In adults, the normal level of COHb is less than 1 to 2 percent, but this low con-

been used as an index of hemolysis, although the difficulty of standardization and the availability of simpler means of assessing red cell destruction have not favored the widespread use of this technique (Coburn et al., 1964, 1966). Further degradation of biliverdin to bilirubin by biliverdin reductase renders a stoichiometry in which one molecule of hemoglobin, by oxidation of the α-methane bridge of the tetrapyrrole ring, generates one molecule of CO and one molecule of biliverdin.

Endogenous CO levels differ among individuals. Caloric restriction, dehydration, and the Asiatic race (Japanese and Amerindians) seem to generate higher endogenous levels of CO. Hemolytic anemia,

centration is rarely found in urban centers. Hemolysis can produce COHb levels of more than 2 percent. Levels more than 3 percent must have an exogenous origin, except for rare conditions as occur in carriers of the abnormal hemoglobin, Hb Zurich (Chapter 44) where because of the amino acid substitution in the heme pocket, CO can bind with higher affinity (Nagel, 1995).

The United States Environmental Protection Agency (EPA) considers an acceptable exposure time to be 1 hour to 25 parts per million (ppm) CO or a 8 hours exposure to 9 ppm. This exposure would raise the COHb by 1.5 percent. Pregnant women and fetuses are particularly at risk (Balster et al., 1991), because they already have higher levels of COHb. In addition, the oxygen affinity of HbF is shifted to the left (Benesch et al., 1972; Engel et al., 1969) owing to its lack of 2,3 BPG binding, making the Darling-Roughton effect particularly pernicious; this is one reason why cigarette smoking during pregnancy is hazardous to the fetus.

Etiology of Chronic CO Intoxication. The most frequent exogenous source of CO is cigarette smoking, which can increase the COHb level to 15 percent. Pregnant women, fetuses, neonates, and infants are particularly susceptible to CO poisoning from smoking (Balster et al., 1991). One, two, or three packets a day may increase COHb levels from 5 to 15 percent. By increasing hemoglobin-O_2 affinity, COHb may cause erythrocytosis in smokers. In patients with chronic lung disease who have perfusion-ventilation mismatch and are exposed to CO, O_2 is transferred from ventilated blood to COHb in blood from perfused but unventilated alveoli, further increasing hypoxemia. Hypoxemia and carboxyhemoglobinemia are a nasty combination.

Houses with defective heating exhaust systems and vehicles that leak CO into the passenger compartment, either because of mechanical failure or driving with the rear hatch-door open, are the second most common cause of chronic CO exposure.

Occupations that involve a high risk for CO intoxication include garage work with improper ventilation, toll booth attendants, tunnel workers, firefighters, and workers exposed to paint remover, aerosol propellent, or organic solvents containing dichloromethane (Stewart et al., 1972).

Treatment. Removing the patient from the source of environmental CO is usually curative. If the COHb level is high, breathing 100 percent O_2 will increase the rate of CO removal. Hyperbaric oxygen, which has complications of its own such as bronchial irritation and pulmonary edema, should be reserved for exceptional cases of CO intoxication. In most cases,

by the time the patient is brought into a hyperbaric chamber, the simple breathing of 100 percent O_2 has reduced COHb sufficiently to make the procedure unnecessary.

Carbon Monoxide Acute Intoxication

COHb levels above 20 percent are usually required before symptoms appear. Accidental exposure to high environmental levels of CO or suicidal attempts by deliberate exposure to a CO source are the most frequent causes of acute poisoning deaths in adults in the United States. CO is responsible for about 4,000 adult deaths per year.

CO rapidly affects the central and peripheral nervous systems and cardiopulmonary functions. Cerebral edema is common, as are alterations of sensory and peripheral nerve function. CO induces increased permeability in the lung resulting in acute pulmonary edema. Cardiac arrythmias, generalized hypoxemia, and respiratory failure are the common causes of CO death. COHb levels more than 40 percent are found in these cases. In survivors, considerable neurologic deficits may remain.

Patients with less severe acute cases have the same type of symptoms as patients with chronic intoxication. In addition to arrythmias, myocardial ischemia, lactic acidosis, and convulsions, coma can sometimes occur. An interesting complication observed several days after the exposure to CO are patches of necrotic skin induced by localized hypoxia. Levels of COHb that can elicit any of these symptoms vary widely among patients.

Acute CO intoxication in children (Gemelli and Cattani, 1985) is responsible for about 400 deaths a year, is more severe, and sometimes has unique symptomatology (resembling gastroenteritis). Children are more likely to have severe sequelae such as leukoencephalopathy, white matter destruction, and severe myocardial ischemia (Lacey, 1981).

Treatment. After identification and removal of the source of CO, 100 percent O_2 should be administered, if necessary after endotracheal intubation. Other support interventions should be cued by the symptomatology. For reasons mentioned, hyperbaric oxygen is often more dramatic than useful.

Instruments for the Diagnosis of COHb

The most commonly used instrument for the detection and quantification of COHb is the CO-oximeter (Mahoney et al., 1993), which in addition provides the levels of oxy, deoxy, and metHb, as well as total hemoglobin. The instrument is reliable at and above 5 percent COHb but becomes progressively less accurate below that level. Bilirubin, methylene blue, and sulfhemoglobin are sources of interference at <5 percent COHb. If low levels need to be measured, gas chromatography, a research tool, is the only alternative.

METHEMOGLOBINEMIA

Background

Auto-Oxidation of Hemoglobin. Circulating methemoglobin levels are determined by the balance between its production, from auto-oxidation and oxidation of hemoglobin, and its enzymatic reduction. Hemoglobin oxidation has been discussed thoroughly by Bunn and Forget (1986).

When left at room temperature, hemoglobin solutions turn brown, the color of methemoglobin. This reaction is more rapid at 37°C. Its chemical basis is probably the generation of superoxide anion (O_2^-). This is an infrequent event because most often, oxyhemoglobin gives up molecular oxygen (O_2) converting itself partially into deoxyhemoglobin (Nagel et al., 1970; Jaffé and Hultquist, 1995).

O_2^- is generated by the transfer of an electron from the heme iron to the unoccupied p2* orbital. The loss of this electron converts iron into the low spin ferric state. These conditions are catalyzed by H^+, Cl^-, and O_2^-, probably by the T state of hemoglobin (generated by 2,3 BPG and other polyphosphates, T-stabilizing mutations, and partial deoxygenation), and they favor auto-oxidation. Totally deoxygenated hemoglobin, although in the "tense" (T) state, has no oxygen to contribute to the reaction and is more stable with respect to auto-oxidation. OxyHbA shows a biphasic auto-oxidation curve containing two rate constants, one for the fast oxidation of α chains and a slow component that corresponds to the auto-oxidation of β chains. Proton-catalyzed auto-oxidation was the dominant effect in α-globin chains as part of a tetramer but did not occur in β-globin chains. Isolated α- and β-globin chains have similar auto-oxidation rates. These findings suggest that the formation of the α1β1 contact induces a conformation restraint in the β chains, thereby inducing a slight tilt of the distal histidine away from the bound oxygen and preventing the proton-catalyzed displacement of O_2 by solvent water molecules. This observation explains why isolated β-globin chains, as seen in the cytosol of α thalassemia, reacquire the capacity for ready auto-oxidation (Perutz, 1978).

Auto-oxidation of hemoglobin is favored by increased temperature, 2,3 BPG, trace metals, and low pH. Oxidation of hemoglobin can also occur as a result exogenous sources. One exogenous source is Cu^{2+}, which binds Cysβ 93 with high affinity and multiple other sites with low affinity converting β-globin

chain heme iron into ferric iron (Nagel et al., 1970). Drugs can also oxidize hemoglobin (see later). Methemoglobin facilitates the denaturation of hemoglobin with hemichrome formation.

Heinz bodies, found in red cells containing an excess of methemoglobin, are the product of hemoglobin denaturation. They contain hemichromes, generated when the heme is dissociated from the heme pocket and rebound elsewhere in globin after the α- or β-globin chains have been denatured. Hemichromes may be reversible or irreversible, but the latter seem to be indispensable in the formation of Heinz bodies. Both α- and β-globin chains are found in Heinz bodies. It is easy to see that any mechanism that weakens the heme-globin bond will accelerate hemoglobin denaturation and promote methemoglobin formation in the remaining hemes (Chapter 44).

NO production from the substrate L-arginine by the several forms of NO synthase (NOS), important as a vasoactive compound, also has an impact on hemoglobin oxidation (see later). In conditions of relative scarcity of the arginine substrate, NOS produce a preponderance of peroxynitrite ion ($ONOO^-$). This very reactive compound readily oxidizes hemoglobin ($2^+ \rightarrow 3^+$). An excess of $ONOO^-$ produces a reduction of ferrilHb ($4^+ \sim 3^+$) with the corresponding spectral change (Alayash et al., 1998). The reaction of $ONOO^-$ and oxyHb yields biphasic curves for the oxidation process. Interestingly, the modification occurs primarily in the β-globin subunits, and $ONOO^-$ is known to nitrate amino acid side chains, particularly tyrosine, producing nitrotyrosine. Depending on the role of the Tyr in the protein of interest, this change can drastically modify the function. Alayash et al. (1998) concluded that $ONOO^-$, locally present during reperfusion injury for example, affects hemoglobin by oxidation and protein modification. This phenomenon could be important for the development of hemoglobin-based blood substitutes, because modified free hemoglobin might be more susceptible to this mechanism.

Entry of $ONOO^-$ into red cells increases the chances of methemoglobin production. Inhibitors of red cell membrane protein Band 3 inhibit $ONOO^-$ permeability, suggesting that it gains access through the anion transporter (Soszynski and Bartosz, 1997). More recently, it was shown that addition of $ONOO^-$ to red cells produced intracellular methemoglobin, with yields of about 40 percent (Denicola et al., 1998). This result confirms earlier studies reputing that DIDS, an inhibitor of Band 3 Cl^- transport, resulted in a 50 percent inhibition of methemoglobin formation (Soszynski and Bartosz, 1997). At pH 5.5, where $ONOO^-$ is converted to its acidic form (ONOOH; pKa = 6.8), there was no effect on inhibition. Nitration of hemoglobin is enhanced in thiol-depleted erythrocytes (Denicola et al., 1988). These data suggest that $ONOO^-$ penetrates the red cells via Band 3, but also by passive diffusion.

Definition. Methemoglobinemia (more precise but more cumbersome would be the designation methemoglobincythemia) is the consequence of the oxidation of iron in the center of the protoporphyrin IX ring that forms the prosthetic group (heme) of hemoglobin from ferrous to ferric. Its reduction in normal erythrocytes is very efficient, and the normal level is less than 1 percent even though its actual production is much higher. At higher levels, methemoglobinemia can induce clinical disease because it renders hemoglobin incapable of binding and delivering oxygen, an exclusive property of ferrous heme.

Classification of Methemoglobinemias. Methemoglobinemia is generally, but not always, benign. Changes of skin color can be dramatic, placing methemoglobinemia in the differential diagnosis of cyanosis.

A modified clinical classification, based on a schema of Jaffé and Hultquist (1995) of hereditary methemoglobinemia, includes the following:

1. Genetically mediated causes
   a. Hereditary deficiency of NADH-dependent cytochrome b_5 reductase (b_5R)
   b. Mutant hemoglobins (HbM) that result in the stabilization of the hemes in the ferric state (Chapter 44)
2. Exogenous oxidizing agents capable of oxidizing hemoglobin (acquired methemoglobinemia)

Hereditary Methemoglobinemia

Clinical Aspects and Classification. Cyanosis is the principal sign of methemoglobinemia. It has been calculated that the degree of cyanosis produced by 5 g/dL of ferrous deoxyhemoglobin is equivalent to 1.5 g/dL of methemoglobin or 0.5 g/dL of sulfhemoglobin (Jaffé and Hultquist, 1995).

Mutations of the b_5R gene associated with methemoglobinemia are recessive, so only homozygotes express the disease. Nevertheless, heterozygotes can be at special risk for acquired methemoglobinemia (see later).

Red Cell Type (Type I Hereditary Methemoglobinemia). Patients with type I hereditary methemoglobinemia are more cyanotic than sick, in the worst cases complaining of fatigue with strenuous exercise. They have normal survival rates and normal pregnancies. Methemoglobin levels vary from 20 to 40 percent. When exposed to methemoglobin-inducing drugs or chemicals, these patients are at risk for developing more severe symptoms.

Activity of the nicotinamide adenine dinucleotide (NADH)-dependent methemoglobin reductase system is reduced in the erythrocyte (Gibson, 1948; Scott, 1960; Passon and Hultquist, 1972). NADH-methemoglobin reductase works in conjunction with cytochrome b_5 to reduce methemoglobin. In red cell progenitors, this same enzyme has a totally different function clipping the hydrophobic C-terminal portion of microsomal cytochrome b_5.

Treatment of hereditary methemoglobinemia is rarely necessary, but methylene blue is effective because it reduces methemoglobin through the NADPH-flavin reductase pathway, bypassing the impaired cytochrome b_5 system.

Generalized Form (Type II). This type of hereditary methemoglobinemia affects 10 to 15 percent of the patients. This is a severe and lethal disease, with a strong neurologic component. Although the methemoglobinemia can be treated, the neurologic syndrome is refractory. The disease is secondary to homozygosity, or compound heterozygosity, for defective cytochrome b_5-reductase in all tissues.

Two NADH-methemoglobin reductases are found in red cells: one attached to the membrane and involved in lipid metabolism and another free in the cytosol. Cytosolic enzyme has been proteolyzed to where it no longer can assemble in the membrane (Schwartz et al., 1983). Because both enzymes are deficient in type II methemoglobinemia, a single gene is believed to code for both enzyme forms. Two different transcripts have been identified in humans, the membrane (M) and soluble (S) types, which differ in their first exon. The S form is undetectable in nonerythroid cells and in induced K562 cells, but is present in terminal erythroblast cultures and represents the major b_5R in reticulocytes. This form seems to be particularly important for late stages of erythroid differentiation.

Prenatal diagnosis for cytochrome b_5 deficiency is feasible. Because of the autosomal recessive basis of cytochrome b_5 reductase deficiency, prenatal diagnosis can be applied to future pregnancies only after a case is identified.

Pathophysiology

Reduction of Methemoglobin. In normal hemolysates, methemoglobin levels are less than 1 percent of total hemoglobin. More methemoglobin is produced, but the intact erythrocyte has an elaborate mechanism by which the ferric hemes are constantly reduced to the ferrous form (Fig. 46.2). These mechanisms include the NADH-dependent enzyme cytochrome b_5 reductase system (b_5R, diaphorase I, NADH-methemoglobin reductase, NADH-dehydrogenase).

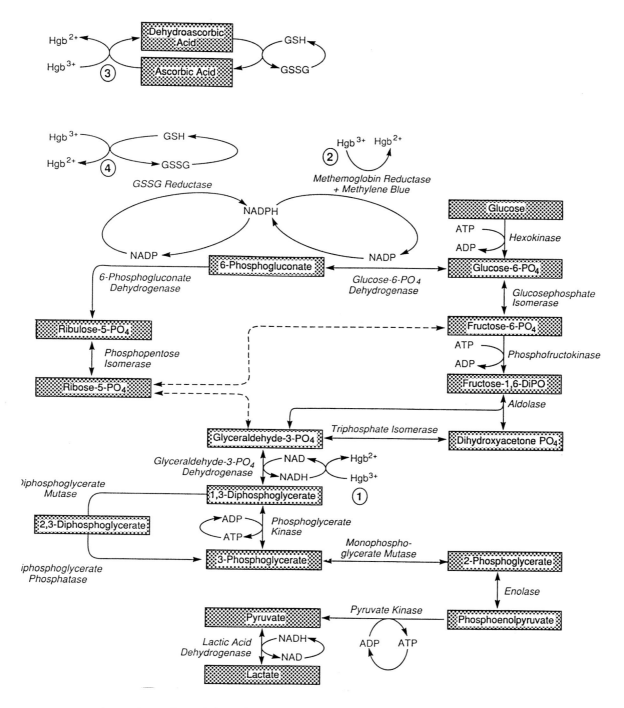

Figure 46.2. Pathways for methemoglobin reduction.

Cellular Biochemistry and Molecular Biology of b₅R. The housekeeping enzyme b_5R is a member of the flavoenzyme family of dehydrogenases/electron transferases. Its central function is to transfer electrons from NADH to cytochrome b_5. In turn, cytochrome b_5 is an electron donor, with different functions in different cells. In red cells, by transferring electrons to methemoglobin, it reduces this form to hemoglobin.

Cytochrome b_5 reductase has been mapped to chromosome 22. Its cDNA has six exons and four promoter regions that lead to the synthesis of cellular-specific isoforms (Bull et al., 1988). One promoter is a typical housekeeping gene promoter and does not contain TATA or CAAT boxes (Tomatsu et al., 1989). The erythroid-specific promoter region contains the GATA-1 binding domains, TATA and CAAT boxes, and a GT box (Pietrini et al., 1992). Two other promoter regions have not been fully characterized.

In immature erythroblasts, membrane-bound b_5R has a N-terminus membrane-binding domain. Membrane-bound enzyme in somatic cells desaturates and elongates fatty acids in cholesterol biosynthesis and in drug metabolism. Although the erythrocyte enzyme was thought to be derived from the membrane-bound form by proteolytic loss of the membrane-binding domain during erythroid maturation, this interpretation must be revised now that the structure of the b_5R gene and its characteristics are known (Tomatsu et al., 1989). Exon 2 is 31 kb long with nine exons and eight introns. It contains the junction of the membrane-binding domain and the catalytic domain of b_5R. This suggests that two forms of b_5R, the S and M form, are generated by posttranslational processing. Although the 5′ untranslated portion lacks the canonical transcriptional regulatory elements, it contains five copies of the GC box sequence GGGCGG. The average GC content of the b_5R gene is 55 percent, but the GC content of the 5′ portion is an extraordinarily high 86 percent, and CpG dinucleotides were present at a very high frequency in this GC rich region. These structural features resemble regulatory elements of constitutively expressed housekeeping genes.

By primer extension analysis, several transcription start points have been identified. Seventeen complete and twelve incomplete Alu family sequences were found in introns. An uncanonical polyadenylation signal, AGTAAA instead of AATAAA, was present in the 3′ untranslated region. Du et al. (1997) have tested the hypothesis that the human-soluble form of b_5R is generated through posttranslational processing of the membrane-bound form. Examination of the 5′ ends of cDNA from human reticulocytes, liver, brain, and HL60 cells revealed the ubiquitous presence of an alternative type of human b_5R mRNA, which can probably be translated into the S form of b_5R directly, but there was no erythroid-specific transcript of the b_5R gene. This b_5R mRNA, which appears to have initiated from at least two sites, contains a new first exon that is noncoding and located between the first two exons of the previously described b_5R gene. This new first exon shares 62 percent homology with the first exon and its 3′ flanking intron sequences of rat erythroid-specific b_5R mRNA. The rat and fly b_5R genes have a structure similar to the human gene (Zenno et al., 1990; Zhang and Scott, 1996).

Meyer et al. (1995) have studied the transient kinetics of reduction and interprotein electron transfer in b_5R by laser flash photolysis in the presence of deazariboflavin and EDTA at pH 7.0. When cytochrome b_5 and b_5R were mixed at low ionic strength, a strong complex was formed, and the dissociation constant for protein-protein transient complex formation was approximately 1 µmol/L. The observed rate constants for interprotein electron transfer decreased 23-fold when the ionic strength was increased to 1 mol/L, indicating an electrostatic interaction between the two proteins. Nicotinamide adenine dinucleotide (NAD) appears to both stabilize and optimize the protein-protein complex with respect to electron transfer. Another effect of NAD is to appreciably slow auto-oxidation and disproportionation of the flavine adenine dinucleotide (FAD) semiquinone.

Kawano et al. (1998) have identified the cytochrome b_5 residues responsible for the electrostatic interaction with b_5R by recombinant technology. They replaced Glu41, Glu42, Glu63, Asp70, and Glu73 by Ala. Apparent K_m values of the wild type b_5R for Glu42Ala cytochrome b_5 and Asp70Ala cytochrome b_5 were approximately threefold and sixfold higher, respectively, than those for the wild recombinant cytochrome b_5. The k_{cat} values for those mutants were not remarkably affected. In contrast, Glu41Ala, Glu63Ala, and Glu73Ala cytochrome b_5 showed almost the same kinetic properties as the wild type cytochrome b_5. Furthermore, kinetic studies of mixtures of cytochrome b_5 and b_5R mutants suggested an interaction between Glu42 and Asp70 of cytochrome b_5 and Lys125 and Lys41 of b_5R, respectively, in the electrostatic interaction between these two proteins.

Mutants b_5R Producing Methemoglobinemia

A cartoon of the b_5R gene and mutants that generate NADH-dependent b_5R variants described according to type in Tables 46.1 and 46.2 is depicted in Figure 46.3. (Prchal et al., 1990). Four missense mutations cause type I methemoglobenemia; type II mutations are more heterogeneous and numerous. Eleven have been reported including missense mutations, deletions, nonsense mutations, and exon-skipping variants.

Using polymerase chain reaction (PCR)-related technology, the b_5R gene of a Chinese patient with hereditary methemoglobinemia type I was found to contain a novel missense mutation, CTC→CCC (Leu→ Pro), at codon 72 in exon 3 (Wu et al., 1998). As the mutation generated an Apa I recognition site, homozygosity for the mutation was confirmed by restriction analysis of PCR-amplified fragments from genomic DNA.

An interesting polymorphism was found in b_5R among African Americans (Jenkins and Prchal, 1997). It consisted of a C→G change in exon 5, which changed Thr to Ser at codon 116. This is the first polymorphism of b_5R. Screening of different ethnic groups revealed that this polymorphism is present in 23 percent of African Americans (n = 112) but absent in 108 European Caucasians, forty-six Asians, forty-four Caucasians from the Indian subcontinent, and fourteen Caucasians of Arabian

Table 46.1. Mutations in Type I Cytochrome b5 Reductase Deficiency

Nucleotide change	Mutation	Protein effect	Exon	Ethnic origin	Comment
T→C	Missense	148 Leu→Pro	5	Japanese	Previously classified as type III
G→A	Missense	57 Arg→Glu	3	Japanese	
G→A	Missense	105 Val→Met	4	Italian	
G→A	Missense	212 Glu→Lys	8	African-American	

Table 46.2. Mutations in Type II Cytochrome b5 Reductase Deficiency

Nucleotide change	Mutation	Protein effect	Exon	Ethnic origin	Comment
T→C	Missense	127 Ser→Pro	5	Japanese	
3bp deletion (in frame)	Deletion	298 Phe, Del	9	Japanese	
G→C	Exon skipping	Truncation	Intron 5	Algerian	Exon 5 skipping; frameshift
C→T	Nonsense	218 Arg→Stop	8	Algerian	
T→C	Missense	203 Cys→Arg	7	French/Spanish	Compound heterozygote
3bp deletion (out of frame)	Deletion	272 Met del, frameshift	9	French/Spanish	Compound heterozygote
G→T at splice acceptor site	Unknown	Unknown	Intron 8	Italian	No detectable b5R in blood cells/fibroblasts
G→C	Missense	60 Arg→Pro	3	Caucasian	
C→A	Nonsense	42 Tyr→Stop	2	Caucasian (UK)	Compound heterozygote
C→A	Missense	95 Pro→His	4	Caucasian (UK)	Compound heterozygote
A→C at splice acceptor site	Exon skipping	Deletion 28 amino acids	Intron 5 not reported		Exon 6 skipping

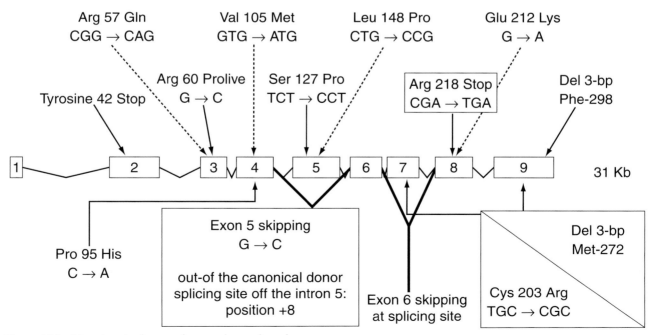

Figure 46.3. Mutations in the gene for cytochrome b₅ reductase.

origin. Preliminary data do not correlate this polymorphism with any change in b_5R activity or phenotype. Nevertheless, it could be relevant in conjunction with other acquired or genetic defects, and the potential selective factors for a polymorphism of this high frequency need to be elucidated.

Type II hereditary methemoglobinemia, with generalized deficiency of NADH b_5R, is a very rare disease characterized by severe developmental abnormalities and often premature death. Although the relationship between the symptoms and the enzyme deficit is not understood, an important cause might be the loss of the lipid-metabolizing activities of the reductase located in the endoplasmic reticulum. However, the b_5R form located on outer mitochondrial membranes was not initially considered. Shirabe et al. (1995) have analyzed the gene of an Italian patient and identified a novel G→T transversion at the splice acceptor site in exon 9, which resulted in the absence of detectable b_5R in blood cells and skin fibroblasts. In cultured fibroblasts, b_5R, ferricyanide reductase, and semidehydroascorbate reductase activities were severely reduced. Because the latter activity is known to be due to b_5R located on outer mitochondrial membranes, these results suggest that the reductase in the endoplasmic reticulum and in the outer mitochondrial membranes are products of the same gene. They suggest that a defect in ascorbate regeneration may contribute to the phenotype of hereditary methemoglobinemia of the generalized type.

Yawata et al. (1992) described a Japanese man with b_5R deficiency (b_5R Kurashiki) in red cells, platelets, lymphocytes, and cultured fibroblasts. Congenital methemoglobinemia was associated with mental and neurologic retardation and spondylosis deformans and finger joint deformations never before described in association with this enzyme deficiency. b_5R deficiency was most severe in red cells and less marked in platelets, lymphocytes, and fibroblasts.

In the b_5R gene from a patient homozygous for hereditary methemoglobinemia, generalized type II, a TCT→CCT (Ser→Pro) mutation was present in codon 127 (Kobayashi et al., 1990). Dot blot hybridization of the amplified DNA samples with allele-specific oligonucleotide probes showed that the proband and her brothers were homozygotes, and their father heterozygous. b_5R activity in lymphoblastoid cells from homozygotes was reduced 10 times below normal levels. RNA blot and protein blot analyses showed that synthesis of b_5R mRNA and the b_5R polypeptide were normal. Ser at residue 127 was presumed to be in an α-helix structure that was part of a nucleotide-binding domain. Pro127 most probably disrupts the α helix, changing the nucleotide-binding domain that affects electron transport from NADH to cytochrome b_5. Functional

enzyme deficiency then resulted in a generalized type of hereditary methemoglobinemia.

Type II hereditary methemoglobinemia also resulted from a single base mutation in position 102 (b_5R Hiroshima), where a serine is replaced by proline. This exon 5 mutation is in a region likely to be an α helix where proline disrupts the secondary structure. Only 21 amino acids downstream from this mutation is the 123 Leu→Pro mutation for type II hereditary methemoglobinemia (b_5R-Kurobe).

A British patient with type II hereditary methemoglobinemia was a compound heterozygote for two novel mutations of the b_5R gene (Manabe et al., 1996). One allele had a nonsense mutation at codon 42 that generated a protein lacking the catalytic portion of the enzyme. The second allele contained a missense mutation at codon 95, CCC→CAC (Pro→His) within the FAD-binding domain. To characterize the effects of this missense mutation on the enzyme function, glutathione S transferase-GST-fused mutant and normal enzymes were compared in *Escherichia coli*. The mutant enzyme showed less catalytic activity and thermostability and a greater susceptibility to trypsin than did the normal counterpart. The absorption spectrum of the mutant enzyme in the visible region differed from that of the wild type. These results suggested that this amino acid substitution influenced both secondary structure and catalytic activity of the enzyme.

Hereditary methemoglobinemia caused by an erythrocytic deficiency of b_5R type I in African Americans was first reported by Prchal et al. (1990). The rarity of reports of hereditary methemoglobinemia in blacks may be related to the difficulty in detecting cyanosis in pigmented skin, although nail bed and mucosa can be useful for this purpose. Biochemical studies on the African-American family with variant enzyme b_5R Shreveport (Jenkins and Prchal, 1996) showed enzyme instability. Transcript size was the same as the control sample, and the nucleotide sequence showed that the proband was homozygous for a G→A transition at codon 212 in exon 8, changing a Glu→ Lys. A C→G transversion was found at codon 116 in exon 5, changing a Thr→Ser. The codon 212 change was found only in the propositus and her heterozygous mother. This mutation was predicted to disrupt an α helix in b_5R, so it is likely to be the disease-causing mutation. In contrast, the codon 116 change is a high frequency polymorphism in blacks (Jenkins and Prchal, 1997).

A patient with hereditary methemoglobinemia associated with a deficiency of the essential cofactor, cytochrome b/5, has been reported (Hegesh et al., 1986). Confirmation of this defect would complete the roster of possible genetic metabolic abnormalities responsible for hereditary methemoglobinemia.

Measurement of b₅R Activity

Two mouse hybridoma cell lines secreting IgG monoclonal antibodies (MAbs) to b₅R were established by using recombinant human red cell b₅R as antigen to immunize BALBc mice (Lan et al., 1996). Reacting specifically with b₅R, antibodies were also capable of capturing enzyme activity from b₅R in solution and in normal human hemolysate. A sensitive sandwich enzyme-linked immunosorbent assay (ELISA) procedure for the determination of b₅R concentration was used to study enzyme concentration in erythrocytes (Lan et al., 1998a). In thirty normal Chinese adults, levels were 25.6 ± 8.54 ng/mg Hb. Red cell soluble b₅R in five newborns was significantly lower than that in normal adults, and soluble b₅R was undetectable in the erythrocytes of four patients with type I hereditary methemoglobinemia. b₅R activity can also be measured in human hemolysates (Lan et al., 1998b). b₅R monoclonal antibodies were dot-blotted on nitrocellulose membranes and used to capture and enrich b₅R from hemolysates. Captured b₅R activity was visualized with the substrate 3,4,5 dimethylthiazoly 1,2,2,5 diphenyltetrazolium bromide. This simple method for the detection of b₅R activity in hemolysates could be useful in the laboratory diagnosis of congenital methemoglobinemia.

The NADH Reductase System (NADH and Cytochrome b₅).

NADH is a cofactor for cytochrome b₅ reductase, generated by glyceraldehyde-3-phosphate dehydrogenase, that reduces NAD to NADH while converting glyceraldehyde-3-phosphate to fructose-1, 3-biphosphate in the glycolytic pathway (Reaction 1, Fig. 46.2). Conversely, lactic acid dehydrogenase converts NADH into NAD, as it converts pyruvate into lactic acid. In the steady state, there is no net accumulation of NADH. Nevertheless, when increased methemoglobin levels need to be reduced, pyruvate accumulates because NADH has been consumed in the reduction of methemoglobin.

Cytochrome b₅ is the electron carrier between NADH and methemoglobin. Electron transfer between cytochrome b₅ and methemoglobin occurs via the formation of a complex between these two molecules. The cytochrome binds to four lysines in the heme pocket in both chains. Figure 46.2 depicts the entire cytochrome b₅ reductase system and the reactions in which this enzyme and its cofactors are involved.

The NADPH-Flavin Reductase System.

This reaction (Reaction 2, Fig. 46.2) is probably not physiologic because glucose-6-phosphate dehydrogenase-deficient patients do not have methemoglobinemia. Nevertheless, in the presence of non-physiologic electron carriers, such as methylene blue, this system becomes active and is the basis for the use of this dye in the treatment of hereditary methemoglobinemia.

Ascorbic Acid. Ascorbic acid can directly reduce methemoglobin at a low rate in red cells (Reaction 3, Fig. 46.2). In the process it is nonenzymatically converted into dehydroascorbic acid.

Reduced Glutathione System. GSH can nonenzymatically reduce methemoglobin (Reaction 4, Fig. 46.2). The resulting oxidized glutathione (GSSG) is reduced by glutathione reductase.

These four metabolic systems generate a reducing capacity 250 times greater than required to reduce physiologically generated red cell methemoglobin (Scott, 1960; Jaffé and Hultquist, 1995).

Protective Mechanisms to Avoid Methemoglobin Formation

Several metabolic processes protect hemoglobin from oxidation to methemoglobin. These include superoxide dismutase whose function is to remove toxic superoxide ion-generating hydrogen peroxide. This compound is also toxic but can be removed by glutathione peroxidase and, in a less efficient way, by the low-affinity enzyme catalase that intervenes only when peroxides reach an excess. This explains why acatalasemia does not involve methemoglobinemia, whereas inherited deficiency of glutathione peroxidase exhibits low levels of methemoglobinemia. Because the latter enzyme has low levels in red cells of newborns, this might explain their susceptibility to acquired methemoglobinemia.

ACQUIRED (TOXIC) METHEMOGLOBINEMIA

Several chemical agents and drugs can induce methemoglobinemia in normal people. Table 46.3 lists the common offenders (Jaffé and Hultquist, 1995). Newborn infants are at increased risk for acquired methemoglobinemia owing to their diminished enzymatic capacity for methemoglobin reduction. Certain cream medications to treat diaper rash that contain benzocaine and resorcinol have been reported to produce methemoglobin levels as high as 35 percent (Griffin, 1997).

Dapsone and primaquine-induced methemoglobinemia at levels of 15 to 33 percent have been reported in patients infected with the human immunodeficiency virus (Sin and Shafran, 1996; Valentovic et al., 1997). Some individuals become symptomatic, requiring hospitalization and treatment with methylene blue and red cell transfusions. Pulse oxymeter or blood gas determinations are useless in the diagnosis, but CO oxymeter measurements can be helpful.

Aniline dyes and aniline reduce molecular oxygen and generate methemoglobin. After reducing oxyhemoglobin, phenylhydroxylamine can generate nitrosoben-

Table 46.3. Some Drugs and Agents That May Cause Methemoglobinemia

Local anesthetics
  Benzocaine
  Lidocaine
  Procaine
  Prilocaine
Analine dyes
Chlorates
Diaminodiphenylsulfone (Dapsone)
Diarylsulfonylureas (Sulofenur)
Primaquine
Nitrite
Nitroglycerin
Amylnitrate
Isobutyl
Nitrobenzine
Nitrofurans
Pyridium
Sulfonamides
Acetaminophen/phenacetin

zene, which is reduced again to phenylhydroxylamine by red cell enzymes. This cycle can then, in turn, generate more methemoglobin.

Nitrites are common offenders, particularly in children, but the mechanism is less well understood. Nitrate-contaminated well water has been suspected of causing spontaneous abortion in livestock in La Grange County, Indiana (Anonymous, 1996). Nitrate-contaminated well-water has also been reported to induce methemoglobinemia in infants.

Methemoglobinemia has been reported in association with the inhalation of NO for treatment of hydrochlorothiazide-induced pulmonary edema (Hovenga et al., 1996) and with premedication for endoscopy (Brown et al., 1994).

Recreational use of amyl, butyl, or isobutyl nitrites is another cause of acquired methemoglobinemia. In addition, infections might release toxins (including nitrites) that produce methemoglobin.

Henna is a natural product used worldwide as a hair dye, but particularly in the Middle East and India to stain skin and nails (Zinkham and Oski, 1996). A chemical, lawsome (2-hydroxy-1,4 naphthoquinone), is present in this natural product. Incubation in vitro of blood from glucose-6-phosphate dehydrogenase (G-6-PD)-normal and G-6-PD-deficient individuals with lawsome, has shown a 0.5 to 12.5 percent increase of methemoglobin in normal individuals and 20 to 54 percent in deficient individuals. Because the incidence of G-6-PD deficiency is high in the areas where henna is popular, outbreaks of methemoglobinemia are possible.

Methemoglobinemia has been found in children with *Plasmodium vivax* malaria (Erel et al., 1997) and in acidotic children in the absence of malaria. In children with *Plasmodium falciparum* malaria mean methemoglobin levels were 16.4 percent. Methemoglobin levels correlated with disease severity and the severity of anemia (Anstey et al., 1996). Because malaria alone produces hypoxia, the additional reduction in oxygen-carrying capacity by the presence of methemoglobinemia might be particularly critical for the subgroup of patients who are anemic or acidotic.

Children with septic shock have increased methemoglobinemia and circulating nitrite/nitrate levels, probably owing to the overproduction of NO (Krafte-Jacobs et al., 1997). Overproduction of NO in septic shock can be blocked experimentally by diasperin cross-linked hemoglobin (Kilbourn, 1997).

Fungicides contain methemoglobinemia-forming compounds, and farmers are often exposed to these agents. Recently, induction of methemoglobinemia by 3,5 dichloroaniline, 4-amino-2,6-dichlorophenol, and 3,5-dichlorophenylhydroxylamine has been studied in laboratory animals and in vitro (Valentovic et al., 1997). None of these compounds induced lipid peroxidation, but all three could induce methemoglobin. The most potent was the N-hydroxy metabolite. Glutathione depletion is associated with methemoglobin formation by 3,5-dichlorophenylhydroxylamine.

Sulofenur, a diarylsulfonylurea antineoplastic drug, produced a dose-limited induction of methemoglobin during phase I trials. One of nine patients had heterozygous cytochrome b_5 reductase deficiency (Molthrop et al., 1994).

Diagnosis of Methemoglobinemia

Recent or sudden clinically apparent cyanosis, in the absence of cardiopulmonary pathology that usually accounts for cyanosis, suggests acquired methemoglobinemia, although sulfhemoglobinemia (see later) should also be considered. Long-standing symptoms or symptoms in siblings is compatible with hereditary methemoglobinemia. Because this condition is recessive, clinical disease should not be expected in the parents. The differential diagnosis includes the HbM variants and low O_2 affinity hemoglobins in which, because of the "dominance" of these genes, one parent often has the same symptoms. Enzymatic assays or spot tests are available for the methemoglobin reductases, and genetic ascertainment is available for the known mutations. Prenatal diagnosis is available for type II hereditary methemoglobinemia. The effect of methylene blue for reversing cyanosis is also diagnostic.

There is an unusual high incidence of hereditary methemoglobinemia among Alaskan Eskimos,

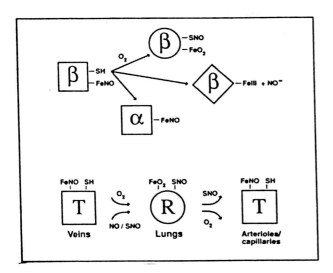

Figure 46.5. NO reactions with hemoglobin. (**Top Panel**) Reactions proposed for the β-globin chain nitosyl heme groups in the T structure include transfer of the NO of the α-globin chain heme iron, an event most likely to happen in the venous system and microcirculation, and charge-transfer at the heme iron producing metHb and nitoxyl ion, an event an event most likely to happen in the venous system and microcirculation when NO synthesis is high. NO exchange with the Cys β93 mediated by the T→R transition forms SNO-Hb Fe^{+2} O_2 in the lung and arterial blood. (**Bottom Panel**) Model of NO binding to heme and thiols of circulating hemoglobin. Partially nitrosylated blood enters the pulmonary circulation in the T or R state. Here it is exposed to more NO and high O_2 tension that couple the allosteric transition with NO exchange from heme to the β thiols. Blood that enters the arterial circulation contains hemoglobin in the R state as SNO-oxyHb. In the microcirculation, where PO_2 is low, the T state is favored, promoting NO release, and vasodilation may occur. Squares represent the T state, circles, the R state, and diamonds, metHb. (For a more complete explanation see Gow and Stamler, 1998.)

that question by studying the kinetics of the reaction in a variety of recombinant sperm whale myoglobins and human hemoglobins. The observed rates of NO-dependent oxidation varied linearly with NO concentration but not with oxygen concentration. Reversible NO binding and NO-induced oxidation occurred in two steps: (1) bimolecular entry of NO into the distal portion of the heme pocket and (2) rapid reaction of noncovalently bound NO with iron, producing Fe^{2+} –N = O, or with Fe^{2+}–O–O– δ, producing Fe^{3+} –OH_2 and nitrate. When the distal histidine was replaced by

Figure 46.6. Structure-function relationships among HbMs and α-nitosylHb in O_2 binding equilibria. $α^-$ represents a metHb-containing α-globin subunit. Reversible four-step O_2 binding in HbS takes place between the T and R states. In HbM the His→Tyr substitutions cause an irreversible shift to the T state. O_2 binding to the β-globin subunits occurs within the T state and is noncooperative and nonallosteric. Ligation of two molecules of NO to the α-heme groups causes a shift toward the T state that is modulated by ligation in the β hemes, pH, and 2,3 BPG. Therefore, O_2 binding of the $α(Fe-NO)_2β(Fe)_2$ occurs between the T and R states and is both cooperative and allosterically sensitive.

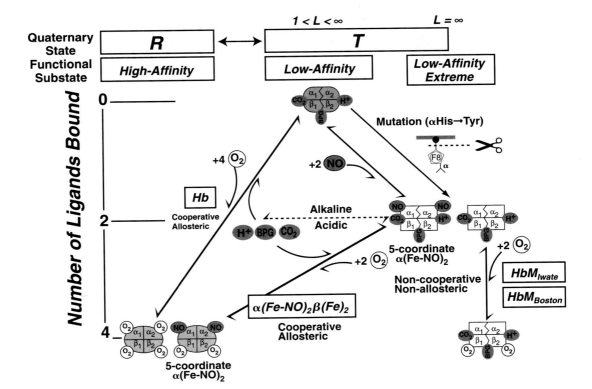

aliphatic residues, oxidation was increased. The mutant hemoglobins lacked polar interactions in the distal pocket that normally hinder NO entry into the protein. Decreasing the volume of the distal pocket by substituting aromatic residues in place of Leu(B10) and Val(E11) markedly inhibited NO-mediated oxidation. Consumption of NO by extracellular hemoglobin and subsequent vasoconstriction have been suggested as the cause of the mild hypertension reported during clinical trials of hemoglobin-based O_2 carriers. The depletion of NO from endothelial cells is most likely due to the oxidative reaction of NO with oxyhemoglobin in arterioles and surrounding tissue. These studies suggest ways of minimizing hypertension when hemoglobin-based blood substitutes are engineered from recombinant proteins (Eich et al., 1996).

CONCLUSIONS

CO–, NO–, and methemoglobins are all present in normal red cells in very low concentrations, in the order NO < Met < < CO. Mutations or environmental conditions can increase the concentrations of all these liganded or oxidized hemoglobins, producing a dyshemoglobinemia. Sometimes increased levels of dyshemoglobins are life-threatening, and because effective treatments are available, their presence should be identified in a timely fashion.

The distinction between environmental and genetic dyshemoglobinemia is often blurred because many acquired dyshemoglobins are, in effect, the consequence of both an environmental challenge and a genetic predisposition. One of the problems in understanding noxious environmental agents is that most of them are dangerous only to a susceptible subset of the population. Without knowing who is at risk, the dangers are not easily identifiable.

References

Afane, Ze, E, Roche, N, Atchou, G et al. (1996). Respiratory symptoms and peak expiratory flow in survivors of the Nyos disaster. Chest 110: 1278–1281.

Alayash, AI, Ryan, BA, and Cashon RE. (1998). Peronitrate-mediated heme oxidation and protein modification of native and chemically modified hemoglobins. Arch. Biochem. Biophys. 349: 65–73.

Anonymous. (1996). Spontaneous abortions possibly related to the ingestion of nitrate-containing well water. La Grange County, Indiana, 1991–1994. Mortal. Wkly. Rep. 45: 569–572.

Antonini, E and Brunori, M. (1971). Hemoglobin and myoglobin in their reactions with ligands. In Neuberger, A, and Tatum, EL, editors. Frontiers of biology. Amsterdam, London: North-Holland Publishing Company.

Anstey, NM, Hassanali, MY, Mlalasi, J et al. (1996). Trans. R. Soc. Trop. Med. Hyg. 90: 147–151.

Balster, RL, Ekelund, LG, and Grover, RF. (1991). Evaluation of subpopulations potentially at risk to carbon monoxide exposure. In EPA 600/8-90/045F: Air quality criteria for carbon monoxide. Research Triangle Park, NC: Environmental Criteria and Assessment Office, Office of Health and Environmental Assessment, Office of Research and Development, US Environmental Protection Agency.

Basch, F. (1926). On hydrogen sulfide poisoning from external application of elementary sulfur as an ointment. Arch. Exp. Pathol. Pharmacol. 111: 126.

Benesch, RE, Maeda, N, and Benesch R. (1972). 2,3-Diphosphoglycerate and the relative affinity of adult and fetal hemoglobin for oxygen and carbon dioxide. Biochim. Biophys. Acta 257: 178–182.

Berzofsky, JA, Peisach, J, and Blumberg, WE. (1971). Sulfheme proteins. II. The reversible oxygenation of ferrous sulfmyoglobin. J. Biol. Chem. 246: 7366–7372.

Bradenburg, RO and Smith, HL. (1951). Sulfhemoglobinemia: A study of 62 clinical cases. Am. Heart. J. 42: 582.

Brown, CM, Levy, SA, and Sussan, PW (1994). Methemoglobinemia: Life-threatening complication of endoscopy premedication. Am. J. Gastroenterol. 89: 1108–1109.

Bull, P, Shephard, E, Povey, J et al. (1988). Cloning and chromosomal mapping of human cytrochorme b_5 reductase (DIA1). Ann. Hum. Genet. 52: 263–268.

Bunn, HF and Forget, BG. (1986). Hemoglobin: Molecular, genetic and clinical aspects. Philadelphia: WB Saunders.

Burnett, E, King, EG, Grace, M, and Hall, WF. (1977). Hydrogen sulfide poisoning: Review of 5 years' experience. J. Can. Med. Assoc. 117: 1277–1280.

Carrico, RJ, Blumberg, WE, and Peisach JJ. (1978). The reversible binding of oxygen to sulfhemoglobin. J. Biol. Chem. 253: 7212–7215.

Cheng, X and Schoenborn, BP. Neutron diffraction study of carbon-monoxymyoglobin. (1991). J. Mol. Biol. 220: 381–399.

Coburn, RF, Danielson, GK, Blakemore, WS et al. (1964). Carbon monoxide in blood: Analytical method and sources of error. J. Appl. Physiol. 19: 510–515.

Coburn, RF, Williams, WJ, and Kahn, SB. (1966). Endogenous carbon dioxide production in patients with hemolytic anemia. J. Clin. Invest. 44: 460–468.

Coleman, MD and Coleman, NA. (1996). Drug induced methemoglobinaemia. Treatment issues. Drug Saf. 14: 394–405.

Cumming, RLC and Pollock, A. (1967). Drug induced sulphaemoglobinemia and Heinz body anemia in pregnancy with involvement of the foetus. Scott. Med. J. 12: 320–322.

Darling, RC and Roughton, FJW. (1942). The effect of methemoglobin on the equilibrium between oxygen and hemoglobin. Am. J. Physiol. 137: 56.

Denicola, A, Souza, JM, and Radi, R. (1988). Diffusion of peroxynitrate across erythrocyte membranes. Proc. Natl. Acad. Sci. U.S.A. 95: 3566–3571.

Du, M, Shirabe, K, and Takeshita, M. (1997). Identification of alternative first exons of NADH-cytochrome b_5 reductase gene expressed ubiquitously in human cells. Biochem. Biophys. Res. Commun. 235: 779–783.

Eich, RF, Li, T, Lemon, DD et al. (1996). Mechanism of NO-induced oxidation of myoglobin and hemoglobin. *Biochemistry* 35: 976–983.

Engel, RR, Rodkey FL, O'Neal, JD et al. (1969). Relative affinity of human fetal hemoglobin for CO and O_2. *Blood* 33: 37–45.

EPA 600/8-90/045F. (1991). *Air quality criteria for carbon monoxide.* Research Triangle Park, NC: Environmental Criteria and Assessment Office, Office of Health and Environmental Assessment, Office of Research and Development, US Environmental Protection Agency.

Erel, O, Kocyigit, A, Avci, S et al. (1997). Oxidative stress and antioxidative status of plasma and erythrocytes in patients with vivax malaria. *Clin. Biochem.* 30: 631–639.

Evans, As, Enzer, N, Eder, HA, and Finch, CA. (1950). Hemolytic anemia with paroxymal methemoglobnemia and sulfhemoglobinemia. *Arch. Intern. Med.* 86: 22.

Fallstrom SP. Endogenous formation of carbon monoxide in newborn infants. (1968) *Acta Paediatr Scand* 57: 321–329.

Ford, R, Shkov, J, Akman, WV et al. (1978). Deaths from asphyxia among fisherman. *Mor. Mortal. Wkly. Rep.* 27: 309.

Gemelli, F and Cattani, R. (1985). Carbon monoxide poisoning in childhood. *Br. Med. J.* 291: 1197.

Gibson, QH. (1948). The reduction of methaemoglobin in red blood cells and studies on the cause of idiopathic methaemoglobinaemia. *Biochem. J.* 42: 13–23.

Gibson, GA and Douglas, CC. (1966). Microbic cyanosis. *Lancet* 2: 72.

Glud, TK. A case of enterogenic cyanosis? Complete recovery from acquired met-and sulfhemoglobinemia following treatment with neomycin and bacitracin. *Ugeskr Laeger* 141: 1410–1411.

Golden, PJ and Weinstein, R. (1998). Treatment of high-risk, refractory acquired methemoglobinemia with automated red cell exchange. *J. Clin. Apheresis* 13: 28–31.

Gow, AJ and Stamler, JS. (1998). Reactions between nitric oxide and haemoglobin under physiological conditions. *Nature* 391: 169–173.

Griffin, JP. (1997). Methaemoglobinemia. *Adv. Drug React. Toxicol.* 16: 46–53.

Hegesh, E, Hegesh, J, and Kaftory, A (1986). Congenital methemoglobinemis with a deficiency of cytochrome b/5. *N. Engl. J. Med.* 314: 757–61

Holzmann, A. (1997). Nitric oxide and sepsis. (1997). *Respir. Care. Clin. North Am.* 3: 537–550.

Hovenga, S, Koenders, ME, van der Werf, TS et al. (1996). Methaemoglobinaemia after inhalation of nitric oxide for treatment of hydrochlorothiazide-induced pulmonary oedema. *Lancet* 348: 1035–1036.

Ignarro LJ. (1990). A novel signal transduction mechanism for transcellular communication. *Hypertension* 16: 477–483.

Jaffé, ER and Hultquist, DE. (1995). Cytochrome b/5 reductase deficiency and enzymopenic hereditary methemoglobinemia. In Scriver, CR, Beaudet, AL, Sly, WS, and Valle, D, editors. *The metabolic basis of inherited disease* (ed 7). New York: McGraw-Hill.

Jain, KK. (1990). *Carbon monoxide poisoning.* St Louis: Warren H. Green.

Jenkins, MM and Prchal, JT. (1996). A novel mutation found in the 3′ domain of NADH-cytochrome B5 reductase in an African-American family with type I congenital methemoglobinemia. *Blood* 87: 2993–2999.

Jenkins, MM and Prchal, JT. (1997). A high-frequency polymorphism of NADH-cytochrome b5 reductase in African-Americans. *Hum. Genet.* 99: 248–250.

Kachalova, GS, Popov, AN, and Bartunik, HD. (1999). A steric mechanism for inhibition of CO binding of heme proteins. *Science* 284: 473–476.

Kawano, M, Shirabe, K, Nagai, T, and Takeshita, M. (1998). Role of carboxyl residues surrounding heme of human cytochrome b5 in the electrostatic interaction with NADH-cytochrome b5 reductase. *Biochem. Biophys. Res. Commun.* 245: 666–669.

Kiese M. (1966). The biochemical production of ferrihemoglobin-forming derivatives from aromatic amines and mechanisms of ferrihemoglobin formation. *Pharmacol. Rev.* 18: 1091–1161.

Kilbourn, RG. (1997). Nitric oxide overproduction in septic-shock-methemoglobin concentrations and blockade with diaspirin cross-linked hemoglobin. *Crit. Care Med.* 25: 1446–1447.

Kindwall, EP. (1992). Uses of hyperbaric oxygen therapy in the 1990s. *Clev. Clin. J. Med.* 59: 517–528.

Kneezel, LD and Kitchens, CS. (1967). Phenacetin-induced sulfhemoglobinemia: Report of a case and review of the literature. *Johns Hopkins Med. J.* 139: 175–180.

Kobayashi, Y, Fukumaki, Y, Yubisui, T et al. (1990). Serine-proline replacement at residue 127 of NADH-cytochrome b5 reductase causes hereditary methemoglobinemia, generalized type. *Blood* 75: 1408–1413.

Krafte-Jacobs, B, Brilli, R, Szabo, C et al. (1997). Circulating methemoglobin and nitrite/nitrate concnetrations as indicators of nitric oxide overproduction in critically ill children with septic shock. *Crit. Care Med.* 25: 1588–1593.

Lacey, DJ. (1981). Neurologic sequelae of acute carbon monoxide intoxication. *Am. J. Dis. Child.* 135: 145–147.

Lambert, M, Sonnet, J, Mahien, P and Hassoun, A. (1982). Delayed sulfhemoglobinemia after acute dapsone intoxication. *Clin. Toxicol.* 19: 45–49.

Lan, F, Tang, Y, Huang, C, and Zhu, Z. (1996). Establishment of monoclonal antibodies against human erythrocyte NADH-cytochrome b5 reductase. *Hybridoma* 15: 295–298.

Lan, F, Tang, Y, Huang, C, and Zhu, Z. (1988a). Determination of concentration of cytosolic NADH-cytochrome b5 reductase in erythrocytes from normal Chinese adults, neonates and patients with hereditary methemoglobinemia by double-antibody sandwich ELISA. *Acta Haematol.* 100: 44–48.

Lan, FH, Tang, YC, Huang, CH et al. (1998b). Antibody-based spot test for NADH-cytochrome b5 reductase activity for the laboratory diagnosis of congenital methemoglobinemia. *Clin. Chim. Acta* 273: 13–20.

Liu, X, Miller, MJ, Joshi, MS et al. (1998). Diffusion-limited reaction of free nitric oxide with erythrocytes. *J. Biol. Chem.* 273: 18709–18713.

McCutcheon, AD. (1960). Sulphaemoglobinaemia and glutathione. *Lancet* 2: 290.

McGrath, JJ. (1992). Effects of altitude on endogenous carboxyhemoglobin levels. *J. Toxicol. Environ. Health* 35: 127–133.

Mahoney, JJ, Vreman, HJ, Stevenson, DK et al. (1993). Measurement of carboxyhemoglobin and total hemoglobin by five specialized spectrophotometers (CO-oximeters) in comparison with reference methods. *Clin. Chem.* 39: 1963–1700.

Manabe, J, Arya, R, Sumimoto, H et al. (1996). Two novel mutations in the reduced nicotinamide adenine dinucleotide (NADH)-cytochrome b5 reductase gene of a patient with generalized type, hereditary methemoglobinemia. *Blood* 88: 3208–3215.

Mansouri, A and Nandy, I. (1998). NADH-methemoglobin reductase (cytorchrome b5 reductase) levels in two groups of American blacks and whites. *J. Invest. Med.* 46: 82–86.

Marks, GS, Brien, JF, Nakatsu, K, and McLaughlin, BE. (1991). Does carbon monoxide have a biological function? *Trends Pharmacol. Sci.* 12: 185–188.

Madeiros, MH, Bechara, EJ, Naoum, PC, and Mourao, CA. (1983). Oxygen toxicity and hemoglobinemia in subjects from a highly polluted town. *Arch. Environ. Health* 38: 11–15.

Meyer, TE, Shirabe, K, Yubisui, T et al. (1995). Transient kinetics of intracomplex electron transfer in the human cytochrome b5 reductase-cytochrome b5 system: NAD + modulates protein-protein binding and electron transfer. *Arch. Biochem. Biophys.* 318: 457–464.

Molthrop, DC Jr, Wheeler, RH, Hall, KM, and Prchal, JT. (1994). Evaluation of the methemoglobinemia associated with sulofur. *Invest. New Drugs* 12: 99–102.

Nagel, RL, Bemski, G, and Pincus, P. (1970). Some aspects of the binding of Cu (II) to human hemoglobin and its subunits. *Arch. Biochem. Biophys.* 137: 428–431.

Nagel, RL. (1995). Disorders of hemoglobin function and stability. In Handon, RI, Lux, SE, and Stossel, TP, editors. Blood: *Principles and practices of hematology*. Philadelphia: J.B. Lippincott.

Nichol, AW, Hendry, I, Movell, DB, and Clezy, PS. (1968). Mechanism of formation of sulfhemoglobin. *Biochim. Biophys. Acta* 156: 97–103.

Park, CM and Nagel, RL. (1984). Sulfhemoglobinemia. Clinical and molecular aspects. *N. Engl. J. Med.* 310: 1579–1584.

Park, CM, Nagel, RL, Blumberg, WE et al. (1986). Sulfhemoglobin. Properties of partially sulfurated tetramers. *J. Bio. Chem.* 261: 8805–8810.

Passon, PG and Hultquist, DE. (1972). Soluble cytochrome b5 reductase from human erythrocytes. *Biochim. Biophys. Acta* 275: 62–69.

Pawloski, JR, Swaminahan, RV, and Stamler, JS. (1998). Cell free and erythrocytic S-nitrohemoglobin inhibits platelet aggregation. *Circulation* 97: 263–267.

Perutz, MF. (1978). Electrostatic effects in proteins. *Science* 201: 1187–1188.

Pietrini, G, Aggujaro, D, Carrera, P et al. (1992). A single mRNA, transcribed from an alternative erythroid-specific promoter, codes for two non-myristylated forms of NADH-cytochrome-b5 reductase. *J. Cell Biol.* 117: 975–986.

Prchal, JT, Borgese, N, Moore, MR et al. (1990). Congenital methemoglobinemia due to methemoglobin reductase deficiency in two unrelated American black families. *Am. J. Med.* 89: 516–521.

Reynolds, TB and Ware, AG. (1952). Sulfhemoglobinemia following habitual use of acetanilid. *JAMA* 149: 1538–1542.

Schwartz, JM, Reiss, AI, and Jaffé, ER. (1983). Hereditary methemoglobinemia with deficiency of NADH-cytochrome reductase b5 reductase. In Stanbury, JB, Wyngaarden, JB, Goldstein, JL, and Brown, MS, editors. *The molecular basis of disease* (ed 5). New York: McGraw-Hill.

Scott, EM. (1960). The relation of diaphorase of human erythrocytes to inheritance of methemoglobinemia. *J. Clin. Invest.* 39: 1176–1182.

Shirabe, K, Landi, MT, Takeshita, M et al. (1995). A novel point mutation in a 3′ splice site of the NADH-cytochrome b5 reductase gene results in immunologically undetectable enzyme and impaired NADH-dependent ascorbate regeneration in cultured fibroblasts of a patient with type II hereditary methemoglobinemia. *Am. J. Hum. Genet.* 57: 302–310.

Sin, DD and Shafran, SD. (1996). Dapsone- and primaquine-induced methemoglobinemia in HIV-infected individuals. *J. Acquir. Immune Defic. Syndr. Hum. Retrovirol.* 12: 477–481.

Sjostrand T. (1949). Endogenous formation of carbon monoxide in man. *Nature* 164: 580–581.

Soszynski, M and Bartosz, T. (1997). Penetration of erythrocyte membrane by peroxynitrate: Participation of the anion exchange protein. *Biochem. Mol. Biol. Int.* 43: 319–325.

Stamler, JS, Jia, L, Eu, JP et al. (1997). Blood flow regulation by S-nitrosohemoglobin in the physiological oxygen gradient. *Science* 276: 2034–2037.

Stewart, RD, Fisher, TN, Hosko, MJ et al. (1972). Carboxyhemoglobin elevation after exposure to dichloromethane. *Science* 176: 295–296.

Suzuki, T, Hayshi, A, Shimizu, A, and Yamamura, Y. (1966). The oxygen equilibrium of hemoglobin M Saskatoon. *Biochim. Biophys. Acta* 127: 280–282.

Tomatsu, S, Kobayashi, Y, Fukumaki, Y et al. (1989). The organization and the complete nucleotide sequence of the human NADH-cytochrome b5 reductase gene. *Gene* 80: 353–361.

Valentovic, MA, Rogers, BA, Meadows, MK et al. (1997). Characterization of methemoglobin formation induced by 3,5 dichloroanaline, 4-amino-2,6-dichlorophenol and 3,5-dichlorophenylhydroxamine. *Toxicology* 118: 23–36.

Vreman, HJ, Mahoney, JJ, and Stevenson, DK. (1995). Carbon monoxide and carboxyhemoglobin. *Adv. Pediatr.* 42: 303–325.

Yawata, Y, Ding, L, Tanishima, K, and Tomoda, K. (1992). A new variant of cytochrome b5 reductase deficiency (b5R Kurashiki) in red cells, platelets, lymphocytes, and cultured fibroblasts with congenital methemoglobinemia, mental and neurological retardation, and skeletal anomalies. *Am. J. Hematol.* 40: 299–305.

Yonetani, T. (1998). Nitric oxide and hemoglobin. *Nippon Yakurigaku Zasshi* 112: 155–160.

Wu, YS, Huang, CH, Wan, Y et al. (1998). Identification of a novel point mutation (Leu72Pro) in the NADH-cytochrome b5 reductase gene of a patient with hereditary methaemoglobinaemia type I. *Br. J. Haematol.* 102: 575–577.

Zenno, S, Hattori, M, Misumi, Y et al. (1990). Molecular cloning of a cDNA encoding rat NADH-cytochrome b5 reductase and the corresponding gene. *J. Biochem. (Tokyo)* 107: 810–816.

Zhang, M and Scott, JG. (1996). Purification and characterization of cytochrome b5 reductase from the house fly, Musca domestica. *Comp. Biochem. Physiol. B Biochem. Mol. Biol.* 113: 175–183.

Zinkham, WH and Oski, FA. (1996). Henna: A potential cause of oxidative hemolysis and neonatal hyperbilirubinemia, *Pediatrics* 97: 707–709.

Index

Abdominal pain in sickle cell anemia, 649, 650t
  management of, 650f
ABH,iI blood group antigen on erythroid progenitors, 54t
AC133 antigen on erythroid progenitors, 54t, 55
Acetaldehyde adducts in hemoglobin, 220–221
Acetaminophen
  in sickle cell disease painful episodes, 678t, 679
  sulfhemoglobinemia from, 1226
Acetanilid, sulfhemoglobinemia from, 1226
N-Acetyl cysteine as antioxidant, 1129
Acetylated hemoglobin, 220, 1199
Acidity, and potassium-chloride cotransport in red cells, 559, 559f, 560f
Acidosis, and sickle cell disease painful episodes, 673
Acosta, Joseph, 6
Acquired hemoglobin disorders, 1213–1230. *See also* Dyshemoglobins
Activin A affecting erythroid development, 55t
Acute phase proteins in sickle cell disease painful episodes, 689
Adeno-associated virus, recombinant, as vectors in gene therapy, 1089–1091, 1090f
  for globin gene transfer, 1105
Adenoviral vectors for gene therapy, 1091
Adherence of sickle cells
  to endothelium. *See* Sickle cell disease, and adherence of cells to endothelium
  to monocytes or macrophages, membrane damage affecting, 557
Adjuvant drugs in sickle cell disease painful episodes, 694t, 695

Adolescence, sickle cell disease in, 634
  growth and development in, 617
Adrenal function
  in sickle cell anemia, 641
  in β thalassemia major, 291
α-Adrenergic agonists in priapism, 647–648
Adult blood
  CD34 and CD38 cells in, 54–55, 55t, 60
  erythropoiesis features, 61–65, 62t
    definitive erythrocytes in, 72
    globin gene expression in, 26, 33
  hemoglobin in. *See* Hemoglobin A
  progenitor cells in, 61t
Afghanistan, β thalassemia in, 862t
Africa
  hemoglobin S β-globin gene, 712–719
  prevalence of hemoglobinopathies, 18, 18t
  sickle cell disease in West Africa, 900
  sickle cell trait, 817, 817t, 818
  α thalassemia in sub-Saharan region, 880, 881t
  β thalassemia, 862t, 951t
    in Central and South Africa, 872–873
    in North Africa, 868, 869t
African-Americans
  hemoglobin S β-globin haplotypes in, 716f, 725–726
  hereditary persistence of fetal hemoglobin in, 359f, 366t, 369t, 375, 376t, 378
  sickle cell disease in, 900–901
  sickle cell trait in, 817t
  β thalassemia in, 863t, 873, 873t, 947t
  δβ thalassemia in, 359f, 362, 363, 366t, 368t
Age
  and alloimmunization from transfusion therapy, 990
  and desferrioxamine therapy initiation, 1005

and hemoglobin A$_2$ levels, 211
and hemoglobin levels in sickle cell disease, 494–495
and retinopathy in hemoglobin SC disease, 778t
and sickle cell disease prognosis, 899–900
Agranulocytosis from deferiprone, 1013
AIDS. *See* HIV infection
Aircraft travel, effects in sickle cell trait, 820
Albania
  hemoglobin S β-globin gene in, 722
  β thalassemia in, 865t, 866
Aldehyde compounds, cyclic, in sickle cell disease, 1120–1121
Algae, hemoglobin in, 96, 97f
Algeria
  hemoglobin S β-globin gene in, 722
  α thalassemia in, 884t
  β thalassemia in, 863t, 868, 869t, 951t
Alkali resistance of fetal hemoglobin, 194, 198
Alkyltransferase genes in selection of stem cells, 1098
Allergic reactions to desferrioxamine, 1004
Alloimmunization from transfusion therapy, 990–991
Allopurinol as antioxidant, 1129
Allosteric enzymes, 180
Allostery, 180–182, 181f
  and hemoglobin structure changes, 190–192
N-Allylsecoboldine as antioxidant, 1130
α$_2$β$_1$ phenotype in fetal, neonatal, and adult cells, 62t
Altitude
  and adaptation to hypoxia, 1165
  effects in sickle cell trait, 820
  and erythropoiesis, 6
Amenorrhea in β thalassemia major, 289–290